MELMON AND MORRELLI'S

*C*LINICAL
*P*HARMACOLOGY

NOTICE

Medicine is an ever-changing science. As new research and clinical experience broaden our knowledge, changes in treatment and drug therapy are required. The editors and the publisher of this work have checked with sources believed to be reliable in their efforts to provide information that is complete and generally in accord with the standards accepted at the time of publication. However, in view of the possibility of human error or changes in medical sciences, neither the editors nor the publisher nor any other party who has been involved in the preparation or publication of this work warrants that the information contained herein is in every respect accurate or complete, and they are not responsible for any errors or omissions or for the results obtained from use of such information. Readers are encouraged to confirm the information contained herein with other sources. For example and in particular, readers are advised to check the product information sheet included in the package of each drug they plan to administer to be certain that the information contained in this book is accurate and that changes have not been made in the recommended dose or in the contraindications for administration. This recommendation is of particular importance in connection with new or infrequently used drugs.

MELMON AND MORRELLI'S

CLINICAL PHARMACOLOGY

BASIC PRINCIPLES IN THERAPEUTICS

THIRD EDITION

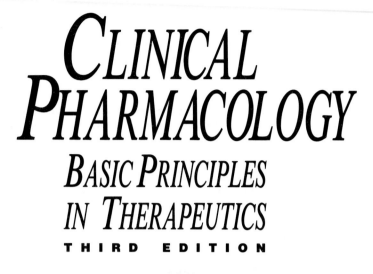

Editors

Kenneth L. Melmon, M.D.
Professor of Medicine and Pharmacology
Stanford University School of Medicine
Stanford, California

Howard F. Morrelli, M.D.
Professor of Medicine, Pharmacology, and Psychiatry
Veterans Administration Medical Center Fresno
Fresno, California

Brian B. Hoffman, M.D.
Associate Professor of Medicine and Pharmacology
Veterans Administration Medical Center
Palo Alto, California

David W. Nierenberg, M.D.
Associate Professor of Medicine and Pharmacology
Dartmouth-Hitchcock Medical Center
Lebanon, New Hampshire

McGRAW-HILL, INC.
Health Professions Division
New York • St. Louis • San Francisco •
Auckland • Bogatá • Caracas • Lisbon •
London • Madrid • Mexico • Milan •
Montreal • New Delhi • Paris • San Juan •
Singapore • Sydney • Tokyo • Toronto

MELMON AND MORRELLI'S CLINICAL PHARMACOLOGY:
Basic Principles in Therapeutics

ISBN 0-07-105385-9

1234567890   HALHAL   98765432

This book was set in English Times by Bytheway Typesetting Services, Inc.
The index was prepared by Barbara Long.
Arcata Graphics/Halliday was printer and binder.

Library of Congress Cataloging-in-Publication Data

Melmon and Morrelli's clinical pharmacology : basic principles in
    therapeutics / edited by Kenneth L. Melmon . . . [et al.]. — 3d ed.
        p.   cm.
    Rev. ed. of: Clinical pharmacology. 2d ed. c1978.
    Includes bibliographical references and index.

    1. Clinical pharmacology.   I. Melmon, Kenneth L.
II.   Clinical pharmacology.
    [DNLM: 1.   Drug Therapy.   WB 330 M5272]
RM301.28.M45   1992
615.5′8 — dc20
DNLM/DLC
for Library of Congress   90-14355
                                                                      CIP

*This book is dedicated
to the
proposition
that the
quality of therapeutics
should and can be improved,
and to
the people who have tolerated and assisted us
during
its preparation.
This edition also is dedicated to
the memory of
a standard bearer
for Clinical Pharmacology—
Leon Goldberg, M.D., Ph.D.*

Contents

Section II CORE MATERIAL OF CLINICAL PHARMACOLOGY

Contributors

Gregory W. Albers, M.D. Assistant Professor of Neurology and Neurological Sciences, Stanford University School of Medicine, Stanford, CA

Peter J. Barnes, M.A., D.M., D.Sc. Professor and Chairman of Thoracic Medicine and Honorary Consultant Physician, National Heart and Lung Institute (University of London), and Royal Brompton and National Heart Hospital, London, England

Neal L. Benowitz, M.D. Professor of Medicine, Psychiatry and Pharmacy, University of California, San Francisco, San Francisco General Hospital Medical Center, San Francisco, CA

Elliot M. Berry, M.D. Professor of Medicine, Department of Medicine, Hadassah University Hospital, Jerusalem, Israel

J. R. Bertino, M.D. Professor and Chairman of Medicine and Pharmacology, Cornell University School of Medicine, New York, NY

Terrence F. Blaschke, M.D. Professor of Medicine and Pharmacology, Stanford University School of Medicine, Stanford, CA

D. Craig Brater, M.D. Professor and Chairman of Medicine, Professor of Pharmacology, Indiana University School of Medicine, Indianapolis, IN

Deborah Cook, M.D., M.Sc. Assistant Professor of Medicine and Clinical Epidemiology and Biostatistics, McMaster University Medical Centre, Hamilton, Ontario, Canada

Robert F. DeBusk, M.D. Professor (Clinical) of Medicine (Cardiovascular Medicine), Stanford University School of Medicine, Stanford, CA

Fredrick L. Dunn, M.D. Associate Professor of Medicine (Metabolism, Endocrinology and Genetics), Duke University Medical Center, Durham, NC

Elliott Ehrich, M.D. Fellow, Department of Medicine (Immunology and Rheumatology), Stanford University School of Medicine, Stanford, CA

Gary Francis, M.D. Professor of Medicine (Cardiology), University of Minnesota Hospital, Minneapolis, MN

Gabriel Garcia, M.D. Assistant Professor of Medicine (Gastroenterology), Stanford University School of Medicine, Stanford, CA

Frederic S. Glazener, M.D. Clinical Professor of Medicine (Clinical Pharmacology), Stanford University School of Medicine; and Clinical Professor of Medicine, University of California School of Medicine, San Francisco, San Francisco, CA

Marc E. Goldyne, M.D., Ph.D. Associate Professor of Dermatology and Medicine, University of California, San Francisco, San Francisco, CA

Steven R. Goldsmith, M.D. Associate Professor of Medicine and Cardiology, University of Minnesota, Minneapolis, MN

Peter L. Greenberg, M.D. Professor of Medicine (Hematology), Stanford University School of Medicine, Palo Alto, CA

Gordon H. Guyatt, M.D. Professor of Medicine and Clinical Epidemiology and Biostatistics, McMaster University, Hamilton, Ontario, Canada

Andrew R. Hoffman, M.D. Associate Professor of Medicine (Endocrinology, Gerontology and Metabolism), Stanford University School of Medicine, Palo Alto, CA

Nick Holford, M.Sc. Senior Lecturer, Department of Pharmacology and Clinical Pharmacology, University of Auckland, Auckland, New Zealand

Leo E. Hollister, M.D.   Professor of Psychiatry and Pharmacology, University of Texas Medical School, Houston, Harris County Psychiatric Center, Houston, TX

Halsted Holman, M.D.   Professor of Medicine (Immunology and Rheumatology), Stanford University School of Medicine, Stanford, CA

Mark Holodniy, M.D.   Clinical Assistant Professor of Medicine (Infectious Diseases), Stanford University School of Medicine, Palo Alto, CA

Fredric B. Kraemer, M.D.   Associate Professor of Medicine (Endocrinology, Gerontology and Metabolism), Stanford University School of Medicine, Palo Alto, CA

R. Elaine Lambert, M.D.   Acting Assistant Professor of Medicine (Immunology and Rheumatology), Stanford University School of Medicine, Stanford, CA

Steven A. Lieberman, M.D.   Fellow, Department of Medicine (Endocrinology, Gerontology and Metabolism), Stanford University School of Medicine, Stanford, CA

Richard D. Mamelok, M.D.   Senior Director, Biomedical Research, ALZA Corporation, Palo Alto, CA

Robert Marcus, M.D.   Professor (Clinical) of Medicine (Endocrinology, Gerontology and Metabolism), Stanford University School of Medicine, Palo Alto, CA

James L. McGuire, M.D.   Associate Professor of Medicine (Immunology and Rheumatology), Stanford University School of Medicine, Palo Alto, CA

Diana B. McNeill, M.D.   Assistant Professor of Medicine (Metabolism, Endocrinology and Genetics), Duke University Medical Center, Durham, NC

Kenneth L. Melmon, M.D.   Professor of Medicine and Pharmacology (Clinical Pharmacology), Stanford University School of Medicine, Stanford, CA

Urs A. Meyer, M.D.   Professor and Chairman of Pharmacology, Biocenter of the University of Basel, Switzerland

Stephen C. Montamat, M.D.   Assistant Professor of Medicine (Clinical Pharmacology and Hematology), University of Washington School of Medicine, Veterans Administration Medical Center, Boise, ID

Stanley Nattel, M.D.   Associate Professor of Medicine, University of Montreal; Associate Professor of Medicine and Pharmacology, McGill University, Montreal, Quebec, Canada

Robert Negrin, M.D.   Assistant Professor of Medicine (Hematology), Stanford University School of Medicine, Stanford, CA

Christopher P. Nielson, M.D.   Associate Professor of Medicine (Clinical Pharmacology and Gerontology), University of Washington School of Medicine, Veterans Administration Medical Center, Boise, ID

David W. Nierenberg, M.D.   Associate Professor of Medicine and Pharmacology (Clinical Pharmacology), Dartmouth-Hitchcock Medical Center, Lebanon, NH

Alan Nies, M.D.   Professor of Medicine and Pharmacology (Clinical Pharmacology), University of Colorado Health Sciences Center, Denver, CO

Peter D. O'Hanley, M.D., Ph.D.   Assistant Professor of Medicine (Infectious Diseases and Microbiology and Immunology), Stanford University School of Medicine, Palo Alto, CA

Jack Onrot, M.D.   Clinical Assistant Professor of Medicine, University of British Columbia, Vancouver, BC, Canada

Ronald Pearl, M.D., Ph.D.   Assistant Professor of Anesthesia, Stanford University School of Medicine, Stanford, CA

Stephen J. Peroutka, M.D., Ph.D.   Director, Department of Neuroscience, Genentech, Inc., South San Francisco, CA

Robert E. Rangno, M.D.   Associate Professor of Medicine and Pharmacology, University of British Columbia, Vancouver, BC, Canada

David Robertson, M.D.   Professor of Medicine and Pharmacology, Vanderbilt University Medical Center, Nashville, TN

Dan M. Roden, M.D. Professor of Medicine and Pharmacology (Clinical Pharmacology), Vanderbilt University Medical Center, Nashville, TN

George M. Rodgers, M.D., Ph.D. Associate Professor of Medicine and Pathology (Hematology and Oncology), University of Utah School of Medicine, Salt Lake City, UT

Michael F. Roizen, M.D. Professor and Chairman of Anesthesia and Critical Care; Professor of Medicine, University of Chicago, Pritzker School of Medicine, Chicago, IL

Irwin H. Rosenberg, M.D. Professor of Medicine (Nutrition and Physiology), Tufts University, Boston, MA

Douglas S. Ross, M.D. Assistant Professor of Medicine (Endocrinology), Harvard Medical School, Boston, MA

Peter C. Rubin, Ph.D. Professor of Therapeutics, University of Nottingham, Nottingham, England

David L. Sackett, M.D. Professor of Medicine and Clinical Epidemiology and Biostatistics, McMaster University, Hamilton, Ontario, Canada

Gregory Scott, Pharm.D. Instructor, Department of Medicine (Clinical Pharmacology), Dartmouth–Hitchcock Medical Center, Lebanon, NH

Tammi L. Shlotzhauer, M.D. Fellow, Department of Medicine (Immunology and Rheumatology), Stanford University School of Medicine, Stanford, CA

Wayne R. Snodgrass, M.D., Ph.D. Professor and Head, Clinical Pharmacology-Toxicology Unit, University of Texas Medical Branch, Galveston, TX

Donald R. Stanski, M.D. Professor of Anesthesia and Medicine (Clinical Pharmacology), Stanford University School of Medicine, Palo Alto, CA

Brian L. Strom, M.D., M.P.H. Associate Professor of Medicine and Pharmacology, University of Pennsylvania School of Medicine, Philadelphia, PA

Janice Tam, Pharm.D. Pharmacist, Department of Medicine (Infectious Diseases), Stanford University School of Medicine, Stanford, CA

Hugh Tilson, M.D. Adjunct Professor of Epidemiology, School of Public Health, University of North Carolina, Research Triangle Park, NC

Robert E. Vestal, M.D. Professor of Medicine and Adjunct Professor of Pharmacology, University of Washington School of Medicine; Veterans Administration Medical Center, Boise, ID

Brian Whiting, M.D. Professor of Clinical Pharmacology, Department of Medicine and Therapeutics, University of Glasgow, Glasgow, Scotland

J. M. Wright, M.D., Ph.D. Associate Professor of Pharmacology and Therapeutics and Medicine, University of British Columbia, Vancouver, BC, Canada

Preface to the Third Edition

The goals and objectives for revising this book were not only to update material previously covered, but also to deliberately shift emphasis to deal with most of the therapeutic decisions commonly made by practicing physicians. We hope that this edition attracts the student and practitioner into wanting to learn core facts, skills, and the most basic principles of clinical pharmacology by drawing them into the subject via discussions of routine as well as difficult therapeutic decisions encountered in the practice of medicine. We have tried to avoid the Charybdis of cookbook practicality and the Scylla of excessive dry theory.

We present what we believe is mandatory to know about decisions about drugs in brief introductory form in the first chapter. The rest of the first section of the book builds on these principles in specific clinical settings to ensure that most common therapeutic problems are discussed. To learn what the most common decisions were, we reviewed the list of 100 most used drugs and 100 most common diagnoses for which prescriptions were written in North America and Western Europe. The list for the U.S. was obtained from IMS America. It probably covers about 80% or more of the volume of prescription drugs used in North America and Europe today. Individual authors were assigned to cover each of those diagnoses and the drugs used to treat them. All are covered in the first section of the book as minimum subject matter. Thus, this section should be more useful as a reference text to clinicians than were the previous editions. For heuristic purposes, essential principles are highlighted throughout the text as they have been in previous editions.

Section II contains the basic subject material that is the core of clinical pharmacology without reference to specific diseases. Chapters in Section I consistently refer to chapters in Section II as the basis of most therapeutic decisions. This book continues to be a supplement to, not a substitute for, the basic textbooks of medicine and pharmacology.

The editors are very grateful for the editorial and secretarial assistance, patience, and dedication of Wallace Waterfall and Dana O'Neill.

Preface to the Second Edition

The objectives of this book have not changed since the first edition. *Clinical Pharmacology: Basic Principles in Therapeutics* is designed to illustrate a consistency of approach to qualitative and quantitative decision making in therapeutics. Its use should allow the therapist to distinguish drug-related events from spontaneous alterations in disease and provide general knowledge about objective therapeutics that will allow him/her to individualize therapy. The text is written with medical, osteopathy, pharmacy, and allied health students uppermost in mind; such students are the best candidates to evolve therapeutics from an "art" to a rational and objective science.

Readers might legitimately ask why a textbook of "principles" requires revision, since true principles remain constant. In short, the editors are students in a rapidly evolving and novel discipline. Although a number of useful principles were identified in the first edition, some that were designated as principles were not fundamental concepts and, because the field of clinical pharmacology has grown rapidly in recent years, a number of new principles have evolved. Many factors that now impact on therapeutic decisions were not known in 1972, nor were data related to the psychology of the doctor-patient "therapeutic contract" necessarily widely available or easily summarized (Chapter 4). The science of pharmacokinetics was not as aggressively applied to man as it has been in the last 5 to 10 years. Furthermore, the mathematical concepts necessary to make precise and therefore biologically useful decisions during use of high-risk drugs had not been tested in therapeutic settings (Chapters 2 and 3). Clinical pharmacologists had not developed a useful, defensible, and systematic approach about placebos, about how to make therapeutic decisions in circumstances of uncertainty, or about the economic factors that overtly or covertly influence therapeutic decisions and the epidemiology of drug use (Chapters 24 to 26). Only in the last few years has consideration been given to therapeutic decisions affecting women of child-bearing age, pregnant women, the fetus, and the neonate (Chapter 5). Patients with dermatologic disorders can be rationally as well as empirically approached (Chapter 19). The therapeutics of some hepatic, respiratory, endocrine, and inflammatory disorders have become much more specific and effective, and this has allowed the description of new "principles."

The organization of this second edition is similar to that of the first edition. Unit I presents general principles that apply to all therapeutic decisions; Unit II emphasizes the specific factors about a disease and a drug that justify the setting of therapeutic objectives in their coordination; and Unit III stresses the obvious and less overt factors that impact on therapeutic decisions and the observations that can be made and attributed to the drug per se. Unit IV has been deleted from this revision; although the programmed cases were popular, they were too individualized in some respects to justify the space they occupied.

As in the first edition, successful use of this book requires knowledge of both pharmacology and medicine. It should serve as a supplement to, rather than a replacement of, the basic textbooks of medicine and pharmacology. We hope that *Clinical Pharmacology: Basic Principles in Therapeutics* will not foster dogma, recipes, or folklore about drugs, but will help to stimulate scholarly and rational thought about therapeutics that is applicable to individualized settings.

We deeply appreciate the persistent, imaginative, and sometimes exciting writing of our contributors as well as the assistance of our editors, Elyce Melmon and Emma Ponick. We also gratefully acknowledge the thoughtful suggestions made by our fellows and students and the secretarial help of Ms. Vivian Abe.

KENNETH L. MELMON
HOWARD F. MORRELLI

Preface to the First Edition

Even in medicine, though it is easy to know what honey, wine and hellebore, cautery and surgery are, to know how and to whom and when to apply them so as to effect a cure is no less an undertaking than to be a physician.

ARISTOTLE, *Nicomachean Ethics,* Vol. IX

Detailed pharmacologic knowledge stands alone as a basic science, but successful therapeutics requires application of this information to disease-induced abnormalities in individual patients. Aristotle did not claim that physicians were successful, only that they attempted to be. There is abundant information that physicians generally are poor therapists, despite their detailed knowledge of the pathogenesis of disease and the pharmacology of specific drugs that can alter a disease. The consequences of poor therapy include both toxic reactions to drugs and unchecked or even exacerbated disease. No longer can it be said, "The diagnosis is always more important than the treatment." Therapeutics must not continue to lag so far behind pharmacology, physiology, biochemistry, and pathophysiology, which serve as its foundation. Much information must be applied to clinical settings to allow major improvements in the management of disease and decreases in the incidence, morbidity, and mortality of drug toxicity.

This textbook was written (1) to help medical students understand how to approach the problems of administration of drugs to man, and (2) to show house staff and practicing physicians who learned therapeutics in a "hand-me-down" fashion that this instructional approach at best fosters mediocrity in therapeutics and should be replaced by a more efficacious and satisfying method. A consistent approach to therapeutic settings is possible, and the organization of the book generally describes the rationale for therapeutic decisions. An underlying principle herein is that the pathophysiology of disease and basic facts of pharmacology must be interdigitated in order to select drugs and establish therapeutic objectives. Once a category of drug is considered, the therapist must recall and use the basic principles of drug administration (Unit I); then the specific factors of disease and drug that justify bringing them together must be contemplated, so that the dynamics of pharmacology and pathophysiology can be put into perspective in the therapeutic plan (Unit II). Once the therapeutic objectives have been set, a plan must be made and implemented to observe, recognize, and evaluate the effects of drug administration (Unit III). The student may then evaluate his ability to recognize and apply principles in programmed problem-solving situations, taken from actual cases of the clinical pharmacology consultation service, University of California Medical Center, San Francisco (Unit IV).

Successful use of this book requires knowledge of both pharmacology and medicine. It does not replace the basic textbook in either discipline; rather, it is a supplement to both. Unit II does not include all, or even most, of the important diseases or drugs that might be discussed. The approach described in each chapter—physiology, pathophysiology, pharmacology, and, finally, the integration of these subjects—is consistent, can be applied at the bedside, and constitutes what the editors consider to be active clinical pharmacology. Such an approach can be subdivided into guidelines (principles), and some clinical states lend themselves more readily than others to illustration of principles that can be applied broadly. We hope the reader will find that principles applicable to one disease also apply to other disorders, for that is what makes them principles. They should help to stimulate thought rather than to propagate dogma or provide further recipes for therapeutics.

The contributors have demonstrated extraordinary diligence and patience in writing this innovative textbook. The editors thank their colleagues, fellows, house staff, and students for encouragement, criticism, and help during the long gestation period. They are greatly indebted for the thoughtful criticism and suggestions made by Arthur P. Grollman, Jr., M.D., associate professor of pharmacology and medicine, Albert Einstein College of Medicine, Bronx, New York. They are also indebted to Peggy Langston for editorial assistance in preparing the final manuscript.

KENNETH L. MELMON
HOWARD F. MORRELLI

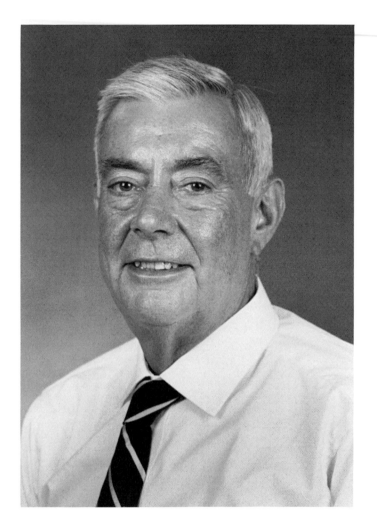

On December 15, 1991, just as the hard work for this third edition ended, news of Howard Morrelli's unexpected and untimely death arrived. Howard was deeply committed to learning and teaching scientifically sound clinical medicine and to practicing the universal, compassionate philosophy that became a touchstone for his therapeutic decisions. He warmly befriended and sternly nurtured a generation of students, housestaff, fellows, and colleagues. His effectiveness at distilling the significant from the complex earned him a reputation as one of the best of the first generation of clinical pharmacologist-therapeutic decision makers. He constantly reminded the more than 125 fellows he helped to train that their sound decisions about treatment had to match the quality of their scientific inquiries. Howard had faith in his students and in the future of this discipline.

We have lost an important contributor to and forthright practitioner of Clinical Pharmacology. We have lost a cherished friend, colleague, and teacher.

Section I
ESSENTIALS IN COMMON THERAPEUTIC DECISIONS

1

Introduction to Clinical Pharmacology

David W. Nierenberg and Kenneth L. Melmon

HISTORICAL PERSPECTIVE ON CURRENT PROBLEMS WITH THERAPEUTICS

The progressive improvement in physicians' diagnostic capabilities does not seem to be matched by improvement in therapeutic decisions. Those decisions often appear to be guided by personal impression, tradition, sentiment, or uncritical acceptance of advertising claims.

Relative inattention to therapy and the therapeutic decision process is not new. In 1903, a clinical pharmacologist observed that "the day has come when something more is demanded of the practitioner or physician-consultant than a diagnosis. . . . Our obligation will not be satisfied until general principles have been fitted to the particular patient. The *what* may be the easiest determined; the *how much*, the *when* and *in what form* and *under what precautions*, must be fully stated" (Wilcox, 1903). In 1905, the president of the American Therapeutic Society asserted that "every medical school should have a special chair of applied therapeutics, held by a clinical man who is a specialist in internal medicine" (Osborne, 1905). And yet, today's medical students and residents continue to be undermotivated to and have inadequate opportunity to develop therapeutic skills, because even today as in the past "most teachers of clinical medicine, though brilliant in diagnosis and learned in pathology, glide over the therapy of disease" (Osborne, 1916). This earlier concern over instruction in rational therapeutics remains appropriate. It has been emphasized that the clinical pharmacologist "must teach students at all levels the basic concepts of an approach to rational therapeutics. Although new specific therapeutic agents will be discovered, the new agents will be used properly only if the student has developed a critical approach to the choice and use of drugs" (Melmon and Morrelli, 1969). Other arguments for the importance of teaching such an approach to rational therapeutics were summarized in a commentary pointing out the need for instruction in clinical pharmacology for all medical students (Nierenberg, 1986). Such instruction has been adopted in countries such as the United Kingdom, where all medical schools include obligatory courses in clinical pharmacology (Anglo-American Workshop, 1986).

Many physicians generally have not felt a great need to improve their knowledge of therapeutics. The need may be masked by patients improving while taking their prescribed drugs, perhaps because most drugs have a large margin of safety, or because many conditions are self-limited, and because problems caused by drugs often can be attributed to the disease for which they are prescribed. Nevertheless, most physicians would agree that depending on homeostatic mechanisms to overcome the effects of poor therapeutic decisions is no way to practice medicine. Suboptimal therapeutics have begun to receive attention. Pharmacists have been very active in highlighting the extent of therapeutic misadventures (Manasse, 1989). In the past 2 years, both the American College of Physicians and the U.S. federal government have urged that measures be taken to help correct the widespread problem of poor prescribing by physicians (Meyer, 1988; Kusserow, 1989).

Consider the following regarding overall drug use in the United States alone:

• Many entirely new classes of drugs have been introduced during the past 15 years.
• The U.S. Food and Drug Administration (FDA) approves an average of 21 new molecular entities per year (Manasse, 1989).
• Many medications had not been discovered at the time the prescribing physician graduated from medical school.
• By 1988, about $30 billion was spent on prescription drugs, and another $8 billion on nonprescription products, for a total per capita expenditure of almost $160 (Manasse, 1989).
• By the late 1980s, more than 1.5 billion outpatient prescriptions were filled annually in the United States, an average of about six prescriptions per person per year (Meyer, 1988; Manasse, 1989).
• People over age 65 make up only about 12% of the population, but they receive about 30% of prescription drugs and purchase about 40% of nonprescription drugs (Kusserow, 1989).
• In 1986, elderly Americans received 613 million prescriptions (an average of 15.5 prescriptions per person) from retail outlets. These data do not include prescriptions filled by other suppliers (Public Citizen Health Research Group, 1988; Kusserow, 1989).
• Hospitalized patients receive an average of 15 drug administrations per day, costing about $5 billion per year (Manasse, 1989).
• About two thirds of all physician visits lead to a prescription (Meyer, 1988).
• As many as 64% of prescriptions for antibiotics in hospitalized patients may be unnecessary or are otherwise flawed (Moss and McNicol, 1983; Meyer, 1988).
• As drug use has increased, adverse drug reactions (ADRs) also have increased. Up to 15% of hospitalized patients experience an ADR. What proportion of these are avoidable without compromising the efficacy of the drug has never been determined.
• About 5% of all admissions to hospitals are to manage ADRs. Again, what portion of these ADRs could have been avoided without compromising efficacy is not known.
• Elderly patients may be especially prone to develop ADRs. In 1985, an estimated 243,000 older adults were hospitalized because of ADRs.
• In 1988, the diuretic furosemide was the second most used drug in the United States, and folic acid and vitamin B_{12} appeared on the list of the 100 most used drugs. Could these be patterns of rational use of drugs? Such might be true for furosemide, but in the case of vitamin B_{12}, there are not enough patients with pernicious anemia to justify the quantities used.

Better understanding of the medical meaning of the above statements depends on systematic studies of use patterns and effects of marketed drugs. Better education can be based on the results of those studies. Physicians often learn about new drugs from colleagues, advertisements, drug detail persons, or other sources that may lack scientific foundations and objectivity (Avorn et al., 1982). In 1985, only 14% of American medical schools offered formal courses in clinical pharmacology (Nierenberg, 1986), compared with 100% of medical schools in the United Kingdom. Medical students are not exposed to the challenge and satisfaction of considering each drug prescription as a therapeutic experiment.

This book is dedicated to a deliberate, thoughtful approach to drug therapy as a basis for rational therapeutics. Rational therapeutics means *prescribing drugs to maximize the chances of efficacy and to minimize drug-induced illness*. Rational therapeutics strives to individualize the therapeutic plan to match the needs of a particular patient by following the scientific principles of medicine and pharmacology. The core of information needed to practice rational therapeutics is introduced in this chapter. The principles of rational therapeutics will be illustrated in specific settings with the challenge to test the validity of these principles by applying them in a host of settings encountered in clinical practice.

AN APPROACH TO RATIONAL THERAPEUTICS

What are the key components of a rational approach to medical therapeutics that can be applied to most situations? Consider a case gone awry, and try to envision the important steps that could have been taken to make this patient's management more rational and effective.

Case History

A 54-year-old woman developed new onset of mild-to-moderate seropositive rheumatoid arthritis. Her symptoms were not relieved by the ingestion of eight aspirin tablets per day, so her physician prescribed a drug recently approved for the treatment of rheumatoid arthritis—oral methotrexate, 7.5 mg each week.

This regimen worked well for several months until the physician prescribed oral probenecid to treat her asymptomatic hyperuricemia. The next dose of methotrexate was followed by profound pancytopenia and sepsis. The probenecid was discontinued; the patient recovered; and methotrexate was successfully continued for several more months with clear clinical benefit and no clinical toxicity. However, the patient began to complain of fevers, dyspnea on exertion, and a dry nonproductive cough. Her physical examination was remarkable only for dry rales throughout both lungs, and her chest film showed a bilateral and symmetric interstitial pattern. The physician treated her presumed mild congestive heart failure with furosemide, and the methotrexate was continued.

The next week her symptoms were worse, and, as an outpatient, she was given cefalexin orally to treat a possible pneumonia. Her other medications were continued. Finally, her symptoms became so severe that she required hospitalization. All her medications were discontinued. Her laboratory studies confirmed severe hypoxemia, hyperventilation, and bilateral and symmetric interstitial pneumonitis. She received folinic acid to treat a possible methotrexate-induced interstitial pneumonitis, but she deteriorated rapidly and required intubation. Results of a lung biopsy were consistent with the diagnosis of methotrexate-induced interstitial pneumonitis. Corticosteroids were begun, but the patient died several days later.

Discussion: This case illustrates a number of ways that uninformed therapeutics may silently creep up on a physician. Sometimes the results can be severe and irreversible. Initially, the patient's diagnosis was rheumatoid arthritis. The physician considered the drugs that were available to treat this disease and appropriately chose aspirin as a first-line drug. Aspirin is relatively safe and efficacious, has minimal and usually predictable toxicity, and is not costly. In this case, aspirin may have been used suboptimally. If a target effect had been chosen and followed and if a target concentration of salicylate in blood had been established, the efficacy–toxicity profile of the drug could have been optimized. The use of an arbitrary dose of aspirin may not have achieved optimal plasma concentrations of the drug in this patient. Instead, the physician prematurely gave up on aspirin without considering the need to possibly increase the dose. His prescription of methotrexate, a powerful but frequently toxic drug, should probably have been reserved for very severe disease that was refractory to maximally tolerated anti-inflammatory drugs. ***Principle: Set the legitimately expected results of therapy (as to efficacy and lower limits of toxicity) before beginning. Use those objectives to monitor drug effects and to signal the need for qualitative or quantitative changes in therapy.***

The physician prescribed methotrexate without fully understanding its pharmacokinetics or profile of adverse reactions. Then, when he inappropriately treated the patient's asymptomatic mild hyperuricemia with probenecid, he unwittingly caused a drug–drug interaction. Probenecid is a potent inhibitor of the renal tubular secretion of weak organic acids. It can similarly inhibit the tubular secretion (and thereby the renal clearance) of methotrexate. The decreased clearance of methotrexate led to drug accumulation and increased concentrations of the drug in plasma, thereby leading to systemic toxicity. Fortunately the physician recognized this mistake, and the patient recovered from a near-fatal episode of methotrexate-induced pancytopenia.

Finally, the patient developed an unusual but by no means rare idiosyncratic reaction to methotrexate, an inflammatory interstitial pneumonitis. Because the possibility of an adverse drug reaction was not considered seriously, both congestive heart failure and pneumonia were treated. By the time the correct drug-induced problem was recognized, the condition was irreversible, and the patient died. ***Principle: A logical approach to therapy results in rational prescribing of even the most common medications. Requirements for rational therapy include***

1. Reasonable certainty of the diagnosis

2. Understanding the pathophysiology of the disease

3. Understanding the pharmacology of the drugs that could be used

4. Choosing the drug and dose that are likely to be optimal for the specific patient

5. Picking end points of efficacy and toxicity, and vigorously monitoring the patient to check for those end points

6. Developing a contract or alliance with the patient and keeping it; being willing to alter the therapeutic regimen if objective evidence of drug efficacy is not seen or if unacceptable toxicity is encountered

In retrospect, the physician's failure in each of these requirements, sometimes more than once, is easy to spot. Even a seemingly trivial decision, such as how to administer aspirin to a patient with arthritis, or deciding to treat a patient with asymptomatic mild hyperuricemia, can have very important implications.

Case histories in this book will reinforce the value of the fundamental steps that should be considered whenever the physician prescribes a medication, uses a device, or performs a procedure. However, the steps can be applied only when the physician has adequate knowledge of the core of clinical pharmacology. This entails understanding how the body handles drugs (pharmacokinetics) and how drugs affect the body (pharmacodynamics). Also, the physician must be aware that many patients require special consideration when drugs are prescribed. For example, patients with renal or hepatic disease, the very young, the very old, and pregnant or nursing women may not be able to receive the usual medications in the standard doses. Further, the physician-pharmacologist must know how to distinguish symptoms of drug toxicity from symptoms due to disease and must be able to recognize—or better yet predict—which drugs are likely to interact adversely with others. In addition, there are legal rules and regulations that govern prescribing, and the physician must also be aware of the complex and perhaps subconscious forces that are at work in the writing of a prescription. All these factors will be introduced in this chapter and discussed in more detail in section II. The chapters in section I will illustrate how these principles of rational therapeutics can and should be applied to the treatment of common, serious diseases.

AN OVERVIEW OF DRUG ACTION

To understand the principles of rational therapeutics, the principles of drug action must be understood. The most important concepts of administering drugs have to do with the dose-response relationship (Fig. 1–1). Most physicians assume that there is a rough but proportionate relation between the dose of a drug ingested and the intended pharmacologic effect. Figure 1–2 illustrates such a relation between the dose of aspirin and relief of headache in a hypothetical patient.

In panel A, one tablet (325 mg) relieves about 40% of this patient's pain. Two tablets (650 mg) relieve more of the pain. But increasing the dose to three or even four tablets produces little additional relief; *more* is not *better* when the top of the dose-response curve has been reached. In fact, even after large doses of aspirin, this patient cannot achieve greater than 80% relief of his pain. This maximal effect is sometimes referred to as a *ceiling* effect. The 325-mg dose relieved about 40% of his pain, about half the maximal, or ceiling, effect. The dose that produces half the maximal effect in a patient is called the ED_{50}. While the shape of this curve may not look familiar when plotted linearly in panel A, the semilogorithmic (semilog) plot in panel B gives the dose-response curve its characteristic sigmoid shape.

Figure 1–3 looks very much like a dose-response curve for a single patient (Fig. 1–2) but has quite a different meaning. This figure represents the cumulative percentage of patients who achieve a specific and measurable therapeutic end point after receiving various doses of aspirin. Of all patients who will achieve "substantial relief" of pain from headache (perhaps 90%), about half (45%) will achieve such benefit after taking a dose of 650 mg. In this group of patients, the ED_{50} is 650 mg. Whether dose-response curves are applied to individual patients or groups of patients, the characteristics of the semilog curve, the concept of the ED_{50}, and the concept of a ceiling effect are valid.

For many drugs, the dose-response relationship in a population of patients is well defined and can act as a therapeutic guideline helping the physician choose appropriate first doses for patients. For other drugs, the population dose-response relationship is not as smooth and predictable as are the data for aspirin. Wide interindividual variation in the concentration of drug in plasma following equivalent doses can distort the population-derived dose-response curve.

In such cases, the relation of concentration of drug in plasma to the effect of the drug is often more "precise" than dose-effect relations because the former eliminates many factors that lead to large interpatient variability in the dose-response relationship (see Fig. 1–1). Figure 1–4 illustrates a typical concentration-response curve for a single

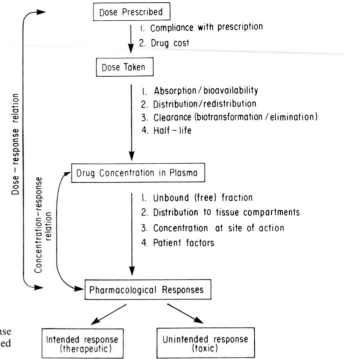

Fig. 1-1. Determinants of the dose–response and concentration–response relations. (Modified from Koch-Weser, 1972.)

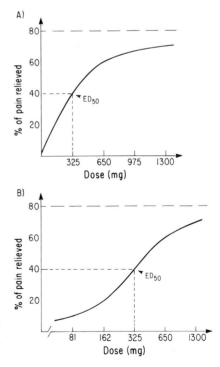

Fig. 1-2. A dose–response curve obtained in one patient relating the dose of aspirin ingested to the percentage of headache pain relieved. (A) A linear plot: the abscissa (dose in milligrams) has a linear scale. (B) A semilog plot: the abscissa (dose in milligrams) has a logarithmic scale.

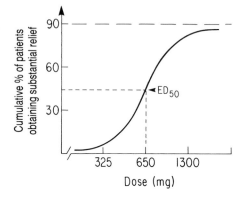

Fig. 1-3. A dose-response curve obtained in a group of patients. The ordinate plots the cumulative percentage of patients achieving "substantial" relief of headache pain after ingesting aspirin. Note that the abscissa has a logarithmic scale.

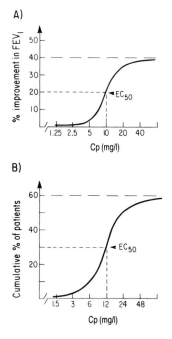

Fig. 1-4. Concentration-response curves describing theophylline's ability to increase the FEV_1. (A) A concentration-response curve obtained in a single patient. In this patient, the EC_{50} appears to be about 10 mg/l. (B) A concentration-response curve obtained in a group of asthmatic patients. In this group, the EC_{50} appears to be about 12 mg/l.

patient (panel A) versus that for a group of patients (panel B) receiving theophylline.

In panel A, ceiling effect for the single patient is 40% improvement in forced expiratory volume in 1 second (FEV_1), and half the maximal benefit occurs at a concentration of 10 mg/l (the EC_{50}). For this patient, concentrations of drug in plasma of less than 5 mg/l are associated with little, if any, benefit, while concentrations in plasma greater than 20 mg/l produce little additional benefit. Panel B represents similar data for a group of asthmatic patients. For this group, about 60% will eventually show at least moderate improvement from theophylline, and half of these responders will show improvement at concentrations of 12 mg/l or less (the EC_{50}). *Principle: Dose-response curves derived from populations can be used to approximate the first dose in a patient who has had no previous experience with the drug. The best curves for that patient's future management with the same drug will come from careful observation of what the first doses actually accomplish. Even when population data predict individual responses, the challenge to individualize doses remains if therapy is to be optimized.* We will refer to dose-response and concentration-response curves throughout the book. They are fundamental to understanding clinical pharmacology.

Figure 1-5 illustrates several additional features of dose-response relations—potency and overall efficacy. *Potency* of a drug refers to the dose required to have a specific effect; the more potent a drug, the smaller the dose. In this context, *efficacy* refers to the maximal effect achievable with a particular drug. Potency and efficacy are entirely separate concepts. For example, a drug that is not very potent (large doses must be used) may nonetheless be highly efficacious.

Consider two drugs that may be used in the treatment of migraine headaches in a group of patients. Aspirin, even at high doses, produces

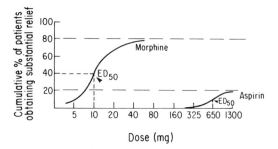

Fig. 1-5. Dose-response curves describing the ability of aspirin and morphine to relieve pain in patients with migraine headache. Note that morphine is both more potent (has a lower ED_{50}), and has a greater overall efficacy (ceiling effect).

substantial relief in only about 20% of such patients. In contrast, morphine produces substantial relief in about 80% of patients. Thus, morphine has a greater overall (relative) efficacy, effectiveness, or ceiling effect. These terms *often are used synonymously*. In addition, the ED_{50} for morphine is about 10 mg, while the ED_{50} for aspirin is about 650 mg. Thus, morphine is more potent. However, there may be no clinical advantage between two drugs with equal efficacy for the same indication but widely different potencies. As long as the patient can conveniently take the needed dose of each and as long as toxicities of each are rare when the needed doses are taken, one preparation can be used as readily as the other. These drugs illustrate how potency and efficacy are not synonymous. For example, morphine (usual dose 1(mg) is more potent than meperidine (usual dose 100 mg) for treatment of pain. Yet if a patient's headache was caused by fungal meningitis or encephalitis and he or she also required amphotericin, these two drugs would have similar efficacies in suppressing pain. However, meperidine can have an clinical advantage over morphine because meperidine may relieve the rigors caused by amphotericin when morphine fails to do so. On the other hand, if the patient had renal insufficiency, morphine might be safer since a toxic metabolite of meperidine may accumulate in such patients. Here the choice between the drugs has nothing to do with their relative potencies as analgesics.

We could generate similar dose–response curves for toxic effects of morphine, such as somnolence or respiratory depression. If 50% of patients fall asleep at a cumulative dose of 20 mg, then this dose is the TD_{50} (dose causing toxicity in 50% of patients) for sleep. The TD_{50} for morphine-induced respiratory depression might be 60 mg. Thus, dose–response curves (or concentration–response curves) also demonstrate when a drug's efficacy will be attended by its toxic effects. The therapeutic index is a measure of how far apart the dose that produces a desired efficacious effect is likely to be from the dose that will likely produce a serious unwanted but predictable toxic effect. The therapeutic index is defined as the ratio of the TD_{50} to the ED_{50}. Clearly, a drug with a therapeutic index of 4 is considerably safer than a drug with a therapeutic index of 1. *Principle: The therapeutic index is not a constant. Most chemical entities have several pharmacologic effects with different dose-response relationships. Depending upon the efficacy needed or intended in a given patient, the therapeutic index will vary.*

The fact that there are different legitimate reasons for giving the same drug to different people, variation in the dose–response relationships for different effects in the same patient, and between-patient variation in dose–response relationships for the same effects creates the need for individualization of drug therapy. In contrast to the examples used above, morphine's central anesthetic effect may be needed and desired as a component of balanced anesthesia for patients undergoing open heart surgery. In this situation, the ED_{50} might be 80 mg or higher. Concern about the TD_{50} with respect to respiratory depression would not be great, because the patient is intubated to maintain ventilation. Thus, depending on the desired pharmacologic effect and toxicity assessed, the calculation of the therapeutic index may vary greatly from patient to patient. *Principle: Every qualitative (choosing a drug) and quantitative (doses: how often and how much) therapeutic decision should be individualized and optimized.*

THE ESSENTIAL COMPONENTS OF PHARMACOKINETICS

Definition

After systemic administration, a drug achieves a certain concentration in the blood (or plasma or serum) that changes over time. The usual determination is the peak concentration of drug in serum or plasma (C_p) rather than in whole blood. The concentration of drug in plasma ultimately determines and is in equilibrium with the concentration of drug at its sites of action. The relation between the dose of the drug and its concentration in plasma is described by the pharmacokinetics of the drug. Figure 1–1 emphasizes the key variables that determine the pharmacokinetic properties of each drug.

The pharmacokinetics of a drug describes what the body does to the drug. Once a drug is administered, a number of processes occur that make up the body's handling of the drug. First, the drug is absorbed from its site of administration; then it passes into the systemic circulation and is distributed throughout the body. The speed and pattern of distribution can vary widely from one drug to another. Finally, the drug is removed or cleared from the plasma and eliminated from the body by metabolic biotransformation and/or direct excretion of unchanged drug. Each of these processes has been analyzed and modeled in considerable detail (see chapters 37 and 38), but it is necessary for any physician who prescribes drugs to understand the basic concepts of clinical pharmacokinetics and how to apply them to patients. With that understanding, the physician can titrate any drug to obtain appropriate pharmacologic effects and to optimize dosage and dosage intervals to maximize the therapeutic index in a given patient.

Drug Absorption and Bioavailability

Drugs are absorbed from most sites of administration, but each route provides different access of the drug to the systemic circulation. A choice must be made among the oral, transdermal, intravenous, intraarterial, intramuscular, or rectal routes to ensure the drug's absorption into the body as a whole. Entry of the drug into the systemic circulation can be lessened by administering it locally as in eye drops (e.g., sulfacetamide), nose sprays (e.g., phenylephrine), inhalants (e.g., albuterol), or topical creams (e.g., vaginal estrogens). These maneuvers can maximize the percentage of the dose that concentrates on a desired target organ, but they rarely prevent at least a portion of the dose from entering the systemic circulation and producing effects distant from the target tissue.

Absorption of the drug from the site of administration depends on properties of the drug, the vehicle in which it is administered, and conditions (e.g., adiposity of the tissue, rates of blood flow) at the site of administration. For drugs administered orally, the rate of absorption often is deliberately controlled by altering the pharmaceutical properties of the tablet or capsule itself. For example, Fig. 1–6 demonstrates profiles of absorption following two different pharmaceutical forms—rapid-release capsules and sustained-release capsules—of the same drug given in the same dosage.

The rate of absorption is reflected in the time it takes to achieve the maximal concentration of drug in plasma. These variables are referred to as the T_{max} and C_{max}, respectively. The rapid-release product produces a higher peak concentration (C_{max}) within a shorter time (T_{max}). The sustained-release product produces a lower peak that is reached considerably later. Theophylline, mor-

phine, and procainamide are three of many drugs available in sustained-release formulations. These preparations enable the patient to take the drug fewer times per day than would be needed if only the rapidly absorbed formulations were available. The fewer doses of drug needed per day, the better the compliance with a therapeutic regimen. But these preparations may be used with additional objectives in mind. If the desired efficacy of a drug is achieved at lower plasma concentrations than is toxicity, then one strategy for widening a therapeutic index would be to deliver the full dose over long periods to avoid high peak concentrations (i.e., lower C_{max}). Before going to chapters 37 and 38, think about what other advantages there may be in absorbing a given dose of a drug slowly.

The three parenteral formulations of penicillin G serve as a useful example of important formulation-dependent differences in drug absorption. Crystalline penicillin G aqueous is administered intravenously (IV) and is "absorbed" into the systemic circulation essentially as rapidly as it is infused into the vein. It produces very high concentrations of drug in plasma. After a single injection, the concentration declines rapidly because of rapid excretion of the drug by the kidneys. In contrast, the suspension of procaine penicillin G is only moderately water-soluble. Following its intramuscular (IM) injection, absorption continues over several hours, producing lower peak concentrations of penicillin than would be obtained by giving the same dose of crystalline penicillin IV. However, these concentrations are sustained for several hours. Finally, the suspension of benzathine penicillin G is very poorly soluble in water and very slowly absorbed from an IM depot site. In fact, this formulation produces low but sustained concentrations of penicillin G in plasma over *4 weeks*. The pharmacokinetic properties of absorption of these three formulations of penicillin G make them useful for different diseases—for example, crystalline aqueous for meningococcal meningitis, procaine suspension for urethral gonorrhea, and benzathine suspension for prophylaxis of rheumatic fever.

Patient factors also are important in determining absorption of drug. Patients in shock have decreased blood flow to subcutaneous tissues and highly variable rates of flow through skeletal muscle. Therefore these sites should not be used for prompt or reliable drug absorption. For example, a patient in anaphylactic shock may need epinephrine, but its administration via the subcutaneous route (routinely used in the treatment of patients with asthma) would not be advisable. The immunogenicity of hepatitis B vaccine can be different when it is given intramuscularly (IM) in the deltoid muscle compared with the gluteal

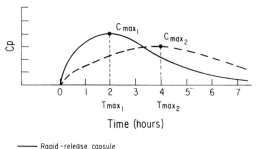

Time (hours)

—— Rapid-release capsule

— — Sustained-release capsule

Fig. 1–6. The plasma concentration of an idealized drug over time following oral administration. Note that the rapid-release capsule has a higher peak concentration (C_{max}) and an earlier peak concentration (T_{max}) than does the sustained-release capsule.

muscle, perhaps because gluteal injections are often made into fat tissue rather than muscle. *Principle: Absorption of drugs is a complex process that depends on factors related to the drug itself, the vehicle of administration, the site of administration, and the state of the patient. The choice of a route or site of administration of a drug should be made deliberately as part of a carefully considered therapeutic program.*

When a drug is given by direct IV injection or infusion, 100% is delivered to the systemic circulation (barring inactivation of the drug by light, incompatible substances in IV fluids, or adsorption of the drug to the plastic tubing). Drugs delivered via any other route result in less than 100% bioavailability (i.e., less than 100% of the administered dose is delivered to the systemic circulation in its original form). For example, 35% or less of lidocaine administered by mouth is bioavailable. Some of the drug is destroyed in the stomach, and a large portion of the lidocaine that is absorbed from the intestine into the portal blood is metabolized by the liver before the portal blood reaches the inferior vena cava (the so-called first-pass effect). Less than 5% of neomycin is bioavailable by the oral route. Many other drugs taken orally, such as salicylic acid or sulfisoxazole, have bioavailabilities that approach 100%. *Principle: When drugs are given by any route other than the IV route, the extent of absorption and bioavailability must be understood to prescribe it rationally and to make appropriate quantitative adjustments if the route of administration needs to be changed.*

Distribution and Redistribution of Absorbed Drug

After a drug has been absorbed and reaches the systemic circulation, the process of distribution begins. Usually, the drug appears to be rapidly mixed in the intravascular space and comes to a rapid equilibrium with other tissues in the body. Drugs that are tightly bound to plasma proteins, or drugs that have very high molecular weight (large proteins, dextrans, etc.) tend to be confined to the intravascular space (about 5 liters). Most drugs are sufficiently small and lipid-soluble that much of the dose is distributed to tissues outside the vascular space.

After an IV dose of most drugs, a concentration-of-drug-over-time curve similar to that illustrated in Fig. 1–7 is seen. In this example, 1000 mg of a drug was given IV. It appeared to be rapidly mixed in the blood and rapidly distributed throughout the body. The C_p of the drug was 40 mg/l. Thus, the apparent volume of distribution (V_d) was 25 liters, that is, the dose of 1000 mg behaved as if it were rapidly distributed into a

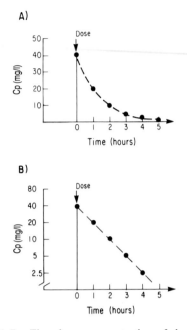

Fig. 1–7. The plasma concentration of drug at various times following an IV bolus injection. (A) Note that the ordinate (C_p) has a linear scale, and the curve demonstrates a shape characteristic of *exponential decay*. (B) Note that the ordinate has a logarithmic scale, and the curve appears to be a straight line.

25-liter compartment (derived by dividing the total dose, D, by the initial plasma concentration, C_0). The V_d of a drug may be calculated as

$$V_d = D/C_0$$

There is no real 25-liter compartment in the human body, but the term "*apparent* volume of distribution" is a useful way to think about how drugs seem to be distributed. By making this approximation, we can make quick approximations of the appropriate doses to give patients in order to arrive at a desired C_0. The two panels in Fig. 1–7 demonstrate the rapid distribution of the 1000-mg dose into a V_d of 25 liters, with a C_0 of 40 mg/l. The subsequent decline in C_p over time (plotted on a linear scale and a log-linear scale) is caused by clearance (or removal) of the drug from the plasma. Knowing any two of three variables (D, V_d, or C_0), enables one to calculate the third. For example, the V_d can be calculated by knowing D and C_0 plasma. From this information, pause to calculate a dose of drug that will produce a desired C_0 if you are given its V_d and the desired C_0. When most drugs are administered, they seem to be rapidly distributed into a volume that represents the blood volume plus other tissues but appears as a single compartment analogous to a pool of water (Fig. 1–7). How large the apparent V_d is depends on a number of factors intrinsic to the drug. Properties of molecular weight, lipophilicity, and affinity for binding to plasma and tissue proteins all are factors that enter into a drug's apparent V_d; this is discussed in greater detail in chapter 37. Knowing the simple factors can help you predict how disease states may affect the pharmacokinetics of a drug and the modification of dosing that will be needed to compensate for these changes. ***Principle: Drugs with a large V_d often bind reasonably avidly to tissue sites, are lipophilic, and will require hepatic metabolism before they can be eliminated.*** Consider then the value of knowing a likely V_d when two drugs with widely discrepant V_d's can be chosen for treating the same indication in patients with or without severe liver disease. ***Principle: A low V_d often means that the drug is large or bound to plasma proteins, is hydrophilic, shows no special predilection for distribution to lipid-laden tissues (including the brain), and is eliminated predominantly by the kidney in an unchanged form.*** Think about the impact of renal disease upon such drugs.

Some drugs, such as diazepam and thiopental, demonstrate complex concentration-of-drug-over-time curves. Figure 1–8 illustrates what such a curve might look like in a 70-kilogram (kg) patient receiving a 10-mg IV dose of diazepam. On this semilog plot, the decline in concentration of drug over time has two phases. The initial phase lasts several hours, during which the concentration of drug declines relatively rapidly. This is followed by a more prolonged phase of gradual decline in C_p that lasts for days. The initial phase is called the α phase of redistribution. The rapid decline in C_p is caused mainly by the prompt redistribution of drug from the small central compartment of well-perfused tissues (including the blood, brain, and heart) into a much larger peripheral compartment of more poorly perfused tissues (fat, muscle, other tissues) rather than by actual disappearance of the drug from the body. The second phase is called the β phase of elimination, in which the decline in C_p is caused predominantly by the gradual clearance (removal) of diazepam from the plasma, in this case by hepatic biotransformation.

Concentrations of diazepam in plasma following an injection closely resemble data displayed in Fig. 1–8 (Greenblatt et al., 1989). Diazepam works quickly to suppress grand mal seizures because the small central compartment includes the blood and brain. Thus a high concentration of drug is achieved quickly in the brain (usually within a few seconds of a rapid IV injection), and seizures usually are rapidly controlled. However, seizures may recur after 15 to 60 minutes, not

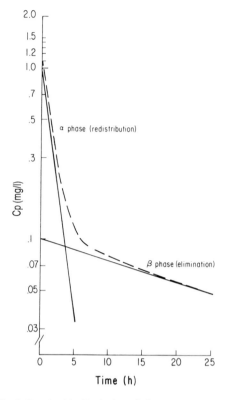

Fig. 1–8. An idealized plot of plasma concentration of diazepam over time following a rapid IV injection of 10 mg. Note that the ordinate (C_p) has a logarithmic scale. The decay curve (dashed line) is the sum of two straight lines, each representing a different exponential process.

because the drug is cleared from plasma and eliminated from the body (which takes many hours to occur) but because the drug is rapidly redistributed from the small central compartment into the larger peripheral compartment. When this happens, C_p falls to a value that is subtherapeutic for controlling seizures. Thus, acute management of grand mal seizures usually consists of rapidly controlling the seizures with intravenous diazepam, and then "loading" the patient with a second drug such as phenytoin or phenobarbital. While a loading dose of phenytoin may take 30 minutes to administer, it should begin to work as the beneficial effects of diazepam are waning.

Other commonly used drugs that exhibit such prominent, rapid, and clinically important redistribution include midazolam and thiopental. These drugs all have the same property: their clinical effects decline much more rapidly than could be accounted for by their elimination from the body. In the case of diazepam, the half-life of redistribution is about 1 hour, but the half-life of elimination is 24 to 36 hours (up to 72 hours in some elderly patients).

Drugs that exhibit clinically important redistribution and have concentration-over-time curves as illustrated in Fig. 1–8 are described mathematically by a *two-compartment model*. Drugs that do not exhibit such clinically important redistribution are described by a *one-compartment model*. Most drugs have some redistribution effect, but the redistribution often is small enough to be clinically insignificant. For most drugs, a one-compartment model is sufficiently accurate to represent the clinically observed effects and behavior of the drug.

Plasma Clearance

Clearance, in its simplest terms, is the body's ability to rid itself of a drug, xenobiotic, or waste product (such as creatinine). In therapeutics, this is thought of as clearance of the drug from plasma. One way to begin to understand this process is to consider the body to be a swimming pool connected to a pump and filter unit. The pump circulates water at a constant rate through a filter designed to be 100% efficient in removing particulates and unwanted chemicals or substances. Clearance from the swimming pool water would be expressed as gallons per minute. In human beings, we can think of the central compartment (pool) being connected to at least two important pump and filter systems—the liver and kidneys. We measure their contributions to total plasma clearance in milliliters per minute. As the volume of distribution is an apparent volume, so clearance of drug from plasma corresponds to the (apparent) volume of plasma that appears to be completely cleared of all its drug in 1 minute. In addition, if both the liver and kidney are active in the clearance process, then the total clearance is equal to the sum of the clearance of both units. If other organs contribute to plasma clearance, these effects are added to those of the major organs of elimination.

In a healthy adult man weighing about 70 kg, the flow of blood through the liver and kidneys may be estimated. From this figure for total blood flow, the total plasma flow (assuming a hematocrit of 40%) can be calculated. Because most drugs are carried predominantly in plasma (as opposed to formed elements of the blood), it is customary to measure concentrations of drug in plasma (C_p), and to state clearance of drugs in terms of plasma clearance (Cl_p). Maximal figures for the contributions of the liver and kidneys to plasma clearance are illustrated in Table 1–1. Clearance of drugs from the plasma of patients with hepatic or renal disease may decrease if the drug in question usually is cleared mainly by the

Table 1-1. MAXIMAL CONTRIBUTIONS TO TOTAL PLASMA CLEARANCE BY THE LIVER AND KIDNEYS

ORGAN	TOTAL BLOOD FLOW (ML/MIN)	TOTAL PLASMA FLOW (ML/MIN)	MAXIMAL PLASMA CLEARANCE (ML/MIN)
Liver	1500	900	900
Kidney	1200	720	720

liver (e.g., lidocaine, theophylline) or the kidneys (e.g., gentamicin, penicillin), respectively.

The concept of plasma clearance of drugs is highly analogous to the familiar creatinine clearance, the ability of the kidneys to remove creatinine from plasma via renal excretion. The average healthy man weighing 70 kg produces about 1500 mg of creatinine per 24 hours. While creatinine is a waste product produced by skeletal muscle, we can think of it as being continuously infused from muscle into the central compartment. The resultant concentration of creatinine in plasma is about 1 mg/dl or 10 mg/l. If we know the rate of administration for either creatinine or drugs and the steady-state plasma concentration (C_{pss}), we can calculate the Cl_p of either. Using creatinine as our example (where Cl_{creat} is the creatinine clearance):

$$Cl_{creat} = \frac{\text{Rate of administration}}{C_{pss}}$$

$$Cl_{creat} = \frac{1500 \text{ mg/24 h}}{10 \text{ mg/l}} = \frac{150 \text{ l}}{24 \text{ h}} = \frac{100 \text{ ml}}{\text{min}}$$

The units of clearance are volume of plasma per unit time.

The concept of clearance also is important in explaining the shape of the plasma-concentration-over-time curves as illustrated in Fig. 1–7. After a single dose of a drug is administered (as opposed to a continuous infusion), its concentration in plasma declines in a characteristic fashion referred to as *exponential decay* (Fig. 1–7, panel A). The C_p declines by a constant percentage per unit time. [For most drugs, patients eliminate a constant percentage of the drug's concentration per unit time rather than a fixed amount (in milligrams) of drug per unit time.] In Fig. 1–7, panel B, C_p is plotted on a logarithmic scale that linearizes this relationship. In this example, the value of C_p falls about 50% every hour.

The process of clearance by the kidney involves a combination of glomerular filtration, tubular secretion, and sometimes tubular reabsorption as well. Drug clearance by the liver involves biotransformation, biliary excretion, or both. Many drugs undergo both renal and hepatic clearance. Some drugs are cleared from plasma by other routes as well, such as via exhalation (halothane), renal metabolism (imipenem), fecal excretion (charcoal), metabolism in plasma (succinylcholine). As discussed above, the total plasma clearance of a drug equals the sum of each individual clearance term contributed by each organ of biotransformation (most often the liver) or elimination (most often the kidney). For example, the total plasma clearance of procainamide in a healthy adult is about 500 ml/min, of which about one third is contributed by hepatic biotransformation and the rest by renal filtration and secretion.

The processes of hepatic biotransformation and renal excretion are discussed in greater depth in chapters 9, 11, 37, and 39. As a general rule, most drugs that are highly lipophilic (lipid-soluble) are not rapidly cleared by the kidneys. Even when these drugs are present in renal tubular fluid, they are very likely to be reabsorbed back into blood. Thus, *most lipophilic drugs must first be biotransformed in the liver to more hydrophilic metabolites*. The kidneys generally clear hydrophilic (water-soluble) drugs and drug metabolites. There are many different types of biotransformation reactions that occur in the liver. The enzymatically mediated reactions that oxidize, reduce, hydrolyze, hydroxylate, or dealkylate at active sites often occur in microsomal fractions of liver cells. These reactions are mediated by a class of enzymes called the mixed-function monooxygenase system, also known as the cytochrome P450 system. The metabolites of drugs that undergo these types of reactions (also called phase I, or nonsynthetic, reactions) are more hydrophilic than the progenitor drugs, and therefore are more likely than the progenitor to be cleared by the kidneys. *Principle: Analysis of the chemical characteristics of drugs can aid in choices between chemical entities used for the same indication. If inspection of a molecule's structure allows sensible estimates of hepatic versus renal excretion of a drug, make a point of that analysis for drugs you use often. Basic pharmacology texts infrequently make this analysis for you. An excellent resource is The Merck Index.* In addition, since these types of phase I changes in the drug often are sterically small, the metabolites frequently are pharmacologically active. *Principle: The pharmacologic profile of an active metabolite can be very different from that of its progenitor. The "purpose" of liver metabolism of drugs is generally to make them more polar and thus water-soluble, not to "inactivate" the drug's pharmacologic effects.*

The amount and activity of the drug-metabolizing enzymes in the liver may be increased (induced) by a variety of conditions, including smoking or administration of enzyme-inducing drugs such as phenytoin, phenobarbital, or rifampin. The activity or amount of these enzymes may also be inhibited or reduced because of hepatic disease (cirrhosis, hepatitis) or because of administration of drugs such as cimetidine. The large potential for drug–drug interactions at the level of hepatic drug-metabolizing enzymes is described in chapters 39 and 40. Finally, there are large pharmacogenetic differences between patients in their ability to biotransform drugs (see chapters 29–32).

Biotransformation of drugs in the liver can also be accomplished by addition of large donor groups to the parent drug (conjugation reactions). A variety of enzymes called transferases or conjugases facilitate the covalent transfer of groups such as glucuronic acid, glycine, sulfate, acetyl, or glutathione to the drug itself. These reactions are all enzymatically mediated, require a donor group, and consume energy. They are referred to as phase II, or synthetic, reactions. Phase II changes to the drug molecule often are pharmacologically more substantive than are phase I reactions; in fact, the metabolites of phase II reactions usually are pharmacologically inactive. *Principle: Both phase I and phase II reactions convert lipophilic drugs to more hydrophilic metabolites as a means to facilitate subsequent renal excretion.* Many drugs undergo a series of phase I and phase II reactions before they are eliminated from the body. Consider the biotransformation pathways of two commonly prescribed benzodiazepines—diazepam and lorazepam (Fig. 1-9). The parent drug is cleared predominantly by hepatic biotransformation in a series of phase I reactions ending in a phase II conjugation to glucuronic acid to form the glucuronide. The glucuronide is pharmacologically inactive, hydrophilic, and excreted by the kidneys. The metabolic fate of lorazepam is considerably simpler. It requires one phase II reaction to form the glucuronide that is excreted renally. Since cimetidine can inhibit phase I but not phase II reactions, it becomes clear why cimetidine can slow the biotransformation and clearance of diazepam (or chlordiazepoxide) but not lorazepam (or oxazepam).

Some metabolites have complex pharmacokinetic or pharmacodynamic properties. For example, some of the metabolites of the hypnotic flurazepam are pharmacologically active and are cleared much more slowly than the parent drug. These metabolites contribute to the drug's tendency to cause daytime somnolence. Drug metabolites may be cleared at different rates than is their progenitor drug. Azathioprine, cyclophosphamide, and enalapril are prodrugs that are pharmacologically inactive. They gain pharmaco-

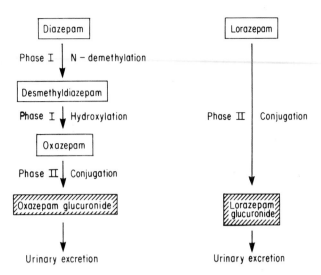

Fig. 1–9. Important pathways of hepatic biotransformation of two benzodiazepines, diazepam and lorazepam. Each arrow represents an enzyme-mediated reaction. Drugs and metabolites in white boxes are those that have pharmacologic activity. Metabolites in gray boxes have undergone conjugation reactions and are pharmacologically inactive.

logic activity only after active metabolites are formed. *Principle: Drug metabolites may exhibit pharmacokinetic or pharmacodynamic properties quite unlike those of the progenitor drugs.* When metabolism is predictable and has little interpersonal variation, we often attribute the pattern of pharmacologic effects to the parent drug. That attribution is dangerous if metabolism is genetically dependent, or if the patient develops disease of the organ of elimination of the metabolite or takes drugs that interfere (by acceleration or inhibition) with metabolism of the parent drug or excretion of the metabolites.

The pathways of renal clearance are discussed in chapters 11 and 37. The kidney can excrete drug present in the protein-free ultrafiltrate (glomerular filtration) and can actively secrete weak organic acids (anionic drugs such as penicillin or methotrexate) or weak organic bases (cationic drugs such as procainamide or quinidine) into the renal tubules. Reabsorption of the drug or metabolite from the tubular fluid can also occur. The active secretory processes may be inhibited by other drugs that bind to the transport carrier protein and act as a competitive inhibitor of the transport process. Probenecid is the prototype inhibitor of active secretion of weak organic acid drugs (e.g., penicillin, methotrexate, furosemide), and cimetidine appears to inhibit the tubular secretion of several weak organic cations (e.g., procainamide, quinidine).

Many drugs are cleared by both the liver and kidneys. For example, phenobarbital is cleared by both the liver (75% of total clearance) and the kidney (25%), but the total clearance rate of the drug is only 6 ml/min. Such a low rate of plasma clearance is less than 1% of the rate of plasma flow to these organs, implying a very low efficiency of these organs as pump and filter units

with respect to phenobarbital. The importance of both hepatic and renal clearance is illustrated when drugs are first biotransformed by the liver to active metabolites that are themselves cleared by the kidney. This type of pattern can have serious consequences, as seen in the following case.

Case History

A 68-year-old woman with metastatic breast cancer was admitted to the hospital for radiation therapy of painful bone metastases. She was given large doses of meperidine, up to 100 mg every 2 hours, to control her pain. Because of unrecognized prerenal azotemia and hypercalcemia, she developed progressive renal failure, and her creatinine concentration increased from 1.4 mg/dl on admission to 4.2 mg/dl 4 days later. On her fifth hospital day she had severe myoclonic jerking movements of her extremities. By the next day, she had severe and refractory grand mal seizures.

Discussion: The intense pain of bone metastases may be difficult to control. In this patient, meperidine was a poor choice of analgesic for several reasons. Meperidine is cleared predominantly (about 85%) by hepatic biotransformation to normeperidine, a phase I (nonsynthetic) demethylation reaction. Normeperidine is not very active as an analgesic, but it stimulates CNS activity that can result in myoclonus and seizures. Normally, this metabolite is readily excreted by the kidneys. However, in patients receiving high doses of meperidine who develop renal dysfunction, large amounts of normeperidine will be formed in the liver and slowly cleared by the kidneys. The resultant accumulation of this metabolite can lead to severe seizures, as was demonstrated in this patient. Another disadvantage of using meperidine is that it has a short half-life, requiring administration every 2 to 3 hours.

Principle: The balance of hepatic and renal clearance, both of the parent drug and any active metabolites, must be understood in order to prescribe a drug wisely.

The Half-Life of Elimination

For most drugs, a certain constant percentage of the drug is eliminated from the body per unit time. The time it takes a patient to eliminate half the drug from the body or decrease the concentration of drug in plasma by 50% is known as a drug's elimination half-life.

The half-life of elimination is determined by the drug and the patient. The average half-life of elimination of penicillin G is about 30 minutes. Diazepam has an elimination half-life of about 24 hours in young adults, thyroxine about 7 days, and amiodarone more than 1 month! The elimination half-life of a drug is not determined by its route of clearance. It can be long or short whether it is cleared by the kidney, liver, or lung, and so forth.

Why do drugs exhibit such marked differences in elimination half-life? The half-life of elimination is determined by both the clearance and the volume of distribution of the drug. Figure 1–10 illustrates this concept.

Consider two swimming pools attached to pump and filter units. The volume of one is 1000 liters, and it is connected to a small pump and filter unit capable of a clearance rate of 10 l/min. The second pool is a smaller pool (500 liters), but it is connected to a pump and filter unit that can clear 25 l/min. The drug would be eliminated (cleared) more rapidly from the pool with the smaller volume and the larger clearance rate. That is, the longer half-life of elimination is associated

with the larger volume of distribution and the lower clearance. The half-life of elimination ($t_{1/2}$) is proportional to the volume of distribution of the drug, and inversely proportional to the clearance:

$$t_{1/2} \propto \frac{V_d}{Cl}$$

As described in chapter 37, $t_{1/2} = 0.7 \times V_d/Cl$. *Principle: The half-life of elimination of a drug is determined by both the drug's volume of distribution and its clearance.*

The half-life of elimination is important in understanding three important concepts:

1. Half-life is used to determine how much time will be needed to achieve the ultimate steady-state concentration of drug in plasma. For example, consider a continuous infusion of theophylline begun in an asthmatic patient. If no loading dose is given, the plasma concentration will increase over time until a plateau, or steady-state, concentration is approached that occurs when as much drug is going into the body as is being eliminated (see Fig. 1–11). A typical value for the elimination half-life of theophylline is about 9 hours. The plasma concentration will move 50% closer to its ultimate steady-state concentration every 9 hours. After 1 half-life, the plasma concentration will equal 50% of the eventual steady-state concentration (panel A). After 3 half-lives, the plasma concentration will be about to 87% of the eventual steady-state concentration.

2. The half-life of elimination also is used to determine how long it will take for the concentration of drug in plasma to fall once drug administration is stopped. When the theophylline infu-

A   **B**

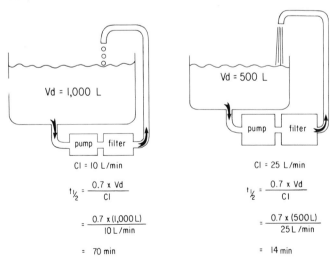

Fig. 1–10. The influence of the V_d and Cl on the half-life of elimination. (A) For this pool, the large volume of distribution ($V_d = 1000$ liters) combined with the low clearance ($Cl = 10$ l/min) define a half-life of elimination of 70 minutes. (B) For this pool, the smaller volume of distribution ($V_d = 500$ liters) and the higher clearance ($Cl = 25$ l/min) define a half-life of elimination of only 14 minutes.

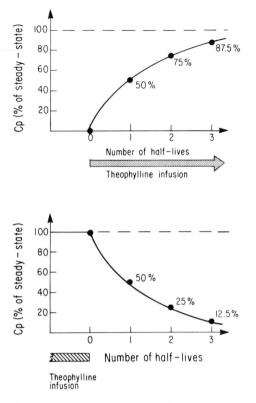

Fig. 1–11. (A) The approach of the plasma concentration (C_p) of theophylline to its eventual steady-state concentration (C_{pss}) during a continuous IV infusion. After two half-lives, C_p has climbed to about 75% of the eventual steady-state concentration. (B) The decay of C_p of theophylline after a continuous infusion has been abruptly discontinued. After two half-lives, C_p has fallen to about 25% of the original value.

sion is abruptly discontinued (illustrated in panel B), the plasma concentration will fall toward zero by 50% every half-life. After 3 half-lives (about 27 hours), about 87% of the drug will have been eliminated from the body.

3. The half-life is useful in designing an appropriate dosing interval. For a drug with a very short half-life of elimination (e.g., insulin, dopamine, heparin) a continuous infusion may be required. When the half-life of elimination is about 30 minutes (e.g., penicillin G) the drug may have to be given every 2 to 4 hours. For a drug with a half-life of elimination of about 33 hours (e.g., digoxin), once daily administration is usually adequate.

APPLIED PHARMACOKINETICS

Target Concentration

The concepts of the EC_{50}, the TC_{50}, the concentration–response curves associated with those values, and the "therapeutic range" all enter into the quantitative therapeutic decision process. Usually, the concentration of drug in plasma correlates better with the pharmacologic effects of a drug than does the dose of the drug administered to the patient. For many drugs, pharmacologic efficacy and clinical responses are delayed or harder to measure than is the concentration of a drug in plasma. In such cases, a surrogate end point for approximating the appropriate use of a drug is the concentration of a drug in plasma rather than the clinical response. Population-based data often can be used to establish a range of plasma concentrations that correlate with therapeutic efficacy or toxicity of a drug (see chapter 38). Therefore, plasma concentrations of drugs are one checkpoint for the quantitative adequacy of a therapeutic regimen. These measurements are also useful in changing dosages when the response is not as intended.

Different plasma concentrations of drug within the therapeutic range may be appropriate for different patients, or for the same patient at different times (see chapters 37 and 38). However, when the physician begins to treat a specific patient, an initial target concentration should be chosen when using a drug whose concentration helps predict therapeutic effects.

For example, we usually think of the therapeutic range of theophylline as from 5 to 20 mg/l. Most patients receive minimal benefit from the drug when concentrations are below 5 mg/l; concentrations greater than 20 mg/l are often associated with unacceptable toxicity. About half the maximal benefit from the drug (the EC_{50}) is achieved at a concentration of 10 mg/l. For a relatively stable asthmatic patient, an appropriate target concentration might well be 10 mg/l. The added benefit achieved with higher concentrations may not be needed, and staying at relatively low plasma concentrations minimizes the associated risks of toxicity. For a very sick asthmatic patient who has tight bronchospasm that has failed to respond adequately to otherwise optimal management with theophylline and other agents, the target concentration might be increased to 20 mg/l. The added efficacy associated with the higher concentration may be necessary, even though the risk of greater systemic toxicity at these concentrations is enhanced. ***Principle: The target concentration of a drug in plasma is determined not only by the properties of the drug, but also by the balance of risks to benefits in the specific patient.***

The first step in applying pharmacokinetics to the therapy of a specific patient is to determine from population information whether the therapeutic range of the proposed drug is known. The next step is to pick a specific target concentration based on the patient's clinical condition and the presence of concurrent illnesses or concurrent drugs that might affect the pharmacodynamics or pharmacokinetics of the intended drug. To illustrate how to proceed once a target concentration is chosen, an example is given of prescribing theophylline to a 35-year-old male patient weighing 70 kg with a severe acute asthmatic attack that has not responded adequately to therapy in the emergency room.

Loading Dose

The essential pharmacokinetic data concerning theophylline in the "average" adult patient is widely available (see chapter 7 and Appendix I). The appendix describes the following values for theophylline:

$$V_d = 0.5 \text{ l/kg} \times 70 \text{ kg} = 35 \text{ liters}$$

$$Cl = 50 \text{ ml/min (or 3 l/h)}$$

$$t_{1/2} = 8.2 \text{ hours}$$

One way to initiate theophylline therapy would be an IV infusion of the drug at a constant rate sufficient to produce an eventual steady-state target concentration of 15 mg/l. However, such a continuous infusion would require about 3.3 half-lives (or about 3.3×8.2 hours $= 25$ hours) before the plasma concentration rose to 90% of the ultimate steady-state concentration. In a patient with severe asthma, we would like to achieve a therapeutic plasma concentration much more quickly. Administering a loading dose of the drug before starting the infusion is a way to get to the target concentration rapidly. ***Principle: A loading dose of a drug should be administered when the patient's condition requires the prompt achievement of the chosen target concentration.***

Given our knowledge of the drug's distribution, the loading dose (LD) can be calculated as the product of the estimated V_d and the target concentration:

$$LD = V_d \times C_{\text{target}}$$

$$LD = 35 \text{ liters} \times 15 \text{ mg/l} = 525 \text{ mg}$$

In this case the loading dose is given IV so that the peak plasma concentration will be achieved shortly after the end of the loading infusion, rather than in the 1 to 2 hours that would be required following oral administration of the same dose. Because the bioavailability of IV theophylline is by definition 100% ($F = 1.0$), no dose adjustment is needed to compensate for the incomplete bioavailability that would occur if the drug were to be given by the oral route. If we had chosen aminophylline rather than theophylline,

the dose would be different, because only 85% of the weight of aminophylline is theophylline. The other 15% is ethylenediamine, added to increase theophylline's solubility in water. Using aminophylline, the correct loading dose would be

$$LD_{\text{aminophylline}} = 525 \text{ mg}/0.85 = 618 \text{ mg}$$

The dose is not given as a bolus, rather it is infused over 20 to 30 minutes. The slower infusion keeps the maximal concentration in plasma at an acceptable level in the blood perfusing the CNS, heart, and kidneys to minimize transient toxicity at those sites. The full loading dose must be given to a patient who has not previously received the drug on a chronic basis. If the patient has been taking theophylline before coming to the emergency room, then the loading dose must be reduced appropriately to allow for the theophylline concentration already present in the patient's plasma. In that case,

$$LD = V_d \times (C_{\text{target}} - C_i)$$

where C_i is the initial concentration of the drug.

Maintenance Dose by IV Infusion

Once the infusion of the loading dose of theophylline is completed, the concentration in plasma will be approximately 15 mg/l. A maintenance infusion of the drug should be started, or the concentration will decline with a half-life of approximately 8.2 hours. The goal of the maintenance infusion is to supply theophylline at the same rate that it is being cleared from the plasma (largely by hepatic biotransformation). When the rate of administration equals the rate of elimination of drug, the drug concentration in plasma will remain constant, that is, at a steady state. The rate of administration of drug is called the maintenance dose. The rate of elimination of drug is the product of the clearance of drug from plasma and its concentration in plasma at steady state (C_{pss}), as was discussed above. Consequently, at steady state:

Rate of administration of drug =
rate of elimination of drug

$$\text{Maintenance infusion rate} = Cl \times C_{\text{pss}}$$
$$= 3 \text{ l/h} \times 15 \text{ mg/l}$$
$$= 45 \text{ mg/h}$$

Maintenance Dose by Repeated Doses

If the patient remains critically ill, continuing to administer theophylline as a continuous IV infusion is generally necessary. The target concentration can be changed depending on the patient's clinical condition or improvement and the drug's observed efficacy or toxicity. A continuous infusion avoids both the peak and trough concentrations associated with intermittent dosing regimens.

As the patient improves, the maintenance regimen usually is changed to drug doses delivered orally at fixed intervals. Since oral theophylline has a bioavailability of about 90% ($F = 0.9$), a regimen of 50 mg/h would offer the closest approximation of the continuous IV infusion. But hourly oral administration of theophylline is inconvenient and not necessary because the drug's elimination half-life is about 8 hours. For standard oral theophylline preparations, a dosing interval of about 6 hours usually is employed. In this situation, the dose most equivalent to the infusion would be 50 mg/h × 6 hours = 300 mg every 6 hours.

For many years, most patients taking theophylline had to remember to take it four times a day. However, theophylline was one of the earliest drugs to become available in a sustained-release (delayed-release or continuous-release) formulation. Such sustained-release products approximate an oral infusion of the drug, with delayed absorption of drug and larger values of T_{max}. These pharmaceutical properties allow the drug to be administered every 12 hours to most patients rather than every 6 hours. Oral bioavailability may not be consistent with different sustained-release products, but assuming equivalent bioavailability, an equivalent dose would be 50 mg/h × 12 hours = 600 mg by mouth every 12 hours. Such a dosage regimen should allow the plasma theophylline concentration to hover about the desired concentration of 15 mg/l, with peaks a bit higher than that value, and trough values a bit lower. (The peaks and troughs can be predicted using information discussed in chapters 37 and 38). As the patient continues to improve, a new target concentration of only 10 mg/l may be appropriate. In that situation, the maintenance dose would be two thirds of the 600 mg, or about 400 mg by mouth every 12 hours.

The logic and equations needed to calculate appropriate loading doses, maintenance infusions, and changes to chronic maintenance therapy with intermittent oral dosing is theoretically straightforward. However, variability within patients and even more variability between patients for volumes of distribution, drug clearance, oral bioavailability, half-lives, and so forth, make it necessary to check the predicted drug concentrations at reasonable intervals to determine whether individual variations require dosage adjustment. Review is particularly germane when the drug has a narrow therapeutic index or is being used in an effort to achieve maximal efficacy. Patients require different target concentrations at different stages of their disease. Analysis of benefits and risks dictates different choices for target concentrations in different patients. For many drugs, including theophylline, measurement of the concentration of drug in the patient's plasma allows calculation of an accurate value of the patient's own V_d, Cl, or $t_{1/2}$, rather than relying on an average calculated from a population of patients. Calculating the patient's own pharmacokinetic values allows greater accuracy in achieving the desired target concentration. A more detailed discussion of these pharmacokinetic approaches to therapeutic drug monitoring is included in chapters 37 and 38. *Principle: The physician always should set explicit expectations of specific drug therapy before the regimen is initiated. Clearly defined measures of efficacy and lower levels of acceptable toxicity should be considered. If* **direct** *measurement of pharmacologic effects is not feasible, surrogate end points should be used. One such surrogate end point is a blood or plasma concentration of drug. The plasma concentration rarely is sufficient as the only measurement of drug effect and never preempts the actual measurement of direct pharmacologic effects where this is possible.*

PATIENTS WITH "SPECIAL" FEATURES

In the case of the asthmatic patient described above, we assumed that the patient had pharmacokinetic values (F, V_d, Cl, $t_{1/2}$) similar to those of previously studied normal volunteers or asthmatic patients, and that the patient would respond to theophylline similarly to "typical" patients. However, every patient is an individual, and differences in response to drugs (pharmacodynamic differences) and in the way that the drug is "handled" (pharmacokinetic differences) are to be expected. "Average" figures for F, V_d, and Cl obtained from cohorts of patients offer a good base from which to initiate therapy. But the prescriber should expect to encounter many between-patient differences that will require revision both in the qualitative and quantitative therapeutic decisions.

Theophylline can also serve as an example for consideration of patient demographics that affect therapeutic strategy. Clinical studies have demonstrated that the clearance of theophylline may be increased in smokers and significantly decreased in infants, the elderly, and those with cirrhosis, with severe liver disease, with congestive heart failure, or using cimetidine. The V_d of theophylline may be increased in premature infants and cirrhotic patients. Pregnant women (lack of established safety to the fetus) and nursing mothers (documented adverse reactions in nursing babies) have special contraindications for theophylline.

Patients allergic to ethylenediamine should avoid aminophylline, which can contain 15% ethylenediamine by weight.

Although each patient stands alone with respect to the pharmacodynamics and pharmacokinetics of a given drug, several key variables such as age, organ function, concomitant use of other medications, and so forth, present predictable factors to consider before using many medications. These important "special features" are briefly discussed in this section. Detailed presentations of some of these special features are included in chapters 29 to 32.

Pediatric Patients

Premature infants, neonates, infants, children, and adolescents should not be considered small adults. Not only are their diseases and treatments often different (e.g., artificial surfactant for respiratory distress syndrome, use of specific antibiotics to treat necrotizing enterocolitis), but also such patients may exhibit substantially altered pharmacokinetics and pharmacodynamics when compared with adults. The pharmacokinetics of drugs may change rapidly as a neonate becomes an infant and toddler. In addition, the premature infant may handle drugs differently from the normal neonate. The FDA has approved many drugs on the basis of data concerning efficacy, toxicity, and pharmacokinetics obtained in healthy adults, but with little or no drug experience in neonates, infants, and children. Thus, optimal drug treatment of infants and children poses an even greater challenge than optimal treatment of mature adults (Roberts, 1984).

Differences in Pharmacokinetics. Changes in pharmacokinetics of drugs in pediatric patients cannot be generalized. Although absorption of most drugs by the healthy neonate is often similar to that of the adult, premature neonates may secrete relatively small quantities of bile into the gut, thus decreasing the absorption of highly lipid-soluble drugs such as vitamins A, D, E, and K. Drug distribution may change rapidly as body water (expressed as the percentage of body weight) drops from 85% in premature infants to 75% in full-term infants. (For adults, 60% of body weight is water.) Total body fat content in the premature infant may be as low as 1%, contrasted to 15% in the normal full-term neonate. The implications of these differences for the distribution of water-soluble and lipid-soluble drugs are easy to understand. In addition, drug binding to plasma proteins may be much less in the fetus and neonate than it is in the adult, thereby increasing the free fraction (percentage unbound) for many drugs.

Although there are many different pathways for hepatic biotransformation, enzyme activity for them may be substantially less in the neonate. Decreased hepatic clearance (associated with increased steady-state plasma concentrations and prolonged half-life of elimination) of drugs such as acetaminophen, diazepam, tolbutamide, phenobarbital, theophylline, and many others is observed in the neonate but becomes closer to adult values as the infant matures. Perhaps the most widely publicized example of decreased hepatic biotransformation in the neonate involves chloramphenicol.

Case History

A 1-week-old, 4-kg infant develops neonatal septicemia and meningitis. A broad-spectrum antibiotic that penetrates the cerebrospinal fluid is desired. Chloramphenicol is chosen because it meets both criteria; the dose is 100 mg/kg per day. After about 4 days, the baby develops listlessness, refusal to suck, abdominal distension, and irregular and rapid respirations. This syndrome progresses to periods of cyanosis, flaccidity, hypothermia, and an ashen gray color. The antibiotic is stopped and the infant recovers. What happened?

Discussion: This syndrome is known as the *gray syndrome* or the *gray baby syndrome*. It was first recognized in 1959. The explanation of the syndrome became clear by 1963. Babies receiving the drug in conventional doses (on a milligram per kilogram basis) accumulated the antibiotic until it reached extremely high concentrations in plasma by about the fourth day of treatment. (Because the half-life of elimination was prolonged, it took several days to achieve a steady-state concentration in plasma.) Neonates display altered pharmacokinetics of this drug for two reasons. First, their livers have inadequate activity of the phase II biotransformation enzyme glucuronyl transferase for the first 3 to 4 weeks of life. Thus, the metabolism of the drug by glucuronidation is slow. Second, the immature kidney inadequately excretes both the unconjugated drug and the glucuronide conjugate of the drug. Elimination half-life in infants under 1 week of age is as long as 26 hours, compared with 4 hours in older children. So practitioners learned to avoid administering chloramphenicol during the first 4 weeks of life, or to use it in reduced doses (e.g., 25 mg/kg per day) if it is a drug of choice. When the drug must be used in children, close clinical monitoring of its efficacy and toxicity and measurement of its concentrations in plasma are mandatory.

Renal function (both glomerular filtration and tubular secretion) in the premature and full-term neonate is significantly reduced in comparison with that of older children and adults. When compared on the basis of body surface area, drugs such as penicillin G are cleared at only 7% of the rates in adults. Other drugs cleared by either tubular secretion or glomerular filtration (e.g., aminoglycosides, salicylate, and digoxin) behave similarly to penicillin G in neonates.

Practical problems in therapy also may be posed by children. Oral liquid suspensions and elixirs may be refused or spit out; tablets and capsules are impractical to administer. The small muscle mass of a child may make IM injections difficult. Limits on IV fluid volumes often require drugs to be prepared in relatively concentrated solutions. Flow rates through IV lines may be so low (several milliliters per hour) that an IV dose of a drug may take hours.

Pharmacodynamic Changes. Drugs may produce different pharmacodynamic effects in children than in adults. Amphetamine-like drugs usually produce CNS stimulation and excitement in an adult but can be efficacious in treating hyperactive (hyperkinetic) children with attention disorders. Glucocorticoids may produce problems with bone growth and epiphyseal maturation in children. Many features of the pharmacodynamics of drugs are seen only in children because diseases such as infant respiratory distress syndrome, necrotizing enterocolitis, and kernicterus occur predominantly or exclusively in them.

Although the problems encountered in treating pediatric patients may seem unusual when compared with those encountered in treating adults, the same principles of rational therapeutics apply. Close attention to the scientific basis of treatment and deliberate attempts to individualize therapy should result in increased drug efficacy and decreased drug toxicity.

Elderly Patients

Overview of Problem. In many ways, the elderly are at increased risk when they receive medications (see chapter 31). Recent review articles suggest that the special problems of elderly patients are beginning to be appreciated (Everitt and Avorn, 1986; Lamy, 1986; Beers and Ouslander, 1989; Montamat et al., 1989). Although Americans aged 60 years or greater make up about 17% of the U.S. population, they account for 39% of all hospitalizations and 51% of deaths from drug reactions (Kusserow, 1989). While those over 65 years (sometimes referred to as "the elderly") constitute about 12% of the population, they received about 30% of prescription drugs and about 40% of nonprescription drugs in 1986 (Kusserow, 1989). The taking of multiple medications is a particular problem in elderly patients. For elderly patients who are institutionalized, 61% receive three or more prescription drugs within 1 year;

37% receive five or more drugs; and 19% receive seven or more drugs (Kusserow, 1989). In a recent study of almost 473 outpatients in 19 family medicine and internal medicine practices in New England, patients were taking an average of 2.9 prescription drugs and 0.3 nonprescription drugs (J. Wasson, M.D., personal communication, December 1990).

In 1985 perhaps as many as 243,000 older adults were hospitalized because of adverse drug reactions. A recent report noted that "a growing body of evidence accumulated over the past 10 years indicates that mismedication of the elderly has become a critical health care issue" (Kusserow, 1989). Such mismedication can include the prescription of higher dosages than needed for adequate effects, the prescription of more dangerous drugs when less toxic preparations would be equally effective, the prescription of drugs that are unnecessary, or the use of drug combinations that produce adverse effects. Because elderly patients are a large subset of hospitalized patients, they are at most risk for the adverse drug reactions that occur during the course of hospitalization. As mentioned earlier, the largest risk factor for developing an adverse drug interaction is the number of drugs being taken. In addition, understanding instructions may be difficult for the elderly. Consequently problems with compliance (over- and underuse of medications) ensues; this important issue was recently addressed (Stewart and Caranasos, 1989). As many as from 14% to 21% of patients never fill their prescription, and drugs may not have their desired effects in 50% of patients because of improper use. Compliance with drug regimens may be especially difficult for many elderly patients because of poor vision or hearing, decline in cognitive function, use of complicated drug regimens with large numbers of medications, or even difficulty opening child-proof containers.

A large number of syndromes are present either predominantly or uniquely in the elderly. They include orthostatic hypotension, stroke, dementing illness, urinary incontinence, osteoporosis, constipation, and poor nutrition (Bender and Caranasos, 1989). These problems are often treated with prescription drugs rarely used in younger patients. The following case illustrates this double jeopardy that often is the elderly patient's plight.

Case History

A 70-year-old man was living in a nursing home because of complications of Alzheimer's disease, mild urethral obstruction, and congestive heart failure. With the death of a roommate, his room was changed and he became disoriented, especially at night. Thioridazine was prescribed to help control his agitated behavior. During the next several weeks he developed increasing symptoms of slow and diminished movement, tremor, and stiffness. A diagnosis of parkinsonism was made, and benzotropine was added to his regimen. During the next several days, his course deteriorated and was marked by difficulty with his vision, dry skin, fever, constipation, difficulty voiding, and increasing confusion and agitation. He was transferred to the hospital for management of an episode of acute urinary retention.

Discussion: The patient's initial episodes of disorientation late in the day ("sundowning") precipitated by recent disorienting events (e.g., loss of a roommate, change in rooms and nurses, etc.) is a common problem. The prescribing of a neuroleptic agent may have been overly aggressive, because the likelihood of toxicity often outweighs the minimal benefit. The overuse of neuroleptics in this setting and the relation between neuroleptic use and risk of hip fracture have been demonstrated (Ray et al., 1987; Avorn et al., 1989). In this case, toxicities such as increased sedation and the anticholinergic or antidopaminergic properties of thioridazine could have been expected. Pseudoparkinsonism is one such common effect but was not recognized as a drug-induced effect that indicated discontinuing the drug. Rather, the adverse reaction was treated with another new drug, benztropine, that also has anticholinergic activity.

A large variety of drugs that are commonly prescribed to the elderly have anticholinergic effects. In addition to antiparkinsonian drugs such as benztropine, the tricyclic antidepressants, antiemetics such as promethazine, antipsychotics, antiarrhythmics such as disopyramide, antihistamines, and drugs for dizziness such as meclizine all have anticholinergic properties in addition to their intended pharmacologic effects (Peters, 1989). The elderly may be especially vulnerable to the adverse effects of constipation, difficulty with vision (pupillary dilation, cycloplegia), decreased bladder tone, and confusion caused by such drugs. The episode of acute urinary retention in this patient likely was precipitated by the two drugs with anticholinergic properties superimposed on the patient's underlying symptoms of benign prostatic hypertrophy. The elderly patient is at risk of entering a vicious cycle in which he or she is more likely to receive drugs, more likely to develop adverse drug reactions, and potentially more likely to receive even more drugs to treat the adverse drug effects that are not recognized as such.

Altered Pharmacokinetics in the Elderly. Elderly patients may have altered drug pharmacokinetics. This should not be surprising because most drugs released to marketing have their pharmacokinetics investigated in younger volunteers or patients (see chapters 31, 34, 35, and 41). Only recently has the FDA in the United States required that new drugs that may be prescribed in elderly patients must have their kinetics and dynamics evaluated in the elderly before approval.

Age-related changes in drug pharmacokinetics are complex and often difficult to predict. Age-related changes in the bioavailability, distribution, hepatic biotransformation, and renal clearance of drugs are discussed in chapters 29 to 32. Absorption of most drugs is intact in the elderly. Decreased hepatic function may reduce the first-pass effect for some drugs with large first-pass effects and thereby increase oral bioavailability of some drugs. More changes are seen with respect to distribution of drugs. Tendencies to decreased total body water and increased total body fat, along with a fall in concentration of albumin in plasma leads to alterations in the V_d of some drugs. For example, there may be a decreased V_d for water-soluble drugs such as ethanol and lithium, and increased V_d for lipid-soluble drugs such as diazepam.

Decreased blood flow to the liver and kidney (with decreased renal plasma flow, glomerular filtration, and tubular secretion) can be associated with decreased drug clearance. While many elderly persons preserve good renal function into old age, as a group, elderly patients are at increased risk of having decreased renal function. Some drugs cleared by the liver (e.g., lidocaine, theophylline, diazepam), and most drugs cleared by the kidney (e.g., gentamicin, lithium) must be especially carefully monitored when given to older patients.

Several nomograms or formulas that are easy to use can predict renal function (glomerular filtration rate, or GFR) once the patient's age and serum creatinine concentration are known (Paladino et al., 1986). One of the more common of these is based on the following formula:

$$Cl_{\text{creatinine}} \text{ in ml/min} = \left[\frac{114 - (0.8 \times \text{age})}{C_{\text{creatinine}} \text{ in mg/dl}} \right]$$
$$\times \; [1.00 \text{ or } 0.85]$$

where a multiplicative correction factor of 1.0 is assigned for men and 0.85 for women. The formula illustrates that an 80-year-old man with a "normal" creatinine concentration of 1.0 mg/dl would likely have a creatinine clearance of only about 50 ml/min. Between-patient differences in organ function in patients of the same age are often large. Nomograms and formulas help estimate initial maintenance doses of drugs in the elderly, but they do *not* substitute for clinical judgment and measurement of plasma concentrations of drug.

Changes in drug distribution and drug clearance may combine to cause large changes in elimination half-life for certain drugs. For example, the elimination half-life of diazepam may be prolonged from 24 hours in a young man to 96 hours in an octogenarian who has increased V_d and decreased hepatic clearance.

Altered Pharmacodynamics in the Elderly. Even when medications are not overprescribed or misused in this population, elderly patients experience changes in their physiology that are partially responsible for altered pharmacodynamic responses to some medications.

Case History

An 83-year-old man had been in good health until he suffered a compression fracture of his thoracic spine. The nocturnal pain had made it difficult for him to fall asleep. His physician prescribed chlorpromazine 50 mg taken orally (p.o.) before bed to help him sleep. Over the next few days he noted increasing faintness when he stood up, had increasing difficulty urinating, and fell twice, injuring his right hip and wrist.

Discussion: There are many important issues hidden in this very brief case history. While the cause of the compression fracture could be simple osteoporosis, other causes such as bony metastatic disease need to be considered. Difficulty falling asleep was probably caused by pain. Therefore, if a drug were needed, an analgesic would probably make more sense than a hypnotic. The phenothiazines cause adverse reactions in many patients regardless of age. But in the elderly, pharmacologic actions in addition to sedating effects may cause special problems. The α-adrenergic receptor blocking effects cause orthostatic hypotension that can lead to a spectrum of problems from faintness to frank syncope. Their anticholinergic effects may lead to acute urinary retention, especially when underlying prostatic hypertrophy and mild-to-moderate urethral obstruction are already present. Epidemiologic studies have shown that the phenothiazines, like other drugs with CNS depressant properties, significantly increase the risk of falling and hip fractures in the elderly (Ray et al., 1987). In addition, a spectrum of acute and chronic extrapyramidal neurologic adverse reactions may develop, some of which (e.g., parkinsonism, neuroleptic malignant syndrome; see chapter 26) may occur more commonly in elderly patients than in young adults.

Elderly patients may experience altered pharmacodynamic effects of medications (compared with effects observed in younger and healthier patients), but clearly documented examples have only recently been described and mechanisms for the alterations are not well understood. Examples include greater anticoagulation in response to similar concentrations of warfarin in plasma; increased risk of bleeding while receiving ordinarily therapeutic doses of heparin; increased analgesic effects from opioids; increased sedation from longer-acting benzodiazepines (and paradoxical agitation from shorter-acting agents); and decreased tachycardia in response to β-adrenergic agonists. More detailed discussion of these and other pharmacodynamic changes in the elderly is presented in chapters 29 to 32.

Adverse Drug Reactions and Drug Interactions. The elderly experience an excessive number of adverse drug reactions and drug interactions. However, age itself may not be an independent risk factor. Rather, the presence of more diseases, more severe disease, altered pharmacodynamics, and more justified medications all act together to increase the probability of an adverse reaction. In other words, some adverse effects of medication may often be unavoidable without also avoiding efficacy. Similarly, an increased number of total medications increases the chances of an unintended drug interaction. For example, since elderly patients are more likely to receive both digoxin and quinidine, they are more likely to experience the common interaction of quinidine increasing the steady-state plasma concentration of digoxin. Other drug pairs at high risk of producing clinically important interactions include diuretics with digoxin (hypokalemia increasing the risk of digoxin toxicity), tricyclic antidepressants with guanethidine (decreased control of blood pressure), or oral hypoglycemic agents with β-adrenergic antagonists (more prolonged episodes of hypoglycemia, etc.).

Certain drugs may have such excessive risk profiles when given to the elderly that they should rarely be prescribed for such patients. For example, drugs such as amitriptyline (excessive anticholinergic effects), antipsychotics (movement disorders), chlorpropamide (long half-life with risk of prolonged hypoglycemia), disopyramide (highly anticholinergic), or long-acting benzodiazepines (confusion, sedation, falls, and even increased risk of hip fracture) are all less than ideal in the elderly. Equally effective and safer alternatives are usually available for each (Beers and Ouslander, 1989).

Summary. An effective approach to prescribing for the elderly patient requires considerable judgment. Recently approved drugs usually have not been given to many elderly patients during phase III testing. Data concerning dosing and adverse reactions in elderly patients are often lacking, even for many established drugs. The principles of rational therapeutics outlined early in this chapter should serve the practitioner well when prescribing for any patient, including an elderly one. Attention should be paid to the following points.

1. **Be sure the drug history is thorough.** The elderly take many prescriptions, as well as over-the-counter (OTC) and topical agents that could contribute to systemic effects. Know all the agents a patient is receiving in order to assess the possibility of an adverse reaction and to plan the rational introduction of a new agent.

2. **Reevaluate drug use at frequent intervals.** Most physicians feel more comfortable starting a new drug than discontinuing medication that has been given over time. Drugs should be discontinued when they are no longer necessary. Antihypertensives, antiseizure medications, sedative-hypnotics, neuroleptics, and digoxin all can be safely discontinued in patients whose indications for them have passed. Because the number of medications being taken is a major determinant of the likelihood of drug toxicity and drug interactions, reducing the number of medications is important.

3. **Make all feasible attempts to establish the diagnosis.** Some drugs are more likely to produce adverse effects in the elderly, but therapy that does not have a good chance of efficacy is more risky in the elderly. Establishing a firm working diagnosis allows the formation of a sound therapeutic strategy.

4. **Understand nonpharmacologic as well as pharmacologic approaches to treating diseases.** Many of the problems of the elderly may respond to nonpharmacologic treatment. Examples include exercise and dietary changes to help relieve hyperglycemia or constipation, or weight loss to help lower blood pressure, reduce exertional dyspnea, or improve claudication. Usually such nonpharmacologic interventions are safer than using drugs. If they are not adequate to accomplish a therapeutic end point, they still may permit the use of lower doses of necessary drugs.

5. **Make extra efforts to know the clinical pharmacology of prescribed drugs.** Understand both the intended and unintended pharmacologic actions of drugs. For example, a neuroleptic drug not only may act as a "tranquilizer," but may simultaneously cause unacceptable orthostatic hypotension, anticholinergic effects, sedation, ataxia and/or extrapyramidal syndromes. Different neuroleptics differ widely in these adverse effects.

6. **Make extra efforts to individualize treatment.** Individualization of treatment of the elderly must be based upon knowledge of the other drugs the patient is taking, the full constellation of diseases the patient may have, and the altered pharmacokinetics or pharmacodynamics the drug may have. The loading dose or especially the maintenance dose of drugs may need unusually careful adjustment. Each of these factors is more likely to be a relevant concern in the elderly patient.

7. **Pick end points to follow carefully.** The end points may not be the same ones followed in younger patients. The use of a neuroleptic in an older patient requires the physician to be sensitive to the earliest complaints of dizziness upon standing, sedation, falling, ataxia, constipation, urinary retention, stiffness, or difficulty moving because compensatory responses are not as reliable in the old as they are in younger adult patients.

8. **Emphasize the contract or alliance with the patient.** The physician must take extra steps to ensure compliance with his or her prescription. The fewer the drugs and the simpler the drug regimen, the more likely the patient will be to take all drugs correctly. Clear drug labeling and accompanying patient information inserts may be especially important for patients with poor hearing, vision, or memory. The instruction of a spouse, relative, or friend in addition to the patient may be useful. A medication schedule, calendar, or aid may be necessary to ensure adequate compliance. The patient and responsible caregivers or family members must be encouraged to call the physician and report problems whether or not they are thought to be drug-related.

Pharmacogenetic Factors

Genetic differences in genotype and phenotype modify a patient's pharmacokinetic or pharmacodynamic response to a medication. Although some interpatient differences are expected in the pharmacokinetics and pharmacodynamics of a drug, an occasional patient will respond in a manner so unusual that the reaction is termed idiosyncratic. As more is learned about influences of pharmacogenetics on drug kinetics and dynamics, more idiosyncratic drug reactions can be explained in molecular terms.

Pharmacogenetic effects are often caused by inheritance of a gene that leads to synthesis of an abnormal protein or deletion of a gene that results in decreased synthesis of a normal protein. In most cases, the protein is an enzyme, but sometimes unusual drug effects are mediated by alterations in receptors, transport carrier proteins, or hemoglobin. Genetic abnormalities often are revealed in one of three circumstances: (1) the patient exhibits altered drug pharmacokinetics, such as enhanced or diminished drug clearance, (2) the patient exhibits altered pharmacodynamics that enhances or reduces the usual pharmacologic effect, or (3) the patient exhibits a novel pharmacologic response that is not anticipated or seen in the average patient.

An example of the first two possibilities was

the observation that a small minority of patients with normal renal and hepatic function who were receiving short courses of low-dose therapy with azathioprine experienced acute and prolonged bone-marrow toxicity. About 1 in every 300 patients has increased susceptibility to the bone-marrow depressant effects of azathioprine caused by an inherited defect. When compared with control patients who tolerate standard doses of azathioprine without such problems, the patients who are unusually sensitive to the drug demonstrate substantially reduced activities of the enzyme thiopurine methyltransferase. This enzyme plays an important role in the catabolism of azathioprine. Low activities lead to unexpected high values of 6-thioguanine nucleotides, which in turn induce myelosuppression (Lennard et al., 1989).

Pharmacogenetic factors also may lead to novel reactions to drugs. One example of this type of pharmacogenetic anomaly is seen in the X-linked genetic trait of a deficiency in the red cell enzyme glucose-6-phosphate dehydrogenase (G-6-PD). Patients with the G-6-PD deficiency develop drug-induced hemolytic anemia when they are exposed to a wide variety of drugs that have in common an ability to oxidize red cell membranes. Red cells normally are protected from oxidization and injury by adequate stores of reduced glutathione generated from reduced nicotinamide adenine dinucleotide phosphate (NADPH). Cells deficient in G-6-PD activity are unable to generate adequate amounts of NADPH. These patients may not know of any abnormality until they take drugs with substantial oxidizing potential such as antimalarials (e.g., primaquine), sulfonamides (e.g., sulfisoxazole), sulfones (e.g., dapsone), nitrofurans (e.g., nitrofurantoin), or analgesics (e.g., aspirin). The subsequent hemolysis can range from mildly annoying to severe and life-threatening.

More pharmacogenetic conditions have been identified that lead to the three types of problems outlined above (see also chapters 29–32). The importance of these pharmacogenetic conditions to the practice of rational therapeutics is illustrated by the following incidents.

Case Histories

Three previously healthy college athletes are scheduled to undergo orthopedic surgery. In each case, the anesthesiologist plans an induction with IV thiopental; initial paralysis with succinylcholine to facilitate endotracheal intubation; maintenance anesthesia and relaxation with oxygen, halothane, and pancuronium; and extubation assisted by neostigmine and glycopyrrolate. In the first case, everything goes smoothly. In the second case, no pancuronium is needed because the patient remains flaccid and paralyzed after receiving only succinylcholine. As the patient awakes from the halothane, he remains paralyzed and requires mechanical ventilation for a further 12 hours after his surgery. The third case proceeds smoothly for the first 45 minutes, until the anesthesiologist notices the patient has developed tachycardia and cyanosis. Further examination reveals that the patient has a core temperature of 41°C and a profound metabolic acidosis. The surgery and anesthesia are abruptly terminated, the patient is actively cooled, and an antidote is administered.

Discussion: The first patient had a normal anesthetic induction, surgical course, and reversal of anesthesia. The second patient demonstrated an exaggerated or prolonged response to succinylcholine. Succinylcholine, a depolarizing muscle relaxant, had a prolonged duration of action leading to paralysis for 12 hours (normal is about 10–15 minutes). The abnormally prolonged response to this drug was pharmacogenetically determined. The patient was unable to metabolize the succinylcholine, which is structurally similar to acetylcholine and is metabolized by pseudocholinesterase. In a small number of patients, this plasma enzyme is abnormal or absent. Such patients will appear normal until challenged with succinylcholine, at which point they will experience normal onset of drug effect but dramatically prolonged time required for elimination of the drug. As long as the cause for such a prolonged response is promptly recognized, the patient can be supported (with mechanical ventilation) until the drug is slowly cleared and the patient regains motor strength.

The third patient also experienced an unusual reaction to succinylcholine and/or halothane. This bizarre and life-threatening reaction, called malignant hyperthermia, includes extreme hyperthermia, acidosis, shock, arrhythmias, and even death. It appears to be caused by a genetically determined membrane defect involving the sarcoplasmic reticulum of skeletal muscle cells (Gronert et al., 1988). This defect results in an unusually massive accumulation of intracellular calcium that leads to severe tetany and consequent increase in heat production when skeletal muscle is exposed to a variety of anesthetic agents.

The two pharmacogenetic conditions illustrate the importance of understanding and recognizing abnormal responses to common medications. Many such responses are sometimes predictable (based on a good family history), treatable if recognized, or preventable if anticipated (see chapters 29–32).

Patients with Renal Disease

A variety of disease states can alter the patient's pharmacokinetics, pharmacodynamics, or both.

Renal disease is especially noteworthy in both regards, because many patients are renally impaired and many drugs (or their active metabolites) are cleared by renal excretion.

Unsuspected Renal Compromise. Both glomerular filtration and active tubular secretion may progressively decline with age. However, this decline in renal function may not be apparent because muscle mass also declines with age. Thus a plasma creatinine concentration that represents a steady-state concentration determined by creatinine production (from skeletal muscle) and clearance (via the kidneys) may be normal. A "normal" plasma creatinine concentration may mask both a decline in production and in renal clearance. Do not assume that renal function in an elderly patient is normal because the creatinine concentration in plasma is normal.

Case History

An 80-year-old woman was admitted to the hospital with a fractured hip. On admission, her blood urea nitrogen (BUN) concentration was 25 mg/dl, and her creatinine concentration was 1.5 mg/dl. Both were at the upper limits of normal. She was assumed to have normal kidney function. She underwent open reduction of the fracture and internal fixation of the femur. She did well for several days. A Foley catheter was placed at the time of surgery.

Discussion: When the physician learned that the creatinine concentration was normal, he mistakenly concluded that the patient's creatinine clearance also was normal. We now know that we can estimate or approximate the patient's GFR using one of several nomograms or formulas. This woman's GFR was calculated to be 28 ml/min. A normal GFR should be from 85 to 100 ml/min for a healthy young woman. This woman's GFR was only about one third of normal. ***Principle: When a number such as a plasma creatinine concentration represents a dynamic balance between two simultaneous processes (e.g., input and clearance), knowledge of the concentration alone is not sufficient to understand the status of an important underlying physiologic process such as glomerular filtration.***

The Effects of Renal Disease on the Pharmacokinetics of Drugs. Renal insufficiency can alter any aspect of pharmacokinetics. Although absorption and bioavailability of drugs are not predictably altered by renal disease, drug distribution can be substantially changed. For example, the free fraction of an acidic drug such as phenytoin is about 10% in healthy patients (i.e., 90% is bound to albumin, 10% is free). In the presence of severe azotemia, the free fraction may double

to 20% as the concentration of albumin falls, especially in patients with nephrotic syndrome. During renal failure, nondialyzable acidic substances accumulate that displace phenytoin from its protein-binding sites. The increase in the free fraction of drug means that at any total concentration of the drug in plasma (as measured by a clinical laboratory), twice as much free drug is present than is usual. The therapeutic range for the drug, measured in terms of total drug concentration (bound plus free), drops from 10–20 mg/l to 5–10 mg/l. This shift in therapeutic range and appropriate target concentrations must be appreciated for proper use of the drug.

Distribution of drug also can be altered by edema, pleural effusion, or ascites. For example, pleural effusion increases the V_d of a water-soluble drug such as methotrexate. The half-life of elimination of this drug may be prolonged in patients with renal failure and pleural effusion, partly because the renal clearance of the drug is reduced and partly because its V_d is increased.

The most frequent and worrisome effect of renal insufficiency on drug pharmacokinetics is the effect on clearance of the drug. Changes in clearance become clinically important in cases where the drug is predominantly cleared by the kidneys and has a narrow therapeutic index. Commonly prescribed drugs that share these properties include aspirin, methotrexate, vancomycin, and the aminoglycosides (Bennett et al., 1987). A patient with renal insufficiency would not be expected to require significantly altered doses of drugs such as lorazepam that are cleared almost entirely by the liver. Likewise low-dose penicillin G that is eliminated almost completely by the kidneys but has a large therapeutic index may not require dosage changes to compensate for mild uremia.

Returning to the patient introduced above, we can see how renal insufficiency alters the safety profile of a drug such as gentamicin.

Case History (continued)

On the fifth postoperative day, the patient appeared septic. Urinalysis obtained through the Foley catheter revealed many leukocytes and gram-negative rods. The urosepsis was most probably due to Escherichia coli. Her physician prescribed the "usual" loading dose of gentamicin (2 mg/kg), and the "usual" maintenance dose (1.5 mg/kg every 8 hours). Peak and trough drug concentrations drawn the next day after the fourth dose were both excessively high and in the toxic range.

Discussion: A patient with urosepsis should receive the first dose of antibiotic quickly to promptly achieve a therapeutic plasma concentration. Because the loading dose of a drug is not affected by expected alterations in its clearance, the loading dose of gentamicin could have been given, even before the physician knew the creatinine concentration. The physician only needs to know the patient's weight (in kilograms), the drug's V_d (in liters per kilogram), and the target concentration for gentamicin to prescribe a loading dose. Using information about the volume of distribution in appendix I ($V_d = 0.25$ l/kg), and aiming for a target concentration of 8 mg/l, an appropriate loading dose was 2 mg/kg (LD = $V_d \times C_{target}$ = (0.25 l/kg) × (8 mg/l) = 2 mg/kg).

However, because the drug is almost entirely (>95%) cleared by the kidneys, the maintenance dose should be determined by the target steady-state concentration selected and the renal clearance of the drug. Renal drug clearance parallels the creatinine clearance. Because this patient's creatinine clearance is only about one third normal, the maintenance dose of gentamicin should be only about one third the usual (e.g., about 1.5 mg/kg every 24 hours instead of every 8 hours). But because the maintenance dose of gentamicin was not reduced in this case, toxic steady-state concentrations developed, raising the risk of ototoxicity, nephrotoxicity, or both.

Appendix I lists the contribution of renal clearance to the total plasma clearance of many drugs. The effect of end-stage renal disease upon the half-life of elimination of drugs also is tabulated. For a few drugs, V_d also may be altered. In general, the decline in a drug's renal clearance closely parallels the decline in renal function, whether the drug is eliminated by glomerular filtration or tubular secretion. Thus to the extent that creatinine clearance can act as a marker of overall renal function, it also can act as a marker for changes in drug clearance.

A detailed approach to adjusting maintenance doses of drugs in patients with renal insufficiency is presented in chapters 37 and 38. Adjustment of dose in patients with renal failure is especially important when the drug can accumulate and cause further renal failure. For example, drugs such as ibuprofen, methotrexate, vancomycin, and gentamicin all are predominantly cleared by the kidneys. In patients with renal insufficiency, their clearances decrease and their steady-state concentrations rise. At higher concentrations in plasma the drugs can cause severe renal toxicity, thereby exacerbating the preexisting renal insufficiency. A vicious cycle is established (see chapter 11). *Principle: The renal status of a patient must be known in order to prescribe drugs wisely. For some drugs, dosing is not affected; for others, the maintenance dose of the drug must be reduced; and for yet others, the presence of renal insufficiency is a relative contraindication to the use of the drug at all.*

Even when the pharmacokinetics of a parent drug are not altered by renal disease, the pharmacokinetics of active metabolites may be different. Recall the patient presented earlier in this chapter, an elderly woman receiving high doses of meperidine to treat painful metastatic cancer. After several days, she began to exhibit myoclonic jerks that progressed to severe and refractory grand mal seizures.

Meperidine is cleared almost entirely by the liver. A metabolite of meperidine arises by demethylation to form normeperidine, which has minimal analgesic properties but is much more likely than the parent drug to cause myoclonus and seizures. Like many metabolites of drugs, normeperidine is cleared primarily by *the kidney*. High doses of meperidine given to patients with renal insufficiency result in normal production but abnormal accumulation of normeperidine, whose concentration in plasma reaches toxic levels. Other drugs that have active and/or toxic metabolites that can accumulate during renal insufficiency include procainamide (N-acetylprocainamide), nitroprusside (thiocyanate), and allopurinol (oxipurinol). *Principle: Understanding the routes of clearance of a drug and its metabolites is necessary for appropriate use of the drug.*

Drugs with Altered Pharmacodynamics in Patients with Renal Insufficiency. The pharmacodynamics of a number of different classes of drugs change with renal insufficiency. Potassium salts, potassium-sparing diuretics, nonsteroidal anti-inflammatory drugs, and angiotensin-converting-enzyme inhibitors all are more likely to cause hyperkalemia in patients with renal disease. Diuretics may exhibit decreased overall efficacy or produce a slower or more delayed diuresis in patients with renal disease. Nonsteroidal anti-inflammatory drugs may be more likely to cause gastrointestinal (GI) bleeding from gastritis or ulcer disease, possibly because such patients with underlying renal disease are already at higher risk for these problems.

Drug-Induced Nephrotoxicity. The kidneys receive about 20% of the total resting cardiac output and actively concentrate drugs and metabolites in tubular fluid and parenchymal cells (see chapter 11). This function may contribute to the special risk that the kidneys face from some drugs. Any anatomic area of the kidney can be adversely affected by drugs. Prerenal azotemia related to drug-induced hypovolemia or other low-output states, renal parenchymal disease (glomerulonephritis, interstitial nephritis, tubular necrosis), and postrenal disease (ureteral obstruction, bladder outlet obstruction) are all possible manifestations of drug-induced renal disease.

Other rare but serious syndromes may markedly impair renal function, such as methysergide-induced retroperitoneal fibrosis that obstructs the ureters, or mitomycin C–induced acute renal failure and hemolysis. While certain drugs are notorious for frequently causing nephrotoxicity (e.g., aminoglycosides and tubular necrosis, methicillin and interstitial nephritis) many other drugs have a lower incidence but still significant capacity for causing toxicity.

A variety of fluid and electrolyte abnormalities can be caused by drugs because of their effects on the kidneys. Fluid retention (nonsteroidal anti-inflammatory drugs, NSAIDs), nephrogenic diabetes insipidus (lithium), the syndrome of inappropriate secretion of antidiuretic hormone, or ADH (chlorpropamide), potassium depletion (thiazide diuretics, amphotericin), hyperkalemia (NSAIDs, potassium-sparing diuretics), metabolic acidosis (acetazolamide), and metabolic alkalosis (loop diuretics) are all fluid and electrolyte abnormalities that can be drug-induced. *Principle: Because renal disease can drastically alter the pharmacokinetics and pharmacodynamics of many drugs and its presence must modulate the choice and dose of drugs, the physician should generally know about a patient's renal function before making therapeutic decisions.*

Patients with Hepatic Disease

Many of the same concerns that influence therapeutics in the presence of renal disease also arise when similar decisions need to be made in patients with hepatic disease. The pharmacokinetics of drugs in patients with diseases such as hepatitis or cirrhosis may be abnormal. Altered pharmacodynamics of drugs also result from liver disease. Some of these points are illustrated in the following case history.

Case History

A 38-year-old man was admitted to the hospital for treatment of gastritis and alcohol abuse. He had end-stage cirrhosis and in addition was believed to have acute alcoholic hepatitis superimposed by his recent binge. He received thiamine prophylactically and 650 mg of acetaminophen every 4 hours for pain from a painful abscess in his arm. As he began to experience withdrawal from alcohol, hallucinations became apparent. He received increasing doses of oral diazepam that over 24 hours totaled 650 mg. He then became obtunded. Further use of diazepam was discontinued. Over the next 6 days, he very slowly regained consciousness, and his hepatitis dramatically worsened.

Discussion: There are several problems with the treatment this patient received. The patient required relatively high doses of diazepam to treat his withdrawal from alcohol because his high tolerance to ethanol led to cross-tolerance to benzodiazepines. However, his slow recovery from the obtundation induced by diazepam was due to the slow rate of hepatic clearance of that drug. In a healthy young adult, diazepam has a half-life of about 24 hours. However, in this patient with both cirrhosis and active hepatitis, it is likely that clearance of diazepam would be decreased because of impaired activity of microsomal (P450) enzymes. These enzymes are responsible for the first two steps of metabolism of diazepam. In this patient, the prolonged half-life of diazepam probably was caused by the effects of his liver disease upon the hepatic clearance of the drug (Klotz et al., 1975). To avoid problems of calculating the precise dose needed or guessing what it might be, such patients often are treated with lorazepam rather than diazepam. Lorazepam is cleared by the liver by a conjugation (phase II) reaction to form a glucuronide; this pathway is generally relatively intact in patients with moderately severe liver disease. In other words, conjugation reactions seem less affected than are P450 enzymes.

Unfortunately there are few helpful generalizations about the effects of hepatic disease on the pharmacokinetics of drugs, even those predominantly cleared by the liver. Although clearance of some drugs such as propranolol, cimetidine, meperidine, and lidocaine may be predictably impaired whenever liver blood flow is compromised, the situation can become quite complex (Thomson et al., 1973; Klotz et al., 1974). Liver impairment often is associated with hypoalbuminemia, which leads to decreased binding of drug to plasma proteins and thereby increased hepatic extraction. But if blood flow and the concentration of albumin are reduced, it would be likely that hepatocellular functions of varying sorts would be compromised to varying extents. Predicting that a patient with acute viral hepatitis should have altered pharmacokinetics of phenytoin is plausible, but such was not found (Blaschke et al., 1975). Enalapril may exhibit altered pharmacokinetics (bioactivation of enalapril to enalaprilat is impaired in patients with cirrhosis), but its pharmacodynamic effects do not appear to be blunted in those patients (Ohnishi et al., 1989). *Principle: Liver disease produces so many alterations in physiology that it is difficult to predict accurately its effects upon a particular drug's pharmacokinetics in a given patient. Extra attention to the effects of all drugs given to patients with liver disease is fundamental to their optimal use.*

This same patient also illustrates two other examples of altered pharmacodynamics. First, he had an abnormal response to a customary dose of acetaminophen. Although acute severe hepatitis is a well-known toxic reaction in patients taking large overdoses, such a low dose of acetaminophen rarely causes hepatotoxicity in healthy patients. The liver metabolizes acetaminophen to a toxic intermediate that is itself detoxified by conjugation to glutathione. Patients with preexisting liver disease or severe nutritional deficiencies (this patient had both) have decreased stores of glutathione and therefore are more susceptible to disproportionate accumulation of the unconjugated hepatotoxic metabolite. Similarly, patients with liver disease may be more sensitive to toxic effects of aspirin (hepatitis, prolonged prothrombin time, gastritis and ulcer disease, upper GI hemorrhage, etc.).

Finally, this case is a reminder that almost every type of liver disease can be caused by medications. Acute fulminant hepatitis (e.g., acetaminophen), chronic active hepatitis, cholestasis, hepatitis and cholestasis, fatty changes, and prolongation of the prothrombin time all can be caused by drugs (see chapter 9). As is true of the kidney, the liver is especially susceptible to the toxic effects of medications. It receives substantial blood flow (1.5 l/min), and drugs given orally first pass through the liver in the portal venous blood. Some drugs are so predictably toxic to an already diseased liver that they are not advisable in patients with preexisting liver disease. Halothane, isoniazid, rifampin, erythromycin, tetracycline, and high doses of acetaminophen should be avoided if at all possible in patients with moderate or severe liver disease. *Principle: The presence of an underlying disease may change the relative contraindications to the use of a drugs or convert a relative contraindication to an absolute one. Estimation of benefits and risks of drug administration is a dynamic process that changes from patient to patient, and in the same patient as the condition improves or deteriorates.*

Pregnant Patients

The pregnant patient poses a set of problems to the physician that must be considered before prescribing medications. She may exhibit altered pharmacokinetic or pharmacodynamic response to medications. Some diseases such as eclampsia occur only in pregnant patients. Perhaps most important, all drugs administered to the pregnant patient have the potential to cross the placenta and cause a variety of pharmacologic and teratogenic effects. Many drugs have known potential for causing teratogenesis during the first trimester and other problems if given later in the pregnancy, especially just before term. However, the risks of taking most drugs during pregnancy, especially newer drugs, not only is unknown, but

will be very difficult ever to determine (see chapter 29).

Placental Transfer of Drugs.   Whether medications cross the placenta depends on several factors. Drugs that have low molecular weight, are uncharged at physiologic pH, and are highly lipid-soluble (such as thiopental) rapidly cross the placenta. Charged drugs such as succinylcholine that are weak acids and are highly ionized at physiologic pH diffuse slowly across the placenta. Diffusion is even slower if the drug is highly bound to plasma proteins. However, in the presence of large maternal-to-fetal concentration gradients that are prolonged by chronic therapy, even highly polar compounds eventually cross the placenta.

Altered Pharmacokinetics and Pharmacodynamics.   During pregnancy, the mother's cardiac output increases up to 40%; renal blood flow, glomerular filtration, and plasma volume increase, and plasma albumin concentration decreases. These physiologic changes can alter the pharmacokinetics or pharmacodynamics for some drugs. For example, IV terbutaline may be administered as a tocolytic agent in women presenting with premature labor. However, the drug also can create unusual toxicity in pregnant patients that may lead to chest pain, pulmonary edema, tachycardia, ischemic changes on the electrocardiogram (ECG), and even myocardial infarction. Such toxicity is more likely to occur with excessive infusion rates, but the underlying hyperdynamic state of the cardiovascular system of the pregnant patient also may predispose her to such toxicity.

Risks to the Fetus of Drug Administration. There are few situations in which it is more important to know that a drug truly is needed than before prescribing for a pregnant patient. The difficulty is of knowing about drug effects in a population that is almost never involved in premarketing testing of a drug (see chapters 29–32, 34, 35, and 41). What is believed known about drugs and the fetus, in fact, has been based upon risks assessed in animal preclinical research, clinical reports, and event monitoring as available. Data from human pregnancy is scanty.

A rating scale and supporting references for many drugs that have been studied is described in several reference texts (Berkowitz et al., 1986; Briggs et al., 1986). These five categories of drug risks are as follows:

Category A: There are considerable data available concerning use in pregnant patients, and risk to the fetus appears to be remote. Safest category of drugs to use during pregnancy.

Category B: Either animal studies have shown no risk and there are few human data, or animal studies showed some risk, but human data did not confirm that risk.

Category C: Either studies in animals revealed risk and there are no human studies, or there are no animal or human studies.

Category D: There is positive evidence of risk to the human fetus, but benefits of the drug may still outweigh those risks in certain situations.

Category X: There is animal or human experience that shows risk to the fetus. This risk clearly outweighs any potential benefit to the mother. Drugs in this category pose definite high risk if used during pregnancy, and should rarely if ever be prescribed.

Drugs should be prescribed for the pregnant patient only after careful consideration leads to the conclusion that the potential benefits from the drug outweigh the potential maternal and fetal risks, regardless of how vague these risks may seem. There is more than simply teratogenic risk caused by drugs administered during the first trimester of pregnancy. Drugs can be toxic to the fetus if they are given just prior to delivery. Narcotics given to the mother can cause CNS depression, apnea, and low Apgar scores. These harmful effects usually are the same classic pharmacologic effects seen in the adult but are now produced in an immature human who lacks the homeostatic mechanisms seen in the older child or adult.

Drugs of abuse such as ethanol and cocaine can cause both teratogenic effects and toxic effects at birth, as well as withdrawal syndromes in the newborn infant. Recent work has laid out the syndrome of abnormalities we now refer to as the fetal alcohol syndrome, and the fetal and perinatal toxicity of other drugs of abuse is becoming increasing well described (Braude et al., 1987).

Choosing the Best Drug When Therapy Is Indicated. Several diseases commonly occur during pregnancy. Consider the table of diseases and their recommended treatment for pregnant patients, below.

Not only is pregnancy a condition that distinctly alters the patient's pharmacokinetic and pharmacodynamic response to medications, but also the additional element of fetal toxicity makes prescribing during pregnancy especially difficult.

Nursing Patients

Prescribing medications for a mother who is breast-feeding can be complicated. As recently as 1970, only about 28% of American mothers chose to breast-feed. By 1985, this proportion had risen to about 50%. While the nursing mother's physiology has returned almost to pre-pregnancy condition, she still can pass drugs in her breast milk to the newborn; the baby becomes exposed to risks from the mother's medications.

Drug Secretion into Breast Milk. Most drugs are secreted into breast milk to some extent. However, the rate of secretion and the relative concentrations of drug in milk and maternal plasma are determined by a variety of factors. The molecular weight of the drug, its lipophilicity, its charge at physiologic pH, and its concentration in maternal plasma all are key determinants of the concentrations of the drug in breast milk. Because the mother produces approximately 600 ml of milk per day, the nursing infant could ingest substantial amounts of drug if it were present in high concentrations in breast milk. Nursing infants might also be at increased risk for drug toxicity because their renal and hepatic pathways of drug excretion and biotransformation are not fully developed at birth. Fortunately, many drugs are well tolerated by both the mother and the nursing baby. However, certain drugs can be toxic to the nursing infant.

Drugs Likely to Cause Toxicity in the Infant. Drugs with greatest potential for toxicity are usually secreted into breast milk, well absorbed by the infant, and have low therapeutic in-

DISEASE	RECOMMENDED TREATMENT FOR THE PREGNANT PATIENT	NOT RECOMMENDED DURING PREGNANCY
Diabetes	Insulin	Sulfonylureas
Hypertension	Methyldopa, hydralazine	Diuretics
Urinary infections	Ampicillin, cephalosporins	Sulfonamides
Thrombophlebitis	Heparin	Warfarin during first and third trimesters
Hyperthyroidism	Propylthiouracil	Surgery, radioactive iodine

dices. Some of the better described examples include

Antithyroid drugs: propylthiouracil, methimazole, iodine
Radiopharmaceuticals: technetium, iodine, gallium
Cytotoxic agents: methotrexate, cyclophosphamide
Antibiotics: sulfonamides, isoniazid, metronidazole, chloramphenicol
Hormones: estrogens, androgens
Lithium
CNS depressants: ethanol, barbiturates
Opioids: morphine, heroin

Approach to Drug Treatment in Nursing Women. As with therapy for pregnant patients, therapy for nursing mothers requires careful planning (Briggs et al., 1986). Even close attention to weighing risks and benefits may produce different "right" answers for similar patients. For example, continuation of phenobarbital in a woman with well-controlled epilepsy would be beneficial to the mother but could mildly sedate the infant. However, continuation of use of phenobarbital or diazepam in a woman who takes it only for intermittent difficulty falling asleep likely would lead to a different analysis of risks and benefits, and using the drug would not be justified.

If the physician and woman agree that both drug treatment and continued breast-feeding are indicated, there are several strategies that can be followed to minimize the potential for drug toxicity in the infant. Milk can be expressed and discarded in the period immediately following the administration of a toxic drug. If a drug deteriorates while standing, the milk can be stored. If technetium-containing radionuclide must be administered, the mother may need to discontinue breast-feeding for several days, while storing her milk, because the radionuclide has a relatively short half-life. If more than one drug alternative is possible for the same indication, the drug with the fewest effects on the infant should be chosen.

Patients with Drug Interactions

Any patient receiving two or more medications is at risk for a drug interaction, which is simply a response to both drugs given together that would not be seen if either drug were given alone. Drug interactions may be beneficial or harmful, deliberate or unexpected. For example, the deliberate prescription of probenecid before a dose of penicillin (given to inhibit the tubular secretion of penicillin and thereby prolong its half-life) is an example of a beneficial drug interaction. Other examples of beneficial drug interactions are the deliberate administration of penicillin plus gentamicin to treat enterococci, and hydrochlorothiazide plus propranolol to treat hypertension.

Harmful drug interactions are most likely to occur when the physician does not anticipate their significance and does not plan for them. *Principle: When drug interactions are anticipated in advance, they can be used to advantage, or their negative impact can often be avoided or reduced. Dangerous drug interactions usually occur when the prescribing physician does not recognize or anticipate their occurrence.*

Drug interactions generally occur because of pharmacokinetic or pharmacodynamic interactions. Pharmacokinetic drug interactions may be most clearly illustrated with a case study.

Case History

A 23-year-old nurse was involved in the care of an infant with meningococcal meningitis. The hospital infection control nurse recommended that all health care workers closely involved in the patient's care receive 4 days of treatment with rifampin to reduce their chances of carrying or developing meningococcal disease. The patient used a low-dose oral contraceptive (containing an estrogen and a progestin) for birth control. She had used this method of birth control successfully for 4 years, but she became pregnant following the course of treatment with rifampin, even though her compliance with the pill remained excellent.

Discussion: Over the years both the estrogen and the progestin component of the oral contraceptive pill have been reduced to minimize the toxic side effects of the drugs. The current low-dose formulations contain one of several estrogens, but in a dose as low as 35 μg/day of ethinyl estradiol. At this low dose, there is little margin for error, and a few missed doses can result in breakthrough bleeding or pregnancy. In addition, most of the estrogens are metabolized in the liver by the P450 (microsomal) enzyme system. This enzyme system is inducible by a number of environmental factors (e.g., smoking) and drugs (e.g., phenobarbital, phenytoin). One of the most potent enzyme inducers is the drug rifampin. In this case, the administration of only 4 days of oral rifampin caused an induction of the nurse's hepatic P450 drug-metabolizing enzymes. The induction developed over several days, and it can persist for several weeks. The induced enzymes led to enhanced clearance of the estrogens contained in the low-dose pill, and loss of efficacy, hence the undesired pregnancy (Skolnick et al., 1976; Tatro, 1990). This is an example of a pharmacokinetic type of drug interaction, in which one drug alters the pharmacokinetic behavior of a second drug. Other examples of this type of interaction are listed below.

DRUG A	DRUG B	EFFECT OF DRUG B ON DRUG A
Estrogens	Rifampin	Increased hepatic metabolism of estrogens
Phenytoin	Cimetidine	Decreased hepatic metabolism of phenytoin
Penicillin	Probenecid	Decreased tubular secretion of penicillin
Digoxin	Quinidine	Decreased renal and nonrenal clearance of digoxin, and decreased V_d of digoxin

Such pharmacokinetic interactions are quite common and can alter any aspect of a drug's pharmacokinetics, including absorption, distribution, protein binding, biotransformation, or excretion (see chapter 40).

The second type of drug interaction may be the most common, the pharmacodynamic interaction. These interactions result in two drugs combining their known pharmacologic effects in a predictable fashion that results either in increases or decreases of their effects. Drugs may affect the same receptor, tissue, or organ system to produce enhanced or antagonistic effects. There are many examples of such pharmacodynamic interactions. Many are used to clinical advantage (e.g., treatment of hypertension with a diuretic plus a β-adrenergic antagonist). Other examples include:

teractions are most likely to occur between drugs with narrow therapeutic indices. *Principle: The best treatment for unwanted adverse drug interactions is prevention. If there is need to use more than one drug at a time, sequencing their initiation may lessen risk. Establish pharmacologically legitimate qualitative and quantitative indications of efficacy and lower limits of acceptable toxicity that can be expected of each drug. Consider an unexpected change in the course of the disease (good or bad) as possibly being caused by a drug interaction.*

Patients with Adverse Drug Reactions

Definition of an Adverse Drug Reaction. A broad definition of an ADR is any unwanted consequence of drug administration, even ad-

DRUG A	DRUG B	INTERACTION (LEVEL OF INTERACTION)
Ethanol	Benzodiazepines	Increased CNS depression (organ)
Phenothiazines	Opioids	Increased CNS depression (organ)
Scopolamine	Diphenhydramine	Increased anticholinergic effects (receptors)
Atropine	Physostigmine	Decreased anticholinergic effect (receptors)
Morphine	Naloxone	Decreased pain relief, and decreased sedation (receptor)
KCl	Triamterene	Increased risk of hyperkalemia (tissue)
Thiazides	Amphotericin	Increased risk of hypokalemia (tissue)

The two simplest ways of avoiding adverse drug interactions are straightforward, but not often considered. First, keep the number of medications the patient receives to the minimum required. Several epidemiologic studies have shown that the frequency of drug interactions rises almost exponentially as the total number of drugs the patient receives increases (see chapters 39 and 40). Try to discontinue drugs no longer necessary, reduce doses of drugs when that is feasible, and begin treatment with new agents only when there is evidence that adequate doses of drugs already being used have been given.

Second, before adding a new drug to a patient's regimen, carefully review the drugs the patient is already receiving. If there are doubts about whether the new drug might interact with an agent already being used, first consult one of the several excellent reference sources (for example, Hansten, 1985; Tatro, 1990). Serious adverse drug interactions will most likely be known although not all have been discovered, even for "old drugs" (see chapters 39 and 40 and Appendix II). Serious in-

ministration of the wrong drug to the wrong patient, in the wrong dosage, or at the wrong time. Any of these errors can cause an adverse reaction.

A narrower definition of an ADR is more useful. Most physicians assume that the right drug is being given to the right patient, but it pays to doubt such assumptions. A more useful definition of an ADR is "any response to a drug that is noxious and unintended and that occurs at doses of an appropriately given drug used in man for prophylaxis, diagnosis, or therapy excluding therapeutic failures" (Karch and Lasagna, 1975). Many recent studies of the incidence of ADRs use definitions similar to this one, and some studies try to distinguish "acceptable" ADRs (e.g., neutropenia from chemotherapy) from unintended ADRs (e.g., penicillin-induced anaphylaxis).

Dimensions of the Problem. These unintended, adverse drug-induced events can be frequent and severe. Exact rates of incidence and prevalence of ADRs are not known. However, approximate rates have been reported in a number of studies for outpatients, hospital inpatients on various services, and in nursing homes. Some observers believe that the rate of occurrence is increasing, possibly because the number of drugs per patient, the number of drugs available, and the potential toxicity of both prescription and nonprescription medications are increasing.

Many studies suggest that up to 30% of hospitalized patients will have one or more ADRs while they are in the hospital. On the order of 3% of patients will have an ADR of considerable severity, and about 0.3% of patients will die as a result of an ADR. In addition, approximately 5% of admissions to the medical service of many hospitals are caused by the development of an ADR in an outpatient (Lakshmanan et al., 1986). Unfortunately, there are almost no data that segregate patients who inevitably and predictably sustain ADRs in order to obtain efficacy from their drugs, from those who could have been treated in a way that avoids the toxicity without compromising efficacy.

Separating avoidable from unavoidable ADRs in epidemiologic studies is difficult. It is well established that drug-induced adverse reactions cause significant morbidity and mortality in both inpatients and outpatients and are a frequent cause of hospital admissions. Furthermore it is likely that only a fraction of the ADRs are actually being detected; many are missed completely, and others are attributed to the natural progress of the patient's disease or development of a new illness.

Blaming an Innocent Drug. It is important to detect ADRs when they occur, but it is equally important not to blame a drug for toxicity it did not cause. For some diseases, the best or most effective drug may be denied to a patient because of a false conclusion that the patient cannot tolerate that drug. A case illustrates this problem.

Case History

A 65-year-old man developed enterococcal endocarditis on his prosthetic mitral valve. Because of a prior anaphylactic reaction to penicillin, he was treated with vancomycin and gentamicin. Appropriate target concentrations of drug in plasma were chosen, and doses of both drugs were adjusted to keep the plasma concentrations (peak and trough) in the desired range. He required valve replacement after several days, when his first prosthetic valve failed. The open heart surgery was technically difficult with substantial intraoperative and postoperative blood loss. His physicians planned to administer 6 weeks of vancomycin and gentamicin from the date of the surgery. Approximately 3 weeks postoperatively, the patient complained of anorexia and nausea, and

occasional vomiting. BUN and creatinine concentrations were found to have climbed from 25 mg/ dl and 1.2 mg/dl 1 week earlier to 80 mg/dl and 2.4 mg/dl, respectively. His physicians concluded that he was becoming progressively uremic from the combination of gentamicin and vancomycin. Both drugs were discontinued, but there was no clear alternative left to choose.

Discussion: In this case, his physicians falsely accused vancomycin for causing the patient's azotemia. When the patient was interviewed and examined more carefully, the anorexia and nausea were found to have been preceded and accompanied by mild right upper quadrant abdominal pain, slight jaundice, and decreased oral intake of both liquids and solids. Laboratory studies revealed moderately severe hepatitis in a pattern suggesting viral hepatitis; urinary sediment, specific gravity, and the sodium concentration suggested the presence of prerenal azotemia without acute tubular necrosis. The timing was consistent with classic transfusion-acquired non-A non-B viral hepatitis. The patient was given IV and oral fluids, and the vancomycin and gentamicin were reinstituted (at reduced doses). Within 24 hours, the BUN concentration, creatinine concentration, and specific gravity were back to normal. Both antibiotics were continued uneventfully for the last 3 weeks.

Blaming the azotemia on his two antibiotics would have deprived the patient of the best drugs for his bacterial prosthetic valve endocarditis, would have postponed appropriate treatment of the prerenal azotemia, and perhaps would have resulted in failure to clear the serious infection from his new prosthetic valve, with catastrophic results.

Failure to Detect True ADRs When They Are Present. A reasonable approach to ADRs is to determine which drugs have been associated with the patient's problem and which ones are unlikely to cause the clinical findings you are concerned with. Discontinue the former. "Justice" with respect to ADRs requires that innocent drugs be cleared of suspicion. However, in a patient with a serious ADR, it may be prudent to discontinue likely innocent drugs if they are not essential for the patient's care. Failure to recognize the presence of a true ADR can lead to continued administration of a damaging drug and worsening of the problem, as in the next case.

Case History

A 48-year-old woman had mild rheumatoid arthritis, easily controlled with moderate doses of naproxen begun about 4 months earlier. Her other medications included propranolol for treatment of hypertension, and an oral antacid when needed for "heartburn." Her annual physical exam was unremarkable, but her physician ordered a chemistry panel "just to check on things." Electrolyte, BUN, and creatinine concentrations all were normal, but her liver function tests revealed a picture of moderate elevation of transaminase concentrations, with the aspartate aminotransferase (AST) and alanine aminotransferase (ALT) concentrations about three times normal, and a slight elevation of her bilirubin concentrations. Further questioning revealed that she was asymptomatic. The physician pursued the biochemical abnormality with a liver-spleen scan that was normal, and an ultrasound examination of the liver that showed the common bile duct to be at upper limits of normal. The head of the pancreas was not visualized. The patient was transferred to a university hospital where a 4-day admission yielded a normal computed tomography (CT) scan of the abdomen, and a normal ERCP (endoscopic retrograde cannulation of the pancreatic duct) study. At this point in her workup, a medical student added to the differential diagnosis the possibility that her abnormal liver function tests might be caused by one of her medications.

Discussion: Review of the literature revealed that this pattern of mild-to-moderate hepatitis is ocassionally seen during treatment with NSAIDs, including naproxen. Propranolol appeared to be less likely to cause such a syndrome. The timing of the reaction usually is weeks or months into therapy. While rare cases of fatal hepatotoxicity have been reported, most patients improve over several weeks when the drug is discontinued. A tentative diagnosis of drug-induced hepatitis was made, and the patient was discharged home on the fifth hospital day. Over the next 4 weeks, subsequent to discontinuing naproxen, her liver function tests returned to normal and she remained asymptomatic.

The failure to recognize the possibility of an ADR caused by naproxen resulted in unnecessary morbidity, inconvenience, and expense. A more rational strategy would have been to consider the possibility of an ADR in the first instance and discontinue the most likely potentially offending drug(s). If the problem improved, then the probability of a drug-induced syndrome would have been enhanced. No further workup would have been necessary. If the problem did not improve, then an appropriate workup could have commenced with little risk caused by the delay to an otherwise asymptomatic patient.

How to Evaluate Potential Adverse Drug Reactions. The two cases described above illustrate the importance of having a rational approach to evaluating a patient who has a syndrome that might be caused by a drug. There is a large litera-

ture on this subject with algorithms that can be used, and that have been formally evaluated and tested (see chapters 39 and 40). Consider a simple sequence of questions whose answers will aid in the identification of true-positive ADRs. Responses can be set to vary from 0 (clearly no), to 1 (equivocal response), to 2 (clearly yes). Total point scores can be obtained to help sort possible ADRs into those that appear to be very likely (10–12 points), probable (7–9 points), possible (4–6 points), or highly unlikely (0–3 points).

1. Has this drug ever caused this type of reaction as reported in the literature?
2. Is the timing of the patient's response to the drug typical of previous reports?
3. Can other likely reasons or causes for the patient's syndrome be eliminated?
4. Has the patient ever had a similar response to this drug?
5. If the drug is discontinued, does the patient improve (dechallenge)?
6. If the drug is restarted, does the syndrome recur (rechallenge)?

Application of these simple questions to the two cases would have generated concern about simply blaming vancomycin and gentamicin for the first patient's renal compromise, and would have confirmed the validity in thinking about naproxen as a cause of the second patient's hepatitis. In the first case, the key points that would have been discovered were that vancomycin and gentamicin do not cause pre-renal azotemia; that there was another likely cause for the azotemia (dehydration); and that renal function improved while both drugs were continued (2 total points). For the second case, the key points included the recognition that naproxen can cause this type of hepatic dysfunction, that the timing was typical of such ADRs, that there were no other likely causes in an asymptomatic patient, and that drug dechallenge resulted in prompt improvement (8 total points).

Uncertainty Concerning ADRs. Several important sources of uncertainty exist concerning whether a particular patient is experiencing an ADR. Clearly if you do not suspect an ADR, you will not find it. The frequency of ADRs is underestimated when based on spontaneous reports by physicians. In several studies in hospitalized patients, the more vigorously the investigators searched for the presence of an ADR (often using specially trained nurses or pharmacists), the more true ADRs were identified (Koch-Weser et al., 1969; Karch and Lasagna, 1975).

Other less obvious sources of uncertainty include the ADRs that occur infrequently and thus may not be noted during clinical drug testing prior to marketing (see chapters 34, 35, and 39–41). Recently, the incidence of intracranial hemorrhage in patients receiving tissue plasminogen activator for coronary thrombolysis has been estimated to be higher than thought in the original studies (Kase et al., 1990). Pharmacoepidemiologic studies may reveal ADRs when none were previously known. For example, recent studies have suggested that sedatives with long half-lives, tricyclic antidepressants, and antipsychotic agents all are associated with increased risk of hip fractures in the elderly (Ray et al., 1987). Finally, the physician should remember that he or she may be the first to spot a rare drug-induced adverse effect or drug interaction and should try to believe what he or she sees (Melmon and Nierenberg, 1981; Melmon, 1984).

Increased experience with new drugs sometimes leads to recognition of new ADRs. For example, when cisplatin was initially released, the most feared dose-limiting toxicity was renal failure. Careful clinical attention to its use resulted in a dramatically lower incidence and severity of this ADR. A drug-induced peripheral neuropathy replaced nephrotoxicity as the leading dose-dependent toxicity. Recent studies with an adrenocorticotropic hormone (ACTH) analog have suggested that the neurotoxicity of cisplatin can be delayed until a large total dose has been administered (Mollman, 1990).

Mechanisms of ADRs and Their Prevention. Many studies have suggested that most ADRs (70% to 80%) are caused by expression of the known pharmacologic effects of the drugs. Fewer ADRs are caused by mechanisms that make them unpredictable, such as drug allergy (e.g., penicillin-induced anaphylaxis), abnormal pharmacogenetics (e.g., G-6-PD deficiency), or idiosyncratic reactions (e.g., anaphylactoid reaction to IV contrast media). Patients at highest risk for ADRs appear be those receiving many drugs, those receiving high doses of drugs, those who have renal insufficiency, and those who are more than 60 years old. Many ADRs can be prevented by considering the particular patient and drug carefully before initiating a new drug regimen. *Principle: Reducing the incidence of ADRs requires the use of sound knowledge of the pharmacology of the drugs and constant evaluation of the changing risk/benefit ratio of each drug in a particular patient.*

If despite all caution a true ADR is identified, try to stop the drug if alternatives are available. However, some patients may need to be treated with a toxic drug that offers unique efficacy. Record the event in the patient's chart, thoroughly inform the patient of the event, and, if appropriate, arrange for an alert bracelet or necklace with an applicable warning. *Principle: Adequate documentation that an ADR occurred is essential to the patient and to further knowledge of the true incidence and severity of ADRs.*

Patients with Allergies to Drugs

Definition and Features. Allergy to medications is a subset of ADRs. Understanding the pathophysiology and presenting symptoms of such reactions is essential to recognizing and avoiding them. Drug allergies are fundamentally different from the 80% or more of all ADRs that are caused by undesired, dose-dependent, pharmacologic responses to drugs. They are adverse effects mediated by humoral or cell-mediated immunologic mechanisms. Drug allergies are a reaction to the drug as an immunogen. Although they can represent true "hypersensitivity," some reactions to drugs mimic drug allergy closely, but there is no evidence that the immune system is involved.

Allergies to drugs often have distinctive features that aid in their identification (Parker, 1975; Assem, 1985). The consequences of allergy have no relation to the intended effects of the drug or its adverse pharmacologic properties. For example, the development of systemic lupus erythematosus following exposure to procainamide has no relationship to that drug's properties as an antiarrhythmic agent. The allergy is not dose-related. Microgram quantities of a drug can trigger a drug allergy, whereas most drugs are administered in milligram or gram amounts to achieve their intended pharmacologic effect. Drug allergy sometimes is associated with symptoms typical of other allergies, such as a maculopapular rash, hives, or eosinophilia. Usually there is a delay after the initial exposure to the drug before the allergy appears. Subsequent exposures to the same or smaller doses of the drug may trigger the reaction more quickly or with greater severity. Drug allergies usually disappear upon cessation of administration of the drug. In some cases deliberate desensitization is possible. However, since desensitization is inherently risky, this time-consuming procedure is undertaken only when the benefits clearly outweigh the risks (Condemi, 1986). This might be appropriate in a penicillin-allergic patient with a serious infection for which no effective alternative antibiotic were available.

Allergies to drugs can present at various times after exposure to the drug. Reactions that occur in less than 1 hour following exposure are usually called *immediate reactions*. Those developing from 1 to 72 hours following exposure are termed *accelerated reactions*, and those developing more than 3 days following exposure are termed *late reactions*. Drug allergies can present in trivial or life-threatening forms and can involve essentially any body part (Assem, 1985). Minor reactions such as macular rashes and asymptomatic eosinophilia are at the benign end of the spectrum. Reactions with more pronounced toxicity such as major skin eruptions, serum sickness, immune cytopenias, hectic fever, hepatitis, or nephritis are severe presentations. Drug allergy can be life-threatening involving acute renal failure, acute hepatitis, acute pulmonary infiltrates, vasculitis, and/or anaphylaxis. *Principle: A variety of reactions caused by drug allergies are possible. They range from acute to chronic, trivial to life-threatening, restricted to one organ system or involving many.*

Drug allergies often are unpredictable but many can be averted by obtaining a careful drug history. A patient who has been exposed to streptokinase a few weeks earlier is more likely to develop an acute allergic reaction if it is readministered than is a patient who has never received the drug. A patient with a previous history of an anaphylactic reaction to penicillin is likely to have a similar reaction on reexposure even though those chances are less than 100% (Condemi, 1986; Saxon et al., 1988). For a few drugs such as penicillin, the predictive value of positive or negative skin tests prior to readministration of drug has been fairly well established. This makes it somewhat easier to interpret the implications of a prior allergic reaction (Condemi, 1986; Saxon et al., 1988). However, skin tests are not always useful for identifying patients at high risk for acute allergic reactions to other drugs (VanArsdel and Larson, 1989). For a few drugs such as sulfonamide, in vitro tests identifying patients with decreased ability to detoxify reactive metabolites may help identify patients at risk for developing "hypersensitivity" reactions (Rieder et al., 1989).

Knowledge of a prior anaphylactic reaction to penicillin should compel selection of an alternative antibiotic. In addition, patients with a prior history of drug allergy (not anaphylaxis) to penicillin are at increased risk for developing allergic reactions to other drugs. Finally, there is some cross-reactivity of antipenicillin antibodies with drugs from the cephalosporin, monobactam, and carbapenem classes (Saxon et al., 1988). In summary, a detailed drug history is the best strategy for reducing the risk of drug allergy. For a few drugs, appropriate skin testing can further reduce the risk of drug administration. Given the current state of knowledge of drug allergy, it is difficult to eliminate this risk completely.

Mechanisms of Allergic Reactions. Why some drugs frequently cause allergic responses while others almost never do is not understood. The molecular weight of a drug is one important factor. Some drugs or their metabolites are allergenic only when complexed to larger molecules such as proteins. Such drugs and metabolites are called haptens. The hapten property is utilized when penicilloyl-polylysine (PPL) is utilized to perform skin tests for penicillin allergy. This commercially available diagnostic agent is a metabolite of penicillin that is complexed to a polypeptide, to mimic one of the important naturally occurring haptens in patients receiving penicillin.

Prior exposure to a drug is a requirement to develop allergy to it. But the patient may not be aware of such an exposure. In the case of antibiotics, perhaps the patient was exposed to the antibiotic as a child, or perhaps the antibiotic was present in dairy products, beef, or poultry. In the case of streptokinase, a prior streptococcal infection may have exposed the patient to this bacterial enzyme. Insulin-requiring diabetics receiving protamine insulin are at increased risk of serious allergic reactions when IV protamine is administered to reverse the effects of heparin (Weiss et al., 1989). Patients with an "allergic" or atopic history appear to be more likely to develop drug allergies, while the presence of kidney or liver disease does not appear to predispose to drug allergies. A previous allergic reaction to penicillin appears to increase the chances for a subsequent allergic reaction to many classes of drugs, not just those that are structurally similar (Saxon et al., 1988).

Type I (Acute, Anaphylactic) Reactions. Perhaps the most morbid are the type I or acute allergic reactions. Anaphylaxis is the most extreme example. Other less severe type I reactions include hives or urticaria, angioedema, bronchospasm, laryngospasm, and so forth. These reactions develop quickly (immediate reactions usually in minutes, but accelerated reactions may occur in up to 72 hours) after reexposure. The reaction is mediated by the release of a variety of vasoactive substances (kinins, leukotrienes, histamine, serotonin) from mast cells that are coated with immunoglobulin E (IgE) (and sometimes IgG). There must be more than one antibody molecule per cell, and they must be bridged by an antigen (allergen) having at least two haptens. Inhibition by monovalent hapten is possible, as is deliberate desensitization. Treatment is determined primarily by the severity of the reaction, ranging from observation alone (mild hives), to diphenhydramine (moderate hives, mild bronchospasm) to maximal therapy with epinephrine, diphenhydramine, IV fluids, and possibly corticosteroids for anaphylactic shock (Assem, 1985). The importance of preventing such reactions if at all possible is illustrated by the following case history.

Case History

A 75-year-old man with severe angina was scheduled to undergo elective coronary artery bypass graft surgery. Several years earlier he had been given oral penicillin for local cellulitis. He had developed a mild anaphylactic reaction. Knowing this, the surgical team avoided prophylactic nafcillin prior to surgery and prescribed cefamandole in the induction room to prevent infection of the sternal wound. Within 4 minutes of beginning the rapid infusion, the patient developed hives, angioedema, bronchospasm, hypotension, and angina. Epinephrine and diphenhydramine were given promptly in appropriate doses, but the patient's hypotension persisted and ischemic changes appeared on his ECG. He complained of chest pain and then became unconscious and profoundly hypotensive.

Given his dire situation and the inability to stabilize his condition, bypass surgery was begun. He underwent general anesthesia, was placed on cardiopulmonary bypass, and received a triple bypass. During the case, he required almost 20 liters of crystalloid to maintain his intravascular volume. His lungs were markedly edematous and stiff, and he developed profound edema. He could not be weaned off bypass, and he died. At autopsy, a large acute myocardial infarction that was several hours old was found.

Discussion: There are several important and instructive aspects to this case. First, the team did well to take a complete drug history and discover the patient's prior type I (acute, anaphylactic) reaction to penicillin. Such a history implies that the patient is at a greater than usual risk of developing a severe anaphylactic reaction if challenged again with penicillin. In patients with no prior history of such an allergic reaction, about 1/10,000 patients will develop a systemic type I reaction; this will be fatal in about 10% of cases (overall about 1/100,000). A mild urticarial reaction will occur in about 5% of patients who have no prior history of penicillin allergy, and about 10% of such patients will develop a morbilliform rash from ampicillin (Saxon et al., 1988). All these chances are increased considerably (exact risk unknown) in patients who report a previous history of a type I reaction to penicillin.

Prior history of an allergic reaction to a penicillin increases the chances of subsequent allergic reactions to other drugs, and cephalosporins are structurally similar to penicillin; therefore, the same patients are at increased risk for developing type I reactions to cephalosporins. In this patient, if prophylactic antibiotics were used at all, a structurally dissimilar drug (e.g., vancomycin) active against staphylococci would have been preferable.

For drugs such as streptokinase or penicillin, skin tests may help identify patients who are at high risk for reactions. Of patients who report previous allergic reactions to penicillin, between 9% and 63% will have positive reactions to skin tests with benzylpenicillin (penicillin G) or the metabolite PPL. Of those who are skin-test negative, less than 1% will develop a systemic type I reaction upon reexposure to penicillin within from 24 to 72 hours. Of those patients with a positive skin test, two thirds will develop a systemic acute reaction if reexposed (Condemi, 1986; Saxon et al., 1988). Therefore, skin-testing results have useful positive and negative predictive values for this drug.

Type II (Cytotoxic, Autoimmune) Reactions. In type II reactions, the drug (or drug hapten) induces development of antibodies directed against the drug, a similar antigen on a cell, or even an unrelated antigen in the patient. The antibody–allergen complex can fix complement leading to cell lysis and death. A common example of the first type is the hemolytic reaction induced by penicillin. The penicillin is bound to the erythrocyte membrane; antibodies then bind to the membrane-bound penicillin, fix complement, and lyse the erythrocyte. Because penicillin is essential for antibody binding and complement activation, hemolysis ceases as soon as the drug is cleared from the blood.

A slightly different reaction is seen with methyldopa-induced positive Coombs reaction or hemolytic anemia. In this case, the drug somehow tricks the body into developing antibodies against an antigen on the erythrocyte membrane itself. Although a positive Coombs test is a relatively common occurrence (perhaps 30% of patients develop this while taking methyldopa), clinically significant hemolytic reactions fortunately are relatively rare (developing in less than 1% of patients receiving the drug). In this situation, the binding of antibody to the red cell antigen continues even after all the methyldopa is cleared from the body.

Drug-induced systemic lupus erythematosus also is a type II reaction. For some drugs such as hydralazine or procainamide, the chances of developing this drug allergy are increased in individuals with a slow acetylation phenotype. Perhaps other subtle defects in the metabolism of the parent drug or a toxic metabolite will eventually be shown to be responsible for the development of this form of drug allergy, as it has been with allergic responses to sulfa derivatives (Rieder et al., 1989).

Type III (Serum Sickness, Immune Complex) Reactions. These reactions were first observed when horse serum containing horse antibodies (antiserum) was administered to patients with an infectious disease such as diphtheria. Because the horse serum contained horse proteins, many patients developed antibodies to the foreign horse proteins. The symptoms that developed from 7 to 14 days after the initial exposure to horse antiserum was known as serum sickness. Reexposure to the allergen resulted in disease that developed in just a few days, an anamnestic response.

Serum sickness consists of a combination of general malaise, fever, rash, arthralgias, lymphadenopathy, hepatitis, and a peculiar serpiginous petechial rash that develops along the lateral aspects of the palms and feet. The reaction develops as immune complexes between foreign proteins and human antibodies are formed in the circulation and then deposited in various tissues, leading to end-organ damage. Other examples of this type of reaction appear to include drug-induced vasculitis and penicillin-induced serum sickness. Other names for this reaction include Arthus reaction and immune-complex disease.

Usually serum sickness gradually improves over several days as long as the offending drug is discontinued, and no other treatment is needed. However, the existence of this syndrome must be recognized in order to administer appropriate therapy, as demonstrated in the following case.

Case History

A 45-year-old man underwent elective open repair of a poorly healed tibial fracture. While recovering at home 3 weeks after surgery, he developed classic symptoms of deep venous thrombophlebitis and pulmonary thromboembolism. He was admitted to the hospital, where studies confirmed the presence of two segmental pulmonary emboli, and extensive clot in the deep venous system of his injured leg. He was treated with 48 hours of streptokinase, followed by IV heparin. All went well, and on the fourth day of heparin therapy (day 6 after admission) oral warfarin was begun. His heparin was discontinued on the tenth hospital day, when his prothrombin time was controlled by warfarin. Plans were made for discharge on the eleventh hospital day. On that day, he suddenly developed fever, malaise, arthralgias, a macular rash, mild hepatitis, and a peculiar petechial rash on the lateral aspect of his feet and palms. Fearing an unusual reaction to warfarin, that drug was stopped and heparin was restarted. His heparin was continued, and he was evaluated for placement of an inferior vena caval "umbrella" to prevent further episodes of pulmonary embolism, given his adverse reaction to his most recent drug, warfarin.

Discussion: While both warfarin and heparin can cause adverse effects other than simple bleeding (e.g., blue toes syndrome or thrombocytopenia, respectively), the reaction described in this patient is a classic case of serum sickness. This reaction has not been previously described following administration of either heparin or warfarin. While the full syndrome had not been described following administration of streptokinase, each of the elements of the reaction had been previously described. In addition, streptokinase was a foreign protein given 11 days before the reaction occurred. Heparin did not seem involved since it had been restarted without worsening of the patient's syndrome. The decision was made to warn the patient of future use of streptokinase, continue heparin, and reintroduce warfarin. This was done uneventfully, and the patient was able to be discharged home several days later. Interruption of the inferior vena cava was avoided by the prompt recognition of this drug allergy. *Principle: Sometimes the value of recognizing an ADR or drug allergy is not that it leads to specific treatment, but that inappropriate, more toxic, or risky therapeutic procedures may be avoided.*

Type IV (Delayed Hypersensitivity, Cell-Mediated) Reactions. The delay in onset of these immune-mediated reactions is related to the fact that they are mediated by sensitized lymphocytes rather than humoral antibodies. This is the type of reaction that is evaluated when certain intradermal skin tests are placed [e.g., mumps, *Candida*, purified protein derivative (PPD)], or when a patient develops a delayed reaction to topical exposure to poison ivy oil. Drugs that can cause this type of delayed reaction include ethylenediamine (combined with theophylline to form aminophylline), or its closely related derivative ethylenediamine tetraacetic acid (EDTA), a preservative used in many topical and ophthalmic preparations.

Reactions Mimicking Drug Allergy. In many cases, reactions to drugs appear to be allergic but no firm evidence of immune response has been uncovered. Skin rashes of various types, ranging from a benign macular eruptions to toxic epidermal necrolysis or erythema multiform major, fit this description. Drug fevers often are assumed to be caused by drug allergy, since they usually develop after days or weeks of therapy, develop almost immediately upon reexposure, are not dose-related, and are occasionally accompanied by eosinophilia. However, direct involvement of the immune system has not been documented (Mackowiak and LeMaistre, 1987).

Drugs such as vancomycin and morphine can cause sudden itching and hypotension, probably caused by a direct release of histamine rather than drug allergy. Intravenous contrast agents, especially the ionic variety, can cause a reaction mimicking an anaphylactic reaction. These responses are called *anaphylactoid reactions*. They can be quite severe and are treated in the same fashion as true IgE-mediated anaphylactic reactions. Aspirin can appear to cause an "allergic" reaction, with hypotension and bronchospasm, especially in patients with nasal polyposis and asthma. All the NSAID agents can cause a similar reaction. The reaction has been characterized as being mediated by the ability to inhibit cyclooxygenase. Yet nonacetylated salicylates are good inhibitors of cyclooxygenase but do not cause the syndrome.

Many drug-induced cytopenias seem to be mediated by drug-induced antibody formation against circulating cells or bone marrow precursors. Other similar reactions have not been linked to the development of specific antibodies. Drug-induced liver or renal disease sometimes can have the appearance of a drug allergy with a peripheral eosinophilia, even though direct involvement of the immune system is hard to demonstrate. Phenothiazine- and halothane-induced hepatitis, and methicillin-induced interstitial nephritis, appear to be allergic reactions, although debate continues on this point.

In summary, allergies to medications constitute a small percentage of total ADRs. Because they are not dose-dependent and not related to the pharmacologic effects of their respective drugs, they are viewed as being idiosyncratic or unpredictable. Nevertheless, a detailed drug history often enables the physician to identify patients with known previous drug allergies, or an atopic history, making drug allergy in general more likely. Some allergic reactions may be avoided by a detailed history or appropriate skin testing. Even when drug allergies cannot be avoided, prompt recognition is essential to minimize toxicity and avoid a new round of treatments for the "new" disease. *Principle: Rare events become important when they contribute to patient morbidity and mortality. Lack of predictability of occurrence does not lead to lack of responsibility for prompt recognition and management, or even better, prevention.*

FACTORS THAT AFFECT THE PRACTICE OF RATIONAL THERAPEUTICS

What is the explanation for our failure as a profession to optimize therapeutics? (Meyer, 1988; Kusserow, 1989; Manasse, 1989). Mismedication of the elderly has become a critical health care issue and occurs mostly in one of four ways: (1) prescribing higher doses of a medication when lower doses would be equally effective and less toxic, (2) using more dangerous drugs when less toxic ones could achieve equivalent efficacy, (3) using a drug that is unnecessary, and (4) prescribing two our more medications that produce an unintended and unnecessary drug interaction

(Kusserow, 1989). These errors can be compounded by a more basic problem. Even if a doctor has chosen an appropriate drug to prescribe, the prescription frequently is illegible, incoherent, or incomplete (Walson et al., 1981).

These errors appear to be avoidable. In fact, most physicians probably feel that they rarely make such basic and fundamental errors in prescribing. There probably are a large number of factors that influence prescribers at both conscious and unconscious levels. Some promote irrational therapeutic decisions (Kroenke, 1985). These include the apparent need to use many drugs in treating patients with multiple complaints; the problem of multiple physicians' prescribing to the same patient without full knowledge of one another's therapeutic decisions; prescribing that is promoted in part by the latest fad; prescribing an older medicine out of habit without considering the use of alternatives available for the same indication; prescribing to satisfy the expectation (no matter how illogical) of the patient; inaccurately generalizing the conclusions of a study used to base a therapeutic decision; and salesmanship exerted by pharmaceutical companies (detailing), other physicians, or the media that may be incomplete or out of context. Others have commented on internal pressures or conflicts of interest experienced by physicians trying to conduct unbiased research (Healy et al., 1989). Similar types of conflicts of interest can interfere with the ability of physicians to prescribe in a scientifically sound and unbiased fashion.

Take another look at the six steps presented earlier as the foundation of an approach to rational therapeutics. For each step, consider some of the more subtle factors that may work to prevent you from achieving a rational, objective, medically and scientifically sound therapeutic decision.

Knowing the Diagnosis with Reasonable Certainty

Problems that Lead to Empiric Therapy. Making a correct diagnosis appears obviously enough as the first step toward rational therapy. However, consider the febrile leukemic patient, neutropenic from chemotherapy, who is appropriately and empirically started on broad-spectrum antibiotics. The action is justified in the absence of a definitive diagnosis because the risks of not treating a real infection in such patients are so great, despite the fact that only a minority (perhaps as low as 37% of those treated) will turn out to have a documented infection. Uncertainty about the diagnosis results in strong pressure on the physician to use the newest and the most expensive antibiotics. In one study, an average of

4.9 antimicrobials were used in each course of treatment (O'Hanley et al., 1989). Yet analysis of the data indicates that the greater number of antibiotics prescribed, the greater the toxicity (especially renal and hepatic toxicity). Those patients who developed renal or hepatic toxicity had a higher mortality than did patients who did not develop such toxicity (39% vs. 7.5%). Yet a substantial percentage of toxicity might have been avoided without compromising efficacy by better choice of antibiotics. *Principle: Failure to be able to establish a firm diagnosis makes therapeutic plans difficult (especially in critically ill patients) but not impossible. Data can be carefully gathered and be the basis of sound therapeutic decisions involving empiric treatment.*

Inappropriate Acceptance of Empiric Treatment. The customary goals of treating fever of unknown origin in an immunosuppressed patient (treat early, empirically, with multiple agents that convey broad-spectrum coverage) often are sound. But there is no justification in generalizing and applying these goals to populations of patients with entirely different demography (i.e., those who do not have cancer, have not received chemotherapy, are not immunosuppressed, and are not neutropenic). The irrational overuse of antibiotics has been documented repeatedly and appears to be an international problem (Moss and McNicol, 1983). In fact, the causes of such irrationality and reasons for its growth in spite of its perils have been specifically addressed (Kim and Gallis, 1989). A common situation is that of a surgical patient, recovering nicely from his or her operation, who develops a low-grade fever. Even before a thorough workup of the patient's fever is completed, antibiotics appropriate for the febrile neutropenic patient sometimes are begun. In fact, a rigorous fever workup itself may never be attempted, because physicians have become so used to obtaining unrevealing cultures from the febrile neutropenic patient. The necessity for treating neutropenic febrile cancer patients with antibiotics has conditioned physicians to accept the same behavior when it may be inappropriate. For example, consider an immunosuppressed patient (perhaps receiving methotrexate) who develops a cough, hypoxemia, and pulmonary infiltrates. The differential diagnosis is long and includes drug reactions (possibly requiring steroids), typical bacterial pneumonia (requiring one or more of several antibiotics), atypical bacterial pneumonia (requiring erythromycin), mycobacterial pneumonia (requiring two antimycobacterial drugs), viral pneumonia (requiring acyclovir), *Pneumocystis* pneumonia (requiring co-trimoxazole), fungal pneumonia (requiring amphotericin), interstitial pneumonitis, and so forth. The clinician may speak of employing a "shotgun" approach to treating the patient when sputum samples have been nondiagnostic. Indeed, for nonneutropenic cancer patients with diffuse infiltrates, there is some evidence that treatment with co-trimoxazole plus erythromycin may be successful in up to 71% (Rubin et al., 1988).

However, neutropenic patients pose a larger problem, and for patients who fail to improve, an "adequate shotgun" ultimately may require 10 barrels! In such a situation, the physician is likely to overestimate the risks of diagnostic procedures (such as bronchial aspirate or lavage with transbronchial biopsy, or even open lung biopsy) and underestimate their frequent success in providing a definitive diagnosis (Greenman et al., 1975; Stover et al., 1984; Cockerill et al., 1985; Masur et al., 1985). This error is compounded when the physician underestimates the risks of drug toxicity resulting from a shotgun approach.

Understanding the Pathophysiology of the Patient's Disease

Difference between Syndrome and Disease. The identification of an abnormality may require attempts to understand the pathophysiology of the disease process before therapy can be correctly chosen. One situation in which failure to understand the disease process leads to poor therapeutic decisions occurs when the disease is really a syndrome that can result from several different pathophysiologic mechanisms.

For example, a patient with metastatic bronchogenic carcinoma and hyponatremia is likely to respond best to restriction of fluid and to drugs that counter the effects of ADH. A patient with hyponatremia resulting from severe losses of salt and water and some oral replacement with free water may respond best to therapy with IV solutions of isotonic and hypertonic saline, and treatment of the underlying condition causing such losses. In such hyponatremic patients, the understanding of the pathophysiology of the observed state of hyponatremia is paramount in selecting the most appropriate therapeutic option (see chapter 11).

Being Misled by a Name. Sometimes the name or presentation of the disease itself may fool the physician into misunderstanding both the underlying pathophysiology of the disease and the optimal therapeutic plan. A patient with systemic lupus erythematosus and a circulating "lupus anticoagulant" may present with a slightly prolonged prothrombin time. The implications of the name *lupus anticoagulant* and the abnormal prothrombin time it produces may conceal the fact that such patients actually are in a hypercoagulable state, are at increased risk for thromboembolic events, and require anticoagulant therapy in spite of the circulating anticoagulant. Thus, the introduction of heparin or warfarin may be unduly delayed because of attribution of a characteristic to a disease that is not there. *Principle: Too often the profession substitutes a name of a disease for an understanding of pathogenesis. Although such practices are understandable in the face of limited information and practical in helping with a diagnosis and prognosis, they often are counterproductive elements in planning therapeutic strategy.*

Further Advantages of Understanding the Disease. At times the proper understanding of the disease leads not only to appropriate therapeutic plans but also to appropriate preventive measures as well. For example, consider a hospital that identified a cluster of patients with urinary tract infections caused by *Pseudomonas aeruginosa*. All the patients in this cluster were on the orthopedic service recovering from hip surgery. All had unremarkable urinalyses the day prior to surgery. The positive urine cultures were obtained on the fourth postoperative day as the Foley catheter was being removed. In each case, the clinician correctly deduced that the infection was related to the presence of the Foley catheter and prescribed an appropriate antibiotic with excellent coverage of the pathogen. The urinary catheters increased the risk of developing cystitis by facilitating entry of pathogens into the bladder. *Pseudomonas aeruginosa* is a relatively uncommon pathogen for such infections, and the cluster of cases in time and space suggested a common vector. This more sophisticated approach to the disease eventually led to the discovery that one of the nurses on the floor responsible for catheter care was not washing her hands between patients and was spreading the organism from one patient to the next. In this situation, understanding the pathogenesis and epidemiology of the disease led to the most appropriate response: a conference for the floor nurses, and increased emphasis on hand washing and improved catheter care. The efficacy of the approach was obvious. Postoperative bladder infections in patients on the orthopedic service rapidly decreased. The few that did occur were caused mostly by *E. coli*, the usual pathogen in this situation. *Principle: The name of a patient's disease does not automatically spell out its pathogenesis. Time spent rigorously defining the most likely pathophysiologic sequence of a patient's disease often pays dividends in planning optimal therapeutic interventions.*

Some diseases, particularly chronic and incurable ones, pose a major challenge to the therapist. Consider, for example, the rheumatic diseases. In the rest of the chapter, notice how the author (Halsted Holman, M.D.) "uses" time as a factor that affects therapeutic strategies. What and how much of a drug must be used for an incurable disease require very different approaches to therapy than decisions that would affect a very morbid or lethal curable illness.

Editor's Note: The rest of this section was contributed by Halsted Holman, M.D., Department of Medicine, Stanford University.

The present classification of rheumatic diseases (rheumatoid arthritis, systemic lupus erythematosus (SLE), dermatomyositis, progressive systemic sclerosis, vasculitis) was established decades ago, when only the most severe forms of these diseases were recognized clinically. Since then, clinical experience and laboratory investigation have combined to identify many forms of rheumatic disease not captured by the original classification. Also, contemporary treatments have prolonged life with further diversification of the clinical appearances of rheumatic diseases. As a consequence, the original classification has lost considerable utility and, it can be argued, constitutes a significant barrier to accurate clinical and biological understanding of the diseases.

The disutility of the prevailing classification is evident in a number of ways. First, each of the original diagnoses encompasses a range of different manifestations and severities that can be depicted as a normal curve of characteristics (Fig. 1–12). However, the curves of characteristics are not separate from one another; they overlap significantly. Thus patients are commonly found who exhibit characteristics of more then one of the original diagnoses. Second, while certain serologic abnormalities are associated more frequently with one rheumatic disease or a particular manifestation (e.g., rheumatoid factor with rheumatoid arthritis, anti-DNA antibody with SLE nephritis), none is exclusively associated with, or diagnostic of, a particular rheumatic disease. Third, within a given rheumatic disease, the target organ may change partially or completely as time progresses. For instance, a patient with SLE may at one time have serositis and rash, later only thrombocytopenia, and, still later, nephritis. Occasionally, patients with one diagnosis will transform totally to the characteristics of another of the classic categories.

The present discrete and static classification system cannot accommodate these clinical attributes of rheumatic disease. An alternative conceptualization, which has two central components, serves far better. The first component asserts that the classic diagnoses are but a few of the many patterns of rheumatic disease. Because all the classic diseases can overlap with one another, a broad array of clinical patterns is seen in

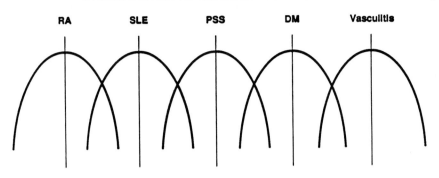

Fig. 1–12. A representation of five rheumatic diseases (rheumatiod arthritis, RA; systemic lupus erythematosus, SLE; progressive systemic sclerosis, PSS; dermatomyositis, DM; and vasculitis), illustrating the overlap of one syndrome with several others.

practice; patterns often are not static, shifting and blending into one another. Thus, an individual patient's rheumatic disease, at the outset, can have one of a large array of biological appearances and, over time, can pass into and out of additional appearances. Further, when one adds therapeutic adversities plus the multiple psychological and social consequences of chronic disease, the number of factors that might contribute to a clinical illness pattern can be huge. Experienced clinicians become quite adept at recognizing both the differences and the commonalities in the illness patterns and at identifying those attributes that are most influential in creating a pattern. Clinically meaningful diagnosis in the rheumatic diseases is thus a process of pattern recognition and interpretation, not simply matching characteristics to a criterion list.

The second component of the alternative conceptualization emphasizes a long-recognized characteristic of rheumatic disease, namely, undulation in the severity of disease. This undulation occurs both spontaneously and in response to therapy. Thus, for any particular patient, both the disease pattern and its severity may be in continuous change. Why the undulation in severity? The existence of a spontaneous reduction in severity implies a biological recovery or healing process. That is, the fluctuating disease intensity results from a continuous interaction between the pathogenic force and the patient's recovery capacity. Treatment often, but not always, affects the balance between them.

Taken together, these two conceptual components create an image of rheumatic disease as an aberrant biological process wending its way across a landscape only roughly delineated by the classic definitions of disease. En route it experiences changes in direction, characteristics, and intensity.

The changing patterns and undulating severity of rheumatic diseases have significant implications for treatment. Because rheumatic diseases are chronic diseases for which the cause and cure are unknown, management over time, not cure, is the goal. Management involves attention not only to the biological consequences of the disease but to other components of the illness created by the disease (psychological, social, economic consequences), and to the interactions among them. Appropriate management entails an accurate characterization of the patient's state and direction of change followed by judicious application of interventions intended to influence favorably that state and its direction. For example, at any given moment when seen by a physician, a patient's clinical characteristics could represent a state of worsening, a state of improvement, or a state of stability (points A, B, or C respectively on Fig. 1–13). Though the severity of these states is comparable, the three individuals would likely require different management: increased intensity for individual A, reduced intensity for individual B, and watchful waiting for individual C.

Three types of information are critical for management decisions: the patient's present clinical state, the direction or trajectory of the disease (arrows in Fig. 1–13), and the pace or tempo with which the state is moving along the trajectory. The clinical state is determined by conventional clinical assessment employing historical, physical, and laboratory data. However, because of the pleomorphism and chronicity of rheumatic diseases, the critical factors defining a present state can be quite variable. For instance, an individual may be asymptomatic while renal disease worsens; here laboratory information is crucial. For another individual with chronic arthritis who depends upon hands for employment and is threatened with a job loss, nonmedical considerations may be the primary determinant.

The trajectory and tempo of a patient's disease are defined by change over time. Therefore, the clinician uses time as a tool to gather the information that reveals the trajectory and its tempo. Indeed, the appropriate use of time is often the most

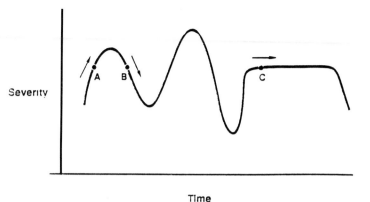

Fig. 1-13. A representative general relationship of time and severity of chronic rheumatic diseases.

important tool in the clinician's hands for the management of a chronic disease. Three aspects of the wise use of time merit mention. First, the physician must select the variables that will reveal the disease trajectory. Among the wide range of abnormalities in a rheumatic disease, usually only a central few are necessary to define trajectory. Examples would be the creatinine concentration in the first case above, and measures of the activity and severity of the arthritis plus the employer's flexibility in the second case. The second aspect of the use of time is determining the length of time necessary to identify accurately the trajectory and the tempo of movement. How long can or should one take to interpret the evidence? The choice is affected by fluctuations in symptoms and laboratory values that are independent of the basic disease or illness state. Such fluctuations reflect variations in measurements and symptom perceptions around the true mean. A symptom such as pain normally varies over the course of the day as circumstances and environments change. Therefore, the smooth undulation of the severity of disease depicted in Fig. 1-13 is erroneous. The real circumstance is much more like that shown in Fig. 1-14, with a series of secondary, semichaotic variations around the mean

of the true disease course. In order to identify and discount the secondary fluctuations, the patient must play a role in selecting and interpreting the information that is gathered. In the case of the creatinine concentration, ambiguity is minimal. However, when judging pain or ability to perform an employment function, the ambiguity is potentially large. In the latter instance, the patient's interpretation of the impact of the pain and its effect on work capacity is central. Thus the third aspect of the use of time is securing a knowledgeable and confident patient who can work effectively in partnership with the physician. In general, it is the physician's task to ensure that the patient becomes such an individual.

In emphasizing the centrality of the use of time to determine trajectory and tempo of a disease or its illness, the value of prediction is commensurately diminished. That is deliberate. While it would be highly desirable to have one or two clinical or laboratory indicators that accurately predict the future for an individual patient, such rarely exist. Decades of clinical experience and years of laboratory studies have failed to reveal abnormalities that, by themselves, yield an accurate diagnosis or prognosis. The biology of the disease and the characteristics of the illness it

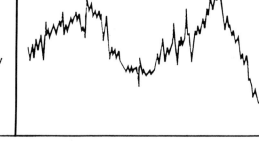

Fig. 1-14. A representation of severity of chronic rheumatoid arthritis over time in a single patient.

causes are revealed only by the pattern, created by the various abnormalities, the trajectory of that pattern, and the tempo with which it moves.

Once the disease pattern, its severity, its trajectory, and its tempo have been determined, the issue in management is selecting the appropriate intervention. Here matters have changed significantly in recent years. Not long ago each classic rheumatic diagnosis was, in general, thought to require a particular type of therapy. Examples were aspirin or other NSAIDs for rheumatoid arthritis, corticosteroids for SLE, and no medicine for scleroderma. While these generalities still retain validity, virtually all drugs now employed in treating rheumatic diseases are used, under one circumstance or another, in each of the rheumatic diseases. Formal diagnosis is no longer the determinant of treatment. Rather, the nature of organ involvement, its trajectory, and its tempo dictate the type and intensity of therapy. Whatever the formal diagnosis, when essential parenchymal organs are not involved, less intensive symptomatic therapy is appropriate; more intensive and more dangerous treatment is applied when major organs are affected and/or the course is unfavorable.

To illustrate this concept of rheumatic diseases and their management, an example may be helpful. Pain, the most common concern of patients with chronic rheumatic diseases, can have many origins: active synovitis, joint deformity from previous synovitis, gait change from favoring a limb, physical deconditioning, adverse effects of medication, intercurrent illness, comorbidity, and psychological distress from the chronic illness or from an unrelated source. Management of each is likely to be different. Sometimes more than one cause is present, requiring combinations of therapies. In both instances, severity of the pain may be quite variable. Accurate identification of the cause of the pain and its severity is essential. But how? Often, neither the physical examination nor the laboratory will yield an unequivocal answer. Historical information from both the patient and the physician may come closer, but ambiguity is likely to remain. In this setting the practical clinical answer is an agreement between the patient and the physician on a probable cause and a trial of observation, or of therapy with careful determination of the effects on the pain. In a sense, this is a negotiated settlement. Negotiated settlements are pervasive in the management of chronic disease. They are particularly evident when subjective symptoms exceed objective evidence of a disease flare, and emotional sources of the pain are suspected by the physician. Again, the physician must seek to persuade the patient and to obtain agreement on a plan of management. Throughout this example one sees the persistence of uncertainty, the importance of identifying the trajectory of the symptom, the use of time to assess validity of interpretations, and the essential role of the patient in the process. *Principle: Especially for chronic diseases, understanding disease pathophysiology requires identifying illness trajectories and the variety of factors that can influence them. The wise use of time to detect trajectories and their tempos, with attention to the patient's perceptions and wishes, is central to that process.*

Understanding the Pharmacology of Useful Drugs

Drugs That Have No Evidence of Efficacy. Drug therapy should generally be used only with a drug that has been shown to have efficacy in appropriately designed clinical trials. While it might be imagined that cerebrovascular senile dementia or peripheral arterial insufficiency might be improved if treated with vasodilating drugs, clinical studies have not found any presently available drug useful in these two conditions (Avorn et al., 1982). In the usual doses employed, such drugs have negligible ability to effect vasodilation in vessels that have been narrowed by fixed atherosclerotic lesions. To the extent that they lower mean arterial pressure, vasodilators may even reduce flow to ischemic areas by creating a shunt through areas that do vasodilate (Avorn et al., 1982).

In a study of primary care physicians picked at random in the greater Boston area, 71% believed that "impaired cerebral blood flow is a major cause of senile dementia," and 32% said that they found "cerebral vasodilators useful in managing confused geriatric patients". Reports of clinical trials were not likely the source of these opinions. However, only 4% of these physicians felt that drug advertisements were very important in influencing their prescribing; 20% felt that detail people were very important; and 62% felt that scientific papers were very important. The authors of the study concluded that these data demonstrated a predominance of commercial rather than scientific sources of drug information, *even while the physicians themselves were not aware of sources of their information.* Of course, other sources of influence (patient preference, advice from colleagues, personal experience) could have led to this irrational prescribing as well. *Principle: When a physician believes a drug is effective in the management of a disease in spite of strong scientific evidence to the contrary, irrational prescribing results. Nonscientific factors influence physician prescribing even while the physician may be unaware of the power of those factors.*

In some cases, a physician may wish to conduct

an *n* = 1 clinical trial in an individual patient to determine the efficacy of a specific treatment. This approach is discussed in chapter 36.

Prescribing Drugs Because It "Makes Sense". Clinicians may have difficulty accepting that a drug lacks clinical efficacy if they have been using the drug for a particular indication. Consider the controversy about using antiseizure medications to control new-onset seizures related to withdrawal from alcohol in nonepileptic alcoholics (see chapters 12 and 27). Patients who have experienced one such seizure related to alcohol withdrawal are at risk of sustaining further seizures during their course of detoxification. Phenytoin is an antiseizure medication with a wide spectrum of activity for a variety of seizures. It seems reasonable that administration of phenytoin to patients experiencing alcohol withdrawal seizures might reduce the chances of their sustaining further seizures. Nevertheless, rigorous clinical studies have failed to demonstrate a significant benefit over placebo in the prevention of subsequent seizures in this specific situation (Alldredge et al., 1989). In addition, the toxicity of rapid IV phenytoin (e.g., hypotension, arrhythmias) appears to outweigh the benefits of the drug during alcohol withdrawal.

There are a number of examples in therapeutics that on the surface are hard to understand. For example, why do some physicians use propoxyphene as an analgesic after it has been shown to less effective and more toxic than other analgesics (see chapters 12, 25, and 27)? Why do doctors treat some types of lymphoma when treatment can actually accelerate mortality (see chapter 23)? *Principle: The temptation to treat for no other reason than "it makes sense" is very hard to resist, even in the face of strong evidence that contradicts the therapeutic strategy. Although the psychology of such behavior may be understandable, all the consequences are borne by the unfortunate patient.*

Factors That Perpetuate Incorrect Information about Drugs. There are many examples that demonstrate how use of drugs can begin with a reasonable hypothesis that is eventually not confirmed in careful clinical trials. However, once such therapy becomes established, it can be perpetuated by many factors that affect the prescribing habits of physicians. More than 20 years ago, Cluff (1967) summarized these nonscientific factors, which included the example of a teacher or respected peer, testimonials of colleagues, extrapolation of a perfectly legitimate use of a drug to an incorrect situation, satisfaction of doing something for the patient, persuasiveness of advertising, and availability of liberal samples. Thus, pre-

scribing habits lacking in scientific justification can be passed on from one generation of physicians to the next for years before such habits are scrutinized under the light of appropriate clinical trials.

Optimizing Selection of Drug and Dose

The Option of Not Using a Drug. For many diseases ranging from viral infection to cancer, no drug treatment may be the best treatment, as long as other strategies for managing symptoms are discussed. However, the physician's prescribing of a medication has taken on roles and connotations far beyond recommending a specific drug to the patient (see chapter 33). The prescription itself has come to be viewed as an expected and essential transaction that formally concludes the exchange between the patient and the physician (Manasse, 1989). The patient may feel that he or she has not received his or her money's worth unless a prescription is given. The physician may feel pressed to provide a prescription to keep the patient satisfied with the care. In addition, writing a prescription may be quicker and simpler than taking time to explain to the patient why no drug is indicated for this particular problem. *Principle: What may be the most expedient maneuver for the physician may be quite costly and morbid for the patient without either party realizing it.*

New Drug Information Not Provided by the Manufacturer. By the time a drug is approved by the FDA for marketing in the United States, a large amount of information about it has been provided by the company, reviewed by the FDA, and finally synthesized into the standard package insert that is contained in the *Physicians' Desk Reference*. However, even this large amount of reviewed and approved information is incomplete and in many ways inadequate to permit the prescriber to make adequately informed therapeutic decisions (see chapters 33–36 and 39–41). This deficiency in information provided to prescribers has been briefly but elegantly described (Herxheimer, 1987). Data comparing a new drug to older drugs of the same class are distinctly missing from the information provided by the manufacturer. The clinician must look elsewhere (primary clinical trials, review articles, books, etc.) for such comparisons.

There also are other gaps in the information provided to physicians. The physician likely will not know how the maximum recommended dose was determined, nor how "safe" the drug is likely to be in pregnant women, children, or the elderly. Warnings and adverse effects tend to be nonquantitative and difficult to translate into practical strategies. The physician will likely not know exactly what to communicate to the patient as well. For older, established, commonly used drugs, patient information sheets are available from organizations such as the American Medical Association (AMA) and the U.S. Pharmacopeial (USP) Convention.

With time, additional clinical trials often will be done, increasing knowledge of how to use the drug for old and new indications. For example, the standard target concentration of lithium for maintenance treatment of bipolar disorder has been from 0.8 to 1.0 millimols per liter (mmol/l), although concern about the drug's toxic effects have led some physicians to aim for a lower target concentration of lithium (see chapter 13). Only recently has a clinical trial been conducted that clearly shows that the risk of relapse was 2.6 times higher among patients in the low-range group (median concentration 0.54 mmol/l) than it was in the standard-range group (median 0.83 mmol/l) (Gelenberg et al., 1989). Adverse effects were more common in the standard-range group as well, but this type of study makes it possible to choose an optimal target concentration.

Increasing Knowledge of a Drug's Adverse Effects. As discussed in chapters 34 and 41, when a new drug is approved by the FDA it may have been used in from only 1000 to 3000 patients or fewer. Therefore, the likelihood of identifying infrequent adverse effects prior to approval is low (see chapters 34, 35, and 41). However, it is not commonly appreciated that new adverse and beneficial effects may be noted in "old" drugs that have been in frequent use for years (see chapter 41). For example, phenobarbital has been used in children with new-onset febrile seizures who were at increased risk of sustaining subsequent seizures. Although some reports suggested possible behavioral and cognitive effects of the drug, it remained commonly used for this indication. A recent placebo-controlled trial demonstrated that after 2 years of therapy, the mean IQ in the group assigned to phenobarbital was 8.4 points lower than that in the placebo group. A trend toward lower IQ in the treatment group persisted even 6 months after the drug was discontinued. Finally, the study failed to demonstrate any benefit of reduced risk of subsequent seizures in the treated group (Farwell et al., 1990; chapter 8). A well-performed study documented significant toxicity not balanced by any measurable efficacy.

A recent case-control study was performed to assess the risk of hip fracture associated with the use of four classes of psychotropic drugs (Ray et al., 1987). Patients treated with short-acting hypnotics had no increased risk of hip fracture, but patients who received long-acting hypnotics (odds ratio 1.8), tricyclic antidepressants (odds ratio 1.9), and antipsychotics (odds ratio 2.0) were at increased risk. The additional risk associated with these classes of drugs appeared to be dose-related as well. The study did not prove a causal relationship, but it suggests the possibility that these classes of drugs increase the risk of hip fractures in elderly patients, possibly because of their sedative or hypotensive effects. *Principle: Even when a drug has been used for years for approved indications, the physician should not be surprised when new data document a new form of drug-related efficacy or toxicity. Increased experience with a drug likely will lead not only to new indications for the drug but also provide data that modify older indications.*

Impact of Drug Costs. For some patients, the cost of a prescription is not a factor in determining whether the prescription will be filled. However, for many patients, cost is often a major factor in compliance (Babington et al., 1983). One implication of this is that physicians should have an idea how much a prescription really costs. A recent study compared patterns of patient behavior in two states in filling prescriptions for 16 different drugs (Soumerai et al., 1987). In New Hampshire, the state Medicaid program began a policy of limiting patients to three paid prescriptions per month. This policy resulted in a 30% drop in the number of such prescriptions filled, while no change was observed in the comparison state. In the elderly, a group that often requires many drugs, the number of prescriptions filled per month fell from an average of 5.2 to 2.8 drugs. While much of this decrease was accounted for by a drop in "ineffective drugs," decreases in the purchases of "essential" medications such as insulin and diuretics also were observed. The next year, New Hampshire changed its policy by replacing the three-prescription cap with a $1 co-payment policy. Prescriptions increased almost to precap levels for most drugs. Savings to Medicaid on drug costs were comparable under both policies. *Principle: The cost of filling a prescription definitely affects patient compliance in filling the prescription in some patient groups.*

A recent study of 54 residents in internal medicine and primary care medicine documented that residents did not know actual drug prices. The total mean percentage deviation of their estimates from actual drug price was about 63%. Surprisingly, even when the residents were given a price guide booklet, they did not use it (Babington et al., 1983). Another study asked medical students, pediatric residents, and pediatricians to evaluate the cost of commonly prescribed medications (Weber et al., 1986). The cost estimates of that group were considered adequate in only 40%,

52%, and 62% of the cases, respectively. These data suggest that when physicians try to pick an optimal drug for a given patient, the price of the medication and the patient's ability to pay for the medication are important factors for the prescriber to consider.

Adding a new drug to a patient's regimen frequently leads to potential or real drug interactions (Beers et al., 1990). In a survey of 424 randomly selected adults seeking care at a university-affiliated hospital emergency department, 47% of visits led to the addition of one or more new medications. In 10% of the visits in which one or more medications were added, a new medication produced the potential for an adverse interaction that was clinically important. The best predictor of a potential interaction was the number of medications used by the patient at the time of presentation to the emergency room. Perhaps most discouraging, a medication history was recorded for every patient at admission to the emergency room (presumably by an admitting nurse) and was available to the treating physician, but the treating physician did not routinely screen for potential drug interactions. *Principle: More than knowledge about probable drug interactions is needed to prevent them. An attitude that encourages anticipation of the possible effects of any change in a patient's drug regimen should be developed.*

Irrational Beliefs. In an editorial, Burnham (1987) describes fads and fashions in medical science. Many of his examples focus on the influence of fads on prescribing habits. What can account for the fact that Atarax^{TM} is usually prescribed for itching and Vistaril^{TM} for nausea, even though they are the same drug (hydroxyzine)? Burnham points out that therapies and even diagnoses come in and out of fashion, often for no clear or rational reason. He concludes that "medical fashions have a powerful effect on how we treat, whom we treat, and what we treat, on how patients take care of themselves, and even on the directions of medical science."

Recent work has begun to unravel the factors accounting for large differences in practice patterns. Rates of hospitalization of children for illnesses such as asthma or toxic ingestions, and rates of surgical procedures such as hysterectomy or prostatectomy, can vary widely from county to county, or city to city (Wennberg and Gittelsohn, 1982; Perrin et al., 1989). The amount and cost of hospital care for patients in a community may have more to do with factors such as the number of physicians, their specialties, and their preferred procedures than with the health status or needs of the inhabitants (Wennberg and Gittelsohn, 1982).

Differences in physician choices for therapy are

evident. For example, physicians confronting similar nonrheumatic patients with chronic atrial fibrillation make different decisions about whether to anticoagulate such patients. In one study, physicians with different training (family physicians, general internists, and cardiologists) behaved similarly when confronted with patients with mitral valve disease or those with a history of chronic alcohol abuse but behaved differently when confronted with patients in atrial fibrillation (Chang et al., 1990). A physician's treatment decision was strongly related to his or her assessment of the relative risk of embolism compared with hemorrhage derived for each case. Cardiologists were least likely to initiate chronic anticoagulation (they judged the risk of embolism to be lower), and family practitioners were most likely to institute anticoagulation (they judged the risk of embolism to be higher). Although these groups of physicians differed in their assessment of the risk of hemorrhage, none of the groups' estimates of the risk of embolization was close to the best estimate published in recent literature.

When "local" prescribing patterns seem out of step with generally accepted and validated prescribing practices, other nonmedical factors may be playing a role. Several such examples were provided in a study of drug prescribing on a Yugoslavian pediatric service (Stanulovic et al., 1984). For example, an unexpected reduction in the appropriate use of penicillin was triggered by two recent deaths of patients thought to be caused by procaine penicillin–induced rhabdomyolysis. Less effective or more toxic drugs were used in place of penicillins. *Principle: A physician's recent personal experience is important, but it may lead to overestimation of the frequency of the most recently recognized adverse drug reactions and underestimation of what he or she has not seen.*

Detailing and Counterdetailing. One influence that modifies prescribing by physicians is unbalanced, inaccurate, or frankly misleading information provided by colleagues, investigators, or drug companies in the form of the detail person. The pharmaceutical industry spends about $5000 per year per physician in the United States on detailing activities designed to acquaint physicians with specific drug products and encourage their prescription (Silverman and Lee, 1974; *Wall Street Journal*, 1984; Soumerai and Avorn, 1990). Industry uses approximately 1 representative for every 10 office-based practitioners. This amount is more than half of the estimated $3 billion spent each year on drug promotion, which also includes activities such as journal advertising, direct mail, free samples, conventions, and so forth. Drug detailing and advertising can cause physicians to change their beliefs and prescribing habits, even when they are not aware of the impact of the advertising or detailing itself, and even when they deny the importance of such factors in their therapeutic decisions (Avorn et al., 1982).

Subtle and effective combinations of printed advertisements and personal contact during visits from detail persons can constitute messages that are difficult to counteract or reverse. However, several investigators have explored educational strategies that offer various degrees of success. In one study of three educational methods designed to improve antibiotic prescribing in office practice, a mailed brochure had no detectable effect; a drug educator had only a modest effect; but personal visits by a physician produced strong attributable changes in prescribing behavior (Schaffner et al., 1983). This beneficial effect was seen with respect to improving the quality of care and to reducing the cost of care.

A second study also demonstrated improved therapeutic decisions achieved through educational outreach programs termed *academically based detailing* (Avorn and Soumerai, 1983). In this study, two separate interventions (and a control group) were used in an effort to reduce the excessive use of three groups of drugs. Physicians who received only mailed printed materials did not reduce their prescribing of the target drugs relative to controls. However, physicians who received a series of mailed "unadvertisements" along with personal educational visits by specially trained clinical pharmacists reduced their prescribing of the target drugs by 14% compared with controls. In a subsequent report, the same authors enumerated some of the key factors that make such "academic detailing" successful (Soumerai and Avorn, 1990).

Conflicts of Interest. Although well-intentioned clinicians may be unwittingly influenced by pharmaceutical companies, an even more subtle but effective process might also contribute to inappropriate prescribing. Physicians' decisions concerning which drug to prescribe for a given patient may be increasingly affected by unrecognized conflicts of interest on the part of the physician-prescriber. One physician has framed the problem as follows: "The charge against us is that, in many of our dealings with the industry, we have become corrupt; that in return for needlessly (and sometimes recklessly) prescribing their expensive products, we accept (or even demand) rewards on a breathtaking scale" (Rawlins, 1984). When challenged with this idea, most physicians believe that *they* are not affected by promotional activities, and that they can receive gifts from drug companies without prescribing that company's products. These earnest denials of conflict

of interest may be sincere but they also are incorrect. "The degree to which the profession, mainly composed of honorable and decent people, can practice such self-deceit is quite extraordinary" (Rawlins, 1984).

It is tempting to view such harsh judgments on clinicians as being extreme, biased, or inaccurate. Nevertheless, such statements seem to be credible. Physicians accept gifts from pharmaceutical companies in many forms, perhaps without recognizing the general rule that accepting a gift has complex practical and ethical repercussions (Chen et al., 1989). In an interesting analysis of doctors receiving gifts from drug companies, the authors point out that such gifts cost patients money and are likely to influence the way society perceives the medical profession. In an extreme situation, physicians may substantially alter their prescribing practices in order to obtain additional gifts such as free airline tickets, money, or vacations (Wilkes and Shuchman, 1989).

Potential and real conflicts of interest have led to the interesting situation in which most physicians maintain that they can accept gifts without becoming biased, but several organizations have proposed new guidelines for physician–industry relations. The Royal College of Physicians has proposed that "the overriding principle is that any benefit in cash or kind, any gifts, any hospitality or any subsidy received from a pharmaceutical company must leave the doctor's independence of judgment manifestly unimpaired. When it comes to the margin between what is acceptable and what is unacceptable, judgment may sometimes be difficult: a useful criterion of acceptability may be 'Would you be willing to have these arrangements generally known?'" (Royal College of Physicians, 1986). The American College of Physicians (ACP) also felt compelled to issue a position paper concerning the relation of physicians to the pharmaceutical industry. The ACP was concerned that physicians receiving excessive or inappropriate gifts impair public confidence in the integrity of the profession and could compromise the physician's clinical judgment. The ACP's primary position was similar to that advocated by its British counterpart, namely that a useful criterion in determining which activities are acceptable is whether the physician would be willing to have such arrangements generally known (Goldfinger, 1990).

Another physician activity that can produce an inherent conflict of interest occurs when clinicians sell prescription drugs to their patients. A recent bill in the U.S. Congress dealt with this issue, and a recent editorial posed both sides of the argument (Relman, 1987). This is yet another activity in which physician conflict of interest can lead to irrational or suboptimal prescribing. ***Principle:***

The physician must put the patient's welfare first and practice rational therapeutics. The physician cannot do either when he or she consciously or unconsciously has a material interest in which drug is prescribed. Such real and potential conflicts of interest not only can undermine the doctor–patient relationship, but also can undermine public confidence in the profession.

Selection of Appropriate Therapeutic End Points

Appropriate End Points of Efficacy. When a physician prescribes a new drug, what end points should be followed to assess the drug's effects? In some situations, the patient should help the physician pick the most appropriate effects. For example, a recent study of the use of methotrexate in rheumatoid arthritis demonstrated statistically significant but clinically small (5%–11%) differences in patients treated with methotrexate versus placebo with respect to standard measures of physical, social, and emotional function (Tugwell et al., 1990). Yet when patients specified in advance a set of measurements that best described the functions they most wanted the treatment to improve, patients receiving methotrexate fared about 29% better than patients receiving placebo.

This type of study suggests that end points for certain drugs can be easily picked by the physician (e.g., prothrombin time in the patient receiving warfarin) but that in some situations a combination of end points of efficacy must be chosen based on discussions between the patient and the physician. However, even a "simple" end point of efficacy may turn out to be difficult to use wisely. Consider the monitoring of prothrombin time. Recent work has suggested that the intensity of anticoagulation in the treatment of patients with proximal-vein thrombosis (Hull et al., 1982) or mechanical prosthetic heart valves (Saour et al., 1990) can be lower than originally believed and yet have equal efficacy and less toxicity. In addition, it now appears that different intensities of anticoagulation are required for different underlying thromboembolic conditions (e.g., prophylaxis during hip surgery, treatment of thrombophlebitis, prevention of embolism in patients with cardiac dysfunction, prevention of thrombus formation in patients with prosthetic heart valves, etc.). It has been demonstrated that very low doses of warfarin (1 mg/day) can help prevent thrombosis in patients with central venous catheters without producing change in the prothrombin time (Bern et al., 1990). In addition, the method of laboratory determination of prothrombin time has changed over time with growing international standardization of the thromboplastin reagents used in the assay. *Principle: Choosing appro-priate end points of efficacy may not be straightforward. Targets and goals may change as understanding of the disease or the drugs changes.*

End Points Reflecting Toxicity. Physicians frequently recognize ADRs in patients (Koch-Weser et al., 1969; Rogers et al., 1988). How often physicians fail to appreciate the occurrence of ADRs when they occur is not known. Because most drugs can cause a wide variety of adverse effects, it is difficult for the physician to consider them all and look for them all. For example, many physicians prescribing an NSAID ask the patients about abdominal pain symptoms during subsequent visits but do not think to check for the development of renal toxicity, which appears more commonly than is generally appreciated (Murray and Brater, 1990; Whelton et al., 1990; chapter 11). Physicians prescribing an aminoglycoside generally check for the development of nephrotoxicity but fail to check for the development of cochlear or vestibular ototoxicity. Physicians must anticipate the most likely toxic effects of a drug, develop a plan to follow the patient to see whether those adverse reactions develop, and recruit the patient's help and cooperation in carrying out the plan.

The Prescription as an Experiment. Perhaps 75% of all office visits to a physician end with one or more new prescriptions (Soumerai et al., 1990). However, although the writing of the prescription may terminate the office visit, it only serves to begin a new experiment for each patient. There is no certainty that the desired pharmacologic effect will occur. Undesired pharmacologic, immunologic, or idiosyncratic reactions—drug toxicity—also may occur. Thus the prescription represents the beginning of an experiment that may last for hours (e.g., one dose of subcutaneous terbutaline) or years (chronic daily use of penicillamine). The physician must pick appropriate end points of drug efficacy and toxicity and follow those end points over the course of the experiment. The appropriate end points should take into account patient preferences, common reactions, and less common but potentially severe reactions. *Principle: Only when the physician approaches each prescription as the beginning of a therapeutic experiment of uncertain outcome, and not as a concluding act to an office visit, will the chances that the experiment will be as safe, effective, and fruitful as possible be optimized.*

The Physician–Patient Relationship

How can the relationship between the prescribing physician and the patient be improved so that it results in a bond that is maximally satisfying for both parties? This relationship is a complicated one because it is dynamic, reciprocal, and constantly evolving (Kaplan et al., 1989). The patient–physician relationship has been extensively examined and discussed. Interesting contradictions have been observed. The patient may desire to tell a physician about a particular problem, but the physician feels he or she is too busy to really listen to the patient (Baron, 1985). The patient comes seeking advice and guidance, but the physician does not ask about or ignores patient preferences in making difficult choices between therapeutic options. The problem has been blamed by some on high technology and the science of modern medicine, but others have pointed out that the apparent dichotomy between science and humanism in medicine is false. An inclusive scientific model for medicine must acknowledge the science of the human domain as well (Engel, 1987). Other factors modulate the patient–physician relationship; for example, the current pattern of physician remuneration tends to reward doing things to rather than talking with and thinking about patients (Almy, 1980).

Patient–Physician Communication Can Affect the Choice of Therapy and Its Outcome. There is a relationship between the way in which patients and physicians behave and communicate during an office visit, and the patients' subsequent health status (Greenfield et al., 1985; Kaplan et al., 1989). One of the largest problems is noncompliance with recommended therapy which, in various studies, has ranged from 10% to 95% (Bond, 1990). Even if the physician takes time to educate his patient about medications, perhaps 50% of the statements made about the medication are quickly forgotten by the patient (Bond, 1990). Results of patient noncompliance can range from minor to severe. For example, one study found that patients who had recently stopped using a β-adrenergic antagonist had a transient, fourfold increase in the relative risk of angina and myocardial infarction (Psaty et al., 1990). Compliance can be very low even when patients have potentially curable malignant disease (Levine et al., 1987; chapter 23).

Recent work suggests that patient compliance, and even outcomes of chronic disease, are positively correlated with certain types of physician-patient communication (Kaplan et al., 1989). After analyzing communication patterns during office visits (based on three broad categories of control, communication, and affect), these researchers found that better patient health status was positively related to more patient and less physician control, more affect (positive or negative) expressed by physician and patient, and more information provided by the physician in response to questions from patients. An intact

and dynamic patient–physician bond is necessary for the physician to have the greatest chance of making an accurate diagnosis. The patient and physician should jointly select an optimal therapeutic plan. When the patient or physician does not uphold his or her end of the relationship, mistakes can be costly.

Attention to Rational Therapeutics. All physicians want an optimal outcome for their patients. However, to achieve this goal the physician must master the facts, skills, and attitudes that make up the core of clinical pharmacology. Although our undergraduate and postgraduate medical curricula tend to emphasize the importance of diagnostic skills and knowledge over those related to therapeutics, the risk of such an unbalanced approach is now clear. A core curriculum of facts, skills, and attitudes has been mentioned in this chapter. This condensation of clinical pharmacology is expanded in subsequent chapters.

Summary Principle: Appropriate therapeutic choices are not simple, but they can appear to be. Guidelines are available to treat almost everything; the resilience of human physiology frequently makes up for pharmacologic overkill, and when it doesn't, drug-induced complications can mimic and therefore be attributed to disease-induced problems. When therapy fails, we frequently can attribute the failure to the disease and escape blame. Probably nowhere else in professional life are mistakes so easily hidden, even from ourselves. But there is another side to the story. The rewards for appropriate therapeutic decisions, no matter how time-consuming and how expendable others will tell you such tinkering is, can be the biggest ones in medicine. Consider preventing a stroke, relieving pain, curing pneumonia, compensating for threatening imbalances in electrolytes, managing a seizure, relieving depression, curing leukemia, or preventing blindness. These therapeutic acts require unusual skill and time, but they are the essence of why many have entered medicine. These accomplishments do not come from simply following guidelines. They come from individualization of a therapeutic plan that is based on the physician's mastery of the core facts, skills, and attitudes of the discipline of clinical pharmacology.

REFERENCES

Alldredge, B. K.; Lowenstein, D. H.; and Simon, R.: Placebo-controlled trial of intravenous diphenylhydantoin for short-term treatment of alcohol withdrawal seizures. Am. J. Med., 87:645–648, 1989.
Almy, T. P.: The healing bond: Doctor and patient in an era of scientific medicine. Am. J. Gastroenterol., 73:403–407, 1980.
Anglo-American Workshop on Clinical Pharmacology: Clin. Pharmacol. Ther., 39:435–480, 1986.
Assem, E. S. K.: Drug Allergy. In, Textbook of Adverse Drug Reactions, 3rd ed. (Davies, D. M., ed.). Oxford University Press, New York, pp. 611–633, 1985.

Avorn, J.; and Soumerai, S. B.: Improving drug-therapy decisions through educational outreach. N. Engl. J. Med., 308: 1457–1463, 1983.

Avorn, J.; Chen, M.; and Hartley, R.: Scientific versus commercial sources of influence on the prescribing behavior of physicians. Am. J. Med., 73:4–8, 1982.

Avorn, J.; Dreyer, P.; Connelly, K.; and Soumerai, S. B.: Use of psychoactive medication and the quality of care in rest homes. N. Engl. J. Med., 320:227–232, 1989.

Babington, M. A.; Robinson, L. A.; and Monson, R. A.: Effect of written information on physicians' knowledge of drug prices. South. Med. J., 76:328–331, 1983.

Baron, R. J.: An introduction to medical phenomenology: I can't hear you while I'm listening. Ann. Int. Med., 103:606–611, 1985.

Beers, M. H.; and Ouslander, J. G.: Risk factors in geriatric drug prescribing: A practical guide to avoiding problems. Drugs, 37:105–112, 1989.

Beers, M. H.; Storrie, M.; and Lee, G.: Potential adverse drug interactions in the emergency room: An issue in the quality of care. Ann. Int. Med., 112:61–64, 1990.

Bender, B. S.; and Caranasos, G. J. (eds): Geriatric medicine: A problem-oriented approach. Med. Clin. North. Am., 73: (6), 1989.

Bennett, W. M.; Aronoff, G. F.; Golper, T. A.; Morrison, G.; Singer, I.; and Brater, D. C.: Drug Prescribing in Renal Failure. American College of Physicians, Philadelphia, 1987.

Berkowitz, R. L.; Coustan, D. R.; and Mochizuki, T. K.: Handbook for Prescribing Medications during Pregnancy, 2nd ed. Little Brown, Boston, 1986.

Bern, M. M.; Lokich, J. J.; Wallach, S. R.; Bothe, A.; Benotti, P. N.; Arkin, C. F.; Greco, F. A.; Huberman, M.; and Moore, C.: Very low doses of warfarin can prevent thrombosis in central venous catheters. Ann. Int. Med., 112:423–428, 1990.

Blaschke, T. F.; Meffin, P. J.; Melmon, K. L.; and Rowland, M.: Influence of acute viral hepatitis on phenytoin kinetics and protein binding. Clin. Pharmacol. Ther., 17:685–691, 1975.

Bond, W. S.: Medication noncompliance. Drug Newsletter, 9: 33–35, 1990.

Braude, M. C.; Szeto, H. H.; Kuhn, C. M.; Bero, L.; Ignar, D.; Field, E.; Lurie, S.; Chasnoff, I. J.; Mendelson, J. H.; Zuckerman, B.; Hingson, R.; Frank, D.; Parker, S.; Vinci, R.; Kayne, H.; Morelock, S.; Amaro, H.; Kyei-Aboage, K.; and Howard, J.: Perinatal effects of drugs of abuse. Fed. Proc., 46:2446–2453, 1987.

Briggs, G. G.; Bodendorfer, T. W.; Freeman, R. K.; and Yaffe, S. J.: Drugs in Pregnancy and Lactation, 2nd ed. Williams & Wilkins, Baltimore, 1986.

Burnham, J. F.: Medical practice à la mode: How medical fashions determine medical care. N. Engl. J. Med., 317:1220–1222, 1987.

Chang, H. J.; Bell, J. R.; Deroo, D. B.; Kirk, J. W.; and Wasson, J. H.: Physician variation in anticoagulating patients with atrial fibrillation. Arch. Int. Med., 150:81–84, 1990.

Chen, M.; Landefeld, C. S.; and Murray, T. H.: Doctors, drug companies, and gifts. J.A.M.A., 262:3448–3451, 1989.

Cluff, L. E.: The prescribing habits of physicians. Hosp. Practice, 101–104, 1967.

Cockerill, F. R.; Wilson, W. R.; Carpenter, H. A.; Smith, T. F.; and Rosenow, E. C.: Open lung biopsy in immunocompromised patients. Arch. Intern. Med., 145:1398–1404, 1985.

Condemi, J. J.: Allergy to penicillin and other antibiotics. In, A Practical Approach to Infectious Diseases, 2nd ed. (Reese, R. E.; and Douglas, R. G.; eds). Little Brown, Boston, pp. 680–697, 1986.

Engel, G. L.: Physician-scientists and scientific physicians: Resolving the humanism-science dichotomy. Am. J. Med., 82: 107–111, 1987.

Everitt, D. E.; and Avorn, J.: Drug prescribing for the elderly. Arch. Int. Med., 146:2393–2396, 1986.

Farwell, J. R.; Lee, Y. J.; Hirtz, D. G.; Sulzbacher, S. I.; Ellenberg, J. H.; and Nelson, K. B.: Phenobarbital for febrile seizures—Effects on intelligence and on seizure recurrence. N. Engl. J. Med., 322:364–369, 1990.

Gelenberg, A. J.; Kane, J. M.; Keller, M. B.; Lavori, P.; Rosenbaum, J. F.; Cole, K.; and Lavelle, J.: Comparison of standard and low serum levels of lithium for maintenance treatment of biopolar disorder. N. Engl. J. Med., 321:1489–93, 1989.

Goldfinger, S. E.: Physicians and the pharmaceutical industry. Ann. Int. Med., 112:624–626, 1990.

Greenblatt, D. J.; Ehrenberg, B. L.; Gunderman, J. S.; Locniskar, A.; Scavone, J. M.; Harmatz, J. S.; and Shader, R. I.: Pharmacokinetic and electroencephalographic study of intravenous diazepam, midazolam, and placebo. Clin. Pharmacol. Ther., 45:356–365, 1989.

Greenfield, S.; Kaplan, S.; and Ware, J. E.: Expanding patient involvement in care: Effects on patient outcomes. Ann. Int. Med., 102:520–528, 1985.

Greenman, R. L.; Goodall, P. T.; and King, D.: Lung biopsy in immunocompromised hosts. Am. J. Med., 59:488–496, 1975.

Gronert, G. A.; Mott, J.; and Lee, J.: Aetiology of malignant hyperthermia. Br. J. Anaesth., 60:253–267, 1988.

Hansten, P. D.: Drug Interactions, 5th ed., Lea & Febiger, Philadelphia, 1985.

Healy, B.; Campeau, L.; Gray, R.; Herd, J. A.; Hoogwerf, B.; Hunninghake, D.; Knatterud, G.; Stewart, W.; and White, C.: Conflict of interest guidelines for a multicenter clinical trial of treatment after coronary-artery bypass-graft surgery. N. Engl. J. Med., 320:949–951, 1989.

Herxheimer, A.: Basic information that prescribers are not getting about drugs. Lancet, 1:31–32, 1987.

Hull, R.; Hirsh, J.; Jay, R.; Carter, C.; England, C.; Gent, M.; Turpie, A. G. G.; McLoughlin, D.; Dodd, P.; Thomas, M.; Raskob, G.; and Ockelford, P.: Different intensities of oral anticoagulant therapy in the treatment of proximal-vein thrombosis. New Engl. J. Med., 307:1676–1681, 1982.

Kaplan, S. H.; Greenfield, S.; and Ware, J. E.: Assessing the effects of physician-patient interactions on the outcomes of chronic disease. Med. Care, 27:S110–S127, 1989.

Karch, F. E.; and Lasagna, L.: Adverse Drug Reactions in the United States. Medicine in the Public Interest, Washington, D.C., 1975a.

Karch, F. E.; and Lasagna, L.: Adverse drug reactions. J.A.M.A., 234:1236–1241, 1975b.

Kase, C. S.; O'Neal, A. M.; Fisher, M.; Girgis, G. N.; and Ordia, J. I.: Intracranial hemorrhage after use of tissue plasminogen activator for coronary thrombolysis. Ann. Int. Med., 112:17–21, 1990.

Kim, J. H.; and Gallis, H. A.: Observations on spiraling empiricism: Its causes, allure, and perils, with particular reference to antibiotic therapy. Am. J. Med., 87:201–206, 1989.

Klotz, U.; Avant, G. R.; Hoyumpa, A.; Schenker, S.; and Wilkenson, G. R.: The effects of age and liver disease on the disposition and elimination of diazepam in adult man. J. Clin. Invest., 55:347–359, 1975.

Klotz, U.; McHorse, T. W.; Wilkenson, G. R.; and Schenker, S.: The effect of cirrhosis on the disposition and elimination of meperidine (pethidine) in man. Clin. Pharmacol. Ther., 16:667–675, 1974.

Koch-Weser, J.: Serum drug concentrations as therapeutic guides. N. Engl. J. Med., 287:227–31, 1972.

Koch-Weser, J.; Sidel, V. W.; Sweet, R. H.; Kanarek, P.; and Eaton, A. E.: Factors determining physician reporting of adverse drug reactions. N. Engl. J. Med., 280:20–26, 1969.

Kroenke, K.: Polypharmacy: Causes, consequences, and cure. Am. J. Med., 79:149–152, 1985.

Kusserow, R. P.: Medicare Drug Utilization Review. Document OAI-01-88-00980. Washington, D.C., Office of the Inspector General, 1989.

Lakshmanan, M. C.; Hershey, C. O.; and Breslau, D.: Hospital admissions caused by iatrogenic disease. Arch. Int. Med., 146:1931–1934, 1986.

Lamy, P. P.: The elderly and drug interactions. J. Am. Geriatr. Soc., 34:586–592, 1986.

Lennard, L.; Van Loon, J. A.; and Weinshilboum, R. M.: Pharmacogenetics of acute azathioprine toxicity: Relationship to thiopurine methyltransferase genetic polymorphism. Clin. Pharmacol. Ther., 46, 149–154, 1989.

Levine, A. M.; Richardson, J. L.; Marks, G.; Chan, K.; Graham, J.; Selser, J. N.; Kishbaugh, C.; Shelton, D. R.; and Johnson, C. A.: Compliance with oral drug therapy in patients with hematologic malignancy. J. Clin. Oncol., 5: 1469–1476, 1987.

Mackowiak, P. A.; and LeMaistre, C. F.: Drug fever: A critical appraisal of conventional concepts. Ann. Int. Med., 106:728–733, 1987.

Manasse, H. R.: Medication use in an imperfect world: Drug misuse of public policy. Am. J. Hosp. Pharmacy, 46:929–944, 1141–1152, 1989.

Masur, H.; Shelhamer, J.; and Parrillo, J. E.: The management of pneumonias in immunocompromised patients. J.A.M.A., 253:1769–1773, 1985.

Melmon, K. L.: Will the sighted physician see? Pharos, 47:2–6, 1984.

Melmon, K. L.; and Morrelli, H. F.: The need to test the efficacy of the instructional aspects of clinical pharmacology. Clin. Pharmacol. Ther., 10:431–435, 1969.

Melmon, K. L.; and Nierenberg, D. W.: Drug interactions and the prepared observer. N. Engl. J. Med., 304:723–725, 1981.

Meyer, B. R.: Improving medical education in therapeutics. Ann. Int. Med., 108:145–147, 1988.

Mollman, J. E.: Cisplatin neurotoxicity. N. Engl. J. Med., 322: 126–127, 1990.

Montamat, S. C.; Cusack, B. J.; and Vestal, R. E.: Management of drug therapy in the elderly. N. Engl. J. Med., 321: 303–310, 1989.

Moss, F. M.; and McNicol, M. W.: Audits of antibiotic prescribing. Br. Med. J., 286:1513, 1983.

Murray, M. D.; and Brater, D. C.: Adverse effects of nonsteroidal anti-inflammatory drugs on renal function. Ann. Int. Med., 112:559–560, 1990.

Nierenberg, D. W.: Clinical pharmacology instruction for all medical students. Clin. Pharmacol. Ther., 40:483–487, 1986.

O'Hanley, P.; Easaw, J.; Rugo, H.; and Easaw, S.: Infectious disease management of adult leukemic patients undergoing chemotherapy: 1982–1986 experience at Stanford University Hospital. Am. J. Med., 87:605–13, 1989.

Ohnishi, A.; Tsuboi, Y.; Ishizaki, T.; Kubota, K.; Ohno, T.; Yoshida, H.; Kanezaki, A.; and Tanaka, T.: Kinetics and dynamics of enalapril in patients with liver cirrhosis. Clin. Pharmacol. Ther., 45:657–665, 1989.

Osborne, O. T.: The therapeutic art. Trans. Am. Ther. Soc., 13–16, 1905.

Osborne, O. T.: What therapy means. Trans. Am. Ther. Soc., 43–46, 1916.

Paladino, J. A.; Kapfer, J. A.; and DiBona, J. R.: Bedside estimation of creatinine clearance: Which method is most accurate while least complex. Hosp. Form., 21:709–715, 1986.

Parker, C. W.: Drug allergy. N. Engl. J. Med., 511–514, 732–736, 957–960, 1975.

Perrin, J. M.; Homer, C. J.; Berwick, D. M.; Woolf, A. D.; Freeman, J. L.; and Wennberg, J. E.: Variations in rates of hospitalization of children in three urban communities. N. Engl. J. Med., 320:1183–1187, 1989.

Peters, N. L.: Snipping the thread of life. Arch. Int. Med., 149: 2414–2420, 1989.

Psaty, B. M.; Koepsell, T. D.; Wagner, E. H.; LoGerfo, J. P.; and Inui, T. S.: The relative risk of incident coronary heart disease associated with recently stopping the use of beta-blockers. J.A.M.A., 263:1653, 1990.

Public Citizen Health Research Group: Worst Pills, Best Pills. Washington, D.C., p. 7, 1988.

Rawlins, M. D.: Doctors and the drug makers. Lancet, 2:276–278, 1984.

Ray, W. A.; Griffin, M. R.; Schaffner, W.; Baugh, D. K.; and Melton, L. J.: Psychotropic drug use and the risk of hip fracture. N. Engl. J. Med., 316:363–369, 1987.

Relman, A. S.: Doctors and the dispensing of drugs. N. Engl. J. Med., 317:311–312, 1987.

Rieder, M. J.; Uetrecht, J.; Shear, N. H.; Cannon, M.; Miller, M.; and Spielberg, S. P.: Diagnosis of sulfonamide hypersensitivity reactions by in-vitro "rechallenge" with hydroxylamine metabolites. Ann. Int. Med., 110:286–289, 1989.

Roberts, R. J.: Drug Therapy in Infants. W B Saunders, Philadelphia, 1984.

Rogers, A. S.; Israel, E.; Smith, C. R.; Levine, D.; McBean, A. M.; Valente, C.; and Faich, G.: Physician knowledge, attitudes, and behavior related to reporting adverse drug events. Arch. Intern. Med., 148:1596–1600, 1988.

Royal College of Physicians: The relationship between physicians and the pharmaceutical industry. J. R. Coll. Physicians, 20:235–242, 1986.

Rubin, M.; Hathorn, J. W.; and Pizzo, P. A.: Controversies in the management of febrile neutropenic cancer patients. Cancer Invest., 6:167–184, 1988.

Saour, J. N.; Sieck, J. O.; Mamo, L. A. R.; and Gallus, A. S.: Trial of different intensities of anticoagulation in patients with prosthetic heart valves. N. Engl. J. Med., 322:428–432, 1990.

Saxon, A.; Beall, G. N.; Rohr, A. S.; and Adelman, D. C.: Immediate hypersensitivity reactions to beta-lactam antibiotics. Urology, 31(Suppl):14–27, 1988.

Schaffner, W.; Ray, W. A.; Federspiel, C. F.; and Miller, W. O.: Improving antibiotic prescribing in office practice. J.A.M.A., 250:1728–1732, 1983.

Silverman, M.; and Lee, P. R.: Pills, profits, and politics. University of California Press, Berkeley, pp. 54–57, 1974.

Skolnick, J. L.; Stoler, B. S.; Katz, D. B.; and Anderson, W. H.: Rifampin, oral contraceptives, and pregnancy. J.A.M.A., 236:1382, 1976.

Soumerai, S.; and Avorn, J.: Principles of educational outreach ("academic detailing") to improve clinical decision making. J.A.M.A., 263:549–556, 1990.

Soumerai, S. B.; Avorn, J.; Ross-Degnan, D.; and Gortmaker, S.: Payment restrictions for prescription drugs under Medicaid: Effects on therapy, cost, and equity. N. Engl. J. Med., 317:550–556, 1987.

Soumerai, S. T.; Ross-Degnan, D.; Gortmaker, S.; and Avorn, J.: Withdrawing payment for nonscientific drug therapy: Intended and unexpected effects of a large-scale natural experiment. J.A.M.A., 263:831–839, 1990.

Stanulovic, M.; Jakovljevic, V.; and Roncevic, N.: Drug utilization in paediatrics: Non-medical factors affecting decision making by prescribers. Eur. J. Clin. Pharmacol., 27:237–241, 1984.

Stewart, R. B.; and Caranasos, G. J.: Medication compliance in the elderly. Med. Clin. North. Am., 73:1551–1564, 1989.

Stover, D. E.; Zaman, M. B.; Hajdu, S. I.; Lange, M.; Gold, J.; and Armstrong, D.: Bronchoavolar lavage in the diagnosis of diffuse pulmonary infiltrates in the immunosuppressed host. Ann. Int. Med., 101:j1–j7, 1984.

Tatro, D. S.: Drug Interaction Facts. J B Lippincott, St. Louis, 1990.

Thomson, P. D.; Melmon, K. L.; Richardson, J. A.; Cohn, K.; Steinbrunn, W.; Cudihee, R.; and Rowland, M.: Lidocaine pharmacokinetics in advanced heart failure, liver disease, and renal failure in humans. Ann. Intern. Med., 78:499–508, 1973.

Tugwell, P.; Bombardier, C.; Buchanan, W. W.; Goldsmith, C.; Grace, E.; Bennett, K. J.; Williams, H. J.; Egger, M.; Alarcon, G. S.; Guttadauria, M.; Yarboro, C.; Polisson, R. P.; Szydlo, L; Luggen, M. E.; Billingsley, L. M.; Ward, J. R.; and Marks, C.: Methotrexate in rheumatoid arthritis: Impact on quality of life assessed by traditional standard-item and individualized patient preference health status questionnaires. Arch. Int. Med., 150:59–62, 1990.

VanArsdel, P. P.; and Larson, E. B.: Diagnostic tests for patients with suspected allergic disease: Utility and limitations. Ann. Int. Med., 110:304–312, 1989.

Wall Street Journal. May 25, pp. 31, 49, 1984.

Walson, P. D.; Hammel, M.; and Martin, R.: Prescription-writing by pediatric house officers. J. Med. Educ., 56:423–428, 1981.

Weber, M. L.; Auger, C.; and Cleroux, R.: Knowledge of medical students, pediatric residents, and pediatricians about the cost of some medications. Pediatr. Pharmacol., 5:281–285, 1986.

Weiss, M. E.; Nyhan, D.; Peng, Z; Horrow, J. C.; Lowenstein, E.; Hirshman, C.; and Adkinson, N. F.: Association of protamine IgE and IgG antibodies with life-threatening reactions to intravenous protamine. N. Engl. J. Med., 320:886–892, 1989.

Wennberg, J.; and Gittelsohn, A.: Variations in medical care among small areas. Sci. Am., 246:120–134, 1982.

Whelton, A.; Stout, R. L.; Spilman, P. S.; and Klassen, D. K.: Renal effects of ibuprofen, piroxicam, and sulindac in patients with asymptomatic renal failure. Ann. Int. Med., 112: 568–576, 1990.

Wilcox, R. W.: The teaching of therapeutics. Trans. Am. Ther. Soc., 25–34, 1903.

Wilkes, M. S.; and Shuchman, M.: Pitching doctors. New York Times Magazine, November 5, pp. 88–89, 126–129, 1989.

2

Treatment of Cardiovascular Disorders: Hypertension

Jack Onrot and Robert E. Rangno

Chapter Outline

Therapeutic Rationale for Hypertension
  Definition and Epidemiology
  Risks versus Benefits of Therapy
  Diagnosis
  Pathophysiology
Antihypertensive Drugs
  Diuretics
  Drugs that Inhibit the Effects of the
    Adrenergic Nervous System

Peripherally Acting Agents
Guidelines for Management of the
  Hypertensive Patient
  Clinical Assessment
  Physical Examination
  Investigations
  Treatment
  Special Settings Requiring Consideration
    for Antihypertensive Therapy

THERAPEUTIC RATIONALE FOR HYPERTENSION

This chapter attempts to clarify the following issues:

1. What is hypertension and how does it happen?
2. Why do we treat hypertension?
3. Whom do we treat for hypertension?
4. How do we treat hypertension?
5. What drugs are used, under what circumstances, and what are the expected benefits and risks from these drugs?

The treatment of hypertension is ever changing and covers many disciplines of medicine. Because of the profusion of new drugs available, the practitioner will have to keep abreast of developments in order to be optimally effective. This chapter provides an appropriate foundation for therapy based on sound principles of clinical pharmacology.

Definition and Epidemiology

Hypertension is the most common cardiovascular disorder in North America, affecting more than 1 in 10 persons (Rowland and Roberts, 1982). Hypertension is important because elevated blood pressure confers a greater risk of stroke, heart failure, renal disease, peripheral vascular disease, and coronary artery disease including myocardial infarction and sudden death (Kannel, 1974). There is a continuous, direct relationship between blood pressure and these risks.

Therefore, definitions based on values of pressure are arbitrary. However, these arbitrary values allow us to quantify the potential risks of complications of hypertension and to assess the benefits of therapy in large populations and individuals. The World Health Organization (WHO) defines diastolic hypertension as borderline if it is greater than 90 mm Hg and definite if it is greater than 95 mm Hg. Systolic hypertension is considered to be borderline if it is greater than 140 mm Hg and definite if greater than 160 mm Hg (World Health Organization, 1978). Table 2-1 further subdivides hypertension based on values of pressure. *Principle: The ultimate goal of therapy in a hypertensive patient is to prevent cardiovascular complications with little adverse drug effects on the quality of life. Therefore it is crucial to "treat the patient, not just the blood pressure."*

Lowering blood pressure with pharmacologic agents is just one way to prevent complications. Attention also must be paid to the presence and reversal of other associated risks such as smoking,

Table 2-1. CLASSIFICATION OF HYPERTENSION BASED ON BLOOD PRESSURE*

	SYSTOLIC (MM HG)	DIASTOLIC (MM HG)
Borderline	140–159	90–94
Mild	160–179	95–104
Moderate	180–219	105–114
Severe	>220	>115

* Isolated systolic hypertension is defined as systolic BP > 160 *and* diastolic BP < 95.

Table 2–2. METHODS OF REDUCING CARDIOVASCULAR RISK

LOWER BLOOD PRESSURE	ADDRESS OTHER FACTORS
• Use antihypertensive drugs.	• Stop smoking.
• Restrict sodium.	• Control diabetes.
• Lose weight.	• Lose weight.
• Reduce alcohol intake.	• Lower LDL cholesterol concentrations.
• Exercise.	• Raise HDL cholesterol concentrations.
• Eat high-potassium diet.*	
• Eat high-calcium diet.*	
• Eat high-fiber diet.*	
• Restrict intake of simple carbohydrates.*	
• Use biofeedback, meditation, yoga, etc.*	

* Antihypertensive effects remain unproved and/or are limited.

lipid disorders and diabetes (Table 2–2), since the coexistence of these risk factors greatly increases the likelihood of cardiovascular complications caused by hypertension (Kannel et al., 1979).

Risks versus Benefits of Therapy

Hypertension itself usually is asymptomatic, yet therapy (especially with drugs) may have adverse effects. Several considerations may temper one's enthusiasm for starting drug therapy, especially to treat mild hypertension.

The Veterans Administration Study and others have shown clear benefits from drug therapy in patients with moderate to severe hypertension (Veterans Administration Cooperative Study Group, 1970). However, studies of drug treatment of uncomplicated, mild hypertension are less compelling. Some have shown small but statistically significant reductions in some cardiovascular complications (Hypertension Detection and Follow-Up Program, 1979; Australian Therapeutic Trial, 1980; Medical Research Council Working Party, 1985). Others have failed to show any benefits at all (Helgeland, 1980; Multiple Risk Factor Intervention Trial, 1982). Close examination of these studies allows the practitioner to make decisions based on risk–benefit analyses. Both the Australian and British Medical Research Council (MRC) studies have shown impressive 20% to 45% reductions in complicating events when patients were taking active drug. But the baseline incidence of events in the placebo groups was small, and therefore the absolute number of events prevented also was small. Looking at these data another way, large numbers of patients will have to be treated and tolerate the morbidity of drug therapy over long periods to prevent one morbid event caused by hypertension (Anonymous, 1985; Laupacis et al., 1988). Lower risk

groups are less likely to benefit from therapy. Furthermore although drug therapy of moderate and severe hypertension has been conclusively shown to reduce strokes and heart failure, most studies have failed to show a reduction in the raised incidence of myocardial infarction seen in hypertensive patients (Cutler et al., 1989).

Blood pressure, like other physiologic parameters, varies with time. Blood pressures usually are higher in the clinic than at home and higher when measured by physicians than by nurses (white-coat effect) (Mancia et al., 1983). Blood pressure usually is lower at second or subsequent visits than first visits presumably because the patient becomes more accustomed to the clinic setting and because of the phenomenon of *regression to the mean*. Thus, the patient should be assessed with three supine pressures at three successive visits in order to establish a representative baseline. Despite this preparation for therapy, many patients may become normotensive over long periods without therapy. A disquieting feature of the Australian study was that the pressure normalized over 1 to 2 years in 45% of the placebo group initially diagnosed as "mild (treatable) hypertensives" (Australian Therapeutic Trial, 1982). Labeling a patient *hypertensive* may itself have adverse consequences and lead to increased frequency of somatic complaints and absenteeism from work (Haynes et al., 1978).

Knowledge of the risks of cardiovascular complications at varying levels of blood pressure and the results of clinical drug trials, coupled with the implications of misdiagnosis and labeling, allows a rational risk–benefit analysis to be applied to most patients before institution of drug therapy. The WHO consensus recommendations are reliable and solid and similar to North American recommendations (Logan, 1984; WHO/ISH Meeting Memorandum, 1986). Except in patients with severe hypertension (diastolic blood pressure, BP, equal to or greater than 115 mm Hg), there usually is no rush to treat since the goals for treating are prevention of slowly accruing complications. The severe hypertensive patient, however, is at risk for short-term pressure-related complications. Drug treatment in such patients should probably be instituted promptly after verification of the abnormal blood pressures.

The first step in treating mild-to-moderate hypertensive patients can be to institute proven nonpharmacologic therapies (weight loss, sodium restriction, curtailment of alcohol intake, etc.) for 3 to 6 months. If diastolic pressures then remain above 95 mm Hg, drug therapy can be instituted. This conservative approach will avoid overtreatment of patients in whom benefits from drug therapy are controversial. ***Principle: Discovering a disease does not always justify pharmacologic*** *treatment even when treatment has been proved efficacious.*

Diagnosis

Since the benefits of drug therapy in mild hypertensive patients are limited and the risks and the costs are shared by all those treated, one should carefully measure blood pressures to avoid overdiagnosis and overtreatment. *Principle: Proper therapy begins with proper diagnosis.*

Mercury sphygmomanometers should be used in preference to aneroids. The latter should be used only if they are standardized against the mercury manometer. The appropriate cuff size is based on arm size. For instance, blood pressures in obese hypertensive patients with arm size greater than 33-cm circumference may be overestimated by approximately 10 mm Hg systolic and/or diastolic if a standard-sized cuff is used. When in doubt, the large cuff usually is more appropriate. The cuff should be inflated and systolic pressure first checked by palpation to avoid misinterpreting a patient with an auscultatory gap (Joint National Committee, 1988). Use of phase V Korotkoff sounds (disappearance), if detectable, is preferable to use of phase IV muffling in assigning a diastolic pressure.

The recent availability of 24-hour noninvasive ambulatory blood-pressure-monitoring devices can aid in diagnosis, particularly if office measurements are borderline or the patient shows signs of labile blood pressure (Pickering et al., 1985). Ambulatory blood pressures may be better predictors of cardiovascular risk than clinic pressures (Perloff et al., 1983). Simple home blood pressure devices also can be very useful (Kleinert et al., 1984).

Pathophysiology

Systemic Hemodynamics. "Essential" hypertension was initially so named because clinicians at the time thought that higher levels of pressure were "essential" for adequate tissue perfusion, presumably because of blood vessel narrowing, in certain patients. While the foundation for the term is now viewed as ironically incorrect, its use persists. The cause of essential (or, more appropriately termed, *primary*) hypertension remains elusive, and many different regulatory systems likely contribute. A relatively small number of patients have hypertension due to a known cause, such as pheochromocytoma or renal artery sterosis.

Knowledge of basic hemodynamics provides a rationale for understanding hypertension and its therapy. Blood pressure (BP) is the product of cardiac output (CO) and systemic vascular resistance (SVR) (BP = CO × SVR). Thus, eleva-

tions in either cardiac output or peripheral resistance can produce hypertension (Fig. 2-1). Cardiac output can increase as a function of increased myocardial contractility, heart rate, or venous return. Venous return is a function of the total blood volume (regulated by the kidney) and the percentage of blood volume circulating centrally (regulated by venous tone). Arteriolar smooth muscle tone is the major determinant of systemic vascular resistance. This tone ultimately is proportional to the intracellular free Ca^{2+} concentration that regulates the actin–myosin interactions that in turn determine smooth muscle contraction (Onrot, 1987).

Since early in the course of hypertension there is frequently a high cardiac output and normal peripheral resistance, elevation in cardiac output may be the initial hemodynamic alteration in primary hypertension. When cardiac output increases, autoregulation ensues to maintain blood flow to tissues constant. The increased flow from increased cardiac output is therefore countered by vasoconstriction. This is "functional" autoregulation. As well, however, the vessel wall can hypertrophy slowly in response to increased flow (structural autoregulation). The thickened arteriolar walls will cause disproportionate luminal narrowing for any given constrictor stimulus and "bioamplify" the tendency to hypertension (Folkow, 1984). This concept has therapeutic implications since as pressure is controlled, structural changes may slowly regress, and with increasing length of therapy, lesser degrees of antihypertensive therapy may suffice for maintenance of the reduction in pressure. Theoretically, this concept justifies attempts to decrease or withdraw therapy once pressure has been normalized with drugs for some time.

The Kidney. The kidney can contribute in many ways to control of blood pressure (see chapter 11). Renin released from renal juxtaglomerular cells activates the renin-angiotensin-aldosterone axis. Renal prostaglandins and renomedullary lipids are vasodilators. However, the paramount role of the kidney is regulation of blood volume. When blood pressure rises for any reason, the kidney can adjust; it can excrete more sodium and lower blood volume and hence can reduce cardiac output and restore pressure to normal. Thus, theoretically, blood pressure can always be normalized as long as the kidneys are functioning normally. Guyton (1989) has hypothesized that for hypertension to exist there has to be a defect in the ability of the kidney to excrete sodium appropriately. For any given rise in blood pressure, the abnormal "hypertensive" kidney will excrete less sodium than a normal kidney would, thereby permitting hypertension (Guyton, 1989).

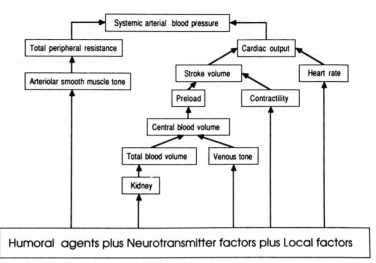

Fig. 2–1. Hemodynamics of blood pressure control (reprinted from Onrot and Ruedy, 1987, with permission).

Transplantation experiments have provided evidence for this hypothesis. Transplanting a kidney from a normotensive to a nephrectomized hypertensive rat normalizes blood pressure, whereas transplantation of a hypertensive rat's kidney into a normotensive control can cause hypertension (Dahl and Heine, 1975).

The Sympathetic Nervous System. The sympathetic nervous system can influence both cardiac output and peripheral resistance. Blood pressure is monitored by arterial baroreceptors with messages transmitted to the brainstem. Here the information is processed and coordinated with information from higher levels in the brain. Brainstem control centers then determine sympathetic efferent tone. Sympathetic nerves travel down the brainstem and through the spinal cord and leave the cord as *preganglionic* neurons. These nerves synapse at sympathetic ganglia, releasing acetylcholine as the neurotransmitter that activates postganglionic neurons. These nerves affect target organs throughout the body, where they release norepinephrine (noradrenaline) and activate adrenergic receptors.

Noradrenergic postganglionic neurons are found in the heart, where they increase contractility and heart rate; in the veins, where they increase tone; and in the kidneys, where they promote retention of salt and water and secretion of renin (Fig. 2–2). Similarly, noradrenergic neurons in the arterioles enhance vasoconstriction. Secretion of renin leads to formation of angiotensin II and further vasoconstriction as well as sodium retention via aldosterone effects (see chapter 11). Elevated sympathetic nervous system activity may result in transient or sustained hypertension.

Other preganglionic nerves synapse in the adrenal medulla and stimulate secretion of epinephrine. Epinephrine then circulates as a hormone exerting direct sympathetic effects on distant tissues. Conceptually, norepinephrine is the sympathetic neurotransmitter and epinephrine is the circulating sympathomimetic hormone.

The catecholamines, norepinephrine and epinephrine, act on adrenergic receptors. These receptors mediate a wide variety of biologic effects. α_1-Adrenergic receptors are located on blood vessels and the heart and when stimulated cause venous and arteriolar constriction and increased inotropy. α_2-Adrenergic receptors are located in the brainstem; when activated, these receptors inhibit sympathetic outflow. Also, presynaptic α_2-adrenergic receptors on postganglionic neurons inhibit release of neurotransmitters. α_2-Adrenergic receptors are also located in the kidney (Na$^+$ retention) and on blood vessels (vasoconstriction). β_1-Adrenergic receptors are located in the heart and the kidney and when stimulated increase heart rate and contractility and secretion of renin. Vasodilator β_2-adrenergic receptors are located on blood vessels. Receptors for catecholamines are also located in other tissues, such as bronchial smooth muscle, that do not contribute to control of blood pressure but are important in terms of the adverse effects of drugs that inhibit the sympathetic nervous system (Table 2–3) (for review, see Motulsky and Insel, 1982; Oates et al., 1983).

A characteristic of essential hypertension is exaggerated vasoconstrictor responses to pressor stimuli. Thus, even normal sympathetic nerve activity may lead to hypertension. Blunted baroreflexes may also contribute to this hyperresponsiveness. For instance, pressure increases normally are sensed by arterial baroreceptors, which transmit impulses to the brainstem leading to a

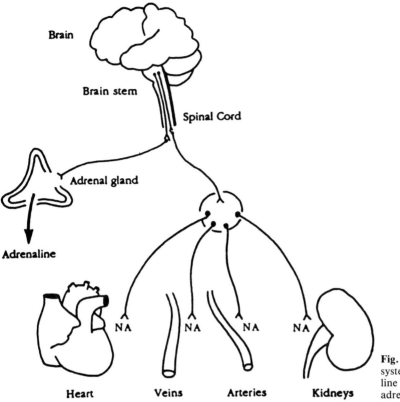

Fig. 2–2. Sympathetic nervous system: efferent limb. Adrenaline = epinephrine; NA = noradrenaline = norepinephrine.

Table 2–3.   SOME ADRENERGIC RECEPTOR FUNCTIONS IN HUMAN TISSUES

	LOCATION	FUNCTION
α_1	Arterioles	Constriction
	Veins	Constriction
	Heart	Inotropy
	Bladder sphincter	Contraction
	Pupil	Mydriasis
	Pilomotor	Contraction
α_2	Arterioles	Constriction
	CNS	Reduction of sympathetic outflow
	Heart	Inotropy
	Presynaptic noradrenergic terminals	Reduction of norepinephrine release
	Platelets	Aggregation
	Adipocytes	Reduction of lipolysis
	Various cells	Opposition to K^+ entry
	Kidney	Na^+ retention
β_1	Heart	Inotropy and chronotropy
	Kidney	Renin release
β_2	Arterioles	Dilation
	Heart	Inotropy and chronotropy
	Islet cells	Insulin release
	Bronchi	Dilation
	Presynaptic noradrenergic terminals	Enhancement of norepinephrine release
	Various cells	K^+ entry
	Uterus	Relaxation
	Leukocytes	Demargination
β_3	Adipocytes	Lipolysis

reduction in sympathetic outflow. This tends to restore pressure to normal. Hypertensive patients can exhibit blunting of this baroreflex. The degree of blunting is proportional to the level of pressure (Goldstein, 1983). However, it is unclear whether blunting of baroreflex responses is a cause of hypertension or an effect of elevated pressures.

Renin-Angiotensin-Aldosterone Axis. Renin is secreted by the kidney in response to a decrease in renal blood flow or delivery of sodium to the kidney for any reason (see chapter 11). Other stimuli to secretion of renin include catecholamines and prostaglandins. Renin then converts renin substrate (angiotensinogen), made by the liver, into angiotensin I, a decapeptide. Angiotensin-converting enzyme (ACE), produced mainly in the lung, then cleaves angiotensin I to angiotensin II, an octapeptide and potent vasoconstrictor. Angiotensin II acts on the zona glomerulosa of the adrenal cortex, causing secretion of aldosterone and hence reabsorption of Na^+ at the distal renal tubule in exchange for H^+ and K^+ that are lost. Activation of the renin system raises blood pressure via enhanced vasoconstriction (angiotensin II) and via increased cardiac output secondary to sodium retention (aldosterone).

A growing body of evidence suggests the presence of local renin-angiotensin systems in other tissues including blood vessels and the brain (Dzau, 1988). Components of this system are either synthesized locally or taken up actively from plasma. For example, prorenin, a precursor of renin, is found in the plasma of nephrectomized animals.

Other Factors. Other mechanisms of blood pressure control include serotonin (van Zwieten, 1987), atrial natriuretic factor (Dietz et al., 1989), neuropeptide Y (Waeber et al., 1988), endothelium-dependent relaxation factor and endothelin (Vane et al., 1990), and factors affecting the sodium-potassium ATP-ase pump (de Wardener and MacGregor, 1983).

ANTIHYPERTENSIVE DRUGS

Diuretics

Pharmacology and Mechanism of Action. The commonly used diuretics include the thiazides, loop diuretics, and aldosterone antagonists (see chapter 11). Diuretics are agents that act upon the kidney to increase urine formation. These agents are also termed *natriuretics* since they increase the excretion of sodium. There is evidence supporting the hypothesis that an inability to excrete appropriate amounts of sodium in the face of hypertension is a factor that contributes to maintenance of elevated blood pressure

(Guyton, 1989). Thus, the rationale for the use of diuretics in hypertensives stems from their ability to augment urinary excretion of sodium. This would of course lead to a decrease in total body sodium, reduce blood volume, and secondarily reduce cardiac output. In additional, improved natriuresis is hypothesized to reduce endogenous secretion of natriuretic factors that are also vasoconstrictor and hence reduce peripheral vascular resistance (de Wardener and MacGregor, 1983).

The first diuretics that were used in clinical practice were mercurial diuretics that are now obsolete. In the 1930s carbonic anhydrase inhibitors (acetazolamide) were synthesized and found to enhance excretion of bicarbonate, sodium, and potassium, resulting in reduction of extracellular fluid volume and metabolic acidosis. These agents are weak diuretics. Experimentation with sulfonamide derivatives led to the discovery of thiazide diuretics in 1950s. These diuretic, natriuretic, and kaliuretic agents act on the cortical diluting segment (Seely and Dirks, 1977). Around 1960 "loop" diuretics (furosemide, ethacrynic acid, bumetanide) were developed. These block the Na^+-K^+-2Cl cotransport system in the ascending limb. Aldosterone antagonists such as spironolactone block the receptors for aldosterone in the distal tubule. This antagonism of aldosterone's actions enhances sodium excretion and reabsorption of potassium and hydrogen. Other potassium-sparing diuretics (triamterene, amiloride) were synthesized in the last 2 decades in order to counteract the distal tubular loss of potassium induced by thiazide and loop diuretics.

Thiazide Diuretics. These are the mainstay of antihypertensive diuretic therapy. Inhibition of sodium reabsorption decreases plasma volume causing reflex increases in renin and aldosterone secretion. This opposes natriuresis by facilitating distal sodium reabsorption in exchange for potassium and hydrogen losses. The decrease in plasma volume causes proximal tubular avidity for salt and water, also limiting natriuresis. The patient then returns to steady state, at a lower extracellular volume. Despite this, blood pressure may continue to fall. Similarly, infusing dextran to restore pretreatment intravascular volumes may not fully return blood pressure to pretreatment levels. Thus, the antihypertensive effects of thiazides are at least partially dissociated from their effects on blood volume. ***Principle: Classification of drugs by their dominant mechanism of action or effects may obscure other useful mechanisms of action and limit understanding of their pharmacology.***

When given orally, thiazide diuretics are absorbed in the intestine with variable bioavailability, are protein-bound, and are excreted in the urine. They act on the luminal side of the tubule after glomerular filtration and/or proximal tubular secretion. Their half lives ($t_{1/2}$) vary, but their antihypertensive effects persist for at least 24 hours, so that all the drugs can be given once daily.

The common agents with equivalent dosages are chlorothiazide 500 mg, hydrochlorothiazide 25 mg, chlorthalidone 25 mg, or bendrofluazide 2.5 mg. Thiazide diuretics, like most other antihypertensive agents, have a steep dose–response curve that plateaus at low doses. Near-maximal antihypertensive effects usually are seen at the doses quoted above. Often, some additional, albeit small, benefit can be gained at double these doses. At higher doses, there is little additional antihypertensive benefit to be gained even though increased diuresis will be seen. The tendency to adverse effects increases markedly at higher doses (Carlsen et al., 1990; see Fig. 2-3). Thus, the risk-benefit of increasing thiazide dosage in the higher ranges becomes increasingly unfavorable.

Clinical Use and Adverse Effects. Thiazides usually are effective when given once daily as monotherapy. They can induce falls in blood pressure of about 25/10 mm Hg in severe hypertension and half that in milder forms (McMahon, 1975). As a group, black patients are more likely to respond to thiazides than white patients. Patients who respond to diuretics are those who would tend to respond to sodium restriction and/or calcium channel blockade (Resnick et al., 1986). In fact, addition of a calcium channel blocker to a diuretic often affords very little increased efficacy, whereas the addition of an ACE inhibitor, α- or β-adrenergic receptor antagonist or direct vasodilator frequently demonstrates additive efficacy (Nicholson et al., 1989). Dietary restriction of sodium may allow a reduction in the dosage of diuretics. This restriction also reduces distal availability of sodium for exchange with hydrogen and potassium and limits the hypokalemic metabolic alkalosis induced by diuretics (for review, see Morgan, 1984).

The multiplicity and frequency of adverse effects of thiazides is well known and used as a reason to curtail their use. However, the adverse effects are dose-dependent and often can be minimized by using appropriate lower doses without compromise of the efficacy of the drug (Carlsen et al., 1990). Patients who are diuresed excessively will experience orthostatic hypotension and fatigue. Exaggerated falls in orthostatic blood pressure, a low jugular venous pressure, and an increase in the blood urea/creatinine ratio suggest overdiuresis. *Principle: Empirical clinical effects of drugs (regardless of their known pharmacology) can be key determinants to dosing and therapeutic index of a drug.*

Diuretics increase plasma triglyceride and low-density lipoprotein (LDL) cholesterol concentrations and lower high-density lipoprotein (HDL) cholesterol concentrations (MacMahon and MacDonald, 1986). Some have suggested that the failure to demonstrate reduction in coronary artery-related mortality in patients taking diuretics stems from the consequences of these effects. Diuretics also can produce glucose intolerance. This effect may partially stem from induction of hypokalemia that causes reduction in insulin secretion. Most likely, the hyperglycemia is a result of peripheral resistance to insulin (Pollare et al., 1989).

Since thiazide diuretics are sulfonamide derivatives, they may cause allergic reactions; particularly skin rashes are common to all the sulfas. Rarely, vasculitis, interstitial nephritis, pancreatitis, and thrombocytopenias have been reported. Impotence is an important adverse effect of thiazide diuretics (Medical Research Council Working Party, 1985).

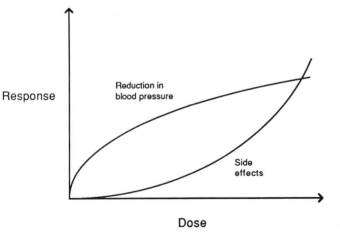

Fig. 2–3. "Plateau" dose–response curve of antihypertensive agents. Schematic representation. For a given dose increment in the higher vs lower dose ranges, a lesser increment in hypertensive effect can be expected. However, adverse effects increase proportionally with dose.

Metabolic complications stem directly from thiazide mechanisms of action. Hypokalemia is the best known. At usual doses, plasma potassium concentrations will fall by less than 0.8 mmol/l and usually remain above 3.4 mmol/l. A potassium concentration below 3 mmol/l in a patient taking diuretics (or less than 3.5 mmol/l when not taking diuretics) should stimulate a search for primary aldosteronism. Some studies have suggested that when thiazide diuretics are taken alone, they may be associated with an increased incidence of sudden death (Multiple Risk Factor Intervention Trial, 1982). This effect has been postulated to be due to a reduction in the plasma potassium concentration that could directly predispose to ventricular arrhythmias and/or sudden death. In addition, if exercise induces shifts of potassium intracellularly, diuretics might predispose to exercise-induced arrhythmias and death. This hypothesis has led to the use of potassium supplementation and/or potassium-sparing diuretics in conjunction with thiazide usage or to the concomitant use of β-adrenergic antagonists with thiazide. It is best to avoid potassium depletion by using a smaller dose of diuretic and/or sodium restriction. Patients with ventricular ectopic activity, or those taking cardiac glycosides or pharmacologic doses of corticosteroids, probably should receive agents to prevent an excessive decrease in the plasma concentration of potassium. ACE inhibitors are particularly useful in this setting since they have additive antihypertensive effect with thiazides and blunt potassium loss. *Principle: Seek drug–drug interactions that not only offer additive efficacy but also decrease the toxicity of one or both drugs.*

Hypomagnesemia results from diuretic-induced enhanced excretion of magnesium. Magnesium depletion predisposes to arrhythmias and muscle weakness and will in itself enhance potassium loss. Metabolic alkalosis is encountered especially during exaggerated volume depletion caused by diuretics. Diuretic-induced hyperuricemia occasionally may be accompanied by gout. While it may be tempting to attribute an episode of gout to the drug-induced hyperuricemia, that change in plasma concentration of uric acid is not accompanied by much of an increase in the total body pool of uric acid. In fact, in some but not all studies the incidence of podagra in patients taking thiazides is no higher than would be predicted by the pretreatment plasma uric acid concentrations. Nonetheless, unless the drug is working exceptionally well, patients with gout should have the thiazide discontinued if podagra occurs. If you wish to continue the use of thiazides, consider using probenecid or allopurinol as you would in other patients with acute gout.

Hyponatremia is a particularly dangerous dose-related side effect of thiazide use. Thiazide-induced hyponatremia is most often seen in the elderly, especially at doses of hydrochlorothiazide 50 mg (or equivalent) or greater. At higher doses of diuretic, potassium-sparing agents can be used to prevent hypokalemia, but correction of the hyponatremia may be overlooked. Increased proximal tubular reabsorption of calcium secondary to decreased plasma volume also will cause enhanced calcium reabsorption. Thiazides can cause frank hypercalcemia (see chapters 11 and 17).

Other Diuretics

The Loop Diuretics. The loop diuretics are more efficacious diuretics than the thiazides. The adverse effects are similar, although the loop diuretics are less likely to induce hypercalcemia or hyponatremia and more likely to induce symptoms of profound hypovolemia. High doses of furosemide may cause hearing loss in patients with renal failure (see chapter 40).

For the treatment of hypertension, thiazides are preferable to loop diuretics. However, when a patient has renal impairment or significant volume overload, the more potent loop diuretics might be needed. Furosemide is used at doses of 20 mg and upward. Patients with renal insufficiency often need higher doses. For a complete discussion of this subject, see chapter 11.

Potassium-Sparing Diuretics. Spironolactone is a competitive blocker of aldosterone at the receptor level. It causes natriuresis with reabsorption of hydrogen and potassium. It is not as useful as thiazides as a first-line antihypertensive but is particularly attractive in treating primary aldosteronism or as an additive to thiazides in order to prevent excessive loss of potassium. Because it is a competitive inhibitor, effective dosages need to be titrated against the stimulus for aldosterone secretion. Spironolactone may cause hyperkalemic metabolic acidosis. Care should be taken in patients with renal insufficiency who already have a predisposition to hyperkalemia or those who are taking potassium supplements or ACE inhibitors. A particular problem with spironolactone in men is gynecomastia and/or breast tenderness. This is dose-related and may occur in up to 30% of men taking the drug. Women may experience reduced libido or menstrual irregularities while taking this drug. GI disturbance may be encountered in both sexes.

Amiloride acts on the collecting tubule to inhibit access of sodium to the transport side independent of aldosterone secretion (see chapter 11). Potassium and hydrogen excretion is reduced, and as with spironolactone, hyperkalemic metabolic acidosis may occur. The drug is not as effective as thiazide in treating hypertension but can be used in conjunction with thiazides to prevent hypokalemia and alkalosis. The same cautions mentioned with spironolactone with respect to hyperkalemia and acidosis apply to amiloride.

Triamterene spares potassium (but less so than spironolactone and amiloride). It has minimal if any antihypertensive effects on its own. Its sole clinical use in this context is to reduce the likelihood and extent of hypokalemia. Triamterene may reduce the bioavailability of thiazides concomitantly administered. It can also cause interstitial nephritis.

Recommendations. Diuretics have been the mainstay of antihypertensive therapy for more than 30 years. They are effective, cheap, and easy to take. Recently, concerns have been raised because of their adverse effects and atherogenic potential. Certain populations (i.e., blacks) are clearly more likely to respond to diuretics, making them first-choice agents in that population (Veterans Administration Cooperative Study Group, 1982).

Diuretics are useful when used in combination with agents that cause salt and water reabsorption. They are still first-line drugs for most hypertension but if possible should be avoided in patients with preexisting glucose intolerance, lipoprotein abnormalities, allergy to sulfa, hypovolemia, hyponatremia, or gout. Because thiazides are relatively ineffective in azotemic states, loop diuretics are preferred in that setting, especially to normalize volume. *Principle: The longer drugs are used, the more useful they become, and the more widespread their use, the more likely that a complete profile on their use and toxicity will become available. Of course, that profile could be more menacing than that of a newer drug, but its completeness should be viewed as an asset not a liability or a reason for preferring drugs that are less well understood.*

Drugs That Inhibit the Effects of the Adrenergic Nervous System

Drugs that inhibit the effects of the adrenergic nervous system were among the first used to treat hypertension. This discussion includes those drugs that are clinically useful today. Adrenergic inhibiting drugs act either to (1) decrease the amount of norepinephrine and epinephrine released from adrenergic terminals and the adrenal medulla, or (2) block the effects of norepinephrine and epinephrine at α- and β-adrenergic receptors. Drugs that reduce catecholamine release may do so by stimulating areas of the brain that inhibit sympathetic outflow or by depleting the peripheral adrenergic neurons of their catecholamine stores (see the section on the sympathetic nervous system).

Drugs That Reduce Sympathetic Activity— Centrally Acting Agents: α-Methyldopa

Pharmacology and Mechanism of Action. α-Methyldopa was introduced in 1960 and for 10 years along with diuretics was a mainstay of antihypertensive therapy. Methyldopa must be activated in the brain by being converted into active α_2-adrenergic agonists (methylnorepinephrine and methylepinephrine) before it exerts its antihypertensive actions. For these reasons it has a slower onset of action (i.e., 4–6 hours) compared with the active α_2-agonist clonidine. The α-agonist metabolites of methyldopa stimulate areas in the brainstem (presumably via α_2 receptors) that inhibit sympathetic nerve discharge. The net effect of the drug is to decrease release of norepinephrine from peripheral adrenergic neurons and consequently decrease blood pressure because of decreased peripheral vascular resistance and inhibition of the reflex increases in heart rate and/or cardiac output.

Methyldopa is variably absorbed (<30% bioavailability). Its $t_{1/2}$ is 2 hours for the parent compound. Elimination is by metabolism and renal excretion. After an IV or oral dose of methyldopa, there is a gradual decrease in blood pressure over 4 to 6 hours. Unexpected hypotension is rare. The effective dose ranges from 125 mg to 3 g may be given as a single daily dose. *Principle: The difference in the pharmacokinetic half-life from pharmacodynamic half-life of drugs that are prodrugs can be particularly striking.* This disparity is explained by the slow elimination of the active metabolites in the brain compared with the rapid clearance of the parent compound from the circulation. Patients in renal failure usually require a lower dose because the drug is eliminated more slowly, thereby allowing a greater percentage of any given dose to be converted into the active metabolites in the brain.

Clinical Use and Adverse Effects. Like other antihypertensive agents, methyldopa reduces blood pressure proportional to pretreatment pressures. In mild hypertension, average reductions are 20/13 mm Hg (using 2 g/day). In more severe hypertension, the average reductions are 38/22 mm Hg (using 3 g/day). Monotherapy may control up to 75% of patients (Bayliss and Harvey-Smith, 1962). Methyldopa's action is additive with that of most other antihypertensives. It can reverse established left ventricular hypertrophy. Its effectiveness is proved not only in lowering blood pressure but also in decreasing adverse cardiovascular events associated with hypertension (Medical Research Council, 1985).

The preeminent and limiting adverse effects of methyldopa are related to depression of CNS function, that is, lassitude, drowsiness, and impotence. As with other central α-adrenergic agonists, dry mouth is dose-related. Autoimmune abnormalities increase with the dose and duration of exposure and include positive Coombs tests (rarely leading to hemolytic anemia), positive antinuclear antibody tests with occasional lupus-like syndrome, and hepatocellular dysfunction. Methyldopa's interference with production of dopamine can sometimes unmask signs of parkinsonism. There are no known adverse effects on glucose or lipid metabolism. Rarely, methyldopa may cause a fever.

Recommendation. Methyldopa remains a proven, effective, comparatively safe and well-tolerated antihypertensive when used in lower dose ranges. Its safety during pregnancy-related hypertension is well established. It can be used on a once- or twice-daily basis and may be given at bedtime to exploit its sedative effects and avoid them during the day (see the discussion of very severe hypertension for more information on IV use; for review, see Reid and Elliott, 1984).

Clonidine

Pharmacology and Mechanism of Action. Clonidine, a partial α_2-agonist, was originally intended to be a nasal vasoconstrictor decongestant. Early studies determined its hypotensive and sedative effects. Fortunately, its high lipid solubility results in predominant concentrations in the brain and a dominant central α_2-agonist-mediated inhibition of sympathetic outflow leading to decreased blood pressure (see the section on α-methyldopa). Guanabenz is a less potent (about 40-fold) more recent derivative of clonidine and has similar actions.

The hemodynamic effects of clonidine include decreased peripheral vascular resistance, heart rate, and cardiac output. All probably are related to decreased sympathetic (and renin) system activity. Also, taken orally, clonidine may enhance vagal tone. A small dose (0.1 mg) decreases blood pressure in 30 minutes with a maximum effect being seen in 2 to 4 hours. The total duration of effect is up to 12 hours. Its plasma $t_{1/2}$ is 6 to 12 hours and doubles in patients with renal failure.

Clonidine should be given at least twice daily for satisfactory control of blood pressure throughout the day. Blood pressure can be further reduced as doses exceed 0.1 mg. But predictable increases in the incidence and severity of adverse effects increase progressively with doses over 0.3 mg. The unique potency of clonidine has allowed it to be delivered by transdermal patches. A single patch can deliver 0.1, 0.2, or 0.3 mg daily continuously for 7 days. This delivery system can substantially enhance efficacy of compliance and may decrease the adverse-effects profile. Unfor-

tunately, the patch causes a high incidence of local skin rash.

Clinical Use and Adverse Effects. Clonidine is effective as monotherapy in divided doses of 0.2 to 1.0 mg/day. Its effect is enhanced when it is combined with diuretics in particular, and with most other agents. Clonidine appears to be most useful when it is used as a second-line, low-dose, antiadrenergic agent to blunt the reflex increase in sympathetic tone caused by diuretics and/or vasodilators. It is also useful in ameliorating the hyperadrenergic-like symptoms of the menopausal syndrome or during alcohol or nicotine withdrawal. Thus clonidine can be used to great benefit in hypertensive menopausal women, especially when estrogens are contraindicated or are not tolerated. Likewise, clonidine may be well employed in the hypertensive patients who are trying to withdraw from use of either alcohol or cigarettes. These all represent "two for one" uses where a single drug can positively impact on more than one indication. ***Principle: Seek settings in which a single drug can positively impact on more than one indication.***

Sedation and dry mouth are common adverse effects. Other toxic effects include bradycardia, orthostatic hypotension, and sexual dysfunction. Abrupt discontinuation of clonidine following chronic use can result in a rebound withdrawal syndrome including marked increase in blood pressure and heart rate plus anxiety, sweating and so forth (Reid et al., 1984). Patients maintained on a β-adrenergic antagonist during clonidine withdrawal may have an exaggerated hypertensive response. ***Principle: The physician should be on special alert whenever a*** **potent, short-acting** ***drug is abruptly (overtly or covertly) withdrawn.***

Recommendations. The antiadrenergic action of central α_2-agonists given in low doses makes them a rational choice for treating hypertension in conjunction with other antihypertensive agents. They also are very useful in treating diseases that tend to enhance autonomic reflexes. Adverse effects may limit them as first-line therapeutic agents. (For review, see Houston, 1981.)

Peripherally Acting Agents

Reserpine

Pharmacology and Mechanism of Action. Reserpine is one of the active extracts of Indian snake root (*Rauwolfia serpentina*). It was first used by the ancient Egyptians to treat snake bite. Reserpine acts primarily by depleting peripheral norepinephrine and serotonin stores, perhaps by increasing the porosity of storage granules in the nerve endings. Lowered sympathetic activity produces a fall in peripheral vascular resistance with little or no change in cardiac output. The observed adverse effect of depression argues for a central action as well that has been shown to be a minor determinant of its hypotensive action.

The pharmacodynamic half-life of the drug can be approximated from the 2 to 3 weeks required to reach its maximum hypotensive effect and the similar time span required to return to baseline pressures after discontinuation of the drug.

Clinical Use and Adverse Effects. Reserpine as monotherapy has efficacy; however, its effectiveness is enhanced with a diuretic or other agents. Low once-daily doses (e.g., 0.05 mg daily) combined with diuretic are as effective as 0.25 mg/day alone (Veterans Administration Medical Centers, 1982). Reserpine was used in the earlier clinical trials that demonstrated that antihypertensive drugs could decrease morbidity and mortality caused by hypertension.

Reserpine can frequently cause severe depression. Suicide was common with the early use of high doses (>2 mg/day) of the drug. Current, lower doses (<0.5 mg/day) are associated with many fewer CNS effects. Adverse effects, especially fatigue, are similar to those encountered with other centrally acting agents. Nasal stuffiness and symptoms of parasympathetic excess (miosis, bradycardia, etc.) can be caused by reserpine. The reluctance to use reserpine was heightened when epidemiologic studies erroneously suggested that the drug caused breast cancer (Goodwin and Bunney, 1971).

Recommendations. Reserpine is an effective, safe, and cheap antihypertensive when used in low doses in combination with low-dose diuretics or other agents that do not inhibit the adrenergic nervous system. Reports of depression and suicide understandably have limited its use but may be greatly exaggerated in view of the efficacy of low dosages.

α-Adrenergic Receptor Antagonists

Pharmacology and Mechanism of Action. Prazosin was developed in the 1960s as a direct-acting vasodilator but was subsequently found to be an α-adrenergic antagonist. The search for α-receptor antagonists with longer duration of action yielded terazosin and doxazosin in the 1980s. Only prazosin will be discussed here since the actions of all three are similar.

α Blockers that are clinically useful to treat hypertension are selective α_1-adrenergic receptor blocking agents. They antagonize the vasoconstrictor actions of norepinephrine and epinephrine. This effect causes arteriolar vasodilatation and lowers peripheral vascular resistance. The action also leads to venodilatation and a fall in venous return. The combination of decreased peripheral vascular resistance with decreased venous return impairs the body's response to upright posture and can result in orthostatic hypotension that can be symptomatic, particularly with initial dosing ("first-dose effect"). The orthostatic effects attenuate over time. There is little tachyphylaxis to the long-term antihypertensive effect of prazosin in contrast to effects in refractory congestive heart failure (see chapter 4).

Given orally, prazosin is well absorbed, but there is a poor relationship between the concentration of the drug in plasma and reduction in blood pressure (Suderman et al., 1981). In patients with renal failure, the hypotensive effect is enhanced.

Clinical Use and Adverse Effects. The average antihypertensive effect of prazosin is not different from the average effects of diuretics, captopril, β antagonists, clonidine, and methyldopa. Falls in blood pressure average about 10/10 mm Hg. Predictably, the antihypertensive effects of prazosin are most marked in the sitting and upright positions (Inouye et al., 1984). Interestingly, in hypertensive patients with left ventricular hypertrophy, prazosin reduced left ventricular mass whereas hydralazine added to a regimen of diuretic plus β-receptor antagonist did not (Leenen et al., 1987). α-Adrenergic antagonists are the only antihypertensive agents that actually lower LDL cholesterol and raise HDL cholesterol. Unfortunately there are no data yet to determine whether this effect translates into a reduction of atherosclerotic disease. Prazosin can be used in asthmatic patients since it has a mild relaxant effect on bronchial smooth muscle and improves exercise-induced asthma. Since α antagonists decrease symptomatic urinary hesitancy and bladder neck spasm associated with prostatic hyperplasia, they are attractive for use in hypertensive elderly men (Kaplan, 1989).

Adverse effects often occur early in therapy using prazosin. Symptomatic orthostatic hypotension is common with initial large doses (10%–50% at 2 mg or more) and in patients who are fasting, volume-depleted, salt-restricted, or elderly, or who are taking any other antihypertensive drug. If the initial dose is about 0.5 mg and is given at bedtime for a few days, this adverse effect may be minimized. This drug has increased risk in the elderly because of the propensity for orthostatic hypotension. Fatigue, weakness, lightheadedness, upset stomach, headaches, dry mouth, and sexual dysfunction can be caused by the drug (Oates et al., 1983).

Recommendations. α-Adrenergic antagonists are useful for patients with lipid abnormalities. They should be reserved as second-line therapy taking advantage of their unique pharmacologic effects in patients with associated asthma, hyperlipidemia, left ventricular hypertrophy, and symptomatic prostatism. (Again the issue of treating multiple indications with one drug arises.) They are useful as the vasodilator "third drug" in a combination with a β-receptor antagonist and a diuretic. Twice-daily dosing is appropriate.

β-Adrenergic Receptor Antagonists

Pharmacology and Mechanism of Action. Propranolol, a nonselective β_1-, β_2-adrenergic receptor antagonist, was born in 1963 and is the grandparent of β-adrenergic antagonists. It was originally used to prevent angina. Its hypotensive action was reported in 1964. Since the marketing of propranolol, a plethora of β-adrenergic blockers has become available.

β-Adrenergic antagonists competitively antagonize the effects of endogenous or exogenous catecholamines at the β receptor. The mechanism or mechanisms responsible for the antihypertensive effects of β-receptor antagonists are uncertain. Interestingly, these drugs do not generally cause hypotension when administered chronically to normal individuals. β-Adrenergic antagonists decrease heart rate and stroke volume and secondarily lower cardiac output. Initially the decreased stroke volume was assumed incorrectly to be completely due to negative inotropy. Newer techniques have also shown a decrease in venous return. The initial increase in peripheral resistance may be related to vascular β_2 blockade, leaving unopposed α-adrenergic vasoconstrictor actions of catecholamines. But with chronic treatment, peripheral vascular resistance decreases to normal or lower.

β-Adrenergic antagonists can inhibit renin secretion and block presynaptic β_2-adrenergic receptors that stimulate norepinephrine release. β-Adrenergic antagonists may also act by an as-yet-undetermined CNS mechanism. *Principle: When a prototype of a class of drugs has multiple mechanisms that contribute to efficacy, it does not necessarily follow that other drugs in the same class will share each of the useful mechanisms. Such similarity must be proved not assumed.*

Manufacturers of β-adrenergic antagonists have placed great stock in developing chemicals with pharmacologic features such as β_1-adrenergic antagonist selectivity, partial agonist activity, and so forth. As theoretically attractive as more selective agents might be therapeutically, one must first determine whether a β-adrenergic blocker should be used, then determine whether there are clinically important differences between the agents, and only then make a therapeutic choice based on the differences within the class. *Principle: Choose the class of drug; then choose within the class.*

Some β-adrenergic blockers have very low affinity for the β_2 receptor. They are therefore called β_1 selective; however, at clinically useful doses they substantially block both classes of β receptors. β_1-Receptor blockade seems essential for antihypertensive effects. Experimental β_2-selective blockers have no appreciable antihypertensive effects (Jefferson et al., 1987). Table 2–3 shows the presence and functions of β_1 and β_2 receptors in human tissues.

While it would be tempting to use a β_1-selective blocker in an asthmatic patient because that agent has the *potential for* leaving β_2 bronchodilator receptors unblocked, unless that potentiality has been proved feasible in clinical settings, one should recognize that the potential for any β-adrenergic antagonist to produce some β_2 blockade exists. Therefore, all β blockers should be avoided in that patient.

Some β blockers bind to the β_2 receptor and stimulate it, albeit with less agonist effect than would endogenous epinephrine. These entities are said to be partial agonists or to possess intrinsic sympathomimetic activity (ISA). Table 2–4 shows the categorization of the available β-adrenergic antagonists according to their various pharmacologic properties.

The human heart has both β_1 and β_2 receptors (Motomura et al., 1990). In patients with coronary artery disease, damping the effects of endogenous adrenergic agonists is best achieved with blockade of both β_1 and β_2 receptors. Nonselective β-receptor antagonists propranolol and timolol are effective in preventing fatal and nonfatal cardiac events after myocardial infarction (Beta-Blocker Heart Attack Trial, 1982). Relatively high doses of β_1-selective adrenergic blockers are also beneficial, but partial agonist β-adrenergic blockers have not been demonstrated to be effective (Frishman et al., 1984). The higher resting heart rate with partial agonist β blockers may account for the ineffective control of rest or nocturnal angina. The ability of nonselective β-adrenergic antagonists to attenuate epinephrine-mediated hypokalemia theoretically may raise the threshold for the arrhythmias and reduce the incidence of sudden death in all patients but particularly those taking kaluretic diuretics. β_2-Adrenergic receptors also relax bronchial and vascular smooth muscle and stimulate release of insulin. Thus β_1-selective agents theoretically would seem preferable in patients with associated problems involving these systems. Whether theory becomes fact depends on the degree of selectivity of the chemical entities and the ability to demonstrate the selectivity in vivo.

The "membrane-stabilizing activity" or "local anesthetic effect" of some β-adrenergic antagonists is most prominent with propranolol. However, this property is not important when these drugs are administered systemically in the usual doses. Only agents such as timolol, devoid of this

Table 2–4. **CHARACTERISTICS OF ADRENERGIC ANTAGONISTS**

β BLOCKERS	USUAL DAILY DOSAGE (MG)	β_1-SELECTIVE	WATER-SOLUBLE	ISA*
Acebutolol	200–800	+	+	+
Atenolol	25–100	+	+	−
Labetalol	200–800	−	−	−
Metoprolol	25–200	+	−	−
Nadolol	20–80	−	+	−
Oxprenolol	60–320	−	−	+
Pindolol	5–30	−	−	+
Propranolol	40–320	−	−	−
Sotalol	160	−	+	−
Timolol	5–40	−	−	−

* ISA = Intrinsic sympathomimetic activity (partial agonist activity).

action, can be used to treat glaucoma while avoiding paralyzing the corneal pain reflex. β-Adrenergic antagonists without local anesthetic activity, that is, atenolol, nadolol, timolol, appear to have far fewer fatalities related to overdose than those β antagonists with this property (Henry and Cassidy, 1986).

The only β-adrenergic antagonist with combined α- and β-adrenergic blockade activity is labetalol. Its relative potency of β- to α-adrenergic blockade is about 8 : 1. There may be diminished α blockade with time in humans after 6 months of dosing (Semplicini et al., 1983).

Propranolol is generally about 30% to 50% bioavailable. However, the concentration of drug in plasma and effects of a given dose can vary as much as 20-fold between subjects. Absorption is nearly complete, but a large fraction is avidly extracted by the liver during its "first-pass" transit (see chapters 1 and 37). Timolol has much higher and predictable absorption. It is also the only β-adrenergic antagonist formulated as the pure active L isomer. Most of the other β-adrenergic antagonists are mixtures of D and L isomers. β-Adrenergic blockers with a long $t_{1/2}$ achieve fairly predictable plateau concentrations. Those more water-soluble agents (atenolol, nadolol, and sotalol) have substantial elimination by the kidneys. These drugs have $t_{1/2}$'s of about 10, 20, and 15 hours, respectively, in contrast to the usual $t_{1/2}$ of 3 hours for propranolol and other more lipid-soluble agents that are extensively metabolized by the liver. The water-soluble agents may have a lower rate of penetration into the CNS. It is possible that these drugs have lower rates of prevalence of sleep disturbance and lassitude, although there are few comparative data currently available.

Clinical Use and Adverse Effects.   The largest clinical experience using β-adrenergic antagonists has been with propranolol. The drug produced benefits in the large-scale trials when mortality was the end point. As monotherapy, β-adrenergic antagonists have similar efficacy to most other agents when studied in direct comparison (Inouye et al., 1984). Studies comparing the various

β-adrenergic antagonists usually reveal no difference in their antihypertensive effects. β-Adrenergic blockers have limited effectiveness as monotherapy in blacks (Veterans Administration Cooperative Study Group, 1982). However in the black population they are useful when combined with other agents. The Medical Research Council (MRC) trial failed to show a benefit of propranolol in smokers, but this subgroup analysis must be interpreted with caution. Similar results were seen with oxprenolol in the International Prospective Primary Prevention Study on Hypertension Collaborative Group (IPPPSH, 1985). As already noted, large-scale trials in hypertensive patients have not shown reduction in coronary artery-related events. However, some, but not all, β-adrenergic antagonists are efficacious in reducing mortality in patients who have already had a myocardial infarction (Beta-Blocker Heart Attack Trial, 1982; Frishman, 1984). β-Adrenergic antagonists may retard atherosclerosis (Kaplan et al., 1987). ***Principle: Do not attribute the claims of one drug to the class of agents it belongs to, until and unless those medically crucial claims have been proved for each agent under consideration.***

As can be seen from Table 2–5, β-adrenergic antagonists have by far the longest list of indications and relative contraindications of any other antihypertensive agents. A careful search for any of these factors might unearth them in an individual patient, facilitating a decision regarding the choice of which agent to use. β-Adrenergic antagonists may be used with other agents (with the emphasis on those that do not affect the adrenergic system). Theoretically, combination of β-adrenergic antagonists and ACE inhibitors might not be efficacious since they both dampen the renin-angiotensin system. In practice, β-adrenergic antagonists are especially useful in combination therapy for patients taking vasodilators. In such a setting, the β-adrenergic antagonists interfere with the reflex sympathetic effects stimulated by the vasodilation.

Adverse effects of propranolol and other β-

Table 2–5. **INFLUENCE OF CONCOMITANT DISEASE ON CHOICE OF THERAPY**

	USE IN	AVOID IN*
• Diuretics	Volume overload states Renal failure Heart failure	Hyperlipidemia Gout Diabetes Impotence Electrolyte imbalances
• β Blocker	Angina Postmyocardial infarct Migraine Tachyarrhythmia Mitral valve prolapse Thyrotoxicosis Aortic dissection Essential tremor Glaucoma Hypertrophic cardiomyopathy Anxiety states	Diabetes Asthma/COPD Heart failure Raynaud phenomenon Peripheral vascular disease Bradyarrhythmia/AV block Depression Impotence
• Sympatholytics	Perimenopausal flushing	Impotence Depression CNS disease Orthostatic hypotension
• Vasodilators (excluding calcium antagonists)	Heart failure	
• Calcium-channel blockers	Angina Tachyarrhythmia Hypertrophic cardiomyopathy Raynaud phenomenon Migraine	Bradyarrhythmias Heart failure Constipation (verapamil) Edema states (nifedipine)

* Note that the "avoid in" column provides a partial list of adverse effects.

adrenergic antagonists are well known. They include fatigue, sleep disturbance, and impotence. β_2-Adrenergic blockade can aggravate bronchospasm and potentially worsen peripheral vascular disease including Raynaud phenomenon and intermittent claudication. Decreased cardiac output and inhibition of β_2-adrenergic-mediated vasodilatation in muscles may lead to a reduction in exercise tolerance that may be further impaired by diminished free fatty acid flux to exercising muscles. Because β-adrenergic antagonists antagonize the effects of catecholamines, epinephrine's use in countering severe allergic reactions may require larger than usual doses and may result in severe hypertension in patients receiving nonselective β blockers because of unopposed α-adrenergic receptor–mediated vasoconstriction.

Blockade of β_2-adrenergic receptors may rarely impair release of insulin in type 2 (non-insulin-dependent) diabetic patients. Of more concern is the use of β-adrenergic antagonists in type I diabetic patients (see chapter 16). It is well known that these agents mask the sympathetic responses to hypoglycemia, delaying recognition of the hypoglycemic state by both the patient and the physician. Of more importance, β-adrenergic blockers may impair counterregulatory responses necessary for warding off or minimizing the hypoglycemia. Consequently, β-adrenergic antago-

nists should be used only with considerable caution in diabetic patients on insulin; if absolutely required, β_1-selective compounds may be preferable.

β-Adrenergic blockade can decrease HDL cholesterol concentrations and increase triglyceride concentrations, but the clinical significance of this is unknown. Since impairment of peripheral conversion of T_4 to T_3 occurs with some β-adrenergic receptor antagonists, these drugs can rarely exacerbate borderline hypothyroidism or mask the development of hyperthyroidism (see chapter 14). β_2-Adrenergic receptor stimulation causes entry of potassium into cells. Therefore antagonists of the receptor can increase potassium concentrations in serum. Some observers feel this is a beneficial effect in warding off epinephrine-induced hypokalemia during stress or exercise or while patients are taking diuretics with attendant lowering of the threshold for arrhythmia.

The effects of β-adrenergic antagonists can adversely influence patients susceptible to bradyarrhythmias, atrioventricular (AV) conduction delays, and heart failure. This is a concern in using the drugs in patients taking digitalis or calcium antagonist therapy. Labetolol hepatotoxicity has been reported (Clark et al., 1990).

Abrupt withdrawal of some β-adrenergic blockers may result in a withdrawal syndrome especially in patients with coronary disease (Rangno, 1984). Symptoms may manifest as worsening angina, myocardial infarction, or cardiac arrest. Rebound hypertension is unusual with β-blocker withdrawal. The withdrawal mechanism may be due to unblocking of upregulated β-adrenergic receptors and can last up to 2 weeks. The rebound can be prevented by tapering the drug, or by using β-adrenergic blockers with longer half-lives.

Recommendations. β-Adrenergic antagonists remain first-line therapy for hypertension. The response rate and acceptance of the drugs are excellent, and their value has been proved. The presence of other diseases coexisting with hypertension, or the use of additional antihypertensive agents in a patient, is a determinant of whether β-adrenergic antagonists are appropriate. Once the decision to use a β-adrenergic antagonist has been made, the pharmacologic differences between them should be exploited. β-Adrenergic antagonists are useful in conjunction with other nonsympatholytic agents, especially vasodilators, and have been used effectively during pregnancy. Adverse effects can be avoided by considering patient factors, using the lowest effective doses, and titrating doses appropriately. β-Adrenergic antagonists can be used twice daily; the more water-soluble agents are appropriate for once-daily dosing. The β-adrenergic antagonists are reviewed by Oates et al. (1983).

Angiotensin-Converting Enzyme Inhibitors

Pharmacology and Mechanisms of Action. The renin system is a contributor to the regulation of blood pressure and extracellular volume. Over the last 15 years, angiotensin-converting enzyme (ACE) inhibitors have become available to inhibit this system. Their use results in control of hypertension and heart failure. Presently captopril, enalapril, and lisinopril are on the market, but others are being developed. Pharmacologic differences between these agents are being proclaimed, but their clinical relevance probably will be limited (Williams, 1988).

In 1960, pit viper venom was noted to increase the effect of bradykinin by interfering with its enzymatic degradation. The enzyme is ACE and is responsible for the conversion of angiotensin I to angiotensin II, a potent endogenous vasoconstrictor. ACE inhibitors, by blocking this conversion, reduce the formation of angiotensin II, and in its absence vasodilatation occurs. Other mechanisms that could contribute to reduction in blood pressure may include an ability to decrease aldosterone secretion and hence decrease blood volume, increase concentrations of the potent endogenous vasodilator bradykinin, decrease adrenergic activity, increase vasodilator renal and vas-

cular prostanoids, and inhibit the intracellular renin-angiotensin systems of the heart, vascular smooth muscle, kidney, and brain (Dzau, 1988). Different mechanisms of the drug's effects may contribute to efficacy at different times. For example, the degree of blood pressure reduction correlates very well with the degree of inhibition of the converting enzyme during the first months of therapy with enalapril. Later, while the blood pressure is still controlled, the correlation with inhibition of the enzyme is lost. As with the β-adrenergic antagonists, labeling of a drug class by mechanism does not necessarily define all its important pharmacologic actions.

Intracellular angiotensin II is mitogenic; that is, it contributes to hypertrophy of the cardiac and vascular myocytes. ACE inhibitors can prevent or reverse hypertrophic changes in hypertensive animals and humans. But this effect also is seen with other nonmitogenic agents. Although left ventricular hypertrophy is a risk factor for cardiovascular morbidity, reversal of the hypertrophy has not yet been shown to reduce the cardiovascular morbidity or mortality in human hypertensive patients. *Principle: Many medically important events caused by drugs take major and expensive studies to determine. Not knowing that a drug can cause an event is not equivalent to knowing that it cannot cause such an event. When all else is equal, theoretical, as-yet-unproven effects may be exploited in choosing a drug.*

Captopril, a sulfhydryl-containing compound, was licensed in 1980, and enalapril followed in the mid-1980s. Enalapril is an inactive prodrug that must be converted by the liver to enalaprilat, the active ACE inhibitor. Lisinopril is the active lysine derivative of enalaprilat. Other ACE inhibitors are in development.

ACE inhibitors are well absorbed after oral administration. Food decreases absorption of captopril by 30% but has no effect on absorption of enalapril. Captopril begins its antihypertensive effects within 30 minutes, whereas enalapril and lisinopril act within 90 minutes. The duration of captopril's antihypertensive effect is dose-dependent, with 25 mg lasting 6 hours and 75 mg lasting up to 12 hours. The pharmacokinetic $t_{1/2}$ is 3 hours for captopril, 11 hours for enalapril, and 12 hours for lisinopril. The required conversion of enalapril to enalaprilat in the liver results in the slow accumulation of the active drug and a delayed peak effect. Renal elimination of both enalapril and lisinopril ($t_{1/2}$ of approximately 36 hours) is sufficiently slow to allow once-daily dosing. Elimination of all ACE inhibitors is prolonged in patients with advanced renal failure. Equivalent ACE-inhibiting potencies are captopril : enalapril : lisinopril = 10 : 2 : 1. Table 2–6 shows a comparison of these three ACE inhibitors.

Table 2-6. COMPARISON OF ACE INHIBITORS

	CAPTOPRIL	ENALAPRIL	LISINOPRIL
Activity	Active	Inactive "prodrug"	Active
$t_{1/2}$ (h)	3	11	12
Duration of antihypertensive effect (h)	12	>24	24
Elimination	Renal	Liver metabolism then renal	Renal
Relative potency	10	2	1
Dose (mg/day)	12.5–150	2.5–40	2.5–40
Dosing	b.i.d.	o.d.*	o.d.
Cost in $/day (daily dose)	0.74 (50 mg)	0.88 (10 mg)	0.68 (5 mg)

* Once a day dosing.

Clinical Use and Adverse Effects. As with most other within-class comparisons, captopril, enalapril, and lisinopril have similar capacities to reduce blood pressure in the order of 10–15/5–12 mm Hg. These agents, like a number of antihypertensives, particularly diuretics, have relatively steep dose–response curves at low doses but flatten out at higher doses. These agents used as monotherapy are equally effective as other antihypertensives used as monotherapy (Canadian Enalapril Study Group, 1987). Addition of a diuretic to an ACE inhibitor appears to have synergistic effects in lowering blood pressure. For instance, patients uncontrolled with 25 mg b.i.d. of captopril had a better response to the addition of hydrochlorothiazide 25 mg than to doubling of captopril to 50 mg b.i.d. (Case, 1987). In addition, hypokalemia caused by diuretics is opposed by combination of the diuretic with an ACE inhibitor.

ACE inhibitors are effective as antihypertensive agents in about 70% of patients. The magnitude of the decrease in blood pressure is proportional to the pretreatment values. Clinical trials have shown that the antihypertensive effects are secondary to a decrease in peripheral vascular resistance with little change in cardiac output and no reflex tachycardia. ACE inhibitors reduce overall renal vascular resistance and can increase renal blood flow. Patients with renovascular hypertension respond best to ACE inhibitors, but there are caveats in these patients (see below). These agents are useful in the treatment of severe hypertension (Traub and Levey, 1983) and as vasodilator third-drug therapy added to a regimen of β-adrenergic antagonists and diuretics.

One study on "quality of life" found a lower incidence of adverse effects due to captopril when compared with methyldopa and propranolol (Croog et al., 1986). Excessive declines in blood pressure even leading to orthostatic hypotension can occur, especially when patients are volume depleted or taking diuretics. Lower initial doses (i.e., captopril 12.5–25 mg or equivalent) minimize this adverse effect. Skin rashes, disturbance of taste, and muscosal lesions are more common with captopril because it contains a sulfhydryl moiety. Probably the most common adverse effect is dry cough in up to 10% to 15% (Just, 1989). This is more common in women and is unrelated to bronchospasm or abnormal lung function. The mechanism is unknown but may be due to chemical mediators that can potentiate the cough reflex. Cough occurs with all ACE inhibitors, is dose-dependent, and reverses with discontinuation of the drug. Most patients complain of the cough as dry and nocturnal, sometimes interfering with sleep.

Early reports of neutropenia and proteinuria with captopril appeared when patients were taking very high doses and had other diseases such as renal failure and connective tissue disease that may have predisposed to the lesions. These adverse effects are rare. Angioneurotic edema, which can occur with all ACE inhibitors, can be severe enough to be fatal but occurs in less than 0.1%. The risk of angioneurotic edema is higher in patients in whom drug administration is continued despite the development of mouth ulcers or skin rash.

Because the drug decreases aldosterone concentrations, hyperkalemia can occur, but it is rarely encountered in patients with normal renal function. Caution should be exercised in administering ACE inhibitors to patients with renal impairment, type 4 renal tubular acidosis (hyporeninemic hypoaldosteronism) as is seen in diabetic patients, and in combination with potassium-sparing diuretics or potassium supplementation. ACE inhibitors should not be used during pregnancy because of their potential teratogenic effects (Broughton et al., 1982).

ACE inhibitors can exacerbate renal insufficiency in patients with bilateral renal vascular hypertension. This effect deserves scrutiny. When there is decreased renal blood flow, preferential vasodilatation of the afferent arteriole occurs. Angiotensin II–induced vasoconstriction of the efferent arteriole increases postglomerular resistance to blood flow, which increases hydrostatic pressure in the glomerulus and favors glomerular filtration at any perfusion pressure. In this setting of decreased renal blood flow, the filtration fraction is increased, and thus glomerular filtration can be preserved. Interruption of this compensatory mechanism with an ACE inhibitor can lead to a decrease in glomerular filtration rate (GFR) in the underperfused kidney. In fact, this phenomenon has been exploited with the use of captopril during isotopic renography. The drug exaggerates a difference between the normal (non-angiotensin-II–dependent) and renal arterial stenotic (angiotensin II–dependent) kidney. The normal kidney in a patient with unilateral renovascular hypertension can compensate for the effects of ACE inhibition by increasing GFR and keeping the creatinine concentrations constant. However, when both kidneys are underperfused or when there is a solitary kidney with a stenotic artery, loss of this compensating mechanism leads to rapid reversible rises in serum creatinine concentration (Keane et al., 1989). Administration of an ACE inhibitor in any clinical setting of decreased renal perfusion has the potential for worsening the insufficiency.

The effect of ACE inhibitors on postglomerular tone has a theoretical advantage in patients with diabetic glomerulopathy. Inhibition of postglomerular tone reduces the transglomerular capillary hydraulic pressure gradient that is thought to play a role in development of glomerular basement membrane damage and subsequent diabetic glomerulosclerosis. There are animal models to support this concept, and clinical trials are currently underway in type 1 diabetic patients to see if ACE inhibitors can slow the progression of diabetic renal disease (Anderson and Brenner, 1986). *Principle: Understanding the pharmacology of new drugs may lead to new diagnostic or therapeutic hypotheses. The new indications must be proved, of course.*

Recommendations. ACE inhibitors are valuable as effective and reasonably safe antihypertensive agents. Their adverse effects are generally predictable, avoidable, or reversible. ACE inhibitors may be considered as first-line therapy, especially for patients in whom diuretics and/or β-adrenergic antagonists are contraindicated (Myers et al., 1989). They are especially useful when combined with diuretics. Of course, using ACE inhibitors to treat patients with heart failure and hypertension exploits the two-for-one principle. Because of their additive effects with other agents, they also are useful in treating severe hypertension and as third-drug vasodilator in combined regimens.

Calcium Antagonists

Pharmacology and Mechanism of Action. The first clinically available calcium antagonist (or calcium-entry blocker), verapamil, is a congener of papaverine and was discovered in 1967.

It became available in the 1980s. These agents are not receptor antagonists but block Ca^{2+} influx into smooth muscle and cardiac muscle cells via the slow (voltage-dependent) Ca^{2+} channel. Presumably, blockade of calcium influx reduces intracellular free Ca^{2+} concentrations that ultimately determine myocyte contractility. Blocking calcium movement occurs without perceptible changes in concentrations of calcium in serum. Two other calcium antagonists, nifedipine (a dihydropyridine) and diltiazem, are calcium-channel blockers that bear no structural relationship to verapamil or to each other. They display slight differences in their sites and modes of action on the slow channel. There are many new dihydropyridine compounds (felodipine, nimodipine, nisoldipine, nitrendipine, etc.), but this chapter will focus on nifedipine as the prototype (see chapters 5 and 6).

Since intracellular calcium flux is a final common path for a spectrum of cellular responses to a wide variety of stimuli, since the molecular basis of calcium channels is quite heterogenous, and since existing calcium-channel blockers are chemically heterogenous, the pharmacologic similarities of presently available compounds may be more apparent than real (see the section on clinical use and adverse effects, below). Those developed in the future should be expected to have very different profiles affecting a variety of tissues not now tested against existing blockers. The therapist armed with this information should (1) expect undescribed effects of existing products that are not related to the cardiovascular system, (2) expect future products in the class to be devoid of cardiovascular actions, and (3) seek effects of existing and future products on organs other than the cardiovascular system for new indications for the drug.

As well as effects on calcium channels, calcium-channel antagonists have additional actions that explain the different effects caused by each. In addition to a local anesthetic effect, verapamil and its major active metabolite norverapamil have α- and β-adrenergic receptor antagonist actions, and they deplete cardiac norepinephrine as would reserpine. However, the clinical relevance of these pharmacologic properties is uncertain (Feldman et al., 1985; Zsoter et al., 1988). Verapamil is the most potent negative inotrope (contractility), chronotrope (heart rate), and dromotrope (AV-node conduction) of the three. Nifedipine is the most potent peripheral smooth muscle dilator. Diltiazem lies somewhere in between (Table 2–7). These differences can be exploited by choosing the most appropriate calcium-channel antagonist for individual patients. So far, calcium-channel antagonists decrease cardiac output and peripheral as well as renal vascular resistance with resulting increase in renal blood flow,

Table 2-7. **COMPARISON OF THREE CALCIUM-CHANNEL ANTAGONISTS**

	VERAPAMIL	DILTIAZEM	NIFEDIPINE
Vasodilator	+ +	+ +	+ + + +
Reflex sympathetic*	+	+	+ + +
Negative inotropy	+ + +	+ +	+ + †
Negative chronotropy	+ + +	+ + +	+
Negative dromotropy	+ + +	+ +	+
$t_{1/2}$ (h)	5‡	5	3
Bioavailability (%)	20	25§	40
Metabolism	Liver	Liver	Liver
Dose (mg)	120–480	120–360	20–120

*Reflex activation of the sympathetic nervous system is in proportion to vasodilator effect.
† Direct effects. In practice, because of reflex sympathetic activation and resultant enhanced contractility, nifedipine has a lesser degree of net negative inotropy = direct + reflex effect.
‡ Will increase with chronic dosing due to saturation of hepatic enzymes.
§ Will increase markedly with higher doses (see text).

GFR, and filtration fraction. The combination of effects produces a mild diuretic and natriuretic effect. Renin and aldosterone are unchanged. Some calcium-channel blockers under development have no negative inotropic or chronotropic actions. If they reach the market, they would have a select place in the treatment of hypertensive patients.

All available calcium-channel antagonists have low and widely variable bioavailability (20%–40%). This is due to very high first-pass hepatic extraction similar to that of propranolol. With higher doses, a greater proportion escapes hepatic uptake. A 50% increase in the dose of diltiazem (from 240 to 360 mg) typically triples the area under the dose–time–concentration curve. Conversely the newer sustained-release formulations, designed to overcome the need for three- or four-times-daily dosing, result in much lower average blood concentrations than equivalent standard doses. *Principle: If the rate of absorption of a drug that has saturable first-pass elimination is slowed, the drug will be in the blood longer but at lower concentrations.*

The standard formulations of these three drugs reach a peak concentration and effect in about 0.5 to 2 hours and have a $t_{1/2}$ of 4 to 8 hours, hence the need for t.i.d. dosing. A lower peak with the sustained-release preparations occurs at 6 to 12 hours, creating the feasibility for once- or twice-a-day dosing.

Early reduction of peripheral vascular resistance and blood pressure caused by nifedipine is associated with a reflex increase in heart rate, release of norepinephrine, and secretion of renin as would follow any equally effective vasodilator (e.g., hydralazine, nitroprusside, diazoxide, etc.). This resolves with chronic dosing of constant amounts of drug. These sympathetically mediated changes are not seen with diltiazem and verapamil, nor is the reduction of peripheral vascular resistance as rapid or profound as that caused by nifedipine.

Clinical Use and Adverse Effects. The three agents discussed can be used to induce similar magnitudes of hypotensive effects. When compared with agents used in monotherapy in other classes of drugs, again a similar magnitude of antihypertensive effect was observed. Calcium-channel blockers are effective when combined with β-adrenergic antagonists and ACE inhibitors but show little additional effect when added to diuretics (Nicholson et al., 1989). Nifedipine, as the "vasodilator" in standard triple therapy (β-adrenergic antagonists plus diuretic plus vasodilator), can be useful (Myers et al., 1986). Verapamil combined with a β-adrenergic antagonist therapy is more effective than when either the verapamil or β antagonists are used alone. However, as might be expected the two drugs developed additive effects on the PR interval and left ventricular end-diastolic volume (Dargie et al., 1986).

Addition of sodium restriction for patients taking calcium-channel blockers has little value (Nicholson et al., 1987). Because calcium-channel blockers have other uses, they are ideal in certain two-for-one situations (Table 2–5). Left ventricular hypertrophy may regress while a patient is taking calcium-channel blockers (an effect similar to that shown by methyldopa, β-adrenergic antagonists, and ACE inhibitors).

Many of the adverse effects caused by calcium-channel blockers may be predicted from the differences of the pharmacologic effects of the different chemical entities (Table 2–7). Nifedipine, the more potent vasodilator, has the potential for causing the greatest reflex sympathetic activation that may cause symptoms. The adverse effects that are common to most vasodilators include flushing, headache, tremor, palpitations, sweating, anxiety, and in some patients exacerbation of angina pectoris. Because nifedipine acts more rapidly, especially when given as capsules, symptomatic hypotension and/or orthostatic hypotension can occur. This is more common in the elderly, those who are volume-depleted, and those taking other antihypertensive medications. Bradyarrhythmias and conduction disturbances are more common with verapamil and to a lesser degree with diltiazem. The arrhythmias are particularly prominent when verapamil is taken in combination with other negative chronotropic and dromotropic agents such as β-adrenergic antagonists, quinidine, or digitalis (Maisel et al., 1985).

All three agents can worsen heart failure, but because of its myocardial depressant properties, verapamil is the most worrisome. Relaxation of smooth muscle can lead to esophageal reflux or urinary retention. Constipation is especially common with verapamil and is unusually prominent in patients with an underlying tendency toward constipation. Ankle edema can occur, especially with nifedipine. This may be secondary to hemodynamic alterations across the capillary, changing Starling forces to favor movement of fluid from the capillary into the interstitium. Since the edema is local and not associated with renal salt and water retention, diuretics are of little use. This adverse effect (ankle edema) should not be clinically confused with the development of congestive heart failure.

As with the sudden discontinuation of clonidine or some β-adrenergic blockers, sudden discontinuation of calcium-channel blockers may result in angina or myocardial infarction in patients with underlying coronary disease (Lette et al., 1984). The drugs have no adverse effect on the lipid profile. In fact an antiatherosclerotic effect has been reported in animal models (Henry, 1987).

When used as uncomplicated monotherapy, adverse effects are more common with nifedipine than with the other two. These can be reduced by using the prolonged release tablets as opposed to the capsule. We recommend that as many patients as possible be treated with the tablet for long-term chronic therapy. The capsule also is useful in treating very severe hypertension (see below). Slow release formulations are more expensive but may improve compliance and lead to gradual and prolonged antihypertensive effect.

Recommendations. Calcium-channel blockers are effective as first-line therapy especially in patients in whom diuretics and β-adrenergic antagonists are contraindicated. First-line therapy with the calcium-channel antagonists is limited by their cost and their profile of adverse effects.

Nifedipine also is a useful third-line agent as a *vasodilator.* It is very useful in treating severe hypertension. Since verapamil and diltiazem may have additive adverse effects when used in conjunction with β-adrenergic blockade, nifedipine is the calcium blocker of choice in this setting. Because β-adrenergic antagonists inhibit the reflex sympathetic effects encountered with nifedipine, the combination is sensible and useful. Calcium-channel blockers are useful for hypertensives with other associated conditions in which the two-for-one concept can be exploited. They are very useful as alternatives for β-adrenergic antagonists in patients in whom those agents are contraindicated.

Direct Vasodilators (Hydralazine and Minoxidil)

Pharmacology and Mechanism of Action. These two agents are no more "direct" than any of the other vasodilating drugs, but they differ from the others in that their actual mechanism of action remains unknown. They are considered together because they predominantly relax arteriolar smooth muscle with little or no effect on the venous musculature. As we have discussed above, vasodilators cause reflex sympathetic activation and venoconstriction with attendant increases in venous return. In turn, the cardiac output increases and limits the antihypertensive effectiveness of the vasodilators. The reflex sympathetic effects on the heart increase myocardial contractility and rate and add to the mechanisms of increased cardiac output. At the same time the kidney retains salt and water, further increasing blood volume and secondarily venous return. The renin system also is stimulated by the sympathetic activity. For all these reasons, these agents are not useful as monotherapy and should be combined with a diuretic and an adrenergic-inhibiting agent.

Both hydralazine and minoxidil are well absorbed; their effects start in 15 to 30 minutes and peak around 60 minutes. The plasma half-life is approximately 3 hours for both these agents, but their durations of action are 6 to 12 hours or more. Hydralazine is excreted in the urine mainly as metabolites. Twenty percent of minoxidil is metabolized, 60% to 70% is conjugated and eliminated, and approximately 10% is excreted unchanged.

Clinical Use and Adverse Effects. Since these drugs are almost always used as third-line therapy, this section concentrates on trials of minoxidil and hydralazine as third drugs in a regimen. In comparison with α-adrenergic antagonists, hydralazine produces equal antihypertensive effects with comparatively similar incidences of adverse effects (Veterans Administration Cooperative Study Group, 1981). Trials comparing hydralazine to prazosin showed similar antihypertensive efficacy, but only prazosin was associated with regression of left ventricular mass (Leenen et al., 1987). Nifedipine as the third drug in a regimen is more effective than hydralazine (Myers et al., 1986).

Minoxidil is a very efficacious oral antihypertensive agent. Its use originally was reserved to treat refractory hypertension. In large-scale trials, as a third drug given to patients with resistant hypertension, minoxidil produced effective control of blood pressure in over 70% of patients. Minoxidil is more effective than captopril or hydralazine in double-blind, randomized, control studies of treatment-resistant patients (Connor et al., 1976). Minoxidil may have particular utility in patients with renal insufficiency and hypertension refractory to other drugs (Taverner et al., 1983). Most studies using minoxidil as a third drug have combined it with β-adrenergic antagonists. However, in certain cases, clonidine, methyldopa, or reserpine have been used as the adrenergic inhibitor. There are no data regarding combinations of minoxidil or hydralazine with calcium-channel blockers. Patients refractory to β-adrenergic antagonists plus diuretics and minoxidil have responded to the addition of a converting-enzyme inhibitor as the fourth drug in the regimen (Traub and Levey, 1983).

As with any potent antihypertensive agents, excessive reduction of blood pressure results in orthostatic hypotension. This can be minimized by starting at low doses (e.g., 1.25 mg of minoxidil or 25 mg of hydralazine). Salt and water retention can occur and may manifest as edema or heart failure or loss of control of blood pressure. Diuretic therapy will be needed in almost all patients with functioning kidneys to reverse the effects of plasma volume expansion. Reflex sympathetic effects can occur (see nifedipine) and include flushing, palpitations, anxiety, tremulousness, and headache. These are controlled by β-adrenergic antagonists or other antiadrenergic agents. It may be possible to reduce the dose of β-adrenergic antagonists once the blood pressure is stabilized. Hydralazine and minoxidil in the absence of a sympathetic inhibitor drug can be associated with *increasing* left ventricular wall mass and ECG changes of left ventricular hypertrophy (LVH). Fatigue and sexual dysfunction can occur.

These agents are contraindicated in patients with aortic dissection because they increase cardiac inotropy and lead to increased shear force on the aortic wall. Patients taking hydralazine may develop positive antinuclear antibody (ANA) at doses of 200 mg/day in whites and 300 mg/day in blacks. However drug-induced lupus only occurs in from 5% to 10% of those with positive ANA and is reversible on discontinuation of the drug. *Principle: Many syndromes produced by drugs look alike but do not produce the pathogenesis, morbidity, or mortality of the disease they mimic. Be aware of the differences between simulating the facade of a disease and causing the disease when it comes time to treat the adverse effect or decide on whether the offending drug can be continued.*

Minoxidil may cause pericardial effusion, usually in patients who have renal failure, heart failure, and severe hypertension requiring high doses. Finally, hirsutism is common with minoxidil, is dose-dependent, and is an important limiting factor to using the drug in women. In fact, minoxidil is now used topically to promote hair growth. *Principle: Note how adversity can be put to use for unexpected alternative indications.*

Recommendations. Hydralazine should be started in dosage of 25 mg b.i.d. and increased gradually to a maximum of 200 mg/day in patients who already are taking diuretics and antiadrenergic therapy. The drug is safe, effective, and relatively inexpensive in this setting. Recently, its use has declined because alternative vasodilators such as ACE inhibitors, α-adrenergic antagonists, and calcium blockers have become available. Minoxidil, because it needs to be coadministered with other agents and has the potential toxicity discussed, has been reserved to treat refractory hypertensive patients. Greater consideration should be given to its use in less severe hypertensive patients, especially male patients with moderate-to-severe hypertension and/or renal insufficiency. Use of the more potent agent may allow reduction in dosage of other drugs and improvement in the quality of life of the patients. Initial dose should be from 1.25 to 2.5 mg with titration in 2.5- to 5-mg increments up to a maximum of 40 mg/day.

Patients who are taking direct vasodilators but have inadequate control of their blood pressure should have their plasma volume status carefully evaluated. If the patient is volume-overloaded, diuretics should be increased and euvolemia restored before increasing dosage of the vasodilator.

GUIDELINES FOR MANAGEMENT OF THE HYPERTENSIVE PATIENT

Clinical Assessment

Table 2–8 lists the cardinal objectives of assessment of a hypertensive patient.

History. Obtaining a thorough history is important to determine (1) the duration and severity of hypertension, (2) all drugs and nondrug therapies that were or are being used with documented response, or adverse effects, (3) the presence or absence of target-organ damage, (4) the presence or absence of other risk factors for atherosclerosis, (5) whether findings can be used to reveal secondary hypertension, (6) whether other factors might be influencing or exacerbating blood pressure, and (7) whether drug use or concomitant

**Table 2–8. CARDINAL OBJECTIVES OF
ASSESSMENT OF A
HYPERTENSIVE PATIENT**

- Establish the diagnosis, duration, and severity of the hypertension, as well as prior therapies and their outcomes.
- Identify remedial causes (secondary hypertension).
- Recognize cardiovascular risk factors other then hypertension.
- Establish the presence or absence of target-organ damage.
- Identify modifiable factors that influence pressure.
- Determine other conditions or drugs that may influence the choice of therapy.

conditions in the patient might influence the choice of therapy for hypertension.

The patient with essential hypertension usually is asymptomatic unless target-organ damage occurs. Headache is unusual except when diastolic pressures exceed 120 mm Hg. It is worthwhile to look for signs and symptoms of pheochromocytoma (especially the triad of headaches, palpitations, and excessive perspiration) or aldosteronism (muscle weakness or cramping). Recent weight gain might suggest Cushing syndrome. A long smoking history or other risk factors for accelerated atherosclerosis or a history of angina, myocardial infarction, stroke, claudication, or previous vascular surgery might suggest renovascular hypertension. If hypertension is seen in a pregnancy, especially in a multipara, it often indicates a predisposition to essential hypertension (Fisher et al., 1981).

History of drug use should be recorded. Oral contraceptives, sympathomimetic agents (e.g., OTC cold remedies), NSAIDs, and licorice-containing compounds can all cause or worsen treated and untreated hypertension. Family history is important since a negative family history should suggest the possibility of a secondary cause of the hypertension. Inquiries about diet, especially sodium and alcohol intake, weight change, and patterns of exercise help set priorities for eventual treatment. Assessment of cardiovascular risk factors also may determine when and what to use for drug therapy.

Physical Examination

This must include careful and repeated measurement of blood pressure in the lying and standing positions, recording of body weight, and a complete cardiovascular examination. Special points to seek include a delayed and dampened femoral pulse in a young patient that suggests coarctation of the aorta. Arterial bruits, especially an epigastric bruit, may suggest renal artery stenosis. Blood volume status should be assessed

utilizing supine and upright measurements of blood pressure, measurements of the jugular venous pressure, assessment for edema, or evidence of cardiac failure. The apex should be inspected carefully for possible lateral displacement with a thrusting diffuse impulse suggesting left ventricular hypertrophy. A fourth heart sound as well as an accentuated aortic second sound can be heard in hypertension, and severe hypertension can be associated with a paradoxically split second sound.

The funduscopic exam is crucial in a hypertensive patient. Findings should be described qualitatively rather than graded. Early hypertensive changes are nonspecific and include diffuse segmental arteriolar narrowing, arterial-venous nicking, and an increase in the venule/arteriole ratio with straightening of vessels. However, evidence of hemorrhages, exudates, and papilledema indicates accelerated or malignant hypertension often requiring hospital admission for aggressive treatment.

Investigations

Minimal investigations that should be done in all patients include urinalysis; creatinine, electrolyte, glucose, and cholesterol profiling in plasma; and an electrocardiogram. These data allow assessment of target-organ damage and cardiovascular risks, help to determine the presence of secondary cause of hypertension, and provide some guidelines for therapy. Other investigations of secondary causes of hypertension should be done if indicated.

Treatment

In the ambulatory patient, the goals of treatment are to

1. Prevent progression of the disease to the malignant phase
2. Reduce the incidence of target-organ complications.

Keeping these in mind, a two-pronged approach to both reduce blood pressure and reduce coexistent risk factors is justified (Table 2–2).

Nonpharmacologic Therapy. Keep in mind that these measures are not always benign and should be subjected to the same scrutiny as drug therapy for efficacy and toxicity. For instance about 50% of the hypertensive population responds to salt restriction with reductions in blood pressure. However, it is fruitless to subject a non-salt-sensitive hypertensive to restrictive maneuvers that ultimately may compromise compliance to more useful measures. The typical western diet includes 150 to 300 mEq of sodium per day. Modest salt restriction to 60 to 90 mEq can be used as a 4-week trial of therapy in hypertensive patients (MacGregor et al., 1982). If there is no effect on blood pressure, salt restriction should be discontinued. Periodic 24-hour or spot urinary sodium determinations can help monitor the overall intake of salt and encourage compliance.

Obesity confers an increased risk for cardiovascular disease, either directly or via the association of glucose intolerance, low HDL and high LDL cholesterol, or hypertension (Gordon and Kannel, 1976). Once the pressure has been carefully documented in an obese hypertensive patient, weight reduction should be implemented (or at least attempted). Weight reduction may not work in the mildly obese patient, but patients more than 20% above ideal weight experience an average decrease of 21/12 mm Hg after a 12-kg loss (Horell, 1982).

Other dietary factors are being studied in hypertensive patients, but their effectiveness is controversial. Diets containing high potassium, magnesium, and calcium intakes have been reported to lower pressure (Kaplan, 1985).

As practitioners, we tend to forget that alcohol, caffeine, and nicotine also are drugs. All these can elevate blood pressure. Ethanol intake above 2 oz per day and caffeine intake greater than 4 cups per day can contribute to hypertension. Of course, every smoker should be helped to quit (see chapter 27).

Isotonic exercise such as walking, jogging, or swimming for at least 30 minutes three times weekly can reduce blood pressure. Although experience is limited, recent studies suggest that modest reductions in blood pressure also can be achieved by means of meditation techniques, biofeedback, relaxation therapy, and so forth (for reviews, see Kaplan, 1985; Joint National Committee, 1986; Chockalingam et al., 1990). *Principle: Substantial progress toward a therapeutic end point may be made when multiple maneuvers (no one of which has dramatic efficacy) are combined to accomplish the same end point.*

Drug Therapy.   Intervention with drug therapy is indicated for mild hypertensive patients who have not sufficiently responded to nondrug therapy and in all patients with moderate or severe hypertension. Rational choices can be made based on correct clinical diagnosis, complete assessment of the patient, and a number of other factors (Table 2-9).

Many guidelines for the choice of therapy are available, and some authors continue to recommend *step care* routines. The Canadian Consensus Conference recommends diuretics and β-adrenergic antagonists as first-line agents, with calcium blockers and ACE inhibitors reserved for

Table 2-9.   FACTORS INFLUENCING CHOICE OF DRUG THERAPY

- The likely pathophysiology in individual patients (patient demographic predictors)
- Pharmacology of drugs related to individual pathophysiology
- Anticipated adverse effects—short and long term
- Concomitant diseases
- Other antihypertensives or other drugs in use
- Cost
- Frequency of drug administration and likelihood of compliance
- Proven efficacy in reducing mortality and morbidity
- Patient lifestyle

those with contraindications (Myers et al., 1989). The American recommendations are for either diuretics, β-adrenergic antagonists, calcium blockers, or ACE inhibitors as first-line therapy (Joint National Committee, 1988). The choice of the first drug(s) should be based on patient factors and knowledge of the drug's pharmacology. In practice, one works through a checklist of drugs and considers each in the context of the factors influencing choice of drug therapy (Tables 2-9 and 2-10).

The likely pathophysiology underlying hypertension in any individual patient may guide therapy, but this remains controversial. For instance, early hypertension in the younger patient is characterized by elevated cardiac output. Thus, in this setting, it might be more logical to use a drug that reduces cardiac output rather than a drug that reduces peripheral resistance. Concentrations of renin are lower in blacks and in the elderly. One might thereby predict the response to various drugs that have effects on the renin system. Unfortunately, in practice, there is no way to predict response of a given individual to a given drug. Therefore, one chooses a candidate drug and submits it to an empirical trial starting at low doses (Brunner et al., 1990). The anticipated adverse effects in the individual (both short- and long-term) are a far greater consideration, since all antihypertensive drugs used as monotherapy produce similar degrees of pressure lowering when directly compared in large populations.

The presence of other diseases will certainly affect the choice of therapy. For instance, a drug that predisposes to bronchoconstriction (e.g., any β antagonist) should be avoided in a patient with asthma, whereas a drug that prevents migraines (e.g., some β-adrenergic antagonists, and calcium blockers) should be tried in a patient with the combination of hypertension and migraines. Similarly, patients with symptoms of benign prostatic hypertrophy may respond well to prazosin. *Principle: Search out indications other than primary uses for an agent in a patient who has more than*

Table 2-10. CHECKLIST OF COMMONLY USED DRUGS BY CLASS

DRUG CLASS	GENERIC DRUG
Diuretics	Thiazides, loop, potassium-sparing
β-Adrenergic antagonists	All members
Calcium-channel blockers	Diltiazem, verapamil, nifedipine
ACE inhibitors	Captopril, enalapril, lisinopril
Central adrenergic inhibitors	Methyldopa, clonidine, guanabenz, guanfacine
Peripheral adrenergic inhibitors	Reserpine
α-Adrenergic antagonists	Prazosin, terazosin, doxazosin
"Direct" vasodilators	Hydralazine, minoxidil

one treatable medical problem—"two for the price of one" (Table 2-5).

Cost of therapy should remain a major consideration in choices of drugs. Many patients are not insured for the cost of drugs and will not even fill prescriptions for expensive agents. The cost of medication for those who are insured is shared by society as a whole in taxes, insurance rates, and so forth. Table 2-11 lists costs for commonly used drugs. From the table (see "Minoxidil") one should note that "milligram for milligram" the stronger formulations are cheaper. If tablets can be divided, this fact can be exploited to save money. However, this does not remain true for the more expensive slow-release formulations (see "Inderal LA" or "verapamil SR" [Isoptin]), which are always more expensive than their "regular" counterparts. Finally as a general rule of thumb, generic formulations and "older" drugs are cheaper. *Principle: When the efficacy of therapy is easily monitored, there is little disadvantage in initially choosing the cheapest preparation of a given chemical entity.*

The ease of administration of a drug should be taken into account since it will impact on a patient's quality of life as well as his or her compliance. In general, pharmacodynamic effects on blood pressure are more prolonged than would be expected from the pharmacokinetic half-life of a preparation. Antihypertensive agents as chronic therapy in stable patients need only be administered once or twice a day. Compliance is challenged when drugs are given three or more times daily.

When considering using an antihypertensive drug, the physician should have a working knowledge of its effectiveness in clinical trials. Currently only the older drugs have been shown to reduce morbidity and mortality in the large-scale clinical trials (e.g., diuretics, β-adrenergic antagonists, methyldopa, reserpine, hydralazine). Information should be forthcoming for the newer agents, and there is no reason to suspect that they will be ineffective. Until they are shown to be effective, however, this should remain a consideration in choice of therapy. *Principle: When individual drugs are approved for marketing on the* basis of their efficacy on surrogate end points of therapy, they are rarely compared with other entities used for the same indications on those end points or on the ultimate efficacy for which the drug will be used.

Finally one should consider prior use of antihypertensive drug therapy and current antihypertensive drug therapy. If at all possible, two drugs that are synergistic should be used, and two drugs that have additive adverse effects should be avoided. This common-sense principle is very useful in guiding multiple-drug therapy. An example can be drawn from the *step-care* concept, whereby addition of a vasodilator to a β-adrenergic antagonist plus diuretic regimen is rational since the diuretic will counter the vasodilator-induced salt retention and β blockers the reflex sympathetic actions on the heart and venous systems.

General Principles of Antihypertensive Drug Therapy

1. **Normalize extracellular fluid volume before other pharmacologic manipulations are carried out.** Volume overload is signaled by peripheral edema, elevated jugular venous pulse (JVP), a gain in weight, or signs of heart failure. Volume overload is particularly important in a patient with hypertension caused by primary renal disease and in patients who are taking arteriolar vasodilators (minoxidil, hydralazine) that cause reflex salt and water retention. Conversely, a patient who is volume-depleted may have excessive stimulation of his or her renin and sympathetic systems and exhibit hypertension on that basis.

2. **Use two drugs at low dose, rather than "pushing" the dose of a single drug causing adverse effects.** The effects of most antihypertensive drugs plateau as the dose is increased. That is, in the lower-dosage range, small increments in dosage result in enhanced lowering of pressure. Whereas in the higher-dosage range, even large increments produce relatively little further hypotensive effect (Fig. 2-3). In contrast, the dose-dependent incidence of adverse effects continues to increase in the higher-dose ranges. Using two drugs in low dosage often exploits synergistic effi-

Table 2-11.   COST COMPARISON OF COMMONLY USED AGENTS[a]

	COST/TABLET ($)	COST/WK ($)[b]
Hydrochlorothiazide 25 mg o.d.	0.07	0.49
Spironolactone 25 mg o.d.	0.07	0.49
Dyazide 25–50 mg o.d.	0.06	0.42
Aldactazide 25–25 mg o.d.[c]	0.07	0.49
Moduret 50–5 mg (1/2 tab) o.d.[c]	0.32	1.17
Furosemide 40 mg o.d.	0.03	0.21
Propranolol 80 mg b.i.d.	0.07	0.98
Inderal LA 160 mg o.d.[d]	0.94	6.58
Atenolol 50 mg o.d.	0.43	3.01
Labetalol 200 mg b.i.d.	0.35	4.90
Acebutolol 200 mg b.i.d.	0.17	2.38
Pindolol 10 mg (1/2 tab) b.i.d.	0.43	3.01
Sotalol 160 mg o.d.	0.91	6.37
Nadolol 80 mg o.d.	0.58	4.06
Timolol 10 mg b.i.d.	0.37	5.18
Metoprolol 50 mg b.i.d.	0.09	1.26
Methyldopa 500 mg o.d.	0.27	1.89
Clonidine 0.1 mg b.i.d.	0.25	3.50
Reserpine 0.1 mg o.d.	0.06	0.42
Prazosin 2 mg b.i.d.	0.32	4.48
Terazosin 5 mg o.d.	0.86	6.02
Verapamil SR 240 mg o.d.	1.27	8.59
Verapamil 120 mg b.i.d.	0.37	5.18
Diltiazem SR 120 mg b.i.d.	1.10	15.40
Nifedipine PA* 20 mg b.i.d.	0.55	7.70
Captopril 25 mg b.i.d.	0.47	6.58
Enalapril 10 mg o.d.	0.88	6.16
Lisinopril 5 mg o.d.	0.68	4.76
Hydralazine 50 mg b.i.d.	0.36	5.04
Minoxidil 2.5 mg, (2 tabs) b.i.d.	0.29	8.12
Minoxidil 10 mg, (1/2 tab) b.i.d.[f]	0.64	4.48

[a] At St. Paul's Hospital Pharmacy, Vancouver, Canada, August 1990. These are list prices from manufacturers, and retail pharmacy prices are usually higher.
[b] Excludes prescribing fees.
[c] For comparison with generic hydrochlorothiazide.
[d] For comparison with generic propranolol.
[e] For comparison with slow-release preparation.
[f] Note same dosage = 5 mg b.i.d. but marked difference in price.
*SR = slow release; PA = prolonged action.

cacy between drugs, allowing maintenance of these low doses and avoidance or a minimization of adverse effects. Note that recommended doses in this text are generally lower than those suggested elsewhere.

3. **In severe hypertension, add drugs, rather than substituting one class of agent for another.** When blood pressure is controlled with the use of the added drug, attempts can then be made to reduce or discontinue other agents. In patients with severe hypertension, one may be unsure whether the drug is having an effect and whether the pressure would be much higher in its absence. Withdrawing a useful agent and allowing the pressure to rise might exacerbate the disease and be dangerous to the patient. In treating mild hypertension, sequential use of drugs as monotherapy can help to empirically determine the most effective agent with the least toxicity in the patient (Brunner et al., 1990).

4. **Individualize the target (goal) blood pressure for each patient.** Concomitant medical conditions in the patient may be important factors in considering antihypertensive therapy. For example, a patient with an expected life span of 2 years due to a malignant neoplasm need not be treated aggressively; rather, blood pressure should only be kept out of the severe range to prevent the acute and severe complications of hypertension.

Patients with target-organ damage should be treated more aggressively than others since they are at greater risk and may be more likely to benefit from such treatment strategies. Patients with other risk factors for atherosclerosis should perhaps be treated more vigorously for the same reason. One might have to accept higher blood pressures in patients who have intolerable adverse effects with many drugs. Until more data are available, a conservative approach to treating hypertension is justified in the elderly since they may be less tolerant to lowering their blood pressures than younger people with the same abnormalities.

5. **Use the lowest possible doses to maintain pressure below the target blood pressure.** Once the goal for blood pressure reduction has been attained with drug therapy, attempts should be made to minimize the dosage required to keep the patient at this level. Because of the implications of lifelong therapy of hypertension, maintaining patients on the lowest possible drug dosage for the longest possible time is justified.

6. **Avoid drugs that worsen concomitant disease, and use drugs that are indicated in concomitant disease.** Optimize the two-for-one concept.

7. **Monitor responses to all drugs and evaluate each for its contribution to therapy.**

Special Settings Requiring Consideration for Antihypertensive Therapy

Very Severe Hypertension. Management of patients with very high blood pressure depends on the clinical setting rather than the actual levels of blood pressure. One must be able to distinguish the true hypertensive emergency (Table 2–12) from the noncrisis situation since the risks of lowering blood pressure rapidly are considerable and should be avoided unless absolutely necessary.

A hypertensive emergency (or crisis) is a very high (or rapidly rising) blood pressure in which failure to lower the pressure rapidly can lead to death or irreversible damage to target organs in a short period of time. The setting requires prompt judicious lowering of blood pressure to relieve symptoms and signs and arrest and reverse pathologic changes. The hypertensive patient has decreased cerebral autoregulation and therefore is susceptible to cerebral ischemia at a much higher pressure than the normotensive patient would be (Strandgaard, 1976). Accordingly it is especially important to avoid precipitous drops in blood pressure unless the situation warrants taking such risks. In the treatment of a hypertensive crisis,

Table 2–12. HYPERTENSIVE EMERGENCIES

- Hypertensive encephalopathy
- Retinal lesions (that can lead to blindness)
- Pregnancy or postpartum state (with BP > 160/110 mm Hg)
- Aortic dissection
- Intracranial bleeding (controversial)
- Arterial bleeding
- Severe left ventricular failure
- Prolonged, symptomatic, resistant myocardial ischemia
- Catecholamine crises (pheochromocytoma; abrupt withdrawal of clonidine; abrupt withdrawal of other potent antihypertension drugs with a short half-life, e.g., cocaine, amphetamine, etc.)

blood pressures that are in the mildly hypertensive rather than normal range should be aimed for. This gives a cushion in case one overshoots the target.

Figure 2–4 provides an algorithm for thinking about the management of a patient with crisis hypertension. In the hypertensive emergency, blood pressure is lowered over minutes. Therefore the ideal drugs are given IV, are titratable, have rapid onset and offset of action, are predictable in their effects, and are easily monitored. Therapy should be given in such a manner to maintain blood flow to all vital organs. Sodium nitroprusside is one drug of choice. Other drugs can be considered (see Table 2–13). Use of nitroprusside requires intraarterial monitoring of blood pressure in an intensive care unit (ICU) setting. Other useful IV agents include labetalol, diazoxide, or hydralazine when nitroprusside is not available.

If a hypertensive emergency does not exist, the physician should determine whether accelerated or malignant hypertension is present as evidenced by hemorrhages, exudates, or papilledema. Accelerated hypertension is defined as very high blood pressure with retinal hemorrhages and exudates. Malignant hypertension is defined as very high blood pressure with papilledema. Principles of management of these two entities are the same. Since changes in the retina reflect changes in other vital tissues, it is important to decrease and eventually normalize pressure in order to minimize and possibly reverse these changes. However, these changes have evolved slowly and should be reversed gradually. It must be emphasized that the presence of these ocular findings and a very high blood pressure does *not* necessarily indicate that the blood pressure should be rapidly lowered. Indeed, many patients with these findings are inappropriately treated too aggressively; this may have tragic consequences without providing any benefits. Therefore, one can choose IV or oral therapy and gradually decrease blood pressure over hours rather than minutes. Drugs that are useful for this purpose are also in Table 2–13.

Finally, even in the context of very high pressures, if the patient is asymptomatic and there is no advanced retinopathy, it is safe to slowly decrease blood pressure over days and to use oral agents in an outpatient setting provided that frequent (up to daily) monitoring is feasible if indicated. For review, see Calhoun and Oparil, 1990; Onrot and Rangno, 1990.

Hypertension in the Elderly and Isolated Systolic Hypertension. Systolic blood pressure continues to rise with age, but diastolic pressure rises until 60 to 65 years, when it plateaus (National Health Examination Survey, 1964). With normal aging, there is a fall in cardiac output and a rise

VERY SEVERE OR CRISIS HYPERTENSION

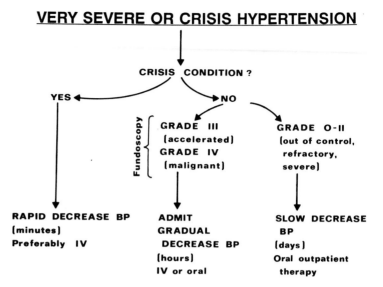

Fig. 2–4. Algorithm for management of patients with severe hypertension. For crisis condition, see Table 2–12. BP = blood pressure (reprinted from Onrot and Rangno, 1990, with permission).

in systemic vascular resistance. In addition, aging reduces the compliance of the great vessels. Normally, ejection of the stroke volume from the left ventricle into the aorta stretches the aortic wall. During diastole, blood flows down the arterial tree as the large vessels contract. This *windkessel* effect is useful in distributing the cardiac output more evenly between systole and diastole. With loss of the windkessel effect, systolic pressure is raised, diastolic pressure is lowered, and more blood is delivered to the peripheral tissues during systole and less during diastole. In the absence of other complicating factors, the pulse pressure (systolic minus diastolic pressure) is a reasonable index of large artery compliance; the index widens with decreased compliance. The mean arterial

Table 2–13.   CLINICAL PHARMACOLOGY OF SOME USEFUL DRUGS

DRUG	DOSE	ONSET	PEAK	DURATION	COMMENT*
Nitroprusside	0.05–10 mg/kg/min titratable infusion	5 sec	2 min	5 min	DOC; thiocyanate toxicity
Diazoxide	50-mg bolus; titrate q. 5–15 min	1–5 min	5–15 min	1–18 h	Alternative DOC; elicits reflex effects
Labetalol	5- to 10 mg bolus; titrate q. 15–20 min or 10–20 mg/h as a titratable infusion	5–10 min	10–30 min	1–12 h	Alternative DOC; useful IV β-adrenergic antagonist
Hydralazine	5–20 mg bolus; titrate q. 20–60 min	10 min	30 min	1–6 h	Useful on ward as p.r.n. medication
Trimethaphan	0.05- to 5-mg/min titratable infusion	1 min	5–10 min	15 min	Useful in aortic dissections; respiratory depression
Phentolamine	1- to 5 mg bolus; titrate q. 2–5 min	< 15 sec	3–5 min	15 min	Useful in catechol crisis; useful in patients who have not eaten (NPO)
Methyldopa	250–1000 mg q6h	2 h	4–6 h	24 h	Not for emergencies
Nifedipine	5–10 mg p.o. or s.l.	5 min	20–30 min	2–6 h	Good if chest pain; rapid-acting oral agent
Clonidine	0.2 mg orally	30 min	90 min	6 h	Outpatient therapy; sedation
Prazosin	0.5–1.0 mg	30 min	120 min	8 h	Outpatient therapy; danger of hypotension
Captopril	6.25–25 mg	45 min	150 min	12 h	Outpatient therapy; danger of hypotension

*DOC = drug of choice; s.l. = sublingual.

pressure is a reasonable index of BP = CO × SVR irrespective of changes in aortic wall compliance (Safar and Simon, 1986). This concept of systemic hemodynamic change during aging accounts for the observed trends in blood pressure.

The elderly therefore are susceptible to isolated systolic hypertension (systolic > 160 and diastolic < 95 mm Hg). In fact, in the elderly, systolic rather than diastolic pressure is better correlated with cardiovascular target-organ damage (Kannel et al., 1981).

There are a paucity of data relating to the effectiveness of drug therapy for isolated systolic hypertension. The European Working Party on Hypertension in the Elderly (EWPHE) Study has demonstrated modest benefits from drug therapy in diastolic hypertension in the elderly population (Amery et al., 1985). The results of further studies such as the U.S. Systolic Hypertension in the Elderly Program (SHEP) are eagerly awaited.

The elderly are much more susceptible to the risks of antihypertensive therapy. Adverse effects are more common, and patients are frequently taking other drugs, so the potential for drug interaction and adverse drug reaction is magnified (see chapters 39 and 40). The elderly also have other diseases that may limit their life span or affect the choice of antihypertensive therapy. Theoretically, treating isolated systolic hypertension might further lower diastolic pressure and jeopardize ischemic areas in the brain and myocardium. All these considerations argue for a conservative approach to antihypertensive therapy in the elderly. Finally, there have been no studies in patients over 75 years of age that show benefits of drug therapy in hypertension.

Recommendations. Although data are not conclusive, we would recommend treating isolated systolic hypertension in the elderly in a fashion similar to treating diastolic hypertension. In both settings, we recommend a conservative approach to therapy. A good rule of thumb is to treat a patient with systolic pressures greater than 200 mm Hg and/or diastolic pressures greater than 105 mm Hg. If the patient has demonstrable target-organ damage, we would be more aggressive and would treat if pressure exceeds 180/100 mm Hg. However, in the over-75 group, we would add 20 mm Hg systolic and 5 mm Hg diastolic before treating. These guidelines are similar to those of the Canadian Consensus Conference on Hypertension in the Elderly (Larochelle et al., 1986). They are flexible and should be individualized. ***Principle: It is frequently necessary to make clinical judgments before the outcome of clinical trials is available.***

The choice of drug therapy in the elderly is similar to that in the younger population. However, one must use lower doses because of the susceptibility to adverse effects. In particular one should watch for hyponatremia when using diuretics, and conduction disturbances when using β-adrenergic antagonists or calcium-channel blockers. Drugs that have potential for affecting the sensorium (e.g., adrenergic-inhibiting agents) should be used with caution in the elderly, who are prone to drug-induced deterioration in their mental status. The tendency to orthostatic hypotension is greater in the elderly than the young, and the consequences may be exaggerated because of concomitant atherosclerosis. In the elderly patient with intolerance to multiple medications, one should accept higher pressures. Compliance with a therapeutic regimen often is a problem, and careful written and verbal instructions as well as liaison with the pharmacist, family, and other health care workers is important. Cost may be a consideration as well.

Secondary Hypertension. There are many causes of secondary hypertension (Table 2–14), but curable secondary hypertension is rarely encountered (much fewer than 2% of all hypertensive patients). Secondary hypertension should always be sought in those patients with severe hypertension, hypertension refractory to medical

Table 2–14. CAUSES OF SECONDARY HYPERTENSION

Renal	Renovascular hypertension
	Renal parenchymal disease
	Polycystic kidney disease
	Obstructive kidney disease
Endocrine	Pheochromocytoma
	Primary aldosteronism
	Hyperthyroidism, hypothyroidism
	Hyperparathyroidism
	Acromegaly
	Cushing disease
Neurologic	Increased intracranial pressure
	Space-occupying lesions
	Brainstem disorders
	Stroke
Vascular	Renovascular hypertension (see "Renal")
	Coarctation of the aorta
	Aortic dissection
Drugs	Estrogen compounds and oral contraceptives
	Sympathomimetic agents (e.g., cold remedies)
	Amphetamines
	Cocaine
	Licorice-containing compounds
	NSAIDS
Miscellaneous	Pregnancy
	Sleep apnea

therapy, the young (less than 35 years), and patients with progressive target damage or advanced retinopathy with hemorrhages, exudates, or papilledema. Other clues to secondary hypertension have been noted in the "Clinical Assessment" section.

Pheochromocytoma.   Since pheochromocytoma (tumor of the sympathetic chain or adrenal gland) is life-threatening, any search for secondary hypertension should begin with determination of 24-hour urine catecholamine, vanillylmandelic acid (VMA) and metanephrine concentrations as the standard screen. Patients suspected and proved to have pheochromocytoma should be treated with α-adrenergic blockade followed by β-adrenergic blockade if necessary. The rapidly acting agent phentolamine is useful for controlling hypertensive crises that complicate pheochromocytoma (Table 2–12). The oral agent phenoxybenzamine is used in preparing patients for surgery as well as for long-term therapy in surgically incurable patients.

Renovascular Hypertension.   Renovascular hypertension is defined as hypertension caused by a narrowing of the renal artery(ies). This disease occurs far more commonly in patients with risk factors for atherosclerosis or evidence of atherosclerosis in the abdominal vessels or elsewhere (e.g., the smoker with peripheral vascular disease). There are still not enough data to determine whether medical or surgical (bypass or angioplasty) therapy is superior in all settings, but surgical therapy appears better when there is renal insufficiency, a small kidney, or bilateral disease, and of course when medical therapy fails. Investigation should not be undertaken unless the decision has been made a priori to fix the renal artery if a lesion is found. ***Basic principle: Do not order tests that will not affect diagnosis or management.***

The most sensitive screening test for renal vascular hypertension is the arteriogram. Unfortunately, about 50% of patients with narrowing on arteriogram do not have renovascular hypertension. In these patients, the narrowing is not hemodynamically significant and does not contribute to the high blood pressure. In the setting of a positive arteriogram, further confirmation of renovascular hypertension is sought by sampling renal venous blood to determine the ratio of renal vein renin on the affected versus contralateral side (positive is greater than 1.5 : 1). Other useful tests to determine if the lesions are of hemodynamic significance include isotopic renography and the IV pyelogram. To detect differences in perfusion between the two kidneys, recent interest has centered upon the use of ACE inhibitors to accentuate the difference between an ischemic and a normal kidney to aid in the diagnosis using renography.

ACE inhibitors are logical therapeutic choices since they interrupt the overstimulated renin system. Multiple drug regimens usually are necessary due to the severity of the hypertension.

Primary Aldosteronism.   Primary aldosteronism should be suspected when a patient eating a regular salt diet has a serum potassium concentration under 3.5 mEq/l in the absence of diuretics or less than 3.0 mEq/l while taking diuretics. However many patients with this entity are normokalemic. There are many useful tests including measurements of renin and aldosterone values (random or on ACE-inhibitor) looking for suppression of renin concentrations with elevated aldosterone concentrations. A principle of endocrine diagnosis is to *diagnose an overactive gland, demonstrate failure of suppression.* To do this one attempts to suppress aldosterone secretion with infusions of saline. Failure to suppress below accepted limits indicates aldosteronism. Subsequent tests differentiate bilateral adrenal hyperplasia from a unilateral tumor (Conn syndrome). These include isotopic iodocholesterol scanning, CT scanning, and bilateral adrenal vein sampling (Weinberger, 1983).

Spironolactone, the specific competitive antagonist of aldosterone, is the medical therapy most useful to treat primary aldosteronism. Patients with bilateral adrenal hyperplasia should not have bilateral adrenalectomies but can be managed with large doses of spironolactone. Patients with unilateral aldosteronomas tumors are best operated upon, but if this is not possible, spironolactone usually is effective therapy.

Hypertension Secondary to Renal Parenchymal Disease.   Hypertension secondary to renal parenchymal disease is suspected on clinical grounds and in patients with abnormal serum creatinine concentrations and urinalysis. Hypertension secondary to renal disease is important to diagnose because its treatment and prognosis are different from those in hypertensive patients without compromise of renal function.

Other endocrinopathies ordinarily are not routinely looked for, but when they are clinically suspected, the appropriate tests should be done (Table 2–14).

Finally *drug-induced hypertension* is an easily reversible cause of secondary hypertension and must never be forgotten.

Hypertension during Pregnancy.   Hypertension during pregnancy is defined as blood pressures greater than 140/90 mm Hg or an increase of 30/15 mm Hg over baseline. It is important to differentiate hypertensive disorders encountered in pregnancy. The patient may have pregnancy-induced hypertension (PIH). PIH usually occurs in nulliparas, usually in the third trimester, and in patients with previously normal blood pressures. It can be associated with proteinuria and generalized edema. PIH is characterized by intense vasoconstriction and may have dire effects on the fetus and mother if left unchecked.

The pregnant hypertensive patient alternatively might have chronic hypertension that is ongoing throughout pregnancy. She may also have chronic hypertension with superimposed PIH. Finally, a patient may develop hypertension late in pregnancy without edema or proteinuria indicating a more benign situation.

Patients with PIH may be asymptomatic or may evidence recent weight gain, edema, headache, and tremors. On physical examination, they may be found to be "small for dates of the pregnancy" and have hypertension and edema. The retina has a glistening sheen, usually with arteriolar narrowing, and the patient is hyperreflexic and may have clonus. Laboratory tests may reveal anemia, changes consistent with microangiopathy or disseminated intravascular coagulation (DIC), abnormal renal function, high uric acid concentrations, proteinuria, mildly abnormal concentrations of liver enzymes in plasma, and/or thrombocytopenia. Treatment of mild PIH involves bed rest in the lateral decubitus position as much as possible. In the setting of disease, mild oral antihypertensive agents such as methyldopa, hydralazine, or β-adrenergic antagonists have proven efficacy. Diuretics are best avoided in PIH because these patients usually exhibit volume contraction. The patient with severe PIH (BP greater than 160/110 mm Hg) should receive IV β-adrenergic antagonists (labetalol), parenteral hydralazine, or oral nifedipine for rapid lowering of her blood pressure. Nitroprusside should not be used. Magnesium sulphate is used to prevent seizures.

The ultimate treatment for PIH is, of course, delivery. Postpartum patients may be hypertensive for up to 6 months after delivery. Recent studies suggest the preventive role for low-dose aspirin (60 mg daily) in PIH to address the potential abnormalities of vasoconstrictor- and thrombosis-promoting prostaglandins (Wallenburg et al., 1986).

Women with chronic hypertension may be suspected before pregnancy or detected during pregnancy. Essential hypertension during pregnancy rather than PIH is suspected when the blood pressure is higher than 140/90 mm Hg before 20 weeks. In this setting, the blood pressure should be maintained below 140/90 mm Hg during the pregnancy. One avoids ACE inhibitors, reserpine, and nifedipine early in pregnancy because of their teratogenic potential. Methyldopa or β-adrenergic antagonists are most useful. Diuretics can be used in this setting in contradistinction to PIH. For review, see Lindheimer and Katz, 1985.

Withdrawal of Antihypertensive Drug. Even gradual, controlled, and well-monitored discontinuation of antihypertensive drugs often provokes anxiety in the minds of most physicians and patients. Concern exists that hypertension will always return to, or exceed, previous untreated values after the drugs are discontinued. This ignores the beneficial changes in lifestyle plus drug-induced damping or reversal of pathophysiology. A recent review of five large studies shows that from 15% to 74% of previously treated "hypertensive" patients remained normotensive for 12 to 36 months after their medication was stopped (Flecter et al., 1988). Additionally, many patients may be maintained normotensive on reduced dose of antihypertensive drugs after prolonged therapy. While misdiagnosis and inappropriate treatment might account for some of this reversal, it surely cannot account for all.

Some predictors of maintained normotension after discontinuation of antihypertensive drugs are pretreatment diastolic pressures < 105 mm Hg, treated pressures < 140/90 mm Hg, a long duration of controlled hypertension, and interim weight loss. When patients have had a taste of the inconvenience, adverse effects, and cost of medication, the offer of reduction or discontinuation of therapy may be an enticement to consider appropriate and useful changes in lifestyle.

Hypertension is a lifelong problem, and temporary loss of control is probably not harmful to the patient as long as severe hypertension is avoided. When the blood pressure increases upon discontinuation of a drug, it is reassuring proof of the drug's continuing efficacy. There may be concern that some drugs, like β-adrenergic antagonists, when taken chronically can result in adaptation with receptor up-regulation. Theoretically this could produce a risky "rebound" withdrawal syndrome if the drug is suddenly stopped. Rebound of blood pressure and heart rate is well documented after withdrawal from clonidine and some short-half-life β-adrenergic antagonists (Rangno, 1984). Most antihypertensive drugs have not been systematically studied after withdrawal, and so one must always be cautious and not stop abruptly. Rebound can be avoided by gradual tapering of the drug.

Recommendation. Once the blood pressure is well controlled at or below target goals, institute a cautious trial of tapering one agent at a time with frequent (e.g., every 2 weeks) monitoring of the blood pressure to ensure that escape from control has not occurred. ***Principle: Periodically reevaluate the need to treat and choice of drug therapy in most chronic diseases.***

REFERENCES

Amery, A.; Birkenhäger, W.; Brixko, P.; Bulpitt, C.; Clement, D.; Deruyttere, M.; de Schaepdryver, A.; Dollery, C.; Fagard, F.; Forette, F.; Forte, J.; Hamdy, R.; Henry, J. F.; Joosens, J. V.; Leonetti, G.; Lund-Johansen, P.; O'Malley, K.; Petrie, J.; Strasser, T.; Tuomilehto, J.; and Williams, B.: Mortality and morbidity results from the European Working Party on High Blood Pressure in the Elderly trial. Lancet, 2: 1349–1354, 1985.

Anderson, S.; and Brenner B. M.: The role of infra-glomerular hypertension in the initiation and progression of renal disease. J. Hypertens., 4(suppl. 5):S236–S238, 1986.

Anonymous: Treatment of hypertension: The 1985 results. Lancet, 2:645–647, 1985.

Australian Therapeutic Trial in Mild Hypertension: A report by the management committee. Untreated mild hypertension. Lancet, 1:185–191, 1982.

Australian Therapeutic Trial in Mild Hypertension: Report by the management committee. Lancet, 1:1261–1267, 1980.

Bayliss, R. I. S.; and Harvey-Smith, E. A.: Methyldopa in the treatment of hypertension. Lancet, 1:763–768, 1962.

Beta-Blocker Heart Attack Trial Research Group: A randomized trial of propranolol in patients with acute myocardial infarction: I. Mortality results. J.A.M.A., 247:1707–1714, 1982.

Broughton, P. F.; Symonds, E. M.; and Turner, S. R.: The effect of captopril (SQ 14,225) upon mother and fetus in the chronically cannulated ewe and on the pregnant rabbit. J. Physiol., 323:415–422, 1982.

Brunner, H. R.; Menard, J.; Waeber, B.; Burnier, M.; Biollaz, J.; Nussberger, J.; and Bellet, M.: Treating the individual hypertensive patient: Considerations on dose, sequential monotherapy and drug combinations. J. Hypertens., 8:3–11, 1990.

Calhoun, D. A.; and Oparil, S.: Treatment of hypertensive crisis. N. Engl. J. Med. 323(17):1177–1183, 1990.

Canadian Enalapril Study Group: Comparison of monotherapy with enalapril and atenolol in mild to moderate hypertension. Can. Med. Assoc. J., 137:803–808, 1987.

Carlsen, J. E.; Kober, L.; Torp-Pedersen, C.; and Johansen, P.: Relation between dose of bendrofluazide, antihypertensive effect, and adverse biochemical effects. Br. Med. J., 300: 975–978, 1990.

Case, D. B.: Angiotensin-converting enzyme inhibitors: Are they all alike? J. Clin. Hypertens., 3:243–256, 1987.

Chockalingam, A.; Laidlaw, J.; Abbott, D.; Bass, M.; Barrista, R.; Cameron, R.; de Champlain, J.; Evans, C. E.; Laidlaw, J.; Lee, B. L.; Leiter, L.; Lessard, R.; MacLean, D.; Nishikawa, J.; Rabkin, S.; Thibaudeau, C.; and Strachan, D.: Recommendations of the Canadian Consensus Conference on non-pharmacological approaches to the management of high blood pressure. Can. Med. Assoc. J., 142:1397–1409, 1990.

Clark, J. A.; Zimmerman, H. J.; and Tanner, L. A.: Labetalol hepatotoxicity. Ann. Intern. Med. 113(3):210–213, 1990.

Connor, G.; Wilburn, R. L.; and Bennett, C. M.: Double blind comparison of minoxidil and hydralazine in severe hypertension. Clin. Sci. Mol. Med., 51(suppl.):593s–595s, 1976.

Croog, S. H.; Levine, S.; Testa, M. A.; Brown, B.; Bulpitt, C. J.; Jenkins, C. D.; Klerman, G. L.; and Williams, G. H.: The effects of antihypertensive therapy on quality of life. N. Engl. J. Med., 314:1657–1664, 1986.

Cutler, J. A.; MacMahon, S. W.; and Furberg, C. D.: Controlled clinical trials of drug treatment for hypertension. A Review. Hypertension, 13(suppl. I):I-36–I-44, 1989.

Dahl, L. K.; and Heine, M.: Primary role of renal homografts in setting chronic blood pressure levels in rats. Circ. Res., 36: 692–696, 1975.

Dargie, H.; Cleland, J.; Findlay, I.; Murray, G.; and McInnes, G.: Combination of verapamil and beta blockers in systemic hypertension. Am. J. Cardiol., 57:80D–82D, 1986.

de Wardener, H. E.; and MacGregor, G. A.: The natriuretic hormone and its possible relationship to hypertension. In,

Hypertension (Genest, J.; Kuchel, O.; Hamet, T.; and Cantin, M.; eds.). McGraw-Hill, New York, pp. 84–94, 1983.

Dietz, R.; Haass, M.; and Kubler, W.: Atrial natriuretic factor. Its possible role in hypertension and congestive heart failure. Am. J. Hypertens., 2:295–335, 1989.

Dzau, V. J.: Evolving concepts of the renin–angiotensin system. Focus on renal and vascular mechanisms. Am. J. Hypertens., 1:334S–337S, 1988.

Feldman, R. D.; Park, G. D.; and Chein-Yu, C. L.: The interaction of verapamil and norverapamil with beta-adrenergic receptors. Circulation, 72:547–554, 1985.

Fisher, K. A.; Luger, A.; Spargo, B. H.; and Lindheimer, M. D.: Hypertension in pregnancy. Clinical-pathological correlations and late prognosis. Medicine, 60:267–268, 1981.

Flecter, A. E.; Franks, P. J.; and Bulpitt, C. J.: The effect of withdrawing antihypertensive therapy: A review. J. Hypertens., 6:431–436, 1988.

Folkow, B.: Early structural changes. Brief historical background and principle nature of process. Hypertension, 6(suppl. III): III-1–III-3, 1984.

Frishman, W. H.; Furberg, C. D.; and Friedewald, W. T.: Beta-adrenergic blockage for survivors of acute myocardial infarction. N. Engl. J. Med., 310:830–837, 1984.

Goldstein, D. S.: Arterial baroreflex sensitivity in essential hypertension. Circulation, 68:234–240, 1983.

Goodwin, F. K.; and Bunney, W. E.: Depressions following reserpine: A reevaluation. Semin. Psychiatr., 3:435–447, 1971.

Gordon, T.; and Kannel, W. B.: Obesity and cardiovascular disease: The Framingham Study. Clin. Endocrinol. Metab., 5:367–375, 1976.

Guyton, A. C.: Dominant role of the kidneys and accessory role of whole body autoregulation in the pathogenesis of hypertension. Am. J. Hypertens., 2:575–585, 1989.

Haynes, R. B.; Sackett, D. L.; Taylor, D. W.; Gibson, E. S.; and Johnson, A. L.: Increased absenteeism from work after the detection and labelling of hypertensive patients. N. Engl. J. Med., 291:741–744, 1978.

Helgeland, A.: Treatment of mild hypertension: A five year controlled drug trial. The Oslo Study. Am. J. Med., 69:725–732, 1980.

Henry, J. A.; and Cassidy S. L.: Membrane stabilizing activity: A major cause of fatal poisoning. Lancet, 1:1414–1417, 1986.

Henry, P. D.: Anti-atherosclerotic effects of calcium antagonists: A brief review. Clin. Invest. Med., 10:601–605, 1987.

Horell, M. F.: The experimental evidence for weight loss treatment of essential hypertension: A critical review. Am. J. Public Health, 72:359–368, 1982.

Houston, M. C.: Clonidine hydrochloride: Review of pharmacological and clinical uses. Prog. Cardiovasc. Dis., 23:337–350, 1981.

Hypertension Detection and Follow-up Program: Five year findings: I. Reduction in mortality of persons with high blood pressure, including mild hypertension. J.A.M.A., 242:2562–2571, 1979.

Inouye, I.; Massie, B.; Benowitz, N.; Simpson, P.; Loge, D.; and Topic, N.: Monotherapy in mild to moderate hypertension: Comparison of hydrochlorothiazide, propranolol and prazosin. Am. J. Cardiol., 53:24A–28A, 1984.

International Prospective Primary Prevention Study on Hypertension Collaborative Group (IPPPSH): J. Hypertens., 3: 379–392, 1985.

Jefferson, D.; Wharrad, H. J.; Birmingham, A. T.; and Patrick, J. M.: The comparative effects of ICI 118551 and propranolol on essential tremor. Br. J. Clin. Pharmacol., 24: 729–734, 1987.

Joint National Committee on Detection, Evaluation, and Treatment of High Blood Pressure: Final report of the subcommittee on nonpharmacological therapy. Hypertension, 8:444–467, 1986.

Joint National Committee: The 1988 report of the Joint National Committee on detection, evaluation, and treatment of high blood pressure. Arch. Intern. Med., 148:1023–1038, 1988.

Just, P. M.: The positive association of cough with angiotensin-converting enzyme inhibitors. Pharmacotherapeutics, 9: 82–87, 1989.

Kannel, W. B.: Role of blood pressure in cardiovascular morbidity and mortality. Prog. Cardiovasc. Dis., 17:5–24, 1974.

Kannel, W. B.; Wolf, P. A.; McGee, D. L.; Dawber, T. R.; McNamara, P.; and Castelli, W. P.: Systolic blood pressure, arterial rigidity, and the risk of stroke: The Framingham study. J.A.M.A., 245:1225–1229, 1981.

Kannel, W. B.; Castelli, W. P.; and Gordon, T.: Cholesterol in the prediction of atherosclerotic disease. New perspectives based on the Framingham study. Ann. Intern. Med., 90:85–91, 1979.

Kaplan, J. R.; Manuck, S. B.; Adams, M. R.; Weingand, K. W.; and Clarkson, T. B.: Inhibition of coronary atherosclerosis by propranolol in behaviorally predisposed monkeys fed an atherogenic diet. Circulation, 76:1364–1372, 1987.

Kaplan, N. M.: Alpha-blockade for hypertension. Lancet, 1: 1448–1449, 1989.

Kaplan, N. M.: Non-drug treatment of hypertension. Ann. Intern. Med., 102:359–373, 1985.

Keane, W. F.; Anderson, S.; Aurell, M.; de Zeeuw, D.; Narins, R. G.; and Povar, G.: Angiotensin converting enzyme inhibitors and progressive renal insufficiency. Ann. Intern. Med., 111:503–516, 1989.

Kleinert, H. D.; Harshfield, G. A.; Pickering, T. G.; Devereux, R. B.; Sullivan, P. A.; Marion, R. M.; Mallory, W. K.; and Laragh, J. H.: What is the value of home blood pressure measurement in patients with mild hypertension? Hypertension, 6:574–578, 1984.

Larochelle, P.; Bass, M. J.; Birkett, N. J.; deChamplain, J.; Myers, M. G.: Recommendations from the Consensus Conference on hypertension in the elderly. Can. Med. Assoc. J., 135:741–745, 1986.

Laupacis, A.; Sackett, D.L; and Roberts, R. S.: An assessment of clinically useful measures of the consequences of treatment. N. Engl. J. Med., 318:1728–1733, 1988.

Leenen, F. H. H.; Smith, D. L.; Farkas, R. M.; Reeves, R. A.; and Marquez-Julio, A.: Vasodilators and regression of left ventricular hypertrophy. Hydralazine versus prazosin in hypertensive humans. Am. J. Med., 82:969–978, 1987.

Lette, J.; Gagnon, R. M.; Lemire, J. G.; and Morissette, M.: Rebound of vasospastic angina after cessation of long-term treatment with nifedipine. Can. Med. Assoc. J., 130:1169–1172, 1984.

Lindheimer, M. D.; and Katz, A. I.: Hypertension in pregnancy. N. Engl. J. Med., 313:675–680, 1985.

Logan, A. G.: Report of the Canadian Hypertension Society's consensus conference on the management of mild hypertension. Can. Med. Assoc. J., 131:1053–1057, 1984.

MacGregor, G. A.; Markandu, N. D.; Best, F. E.; Elder, D. M.; Cam, J. M.; Sagnella, G. A.; and Squires, M.: Double-blind, randomised, crossover trial of moderate sodium restriction in essential hypertension. Lancet, 1:351–356, 1982.

MacMahon, S. W.; and MacDonald, G. J.: Antihypertensive treatment and plasma lipiprotein levels. The associations in data from a population study. Am. J. Med., 80(suppl. 2A): 40–47, 1986.

McMahon, F. C.: Efficacy of antihypertensive agents; comparison of alpha methyldopa plus hydrochlorothiazide in combination and singly. J.A.M.A., 231:155–158, 1975.

Maisel, A. S.; Motulsky, H. J.; and Insel, P. A.: Hypotension after quinidine plus verapamil. N. Engl. J. Med., 312(3):167–170, 1985.

Mancia, G.; Grassi, G.; and Pomidossi, G.: Effects of blood-pressure measurement by the doctor on patient's blood pressure and heart rate. Lancet, 2:695–698, 1983.

Medical Research Council Working Party: MRC trial of treatment of mild hypertension: Principal results. Br. Med. J., 291:97–104, 1985.

Morgan, T.: The use of diuretic drugs and aldosterone antagonists in hypertension. In, Handbook of Hypertension (Doyle,

A. R. E., ed.). Vol. 5, Clinical Pharmacology of Antihypertensive Drugs. Elsevier, Amsterdam, pp. 67–91, 1984.

Motomura, S.; Zerkowski, H. R.; Daul, A.; and Brodde, O. E.: On the physiologic role of beta 2 adrenoceptors in the human heart: In vitro and in vivo studies. Am. Heart J., 119: 608–619, 1990.

Motulsky, H. J.; and Insel, P. A.: Adrenergic receptors in man. Direct identification, physiologic regulation, and clinical alterations. N. Engl. J. Med., 307:18–29, 1982.

Multiple Risk Factor Intervention Trial: Risk factor changes and mortality results. J.A.M.A., 248:1465–1477, 1982.

Myers, M. G.; Carruthers, S. G.; Leenen, F. H. H.; and Haynes, R. B.: Canadian Hypertension Society Consensus Conference on the pharmacological treatment of hypertension. Can. Med. Assoc. J., 140:1141–1146, 1989.

Myers, M. G.; Leenen, F. H. H.; Burns, R.; and Frankel, D.: Nifedipine tablet vs. hydralazine in patients with persisting hypertension who receive combined diuretic and beta-blocker therapy. Clin. Pharmacol. Ther., 39:409–413, 1986.

National Health Examination Survey—United States 1960–1962. Series 2. Bethesda, U.S. Dept. of Health, Education and Welfare, 1964.

Nicholson, J. P.; Resnick, L. M.; and Laragh, J. H.: Hydrochlorothiazide is not additive to verapamil in treating essential hypertension. Arch. Intern. Med., 149:125–129, 1989.

Nicholson, J. P.; Resnick, L. M.; and Laragh, J. H.: The antihypertensive effect of verapamil at extremes of dietary sodium intake. Ann. Intern. Med., 107:329–334, 1987.

Oates, J. A.; Robertson, D.; Wood, A. J. J.; and Woosley, R. L.: Alpha- and beta-adrenergic agonists and antagonists. In: Cardiac Therapy (Rosen, M. R.; and Hoffman, B. F., eds.). Martinus Nijhoff, Boston, pp. 145–169, 1983.

Onrot, J.: The role of calcium ion in human hypertension. Med. North Am., 7(suppl.):3–11, 1987.

Onrot, J.; and Rangno, R. E.: Management of very high blood pressure. Med. North Am., 7:800–806, 1990.

Onrot, J.; and Ruedy, J.: Hypertension: Diagnosis and management. Med. North Am., 7:1370–1385, 1987.

Perloff, D.; Sokolow, M.; and Cowan, R.: The prognostic value of ambulatory blood pressures. J.A.M.A., 249:2792–2798, 1983.

Pickering, T. G.; Harshfield, G. A.; Devereux, R. B.; and Laragh, J. H.: What is the role of ambulatory blood pressure monitoring in the management of hypertensive patients? Hypertension, 7:171–177, 1985.

Pollare, T.; Lithell, H.; and Berne, C.: A comparison of the effects of hydrochlorothiazide and captopril on glucose and lipid metabolism in patients with hypotension. N. Engl. J. Med., 321:868–873, 1989.

Rangno, R. E.: Beta blocker withdrawal syndrome. In, Beta Blockers in the Treatment of Cardiovascular Disease (Kostis, J. B.; and DeFelice, E. A.; eds.). Raven Press, New York, pp. 275–300, 1984.

Reid, J. L.; and Elliott, H. L.: Methyldopa. In, Handbook of Hypertension. Vol. 5, Clinical Pharmacology of Antihypertensive Drugs (Doyle, A. R. E., ed.). Elsevier, Amsterdam, pp. 92–112, 1984.

Reid, J. L.; Campbell, B. C.; and Hamilton, C. A.: Withdrawal reactions following cessation of central alpha-adrenergic receptor agonists. Hypertension, 6(5):71–75, 1984.

Resnick, L. M.; Nicholson, J. P.; and Laragh, J. H.: Calcium metabolism in essential hypertension: Relationship to altered renin system activity. Fed. Proc., 45:2739–2745, 1986.

Rowland, M.; and Roberts, J.: Blood pressure levels in persons 6–74 years: United States 1976–1980. National Center for Health Statistics, Vital and Health Statistics No. 84. U.S. Dept. of Health and Human Services, Public Health Service, October 8, 1982.

Safar, M. E.; and Simon, A. C.: Hemodynamics in systolic hypertension. In, Handbook of Hypertension. Vol. 7, Cardiovascular Aspects (Tarazi, R.; and Zanchetti, A.; eds.). Elsevier, Amsterdam, pp. 225–241, 1986.

Seely, J. F.; and Dirks, J. H.: Site of action of diuretic drugs. Kidney Int., 11:1–8, 1977.

Semplicini, A.; Pessinac A. C.; Rossi, G. P.; Hlede, M.; and Morandin, F.: Alpha-adrenoceptor blockade by labetalol during long-term dosing. Clin. Pharmacol. Ther., 33:278–282, 1983.

Strandgaard, S.: Autoregulation of cerebral blood flow in hypertensive patients. Circulation, 4:720–727, 1976.

Suderman, P.; Grahnen, A.; Haglund, K.; Lindstrom, B.; and von Bahr, C.: Prazosin dynamics in hypertension: Relationship to plasma concentration. Clin. Pharmacol. Ther., 30: 447–454, 1981.

Taverner, D.; Bing, R. F.; Heagerty, A.; Russell, G. I.; Pohl, J. E. F.; Swales, J. O.; and Thurston, H.: Improvement of renal function during long term treatment of severe hypertension with minoxidil. Q. J. Med., 206:280–287, 1983.

Traub, Y. M.; and Levey, B. A.: Combined treatment with minoxidil and captopril in refractory hypertension. Arch. Intern. Med., 143:1142–1144, 1983.

Vane, J. R.; Anggard, E. E.; and Botting, R. M.: Regulatory functions of the vascular endothelium. N. Engl. J. Med. 323: 27–36, 1990.

Van Zwieten, P. A.: Pathophysiological relevance of serotonin. J. Cardiovasc. Pharmacol., 10(suppl. 3):S19–S25, 1987.

Veterans Administration Cooperative Study Group on Antihypertensive Agents: Comparison of propranolol and hydrochlorothiazide for the initial treatment of hypertension: II. Results of long-term therapy. J.A.M.A., 248:2004–2011, 1982.

Veterans Administration Cooperative Study Group on Antihypertensive Agents: Comparison of prazosin with hydralazine in patients receiving hydrochlorothiazide. A randomized double-blind clinical trial. Circulation, 64:772–779, 1981.

Veterans Administration Cooperative Study Group on Antihypertensive Agents: Effects of treatment on morbidity in hypertension: II. Results in patients with diastolic blood pressure averaging 90 through 114 mm Hg. J.A.M.A., 213:1143–1152, 1970.

Veterans Administration Medical Centers: Low dose vs standard dose of reserpine: A randomized, double-blind, multiclinic trial in patients taking chlorthalidone. J.A.M.A., 248: 2471–2477, 1982.

Waeber, B.; Aubert, J. F.; Corder, R.; Evequoz, D.; Nussberger, J.; Gaillard, R.; and Brunner, H. R.: Cardiovascular effects of neuropeptide Y. Am. J. Hypertens., 1:193–199, 1988.

Wallenburg, H. C. S.; Makovitz, J. W.; Dekker, G. A.; and Rotmans, P.: Low-dose aspirin prevents pregnancy-induced WHO/ISH Meeting Memorandum: 1986 guidelines for the treatment of mild hypertension. J. Hypertens., 4:383–386, 1986.

Williams, G. H.: Converting-enzyme inhibitors in the treatment of hypertension. N. Engl. J. Med., 319(23):1517–1525, 1988.

World Health Organization: Arterial Hypertension Report of WHO Expert Committee. Technical report series No. 628. 1978.

Zsoter, T. T.; Nebitko, R. L.; and Chow, R.: The effect of verapamil, diltiazem and nifedipine on baroreceptor reflexes. Clin. Invest. Med., 2(6):430–434, 1988.

3

Treatment of Cardiovascular Disorders: Orthostatic Hypotension

David Robertson

DEFINITION OF ORTHOSTATIC HYPOTENSION

Orthostatic hypotension can be defined as any fall in blood pressure on standing that causes symptoms (Blomqvist and Stone, 1984; Houston et al., 1984; Onrot et al., 1987c; Streeten, 1987). This operational definition avoids the difficulty of specifying an absolute blood pressure below which a pathologic condition is universal and above which normality can be reliably inferred. Some young individuals whose sphygmomanometric blood pressures are routinely near 85/40 mm Hg, whether lying or standing, have no symptoms referable to this supposed "hypotension" (Pemberton, 1989). Conversely, some elderly individuals with significant atherosclerosis in their cerebral vasculature may manifest symptoms of inadequate cerebral perfusion when blood pressure has only fallen from, for example, 150/95 to 130/80 mm Hg. Perhaps the best reason to rely upon an operational definition of orthostatic hypotension is that there is no current justification for the treatment of any patient, however low his or her blood pressure, if it is not causing symptoms or limiting his or her activities in any way.

Although there are probably a number of patients in the early literature whose symptoms were due to chronic hypotension (Beales, 1856), recognition of the syndrome of orthostatic hypotension came slowly. Only in 1925 did a clear description of autonomic failure appear (Bradbury and Eggleston, 1925).

Orthostatic hypotension is a highly variable phenomenon. In many patients, it is completely absent at certain times of the day. In other patients, it may be present in the morning but not later in the day, after a large breakfast but not before breakfast, after climbing a flight of stairs but not before (Robertson et al., 1981; Mathias et al., 1989a). In other individuals, orthostatic hypotension may be present at all times, while its degree remains variable. Other major determinants of the degree of hypotension include hyperventilation (Burnum et al., 1954), fever, and environmental temperature. In the most severely affected patients, admittedly a small subgroup of all patients with orthostatic symptoms, the upright sphygmomanometric blood pressure can be as low as 60/40 mm Hg. Obviously, at this cuff estimate of blood pressure, the sphygmomanometer is inadequate to assess true intraarterial blood pressure (Cohn, 1967). For this reason, in severely affected patients, it is useful to monitor the severity of disease and its response to therapy by the standing time.

The standing time is defined as the length of time a patient can stand motionless before the onset of symptoms of orthostatic hypotension. In patients with autonomic impairment, standing motionless is more stressful than walking since the pumping action of the calf muscles helps venous return during the latter activity. The most common symptoms of orthostatic hypotension are dizziness or lightheadedness, dimming or tunneling of vision, and pain or discomfort in the back of the neck or head. In a small number of patients, slurred speech may be the presenting symptom. As soon as the patient's herald symptom of orthostatic hypotension appears, he or she is allowed to sit down as the number of elapsed seconds is recorded. If a patient is able to stand for 3 minutes without the onset of symptoms, it is assumed that a reliable blood pressure probably is obtainable, and a sphygmomanometric blood pressure determination is made at that time.

The standing time is primarily of value in monitoring individuals who are unable to stand motionless for as long as 3 minutes. The importance of the standing time is that many individuals who have an increase in standing time from 30 to 120 seconds may have a substantial increase in functional capacity, even though they may have no change in their level of upright blood pressure as assessed by the sphygmomanometer. A patient with a standing time under 30 seconds usually cannot live alone, while a patient with a standing time greater than 60 seconds generally can. Thus, the standing-time determination greatly facilitates the management of the most severely affected patients with orthostatic hypotension. *Principle: Understanding the value of a diagnostic test in establishing both the diagnosis and the adequacy of therapy is key to adequate monitoring of the treated and untreated patient.*

Etiology of Orthostatic Hypotension

The differential diagnosis (Table 3–1) of orthostatic hypotension is extensive (Schirger and Thomas, 1976; Schatz, 1984; Tung et al., 1985; Bannister and Mathias, 1988; Mader, 1989). Acute hypotension can occur in paroxysmal autonomic syncopes (Allen et al., 1945) that may be due to parasympathetic activation and sympathetic withdrawal (Engel, 1978; Williams and Bashore, 1980; Robertson and Robertson, 1981; Mark, 1982; Robertson et al., 1985; Onrot et al., 1987a; Sanders and Ferguson, 1989), but there is not usually a strong orthostatic component.

If one limits consideration to chronic orthostatic hypotension, it is convenient to divide the etiologies into those due to impairment of the autonomic nervous system (dysautonomic orthostatic hypotension) and those due to other causes (sympathotonic orthostatic hypotension) (Nylin and Levander, 1948; Bannister, 1971). There is a disproportionate prevalence of orthostatic hypotension in the older age group (Mader, 1988; Lipsitz, 1989a), but the mechanism of this is not yet certain (Shannon et al., 1986; Lipsitz, 1989b). It is known that there is an age-related reduction in cell bodies in the intermediolateral column of the spinal cord (Low et al., 1977). Chronic orthostatic hypotension is frequently due to an adverse

Table 3–1. DIFFERENTIAL DIAGNOSIS OF ORTHOSTATIC HYPOTENSION

Autonomic Disorders
  Primary autonomic failure (Bradbury-Eggleston syndrome)
  Multiple system atrophy (Shy-Drager syndrome)
  Familial dysautonomia (Riley-Day syndrome)
  Dopamine-β-hydroxylase deficiency
  Monoamine oxidase deficiency
  Baroreceptor dysfunction
  Acute pandysautonomia
  Secondary autonomic neuropathies

Hypovolemic Disorders
  Hemorrhage or plasma loss
  Overdiuresis
  Overdialysis
  Idiopathic hypovolemia

Endocrinologic Disorders
  Addison disease
  Hypoaldosteronism
  Pheochromocytoma (see de Gennes et al., 1964)
  Renovascular hypertension

Vascular Insufficiency
  Varicose veins (see Arenander, 1960; Chapman and Asmussen, 1942)
  Absent venous valves
  Arteriovenous malformations

Vasodilator Excess
  Mastocytosis (histamine, prostaglandin D_2)
  Hyperbradykininism (bradykinin and other vasodilators)
  Carcinoid (bradykinin)
  Hypermagnesemia (see Ferdinandus et al., 1981)

Paroxysmal Autonomic Syncopes
  Glossopharyngeal syncope (see Ray and Stewart, 1948; Onrot et al., 1987a)
  Micturition syncope (see Lyle et al., 1961)
  Carotid sinus syndrome (see Draper, 1950)
  Swallow syncope
  Cough syncope (see Sharpey-Schaefer, 1953; Baker, 1949)
  Bezold-Jarisch reflex activation

Miscellaneous
  Drugs (see Benowitz et al., 1980)
  Stokes-Adams attacks (see Barlow and Howarth, 1953)
  Mitral valve prolapse syndrome
  Gastrectomy (see Cohen, 1957)
  Hypokinesia, weightlessness, prolonged bed rest

drug effect. The most common such agents are tricyclic antidepressants, phenylpropanolamine, diuretics, clonidine, and marijuana.

There are many specialized tests for the evaluation of autonomic function at the bedside and these have been extensively reviewed (Thomson and Melmon, 1968; Dobkin and Rosenthal, 1975; Low et al., 1977; Robertson et al., 1984a, 1984b; Eckberg, 1980). Autonomic regulation of the blood pressure is modulated by cardiovascular control nuclei in the brainstem (Resnik et al.,

1936). A complex array of neurotransmitters appear to be involved (Tung et al., 1983; Robertson et al., 1988; Tseng et al., 1988). These sites, if damaged, may lead to the abnormalities characteristic of various forms of autonomic failure (Table 3–2).

SPECIFIC SYNDROMES

Bradbury-Eggleston Syndrome (Idiopathic Orthostatic Hypotension)

The Bradbury-Eggleston syndrome (idiopathic orthostatic hypotension or pure autonomic failure) is a degenerative disorder of the autonomic nervous system present in middle to late life. The

Table 3–2. CAUSES OF AUTONOMIC FAILURE

CAUSE	REFERENCE
Bradbury-Eggleston syndrome (idiopathic orthostatic hypotension, primary autonomic failure)	Bradbury and Eggleston, 1925
Shy-Drager syndrome (multiple system atrophy)	Shy and Drager, 1960
Riley-Day syndrome (familial dysautonomia)	Riley et al., 1949
Dopamine-β-hydroxylase deficiency	Robertson et al., 1986a Man in't Veld et al., 1987a, 1987b
Monoamine oxidase deficiency	Sims et al., 1989
Baroreceptor dysfunction	Robertson et al., 1984b
Parkinsonism	Gross et al., 1972
Porphyria	Perlroth et al., 1966 Barrclough and Sharpey-Shaefer, 1963
Alcoholism	Charness et al., 1989
Carcinoma	Baraclough and Sharpey-Shaefer, 1963
Wernicke-Korsakoff syndrome	Birchfield, 1964
Guillain-Barré syndrome	Birchfield and Shaw, 1964
Diabetes mellitus	
Amyloidosis	
Autoimmune diseases	Edmonds et al., 1979
Pernicious anemia	Gonin et al., 1953
Leprosy	Radnakrishnan et al., 1978
AIDS	Cohen and Laudenslager, 1989
Hemodialysis	Nies et al., 1979
Acute pandysautonomia	
Thoracolumbar sympathectomy	Hammarstrom, 1942 Evelyn et al., 1960 Mathias et al., 1979
Spinal cord lesion	Johnson et al., 1952 Krum et al., 1989
Botulism	Koenig et al., 1964
Tetanus	van Lieshout et al., 1988

disorder appears to be confined to the sympathetic and parasympathetic nervous systems (Table 3–2). The adrenal medulla is relatively spared (Polinsky et al., 1980). The initial feature in men can be impotence (Krane et al., 1989), but more commonly orthostatic hypotension is the symptom that brings patients to their physician. Hypotension may be so severe that seizures supervene in perhaps 3% of affected patients. Such seizures usually are clonic. Some patients find that leg-crossing helps to maintain upright posture (Ghrist and Brown, 1928). About 5% of patients with the Bradbury-Eggleston syndrome have angina pectoris, usually in the absence of significant angiographically demonstrable coronary atherosclerosis (Silverberg et al., 1979). Patients with the Bradbury-Eggleston syndrome do not tolerate high altitude well, perhaps because they hyperventilate in this situation. ***Principle: The forme fruste of a disease can alert the clinician to a less obvious syndrome. If it does not, treatment of the forme fruste alone could be frustrating and counterproductive.*** In this case one should consider the consequence of treating the angina with reducers of preload and afterload. It would likely be unsuccessful and exacerbate other elements of the disease.

Orthostatic hypotension is usually accompanied by supine hypertension, even when the patient is not taking vasopressor medications (Shneider, 1952). However, even when the supine hypertension is quite severe, cardiac function is well preserved and contractility may even be raised (Kronenberg et al., 1990). Usually hypohidrosis or at least an asymmetric distribution of sweating is seen (Hines et al., 1981). Nocturia is an invariable accompaniment of dysautonomic orthostatic hypotension and may cause the patient to get up as many as five to eight times per night to pass substantial volumes of urine. Some patients develop signs of neurogenic urinary retention, and these individuals may have repeated urinary tract infections. It is noteworthy that patients with the Bradbury-Eggleston syndrome do not usually have fevers as high as healthy subjects; nevertheless, any fever will significantly lower their blood pressure and consequently decrease their functional capacity. In the absence of infection, a reduced basal metabolic rate is typical (Korns and Randall, 1937). A sudden decline in functional mobility in a patient with the Bradbury-Eggleston syndrome is suggestive of an intercurrent infection, usually of the urinary tract. There is marked hypersensitivity to all pressor and depressor stimuli, especially sympathomimetic amines (Demanet, 1976; Ibrahim et al., 1979; Robertson, 1979).

The pathology of the Bradbury-Eggleston syndrome has not been completely elucidated, but

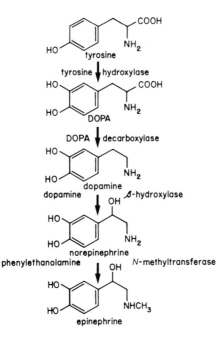

Fig. 3–1. The synthesis of norepinephrine and epinephrine. All these enzymatic steps take place in the cytoplasm except for the conversion of dopamine to norepinephrine. Dopamine-β-hydroxylase is confined to the neurotransmitter vesicles.

there is known to be a loss of cells in the intermediolateral column of the spinal cord and secondarily a loss of catecholamine uptake (Polinsky et al., 1985) and catecholamine fluorescence in sympathetic postganglionic neurons (Pettito and Black, 1978). Plasma and urinary concentrations of norepinephrine usually are greatly reduced, sometimes to 10% of normal (Goldstein et al., 1989). The concentration of norepinephrine in plasma is virtually always less than 200 pg/ml and often less than 100 pg/ml (Ziegler et al., 1977; Robertson et al., 1979). Plasma concentrations of epinephrine are also reduced but usually to a lesser extent than those of norepinephrine. Dopamine (Figure 3–1) concentrations in urine usually are about 50% of normal values.

Patients with the Bradbury-Eggleston syndrome have a generally good prognosis; many live for 20 years or more after the onset of their disease. The most common cause of death in these patients is pulmonary embolus.

Shy-Drager Syndrome
(Multiple System Atrophy)

In the Shy-Drager syndrome (multiple system atrophy), autonomic failure is widespread and is associated with impairment in other neurologic systems (Shy and Drager, 1960). The other neuro-

logic systems may be cerebellar, extrapyramidal, neuromuscular, or cerebral. The autonomic dysfunction in the Shy-Drager syndrome can be viewed predominantly as a central defect with an inability to engage a generally healthy peripheral autonomic system. In these patients, chronic orthostatic hypotension may be a presenting symptom; in other cases, extrapyramidal symptoms or cerebellar symptoms may predominate early in the course. In patients with cerebellar involvement, tremor is worsened by nicotine (Graham and Oppenheimer, 1969), and Shy-Drager patients generally discontinue smoking at the onset of their disease. When the chronic orthostatic hypotension antedates other neurologic involvement, it may be very difficult to differentiate the Shy-Drager syndrome from the more benign Bradbury-Eggleston syndrome (Table 3–3). Clinical symptoms of autonomic failure discussed above in terms of the Bradbury-Eggleston syndrome often apply to the patients with Shy-Drager syndrome. *Principle: Habits (e.g., smoking that delivers nicotine) can exacerbate a disease and often may be used as a diagnostic test. Look for the associations and medical opportunities.*

Pathologically, multiple sites within the brain and spinal cord are involved. Sympathetic and parasympathetic postganglionic neurons, however, appear to be intact. Very likely, the Shy-Drager syndrome will ultimately be found to represent several distinct clinical entities. Some investigators distinguish between a spinocerebellar degeneration and an autonomic dysfunction associated with extrapyramidal involvement. In addition, some investigators have suggested a relationship between the Shy-Drager syndrome and Parkinson's disease, although this is not supported by the pathologic data accumulated to date. Lewy bodies have been absent in several careful autopsies of Shy-Drager patients (Heieren, 1972). At least one family has been reported in whom four members had a Shy-

Table 3–3. CLINICAL FEATURES OF AUTONOMIC FAILURE

Orthostatic hypotension
  Dizziness
  Dimming of vision
  Neck or head discomfort
  Weakness in legs
  Postprandial angina pectoris
  Syncope
  Seizures
Impotence
Hypohidrosis
Nasal stuffiness
Constipation or diarrhea
Bladder dysfunction
Mild anemia

Drager-like syndrome (Lewis, 1964), but there is no other suggestion of a strong genetic component in the disease.

Blood and urinary concentrations of norepinephrine often are near normal in the unstimulated state in patients with the Shy-Drager syndrome, but they do not rise appropriately on assumption of the upright posture (Ziegler et al., 1977). Peripheral norepinephrine concentrations tend to be higher in the Shy-Drager syndrome than in the Bradbury-Eggleston syndrome. Catecholamine metabolites reflect the central nature of the neurologic defect (Polinsky et al., 1981; Kopin et al., 1983; Polinsky et al., 1984; Polinsky et al., 1987). Noteworthy is the biochemical evidence of central abnormalities in the dopamine, acetylcholine, and serotonin systems (Polinsky et al., 1988; Polinsky et al., 1989).

The prognosis is more guarded in the Shy-Drager syndrome than in the Bradbury-Eggleston syndrome. It is rare for a patient to survive 12 years, although the autonomic abnormalities are rarely the direct cause of death. A significant number of Shy-Drager patients develop laryngeal stridor and difficulty in swallowing. This may lead to recurrent episodes of pneumonia, a frequent cause of death. In addition, many patients with the Shy-Drager syndrome experience Cheyne-Stokes or periodic respiration. In some cases this may lead to a critical loss of respiratory drive, so-called Ondine's curse (Craddock et al., 1987). Pulmonary hypertension may occur during apnea (Guilleminault et al., 1977). In spite of the frequency of these two problems, however, one of the most common causes of death in patients with the Shy-Drager syndrome is pulmonary embolus.

Riley-Day Syndrome (Familial Dysautonomia)

The Riley-Day syndrome (familial dysautonomia) is an autosomal recessive disorder that occurs with an incidence of 1 in 5000 in Ashkenazi Jews (Riley et al., 1949). The disorder involves widespread abnormalities in the nervous system with poor motor coordination, a relative indifference to pain, and psychological instability. Autonomic symptoms that have been noted include lability of blood pressure, orthostatic hypotension, altered temperature control, and increased sweating. These patients also have defective production of tears, and recurrent pulmonary infections. The disease has a high mortality, but a significant number of patients reach adulthood. The molecular basis for the disease is currently unknown. There are many other forms of congenital sensory neuropathies, distinct from the Riley-Day syndrome, that also are present with postural hypotension. Only a rudimentary classification of these disorders is available given the limitations of our current understanding of this syndrome.

Dopamine-β-Hydroxylase Deficiency

In 1986, the syndrome of dopamine-β-hydroxylase (DBH) deficiency was first demonstrated (Robertson et al., 1986a; Man in't Veld et al., 1987a, 1987b; Biaggioni et al., 1987a; Biaggioni et al., 1990a, 1990b). In retrospect, there may have been previous patients who had this disorder, but for technical reasons, the diagnosis could not be established (Anlauf et al., 1975; Nanda et al., 1977).

The characteristics of DBH deficiency are different from previously recognized forms of autonomic dysfunction. There is virtual absence of norepinephrine, coupled with a greatly increased dopamine concentration in plasma, cerebrospinal fluid, and urine. It differs from the Riley-Day syndrome and various other autonomic disorders seen in adults in that the peripheral defect can be localized to the noradrenergic and adrenergic tissues. Furthermore, there is no evidence of other neurologic defects, either central or peripheral. The clinical presentation of DBH deficiency is now known to include incapacitating orthostatic hypotension, ptosis, retrograde ejaculation, hyperextensible joints, nasal stuffiness, and a difficult perinatal course with otherwise normal development. There is an absence of pressor responses to exposure to cold, an absence of sustained handgrip, and an inability to perform mental arithmetic. There is also an absence of blood pressure overshoot on release of the Valsalva maneuver. However, sympathetic cholinergic function is intact, as evidenced by normal sweating. Parasympathetic function is also preserved, as assessed by intact sinus arrhythmia, normal heart rate increase during the Valsalva maneuver, and tachycardia after atropine. The clinical characteristics and the response to autonomic maneuvers of patients with DBH deficiency are shown in Tables 3–4 and 3–5.

The most distinguishing feature of these pa-

Table 3–4. CLINICAL FEATURES OF DOPAMINE-β-HYDROXYLASE DEFICIENCY
($n = 6$)

FEATURE	FREQUENCY (%)
Severe orthostatic hypotension	100
Retrograde ejaculation	100
Ptosis	67
Complicated perinatal course	67
Nocturia	67
Hyperextensible joints	50
Nasal stuffiness	50
Behavioral changes	33
Seizures (with hypotension)	33
Sluggish deep tendon reflexes	33
Hypotonic skeletal muscles	33
Atrial fibrillation	16

Table 3-5. AUTONOMIC MANEUVERS IN DOPAMINE-β-HYDROXYLASE DEFICIENCY

FINDING	FREQUENCY (%)
Orthostatic hypotension > 40 mm Hg systolic	100
Absent pressor isometric handgrip > 10 mm Hg	87
Absent cold pressor response > 10 mm Hg	87
Abnormal Valsalva maneuver	100
Sweating present	100
Sinus arrhythmia present	100
Atropine tachycardia > 25 beats/min	100
Pressor clonidine response	100
Absent pressor tyramine response	100
Pressor efficacy of DOPS	100

DOPS = Dihydroxyphenylserine

tients is the virtual absence of plasma, urinary, and cerebrospinal norepinephrine and epinephrine together with the greatly increased plasma concentration of dopa and dopamine. Norepinephrine metabolites are virtually absent (vanillylmandelic acid [VMA], dihydroxyphenyl glycol [DHPG], normetanephrine), while dopamine metabolites (homovanillic acid [HVA], dihydroxylphenylacetic acid [DOPAC]) are increased. These patients have no response to high (8 mg IV) doses of tyramine that would normally increase blood pressure by releasing neuronal norepinephrine. Even the most severely affected patient with the Bradbury-Eggleston syndrome would be expected to respond to high doses of tyramine with at least some increase in blood pressure. Yet, in DBH-deficient patients, norepinephrine remained undetectable following administration of tyramine, while dopamine concentrations were increased. This is consistent with the hypothesis that dopamine, instead of norepinephrine, is present in these patients in presynaptic terminals and is released instead of norepinephrine.

In patients with DBH deficiency, central autonomic control as well as mechanisms that release catecholamines are intact, but dopamine, acting as a false neurotransmitter, is released instead of norepinephrine. Dopamine concentrations increase on assumption of the upright posture, during sustained handgrip, and after administration of tyramine. Furthermore, the concentration of plasma dopamine decreases after administration of clonidine. Also, muscle sympathetic nerve traffic, as measured by direct intraneuronal recordings, is present, perhaps even in excess under basal conditions but is otherwise normally modulated by baroreceptor mechanisms in these patients (Rea et al., 1990). Therefore, primary autonomic neuronal pathways are intact and responsive to appropriate stimuli, but dopamine in-

stead of norepinephrine is present in the noradrenergic neuron terminals.

More than 10 patients with this disorder have now been recognized. While DBH deficiency is no doubt a rare disease in adults, it could be more common in the perinatal period. Adrenergic tissue is comparatively widespread in neonates, but there is involution of some of this tissue in the course of subsequent development. Adult patients with DBH deficiency generally have had near-fatal illness during the neonatal period due to hypotension, hypoglycemia, and hypothermia. It is likely, although specific numbers are unknown, that many DBH-deficient infants die undiagnosed shortly after birth.

Prior to the recognition of patients with DBH deficiency, many investigators would have presumed that norepinephrine was essential for life. With current assays for norepinephrine, it may be that the more severely affected individuals with this disorder are totally deficient in norepinephrine. If any is present, the plasma concentrations are less than 1% of normal. Since norepinephrine and its receptor sites have long been postulated to play a role in a number of psychiatric disorders, the generally normal mood and mental status of DBH-deficient subjects so far encountered has elicited great interest among investigators in the areas of depression and schizophrenia.

Patients with DBH deficiency must be identified as early as possible. There are several reasons for this. First, the disease is likely to be fatal in the neonatal period if it is unrecognized. Patients so far encountered as adults have had unusually meticulous care during illnesses in the neonatal period. Second, unlike other dysautonomias, DBH deficiency has a relatively specific and uniquely effective treatment. The administration of dihydroxyphenylserine results in the endogenous replacement of dopamine by norepinephrine and a remarkable improvement in blood pressure regulation in these patients (discussed in detail below). *Principle: A marvelous reward of understanding the molecular pathogenesis of a disease is devising a disease-specific molecular therapy. In spite of the intellectual attractiveness of such specific intervention, its toxicity relative to nonspecific intervention must be compared before it becomes a "drug of choice."*

The disorder is most easily diagnosed by measuring the ratio of the concentration of norepinephrine to dopamine in plasma. Normally, the norepinephrine/dopamine ratio is approximately 10. In patients with DBH deficiency this ratio has generally been 0.1 or less. In Menkes syndrome, due to abnormal copper metabolism, the ratio is near 1.0 (Hoeldtke et al., 1988b). The biochemical manifestations of DBH deficiency are thus so dramatic that they may be said to be pathognomonic.

Acute Dysautonomia

Several reports document complete autonomic failure developing acutely in an otherwise healthy individual (Owen et al., 1967; Appenzeller and Kornfeld, 1973). Some of these individuals may recover partially or completely. In some cases, the disorder appears to be restricted to the autonomic nervous system, but in other patients neuromuscular symptoms develop; this latter group probably represents a form of the Guillain-Barré syndrome.

The Guillain-Barré syndrome typically presents about 3 weeks after a viral illness, with predominantly motor involvement, especially in the leg muscles. Muscle weakness may become so severe that respiration must be supported. The autonomic involvement usually is relatively minor in the Guillain-Barré syndrome, but in some cases it can dominate the disorder.

Secondary Autonomic Neuropathies

Any pathologic process that can produce peripheral neuropathy potentially can produce autonomic neuropathy (Finley and Tibbles, 1982; Ingall et al., 1990). A large number of these disorders have been identified and studied. Usually the autonomic impairment is mild to moderate and *it seldom dominates the presentation of the primary illness*.

Perhaps the most common cause of secondary autonomic dysfunction is diabetes mellitus (Cryer and Weiss, 1976; Ewing et al., 1980; Schumer et al., 1988; Watkins, 1990). Although sensory fibers usually are affected first, subtle autonomic abnormalities may be discovered quite early in some diabetic patients. Orthostatic hypotension usually is a relatively late development. In some long-term diabetic patients, the autonomic involvement can be widespread and quite severe. All signs and symptoms of autonomic failure may be present, but gastrointestinal manifestations, especially diarrhea and gastroparesis, appear to be relatively more common in diabetic autonomic dysfunction than in other forms of autonomic dysfunction. Gastroparesis in diabetic patients may improve with erythromycin (Janssens et al., 1990).

A practical difficulty in patients with diabetic autonomic neuropathy and orthostatic hypotension is the powerful vasodepressor effect of insulin itself in these subjects (Luft and von Euler, 1953; Christensen, 1983; Brown et al., 1989). It is noteworthy that food also is vasodepressor, and the combined effects of insulin and food may make blood pressure almost impossible to keep under control. Unfortunately, neither of these effects is widely recognized by practicing physicians. *Principle: Get used to believing what you see even if it has not been commonly or widely described.* You will not read about insulin's vascular effects in chapter 16, but the effect occurs and must be reckoned with.

Pathologic study reveals that affected diabetic patients have segmental loss of myelin, axon degeneration, and vacuolization and degeneration in the intermediolateral column of the spinal cord and the sympathetic ganglia. There is also a loss of myelinated fibers. Mononuclear cells and mast cells are sometimes found in the vicinity of local neural involvement. There is hope that pancreatic transplants will have a beneficial impact on the course of autonomic neuropathy in diabetes (Solders et al., 1987; Kennedy et al., 1990).

Many other disorders may present with secondary autonomic neuropathy, including tabes dorsalis, porphyria, pernicious anemia, the Wernicke-Korsakoff syndrome, and amyloidosis. Amyloidosis as a cause of autonomic failure is by no means rare, and any patient with autonomic insufficiency in whom no primary or secondary diagnosis has been made should be evaluated for amyloidosis.

Malignancies, especially bronchogenic carcinoma (Park et al., 1972), may present with autonomic neuropathy and adrenoreceptor hypersensitivity (Hui and Conolly, 1981). The autonomic abnormality may respond to radiation and chemotherapeutic regimens in proportion to the change in tumor size. Finally, patients with a variety of spinal cord lesions, whether induced by disease or injury, may have marked autonomic impairment.

Baroreceptor Dysfunction

Baroreceptor dysfunction results in a disorder characterized by high blood pressure and elevated heart rate on some occasions and low blood pressure and low heart rate on other occasions (Robertson et al., 1984a; Aksamit et al., 1987; Langford et al., 1987). It is probably a heterogeneous entity since current investigative methods do not usually permit one to distinguish a lesion of deafferentation from an intrinsic lesion in the posterior brainstem. Extremes of blood pressure may range from 230/130 to 80/50. The disorder usually is secondary to trauma, tumor, or surgery in the brainstem, neck, or chest and sometimes due to radiation of throat carcinomas. While blood pressure and heart rate are quite labile, orthostatic hypotension is not a systematic feature in patients with baroreceptor dysfunction. Rather, on occasions when blood pressure is high, it usually is high in both upright and supine postures, and when it is low, it is low in both postures. The prevailing level of blood pressure appears to be highly dependent on cerebral stimulation. Anxiety and wakefulness potently raise blood pressure and concentrations of norepinephrine in plasma (sometimes to greater than 2000 pg/ml), while drowsiness and sedation (for example, with low doses of a benzodiazepine) tend to lower blood pressure, heart rate, and the concentration of norepinephrine in plasma. When patients are hypertensive, they are extraordinarily sensitive to clonidine such that doses typically used to treat hypertension may result in precipitous hypotension and bradycardia. This syndrome is clearly distinguished from the paroxysmal hypertension sometimes seen in hypovolemia (Cohn, 1966). The relatively mild baroreceptor abnormalities in essential hypertension do not lead to the dramatic findings seen in patients with full-fledged baroreceptor dysfunction (Floras et al., 1988). A mild baroreceptor dysfunction syndrome may occur following endarterectomy.

Patients with baroreceptor dysfunction sometimes seem "high-strung," and they may present with a volatile temper. The putative relationship of these psychological symptoms to the baroreceptor dysfunction must await study of larger numbers of patients.

Patients with baroreceptor dysfunction can easily be misdiagnosed as having labile hypertension. Indeed, many patients with baroreceptor dysfunction are initially treated as hypertensive patients but do not respond to numerous blood pressure-lowering regimens. Unfortunately, even when the proper diagnosis is recognized, treatment is by no means easy. One approach has been to try to avoid extremes of blood pressure by using diazepam (2 mg) three times daily to reduce the peaks of blood pressure and, when the patient is symptomatic from hypotension, covering the "hypotensive" valleys with low doses of fludrocortisone. This approach leaves much to be desired, but controlled investigative studies are difficult in this relatively rare syndrome.

Mitral Valve Prolapse Syndrome

Orthostatic hypotension is present in approximately 10% of patients with mitral valve prolapse as determined by a click and/or murmur on physical examination or echocardiography (Santos et al., 1981). Usually the orthostatic hypotension is milder than that encountered in the autonomic failure syndromes discussed above. However, occasional patients have very severe orthostatic hypotension requiring treatment.

As many as 30% of patients with the mitral valve prolapse syndrome have dramatic orthostatic tachycardia even though orthostatic hypotension itself may not be present or may be present only after meals. Careful studies have shown that many patients with the mitral valve prolapse syndrome have a 5% to 8% reduction in blood volume (Gaffney et al., 1983; Blomqvist, 1987). This reduction in blood volume may explain the hypotension, tachycardia, and high-normal or slightly raised concentrations of norepinephrine in plasma sometimes found in these subjects. The cause of the reduced blood volume in the mitral valve prolapse syndrome is uncertain, although there has been speculation about a possible role for atrial natriuretic factor. Many patients with similar clinical symptoms do not necessarily have concomitant mitral prolapse (Bjure and Laurell, 1927; Fouad et al., 1986; Hoeldtke et al., 1989b).

There has long been speculation that the mitral valve prolapse syndrome constitutes a dysautonomia (Mares et al., 1990). Indeed, some evidence for β-adrenergic receptor abnormalities has been found in a small number of these patients (Davies et al., 1987). However, it appears that the vast majority of patients with the mitral valve prolapse syndrome do not have any failure in the autonomic nervous system (Schatz et al., 1990) but rather have increased sympathetic activity due to the reduced blood volume. On the other hand, it has been suggested that the enhanced sympathetic activity may be primary in this disorder and that reduction of blood volume is secondary to enhanced sympathetic activity. For this reason, very low doses of clonidine (0.05 mg twice daily) have been employed to suppress sympathetic outflow with apparent symptomatic benefit in occasional patients. More commonly, however, these patients have been treated successfully with fludrocortisone (0.1–1.0 mg daily) and, in individuals in whom the tachycardia is the predominant symptom, pindolol (5 mg three times daily). Through judicious use of these agents, it is usually possible to successfully manage the blood pressure abnormalities in the mitral valve prolapse syndrome.

Mastocytosis

Disorders of abnormal mast cell activation or proliferation (mastocytosis) may be more common than is generally appreciated (Roberts and Oates, 1985). A major reason for this is that many patients with mastocytosis do not manifest the chronic urticaria, and some may also lack the erythematous acneiform papular lesions, even though they may have flushing. Typical symptoms in patients with mastocytosis include flushing, pruritus, and paresthesias; palpitations with or without chest pain; dyspnea and dizziness; syncope (in one third of cases), usually disproportionate to the hypotension measured; headaches;

and intermittent nausea, vomiting, or diarrhea. Blood pressure may be high or low, but chronic abnormalities in blood pressure are not seen. With large mast cell degranulations, there may be sufficient heparin released to affect clotting time and the partial thromboplastin time (PTT).

These symptoms are often provoked by exercise, emotional stimuli, narcotics, and heat. The diagnosis of mastocytosis is made by measuring the concentrations of urinary methylhistamine and urinary prostaglandin D_2; one or both of these are generally dramatically raised in a 4-hour urine collection made immediately following an attack. About 75% of cases develop mastocytosis without an identifiable pattern (i.e., they are sporadic cases), while the rest are familial, and are expressed as autosomal dominant inheritance. For treatment, histamine receptor H_1 and H_2 antagonists should be used initially. If the response to these drugs is insufficient, aspirin is begun with low doses and advanced stepwise until plasma salicylate concentrations of 20 to 30 mg/100 ml are obtained. Occasionally, severe attacks of mastocytosis may result in a profound life-threatening fall in blood pressure. These attacks respond to an IV infusion of epinephrine at 2 to 8 μg/min that acts at least in part by inhibiting mast cell degranulation.

TREATMENT OF ORTHOSTATIC HYPOTENSION

There are significant difficulties in assessing the efficacy of pharmacologic and nonpharmacologic therapy of chronic orthostatic hypotension. Most studies have involved very small sample sizes (typically fewer than four patients), which presents a statistical challenge (see chapter 36). In view of the rarity of patients with orthostatic hypotension and our limited understanding of the appropriate taxonomy of autonomic disorders, there has been a tendency to lump them together in therapeutic studies in spite of their disparate diagnostic categories. Patients with heterogeneity in degree of autonomic involvement are included within the same studies, whereas only a subgroup of these might be the true beneficiaries of the proposed treatment. There have been almost no studies assessing long-term safety, and there are no studies of sufficient duration to allow assessment of the impact of therapy on mortality. Finally, there are few studies that directly compare the efficacy of two potential therapeutic modalities. For all these reasons, therapeutic advice concerning treatment of chronic orthostatic hypotension remains much less well founded than theoretically desirable. *Principle: When the classification of a disease encompasses remarkable demographic heterogenicity, useful therapies often will remain undiscov-* *ered because only a minority subset of the whole will respond well. That good response will be diluted by the nonresponsiveness of the majority. Remember that most "named diseases" truly are multiple diseases, and judge study results accordingly.*

Nonpharmacologic Measures

The purpose of therapeutic interventions in patients with chronic orthostatic hypotension is to increase the patient's functional capacity rather than to achieve any particular level of blood pressure. Factors such as prior ingestion of food and drug as well as the rate of ventilation should be taken into account when assessing the patient's standing time or blood pressure. Hyperventilation lowers (Onrot et al., 1990), and hypoventilation raises blood pressure. Strenuous exercise may markedly lower blood pressure in these patients, but an appropriate exercise program may have long-term benefits. *Principle: Be very careful in evaluation of therapy that a surrogate end point does not replace more substantial end points that are more difficult to measure but more meaningful medically.*

Patient education is the cornerstone of treating individuals with postural hypotension. Many patients discover for themselves that they are less able to carry out vigorous activities following meals. This association may not have been made by other patients, who should be advised to utilize the period before meals for most of their activities and to limit their activities in the hour or so following a large meal.

Maximizing circulating blood volume is extremely important in treating orthostatic hypotension in severely affected patients with autonomic failure. Even healthy young people pool 350 ml of blood in their legs on standing (Barbey et al., 1966), and this pooling is, of course, much more marked in patients with autonomic failure. There is a reduction in central blood volume, and most patients have a reduced total blood volume as well. Low-normal values of central venous pressure, right atrial pressure, and pulmonary wedge pressure are frequently seen in severely affected patients with autonomic failure even in the supine position (Ibrahim et al., 1974). Liver blood flow is reduced considerably by upright posture, and drug metabolism may thus be altered (Feely et al., 1982).

Patients with autonomic failure have inadequately conserved sodium during low salt intake (Bachman and Youmans, 1953). This may be due to decreased noradrenergic activity in the kidney, to relatively enhanced dopamine actions, or to other effects (Slaton and Biglieri, 1967). In addition, renin responses to a low-salt diet and upright posture are reduced or absent during autonomic failure (Gordon et al., 1967; Bliddal and Nielsen, 1970). Virtually all these patients have elevated supine systemic vascular resistance that does not increase with upright posture (Chokroverty et al., 1967; Magrini, 1975). This elevated supine pressure probably also contributes to the failure of the kidney to conserve salt and water. At night, when supine, these patients inappropriately waste sodium in the urine, leading to relative hypovolemia and a degree of orthostatic hypotension that is worse in the morning and improves during the day. Interestingly angiotensin-converting enzyme (ACE) inhibitors can sometimes reduce blood pressure in spite of the very low plasma renin activity levels present in these patients, raising the possibility of the involvement of a kallikrein mechanism (Kooner et al., 1989). *Principle: Oversimplification of the mechanisms of dominant effects of a drug leads to underutilization of the chemical entity.*

Supine hypertension and its attendant diuresis can be minimized by elevating the head of the bed on blocks to approximately 5 to 20 degrees (MacLean et al., 1944). In addition to attenuating nocturnal diuresis, this will reduce the notable worsening of symptoms in the morning. Head-up tilt at night also may minimize nocturnal shifts of interstitial fluid from the legs into the circulation. Interstitial fluid in the legs on standing may exert greater support and oppose the tendency of blood to pool. Supine blood pressure is usually highest just after a person goes to bed at night. Most treatment modalities raise supine as well as upright blood pressure. Thus, head-up tilt can minimize the effect of pressor drugs during the night, a time when pressor actions are no longer necessary and may in fact be harmful. Tilt-table conditioning has led to improved functional capacity in some patients with autonomic failure (Hoeldtke et al., 1988a).

Salt intake should be liberalized in all patients except those few with coexisting congestive heart failure (Wilcox et al., 1984; Kranzler and Cardoni, 1988). Slight pedal edema is well tolerated and implies higher intravascular volume as well as increased interstitial hydrostatic pressure in the legs.

Waist-high, custom-fitted elastic support garments exert graded pressure on the legs and increase interstitial hydrostatic pressure. When the patient stands, this hydrostatic pressure will tend to keep blood from pooling in the legs. However, patients must be cautioned not to wear these stockings at night or when supine, since they will increase central blood volume, contribute to diuresis, and decrease interstitial fluid in the legs. *Note that support stockings are not of much use unless they go at least to the waist.* In fact, an abdominal binder in association with elastic stockings is even more useful. This will serve to augment venous return from the splanchnic bed, a major source of venous pooling. Antigravity suits and shock suits have been used in the past with some success but are quite awkward and bring attention to the patient's problems (Landmark and Kravik, 1979).

Patients should avoid activities that involve straining, such as lifting heavy objects. Increased abdominal and/or intrathoracic pressure at these times significantly compromises venous return and can precipitate hypotension. Coughing and straining at stool or with voiding may particularly bring on hypotension. Working with one's arms above shoulder level (e.g., shaving) can lower pressure dramatically. Ambulation or shifting weight from leg to leg as opposed to standing motionless takes advantage of muscular pumping on the veins. A slightly stooped walking posture may be helpful to the severest patients. Squatting is also a valuable "emergency" mechanism of increasing venous return, particularly when presyncopal symptoms occur. Patients may hang their legs over the side of the bed prior to standing. This minimizes hemodynamic stress, since assumption of the upright posture is broken down into two movements: (1) assumption of the seated posture and (2) standing from the seated posture. *Principle: The appropriate use of measures that are considered adjunctive to drug therapy may be a key determinant of the efficacy of the drug therapy.*

The effect of food on blood pressure in chronic orthostatic hypotension can be important (Sanders, 1932; Robertson et al., 1981; Lipsitz et al., 1986; Bannister et al., 1987; Berne et al., 1989; Mathias et al., 1989b). In normal subjects, there is a slight tachycardia with little or no fall in blood pressure after eating. However, patients with autonomic failure, the elderly, and those taking sympatholytic agents may exhibit large postprandial falls in blood pressure. Digestion shifts blood flow to the hepatic and splanchnic beds, and as already noted, these patients are exquisitely sensitive to changes in circulating blood volume. In addition, several vasoactive substances such as histamine and adenosine, and a variety of vasodilatory gastrointestinal hormones, may be elicited by meals. These substances, acting either as local vasodilators or systemic hormones, might contribute to the hypotensive response, although their role is uncertain. Patients should avoid excessive activity in the 2-hour period after meals, since at these times, especially after breakfast, they are most likely to have symptomatic orthostatic hypotension. Patients should also eat smaller meals and limit confections to minimize this effect.

Adenosine may be partially responsible for splanchnic vasodilatation after meals through either local (Onrot et al., 1986) or central (Mosqueda-Garcia et al., 1989) mechanisms. Simple measures such as a cup of coffee with meals may lessen this hypotensive response, perhaps because of the ability of caffeine to block adenosine receptors. Pressor agents should be administered in such a way that peak effects occur in the postprandial period when they are needed most. The depressor effect of meals can also be exploited in these patients. Those who have supine hypertension benefit from a small meal or snack at bedtime in order to lower their nocturnal blood pressure. This is especially important in those who have been receiving pressor agents during the day. *Principle: Being aware of the effects of routine maneuvers during an average day that can affect the outcome of drug therapy is facilitated by outcome measures that are easy to make and quick to respond. Sophisticated therapy uses rather than fights environmental factors.*

Although exhaustive isometric exercise in normal subjects raises blood pressure via sympathetic activation, it can precipitate hypotension in patients with autonomic failure. A graded program of isotonic exercise such as walking may be beneficial (Youmans et al., 1934; Youmans et al., 1935). More vigorous exercise like jogging is rarely tolerated because decreases in blood pressure occur. Climbing stairs is a common hypotensive stimulus. Exercise, even while a patient is supine, may cause hypotension.

Periods of inactivity and prolonged bed rest should be avoided, since they will worsen tolerance to standing. Prolonged bed rest, even in normal subjects, may cause mild orthostatic hypotension, and even astronauts who are very fit physically experience orthostatic hypotension on return to Earth after the weightlessness of outer space. Even well-trained and healthy young pilots, during the positive G accelerations of aerial maneuvers, may experience quite severe hypotension leading to unconsciousness and seizures (Zarriello, 1960). Small wonder that in severely affected patients with autonomic failure, quite mild accelerations, such as that encountered in an ordinary elevator, can bring on symptoms.

The ideal exercise for patients with autonomic failure is swimming. While the patient is submerged in water, his or her tolerance of upright posture is almost unlimited. In this situation, hydrostatic pressure prevents blood pooling in the legs and abdomen, and blood pressure is well maintained. We recommend that our patients undertake a graded program of swimming. Leaving the swimming pool, however, may pose difficulty. Furthermore, patients with the Shy-Drager syndrome may find swimming more of a challenge if the extrapyramidal disease restricts their mobility.

Other stresses can also worsen orthostatic hypotension. Symptoms are more pronounced in hot weather. This is not so much due to volume loss from sweating (which is usually reduced) as to vasodilatation and increased blood flow to the skin. In addition, fever in patients with autonomic failure may contribute markedly to orthostatic hypotension. Patients are also especially at risk in the shower or arising from a hot bath.

Patients should avoid certain OTC medications such as diet pills containing phenylpropanolamine or nasal sprays containing phenylephrine or oxymetazoline (a congener of clonidine). Although acutely pressor, these agents, when ingested in excess over time, can lead to significant orthostatic hypotension. All prescription medications should be carefully screened for their potential effects on blood pressure. In particular, antihypertensive medicines prescribed for supine hypertension and drugs such as tricyclic antidepressants can cause real trouble (Kranzler et al., 1988). Alcohol tends to lower blood pressure in these patients and can worsen symptoms. On the other hand, alcohol can be exploited in order to treat supine hypertension at night. We often advise our patients to have a glass of wine before retiring. *Principle: Always be aware that patients have multiple sources of drugs, many of which do not require medical supervision. In addition, it often is hard for doctors to remember that nose drops, for example, do not confine their effects to the nose and that some truly produce hypertension or hypotension.*

Patients with autonomic failure are extremely sensitive to venodilating agents. They have increased sensitivity to the effects of sympathomimetic amines and have an exaggerated sensitivity to β_2-agonist stimulation compared with β_1-agonist stimulation (Robertson et al., 1984a). Consequently, β agonists may exert a marked vasodepressor effect in these patients. The dramatic vasoactive effects of many classes of drugs make use of anesthetics especially difficult in these patients (Parris et al., 1984).

Some mechanical aids may allow patients to carry on activities of daily living more easily. For instance, a "derby chair" (a cane when folded, and a small seat when unfolded) can be used by severely affected patients to extend their walking range. Patients may use the cane for support while walking, and when symptoms ensue, they can unfold the chair and sit until they are ready to walk again. Recliner chairs are used so that patients can rest during the day without lying flat. This is especially important when pressor drugs are administered during the day, conferring added risk for supine hypertension. *Principle:*

You can not be an optimal therapist without being a consummate clinician.

While atrial tachypacing has been advocated in the management of autonomic failure, our results have been poor (Goldberg et al., 1980). This approach cannot be recommended except in the face of significant persistent bradycardia.

Pharmacologic Treatment

Drug treatment of orthostatic hypotension can be genuinely beneficial for selected patient populations (Davis and Delafuente, 1989; Ahmad and Watson, 1990; Schatz, 1990). On the whole, however, severely affected patients may prove extremely difficult to manage. The most common limitation in the treatment of patients with orthostatic hypotension is development of unacceptable levels of supine hypertension, which is present in most patients, even in the absence of any treatment. One approach has been to accept relatively high levels of supine blood pressure if that is required to keep the patient functionally mobile, although one must always try to avoid supine blood pressure above 200/120. Most of our patients with autonomic failure given optimal drug treatment maintain their supine blood pressures in the 140–180/90–100 range. There are a number of drugs that can be considered in treating autonomic failure and orthostatic hypotension of diverse causes (Table 3–6).

Fludrocortisone. Fludrocortisone (9α-fluorohydrocortisone, Florinef) is the single most important agent in the treatment of chronic orthostatic hypotension (Chobanian et al., 1979). While other mineralocorticoids have been used, fludrocortisone has become the treatment of choice. The aim is for patients to have a 3-minute standing time. While some patients will respond to 0.1 mg daily, other patients require dosages as high as 1.0 mg daily given orally. An average dose in patients with severe autonomic impairment is probably 0.3 mg once daily given orally. Fludrocortisone should generally be avoided in patients who by physical examination or history are on the verge of congestive heart failure. There are very few such patients. The drug is begun at a dose of 0.1 mg once daily and titrated higher at 1- to 2-week intervals depending on the therapeutic response. We monitor standing time, patient weight, supine blood pressure, the presence or absence of rales and gallop rhythm, and plasma potassium and magnesium concentrations. Most patients develop a reduction in either potassium or magnesium concentration in plasma after 2 to 4 weeks of adequate dosage of fludrocortisone. While this may be mild in some individuals, in others it is quite severe, and potassium concentra-

Table 3–6. DRUG TREATMENT OF AUTONOMIC FAILURE

Fludrocortisone (9α-fluorohydrocortisone)
Caffeine
Sympathomimetic Amines
   Midodrine
   Phenylpropanolamine
   Ephedrine
   Tyramine + MAO inhibition (Davies et al., 1978; Diamond et al., 1970)
Cyclooxygenase Inhibitors
   Indomethacin
   Ibuprofen
Ergot Alkaloids
   Ergotamine (Biaggioni et al., 1990)
   Dihydroergotamine (Lang et al., 1975)
Somatostatin Analogs
   Somatostatin (Hoeldtke et al., 1986a, 1986b)
   Octreotide (Hoeldtke et al., 1989a, 1989b)
Dihydroxyphenylserine (Biaggioni and Robertson, 1987; Man in't Veld et al., 1987b)
Antihistamines
   Diphenhydramine (Stacpoole and Robertson, 1982)
   Cimetidine (Stacpoole and Robertson, 1982)
Other Drugs
   Dopamine antagonists (Kuchel et al., 1985)
      Metoclopramide
      Domperidone
   α₂ Agonists and antagonists
      Clonidine
      Yohimbine
   β Antagonists (Man in't Veld et al., 1982)
   Serotonin antagonists (cyproheptidine) (Mahoudeau et al., 1972)
   Vasopressin analogs (Wagner and Braunwald, 1956)
   Angiotensin (Kipfer, 1959)
   Vasodilators
      Hydralazine
      Minoxidil
   Nonpharmacologic Measures
      Elevated head of bed (Bickelman et al., 1961)
      Antigravity suite (Bevegard et al., 1962)

tions below 2.2 mEq/l can occur. Most patients ultimately require replacement of potassium, while only a minority will require replacement of their magnesium while receiving fludrocortisone. Slow-release preparations of magnesium chloride are available in tablet form containing 64 mg of elemental magnesium. A twice-daily dosage regimen minimizes the problem of diarrhea. Weight gain occurs commonly with fludrocortisone therapy, and indeed, few patients derive much benefit before they have gained 5 lb. In general, we avoid weight gains greater than 10 lb.

Caffeine. Caffeine, in part through blockade of adenosine receptors, raises blood pressure in normal subjects (Robertson et al., 1978) as well as in patients with autonomic impairment (Onrot et al., 1985). The pressor response to caffeine is at least as great in patients with autonomic failure as in normal subjects. More importantly, the fall in blood pressure following a meal can be significantly attenuated by administration of caffeine with the meal (Lenders et al., 1988). Although 250 mg of caffeine is the dosage that has been most widely employed in studies, it is possible that as little as one cup of coffee (100 mg of caffeine) may increase the cardiovascular tolerance to meals of a patient with autonomic impairment. Caffeine is perhaps most valuable as an adjunct to fludrocortisone therapy. *Principle: As in most therapeutic decisions, the right choice of drug at the right time is the key to success. It must have been a pharmacologist who first thought of one man's poison being another's food.*

Sympathomimetic Amines. A great many pressor agents that act directly or indirectly through α-adrenergic receptors have been used for many years with nominal success. It sometimes appears that patients receiving these agents do not benefit functionally as much as their increase in blood pressure would suggest that they should. Another limitation of most of these agents is their short duration of action. Occasional patients benefit from the α-adrenergic receptor agonist midodrine (Schirger et al., 1981; Kaufmann et al., 1988). Ephedrine has been widely used in the treatment of autonomic failure, but comparable success is usually achievable with phenylpropanolamine that is available without prescription in the United States (Biaggioni et al., 1987b) (see chapter 4). Quite low doses of phenylpropanolamine (12.5 mg) may have significant pressor effects in some hypersensitive individuals with severe autonomic impairment. Others may require doses two- to fourfold higher. Although it might have been predicted that this agent would be ineffective in the absence of substantial endogenous stores of norepinephrine, in fact it has pressor effects even in subjects who have no endogenous norepinephrine.

Cyclooxygenase Inhibitors. Indomethacin will raise blood pressure about 20 mm Hg in most (Kochar et al., 1979; Goldberg et al., 1985) but not all (Crook et al., 1981) severely affected patients with autonomic failure. The response is more dramatic in the postprandial period than at other times of the day. Since patients may have troubling gastrointestinal or central nervous system adverse effects with indomethacin, other NSAIDs, such as ibuprofen, have also been successfully employed, although their relative efficacies have not been compared.

Dihydroergotamine. The relatively specific effect of dihydroergotamine on the venous capacitance bed has led this agent to be considered in the treatment of orthostatic hypotension (Tik-

holov, 1976; Benowitz et al., 1980; Hoeldtke et al., 1986a). A major limitation of this drug is its low oral bioavailability, leading to inconsistent plasma concentrations and unreliable pressor effects. However, when it is administered by inhalation, bioavailability appears to be good and patients may respond dramatically (Biaggioni et al., 1990a).

Ergotamine itself has occasionally been employed inasmuch as it has a higher bioavailability than dihydroergotamine (Chobanian et al., 1983). Although serious adverse effects of ergot alkaloids in patients with autonomic impairment have rarely been reported, concern that with increased experience these complications may be encountered is more than legitimate. Angina pectoris, myocardial infarction, and sudden death have been encountered in patients receiving ergot alkaloids for the treatment of migraine headache (Benedict and Robertson, 1979) and at least one patient with autonomic failure developed angina pectoris while taking ergotamine (Nylin and Levander, 1948). On the other hand, a patient with ventricular tachycardia brought on by standing up was improved by ergotamine (Peters and Penner, 1946).

Somatostatin Analogs. Somatostatin has recently been found to be useful in the treatment of postprandial hypotension in autonomic failure (Hoeldtke et al., 1986a). Many gastrointestinal hormones are predominantly vasodilatory, and somatostatin analogs attenuate the secretion of these vasodilatory peptides (Mathias et al., 1988). By other mechanisms, somatostatin decreases the postprandial effect of food on blood pressure (Jansen et al., 1989). If sufficiently high dosages of somatostatin analogs are given, blood pressure is raised even in patients who have not ingested food. *Principle: Very few drugs have all or even their dominant effects caused by a single mechanism of action.*

Recently the interest in octreotide, a somatostatin analog, as a pressor in patients with autonomic failure has increased (Hoeldtke et al., 1989a; Hoeldtke and Israel, 1989). Experimental protocols are being developed that allow patients to control a pump that when activated infuses octreotide subcutaneously. The infusion can be turned off when the patient is sitting down or when the patient wishes to lie down. The advantage of this pressor agent over others such as norepinephrine is that it does not cause local tissue necrosis when it is given subcutaneously, a major limitation of most agents acting through α-adrenergic receptors. Currently, there is still limited experience with octreotide administered in this fashion, however. Now we need a cheap, unobtrusive, and easily manipulable pump to deliver the drug.

Unfortunately, adverse effects of somatostatin analogs can be pronounced. Some patients experience diarrhea and malabsorption of fat. The diarrhea can be sufficient to reduce overall blood volume and hence counteract the beneficial effects that the analog exerts on the cardiovascular system. This problem may be lessened in some patients by the use of initially very low and slowly increasing dosages of the peptide. Gallstones may develop with chronic use of somatostatin analogs. *Principle: A number of the pharmacologic products of biotechnology will be peptides and proteins that are not orally bioavailable. Optimization of their use will depend on novel ways to deliver them by other than oral routes.*

Dihydroxyphenylserine. Dihydroxyphenylserine (L-DOPS) is an analog of norepinephrine to which a carboxyl group has been attached. This agent is uniquely beneficial in patients with DBH deficiency (Biaggioni and Robertson, 1987c; Man in't Veld et al., 1987b). The advantage of this agent in this disorder is that L-DOPS is already β-hydroxylated and can be converted directly into norepinephrine by the enzyme dopa decarboxylase, which lacks substrate specificity.

While this agent has limited use in other forms of autonomic impairment since the synthetic step to norepinephrine synthesis is not limited by DBH, dosages of 250 to 500 mg two or three times daily are dramatically pressor in patients with DBH deficiency. In general, the drug has been well tolerated. Orthostatic tolerance is greatly enhanced during therapy with this agent, and plasma norepinephrine concentrations, previously undetectable, usually rise into the normal range. A concomitant fall in plasma concentrations of dopamine usually occurs, perhaps because the rate-limiting tyrosine hydroxylase activity is decreased by the newly synthesized feedback inhibition actions of norepinephrine now present in the patient's sympathomimetic neurons. *Principle: Undeniably, understanding of the molecular mechanisms of disease ultimately leads to development of disease-specific therapeutics. The challenge is to be aware of the opportunity for discovering such agents and to develop a perspective that optimizes their use.*

Histamine-Receptor Antagonists. While antihistamines have no role in the treatment of chronic orthostatic hypotension due to autonomic failure, they have a modest role in treating diabetic dysautonomia (Stacpoole and Robertson, 1982) and a very important role in treating the hypotension due to mastocytosis. For this purpose, chlorpheniramine (8 mg three times daily) and cimetidine (300 mg four times daily) or comparable H_1- and H_2-receptor antagonists are generally used. In some patients with mastocytosis, combined treatment with H_1 and H_2 antihistamines alone is insufficient. In these settings, gradually increasing doses of aspirin are utilized until salicylate concentrations reach the 20- to 30-mg/100 ml range. In some patients with mastocytosis, aspirin induces secretion from mast cells; it is wise to undertake aspirin therapy incrementally and with great caution. The usefulness of aspirin relates to its inhibition of formation of the otherwise high quantities of prostaglandin D_2 released by many patients with disorders of mast cell activation.

Other Agents. A variety of other drugs have been employed to treat autonomic impairment that for various reasons have been less successful than the agents discussed above. Nevertheless, for an occasional patient they may be useful adjuncts.

While levodopa has been extremely useful in the management of parkinsonism, it lowers pressure (Michelakis and Robertson, 1970), and overall results in patients with the Shy-Drager syndrome have been disappointing (Aminoff et al., 1973).

In individuals in whom dopamine is contributing significantly to the hypotension (Kuchel et al., 1980; Kuchel et al., 1985), dopamine antagonists such as domperidone or metoclopramide may be useful (Lopes de Faria et al., 1988; de Caestecker et al., 1989). Many patients, however, do not respond very well to these agents.

The use of α_2-adrenergic receptor agonists and antagonists has been extensively studied (Goldberg et al., 1983a; Goldberg and Robertson, 1983, 1984; Robertson et al., 1986b; Onrot et al., 1987a, 1987c). In the vasomotor center, α_2-adrenergic receptor stimulation inhibits sympathetic outflow; on the other hand, centrally active α_2-receptor agonists also have direct activity on muscular α_2 receptors in the periphery. In patients with essentially complete sympathetic denervation, clonidine does not decrease blood pressure, and the direct effects of clonidine on vascular smooth muscle α_2-adrenergic receptors promote smooth muscle contraction. This can result in a dramatic elevation in blood pressure, particularly with dosages of 0.4 to 0.8 mg (Robertson et al., 1983). However, the major limitation of clonidine is its depressor effect, observed when this agent is administered to a patient with partial autonomic failure. Sometimes patients with partial autonomic impairment may develop quite severe orthostatic hypotension in response to clonidine. In such patients, although only a low level of sympathetic activity remains, it may be pivotal in the maintenance of blood pressure, and the administration of clonidine, particularly at low doses, may result in incapacitating hypotension. This is especially likely to occur in patients with baroreceptor dysfunction. Finally, some patients given clonidine for the management of low blood pressure have narcotic-like side effects. For all these reasons, clonidine should rarely be used in the management of orthostatic hypotension.

The α_2-adrenergic receptor antagonist yohimbine is sometimes useful in patients with autonomic failure (des Lauriers et al., 1980; LeCrubier et al., 1981; Goldberg and Robertson, 1983; Robertson et al., 1986b; Onrot et al., 1987d; Seibyl et al., 1989). Although it might seem paradoxical that both α_2-adrenergic receptor agonists, such as clonidine, and α_2-adrenergic receptor antagonists, such as yohimbine, would be employed in treating low blood pressure, they are useful in different subgroups of patients. While clonidine should be restricted to patients who have no sympathetic function remaining, yohimbine may be useful in proportion to the amount of sympathetic activity the patient still possesses. In a sense, yohimbine may be a particularly physiologic approach in that it enhances the patient's own sympathetic nervous system activation, whereas most other drugs merely supplement or compensate for it. Adverse effects with yohimbine are predominantly anxiety, nervousness, and diarrhea.

Although β-adrenergic antagonists have been recommended for the treatment of autonomic failure (Chobanian et al., 1977; Man in't Veld et al., 1982), pure antagonists have generally proved to be of limited benefit in enhancing the patient's functional capacity. The partial agonist pindolol has been more useful (Man in't Veld et al., 1981).

Paradoxically, vasodilators such as hydralazine (Jones and Reid, 1980) and minoxidil have been used with apparent functional improvement in patients with severe autonomic failure, perhaps because these agents reduce the raised systemic vascular resistance that characterizes these patients, although the mechanism of improvement in symptoms is unclear.

Finally, vasopressin analogs have been beneficial when administered by nasal spray (Wagner and Braunwald, 1956). Occasional patients achieve long-term, improved control of blood pressure with desmopressin nasal spray (Mathias et al., 1986).

Unfortunately, in spite of the many pharmacologic agents currently available, there still remain patients whose symptoms cannot be adequately relieved. Each patient is a challenge in the individualization of therapy in this recalcitrant syndrome.

Supported by National Institutes of Health grants RR0095 and HL34021, and the Vanderbilt Center for Space Physiology and Medicine. Dr. Robertson is a Burroughs Wellcome Scholar in Clinical Pharmacology.

REFERENCES

Ahmad, R. A. S.; and Watson, R. D. S.: Treatment of postural hypotension. Drugs, 39:75–85, 1990.

Aksamit, T. R.; Floras, J. S.; Victor, R. G.; and Aylward, P. E.: Paroxysmal hypertension due to sinoaortic baroreceptor denervation in humans. Hypertension, 9:309–314, 1987.

Allen, S. C.; Taylor, C. L.; and Hall, V. E.: A study of orthostatic insufficiency by the tiltboard method. Am. J. Physiol., 143:11–20, 1945.

Aminoff, M. J.; Wilcox, C. S.; Woakes, M. M.; and Kremer, M.: Levodopa therapy for Parkinsonism in the Shy-Drager syndrome. J. Neurol. Neurosurg. Psychiatr., 36:350–353, 1973.

Anlauf, M.; Werner, U.; Merguet, P.; Nitsche, T.; Graben, N.; and Bock, K. D.: Klinisch-experimentelle Untersuchungen bei Patienten mit asympathikotoner Hypotonie. Dtsch. Med. Wochenschr., 100:924–933, 1975.

Appenzeller, O.; and Kornfeld, M.: Acute pandysautonomia. Clinical and morphologic study. Arch. Neurol., 29:334–339, 1973.

Arenander, E.: Hemodynamic effects of varicose veins and results of radical surgery. Acta. Chir. Scand., 260(suppl.):1–76, 1960.

Bachman, D. M.; and Youmans, W. B.: Effects of posture on renal excretion of sodium and chloride in orthostatic hypotension. Circulation, 7:413–421, 1953.

Baker, C.: The cough syndrome. Faintness and loss of consciousness from coughing: The so-called syndrome of laryngeal vertigo. Guy's Hosp. Rec., 98:132–167, 1949.

Bannister, R.: Degeneration of the autonomic nervous system. Lancet, 2:175–179, 1971.

Bannister, R.; and Mathias, C.: Testing autonomic reflexes. In, Autonomic Failure: A Textbook of Clinical Disorders of the Autonomic Nervous System, 2nd ed. (Bannister, R., ed.). Oxford Medical, Oxford, pp. 289–307, 1988.

Bannister, R.; daCosta, D. F.; Forster, S.; Fosbraey, P.; and Mathias, C. J.: Cardiovascular effects of lipid and protein meals in autonomic failure. J. Physiol. (Lond), 377:62P, 1987.

Barbey, K.; and Barbey, P.: Die Blutverschiebung in die unteren Extremitäten bei der akuten orthostatischen Kreislaufbelastung. Med. Welt., 33:1693–1698, 1966.

Barlow, E. D.; and Howarth, S.: Effects on blood pressure of ventricular asystole during Stokes-Adams attacks and acetylcholine injections. Br. Med. J., 2:863–864, 1953.

Barraclough, M. A.; and Sharpey-Schaefer, E. P.: Hypotension from absent circulatory reflexes: Effects of alcohol, barbiturates, psychotherapeutic drugs and other mechanisms. Lancet, 1:1121–1126, 1963.

Beales, R.: On syncope senilis. Lancet, 2:102, 1856.

Benedict, C. R.; and Robertson, D.: Angina pectoris and sudden death in the absence of atherosclerosis following ergotamine therapy for migraine. Am. J. Med., 67:177–178, 1979.

Benowitz, N. L.; Byrd, R.; Schambelan, M.; Rosenberg, J.; and Roizen, M. F.: Dihydroergotamine treatment for orthostatic hypotension from Vacor rodenticide. Ann. Int. Med., 92:387–388, 1980.

Berne, C.; Fagius, J.; and Niklasson, F.: Sympathetic response to oral carbohydrate administration. J. Clin. Invest., 84:1403–1409, 1989.

Bevegard, S.; Jonsson, B.; and Karlof, I.: Circulatory response to recumbent exercise and head-up tilting in patients with disturbed sympathetic cardiovascular control (postural hypotension). Acta Med. Scand., 172:623–636, 1962.

Biaggioni, I.; and Robertson, D.: Endogenous restoration of noradrenaline by precursor therapy in dopamine-beta-hydroxylase deficiency. Lancet, 2:1170–1172, 1987.

Biaggioni, I.; Zygmunt, D.; Haile, V.; and Robertson, D.: Pressor effect of inhaled ergotamine in orthostatic hypotension. Am. J. Cardiol., 65:89–92, 1990a.

Biaggioni, I.; Goldstein, D. S.; Atkinson, T.; and Robertson, D.: Dopamine-beta-hydroxylase deficiency in man. Neurology, 40:370–373, 1990b.

Biaggioni, I.; Hollister, A. S.; and Robertson, D.: Dopamine-beta-hydroxylase deficiency and dopamine. N. Engl. J. Med., 314:1415–1416, 1987a.

Biaggioni, I.; Onrot, J.; Stewart, C. K.; and Robertson, D.: The potent pressor effect of phenylpropanolamine in patients with autonomic impairment. J.A.M.A., 258:236–239, 1987b.

Bickelman, A. G.; Lippschutz, E. J.; and Brunjes, C. F.: Hemodynamics of idiopathic orthostatic hypotension. Am. J. Med., 30:26–38, 1961.

Birchfield, R. I.: Postural hypotension in Wernicke's disease: A manifestation of autonomic nervous system involvement. Am. J. Med., 36:404–414, 1964.

Birchfield, R. I.; and Shaw, C. M.: Postural hypotension in the Guillain-Barré syndrome. Arch. Neurol., 10:149–157, 1964.

Bjure, A.; and Laurell, H.: Om abnorma statiska cirkulationsfenomen och darmed sammanhängande sjukliga symptom. Lakareforen. Forhandl., 33:1–23, 1927.

Bliddal, J.; and Nielsen, I.: Renin, aldosterone, and electrolytes in idiopathic orthostatic hypotension. Dan. Med. Bull., 17:153–157, 1970.

Blomqvist, C. G.: Orthostatic hypotension. Hypertension, 8:772, 1987.

Blomqvist, C. G.; and Stone, H. L.: Cardiovascular adjustments to gravitational stress. In, Handbook of Physiology (Shepherd, J. T.; and Abboud, F. M.; eds.). Sect. 2, The Cardiovascular System. American Physiological Society, Washington, D.C., pp. 968–1025, 1984.

Bradbury, S.; and Eggleston, C.: Postural hypotension: A report of three cases. Am. Heart J., 1:73–86, 1925.

Brown, R. T.; Polinsky, R. J.; and Baucom, C. E.: Euglycemic insulin-induced hypotension in autonomic failure. Clin. Neuropharmacol., 12:227–231, 1989.

Burnum, J. F.; Hickam, J. B.; and Stead, E. A.: Hyperventilation in postural hypotension. Circulation, 10:362–365, 1954.

Chapman, E. M.; and Asmussen, E.: On the occurrence of dyspnea, dizziness, and precordial distress occasioned by the pooling of blood in varicose veins. J. Clin. Invest., 21:393–399, 1942.

Charness, M. E.; Simon, R. P.; and Greenberg, D. A.: Ethanol and the nervous system. N. Engl. J. Med., 321:442–454, 1989.

Chobanian, A. V.; Tifft, C. P.; Faxon, D. P.; Creager, M. L. A.; and Sackel, H.: Treatment of orthostatic hypotension with ergotamine. Circulation, 67:602–609, 1983.

Chobanian, A. V.; Volicer, L.; Tifft, C. P.; Gavras, H.; Liang, C. S.; and Faxon, D.: Mineralocorticoid-induced hypertension in patients with orthostatic hypotension. N. Engl. J. Med., 301:68–73, 1979.

Chobanian, A. V.; Volicer, L.; Liang, C. S.; Kershaw, G.; and Tifft, C.: Use of propranolol in the treatment of idiopathic orthostatic hypotension. Trans. Assoc. Am. Physicians, 90:324–334, 1977.

Chokroverty, S.; Barron, K. D.; Arieff, A. J.; and Rovner, R. N.: A case of severe orthostatic hypotension. Trans. Am. Neurol. Assoc., 92:216–219, 1967.

Christensen, N. J.: Acute effects of insulin on cardiovascular function and noradrenaline uptake and release. Diabetologia, 25:377–381, 1983.

Cohen, E. I.: L'Hypotension orthostatique des gastrectomises. Presse. Med., 65:688–690, 1957.

Cohen, J. A.; and Laudenslager, M.: Autonomic nervous system involvement in patients with human immunodeficiency virus infection. Neurology, 39:1111–1112, 1989.

Cohn, J. H.: Blood pressure measurement in shock. J.A.M.A., 199:118–121, 1967.

Cohn, J. N.: Paroxysmal hypertension and hypovolemia. N. Engl. J. Med., 275:643–646, 1966.

Craddock, C.; Pasvol, G.; Bull, R.; Protheroe, A.; and Hopkin, J.: Cardiorespiratory arrest and autonomic neuropathy in man. Lancet, 2:16–18, 1987.

Crook, J. E.; Robertson, D.; and Whorton, A. R.: Prostaglandin suppression: Inability to correct severe idiopathic orthostatic hypotension. South. Med. J., 73:318–320, 1981.

Cryer, P. E.; and Weiss, S.: Reduced plasma norepinephrine response to standing in autonomic dysfunction. Arch. Neurol., 33:275–277, 1976.

Davies, A. O.; Mares, A.; Pool, J. L.; and Taylor, A. A.: Mitral valve prolapse with symptoms of beta-adrenergic hypersensitivity—Beta2-adrenergic receptors supercoupling with desensitization on isoproterenol exposure. Am. J. Med., 82:193–201, 1987.

Davies, B.; Bannister, R.; and Sever, P.: Pressor amines and monoamine oxidase inhibitors for treatment of postural hypotension in autonomic failure: Limitations and hazards. Lancet, 1:172–175, 1978.

Davis, T. A.; and Delafuente, J. C.: Orthostatic hypotension: Therapeutic alternatives for geriatric patients. D.I.C.P., 23:750–756, 1989.

de Caestecker, J. S.; Ewing, D. J.; Tothill, P.; Clarke, B. F.; and Heading, R. C.: Evaluation of oral cisapride and metoclopramide in diabetic autonomic neuropathy: An eight week double-blind crossover study. Aliment. Pharmacol. Therap., 3:69–81, 1989.

de Gennes, L.; Bricaire, H.; Moreau, L.; Courjaret, J.; Blanc, G.; and Pasquier, P.: Les phéochromocytomes avec hypotension orthostatique: à propos d'une observation personnelle. Presse. Med., 72:1413–1418, 1964.

Demanet, J. C.: Usefulness of noradrenaline and tyramine infusion tests in the diagnosis of orthostatic hypotension. Cardiology, 61(suppl. 1):213–224, 1976.

des Lauriers, A.; Widlocher, D.; Allilaire, J. F.; Lecrubier, Y.; and Simon, P.: Effects correcteurs de la yohimbine sur l'hypotension orthostatique induite par les antidepresseurs tricycliques. Ann. Med. Interne., 131:508–509, 1980.

Diamond, M. A.; Murray, R. H.; and Schmid, P. G.: Idiopathic postural hypotension: Physiologic observations and report of a new mode of therapy. J. Clin. Invest., 49:1341–1348, 1970.

Dobkin, B. H.; and Rosenthal, N. P.: Clinical assessment of autonomic dysfunction: An approach to the Shy-Drager syndrome. Bull. Los Angeles Neurol. Soc., 40:101–110, 1975.

Draper, A. J.: The cardioinhibitory carotid sinus syndrome. Ann. Intern. Med., 32:700–716, 1950.

Eckberg, D. L.: Parasympathetic cardiovascular control in human disease: A critical review of methods and results. Am. J. Physiol., 239:H581–H593, 1980.

Edmonds, M. E.; Jones, T. C.; Saunders, W. A.; and Sturrock, R. D.: Autonomic neuropathy in rheumatoid arthritis. Br. Med. J., 2:173–175, 1979.

Engel, G. L.: Psychologic stress, vasodepressor (vasovagal) syncope, and sudden death. Ann. Intern. Med., 89:403–412, 1978.

Evelyn, K. A.; Singh, M. M.; Chapman, W. P.; Perera, G. A.; and Thaler, H.: Effect of throacolumbar sympathectomy on the clinical course of primary (essential) hypertension. A ten-year study of 100 sympathectomized patients compared with individually matched, symptomatically treated control subjects. Am. J. Med., 28:188–221, 1960.

Ewing, D. J.; Campbell, I. W.; and Clarke, B. F.: The natural history of diabetic autonomic neuropathy. Q. J. Med., 49:95–108, 1980.

Feely, J.; Wade, D.; McAllister, C. B.; Wilkinson, G. R.; and Robertson, D.: Effect of hypotension on liver blood flow and lidocaine disposition. N. Engl. J. Med., 307:866–869, 1982.

Ferdinandus, J.; Pederson, J. A.; and Whang, R.: Hypermagnesemia as a cause of refractory hypotension, respiratory depression, and coma. Arch. Intern. Med., 141:669–670, 1981.

Finley, J. P.; and Tibbles, J. A. R.: Severe postural hypotension in childhood with autonomic neuropathy and occult systemic neuropathy. J. Pediatr., 100:409–412, 1982.

Floras, J. S.; Hassan, M. O.; Jones, J. V.; Osikowska, B. A.; Sever, P. S.; and Sleight, P.: Consequences of impaired arterial baroreflexes in essential hypertension: Effects on pressor responses, plasma noradrenaline and blood pressure variability. J. Hypertens., 6:525–535, 1988.

Fouad, F. M.; Tadena-Thome, L.; Bravo, E. L.; and Tarazi,

R. C.: Idiopathic hypovolemia. Ann. Intern. Med., 104:298–303, 1986.

Gaffney, F. A.; Bastian, B. C.; Lane, L. B.; Taylor, W. F.; Horton, J.; Schutte, J. E.; Graham, R. M.; Pettinger, W.; and Blomqvist, C. G.: Abnormal cardiovascular regulation in the mitral valve prolapse syndrome. Am. J. Cardiol., 52: 316–320, 1983.

Ghrist, D. G.; and Brown, G. E.: Postural hypotension with syncope: Its successful treatment with ephedrine. Am. J. Med. Sci., 175:336–349, 1928.

Goldberg, M. R.; and Robertson, D.: Evidence for the existence of vascular α2-adrenergic receptors in humans. Hypertension, 6:551–556, 1984.

Goldberg, M. R.; and Robertson, D.: Yohimbine: A pharmacological probe for study of the α2-adrenoreceptor. Pharmacol. Rev., 35:143–180, 1983.

Goldberg, M. R.; Robertson, D.; and FitzGerald, G. A.: Prostacyclin biosynthesis and platelet function in autonomic dysfunction. Neurology, 35:120–123, 1985.

Goldberg, M. R.; Hollister, A. S.; and Robertson, D.: Influence of yohimbine on blood pressure, autonomic reflexes and plasma catecholamines in humans. Hypertension, 5:772–778, 1983.

Goldberg, M. R.; Robertson, R. M.; and Robertson, D.: Atrial tachypacing for primary orthostatic hypotension. N. Engl. J. Med., 303:885–886, 1980.

Goldstein, D. S.; Polinsky, R. J.; Garty, M.; Biaggioni, I.; Robertson, D.; Brown, R. T.; Stull, R.; and Kopin, I. J.: Patterns of plasma levels of catechols in idiopathic orthostatic hypotension. Ann. Neurol., 26:558–563, 1989.

Gonin, A.; Mornex, R.; and Dissard, P.: Hypotension orthostatique, secondaire à une anémie hypochrome. Arch. Mal. Coeur., 46:911–921, 1953.

Gordon, R. D.; Kuchel, O.; Liddle, G. W.; and Island, D. P.: Role of the sympathetic nervous system in regulating renin and aldosterone production in man. J. Clin. Invest., 46:599–605, 1967.

Graham, H. G.; and Oppenheimer, D. R.: Orthostatic hypotension and nicotine sensitivity in a case of multiple system atrophy. J. Neurol. Neurosurg. Psychiatry, 32:28–34, 1969.

Gross, M.; Bannister, R.; and Godwin-Austen, R.: Orthostatic hypotension in Parkinson's disease. Lancet, 1:174–176, 1972.

Guilleminault, C.; Tilkian, A.; Lehrman, K.; Forno, L.; and Dement, W. C.: Sleep apnoea syndrome: States of sleep and autonomic dysfunction. J. Neurol. Neurosurg. Psychiatry, 40:718–725, 1977.

Hammarstrom, S.: Orthostatic hypotension after sympathectomy in hypertensives—The possible key to the beneficial effect of the operation. Acta. Med. Scand., 110:126–137, 1942.

Heieren, E.: Primaer postural hypotensjon: To tilfelle av Shy-Dragers syndrom. Tidsskr. Nor. Laegeforen., 92:1115–1119, 1972.

Hines, S.; Houston, M.; and Robertson, D.: The clinical spectrum of autonomic dysfunction. Am. J. Med., 70:1091–1096, 1981.

Hoeldtke, R. D.; and Israel, B. C.: Treatment of orthostatic hypotension with octreotide. J. Clin. Endocrinol. Metab., 68: 1051–1059, 1989.

Hoeldtke, R. D.; Dworkin, G. E.; Gaspar, S. R.; Israel, B. C.; and Boden, G.: Effect of the somatostatin analogue SMS-201-995 on the adrenergic response to glucose ingestion in patients with postprandial hypotension. Am. J. Med., 86: 673–677, 1989a.

Hoeldtke, R. D.; Dworkin, G. E.; Gaspar, S. R.; and Israel, B. C.: Sympathotonic orthostatic hypotension. Neurology, 39:34–40, 1989b.

Hoeldtke, R. D.; Cavanaugh, S. T.; Hughes, J. D.; and Polansky, M.: Treatment of orthostatic hypotension with dihydroergotamine and caffeine. Ann. Int. Med., 105:168–173, 1989c.

Hoeldtke, R. D.; Cavanaugh, S. T.; and Hughes, J. D.: Treatment of orthostatic hypotension: Interaction with pressor drugs and tilt table conditioning. Arch. Phys. Med. Rehabil., 69:895–898, 1988a.

Hoeldtke, R. D.; Cavanaugh, S. T.; Hughes, J. D.; Mattis-Graves, K.; Hobnell, E.; and Grover, W. D.: Catecholamine metabolism in kinky hair disease. Pediatr. Neurol., 4:23–26, 1988b.

Hoeldtke, R. D.; Boden, G.; and O'Dorisio, T. M.: Treatment of postprandial hypotension with a somatostatin analogue. Am. J. Med., 81:83–87, 1986a.

Hoeldtke, R. D.; O'Dorisio, Th. M.; and Boden, G.: Treatment of autonomic neuropathy with a somatostatin analog SMS 201-995. Lancet, 2:602–605, 1986b.

Houston, M.; Thompson, W. L.; and Robertson, D.: Shock: Diagnosis and management. Arch. Int. Med., 144:1433–1439, 1984.

Hui, K. K. P.; and Conolly, M. E.: Increased numbers of beta receptors in orthostatic hypotension due to autonomic dysfunction. N. Engl. J. Med., 304:1473–1476, 1981.

Ibrahim, M. M.; Tarazi, R. C.; Shafer, W. H.; Bravo, E. L.; and Dustan, H. P.: Unusual tyramine responsiveness in idiopathic orthostatic hypotension. Med. J. Cairo Univ., 47:49–55, 1979.

Ibrahim, M. M.; Tarazi, R. C.; Dustan, H. P.; and Bravo, E. L.: Idiopathic orthostatic hypotension: Circulatory dynamics in chronic autonomic insufficiency. Am. J. Cardiol., 34:288–294, 1974.

Ingall, T. J.; McLeod, J. G.; and Tamura, N.: Autonomic function and unmyelinated fibers in chronic inflammatory demyelinating polyradiculoneuropathy. Muscle Nerve, 13: 70–76, 1990.

Jansen, R. W. M. M.; Peeters, T. L.; Lenders, J. W. M.; van Lier, H. J. J.; V't Laar, A.; and Hoefnagels, W. H. L.: Somatostatin analog octreotide (SMS 201-995) prevents the decrease in blood pressure after oral glucose loading in the elderly. J. Clin. Endocrinol. Metab., 68:752–756, 1989.

Janssens, J.; Peeters, T. L.; Vantrappen, G.; Tack, J.; Urbain, J. L.; De Roo, M.; Muls, E.; and Bouillon, R.: Improvement of gastric emptying in diabetic gastroparesis by erythromycin. N. Engl. J. Med., 322:1028–1031, 1990.

Johnson, D. A.; Roth, G. M.; and Craig, W. M.: Orthostatic hypotension following chordotomy for intractable pain. Mayo Clin. Proc., 27:131–136, 1952.

Jones, D. H.; and Reid, J. L.: Volume expansion and vasodilators in the treatment of idiopathic postural hypotension. Postgrad. Med., 56:234–235, 1980.

Kaufmann, H.; Brannan, T.; Krakoff, L.; Yahr, M. D.; and Mandeli, J.: Treatment of orthostatic hypotension due to autonomic failure with a peripheral alpha-adrenergic agonist (midodrine). Neurology, 38:951–956, 1988.

Kennedy, W. R.; Navarro, X.; Goetz, F. C.; Sutherland, D. E. R.; and Najarian, J. S.: Effects of pancreatic transplantation on diabetic neuropathy. N. Engl. J. Med., 322:1031–1037, 1990.

Kipfer, K.: Postural Hypotension: Ein Therapieversuch mit synthetischen Hypertensin II. Cardiologia, 34:131–138, 1959.

Kochar, M. S.; Itskowitz, H. D.; and Albers, J. W.: Treatment of orthostatic hypotension with indomethacin. Am. Heart J., 98:271, 1979.

Koenig, M. G.; Spickard, A.; Cardella, M. A.; and Rogers, D. E.: Clinical and laboratory observations on type E botulism in man. Medicine, 43:517–545, 1964.

Kooner, J. S.; Raimbach, S.; Bannister, R.; Peart, S.; and Mathias, C. J.: Angiotensin converting enzyme inhibition lowers blood pressure in patients with primary autonomic failure independently of plasma renin levels and sympathetic nervous activity. J. Hypertens., 7(suppl. 6):S42–S43, 1989.

Kopin, I. J.; Polinsky, R. J.; Oliver, J. A.; Oddershede, I. R.; and Ebert, M. H.: Urinary catecholamine metabolites distinguish different types of sympathetic neuronal dysfunction in patients with orthostatic hypotension. J. Clin. Endocrinol. Metab., 57:632–637, 1983.

Korns, H. M.; and Randall, W. L.: Orthostatic hypotension treated with Benzedrine. Am. Heart J., 13:114–118, 1937.

Krane, R. J.; Goldstein, I.; and Saenz de Tejada, I.: Impotence. N. Engl. J. Med., 321:1648–1659, 1989.

Kranzler, H. R.; and Cardoni, A.: A sodium chloride treatment of antidepressant-induced orthostatic hypotension. J. Clin. Psychol., 49:366–368, 1988.

Kronenberg, M. W.; Forman, M. B.; Onrot, J.; and Robertson, D.: Enhanced left ventricular contractility in autonomic failure: Assessment using pressure-volume relations. J. Am. Coll. Cardiol., 15:1334–1342, 1990.

Krum, H.; Howes, G. L.; Brown, D. J.; and Louis, W. J.: Blood pressure variability in tetraplegic patients with autonomic hyperreflexia. Paraplegia, 24:284–288, 1989.

Kuchel, O.; Buu, N. T.; Hamet, P.; LaRochelle, P.; Gutkowska, J.; Schiffrin, E. L.; Borque, M.; and Genest, J.: Orthostatic hypotension: A posture-induced hyperdopaminergic state. Am. J. Med. Sci., 289:3–11, 1985.

Kuchel, O.; Buu, N. T.; Gutkowska, J.; and Genest, J.: Treatment of severe orthostatic hypotension by metoclopramide. Ann. Intern. Med., 93:841–843, 1980.

Landmark, K.; and Kravik, S.: Bruk av anti-G-drakt: Behandlingen av idiopatisk ortostatisk hypotensjon. Tidsskr. Nor. Laegeforen., 99:1530–1531, 1979.

Lang, E.; Jansen, W.; and Pfaf, W.: Orthostatische Hypotonie bei ältern Menschen. Med. Klin., 70:1976–1981, 1975.

Langford, H. G.; Sanford, R.; Smith, R.; Currier, R.; Johnson, W.; Klein, R.; and Bagget, J.: Neurogenic hypertension in man: Reis, Barman-Gebber, or Carey Syndrome. J. Hypertens., 5 (suppl. 5):S467–S469, 1987.

LeCrubier, Y.; Puech, A. J.; and Des Lauriers, A.: Favourable effects of yohimbine on clomipramine-induced orthostatic hypotension: A double-blind study. Br. J. Clin. Pharmacol., 12:90–93, 1981.

Lenders, J. W. M.; Morre, H. L. C.; Smits, P.; and Thien, T.: The effects of caffeine on the postprandial fall of blood pressure in the elderly. Age Ageing, 17:236–240, 1988.

Lewis, P.: Familial orthostatic hypotension. Brain, 87:719–728, 1964.

Lipsitz, L. A.: Minireview: Altered blood pressure homeostasis in advanced age: Clinical and research implications. J. Gerontol., 44:M179–M183, 1989a.

Lipsitz, L. A.: Orthostatic hypotension in the elderly. N. Engl. J. Med., 321:952–957, 1989b.

Lipsitz, L. A.; Pluchino, F. C.; Wei, J. Y.; Minaker, K. L.; and Rowe, J. W.: Cardiovascular and norepinephrine responses after meal consumption in elderly (older than 75 years) persons with postprandial hypotension and syncope. Am. J. Cardiol., 58:810–815, 1986.

Lopes de Faria, S. R. G. F.; Zanella, M. T.; Amoriolo, A.; Ribiero, A. B.; and Chacra, A. R.: Peripheral dopaminergic blockade for the treatment of diabetic orthostatic hypotension. Clin. Pharmacol. Ther., 44:670–674, 1988.

Low, P. A.; and Dyck, P. J.: Splanchnic preganglionic neurons in man. II. Morphometry of myelinated fibers of T7 ventral spinal root. Acta Neuropath. (Berl.), 40:55–61, 219–225, 1977.

Luft, F.; and von Euler, U. S.: Two cases of postural hypotension showing a deficiency in release of norepinephrine and epinephrine. J. Clin. Invest., 32:1065–1069, 1953.

Lyle, C. B.; Monroe, J. T.; Flinn, D. E.; and Lamb, L. E.: Micturition syncope: Report of 24 cases. N. Engl. J. Med., 265:982–986, 1961.

MacLean, A. R.; Allen, E. V.; and Magath, T. B.: Orthostatic tachycardia and orthostatic hypotension: Defects in the return of venous blood to the heart. Am. Heart J., 24:145–163, 1944.

Mader, S. L.: Orthostatic hypotension. Geriatr. Med., 73:1337–1349, 1989.

Mader, S. L.: Diurnal measurement of postural blood pressure responses in healthy old and young subjects. J. Am. Geriatr. Soc., 36:655, 1988.

Magrini, F.: Funzione cardiaca e vascolare dell'ipotensione ortostatica idiopatica. Boll. Soc. Ital. Cardiol. (Roma), 20:1183–1192, 1975.

Mahoudeau, D.; Singer, B.; Gilbert, J. C.; Goulon, M.; and Gajdos, P.: À propos d'un cas de maladie de Shy et Drager: Études hemodynamiques et pharmacodynamiques: interêt de la cyproheptadine. Rev. Neurol., 126:410–414, 1972.

Man in't Veld, A. J.; and Schalekamp, M. A. D. H.: Pindolol acts as a beta-adrenoceptor agonist in orthostatic hypotension: Therapeutic implications. Br. Med. J., 282:929–931, 1981.

Man in't Veld, A. J.; Boomsma, F. V. D.; Mieracker, A. H.; and Schalekamp, M. A. D. P.: Effect of an unnatural noradrenaline precursor on sympathetic control and orthostatic hypotension in dopamine-beta-hydroxylase deficiency. Lancet, 2:1172–1175, 1987a.

Man in't Veld, A. J.; Boomsma, F.; Moleman, P.; and Schalekamp, M. A. D. H.: Congenital dopamine-beta-hydroxylase deficiency. A novel orthostatic syndrome. Lancet, 1:183–187, 1987b.

Man in't Veld, A. J.; Boomsma, F.; and Schalekamp, M. A. D. H.: Effects of beta-adrenoreceptor agonists and antagonists in patients with peripheral autonomic neuropathy. Br. J. Clin. Pharmacol., 13:367S–374S, 1982.

Mares, A.; Davies, A. O.; and Taylor, A. A.: Diversity in supercoupling of beta2-adrenergic receptors in orthostatic hypotension. Clin. Pharmacol. Ther., 47:371–381, 1990.

Mark, A. L.: The Bezold-Jarisch reflex revisited: Clinical implications of inhibitory reflexes originating in the heart. Br. Med. J., 285:1599–1601, 1982.

Mathias, C. J.; daCosta, D. F.; Fosbraey, P.; Bannister, R.; Wood, S. M.; Bloom, S. R.; and Christensen, N. J.: Cardiovascular, biochemical and hormonal changes during food-induced hypotension in chronic autonomic failure. J. Neurol. Sci., 94:255–269, 1989a.

Mathias, C. J.; daCosta, D. F.; McIntosh, C. M.; Fosbraey, P.; Bannister, R.; Wood, S. M.; Bloom, S. R.; and Christensen, N. J.: Differential blood pressure and hormonal effects after glucose and xylose ingestion in chronic autonomic failure. Clin. Sci., 77:85–92, 1989b.

Mathias, C. J.; Raimbach, S. J.; Cortelli, P.; Kooner, J. S.; and Bannister, R.: The somatostatin analogue SMS 201-995 inhibits peptide release and prevents glucose-induced hypotension in autonomic failure. J. Neurol., 235:S74–S75, 1988.

Mathias, C. J.; Fosbraey, P.; daCosta, D. F.; Thornely, A.; and Bannister, R.: Desmopressin reduces nocturnal polyuria, reverses overnight weight loss and improves morning postural hypotension in autonomic failure. Br. Med. J., 293:353–354, 1986.

Mathias, C. J.; Christensen, N. J.; Frankel, H. L.; and Spalding, J. M. K.: Cardiovascular control in recently injured tetraplegics in spinal shock. Q. J. Med., 48:273–287, 1979.

Michelakis, A. M.; and Robertson, D.: Plasma renin activity and levodopa in Parkinson's disease. J.A.M.A., 213:83–85, 1970.

Mosqueda-Garcia, R.; Tseng, C. J.; Appalsamy, M.; and Robertson, D.: Modulatory effects of adenosine on baroreflex activation in the brainstem of the normotensive rat. Eur. J. Pharmacol., 174:119–122, 1989.

Nanda, R. N.; Boyle, F. C.; Gillespie, J. S.; Johnson, R. H.; and Keogh, H. J.: Idiopathic orthostatic hypotension from failure of noradrenaline release in a patient with vasomotor innervation. J. Neurol. Neurosurg. Psychiatry, 40:11–19, 1977.

Nies, A. S.; Robertson, D.; and Stone, W. J.: Hemodialysis hypotension is not the result of uremic peripheral autonomic neuropathy. J. Lab. Clin. Med., 94:395–402, 1979.

Nylin, G.; and Levander, M.: Studies on the circulation with the aid of tagged erythrocytes in a case of orthostatic hypotension (asymphaticotonic hypotension). Ann. Intern. Med., 28:723–746, 1948.

Onrot, J.; Bernard, G. R.; Biaggioni, I.; Hollister, A. S.; and Robertson, D.: Cardiovascular effects of hypertension and alterations in PaCO2 in patients with autonomic failure. Am. J. Med. Sci., Submitted, 1990.

Onrot, J.; Fogo, A.; Biaggioni, I.; Robertson, D.; Hollister, A. S.; and Wiley, R. G.: Neck tumor with syncope due to paroxysmal sympathetic withdrawal. J. Neurol. Neurosurg. Psychiatry, 50:1063–1066, 1987a.

Onrot, J.; Goldberg, M. R.; Biaggioni, I.; Hollister, A. S.; Kincaid, D.; and Robertson, D.: Postjunctional vascular smooth muscle alpha-2 adrenoreceptors in human autonomic failure. Clin. Invest. Med., 10:26–31, 1987b.

Onrot, J.; Goldberg, M. R.; Hollister, A. S.; Biaggioni, I.; Robertson, R. M.; and Robertson, D.: Management of chronic orthostatic hypotension. Am. J. Med., 80:454–464, 1987c.

Onrot, J.; Goldberg, M. R.; Biaggioni, I.; Wiley, R.; Hollister, A. S.; and Robertson, D.: Oral yohimbine in human autonomic failure. Neurology, 37:215–220, 1987d.

Onrot, J.; Shaheen, O.; Biaggioni, I.; Goldberg, M. R.; Feely, J.; Wilkinson, G. R.; Hollister, A. S.; and Robertson, D.: Reduction in liver blood flow in many by caffeine and theophylline. Clin. Pharmacol. Ther., 40:506–510, 1986.

Onrot, J.; Goldberg, M. R.; Biaggioni, I.; Hollister, A. S.; Kincaid, D.; and Robertson, D.: Hemodynamic and humoral effects of caffeine in human autonomic failure. N. Engl. J. Med., 313:549–554, 1985.

Owen, C.; Dodson, W. H.; and Hammack, W. J.: Medical grand rounds from the University of Alabama Medical Center. South. Med. J., 60:289–296, 1967.

Park, D. M.; Johnson, R. H.; Crean, G. P.; and Robinson, J. F.: Orthostatic hypotension in bronchial carcinoma. Br. Med. J., 3:510–511, 1972.

Parris, W. C.; Goldberg, M. R.; and Robertson, D.: The anesthetic management of autonomic dysfunction. Anesthesiol. Rev., 11:17–23, 1984.

Pemberton, J.: Does constitutional hypotension exist? Br. Med. J., 298:660–662, 1989.

Perlroth, M. G.; Tschudy, D. P.; Marver, H. S.; Bernard, C. W.; Zeigel, R. F.; Rechgigl, M.; and Collins, A.: Acute intermittent porphyria. Am. J. Med., 41:149–162, 1966.

Peters, M.; and Penner, S. L.: Orthostatic paroxysmal ventricular tachycardia. Am. Heart J., 32:645–652, 1946.

Petito, C. K.; and Black, I. B.: Ultrastructure and biochemistry of sympathetic ganglia in idiopathic orthostatic hypotension. Ann. Neurol., 4:6–17, 1978.

Polinsky, R. J.; Holmes, K. V.; Brown, R. T.; and Weise, V.: CSF acetylcholinesterase levels are reduced in multiple system atrophy with autonomic failure. Neurology, 39:40–44, 1989.

Polinsky, R. J.; Brown, R. T.; Burns, R. S.; Harvey-White, J.; and Kopin, I. J.: Low lumbar CSF levels of homovanillic acid and 5-hydroxyindoleacetic acid in multiple system atrophy with autonomic failure. J. Neurol. Neurosurg. Psychiatry, 51:914–919, 1988.

Polinsky, R. J.; Brown, R. T.; Lee, G. K.; Timmers, K.; Culman, J.; Foldes, O.; Kopin, I. J.; and Recant, L.: Beta-endorphin, ACTH and catecholamine responses in chronic autonomic failure. Ann. Neurol., 21:573–577, 1987.

Polinsky, R. J.; Goldstein, D. S.; Brown, R. T.; Keiser, H. R.; and Kopin, I. J.: Decreased sympathetic neuronal uptake in idiopathic orthostatic hypotension. Ann. Intern. Med., 18: 48–53, 1985.

Polinsky, R. J.; Jimerson, D. C.; and Kopin, I. J.: Chronic autonomic failure: CSF and plasma 3-methoxy-4-hydroxyphenylglycol. Neurology, 34:979–983, 1984.

Polinsky, R. J.; Kopin, I. J.; Ebert, M. H.; and Weise, V.: Pharmacologic distinction of different orthostatic hypotension syndromes. Neurology, 31:1–7, 1981.

Polinsky, R. J.; Kopin, I. J.; Ebert, M. H.; and Weise, V.: The adrenal medullary response to hypoglycemia in patients with orthostatic hypotension. J. Endocrinol. Metabol., 51:1401–1406, 1980.

Radnakrishnan, K.; Shenoy, K. T.; Kumar, B.; Kaur, S.; and Khattri, H. N.: Orthostatic hypotension in lepromatous leprosy. Neurol. India, 26:25–27, 1978.

Ray, B. S.; and Stewart, H. J.: Glosspharyngeal neuralgia: A cause of cardiac arrest. Am. Heart J., 35:458–462, 1948.

Rea, R. F.; Biaggioni, I.; Robertson, R. M.; Haile, V.; and Robertson, D.: Reflex control of muscle sympathetic nerve activity in dopamine-beta-hydroxylase deficiency. Hypertension, 15:107–112, 1990.

Resnik, H. Jr.; Mason, M. F.; Terry, R. T.; Pilcher, C.; and Harrison, T. R.: The effect of injecting certain electrolytes

into the cisterna magna on the blood pressure. Am. J. Med. Sci., 191:835–850, 1936.

Riley, C. M.; Day, R. L.; Greeley, D. M.; and Langford, W. S.: Central autonomic dysfunction with defective lacrimation: I. Report of five cases. Pediatrics, 3:468–478, 1949.

Roberts, L. J.; and Oates, J. A.: Mastocytosis. In, Williams Textbook of Endocrinology (Wilson J. D.; and Foster, D. W.; eds.). Saunders, Philadelphia, pp. 1363–1379, 1985.

Robertson, D.: Contraindication to the use of ocular phenylephrine in idiopathic orthostatic hypotension. Am. J. Ophthalmol., 87:819–822, 1979.

Robertson, D.; and Robertson, R. M.: The Bezold-Jarisch reflex: Possible role in limiting myocardial ischemia. Clin. Cardiol., 4:75–79, 1981.

Robertson, D.; Tseng, C. J.; and Appalsamy, M.: Effects of smoking and nicotine on the cardiovascular system. Am. Heart J., 115:258–263, 1988.

Robertson, D.; Goldberg, M. R.; Onrot, J.; Hollister, A. S.; Thompson, J. C.; Wiley, R.; and Robertson, R. M.: Isolated failure of autonomic noradrenergic neurotransmission: Evidence for impaired beta-hydroxylation of dopamine. N. Engl. J. Med., 314:1494–1497, 1986a.

Robertson, D.; Goldberg, M. R.; Tung, C. S.; Hollister, A. S.; and Robertson, R. M.: Use of α2 adrenoreceptor agonists and antagonists in the functional assessment of the sympathetic nervous system. J. Clin. Invest., 78:576–581, 1986b.

Robertson, D.; Hollister, A. S.; Forman, M.; and Robertson, R. M.: Reflexes unique to myocardial ischemia and infarction. J. Am. Coll. Cardiol., 5:99B–104B, 1985.

Robertson, D.; Hollister, A. S.; Carey, E. L.; Tung, C. S.; Goldberg, M. R.; and Robertson, R. M.: Increased vascular beta2-adrenoceptor responsiveness in autonomic dysfunction. J. Am. Coll. Cardiol., 3:850–856, 1984a.

Robertson, D.; Goldberg, M. R.; Hollister, A. S.; Wade, D.; and Robertson, R. M.: Baroreceptor dysfunction in man. Am. J. Med., 76:A49–A58, 1984b.

Robertson, D.; Goldberg, M. R.; Hollister, A. S.; Wade, D.; and Robertson, R. M.: Clonidine raises blood pressure in idiopathic orthostatic hypotension. Am. J. Med., 74:193–199, 1983.

Robertson, D.; Wade, D.; and Robertson, R. M.: Postprandial alterations in cardiovascular hemodynamics in autonomic dysfunctional states. Am. J. Cardiol., 48:1048–1052, 1981.

Robertson, D.; Johnson, G. A.; Robertson, R. M.; Nies, A. S.; Shand, D. G.; and Oates, J. A.: Comparative assessment of stimuli that release neuronal and adrenomedullary catecholamines in man. Circulation, 59:637–643, 1979.

Robertson, D.; Frolich, J. C.; Carr, R. K.; Shand, D. G.; and Oates, J. A.: Effect of caffeine on plasma renin activity, catecholamines, and blood pressure. N. Engl. J. Med., 298: 181–186, 1978.

Sanders, A. O.: Postural hypotension with tachycardia. A case report. Am. Heart J., 7:808–813, 1932.

Sanders, J. S.; and Ferguson, D. W.: Profound sympathoinhibition complicating hypovolemia in humans. Ann. Intern. Med., 111:439–441, 1989.

Santos, A. D.; Mathew, P. K.; Hilal, A.; and Wallace, W. A.: Orthostatic hypotension: A commonly unrecognized cause of symptoms in mitral valve prolapse. Am. J. Med., 71:746–750, 1981.

Schatz, I. J.: Orthostatic hypotension: II. Clinical diagnosis, testing and treatment. Arch. Intern. Med., 144:1037–1041, 1990.

Schatz, I. J.: Orthostatic hypotension: Functional and neurogenic causes. Arch. Intern. Med., 144:773–777, 1984.

Schatz, I. J.; Ramanathan, S.; Villagomez, R.; and MacLean, C.: Orthostatic hypotension, catecholamines, and α-adrenergic receptors in mitral valve prolapse. West. J. Med., 152: 37–40, 1990.

Schirger, A.; and Thomas, J. E.: Idiopathic orthostatic hypotension: Clinical spectrum and prognosis. Cardiology, 61(suppl. 1):144–149, 1976.

Schirger, A.; Sheps, S. G.; Thomas, J. E.; and Fealy, R. D.:

Midodrine. A new agent in the management of idiopathic orthostatic hypotension and Shy-Drager syndrome. Mayo Clin. Proc., 56:429–433, 1981.

Schumer, M.; Burton, G.; Burton, C.; Crum, D.; and Pfeifer, M. A.: Diabetic autonomic neuropathy—Part I, II. Am. J. Med., 85:137–146, 1988.

Seibyl, J. P.; Krystal, J. H.; Price, L. H.; and Charney, D. S.: Use of yohimbine to counteract nortriptyline-induced orthostatic hypotension. J. Clin. Psychopharmacol., 9:67–68, 1989.

Shannon, R. P.; Wei, J. Y.; Rosa, R. M.; Epstein, F. H.; and Rowe, J. W.: The effect of age and sodium depletion on cardiovascular response to orthostasis. Hypertension, 8:438–443, 1986.

Sharpey-Schaefer, E. P.: The mechanism of syncope after coughing. Br. Med. J., 2:860–863, 1953.

Shneider, M. S.: Sindrom nedostatochnosti aortal'nosinokarotidnovo reflektornovo mekhanisma. Ter. Arkh., 34: 49–56, 1952.

Shy, G. M.; and Drager, G. A.: A neurological syndrome associated with orthostatic hypotension. Arch. Neurol., 2:511–527, 1960.

Silverberg, R.; Naparstek, Y.; Lewis, B. S.; and Levy, M.: Angina pectoris with normal coronary arteries in Shy-Drager syndrome. J. Neurol. Neurosurg. Psychiatry, 42:910–913, 1979.

Sims, K. B.; de la Chapelle, A.; Norio, R.; Sankila, E. M.; Hus, Y. P.; Rinehart, W. B.; Corey, T. J.; Ozelius, L.; Powell, J. F.; Bruns, G.; Gusella, J. F.; Murphy, D. L.; and Breakefield, X. O.: Monoamine oxidase deficiency in males with an X chromosome deletion. Neuron, 2:1069–1076, 1989.

Slaton, P. E.; and Biglieri, E. G.: Reduced aldosterone excretion in patients with autonomic insufficiency. J. Clin. Endocrinol., 27:37–45, 1967.

Solders, G.; Wilczek, H.; Gunnarson, R.; Tyden, G.; Persson, A.; and Groth, C. G.: Effects of combined pancreatic and renal transplantation on diabetic neuropathy: A two-year follow-up study. Lancet, 2:1232–1235, 1987.

Stacpoole, P.; and Robertson, D.: Combination H1 and H2 receptor antagonist therapy in diabetic autonomic neuropathy. South. Med. J., 75:634–635, 1982.

Streeten, D. P.: Orthostatic Disorders of the Circulation: Mechanisms, Manifestations, and Treatment. Plenum Publishing, New York, 1987, p. 167.

Thomson, P. D.; and Melmon, K. L.: Clinical assessment of autonomic function. Anaesthesiol. 29:724–731, 1968.

Tikholov, K.: Lechenie na ortostatichnaya khipotoniia s dikhidrirani ergotaminovi proizvodni. Vatr. Bol., 15:82–86, 1976.

Tseng, C. J.; Appalsamy, M.; Biaggioni, I.; and Robertson, D.: Purinergic receptors in the NTS and area postrema mediate hypotension and bradycardia. Hypertension, 11:191–197, 1988.

Tung, C. S.; Luk, H. N.; and Robertson, D.: The causes of chronic orthostatic hypotension. Anesth. Sinica., 23:124–130, 1985.

Tung, C. S.; Onuora, C. O.; Robertson, D.; and Goldberg, M. R.: Hypertensive effect of yohimbine following selective injection into the nucleus tractus solitarii of normotensive rats. Brain Res., 277:193–195, 1983.

van Lieshout, J. J.; Wieling, W.; Romijn, J. A.; and Stam, J.: Hyperadrenergic syndrome with hypertension, hypotension and myocardial necrosis in tetanus. Neth. J. Med., 33:33–36, 1988.

Wagner, H. N.; and Braunwald, E.: The pressor effect of the antidiuretic principle of the posterior pituitary in orthostatic hypotension. J. Clin. Invest., 35:1412–1418, 1956.

Watkins, P. J.: Diabetic autonomic neuropathy. N. Engl. J. Med., 322:1078–1079, 1990.

Wilcox, C. S.; Puritz, R.; Lightman, S. L.; Bannister, R.; and Aminoff, M. J.: Plasma volume regulation in patients with progressive autonomic failure during changes in salt intake and posture. J. Lab. Clin. Med., 104:331–339, 1984.

Williams, R. S.; and Bashore, T. M.: Paroxysmal hypotension associated with sympathetic withdrawal: A new disorder of autonomic vasomotor regulation. Circulation, 62:901–908, 1980.

Youmans, J. B.; Akeroyd, J. H.; and Frank, H.: Changes in the blood and circulation with changes in posture. The effect of exercise and vasodilatation. J. Clin. Invest., 14:739–753, 1935.

Youmans, J. B.; Wells, H. S.; Donley, D.; and Miller, D. G.: The effect of posture (standing) on the serum protein concentration and colloid osmotic pressure of blood from the foot in relation to the formation of edema. J. Clin. Invest., 13: 447–459, 1934.

Zarriello, J. J.: Idiopathic orthostatic hypotension and its relation to positive G tolerance. Armed Forces Med. J., 11:535–541, 1960.

Ziegler, M. G.; Lake, C. R.; and Kopin, I. J.: The sympathetic-nervous-system defect in primary orthostatic hypotension. N. Engl. J. Med., 296:293–297, 1977.

4

Treatment of Cardiovascular Disorders: Congestive Heart Failure

Gary Francis and Steven R. Goldsmith

SYNDROME OF CONGESTIVE HEART FAILURE

Physiology of Heart Failure

Congestive heart failure (CHF) is a common and highly lethal condition. Despite recent advances in the treatment of CHF, mortality remains high, in the range of 30% to 50% per year at the more advanced stages (Franciosa et al., 1983). Clearly, more effective measures are needed for treatment of CHF if significant additional progress is to be made in reducing the overall mortality and morbidity from this disease.

Prevention and treatment of CHF require insight into the pathophysiologic processes that underlie the initiation, maintenance, and progression of the disease. Treatment of CHF requires a sound knowledge of the pharmacologic therapy currently available, as well as of experimental approaches that show promise. This chapter will review the pathophysiology of CHF due to congestive cardiomyopathy with an emphasis on the implications of the various pathophysiologic mechanisms for therapy. An overview of the various classes of pharmacologic therapy for CHF with additional specific information regarding the major agents within each class will then be presented. The chapter should serve as a concise summary of our current level of insight into both the pathophysiology and treatment for CHF and should leave the reader prepared to appreciate the bases for the next series of advances in the therapy for CHF, some of which may be implemented widely in the near future.

Congestive heart failure is a term that encompasses many diseases if broadly construed. Literally, it may refer to vascular congestion (in the pulmonary or systemic circulations) due to failure of any component of the heart. Considering the pathophysiology and therapy of CHF in the broadest sense would therefore include discussion of diseases as diverse as congestive cardiomyopathy; diastolic heart failure due to either hypertrophy, infiltrative disease, or ischemia; valvular stenosis and insufficiency; several forms of congenital heart disease; cor pulmonale; and also the various acute and chronic constrictive processes originating in the pericardium. While the clinical presentation of many of these diseases may be similar, the causes and specific treatment of each problem may differ widely. Indeed, optimal therapy for CHF due to congestive cardiomyopathy may be contraindicated in the presence of significant valvular stenosis. This chapter will focus on CHF due to systolic failure of the left ventricle (LV). While some of the pathophysiologic processes involving the peripheral circulation in this syndrome may also be applicable to other forms of CHF, the relationship of peripheral circulatory factors to ventricular function in these other diseases and their implications for therapy may be substantially different. Therefore, the remaining discussion will be relevant primarily to CHF in the setting of impaired ventricular systolic function. Where appropriate, contrasts will be made with CHF caused by diastolic dysfunction, since this appears to be a common entity requiring pharmacologic therapy. No attempt will be made to discuss the other disease processes mentioned as they frequently require therapy directed at other problems such as ischemia or valve replacement.

We also note that *CHF* may not necessarily be the most accurate term to describe the syndrome primarily discussed in this chapter. Frequently, fatigue is the dominant symptom in patients with CHF, particularly in the early stages of the illness. Frank *congestion* may not be present at that stage. Many formulations have been put forward to describe the syndrome of CHF; none is perfect. In the simplest operational terms, CHF due to congestive cardiomyopathy is a syndrome in which there is a functional deficit in the contractile function of the left ventricle, which leads at first to diminished exercise capacity, and later, on the basis of both progressive LV dysfunction and various peripheral circulatory factors, to fluid retention and the development of frank circulatory congestion. This description implies that CHF is not just a disease of the heart. Indeed, as we shall emphasize, the full expression of the syndrome of CHF depends upon a highly complex interplay among the heart, the kidney, the peripheral circulation, and various neuroendocrine factors. The need to view CHF in this fashion is crucial if one is to understand fully contemporary therapy for CHF, which depends on modifying the milieu in which the LV functions to a much greater degree than treating the dysfunctional LV directly.

Pathophysiology of CHF

In this section, we focus on the pathophysiologic processes of CHF. We first consider factors directly affecting LV function and then discuss the importance of ventricular-loading conditions in congestive failure, emphasizing the disordered relationships between preload, afterload, and LV function. Finally, we discuss the neuroendocrine factors involved in exacerbating the peripheral circulatory abnormalities in CHF. This discussion should provide the reader with a background for understanding the rationale for the use of the various classes of pharmacologic agents, including diuretics, vasodilators, neurohumoral antagonists, inotropic agents, and β-adrenergic antagonists in the therapy of CHF.

Myocardial Dysfunction in CHF. Myocardial dysfunction in congestive cardiomyopathy is due to an irreversible loss of viable myocytes and other changes that may progress to dysfunction in initially normal myocardium. Loss of myocytes is irreversible since myocytes do not usually divide in adult hearts. Cell death may be a result of infarction in ischemic cardiomyopathy, but the cause is poorly understood in the idiopathic dilated cardiomyopathies. Although difficult to demonstrate convincingly in individual patients, many of these cases may be due to direct or immunologically mediated consequences of viral myocarditis. Hereditary, metabolic, and environmental factors also may contribute significantly to the causes of idiopathic dilated cardiomyopathy. While ethanol abuse seems to be a consistent environmental association, the explanation for this is not clear. A greater understanding of the causes of idiopathic dilated cardiomyopathy could allow specific therapeutic intervention prior to irreversible damage to large numbers of myocytes. At present, no such interventions are available, and we are left to treat the consequences of the destructive process or processes, whatever they may be.

Most of our current knowledge concerning contractile abnormalities in the residual myocardium in failing ventricles relates to disturbances in the adrenergic control of myocardial function. The basic components of the β-adrenergic pathway involved in stimulating myocardial contractility are shown in Fig. 4–1. Endogenous norepinephrine or adrenergic agonists when used as drugs interact with β-adrenergic receptors located on the cell surface. The human heart contains both β_1 and β_2 subtypes (as well as α_1-adrenergic receptors). β-Adrenergic agonists lead to an increase in the concentration of cytoplasmic calcium, which enhances contractility.

In CHF, there are several abnormalities in the β-adrenergic control of myocardial function. As a consequence of increased sympathetic stimulation, β_1 receptors are down-regulated (Bristow et al., 1982) in the hearts of patients with CHF compared with controls. In addition, there may be uncoupling of β_2 receptors from distal events in the contractility pathway (Bristow et al., 1986). These changes, as well as possible alterations in regulatory G proteins, may contribute to blunted responses to β-adrenergic agonists in CHF (Feldman et al., 1988; Neumann et al., 1988; Bohm et al., 1989). Interestingly, there is some evidence for preserved responses to forskolin (which causes maximal accumulation of cAMP independent of cell-surface receptors) or calcium in hearts from patients with CHF (Ginsburg et al., 1983; Fowler et al., 1986).

These observations have considerable importance for therapeutics in CHF, since benefit from β-adrenergic agonists would likely be limited acutely and could well exacerbate adrenergic receptor down-regulation that would contribute to tolerance developing during continuous exposure to adrenergically active agents. Conversely, β-adrenergic blockade *theoretically* could be useful in CHF by protecting the β-adrenergic receptors from excess chronic adrenergic stimulation. Up-regulation of the receptors would be the result (Heilbrunn et al., 1989). These biochemical

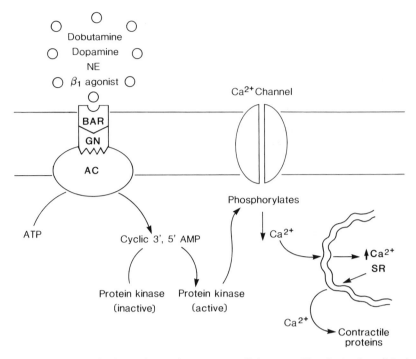

Fig. 4–1. Mechanism of β-adrenergic agonists on myocardial contractility. Activation of β-adrenergic receptors (BAR) stimulates adenylate cyclase (AC) via G_s, the stimulatory guanine nucleotide (GN) regulatory protein that leads to an increased concentration of cAMP. The cAMP activates a cAMP-dependent protein kinase that phosphorylates substrate proteins, including sarcolemma-bound Ca^{2+} transport channels and transport systems of sarcoplasmic reticulum (SR). This results in an influx of extracellular Ca^{2+}, which then activates the SR transport system to further increase the amount of Ca^{2+} available to contractile proteins. Also there is evidence that the α subunit of G_s may directly activate calcium channels. (Modified with permission from Francis, G. S.: Inotropic agents in the management of heart failure. In Drug Treatment of Heart Failure (Cohn, J. N., ed.). Adv. Ther. Com., Secaucus, NJ, 1988, pp. 179–197.)

considerations also imply that the most effective inotropic agents for chronic use in CHF might be directed at pathways distal to cell-surface receptors. However, phosphodiesterase inhibition, which increases the concentration of cAMP by slowing its rate of metabolism, has limited utility. An active area of investigation relates to the design of compounds that may directly affect calcium flux or sensitize contractile proteins to calcium.

Apart from the primary etiologic factors in CHF, other abnormalities may include ischemia, the consequences of compensatory cellular hypertrophy, depletion of high-energy phosphate stores, abnormalities in calcium transport, and abnormalities in coronary vasodilation (Hittinger et al., 1987). These abnormalities may be exacerbated by increased cardiac filling pressures that reduce coronary perfusion pressure for any given value of diastolic blood pressure (Salisbury et al., 1963). In the setting of increased myocardial oxygen demands, with increased cardiac filling pres-

sure (a situation typical of exercise in CHF, even if pressures are normal at rest), subendocardial ischemia may occur. Even without infarction, chronic ischemia may decrease LV function over time. This setting provides some rationale for the use of diuretic and venodilating drugs in CHF in order to maintain LV end-diastolic pressures as low as is feasible.

As a response to the loss of functional myocytes, hypertrophy occurs in the remaining myocardial tissue. Initially this response helps to maintain contractile function; however, over the long term, anatomic and biochemical changes in hypertrophied cells may actually contribute to further deterioration in myocardial performance. Current understanding of this process has been reviewed and termed *the cardiomyopathy of overload* (Katz, 1990). An important unresolved issue for therapeutics is whether chronic inotropic therapy exaggerates this process, thereby actually worsening myocardial function in the long term.

In some models of CHF, the myocardium has

been characterized by diminished stores of high-energy phosphate (Sievers et al., 1983). The explanation for this finding is unclear but is of potential concern since inotropic drugs can potentially enhance energy demands. However, the relevance of these findings to human CHF is uncertain (Katz, 1973).

Finally, there have been suggestions that calcium handling by failing myocardium is abnormal (Harigaya and Schwartz, 1969), resulting in impaired myocardial contractility and relaxation. There are also data that suggest that there is no clear abnormality of calcium handling (Movesesian et al., 1989; Wiegand et al., 1989). It is not clear whether this abnormality, if it exists, is a true etiologic factor contributing to the progression of CHF or actually a consequence of the already-established CHF.

Preload and Afterload. An understanding of the pathophysiology and therapy of CHF requires an appreciation of the relationships between ventricular function and conditions of cardiac loading, as well as identification of the primary abnormalities in myocardial function. Abnormalities in cardiac loading govern much of the clinical presentation of CHF and are the major therapeutic targets of current pharmacologic therapy for CHF. In this section, preload and afterload as they relate to LV function in CHF are discussed.

Preload. From the standpoint of muscle mechanics, preload is defined as end-diastolic fiber length. In the intact patient, preload is most closely correlated with LV volume. Since LV volume is difficult to measure accurately on a repetitive basis, end-diastolic pressure and pulmonary capillary wedge pressure often are used as surrogate measurements of preload. If the compliance of the LV is normal, this substitution usually is reasonable. However, if there is a primary reduction in compliance of the LV, then changes in pressure may not reflect expected changes in volume. This is an important issue in "diastolic" congestive heart failure in which filling pressures may be high despite low or normal preload; this may lead to dyspnea even with normal cardiac contractile function. In diastolic congestive failure, the fact that preload is normal despite an increase in cardiac filling pressure helps explain the sometimes deleterious effects of diuretics. Tachycardia may be increased in these patients because of diuretic-induced volume contraction. However, in congestive cardiomyopathy, preload is elevated due to a markedly dilated LV. Changes in pressure more accurately parallel changes in volume in this setting; nonetheless, care should be taken in relying too heavily on this pressure measurement as a true reflection of preload. Filling pressure may fall, with relief of vascular congestion,

while preload fails to change markedly due to a highly compliant, distended chamber.

The cardinal abnormality in preload in congestive heart failure, beyond the fact that it is increased, is expressed by the downward shift of the Frank-Starling relationship (Fig. 4–2). The Frank-Starling relationship relates LV volume to systolic function at constant contractility and afterload (Patterson et al., 1914). For a given increase in cardiac volume in CHF, less increase in cardiac output occurs than would be expected in a subject with a normal heart. This abnormality has several implications for patients with CHF. First, it is less possible for these patients to rely on increased cardiac volume to increase systolic function; indeed, these patients typically operate on a fairly flat, as well as depressed, Frank-Starling curve. As a result, when cardiac volume expands, there is little or no increase in ventricular performance; as volume continues to expand, pressure rises with pulmonary venous congestion, and dyspnea is the result. On the other hand, whereas a reduction in preload in a normal individual operating on a fairly steep normal curve results in a fall in cardiac output, a fall in preload in a patient with congestive heart failure can be accomplished without compromising cardiac performance. The "descending limb" of the Frank-Starling curve probably is not a relevant consideration over clinically encountered pressures and volumes (MacGregor et al., 1974), but improvements in ventricular function can result from a decreased preload in heart failure. A fall in cardiac volume and pressure decreases myocardial wall stress, which lessens myocardial oxygen demand. It also improves subendocardial perfusion pressure for any given arterial diastolic pressure. Less oxygen demand and better myocardial perfusion may then lead to improved systolic function. Since wall stress is a component of afterload, a decrease in preload also may lead to a fall in afterload with secondary improvement in systolic function (see below). Consequently, a fall in preload in a normal individual essentially moves the heart to a lower position on a normal Frank-Starling curve; reducing preload in a patient with congestive heart failure may lead to a shift to a more normal Starling curve, because of both decreased afterload and improved function. In patients with overt pulmonary edema, the sympathetic nervous system often is activated, leading to greatly increased afterload. In this setting, decreasing preload will lead to a decrement in afterload as well.

Afterload. Afterload can be thought of as the work done by the LV to eject blood. Put another way, afterload comprises the forces that oppose emptying of the LV during systole. While we often approximate afterload by the readily defined

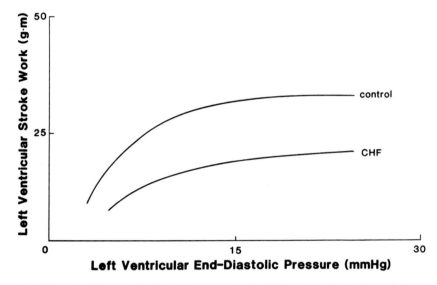

Fig. 4–2. Schematic left ventricular function curves plotting left ventricular stroke work (g · m) as a function of left ventricular end-diastolic filling pressure. Patients with CHF have a downward displacement of the curve. For any given filling or distending pressure, there is less stroke work, a fundamental hemodynamic abnormality of the failing heart. (From Francis, G. S.; and Archer, S. L.: J. Int. Care. Med., 4:84–92, 1989, by permission of Blackwell Scientific Publications, Inc.)

systemic vascular resistance, afterload is actually much more complex. Systemic vascular resistance is a static quantity—the instantaneous ratio of mean arterial pressure to cardiac output. But a true appreciation of afterload includes recognition of other influences that contribute to the total impedance to LV ejection. These factors include elastic properties of the great vessels and systolic wall stress. Systolic wall stress is modified by arterial pressure, which is influenced by systemic vascular resistance. Systolic wall stress is also dependent upon the volume of the LV and is therefore related to preload.

In CHF, the LV is exquisitely sensitive to small changes in afterload that would not greatly affect the function of the normal heart (Fig. 4–3) (Cohn, 1973). Very small increases in afterload may substantially decrease LV function; conversely, very small decreases in afterload may improve LV function considerably in patients with CHF. The sensitivity of the failing ventricle to changes in afterload may contribute to the efficacy of drugs that decrease afterload in patients with CHF. While we commonly think of such drugs primarily as vasodilators acting on the arterial side of the circulation, it is important to realize that since afterload is in fact a complex quantity, agents that act at sites other than the arterial resistance vessels also may influence afterload. For example, since preload actually modifies afterload through its impact on systolic wall stress, a fall in preload tends to reduce afterload to some extent.

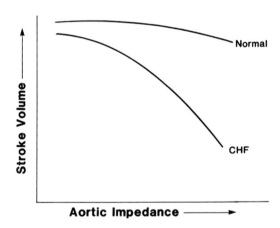

Fig. 4–3. Schematic left ventricular stroke volume is plotted as a function of aortic impedance in normal persons and in a theoretical patient with CHF. The normal left ventricle will call upon "preload reserve" to maintain stroke volume when impedance to left ventricular ejection is increased. However, the failing left ventricle is exquisitely sensitive to heightened aortic impedance, which leads to a prompt and substantial reduction in stroke volume. (From Francis, G. S.; and Archer, S. L.: J. Int. Care Med., 4:84–92, 1989, by permission of Blackwell Scientific Publications, Inc.)

In a normal ventricle, this is not very important since the function of the LV is not sensitive to small changes in afterload (Fig. 4–3). However, in the setting of a large heart with an increased sensitivity to changes in afterload, the fall in afterload accomplished solely by decreased preload may be considerable. Reliable data to directly support this contention are lacking in human heart failure, but the dependence of afterload on cardiac size has been shown in canine hearts (Weber and Janicki, 1979). Consequently, in CHF, the improvement in LV function due to a fall in afterload may require understanding a number of different variables that may be influenced to a greater or lesser degree by a number of different types of pharmacologic intervention. Also, one should be aware that improvement in LV function due to diminished afterload may not be immediate. Time may be required for the LV to derive maximum improvement from functioning in the milieu of diminished impedance. This time dependence in the adaptation of ventricular function to a decreased afterload may explain in part why the acute hemodynamic response of the LV to vasodilators does not always correlate with long-term clinical outcome.

The relationships between preload, afterload, and LV contractility are significantly altered during CHF. Understanding the factors that lead to and perpetuate increased preload and afterload is important. Modification of these factors may lead to a reduction in preload and afterload with improvements in LV function and the clinical state of the patient.

Abnormalities of preload initially develop as a consequence of reduced LV ejection. Diminished systolic function leads to cardiac enlargement, and as failure progresses, the heart may continue to dilate. The progression of cardiac dilatation may be markedly accentuated by salt and water retention. Indeed, if salt and water were not retained and the circulation were not expanded, very little actual change in preload would occur. Congestive heart failure reflects a complex state associated with avid sodium retention. If cardiac output or arterial pressure falls, the kidney may sense this as volume "depletion" and act via normal homeostatic mechanisms to retain salt and water in an effort to compensate for circulatory inadequacy. The problem with invoking this explanation as the sole mechanism to explain salt and water retention in CHF is that retention of salt frequently is seen even when the resting cardiac output and arterial pressures are normal.

Afterload becomes abnormal during LV systolic failure in part as a consequence of increased wall stress due to the expansion of preload. Remodeling and hypertrophy of the ventricle in response to volume expansion (and possibly neuro-endocrine influences) also contribute to changes in wall stress. However, increased impedance to ventricular ejection depends largely on extracardiac factors. Salt and water retention lead to stiffness in the vasculature that may decrease responsiveness to vasodilating stimuli (Zelis et al., 1968). Also, since an increased systemic vascular resistance is characteristic of many patients with congestive failure, it may be that activation of various endogenous vasoconstrictor systems underlies much of the increased vascular impedance in patients with CHF.

Neuroendocrine Factors in CHF. Maladaptive worsening of the abnormalities in ventricular loading conditions that occur in CHF may depend in part upon an imbalance of vasoconstrictors and vasodilator mechanisms in the peripheral circulation. Progressively increased preload and afterload may lead to a further deterioration in ventricular function; consequently, the activation of vasoconstrictor forces in the periphery in CHF may tend to exacerbate the fundamental abnormality in congestive cardiomyopathy. This view is supported by the observation that improvements in clinical outcome, including survival, may occur with drugs that either are vasodilators or can interrupt specific neuroendocrine pathways.

The major components of the neuroendocrine axis involved in chronic CHF include atrial natriuretic factor, the sympathetic nervous system, the renin-angiotensin system, and arginine vasopressin (Fig. 4–4). Imbalances in prostaglandins regulating vasoconstriction and vasodilation also have been reported (Dzau et al., 1984) but are less well studied than these other systems.

The major endogenous vasodilator-natriuretic substance likely to be of clinical significance in CHF is atrial natriuretic factor. Atrial natriuretic factor has both saluretic (Needleman and Greenwald, 1986) and vasodilating actions (Bolli et al., 1987) as well as a potent inhibitory effect on renin secretion (Burnett et al., 1984). The magnitude and importance of these effects in human physiology are uncertain. Atrial natriuretic factor concentrations are elevated in chronic CHF (Cody et al., 1986). Increased atrial natriuretic factor concentrations in plasma, particularly early in CHF, may exert a protective effect by promoting salt excretion, dilating the peripheral vasculature, and inhibiting release of renin. However, it is likely that once CHF is established, both the saluretic and vasodilating effects of atrial natriuretic peptide are markedly attenuated, possibly because of contracting vasoconstrictor systems.

Vasoconstricting systems of importance in CHF include elevated activity of the sympathetic nervous system, increased activity of the renin-

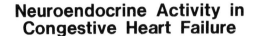

Neuroendocrine Activity in Congestive Heart Failure

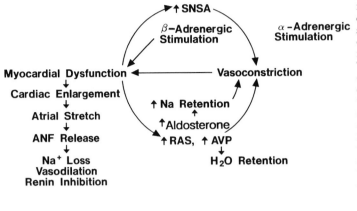

Fig. 4-4. Schematic representation of the neuroendocrine milieu in CHF. Atrial stretch leads to increased secretion of atrial natriuretic factor (ANF), which promotes salt excretion, vasodilation, and inhibition release of renin. In established CHF, however, there is activation of vasoconstrictor mechanisms that feedback negatively on myocardial function. This feedback may be direct, from possible adverse consequences of excessive adrenergic stimulation, and indirect, as a result of the contribution of vasoconstrictor mechanisms to ventricular afterload. The most likely effectors of neuroendocrine-related vasoconstriction include the α-adrenergic system, angiotensin II, and arginine vasopressin (AVP). Angiotensin II also stimulates aldosterone secretion. This in turn leads to retention of salt that may further contribute to vasoconstriction by impairing vascular reactivity. Finally, vasopressin also may contribute to expansion of intravascular volume by facilitating retention of water by the kidney. RAS refers to the renaangiotensin system. SNSA refers to the activity of the sympathetic nervous system.

angiotensin system, and increased plasma concentrations of arginine vasopressin (Francis et al., 1984). The sympathetic nervous system exerts vasoconstrictor effects via activation of peripheral α-adrenergic receptors. Both angiotensin II and arginine vasopressin (AVP) are vasoconstrictors with additional complex effects on circulatory regulation. These systems may have evolved as short-term regulators of the circulation in response to increases and decreases in blood volume and arterial pressure. The activity of the sympathetic nervous system and of vasopressin secretion are inhibited by the low-pressure cardiopulmonary mechanoreceptors (located within the ventricles and atria) and the high-pressure sinoaortic baroreceptors (Fig. 4-5). When pressure falls within the heart or the carotid sinus, this inhibition is diminished, leading to increased sympathetic nervous systemic activity and increased secretion of vasopressin. Conversely, when pressure is increased within the heart or in the region of the sinoaortic baroreceptor, additional suppressive activity is exerted on both these systems. In humans, hemodynamic determinants of secretion of arginine vasopressin are relatively unimportant; marked hypotension likely is required to stimulate release of AVP by nonosmotic means (Goldsmith et al., 1982). Activation of this system in CHF also does not seem to correlate with hemodynamic abnormalities (Goldsmith, 1983) and

may therefore be in part a response to the activation of the renin-angiotensin system and/or high circulating atrial natriuretic factor (ANF) concentrations. In many patients with chronic CHF, the arterial pressure is normal, the cardiac output may be normal at rest, and the intracardiac volume is typically expanded. Consequently, the explanation for elevated activity of the sympathetic nervous system in patients with CHF is not clear. Abnormalities may be present in the atrial receptor function, which could lessen tonic inhibition of the sympathetic nervous system (Zucker and Gilmore, 1985).

Plasma renin activity also is governed in part by hemodynamic factors. A fall in renal perfusion pressure promotes renin release; whether there is a specific link between the low-pressure cardiopulmonary receptors and renin release is unclear. There also are several other important determinants of plasma renin activity separate from baroreflex mechanisms—increased sympathetic drive to the kidney stimulates release of renin that could be important in the earlier stages of heart failure before any reduction in perfusion pressure is evident. Reduction in sodium chloride delivery to the macula densa also stimulates release of renin independently of the perfusion pressure and the level of sympathetic activity. The complexity of the control systems for renin likely accounts for the relative heterogeneity of plasma renin ac-

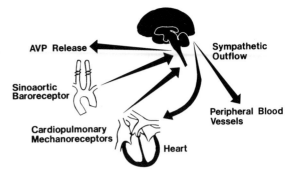

Fig. 4–5. Schematic representation of the baroreflex pathways that regulate the activity of the sympathetic nervous system and the release of AVP. Tonic inhibitory input from both the low-pressure cardiopulmonary mechanoreceptors and the high-pressure sinoaortic baroreceptors restrains activity of both systems. A rise in arterial pressure or expansion of cardiac volume increases receptor activity, enhances the inhibitory input, and decreases sympathetic activity and secretion of AVP. Conversely, a decrease in arterial pressure or cardiac volume decreases receptor activity, diminishes the inhibitory input, and increases sympathetic activity and secretion of AVP. In humans, only severe hypotension will increase secretion of AVP under isosmotic conditions, although the baroreceptor networks may be important in modulating the osmotic control of AVP.

tivity in patients with CHF compared with the consistent increase in measured sympathetic nervous system activity, the atrial natriuretic factor, and concentrations of vasopressin in plasma.

The afferent signals for neuroendocrine activation are not always evident. To state that increased sympathetic activity, increased renin-angiotensin system activity, and high concentrations of AVP are all present in order to maintain perfusion in the periphery in a patient with chronic CHF probably is an oversimplification. All these events may occur when cardiac output falls acutely, and this may occur in the end stages of the disease when the perfusion of vital organs requires activation of powerful vasoconstrictive mechanisms. However, these systems often are activated even at mild and moderate stages of the disease (Francis et al., 1990). Whether these changes represent useful adaptations to decreased cardiac function or are deleterious alterations is unclear.

In CHF, excessive sympathetic activity is reflected in an increased plasma norepinephrine concentration (Thomas and Marks, 1978; Levine et al., 1982), in increased norepinephrine spillover into plasma as assessed by kinetic techniques (Hasking et al., 1986), and by direct recordings of muscle sympathetic nerve activity (Leimbach et al., 1986). Plasma renin activity is increased in most patients with CHF, especially in more severely ill patients, and this could lead to increased concentrations of angiotensin II (Levine et al., 1982; Lilly et al., 1984). Finally, AVP concentrations also are frequently increased in congestive heart failure to an extent that may be associated with potential hemodynamic as well as renotubular effects (Goldsmith et al., 1986). These changes in CHF taken together suggest that norepinephrine, angiotensin II, and AVP all could contribute to both increased preload and increased afterload in heart failure by increasing systemic vascular resistance directly, and by pro-

moting renal salt and water retention via vasoconstriction in the renal circulation. Because of its role in regulating aldosterone secretion, angiotensin II also may exert indirect circulatory effects by enhancing sympathetic nervous system activity, releasing vasopressin, and increasing salt retention (Fig. 4-6). Arginine vasopressin may also directly increase water retention by virtue of its actions on the kidney.

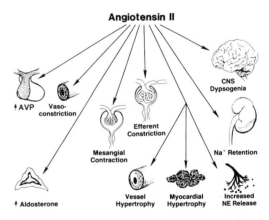

Fig. 4–6. The multiple actions of angiotensin II. This peptide is believed to have evolved to defend against volume loss and inadequate blood pressure. It is found circulating in blood and is also produced locally in a number of organs. In patients with CHF, angiotensin II directly constricts resistance vessels, the renal mesangium, and the postglomerular efferent arterioles and also stimulates release of aldosterone from the adrenal cortex. Angiotensin II also may promote vascular and myocardial hypertrophy, directly promote sodium retention, increase thirst via central nervous system actions, facilitate the release and/or the effects of norepinephrine (NE), and enhance vasopressin release. (From Francis, G. S.: Am. Heart J., 118:642–648, 1989, with permission.)

The extent to which these neuroendocrine changes actually explain the vasoconstriction found in patients with chronic CHF is not fully understood. The correlation between plasma concentrations of these substances and hemodynamic alterations has been consistently found but is not highly predictive (Levine et al., 1982). The best evidence for the contribution of neuroendocrine activation to vasoconstriction in CHF has been obtained by experiments that antagonize the actions of these systems. In terms of the sympathetic nervous system, α-adrenergic antagonists produce an acute fall in systemic vascular resistance and a rise in cardiac output (Creager et al., 1986; Kluger et al., 1982). However, chronic therapy with the α_1-receptor-selective antagonist prazosin does not appear to have efficacy, although the explanation for this loss in effect is not clear. Interestingly, β-adrenergic receptor antagonists may be useful in chronic therapy of selected patients with CHF, suggesting the possibility that continued stimulation of β-adrenergic receptors may have deleterious consequences in some patients with CHF.

The possible role of AVP in the vasoconstriction of chronic CHF is uncertain. Acutely, infusions of AVP cause a deterioration in hemodynamics in patients with CHF (Goldsmith et al., 1986). Administration of a selective antagonist of the V_1 receptor (the AVP-receptor subtype that mediates the vascular effects of AVP) produces some hemodynamic benefit in patients with elevated concentrations of AVP (Creager et al., 1986). However, there is no information regarding the effects of chronic administration of this antagonist to patients with CHF. Arginine vasopressin also may aggravate hyponatremia in CHF by activating the renal V_2-receptor subtype that promotes water retention; to what extent a V_2 antagonist might ameliorate this problem is not known. The largest body of data regarding the impact of neuroendocrine abnormalities in the vasoconstriction of CHF relates to the renin-angiotensin system. Angiotensin II may directly increase impedance to ejection in CHF by inducing vasoconstriction. Angiotensin II also may activate the sympathetic nervous systems and potentiate the effects of norepinephrine (Zimmerman et al., 1984) as well as stimulate secretion of vasopressin (Brooks et al., 1986) and release of aldosterone (Fig. 4–6). Consequently, excessive effects of angiotensin II may have an adverse impact on the course of CHF. There is a large clinical experience with angiotensin-converting enzyme (ACE) inhibitors, drugs that decrease plasma concentrations of angiotensin II. While not all the effects of inhibition of converting enzyme may be accounted for by a decrease in concentrations of angiotensin II in plasma, the acute effects of ACE inhibitors do relate to baseline renin activity in plasma (Kluger et al., 1982).

There is a great deal of evidence that neuroendocrine activation is found in patients with CHF and leads to enhanced vasoconstriction. The actual degree to which α-adrenergic receptor activity and vasopressin contribute to vasoconstriction and so to abnormalities in cardiac loading conditions during chronic CHF remains to be determined. Activation of the renin-angiotensin system over time is likely to have deleterious consequences. It appears that the homeostatic mechanisms activated by CHF may be maladaptive in the long term since these responses presumably evolved to cope with dehydration or blood loss rather than a chronic disease such as CHF. From a clinical standpoint, the most important aspect of activation of neuroendocrine mechanisms in CHF is that they provide specific targets for therapeutics. If indeed the imbalance between vasodilator and vasoconstrictor mechanisms is an important part of the syndrome, then pharmacologic agents that promote the activation of vasodilator mechanisms or prolong their effectiveness could be efficacious. Similarly, pharmacologic therapy based on a reduction in the activity of vasoconstrictor systems, or on the antagonism of the effect of these vasoconstrictor systems, might also be useful. A major component of our current therapy for CHF is in fact based on interference with the renin-angiotensin system. In the future, additional benefits may perhaps be derived through manipulation of the atrial natriuretic factor, the sympathetic nervous system, and AVP.

THERAPY FOR CHF

Acute heart failure often is due to myocardial infarction or decompensation of previously stable chronic heart failure. The treatment of *acute* CHF generally mandates that the patient be admitted to the hospital. Treatment often is initiated and carried out in the emergency ward and in the intensive care unit. With the benefit of hospitalization, patients usually can be stabilized with diuretics and vasodilators and the use of IV inotropic agents. The first part of this section will focus on therapy for the acutely ill patient with severe congestive heart failure or with pulmonary edema. The latter part of the section will present the treatment of stable, chronic CHF.

Treatment of Acute CHF

Acute heart failure, or acute pulmonary edema, represents a medical emergency. Patients often are breathless and unable to give a detailed history. The physical examination often reveals the cardinal features of circulatory congestion, including pulmonary rales, jugular venous distension, peripheral edema, diaphoresis, tachypnea, and cyanosis. The extent of physical findings is related to the acuteness of the onset of the syndrome as well as to the severity of pulmonary congestion. Vigorous therapy usually is needed and will depend to some extent on the cause of the heart failure. Generally, IV loop diuretics, nasal oxygen, morphine sulfate, and often IV nitroprusside or nitroglycerin are required. Selected patients will require inotropic support either with dobutamine or dopamine or a combination of these agents (Francis and Archer, 1989). In occasional instances, amrinone, an IV phosphodiesterase inhibitor, is useful. Each of these drugs will be discussed individually with reference to patients with severe and acute CHF in need of urgent therapy.

Diuretics. The usual therapeutic approach to the patient with acute pulmonary edema is to give IV furosemide as soon as the clinical diagnosis is suspected. The recommended dose is from 40 to 80 mg IV given over several minutes. Oral diuretics are not particularly useful in acute heart failure because they may not be readily absorbed by the edematous bowel, and their onset of action is much slower than that of IV agents (Vasko et al., 1985). The pharmacology of diuretics is presented in more detail in chapter 11.

Administration of loop diuretics generally results in a prompt and marked diuresis. At the time of peak diuresis, as much as from 40% to 50% of the filtered load of sodium is excreted, with chloride as the accompanying anion. Potassium, magnesium, and calcium excretion also are increased. The increased excretion of potassium is due to the increased distal secretion and correlates with the increased flow rate and exchange for sodium in this segment of the kidney.

Prior to the diuresis, IV furosemide produces acute systemic arteriolar constriction (Francis et al., 1985). This may be due to the capacity of the drug to release renin from the kidney. The action of renin in combination with angiotensinogen produces angiotensin I, which is rapidly converted by ACE to angiotensin II. Angiotensin II is likely responsible for most of the immediate pressor effects of IV furosemide, because they can be blocked by pretreatment with captopril, an ACE inhibitor (Goldsmith et al., 1989). The acute increase in afterload can raise pulmonary capillary wedge pressure and transiently reduce cardiac output (Fig. 4–7). This action is generally not clinically significant, although rarely patients may have a brief period of clinical deterioration following IV furosemide. Within 30 minutes there generally is a prompt diuresis with a fall in left

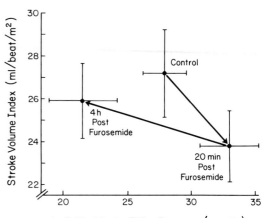

Fig. 4–7. The stroke volume index is plotted as a function of left ventricular filling pressure following 1 mg/kg of IV furosemide in 15 patients with CHF. The initial peripheral vasoconstriction likely is mediated by angiotensin II that transiently reduces left ventricular function. Hours later, following a diuresis, there is a marked reduction in left ventricular filling pressure and a modest increase in stroke volume index. (Reproduced with permission from Francis, G. S.; et al.: Acute vasoconstrictor response to intravenous furosemide in patients with chronic congestive heart failure. Ann. Intern. Med., 103:1–6, 1985.)

ventricular filling pressure accompanied by a slight increase or no change in cardiac output (Fig. 4–7). The mechanism of the early reduction in left ventricular filling pressure is not completely understood but possibly is secondary to a direct venodilator effect or secondary to furosemide-stimulated prostaglandin-induced venodilation resulting in an increase in capacitance of the venous bed (Dikshit et al., 1973). The later reduction in left ventricular filling pressure results from the diuresis. Consequently, the efficacy of furosemide in acute pulmonary edema may be due to both venodilation and its well-known diuretic effects.

The usual therapeutic strategy is to employ IV furosemide or bumetanide as needed to control symptoms of pulmonary congestion. Repeated dosing may be necessary to maintain clinical stability and afford a diuretic response. Once the patient has stabilized clinically, usually after 1 or 2 days, oral loop diuretics can be effectively employed. The usual dose of oral furosemide is 40 to 100 mg/day or bumetanide 0.5 to 2 mg/day. Bumetanide is a substantially shorter acting agent and is sometimes employed at 4- to 5-hour intervals up to a maximum of 10 mg daily.

Patients with underlying renal insufficiency will sometimes require larger doses of furosemide, in the range of 250 to 4000 mg/day (Gerlag and van-Meijel, 1988). Patients who remain refractory to IV furosemide may respond to bumetanide, the usual dose being 0.5 to 2 mg IV.

The loop diuretics can cause dehydration and serious loss of electrolytes leading to hypokalemia, hypotension, and hypochloremic alkalosis. Asymptomatic hyperuricemia also can occur. Ototoxicity is an additional adverse effect of loop diuretics, and deafness, both transient and permanent, is a rare but serious effect. Nonsteroidal anti-inflammatory agents will block prostaglandin secretion, the increase in renal blood flow, and the venodilation normally promoted by furosemide, thereby potentially reducing its effectiveness. In general, the use of NSAIDs should be avoided when treating patients with chronic or acute congestive heart failure (Dzau et al., 1984). *Principle: We are frequently limited in therapeutics by our prejudices that favor the "most potent" drugs for the "worst disease." There is little information on the relative efficacy and toxicity of furosemide compared with other diuretics used for the same indication in patients with equivalent severity of CHF.*

Morphine Sulfate. Morphine is efficacious in the management of acute pulmonary edema. Its beneficial effects are related to its direct vasodilator action and perhaps both a central and peripheral sympathetic effect. In monkeys and probably in humans it can selectively increase blood flow to the brain and coronary blood vessels while decreasing actual flow only to bronchial vessels and the diaphragm. Arteriolar and venous dilation cause pooling of blood in the peripheral circulation, thereby decreasing venous return, cardiac work, and pulmonary venous pressure and shifting blood from the central to the peripheral circulation. The inotropic effect of morphine, sometimes seen in experimental animals, is an indirect effect related to release of catecholamines. Morphine should be used carefully in patients with myocardial infarction or with limited myocardial contractile reserve since a marked fall in cardiac output and blood pressure may attend the drug-induced peripheral vasodilation and bradycardia. Such a fall in blood pressure was attributed previously to release of histamine by morphine but more likely is due to direct effects of morphine. Morphine leads to the redistribution of blood flow even before major changes in hemodynamics can be measured.

Sensitization of the vestibular apparatus by morphine may lead to nausea and vomiting, and histamine release by morphine may trigger bronchospasm in asthmatic individuals. The effects of morphine on the blood pressure and vestibular apparatus are most obvious when the patient is in the upright position, which is favored for the treatment of pulmonary edema.

The use of morphine sulfate for acute pulmonary edema is time-honored and has proved to be extremely useful in relieving both the pulmonary vascular congestion and the acute anxiety that usually occurs as a result of the syndrome. Arterial blood gas concentrations should be monitored prior to the use of morphine sulfate to ensure that the patient's respiratory drive is not unduly suppressed — leading to drug-induced elevated levels of P_{CO_2}. The usual blood-gas profile in the setting of acute pulmonary edema includes a *low* P_{CO_2} secondary to hyperventilation, although CO_2 retention may occur in severely ill patients.

The average dose of morphine sulfate for the adult patient is from 2 to 4 mg IV repeated as necessary to control respiratory distress. Should respiratory depression occur, the first step is to establish a patent airway and ventilate the patient. Opiate antagonists such as naloxone can produce dramatic reversal of severe respiratory depression caused by morphine. The safest approach usually is to administer small (0.4 mg) doses of IV naloxone to be repeated after 2 to 3 minutes as necessary to establish normal ventilation.

Vasodilators. Dilators of the resistance and capacitance vessels can improve the pumping performance of the heart. This approach to the treatment of heart failure does not directly affect the myocardium but decreases the external factors that oppose ejection of blood. Vasodilators decrease both preload (the stretch on myocardial fibers) and afterload (the tension developed during contraction). The resultant shift of the cardiac function curve is upward and to the left so that increased cardiac output is accomplished at lower filling pressures without direct drug-induced increases in inotropism. Since the heart decreases in size, myocardial oxygen demands decrease as stroke work increases.

With careful use of vasodilators, there is the potential that the increases in cardiac output balance with the decreases in total peripheral resistance in some patients, leading to little change in mean arterial pressure. Consequently, CHF is improved and diuresis may occur. In a normal individual, combined venous and arteriolar dilation triggers an increase in sympathetic tone resulting in tachycardia. In patients with severe heart failure, the sympathetic tone is already high and the venous and arteriolar dilators usually cause little or no change in heart rate. The vasodilators effective in patients with heart failure are those that dilate both arterioles and veins. Therefore, hydralazine and diazoxide, which predominantly dilate arterioles, are not primary drugs of choice in heart failure. These arteriolar dilators may increase myocardial oxygen demands because the heart's size does not decrease, and angina or myocardial infarction can result. In contrast, the vasodilators of both arterioles and veins (e.g., nitroprusside and nitrates) decrease heart size and myocardial oxygen demands.

Selection of patients for vasodilator therapy of acute heart failure is critical. Optimum use of vasodilators requires catheterization of the right heart and continuous monitoring of the pulmonary artery pressures. Patients must have elevated pulmonary capillary wedge pressures; those with wedge pressure <15 mm Hg will not improve with vasodilators and may deteriorate. In selected patients, vasodilators can improve myocardial performance and have successfully aided managing CHF that is refractory to standard treatment with digitalis and diuretics. Also, in the presence of functional or valvular mitral regurgitation, reduction of afterload can result in improved forward ejection of regurgitant flow.

The ideal vasodilator has yet to be developed. Sodium nitroprusside has been used successfully for the management of acute heart failure as has IV nitroglycerin. The ganglionic blocker trimethaphan and the α-adrenergic antagonist phentolamine were used more frequently in the past to decrease preload and afterload but cause many adverse effects. Comparative studies of nitroprusside and nitroglycerin indicate that the major action of nitroglycerin is on the capacitance bed; preload is decreased more than afterload. With nitroprusside, arteriolar vasodilation and venodilation produce substantial reductions in both preload and afterload. The increase in cardiac index appears to be greater with nitroprusside than it does with nitroglycerin, which may actually decrease cardiac output. For chronic maintenance of vasodilation, nitroglycerin ointment and isosorbide dinitrate have been used with some success.

Nitroprusside. Nitroprusside is a highly efficacious venous and arteriolar dilator that acts very quickly to lower filling pressure and improve cardiac output (Franciosa et al., 1972). Its rapid onset of action and short half-life make it an ideal agent for the treatment of acute heart failure. Intravenous sodium nitroprusside is particularly useful in the syndrome of acute CHF because it does not increase myocardial oxygen demand. Myocardial contractility is not influenced by nitroprusside, and heart rate usually is unchanged. Nitroprusside decreases systemic vascular resistance; however, since cardiac output usually increases in response to the decrement in systemic vascular resistance, mean arterial pressure generally is maintained or falls only modestly. However, some patients may develop unacceptable hypotension with systolic blood pressure less than 50 mm Hg requiring a decrement in rate of infusion of the drug. Careful monitoring of arterial pressure is mandatory, usually from an arterial line. The usual starting dose of nitroprusside is 3 to 10 μg/min with a rapid titration up to whatever dose is necessary to adequately reduce filling pressure and improve cardiac output. The dose can vary from 10 to 300 μg/min. Patients who are unresponsive to 300 μg/min of nitroprusside are not likely to respond to higher doses. The usual strategy is to employ nitroprusside as a continuous infusion for 48 to 72 hours as needed to control left ventricular filling pressure and cardiac output. The usual effective dose is in the range of 40 to 150 μg/min. Toxicity to nitroprusside can occur in the form of increased concentrations of thiocyanate in the blood. Nitroprusside toxicity is more likely to occur when high doses are used for prolonged periods of time in patients with renal insufficiency. This problem is discussed in more detail in chapter 26.

Nitroglycerin. Nitroglycerin is useful in treating the syndrome of acute CHF. Like nitroprusside, nitroglycerin is used most safely in the setting of the intensive care unit with careful monitoring of arterial pressure. Measurement of left ventricular filling pressure and cardiac output may be very useful in monitoring responses to nitroglycerin in selected patients. Nitroglycerin is primarily a venodilator and causes a prompt and sustained reduction in left ventricular filling pressure. Doses in excess of 40 to 50 μg/min may decrease systemic vascular resistance that may augment cardiac output as described above. Intravenous nitroglycerin has some advantage over nitroprusside in patients with acute myocardial infarction as nitroglycerin may improve the intramyocardial distribution of coronary blood flow and decrease myocardial ischemia. In the setting of acute myocardial infarction with associated pulmonary edema, nitroglycerin is preferred over IV nitroprusside for these reasons.

Patients who do not respond promptly to IV loop diuretics and nitroprusside or nitroglycerin should be considered for treatment with inotropic drugs such as dobutamine or dopamine. When blood pressure is adequate but the patient remains in a state of low cardiac output, dobutamine is the preferred agent (Francis et al., 1982).

Dobutamine. Dobutamine was synthesized from dopamine as part of a project that sought a pure β_1-adrenergic agonist (Sonnenblick et al., 1979). The goal was never reached. The molecule has a major substitution at the amino group that appears to be responsible for the drug's strong β_1-adrenergic activity. However, dobutamine is a mixture of two enantiomeric forms; the (−)-isomer is a potent α_1-receptor agonist that is capable of substantial pressor effects in animals. The net effect of the racemic mixture is to develop substantial β_1-, less β_2-, and probably even less α_1-adrenergic activity. Dobutamine activates β_1-adrenergic receptors in the myocardium to stimulate the production of cAMP that subsequently leads to a heightened inotropic state and modest increases in heart rate. Compared with isoproterenol, dobutamine has more prominent inotropic and less chronotropic effects on the heart, has less prominent effects on the sinus node for equivalent inotropic actions, has equivalent effects on the atrioventricular and intraventricular conduction systems, and causes less reduction of peripheral resistance. The usual practice is to initiate therapy with dobutamine at a dose of 2 to 3 μg/kg per minute in patients with CHF due to acute causes (myocardial infarction or postsurgically). The dose is then increased every 30 minutes until the optimal balance between desired hemodynamic effects (inotropic, chronotropic, and peripheral vascular effects) and adverse effects are seen (Leier et al., 1977). The half-life is about 2 minutes (Kates and Leier, 1978). Therefore, adjustments in dosage are followed rapidly by changes in response. Adverse effects include sinus tachycardia, angina pectoris, headache, nausea, tremor, and ventricular ectopy (Leier and Unverferth, 1983). Because dobutamine enhances atrioventricular nodal conduction, it can increase ventricular response to atrial fibrillation or flutter. Because its half-life is so short, termination of therapy results in rapid reversal of toxicity.

Dobutamine raises cardiac output by increasing stroke volume and modestly increasing heart rate. Its lack of peripheral vasoconstrictor effects make it unsuitable for the patient with severe hypotension or shock (Francis et al., 1982). Although dobutamine can increase blood pressure, this effect is mainly due to its ability to increase stroke volume. This latter results in an increase in systolic pressure with little or no change in diastolic or mean arterial pressure.

A frequent practice is to combine dobutamine with nitroprusside or nitroglycerin to augment cardiac output maximally and lower left ventricular filling pressure with only a minimal increase in myocardial oxygen demand (Mikulic et al., 1977). Dobutamine infusions can be maintained for periods of 48 to 72 hours, at which time a relative tolerance to the drug may occur. The decreased efficacy may be due to desensitization of β-adrenergic receptors.

Dopamine. Unlike dobutamine, dopamine is a naturally occurring catecholamine and has effects in low doses on vascular DA_1 (dopaminergic) receptors (Goldberg, 1974). When used in doses of 2 μg/kg per minute or less, dopamine preferentially activates vascular DA_1 receptors.

The interaction promotes vasodilation within the renal, coronary, mesenteric, and cerebrovascular beds (Goldberg, 1974); dopamine at these rates of infusion may cause a transient but modest fall in blood pressure. These low doses of dopamine enhance renal blood flow and promote a natriuretic effect (Goldberg, 1974). These pharmacologic effects may be useful in patients who do not respond to furosemide. Larger doses of dopamine, in excess of 2 μg/kg per minute, have β_1-adrenergic activity producing positive inotropic and chronotropic effects (Rajfer et al., 1988). Stroke volume and heart rate tend to increase markedly with larger doses.

Doses of dopamine in the range of 5 to 20 μg/kg per minute also activate α_1-adrenergic receptors resulting in peripheral vasoconstriction. This may help elevate blood pressure in patients who are hypotensive or in shock (MacCannell et al., 1966). In patients with CHF who demonstrate hypotension or shock, dopamine can be used to restore adequate perfusion pressure. Unlike dobutamine, dopamine in higher doses (5–20 μg/kg per minute) can increase left ventricular filling pressure further in patients with CHF (Loeb et al., 1977; Leier et al., 1978) (Fig. 4–8). Therefore, dopamine should be combined with a vasodilator agent such as IV nitroglycerin or nitroprusside (Fig. 4–9), if blood pressure is adequate (Miller

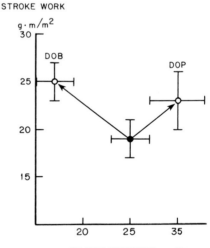

LEFT VENTRICULAR FUNCTION

Fig. 4–8. The contrasting effects of dobutamine (DOB) and dopamine (DOP) on left ventricular function in patients with severe CHF. Both DOB and DOP increase cardiac stroke work. Dopamine tends to increase left ventricular filling pressure. (Reproduced from Loeb, H. S.; et al.: Circulation, 55:375–381, 1977, with permission of the American Heart Association, Inc.)

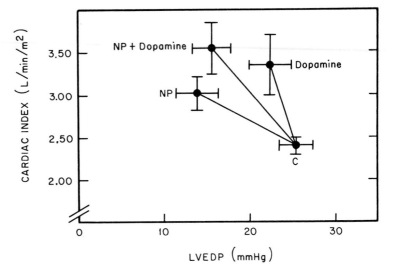

Fig. 4–9. The effects of nitroprusside (NP) and dopamine, alone and in combination, on left ventricular end-diastolic pressure (LVEDP) in patients with advanced heart failure. The combination of nitroprusside and dopamine is augmentative. (Reproduced from Miller, R.; et al.: Circulation, 55:881–884, 1977, with permission of the American Heart Association, Inc.)

et al., 1977; Stemple et al., 1978; Awan et al., 1983).

Amrinone. Amrinone is a positive inotropic drug and peripheral vasodilator, possibly in part because it is a phosphodiesterase inhibitor. Amrinone does not activate β-adrenergic receptors directly (LeJemtel et al., 1979). The drug increases the peak tension developed, the maximal rate of development of tension, and the maximal rate of myocardial relaxation. Intravenous administration of amrinone causes a marked increase in cardiac output and a modest reduction in left ventricular filling pressure (Benotti et al., 1978). While its hemodynamic profile is reminiscent of that of dobutamine (Klein et al., 1981), the improvement in inotropic state with amrinone may occur without increasing myocardial oxygen demand as greatly. The relative diminished myocardial oxygen demand is likely due to the potent peripheral vasodilator effects of amrinone that contributes to improved left ventricular performance with little or no additional consumption of oxygen (Jentzer et al., 1981). Amrinone is particularly effective in the rare patient who no longer responds to dobutamine or dopamine, but in whom blood pressure and perfusion to vital organs remain inadequate unless inotropism is augmented. Prolonged use of catecholamines in patients with severe CHF may lead to ineffective responses to β-adrenergic agonists such as dobutamine. In the setting of desensitized β-adrenergic receptors, amrinone may still have efficacy.

Therapy with amrinone usually is initiated with 0.75 mg/kg given IV over 2 to 3 minutes with a maintenance infusion of 5 to 10 μg/kg per minute. The dose is then titrated according to the patient's clinical hemodynamic needs. The total daily dose should not exceed 10 mg/kg. As with

dobutamine and dopamine, hemodynamic monitoring is required when using IV amrinone. Tolerance to IV amrinone can occur after 48 to 72 hours of treatment (Maisel et al., 1989). Amrinone can be combined with dobutamine to further augment myocardial performance (Gage et al., 1986). Knowledge of the rather distinctive effects of dobutamine, dopamine, nitroprusside, amrinone, and furosemide on the failing myocardium are essential when using combination therapy (Fig. 4-10). *Principle: The nonoverlapping mechanism of useful effect of amrinone, digitalis, catecholamines, and vasodilators in treating CHF makes combining them when needed very rational. But the toxicity of these drugs makes combination difficult. Monitoring is often needed to develop an optimal dosage regimen for drugs used in very dynamic disease states (chapter 26). Generally speaking, drugs should not be given without a predetermined goal.*

Therapy for Chronic CHF

Digitalis Glycosides

Inotropic and Extracardiac Effects. Digitalis exerts positive inotropic effects in both normal and diseased hearts, resulting in an upward shift of the cardiac function curve. The effect on cardiac output, however, is modulated by the extracardiac effects of digitalis as well as by normal homeostatic mechanisms. In the normal subject, arteriolar and venous constriction is produced by digitalis, and the increased peripheral vascular resistance and bradycardia (see below) tend to negate the effects of increased contractility. The cardiac output in normal subjects may remain unchanged or may actually decrease. Vasoconstriction is not a prominent effect of digitalis

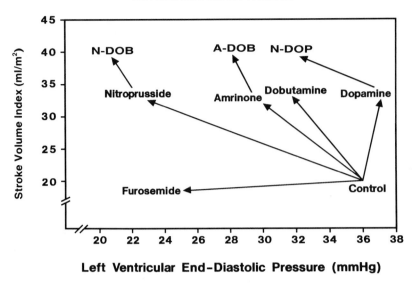

Fig. 4–10. Stroke volume index and left ventricular end-diastolic pressure are plotted according to the usual and expected responses to maximal dose dopamine (DOP), dobutamine (DOB), amrinone (A), nitroprusside (N), and furosemide in patients with severe CHF. These responses represent theoretical individual patients and are not actual data points. (From Francis, G. S.; and Archer, S. L.: J. Int. Care Med., 4:84–92, 1989, by permission of Blackwell Scientific Publications, Inc.)

in patients with heart failure because vascular tone is already increased by adrenergic activity.

As cardiac function improves following the administration of digitalis, the compensatory mechanisms to maintain cardiac output are no longer required; a diuresis occurs, and sympathetic tone to the heart and vasculature decreases. By relieving CHF, digitalis indirectly produces vasodilation of arterioles and veins as enhanced sympathetic tone is withdrawn; these indirect effects counter the primary effects of digitalis on the vasculature. Thus, although patients with CHF respond to digitalis with increased cardiac output, the result depends on the interplay of cardiac and extracardiac effects of the glycosides. Experimentally the inotropic effects of digitalis increase linearly with increasing dose. Indeed, the inotropic effects seen at low doses may be sufficient clinically without risking toxicity.

The proper use of digitalis was well described 175 years ago:

The proper dose of a medicine is undoubtedly that quantity which produces the effect required, whatever be its numerical denomination. A full dose of foxglove is, therefore, merely a relative term.

To one patient one-half grain may be a full dose; to another, six or eight grains may be given, not only without inconvenience, but without producing any sensible effect.

These varieties of sensibility and habit can only be ascertained by beginning with the lowest dose and increasing it with the most scrupulous care.

The patient's pulse must be examined from hour to hour, and on its first tendency to flag, or on the slightest indication of sickness, the exhibition of the medicine must be suspended (Ferriar, 1816).

The inotropic effect of digitalis can increase myocardial oxygen demands. However, the actual effect of digitalis on myocardial oxygen consumption depends on the relationship of the three major determinants of oxygen requirements: (1) ventricular tension, (2) heart rate, and (3) contractility. In the nonfailing heart, the increase in contractility increases overall myocardial oxygen demand. However, in the failing heart, digitalis decreases overall oxygen demands by decreasing heart rate and intramyocardial tension (which is related to ventricular pressure and radius) by making the heart smaller.

Effects of Digitalis on Heart Rate. Digitalis can slow ventricular rates during normal sinus rhythm or during supraventricular tachyarrhythmias by several mechanisms. Sinus tachycardia is common during CHF because of enhanced sympathetic nervous system activity. Because digitalis improves myocardial function and cardiac output in these patients, sympathetic activity decreases, as does nerve discharge to the sinoatrial node. This mechanism of cardiac slowing is indirect and does not occur if the sinus tachycardia is due to some other cause. Thyrotoxic patients, for example, continue to have sinus tachycardia even when receiving digitalis.

Digitalis also indirectly slows the sinus rate by a vagomimetic action. This may be due in part to an increased sensitivity of the carotid sinus baroreceptors, so that at any level of blood pressure there is increased vagal activity and decreased sympathetic tone. In the normal individual, these effects of digitalis, along with the extracardiac effects, can negate the expected increase in cardiac output caused by its inotropic action.

Another mechanism for cardiac slowing involves the direct action of digitalis to depress atrioventricular (AV) nodal conductivity (negative dromotropic effect). Digitalis decreases AV conduction velocity and lengthens the functional refractory period of the AV node. Therapeutic doses of digitalis may prolong the PR interval, but this effect is not ordinarily of clinical consequence. Larger doses can cause second- or third-degree heart block. In atrial fibrillation with rapid ventricular response, the effect of digitalis to prolong the functional refractory period of the AV node slows the ventricular response and may be the major therapeutic effect. This is particularly true in patients with mitral stenosis and no left ventricular disease; slowing the ventricular rate greatly enhances diastolic filling of the left ventricle and increases cardiac output.

Conductivity in the AV node is determined by the interplay of multiple factors. Vagal stimulation depresses conductivity and prolongs the functional refractory period of the AV node; sympathetic stimulation has the opposite effect. Although there is no doubt that digitalis has direct effects on the AV node, there is continuing uncertainty as to the relative importance of the direct effects of digitalis versus the vagotonic effects. The effects of digitalis on the AV node are clinically influenced by the autonomic nervous system, electrolyte concentrations, and other drugs. For example, in the patient with atrial fibrillation, CHF, and excess sympathetic stimulation, digitalis can decrease the ventricular response both by directly depressing AV conduction and by indirectly decreasing sympathetic stimulation as the CHF is corrected. In such patients, sufficient ventricular slowing can be produced with "therapeutic" concentrations of glycosides in plasma. However, in patients with atrial fibrillation who have complicating serious illnesses, the effects of digitalis on the AV node may be insufficient to slow the ventricular response to less than 100/min even at very high, potentially toxic concentrations of drug in plasma. In these patients other influences on the AV node, including persistent excessive sympathetic stimulation and lack of vagal tone, appear to counteract some of the effects of digitalis. Thus in patients with fever, sepsis, major surgery, hypoxemia, thyrotoxicosis, and other situations where a tachycardia would be appropriate, digitalis has a lesser effect on the AV node than it does in the uncomplicated patient. As a corollary to these considerations, it should not be surprising that excessive effects of digitalis-induced heart block may be overcome by atropine or isoproterenol, whereas potassium administration may induce hyperkalemia, which may increase the degree of heart block. *The AV node is subject to multiple influences. The expected effects of digitalis can be modulated by the autonomic nervous system, serum potassium concentrations, and the presence of other drugs.*

Cellular Effects. Considerable information is available on the cellular effects of digitalis and the relationship of these effects to the inotropic and toxic manifestations of the drug. Digitalis probably has no direct effect on the contractile proteins or on myocardial intermediary metabolism; the mechanism of the inotropic action of digitalis is still incompletely understood. Digitalis enhances excitation–contraction coupling, that process by which chemical energy is converted into mechanical energy when triggered by membrane depolarization. Evidence relates this process to entry of calcium ions into the cell during depolarization of the membrane and/or to release of calcium from intracellular storage sites on the sarcoplasmic reticulum. The free calcium ion binds to troponin, which releases the inhibition by the troponin–tropomyosin complex of the interaction of actin and myosin, thereby allowing contraction. The way that digitalis affects calcium balance is still unknown. The evidence for a direct effect on calcium flux across the cell membrane or on release of calcium from the sarcoplasmic reticulum is inconsistent and has little support. Catecholamines are not required for the inotropic effects of digitalis.

In the absence of other discernible effects, attention has focused on the unquestioned ability of digitalis to inhibit the transport of sodium and potassium across the cell membrane by the magnesium-dependent, sodium- and potassium-activated adenosinetriphosphatase (Na^+, K^+-ATPase) (Smith, 1988). The earliest observations were related to the inhibition of the Na^+, K^+-ATPase by toxic doses of glycoside, resulting in profound loss of intracellular potassium and increase in intracellular sodium. The inhibition of the Na^+, K^+-ATPase occurs even at therapeutic concentrations of digitalis, resulting in loss of myocardial potassium. Impressive circumstantial evidence indicates that Na^+, K^+-ATPase may be the digitalis receptor. Binding to the Na^+, K^+-ATPase is specific for active glycosides and correlates with the glycoside's inotropic potency. There is a correlation between species sensitivity to glycosides and the binding to the Na^+, K^+-ATPase of that species. The time course of Na^+, K^+-ATPase inhibition and the inotropic effect of digitalis are also correlated in most studies.

Lowering the temperature or increasing extracellular potassium concentration inhibits the glycoside's binding to the Na$^+$, K$^+$-ATPase and decreases digitalis's inotropic effects. If the receptor for digitalis's effect is the Na$^+$, K$^+$-ATPase, then the mechanism linking this interaction with the inotropic effect must be explained. There is considerable evidence suggesting that the final pathway involves increased calcium availability. The effects on calcium likely are indirectly mediated by shifts in sodium and/or potassium that occur as a consequence of inhibition of the Na$^+$, K$^+$-ATPase. The increase in intracellular sodium concentration may activate the calcium–sodium exchange mechanisms in myocytes. The change in intracellular calcium concentrations appears to activate release of calcium from the sarcoplasmic reticulum. These mechanisms allow more calcium to interact with contractile proteins and increase inotropism. Calcium ion and digitalis have additive inotropic and toxic effects. Administration of calcium is contraindicated during digitalis toxicity; administration of digitalis is dangerous during hypercalcemia.

Many of the toxic effects of digitalis are directly related to inhibition of the Na$^+$, K$^+$-ATPase and the subsequent loss of intracellular potassium.

Whether digitalis toxic tachyarrhythmias are due to enhanced automaticity, triggered automaticity, and/or reentry is unknown (see chapter 6). Since the major known biochemical defect in digitalis intoxication is intracellular potassium depletion and since the binding to myocardium and the effects of digitalis are enhanced by hypokalemia, potassium replacement is a useful therapy for digitalis toxicity. Potassium must be given with care, however, lest hyperkalemia be produced. In massive digitalis toxicity, hyperkalemia is the rule, as potassium leaks from intracellular stores. In such cases a digitalis-binding antibody can reverse toxicity.

There are additional mechanisms whereby digitalis may improve myocardial performance in patients with CHF. Digitalis glycosides exert excitatory influences on sympathetic mechanisms when administered into the CNS in animals. Patients with CHF may have impairment of reflex control of the peripheral circulation; these patients may respond to digitalis with a sympathoinhibitory action due to sensitization of afferent baroreceptor mechanisms that inhibit sympathetic outflow for a given cardiac volume (Thames et al., 1980). This possibility is supported by the observation that patients with heart failure treated with digitalis have a substantial reduction in plasma catecholamines as well as a reduction in directly measured efferent sympathetic nerve activity to muscle (Ferguson et al., 1989).

The direct inotropic effect may account for the hemodynamic efficacy of digitalis in patients with heart failure. However, the long-term consequences of these effects in patients with CHF are still not clear.

Pharmacokinetics. The cardiac glycosides vary widely in their kinetic properties including GI absorption, distribution, and route of elimination.

DIGOXIN. Digoxin is 55% to 65% absorbed from orally administered tablets and nearly 100% from capsules. It is not appreciably bound by plasma proteins ($<30\%$), and it is excreted largely unchanged in the urine with a half-life of about 36 hours.

Malabsorption of digoxin may occur in patients with GI mucosal defects and to lesser extent on the basis of pancreatic insufficiency without primary bowel disease.

The mechanisms of renal excretion of digoxin include glomerular filtration, tubular secretion, and, at low urinary flow rates, passive tubular reabsorption. The plasma clearance of digoxin in patients with normal renal function is about 136 ml/min, of which 100 ml/min is renal and 36 ml/min is nonrenal clearance. Over a wide range of renal function, the renal clearance of digoxin correlates directly with the creatinine clearance. However, at low urinary flow rates or in the presence of prerenal azotemia, urea clearance appears to be slightly superior in predicting digoxin clearance, probably because both urea and digoxin are passively reabsorbed. In the presence of renal failure, the renal clearance of digoxin is reduced in proportion to the reduction in creatinine clearance whereas the nonrenal clearance is unchanged. In many cases, the half-life of digoxin becomes prolonged as digoxin clearance decreases in renal failure. However, the apparent volume of distribution of digoxin (about 7 l/kg) also is decreased in some patients with renal failure. In these circumstances, half-life does not correlate with the change in drug clearance. Therefore, determination of half-life may be an inadequate guide to the required dosage adjustment in patients with renal failure. Hemodialysis does not appreciably remove digoxin from the body because of the drug's large apparent volume of distribution.

Occasional patients are resistant to the usual therapeutic doses of digoxin. In some of these patients the drug is metabolized to inactive compounds, primarily dihydrodigoxin by an intestinal bacterium. This does not occur with the capsule form of digoxin, which is absorbed completely in the upper small intestine.

DIGITOXIN. Digitoxin is less polar (i.e., it is more lipid-soluble) than digoxin. It is essentially 100% absorbed from the GI tract; it is 90% to

97% bound to plasma proteins; and it is extensively metabolized by the liver. The half-life of digitoxin is 5 to 7 days. Renal insufficiency does not appreciably alter the kinetics of digitoxin, but binding to plasma proteins may be slightly decreased in such patients. In patients with severe liver disease, caution in the use of digitoxin has been advised, but no studies in humans have shown abnormalities of digitoxin disposition in such patients. In animals, and probably in humans, an enterohepatic circulation exists for digitoxin and/or its active metabolites. Cholestyramine, which can bind cardiac glycosides in the gut and prevent their absorption, has been used to interrupt the enterohepatic circulation of digitoxin and has resulted in a small reduction in serum half-life in normal individuals.

The elimination of digitoxin is enhanced by treatment with phenobarbital, phenytoin, and phenylbutazone, perhaps due to induction of hepatic microsomal enzymes. In some patients, concentrations in plasma dropped by half during simultaneous treatment with phenobarbital. No studies have correlated the decreased concentrations in plasma with diminished effect of the glycoside, and the clinical importance of the interaction is unknown.

Concentrations of Drug in Plasma. To be useful in clinical medicine, concentrations in plasma must be related to the pharmacologic effect of the drug. There is considerable evidence that this is the case for the inotropic effects, and for effects on the AV node and electrocardiogram, provided at least 4 hours has elapsed after the last dose before the blood sample is drawn. Although there is overlap when the concentrations of drug in plasma from patients with digoxin toxicity are compared with those of individuals who do not have toxicity, there is, nonetheless, a relationship between the concentration of digoxin in plasma and the presence or absence of clinical toxicity.

The overlap of plasma concentrations in the toxic and nontoxic groups is not surprising when the multiple factors influencing sensitivity to digitalis are considered. The concentration of digoxin in plasma correlates better with drug effects and toxicity than does the dose of digoxin. Therefore, the concentration of digoxin can be useful in explaining an unanticipated clinical response and in assessing compliance of a patient to his or her regimen. The concentration of digoxin in plasma can also be a guide to regulation of dosage, particularly in patients who have renal dysfunction, and often can obviate the common practice of producing toxicity in order to be certain that digitalization is adequate in patients with sinus rhythm. There is retrospective evidence that the incidence of digitalis toxicity is reduced when the concentration of digoxin in plasma is used to guide therapy. It is inappropriate to use digoxin concentrations to establish the diagnosis of digitalis toxicity in a patient who is clinically toxic. If the concentration of digoxin is in the "nontoxic" range in such a patient, there is still a real possibility of the patient's having digitalis intoxication. This in no way negates the rational use of digoxin concentrations in plasma to aid in the regulation of therapy in patients who are clinically nontoxic and in whom the end points of therapy, short of toxicity, are indistinct.

Effects in Patients. There has been a longstanding controversy regarding the effectiveness of digitalis glycosides for the treatment of CHF, particularly for patients who have normal sinus rhythm (Fleg and Lakatta, 1984). Although numerous studies document the short-term efficacy of digitalis (Gheorghiade et al., 1987; Captopril-Digoxin Multicenter Research Group, 1988; Guyatt et al., 1988), a number of studies on the effects of withdrawal of the glycosides have reported mixed results with regard to the usefulness of digoxin in patients with heart failure and normal sinus rhythm (Fleg et al., 1982; Gheorghiade and Beller, 1983; Taggart et al., 1983). On the other hand, several well-controlled studies have indicated clear evidence of sustained clinical or hemodynamic improvement when digitalis is added to diuretic therapy (Arnold et al., 1980; Lee et al., 1982). However, no randomized double-blinded, placebo-controlled study has yet addressed the issue of whether digitalis, when added to a regimen of diuretics and vasodilators, improves exercise capacity or long-term survival. A large multicenter trial is currently being planned to test the hypothesis that digoxin improves survival in patients with chronic congestive heart failure (Francis, 1988a).

Patients who are most likely to derive benefit from digoxin therapy include those with large dilated hearts, a third heart sound, and resting tachycardia. Moreover, patients with congestive heart failure who are prone to supraventricular tachycardia or have atrial fibrillation are excellent candidates for digoxin therapy. The usual maintenance dose of digoxin is 0.25 to 0.375 mg/day, although the maintenance dose varies widely and is dependent on body surface area and renal function. It is common practice to begin therapy with a simple maintenance dose of digoxin, for example 0.25 mg/day, and allow the patients to "digitalize" themselves over a period of several days. Alternatively, a loading dose of digoxin can be given as a total dose of from 7 to 14 μg/kg over an 18- to 24-hour period. It is generally safer to employ simple once-a-day maintenance therapy unless rapid digitalization is clinically required (e.g., rapid atrial fibrillation) as using loading doses increases the risk of inducing toxicity. Risk of toxicity may be increased in patients with renal failure, hypokalemia, hypercalcemia, hypothyroidism, advanced age, and hypoxemia.

The value of routine therapeutic monitoring of plasma digoxin concentrations is uncertain. Measurement of plasma concentrations may be useful in the setting of possible clinical toxicity or when there is an inadequate therapeutic response. The recommended therapeutic range for digoxin is 0.5 to 2 ng/ml. It is important to emphasize that there is no unambiguous relationship between the plasma concentration of digoxin and the presence of a therapeutic response or of drug toxicity. The presence of a concentration higher than 2 ng/ml in patients with atrial fibrillation and no signs of toxicity, or lower than 0.5 ng/ml in patients with an adequate clinical response, does not indicate that the dose of digoxin should be changed. When toxicity is suspected, the finding of a high plasma concentration should lead to dosage reduction. On the other hand, a low plasma concentration in the presence of a poor therapeutic response should lead to an increase in recommended dose or questioning whether bioavailability is low or compliance with therapy is inadequate. Measurement of plasma digoxin concentrations is particularly important in dosing adjustments in patients with changing renal function.

Vasodilator Agents. Vasodilator therapy has now gained widespread acceptance in the routine management of patients with congestive heart failure (Cohn and Franciosa, 1977). The overall explanation for efficacy may be that heart failure is characterized by excessive peripheral vasoconstriction and an increase in the impedance to left ventricular ejection (Francis et al., 1984). Drugs that reduce afterload by promoting arteriolar dilation and reducing heart volume consistently improve cardiac function in chronic heart failure (Fig. 4-3) (Cohn, 1973).

Several large placebo-controlled trials have documented that some vasodilator drugs not only provide symptomatic improvement but also actually increase survival in patients with congestive heart failure. The Veterans Administration's Vasodilator Heart Failure Trial (V-HeFT) I demonstrated that patients with New York Heart Association (NYHA) functional class II and III heart failure assigned to a combination of hydralazine and isosorbide dinitrate (added to baseline therapy with diuretics and digitalis in all patients) had a 38% reduction in overall mortality during the first year of treatment compared with patients treated with placebo or with the α_1-receptor antagonist prazosin (Fig. 4-11) (Cohn et al., 1986). The CONSENSUS Trial reported that patients with class IV congestive heart failure already on

therapy with digitalis and diuretics (and in some cases various vasodilators) had a highly significant improvement in survival when treated with enalapril compared with placebo (Fig. 4-12) (CONSENSUS Trial Study Group, 1987). Based on the results of these two large, controlled studies, vasodilator therapy has now become incorporated as standard treatment for patients with severe CHF. However, important questions have not yet been resolved: Which type of vasodilator therapy is preferable? When in the natural history of CHF should vasodilator therapy be introduced? And what is the role of diuretics and digoxin in the efficacy of vasodilator therapy (Francis, 1988a)?

Hydralazine. Hydralazine is a direct-acting vasodilator that relaxes smooth muscle primarily in the precapillary resistance arterioles (Koch-Weser, 1976). It is relatively selective for arterial smooth muscle, producing little or no change in venous capacitance. Vasodilation caused by hydralazine in patients with heart failure is primarily directed to the renal and limb vascular beds without change in hepatic blood flow (Magorien et al., 1984).

Hydralazine is rapidly and nearly completely absorbed from the GI tract and is acetylated by the liver. There is substantial first-pass bowel and/or hepatic biotransformation. The bioavailability is dependent on the acetylator phenotype and is greater for the slow than for the fast acetylators (Reece et al., 1980). Peak serum concentrations usually are attained within 30 minutes to 2 hours, depending on whether the patient is a fast or slow acetylator. The drug is nearly completely protein-bound in the serum.

The major hemodynamic effect of hydralazine is an increase in cardiac output due to marked arteriolar dilation (Franciosa et al., 1977). Left ventricular filling pressure usually is not changed by hydralazine since venodilation does not occur. In healthy volunteers or hypertensive patients, reflex tachycardia is a prominent adverse effect of hydralazine; however, this does not generally occur in patients with advanced CHF. Hydralazine has been used primarily in combination with nitrates, which has the advantage of reducing left ventricular filling pressure (Franciosa and Cohn, 1979b). Sustained beneficial hemodynamic and clinical effects have been observed with hydralazine, but occasionally patients appear to develop tolerance to the drug, although the mechanism for this is unknown (Packer et al., 1982).

Hydralazine can be a difficult drug to use in patients with heart failure because of marked variability in dosing requirements (Packer et al., 1980), its relatively high incidence of adverse effects, its stimulatory effects on the renin-angiotensin system, and the occasional provoca-

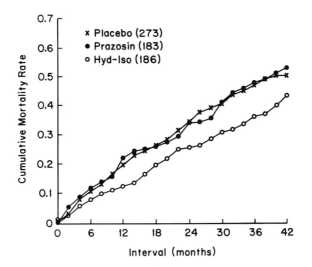

Fig. 4–11. Cumulative mortality from the time of randomization in three treatment groups of 642 men with CHF on treatment with digitalis and diuretics. Patients assigned to hydralazine and isosorbide dinitrate (Hyd-Iso) had a mortality-risk reduction of 38% in 3 years. (From Cohn, J.;et al.: N. Engl. J. Med., 314:1547–1552, 1986, by permission of the New England Journal of Medicine.)

tion of myocardial ischemic events (see below). Therefore, no standard dosage regimen for patients in CHF is available. The V-HeFT I study used a dose of 75 mg of hydralazine four times a day in combination with isosorbide dinitrate. The usual dose of oral hydralazine for the treatment of chronic heart failure is in the range of 200 to 400 mg/day, although larger doses up to 1200 mg/day occasionally are used.

In spite of the fact that hydralazine improves coronary blood flow and the myocardial oxygen supply/demand ratio, patients can develop worsening of angina pectoris (Packer et al., 1981; Magorien et al., 1982). Additionally, the drug tends to stimulate the renin-angiotensin-aldosterone system, adding to peripheral edema and circulatory congestion. Gastrointestinal adverse effects, including nausea and anorexia, also frequently are experienced with hydralazine. Although many patients develop a positive fluorescent antinuclear antibody test, overt clinical lupus erythematosus is relatively unusual, particularly at doses of less than 150 mg/day. The lupus syndrome occurs almost exclusively in white slow acetylators. When the lupus syndrome does occur in the setting of use of hydralazine, it generally does not compromise renal function but usually is restricted to the pericardium, pleura, joints, and skin. The lupus

Fig. 4–12. Cumulative probability of death in the placebo and enalapril groups in 253 patients with class IV CHF on conventional therapy with digitalis and diuretics. There was a 27% reduction in mortality at the end of the study in patients treated with the addition of enalapril. (From the CONSENSUS Trial Study Group (CONSENSUS): N. Engl. J. Med., 316:1429–1435, 1987, by permission of the New England Journal of Medicine.)

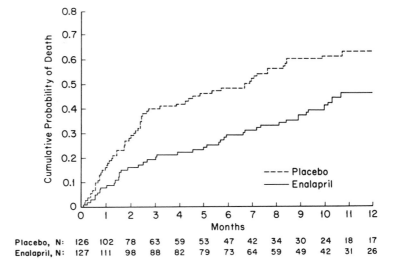

Months	0	1	2	3	4	5	6	7	8	9	10	11	12
Placebo, N:	126	102	78	63	59	53	47	42	34	30	24	18	17
Enalapril, N:	127	111	98	88	82	79	73	64	59	49	42	31	26

syndrome is reversible on discontinuation of the drug (Perry, 1973).

Long-acting Nitrates. Long-acting oral nitrates have been used frequently in the treatment of chronic CHF in the belief that venodilation reduces left ventricular filling pressure and therefore relieves signs and symptoms of pulmonary vascular congestion (Franciosa et al., 1978b). Nitroglycerin and other organic nitrates relax the vascular smooth muscle of the venous capacitance and pulmonary vascular beds. Large doses can result in vasodilation of the arterial resistance bed as well (Franciosa et al., 1978a). Nitrovasodilators stimulate a dose-dependent increase in smooth muscle cell guanosine-3′5′-monophosphate (cGMP) by activation of soluble guanylate cyclase (Murad, 1986). Nitroglycerin reacts with thiols to form *S*-nitrosothiols that in turn are a likely source of nitric oxide (NO). It is the NO that activates the soluble guanylate cyclase to produce cGMP and vasodilation (Moncada et al., 1988).

The administration of oral isosorbide dinitrate, a prototype long-acting oral nitrate, in doses of 20 to 40 mg, results in a prompt reduction in pulmonary capillary wedge pressure and right atrial pressure (Franciosa et al., 1974). Isosorbide dinitrate, when given orally, improves exercise tolerance in patients with chronic heart failure (Franciosa and Cohn, 1979a). The usual duration of action of isosorbide dinitrate on the reduction in pulmonary vascular wedge pressure is from approximately 4 to 6 hours.

Patients develop tolerance to oral nitrates (Abrams, 1989). Dosing strategies using a nitrate-free interval appear to be effective and safe and may prevent the induction of nitrate tolerance (Silber et al., 1987). The exact length of the necessary nitrate-free interval is not known and is probably different in different subjects and varies among different formulations. Tolerance occurs with transdermal, oral, and IV preparations (Axelsson et al., 1987). Generally speaking, the more continuous the delivery of the drug, the more likely is it that tolerance will develop. Consequently, the transdermal delivery forms that were designed to deliver drug continuously in fact do so but tend to lose their effectiveness because this resistance is common in patients with the most severe signs and symptoms of heart failure. Clearly because the drug has efficacy for uncertain periods, some parameter of hemodynamic effect should be monitored frequently to assure that there is value in ongoing drug administration. In patients with very elevated right atrial pressures, the hemodynamic response is somewhat unpredictable; almost 50% of patients respond to the 40-mg dose whereas about 25% require a higher dose, usually in the range of 80 to 120 mg/dose

(Kulick et al., 1988). Occasionally, patients do not respond even to 120 mg of isosorbide dinitrate. Although the reduction in pulmonary artery wedge pressure is an adequate marker for the hemodynamic response to isosorbide dinitrate, the long-term effects of the drug on symptoms, particularly exercise capacity, do not correlate well with changes in the hemodynamic variables. This is true of virtually all the vasodilator agents studied to date (Franciosa et al., 1984). The usual dose of isosorbide dinitrate for patients with CHF probably should be in the range of 40 to 60 mg given two or at most three times per day, with a minimum 6- to 12-hour nitrate-free interval between doses. Sublingual, transdermal, and other preparations of nitrates have not been demonstrated to improve survival in patients with CHF when used as monotherapy or in combination with digoxin and diuretics. However, the issue of monotherapy with nitrates has not yet been studied in a large, controlled trial. It is unclear from the V-HeFT data whether the benefit from the combination of isosorbide dinitrate and hydralazine was due to either drug alone or the combination of the two drugs.

ACE Inhibitors. Captopril was the first ACE inhibitor approved for the treatment of chronic CHF. Subsequently, enalapril has been approved for the same indication, and lisinopril, though not yet approved for heart failure, is also widely used. The results of numerous controlled and uncontrolled studies support their current widespread use for patients with heart failure (Captopril-Digoxin Multicenter Research Group, 1988; CONSENSUS Trial Study Group, 1987).

Congestive heart failure is characterized, at least in the later stages, by activation of the circulating renin-angiotensin-aldosterone system. Although the precise mechanisms responsible for the activation of this system are unknown, it is very likely that excessive angiotensin II contributes to the pathophysiology of advanced, chronic CHF (Francis et al., 1984; Francis, 1986b; Francis, 1989). The efficacy of ACE inhibitors is primarily related to their ability to block the formation of angiotensin II, although other effects of these drugs could be involved.

Within a half-hour of ingestion of a single dose of 6.25 mg of captopril, patients with heart failure generally demonstrate a marked fall in left ventricular filling pressure and right atrial pressure with a modest improvement in cardiac output and no change or a slight reduction in heart rate. Blood pressure usually falls modestly, concomitant with the fall in left ventricular filling pressure (Heel et al., 1980; Kubo and Cody, 1985; Packer et al., 1986). Because this small dose almost completely blocks the ACE, increasing the dose has little influence on the intensity of the hemodynamic response. However, higher doses do tend to prolong the duration of action. The usual maintenance dose of captopril is from 25 to 50 mg three times a day.

Acute administration of captopril in patients with heart failure usually decreases renal vascular resistance and increases renal blood flow, although this is not a consistent finding (LeJemtel et al., 1986). An increase in sodium excretion and potassium retention usually accompanies these changes. The effect on renal function is variable, but serum creatinine and BUN concentrations can increase following the use of ACE inhibitors or other antihypertensives. With ACE inhibitors, the renal dysfunction is likely related to a reduction in angiotensin II–mediated vasoconstriction of the postglomerular efferent arteriole (Hall et al., 1977a and 1977b; Ichikawa et al., 1984). The net result is a reduction in intraglomerular hydraulic pressure that is particularly pronounced when renal perfusion pressure is marginal, as often occurs in severe heart failure, particularly in patients treated with high doses of diuretics. The renal dysfunction can usually be corrected by either reducing the dose of diuretic or discontinuing it. Reducing the dosage of diuretic usually is preferable to discontinuing the ACE inhibitor. Recent studies comparing short- and long-acting ACE inhibitors used with clinical dose titration have not shown marked differences in the incidence or severity of renal failure (Giles et al., 1989).

Captopril has been evaluated in a large number of studies in patients with chronic CHF. It consistently improves exercise tolerance and patient well-being. Left ventricular ejection fraction tends to improve only slightly or remain unchanged. Interestingly, recent reports with long-acting ACE inhibitors (see below) have confirmed a small but consistent rise in ejection fraction after chronic therapy (Giles et al., 1989).

Because ACE inhibitors decrease angiotensin II activity and therefore reduce aldosterone secretion from the adrenal cortex, these drugs tend to increase the concentration of potassium in plasma. Potassium-sparing agents such as spironolactone, triamterene, or amiloride should not be used in conjunction with ACE inhibitors because of the risk of inducing marked hyperkalemia. If supplemental potassium is required, it is generally safer to use the shorter-acting oral potassium chloride preparations than potassium-sparing agents. *Principle: When a common therapeutic measure has real risk associated with it, consider ways of circumventing the risk.*

Enalapril is a long-acting inhibitor of ACE that is widely used for the treatment of CHF. The longer duration of action is because enalapril is a prodrug that must be biotransformed by the liver into the active chemical enaliprilat; the transfor-

mation requires approximately 4 to 6 hours (Ulm, 1983). The usual starting dose of enalapril is 2.5 or 5 mg b.i.d., and the usual maintenance dose is 10 mg b.i.d. The mechanism of action is similar to that of captopril, and the profiles of the adverse effects of the two drugs are comparable. Lisinopril is also a long-acting ACE inhibitor but does not require conversion to an active metabolite. It is given once per day in doses ranging from 5 to 20 mg with a peak effect on blood pressure 4 to 6 hours after the dose.

The usual limiting side effects of ACE inhibitors are hypotension, renal insufficiency, and a chronic, dry nonproductive cough. Patients with hyponatremia appear to be at much higher risk of having a large fall in blood pressure with the first dose of an ACE inhibitor (Packer et al., 1984). A possible explanation is that patients with hyponatremia and CHF generally have a very high concentration of circulating angiotensin II. Such patients may be dependent on angiotensin II for maintenance of their blood pressure. Consequently, these patients should be given their initial dose of an ACE inhibitor in the recumbent position to decrease the risk of hypotension. Also, initial doses for patients with CHF should be much lower than the anticipated maintenance dose.

TREATMENT OF VENTRICULAR ARRHYTHMIAS IN PATIENTS WITH CHF

Patients with advanced CHF often have frequent, complex ventricular premature beats; indeed, 30% to 40% of patients have short runs of nonsustained asymptomatic ventricular tachycardia observed on 24-hour Holter monitoring (Francis, 1986a). Moreover, approximately 40% of all deaths in patients with CHF are sudden and unexpected, presumably due to ventricular fibrillation, although some of these deaths are due to malignant bradyarrhythmias and electrical-mechanical dissociation. Indeed, patients with CHF represent the single largest reservoir of patients at high risk for sudden cardiac death. In spite of this, there is little evidence that antiarrhythmic therapy prolongs survival in this group of patients.

The therapy of life-threatening ventricular arrhythmias in patients with CHF is controversial (Francis, 1988b). Small, uncontrolled studies have indicated that amiodarone decreases the frequency of ventricular premature beats and nonsustained ventricular tachycardia and may possibly improve survival (Cleland et al., 1987; Neri et al., 1987). However, amiodarone has many severe adverse effects (see chapter 6), and its influence on survival has not yet been rigorously tested (Heger et al., 1981; Neri et al., 1987; Mason,

1987). Patients with CHF and *asymptomatic* ventricular arrhythmias, including short runs of nonsustained ventricular tachycardia, do not seem to benefit from antiarrhythmic therapy. There is always the risk that antiarrhythmic therapy can be proarrhythmic and cause other adverse effects. Until there are firm data to indicate that antiarrhythmic drugs will influence long-term survival in patients with heart failure, one should be aware of the controversy regarding their use.

On the other hand, if patients have *symptomatic* ventricular tachycardia or have experienced a cardiac arrest and have been successfully resuscitated, antiarrhythmic therapy probably is indicated, although efficacy data are lacking. Electrophysiology studies may be useful in selecting drug therapy in these patients. Some patients will need implantation of automatic cardioverter defibrillator devices, particularly if they are unresponsive to conventional antiarrhythmic therapy.

EXPERIMENTAL THERAPY OF CHF

β-Adrenergic Receptor Antagonists

There has been recent interest in the use of β-adrenergic receptor blockade in the treatment of congestive cardiomyopathy (Alderman and Grossman, 1985; Shanes, 1987). To date, nearly all the clinical trials with this type of therapy have been uncontrolled and anecdotal. While some have reported clinical improvement with β-antagonist therapy (Waagstein et al., 1975, 1989; Swedberg et al., 1979, 1980a, 1980b), other studies have noted no improvement or even a worsening of the signs and symptoms of CHF (Ikram and Fitzpatrick, 1981; Taylor and Silke, 1981; Currie et al., 1984). At least one relatively well controlled but small study did indicate that low-dose metoprolol improved the NYHA functional class as well as exercise tolerance in patients with chronic idiopathic dilated congestive cardiomyopathy (Engelmeier et al., 1985).

While the mechanism of improvement is not clear, there are data to indicate that chronic treatment with metoprolol increases β-adrenergic receptor density and responsiveness to inotropic therapy (Heilbrunn et al., 1989). Possibly this innovative form of therapy will prove useful for selected patients with chronic CHF. Until the results of the currently ongoing multicenter dilated cardiomyopathy trial comparing metoprolol to placebo is completed, physicians and patients should reserve judgment about this form of treatment. Indeed, in many patients with CHF, β-adrenergic antagonists will worsen heart failure!

Milrinone

Milrinone is a potent phosphodiesterase inhibitor that has both positive inotropic and vasodilator activity (chapter 6). It increases cardiac output and lowers left ventricular filling pressure (Simonton et al., 1985). It is similar in action to amrinone but is about 20 times more potent (Baim et al., 1983). Milrinone has been found to improve exercise tolerance in patients with heart failure when compared with placebo, but not more than digitalis (DiBianco et al., 1989). *Principle: The theoretic or intellectual appeal of a new drug must be balanced against the enormous usefulness of meaningful data that have been acquired during the use of "standard" therapy.*

Milrinone is a bipyridine that improves both the systolic and the diastolic performance of the heart. However, until recently there were no controlled data regarding the influence of this drug on long-term survival rates (Baim et al., 1986). A large multicenter trial designed to test the hypothesis that milrinone, when added to baseline therapy of digitalis, diuretics, and an ACE inhibitor, will improve the survival of patients with class III and IV heart failure was recently prematurely terminated because of a statistically significant excessive number of deaths in the milrinone group.

Flosequinan and Pimobendan

The clinician is well advised to look ahead when treating a disease that has no obvious drug of choice or when there is less-than-definitive treatment available. At no time is the ability to use the literature more important. Flosequinan is a relatively new direct-acting vasodilator agent that increases cardiac output and reduces left ventricular filling pressure (Haas et al., 1989). The mechanism of the direct vasodilator activity is unknown. It also possesses some positive inotropic properties. It has a relatively long duration of action and apparently does not cause tolerance. Studies to date indicate that flosequinan shows promise as a vasodilator agent for the treatment of patients with chronic CHF. Until placebo-controlled, blinded studies are reported, its role in the management of patients with CHF will remain unknown.

Pimobendan is a new oral agent that sensitizes myocardial contractile proteins to calcium (Ruegg, 1987; Fujino et al., 1988). Additionally, it has some inhibitor activity on phosphodiesterase. When given to patients with chronic CHF, the drug modestly improves cardiac output and reduces pulmonary capillary wedge pressure (Hagenmeijer et al., 1989; Hasenfuss et al., 1989). Preliminary data suggest that this agent may improve exercise tolerance and survival in cardiomyopathic hamsters (van Meel et al., 1989). Pimobendan does not act through the β-adrenergic receptor pathway. Its ability to enhance the effects of calcium on the contractile proteins repre-

Fig. 4–13. Once myocardial dysfunction is present from any cause, vasoconstriction exacerbates this dysfunction by raising afterload. Neuroendocrine influences may lead to vasoconstriction, which leads to (and is exacerbated by) salt and water retention. Neuroendocrine influences also may directly exacerbate myocardial dysfunction. The role of inotropic agents in the therapy of ventricular dysfunction is constantly being defined. Acutely, inotropic agents may be of value in severe CHF, and digitalis may be beneficial in chronic CHF. Neurohumoral activation can be partially attenuated with ACE inhibitors, with resultant beneficial clinical effects. Diuretics can dramatically enhance salt and water excretion, with resultant secondary benefits to preload and afterload and so indirectly to ventricular function. The role of experimental therapy with β-adrenergic antagonists requires further definition, as does the use of novel compounds such as flosequinan.

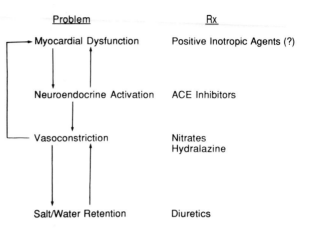

DIASTOLIC HEART FAILURE

A substantial proportion of patients, perhaps 30%, who have signs and symptoms of CHF have normal left ventricular *systolic* function. These patients are classified by the term *diastolic heart failure*. The failure is due to impairment of left ventricular relaxation and filling (Dougherty et al., 1984; Soufer et al., 1985). Such patients frequently have a history of hypertension, left ventricular hypertrophy, high left ventricular filling pressure, and a hypercontractile left ventricle. There presently is no uniformly agreed upon therapy for diastolic heart failure. Control of hypertension is very important. It has been suggested that there may be some role for calcium-channel blockers in patients with diastolic heart failure, but this is not yet defined adequately.

GENERAL STRATEGIES FOR TREATMENT OF CHRONIC CHF

There is substantial heterogeneity in how physicians treat chronic CHF as controlled clinical trials have not yet evaluated many of the approaches to therapy that have been used empirically for many years. Figure 4–13 summarizes a general strategy. Based on currently available information, it is generally reasonable to use digoxin and a loop diuretic in most patients with chronic CHF, particularly if cardiomegaly and a third heart sound are present. Additionally, on account of the results of the CONSENSUS and V-HeFT trials, most patients with CHF should be treated with vasodilators since these drugs have been demonstrated to prolong life. It is not known if

sents a new class of inotropic therapy. We must await the results of further clinical studies before jumping on the bandwagon!

ACE inhibitors are preferable to direct-acting vasodilators or not. In any case, either an ACE inhibitor or a combination of hydralazine and isosorbide dinitrate should be considered for patients who have chronic class II or III congestive heart failure. This recommendation is based on the results of the V-HeFT I trial. For patients with severe CHF (class IV), ACE inhibitors are indicated based on the results of the CONSENSUS Trial.

There is substantial controversy about when to introduce treatment in patients with asymptomatic left ventricular dysfunction. Experimental data (Pfeffer et al., 1985 and 1987) and two clinical trials (Sharpe et al., 1988; Pfeffer et al., 1988) suggest that early intervention with ACE inhibitors following myocardial infarction may prevent left ventricular dilation or remodeling and thereby forestall the onset of heart failure. To what extent, if any, this approach prolongs life is not yet known.

REFERENCES

Abrams, J: Interval therapy to avoid nitrate tolerance: Paradise regained? Am. J. Cardiol., 64:931–934, 1989.

Alderman, J.; and Grossmann, W.: Are β-adrenergic-blocking drugs useful in the treatment of dilated cardiomyopathy? Circulation, 71:854–857, 1985.

Arnold, S. B.; Byrd, R. C.; Meister, W.; Melmon, K.; Cheitlin, M. D.; Bristow, J. D.; Parmley, W. W.; and Chatterjee, K.: Long-term digitalis therapy improves left ventricular function in heart failure. N. Engl. J. Med. 303:1443–1448, 1980.

Awan, N. A.; Evenson, M. K.; Needham, K. E.; Beattie, J. M.; and Mason, D. T.: Effect of combined nitroglycerin and dobutamine infusion in left ventricular dysfunction. Am. Heart J., 106:35–40, 1983.

Axelsson, K. L.; and Ahlner, J.: Nitrate tolerance from a biochemical point of view. Drugs, 33(suppl. 4):63–68, 1987.

Baim, D. S.; Colucci, W. S.; Monrad, S.; Smith, H. S.; Wright, R. F.; Lanoue A.; Gauthier, D. F.; Ransil, B. J.; Grossman, W.; and Braunwald, E.: Survival of patients with severe congestive heart failure treated with oral milrinone. J. Am. Coll. Cardiol., 7:661–670, 1986.

Baim, D. S.; McDowell, A. V.; Cherniles, J.; Monrad, E. S.; Parker, J. A.; Edelson, J.; Braunwald, E.; and Grossman, W.: Evaluation of a new bipyridine inotropic agent — milrinone — in patients with severe congestive heart failure. N. Engl. J. Med., 309:748–756, 1983.

Benotti, J. R.; Grossman, W.; Braunwald, E.; Davolos, D. D.; and Alousi, A. A.: Hemodynamic assessment of amrinone. A new inotropic agent. N. Engl. J. Med. 299:1373–1377, 1978.

Böhm, M.; Gierschik, P.; Jakobs, K-H.; Pieske, B.; Schnabel, P.; Ungerer, M.; and Erdmann, E.: Increase of G_{ia} in human hearts with dilated but not ischemic cardiomyopathy. Circulation, 82:1249–1265, 1990.

Bolli, P.; Muller, F. B.; Linder, L.; Raine, A. E. G.; Resnick, T. J.; Erne, P.; Kiowski, W.; Ritz, R.; and Bühler, F. R.: The vasodilatory potency of atrial natriuretic peptide in man. Circulation, 75:221–228, 1987.

Bristow, M. R.; Ginsburg, R.; Umans, V.; Fowler, M.; Niminobe, W.; Rasmussen, R.; Zera, P.; Menlove, R.; Shah, P.; Jamieson, S.; and Stinson, E. B.: B1- and B2-adrenergic-receptor subpopulations in nonfailing and failing human ventricular myocardium: Coupling of both receptor subtypes to muscle contraction and selective B1-receptor down-regulation in heart failure. Circ. Res., 59:297–309, 1986.

Bristow, M. R.; Ginsburg, R.; Minobe, W.; Cubicciotti, R. S.; Sageman, W. S.; Lurie, K.; Billingham, M. E.; Harrison, D. C.; and Stinson, E. B.: Decreased catecholamine sensitivity and beta-adrenergic-receptor density in failing human hearts. N. Engl. J. Med. 307:205–211, 1982.

Brooks, V. L.; Keil, L. C.; and Reid, I. A.: Role of the renin-angiotensin system in the control of vasopressin secretion in conscious dogs. Circ. Res., 58:829–838, 1986.

Burnett, J. C.; Granger, J. P.; and Opgenorth, T. S.: Effects of synthetic atrial natriuretic factor on renal function and renin release. Am. J. Physiol., 247:F863–F866, 1984.

Captopril-Digoxin Multicenter Research Group: Comparative effects of therapy with captopril and digoxin in patients with mild to moderate heart failure. J.A.M.A., 259:539–544, 1988.

Cleland, J. G. F.; Dargie, H. J.; Findlay, I. N.; and Wilson, J. T.: Clinical, haemodynamic, and antiarrhythmic effects of long term treatment with amiodarone of patients in heart failure. Br. Heart J., 57:436–445, 1987.

Cody, R. J.; Atlas, S. A.; Laragh, J. H.; Kubo, S. H.; Covit, A. B.; Ryman, K. S.; Shaknovich A.; Pondolfino, K.; Clark, M.; Camargo, M. J. F.; Scarborough, R. M.; and Lewicki, J. A.: Atrial natriuretic factor in normal subjects and heart failure patients. Plasma levels and renal, hormonal, and hemodynamic responses to peptide infusion. J. Clin. Invest., 78:1362–1374, 1986.

Cohn, J. N.: Vasodilator therapy for heart failure. The influence of impedance on left ventricular performance. Circulation, 48:5–8, 1973.

Cohn, J. N., and Franciosa, J. A.: Vasodilator therapy of cardiac failure. N. Engl. J. Med., 297:27–31, 254–258, 1977.

Cohn, J. N.; Archibald, D. G.; Phil, M.; Ziesche, S.; Franciosa, J. A.; Harston, W. E.; Tristani, F. E.; Dunkman, W. B.; Jacobs, W.; Francis, G. S.; Flohr, K. H.; Goldman, S.; Cobb, F. R.; Shah, P. M.; Saunders, R.; Fletcher, R. D.; Loeb, H. S.; Hughes, V. C.; and Baker, B.: Effect of vasodilator therapy on mortality in chronic congestive heart failure. Results of a Veterans Administration cooperative study. N. Engl. J. Med., 314:1547–1552, 1986.

CONSENSUS Trial Study Group: Effects of enalapril on mortality in severe congestive heart failure. Results of the cooperative north scandinavian enalapril survival study (CONSENSUS). N. Engl. J. Med., 316:1429–1435, 1987.

Creager, M. A.; Faxon, D. P.; Cutler, S. S.; Kohlman, O.; Ryan, T. J.; and Gavras, H.: Contribution of vasopressin to vasoconstriction in patients with congestive heart failure: Comparison with the renin-angiotensin system and the sympathetic nervous system. J. Am. Coll. Cardiol., 7:758–765, 1986.

Currie, P. J.; Kelly, M. J.; McKenzie, A.; Harper, R. W.; Lim, Y. L.; Federman, J.; Anderson, S. T.; and Pitt, A.: Oral beta-adrenergic blockade with metoprolol in chronic severe dilated cardiomyopathy. J. Am. Coll. Cardiol., 3:203–209, 1984.

DiBianco, R.; Shabetai, R.; Kostuk, W.; Moran, J.; Schlant, R. C.; and Wright, R.: A comparison of oral milrinone, digoxin and their combination in the treatment of patients with chronic heart failure. N. Engl. J. Med., 320:677–683, 1989.

Dikshit, K.; Vyden, J. K.; Forrester, J. S.; Chatterjee, K.; Prakash, R.; and Swan, H. J. C.: Renal and extrarenal hemodynamic effects of furosemide in congestive heart failure after acute myocardial infarction. N. Engl. J. Med., 288:1087–1090, 1973.

Dougherty, A. H.; Naccarelli, G. V.; Gray, E. L.; Hicks, C. H.; and Goldstein, R. A.: Congestive heart failure with normal systolic function. Am. J. Cardiol., 54:778–782, 1984.

Dzau, V. J.; Packer, M.; Lilly, L. S.; Swartz, S. L.; Hollenberg, N. K.; and Williams, G. H.: Prostaglandins in severe congestive heart failure. Relation to activation of the renin-angiotensin system and hyponatremia. N. Engl. J. Med., 310:347–352, 1984.

Engelmeier, R. S.; O'Connell, J. B.; Walsh, R.; Rad, N.; Scanlon, P. J.; and Gunnar, R. M.: Improvement in symptoms and exercise tolerance by metoprolol in patients with dilated cardiomyopathy: A double-blind, randomized, placebo-controlled trial. Circulation, 72:536–546, 1985.

Ferriar, J.: Medical History and Reflections. Vol. 2. Thomas Dobson, Philadelphia, p. 253, 1816.

Feldman, A. M.; Cates, A. E.; Veazey, W. B.; Hershberger, R. E.; Bristow, M. R.; Baughman, K. L.; Baumgartner, W. A.; and Van Dop, C.: Increase of the 40,000-mol wt pertussis toxin substrate (G protein) in the failing human heart. J. Clin. Invest., 82:189–197, 1988.

Ferguson, D. W.; Berg, W. J.; Sanders, J. S.; Roach, P. J.; Kempf, J. S.; and Kienzle, M. G.: Sympathoinhibitory responses to digitalis glycosides in heart failure patients. Direct evidence from sympathetic neural recording. Circulation, 80:65–77, 1989.

Fleg, J. L.; and Lakatta, E. G.: How useful is digitalis in patients with congestive heart failure and sinus rhythm? Int. J. Cardiol., 6:295–305, 1984.

Fleg, J. L.; Gottlieb, S. H.; and Lakatta, E. G.: Is digoxin really important in treatment of compensated heart failure? A placebo-controlled crossover study in patients with sinus rhythm. Am. J. Med., 73:244–250, 1982.

Fowler, M. B.; Laser, J. A.; Hopkins, G. L.; Minobe, W.; and Bristow, M. R.: Assessment of the β-adrenergic receptor pathway in the intact failing human heart: Progressive receptor down-regulation and subsensitivity to agonist response. Circulation, 74:1290–1302, 1986.

Franciosa, J. A.; and Cohn, J. N.: Effect of isosorbide dinitrate on response to submaximal and maximal exercise in patients with congestive heart failure. Am. J. Cardiol., 43:1009–1014, 1979a.

Franciosa, J. A.; and Cohn, J. N.: Immediate effects of hydralazine-isosorbide dinitrate combination on exercise capacity and exercise hemodynamics in patients with left ventricular failure. Circulation, 59:1085–1091, 1979b.

Franciosa, J. A.; Dunkman, W. B.; and Leddy, C. L.: Hemodynamic effects of vasodilators and long-term response in heart failure. J. Am. Coll. Cardiol., 3:1521–1530, 1984.

Franciosa, J. A.; Wilen, M.; Ziesche, S.; and Cohn, J. N.: Survival in men with severe chronic left ventricular failure due to either coronary heart disease or idiopathic dilated cardiomyopathy. Am. J. Cardiol., 51(5):831–836, 1983.

Franciosa, J. A.; Blank, R. C.; and Cohn, J. N.: Nitrate effects on cardiac output and left ventricular outflow resistance in chronic congestive heart failure. Am. J. Med., 64:207–213, 1978a.

Franciosa, J. A.; Nordstrom, L. A.; and Cohn, J. N.: Nitrate therapy for congestive heart failure. J.A.M.A., 240:443–446, 1978b.

Franciosa, J. A.; Pierpont, G.; and Cohn, J. N.: Hemodynamic improvement after oral hydralazine in left ventricular failure. A comparison with nitroprusside infusion in 16 patients. Ann. Intern. Med., 86:388-393, 1977.

Franciosa, J. A.; Mikulic, E.; Cohn, J. N.; Jose, E.; and Fabie, A.: Hemodynamic effects of orally administered isosorbide dinitrate in patients with congestive heart failure. Circulation, 50:1020-1024, 1974.

Franciosa, J. A.; Limas, C. J.; Guiha, N. H.; Rodriguera, E.; and Cohn, J. N.: Improved left ventricular function during nitroprusside infusion in acute myocardial infusion. Lancet, 1:650-654, 1972.

Francis, G. S.: The relationship of the sympathetic nervous system and the renin-angiotensin system in congestive heart failure. Am. Heart J., 118:642-648, 1989.

Francis, G. S.: Heart failure management: The impact of drug therapy on survival. Am. Heart J., 115:699-702, 1988a.

Francis, G. S.: Should asymptomatic ventricular arrhythmias in patients with congestive heart failure be treated with antiarrhythmic drugs? J. Am. Coll. Cardiol., 12:274-283, 1988b.

Francis, G. S.: Inotropic agents in the management of heart failure. In, Drug Treatment of Heart Failure (Cohn, J. N., ed.). Adv. Ther. Com., Secaucus, NJ, pp. 179-197, 1988c.

Francis, G. S.: Development of arrhythmias in the patient with congestive heart failure: Pathophysiology, prevalence and prognosis. Am. J. Cardiol., 57:3B-7B, 1986a.

Francis, G. S.: Sodium and water excretion in heart failure: Efficacy of treatment has surpassed knowledge of pathophysiology. Ann. Intern. Med., 105:272-274, 1986b.

Francis, G. S.; and Archer, S. L.: Diagnosis and management of acute congestive heart failure in the intensive care unit. J. Int. Care Med., 4:84-92, 1989.

Francis, G. S.; Benedict, C.; Johnstone, D. E.; Kirlin, P. C.; Nicklas, J.; Liang, C. S.; Kubo, S. H.; Rudin-Toretsky, E.; and Yusuf, S.: Comparison of neuroendocrine activity in patients with left ventricular dysfunction with and without congestive heart failure. A substudy of the studies of left ventricular dysfunction (SOLVD). Circulation, 82:1724-1729, 1990.

Francis, G. S.; Siegel, R. M.; Goldsmith, S. R.; Olivari, M. T.; Levine, B.; and Cohn, J. N.: Acute vasoconstrictor response to intravenous furosemide in patients with chronic congestive heart failure. Ann. Intern. Med., 103:1-6, 1985.

Francis, G. S.; Goldsmith, S. R.; Levine, T. B.; Olivari, M. T.; and Cohn, J. N.: The neurohumoral axis in congestive heart failure. Ann. Intern. Med., 101:370-377, 1984.

Francis, G. S.; Sharma, B.; and Hodges, M.: Comparative hemodynamic effects of dopamine and dobutamine in patients with acute cardiogenic circulatory collapse. Am. Heart J., 103:995-1000, 1982.

Fujino, K.; Sperelakis, N.; and Solaro, R. J.: Sensitization of dog and guinea pig heart myofilaments to Ca^{2+} activation and the inotropic effect of pimobendan: Comparison with milrinone. Circ. Res., 63:911-922, 1988.

Gage, J.; Rutman, H.; Lucido, D.; and LeJemtel, T. H.: Additive effects of dobutamine and amrinone on myocardial contractility and ventricular performance in patients with severe heart failure. Circulation, 74:367-373, 1986.

Gerlag, P. G. G.; and vanMeijel, J. J. M.: High-dose furosemide in the treatment of refractory congestive heart failure. Arch. Intern. Med., 148:286-291, 1988.

Gheorghiade, M.; and Beller, G. A.: Effects of discontinuing maintenance digoxin therapy in patients with ischemic heart disease and congestive heart failure in sinus rhythm. Am. J. Cardiol., 51:1243-1250, 1983.

Gheorghiade, M.; St. Clair, J.; St. Clair, C.; and Beller, G. A.: Hemodynamic effects of intravenous digoxin in patients with severe heart failure initially treated with diuretics and vasodilators. J. Am. Coll. Cardiol., 9:849-857, 1987.

Giles, T. D.; Katz, R.; Sullivan; Wolfson, P.; Haugland, M.; Kirlin, P.; Powers, E.; Rich, S.; Hackshaw, B.; Chiaramida, A.; Rouleau, J-L.; Fisher, M. B.; Pigeon, J.; and Rush, J. (The Multicenter Lisinopril-Captopril Congestive Heart Failure Study Group): Short- and long-acting angiotensin converting enzyme inhibitors. A randomized trial of lisinopril vs captopril in the treatment of congestive heart failure. J. Am. Coll. Cardiol., 13:1240-1248, 1989.

Ginsberg, R.; Esserman, L. J.; and Bristow, M. R.: Myocardial performance and extracellular ionized calcium in a severely failing human heart. Ann. Intern. Med., 98(Part 1):603-606, 1983.

Goldberg, L. I.: Dopamine—Clinical uses of an endogenous catecholamine. N. Engl. J. Med., 291:707-710, 1974.

Goldberg, L. I.: Cardiovascular and renal actions of dopamine: Potential clinical applications. Pharmacol. Rev., 24:1-29, 1972.

Goldsmith, S. R.; Francis, G. S.; and Cohn, J. N.: Attenuation of the pressor response to intravenous furosemide by angiotensin converting enzyme inhibitor in congestive heart failure. Am. J. Cardiol. 64:1382-1385, 1989.

Goldsmith, S. R.; Francis, G. S.; Cowley, A. W.; Goldenberg, I.; and Cohn, J. N.: Hemodynamic effects of infused arginine vasopressin in congestive heart failure. J. Am. Coll. Cardiol., 8:779-783, 1986.

Goldsmith, S. R.; Francis, G. S.; Cowley, A. W.; Levine, T. B.; and Cohn, J. N.: Increased plasma arginine vasopressin levels in patients with congestive heart failure. J. Am. Coll. Cardiol., 1:1385-1390, 1983.

Goldsmith, S. R.; Francis, G. S.; Cowley, A. W.; and Cohn, J. N.: Response of vasopressin and norepinephrine to lower body negative pressure in humans. Am. J. Physiol., 272: H970-H973, 1982.

Guyatt, G. H.; Sullivan, M. J. J.; Fallen, E. L.; Tihal, H.; Rideout, E.; Halcrow, S.; Nogradi, S.; Townsend, M.; and Taylor, D. W.: A controlled trial of digoxin in congestive heart failure. Am. J. Cardiol., 61:371-375, 1988.

Haas, G. J.; Binkley, P. F.; Carpenter, J. A.; and Leier, C. V.: Central and regional hemodynamic effects of flosequinan for congestive heart failure. Am. J. Cardiol., 63:1354-1359, 1989.

Hagemeijer, F.; Brand, H. J.; and van Mechelen, R.: Hemodynamic effects of pimobendan given orally in congestive heart failure secondary to ischemic or idiopathic dilated cardiomyopathy. Am. J. Cardiol., 63:571-576, 1989.

Hall, J. E.; Guyton, A. C.; Jackson, T. E.; Coleman, T. G.; Lohmeier, T. E.; and Trippodo, N. C.: Control of glomerular filtration rate by renin agiotensin system. Am. J. Physiol., 233(5):F366-F372, 1977a.

Hall, J. E.; Guyton, A. C.; and Cowley, A. W.: Dissociation of renal blood flow and filtration rate autoregulation by renin depletion. Am. J. Physiol., 232(2):F215-F221, 1977b.

Harigaya, S.; and Schwartz, A.: Rate of calcium binding and uptake in normal animal and failing human cardiac muscle. Circ. Res., 25:781-787, 1969.

Hasenfuss, G.; Holubarsch, C.; Heiss, H. W.; and Just, H.: Influence of UDCG-115 on hemodynamics and myocardial energetics in patients with idiopathic dilated cardiomyopathy. Am. Heart J., 118:512-519, 1989.

Hasking, G. J.; Esler, M. D.; Jennings, G. L.; Burton, D.; and Korner, P. I.: Norepinephrine spillover to plasma in patients with congestive heart failure: Evidence of increased overall and cardiorenal sympathetic nerve activity. Circulation, 73: 615-621, 1986.

Heel, R. C.; Brogden, R. N.; Speight, T. M.; and Avery, G. S.: Captopril: A preliminary review of its pharmacological properties and therapeutic efficacy. Drugs, 20:409-452, 1980.

Heger, J. J.; Prystowsky, E. N.; Jackman, W. M.; Naccarelli, G. V.; Warfel, K. A.; Rinkenberger, R. L.; and Zipes, D. P.: Amiodarone. Clinical efficacy and electrophysiology during long-term therapy for recurrent ventricular tachycardia or ventricular fibrillation. N. Engl. J. Med., 305:539-545, 1981.

Heilbrunn, S. M.; Shah, P.; Bristow, M. R.; Valantine, H. A.; Ginsburg, R.; and Fowler, M. B.: Increased B-receptor density and improved hemodynamic response to catecholamine stimulation during long-term metoprolol therapy in heart failure from dilated cardiomyopathy. Circulation, 79: 483-490, 1989.

Hittinger, L.; Gelpi, R. J.; Fujii, A. M.; and Vatner, S. F.:

Impairment of subendocardial coronary reserve in conscious dogs with heart failure. Circulation, 76:IV-147, 1987. (Abstract.)

Ichikawa, I.; Pfeffer, J. M.; Pfeffer, M. A.; Hostetter, T. H.; and Brenner, B. M.: Role of angiotensin II in the altered renal function of congestive heart failure. Circ. Res., 55:669–675, 1984.

Ikram, H.; and Fitzpatrick, D.: Double-blind trial of chronic oral beta blockade in congestive cardiomyopathy. Lancet, 2(8245):490–493, 1981.

Insel, P. A.; and Ransnas, L. A.: G proteins and cardiovascular disease. Circulation, 78:1511–1513, 1988.

Jentzer, J. H.; Lejemtel, T. H.; Sonnenblick, E. H.; and Kirk, E. S.: Beneficial effect of amrinone on myocardial oxygen consumption during acute left ventricular failure in dogs. Am. J. Cardiol., 48:75–83, 1981.

Kates, R. E.; and Leier, C. V.: Dobutamine pharmacokinetics in severe heart failure. Am. Heart J., 24:537–541, 1978.

Katz, A. M.: Cardiomyopathy of overload: A major determinant of prognosis in congestive heart failure. N. Engl. J. Med., 322:100–110, 1990.

Katz, A. M.: Biochemical "defect" in the hypertrophied and failing heart. Circulation, 47:1076–1082, 1973.

Klein, N. A.; Siskind, S. J.; Frishman, W. H.; Sonnenblick, E. H.; and LeJemtel, T. H.: Hemodynamic comparison of intravenous amrinone and dobutamine in patients with chronic congestive heart failure. Am. J. Cardiol., 48:170–175, 1981.

Kluger, J.; Cody, R. J.; and Caragh, J. H.: The contributions of sympathetic tone and the renin-angiotensin system to severe chronic heart failure. Am. J. Cardiol., 49:1667–1673, 1982.

Koch-Weser, J.: Hydralazine. N. Engl. J. Med., 295:320–323, 1976.

Kubo, S. H.; and Cody, R. J.: Clinical pharmacokinetics of the angiotensin converting enzyme inhibitors. A Review. Clin. Pharmacokin. 10:377–391, 1985.

Kulick, D.; Roth, A.; McIntosh, N.; Rahimtoola, S. H.; and Elkayam, U.: Resistance to isosorbide dinitrate in patients with severe chronic heart failure: Incidence and attempt at hemodynamic prediction. Am. Coll. Cardiol., 12:1023–1028, 1988.

Lee, D. C. S.; Johnson, R. A.; Bingham, J. B.; Leahy, M.; Dinsmore, R. E.; Goroll, A. H.; Newell, J. B.; Strauss, W.; and Haber, E.: Heart failure in outpatients. A randomized trial of digoxin versus placebo. N. Engl. J. Med., 306:699–705, 1982.

Leier, C. V.; and Unverferth, D. V.: Dobutamine. Ann. Intern. Med., 99:490–496, 1983.

Leier, C. V.; Heban, P. T.; Hass, P.; Bush, C. A.; and Lewis, R. P.: Comparative systemic and regional hemodynamic effects of dopamine and dobutamine in patients with cardiomyopathic heart failure. Circulation, 58:466–475, 1978.

Leier, C. V.; Webel, J.; and Bush, C. A.: The cardiovascular effects of the continuous infusion of dobutamine in patients with severe cardiac failure. Circulation, 56:468–472, 1977.

Leimbach, W. N.; Wallin, B. G.; Victor, R. G.; Aylward, P. E.; Sundlof, G.; and Mark, A. L.: Direct evidence from intraneural recordings for increased central sympathetic outflow in patients with heart failure. Circulation, 73:913–919, 1986.

LeJemtel, T. H.; Maskin, C. S.; and Chadwick, B.: Effects of acute angiotensin converting enzyme inhibition on renal blood flow in patients with stable congestive heart failure. Am. J. Med. Sci., 292:123–126, 1986.

LeJemtel, T. H.; Keung, E.; Sonnenblick, E. H.; Ribner, H. S.; Matsumoto, M.; Davis, R.; Schwartz, W.; Alousi, A. A.; and Davolos, D.: Amrinone: a new non-glycosidic, non-adrenergic cardiotonic agent effective in the treatment of intractable myocardial failure in man. Circulation, 59:1098–1104, 1979.

Levine, T. B.; Francis, G. S.; Goldsmith, S. R.; Simon, A. B.; and Cohn, J. N.: Activity of the sympathetic nervous system

and renin-angiotensin system assessed by plasma hormone levels and their relationship to hemodynamic abnormalities in congestive heart failure. Am. J. Cardiol., 49:1659–1666, 1982.

Loeb, H. S.; Bredakis, J.; and Gunnar, R. M.: Superiority of dobutamine over dopamine for augmentation of cardiac output in patients with chronic low output cardiac failure. Circulation, 55:375–381, 1977.

Lilly, L.; Dzar, V. J.; Williams, G. H.; Rydstedt, L.; and Hollenberg, N. K.: Hyponatremia in congestive heart failure: Implications for neurohumoral activation and responses to orthostasis. J. Clin. Endocrinol. Metab., 59:924–930, 1984.

MacCannell, K. L.; McNay, J. L.; Meyer, M. B.; and Goldberg, L. I.: Dopamine in the treatment of hypotension and shock. N. Engl. J. Med., 275:1389–1398, 1966.

MacGregor, D. C.; Covell, J. W.; Mahler, F.; Dilley, R. B.; and Ross, J.: Relationships between afterload, stroke volume, and the descending limb of Starling's curve. Am. J. Physiol., 227:884–889, 1974.

Magorien, R. D.; Unverferth, D. V.; and Leier, C. V.: Hydralazine therapy in chronic congestive heart failure. Sustained central and regional hemodynamic responses. Am. J. Med., 77:267–274, 1984.

Magorien, R. D.; Brown, G. P.; Unverferth, D. V.; Nelson, S.; Boudoulas, H.; Bambach, D.; and Leier, C. V.: Effects of hydralazine on coronary blood flow and myocardial energetics in congestive heart failure. Circulation, 65:528–533, 1982.

Maisel, A. S.; Wright, M.; Carter, S. M.; Ziegler, M.; and Motulsky, H. J.: Tachyphylaxis with amrinone therapy: Association with sequestration and down-regulation of lymphocyte beta-adrenergic receptors. Ann. Intern. Med., 110:195–201, 1989.

Mason, J. W.: Amiodarone. N. Engl. J. Med., 316:455–466, 1987.

Mikulic, E.; Cohn, J. N.; and Franciosa, J. A.: Comparative hemodynamic effects of inotropic and vasodilator drugs in severe heart failure. Circulation, 56:528–533, 1977.

Miller, R. R.; Awan, N. A.; Joye, J. A.; Maxwell, K. S.; DeMaria, A. N.; Amsterdam, E. A.; and Mason, D. T.: Combined dopamine and nitroprusside therapy in congestive heart failure. Greater augmentation of cardiac performance by addition of inotropic stimulation to afterload reduction. Circulation, 55:881–884, 1977.

Moncada, S.; Palmer, R. M. J.; and Higgs, E. A.: The discovery of nitric oxide as the endogenous nitrovasodilator. Hypertension, 12:365–372, 1988.

Movesesian, M. A.; Bristow, M. R.; and Krall, J.: Ca^{2+} uptake by cardiac sarcoplasmic reticulum from patients with idiopathic dilated cardiomyopathy. Circ. Res., 65:1141–1144, 1989.

Murad, F.: Cyclic guanosine monophosphate as a mediator of vasodilation. J. Clin. Invest., 78:1–5, 1986.

Needleman, P.; and Greenwald, J. E.: Atriopeptin: A cardiac hormone intimately involved in fluid, electrolyte, and blood pressure hemeostasis. N. Engl. J. Med., 314:828–834, 1986.

Neri, R.; Mestroni, L.; Salvi, A.; Pandullo, C.; and Camerini, F.: Ventricular arrhythmias in dilated cardiomyopathy: Efficacy of amiodarone. Am. Heart J., 113:707–715, 1987.

Neumann, J.; Scholz, H.; Doring, V.; Schmitz, W.; von Meyerinck, L.; and Kalamar, J.: Increase in myocardial G_i-proteins in heart failure. Lancet, 2(8617):936–937, 1988.

Packer, M.: Sudden unexpected death in patients with congestive heart failure: A second frontier. Circulation, 72:681–685, 1985c.

Packer, M.; Lee, W. H.; Yushak, M.; and Medinea, N.: Comparison of captopril and enalapril in patients with severe chronic heart failure. N. Engl. J. Med., 315:847–853, 1986.

Packer, M.; Medine, N.; and Yushak, M.: Relation between serum sodium concentration and the hemodynamic and clinical responses to converting enzyme inhibition with captopril in severe heart failure. J. Am. Coll. Cardiol., 3:1035–1043, 1984.

Packer, M.; Meller, J.; Medina, N.; Yushak, M.; and Gorlin, R.: Hemodynamic characterization of tolerance to long-term hydralazine therapy in severe chronic heart failure. N. Engl. J. Med., 306:57–62, 1982.

Packer, M.; Meller, J.; Medina, N.; Yushak, M.; and Gorlin, R.: Provocation of myocardial ischemic events during initiation of vasodilator therapy for severe chronic heart failure. Clinical and hemodynamic evaluation of 52 consecutive patients with ischemic cardiomyopathy. Am. J. Cardiol., 48: 939–946, 1981.

Packer, M.; Meller, J.; Medina, N.; Gorlin, R.; and Herman, M.: Dose requirements of hydralazine in patients with severe chronic congestive heart failure. Am. J. Cardiol., 45:655–660, 1980.

Patterson, S. W., Piper, H.; and Starling, E. H.: The regulation of the heart beat. J. Physiol., 48:465–513, 1914.

Perry, H. M.: Late toxicity to hydralazine resembling systemic lupus erythematosus or rheumatoid arthritis. Am. J. Med., 54:58–71, 1973.

Pfeffer, M. A.; and Pfeffer, J. M.: Ventricular enlargement and reduced survival after myocardial infarction. Circulation, 75(suppl. 4):493–497, 1987.

Pfeffer, J. M.; Pfeffer, M. A.; and Braunwald, E.: Influence of chronic captopril therapy on the infarcted left ventricle of the rat. Circ. Res., 57:84–95, 1985.

Pfeffer, M. A.; Lamas, G. A.; Vaughan, D. E.; Parisi, A. F.; and Braunwald, E.: Effect of captopril on progressive ventricular dilatation after anterior myocardial infarction. N. Engl. J. Med., 319:80–86, 1988.

Rajfer, S. I.; Borow, K. M.; Lang, R. M.; Neumann, A.; and Carroll, J. D.: Effects on dopamine on left ventricular afterload and contractile state in heart failure: Relation to the activation of beta-1-adrenoceptors and dopamine receptors. J. Am. Coll. Cardiol., 12:498–506, 1988.

Reece, P. A.; Cozamanis, I.; and Zacest, R.: Kinetics of hydralazine and its main metabolites in slow and fast acetylators. Clin. Pharmacol. Ther., 28(6):769–778, 1980.

Ruegg, J. C.: Dependence of cardiac contractility on myofibrillar calcium sensitivity. N.I.P.S., 2:179–182, 1987.

Salisbury, P. F.; Cross, C. E.; and Rieban, P. A.: Acute ischemia of inner layers of ventricular wall. Am. Heart J., 66:650–656, 1963.

Shanes, J. G.: β-blockade—rational or irrational therapy for congestive heart failure? Circulation, 76:971–973, 1987.

Sharpe, N.; Smith, H.; Murphy, J.; and Hannan, S.: Treatment of patients with symptomless left ventricular dysfunction after myocardial infarction. Lancet, 1(8580):255–259, 1988.

Sievers, R.; Parmley, W.; James, T.; and Coffelt-Whilman.: Energy levels at systole vs diastole in normal hamster hearts vs myopathic hamster hearts. Circ. Res., 53:759–765, 1983.

Silber, S.; Vogler, A. C.; Krause, K. H.; Vogel, M.; and Theisen, K.: Induction and circumvention of nitrate tolerance applying different dosage intervals. Am. J. Med., 83:860–870, 1987.

Simonton, C. A.; Chatterjee, K.; Cody, R. J.; Kubo, S. H.; Leonard, D.; Daly, P.; and Rutman, H.: Milrinone in congestive heart failure: Acute and chronic hemodynamic and clinical evaluation. J. Am. Coll. Cardiol., 6:453–459, 1985.

Smith, T. W.: Mechanisms of action and clinical use. N. Engl. J. Med., 318:358–365, 1988.

Sonnenblick, E. H.; Frishman, W. H.; and LeJemtel, T. H.: Dobutamine: A new synthetic cardioactive sympathetic amine. N. Engl. J. Med., 300:17–22, 1979.

Soufer, R.; Wohlgelernter, D.; Vita, N. A.; Amuchestegui, M.; Sostman, H. D.; Berger, H. J.; and Zaret, B. L.: Intact systolic left ventricular function in clinical congestive heart failure. Am. J. Cardiol., 55:1032–1036, 1985.

Stemple, D. R.; Kleiman, J. H.; and Harrison, D. C.: Combined nitroprusside-dopamine therapy in severe chronic congestive heart failure. Dose-related hemodynamic advantages over single drug infusions. Am. J. Cardiol., 42:267–275, 1978.

Swedberg, K.; Hjalmarson, A.; Waagstein, F.; and Wallentin, I.: Beneficial effects of long-term beta-blockade in congestive cardiomyopathy. Br. Heart J., 44:117–133, 1980a.

Swedberg, K.; Hjalmarson, A.; Waagstein, F.; and Wallentin, I.: Adverse effects of beta-blockade withdrawal in patients with congestive cardiomyopathy. Br. Heart J., 44:134–142, 1980b.

Swedberg, K.; Waagstein, F.; Hjalmarson, A.; and Wallentin, I.: Prolongation of survival in congestive cardiomyopathy by beta-receptor blockade. Lancet, 1(8131):1374–1376, 1979.

Taggart, A. J.; Johnston, G. D.; and McDevitt, D. G.: Digoxin withdrawal after cardiac failure in patients with sinus rhythm. J. Cardiovasc. Pharmacol., 5:229–234, 1983.

Taylor, S. H.; and Silke, B.: Haemodynamic effects of beta-blockade in ischaemic heart failure. Lancet, 2(8251):835–838, 1981.

Thames, M. D.; Waickman, L. A.; and Abbout, F. M.: Sensitization of cardiac receptors (vagal afferents) by intracoronary acetylstrophanidly. Am. J. Physiol., 239:H628–H635, 1980.

Thomas, J. A.; and Marks, B. H.: Plasma norepinephrine in congestive heart failure. Am. J. Cardiol., 41:233–243, 1978.

Ulm, E. H.: Enalpril maleate (MK-421), a potent, non-sulfhydryl angiotensin converting enzyme inhibitor: Absorption, disposition, and metabolism in man. Drug Metab. Rev., 14: 99–110, 1983.

van Meel, J. C. A.; Mauz, A. B. M.; Wienen, W.; and Diederen, W.: Pimobendan increases survival of cardiomyopathic hamsters. J. Cardiovasc. Pharmacol., 13:508–509, 1989.

Vasko, M. R.; Brown-Cartwright, D.; Knochel, J. P.; Nixon, J. V.; and Brater, D. C.: Furosemide absorption altered in decompensated congestive heart failure. Ann. Intern. Med., 102:314–318, 1985.

Waagstein, F.; Caidahl, K.; Wallentin, I.; Bergh, C. H.; and Hjalmarson, A.: Long-term β-blockade in dilated cardiomyopathy. Effects of short- and long-term metoprolol treatment followed by withdrawal and readministration of metoprolol. Circulation, 80:551–563, 1989.

Waagstein, F.; Hjalmarson, A.; Varnauskas, E.; and Wallentin, I.: Effect of chronic beta-adrenergic receptor blockade in congestive cardiomyopathy. Br. Heart J., 37:1022–1036, 1975.

Weber, K. T.; and Janicki, J. S.: The heart as a muscle-pump system and the concept of heart failure. Am. Heart J., 98: 371–381, 1979.

Wiegand, V.; Ebecke, M.; Figulla, H.; Schüler, S.; and Kreuzer, H.: Structure and function of contractile proteins in human dilated cardiomyopathy. Clin. Cardiol., 12:656–660, 1989.

Zelis, R. D.; Mason, D. T.; and Braunwald, E.: A comparison of the effects of vasodilator stimuli on peripheral resistance vessels in normal subjects and in patients with congestive heart failure. J. Clin. Invest., 47:960–970, 1968.

Zimmerman, B. G.; Sybertz, E. J.; and Wong, P. C.: Interaction between the sympathetic and renin-angiotensin system. J. Hypertens., 2:581–587, 1984.

Zucker, I. H.; and Gilmore, J. P.: Aspects of cardiovascular reflexes in pathologic status. Fed. Proc., 44:2400–2407, 1985.

5

Treatment of Cardiovascular Disorders: Ischemic Heart Disease

Robert F. DeBusk

OVERVIEW OF CONTEMPORARY MANAGEMENT OF ACUTE ISCHEMIC HEART DISEASE

Until the 1980s, the management of acute ischemic heart disease (IHD) was almost entirely pharmacologic and was focused on the prophylaxis and treatment of arrhythmias, alleviation of chest pain, and mitigation of mechanical consequences of myocardial infarction (MI), that is, shock and pulmonary edema. Nonpharmacologic measures such as defibrillators and pacemakers were useful adjuncts in patients whose left ventricular dysfunction was not overwhelming. Mechanical circulatory-assist devices were occasionally helpful in patients with severe left ventricular dysfunction.

Emergency coronary artery surgery to alleviate ongoing myocardial ischemia and interrupt the process of MI was first applied in the 1980s. Operative mortality was high, but many patients survived who would not have survived with pharmacologic therapy alone. However, the application of emergency coronary artery surgery was limited by logistical factors including the dangers of transporting critically ill patients from community hospitals to tertiary centers.

In the mid-1980s, attention began to shift from treating the complications of acute MI to interrupting the natural history of acute MI. Elucidation of the critical role of intracoronary thrombosis in acute ischemic chest pain syndromes (Dewood et al., 1980) and demonstration of clot lysis after administration of intracoronary fibrinolytic agents (Rentrop et al., 1979) was soon followed by results of the first clinical trials of thrombolytic therapy (Gruppo Italiano, 1986; ISAM, 1986). The earlier these therapies were applied, the greater was their impact on morbidity and mortality. Although many of the early studies employed intracoronary thrombolysis with recombinant tissue-type plasminogen activator (r-TPA), IV administration proved equally efficacious (Tiefenbrunn and Sobel, 1989). The potential for earlier application established IV therapy as the preferred mode of delivery.

The potential to interrupt the natural history of acute MI provided an enormous impetus to the widespread use of antithrombotic and thrombolytic therapy. However useful these pharmacologic agents were for the lysis of intracoronary thromboses, they did not influence the underlying coronary atherosclerosis. The incidence of coronary artery reocclusion during hospitalization ranged from 20% to 30% (Chesebro et al., 1987). The potential for revascularization within 1 week of hospitalization using coronary artery surgery in patients with recurrent myocardial ischemia is limited by logistical factors (Kereiakes, 1989). However, this procedure is used for revascularization in the posthospital phase of treatment.

The combination of initial pharmacologic therapy with antithrombotic and thrombolytic agents followed within 1 week by mechanical therapy with percutaneous transluminal coronary angioplasty (PTCA) has profoundly influenced the management of patients with acute MI. Because they are applied at the very onset of acute MI, these therapies reduce not only in-hospital mortality but long-term mortality as well. Studies that established the efficacy of prophylactic therapy with β-adrenergic receptor antagonists after acute MI were conducted in the 1960s and 1970s prior to the widespread application of thrombolytic and revascularization therapies. Because β antagonists were introduced earlier in time, they were applied to a population of patients in whom the extent of myocardial necrosis and left ventricular dysfunction was relatively great and mortality relatively high. For example, in-hospital mortality after acute MI approximated 12%, and first-year posthospital mortality approximated 8% (Yusuf et al., 1985). In contrast, a large contemporary trial comparing routine PTCA versus elective PTCA after thrombolytic therapy of acute MI documented a *first-year* mortality of 7% (TIMI Study Group, 1989)! Because thrombolysis and revascularization have reduced short- and long-term mortality, they have diminished the potential of prophylactic agents introduced hours or days after the acute event to lower mortality still further. Consequently, very large numbers of patients are required to demonstrate the efficacy of such agents. Since contemporary clinical trials often employ multiple drugs concurrently with revascularization, the possibility of determining the prophylactic value of individual drugs given after acute MI is increasingly difficult.

Contemporary management of acute MI is characterized by the use of *both* pharmacologic and mechanical therapies designed to prevent myocardial necrosis rather than to treat its consequences. In general, the shift in emphasis of management away from acute MI and its complications to the prevention of acute MI has dramatically reduced mortality from acute MI.

PRINCIPLES OF MANAGEMENT OF ACUTE ISCHEMIC CHEST PAIN SYNDROMES

During the past 2 decades acute IHD has been considered synonymous with acute MI. However, natural history studies and intervention trials conducted during this time clearly have shown that the spectrum of acute ischemic chest pain syndromes encompasses not only acute MI but unstable angina and "acute MI ruled out." Indeed, the number of patients hospitalized for acute ischemic chest pain syndromes in which MI is not documented ("acute MI ruled out") outnumber those in whom MI is documented by a ratio of nearly 2 : 1 (Nordlander and Nyquist, 1979). Moreover, the prognosis of patients with "MI ruled out" is in general no better than that of patients with documented MI who survive hospitalization (Schroeder et al., 1980). The distinction between "MI ruled out" and non-Q-wave MI associated with relatively small elevation of cardiac enzymes is not clinically meaningful, and in many studies those groups of patients have been classified together.

Each of the syndromes of acute ischemic chest pain results from coronary atherosclerosis; but the severity of symptoms and hemodynamic derangements, and the short- and long-term outcomes, are influenced by the degree of restriction of coronary blood flow. *Stable angina* results primarily from fixed atherosclerotic coronary artery narrowing. *Unstable angina* and *non-Q-wave MI* usually are precipitated by incomplete occlusion of a coronary artery by platelet thrombi superimposed on a fixed atherosclerotic coronary artery narrowing. In contrast, *Q-wave MI* usually results from total occlusion of a coronary artery by thrombosis at the site of fixed atherosclerotic coronary narrowing. Therapy with antiplatelet agents, anticoagulants, and thrombolytic agents commencing within 4 to 6 hours after the onset of acute ischemic chest pain syndromes may limit the extent of infarction or even prevent infarction altogether.

THERAPY OF ACUTE MI—EARLY PHASE

The taxonomy of acute MI in the prethrombolytic era depended largely on the diagnostic implications of elevation of the concentration of cardiac enzymes in plasma and evolution of ECG changes within 72 hours after the onset of ischemic chest pain. Since there was no definitive therapy to interrupt the natural history of the disease, therapy was generally directed at the complications of acute MI such as congestive heart failure, ventricular ectopic activity, and heart block. In the thrombolytic era, the chief objective of therapy is to prevent myocardial necrosis and its electrical and mechanical complications. Salvage of the myocardium depends on the application of thrombolytic therapy even before a definitive diagnosis of acute MI is established. Indeed, criteria for thrombolytic therapy depend on electrocardiographic criteria for severe myocardial ischemia rather than on elevation of cardiac enzymes.

The use of pharmacologic therapy for prophylaxis of recurrent infarction and death in the post-acute phase of acute MI has been significantly influenced by the availability of PTCA and coronary artery bypass graft (CABG) surgery. Indeed, recanalization trials indicate that as many as 30% of occluded vessels responsible for the infarction and opened by thrombolysis become reoccluded within the next 14 days. Thereby patients are exposed to the hazards of reinfarction and death. Naturally, clinicians wish to reduce this risk.

At present there are three major options for prognostic stratification of asymptomatic patients who have undergone thrombolysis:

1. Coronary angiography followed by revascularization of "infarct vessels" with anatomically "significant" stenosis. Routine post-MI revascularization would be reasonable if patency of the infarct vessel determined by angiography were the sole basis of management. However, reliance upon patency of the infarct vessel as a guide to management has at least two major limitations: (a) a variable relationship exists between the extent of stenosis of the infarct vessel and the extent of myocardial necrosis and residual myocardial ischemia, and (b) the degree of stenosis in other coronary vessels influences the degree of residual myocardial ischemia and ischemic left ventricular dysfunction.

2. Coronary angiography followed by physiologic testing (exercise testing with or without radionuclide ventriculography or thallium scintigraphy) to determine the extent of ischemia or reperfusion in the distribution of "significant" stenoses of infarct vessels. Revascularization is performed if physiologic testing is "positive" for ischemia, and medical therapy is provided if physiologic testing is "negative" for ischemia.

3. Physiologic testing followed by coronary angiography and revascularization in patients whose tests are "positive" for ischemia and medical therapy in those whose tests are "negative" for ischemia.

One of the most helpful of the clinical trials in selecting from among these options was the TIMI II trial that compared invasive with conservative management after thrombolysis to treat acute MI (TIMI Study Group, 1989). A total of 3262 patients aged 76 years or less receiving r-TPA within 4 hours of acute ischemic chest pain were randomized to an *invasive strategy* of coronary angiography followed by PTCA if the anatomy was suitable or a *conservative strategy* consisting of coronary angiography and PTCA only for spontaneous or exercise-induced ischemia.

To summarize the major findings of this trial, coronary angiography was performed in virtually all patients of the invasively treated group but in only one third of the conservatively treated group. PTCA was performed in 60% of the invasive group but in only one sixth of the conservatively treated group. Nonetheless, the clinical outcome in regard to death and reinfarction was virtually identical in the invasive and conservative groups: death within 42 days occurred in 5.2% of those treated invasively and 4.7% of those treated conservatively, and fatal or nonfatal reinfarction occurred in 6.4% of those treated invasively and 5.8% of those treated conservatively.

The TIMI II results obviate much of the urgency attached to revascularization after thrombolysis. Removing the need for routine immediate PTCA after thrombolysis also removes the need for routine coronary angiography at any time, early or late. Angiography can then be reserved, as in the TIMI II trial, for patients with clinical episodes of recurrent ischemia (Baim et al., 1990). Although supine submaximal cycle ergometry was performed prior to hospital discharge, this test identified few patients with clinically important ischemia warranting PTCA.

In the prethrombolytic era a stepwise approach to prognostic stratification utilized clinical variables and specialized tests such as treadmill exercise tests performed in the 3 weeks after acute MI to identify high-risk patients (DeBusk et al., 1983). Coronary arteriography was performed as a prelude to CABG surgery in these high-risk patients. Thrombolysis engendered a perceived need for immediate routine revascularization necessitating immediate routine coronary angiography. The results of the TIMI II trial indicate that clinical variables such as recurrent pain and specialized test results such as exercise-induced myocardial ischemia can once again generate informed decisions about revascularization after thrombolysis. Coronary angiography can be performed as an adjunct or prelude to revascularization rather than the basis for the decision to revascularize. Indeed, specialized tests including exercise testing with or without radionuclide imaging have proved more sensitive than coronary angiography in prognostic stratification after acute MI (Gibson et al., 1983; Hung et al., 1984).

Although the prognostic value of exercise testing, with or without radionuclide imaging, was first established 2 to 3 weeks after acute MI, beginning in the early 1980s such testing was increasingly performed prior to hospital discharge. This is because of the perceived risk that recurrent cardiac events would occur immediately after discharge from the hospital, before exercise testing could be carried out. However, the risk of recurrent infarction and death between days 7 to 21 can be accurately predicted on clinical grounds. In one study (DeBusk and Dennis, 1985), 1000 patients were classified on the seventh hospital day as clinically low-risk and hence eligible for symptom-limited treadmill testing at 21 days. Among these 1000 patients, only 2 died and 3 experienced nonfatal MI between 7 and 21 days — an incidence of 0.5%. Moreover, these 1000 clinically low-risk patients comprised 50% of the entire post-MI population aged 70 or less.

In the era of reperfusion, the risks of recurrent infarction and death within 14 days is lower than ever before. In the TIMI II trial, total mortality was only 5% at 6 weeks and 7% at 52 weeks — *a much better outcome than before thrombolysis and PTCA.*

Randomized trials such as TIMI II have shown that elective revascularization can be performed safely and effectively in most patients who exhibit recurrent myocardial ischemia. Concerns about reocclusion and reinfarction after thrombolysis, which have engendered strategies for immediate revascularization after thrombolysis, seem to be overstated. *Principle: Advances in either diagnostics or the breadth of therapy can alter the expectations and applications of therapy.*

THERAPY OF ACUTE MI—LATE PHASE

Therapy of acute MI 14 or more days after the acute event is determined primarily by the prognosis or likelihood of subsequent cardiac events. General principles of prognostic stratification established over the past 20 years (DeBusk, 1989) still are relevant in the era of thrombolysis: (1) clinical characteristics and routine tests (ECG, chest x-ray films, cardiac enzymes) identify subsets of patients at highest risk, (2) specialized tests are of greatest independent value in subsets of patients whose risk based on clinical characteristics and routine tests is moderate, and (3) the goal of specialized testing in such individuals is to distinguish the few high-risk patients who may benefit from medical or surgical therapy from the many low-risk patients who require little or no medical therapy.

Studies of natural history have demonstrated the capacity to identify the substantial majority of patients whose risk of subsequent cardiac events is very low. However, persuading physicians to pursue less extensive diagnostic evaluation or apply less aggressive medical or surgical treatment even to putatively low-risk patients is difficult in the absence of explicit reassurance that the patient's risk actually is low. In one study (Dennis et al., 1988) of clinically low-risk patients

after acute MI physicians' use of diagnostic tests and medical and surgical therapy was significantly lower when they received a consultation in which the risk of cardiac death within the next year was explicitly stated to be as low as 1.5%. Actual mortality in these patients was in fact 1.5%, and such patients constituted 40% of all patients aged 70 years or less.

Identification of very-low-risk-patient subsets is important because they have least to gain from medical or surgical therapy (DeBusk, 1989). For example, although β-adrenergic receptor antagonists improve post-MI prognosis in general, their therapeutic efficacy is least well established in patients whose risk is very low. Among the 23% of patients classified as clinically low-risk in the Timolol trial (Norwegian Multicenter Study Group, 1981), those receiving this agent experienced no significant benefit compared with those receiving placebo. (This observation was equivalent to the benefit of treatment of hypertensive patients with borderline or inconsistent elevations in blood pressure.) Thrombolytic therapy of acute MI not only has decreased acute mortality but has increased the proportion of patients who are at low risk for late death. Consequently, demonstrating the effect of pharmacologic therapy with β-adrenergic receptor antagonists or calcium antagonists given in the late phase of recovery from MI has become more difficult. *Principle: Assessing a patient for therapy by deciding where in the spectrum of disease he or she stands allows better opportunity for appropriate qualitative decisions about therapy (to treat or not to treat) than when the patient is classified only by the rubric of the diagnostic (e.g., a hypertensive patient or a patient with asthma, chronic obstructive pulmonary disease (COPD), or atherosclerotic heart disease).*

MANAGEMENT OF UNSTABLE ANGINA PECTORIS

Angina that becomes more frequent, severe, or less responsive to medical therapy or occurs at rest or at night generally is classified as *unstable.* Many such patients undergo immediate coronary arteriography to identify "high-risk" lesions amenable to revascularization with PTCA or CABG surgery (Ambrose et al., 1985). However, unstable angina in hospitalized patients usually responds to intensive IV or orally administered antianginal drug therapy. This enables prognostic stratification to be performed on an elective basis using clinical variables and specialized techniques such as treadmill exercise testing performed with or without radionuclide imaging (DeBusk, 1989).

Treadmill testing is valuable in distinguishing high-risk and low-risk subsets of hospitalized patients whose chest pain has been controlled with pharmacologic therapy (Butman et al., 1984). Most patients with unstable angina pectoris can be stabilized with medical therapy and undergo specialized testing later. Only when such tests are significantly abnormal is coronary arteriography warranted. As in the case of acute MI, coronary arteriography should be performed as an adjunct to CABG surgery in patients with severely abnormal exercise tests.

MANAGEMENT OF CHRONIC ANGINA PECTORIS

Percutaneous transluminal angioplasty and coronary artery surgery all have exerted a marked influence on chronic angina pectoris. Indeed, many patients have undergone multiple revascularization procedures for relief of angina pectoris. Consequently, patients currently receiving pharmacologic therapy for the relief of angina pectoris often have advanced coronary artery disease and severely limiting angina pectoris. Many have experienced one or more acute MIs and exhibit moderate to severe left ventricular dysfunction. Consequently, many patients receiving antianginal drug therapy today can be considered to have end-stage heart disease. Success in alleviating their angina often is limited not only by the severity of their underlying coronary artery disease but by the extent of their left ventricular dysfunction.

The need for evaluation of drug therapy has been profoundly influenced by the complex interactions between drug and nondrug treatments for acute ischemic chest pain. *Principle: Drug and nondrug interventions must be integrated if each component of therapy is to be used optimally.*

SILENT ISCHEMIA

Electrocardiographic studies conducted on ambulatory patients during the past decade indicate that most episodes of "ischemic" ST-segment depression in patients with known ischemic heart disease are unaccompanied by angina (Uretsky et al., 1977). However, only patients with exercise-induced ischemic ST-segment depression manifest "silent ischemic" ST-segment depression during ambulatory electrocardiographic monitoring (Weisfeldt, 1986). Thus, patients with silent ischemia represent a subset of patients with ischemic heart disease. The prognostic value of ST-segment changes in patients without clinically manifest ischemic heart disease has not been documented.

Among patients hospitalized for treatment of unstable angina pectoris, those with silent ischemia experience greater refractoriness to drug therapy, more frequent death, and a greater need for coronary surgery (Gottlieb et al., 1986). Antianginal drugs and revascularization with PTCA and CABG surgery have been shown to be effective in alleviating silent ischemia. However, whether silent ischemia alone, separate from other prognostically important clinical characteristics such as left ventricular dysfunction and symptomatic myocardial ischemia, is an indication for such therapies in patients with ischemic heart disease presently is unknown.

CLINICAL APPLICATIONS OF PHARMACOLOGIC AGENTS IN ISCHEMIC HEART DISEASE

Thrombolytic Therapy in Acute MI

Among patients with ECG evidence of transmural injury, that is, ST-segment elevation within 5 hours of onset, 80% will have total coronary artery occlusion (O'Neill et al., 1988). From 6 to 24 hours from the onset of symptoms, approximately two thirds of vessels remain occluded, and at approximately 10 days after infarction approximately 75% of infarct-related arteries remain occluded (O'Neill et al., 1988). Spontaneous reperfusion can occur after acute MI. Moreover, even coronary artery occlusion accompanied by ST-segment elevation often is subtotal (Dewood et al., 1980). Collateral vessels may sustain myocardial perfusion even in the setting of total abrupt coronary artery occlusion. Finally, even total coronary artery occlusion may occur in a gradual or "stuttering" fashion. Although a general relationship exists between the extent of intracoronary thrombosis, the magnitude of electrocardiographic abnormalities, the clinical severity of pain, and the magnitude of myocardial enzyme elevation and left ventricular dysfunction, many factors modify each of these parameters and contribute to the conflicting results observed in clinical trials.

In nearly 75% of cases, coronary thrombosis is caused by rupture of a coronary plaque into the coronary artery lumen (Davies and Thomas, 1981; Davies, 1989). The atherosclerotic plaque, which is situated within the intima, is filled with lipid material. A tear in the cap of the plaque enables blood to enter the lipid pool, and a thrombus forms within the intima as shown in Fig. 5-1. The plaque fissure may subsequently heal or may progress to mural thrombosis, which may be complete or incomplete. Even when the plaque fissure heals without significant intraluminal thrombosis, tissue proliferation occurring within the intima may further enlarge the coronary artery plaque.

Effects of Thrombolytic Agents on Coronary Patency. Three major types of studies have elu-

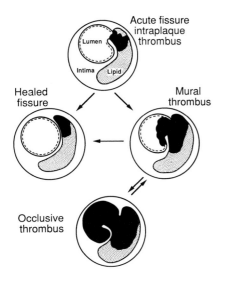

Fig. 5–1. Mechanisms of coronary thrombosis. Reprinted from Davies, M. J.: Thrombosis and coronary atherosclerosis. In Acute Coronary Intervention (Topol E. J., ed.). Marcel Dekker, Inc., New York, p. 29, 1989 by courtesy of Marcel Dekker, Inc.

:idated the therapeutic efficacy of thrombolytic agents (Tiefenbrunn and Sobel, 1989):

1. Recanalization trials require angiographic documentation of occlusive thrombus prior to :reatment as well as angiographic documentation of lysis after treatment. However, pretreatment coronary arteriography delays therapy and can compromise myocardial salvage and clinical outcome. Hence, although these studies were crucial for demonstrating and quantifying the effects of coronary thrombolysis, they are not performed today.

2. In "patency trials" angiography is performed 18 to 24 hours after initiation of thrombolysis. Such studies document the rate of coronary patency, but they are less definitive than recanalization trials in documenting thrombolysis, for they cannot distinguish patients with spontaneous thrombolysis from those without thrombotic occlusion.

3. Studies that do not define the patency of infarct-related arteries rely upon proxy or surrogate data such as left ventricular function and mortality. Because they are less demanding of diagnostic resources, contemporary clinical trials primarily utilize this design.

Mechanisms of Action of Thrombolytic Agents. Syndromes of acute ischemic chest pain reflect a critical reduction in coronary blood flow resulting from partial or complete occlusion of the coronary arteries. This occlusion results from thrombosis secondary to fissuring or rupture of an atherosclerotic coronary plaque that results in exposure of collagen and vessel media to platelets and other hemostatic constituents (Davies and Thameer, 1977). Thrombosis typically occurs in sites of high-grade atherosclerotic occlusion and diminished coronary blood flow (O'Neill et al., 1988).

Thrombolytic agents infused IV convert plasminogen, the inactive proenzyme of the fibrinolytic system, to the proteolytic enzyme plasmin, which lyses the fibrin in coronary artery thrombi. The therapeutic goal of thrombolysis is achieved through degradation of the fibrin constituent of the pathologic thrombus that also incorporates aggregations of platelets and erythrocytes (Marder and Sherry, 1988). Thrombolytic agents attach to and activate fibrin-bound plasminogen. Tissue plasminogen activator and single-chain urokinase plasminogen activator (SCU-PA) have a high affinity for fibrin-bound plasminogen compared with plasma plasminogen. These agents are termed *fibrin-selective*. In contrast, streptokinase and acylated streptokinase (APSAC) have a low ratio of activity for fibrin-bound plasminogen compared with plasma plasminogen and result in a *lytic state*.

The relative selectivity for fibrin of currently available thrombolytic agents shown in Table 5–1 is an important consideration in their clinical use (Marder and Sherry, 1988). The half-life of thrombolytic agents in plasma is a second important consideration in therapy: streptokinase, APSAC, and urokinase have a half-life ranging from 16 to 90 minutes compared with 5 to 8 minutes for r-TPA and recombinant SCU-PA. A short half-life necessitates a prolonged infusion of the latter agents over several hours compared with infusion over 2 to 5 minutes for APSAC and 5 minutes for streptokinase. Moreover, streptokinase, APSAC, and urokinase do not require simultaneous treatment with heparin, whereas SCU-PA and r-TPA require the simultaneous administration of heparin.

A third important consideration in choosing between thrombolytic agents is the time at which therapy is initiated. When therapy is instituted within 3 hours of symptoms, the incidence of reperfusion is similar with all agents. However, r-TPA provides a significant advantage when treatment begins 4 or more hours after the onset of chest pain. This reflects its avidity for fibrin clots, which become more resistant to lysis over time (TIMI Study Group, 1985). Much better studies of comparative efficacy are needed to make very clear choices between available choices.

A fourth consideration in therapy is the risk of rethrombosis. The incidence of rethrombosis

Table 5-1. **PHARMACOLOGIC AND CLINICAL FEATURES OF THROMBOLYTIC PREPARATIONS***

	SK	APSAC	UK	SCU-PA	R-TPA 2-CHAIN	R-TPA 1-CHAIN
Half-life (min)	23	90	16	7	8	5
Fibrin enhancement	1+	1+	2+	4+	4+	3+
Plasma proteolytic state	4+	4+	3+	2+	2+	1+
Duration of infusion	60 min	2–5 min	5–15 min	Several hours	Several hours	Several hours
Thrombus specificity (vs. hemostatic plug)	0	0	0	0	0	0
Incidence of reperfusion (% within 3 h)	60–70	60–70	60–70	60–70	60–70	60–70
Speed of reperfusion (min)	45	45	45	45	45	45
Frequency of reocclusion (estimated %)	15	10	10	NA	20	20
Simultaneous administration of heparin	No	No	No	Yes	Yes	Yes
Bleeding complications	4+	4+	4+	4+	4+	4+
Allergic side effects	Yes	Yes	No	No	No	No
Antigenicity	Yes	Yes	No	NK	NK	NK
Expense	1+	2+	3+	4+	4+	4+

* SK denotes streptokinase, APSAC acylated plasminogen-streptokinase activator complex, UK urokinase, SCU-PA recombinant single-chain urokinase plasminogen activator, RT-PA recombinant tissue-type plasminogen activator, NA data not available, NK not known, 0 none, and 4+ highest. The clinical data were derived mostly from reported experience with current IV dosages in the treatment of acute myocardial infarction. (Reprinted by permission of the New England Journal of Medicine, from Marder, V. J.; Sherry, S.: Thrombolytic therapy: Current status. N. Engl. J. Med., 318:1514, 1988.)

after reperfusion is inversely proportional to the plasma half-life of the drug used: the lowest incidence of rethrombosis is associated with APSAC (Marder et al., 1986), urokinase (Mathey et al., 1985), and streptokinase (Chesebro et al., 1987) and the highest incidence with r-TPA (Collen et al., 1984). The clinical efficacy of thrombolysis may be decreased because of extensive organization of a thrombus, impaired access of the lytic agent to the clot due to proximal coronary artery disease, or a deficiency of circulating plasminogen. Studies of recanalization with intracoronary streptokinase demonstrated efficacy in approximately 75% of patients; the comparable figure for IV streptokinase is approximately 50% (Tiefenbrunn and Sobel, 1989).

Dosage Regimens. The therapeutic objective of thrombolysis is to attain a high concentration of tissue plasminogen activator as soon as possible and to maintain the high level for a sufficiently long period to dissolve the thrombus without causing bleeding complications. Defining dosage regimens that maximize therapeutic efficacy and minimize side effects is a subject of intensive research, and the regimens described below should be considered approximations. Combination therapy with r-TPA and SCU-PA has shown promise (Collen et al., 1986), and doubtless other effective combinations will evolve. More rapid IV infusion of a higher weight-adjusted dose of r-TPA was more effective than the standard regimen of 100 mg over 3 hours in

restoring infarct-related artery patency (Smalling et al., 1990). Moreover, the efficacy of any regimen of thrombolytic agents may be substantially influenced by concurrent antithrombotic drug therapy. For example, failure to administer heparin IV within 1 hour of the initiation of r-TPA therapy may be responsible for the comparable clinical effects on mortality exerted by r-TPA and streptokinase in the GISSI II trial of thrombolysis in acute MI (Collen, 1990).

Regimens in common practice as of the spring of 1989 are as follows: for streptokinase a dose of 1.5 million units is infused over 60 minutes. For urokinase, 3 million units are administered over 90 minutes with half the dose given as a bolus. For APSAC, 30 units are given over a 2- to 5-minute period. For r-TPA the dose ranges from 60 to 100 mg given over the first hour with a total of 100 mg over 3 hours. A weight-adjusted dose regimen of r-TPA that may reduce fibrinogen breakdown and bleeding complications is 1 mg/kg over the first hour with 10% of the dose administered as a bolus and a prolonged low-dose infusion of 10 to 20 mg/h over the following 4 to 8 hours. This regimen may reduce the incidence of reocclusion.

Characteristics of Individual Thrombolytic Agents

Streptokinase. Streptokinase, derived from β-hemolytic streptococci, is a foreign protein that causes allergic reactions in approximately 5% of patients. The reaction consists of fever, drug rash, and anaphylactic reactions in decreasing order of frequency (Smith and Kennedy, 1987). Because of these characteristics, *this agent can be given only once.* Hypotension in patients receiving high-dose IV streptokinase therapy is observed in 2% to 15% of cases (Lew et al., 1985). *Principle: Comparisons of the value of drugs that can be used for the same indications must take into account the character of the disease. If episodes are likely to be recurrent and the drug can only be used in one episode but others can be used repeatedly, an important restriction has been introduced.*

Urokinase. The clinical efficacy of IV urokinase for coronary artery thrombolysis approximates that of streptokinase, but experience with this agent is much less extensive than with streptokinase. Urokinase is not associated with significant hypotension or with allergic reactions. Patency rate after intracoronary or IV administration of urokinase is approximately 60% (Mathey et al., 1985).

r-TPA. Because of its short half-life, r-TPA may be quickly discontinued in the event of untoward bleeding. This rapid management of significant bleeding complications is more feasible with r-TPA than with agents such as streptokinase and urokinase that have a longer half-life (Marder and Sherry, 1988). Because like urokinase, r-TPA is a human protein, allergic phenomena have not been observed. Bleeding after r-TPA administration usually is due to fibrinolysis and is more likely to occur acutely at arterial puncture sites, in the gingival mucosa, or in GI sites within 1 hour after the onset of therapy. In contrast, bleeding induced by nonselective agents is due to fibrinogenolysis and generally occurs hours to days after therapy is initiated.

The r-TPA is equally effective when given either by IV or intracoronary routes, with patency rates of 70% to 80%. The efficacy of r-TPA given IV is equivalent to the maximal recanalization rate seen with intracoronary administration of any fibrinolytic agent (Tiefenbrunn and Sobel, 1989). With respect to initiation and rapidity of lysis, r-TPA is superior to streptokinase. In the TIMI I trial, a recanalization trial, 62% of thrombotically occluded infarct-related coronary arteries were open within 90 minutes of onset of treatment with r-TPA compared with 31% after treatment with streptokinase (Chesebro et al., 1987). Moreover, recanalization rates with r-TPA were greater than with streptokinase regardless of the interval between the onset of symptoms and the onset of treatment. Nonetheless, there has been no demonstrated difference in clinical outcome. *Principle: In comparing the effects of alternative drugs for the same indication, be sure measurements that relate to clinical outcome are being compared.*

Acylated Streptokinase (APSAC). This agent has less hypotensive and allergic potential than streptokinase. The thrombolytic efficacy of 30 mg of APSAC, the currently used dose, is similar to that of standard doses of intracoronary-administered streptokinase (Anderson et al., 1986). Intravenous APSAC results in patency rates of 50% to 60%. As with streptokinase, the efficacy of APSAC is significantly dependent upon the time it is given after the symptoms start. The patency rate is 70% when the drug is given within 4 hours of the onset of symptoms compared with 33% when it is given later (Anderson et al., 1988).

Reocclusion is a problem with all thrombolytic agents. Several types of agents reduce the incidence of rethrombosis: (1) thrombolytic agents that can be infused over an extended period, (2) antithrombotic agents including anticoagulants and antiplatelet agents, or (3) vasodilators such as nitroglycerin. A combination of heparin and aspirin is commonly employed, especially in conjunction with r-TPA therapy. In the TIMI trial, 24% of patients treated with r-TPA who were studied before hospital discharge exhibited reocclusion (Chesebro et al., 1987). The use of heparin and aspirin does not appear to diminish these rates markedly. Similar rates of reocclusion (19%) have been noted with the use of streptokinase (Rao et al., 1988). *Principle: When the logic of combining drugs for an indication is compelling but the data are disappointing—either the logic is incorrect or the agents have not been tested optimally.*

Complications of Thrombolytic Agents

Thrombolytic agents induce a hemostatic defect through their combined actions on blood components, the vessel wall, and the hemostatic plug (Table 5–1; Marder and Sherry, 1988). Despite the fact that streptokinase depresses plasma fibrinogen concentrations to a substantially greater extent than r-TPA, the incidence of hemorrhagic events with these two agents is comparable (Rao et al., 1988). Moreover, the incidence of intracranial hemorrhage with r-TPA appears to be greater than that with streptokinase (Braunwald et al., 1987). Even though r-TPA is relatively clot-specific, it has no way to discriminate between a coronary thrombus and a protective hemostatic plug. Even though r-TPA generates less of a systemic lytic state, that is, depletes fibrinogen to a lesser extent than other agents, there appears to be little correlation between markers of systemic lysis and clinically noticed bleeding events (Marder and Sherry, 1988).

Management of serious bleeding requires cessation of therapy and rapid reversal of the hypocoagulable state. Plasma or cryoprecipitate is used for this reversal. Life-threatening complications including intracerebral hemorrhage may require treatment with antifibrinolytic agents such as ε-aminocaproic acid. The principal site of hemorrhage following thrombolytic therapy is where invasive procedures have taken place. In the TIMI trial (Loscalzo and Brownwald, 1989), major bleeding events were noted in 15% of patients receiving streptokinase *or* r-TPA (Rao et al., 1988). Major bleeding was defined as either intracranial hemorrhage, events associated with a decrease in hematocrit of more than 15%, or a decrease in the hemoglobin level of more than 5 g/dl. Major or minor bleeding was noted in approximately 30% of patients treated with each of these agents. More than 80% of bleeding events in both groups were associated with vascular catheterization sites. Among patients receiving r-TPA in the TIMI II trial, the incidence of intracerebral hemorrhage ranged from 1.6% in patients receiving 150 mg over 6 hours to 0.6% in those who received 100 mg over 6 hours (Braunwald et al., 1987). In the GISSI trial (Gruppo Italiano, 1986), the incidence of stroke was 0.2%. In that study no distinction was made between thrombotic and hemorrhagic stroke. Among patients with acute MI, the incidence of cerebrovascular accidents even without therapy has been reported as high as from 1.7% to 1.9% (Thompson and Robinson, 1978).

Contraindications to Thrombolytic Therapy

Thrombolytic agents are contraindicated in patients who have had internal bleeding within the prior 3 months; a known hemorrhagic diathesis; a history of stroke; intracranial venous malformation or aneurysm; hypertension with systolic pressure of 200 mm Hg or greater or diastolic blood pressure 110 mm Hg or greater; recent intracranial, intraspinal, or intraocular surgery; or trauma within 3 months (Loscalzo and Braunwald, 1989). Patients with major trauma within the previous week and those with traumatic cardiopulmonary resuscitation also should be excluded from treatment with r-TPA.

Age greater than 75 years is associated with more extensive coronary artery disease and left ventricular dysfunction and is an increased risk factor independent of the listed abnormalities. Moreover, the morbidity and mortality of thrombolysis, invasive procedures, coronary surgery, emergency PTCA, and thrombolytic therapy also are significantly higher in such patients (O'Neill et al., 1988). However, the absolute reduction in mortality is greater in these elderly patients than in those who are younger. The decision to use thrombolytic agents in the elderly must therefore be individualized.

ANTITHROMBOTIC THERAPY DURING AND FOLLOWING ACUTE MI

Pathogenesis of Coronary Artery Thrombosis

Disruption of the endothelial surface resulting from ulceration of an atherosclerotic plaque leads to arterial thrombosis in three steps (Fuster et al., 1987): (1) platelet adhesion, (2) platelet aggregation, and (3) activation of clotting mechanisms. Activated platelets release adenosine diphosphate, thomboxane A_2, and serotonin, which promote the formation of thrombosis through the stimulation of adjacent platelets. Moreover, platelet aggregation facilitates the coagulation cascade by providing a suitable surface for interaction of clotting factors. In turn, the coagulation system favors further platelet aggregation through the generation of thrombin, a powerful platelet activator, and fibrin, which stabilizes the platelet mass.

Characteristics of the underlying atherosclerotic plaque and the degree of arterial stenosis determine the magnitude and type of coronary artery occlusion. Thrombi forming in the area of atherosclerotic occlusion, where shear rates are high, are composed predominately of platelets, whereas thrombi forming distal to coronary stenoses, where the shear rate is low, contain primarily fibrin and erythrocytes (Davies and Thomas, 1981). Rupture of an atherosclerotic coronary plaque leads not only to exposure of thrombogenic surfaces but to an increase in shear rate, both of which facilitate platelet and clotting activation and thrombus formation.

Mechanisms of Action of Antithrombotic Agents

Heparin acts indirectly, in vitro as well as in vivo, through a plasma cofactor, antithrombin III, which neutralizes the following activated clotting factors: II, IX, X, XI, and XII. Antithrombin III and heparin cofactor II form an irreversible complex with thrombin, inactivating the proteins (O'Reilly, 1985). Low concentrations of heparin increase the activity of the antithrombin III and the activity of this cofactor against activated clotting factors. In contrast, continuous heparin therapy reduces the activation of antithrombin III, which may paradoxically increase the tendency to thrombosis. Concurrent therapy with aspirin helps to reduce this tendency. Intravenous heparin therapy designed to complement the effects of IV thrombolytic agents is usually given in a dose sufficient to increase the activated partial thromboplastin time (PTT) to 1.5 to 2 times the control value.

Spontaneous lysis of thrombus occurs in both "non-Q" and "Q-wave" infarction. Aspirin presumably exerts its beneficial effects by preventing coronary reocclusion after spontaneous recanalization of the vessel. In the ISIS-2 study (1988), patients with suspected MI were treated with either aspirin (160 mg/day), streptokinase (1.5 million units IV), both, or neither within 24 hours of the onset of symptoms. Compared with placebo, aspirin alone reduced early cardiovascular mortality by 23% and the rate of nonfatal reinfarction by 50%.

As noted previously, reocclusion is common among patients undergoing thrombolysis for acute MI. In general, the risk of reocclusion is higher in patients with severe residual luminal stenosis or poor perfusion (Harrison et al., 1984; Gash et al., 1986). In the ISIS-2 trial, streptokinase reduced 5-week cardiac mortality by 25% and the combination of aspirin and streptokinase reduced mortality by 42%. Because the residual clot is markedly thrombogenic, high-dose IV heparin is helpful in interrupting the process of intracoronary thrombosis. In reducing thrombin generation, heparin inhibits not only fibrin formation but thrombin-dependent platelet activation.

These data have led to the following suggestions about therapy: administer aspirin 160 to 325 mg/day in acute MI. In patients undergoing thrombolysis, heparin should be continued for approximately 3 to 7 days.

PREVENTION OF RECURRENT MI AND SUDDEN CARDIAC DEATH

During the past 15 years, nine large, randomized trials have been conducted to evaluate the effect of platelet inhibitor drugs on prognosis after acute MI. A meta-analysis of these trials (Antiplatelet Trialists' Collaboration, 1988) indicated a significant reduction in cardiac events among patients receiving long-term antiplatelet therapy: cardiovascular mortality was reduced by 13%, nonfatal reinfarction by 31%, nonfatal stroke by 42%, and all vascular events by 25%. Aspirin alone was found as efficacious as dipyridamole or sulfinpyrazone and was associated with lesser cost and toxicity. *Principle: Vital data about how to use drugs optimally in complex combinations or sequences most often become available only after the drugs have been on the market for extensive periods* (see chapters 34 and 39–41).

In an extensive review of the subject, Stein and Fuster (1989) concluded that trials of chronic anticoagulation after acute MI produced a significant reduction in mortality and reinfarction. In the Report on the Sixty Plus Reinfarction Study (1980), patients continuing anticoagulants over a 2-year period exhibited a 26% lower death rate and a 55% lower reinfarction rate.

Among patients recovering from acute MI, chronic use of aspirin at a dose of 325 mg/day is associated with a reduction in cardiovascular events and is associated with a low rate of toxicity. Long-term anticoagulant therapy also is associated with lower rates of reinfarction and mortality but is associated with a greater cost, discomfort, and rate of side effects than aspirin (Stein and Fuster, 1989). *Principle: Insist on familiarizing yourself with data on relative efficiency and toxicity when multiple agents are available with a similar mechanism of positive effects.*

Prevention of Left Ventricular Thrombus and Systemic Embolization

The overall incidence of left ventricular mural thrombosis following acute MI is about 20% (Stein and Fuster, 1989). This figure doubles in the setting of anterior infarction and triples when the infarction is associated with large anterior infarction. Among patients with mural thrombosis, systemic embolization occurs in approximately 10% (Meltzer et al., 1986). Patients at highest risk of embolization exhibit not only large anterior infarction but congestive heart failure, atrial fibrillation, and echocardiographic evidence of protruding or mobile thrombi (Meltzer et al., 1986). In three large randomized controlled trials, the rate of systemic embolization was 2.3% to 5.4% in patients not receiving anticoagulants compared with 0.8% to 1.7% in those receiving these agents (Stein and Fuster, 1989). In these trials, short-term anticoagulation therapy reduced the risk of systemic and pulmonary embolization by at least one half.

Intravenous or subcutaneous heparin in a dosage sufficient to produce an increase in PTT of 1.5 to 2.0 times control is recommended for patients with large anterior infarction, whether or not they exhibit echocardiographic evidence of mural thrombi (Stein and Fuster, 1989). At the time of hospital discharge, patients with persistent mural thrombi or large akinetic regions of the myocardium documented by echocardiography should be treated with warfarin at a dose sufficient to prolong the prothrombin time to 1.3 to 1.5 times control (international normalized ratio of 2.0–3.0) for 3 months and for a longer period in the setting of decompensated heart failure, atrial fibrillation, or prior systemic or pulmonary emboli (Stein and Fuster, 1989). The oral anticoagulants act indirectly to interfere with the hepatic production of the vitamin K–dependent clotting factors II, VII, IX, and X.

β-Adrenergic Antagonists in Acute MI

The beneficial effects of β-adrenergic antagonists in the treatment of acute MI may possibly be mediated by (1) the reduction of myocardial oxygen consumption through reduction of heart rate, blood pressure, and myocardial contractility, (2) redistribution of blood flow preferentially to subendocardial regions where ischemia is most severe, and (3) shift in myocardial metabolism from fatty acids to glucose through a reduction in adrenergic activity (Yusuf et al., 1985).

Individual agents within this class of drugs exhibit distinctive pharmacologic and pharmacodynamic attributes. The differences between the agents reflect primarily the degree of selectivity for β_1 cardiac receptors of these agents: alprenolol, nadolol, pindolol, propranolol, and timolol are nonselective, whereas atenolol and metoprolol are relatively selective (Marder and Sherry, 1988). Other distinctive pharmacologic attributes of these agents include the extent of intrinsic sympathominetic activity: alprenolol and pindolol exhibit such activity. Other attributes distinguishing these agents relate primarily to their plasma half-life: "short" (2–4 hours) with alprenolol, metoprolol, pindolol, and propranolol, and "long" (6–18 hours) with atenolol and nadolol.

Despite these differences, the clinical efficacy of these agents in enhancing prognosis and alleviating angina pectoris is quite similar. For example, both cardioselective agents such as metoprolol and nonselective agents such as propranolol and timolol have been shown to reduce cardiac mortality after acute MI (Yusuf et al., 1985).

Clinical evidence of the therapeutic efficacy of β-adrenergic antagonists administered IV within 6 hours of the acute event include the following: (1) reduction in the degree of ST-segment elevation, (2) preservation of R waves, (3) reduction in development of Q waves, (4) reduction in cardiac enzyme release, (5) reduction in the frequency and complexity of ventricular ectopic activity, (6) reduction in the incidence of ventricular fibrillation, and (7) reduction in chest pain (Yusuf et al., 1985).

Clinical Benefit of IV Administered β-Adrenergic Antagonists. Two large randomized trials have demonstrated a reduction in the mortality of early infarction by approximately 15% (MIAMI Trial Research Group, 1985; ISIS-1, 1988). One of the most relevant contemporary studies evaluating the effects of IV administered β-adrenergic antagonists, the TIMI II trial, demonstrated a significant reduction in nonfatal reinfarction and recurrent ischemic episodes during hospitalization (The TIMI Study Group, 1989). Compared with patients receiving oral metoprolol commencing on the sixth hospital day, patients who received 15 mg of metoprolol IV immediately upon admission followed by oral metoprolol experienced a significantly lower rate of adverse cardiac events. Results of this trial are particularly important inasmuch as patients received IV thrombolytic therapy within 3 hours of the onset of chest pain. The benefits of IV metoprolol were particularly evident in patients classified as clinically low-risk, in contradistinction to previous trials of orally administered β-adrenergic antagonist therapy given to prevent recurrent infarction and sudden cardiac death.

β-Adrenergic Antagonists Administered after Acute MI

β-Adrenergic antagonists reduce total mortality including the incidence of sudden and nonsudden cardiac death and the incidence of nonfatal reinfarction (Yusuf et al., 1985). Mechanisms through which these agents reduce mortality after acute MI include primarily a beneficial antiarrhythmic effect and an anti-ischemic action. Analysis of randomized clinical trials reveals a marked disparity in the efficacy of β-adrenergic antagonists in specified subsets of patients. For example, among the 55% of patients in the Beta Blocker Heart Attack Trial who had neither electrical nor mechanical abnormalities after acute MI, the numerical reduction in mortality was 0.4/100, that is, less than one half of one life was prolonged per 100 patients treated over a 25-month period (Beta-Blocker Heart Attack Trial Research Group, 1982). In contrast, among the 23% of patients with electrical abnormalities only, the numerical difference in mortality was 5.7/100 patients, a 57% reduction in mortality. Among the 10% of patients with mechanical complications only, the mortality difference was 6.4/100, a 47% reduction, and among the remaining 11%, the mortality reduction was 4.2/100, or a 30% reduction. *Principle: One often analyzes the effects of drugs on a disease described by a rubric (e.g., myocardial infarction) that covers a spectrum of pathogenesis and severities. Very often when the disease can be subdivided into subgroups based on severity, it is possible to identify highly effective therapies whose efficacy is diluted if the treatment group is more heterogeneous. The exercise of looking for subgroups that are predictably responsive or nonresponsive to specific therapy is an important step in individualizing therapy.*

The dramatic differences in mortality among different clinical subsets of patients with MI has engendered controversy about whether all post-MI patients should receive β-adrenergic antagonists. The debate focuses particularly on low-risk subsets who constitute the majority of patients with MI. In their meta-analysis of randomized trials of β blockade during and after MI, Yusuf et al. (1985) projected that 12 patients would die during hospitalization for acute MI and an additional 8 patients would die within the next year (see chapters 34 and 41). Assuming that mortality was reduced approximately 25% in the two thirds of patients who could tolerate β-antagonist therapy, mortality would be expected to decline by approximately 16%, that is, only 7 rather than 8 patients would die, or a saving of 1 life per 100 patients treated. However, contemporary therapy with thrombolytic agents, antithrombotic agents, and elective PTCA and CABG surgery has reduced *total* first-year mortality, in-hospital as well as posthospital, to as low as 7% (Baim et al., 1990). This efficacy of treatment with these agents diminishes the overall impact of β-antagonist therapy, especially in clinically low-risk patient subsets. *Principle: Analysis of the effects of only one among many competing therapeutic interventions that may be given singly or in combination can produce major distortion of the efficacy of any of the interventions.*

The reduction in acute and long-term mortality resulting from thrombolysis, antithrombotic therapy, and revascularization has important implications for the contemporary usage of β-adrenergic antagonists. For example, Goldman et al. (1988) conducted a study of the cost benefit of routine β-adrenergic blockade in acute MI based upon 23 published studies. On the assumption that the benefit of 6 years of β-adrenergic antagonist therapy wears off over the subsequent 9 years, the estimated cost of therapy per life saved was estimated to be $13,000 in low-risk patients, $3600 in medium-risk patients, and $2400 in high-risk patients. Contemporary therapy probably has the effect of increasing the proportion of clinically low-risk patients and hence the costs of saving life with β-adrenergic blockers. The increase in life expectancy attributable to β-blocker therapy ranged from a low 0.4% in clinically low-risk patients aged 45, to 5.5% in clinically high-risk patients aged 65 or greater. As with many therapies, there are no clear-cut answers in regard to the efficacy of β-adrenergic blocker therapy after acute MI, particularly in patients with low risk. *Principle: When the efficacy of a drug in a specific group of patients becomes dubious, the risk of using the drug becomes a very important determinant of whether the drug should be used.*

The most serious adverse effect of β-adrenergic antagonists in acute MI is precipitation of congestive heart failure (CHF). This is most common in patients with significant left ventricular dysfunction. In the Beta-Blocker Heart Attack Trial (BHAT), CHF was noted in 14.9% of patients receiving propranolol compared with 8.9% of those receiving placebo (Beta-Blocker Heart Attack Trial Research Group, 1982). A similar proportion of patients with electrical and mechanical abnormalities experienced CHF. Sinus bradycardia leading to discontinuation of β blockers was significantly more common among patients receiving propranolol than in patients receiving placebo irrespective of the clinical risk group, but the absolute incidence was highest in patients with electrical or mechanical abnormalities. However, the greatest potential benefit from β-adrenergic blockers is also in these patients with electrical and/or mechanical complications of MI.

Calcium-Channel Antagonists in Acute MI

Among survivors of acute MI who are free of left ventricular dysfunction, the favorable effect of calcium-channel antagonists on prognosis may depend on the anti-ischemic mechanisms mediated through coronary vasodilation, and negative chronotropic and ionotropic actions or a combination of these (The Multicenter Diltiazem Post-Infarction Research Group, 1988). However, among patients surviving acute MI who exhibited left ventricular dysfunction, calcium antagonists in the Multicenter Diltiazem Post-Infarction Trial actually *increased* mortality through mechanisms that are not clear (The Multicenter Diltiazem Post-Infarction Research Group, 1988). In that trial, the rate of cardiac events was significantly decreased among the 80% of patients without pulmonary congestion, whereas the rate of such events was significantly increased among the 20% of patients with pulmonary congestion. This unfavorable effect on the prognosis of higher-risk patients with left ventricular dysfunction is the opposite of that observed using β-adrenergic antagonists (Yusuf et al., 1985). Inasmuch as both agents depress left ventricular function, the unfavorable effect of calcium antagonists is unexplained.

Patients with non-Q-wave infarction generally exhibit less mechanical damage and a lower in-hospital mortality than patients with Q-wave infarctions (Gibson, 1989). As a group, patients with non-Q-wave MI treated with diltiazem experienced a better outcome than those who did not receive this agent: the cumulative incidence of cardiac death and nonfatal reinfarction was 9% and 15%, respectively (Boden et al., 1988).

There are 13 published clinical trials of nifedipine given after acute MI that include nearly 10,000 patients (Gibson, 1989). There was no evidence that this agent favorably affected electrocardiographic, scintigraphic, or other parameters of myocardial necrosis; progression of Q-wave infarction; or the rate of unstable angina, reinfarction, or mortality. Indeed, several trials reflected the harmful effects of the drug.

Clinical experience with verapamil after acute MI also suggests that the drug has little if any beneficial effects (Gibson, 1989). *Principle: There are very few drugs whose complete pharmacologic profile is known. It is almost inconceivable that drugs in different categories (e.g., β-adrenergic antagonists and calcium-channel antagonists) have the same profiles even if they have some overlapping qualities. Therefore proof of equivalent efficacy among such drugs for the same indication is required and cannot be assumed.*

Calcium-Channel Antagonists Administered after Non-Q-Wave MI. As noted previously, patients with non-Q-wave MI have incomplete infarction because occlusion of the vessel that causes infarction is incomplete. Although in-hospital mortality in these patients is lower compared with that of those with completely occluded infarct vessels and Q-wave infarction, posthospital mortality is high (Gibson, 1989). This reflects the continuing vulnerability of patients with viable but underperfused myocardium to reinfarction. Among patients in the diltiazem reinfarction study (Gibson et al., 1987), 43% had one or more episodes of angina at rest or with minimal effort during the first 10 days after non-Q-wave infarction. Reinfarction or death was more likely to occur in these patients than in those without angina: reinfarction in 12.2% versus 3.6% and death in 6.1% versus 1.5%. Among patients with angina, those exhibiting electrocardiographic evidence of ischemia exhibited a substantially higher rate of reinfarction (20% versus 5.3%), more extensive myocardial necrosis (peak m band creatinine phosphokinase [MB CPK] concentrations 91 IU/l versus 37 IU/l), and higher mortality (11.3% versus 1.5%) within the first 14 days after infarction. Angina associated with transient ST-T changes occurred in 24% of patients in the placebo group versus 16% in the diltiazem-treated group. No reduction in mortality was attributable to treatment with diltiazem during this brief follow-up period (Gibson et al., 1987).

Although the short-term clinical benefits of diltiazem therapy in this study are clear, the clinical utility of this agent must be judged in relationship to other competing therapies including PTCA and CABG surgery. Especially in subsets of patients with both angina and labile electrocardiographic abnormalities, revascularization is likely to prove superior to diltiazem over the long term not only for relief of angina pectoris but for reduction in mortality.

A related question concerns the clinical utility of classifying patients as "Q-wave" versus "non-Q-wave" MI. Although such a classification has the advantage of simplicity, it adds little to previous classification systems that rely upon the presence and extent of myocardial ischemia and left ventricular dysfunction as the basis for prognostic stratification (DeBusk et al., 1986). Particularly among patients with non-Q-wave MI, post-MI treadmill exercise testing reveals a high incidence of myocardial ischemia: not only is the incidence of exercise-induced angina high in such patients, but exercise-induced ST-segment shifts on the exercise electrocardiogram are readily interpretable.

Drugs useful in the management of acute myocardial infarction are summarized in Table 5–2.

TREATMENT OF UNSTABLE ANGINA PECTORIS

Aspirin Therapy

Mechanisms of action of antiplatelet and antithrombotic agents in acute MI have been described above. The same pathophysiologic processes are responsible for unstable angina pectoris and non-Q-wave infarction. The syndrome of unstable angina pectoris usually is characterized by an accelerating pattern of chest pain occurring at rest or with minimal effort, or is associated with chest pain lasting 20 minutes or longer.

Two large double-blind, randomized trials have documented the efficacy of aspirin in reducing the rate of death and reinfarction after hospital admission for patients with unstable angina pectoris. Lewis et al. (1983) documented a 51% reduction in the rate of combined events during a 12-week follow-up period among 1266 men receiving 325 mg/day of aspirin commencing 48 hours after admission to the hospital. Cairns et al. (1985) noted a 30% reduction in cardiac risk among 555 men and women receiving aspirin 325 mg 4 times daily commencing 8 days after hospitalization and continuing for 18 months.

Théroux et al. (1988) documented a 72% reduction in combined events among patients hospitalized with unstable angina who received aspirin 325 mg/day commencing 8 hours after the last episode of pain and a 48% reduction compared with placebo administered with or without heparin. The incidence of refractory angina was not significantly reduced with aspirin.

It is important to emphasize that study patients received intensive antianginal therapy in addition to aspirin alone, heparin alone, or the combination of aspirin and heparin: all patients received nitrates, 96% received β-adrenergic blockers, and

Table 5–2.   DRUGS USEFUL IN THE MANAGEMENT OF ACUTE MYOCARDIAL INFARCTION

DRUG	PHASE OF INFARCTION*	CLINICAL EFFECTS
Nitrates	Early	Alleviate angina, attenuate or abolish myocardial ischemia and infarction
Aspirin, heparin	Early, mid	Attenuate continuing coronary thrombosis; prevent rethrombosis of coronary arteries
β-Adrenergic antagonists	Early	Attenuate or abolish myocardial ischemia and infarction; attenuate or abolish ventricular arrhythmias
Calcium-channel antagonists	Early	Attenuate or abolish myocardial ischemia and infarction
Thrombolytic agents	Early	Lyse intracoronary thromboses, restore myocardial perfusion, attenuate or abolish myocardial ischemia and infarction
β-Adrenergic antagonists	Mid, late	Attenuate severity of reinfarction; prevent reinfarction and sudden cardiac death; alleviate angina pectoris
Calcium-channel antagonists	Mid, late	Attenuate severity of reinfarction; prevent reinfarction and sudden cardiac death; alleviate angina pectoris
Warfarin	Mid, late	Prevent left ventricular mural thrombosis and systemic embolization
Aspirin	Late	Prevent rethrombosis of coronary arteries; prevent left ventricular mural thrombosis and systemic embolization

* Early = minutes to hours; mid = hours to days; late = days to weeks up to 3 years.

67% received calcium antagonists. *Principle: Initial drug efficacy studies often have to pick dose and duration of therapy empirically. Optimal therapy may depend on refinement of each. Look for the optimization by extrapolating information from successive studies.*

Heparin Therapy

Two studies in which heparin was administered to patients hospitalized with unstable angina pectoris demonstrated a beneficial effect (Théroux et al., 1988; Williams et al., 1986). Théroux et al. noted a 63% reduction in the incidence of refractory angina compared with placebo and a 15% reduction compared with placebo administered with or without aspirin. No statistically significant differences between the three treatment groups with respect to any of the end points of the study were noted. Clinically significant bleeding was more frequent with heparin or heparin and aspirin compared with placebo. However, complications were relatively infrequent, and most were related to cardiac catheterization puncture sites.

TREATMENT OF STABLE ANGINA PECTORIS

Nitrates

Nitrates relieve angina pectoris, although the mechanisms are not completely clear. Nitrates promote venodilation (Mason and Braunwald, 1965) and, to a lesser extent, arteriolar dilation (Gorlin et al., 1959). Venodilation decreases left ventricular filling pressure by limiting return of blood to the heart. Arteriolar dilation reduces peripheral resistance and impedance to left ventricular outflow (Williams et al., 1965). These combined effects reduce myocardial oxygen consumption. Nitrates also tend to enhance coronary blood flow through dilation of small- and medium-sized coronary arteries (Brown et al., 1981).

Modes of Administration. For the relief of individual episodes of angina, nitroglycerin (glyceryl trinitrate) is administered sublingually in doses of 0.2 to 0.4 mg, as an ointment 0.5 to 2 in. applied to the skin every 4 to 8 hours, and as a transdermal disc applied once per day providing 2.5 to 15 mg/24 h. Intravenous preparations for stabilization of unstable angina pectoris are usually infused at 5 μg/min with increments of 5 μg/min until angina is relieved or blood pressure falls excessively. Prophylaxis of angina pectoris is achieved through longer-acting agents including isosorbide dinitrate given sublingually in doses of 5 to 20 mg every 2 hours, as a chewable tablet of 5 to 10 mg every 2 to 3 hours, as a sustained-release capsule or tablet containing 40 mg given every 6 to 12 hours, and as an oral tablet containing 5 to 30 mg given every 6 hours; erythrityl tetranitrate of 5 to 10 mg given sublingually three times daily or as a chewable tablet of 10 mg three times daily; or pentaerythritol tetranitrate given as an oral tablet of 10 to 40 mg four times daily or as a sustained-release capsule or tablet of 30 to 80 mg given every 12 hours (Needleman et al., 1985).

The clinical efficacy of nitrates is limited by tolerance to the pharmacologic effects of the drug. When the drug is taken intermittently, the tolerance does not occur because a nitrate-free period of 6 to 8 hours per day allows regeneration of responsiveness. A very interesting dichotomy has developed around dosage forms of nitroglycerin. In hopes of enhancing the convenience of administration over sublingual or oral forms, the industry first provided a paste to be used in hospitals and later the transdermal delivery forms to be used in ambulatory settings. The latter first became available in forms that were delivered for 24 hours. Then longer periods of delivery were found to be feasible periods. The regulatory agency approved the long-acting form of the drug on the basis of bioavailability studies alone. Proof of successful systemic delivery for many days was considered synonymous with proof that the long-acting transdermal patch could be marketed. But the agency fell into a trap for not also having been concerned about the pharmacologic tolerance that could develop to prolonged concentrations of the drug in plasma. Physicians also fell into the same trap! The market for long-acting transdermal patches is very sizable. The product is aggressively sold by many manufacturers. But although the dosage form works for 24 hours, recent studies not surprisingly show that it loses its efficacy beyond that period. Because the clinical manifestations of the disease are so variable and the loss of efficacy can be interpreted as a worsening of disease, it took too long to notice that the preparation was not working *because* the drug was being constantly delivered! *Principle: Bioavailability of the drug is only one determinant of its clinical efficacy. Knowledge of the pharmacology of the agent can help to predict whether simple continuous delivery of the drug is appropriate to achieve a desirable clinical effect.*

Headache is common with nitrates and often is a limiting factor in using the drug. Likewise hypotension is sometimes a problem, especially in elderly patients. Nitrates are rarely administered alone. However, they are useful adjuncts to the antianginal effects of β-adrenergic antagonists and calcium-channel antagonists.

β-Adrenergic Antagonists

The primary effect of β-adrenergic antagonists is to decrease myocardial oxygen consumption through reduction in heart rate, contractility, and blood pressure (Wolfson and Gorlin, 1969). However, reduced contractility may paradoxically increase myocardial oxygen consumption through an increase in left ventricular volume and wall tension. Factors guiding the choice of β-adrenergic antagonists are shown in Table 5–3.

Relief of myocardial ischemia by β-adrenergic antagonists may more than offset the nonspecific depression of left ventricular function by these agents. All β antagonists must be used cautiously in patients who have left ventricular dysfunction or bronchospastic lung disease (Shand, 1975). Sudden discontinuation of these agents in patients with moderately severe angina pectoris may precipitate unstable angina pectoris and myocardial infarction (Alderman et al., 1974).

Cardioselective agents that theoretically have more effect on the heart than other sites include atenolol and metoprolol. Atenolol is given in a dosage of 50 mg once daily and may be increased to 100 mg once daily. Metoprolol is administered in a dose of 100 mg daily in single or divided dose and may be increased to 400 mg daily depending on the response. Cardioselective agents are preferred in patients with diabetes who are receiving insulin. Although all β-adrenergic blockers can mask the signs and symptoms of hypoglycemia, the nonselective β-adrenergic blockers can also decrease the rate of recovery from hypoglycemia.

Nonselective agents and their mode of administration are: nadolol 40 mg once daily, at increments of 40 to 80 mg/day to a maximum daily dosage of 80 to 240 mg; pindolol 10 mg twice daily with increments of 10 mg/day at biweekly intervals to a maximal daily dose of 60 mg/day; propranolol 40 mg twice daily or 80 mg once daily in a sustained release capsule, with the dosage gradually increased to a maximal daily dose of 320 mg; and timolol 10 mg twice daily with a gradual increase to a maximal daily dose of 20 to 40 mg.

Principle: Be careful in ascribing clinical value to the basic pharmacologic differences between drugs. These differences may be pharmacologically real but only clinical nuances.

The affinity of cardioselective β_1 antagonists for β_1-adrenergic receptors is not much different than that of the nonselective antagonists. If the doses of cardioselective agents cannot be kept relatively low, the drug will have little clinical β-selective action (see also chapter 4).

Calcium-Channel Antagonists

The antianginal effects of calcium-channel antagonists are mediated primarily by their ability to alter myocardial oxygen supply–demand relationships (Braunwald, 1983). Verapamil, diltiazem, nifedipine, and nicardipine diminish myocardial oxygen demand by reducing systolic pressure and heart rate (except for nifedipine and nicardipine, which stimulate reflex tachycardia). The effect of diltiazem on atrioventricular and sinoatrial nodes is similar to that of verapamil (Lewis, 1983). Verapamil and diltiazem also reduce myocardial contractibility. Nicardipine has a potent vasodilating effect that increases heart rate to a somewhat lesser extent than nifedipine. Small doses of β-adrenergic blocking drugs, which reduce heart rate, enhance the efficacy of these agents (Subramanian, 1984). These agents increase myocardial oxygen supply by enhancing coronary blood flow, reducing coronary vascular

Table 5–3. FACTORS GUIDING THE CLINICAL USE OF β-ADRENERGIC ANTAGONISTS IN ISCHEMIC HEART DISEASE

Asthma, diabetes mellitus	Cardioselective agents preferred to noncardioselective, but selectivity is only relative: all agents must be given with caution to patients with these conditions.
Left ventricular dysfunction, sinus bradycardia	Partial agonist activity of pindolol may recommend it over other agonists without such activity.
CNS effects: depression, nightmares, insomnia	More prevalent in agents with high lipid solubility: propranolol > metoprolol, pindolol > atenolol, nadolol, timolol.

resistance and spasm, and enhancing collateral blood flow (Singh et al., 1982). Of the four agents, nicardipine exerts the strongest vasodilator effect (Scheidt, 1988).

Nifedipine, verapamil, diltiazem, and nicardipine are equally effective in alleviating variant or Prinzmetal angina (Gelman et al., 1985). Variant angina is due to spasm of coronary arteries that are partially occluded by atherosclerotic disease (Prinzmetal et al., 1959). It is relieved by the effect of these agents in alleviating coronary spasm and increasing coronary blood flow (Opie, 1987). This mechanism differs from that by which these agents relieve classical or exertional angina pectoris. In the latter setting these agents reduce myocardial oxygen demand primarily by reducing systolic blood pressure, heart rate, and left ventricular contractility (Braunwald, 1983).

The clinical utility of these agents for alleviating angina pectoris and enhancing prognosis in acute ischemic chest pain syndromes is determined primarily by the degree of impairment of left ventricular contractility, atrioventricular conduction, and sinoatrial node function as shown in Table 5–4. These agents possess distinctive pharmacologic and pharmacokinetic properties (Needleman et al., 1985). Notwithstanding these differences, the therapeutic effects of the calcium-channel antagonists are mediated primarily through an increase in coronary blood flow, a decrease in coronary vascular resistance, and a reduction in myocardial consumption.

Unlike β-adrenergic antagonists, calcium-channel antagonists can be withdrawn abruptly without precipitating unstable angina pectoris,

myocardial infarction, and death (Alderman et al., 1974) and are more effective than β-adrenergic antagonists in alleviating angina at rest (Parodi et al., 1982).

The initial dose of verapamil for the treatment of angina pectoris is 80 mg three or four times daily with a gradual increase to a maximal daily dose of 320 to 480 mg. The initial dose of diltiazem for the treatment of angina pectoris is 30 mg four times daily. The dosage can be gradually increased to a maximal level of 60 mg three to four times daily. The initial dose of nicardipine is 20 mg three times daily. The dosage can be gradually increased to a maximal leval of 40 mg three times daily.

Nifedipine is uniquely useful in the management of hypertension, including hypertensive emergencies (Frishman et al., 1987), inasmuch as it exerts the greatest vasodilating effect on coronary and systemic arteries. Like nicardipine, it exerts little negative ionotropic effect on myocardial function (Frishman et al., 1988). *Principle: The heterogeneity of calcium channels makes it theoretically possible to develop a number of drugs that antagonize different populations of channels. Don't be surprised if different antagonists exhibit not only very distinctive pharmacologic properties but different clinical efficacy.*

Nifedipine usually is administered orally with a beginning dose of 10 mg three times per day with subsequent increases to 10 to 30 mg three or four times daily, and to a maximal dose of 180 mg. This agent also can be administered IV or sublingually because the drug is poorly absorbed across buccal membranes and is readily absorbed only

Table 5–4. FACTORS GUIDING THE CLINICAL USE OF CALCIUM-CHANNEL ANTAGONISTS IN ISCHEMIC HEART DISEASE

Left ventricular (LV) dysfunction	Nifedipine and nicardipine enhance LV contractility by marked peripheral vasodilation that stimulates asympathetic reaction accompanied by reflex tachycardia. However, angina pectoris may result when peripheral arteriolar vasodilation is intense. Verapamil and diltiazem both substantially decrease LV contractility and may precipitate congestive heart failure.
Impaired AV conduction due to intrinsic disease or β-adrenergic blockers	Verapamil, especially administered IV, and diltiazem may further compromise impaired AV conduction, whereas nifedipine and nicardipine have little effect on AV conduction.
Impaired sinoatrial (SA) node function ("sick sinus")	Same as for impaired AV conduction: verapamil and diltiazem may further compromise impaired SA function resulting in profound bradycardia, whereas nifedipine and nicardipine may induce a reflex tachycardia.

when it is swallowed. The antianginal effect of 1 mg of nifedipine given IV is comparable to that of 20 mg given sublingually. The duration of the effect of the IV dose is 1 hour compared with several hours when sublingual administration is used. The most common side effects limiting the efficacy of this agent are headache, dizziness, flushing, and a pounding sensation in the head (Frishman et al., 1988). Hypotension is common; for this reason this agent is better avoided in the treatment of acute MI. Pedal edema resulting either from venodilation or more likely from arteriolar dilation with increased capillary pressure and transudation may be confused with CHF. These symptoms usually subside after the dose is reduced or the medication is discontinued.

Combination Therapy

Combinations of nitrates, β-adrenergic antagonists, and calcium antagonists often are required to limit severe angina pectoris. Patients who are likely to require such combinations often exhibit left ventricular dysfunction, atrial and ventricular arrhythmias, and atrioventricular block. The clinical rationale for combining these therapies is the same as when other therapy is combined to achieve equal or greater therapeutic effects while limiting the adverse effects of monotherapy: lower doses of each medication in combination may achieve a better efficacy level than is possible with any agent alone. Moreover, unfavorable attributes of single agents may be offset by combination therapy. For example, depression of sinus node function by β-adrenergic antagonists may be offset by the reflex tachycardia induced by nifedipine or the nitrates. The tendency of β-adrenergic antagonists to increase left ventricular volume may be offset by the tendency of nifedipine to reduce left ventricular volume. The tendency of β-adrenergic antagonists to increase coronary resistance may be offset by any of the calcium antagonists. However, both types of agents depress left ventricular function, sinoatrial node function, and atrioventricular conduction. Therefore combination therapy can induce heart block, severe bradycardia, and CHF.

One controlled clinical trial demonstrated that the addition of nifedipine to nitrates and propranolol reduced the number of patients with unstable angina requiring surgery for relief of pain. However, the incidence of sudden death and MI was similar in the two groups (Gerstenblith et al., 1982). *Principle: Combined therapy is particularly attractive when the drugs combined do not share similar mechanisms of either efficacy or toxicity. Then smaller doses of each would be expected to have additive effects on efficacy and insufficient concentrations to produce the toxicity expected of effective monotherapy.*

REFERENCES

Alderman, E. L.; Coltart, D. J.; Wetlach, G. E.; and Harrison, D. C.: Coronary artery syndromes after sudden propranolol withdrawal. Ann. Intern. Med., 81:625–627, 1974.

Ambrose, J. A.; Winters, S. L.; Stern, A.; Eng, A.; Teichholz, L. E.; Gorlin, R.; and Fuster, V.: Angiographic morphology and the pathogenesis of unstable angina pectoris. J. Am. Coll. Cardiol., 5:609–616, 1985.

Anderson, J. L.; Rothbard, R. L.; Hackworthy, R. A.; Sorenson, S. G.; Fitzpatrick, P. G.; Dahl, C. F.; Hagan, A. D.; Browne, K. F.; Symkoviak, G. P.; Menlove, R. A.; Barry, W. H.; Eckerson, H. W.; Marder, V. J. (for the APSAC Multicenter Investigators 1988 Multicenter Reperfusion Trial of intravenous anisoylated plasminogen streptokinase activator complex (APSAC) in acute myocardial infarction): Controlled comparison with intracoronary streptokinase. J. Am. Coll. Cardiol., 2:1153–1163, 1988.

Anderson, J. L.; Rothbard, R. L.; Hackworthy R. A.; Sorensen, S. G.; Dahl, C. F.; Hagan, A. D.; Wagner, J. M.; Symkoviak, G. P.; Menlove, R. A.; Fitzpatrick, P. G.; Marker, V. J.; APSAC-Coinvestigators; University of Utah, Salt Lake City, Utah; University of Rochester, Rochester, New York: Randomized reperfusion trial of intravenous anisoylated plasminogen streptokinase activator complex (APSAC) versus intracoronary streptokinase in acute myocardial infarction: Interim report. Circulation, 74(suppl. 2):11–16, 1986.

Antiplatelet Trialists' Collaboration: Secondary prevention of vascular disease by prolonged antiplatelet treatment. Br. Med. J., 296:320–331, 1988.

Baim, D. S.; Braunwald, E.; Feit, F.; Knatterud, G. L.; Passamani, E. R.; Robertson, T. L.; Rogers, W. J.; Solomon, R. E.; and Williams, D. O.: The thrombolysis in myocardial infarction (TIMI) Trial Phase II: Additional information and perspectives. J. Am. Coll. Cardiol., 15(5): 1188–1192, 1990.

Beta-Blocker Heart Attack Trial Research Group: A randomized trial of propranolol in patients with acute myocardial infarction: 1. Mortality results. J.A.M.A., 247:1707–1714, 1982.

Boden, W. E.; Krone, R. J.; Kleiger, R. E.; Miller, J. P.; Hager, W. D.; Moss, A. J.; and the MDPIT Research Group: Diltiazem reduces long-term cardiac event rate after non-Q wave infarction: Multicenter Diltiazem Post-Infarction Trial (MDPIT). Circulation, 78(suppl. 4):4–579, 1988.

Braunwald, E.: Mechanism of action of calcium-channel blocking agents. N. Engl. J. Med., 307:1618–1627, 1983.

Braunwald, E.; Knatterud, G. L.; Passamani, E.; Robertson, T. L.; and Solomon, R.: Update from the Thrombolysis in Myocardial Infarction Trial. J. Am. Coll. Cardiol., 10:970, 1987.

Brown, B. G.; Boson, E.; Peterson, R. B.; Pierce, C. D.; and Dodge, H. T.: The mechanisms of nitroglycerin action: Stenosis vasodilation as a major component of the drug response. Circulation, 64:1089–1097, 1981.

Butman, S. M.; Olson, H. G.; Gardin, J. M.; Piters, K. M.; Hullett, M.; and Butman, L. K.: Submaximal exercise testing after stabilization of unstable angina pectoris. J. Am. Coll. Cardiol., 4(4):667–673, 1984.

Cairns, J. A.; Gent, M.; Singer, J.; Finnie, K. J.; Froggatt, G. M.; Holder, D. A.; Jablonsky, G.; Kostuk, W. J.; Melendez, L. J.; Myers, M. G.; Sackett, D. L.; Sealey, B. J.; and Tanser, P. H.: Aspirin, sulfinpyrazone, or both in unstable angina: Results of a Canadian multicenter trial. N. Engl. J. Med., 313:1369–1375, 1985.

Chesebro, J. H.; Knatterud, G.; Roberts, R.; Borer, J.; Cohen, L. S.; Dalen, J.; Dodge, H. T.; Francis, C. K.; Hillis, D.; Ludbrook, P. A.; Markis, J. E.; Mueller, H.; Passamani, E. R.; Powers, E. R.; Rao, A. K.; Robertson, T.; Ross, A.; Ryan, T. J.; Sobel, B. E.; Willerson, J.; Williams, D. O.; Zaret, B. L.; and Braunwald, E.: Thrombolysis in myocardial infarction (TIMI) trial, phase I: A comparison between intravenous tissue plasminogen activator and intravenous streptokinase. Circulation, 76:142–154, 1987.

Collen, D.: Coronary thrombolysis: Streptokinase or recombinant tissue-type plasminogen activator? Ann. Int. Med., 112: 529–538, 1990.

Collen, D.; Stassen, J-M.; Stump, D. C.; and Verstraete, M.: Synergism of thrombolytic agents in vivo. Circulation, 74: 838–842, 1986.

Collen, D.; Topol, E. J.; Tiefenbrunn, A. J.; Gold, H. K.; Weisfeldt, M. L.; Sobel, B. E.; Leinbach, R. C.; Brinker, J. A.; Ludbrook, P. A.; Yasuda, I.; Bulkley, B. H.; Robison, A. K.; Hutter, A. M.; Bell, W. R.; Spadaro, J. J.; Khaw, B. A.; and Grossbard, E. B.: Coronary thrombolysis with recombinant tissue-type plasminogen activator: A prospective, randomized, placebo-controlled trial. Circulation, 70: 1012–1017, 1984.

Davies, M. J.: Thrombosis and coronary atherosclerosis. In, Acute Coronary Intervention (Topol, E. J., ed.). Marcel Dekker, New York, p. 29, 1989.

Davies, M. J.; and Thameer, A. C.: Plaque fissuring: The cause of acute myocardial infarction, sudden ischemic death and crescendo angina. Br. Heart J., 53:363–374, 1977.

Davies, M. J.; and Thomas, T.: The pathological basis and microanatomy of occlusive coronary thrombus formation in human coronary arteries. Philos. Trans. R. Soc. Lond., 294: 225–229, 1981.

DeBusk, R. F.: Specialized testing after recent acute myocardial infarction. Ann. Intern. Med., 110:470–481, 1989.

DeBusk, R. F. (for the Clinical Efficacy Assessment Project of the American College of Physicians): Evaluation of patients after recent acute myocardial infarction. Ann. Intern. Med., 110:485–488, 1989.

DeBusk, R. F.; and Dennis, C. A.: "Submaximal" predischarge exercise testing after acute myocardial infarction: Who needs it? Am. J. Cardiol., 55:299–300, 1985.

DeBusk, R. F.; Blomqvist, C. G.; Kouchoukos, N. T.; Luepker, R. V.; Miller, H. S.; Moss, A. J.; Pollock, M. L.; Reeves, T. J.; Selvester, R. H.; Stason, W. B.; Wagner, G. S.; and Willman, V. L.: Identification and treatment of low-risk patients after acute myocardial infarction and coronary-artery bypass graft surgery. N. Engl. J. Med., 314: 161–166, 1986.

DeBusk, R. F.; Kraemer, H. C.; Nash, E.; Berger, W. E. III; and Lew, H.: Stepwise risk stratification soon after acute myocardial infarction. Am. J. Cardiol., 52:1161–1166, 1983.

Dennis, C.; Houston-Miller, N.; Schwartz, R. G.; Ahn, D. K.; Kraemer, H. C.; Gossard, D.; Juneau, M.; Taylor, C. B.; and DeBusk, R. F.: Early return to work after uncomplicated myocardial infarction. Results of a randomized trial. J.A.M.A., 260:214–220, 1988.

Dewood, M. A.; Spores, J.; Notske, R. N.; Mouser, L. T.; Burroughs, R.; Golden, M. S.; and Lang, H. T.: Prevalence of total coronary occlusion during the early hours of transmural myocardial infarction. N. Engl. J. Med., 303:897–903, 1980.

Frishman, W. H.; Stroh, J. A.; Greenberg, S. M.; Suarez, T.; Karp, A.; and Peled, H. B.: Calcium-channel blockers in systemic hypertension. Med. Clin. North Am., 72:449–499, 1988.

Frishman, W. H.; Stroh, J. A.; Greenberg, S. M.; Suarez, T.; Karp, A.; and Peled, H. B.: Calcium-channel blockers in systemic hypertension. Curr. Probl. Cardiol., 12(5):1–346, 1987.

Fuster, V.; Adams, P. C.; Badimon, J. J.; and Chesebro, J. H.: Platelet-inhibitor drugs' role in coronary artery disease. Prog. Cardiovasc. Dis., 29:325–346, 1987.

Gash, A. K.; Spann, J. F.; Sherry, S.; Belber, A. D.; Carabello, B. A.; McDonough, M. T.; Mann, R. H.; McCann, W. D.; Gault, J. H.; Gentzler, R. D.; and Kent, R. L.: Factors influencing reocclusion after coronary thrombolysis for acute myocardial infarction. Am. J. Cardiol., 57:175–177, 1986.

Gelman, J. S.; Feldman, R. L.; Scott, E.; and Pepine, C. J.: Nicardipine for angina pectoris at rest and coronary arterial spasm. Am. J. Cardiol., 56:232–236, 1985.

Gerstenblith, G.; Ougang, P.; Achuff, S.; Bulkley, B. H.; Becker, L. C.; Mellits, E. D.; Baughman, K. L.; Weiss, J. L.; Flaherty, J. T.; Kallman, C. H.; Llewellyn, M.; and Weisfeldt, M. L.: Nifedipine in unstable angina: A double-blind randomized trial. N. Engl. J. Med., 306:885–889, 1982.

Gibson, R. S.: Current status of calcium channel-blocking drugs after Q wave and non-Q wave myocardial infarction. Circulation, 80:107–119, 1989.

Gibson, R. S.; Young, P. M.; Boden, W. E.; Schechtman, K.; Roberts, R. (the Diltiazem Reinfarction Study Group): Prognostic significance and beneficial effect of diltiazem on the incidence of early recurrent ischemia after non-Q wave myocardial infarction: Results from the Multicenter Diltiazem Reinfarction Study. Am. J. Cardiol., 60:203–209, 1987.

Gibson, R. S.; Watson, D. D.; Craddock, G. B.; Crampton, R. S.; Kaiser, D. L.; Denny, M. J.; and Beller, G. A.: Prediction of cardiac events after uncomplicated myocardial infarction: A prospective study comparing pre-discharge exercise thallium-201 scintigraphy and coronary arteriography. Circulation, 68:321–336, 1983.

Goldman, L.; Sia, B. S. T.; Cook, E. F.; Rutherford, J. D.; and Weinstein, M. C.: Costs and effectiveness of routine therapy with long-term beta-adrenergic antagonists after acute myocardial infarction. N. Engl. J. Med., 319:152–158, 1988.

Gorlin, R.; Brachfeld, N.; MacLeod, D.; and Bopp, P.: Effect of nitroglycerin on the coronary circulation in patients with coronary artery disease or increased left ventricular work. Circulation, 19:705–718, 1959.

Gottlieb, S. O.; Weisfeldt, M. L.; Ouyang, P.; Mellits, E. D.; and Gerstenblith, G.: Silent ischemia as a market for early unfavorable outcomes in patients with unstable angina. N. Engl. J. Med., 314:1214–1219, 1986.

Gruppo Italiano per lo studio della streptochinasi nell'infarto miocardico (GISSI): Effectiveness of intravenous thrombolytic treatment in acute myocardial infarction. Lancet, 1:397–401, 1986.

Harrison, D. G.; Ferguson, D. W.; Collins, S. M.; Skorton, D. J.; Erickson, E. E.; Kioschos, J. M.; Marcus, M. L.; and White, C. W.: Rethrombosis after reperfusion with streptokinase: Importance of geometry of residual lesions. Circulation, 69:991–999, 1984.

Hung, J.; Goris, M. L.; Nash, E.; and DeBusk, R. F.: Comparative value of maximal treadmill testing, exercise thallium myocardial perfusion scintigraphy and exercise radionuclide ventriculography for distinguishing high and low risk patients soon after myocardial infarction. Am. J. Cardiol., 53:1221–1227, 1984.

The ISAM Study Group: A prospective trial of intravenous streptokinase in acute myocardial infarction (ISAM): Mortality, morbidity and infarct size at 21 days. N. Engl. J. Med., 314:1465–1472, 1986.

ISIS-1 Collaborative Group: Mechanisms for the early mortality reduction produced by beta-blocking started early in acute myocardial infarction: ISIS-1. Lancet 1:921–923, 1988.

ISIS-2 (Second International Study of Infarct Survival) Collaborative Group: Randomized trial of intravenous streptokinase, oral aspirin, both, or neither among 17,187 cases of suspected acute myocardial infarction: ISIS-2. Lancet 2: 349–360, 1988.

Kereiakes, D. J.: The role of emergency surgical revascularization in acute myocardial infarction. In, Acute Coronary Intervention (Topol, E. J., ed.). Marcel Dekker, New York, pp. 107–121, 1989.

Lew, A. S.; Laramee, P.; Cercek, B.; Shah, P. K.; and Ganz, W.: The hypotensive effect of intravenous streptokinase in patients with acute myocardial infarction. Circulation, 72: 1321–1326, 1985.

Lewis, H. D. Jr.; Davis, J. W.; Archibald, D. G.; Steinke, W. E.; Smitherman, T. C.; Dollery, J. E. III; Schnaper, H. W.; LeWinter, M. M.; Linares, E.; Pouget, J. M.; Sabharwal, S. C.; Chesler, E.; and DeMots, H.: Protective effects of aspirin against acute myocardial infarction and death in men with unstable angina: Results of a Veterans Administration Cooperative Study. N. Engl. J. Med., 309:396–403, 1983.

Lewis, J. G.: Adverse reactions to calcium antagonists. Drugs, 25:196–222, 1983.

Loscalzo, J.; and Braunwald, E.: Tissue plasminogen activator. N. Engl. J. Med., 319:925–931, 1989.

Marder, V. J.; and Sherry, S.: Thrombolytic therapy: Current status (two parts). N. Engl. J. Med., 318:1512–1520, 1585–1594, 1988.

Marder, V. J.; Rothbard, R. L.; Fitzpatrick, P. G.; and Francis, C. W.: Rapid lysis of coronary artery thrombi with anisoylated plasminogen: Streptokinase activator complex: Treatment by bolus intravenous injection. Ann. Intern. Med., 104:304–310, 1986.

Mason, D. T.; and Braunwald, E.: The effects of nitroglycerin and amyl nitrite on arteriolar and venous tone in the human forearm. Circulation, 32:755–766, 1965.

Mathey, D. G.; Schofer, J.; Sheehan, F. H.; Becher, H.; Tilsner, V.; and Dodge, H. T.: Intravenous urokinase in acute myocardial infarction. Am. J. Cardiol., 55:878–882, 1985.

Meltzer, R. S.; Visser, C. A.; and Fuster, V.: Intracardiac thrombi and systemic embolization. Ann. Intern. Med., 104:689–698, 1986.

The MIAMI Trial Research Group: Mortality. Am. J. Cardiol., 56(suppl. G):12–22, 1985.

The Multicenter Diltiazem Post-Infarction Research Group: The effect of diltiazem on mortality and reinfarction after myocardial infarction. N. Engl. J. Med., 319:385–393, 1988.

Needleman, P.; Corr, P. B.; and Johnson, E. M. Jr.: Drugs used for the treatment of angina: Organic nitrates, calcium channel blockers, and β-adrenergic antagonists. In, The Pharmacological Basis of Therapeutics, 7th ed. (Gilman, A. G.; Goodman, L. S.; Rall, T. W.; and Murad, F.; eds.). Macmillan, New York, pp. 813–818, 1985.

Nordlander, R.; and Nyquist, O.: Patients treated in a coronary care unit without acute myocardial infarction. Br. Heart J., 41:647–653, 1979.

Norwegian Multicenter Study Group: Timolol-induced reduction in mortality and reinfarction in patients surviving acute myocardial infarction. N. Engl. J. Med., 304:801–807, 1981.

O'Neill, W. W.; Topol, E. J.; and Pitt, B.: Reperfusion therapy of acute myocardial infarction. Prog. Cardiovasc. Dis., 30(4):235–266, 1988.

Opie, L. H. (ed.): Drugs for the Heart, 2nd ed. Grune & Stratton, Orlando, p. 45, 1987.

O'Reilly, R. A.: Anticoagulant, antithrombotic, and thrombolytic drugs. In, The Pharmacological Basis of Therapeutics, 7th ed. (Gilman, A. G.; Goodman, L. S.; Rall, T. W.; and Murad, F.; ed.). Macmillan, New York, p. 1340, 1985.

Parodi, O.; Simonetti, I.; L'Abbate, A.; and Maseri, A.: Verapamil versus propranolol for angina at rest. Am. J. Cardiol., 50:923–928, 1982.

Prinzmetal, R.; Kennamer, R.; Merliss, R.; Wada, T.; and Bor, N.: Angina pectoris: I. A variant form of angina pectoris: Preliminary report. Am. J. Med., 27:375–388, 1959.

Rao, A. K.; Pratt, C.; Berke, A.; Jaffe, A.; Ockene, I.; Schreiber, T. L.; Bell, W. R.; Knatterud, G.; Robertson, T. L.; and Terrin, M. L.: Thrombolysis in Myocardial Infarction (TIMI) Trial—Phase 1: Hemorrhagic manifestations and changes in plasma fibrinogen and the fibrinolytic system in patients treated with recombinant tissue plasminogen activator and streptokinase. J. Am. Coll. Cardiol., 11:1–11, 1988.

Rentrop, P.; Blanke, H.; Karsch, K. R.; Wiegand, V.; Kostering, K.; Oster, H.; and Leitz, K.: Acute myocardial infarction: Intracoronary application of nitroglycerin and streptokinase in combination with transluminal recanalization. Clin. Cardiol., 2:354–363, 1979.

Report on the Sixty Plus Reinfarction Study Research Group: A double-blind trial to assess long-term oral anticoagulant therapy in elderly patients after myocardial infarction. Lancet, 2:989–993, 1980.

Scheidt, S.: Therapy for angina pectoris: Comparison of nicardipine with other antianginal agents. Am. Heart J., 116:254–259, 1988.

Schroeder, J. S.; Lamb, I. H.; and Hu, M.: Do patients in whom myocardial infarction has been ruled out have a better prognosis after hospitalization than those surviving infarction? N. Engl. J. Med., 303(1):1–5, 1980.

Shand, D. G.: Drug therapy: Propranolol. N. Engl. J. Med., 293(6):280–285, 1975.

Singh, B. N.; Chew, C. Y. C.; Josephson, M. A.; and Packer, M.: Pharmacologic and hemodynamic mechanisms underlying the antianginal actions of verapamil. Am. J. Cardiol., 50: 886–893, 1982.

Smalling, R. W.; Schumacher, R.; Morris, D.; Harder, K.; Fuentes, F.; Valentine, R. P.; Battey, L. L.; Merhige, M.; Pitts, D. E.; Lieberman, H. A.; Nishikawa, A.; Adyanthaya, A.; Hopkins, A.; and Grossbard, E.: Improved infarct-related arterial patency after high dose, weight-adjusted, rapid infusion of tissue-type plasminogen activator in myocardial infarction: Results of a multicenter randomized trial of two dosage regimens. J. Am. Coll. Cardiol., 15:915–921, 1990.

Smith, B.; and Kennedy, J. W.: Thrombolysis in the treatment of acute transmural myocardial infarction. Ann. Intern. Med., 106:414–420, 1987.

Stein, B.; and Fuster, V.: Antithrombotic therapy in acute myocardial infarction: Prevention of venous, left ventricular and coronary artery thromboembolism. Am. J. Cardiol., 64:33B–40B, 1989.

Subramanian, V.: Bala: Comparative evaluation of four calcium antagonists and propranolol with placebo in patients with chronic stable angina. Cardiovasc. Rev. Rep., 5:91–104, 1984.

Telford, A. M.; and Wilson, C.: Trial of heparin versus atenolol in prevention of myocardial infarction in intermediate coronary syndrome. Lancet, 1:1225–1228, 1981.

Théroux, P.; Ouimet, H.; McCans, J.; Latour, J.; Joly, P.; Lévy, G.; Pelletier, E.; Juneau, M.; Stasiak, J.; deGuise, P.; Pelletier, G. B.; Rinzler, D.; and Waters, D. D.: Aspirin, heparin, or both to treat acute unstable angina. N. Engl. J. Med., 319:1105–1111, 1988.

Thompson, P. L.; and Robinson, J. S.: Stroke after acute myocardial infarction: Relation to infarct size. Br. Med. J., 2: 457–459, 1978.

Tiefenbrunn, A. J.; and Sobel, B. E.: The impact of coronary thrombolysis on myocardial infarction (invited review). Fibrinolysis, 3:1–15, 1989.

The TIMI Study Group: Comparison of invasive and conservative strategies after treatment with intravenous tissue plasminogen activator in acute myocardial infarction—Results of the thrombolysis in myocardial infarction (TIMI) Phase II Trial. N. Engl. J. Med., 320:618–627, 1989.

The TIMI Study Group: The thrombolysis in myocardial infarction (TIMI) trial: Phase I findings. N. Engl. J. Med., 312: 932–936, 1985.

Uretsky, B. F.; Farquhar, D. S.; Berezin, A. F.; and Hood, W. B. J. Jr.: Symptomatic myocardial infarction without chest pain: Prevalence and clinical course. Am. J. Cardiol., 40:498–503, 1977.

Weiner, N.: Drugs that inhibit adrenergic nerves and block adrenergic receptors. In, The Pharmacological Basis of Therapeutics, 7th ed. (Gilman, A. G.; Goodman, L. S.; Rall, T. W.; and Murad, F.; eds.). Macmillan, New York, pp. 181–192, 1985.

Weisfeldt, M. L.: Exploring myocardial ischemia: Silent and symptomatic. Am. J. Med., 80(4C):48–55, 1986.

Williams, D. O.; Kirby, M. G.; McPherson, K.; and Phear, D. N.: Anticoagulant treatment of unstable angina. Br. J. Clin. Pract., 40:114–116, 1986.

Williams, J. F. Jr.; Glick, G.; and Braunwald, E.: Studies on cardiac dimensions in intact unanesthetized man: V. Effects of nitroglycerin. Circulation, 32:767–771, 1965.

Wolfson, S.; and Gorlin, R.: Cardiovascular pharmacology of propranolol in man. Circulation, 40:501–511, 1969.

Yusuf, S.; Peto, R.; Lewis, J.; Collins, R.; and Sleight, P.: Beta blockade during and after myocardial infarction: An overview of the randomized trials. Prog. Cardiovasc. Dis., 27:335–371, 1985.

6

Treatment of Cardiovascular Disorders: Arrhythmias

Dan M. Roden

Therapy for cardiac arrhythmias traditionally has relied on empiricism, scientifically justified or not. This unfortunate situation has reflected the small number of available antiarrhythmic drugs, the lack of clear understanding of mechanisms underlying the efficacy of the drugs, the pathogenesis of various disorders of cardiac rhythm (despite the ease with which they can be detected), and, above all, the lack of any sort of reliable information on whether the benefits of antiar-hythmic treatment in specific situations outweigh the risks. The past decade has seen striking changes in each of these areas: a large number of new drugs is now available; a variety of techniques have been used to develop improved understanding of the mechanisms of various cardiac arrhythmias, and new information is becoming available on the benefits and risks of treatment in various subgroups of patients.

NORMAL ELECTRICAL BEHAVIOR OF THE HEART

The Action Potential

In general, movement of ions that generate currents across excitable membranes such as those in the heart occurs through specific pore-forming ion-channel proteins (Hille, 1984). In response to changes in their local environment (such as a change in membrane potential or occupancy of an adjacent receptor), these large membrane-spanning macromolecules can form a transmembrane pore. These "pores" generally are fairly specific for one ion species; that is, sodium channels conduct sodium and not potassium, and so forth. Like calcium channels, other ion channels are heterogeneous: different subtypes of other ion channels have been identified. For example, several different potassium channels are present in heart, each of which opens and closes under different conditions (Roden et al., 1989). One subtype of potassium channel controls the resting potential, others may be important in early and late repolarization, and still others may play a role in pacemaker activity. With advancing understanding of the basic determinants of cardiac electrophysiology, drugs may be targeted more specifically for such different ion channels, perhaps producing safer and more effective treatments.

When the voltage difference between the interior and exterior of an atrial or ventricular cell is measured, a value of about − 80 mV (the cell interior being negative) is normally obtained. The major mechanism maintaining this electrical gradient is thought to be potassium ion channel function. Under normal circumstances, even a minor degree of depolarization of the cell interior (e.g., to − 70 mV) results in outward movement of potassium ions that restores the normal resting potential. Similarly, hyperpolarization (e.g., to − 90 mV) produces inward movement of potassium ions, resulting in depolarization back to the normal resting potential.

When an atrial or ventricular cell is at rest, there is both a concentration and an electrical gradient for sodium to enter the cell. However, sodium-channel proteins are not open at − 80 mV, and consequently there is no sodium current. When a cell is transiently depolarized to a threshold value by normal pacemaker activity or by propagation of an electrical impulse from an adjacent cell, sodium channels open. This leads to many sodium ions (10^7 ions per second) entering the cell, which depolarizes it to approximately + 30 mV; this is termed *phase 0* of the action potential. The maximum slope of phase 0 is a widely used indicator of the magnitude of the sodium current. Once depolarization caused by sodium entry has occurred, a stereotypical series of changes (Fig. 6–1) occurs in the function of other

ion channels. The events result in fairly rapid initial repolarization to approximately 0 mV (phase 1), maintained depolarization for several hundred milliseconds (phase 2), and, finally, repolarization back to the resting potential (phase 3). Phase 1 is thought to reflect activation of an outward potassium current or an inward chloride current. The fact that voltage does not change during phase 2 indicates that there is no net membrane current; there is a balance between inward current (through calcium channels) and outward current (through potassium channels). Ultimately the inward current declines and the outward current increases, which results in phase 3 repolarization. Since this cycle is repeated over a 100,000 times per day, it is clear that the cell must have mechanisms to eliminate the sodium and calcium flowing in during each action potential and to restore the intracellular potassium concentration. Adenosine triphosphate (ATP)-requiring pumps that exchange intracellular sodium ions for extracellular potassium ions and intracellular calcium ions for extracellular sodium ions are activated during each cardiac cycle. These pumps are a particularly important component of the cells' defense mechanisms against intracellular calcium overload and, as discussed in chapter 4, the sodium-potassium pump is the target for binding digitalis.

Action potentials from atrial and ventricular tissue, and, indeed action potentials from different parts of the atria or ventricles, differ somewhat in their configuration. These differences presumably reflect differences in the numbers or function of individual ion channels that make up the action potential. Similarly, tissues from other parts of the heart display different action potential configurations that are thought to be important for their individualized specialized functions. For example, action potentials from the conducting system located on the endocardial surface of the ventricles (the His-Purkinje system) are longer

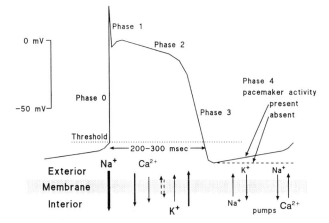

Fig. 6–1. Phases of a cardiac action potential and the ion currents that produce it. See text for details. The ionic mechanism underlying pacemaker activity, which is seen in selected cells, is not fully understood.

and the sodium current larger than in ventricular tissue; the larger sodium current accounts for the faster impulse propagation in these specialized tissues, described in more detail below.

Under normal circumstances, atrial and ventricular muscle reach the resting potential at the end of phase 3 and remain at rest until restimulated. Other tissues, such as His-Purkinje tissue, sinoatrial (SA) node tissue, and atrioventricular (AV) node tissue display spontaneous phase 4 depolarization whose ionic mechanism is not well understood. In addition, sodium channels are inconspicuous in SA and AV nodal tissue; resting potentials are in the depolarized range (-60 to -70 mV) and phase 0 upstroke slope, largely a function of the inward current through calcium channels, is much lower than it is in other parts of the heart. Spontaneous phase 4 depolarization results in gradual depolarization of the membrane potential, opening of sodium (or, in SA or AV node, calcium) channels, and repeated generation of spontaneous action potentials. The rate of repetitive generation of the action potential (pacemaker rate) ordinarily is fastest in the SA node, but, as described further below, any tissue displaying such automatic behavior can theoretically act as the dominant pacemaker of the heart.

Impulse Propagation and the Surface ECG. The magnitude of the inward current accounting for phase 0 depolarization is the most important determinant of conduction velocity (Cranefield, 1985). Thus, impulse propagation is fastest in the His-Purkinje specialized conducting system and slowest within the SA and AV nodes. Impulses normally exit from the SA node and spread very rapidly through both atria, resulting in atrial depolarization that leads to the P wave of the electrocardiogram. Following atrial depolarization (electrical systole), impulses propagate through the AV node; however, since the slope of phase 0 in the AV node is relatively flat, impulse propagation proceeds very slowly. This pause between atrial depolarization and the subsequent ventricular depolarization allows the atria and ventricles to contract sequentially, thus providing time for blood to move from the atria to the ventricles before the atrio-ventricular valves close. Following slow propagation through the AV node, the impulse then reaches the common bundle of His, the bundle branches, and spreads ultimately through the endocardial conducting system. This process ordinarily takes no more than 50 to 60 msec, as assessed by specialized intracardiac recordings (His bundle electrocardiography). The ventricle depolarizes in an endocardial-to-epicardial direction, resulting in calcium entry into ventricular cells, calcium-triggered calcium release from sarcoplasmic reticulum, and mechanical

contraction of the heart (see chapter 4). The QRS complex of the surface electrocardiogram corresponds to ventricular depolarization. Ventricular repolarization occurs in an epicardial-to-endocardial direction; the end of the T wave generally is thought to represent the end of ventricular repolarization. Prominent U waves, which are discussed further below, may arise from delayed repolarization within the His-Purkinje network (Watanabe, 1975).

Slowing of impulse propagation, which may result from treatment with drugs, electrolyte abnormalities, or disease, is an important predisposing factor to certain types of arrhythmias, described below.

States of the Sodium Channel. Although depolarization opens sodium channels, maintained depolarization during phases 1 to 3 of the action potential is not accompanied by a large maintained inward current through sodium channels. The explanation is that the probability that a sodium channel will be open is regulated by two separate processes: (1) activation (opening) that occurs very rapidly as the tissue is depolarized and (2) inactivation that is slower and acts to close sodium channels at depolarized potentials (Hille, 1984; Hondeghem and Katzung, 1984). Sodium-channel proteins open to permit the rapid inward movement of sodium in phase 0 and then are inactivated to terminate this process (Fig. 6-2). Inactivated sodium channels cannot be opened as the membrane repolarizes until they recover from the inactivated state back to the resting state from which opening is again possible. Recovery of sodium channels to the resting state is primarily a function of the membrane potential (see the following section).

Refractoriness. If a ventricular cell is stimulated (by an investigator inserting an artificial pacing stimulus or by adjacent cells depolarizing) during phase 4, a normal action potential will result. If, on the other hand, a cell is stimulated early during phase 2, the sodium channels will all

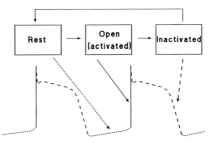

Fig. 6-2. States of the sodium channel during the cardiac action potential. See text for details.

be in the inactivated state, and consequently, no action potential will occur. Extrastimuli inserted early during phase 3 may result in a small inward sodium current, but insufficient to result in propagated excitation. As can be seen in Fig. 6–3, extrastimuli inserted later in phase 3, at a time when sodium channels have recovered to a greater extent from inactivation, produce a larger sodium current that is quite likely to propagate. The relationship between extrastimulus prematurity and the magnitude of the resultant sodium current is thus a reflection of voltage-dependent recovery from inactivation of the sodium channels. The time at which an extrastimulus results in a propagated action potential is often referred to as the end of the *effective refractory period*. As described further below, prolongation of the effective refractory period is one potential mechanism for action of antiarrhythmic drugs. The antiarrhythmic effect can be produced by at least two different mechanisms (Fig. 6–4): either drug may interfere with sodium-channel availability at any given voltage to prolong the effective refractory period or, alternatively, drugs may have no primary effect on sodium channels but merely delay the time course of repolarization (e.g., by interfering with potassium-channel function). In the latter case, perturbing the time course of repolar-

ization will necessarily prolong the time at which the voltage associated with recovery from inactivation occurs.

Fast- versus Slow-Response Tissues. The atria, the ventricles, and the His-Purkinje system are considered fast-response tissues. In the AV node ("slow response" tissue), calcium-channel function is paramount and calcium channels recover from inactivation much more slowly than do sodium channels (Fig. 6–5). Thus, an extra stimulus inserted during phase 4 in AV nodal tissue may not necessarily result in a normal action potential. Here, in contrast to sodium-channel-dependent tissue, the time since the last repolarization, and not the voltage at which the extrastimulus is inserted, is the major factor governing refractoriness. Sodium-channel-dependent tissues display *all-or-nothing conduction*, that is, impulses delivered after the effective refractory period will be conducted through the tissue or they will not be conducted at all. On the other hand, increasingly premature impulses delivered to the AV node result in increasingly slow impulse conduction such that conduction may fail within the AV node, and the impulse is therefore extinguished (*decremental conduction*).

These descriptions of normal electrical behav-

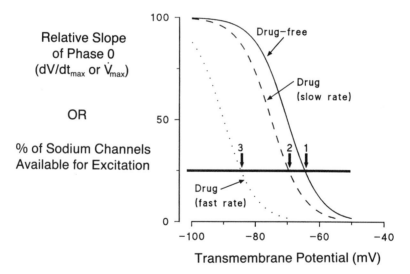

Relative Slope
of Phase 0
$(dV/dt_{max}$ or $\dot{V}_{max})$

OR

% of Sodium Channels
Available for Excitation

Transmembrane Potential (mV)

Fig. 6–3. Membrane responsiveness. The relationship between the upstroke slope of a premature stimulus arising during phase 3 and the voltage at which it arises is the *membrane responsiveness* relationship and is a measure of sodium-channel availability at that voltage. Sodium-channel blocking drugs depress membrane responsiveness, that is, they shift this relationship to more negative potentials. As discussed in the text, sodium-channel block is a function of stimulation rate. Thus, depression of membrane responsiveness by a sodium-channel blocking drug will be greater at fast rates (dotted line) than at slow rates (dashes). In the presence of drug, the point at which enough sodium channels become available to permit propagated excitation to occur (arbitrarily set here at 25%, heavy line) is shifted in a negative direction as indicated by the heavy arrows from (1) − 64 mV in the absence of drug to (2) − 68 mV in the presence of a small amount of drug and/or slow rate to (3) − 84 mV with more sodium-channel block.

Block of sodium channels prolongs refractoriness...

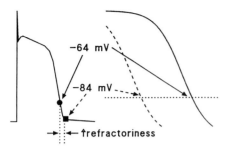

...and so does action potential prolongation

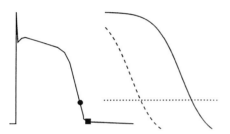

Fig. 6-4. Mechanisms of increased refractoriness. As shown in Fig. 6-3, the point at which sufficient sodium channels become available for propagated excitation is determined by the membrane-responsiveness curve and in the example is −64 mV (•, top panel) in the absence of drug. As discussed in Fig. 6-3, this is shifted in a negative direction, to −84 mV (■), in the presence of drug. In this way, time during which the cell is refractory is prolonged as indicated. If a drug does not alter sodium-channel physiology but prolongs the duration of action potential (a "class III" action), refractoriness also will be prolonged (•, bottom panel). In the presence of a sodium-channel-blocking, action potential–prolonging drug (e.g., quinidine), refractoriness will be prolonged further (■, bottom panel).

ior provide a framework for analysis of the mechanisms underlying the genesis of cardiac arrhythmias and the ways in which drugs might suppress arrhythmias. In addition, other processes can alter normal cardiac physiology and response to drugs. For example, elevation of the extracellular potassium concentration results in depolarization of the resting potential. Thus, some sodium channels will be inactivated at the beginning of an action potential, and the magnitude of the sodium current during phase 0 will be correspondingly decreased. Impulse propagation in the ventricles will therefore slow: the resultant QRS widening is

one electrocardiographic hallmark of hyperkalemia. The effects of ischemia are much more complicated and include membrane depolarization with resultant slowing of conduction as well as induction of abnormal forms of automaticity; either mechanism can result in arrhythmias. *Principle: The effect of antiarrhythmic drugs depends on many factors including the state of the conduction system and myocardium but is not limited to the heart. The effect also will depend on the extramyocardial environment, the extracardiac effects of the drug, and the general state of electrolyte and endocrine balance in the body.*

MECHANISMS OF CARDIAC ARRHYTHMIAS

Three major mechanisms that contribute to cardiac arrhythmias are recognized: abnormalities of normal automaticity, "triggered" automaticity, and reentry (Hoffman et al., 1975; Cranefield and Aronson, 1988). *Principle: Understanding the pathophysiology of individual arrhythmias at the cellular and subcellular levels can directly contribute to rational treatment.*

Abnormal Automaticity

Under normal circumstances, the rate of pacemaker firing in the SA node is faster than that of other pacemakers in the heart. The "arrhythmia" sinus tachycardia represents an increased rate of discharge in the SA nodal pacemaker; obviously, therapy directed at this "arrhythmia" should primarily involve a search for underlying causes (thyrotoxicosis, congestive heart failure, anemia, etc.). Under pathologic conditions, pacemaker activity in tissues normally displaying spontaneous phase 4 depolarization (AV node, His-Purkinje system) may become sufficiently fast to become the predominant pacemaker; in this case, junctional or ventricular tachycardia will result. In addition, automatic behavior may also be seen in diseased atria or ventricles that do not ordinarily display pacemaker activity. Ectopic atrial tachycardia and, possibly, some forms of ischemia-mediated ventricular tachycardia are examples. In isolated tissues, automatic behavior generally starts slowly, can have variable rates, often slows before stopping, and tends to suppress other automatic tissue (Dangman and Hoffman, 1983). These behaviors are often seen in arrhythmias thought to represent abnormal automaticity. Ectopic atrial tachycardia, for example, starts slowly, has a variable rate, often stops slowly, and may be followed by several seconds of asystole while normal SA nodal pacemakers recover from "overdrive suppression" (Josephson and Kastor, 1977). Such parallels between studies in isolated tissue and patterns of clinical arrhythmia

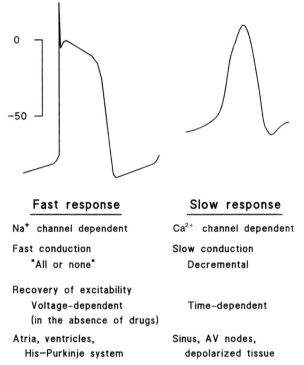

Fast response

Na$^+$ channel dependent

Fast conduction
  "All or none"

Recovery of excitability
  Voltage-dependent
  (in the absence of drugs)

Atria, ventricles,
  His−Purkinje system

Slow response

Ca^{2+} channel dependent

Slow conduction
  Decremental

Time−dependent

Sinus, AV nodes,
  depolarized tissue

Fig. 6–5. Comparison between fast-response and slow-response action potentials.

have been a major clue to understanding the underlying mechanisms of diverse arrhythmias. Similarly, rapid pacing of automatic foci results in transient suppression of arrhythmia (during which other pacemakers such as the SA node may emerge), followed by warm-up and resumption of the arrhythmia. Pacing techniques are not particularly effective for arrhythmias related to abnormal automaticity.

Triggered Automaticity

Triggered automaticity is a special form of abnormal automaticity related to perturbations during repolarization termed *afterdepolarizations* (Fig. 6–6; Cranefield, 1977; Cranefield and Aronson, 1988). One well-studied example of triggered automaticity is delayed afterdepolarizations due to intoxication with digitalis. Preparations exposed to high concentrations of digitalis and paced at normal rates do not display automatic behavior in vitro. However, with premature beats or with rapid pacing, afterdepolarizations may develop during phase 4. Should these reach threshold, single or multiple beats can develop. Thus, the afterdepolarization-mediated arrhythmia only occurs when a normal heartbeat provides the "trigger" in the appropriate environment (Wit and Rosen, 1983). Therefore some arrhyth-

mias that display similar biologic behaviors in patients are thought to reflect delayed afterdepolarizations (Rosen and Reder, 1981). Calcium-channel blockers can abolish delayed afterdepolarizations in vitro and have, as described below, been used in some arrhythmias theoretically related to this mechanism.

Early afterdepolarizations occur during phase 3 (i.e., terminal repolarization). Interventions that prolong cardiac action potentials, such as treatment with quinidine or other action potential-prolonging drugs, hypokalemia, and slow-paced or spontaneous drive rates, all promote prolongation of the action potential and development of early afterdepolarizations in Purkinje tissues (Roden and Hoffman, 1985). Since marked prolongation of the QT interval can be associated with polymorphic ventricular tachycardia (termed *torsades de pointes*) that develops most often in the setting of bradycardia and hypokalemia, it is now widely hypothesized that triggered activity associated with early afterdepolarizations is the underlying mechanism (Roden et al., 1986; Cranefield and Aronson, 1988; Jackman et al., 1988). Interventions that increase heart rate, such as rapid pacing or administration of catecholamines, prevent early afterdepolarizations in vitro and have become the treatment of choice for torsades de pointes. Similarly, raising extracellular concentra-

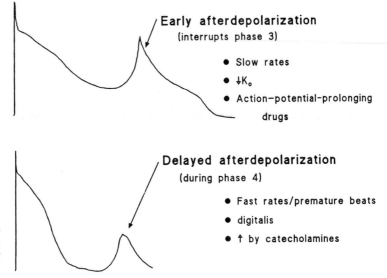

Early afterdepolarization
(interrupts phase 3)

- Slow rates
- $\downarrow K_o$
- Action–potential–prolonging
  drugs

Delayed afterdepolarization
(during phase 4)

- Fast rates/premature beats
- digitalis
- ↑ by catecholamines

Fig. 6-6. Two different types of afterdepolarizations. Both have been implicated in the genesis of certain arrhythmias (see text).

tions of potassium shortens duration of the action potential and is an invaluable adjunct to the management of torsades de pointes. Administration of magnesium also is effective (Tzivoni et al., 1988); interestingly, administration of magnesium in vitro tends to reverse the triggered activity but does not markedly shorten the duration of the action potential (Bailie et al., 1988). Administration of magnesium in patients with torsades de pointes tends to reverse the arrhythmia without markedly shortening the QT interval. The striking parallels between triggered activity related to early afterdepolarizations in vitro and torsades de pointes provide an excellent example of how understanding basic mechanisms can help guide rational therapy. *Principle: The true test of a hypothesis comes when a new chemical entity has the in vivo affects that its in vitro effects predict. Retrofitting drugs into categories of in vivo efficacy that is not predicted by in vitro tests is not a test of the validity of the hypothesis.*

Reentry

Three critical determinants for a reentrant arrhythmia were described by Mines (1914) in his work on circulating impulses in rings of turtle heart tissue. He found that (1) more than one pathway connecting two points (i.e., appropriate anatomy), (2) sufficient heterogeneity in the electrophysiologic properties of the tissue so that impulse propagation can transiently block in one direction yet proceed in another (*unidirectional block*), and (3) prompt termination of the arrhythmia when the pathway is interrupted formed

the criteria. The prototypical reentrant arrhythmias in humans that satisfy all three of Mines's criteria are those seen in the Wolff-Parkinson-White syndrome (Fig. 6–7). In this condition, an accessory pathway connecting atrium and ventricle is present (meeting criterion 1). In sinus rhythm, a portion of the ventricle is excited by normal impulse propagation via the AV node and another portion of the ventricle may be excited prematurely (*preexcitation*) by propagation from the atrium to the ventricle via the accessory pathway. A premature beat arising in the atrium may find the accessory pathway refractory, and all impulse propagation will then occur through the AV node (criterion 2). If the excitatory wave front propagates to the ventricular insertion of the accessory pathway slowly enough, it may find it nonrefractory, and impulses will reenter the atrium, establishing a *circus movement tachycardia* or *orthodromic reciprocating tachycardia* (Josephson and Kastor, 1977). Thus, heterogeneity of refractory periods and conduction slowing contribute to the development of this (and other) reentrant arrhythmia(s). This is the most common type of arrhythmia observed in patients with the Wolff-Parkinson-White syndrome, and, with the demonstration that surgical sectioning of the bypass tract prevents recurrence of the arrhythmia (criterion 3), this is one of the few arrhythmias in humans that meets all three of Mines's criteria for reentry. In the classic form of Wolff-Parkinson-White syndrome, patients may have a variety of other arrhythmias including *antidromic reciprocating tachycardia* (conduction from the atrium to the ventricle via the accessory pathway and

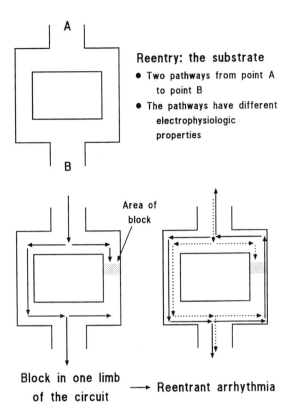

Reentry: the substrate
- Two pathways from point A to point B
- The pathways have different electrophysiologic properties

Area of block

Block in one limb of the circuit ⟶ Reentrant arrhythmia

Fig. 6–7. Reentry. The upper panel shows the "anatomic substrate" necessary to support reentry: two pathways with different electrophysiologic properties form a potential reentry circuit. Points A and B could be the atrium and ventricle and the two pathways could be the AV node and an accessory pathway (as in the Wolff-Parkinson-White syndrome), or the circuit may be as small as the AV node (AV nodal reentry tachycardia) or several millimeters of tissue at the rim of an old myocardial infarction (recurrent sustained ventricular tachycardia). As indicated in the bottom panel, the different electrophysiologic properties of the two pathways of the potential circuit can, under appropriate circumstances, result in block of impulse propagation in one limb (left). As this initially blocked impulse (dotted lines on the right) continues to propagate, reentry can occur (solid arrows) with the establishment of a tachycardia related to a continuously circulating wavefront.

from ventricle to atrium by the AV node), arrhythmias utilizing multiple bypass tracts, and atrial fibrillation. Atrial fibrillation can be particularly dangerous in patients with the Wolff-Parkinson-White syndrome since the normal decremental conduction seen in the AV node is absent in the accessory pathway and extraordinarily rapid ventricular rates can occur and lead to ventricular fibrillation (Klein et al., 1979).

Generally, it is not possible to identify those patients known to have Wolff-Parkinson-White syndrome (WPW) who are at high risk for life-threatening arrhythmias unless they have already had them (Hammill et al., 1986; Wellens et al., 1987; Sharma et al., 1987; Klein et al., 1989). The manifestations of the Wolff-Parkinson-White syndrome in a particular patient depend on the heterogeneity of refractory periods between the accessory pathway and the AV node (i.e., the likelihood an impulse can block in one route and be propagated in the other), the presence of multiple pathways, existing autonomic tone (which can affect predominantly AV nodal refractoriness), and the ventricular rate at which atrial fibrillation can be conducted via the accessory pathway. It is rarely simple to choose the right drugs to treat the arrhythmias of patents with WPW (McGovern et

al., 1986; Rickenberger, et al., 1988). Knowledge of the particular pathophysiology determining the type of arrhythmia in such patients is crucial for deciding upon appropriate therapy. Using this knowledge is especially important in those individuals subject to atrial fibrillation, since drugs usually used in this situation (e.g., digitalis, verapamil) decrease impulse propagation via the AV node but may paradoxically increase ventricular rate (Klein et al., 1979; Gulamhusein et al., 1982). *Principle: Drugs may be efficacious in some patients but produce toxicity in others because of special pathophysiologic considerations. It may be difficult for the physician to recognize that a drug usually effective in a disease actually exacerbates the clinical problem in an unusual patient. Unless the physician is aware of this possibility, he or she may naturally increase the dose of drug when symptoms worsen when discontinuing it would be the correct approach.*

Other sites at which arrhythmias thought to be caused by reentry may commonly occur are within the AV node (AV nodal reentrant tachycardia, often erroneously termed "paroxysmal atrial tachycardia" or PAT), at the rim of a healed myocardial infarction (sustained ventricular tachycardia), and macroreentry within the atrium (atrial flutter). Atrial fibrillation and ventricular fibrillation probably are specialized forms of reentry. One way of thinking about fibrillation is that each cell is immediately depolarized by electrical activity in its neighborhood as soon as it has repolarized sufficiently in phase 3 to be excited. Thus, cells are continuously being reexcited in random order, giving rise to typical electrocardiographic fibrillatory activity. In atrial fibrillation, the ventricular response is a primary determinant of symptoms and most often reflects AV nodal function. Rates in excess of 180 to 200 beats per minute are unusual in adults unless drugs that enhance AV nodal conduction are present (theophylline, catecholamines) or some structural electrophysiologic abnormality such as a bypass tract is present. On the other hand, atrial fibrillation with a ventricular response under 100 to 120 per minute in the absence of drugs suggests advanced conduction-system disease and is a warning to use special caution when drug therapy to reduce the rate is instituted. Ventricular fibrillation is the catastrophic lack of coordinated electrical activity that unless treated promptly by electrical defibrillation will result in death. Sudden cardiac death due to ventricular fibrillation occurs in 500,000 Americans every year. In some patients, ventricular fibrillation is the initial manifestation of an acute myocardial infarction, while in other patients, no underlying cause can be identified. If a patient with ventricular fibrillation is resuscitated, the risk of recurrence depends on why it occurred (Schaffer and Cobb, 1975). In patients with ischemia-mediated ventricular fibrillation, therapy directed at reversing myocardial ischemia is indicated while in patients with a primary arrhythmia, and antiarrhythmic drugs as well as mechanical devices such as the automatic implantable cardioverter defibrillator and specialized surgical procedures may be effective. This is another example of advances in the understanding of mechanisms having contributed to a rational approach to specific arrhythmias.

PRINCIPLES IN THE MANAGEMENT OF ARRHYTHMIAS

Identify Reversible Causes of Arrhythmias

Therapy with antiarrhythmic drugs is generally inappropriate if a readily reversible cause of an arrhythmia can be identified (Table 6–1). Several syndromes of antiarrhythmic-drug-induced arrhythmias have been extensively characterized at the clinical and basic levels and are discussed below. In addition, digitalis is a notorious precipitator of arrhythmias. *Principle: The physician should always remember that a chosen therapy may itself be responsible for an apparent failure to control a patient's arrhythmia.*

Table 6–1. REVERSIBLE CAUSES OF ARRHYTHMIAS

Drugs
  Digitalis
  Antiarrhythmics
  Theophylline
  Catecholamines
  Tricyclic antidepressants
  Phenothiazines
  Anorexiants
  Anesthetic agents
Myocardial Factors
  Ischemia
  Congestive heart failure
Other Disease
  Thyrotoxicosis
  Lung disease
  Cardiovascular injury
Metabolic Abnormalities
  Hypokalemia
  Hyperkalemia
  Hypomagnesemia
  Acidosis
  Alkalosis
  Hypoxia

Identify the Arrhythmia

There are very few arrhythmias for which urgent intervention in the absence of a diagnosis is ever justified. The most striking example is a patient who presents to an emergency room with wide-complex tachycardia (Fig. 6–8). In patients with coronary artery disease, wide complex tachycardia is almost always ventricular tachycardia, but it is very commonly misdiagnosed as supraventricular tachycardia with functional bundle branch block (Stewart et al., 1986; Buxton et al., 1987; Steinman et al., 1989). The misdiagnosis almost certainly stems from the widespread and mistaken impression that ventricular tachycardia causes immediate cardiovascular collapse. *Principle: Symptoms due to an arrhythmia do not provide information on underlying mechanisms.*

The distinction between supraventricular and ventricular mechanisms is critical because the use of verapamil (aimed against supraventricular mechanisms of arrhythmias) will result in cardiovascular collapse in patients with sustained ventricular tachycardia. Intravenous adenosine (which has recently become available) can terminate various supraventricular tachycardias, and, because it is eliminated with a half-life of seconds, may be safer than (and hence replace) verapamil in this setting (Rankin et al., 1989). The most important maneuver to help establish a diagnosis in a patient with wide complex tachycardia is an assessment of atrial electrical activity using 12-lead electrocardiography, esophagal electrocardiography, recording from the right atrium

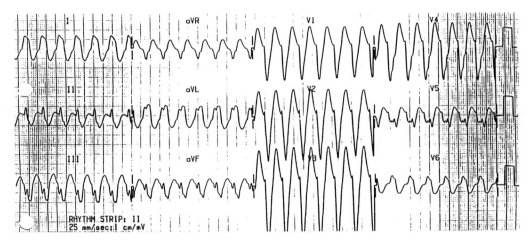

Fig. 6-8. Wide complex tachycardia. This rhythm could be ventricular tachycardia or any one of a number of mechanistically different supraventricular tachycardias with an unusual sequence of intraventricular activation. The distinction cannot be made from this electrocardiogram; likewise, the patient's clinical status (blood pressure, etc.) is not helpful. Treatment with verapamil should be avoided in this situation.

with an electrode catheter, or carotid sinus massage (Wellens, 1986). Finding atrial activity at a rate slower than the ventricular rate makes the diagnosis of ventricular tachycardia; on the other hand, atrial activity at twice the ventricular rate is characteristic of atrial flutter with 2:1 AV conduction. If the atrial rate is exactly the same as the ventricular rate, supraventricular arrhythmias or ventricular tachycardia are both possible. In patients with ventricular tachycardias, examination of the patterns of the QRS complex on the electrocardiogram can be helpful, although specialized intracardiac electrophysiologic evaluation may be required. If the patient is hypotensive or appears near hemodynamic deterioration, electrical cardioversion is the treatment of choice. If the patient appears stable, empiric treatment with procainamide (that often is effective in both ventricular and supraventricular arrhythmias) after collection of as much electrophysiologic data during the tachycardia as logistically feasible should be performed. *Principle: If time is available, do not guess (basis: a nondiagnostic standard ECG) if you can be certain (basis: esophageal or intracardiac leads). Drug therapy based on improper diagnosis could be ineffective and more dangerous than no therapy at all. On the other hand, in an emergency therapy that is least likely to be deleterious is the most appropriate strategy.*

Quantify the Arrhythmia

Prior to initiating therapy, it is important to establish the frequency and reproducibility of an arrhythmia. In general, arrhythmias are highly

sporadic events (Morganroth et al., 1978). In addition, the phenomenon of "ascertainment bias" will confound interpretation of any drug trial; that is, if arrhythmias increase and decrease in frequency spontaneously, it is likely that patients will present for clinical care at a time when their arrhythmia is increasing in frequency. Initiation of drug therapy is thus more likely to occur at a time when a natural "waning" of the frequency of arrhythmia is likely. Therapeutic trials involving antiarrhythmic drugs should include a placebo (see chapter 35). For example, patients presenting to an emergency room with acute-onset atrial fibrillation are frequently treated with digitalis. However, when the efficacy rate of digitalis was compared with that of placebo in this setting, both interventions were found to result in a 50% incidence of restoration of sinus rhythm within 4 hours (Falk et al., 1987).

Three methods generally are available to guide treatment: ambulatory monitoring, exercise testing, or electrophysiologic testing. In some instances, arrhythmias are sufficiently frequent that ambulatory monitoring for from 24 to 72 hours will establish baseline frequency of the arrhythmia, and treatment can then be guided by serial monitoring in the ambulatory setting. In other instances, arrhythmias are more infrequent. In some of these patients, exercise testing can provoke the arrhythmias and thus serve to guide drug therapy. In patients in whom paroxysms of sustained arrhythmias have been documented but in whom ambulatory monitoring and exercise testing are unhelpful, electrophysiologic techniques using multiple electrode catheters can be used to reproduce the patient's arrhythmia. Suppression of inducible arrhythmia can then serve as a surrogate end point to guide drug therapy (see chapter 41).

Assess the Potential Benefit of Treatment

Patients with a history of hemodynamic collapse due to ventricular tachycardia or who had an episode of cardiac arrest due to ventricular fibrillation are at high risk for sudden death. Treatment aimed at preventing recurrences and prolonging life is indicated. Patients with highly symptomatic supraventricular tachycardias may benefit from treatment due to symptomatic improvement. Similarly, patients with atrial fibrillation or atrial flutter, or even some patients with chronic ventricular ectopic beats, may benefit from drug treatment by a reduction of symptoms, although their long-term prognosis is probably unchanged (at best) by drug treatment.

Is the Benefit Greater Than the Risk?

The best-studied example here is treatment of minimally symptomatic ventricular ectopic beats in patients who have had a myocardial infarction. The presence of such ventricular ectopic beats is known to be a marker for an increased risk for sudden death (presumably ventricular fibrillation–related) (Ruberman et al., 1981). The Cardiac Arrhythmia Suppression Trial (CAST) tested the hypothesis that suppression of these ventricular arrhythmias in patients with a history of myocardial infarction would reduce the risk for sudden cardiac death. Patients whose arrhythmias were known to be responsive to drugs were assigned to drug treatment or a corresponding placebo, in a double-blind fashion. After less than 1 year of treatment, patients randomized to encainide or flecainide had a 2.5-fold increase in cardiovascular mortality compared with those randomized to placebo (CAST Investigators, 1989)! *Principle: Although many subsets of patients who might potentially benefit from antiarrhythmic therapy can be identified, in some the risk clearly outweighs the benefit.* A third drug, moricizine, continues to be tested in this population in CAST-II.

In other trials, antiarrhythmic drugs caused similar trends of increased mortality or too many side effects to test the utility of suppressing premature ventricular contractions. (Hine et al., 1989). Thus, treatment for these common arrhythmias cannot be justified by currently available data. The risks of antiarrhythmic therapy include adverse cardiac effects (arrhythmia aggravation, heart block, heart failure) and adverse noncardiac effects. Consideration of the potential

for such adverse noncardiac effects often is primary in selection of a drug (Table 6–2). For example, patients with inflammatory arthritis probably should not receive procainamide, since it would be difficult or impossible to distinguish an exacerbation of inflammatory arthritis from procainamide-induced lupus. Similarly patients with gastrointestinal disease probably should avoid quinidine, patients with prostatism should avoid disopyramide, patients with tremors should avoid mexiletine, and so forth. In addition to common adverse drug reactions such as those described above, some antiarrhythmic agents carry substantial risk: agranulocytosis with procainamide or tocainide, or quinidine-induced hepatitis or thrombocytopenia are examples.

How to Decide If a Drug Doesn't Work

Once a decision to initiate drug therapy is made, the physician should use all available means to assess the effects of treatment. This will include frequent evaluation of the patient, monitoring cardiac rhythm, electrocardiographic interval determinations, and measurement of drug concentrations in plasma. Ultimately, a drug can only be said to be ineffective if arrhythmias recur in the face of unacceptable drug-induced side effects. Drug-induced adverse effects may range from asymptomatic but prognostically ominous electrocardiographic changes, such as marked

Table 6–2. RELATIVE CONTRAINDICATIONS TO SPECIFIC ANTIARRHYTHMIC DRUGS

Noncardiac:	
GI disease	Quinidine
Prostatism, urinary retention, glaucoma	Disopyramide Procainamide
Inflammatory arthritis	Mexiletine, tocainide,
Tremor	lidocaine
Bronchospasm	β Blockers, propafenone
Pulmonary disease	Amiodarone
Young patient	Amiodarone, procainamide
Cardiac*	
Heart failure†	Disopyramide, flecainide,
Aortic stenosis, hypertrophic cardiomyopathy, pulmonary hypertension	β antagonists, verapamil Bretylium Class Ia, III
Long QT‡	

* All antiarrhythmics (especially class Ic agents) must be used cautiously in patients with disease of the conduction system in whom bradycardia and heart block with slow (unstable) escape rates can occur. In addition, *all antiarrhythmics have the potential to provoke arrhythmias.*

† *Development of heart failure can occur as well during treatment with any of the agents discussed in this chapter.*

‡ Amiodarone may be less likely to produce torsades de pointes than other QT-prolonging drugs.

increases in the QT interval with quinidine, to highly symptomatic drug-induced congestive heart failure, heart block, ventricular arrhythmias, or noncardiac adverse effects. If a patient is asymptomatic, no ominous electrocardiographic interval changes are recorded, and concentrations of drug in plasma are at the upper limits of the usual "therapeutic" range, dosages can be cautiously increased. An exception may be drugs whose most prominent and early toxicity is dose-related provocation of an arrhythmia (e.g., flecainide). In such a situation, the advised upper limits on dosages and plasma concentrations should be respected even in the absence of side effects.

Optimize Treatment By Use of Pharmacokinetic Principles

Urgent treatment of immediately life-threatening arrhythmias involves the use of drugs administered IV, usually with loading doses. In less urgent settings, loading doses should be avoided since they may increase the risk of an adverse drug effect. On account of wide interindividual variability in response to drugs, starting dosages (adjusted for concomitant disease if necessary) should always be as low as possible and the response of the patient evaluated at steady state prior to any increase in dose. The frequency of dosing of a drug is influenced both by the elimination half-life of the parent drug and active metabolites (if any) and by the width of the therapeutic range (see chapters 36 and 37). As mentioned above, the physician should also be aware of the drug toxicity anticipated beyond the upper limit of the usual therapeutic range, as well as that which may occur (particularly in susceptible individuals) at usual doses or concentrations in plasma (see chapter 37).

MECHANISMS OF ACTION OF ANTIARRHYTHMIC DRUGS

Most antiarrhythmic drugs block one or more cardiac ion channels as their primary mode of antiarrhythmic action. However, drugs may perturb autonomic function or produce noncardiac effects that can profoundly alter the response of an individual patient to drug therapy. A number of schemes have been developed to group antiarrhythmic drugs with common basic electrophysiologic effects or common clinical actions; the most common grouping (Table 6-3) is that proposed by Vaughan Williams (1989). Such schemes have some utility since the basic electrophysiologic effects of antiarrhythmic drugs can be used to predict clinical situations in which specific drugs are likely to be effective, as well as some cardiac side effects (in particular the aggravation of arrhythmia). *Principle: The connotation of a name—for example, antiarrhythmic drug, β blocker, "H₂ blocker"—should not lead the therapist to expect a priori identical pharmacologic, therapeutic, or toxic effects of all drugs similarly classified. The differences between these drugs may be clinically as important as or more important than their similarities.*

Blockade of cardiac sodium channels is the major electrophysiologic effect of the *class I* antiarrhythmic drugs. Sodium-channel blockade shifts the voltage dependence for recovery from inactivation to more negative potentials: this means that at any given voltage during phase 3 of the action potential, fewer sodium channels will have recovered from inactivation in the presence of drug than in the absence of drug. The time in phase 3 of an action potential at which enough sodium channels have recovered to allow impulse propagation (the effective refractory period) will be prolonged by these drugs. Some drugs, such as quinidine, also increase action potential duration; in this case, refractoriness will be even more greatly prolonged. On the other hand, lidocaine tends to shorten action potentials and therefore does not alter refractoriness to any great extent in normal tissue. Another in vivo effect of sodium-channel blockade is slowed propagation of impulses. Sufficient slowing of impulse propagation in reentrant circuits may result in failure of propagation and termination of the arrhythmia; on the other hand, conduction slowing promotes reentry and can also worsen arrhythmias. Sodium-channel blockers also depress automaticity in the His-Purkinje system and may suppress some arrhythmias related to abnormal automaticity. Finally, experimental evidence suggests that some sodium-channel blockers can be effective in certain types of abnormal automaticity seen in depolarized preparations.

Increasingly sophisticated methodology has allowed insights into the molecular mechanisms of blockade of the sodium channel. Experimental evidence suggests that drugs bind to a specific receptor-like site on proteins of the sodium channel to block the channel. The affinity of binding varies with the state (rest, open, inactivated) of the channel (Hille, 1977; Hondeghem and Katzung, 1977). Sodium-channel-blocking antiarrhythmic drugs may have high affinity for the open state (e.g., quinidine), the inactivated state (e.g., amiodarone), or both (e.g., lidocaine), but all available drugs have very low affinity for channels in the resting state. Thus at sufficiently slow rates, any of these drugs will dissociate from the channel between action potentials. If, on the other hand, the rate of stimulation is faster, some channels will remain blocked between action potentials. Therefore, blockade will increase at faster rates. This cumulation effect is termed

Table 6-3. CLASSIFICATION OF ANTIARRHYTHMIC DRUG ACTION

CLASS	DRUG	CLASS TOXICITY*	EFFICACY	ECG
I. *Sodium-Channel Blockers*				
Ia (recovery time constant 2–5 sec)	Quinidine Procainamide Disopyramide	Torsades de pointes	Atrial fibrillation Ventricular arrhythmias	↑QRS
Ib (recovery time constant <1 sec)	Lidocaine Mexiletine Tocainide	Tremor Psychosis	Ventricular arrhythmias	
Ic (recovery time constant <5 sec)	Flecainide Encainide Propafenone Moricizine Recainam	Incessant ventricular tachy- cardia Metallic taste	AV nodal reentry WPW-related arrhythmias Ventricular arrhythmias†	↑PR, ↑QRS
Incompletely categorized				
II. *β-Adrenergic Antagonists*	Propranolol and others Sotalol Propafenone	Heart failure Bronchospasm, etc. (see chapter 7)	Atrial fibrillation/flutter (Ventricular arrhythmias)	↑PR ↓heart rate
III. *Prolongation of the Action Potential*	Sotalol Amiodarone Bretylium	Torsades de pointes	Atrial fibrillation/flutter Ventricular arrhythmias	↑QT
IV. *AV Nodal Calcium-Channel Blockers*	Verapamil Diltiazem	Heart failure	Atrial fibrillation/flutter Atrial (and rare ventricular) automaticity AV nodal entry	↑PR ↓heart rate
Others				
Amiodarone			Atrial arrhythmias Ventricular arrhythmias	↑PR, ↑QRS ↑QT, ↓heart rate
Adenosine			AV nodal reentry Orthodromic tachychardia	
Digitalis			AV nodal reentry Atrial fibrillation/flutter	↑PR ↓heart rate

* See text for details.
† Can increase mortality despite suppressing arrhythmia (encainide, flecainide).
WPW = Wolff-Parkinson-White syndrome.

163

frequency- or use-dependent blockade. The net blockade at any given heart rate is a function of the rate at which drugs dissociate from open and/ or inactivated channels. The rate of dissociation, which is conveniently measured as a time constant of recovery from blockade (slower recovery (longer time constant) is also slower at depolarized potentials (*voltage-dependent* block). Thus, sodium-channel blockers exert their greatest electrophysiologic effects in tissue that is depolarized and rapidly driven (e.g., ischemic ventricular tachycardia). Subclassifying sodium-channel blockers by their time constants of recovery (Table 6–3) from blockade provides a workable scheme that groups drugs with similar electrophysiologic effects (Campbell, 1983). This approach of relating basic electrophysiologic effects to the clinical actions of antiarrhythmic drugs may require revision. In each section that follows, general actions (including toxicity) of each subclass are outlined, followed by a discussion of the pharmacology, pharmacokinetics, drug interactions, and toxicity of the individual agents. *Principle: The large number of antiarrhythmic agents makes the challenge to classify them irresistible. Nevertheless, the classifications are based on the dominant but by no means the full spectrum of efficacious actions of each drug. While the classifications are helpful in primary selection of a given drug for a given setting, they are based primarily on observations of in vitro electrophysiology and cannot lead to definitive decisions about the utility of most drugs in complex or drug-resistant arrhythmias.*

THE DRUGS

Class Ia: Quinidine, Procainamide, Disopyramide

The time constants for recovery from blockade for this subclass of drug are 2 to 5 seconds. As a consequence of their sodium-channel-blocking properties, treatment with class Ia drugs may result in mild degrees of prolongation of the QRS interval, particularly during fast heart rates, at high concentrations of drug in plasma, or in the presence of underlying disease in the conduction system (Tables 6–4 and 6–5). Class Ia drugs also prolong cardiac repolarization, probably by interfering with outward (repolarizing) potassium currents (Roden et al., 1989). As a consequence, prolongation of the QT interval also occurs with this group of drugs. Class Ia drugs are useful in a wide range of supraventricular and ventricular tachyarrhythmias. In particular, these are among the drugs of choice for conversion to or maintenance of sinus rhythm in patients with atrial flutter or atrial fibrillation (Table 6–6).

Toxicity of Class Ia Drugs. The use of very high doses of quinidine or procainamide, as was the practice for the conversion of atrial fibrillation in the 1950s, may be accompanied by marked widening of the QRS and induction of ventricular tachycardia that may be difficult to convert to normal rhythm (Wetherbee et al., 1951). In experimental animals and in some anecdotes in humans, infusions of sodium (lactate, bicarbonate, or chloride) are effective in treating the drug-induced ventricular arrhythmia (Cox et al., 1961). This tachycardia may result from excess slowing of conduction with resultant establishment of re-entrant tachycardia circuits. This syndrome is very rarely seen with the contemporary use of class Ia drugs since the agents are no longer "pushed" to toxicity to convert atrial fibrillation and since guidelines for monitoring the concentration of drug in plasma are now available to avoid extremely high concentrations. A similar syndrome has, however, reemerged with the class Ic agents.

Class Ia drugs used in patients with advanced conduction system disease may precipitate second- or third-degree heart block with very slow ventricular responses. Treatment of atrial flutter with quinidine alone can also result in a largely predictable and avoidable form of electrophysiologic toxicity. The untreated patient with atrial flutter most often has atrial rates of approximately 300/min with ventricular responses in a 2 : 1 ratio, approximately 150/min. Use of quinidine alone in this setting results in slowing of atrial flutter to rates of approximately 200/min. Since quinidine has vagolytic actions in humans, AV nodal conduction is not perturbed and may actually be enhanced by quinidine. In addition decremental conduction in the AV node is less at an impulse entry rate of 200/min. As a result, atrial flutter at 200/min will be conducted to the ventricle in a 1 : 1 ratio, increasing the ventricular rate from 150/min to 200/min. This form of electrophysiologic toxicity can be avoided by administering an AV nodal blocking agent, such as digitalis, verapamil, or a β-adrenergic antagonist, before using quinidine. Similar aggravation of arrhythmia is a theoretical risk with procainamide and disopyramide and has been reported with lidocaine.

Torsades de pointes is a distinctive polymorphic ventricular tachycardia seen with prolongation of the action potential. As discussed above, this syndrome appears to be most closely related to development of early afterdepolarizations and triggered automaticity in the Purkinje network (Roden et al., 1986; Cranefield and Aronson, 1988; Jackman et al., 1988). Heterogeneity of refractoriness also may be important particularly for the maintenance of the tachycardia following

Table 6–4.   DRUGS FOR IV THERAPY FOR ARRHYTHMIAS

DRUG	ADMINISTRATION		"THERAPEUTIC" PLASMA CONCENTRATION (μg/ml)	DOSAGE ADJUSTMENT
	LOADING	MAINTENANCE		

Lidocaine	3–4 mg/kg (see text and Fig. 6–10)	1–4 mg/min (see Fig. 6–11)	1.5–5	↓loading: heart failure
				↓maintenance:
				    Heart failure
				    Liver disease
				    Infusion >24 h
				    Cimetidine
				    Propranolol

Bretylium	5–30 mg/kg	1–4 mg/min		? Renal disease
Procainamide	10–20 mg/kg (20 mg/min)	1–4 mg/min	4–10	↓maintenance: Renal disease
Verapamil	1–10 mg			
Adenosine	2–20 mg			
Esmolol	500 μg/kg (in-fused at 50 μg/kg/min)	100–300 μg/kg		Infusion rate can be increased to 100–300 μg/kg/min at increments of 50 with a bolus dose (500 μg/kg) preceding each increment.
Propranolol	1–5 mg			

its initiation (Kuo et al., 1985). The most common clinical situations associated with torsades are quinidine therapy, diuretic-associated hypokalemia, or hypomagnesemia. About half the patients who develop drug-induced torsades are receiving antiarrhythmic therapy for management of atrial fibrillation or flutter and the other half for ventricular arrhythmias. In patients with atrial fibrillation or flutter who develop torsades, the arrhythmia almost inevitably develops after conversion to normal rhythm. The electrocardiogram shows stereotypical changes at the initiation of the tachycardia (Fig. 6–9). A ventricular ectopic beat or an episode of tachycardia is followed by an appropriate posttachycardia pause and a (normal) supraventricular beat. This supraventricular beat is then followed by a markedly prolonged QT interval, and the tachycardia almost inevitably develops after the peak of the T wave; in some cases, the repolarization complex on the surface electrocardiogram assumes a bizarre appearance with multiple "late diastolic" waves that may represent multiple giant U waves. Most episodes of torsades de pointes are self-limited, but the arrhythmia occasionally becomes sustained or may degenerate to sustained monomorphic ventricular tachycardia or to ventricular fibrillation.

The most important step in the management of a patient with torsades is to recognize the arrhythmia. Appropriate treatment then consists of withdrawal of the offending agent, correction of hypokalemia, administration of magnesium (even to the nonhypomagnesemic patient), and, if necessary, maneuvers to increase heart rate (pacing, infusion of isoproterenol). Prolonged episodes respond to DC cardioversion.

Interestingly, high concentrations of quinidine in plasma are not necessary to elicit torsades; the mechanism whereby some patients happen to be particularly sensitive to the QT-interval prolonging effects of quinidine is uncertain. For

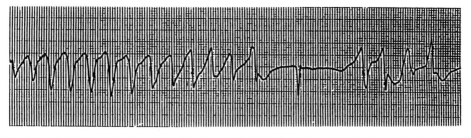

Fig. 6–9. Quinidine-related torsades de pointes. The initiation of an episode of torsades de pointes is shown here. A four-beat run of tachycardia is followed by an appropriate posttachycardia pause, and a sinus beat. The QT of this sinus beat is very long (almost 0.8 sec), and the episode of torsades de pointes starts after the peak of this prolonged T wave.

Table 6-5. DRUGS FOR CHRONIC ORAL THERAPY FOR ARRHYTHMIAS

DRUG	USUAL DOSAGES	MAJOR ROUTES OF ELIMINATION	ELIMINATION $t_{1/2}$	RANGE OF THERAPEUTIC PLASMA CONCENTRATION (µg/ml)	MAJOR DOSE ADJUSTMENT	
					LOWER DOSE	MAY REQUIRE ↑ DOSE
Quinidine	200-600 mg q8h (sulfate) 324-648 mg q8h (glucuronide)	Hepatic (20% renal)	6-12 h	2-5	(Cimetidine)	Inducers of hepatic metabolism* Acute MI (↑ protein binding)
Procainamide	500-1500 mg q6h (slow-release formation) N-acetyl procainamide† (NAPA)	Hepatic/renal Renal	3 h 6-10 h	4-10 10-20	Renal disease	
Disopyramide	100-200 mg q6h (300 mg q12h slow-release)	Renal/hepatic	6 h	2-5 (variable free fraction)	Renal disease	Inducers of hepatic metabolism*
Mexiletine	100-300 mg q8h	Hepatic	11-15 h	0.5-2.0	Hepatic disease	Inducers of hepatic metabolism*
Tocainide	200-800 mg q8-12h	Renal/hepatic	8-20 h	3-11	Renal disease	Inducers of hepatic metabolism*
Flecainide	100-200 mg q12h	Renal	20 h	0.2-1.0	Renal disease	
Encainide‡	25-50 mg q8h	Hepatic/renal			Renal disease	
Propafenone†	150-300 mg q8h	Hepatic/renal				
Amiodarone	1-2 g/day initially tapering to 200-400 mg/day over several months		≥weeks	1-2		
Sotalol	80-480 mg q12h	Renal	8-12 h	0.5-3.0	Renal disease	

* Phenytoin, rifampin, barbiturates.
† NAPA has different electrophysiologic properties from procainamide, and its concentrations during procainamide therapy should be considered separately.
‡ Drug disposition depends on genetically determined oxidative phenotype (see text), although similar doses are effective in extensive and poor metabolizers.

Table 6–6.   DRUGS OF CHOICE FOR MANAGING ARRHYTHMIAS

	ACUTE*	CHRONIC
Atrial fibrillation or flutter		
Rate control	Digitalis, verapamil, β Blockers	Same
Maintenance of sinus rhythm		Quinidine,† procainamide disopyramide, flecainide,† encainide,† propafenone, sotalol, amiodarone
AV Nodal Reentry	Adenosine Verapamil β Blockers	Digitalis, verapamil, β blockers, class Ic agents
Arrhythmias in the Wolff-Parkinson-White Syndrome		
Orthodromic reciprocating	Adenosine Verapamil β Blockers	Class Ia ± AV nodal blocker Class Ic Avoid digitalis or verapamil alone as empiric therapy
Atrial fibrillation with preexcited ventricular complexes	Procainamide	Procainamide Quinidine Class Ic Bypass tract ablation
Automatic Atrial Tachycardia		
Rate control	AV nodal blockers	Verapamil
Restoration of sinus rhythm		Class Ia Class Ic
Premature Ventricular Beats and Nonsustained Ventricular Arrhythmias		
Asymptomatic		None
Symptomatic		β blockers Class Ia‡ Class Ic‡
Sustained ventricular tachycardia	Lidocaine Procainamide Bretylium	Class Ia (alone or with β blocker or with Class Ib) Amiodarone Class Ic
Ventricular fibrillation	Lidocaine Procainamide Bretylium	None if episode caused by acute ischemia; as for sustained ventricular tachycardia if unassociated with ischemia
Undiagnosed wide complex tachycardia	Procainamide Lidocaine ?Adenosine Avoid verapamil	
Narrow complex tachycardia	Adenosine Verapamil	

* Acute treatment can include DC cardioversion for sustained arrhythmias causing hemodynamic compromise. Exacerbating factors should always be sought and eliminated. Pacing therapies may also be effective for regular (nonfibrillatory) rhythms.
† Therapy with quinidine, flecainide, or encainide in atrial flutter can increase ventricular rate if AV nodal blockers are not used as well prior to conversion to sinus rhythm (see text).
‡ Class I agents (especially Ic) may increase mortality despite suppressing symptoms.

procainamide, accumulation of high concentrations of the active metabolite *N*-acetyl procainamide, discussed further below, appears to be important in the genesis of torsades.

Quinidine. The Dutch physician Wenckebach (1923) related that he had been consulted by a merchant with paroxysmal atrial fibrillation who had frequented the far east and had found that an extract of the bark of the antimalarial cinchona plant was effective in preventing his episodes of arrhythmia. Subsequent work (Frey, 1918) demonstrated that quinidine, an isomer of the antimalarial quinine, was the most effective of the agents extracted in suppressing experimental arrhythmias. ***Principle: Listen to what the patient tells you.***

A number of formulations of quinidine are available, and some have the advantage that they maintain concentrations of drug in plasma at the therapeutic range even when taken twice daily. Most patients will not have an antiarrhythmic effect with concentrations of quinidine in plasma of less than 1 to 1.5 μg/ml, while dose-related toxicity, including a syndrome known as *cinchonism* (tinnitus, headache), and ventricular tachycardia are increasing risks at drug concentrations in plasma greater than 5 μg/ml. Quinidine is biotransformed in the liver to at least four metabolites, all of which have pharmacologic activities similar to that of the parent drug but appear less potent (Thompson et al., 1987). Approximately 20% of the parent drug is excreted by the kidneys (Conrad et al., 1977). The doses required to achieve concentrations in the therapeutic range and to suppress arrhythmias in patients with congestive heart failure or in patients with advanced renal disease do not appear substantially different from those required in patients without disease (Kessler et al., 1974). Quinidine is bound to both albumin and α_1 acid glycoprotein. The concentration of α_1 acid glycoprotein, an acute-phase reactant, rises in acute illnesses such as myocardial infarction, cardiac surgery, and trauma; consequently, protein binding of quinidine is increased, the free fraction is decreased, and the pharmacologic effects may be absent or blunted at "usual" plasma concentrations in these acute settings (Kessler et al., 1984).

QUINIDINE DRUG INTERACTIONS. One of the most spectacular drug interactions in cardiovascular medicine is that between quinidine and digitalis (Bigger, 1982). Although quinidine has been used since the 1920s and digitalis glycosides for over 2 centuries, it was only in the late 1970s that the significant interaction between the two was recognized and described. When quinidine therapy is initiated in a patient receiving digitalis, digoxin clearance falls and digoxin accumulates in plasma; in general, plasma concentrations of digoxin can be expected to double with an attendant risk of toxicity, most often manifest as nausea and ventricular bigeminy. The interaction also occurs with digitoxin. ***Principle: Drugs can interact at many sites (protein binding, elimination, receptors, etc); assuming that a drug interaction is not present because it hasn't yet been reported is naive and ignores one of the more important and rewarding challenges in therapeutics.***

Quinidine recently has been shown to be a potent inhibitor of one particular hepatic cytochrome, $P450_{db1}$ (Speirs et al., 1986). This enzyme catalyzes the oxidation of a number of β-adrenergic antagonists (including metoprolol and propranolol), antiarrhythmics (encainide and propafenone, discussed further below), and the model substrate debrisoquin, an antihypertensive drug (Eichelbaum, 1982; Eichelbaum, 1988; Roden, 1988). At doses as low as 50 mg every 8 hours, quinidine inhibits $P450_{db1}$-mediated biotransformation of these substrates. The accumulation of parent drug can lead to altered pharmacologic effects. In the case of propranolol, coadministration of low-dose quinidine resulted in increased β

blockade (Zhou et al., 1989). For encainide and propafenone, the situation is more complicated, since both drugs have active metabolites (Funck-Brentano et al.; 1989a, 1989b); in this case, inhibition biotransformation of parent drug biotransformation by quinidine results in accumulation of parent drug that partially offsets the decrease in formation of active metabolites. As discussed further below, a small subset of patients has been identified who lack functional $P450_{db1}$ on a genetic basis. In this group, quinidine has no effect on drug disposition.

Quinidine clearance is strikingly increased when agents that induce hepatic metabolism (phenytoin, phenobarbital, rifampin) are administered (Data et al., 1975; Twun-Barima and Carruthers, 1981). In this case, therapeutic plasma concentrations can be achieved only by using very high dosages of quinidine. If this is done, the dose of quinidine must be decreased if the hepatic enzyme-inducing agent is subsequently discontinued. Clearance of quinidine is decreased by cimetidine; the magnitude of this effect appears modest in normal human volunteers, and its clinical implications are not yet apparent (Hardy et al., 1983). Verapamil also appears to inhibit clearance of quinidine, which may partially account for a reported beneficial effect of combining verapamil with quinidine (Hunt et al., 1989).

QUINIDINE TOXICITY. Aside from the electrophysiologic toxicities described above, diarrhea is the major limiting factor during chronic therapy with quinidine. The mechanism of quinidine-induced diarrhea is unknown, and the effect appears to be unrelated to dose. Quinidine can also cause immune-based hepatitis and thrombocytopenia. The latter generally recurs upon rechallenge with quinidine or quinine.

Procainamide. Procainamide was introduced into clinical practice in the 1950s and has electrophysiologic properties in common with quinidine. Concentrations in plasma less than 4 μg/ml generally are not associated with an antiarrhythmic effect, while concentrations greater than 8 to 10 μg/ml are associated with increasing incidences of primarily GI side effects. In addition to its use as chronic oral therapy, procainamide can be administered IV for prompt control of arrhythmias that require acute termination.

Procainamide undergoes hepatic N-acetylation to the major metabolite N-acetyl procainamide (NAPA). The distribution of hepatic N-acetyl transferase activity is polymorphic, and about half of whites can be classified as "rapid" acetylators while the other half are "slow" acetylators (Drayer and Reidenberg, 1977). A NAPA/procainamide concentration ratio greater than 1.0 at the end of a dosing interval during chronic oral therapy in the absence of renal disease classifies a patient as "rapid" acetylator. Both procainamide and NAPA are eliminated by the kidney and probably compete with each other for renal elimination by the base transport system (Funck-Brentano et al., 1989c). Because procainamide has a very short elimination half-life (2–3 hours), and because of the relatively narrow range between concentrations that are associated with efficacy and those that are associated with toxicity, the drug must be administered about every 3 hours to maintain therapeutic plasma concentrations. The development of sustained-release formations now permits dosing every 6 to 8 hours. Dosages of procainamide dosages must be reduced and the dosing interval increased in patients with renal failure. Indeed, in patients with renal insufficiency, therapeutic monitoring of procainamide plasma concentrations should be combined with measurements of NAPA since the concentration of NAPA may be unpredictably high in this setting.

The antiarrhythmic activity of NAPA (also known as acecainide) has been evaluated in humans (Roden et al., 1980a). At concentrations greater than 9 μg/ml, NAPA suppresses chronic ventricular arrhythmias, while GI side effects are very common at concentrations greater than 20 μg/ml. Arrhythmias that are responsive to procainamide do not necessarily respond to NAPA, and vice versa; this lack of concordance is likely due to the fact that NAPA has different electrophysiologic effects than procainamide (much weaker sodium-channel blocker). Most importantly, the N-acetyl substitution appears to eliminate the propensity for procainamide-induced lupus, discussed further below. Hence, although NAPA is not particularly well tolerated during chronic therapy, its structure has served as a template for synthesis of other agents with similar electrophysiologic properties that currently are in clinical trials (Lumma et al., 1987).

PROCAINAMIDE TOXICITY. High concentrations of procainamide are associated with GI upset and malaise. Procainamide also appears to be associated with a 0.2% incidence of agranulocytosis that, if untreated, can be fatal. The most prominent immunologic side effect of procainamide therapy is the development of a lupus syndrome. Procainamide-induced lupus is significantly more common among patients with the slow-acetylator phenotype (Woosley et al., 1978). The biochemical mechanism underlying the lupus syndrome is uncertain, but oxidation at the aromatic amine of procainamide appears to be important. Thus, N-acetylation at this site (to NAPA) is protective and accounts for the lower incidence of lupus among rapid acetylators. Antinuclear antibodies are ubiquitous during procainamide therapy and are not themselves an indication to discontinue the drug. The most common symptoms of procainamide-induced lupus are malaise, rash, and arthralgias. If the drug is not stopped at this point, other manifestations of the lupus syndrome such as arthritis, pleuropericarditis, and so forth, may develop, although nephritis is distinctly unusual.

Disopyramide. Disopyramide became available in the United States in the late 1970s (Koch-Weser, 1979b). It undergoes hepatic metabolism and renal excretion, and both hepatic disease and renal dysfunction require reduction of dosage. A tentative therapeutic range of 2 to 5 μg/ml has been proposed. However, disopyramide is bound to plasma proteins in a concentration-related fashion (Lima et al., 1981). Thus, *small increments in dose may lead to large increments in the free fraction.* It has been suggested that sustained-release formulations of the drug may reduce the incidence of side effects by preventing large swings in free plasma concentrations in a dosing interval, although this has not been clearly established.

DISOPYRAMIDE TOXICITY. Disopyramide has prominent anticholinergic side effects that account for most of its dose-limiting adverse effects. These include dry mouth, dry eyes, precipitation of glaucoma, constipation, and urinary retention. The latter is most often seen in males with prostatism, although it can occur in women. Congestive heart failure has been reported to occur in over 50% of patients treated with disopyramide who had a previous history of congestive heart failure. The incidence of congestive heart failure is approximately 3% in patients without a history of failure (Podrid et al., 1980).

Class Ib: Lidocaine, Mexiletine, Tocainide

These agents have short time constants (200–800 msec) of recovery from sodium-channel blockade, so that prolongation of the QRS interval is not a characteristic feature of therapy with class Ib agents. The drugs tend to shorten action potentials and are useful in ventricular, but not supraventricular, arrhythmias. Concentration-related CNS side effects (dysarthria, dizziness, nausea, convulsions, tremor, psychosis) occur with all three, and aggravation of the arrhythmia is unusual. The anticonvulsant phenytoin (chapter 12) also appears to have "class Ib" electrophysiologic properties. Carefully administered IV phenytoin can effectively control some ventricular arrhythmias and has been proposed as a "specific" treatment for digitalis-related arrhythmias (Stone et al., 1971). However other therapies, such as lidocaine, may be equally effective and have less potential for hemodynamic destabilization.

Lidocaine. Lidocaine has traditionally been considered the drug of first choice for the acute management of life-threatening ventricular tachyarrhythmias. In addition, IV lidocaine clearly reduces the incidence of ventricular fibrillation in patients admitted to a coronary care unit with known or suspected myocardial infarction (Lie et al., 1974). However, although lidocaine reduces the incidence of ventricular fibrillation, recent reanalyses of the effects of lidocaine have strongly suggested that therapy is associated with increased mortality (Yusuf et al., 1988). The reason for this outcome is not known. Since patients who develop ventricular fibrillation in the coronary care unit are readily treated, an argument might be made to avoid prophylactic lidocaine. *Principle: Drugs have multiple actions. Acute suppression of an obvious threat (arrhythmia) cannot simply be assumed to equate with an improved overall prognosis. Controlled trials are necessary to evaluate the risk/benefit ratio. Lacking proper studies, physicians must recognize that their own and others' "clinical experience" is biased.*

Relevant Clinical Pharmacokinetics. Following the rapid IV administration of lidocaine, its concentrations in plasma decline biexponentially (Boyes et al., 1971); this observation is consistent with a two-compartment open model of drug disposition, with elimination occurring from the central compartment. The initial half-life, that thought to correspond to drug distribution from the central to the peripheral compartment, is approximately 8 minutes in normal volunteers, while the terminal-phase half-life corresponding to drug elimination is 120 minutes.

Lidocaine is one of the few drugs with which loading doses are generally used; this is the case since lidocaine is frequently administered for prompt control of arrhythmias (Fig. 6–10). When a loading dose is used, a maintenance infusion should be started at the same time. If single loading doses of 75 to 100 mg are used, concentrations in plasma attain the therapeutic range (1.5–5 μg/ml) promptly, but "dip" into the theoretically subtherapeutic range prior to attaining steady state determined by the maintenance infusion. If a larger loading dose, such as 300 mg is used, toxic concentrations in plasma that are most often associated with convulsions can result. Thus, for optimal lidocaine loading, a reasonable scheme is to administer the 200- to 300-mg "loading dose" as intermittent small boluses every distribution half-life (e.g., 100 mg initially, followed by 50 mg at 8, 16, and 24 minutes) or as a single small bolus (100 mg) followed by a rapid infusion (e.g., 8 mg/min for 20 minutes) followed by a maintenance infusion. Regardless of the exact method by which the total loading dose is administered, the physician should remain with the patient so that early lidocaine toxicity, such as dysarthria or dizziness, can be recognized and the loading regimen modified appropriately (Riddell et al., 1983). *Principle: Toxicity appearing after prolonged administration of a drug is likely to last longer than toxicity occurring after the first or second dose (when redistribution rather than elimination can play a determining role).*

The steady-state plasma concentration (C_{pss}) achieved during maintenance infusion is a function solely of the maintenance dose and clearance of lidocaine (C_{pss} = infusion rate/clearance). Assuming that the volume of distribution remains constant, the aim of the loading strategies is to rapidly achieve and maintain concentrations at a desired C_{pss}. If, however, the maintenance infusion rate is excessive, concentrations in the plasma will gradually increase, attaining a steady state after 8 to 10 hours (4–5 elimination half-lives). In this case, lidocaine toxicity frequently manifests as mental disturbance and can be misdiagnosed as "CCU psychosis." If, on the other hand, the maintenance infusion rate is too low, arrhythmias may recur 8 to 10 hours after initiation of apparently effective therapy; in this case, resistance to lidocaine may be misdiagnosed. In either case, the appropriate therapeutic maneuver is to recognize the potential contribution of fluctuating concentrations of lidocaine in plasma to the clinical picture, measure those concentrations, and adjust lidocaine therapy appropriately (Fig. 6–11). *Principle: Use an understanding of the determinants of drug disposition to help form a mental picture of the time course of drug concentrations, which can then be used to help interpret a patient's clinical state and suggest need for monitoring drug concentrations.*

Congestive heart failure reduces the central volume of distribution and the clearance of lidocaine; in this instance, both the magnitude of the loading dose and the size of the maintenance infusion should be decreased (Thompson et al., 1973). Advanced liver disease alters lidocaine clearance. In this case, the maintenance dose should be decreased, but no adjustment of the loading regimen is required. Lidocaine's clearance falls during prolonged infusion of lidocaine; the explanation is uncertain, but competition by metabolites for lidocaine-metabolizing sites on hepatic oxidizing enzymes may play a role (LeLorier et al., 1977). Alternatively, liver blood flow may be reduced by chronic infusion of lidocaine. Propranolol reduces liver blood flow and decreases lidocaine's clearance, mandating the use of smaller maintenance infusions to avoid toxicity. Lidocaine is bound to α_1 acid glycoprotein, so, as with quinidine, the free fraction of lidocaine falls in acute myocardial infarction. As well, in some patients,

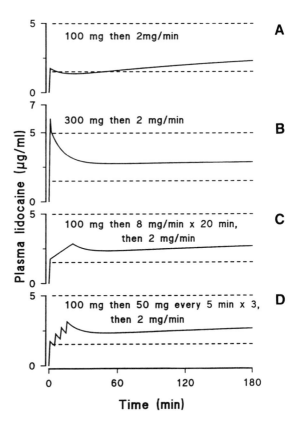

Fig. 6-10. Strategies for loading dose of lidocaine. In each of the four panels, the loading dose is shown; each loading dose was followed by a maintenance infusion of 2 mg/min. The range of usually therapeutic concentrations of lidocaine in plasma (1.5–5 mg/ml) is indicated by the dashed lines. (A) A single loading dose of 100 mg transiently achieves concentrations in the usual therapeutic range but is followed by a "dip" before the maintenance infusion reestablishes therapeutic concentration. If a larger single bolus is used (B), the "dip" is avoided, but toxic plasma concentrations may result. Two different methods (C and D) for administering an appropriate loading regimen over 20 to 25 minutes.

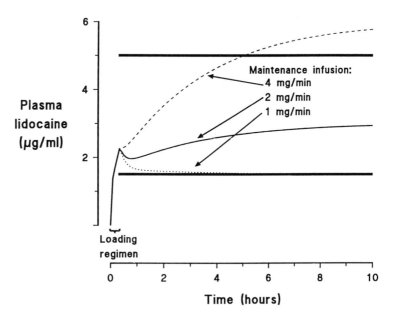

Fig. 6-11. The use of a loading dose does not alter the steady state achieved by a maintenance infusion (see chapters 37 and 38). Lidocaine is used as an example here. If concentrations within the usual therapeutic range (indicated by the heavy bars) are promptly established by a loading regimen, an excessive maintenance infusion rate may result in toxic concentrations several hours later (dashed line). Alternatively, if the maintenance infusion rate is too low (dotted line), plasma concentrations may fall into the subtherapeutic range several hours after the initiation of apparently effective therapy. The effect of a given infusion rate will not be completely expressed until at least 4 to 5 half-lives of the drug pass.

plasma concentrations of lidocaine well above the upper limit of the usual therapeutic range (e.g., 5–9 μg/ml) are required to suppress arrhythmias and yet do not produce adverse effects (Alderman et al., 1974).

Lidocaine undergoes extensive hepatic metabolism to the deethylated metabolites monoethylglycinexylidide and glycinexylidide (GX) that probably contribute to some of the toxicity of acute lidocaine therapy. The metabolites are themselves weak sodium-channel blockers, and there is some evidence that GX may displace lidocaine from binding sites on sodium channels (Bennett et al., 1988). Thus, prolonged infusion of lidocaine may be associated with decreased efficacy via this mechanism. *Principle: A lack of linearity between drug dose and steady-state concentrations of pharmacologically active drug in plasma require careful clinical assessment of the clinical response when changes in dosage are made. This becomes particularly true when factors of therapy or the dynamics of the disease itself contribute to the nonlinearity.*

Mexiletine and Tocainide. Lidocaine at acceptable doses is not effective after oral administration because of extensive first-pass hepatic metabolism. However, there are structural analogs of lidocaine that do not undergo extensive first-pass hepatic metabolism and also have longer elimination half-lives (8–12 hours). As a consequence, chronic oral therapy with these analogs (2–4 doses per day) is feasible (Roden, 1985). Their electrophysiologic properties are similar to those of lidocaine. Mexiletine undergoes hepatic metabolism (which is inducible by agents such as phenytoin, etc.), while tocainide is partially metabolized and partially cleared by the kidney. Dosage adjustments in patients with hepatic and renal disease, respectively, are required. Neither drug has prominent active metabolites. Mexiletine and tocainide have similar toxicities that include tremor, dizziness, and disturbances of CNS function. In addition, tocainide is associated with approximately 0.2% incidence of potentially fatal agranulocytosis.

Class Ic: Encainide, Flecainide, Propafenone

These sodium-channel blockers have very long time constants for recovery from frequency-dependent block (greater than 10 seconds). From a practical point of view, therefore, very little recovery from block occurs during a diastolic interval, even at physiologically slow heart rates. Widening of the PR and QRS intervals are the electrocardiographic hallmarks of therapy. Minor degrees of prolongation of the QT interval may also be seen. Class Ic drugs generally prolong atrial and ventricular refractoriness modestly (Roden and Woosley, 1986; Woosley et al., 1988; Funck-Brentano et al., 1990).

In addition to these electrophysiologic effects, class Ic agents also have similar antiarrhythmic activity. Chronic nonsustained ventricular arrhythmias are readily suppressed by class Ic drugs. Sustained ventricular tachycardia is less responsive to treatment. Moreover, as outlined further below, it is in patients receiving class Ic drugs for sustained ventricular tachycardia that one form of aggravation of the arrhythmia is most likely to occur. Class Ic drugs are also highly effective in automatic atrial tachycardia, AV nodal reentrant tachycardia, and arrhythmias related to the Wolff-Parkinson-White syndrome and appear to be as effective as quinidine-like drugs for maintenance of sinus rhythm in patients with atrial fibrillation.

Class Ic Electrophysiologic Toxicity. Interestingly, electrophysiologic toxicity accompanying class Ic therapy usually is not accompanied by marked widening of the QRS complex. Even when widening occurs, most patients tolerate 25% widening of their QRS complex without symptoms. There are no firm guidelines on what degree of QRS complex widening is unacceptably dangerous. Most would limit the widening to less than 30% to 40% over control. Therapy with class Ic drugs is regularly accompanied by marked prolongation of the PR interval. In individuals with conduction-system disease, these drugs can cause bundle-branch block and advanced degrees of AV block. Exercise-related bundle branch block that may be a manifestation of frequency-dependent sodium-channel block also can also occur.

Patients with recurrent sustained ventricular tachycardia are particularly susceptible to class Ic–induced aggravation of their arrhythmia. This is manifest as a marked increase in episodes of tachycardia, change in hemodynamic symptoms with tachycardia (i.e., hypotension in the presence of drug when it was not present in the absence of drug), and difficulty with cardioversion. Deaths due to nonresuscitable ventricular tachycardia have been reported (Winkle et al., 1981; Morganroth and Horowitz, 1984). A likely mechanism is slowing of conduction without commensurate increases in refractoriness, enabling reentrant circuits. Some series have reported an incidence of up to 20% with encainide or flecainide. The complication appears to be dose-related (>400 mg/day for flecainide; greater than 200 mg/day for encainide) but can occur in patients receiving "usual" dosages and with "usual" concentrations in plasma. Preliminary data suggest a role for sodium loading (Chouty et al., 1987) or

β-adrenergic blockade (Myerburg et al., 1989) in the management of this toxicity.

Marked slowing of conduction also underlies two other syndromes of arrhythmia aggravation seen with the class Ic drugs. One is slowing of atrial flutter with resultant 1:1 conduction, similar to that seen with quinidine (Crijns et al., 1988). Since QRS complexes are widened by drug and by the fast rate, this arrhythmia is very frequently misdiagnosed as ventricular tachycardia. The second syndrome is drug-induced slowing of intraventricular conduction in patients with orthodromic reciprocating tachycardia, resulting in increased frequency of episodes of slow tachycardia.

Far and away the most disturbing form of electrophysiologic toxicity produced by encainide and flecainide is the increased death rate with these drugs recorded in the CAST (CAST Investigators, 1989). The increased mortality persisted during 1 year of treatment and was present in all subgroups examined. This syndrome, unlike other forms of arrhythmia exacerbated by drugs discussed in this chapter, did not occur early after initiation of drug. The mechanism of the increased mortality in the CAST is uncertain, but a likely explanation is that transient events, such as recurrent myocardial ischemia, stretch, or neurohormonal activation, interacted with antiarrhythmic drugs and the myocardial scar in these patients to provoke arrhythmias, presumably related to drug-induced slow conduction. From a practical point of view, the use of encainide and flecainide in patients with nonsustained ventricular arrhythmias and a history of myocardial infarction clearly is inappropriate. Very limited data on safety suggest that death rates with these drugs in patients with normal hearts (e.g., those being treated for supraventricular arrhythmias) are small. Nevertheless, the results of the CAST study have dampened the enthusiasm for the use of encainide and flecainide in any setting and, by extension (appropriate or not), for other agents with similar electrophysiologic properties.

Encainide. In most patients, the elimination half-life of encainide is approximately 3 hours. The observation that a small subset of patients have unusually long elimination half-lives (greater than 12 hours) and high plasma concentrations of encainide and yet fail to demonstrate widening of the QRS complex provided the initial clue that encainide biotransformation is under genetic control (Roden et al., 1980b; Woosley et al., 1988). *Principle: Aberrant responses to drug therapy may provide major clues to underlying abnormalities of physiology.*

In most subjects (greater than 90%), encainide undergoes extensive first-pass hepatic metabolism to O-desmethyl encainide (ODE). In less than 10% of patients, the specific hepatic enzyme $P450_{db1}$, which catalyzes encainide O-demethylation, is genetically absent. ODE itself is further biotransformed by $P450_{db1}$ to a second metabolite, 3-methoxy-O-desmethyl encainide (MODE). ODE is approximately an order of magnitude more potent as a sodium-channel blocker than is encainide, while MODE is approximately three times more potent than encainide. In patients who extensively metabolize the drug, its metabolites are present in higher plasma concentrations than the parent drug and therefore responsible for the majority of pharmacologic effects. In poor metabolizers, high plasma encainide concentrations but only very low concentrations of ODE and a third active metabolite, N-desmethyl encainide (NDE) are present, while MODE is undetectable.

Steady-state concentrations of encainide in plasma are attained within 24 hours of initiating therapy. However, the elimination half-lives of the metabolites (ODE: 6 hours; MODE: 20 hours) are much longer than are those of the parent drug. Thus, "steady state" with respect to the metabolites is attained only after 3 to 4 days of encainide therapy. Similarly, in poor metabolizers in whom encainide half-life is prolonged, steady-state plasma concentrations can be assumed to be present only after 3 or 4 days of encainide therapy. Because of the highly variable contribution of encainide and its metabolites to net effects during therapy, no "therapeutic range" for plasma concentrations has been established for this drug.

The parent drug and metabolites are all renally excreted; dosages of encainide should be markedly reduced in patients with renal failure. No major dosage adjustment appears to be required in patients with liver disease. Quinidine is a potent inhibitor of cytochrome $P450_{db1}$, and doses as low as 60 mg every 8 hours markedly impair encainide's O-demethylation and completely abolish ODE 3-methoxylation (Funck-Brentano et al., 1989b). As a result, during chronic treatment with encainide plus quinidine in extensive metabolizers, plasma concentrations of MODE are undetectable, those of encainide rise approximately 13-fold, and those of ODE (whose rates of formation and elimination are both impaired) remain stable (Turgeon et al., 1989). The clinical consequences of combining the two drugs, particularly in patients with sustained ventricular tachycardia, have not been evaluated, but a risk of toxicity due to accumulation of encainide plus ODE should be anticipated. Anecdotal evidence has linked encainide therapy to exacerbation of hyperglycemia or increasing resistance to antidiabetic therapy.

Flecainide. Flecainide is both excreted by the kidney and metabolized by the liver to a meta-Olactam form. The metabolite is not thought to have pharmacologic activity. Preliminary evidence indicates that the metabolism of flecainids also is via $P450_{db1}$. However, since the extent of metabolism is minor, major clinical differences between extensive and poor metabolizers via P450 enzymes have not been noted. Poor metabolizers with renal failure, or extensive metabolizers with renal failure treated with flecainide plus quinidine, theoretically may be at risk for marked increases in the concentrations of flecainide in plasma and consequent toxicity (Beckmann et al., 1988). Clearance of flecainide is reduced in renal failure and in congestive heart failure (Roden and Woosley, 1986). The minimum plasma concentration associated with antiarrhythmic activity appears to be approximately 200 ng/ml. A limited number of cases suggest that the death rate of patients with sustained ventricular tachycardia being treated with flecainide is greater if plasma concentrations are greater than 1000 ng/ml. Some studies have indicated that flecainide can produce minor increases in plasma concentrations of digoxin although not to the extent seen with coadministration of digoxin and quinidine. Flecainide can depress left ventricular performance and precipitate congestive heart failure in patients with underlying left ventricular dysfunction.

Propafenone. This agent has electrophysiologic properties similar to those of encainide and flecainide (Funck-Brentano et al., 1990). Like encainide, propafenone undergoes $P450_{db1}$-mediated metabolism to an active metabolite, 5-hydroxy propafenone. The parent drug and metabolite are approximately equipotent. A second metabolite, N-desalkyl propafenone, has also been identified and has pharmacologic activity. The potency of this metabolite is less than that of the parent drug. Adjustments of propafenone dose in patients with renal and/or hepatic disease may be required.

In extensive metabolizers, propafenone therapy is generally well tolerated and plasma propafenone concentrations should be less than 500 ng/ml. In poor metabolizers, on the other hand, plasma propafenone concentrations greater than 1000 ng/ml are usually required to suppress arrhythmias. These concentrations of parent drug are significantly more frequently associated with side effects (dizziness and nausea) than when the effective concentrations are at the 500-ng/ml range. In addition, high concentrations of propafenone in plasma (as in poor metabolizers) can be shown to produce β-adrenergic blockade. The parent drug alone (and in fact one of its isomers) determines the presence and extent of β-adrenergic blockade. The β-blocking activity of the metabolites is considerably less than is that of the parent

drug. Although quinidine virtually completely inhibits propafenone's 5-hydroxylation, no change in the arrhythmia-suppressing activity of propafenone therapy was seen, presumably reflecting the offsetting effects of increasing parent drug with decreasing formation of metabolite.

Moricizine. This sodium-channel blocker has recently been marketed in the United States for management of ventricular arrhythmias (Morganroth, 1990). Treatment is accompanied by prolongation of the PR and QRS intervals. It can aggravate the arrhythmia, as can encainide and flecainide. However, the kinetics of interaction of moricizine with cardiac sodium channels have not been extensively characterized. Moreover, moricizine was not withdrawn from testing in CAST when encainide and flecainide were withdrawn. Data on the drug's disposition kinetics are not available; data from the sponsor indicate multiple active metabolites. The place of moricizine in therapy awaits the outcome of further testing in CAST-II.

Class II: Antiarrhythmic Activity of β-Adrenergic Antagonists

β-Adrenergic antagonists have their greatest utility in the management of arrhythmias that are functionally related to "slow-response" tissue (Gianelly et al., 1967; Berkowitz et al., 1969). β-Adrenergic antagonists are useful in controlling the ventricular response in patients with atrial arrhythmias such as atrial fibrillation, atrial flutter, or atrial tachycardia. In AV nodal reentrant tachycardia and AV reentrant tachycardias related to accessory pathways, β-adrenergic blockade can terminate the arrhythmias and prevent their recurrence. Esmolol, a $β_1$-selective-adrenergic antagonist that undergoes intravascular hydrolysis with a half-life of approximately 7 min, may be particularly useful in treating the acute arrhythmia. Then, if unacceptable side effects related to the drug develop, they will rapidly resolve with discontinuation of the drug (Sonnenblick, 1985).

In many patients the frequency of ventricular ectopic beats can be reduced by using β-adrenergic antagonists. The mechanism whereby this effect is produced is uncertain. For some drugs, such as propranolol, there is clear evidence that a *non-β-adrenergic mechanism is involved* (Woosley et al., 1979; Duff et al., 1983a). β Antagonists are not particularly effective in treating patients with recurrent sustained ventricular tachycardia. However, large-scale placebo-controlled clinical trials have shown that therapy with a number of β antagonists in patients who are convalescing from a myocardial infarction can reduce the incidence of reinfarction and sudden death (Norwegian Multicenter Study Group, 1981; Beta-Blocker Heart Attack Trial Research Group, 1982). While the mechanism is incompletely understood, animal models have shown a major antifibrillatory effect of β blockade in acutely ischemic tissue (Anderson et al., 1983). The disposition kinetics of individual β-adrenergic antagonists are discussed in further detail in chapter 2 and Appendix I. *Principle: The only drugs discussed in this section that have been proved (up to 1990) to reduce mortality are β-adrenergic blockers. Once again, prejudging all the effects of a drug by its rubric (e.g., β-adrenergic antagonist) may oversimplify the nuances of choice between drugs in a class resulting in underutilization of selected drugs for special efficacy.*

Class III: Prolongation of the Action Potential as a Mode of Action of Antiarrhythmic Drugs

In theory, reentrant arrhythmias should be abolished by maneuvers that decrease the heterogeneity of refractory periods (Singh and Vaughan Williams, 1970). In fact, such an effect is achieved by quinidine-like agents. However, the simultaneous slowing of conduction by such drugs theoretically may actually enable reentrant arrhythmias. Thus, a number of agents that affect cardiac repolarization, without altering sodium-channel function, are available or are under development for treatment of reentrant arrhythmias. In addition to the quinidine-like agents, these include the β-adrenergic antagonist sotalol, NAPA (acecainide), amiodarone, and bretylium.

Sotalol has been available in Europe since the mid-1970s. It is a β-adrenergic antagonist with prominent actions that prolong action potentials. It is as effective as or more effective than are sodium-channel blocking agents in the maintenance of sinus rhythm in patients with atrial fibrillation or flutter, and in the suppression of sustained ventricular tachycardia. In addition to adverse effects related to β blockade, sotalol can, like quinidine, cause torsades de pointes, particularly in hypokalemic or bradycardiac patients (McKibbin et al., 1984). Acecainide (see procainamide, above) suppresses chronic ventricular ectopic beats at plasma concentrations greater than 10 μg/ml. Its GI side effects become particularly prominent at concentrations in plasma greater than 20 μg/ml. Accumulation of acecainide during chronic therapy with procainamide in patients with renal failure may lead to marked prolongation of the QT interval and development of torsades de pointes (Chow et al., 1984). Both sotalol and acecainide appear to prolong the QT interval in a concentration-dependent fashion, and, in fact, patients who develop torsades de pointes

while using sotalol have been successfully managed with lower doses of sotalol (in contrast to the case with quinidine).

Bretylium. This agent has complex electrophysiologic effects including an ability to reduce the heterogeneity of refractory periods between ischemic and normal tissue (Koch-Weser, 1979a). Bretylium is a quaternary ammonium analog and is very poorly bioavailable after oral administration. After IV administration, the drug is taken up into presynaptic neurons in the sympathetic nervous system and promptly releases norepinephrine. In normal volunteers and patients with ventricular ectopic beats, this increase in plasma norepinephrine is associated with tachycardia, hypertension, and, possibly, a transient increase in ventricular ectopic activity. In patients who receive bretylium as part of resuscitative efforts during recurrent ventricular tachycardia or ventricular fibrillation, these transient adrenergic effects may not be as evident.

Following the transient release of norepinephrine, the presynaptic neuron is incapable of releasing catecholamine. Hence, orthostatic hypotension is very common during bretylium therapy and responds to intravascular volume replacement. The postsynaptic neuron demonstrates denervation hypersensitivity, and exogenous catecholamines may produce a marked hypertensive response. In animals, the maximum change in ventricular refractoriness and in ventricular fibrillation threshold is seen several hours following a bolus IV dose of bretylium. This time lag parallels drug uptake into the myocardium (Anderson et al., 1980). Hence, from a practical point of view, bretylium is a complex drug to use in the critically ill patient, where it may transiently worsen hemodynamic status and arrhythmias, and where it may render hypotension (volume depletion versus cardiogenic shock) particularly difficult to diagnose and treat appropriately. Drugs that block the norepinephrine reuptake mechanism, such as tricyclic antidepressants, will block uptake of bretylium into the presynaptic neuron. In fact, pretreatment with tricyclic antidepressants prevents the autonomic effects of bretylium, yet does not interfere with its antiarrhythmic actions (Woosley et al., 1982). Situations in which a profound fall in peripheral vascular resistance might be very detrimental to the patient's overall hemodynamic status (e.g., critical aortic stenosis, critical carotid disease, pulmonary hypertension, hypertrophic cardiomyopathy) are contraindications to the use of bretylium. Torsades de pointes is not a feature of bretylium therapy.

Bretylium does not undergo extensive biotransformation in humans and is excreted unchanged by the kidney. There is no described dose- or concentration-dependent toxicity, so a well-established therapeutic range has not been worked out (Table 6–4). Although it is highly effective as a "holding maneuver," definitive antiarrhythmic therapy in the form of chronic oral treatment or aggressive anti-ischemic measures (which may include coronary artery bypass grafting) is required for the long-term management of patients whose rhythm status has been transiently stabilized by bretylium.

Amiodarone is discussed further below.

Class IV: Drugs with Calcium-Channel-Blocking Properties

Three subclasses of calcium-channel blockers currently are available in the United States: the benzothiazepine class (including diltiazem), the papaverine derivatives (including verapamil), and the dihydropyridines (including nifedipine). Only the first two have utility in patients with cardiac arrhythmias; the pharmacology of the calcium-channel blockers is discussed in further detail in chapter 2.

Verapamil and diltiazem control ventricular response in patients with atrial fibrillation, atrial flutter, and atrial tachycardia (Talano and Tomasso, 1982). Intravenous verapamil is among the drugs of choice for the acute termination of AV nodal reentrant and reentrant tachycardia related to bypass tracts. Chronic oral therapy significantly decreases recurrences of these reentrant arrhythmias. As outlined above, verapamil and digitalis are contraindicated in patients with bypass tracts and atrial fibrillation with very rapid ventricular rates. Verapamil may have particular utility in arrhythmias thought to be related to delayed afterdepolarizations. These include certain forms of abnormal atrial automaticity (including multifocal atrial tachycardia) as well as unusual patients with no apparent structural heart disease and ventricular tachycardia precipitated by critical increases in heart rate (Belhassen and Horowitz, 1984; Levine et al., 1985). Although fewer data are available on the efficacy of diltiazem in these situations, the electrophysiologic profile of this agent suggests it should be as effective as verapamil.

Acute IV therapy with verapamil can produce marked systemic hypotension due to fall in vascular resistance. The most common situation in which this is a clinical problem is in patients with sustained ventricular tachycardia misdiagnosed as supraventricular tachycardia. Use of verapamil in this setting can, as described above, result in disastrous hypotension and cardiac arrest. Depression of contractile function, AV block, and sinus bradycardia can occur. Constipation may be a troubling adverse effect of verapamil. Chronic oral therapy with verapamil and diltiazem is discussed further in chapter 2.

Verapamil is a racemate. The l-isomer is more potent as an AV blocker than is in the d-isomer. After IV therapy, the two isomers are present at similar concentrations. However, after oral therapy, the l-isomer undergoes more extensive first-pass hepatic metabolism. Thus, at any given concentration of verapamil in plasma, AV nodal block is more prominent when the drug has been administered IV rather than orally (Echizen et al., 1985). Verapamil has at least one active metabolite. Therapeutic ranges are not well established for either verapamil or diltiazem. Verapamil therapy increases concentrations of digoxin in plasma, and emerging data suggest that calcium-channel blockers can be potent inhibitors of metabolism of a number of other agents (Hunt et al., 1989). *Principle: Many drug products actually are consistent mixtures of related chemicals that are not readily separated in the synthetic process. Isomers often do not have the same pharmacologic effects, and the balance of their effects may be very dependent on the route of drug administration. Currently the regulatory agencies increasingly examine the wisdom of allowing mixtures of chemicals in the same drug product.*

Drugs with Unclassified or Mixed Actions

Amiodarone. Amiodarone is a structurally unique iodinated agent with electrophysiologic, toxicologic, and pharmacokinetic properties different from those of other drugs (Zipes et al., 1984; Mason, 1987). Although it is frequently lumped with drugs whose predominant electrophysiologic effect is prolongation of the action potential (i.e., "class III"), amiodarone also blocks cardiac sodium and potassium channels. As well, the drug exerts an antiadrenergic effect by binding noncompetitively to adrenergic receptors.

Amiodarone is a highly effective agent in the management of a broad range of cardiac arrhythmias. Amiodarone prevents recurrent atrial fibrillation or flutter probably more often than quinidine. By virtue of its AV nodal blocking properties, it will control the ventricular response when it does not suppress the arrhythmia. It also is effective in management of automatic atrial tachycardia, in a wide range of arrhythmias related to the WPW syndrome, and in preventing ventricular tachycardia or ventricular fibrillation. Low-dose amiodarone is currently being evaluated in survivors of myocardial infarction and in patients with advanced congestive heart failure, subsets who are at risk for sudden arrhythmic death. Amiodarone prolongs PR and QRS intervals and markedly prolongs QT intervals, but interestingly enough, torsades de pointes is unusual. In fact, amiodarone has been used in patients who developed torsades de pointes during treatment with quinidine. All the attractive actions are enticing, but its potential side effects and unusual pharmacokinetics prevent it from being used as a drug of first choice in any setting.

The drug and its monodeethylated active metabolite are widely distributed in the body. The uptake process into the periphery is *very* slow. True steady-state conditions for amiodarone therapy are probably not reached for several months after the initiation of a maintenance regimen. In fact, with chronic therapy, the liver becomes increasingly radiodense, leading at CT scanning to a diagnosis of a deposition disease. Because of the long lag between institution of therapy and attainment of steady-state conditions, a loading regimen is frequently used. The maintenance dose is 100 to 400 mg/day (as a single dose given the drug's very long elimination half-life). Dosages above 400 mg/day have been associated with an increased risk for potentially fatal pulmonary toxicity discussed further below. Loading regimens range from 800 mg/day for a week to higher dosages, such as 1 to 1.5 gm/day for several weeks, with tapering down to the maintenance dose over several months. Concentrations in plasma of greater than 0.5 μg/ml of the parent drug have generally been associated with suppression of the arrhythmia. Limited data suggest that plasma concentrations of greater than 2 μg/ml may be associated with substantial risk of toxicity.

An IV form of the drug currently is under investigation in the United States. Noncontrolled data suggest that IV amiodarone may acutely control serious cardiac arrhythmias, including recurrent ventricular tachycardia or ventricular fibrillation resistant to other agents. One possible explanation for the efficacy of acute IV amiodarone (versus the time lag required for chronic oral therapy) is that the drug is only 30% to 40% bioavailable. However, even when corrections are made for plasma concentrations, IV administration of the drug appears to be unexpectedly effective very soon after administration. Perhaps selective uptake of drug into the heart may be concentration-dependent, and critical concentrations are developed only after IV administration. The electrophysiologic explanation for this route-dependent efficacy is uncertain. *Principle: There are very few drugs whose slow rates of clearance are critical determinants of whether they can be used. Theoretically there should be no drawback in using the drug if its clearance rate could be established, a steady state target established and measured, and replacement for cleared drug feasible as long as the toxicity of the drug were tolerable at steady state.*

Amiodarone Drug Interactions. Amiodarone is a potent inhibitor of the disposition of a number of other drugs, but in an unpredictable fashion. Amiodarone often markedly decreases requirements for coumarin-like drugs, presumably by inhibiting their metabolism. Digoxin concentrations in plasma may rise during treatment with amiodarone. Inconsistent digitalis intoxication has been reported when the two drugs are used simultaneously. Amiodarone decreases the hepatic metabolism and/or renal elimination of a number of other antiarrhythmics, including flecainide, quinidine, procainamide, and acecainide. Since use of other antiarrhythmic agents is common early during amiodarone treatment (when a therapeutic effect may not yet have been achieved), these interactions can be clinically important. The mechanism underlying these drug interactions is likely multifactorial, since both drugs that undergo extensive hepatic metabolism (e.g., oral anticoagulants) and drugs that undergo primary renal excretion (e.g., NAPA) are effected.

Amiodarone Toxicity. By now it must be pretty obvious that major limitation to widespread use of amiodarone is its potential to cause dysfunction of a variety of organ systems during long-term therapy and its impact on the effects of other drugs often used for the same indications. In general, the risk of amiodarone toxicity increases as the time of exposure to it increases. This makes the drug particularly unattractive for long-term therapy in relatively healthy patients (e.g., children). On the other hand, when patients have a very limited life expectancy, treatment with amiodarone may be more reasonable.

Virtually all patients receiving chronic oral amiodarone for greater than 3 months develop corneal microdeposits of the drug. Symptoms are infrequent, although some patients may complain of seeing halos around lights. This usually is an indication to reduce the dose. The most feared complication in using the drug is pulmonary toxicity. Predisposing factors have not been well characterized, although high dosages (greater than 400 mg/day) appear to carry an increased risk. Other "risk factors" for which uncontrolled reports have suggested a role include the presence of underlying chronic pulmonary disease, living at high altitude, and incurring major operative procedures. Pulmonary toxicity can have a variety of presentations, ranging from fulminant adult respiratory distress syndrome with respiratory failure to asymptomatic increases in diffusion capacity. Histopathologic examination of affected lung usually reveals interstitial fibrosis. The chest x-ray film is compatible with that diagnosis. Some authorities recommend serial chest x-ray films and pulmonary function studies to detect incipient toxicity. However, the value of such screening is uncertain. Certainly, patients starting to take amiodarone should have baseline chest x-ray films and measurements of diffusing capacity. Should pulmonary symptoms develop at any point, these assessments should be repeated. Other studies that may be useful include gallium scanning (which generally is positive over the lungs) and right heart catheterization to assess a potential contribution from left heart failure.

Treatment of the pulmonary complications generally consists of withdrawal of amiodarone and initiation of steroid therapy. In some instances, resumption of amiodarone therapy, at lower dosages with or without steroid treatment, has avoided the recurrence of the pulmonary complications. The biochemical mechanism underlying pulmonary toxicity is not known, although production of oxygen-centered free radicals has been proposed. This would be consistent with the development of amiodarone pulmonary toxicity immediately following other forms of pulmonary insult. The incidence of pulmonary toxicity appears to be 5% to 10%.

Other forms of toxicity include sinus bradycardia, abnormal liver function studies, profound peripheral neuropathy and myopathy that may result in gait disturbances, hypo- or hyperthyroidism, photosensitivity, and a peculiar bluish-gray skin discoloration over sun-exposed areas. Side effects such as these that presumably represent the effects of chronic amiodarone deposition in various body tissues usually resolve over time with reduction of the dose. The presence of side effects such as these generally mandates lowering the dose. A major difficulty with long-term management of patients receiving amiodarone is uncertainty over whether the minimum effective dose to prevent recurrence of serious arrhythmias is being maintained while dosages are reduced in the face of obvious organ toxicity.

Digitalis. Digitalis glycosides are indicated not only for the management of congestive heart failure, but for the management of a variety of supraventricular arrhythmias. The pharmacokinetics of digitalis glycosides are discussed further in chapter 4. Digitalis produces prominent vagotonic effects, resulting in bradycardia, decreased atrial refractoriness, and delayed AV conduction. The effects on cardiac rhythm usually require concentrations in plasma that have already produced most of the inotropic effects that the drug can induce. Digitalis glycosides have their most useful role as antiarrhythmic agents in controlling the ventricular response to atrial fibrillation or atrial flutter. In addition, their ability to prolong AV nodal refractoriness also makes digitalis glycosides useful in the management of patients with

AV nodal reentrant tachycardia or orthodromic reciprocating tachycardia. However, digitalis glycosides may accelerate the ventricular response during atrial fibrillation in patients with Wolff-Parkinson-White syndrome. Therefore, the drug should be avoided in these patients.

Digitalis intoxication includes nausea, disturbances in mentation, AV nodal block, and/or ventricular arrhythmias. The new development of *any* arrhythmia in a patient receiving digitalis should prompt a search for digitalis intoxication. Arrhythmias due to digitalis toxicity are more frequent when concentrations in plasma exceed 2 ng/ml but may be seen while concentrations are in the "therapeutic" range. Factors that are known to increase the risk of digitalis toxicity at any concentration include hypokalemia, hypothyroidism, hypomagnesemia, hypocalcemia, or hypercalcemia.

Adenosine. The rapid IV injection of a bolus dose of adenosine transiently prolongs AV nodal refractoriness and is highly effective in terminating supraventricular tachycardias such as AV nodal reentry or orthodromic reciprocating tachycardia. The effective dose is 2 to 20 mg and should be administered as a bolus since the drug undergoes rapid intravascular metabolism and uptake into cells. Adverse effects include shortness of breath and flushing. In addition, chest pain is frequent, although the mechanism is uncertain and may involve transient "air hunger" rather than myocardial ischemia. Since the effects of the drug are so transient, it may well supplant IV verapamil for the management of these supraventricular tachycardias. In fact, preliminary data suggest that administration of adenosine to patients with ventricular tachycardia does not result in severe hypotension, although tachycardias rarely are terminated.

Use of Antiarrhythmic Drugs in Combination

When single agents cause side effects or fail to control arrhythmias, antiarrhythmic drugs can be combined. For example, combining quinidine-like and lidocaine-like agents achieves substantial suppression of early ectopic beats of rapidly driven tissues without affecting normal tissues in vitro (Hondeghem and Katzung, 1980). Clinical trials that combine well-tolerated doses of quinidine or similar agents with mexiletine or similar agents show enhanced suppression of arrhythmia without increasing the incidence of side effects of any agent (Duff et al., 1983b; Barbey et al., 1988). In fact, low doses of quinidine have been used in combination with low doses of procainamide to achieve a similar effect (Kim et al., 1985); although the two drugs exert similar electrophysiologic actions, side effects that so frequently limit dosages can be avoided by the use of this combination strategy.

Considerable data are available to suggest that the combination of quinidine and propranolol results in better management of atrial fibrillation than either drug used alone (Dreifus et al., 1968). Whether this reflects better rate control achieved by addition of propranolol or a synergistic electrophysiologic effect is uncertain. In addition, quinidine's inhibition of propranolol's metabolism in some patients may play a role in the apparent synergistic effects. Similarly, either pharmacokinetic or electrophysiologic interactions may contribute to enhanced efficacy of the combination of quinidine and verapamil. The strategy of targeting two different links of a reentrant circuit (e.g., verapamil for the AV node, quinidine for the accessory pathway) in patients with Wolff-Parkinson-White syndrome may achieve better control of the arrhythmia with fewer side effects than when a single agent is used alone. The role of the sympathetic nervous system in modulating the effects of β-adrenergic antagonists or calcium-channel blockers is well known. Emerging data suggest that the sympathetic nervous system also may also play a role in modulating the effects of sodium- or potassium-channel blocking drugs. Thus, adjunctive therapy with β blockers may be particularly important in maintaining long-term control of arrhythmias in patients who are subject to sympathetic surges that might ordinarily reverse the antiarrhythmic effects of drugs such as quinidine (Morady et al., 1988).

DC Cardioversion

DC cardioversion is the treatment of choice for sustained atrial or ventricular arrhythmias associated with acute hemodynamic compromise (cardiac arrest, hypotension, heart failure, angina). If hemodynamic compromise has not been severe enough to result in loss of consciousness, adequate sedation with short-acting barbiturates or benzodiazepines should be used before the procedure. Cardioversion should never be used in a patient who has not lost consciousness even if the arrythmia is life-threatening. Intubation should be considered in patients who have recently eaten. For organized rhythms, the DC cardioverter should be set to a "synchronized" setting to avoid delivering a random discharge at the peak of the T wave. That event can initiate ventricular fibrillation. The risk of precipitating ventricular fibrillation by DC cardioversion is increased when there are signs of digitalis toxicity.

Elective cardioversion frequently is employed in patients with atrial fibrillation or flutter. Preceding planned cardioversion with a short period of pharmacologic therapy often may result in restoration of sinus rhythm. Even if sinus rhythm does not result from drug therapy, that treatment can increase the chances of maintaining sinus rhythm following cardioversion. In patients with ventricular fibrillation, high-output DC cardioversion should be delivered as soon as possible with the device set to a nonsynchronized mode, since mandating synchronization in this setting may delay the delivery of the shock.

THE ARRHYTHMIAS

General Approach

In treating a patient with abnormal cardiac rhythm, the physician must ask the series of questions outlined above ("Principles in the Management of Arrhythmias"). The arrhythmia should be identified, reversible causes removed, and assessment of the risks and benefits of treatment made. In patients with atrial arrhythmias and AV nodal reentrant tachycardia, treatment is indicated only if the patient is symptomatic, since there are no data to suggest that suppression of these arrhythmias improves long-term prognosis. The same principles apply to the patient with the Wolff-Parkinson-White syndrome. The most common arrhythmia in these patients, orthodromic reciprocating tachycardia, can usually be readily controlled with AV nodal blocking drugs such as digitalis or calcium-channel blockers. However, these treatments can be associated with atrial fibrillation and catastrophically fast ventricular responses in patients with manifest preexcitation (i.e., those with delta waves). Thus, in this situation, further evaluation (including treadmill testing, Holter monitoring, and potentially evaluation by sophisticated electrophysiologic testing) may be indicated to sort out risk and benefit.

Despite a wealth of epidemiologic data indicating that patients with chronic ventricular ectopic beats are at increased risk of sudden death, no evidence currently supports the notion that suppression of these arrhythmias improves prognosis. In patients with acute myocardial ischemia, ventricular ectopic beats are common, but there is again no evidence that suppressing these arrhythmias decreases the risk of ventricular fibrillation. There is, however, evidence that treatment with lidocaine reduces the incidence of ventricular fibrillation in any patient with acute myocardial ischemia. Thus, many clinicians treat patients with acute myocardial infarction or unstable angina (regardless of the presence or absence of ventricular arrhythmias) with lidocaine. As outlined above, while this treatment strategy may result in a decreased incidence of ventricular fibrillation, overall mortality may be increased. Patients with sustained ventricular tachycardia or ventricular fibrillation obviously require therapy and should be treated with parenteral antiarrhythmic drugs, such as lidocaine, procainamide, or bretylium.

Atrial Fibrillation or Flutter

For acute control of rate, AV nodal blocking drugs, such as digitalis, verapamil, or β antagonists are effective. Correction of identifiable causes of the arrhythmia, such as thyrotoxicosis, congestive heart failure, or acute myocardial ischemia may help to restore sinus rhythm. In patients with paroxysmal atrial fibrillation in the absence of predisposing causes, class Ia or Ic agents, sotalol, and amiodarone have all been effective in maintaining sinus rhythm.

The question the physician must answer is whether the patient's symptoms warrant such intervention. In completely asymptomatic individuals, it is reasonable to withhold therapy. In highly symptomatic individuals, treatment for both control of rate and maintenance of sinus rhythm may be required. In extreme instances, ablation of the AV node and placement of rate-responsive pacemakers have been used successfully. Atrial fibrillation is associated with systemic embolization. However, the need for chronic anticoagulation with warfarin is uncertain since benefits are outweighed by the risks in only the highest-risk patients (Petersen, et al., 1989; Special Report, 1990). Aspirin may prove to be an alternative.

Atrial flutter is an inherently "unstable" rhythm in the sense that ventricular responses may change by increments rather than gradually. Very rapid ventricular rates during treatment with class Ia or Ic drugs have been reported. Thus, AV nodal blocking agents should be instituted along with these drugs. Atrial flutter can be readily terminated acutely by pacing techniques, while atrial fibrillation cannot be so managed. Rare cases of atrial flutter are amenable to chronic pacing therapies, but these only are useful if the patient has no history of atrial fibrillation.

Atrial Tachycardia

As with atrial fibrillation and atrial flutter, two drug strategies can be employed: slowing the ventricular response by using AV nodal block or suppression of the arrhythmia. The latter can be accomplished by class Ia drugs, but some data suggest that class Ic drugs may be particularly effective in this setting. As well, occasional patients appear to respond to verapamil. Surgical therapy has rarely been done to remove an automatic "focus."

AV Nodal Reentrant Tachycardia

Acute therapy in this situation is aimed at maneuvers that increase AV nodal refractoriness. These maneuvers historically included vagal stimulants (carotid sinus message, edrephonium, phenylephrine), but drugs that directly affect AV nodal refractoriness (e.g., β-adrenergic antagonists or verapamil) are now preferred. The acute IV administration of verapamil is highly effective in terminating regular, narrow complex, supraventricular tachycardia related to AV nodal reentry or AV reentry using a bypass tract. As discussed above, adenosine may supplant verapamil for treating acute arrhythmias because it may be less likely to produce adverse hemodynamic effects. Chronic oral treatment with digitalis, verapamil, β blockers, or class Ic agents can help maintain sinus rhythm.

Arrhythmias Related to the Wolff-Parkinson-White Syndrome

The most common arrhythmia seen in these patients is orthodromic reciprocating tachycardia that responds to the same maneuvers as AV nodal reentrant tachycardia. However, with AV nodal block, ventricular response during atrial fibrillation can be accelerated. Thus, while acute IV administration of verapamil to a patient with Wolff-Parkinson-White syndrome and orthodromic reciprocating tachycardia is reasonable, continued monitoring should be used afterward to ensure that atrial fibrillation with a rapid ventricular response does not develop. Ultimately, adenosine may be preferable. Long-term treatment with AV nodal blocking drugs should be avoided unless data are available to indicate that the accessory pathway will not permit atrial fibrillation with a rapid ventricular response to develop.

Atrial fibrillation with a very rapid ventricular response is the other major arrhythmia to which these patients are susceptible. In this situation, class Ia or Ic agents, sotalol, and amiodarone, which increase refractoriness of the accessory pathway, can all be considered. The acute therapy for this arrhythmia is IV procainamide and/or electrical cardioversion. Patients with recurrent episodes of symptomatic, drug-resistant supraventricular tachycardia or a single episode of atrial fibrillation with an ultrarapid ventricular response should be considered for surgical ablation of the bypass tract.

Ventricular Ectopic Beats

Chronic ventricular ectopic beats are very commonly found in patients with and without heart disease. Recent development of ventricular arrhythmias should at least prompt a search for potential contributing underlying factors such as ongoing myocardial ischemia or unrecognized structural heart disease. Exercise testing and echocardiography are frequently useful. Ventricular arrhythmias developing during anesthesia should prompt a search for precipitating causes such as abnormal oxygenation or myocardial ischemia. In addition, anesthesia with halothane is a recognized cause of increased myocardial sensitivity to catecholamines and can result in arrhythmias. The presence of frequent ventricular ectopic beats, particularly in pairs or salvos, in patients who have survived a myocardial infarction, indicates an increased risk for sudden death. However, as discussed above, intervention with antiarrhythmic drugs has resulted in increased mortality. Thus, although chronic ventricular ectopic beats make an attractive target for drug intervention, currently available data indicate that the risks outweigh any possible benefits. *Principle: There can be nothing more frustrating to the physician than to be kept from treating a reversible sign. But remember, a sign is often a surrogate end point for an ultimate effect and may not substitute for it. The decision not to treat is a therapeutic decision and often requires more scholastic rigor than the decision to treat!*

Some patients develop and may require therapy for highly symptomatic arrhythmias. In such an instance, the patient should be aware that treatment is aimed at symptoms and not at improving prognosis. In patients with recent myocardial infarction and highly symptomatic nonsustained ventricular arrhythmias, short-term therapy with the class Ic agents is highly effective but should be avoided because of the prognostic long-term implications of CAST. β-Adrenergic antagonists may be useful, and while other sodium-channel blocking drugs such as quinidine may be used, data on their safety in this setting are simply unavailable. Amiodarone may suppress ventricular ectopic beats but should not be used for this indication because the risk of toxicity probably will outweigh any benefit. Patients with symptomatic ventricular ectopic beats and other types of heart disease should be approached in a similar fashion, although in those with structurally normal hearts, treatment with class Ic agents may be considered when other drug therapies have proved ineffective.

Sustained Ventricular Arrhythmias

The distinction between nonsustained and sustained ventricular arrhythmias can become blurred. In practical terms, an episode of ventricular tachycardia that lasts 15 seconds and is associated with near syncope but spontaneously terminates probably is no different from a prognostic or therapeutic point of view from an arrhythmia that lasts hours and requires intervention for termination. It is in this group that electrophysiologically guided therapy is often used. Until reduction of sudden cardiac death from suppression of ventricular arrhythmias has been demonstrated, one of the only indications for antiarrhythmic drug use in sustained ventricular arrhythmias is to reduce hemodynamic (syncope, palpitation, and dizziness) symptoms (Morganroth, 1990). Drugs of choice include class Ia agents (alone or in combination with mexiletine), class Ic agents, sotalol, or amiodarone. Antitachycardia surgery and the placement of automatic implantable cardioverter defibrillators (ICD) also are options. The ICD is a device that is capable of sensing sustained ventricular arrhythmias, including ventricular fibrillation, and delivering an internal shock to restore normal rhythm. The majority of patients with an ICD require concomitant therapy with antiarrhythmic drugs, most often to prevent atrial arrhythmias or nonsustained ventricular arrhythmias that would result in delivery of inappropriate shocks. Some drugs, notably drugs with class Ic properties, can alter ICD function by changing energy requirements for defibrillation or by altering tachycardia rates in such a way as to render the devices inoperative. Thus, adjustment of drug therapy in such patients should be undertaken with caution.

Principles of advanced cardiac life support, as described and taught by organizations such as the American Heart Association, should be familiar to all physicians. Community-wide educational measures have resulted in an increased incidence of successful resuscitation from ventricular fibrillation that occurs out of hospital. The principles of establishing and maintaining an airway and supporting the circulation with external cardiac message cannot be overemphasized. Sustained ventricular tachycardia or ventricular fibrillation should be treated with cardioversion and drugs such as lidocaine, procainamide, or bretylium as outlined above.

Several areas of controversy in resuscitation remain. For example, epinephrine is widely used, but its mechanism of action is uncertain. The drug has β-adrenergically mediated electrophysiologic effects, with an increase in heart rate, increased automaticity, and increased oxygen demand that may be undesirable. The most important salutory effect is α-adrenergically mediated vasoconstriction that redistributes blood flow to the heart and brain, a desirable action in the patients with cardiac arrest (Michael et al., 1984). Calcium is used to augment myocardial contractility, but the potential for adverse effects (presumably related to intracellular calcium overload with attendant arrhythmias and cell death) has led to the recommendation that it not be used. Similarly, bicarbonate is frequently administered to correct lactic acidosis seen during cardiac arrest. However, administration of sodium bicarbonate can result in cerebrospinal fluid acidosis, hypernatremia, and hyperosmolarity (Bishop and Weisfeldt, 1976), all of which may impair post-resuscitation survival. Most recently, it has been shown that although acidosis itself does not alter energy requirements for defibrillation, the increase in defibrillation energy requirements seen with lidocaine is augmented by acidosis and reversed by administration of bicarbonate (Echt et al., 1989). Thus, if defibrillation is unsuccessful in the presence of lidocaine, bicarbonate could theoretically be considered. Similarly, patients with intractable acidosis or preexisting metabolic acidosis might benefit from bicarbonate. Overall, however, the risks of bicarbonate are thought to outweigh its benefits, and thus it should not be administered on a routine basis to patients with cardiac arrest.

REFERENCES

Alderman, E. L.; Kerber, R. E.; and Harrison, D. C.: Evaluation of lidocaine resistance in man using intermittent large-dose infusion techniques. Am. J. Cardiol., 34:342–347, 1974.

Anderson, J. L.; Rodier, H. E.; and Green, L. S.: Comparative effects of beta-adrenergic blocking drugs on experimental ventricular fibrillation threshold. Am. J. Cardiol., 51:1196–1202, 1983.

Anderson, J. L.; Patterson, E.; Conlon, M.; Pasyk, S.; Pitt, B.; and Lucchesi, B. R.: Kinetics of antifibrillatory effects of bretylium: Correlation with myocardial drug concentrations. Am. J. Cardiol., 46:583–592, 1980.

Bailie, D. S.; Inoue, H.; Kaseda, S.; Ben-David, J.; and Zipes, D. P.: Magnesium suppression of early afterdepolarization and ventricular tachyarrhythmias induced by cesium in dogs. Circulation, 77:1395–1402, 1988.

Barbey, J. T.; Thompson, K. A.; Echt, D. S.; Woosley, R. L.; and Roden, D. M.: Tocainide plus quinidine for treatment of ventricular arrhythmias. Am. J. Cardiol., 61:570–573, 1988.

Beckmann, J.; Hertrampf, R.; Gundert-Remy, U.; Mikus, G.; Gross, A. S.; and Eichelbaum, M.: Is there a genetic factor in flecainide toxicity? Br. Med. J., 297:1316–7, 1988.

Belhassen, B.; and Horowitz, L. N.: Use of intravenous verapamil for ventricular tachycardia. Am. J Cardiol., 54:1131–1133, 1984.

Bennett, P. B.; Woosley, R. L.; and Hondeghem, L. M.: Competitive interactions of lidocaine (L) and one of its metabolites, glycine xylidide (GX), with cardiac sodium channels. Circulation, 78:692–700, 1988.

Berkowitz, V. D.; Wit, A. L.; Lau, S. H.; Steiner, C.; and Damatto, A. M.: The effects of propranolol on cardiac conduction. Circulation, 40:854–862, 1969.

Beta-Blocker Heart Attack Trial Research Group: A randomized trial of propranolol in patients with acute myocardial infarction: I. Mortality results. J.A.M.A., 247:1707–1714, 1982.

Bigger, J. T. Jr.: The quinidine-digoxin interaction. Mod. Concepts Cardiovasc. Dis., 51:73–78, 1982.

Bishop, R. L.; and Weisfeldt, M. L.: Sodium bicarbonate administration during cardiac arrest. Effect on arterial pH, pCO$_2$, and osmolality. J.A.M.A., 235:506–509, 1976.

Boyes, R. N.; Scott, D. B.; Jebson, P. J.; Godman, M. J.; and Julian, D. G.: Pharmacokinetics of lidocaine in man. Clin. Pharmacol. Ther., 12:105–116, 1971.

Buxton, A. E.; Marchlinski, F. E.; Doherty, J. U.; Flores, B.; and Josephson, M. E.: Hazards of intravenous verapamil for

sustained ventricular tachycardia. Am. J. Cardiol., 59:1107–1110, 1987.

CAST Investigators: Preliminary Report: Effect of encainide and flecainide on mortality in a randomized trial of arrhythmia suppression after myocardial infarction. N. Engl. J. Med., 321:406–412, 1989.

Campbell, T. J.: Kinetics of onset of rate-dependent effects of class I antiarrhythmic drugs are important in determining their effects on refractoriness in guinea-pig ventricle, and provide a theoretical basis for their subclassification. Cardiovasc. Res., 17:344–352, 1983.

Chouty, F.; Funck-Brentano, C.; Landau, J. M.; and Lardoux, H.: Efficacité de fortes doses de lactate molaire par voie veineuse lors des intoxications au flecainide. Presse Med., 16: 808–810, 1987.

Chow, M. J.; Piergies, A. A.; Bowsher, D. J.; Murphy, J. J.; Kushner, W.; Ruo, T. I.; Asada, A.; Talano, J. V.; and Atkinson, A. J.: Torsade de pointes induced by N-acetylprocainamide. J. Am. Coll. Cardiol., 4:621–624, 1984.

Conrad, K. A.; Molk, B. L.; and Chindsey, C. A.: Pharmacokinetic studies of quinidine in patients with arrhythmias. Circulation, 55:1–7, 1977.

Cox A. R.; and West T. C.: Sodium lactate reversal of quinidine effect studied in rabbit atria by the microelectrode technique. J. Pharmacol. Exp. Ther., 131:212–222, 1961.

Cranefield, P. F; and Aronson, R. S.: Cardiac Arrhythmias: The Role of Triggered Activity and Other Mechanisms. Futura Publishing, Mt. Kisco, N.Y., 1988.

Cranefield P. F.: The Conduction of the Cardiac Impulse. Futura Publishing, Mt. Kisco, N.Y., 1985.

Cranefield, P. F.: Action potentials, afterpotentials, and arrhythmias. Circ. Res., 41:415–423, 1977.

Crijns, H. J.; van Gelder, I. S.; and Lie, K. I.: Supraventricular tachycardia mimicking ventricular tachycardia during flecainide treatment. Am. J. Cardiol., 62:1303–1306, 1988.

Dangman, K. H.; and Hoffman, B. F.: Studies on overdrive stimulation of canine cardiac Purkinje fibers: Maximal diastolic potential as a determinant of the response. J. Am. Coll. Cardiol., 2:1183–1190, 1983.

Data, J. L.; Wilkinson, G. R.; and Nies, A. S.: Interaction of quinidine with anticonvulsant drugs. N. Engl. J. Med., 294: 699–702, 1976.

Drayer, D. E.; and Reidenberg, M. M.: Clinical consequences of polymorphic acetylation of basic drugs. Clin. Pharmacol. Ther., 22:251–258, 1977.

Dreifus, L. S.; Lim, H. F.; Watanabe, Y.; McKnight, E.; and Frank, M. N.: Propranolol and quinidine in the management of ventricular tachycardia. J.A.M.A., 204:736–739, 1968.

Duff, H. J.; Roden, D. M.; Reele, S. B.; Brorson, L.; Wood, A. J. J.; Dawson, A. K.; Primm, R. K.; Oates, J. A.; Smith, R. F.; and Woosley, R. L.: The electrophysiologic actions of high dose propranolol in man. J. Am. Coll. Cardiol., 2:1134–1140, 1983a.

Duff, H. J.; Roden, D. M.; Primm, R. K.; Smith, R. F.; Oates, J. A.; and Woosley, R. L.: Mexiletine in the treatment of resistant ventricular tachycardia: Enhancement of efficacy and reduction of dose-related side effects by combination with quinidine. Circulation, 67:1124–1128, 1983b.

Echizen, H.; Vogelgesang, B.; and Eichelbaum, M.: Effects of d,l-verapamil on atrioventricular conduction in relation to its stereoselective first-pass metabolism. Clin. Pharmacol. Ther., 38:71–76, 1985.

Eichelbaum, M.: Genetic polymorphism of sparteine/debrisoquine oxidation. ISI Atlas Sci., 243–251, 1988.

Eichelbaum, M.: Defective oxidation of drugs: Pharmacokinetic and therapeutic implications. Clin. Pharmacokinet., 7: 1–22, 1982.

Echt, D. S.; Cato, E. L.; and Cox, D. R.: pH-dependent effects of lidocaine on defibrillation energy requirements in dogs. Circulation, 80:1003–1009, 1989.

Falk, R. H.; Knowlton, A. A.; Bernard, S. A.; Gotlieb, N. E.; and Battinelli, N. J.: Digoxin for converting recent-onset atrial fibrillation to sinus rhythm. Ann. Intern. Med., 106: 503–506, 1987.

Frey, W.: Ueber Vorhofflimmern beim Menschen und seine Beseitigung durch Chinidin. Berl. Klin. Wochnschr., 55:417–419, 1918.

Funck-Brentano, C.; Kroemer, H. K.; Lee, J. T.; and Roden, D. M.: Propafenone. N. Engl. J. Med., 322(8):518–525, 1990.

Funck-Brentano, C.; Kroemer, H. K.; Woosley, R. L.; and Roden, D. M.: Genetically-determined interaction between propafenone and low dose quinidine: Role of active metabolites in modulating net drug effect. Br. J. Clin. Pharmacol., 27:435–444, 1989a.

Funck-Brentano, C.; Turgeon, J.; Woosley, R. L.; and Roden, D. M.: Effect of low dose quinidine on encainide pharmacokinetics and pharmacodynamics: Influence of genetic polymorphism. J. Pharmacol. Exp. Ther., 249:134–142, 1989b.

Funck-Brentano, C.; Light, R. T.; Lineberry, M. D.; Wright, G. M.; Roden, D. M.; and Woosley, R. L.: Pharmacokinetic and pharmacodynamic interaction of N-acetyl procainamide and procainamide in man. J. Cardiovasc. Pharmacol., 14: 364–373, 1989c.

Gianelly, R.; Griffin, J. R.; and Harrison, D. G.: Propranolol in the treatment and prevention of cardiac arrhythmias. Ann. Intern. Med., 66:667–676, 1967.

Gulamhusein, S.; Ko, P.; Carruthers, S. G.; and Klein, G. J.: Acceleration of the ventricular response during atrial fibrillation in the Wolff-Parkinson-White syndrome after verapamil. Circulation, 65:348–354, 1982.

Hammill, S. C.; Sugrue, D. D.; Bersch, B. J.; Porter, C. J.; Osbern, M. J.; Wood, D. L.; and Holmes, D. R.: Clinical entracardiac electrophysiologic testing: Technique, diagnostic indications and therapeutic uses. Mayo Clin. Proc., 61:478–503, 1986.

Hardy, B. G.; Zador, I. T.; Golden, L.; Lalka, D.; and Schentag, J. J.: Effect of cimetidine on the pharmacokinetics and pharmacodynamics of quinidine. Am. J. Cardiol., 52:172–175, 1983.

Hille, B.: Ionic Channels of Excitable Membranes. Sinauer Associates, Sunderland, Mass., 1984.

Hille, B: Local anesthetics: Hydrophilic and hydrophobic pathways for the drug-receptor reaction. J. Gen. Physiol., 69: 497–515, 1977.

Hine, L. K.; Laird, N. M.; Hewitt, P.; and Chalmers, T. C.: Meta-analysis of empirical long-term antiarrhythmic therapy after myocardial infarction. J.A.M.A., 262:3037–3040, 1989.

Hoffman, B. F.; Rosen, M. R.; and Wit, A. S.: Electrophysiology and pharmacology of cardiac arrhythmias. III. The causes and treatment of cardiac arrhythmias. Parts A and B. Am. Heart J., 89:115–122; 253–257, 1975.

Hondeghem, L. M.; and Katzung, B. G.: Antiarrhythmic agents: The modulated receptor mechanism of action of sodium and calcium channel-blocking drugs. Annu. Rev. Pharmacol. Toxicol., 24:387–423, 1984.

Hondeghem, L.; and Katzung, B.: Test of a model of antiarrhythmic drug action: Effects of quinidine and lidocaine on myocardial conduction. Circulation, 61:1217–1224, 1980.

Hondeghem L. M.; and Katzung, B. G.: Time- and voltage-dependent interactions of antiarrhythmic drugs with cardiac sodium channels. Biochim. Biophys. Acta, 472:373–98, 1977.

Hunt, B. A.; Self, T. H.; Lalonde, R. L.; and Bottorff, M. B.: Calcium channel blockers as inhibitors of drug metabolism. Chest, 96:393–399, 1989.

Jackman, W. M.; Friday, K. J.; Anderson, J. L.; Aliot, E. M.; Clark, M.; and Lazzara, R.: The long QT syndromes: A critical review, new clinical observations and a unifying hypothesis. Prog. Cardiovasc. Dis., 31:115–172, 1988.

Josephson, M. E.; and Kastor, J. A.: Supraventricular tachycardia: Mechanisms and management. Ann. Intern. Med., 87:346–358, 1977.

Kessler, K. M.; Kissane, B.; Cassidy, J.; Pefkaros, K. C.; Kozlovskis, P.; Hamburg, C.; and Myerburg, R. J.: Dynamic variability of binding of antiarrhythmic drugs during the evolution of acute myocardial infarction. Circulation, 70:472–478, 1984.

Kessler, K. M.; Lowenthal, D. T.; Warner, H.; Gibson, T.;

Briggs, W.; and Reidenberg, M. M.: Quinidine elimination in patients with congestive heart failure or poor renal function. N. Engl. J. Med., 290:706–709, 1974.

Kim, S. G.; Seiden, S. W.; Matos, J. A.; Waspe, L. E.; and Fisher J. D.: Combination of procainamide and quinidine for better tolerance and additive effects for ventricular arrhythmias. Am. J. Cardiol., 56:84–88, 1985.

Klein, G. J.; Yee, R.; and Sharma, A. D.: Longitudinal electrophysiologic assessment of asymptomatic patients with the Wolff-Parkinson-White electrocardiographic pattern. N. Engl. J. Med., 320(19):1229–1233, 1989.

Klein, G. J.; Bashore, T. M.; Sellers, T. D.; Pritchett, E. L. C.; Smith, W. M.; and Gallagher, J. J.: Ventricular fibrillation in the Wolff-Parkinson-White Syndrome. N. Engl. J. Med., 301:1080–1085, 1979.

Koch-Weser, J.: Drug therapy: Bretylium. N. Engl. J. Med., 300:473–477, 1979a.

Koch-Weser, J.: Disopyramide. N. Engl. J. Med., 300:957–962, 1979b.

Kuo, C. S.; Reddy, C. P.; Munakata, K.; and Surawicz, B.: Mechanism of ventricular arrhythmias caused by increased dispersion of repolarization. Eur. Heart J., 6:63–70, 1985.

LeLorier, J.; Grenon, D.; Latour, Y.; Caillé, G.; Dumont, G.; Brosseau, A.; and Solignac, A.: Pharmacokinetics of lidocaine after prolonged intravenous infusions in uncomplicated myocardial infarction. Ann. Intern. Med., 87:700–702. 1977.

Levine, J. H.; Michael, J. R.; and Guarnieri, T.: Treatment of multifocal atrial tachycardia with verapamil. N. Engl. J. Med., 312:1;21–44, 1985.

Lie, K. I.; Wellens, H. J.; van Capelle, F. J.; and Durrer, D.: Lidocaine in the prevention of primary ventricular fibrillation. N. Engl. J. Med., 291:1324–1326, 1974.

Lima, J. J.; Boudoulas, H.; and Blanford, M.: Concentration-dependence of disopyramide binding to plasma protein and its influence on kinetics and dynamics. J. Pharmacol. Exp. Ther., 219:741–747, 1981.

Lumma, W. C. Jr.; Wohl, R. A.; Davey, D. D.; Argentieri, T. M.; DeVita, R. J.; Gomez, R. P.; Jain, V. K.; Marisca, A. J.; Morgan, T. K. Jr.; Reiser, H. J.; Sullivan, M. E.; Wiggins, J.; and Wong, S. S.: Rational design of 4-[(methylsulfonyl)amino] benzamides as class III antiarrhythmic agents. J. Med. Chem., 30:755–758, 1987.

Mason, J. W.: Amiodarone. N. Engl. J. Med., 316:8;455–466, 1987.

McGovern, B.; Garan, H.; and Ruskin, J. N.: Precipitation of cardiac arrest by verapamil in patients with Wolff-Parkinson-White syndrome. Ann. Intern. Med., 104:791–794, 1986.

McKibbin, J. K.; Pocock, W. A.; Barlow, J. B.; Millar, R. N. S.; and Obel, I. W. P.: Sotalol, hypokalaemia, syncope, and torsade de pointes. Br. Heart J., 51:157–162, 1984.

Michael, J. R.; Guerci, A. D.; Koehler, R. C.; Shi, A. Y.; Tsitlik, J.; Chandra, N.; Niedermeyer, E.; Rogers, M. C.; Traystman, R. J.; and Weisfeldt, M. L.: Mechanisms by which epinephrine augments cerebral and myocardial perfusion during cardiopulmonary resuscitation in dogs. Circulation, 69:822–835, 1984.

Mines, G. R.: On circulating excitations in heart muscle and their possible relations to tachycardia and fibrillation. Trans. R. So. Can., 8:43, 1914.

Morady, F.; Kou, W. H.; Kadish, A. H.; Toivonen, L. K.; Kushner, J. A.; and Schmaltz, S.: Effects of epinephrine in patients with an accessory atrioventricular connection treated with quinidine. Am. J. Cardiol., 62:580–584, 1988.

Morganroth, J.: Placement of moricizine in the selection of antiarrhythmic drug therapy. Am. J. Cardiol., 65:65D–67D, 1990.

Morganroth, J.; and Horowitz, L. N.: Flecainide: Its proarrhythmic effect and expected changes on the surface electrocardiogram. Am. J. Cardiol., 53:89B–94B, 1984.

Morganroth, J.; Michelson, E. L.; Horowitz, L. N.; Josephson, M. E.; Pearlman, A. S.; and Dunkman W. B.: Limitations of routine long-term electrocardiographic monitoring to assess ventricular ectopic frequency. Circulation, 58:408–414, 1978.

Myerburg, R. J.; Kessler, K. M.; Cox, M. M.; Huikuri, H.;

Terracall, E.; Interian, A. Jr.; Fernandez, P.; and Castellanos, A.: Reversal of proarrhythmic effects of flecainide acetate and encainide hydrochloride by propranolol. Circulation, 80:1571–1579, 1989.

Norwegian Multicenter Study Group: Timolol-induced reduction in mortality in reinfarction in patients surviving acute myocardial infarction. N. Engl. J. Med., 304:801–807, 1981.

Petersen, P.; Boysen, G.; Godtfredsen, J.; Andersen, E. D.; and Andersen, B.: Placebo controlled, randomized trial of warfarin and aspirin for prevention of thrombombolic complications in chronic atrial fibrillation. Lancet, 1(8631):175–179, 1989.

Podrid, P. J.; Schoeneberger, A.; and Lown, B.: Congestive heart failure caused by oral disopyramide. N. Engl. J. Med., 302:614–618, 1980.

Rankin, A.; Oldroyd; K. G.; Chong, E.; Rae, A. P.; and Cobbe, S. M.: Value and limitations of adenocine in the diagnosis and treatment of narrow and broad complex tachycardias. Br. Heart J., 62:195–203; 1989.

Rickenberger, R. L.; Naccarelli, G. V.; Miles, W. M.; Markel, M. L.; Dougherty, A. H.; Prystowsky, E. N.; Heger, J. J.; and Zipes, D. P.: Encainide for atrial fibrillation associated with Wolff-Parkinson-White syndrome. Am. J. Cardiol., 62: 26L–30L, 1988.

Riddell, J. G.; McAllister, C. B.; Wilkinson, G. R.; Wood, A. J. J.; and Roden, D. M.: Constant plasma drug concentrations – A new technique with application to lidocaine. Ann. Intern. Med., 100:25–28, 1983.

Roden, D. M.: Encainide and related antiarrhythmic drugs. ISI Atlas Sci., 374–380, 1988.

Roden, D. M.: Tocainide and mexiletine: Orally effective lidocaine analogs. Arch. Intern. Med., 145:417–418, 1985.

Roden, D. M.; and Hoffman, B. F.: Action potential prolongation and induction of abnormal automaticity by low quinidine concentrations in canine Purkinje fibers: Relationship to potassium and cycle length. Circ. Res., 56:857–867, 1985.

Roden, D. M.; and Woosley, R. L.: Flecainide. N. Engl. J. Med., 315:36–41, 1986.

Roden, D. M.; Balser, J. R.; and Bennett, P.B.: Modulation of cardiac potassium currents by antiarrhythmic drugs: Present status and future directions. In, Molecular and Cellular Mechanisms of Antiarrhythmic Agents (Hondeghem, L., ed.). Futura Publishing, Mt. Kisco, N.Y., pp. 133–154, 1989.

Roden, D. M.; Thompson, K. A.; Hoffman, B. F.; and Woosley, R. L.: Clinical features and basic mechanisms of quinidine-induced arrhythmias. The proceedings of the Fourth Annual Joint US–USSR Symposium on Sudden Cardiac Death. J. Am. Coll. Cardiol., 8:73A–78A, 1986.

Roden, D. M.; Reele, S. B.; Higgins, S. B.; Smith, R.; Oates, J. A.; and Woosley, R. L.: Antiarrhythmic efficacy, pharmacokinetics and safety of N-acetylprocainamide in man: Comparison to procainamide. Am. J. Cardiol., 46:463–468, 1980a.

Roden, D. M.; Reele, S. B.; Higgins, S. B.; Mayol, R.; Gammans, R.; Oates, J. A.; and Woosley, R. L.: Total suppression of ventricular arrhythmias by encainide. N. Engl. J. Med., 302:877–882, 1980b.

Rosen, M. R.; and Reder, R. F.: Does triggered activity have a role in the genesis of cardiac arrhythmias? Ann. Intern. Med., 94:794–801, 1981.

Ruberman, W.; Weinblatt, E.; Goldberg, J. D.; Frank, C. W.; Chaudhary, B. S.; and Shapiro, S: Ventricular premature complexes and sudden death after myocardial infarction. Circulation, 64:297–305, 1981.

Schaffer, W. A.; and Cobb L. A.: Recurrent ventricular fibrillation and modes of death in survivors of out-of-hospital ventricular fibrillation. N. Engl. J. Med., 293:259–262, 1975.

Sharma, A. D.; Yee, R.; Guiraudon, G.; and Klein, G. J.: Sensitivity and specificy of invasive and noninvasive testing for risk of sudden death in Wolff-Parkinson-White syndrome. J. Am. Coll. Cardiol., 10(2):373–381, 1987.

Singh, B. N.; and Vaughan Williams, E. M.: A third class of anti-arrhythmic action. Effects on atrial and ventricular intracellular potentials, and other pharmacological actions on cardiac muscle, of MJ 1999 and AH 3747. Br. J. Pharmacol., 39:675–689, 1970.

Sonnenblick, E. H. (issue ed.): Esmolol – An ultrashort-acting intravenous beta blocker. Am. J. Cardiol., 56(suppl.):1F–62F, 1985.

Special Report. Preliminary report of the stroke prevention in atrial fibrillation study. N. Engl. J. Med., 322:863–868, 1990.

Speirs, C. J.; Murray, S.; Boobis, A. R.; Seddon, C. E.; and Davies, D. S.: Quinidine and the identification of drugs whose elimination is impaired in subjects classified as poor metabolizers of debrisoquine. Br. J. Clin. Pharmacol., 22: 739–743, 1986.

Steinman, R. T.; Herrera, C.; Schuger, C. D.; and Lehmann, M. H.: Wide QRS tachycardia in the conscious adult. J.A.M.A., 261:1013–1016, 1989.

Stewart, R. B.; Bardy, G. H.; and Greene, H. L.: Wide complex tachycardia: Misdiagnosis and outcome after emergent therapy. Ann. Intern. Med., 104:766–771, 1986.

Stone, N.; Klein, M. D.; and Lown, B.: Diphenylhydantoin in the prevention of recurring ventricular tachycardia. Circulation, 43:420–427, 1971.

Talano, J. V.; and Tommaso, C.: Slow channel calcium antagonists in the treatment of supraventricular tachycardia. Prog. Cardiovasc. Dis., 25:141–156, 1982.

Thompson, K. A.; Blair, I. A.; Woosley, R. L.; and Roden, D. M.: Comparative electrophysiologic effects of quinidine, its major metabolites and dihydroquinidine in canine cardiac Purkinje fibers. J. Pharmacol. Exp. Ther., 241:84–90, 1987.

Thompson, P. D.; Melmon, K. L.; Richards, J.; Cohn, K.; Steinbrunn, W.; Cudihee, R.; and Rowland, M.: Lidocaine pharmacokinetics in advanced heart failure, liver disease and renal failure in man. Ann. Intern. Med., 78:499–508, 1973.

Turgeon, J.; PaVLou] H.; Funck-Brentano, C.; and Roden, D. M.: Genetically-determined interaction of encainide and quinidine in patients with arrhythmias. Circulation, 80:SII–S326, 1989.

Twum-Barima, Y.; and Carruthers, S. G.: Quinidine-rifampin interaction. N. Engl. J. Med., 304:1466–1469, 1981.

Tzivoni, D.; Banai, S.; Schugar, C.; Benhorin, J.; Keren, A.; Gottlieb, S.; and Stern, S.: Treatment of torsade de pointes with magnesium sulfate. Circulation, 77:392–397. 1988.

Vaughan Williams, E. M.: Relevance of cellular to clinical electrophysiology in interpreting antiarrythmic drug action. Am. J. Cardiol., 64:5J–9J, 1989.

Watanabe, Y.: Purkinje repolarization as a possible cause of the U wave in the electrocardiogram. Circulation, 51:1030–1037, 1975.

Wellens, H. J. J.: The wide QRS tachycardia. Ann. Intern. Med., 104(6):879, 1986.

Wellens, H. J. J.; Brugada, P.; and Penn, O. C.: The management of pre-excitation syndromes. J.A.M.A., 257(17):2325–2333, 1987.

Wenckebach, K. F.: Cinchona derivates in the treatment of heart disorders. J.A.M.A., 81:472–474, 1923.

Wetherbee, D. G.; Holzman, D.; and Brown, M. G.: Ventricular tachycardia following the administration of quinidine. Am. Heart J., 42:89–96, 1951.

Winkle, R. A.; Mason, J. W.; Griffin, J. C.; and Ross, D.: Malignant ventricular tachyarrhythmias associated with the use of encainide. Am. Heart J., 102:857–864, 1981.

Wit, A. L.; and Rosen, M. R.: Pathophysiologic mechanisms of cardiac arrhythmias. Am. Heart J., 106:798–811, 1983.

Woosley, R. L.; Wood, A. J. J.; and Roden, D. M.: Encainide. N. Engl. J. Med., 318:1107–1115, 1988.

Woosley, R. L.; Reele, S. B.; Roden, D. M.; Nies, A. S.; and Oates, J. A.: Pharmacologic reversal of the hypotensive effect that complicates antiarrhythmic therapy with bretylium. Clin. Pharmacol. Ther., 32:313–321, 1982.

Woosley, R. L.; Kornhauser, D.; Smith, R.; Reele, S.; Higgins, S. B.; Nies, A. S.; Shand, D. G.; and Oates, J. A.: Suppression of chronic ventricular arrhythmias with propranolol. Circulation, 60:819–827, 1979.

Woosley, R. L.; Drayer, D. E.; Reidenberg, M. M.; Nies, A. S.; Carr, K.; and Oates, J. A.: Effect of acetylator phenotype on the rate at which procainamide induces antinuclear antibodies and the lupus syndrome. N. Engl. J. Med., 298: 1157–1159, 1978.

Yusuf, S.; Wittes, J.; and Friedman, L.: Overview of results of randomized clinical trials in heart disease: I. Treatments following myocardial infarction. J.A.M.A., 260:2088–2093, 1988.

Zhou, H. H.; Anthony, L. B.; Roden, D.; and Wood, A. J.: Quinidine reduces clearance (+)-propranolol more than (−)-propranolol through marked reduction 4 hydroxidation. Clin. Pharm. Ther., 47(6):686–693, 1990.

Zipes, D. P.; Prystowsky, E. N.; and Heger, J. J.: Amiodarone: Electrophysiologic actions, pharmacokinetics and clinical effects. J. Am. Coll. Cardiol., 3(4):1059–1071, 1984.

7

Pulmonary Disorders

Peter J. Barnes

Options for treatment of pulmonary diseases are somewhat limited, but recent advances in our understanding of respiratory disorders and of the mechanisms of drug action should make it possible to apply currently available treatment in a logical and efficacious way. This chapter first reviews the modes of delivery and the categories of drugs that are available for treating pulmonary diseases and then discusses their application in specific respiratory disorders. Several excellent textbooks on respiratory medicine now are available that describe in detail the diagnosis, clinical features, and management of respiratory diseases (e.g., Murray and Nadel, 1988; Baum and Wolinsky, 1989).

ROUTES OF DRUG DELIVERY

Drugs can be delivered to the lungs by inhalation, or by oral or parenteral routes. Inhalation is becoming more effectively and thus more frequently used to deliver drugs to the lung.

Inhaled Route

Inhalation is the preferred mode of delivery of many drugs with a direct effect on airways, particularly when the disease is asthma or chronic obstructive pulmonary disease (COPD) (Newhouse and Dolovich, 1986). Inhalation is the only way to deliver some drugs, such as cromolyn sodium and anticholinergics, and is the preferred route of delivery for β-adrenergic agonists and

corticosteroids. Antibiotics also may be delivered by inhalation to patients with chronic respiratory infection (e.g., those with cystic fibrosis), or to prevent pulmonary infection in high-risk patients [e.g., prevention of *Pneumocystis* pneumonia in patients with acquired immunodeficiency syndrome (AIDS)]. The major advantage of inhalation is that the delivery of drug is directly to the airways and in doses that are effective and pose a low risk of adverse effects from the drug's extra-pulmonary systemic actions. This is particularly important with the use of corticosteroids and may become more important when β-adrenergic agents are incorporated into inhalable liposomes. Bronchodilators have a more rapid onset of action when inhaled than when taken orally so that more rapid control of symptoms is possible.

Particle Size. The size of particles for inhalation is critical in determining the site of their deposition in the respiratory tract (Newman et al., 1981). The optimum size for particles to settle in the airways is 2 to 5 μm. Larger particles settle out in the upper airways, and smaller particles remain suspended and are exhaled. Even in these two extremes, a drug may still have effects because of absorption by mucous membranes.

Pharmacokinetics. Of the total drug delivered by mouth, probably less than 5% enters the lower airways. The fate of the inhaled drug is poorly understood. Drugs are absorbed from the lumen of the airway and have a variety of effects on various cells in the airway. Drugs also may be absorbed into the bronchial circulation and distributed to peripheral airways. Whether drugs are metabolized in the airways often is obscure. Little is known of the factors that influence local absorption and metabolism of inhaled drugs. Nevertheless, several drugs have great therapeutic efficacy when given by inhalation.

Delivery of Inhaled Drugs. Several ways of delivering inhaled drugs have been employed.

Metered dose inhalers (MDIs) deliver drug from a canister with a chlorofluorocarbon propellant (alternative "ozone friendly" propellants are under development). These devices are convenient and portable and usually deliver from 100 to 400 doses of drug. They usually are easy to use, although the patient may have to be taught to coordinate inhalation with triggering of the delivery by the device.

Spacer chambers are large-volume devices placed between the MDI and the patient. They reduce the velocity of particles entering the upper airways and the size of the particles by allowing evaporation of liquid propellant. This reduces the amount of drug that impinges on the oropharynx and increases the proportion of drug that enters the lower airways. The device reduces the need to carefully coordinate drug delivery with inhalation, because the MDI can be activated into the chamber and the aerosol subsequently inhaled from the one-way valve. Perhaps the most useful application of spacer chambers is to reduce the oropharyngeal deposition of inhaled steroids, thereby decreasing the local and systemic adverse effects of these drugs.

Dry-powder inhalers are devices that scatter a fine powder dispersed by air turbulence on inhalation. These devices may be preferred by some patients, because respiratory coordination is not as necessary as with the MDI. But other patients find the dry powder irritating. Some multiple-dose dry-powder inhalers now are available that are convenient to use. The future may bring other particulate delivery systems for delivery of drugs to the lung or even to the alveoli with direct absorption into the systemic circulation.

Nebulizers are available in two types. Jet nebulizers are driven by a stream of gas (air or oxygen), whereas ultrasonic nebulizers employ a rapidly vibrating piezoelectric crystal and thus do not require a source of compressed gas. The nebulized drug may be inspired during tidal breathing and allow high-dose delivery. Nebulizers therefore are useful in treating acute exacerbations of asthma, for delivering drugs when airway obstruction is marked (e.g., in severe COPD), for delivering inhalable drugs to infants and small children who cannot use the other inhalational devices because of inability to cooperate, and for delivering drugs such as antibiotics when relatively high doses are needed.

Oral Route

Drugs to treat pulmonary diseases may be given orally. The oral dose usually is much higher than the inhaled dose required to achieve the same effect (by a ratio of more than 20 : 1); consequently, systemic adverse effects may be more common and severe than with the same drug inhaled. When there is a choice between inhaled or oral route for a drug (e.g., β-adrenergic agonist or corticosteroid), the inhaled route always is preferable and the oral route should be reserved for those few patients unable to use inhalers (e.g., small children, patients with physical problems such as severe arthritis of the hand, etc.) or in severe disease (e.g., asthmatics who required systemic steroids).

Theophylline is ineffective by the inhaled route and therefore must be given orally. Corticosteroids may have to be given orally for parenchymal lung disease (e.g., interstitial lung diseases), although as mentioned above it may be possible in the future to deliver such drugs into alveoli using specially designed inhalation devices that accomplish high local penetration as well as systemic absorption of the drug without a first-pass effect. *Principle: Although there has been considerable emphasis on delivering a drug to a target organ that is diseased, some target organs may not be diseased and can be used to systematically deliver the drug and bypass its early metabolism.*

Parenteral Route

The IV route should be reserved for delivery of drugs to severely ill patients who are unable to absorb drugs from the GI tract and in whom the inhaled route of drug administration is insufficient. Adverse effects with this delivery route generally are more frequent than with the inhaled route because of the higher plasma concentrations of drug achieved following oral administration. *Principle: When a drug such as a glucocorticoid or antibiotic can be administered topically, orally, or parenterally, the optimal route must be determined for each patient. Goals of treatment (e.g., therapy, prophylaxis), severity of illness, and other factors must be weighed, as each route offers a different combination of benefits and risks.*

BRONCHODILATORS

Bronchodilator drugs have an antibronchoconstrictor effect that may be demonstrated directly in vitro by drug-induced relaxation of precontracted airways (Barnes, 1988). Bronchodilators promptly reverse airway obstruction in asthmatics. This action is believed to be mediated by a direct effect on airway smooth muscle. However, additional pharmacologic effects on other airway cells (such as capillary endothelium to reduce microvascular leakage and mast cells to reduce release of bronchoconstrictor mediators) may contribute to the overall reduction in airway narrowing. Only three types of bronchodilators are in current clinical use: β-adrenergic agonists, methylxanthines, and anticholinergics. Drugs such as cromolyn sodium, which prevent bronchoconstriction, have no bronchodilator action and are ineffective once bronchoconstriction has occurred. Corticosteroids, while gradually improving airway obstruction, have no direct effect on airway smooth muscle and are not therefore considered to be bronchodilators.

β-Adrenergic Receptor Agonists

Epinephrine has been used to treat asthma since the beginning of the 20th century. Desiccated adrenal gland originally was given to asthmatic patients in the belief that it would reduce the swelling of the bronchial mucosa in the same way that it produces blanching of the skin. Epinephrine stimulates both α- and β-adrenergic receptors; its bronchodilator effect is mediated by β receptors. Consequently, extensive efforts have been aimed at developing drugs that more specifically stimulate the β receptors of the bronchus. Isoproterenol, a strong β agonist with very weak α-adrenergic potency, was used in the 1940s in the treatment of asthma. However, isoproterenol is a nonselective β agonist that stimulates both β_1 and β_2 receptors. Because bronchodilation is mediated by β_2 receptors, selective β_2 agonists, such as albuterol, or salbutamol, and terbutaline, were introduced in the 1960s. The hope was that bronchodilator action equivalent to that produced by maximally tolerated doses of isoproterenol would not be accompanied by the β_1 cardiovascular effects of isoproterenol (see chapter 6).

Pharmacology. The development of selective β_2 agonists was an outcome of substitutions in the catecholamine structure (McFadden, 1981). The catechol ring consists of hydroxyl groups in the 3 and 4 positions of the benzene ring (Fig. 7–1). Norepinephrine differs from epinephrine (adrenaline) only in the substitution on the terminal amino group. Modification at this site helps confer β-receptor selectivity. Further substitution of the terminal amino group results in the development of β_2-receptor selectivity as for albuterol and terbutaline.

Endogenous catecholamines are rapidly re-

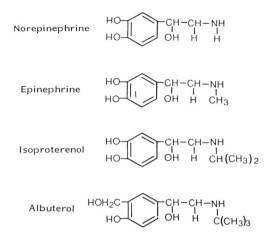

Fig. 7–1. Chemical structure of four adrenergic agonists showing their evolution from catecholamines.

moved by two active uptake processes (Figure 7–2; Iversen, 1971). *Uptake₁* is localized to sympathetic postganglionic nerve terminals, where the catecholamine is rapidly taken up and stored in reusable form in storage vesicles. *Uptake₂* facilitates uptake into nonneural tissue, such as smooth muscle cells, where enzymatic degradation occurs. Isoproterenol is not a substrate for uptake₁. It is rapidly removed by the uptake₂ mechanism. Exogenous noncatecholamine β-adrenergic agonists typically are not taken up by either of these pathways (see chapters 4 and 26). Catecholamines are rapidly metabolized by the enzyme catechol O-methyltransferase (COMT), which methylates the catechol in the 3-hydroxyl position. This step plus the rapid uptake of catecholamines against enormous concentration gradients accounts for the short duration of action of catecholamines. Modification of the catechol ring, as in albuterol and terbutaline, prevents this degradation and therefore prolongs the effect of these drugs compared with catecholamines. Catecholamines also are oxidized by monoamine oxidase (MAO) while stored in sympathetic nerve terminals. Isoproterenol is a substrate for MAO and is extensively metabolized in the gut, leading to very low bioavailability after oral administration. Substitution in the amino group confers resistance to MAO and leads to much greater oral bioavailability. While there are many β_2-selective adrenergic agonists available clinically that have differences in potency, there have been no clinically or therapeutically significant differences demonstrated in their receptor selectivity. Inhaled β_2-selective drugs in current clinical use have similar durations of action. Recently, β_2-selective drugs have been developed that have a very long

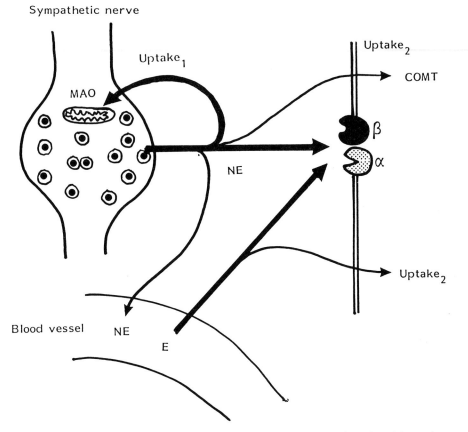

Fig. 7–2. Uptake mechanisms for endogenous catecholamines. Norepinephrine released from adrenergic nerves is taken back up into the nerve ending by a high-affinity active-transport system (Uptake₁). In the nerve ending it can either be stored in retrievable form in granules or be degraded by monoamine oxidase (MAO). Both norepinephrine (NE) and epinephrine (E) are taken up by a lower-affinity mechanism (Uptake₂) in tissues and subsequently degraded by catechol O-methyltransferase (COMT).

duration of effect, such as salmeterol and formoterol.

β-Adrenergic agonists promote bronchodilation by direct stimulation of β-adrenergic receptors in the airway smooth muscle, which leads to relaxation of bronchial smooth muscle. This can be demonstrated in vitro by the relaxant effect of isoproterenol on human bronchi and lung strips (Zaagsma et al., 1983.), and in vivo by a rapid decrease in airway resistance. β-Adrenergic receptors are in airway smooth muscle from the trachea to the terminal bronchioles (Carstairs et al., 1985). The molecular mechanisms by which β-adrenergic agonists relax airway smooth muscle have been extensively investigated. Activation of adenylate cyclase increases the concentration of intracellular cyclic adenosine 3′,5′-monophosphate (cAMP), leading to activation of specific cAMP-dependent protein kinases that cause relaxation by several mechanisms. β-Adrenergic agonists may lower the cytoplasmic concentration of calcium ion by actively removing calcium ions from the cell or by transporting them into intracellular stores. Relaxation may also be due to an inhibition of myosin phosphorylation (Torphy et al., 1982; Silver and Stull, 1984). β-Adrenergic agonists reverse bronchoconstriction irrespective of the contractile agent. This is an important property, because many different bronchoconstrictor mechanisms (neural and mediators) are likely to be operative in asthma.

β-Adrenergic agonists may have several effects on airways other than on smooth muscle that lead to decreased airway resistance (Carstairs et al., 1985). β-Adrenergic agonists have potent effects in preventing release of mediators from a number of cells including isolated human lung mast cells in vitro (Church and Hiroi, 1987) and in vivo (Howarth et al., 1985). By a separate mechanism, β-adrenergic agonists can reduce leakage from the microvasculature and thus the development of bronchial mucosal edema caused by exposure to mediators such as histamine (Erjefalt and Persson, 1986). In addition, β-adrenergic agonists increase mucus secretion from submucosal glands and ion transport across airway epithelium. These effects enhance mucociliary clearance and therefore reverse the defect in clearance caused by asthma (Pavia et al., 1980). β-Adrenergic agonists also may release a putative relaxant factor from epithelial cells. And β-adrenergic agonists reduce neurotransmission in cholinergic nerves by an action at prejunctional β_2 receptors that inhibits release of acetylcholine (Rhoden et al., 1988). This may contribute to the bronchodilator effects of the amines by reducing cholinergic reflex bronchoconstriction.

Although the effects additional to bronchodilation may be relevant to the prophylactic use of these drugs against various challenges, their primary and rapid bronchodilator action is probably due to the direct effect on airway smooth muscle.

Pharmacodynamics. *Epinephrine* is the drug most often used to treat acute anaphylaxis because a combination of α- and β-adrenergic properties may be desirable. However, the lack of β_2 selectivity (resulting in β_1-receptor-mediated cardiac stimulation), short duration of action, and prominent α-adrenergic receptor–mediated vasoconstrictor effects make epinephrine a second-line drug in the treatment of asthma. Epinephrine's effects could be an advantage in reducing microvascular leakage in airways (by a vasoconstrictor effect on bronchial arterioles; Boschetto et al., 1989), but the clinical significance of this effect is not clear. There is no convincing evidence that epinephrine causes bronchoconstriction by activation of α-adrenergic receptors on airway smooth muscle. Nebulized epinephrine offers no advantage over nebulized albuterol, at least in acute severe asthma (Coupe et al., 1987), although some patients may have a better response to epinephrine administered subcutaneously than to aerosolized metaproterenol (Appel et al., 1989).

Isoproterenol is a nonselective β-adrenergic agonist that may have undesired cardiac effects in the treatment of asthma. Dose–response curves obtained with isoproterenol and albuterol (a β_2-selective drug) show no greater bronchodilating effect with isoproterenol (Barnes and Pride, 1983). Isoproterenol has a relatively prompt onset of action and offset (less than 2 hours) in bronchodilator effect.

Several β_2-*selective agonists* now are available (Nelson, 1986). These drugs are as effective as nonselective agonists in their bronchodilator action, because airway effects are mediated only by β_2 receptors. However, they are less likely to pro-

duce cardiac stimulation than isoproterenol because β_1 receptors are stimulated relatively less than the target β_2 receptors. With the exception of rimiterol (which retains the catechol ring structure and is therefore susceptible to the enzyme COMT), they have a longer duration of action because they are resistant to uptake and enzymatic degradation by COMT and MAO. There is little to choose between the various β_2-adrenergic agonists currently available; all are usable by the inhalation and oral routes, have a similar duration of action (usually 3–4 hours, but less in severe asthma) and similar adverse effects. Differences in β_2 selectivity have been claimed but have not been demonstrated to be clinically important. Drugs in clinical use include albuterol, terbutaline, fenoterol, bitolterol, metaproterenol, and isoetharine.

Longer-acting β_2-adrenergic agonists that are effective by inhalation now have been developed and are in clinical trials. Formoterol and salmeterol bronchodilator effects last more than 12 hours and therefore are suitable for twice-daily dosing (Ullman and Svedmyr, 1988; Arvidsson et al., 1989).

Indications and Clinical Use. β-Adrenergic agonists are the most widely used and effective bronchodilators for the treatment of asthma. When inhaled from metered-dose aerosols, they are convenient, easy to use, rapid in onset, and without significant adverse effects. In addition to an acute bronchodilator effect, they are effective in protecting against various bronchoconstrictor challenges, such as exercise, cold air, and allergens. This class of drug is the bronchodilator of choice in treating acute severe asthma; the nebulized route of administration is apparently as effective as IV use (Williams et al., 1981). The inhaled route of administration is preferable to the oral route because adverse effects caused by systemic actions of the drug are less, and also because this route may be more effective. β-Adrenergic agonists are commonly used on a regular basis, but it may be preferable to give them as required by symptoms, since increased usage would then indicate the need for more anti-inflammatory therapy (Barnes, 1989d). Inhaled albuterol is able to prevent exercise-induced asthma, whereas an oral dose with similar bronchodilator effect is not (Anderson et al., 1976). This observation may indicate that the inhaled drug may reach surface cells (e.g., mast cells or epithelial cells) less accessible to the orally administered drug. β-Adrenergic agonists normally are given by MDI, but dry-powder formulations are available.

Oral administration of β-adrenergic agonists provides no advantage over the inhaled route and is more likely to be associated with adverse effects caused by systemic absorption of the drug. Sustained-release preparations may be useful in treating nocturnal asthma. Subcutaneous infusion of a β-adrenergic agonist has proved useful in some asthmatic patients with "brittle" asthma characterized by sudden and unpredictable episodes of bronchoconstriction (O'Driscoll et al., 1988). In settings of cardiovascular-respiratory instability, the circulation in the subcutaneous and skeletal muscle areas may be quite unpredictable. When circulation in these sites is compromised, drug absorption from these sites will be unpredictable.

Tolerance. Continuous treatment with an agonist often leads to tolerance or subsensitivity to the drug that may be due to down-regulation of its receptor. For this reason, many studies of bronchial β-adrenergic receptor function after prolonged therapy with β-adrenergic agonists have been conducted. The studies have shown tolerance to the nonairway β-adrenergic responses, including tremor, cardiovascular, and metabolic effects, that is readily induced in both normal and asthmatic subjects (Tattersfield, 1985). However, tolerance to β-adrenergic receptor–mediated bronchodilation has not been demonstrated in asthmatics. Because tolerance of human airway smooth muscle to β-adrenergic agonists occurs in vitro, it may be that desensitization occurs in some patients. For example, in normal subjects, tolerance has been demonstrated in some, but not all, studies after high-dose inhaled albuterol (Holgate et al., 1977). Similarly, tolerance in asthmatic subjects has been found in some but not all studies; the extent of desensitization has generally been small, and it may not be clinically important. The more readily demonstrable tolerance of extrapulmonary effects actually has clinical benefit because adverse effects tend to decrease with continued use of the drug. The mechanisms for the relative resistance of airway β receptors to desensitization by β agonists remains uncertain.

Glucocorticoids can prevent the development of tolerance to β-adrenergic agonists in airway smooth muscle. Glucocorticoids may prevent or reverse the fall in pulmonary β-adrenergic receptor density seen in lungs of animals after prolonged exposure to β-adrenergic agonists. Similarly, IV hydrocortisone reverses the tolerance of airway β-adrenergic receptors to chronic adrenergic stimulation in normal subjects (Holgate et al., 1977). Thus, any tendency for development of tolerance to high-dose inhaled β-adrenergic agonists should be moderated by concomitant administration of corticosteroids. *Principle: Drugs can produce their beneficial effects on the basis of multiple and different mechanisms, including unexpected but beneficial drug interactions.*

Adverse Reactions and Contraindications. Unwanted effects are dose-related and are due to stimulation of extrapulmonary β receptors. Adverse effects are less common with inhaled therapy than with oral or IV administration.

Muscle Tremor. Muscle tremor is caused by stimulation of the β_2-adrenergic receptors in skeletal muscle and is a common adverse effect (Nelson, 1986). The problem may be most troublesome in elderly patients.

Cardiovascular Effects. Tachycardia and palpitations are caused both by reflex cardiac stimulation secondary to peripheral vasodilation from direct stimulation of the vascular β receptors and by direct stimulation of atrial β-adrenergic receptors. Human heart expresses β_2 receptors that increase heart rate. Tachycardia also may arise from "selective" β_2-adrenergic agonists activating β_1-adrenergic receptors at doses of drug above those that enable selective β_2 effects. These adverse effects tend to disappear with continued use of the drug, reflecting the development of differential tolerance to the less prominent actions of the drug. *Principle: When the mechanisms that are responsible for diminishing both the toxic and the efficacious effects of a drug are the same (e.g., down-regulation of β-adrenergic receptors leading to tolerance to the effects of the drug), special effort must be made to measure efficacy as toxicity wanes.*

Metabolic Effects. Metabolic effects (increase in free fatty acids; release of insulin, glucose, pyruvate, and lactate) in plasma usually are seen only after large doses are given so that high concentrations reach the systemic circulation. Hypokalemia potentially is a serious adverse effect (Haalboom et al., 1985) because of β_2-adrenergic receptor stimulation of potassium entry into skeletal muscle. The effect may be in part secondary to a rise in secretion of insulin, as well as to a direct effect on skeletal muscle (Schnack et al., 1989). Hypokalemia may be serious in the presence of hypoxia, as in acute asthma, and with use of antiarrhythmic or other cardioactive drugs that predispose to cardiac dysrhythmias. The incidence of serious supraventricular or ventricular arrhythmias when these agents are used is difficult to determine because of the risk of arrhythmias associated with the underlying disease.

Hypoxemia. β-Adrenergic agonists may increase ventilation–perfusion mismatch by vasodilation of pulmonary blood vessels previously constricted by hypoxia. The result is a shunt of blood to poorly ventilated areas, causing a fall in arterial oxygen tension. Although in practice the adverse effect of β agonists on PaO_2 usually is very small (less than 5 mm Hg fall); occasionally in patients with severe and chronic airway obstruction it may be much larger. Hypoxemia may be prevented by giving additional inspired oxygen with the adrenergic agonists (Maquire and Nair, 1978). Arterial blood-gas analysis is mandatory when evaluating a patient's Pao_2, Pco_2, and pH because serious abnormalities often are impossible to predict from clinical findings alone. The problem can be compounded when drugs are used whose efficacy can be prominent and easy to measure (e.g., change in FEV_1) and whose toxicity subtly enters, requiring other objective measurements.

Safety. Because of a possible relationship between adrenergic drug therapy and the rise in death rates of patients with asthma in the 1960s in the United Kingdom, doubts have been cast on the safety of β-adrenergic agonists. The apparent increase in mortality might equally well be explained by reduced usage of corticosteroids and delay in seeking medical attention since the introduction of isoproterenol as an effective outpatient bronchodilator sold over the counter (Stolley, 1972). More recently, these doubts have been revived, and the use of high doses of β-adrenergic agonists given by nebulizers at home has been linked to the increase in deaths caused by asthma in New Zealand (Wilson et al., 1981). However, there still is no convincing evidence that the β-adrenergic agonists per se contribute to deaths in asthmatics (Benatar, 1986). Most of these patients have been poorly diagnosed and treated.

The use of β-adrenergic agonists should not preclude concomitant administration of anti-inflammatory drugs. β-Adrenergic agonists (at least those currently available for clinical use) do not suppress the chronic inflammatory process in asthmatic airways (Barnes, 1989b), nor do they reduce bronchial hyperresponsiveness (Kraan et al., 1985; Kerrebijn et al., 1987), or prevent the development of increased bronchial responsiveness after challenge with an allergen (Cockcroft and Murdock, 1987). A rebound increase in bronchial responsiveness has been described after stopping regular use of inhaled β-adrenergic agonists (Vathenen et al., 1988).

Anticholinergics

Background and Pharmacology. Datura plants contain the muscarinic antagonist stramonium and were smoked for relief of asthma 2 centuries ago. Atropine, a related naturally occurring compound, also was introduced for treating asthma, but, because these compounds had prominent systemic adverse effects, particularly drying of secretions, their benefit was doubted. Now less soluble quaternary compounds (e.g., atropine

methylnitrate and ipratropium bromide) have become available. When these drugs are inhaled, they are active and are not significantly absorbed from the respiratory tract. The efficacy of atropine-like drugs in the treatment of asthma has thus emerged again.

Anticholinergics specifically antagonize muscarinic receptors and have no other significant pharmacologic effects when used clinically. In normal animals and humans, a small degree of resting bronchomotor tone is due to tonic vagal nerve impulses that release acetylcholine in the vicinity of airway smooth muscle. This bronchoconstriction can be blocked by anticholinergic drugs (Barnes, 1987a). There is considerable evidence that cholinergic pathways play an important role in regulating acute bronchomotor responses in animals. A wide variety of mechanical, chemical, and immunologic stimuli also are capable of eliciting reflex bronchoconstriction via vagal pathways. All these data suggest that cholinergic mechanisms could underly bronchial hyperresponsiveness and acute bronchoconstrictor responses during asthma attacks. The implication, if the hypothesis were correct, would be that anticholinergic drugs would be effective bronchodilators during asthmatic attacks in humans. Many controlled studies indicate that anticholinergic drugs protect against acute challenge by sulfur dioxide, inert dusts, cold air, and emotional factors (Gross and Skorodin, 1984a; Mann and George, 1985). The drugs are less effective against antigen challenge, exercise, and fog. The results of the studies are not surprising because anticholinergic drugs only inhibit reflex cholinergic bronchoconstriction and do not significantly block the direct effects of inflammatory mediators, such as histamine and leukotrienes, on bronchial smooth muscle and vessels. Furthermore, cholinergic antagonists probably have little or no effect on mast cells.

Pharmacodynamics. Ipratropium bromide is the most widely used anticholinergic inhaler. It is available as an MDI and nebulized preparation (Gross, 1988). The onset of bronchodilation is relatively slow—usually maximal 30 to 60 minutes after inhalation. However, the efficacy may persist for as long as 8 hours. The drug usually is given by MDI four times daily on a regular basis, rather than intermittently to control symptoms. Oxitropium bromide is a novel quaternary anticholinergic bronchodilator similar to ipratropium bromide in terms of muscarinic receptor blockade. It is available in higher doses for inhalation and may lead to more prolonged effects (Frith et al., 1986). Thus, it may be useful in some patients with nocturnal asthma (Coe and Barnes, 1986). *Principle: Diseases, like drugs, have characteristic* *dynamics. Because dose-related response to a drug depends on the severity of the lesion it is to reverse, assessing the dynamics of the disease and matching the kinetics and dynamics of the drug to severity is crucial in preventing worsening of the disease. Proper matching of drugs to disease can simplify overall management, minimizing the need to combine drugs or "push" doses to the point of toxicity.*

Indications and Clinical Use

Asthma. Anticholinergic drugs usually are less effective as bronchodilators in asthmatic subjects than β-adrenergic agonists. Anticholinergic drugs offer less efficient protection against various challenges that lead to bronchial constriction, although their duration of action is significantly longer than that of β-adrenergic agonists (Gross and Skorodin, 1984a; Barnes, 1987b). The anticholinergic drugs may be more effective in older rather than younger patients with asthma (Ullah et al., 1981). Nebulized anticholinergic drugs may be useful in reversing acute severe asthma (Ward et al., 1981; Rebuck et al., 1987), although they appear to be more effective than β-adrenergic agonists for this purpose. Nevertheless, for the acute and chronic treatment of asthma, anticholinergic drugs may have an additive effect with β-adrenergic agonists and should therefore be considered when control of asthma is not adequate using β-adrenergic agonists alone. The combination is particularly useful when problems develop during use of theophylline. *Principle: Even when a type of drug is less effective than another first-line type, it may contribute significantly to overall clinical efficacy and lowered toxicity when utilized to produce a deliberate and rational drug interaction.*

COPD. In patients with COPD, anticholinergic drugs may be as effective as, or even superior to, β-adrenergic agonists (Gross and Skorodin, 1984a and 1984b). Their relatively greater effect in patients with COPD rather than those with asthma may be explained by the exclusive inhibitory effect on vagal tone of anticholinergics. Although such tone may not be vastly increased in patients with COPD, it may be the only reversible element of airway obstruction exaggerated by geometric factors in an airway narrowed by disease (see Fig. 7–3). *Principle: Assessing the potential for reversibility of a preliminary lesion is crucial to making the qualitative decision to treat or not treat. Then the quantitative decisions (how much, how often, and by which route) are measured against actual change in the disease.*

Adverse Reactions and Contraindications. Inhaled anticholinergic drugs usually are well toler-ated, and there is no evidence that their effect diminishes during continued clinical use. When inhaled anticholinergics are discontinued, a small rebound increase in bronchial constriction has been described, although its clinical relevance is uncertain (Newcomb et al., 1985). The adverse effects of atropine are dose-related and are due to cholinergic antagonism in systems other than the lung. These include dryness of the mouth, blurred vision, and urinary retention. However, adverse effects due to ipratropium are very uncommon because the drug is not well absorbed into the systemic circulation from the lung (Gross, 1988).

Because cholinergic agonists stimulate mucus secretion, several studies of anticholinergics have examined their effects on reduction of mucus secretion—the drugs might lead to a more viscous mucous. Atropine reduces mucociliary clearance in normal subjects and in patients with asthma and chronic bronchitis, but the quaternary derivative, ipratropium bromide, even when given in high doses, has no such detectable effect either on normal subjects or in patients with airway disease (Pavia et al., 1980).

A significant unwanted effect of inhaled ipratropium is its unpleasant, bitter taste. This may contribute to poor compliance with this drug. Nebulized ipratropium bromide may precipitate glaucoma in elderly patients because of its direct mydriatic effect on the eye. The complication may be prevented by nebulizing with a mouthpiece rather than a face mask. *Principle: The physician can be deceived when delivering a drug to a local site of interest by not observing effects of the drug beyond that site. An industry has grown from the profession's finally admitting that corticosteroids delivered to the skin actually are absorbed and have systemic effects. Many other drugs that are placed locally have more distant effects, for example, "nonabsorbable antibiotics" delivered to the gut, many drugs "delivered" to the skin, β-adrenergic antagonists "delivered" to the eye, contraceptives "delivered" to the cervix, and so forth.*

Paradoxical bronchoconstriction can occur with ipratropium bromide. This complication is particularly prominent when the drug is given by nebulizer and is largely explained by the hypotonicity of the solution in the nebulizer and the antibacterial additives, such as benzalkonium chloride and EDTA. Nebulizer isotonic solutions free of these additives are less likely to cause bronchoconstriction (Rafferty et al., 1988). Occasionally, bronchoconstriction may occur after ipratropium bromide is given by MDI. This reaction probably is due to blockage of prejunctional muscarinic receptors on cholinergic nerves that normally inhibit acetylcholine release (Barnes, 1989c). *Princi-*

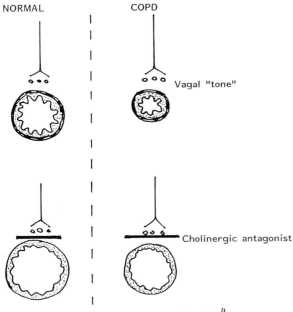

NORMAL

COPD

Vagal "tone"

Cholinergic antagonist

Resistance $\propto 1$ / radius^4

Fig. 7–3. Anticholinergic drugs inhibit vagally mediated airway tone leading to bronchodilation. This effect is small in normal airways but is greater in structurally narrowed airways in patients with COPD.

ple: Drug effects most often are caused by the chemical entity but also have been attributable to the excipients the product is compounded with. If ordinary doses produce paradoxical effects, be particularly concerned about the vehicle or excipient the chemical entity is in.

Theophylline

Background and Pharmacology. The bronchodilator effect of strong coffee was described by Hyde Salter during the last century. Methylxanthines such as theophylline are related to caffeine and have been used to treat asthma since 1930. Indeed, theophylline is widely used in the therapy of asthma worldwide. Theophylline has become easier to use, as its plasma concentrations can be readily determined and reliable slow-release preparations are available. Nonetheless, because β-adrenergic agonists are more effective bronchodilators and inhaled steroids have a much greater anti-inflammatory effect than theophylline, the use of theophylline is declining.

Chemistry. Theophylline is a methylxanthine chemically and structurally similar to the common dietary xanthines, caffeine and theobromine. Several substituted derivatives of natural xanthines have been synthesized, but none have any clinical advantage over theophylline. Only enprofylline, the 3-propyl derivative, is more potent as a bronchodilator and may have fewer toxic effects (Persson, 1986b). In addition, a number

of salts of theophylline have been marketed. Aminophylline is the ethylenediamine salt that was synthesized to increase solubility of the xanthines at neutral pH. Other salts, such as choline theophyllinate, have no therapeutic advantage over theophylline, and acepifylline is virtually pharmacologically inactive (Weinberger, 1984).

Mode of Action. Although theophylline has been used for more than 50 years, its mode of action as a bronchodilator is still uncertain; several mechanisms have been proposed (Persson, 1986a, 1988).

PHOSPHODIESTERASE INHIBITION. The bronchodilator effect of theophylline long has been attributed to inhibition of the enzyme phosphodiesterase (PDE), the enzyme that inactivates cAMP in cells. Accumulation of intracellular cAMP concentrations was thought to be a key determinant of bronchodilation. However, the degree of inhibition of PDE is not very great at concentrations of theophylline that are therapeutically efficacious. There is no evidence that airway smooth muscle cells concentrate theophylline to achieve higher concentrations intracellularly than is seen in plasma. Other drugs that have greater inhibitory effects on PDE, such as dipyridamole and papaverine, are not effective bronchodilators. Furthermore, inhibition of PDE theoretically should lead to synergistic interaction with β-adrenergic agonists because the latter accelerate production of cAMP by activating adenylate cyclase. The synergism has not been convincingly demonstrated in vivo. Several isozymes of PDE now have been identified, and some are much more relevant to smooth muscle relaxation (Torphy, 1989). Several selective inhibitors are now under development as potential antiasthma drugs.

ADENOSINE-RECEPTOR ANTAGONISM. Theophylline at therapeutic concentrations is a potent inhibitor of adenosine receptors. This inhibition could contribute to its bronchodilator effects. Although adenosine has little effect on human airway smooth muscle in vitro, when given by inhalation it causes bronchoconstriction in asthmatic subjects. Bronchoconstriction induced by inhaled adenosine is prevented by therapeutic concentrations of theophylline (Cushley et al., 1984). However, this observation only confirms that theophylline is capable of antagonizing the effects of exogenous adenosine, not that it plays such a role clinically. Enprofylline, which is more potent than theophylline as a bronchodilator, does not block adenosine receptors. Thus, antagonism of adenosine receptors is an unlikely explanation for the bronchodilator effect of theophylline (Persson, 1986a). Nevertheless, adenosine antagonism may account for some adverse effects of theophylline, such as stimulation of the CNS, cardiac arrhythmias, and diuresis.

RELEASE OF ENDOGENOUS CATECHOLAMINES. Theophylline increases the secretion of epinephrine from the adrenal medulla. The increase in plasma concentration is small and insufficient to account for any significant bronchodilator effect.

PROSTAGLANDIN INHIBITION. Theophylline antagonizes the effect of some prostaglandins on vascular smooth muscle in vitro, but there is no evidence that these effects occur at therapeutic concentrations or are relevant to the beneficial effects of the drug on the airway.

CALCIUM INFLUX. Theophylline may interfere with calcium mobilization in airway smooth muscle. The drug does not effect entry of calcium ions via voltage-dependent channels, but it may influence calcium entry via receptor-operated channels or release from intracellular stores, or have some effect on phosphatidylinositol turnover.

UNKNOWN MECHANISMS. Despite extensive study, the molecular mechanism for the bronchodilating or other antiasthma actions of theophylline remain elusive. Its beneficial effect in treating asthma may be related to its action on nonpulmonary cells such as platelets, neutrophils, or macrophages, or in the microvascular leaks and edema in airway tissue, in addition to its direct actions on airway smooth muscle. Interestingly, theophylline is ineffective when given by inhalation. Its effects only are seen when a critical concentration in plasma is reached (Cushley and Holgate, 1985). Such data may indicate that the drug's efficacy also is via important effects on widely scattered cells in addition to those in the airway.

In summary, the primary effect of theophylline seems to be to relax smooth muscle in both large and small airways. However, theophylline at therapeutically relevant concentrations is a rather weak bronchodilator, suggesting that its effects on other targets may be clinically important. Theophylline inhibits release of mediators from mast cells, increases mucociliary clearance, and prevents the development of microvascular leakiness as would an "anti-inflammatory" drug (Persson, 1988). Theophylline also inhibits some functions of T lymphocytes which may be relevant to control of chronic inflammation of the airway. The drug has no effect on degranulation of eosinophils, a finding that agrees with its lack of effect in reducing bronchial hyperactivity (Cockcroft et al., 1989; Yukawa et al., 1989). In addition, aminophylline apparently increases the contractility of the fatigued diaphragm in humans (Aubier et al., 1981). Whether this action is clinically relevant in patients with respiratory failure is uncertain. *Principle: When a prototype drug (e.g., theophylline) has multiple fundamental mechanisms of action that contribute to its efficacy in a complex clinical setting, extrapolation of all these effects to other drugs in the "same class" (e.g., other xanthines) is inappropriate until the extrapolation is demonstrated to be valid. Oversimplifying a drug action by incomplete classification (e.g., theophylline is a PDE inhibitor) removes the opportunity for understanding the pathogenesis of the disease it is used to treat and for the strategies of combining drugs whose different dominant mechanisms could result in excellent efficacy* (see chapters 2, 13, and 23).

Pharmacokinetics. There is a close relationship between improvement in airway function and the serum concentration of theophylline. Below 10 mg/l, therapeutic effects are small. Above 25 mg/l, additional benefits are outweighed by adverse effects. Consequently the therapeutic range usually is taken as 10 to 20 mg/l (Weinberger, 1984). The dose of theophylline required to achieve these therapeutic concentrations varies among subjects, largely because of differences in rates of clearance. In addition, the bronchodilator response to theophylline may be dependent on the severity of constriction. During acute bronchoconstriction, higher than usual concentrations may be required to produce adequate bronchodilation (Vozeh et al., 1982).

Theophylline is rapidly and completely absorbed. The large interindividual variations in its clearance are caused by differences in hepatic metabolism. Theophylline is metabolized in the liver by the cytochrome P450 microsomal enzyme system. A large number of factors may influence hepatic metabolism (Weinberger, 1984). Increased clearance is seen in children (1–16 years), and in cigarette and marijuana smokers. Other drugs also can influence clearance. When patients are receiving phenytoin and phenobarbital, higher than usual doses of theophylline may be required. Reduced clearance is found in patients with liver disease, pneumonia, and heart failure and in patients receiving drugs such as erythromycin, allopurinol, and cimetidine that inhibit cytochrome P450. Thus, if a patient receiving maintenance theophylline also requires a course of erythromycin, the dose of theophylline should be decreased. Viral infections and vaccination also may decrease clearance. Because of these variations in clearance, individualization of the theophylline dosage is required, and plasma concentrations should be measured about 4 hours after dosing with slow-release preparations, and after a steady state has been achieved. There is no significant circadian variation in the metabolism of theophylline (Taylor et al., 1983), although absorption may be delayed at night due to the effects of the supine posture (Warren et al., 1985).

Intravenous aminophylline (85% theophylline by weight) has been used for many years to treat acute severe asthma. The recommended loading dose is 6 mg/kg given over 20 to 30 minutes followed by a maintenance dose of 0.5 mg/kg per hour. If the patient is already taking theophylline, the loading dose should be decreased or omitted depending on the measured or expected concentration of theophylline already present in plasma. In patients in whom the clearance of theophylline may be low, the infusion rate should generally be halved and plasma concentrations measured frequently during therapy (see Table 7–1 and chapter 1).

Theophylline from ordinary tablets or elixir is rapidly absorbed and leads to wide differences between peak and trough concentrations of drug in plasma. This variation in concentrations is undesirable (see chapters 37 and 38). Several effective sustained-release preparations now are available, which lead to slower and more continuous absorption of the drug, providing steady concentrations in plasma over 12 to 24 hours (Weinberger and Hendeles, 1983). Although there are differences among slow-release preparations, they are minor and of little clinical significance. Both slow-release (sustained-release) aminophylline and slow-release theophylline are available and equally effective. However, the ethylenediamine component of aminophylline has been implicated in allergic reactions.

For continuous treatment, twice-daily therapy (approximately 8 mg/kg twice daily) is needed. Some preparations are designed for once-daily administration. For nocturnal asthma, a single dose of slow-release theophylline at bedtime often is effective (Barnes et al., 1982). Once optimal doses have been determined, concentrations of drug in plasma usually remain stable as long as the above-mentioned factors that alter the clearance do not change.

Other theophylline salts, such as choline theophyllinate, offer no advantages over theophylline. Some derivatives, such as acepiphylline, diprophylline, and proxophylline, are less effective than theophylline (Weinberger, 1984). Compound tablets that contain fixed-dose combinations of β-adrenergic agonists and sedatives in addition to theophylline should be avoided. *Principle: The availability of and requirement for dose-dependent, highly effective drugs for a given indication (e.g., bronchoconstriction) should render the use of any fixed-dose combination preparation obsolete.*

Aminophylline can be given as a suppository, but rectal absorption is unreliable, and proctitis may occur; this route of administration should be avoided. Inhalation of theophylline is irritating and ineffective. Intramuscular injections of theophylline are very painful and should never be given. *Principle: Adverse reactions to a drug product may be caused by the base drug, a salt, or an excipient (preservative, coloring agent, etc.); this is yet another reason for the physician*

Table 7–1. **FACTORS THAT MODIFY CLEARANCE OF THEOPHYLLINE**

INCREASED CLEARANCE	DECREASED CLEARANCE
Enzyme induction by rifampin phenobarbital ethanol	Enzyme inhibition by cimitidine erythromycin allopurinol
Smoking tobacco, marijuana	Congestive heart failure
High-protein, low-carbohydrate diet	Liver disease
Barbecued meat	Pneumonia
Childhood	Viral infection and vaccination
	High-carbohydrate diet
	Old age

to be aware of specific formulations being pre-scribed.

Case Study Using Theophylline

An 82.9-kg, 44-year-old woman with chronic asthma entered the hospital with an acute attack of asthma. No other significant medical problems were present. Aminophylline was begun by IV infusion at a rate of 93 mg/h. Approximately 36 hours later, the patient, whose breathing was improving, was found to be agitated and tremulous. The plasma concentration of theophylline was 57 mg/l. The infusion was stopped, and 18 hours later the concentration of theophylline was 26 mg/l (see Fig. 7–4). The infusion was restarted at a rate of 30 mg/h 12 hours later, and after a further 12 hours, the theophylline concentration was 13 mg/l.

Question: Why was the original concentration so high, and what is the appropriate infusion rate to achieve an average concentration of 15 mg/l in the patient?

Answer: The first determination of concentration of theophylline is approximately four times higher than that expected from an IV infusion rate of approximately 1 mg/kg of aminophylline.

Assuming the original 57 mg/l value is at steady state, the high concentration leads to a calculation of drug clearance of 23 ml/min, considerably less than the approximately 1 ml/min per kilogram that is average. The half-life, calculated from the subsequent data, is approximately 16 hours. The estimated half-life and clearance are compatible with a slightly lower-than-average volume of distribution (V_d), but most of the prolongation of half-life appears to be due to the low clearance. The explanation for the reduced clearance in this patient is not known, but clearance is reduced. The concentration of 13 mg/l taken only 12 hours after the new infusion was begun is not a steady-state value. On the basis of the clearance of 23 ml/min, the steady-state concentration likely to result from this regimen is approximately 18 mg/l.

Comment: Given the calculation of $t_{1/2}$ of 16 hours, the original (57 mg/l) concentration was probably not at steady state (only somewhat more than 2 half-lives had elapsed). Nonetheless, the value of 57 mg/l was assumed to be steady state and the clearance was calculated noting that aminophylline is only 85% theophylline. The half-life calculation is indicated on the figure; the 57-mg/l value was assumed to be steady state;

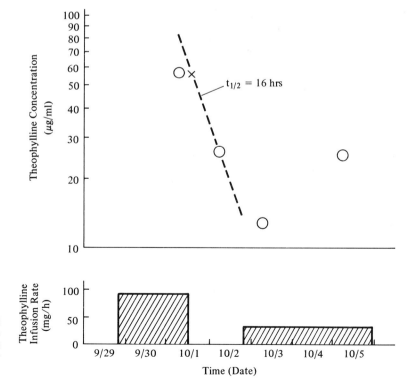

Fig. 7–4. Plot of observed theophylline C_p (○), calculated C_p (×), and theophylline infusion rates. See case study in text.

hence the value at the end of the infusion was the same (point x in Fig. 7–4) and the half-life could be calculated. The prediction of a C_{pss} of 18 mg/l on the subsequent regimen was low by 30% (8 mg/l—see Fig. 7–4), indicating that the true clearance was at least 30% lower than the calculated value of 23 ml/min. This is consistent with the 57 mg/l being approximately 25% lower than the initial true C_{pss} (75% of C_{pss} is attained after 2 half-lives). Even a 30% error is not likely to be serious, however. The 200% to 400% errors are a problem, as illustrated in this case by the initial choice of an "average" aminophylline dose of about 1 mg/kg per hour (although this could not have been known to be a mistake beforehand) (see chapters 1, 37, and 38).

Indications and Clinical Use. Intravenous aminophylline is less effective than nebulized β-adrenergic agonists for treating patients with acute asthma (Rossing et al., 1980). Aminophylline should therefore be reserved for patients who fail to respond adequately to β-adrenergic agonists. Theophylline has little or no effect on normal bronchomotor tone, but reverses bronchoconstriction in asthmatic patients (Weinberger, 1984). It is less effective than inhaled β-adrenergic agonists and for equivalent efficacy is more likely to have unwanted effects (Barnes, 1989a). Theophylline and β-adrenergic agonists have additive, if not synergistic, effects (Shenfield, 1982). Therefore, theophylline may provide bronchodilator effects additional to those from maximally effective doses of β-adrenergic agonists (Barclay et al., 1981). This means that if adequate bronchodilation is not achieved by β-adrenergic agonists alone, theophylline may be added to the maintenance therapy with good chances of added benefit.

Theophylline is useful in the treatment of nocturnal asthma. The slow-release preparations provide therapeutic concentrations overnight and are more effective for this purpose than slow-release β-adrenergic agonists (Barnes et al., 1982; Heins et al., 1988). Although theophylline is less effective than a β-adrenergic agonist plus corticosteroids, only a minority of asthmatic patients appear to derive exceptional benefit from the use of the two drugs. But some patients taking corticosteroids orally may show deterioration in lung function when theophylline is withdrawn (Brennan et al., 1988).

Theophylline can be useful in treating patients with COPD. Taken alone it increases exercise tolerance (Taylor et al., 1985; Murciano et al., 1989) without improving spirometry tests. Theophylline may reduce the volume of trapped gas, suggesting its effect on peripheral airways (Chrystyn et al., 1988). When theophylline is combined with an inhaled β-adrenergic agonist, both exercise tolerance and spirometry improve.

Adverse Reactions and Contraindications. The unwanted effects of theophylline usually are related to concentration in plasma, tending to occur when concentrations exceed 20 mg/l. However, some patients develop adverse effects while concentrations in plasma are lower. Adverse effects may be avoided to some extent by gradually increasing the dose until therapeutic concentrations are achieved. The most common adverse effects are headache, nausea and vomiting, abdominal discomfort, and restlessness. There also may be an increase of gastric acid secretion and enhanced urine output. At high concentrations, cardiac arrhythmias and potentially lethal convulsions may occur. Some of the adverse effects (central stimulation, effects on gastric secretion, diuresis, and arrhythmias) may be due to antagonism of adenosine receptors and may therefore be avoided by drugs such as enprofylline that do not block these receptors at doses sufficient to cause bronchodilation. Theophylline, even at therapeutic concentrations, may lead to behavioral disturbances and learning difficulties in school children (Rachelefsky et al., 1986), although the extent of this potential problem is uncertain.

ANTI-INFLAMMATORY DRUGS

Corticosteroids

Although the type of inflammatory responses may differ among diseases, inflammation is a common denominator of several lung diseases. Anti-inflammatory drugs suppress the inflammatory response by inhibiting infiltration and activation of inflammatory cells as well as their synthesis, or release of mediators and the effects of inflammatory mediators themselves. Several types of anti-inflammatory drugs have been used in the treatment of lung disease, but the most widely used are corticosteroids.

Background and Pharmacology. Corticosteroids are used to treat several lung diseases. They were introduced to treat asthma shortly after they were discovered in the 1950s. They remain the most effective therapy available for asthma but the legitimate fear of their adverse effects makes using them difficult. Therefore, there has been considerable research into discovering new or related agents that retain their beneficial corticosteroid action on airways without imposing as many unwanted effects. *Principle: The most effective drug for a disease may not be the best drug to use. Usefulness of a drug is always determined by both its efficacy and its profile of toxicity. A very difficult dilemma in therapy is whether to* *withhold a drug whose efficacy is better than that of alternative drugs, when the most effective drug is also the most toxic.*

The introduction of inhaled steroids constitutes a major advance in the treatment of chronic asthma. Now that asthma is viewed as a chronic inflammatory disease and we have come to rely on the low toxicity of inhaled corticosteroids, they may be considered as first-line therapy (Barnes, 1989a).

Orally administered steroids are indicated in the treatment of several other pulmonary diseases including sarcoidosis, selected interstitial lung diseases, and pulmonary eosinophilic syndromes.

Chemistry. Modification of the structure of cortisol (hydrocortisone) resulted in derivatives such as prednisolone and dexamethasone. These derivatives have enhanced glucocorticoid effects and reduced mineralocorticoid activity when compared with cortisol. Their potent glucocorticoid actions were effective when they were given systemically to treat asthma, but they had no antiasthmatic activity when they were given by inhalation. Further substitution at the 17α ester position resulted in a new group of extremely potent steroids [e.g., beclomethasone dipropionate (BDP), betamethasone, and budesonide], effective when applied topically for skin diseases and effective in treating asthma when given by inhalation.

The antiasthma potency of an inhaled steroid is approximately proportional to its potency as an anti-inflammatory agent. Thus, budesonide is approximately twice as potent as BDP and 1000 times more potent than prednisolone. More recent studies have shown that although the effects of the steroid may be slow in onset, only a short period of its use may be necessary to achieve maximal effects (Brattsand, 1989). This implies that if topical steroids could be metabolized locally, the full effect might be obtained but the incidence of systemic adverse effects would be reduced. Then higher inhaled doses could be administered without risking serious toxicity. Such local metabolism occurs to some extent with budesonide and BDP, but further improvements may be possible. Budesonide also is extensively metabolized in liver. Therefore, what is not metabolized locally will be as it enters the liver, making it possible to give high doses by inhalation before systemic effects are produced.

Mode of Action

Steroid Receptors. Most effects of steroids are mediated by interaction with specific receptors. At concentrations higher than those usually used therapeutically, nonspecific effects due to insertion into the cell membrane may occur. Steroids enter target cells and combine with their receptors within the cytoplasm. These receptors are specific to certain classes of steroids (such as corticosteroids, androgens, estrogens), but each class is similar in each tissue that contains it (Evans, 1988). The steroid–receptor complex is transported to the nucleus, where it initiates DNA transcription of specific messenger RNAs. These RNAs induce the synthesis of specific proteins that bring about the physiologic or pharmacologic effects of the steroid. This sequence of events explains why the onset of pharmacologic effects of steroids usually is delayed by several hours. The effects of steroids on calcium ion flux and vascular permeability may occur more rapidly and may be independent of protein synthesis.

Lipocortin. Corticosteroids inhibit the release of arachidonic acid metabolites and platelet-activating factor (PAF) from lung and macrophages by enhancing the production of a protein called lipocortin. A lipocortin inhibits phospholipase A_2 in the cell membrane (Flower, 1988). This 37-kd protein now has been cloned and expressed. Understanding its effects provides the basis of a unitary hypothesis for the mode of action of steroids through inhibition of phospholipase A_2, thus inhibiting the formation of prostaglandins, leukotrienes, and PAF (Fig. 7–5). Steroids also may inhibit other phospholipases such as phospholipase C. But it is unlikely that lipocortin can account for all the effects of steroids, and steroids may induce the synthesis of several regulatory proteins through multiple steroid-sensitive genes.

Anti-Inflammatory Effects. The mechanism of action of corticosteroids that modulates airway disease still is poorly understood. There is increasing evidence that inflammation is involved in the pathogenesis of asthma and bronchial hyperresponsiveness. Several components of this inflammatory response, which might be inhibited by steroids and most likely by the anti-inflammatory properties of corticosteroids, are involved in their efficacy (Morris, 1985).

By virtue of their inhibiting the production of chemotactic factors in tissues, corticosteroids potently inhibit the accumulation of neutrophils. They have a number of effects that can be termed anti-inflammatory, including inhibition of secretion by human pulmonary macrophages of leukotrienes and prostaglandins; inhibition of the formation of interleukins (ILs) such as IL-1, IL-2, IL-3, and IL-5; direct actions causing eosinopenia; inhibition of degranulation and adherence of eosinophils; reduction in the number of circulating T lymphocytes; and formation of an IgE-binding suppressive factor. The action of steroids on T lymphocytes also may be important in the control of pulmonary diseases such as fibrosing alveolitis and sarcoidosis. Steroids prevent and reverse the increase in vascular permeability due

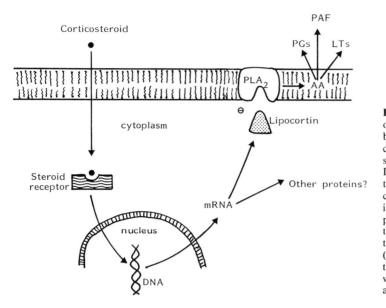

Fig. 7–5. Molecular mechanisms of steroid action. Corticosteroids bind to a cytoplasmic glucocortocoid receptor that interacts with steroid-responsive elements of DNA. This leads to the transcription of mRNA, and translation of certain proteins. One such protein is lipocortin, which inhibits phospholipase A_2 (PLA_2), thus leading to inhibition of formation of prostaglandins (PGs), leukotrienes (LTs), and platelet-activating factor (PAF). Several other proteins, which have not yet been well characterized, also are induced.

to inflammatory mediators and may therefore lead to resolution of airway edema (Erjefalt and Persson, 1986).

Effect on Airway Function. Steroids do not directly affect airway smooth muscle. The improvement in lung function following use of corticosteroids presumably is due to their effects on chronic airway inflammation and bronchial reactivity (Barnes, 1990). In a single dose, inhaled corticosteroids have no effect on the early response to allergens (reflecting their lack of effect on mast cells), but they inhibit the late response that may be due to their effect on macrophages and eosinophils. Inhaled corticosteroids inhibit bronchial reactivity and reduce bronchial hyperactivity, but this latter effect may take several weeks or months to be clearly evident. Presumably, the slow effect is a reflection of the slow healing of inflamed airway (Woolcock et al., 1988). Steroids have no immediate effect on the early bronchoconstrictor response to allergen or exercise, but, if taken over several weeks, they reduce even the acute bronchoconstrictor responses (Dahl and Johansson, 1982). This could be due either to drug-induced reduction of bronchial responsiveness or to reduction in the numbers of mast cells in airway tissue. The effect on the density of mast cells has been demonstrated in the nasal mucosa after topical application of the drug.

Effect on β-Adrenergic Receptors. Corticosteroids increase β-adrenergic responsiveness, but whether this effect contributes to their efficacy in asthma is uncertain. Steroids potentiate the effects of β-adrenergic agonists on bronchial smooth muscle and appear to prevent β-adrenergic receptor down-regulation and therefore tachyphylaxis to the adrenergic agonist in airways in vitro. In vivo steroids similarly reverse tolerance to β-adrenergic agonists in dogs (Stephan et al., 1980) and normal humans (Holgate et al., 1977). Corticosteroids increase the density of β-adrenergic receptors in rat lung membranes, increase the proportion of available receptors in the high-affinity binding state in human leukocytes, and reverse and prevent the fall in leukocyte β-adrenergic receptor density in the presence of β-adrenergic agonists in normal and asthmatic subjects (Davis and Lefkowitz, 1980). These actions may be clinically important in preventing the development of pharmacologic tolerance when high doses of nebulized β-adrenergic agonists are used.

Pharmacokinetics. Prednisone and prednisolone are readily and consistently absorbed (bioavailability near 80%) after oral administration. There is little interindividual variation in their bioavailability. Enteric coatings that are designed to reduce the incidence of dyspepsia delay absorption but do not reduce the total amount of drug absorbed. Prednisone is activated by metabolism to prednisolone, and prednisolone is further metabolized in the liver. Drugs such as rifampin (rifampicin), phenobarbital (phenobarbitone), or phenytoin, which induce hepatic enzymes, increase the clearance of prednisolone (Gambertoglio et al., 1980). The plasma half-life of prednisolone is 1 to 2 hours. However, the half life of its biologic effects is in the range of approximately 24 hours, making it suitable for once-daily dosing. There is no evidence that previous exposure of a patient to steroids changes his or her subsequent metabolism of these drugs. Prednisolone is approximately 92% protein-bound, the majority to the specific binding protein transcortin and the remainder to albumin. Only the unbound fraction (free fraction) is biologically active.

Some patients, usually those with severe asthma, apparently fail to respond to corticosteroids. Steroid-resistant asthma is not due to impaired absorption or metabolism of steroids but may be associated with a defect in responsiveness of certain cells to the drug (Carmichael et al., 1981).

Routes of Administration

Oral. Prednisolone and prednisone are the most commonly used oral corticosteroids. Initial clinical improvement in patients with severe asthma given oral steroids may take several days. The maximal beneficial effects usually are achieved while using 30 mg of prednisone daily. A few patients may need 60 mg daily to achieve adequate control. The usual maintenance dose once the acute episode subsides is on the order of 10 mg/day.

Oral steroids should be given as a single dose in the morning. This timing coincides with the normal diurnal peak of cortisol in plasma and therefore produces less adrenal suppression than if prednisone were given in divided doses or at night. Furthermore, the amount of steroid bound to transcortin is less during the day, resulting in higher concentrations of free drug in plasma and optimal effects for a given dose (Reinberg et al., 1983).

Alternate-day treatment has some advantages over daily dosing. It can produce less adrenal suppression and other adverse effects with control of asthma that is equivalent to what would be produced by the same doses spread evenly on a daily basis. Unfortunately, some patients do not achieve adequate benefit on an alternate day (q.o.d) schedule. *Principle: The schedule of drug administration may significantly alter both the efficacy and the toxicity of the drug. When the demography of patients cannot be used to predict who is susceptible to the most conservative approach, that approach should be used first on all candidates whose clinical severity can tolerate possible failure of the regimen.*

IV. Parenteral steroids are indicated in patients with acute severe exacerbations of asthma. In these circumstances, hydrocortisone is the steroid of choice because it has the most rapid onset of action—5 to 6 hours after administration, versus 8 hours after administration of prednisolone (Ellul-Micallef and Fenech, 1975). The optimal dose is not predictable. Commonly 4 mg/kg of hydrocortisone initially is given, followed by a maintenance dose of 3 mg/kg every 6 hours. These doses are based on the argument that it is necessary to maintain the concentration of cortisol in plasma that would be produced by major physiologic stresses (Collins et al., 1975).

Inhaled. With corticosteroids, inhalation has a great advantage over other routes of administration in managing chronic asthma. Inhalation may permit control of symptoms without causing adrenal suppression or other systemic adverse effects, using total doses of corticosteroid that may be substantially lower than those required when the drug is given orally (Toogood et al., 1985; Ellul-Micallef, 1988). Only when very large doses are inhaled is sufficient steroid absorbed to cause adrenal suppression. Most patients get a maximal response at a dose of 400 μg of BDP per day, but some patients may benefit from higher doses (up to 1500 μg/day). High-dose inhalers have been used four times daily, but twice-daily administration usually is as effective, and compliance is better (Meltzer et al., 1985). Several inhaled preparations are available, including BDP, triamcinolone, flunisolide, and budesonide (the latter has the highest topical potency but is not available in the United States).

Indications and Clinical Use

Acute Asthma. Hydrocortisone or another parenteral formulation such as methylprednisolone is given IV to patients with acute severe asthma. Using corticosteroids in such patients has been debated, but studies demonstrate that they speed the resolution of the acute attacks (Ellul-Micallef, 1988). There is no apparent advantage in giving very high doses of IV steroids such as 1 g of methylprednisolone. IV steroids are indicated in acute asthmatics if their lung function is less than 30% predicted, or if they experience no significant improvement with nebulized β-adrenergic agonists. Also, special caution is required in the management of an acute asthmatic attack in a patient taking maintenance doses of steroids. IV therapy usually is given until a satisfactory response is obtained, and then oral prednisolone or prednisone may be substituted. The effect of oral prednisolone (40–60 mg) is similar to that of IV hydrocortisone, and it is easier to administer (Harrison et al., 1986). Inhaled steroids have no proven value in the management of acute asthma.

Chronic Asthma. Corticosteroids clearly are indicated if asthma is not adequately controlled with bronchodilators alone. Increasingly, inhaled corticosteroids are being advocated as first-line therapy to treat chronic asthma (Barnes, 1989a).

Generally, oral corticosteroids are reserved for patients who cannot be controlled with other therapy. When used orally, the dose should be titrated to the lowest that provides acceptable control of symptoms. Any patient regularly taking oral corticosteroids must show objective evidence of responsiveness to the drug before maintenance therapy is instituted. Short courses of oral corticosteroids (such as 30 mg of prednisolone daily for 1–2 weeks) are indicated for exacerbations of asthma.

Once control of asthma has been achieved using inhaled corticosteroids up to four times daily, compliance can be improved by switching to a twice-daily (b.i.d.) schedule. If a daily dose of more than 500 μg is used, a spacer device should be considered to reduce the risk of oropharyngeal adverse effects. Inhaled steroids also may be used in children, but disodium cromoglycate is the preferred anti-inflammatory drug (see below). In children, the inhaled dose of corticosteroid should be kept under 500 μg daily to reduce the risk of inhibitory effects on growth (Konig, 1988). Patients with chronic bronchitis occasionally respond to steroids, possibly because some have an element of undiagnosed asthma. Steroids produce no objective benefit on airway function in patients with chronic bronchitis. They often may produce subjective apparent benefit because of the euphoria they can produce. *Principle: When objective measurements of the change in severity of disease can be used to monitor the effects of intervention, they are preferable to other types of observations or end points. No matter how tempting it may be to use a subjective compliment from a patient in lieu of objective improvement to therapy, yielding to such temptation often leads to the patient's paying heavy consequences. Think for a moment of the consequences of extending corticosteroid use in order to make a patient with COPD "feel better."*

Interstitial Lung Disease. Oral steroids suppress the chronic inflammation associated with interstitial lung diseases and have been used to treat sarcoidosis, fibrosing alveolitis, pulmonary eosinophilic syndromes, and autoimmune diseases such as scleroderma. To treat these diseases, steroids initially should be given in a high dose (e.g., 40–60 mg of prednisone daily) to establish maximum improvement. Once the response plateaus, the steroid should be slowly tapered to the lowest dose that continues to give optimal control (Crystal et al., 1984). Inhaled steroids are not known to be useful in controlling these diseases.

Adverse Reactions and Contraindications

Adrenal Suppression. Corticosteroids inhibit release of ACTH and secretion of cortisol by a negative-feedback effect on the pituitary gland. This suppression is dose-dependent and usually occurs only when a dose of prednisolone greater than 7.5 to 10 mg daily is used. Significant suppression after short courses (e.g., 1–2 weeks) of steroid therapy usually is not a clinical problem. But prolonged use of corticosteroids can result in adrenal suppression that can endure for several months or years. Therefore, therapeutic strategies for using the drug include frequent assessments to determine the lowest possible dosages that produce adequate clinical effects. When doses are lowered after prolonged oral therapy, this should be done very gradually. Symptoms of "steroid withdrawal syndrome" include lassitude, musculoskeletal pains, and occasionally fever. In addition, patients with adrenal suppression will require supplemental steroid administration if they become physiologically stressed (e.g., trauma, burn, sepsis, etc.).

Systemic Adverse Effects. Adverse effects of long-term therapy with corticosteroids are well described and include fluid retention, increased red cell mass, increased appetite, weight gain, osteoporosis, capillary fragility, hypertension, peptic ulceration, diabetes, cataracts, and psychosis. Very occasionally adverse reactions (such as anaphylaxis) to IV hydrocortisone have been described, particularly in aspirin-sensitive asthmatics (Dajani et al., 1981). *Principle: The pattern, frequency, and severity of adverse effects caused by a drug often may depend on the characteristics of the patient taking the drug* (see chapters 29–32).

Local Adverse Effects. Adverse effects of inhaled steroids are few. The most common problem is oropharyngeal candidiasis (which may occur in 5% of patients). Hoarseness and weakness of voice (dysphonia) may also occur, possibly due to atrophy of the vocal cords. The incidence of these adverse effects may be related to the local concentrations of steroid and may be reduced by the use of various spacing devices that reduce oropharyngeal deposition of the drug (Toogood et al., 1984). There is no evidence for atrophy of the lining of the airway or of an increase in lung infections after inhaled steroids.

Cromolyn Sodium

Cromolyn sodium (sodium cromoglycate) is a derivative of khellin, an Egyptian herbal remedy. The drug was found to protect against challenge with allergen yet had no bronchodilator effects (Altounyan, 1980). It is classified as a chromone.

Mode of Action

Mast Cell Stabilization. Initial investigations indicated that cromolyn inhibited the release of mediators by allergen in passively sensitized animal and human lung preparations (Cox, 1967). It inhibited passive cutaneous anaphylaxis in the rat but had no effect in the guinea pig. The activity was attributed to the drug's ability to stabilize the mast cell membrane. Cromolyn was classified as a mast cell stabilizer in spite of its rather low potency on human lung mast cells (Church and Gradidge, 1980). In fact, other drugs that are more potent than cromolyn as membrane stabilizers have little or no efficacy in treating asthmatics. *Principle: Simple classifications of drugs often confuse their true mechanisms of efficacious actions.*

Interaction with Sensory Nerves. Cromolyn potently inhibits bronchoconstriction induced by sulfur dioxide and bradykinin, both of which are believed to activate sensory nerves in the airway. In dogs, cromolyn suppresses firing of unmyelinated C-fiber nerve endings (Dixon et al., 1979), reinforcing the view that cromolyn might be acting to suppress sensory nerve activation and thus neurogenic inflammation in the airways.

Effect on Other Inflammatory Cells. Cromolyn has variable inhibitory actions on other inflammatory cells including macrophages and eosinophils that may participate in allergic inflammation. In vivo cromolyn can block both the early response that may be mediated by mast cells to allergens and the late response and bronchial hyperresponsiveness that are more likely to be mediated by macrophage and eosinophil interactions (Cockcroft and Murdock, 1987).

Pharmacokinetics and Pharmacodynamics. Cromolyn is neither lipid-soluble nor significantly absorbed after oral administration. It must be delivered by inhalation, either as a dry powder or as an MDI. The doses used in clinical practice are somewhat arbitrary.

Indications and Clinical Use. Cromolyn sodium is used for prophylactic treatment and consequently needs to be taken regularly. The drug protects against various indirect bronchoconstrictor stimuli including exercise. Cromolyn should be given four times daily to provide good protection and should be taken prior to provocative stimuli such as exercise. Cromolyn is effective only in some patients, and these are difficult to identify in advance of treatment. Cromolyn is the first-choice anti-inflammatory drug for children because it has few adverse effects (Bernstein, 1985). In adults, inhalational corticosteroids are first choices because they are effective in most patients. Some adults with mild asthma can respond to cromolyn (Petty et al., 1989). *Principle: Very careful controls and evidence of compliance need to be a part of the study of any drug that is given for prophylaxis of an intermittent disease. Compliance is a particularly important issue when the disease-free interval is asymptomatic and the drug must be given in an inconvenient way (e.g., four times per day) in order to be useful.*

Adverse Reactions and Contraindications. Cromolyn is a very safe drug; its adverse effects are rare. The dry-powder inhaler may cause throat irritation, coughing, and, occasionally, wheezing but this is usually prevented by prior administration of a β-adrenergic agonist via inhaler. Very rarely a transient rash and urticaria are seen, and a few cases of pulmonary eosinophilia have been reported, all of which are due to hypersensitivity.

Other Antiallergy Drugs

Cromolyn sodium is classified as an antiallergic drug because it appears to have a specific effect on allergy-based inflammation. Several other drugs also may be included in this category.

Nedocromil Sodium. Nedocromil sodium is a new drug used for prophylaxis. It has a similar pharmacologic profile of activity to cromolyn, is more potent in various tests, and may have a longer duration of action (Gonzales and Brogden, 1987). It is currently undergoing clinical evaluation for the treatment of chronic asthma, but comparisons with cromolyn or inhaled steroids are not complete (Thomson, 1989). The drug's longer duration of action than cromolyn could make it suitable for twice-daily dosing or perhaps even less.

Ketotifen. Ketotifen also is described as a drug to be used for prophylaxis against asthma (Martin and Baggliolini, 1981). One of its prominent effects is antagonism of the H_1 receptor that may account for its sedative properties. Ketotifen has little effect in modulating bronchial hyperresponsiveness to acute challenges or other clinical symptoms of asthma. A long-term, placebo-controlled trial of oral ketotifen in children with mild asthma showed no clinical benefit (Loftus and Price, 1987).

Antihistamines. H_1-receptor antagonists block the bronchoconstrictor effect of histamine. If histamine were released from airway mast cells in sufficient amounts to contribute to the features of asthma, then antihistamines should be clinically beneficial. But antihistamines have been tried in the past and found not to be efficacious. Because they are competitive antagonists of H_1 effects, it has been speculated that their lack of efficacy was due to limited dosages used in these studies (constrained by the sedative actions of the antihistaminics available at the time). Recently, nonsedating antihistamines such as terfenadine, loratidine, and astemizole have been introduced. These antihistamines are useful in treating the symptoms of allergic rhinitis and reduce the early bronchoconstrictor responses to allergens and exercise (in which mast cell degranulation is involved) (Patel, 1984; Rafferty et al., 1987). However, not even these antihistaminics are useful in the treatment of chronic asthma. Presumably the old hypothesis that histamine plays a minor role in the pathogenesis of human asthma is valid, but other mediators are likely more important (Sly and Kemp, 1988).

Mast Cell Stabilizers. Almost 40 drugs have now been developed as "mast cell stabilizers" (Church, 1978). In vitro these drugs inhibit release of mediators from mast cells triggered by allergens. All of them have been disappointing in tests of their efficacy for treatment of clinical asthma. None has become available for clinical use. Presumably this reflects the fact that mast cells do not play a prominent role in the inflammatory response of chronic asthma and that they do not share the pharmacologic properties that make cromolyn useful.

OTHER DRUGS

Immunosuppressants

Immunosuppressive therapy has been used in a number of pulmonary diseases in which immunologic pathogenetic mechanisms are implicated. These include sarcoidosis, fibrosing alveolitis, pulmonary vasculitides, and asthma. The details of these drugs are covered elsewhere in the book (see chapters 19, 20, and 23).

Methotrexate. Low-dose methotrexate (15 mg weekly) has a steroid-sparing effect when used to treat patients with asthma (Mullarkey et al., 1988). Methotrexate may be indicated when oral steroids are contraindicated because of unacceptable adverse effects (e.g., in postmenopausal women for whom osteoporosis is a problem), or in patients who do not respond adequately to maximally tolerated doses of corticosteroids. However, the potential toxicity of methotrexate needs to be balanced against adverse effects due to steroids.

Cyclophosphamide. Cyclophosphamide is particularly useful in treating the pulmonary vasculitis that may occur in a spectrum of diseases including polyarteritis nodosa, Churg-Strauss syndrome, and Wegener granulomatosis.

Cyclosporin. Cyclosporin A is active against T-helper lymphocytes and might be useful for treating pulmonary diseases, including asthma, in which these cells are implicated. Theoretically, the drug could be useful in treating fibrosing alveolitis and sarcoidosis. Its use is limited by adverse effects, such as nephrotoxicity, and its value in these diseases remains unestablished.

Gold. Gold has long been used to treat chronic arthritis and severe rheumatism (see chapter 19). Anecdotal evidence suggests that it also may be useful in patients with asthma. It has been used in Japan for this purpose for many years (Muranaka et al., 1978). An open study has shown some efficacy of an oral gold preparation in patients with chronic asthma (Bernstein, 1985). But until controlled trials have demonstrated that it is useful, it cannot be recommended. *Principle: Unless the effect of a drug is immediate, unequivocal, and definitive, the value of an open study will be questioned. Even when a drug has dramatic effects (e.g., naloxone antagonizing morphine's action), controlled studies are necessary to develop convincing information about the appropriate indications for it. There is very little excuse for relying on the results of an open study as definitive for establishing an indication for drug use.*

Drugs Acting on Mucus

Many pharmacologic agents influence mucus secretion. Autonomic agonists and several other neurotransmitters and mediators of inflammation increase mucus secretion in experimental animals (Nadel et al., 1985) and speed mucociliary clearance in humans (Pavia et al., 1980). The clinical importance of the effects of β-adrenergic agonists and methylxanthines on mucociliary clearance in asthmatics and patients with COPD is uncertain.

Mucolytics. Several drugs that reduce the viscosity of sputum have been used to treat chronic asthma, COPD, bronchiectasis, and cystic fibrosis. These drugs usually are derivatives of cysteine (such as acetylcysteine and carbocysteine). These drugs reduce the disulfide bridges that bind glycoprotein to other proteins such as albumin and secretory IgA. In addition, these drugs may act as antioxidants to reduce oxidant lung damage in cigarette smokers. Some mucolytics such as bromhexine also affect lysozyme in sputum, whereas others such as ambroxil may stimulate surfactant secretion resulting in reduced viscosity of mucus. While these agents cause a significant reduction in sputum viscosity in vitro, they provide little or no clinical benefit (Minette, 1983).

Inhaled acetylcysteine may cause severe bronchoconstriction in patients with airway obstruction, and there is no evidence that it produces significant improvement in lung function. Oral administration of acetylcysteine, carbocysteine, methylcysteine, and bromhexine are well tolerated, but there is no evidence that they improve pulmonary function in patients with asthma or COPD. Long-term trials of these drugs in patients with chronic bronchitis either have shown no benefit (British Thoracic Society Research Committee, 1985) or only marginal reduction in symptoms. They are effective in reducing exacerbations (Boman et al., 1983). A few patients in these trials appear to show significant benefit; however, there are no clinical features that have been found to identify in advance patients who may respond to these drugs. Mucolytic therapy cannot be recommended for routine use in patients with COPD, asthma, or bronchiectasis. Furthermore, these drugs can produce adverse effects that include disturbance of the GI system, urticaria, and fever.

Expectorants. Expectorants are drugs that are taken orally to enhance clearance of mucus. Although they are commonly prescribed, there is little evidence that they provide any clinical benefit. Such drugs often are emetics (such as quaifenesin, ipecac, ammonium chloride, squill) that are given in subemetic doses on the basis that gastric irritation promotes an increase in mucus secretion by a cholinergic reflex mechanism. However, there is no good evidence for this assumption (Richardson and Phipps, 1978). Expectorants and mucolytic agents have little, if any, clinical value. Instead of reliance on drugs to facilitate removal of secretions, efforts should be directed toward treatment of the underlying disease with adequate hydration (water is an effective expectorant), vigorous bronchial toilet, and respiratory therapy. Whatever a physician decides to do about use of expectorants, they should not be used in lieu of these more helpful measures.

Antitussives

The treatment of cough is unsatisfactory, partly because there are few controlled trials of therapy and partly because of the difficulties in objectively measuring this system. Because cough usually is a protective reflex, suppressing it may not be beneficial. Cough suppressants can cause retention of sputum that could be detrimental in patients with chronic bronchitis or bronchiectasis. Before treatment of cough, its underlying cause should be identified if possible. Specific treatment of those causes is desirable when possible. For example, asthma may present as cough; cough may be a manifestation of bronchial hyperactivity that may be best treated using an inhaled β-adrenergic agonist or steroid (Ellul-Micallef, 1983). The cough resulting from postnasal drip because of sinusitis should respond to antibiotics and nasal decongestants, whereas the cough resulting from gastroesophageal reflux should be treated with antacids. The cough of bacterial pneumonia responds to antibiotics, and transient cough associated with viral infection often needs no therapy. In a prospective study, the use of specific treatments alleviated symptoms in most patients with chronic cough of greater than 3 weeks' duration (Irwin et al., 1981).

Opioids. Symptomatic treatment of chronic cough can be difficult. The cough suppressants in current use usually are opiate derivatives that are presumed to act centrally on the medullary cough center. Codeine and pholcodine commonly are used in spite of little objective evidence that they are clinically effective. Morphine and methadone undoubtedly are effective, but they are indicated only in patients whose cough is intractable because it is associated with irreversible disease such as bronchial carcinoma. Dextromethorphan and noscapine are opioids with less potential for addiction than morphine, but there is little information about the basis for their use as antitussives. Part of their apparent efficacy may be due to reduced perception of the cough, rather than reduced frequency. Opiate analgesics are contraindicated for treating chronic cough in patients with COPD and asthma because they may depress respiration.

Ventilatory Stimulants

Several classes of drugs stimulate ventilation. These drugs have been used when a patient's ventilatory drive is depressed or when ventilation is inadequate. Although nonspecific central stimulants such as amphetamines, ephedrine, and theophylline can act on respiratory centers, they also produce generalized central stimulatory effects that limit their clinical value. Nikethamide and ethamivan were introduced as specific respiratory stimulants, but doses capable of stimulating ventilation are very close to those that cause convulsions (Wong and Ward, 1977). Furthermore, central stimulation increases muscular activity and thereby oxygen demand, creating a disadvantageous physiologic response. The use of these drugs has largely been abandoned.

Safer ventilatory stimulants have been introduced, and their role has been more thoroughly evaluated. Respiratory stimulants may be indicated if ventilation is impaired (i.e., the patient demonstrates CO_2 retention) as a result of overdose with sedatives, postanesthetic respiratory depression, or idiopathic hypoventilation, and in patients with hypercapnia, particularly when it is precipitated by sedatives. The role of these stimulants in COPD is limited because respiratory drive in these patients probably is maximal and the poor alveolar ventilation is due more to inefficient mixing of gas than to reduction in ventilatory drive. Further stimulation of ventilation under these conditions may be counterproductive because of increased energy expenditure produced by the drugs. The increase in oxygen consumption may exceed the increase in oxygen delivery to the systemic circulation.

Doxapram. Doxapram is the first relatively selective analeptic with an acceptable margin of safety to cause stimulation of the respiratory centers. At low doses (0.5 mg/kg IV) doxapram stimulates carotid chemoreceptors, but at higher doses it stimulates medullary respiratory centers. Its onset of action is within 10 minutes, but the effect lasts for only a few minutes when the drug is given IV; consequently, it must be administered by continuous IV infusion. The ventilatory response is linear over the dosage range from 0.3 to 3 mg/kg per minute. Unwanted effects are uncommon but include nausea, sweating, anxiety, and hallucinations. At higher doses, increased systemic and pulmonary arterial pressures may result (Hunt et al., 1979). Hepatic failure and GI hemorrhage are rare effects of the drug. Because doxepram is metabolized in the liver, care should be taken in patients with impaired hepatic function.

Almitrine. Almitrine is a piperazine derivative that recently has been introduced as a respiratory stimulant in Europe. It selectively stimulates carotid chemoreceptors and does not appear to have any central actions (Howard, 1984). The drug has no effect in experimental animals with denervated peripheral chemoceptors or in patients with surgically removed carotid bodies. Its mode of action at a cellular level is uncertain, but the drug is concentrated in the carotid body and may interfere with the release from or action of dopamine in the carotid body. Almitrine increases ventilation in normal subjects only when they are made hypoxic (Stradling et al., 1982) and in patients with COPD at rest (Stradling et al., 1984). When the drug is given acutely by IV injection or chronically by mouth, its long-term effects in patients with COPD include reduction of hypercapnia. As attractive as this result seems to be, its value is uncertain (Howard, 1984). The drug is well tolerated even though it may cause sweating and nausea when used acutely and may lead to increases in pulmonary artery pressure. Unfortunately, long-term use is associated with peripheral neuropathy, so that the routine use of this drug can-

not be recommended. *Principle: As tempting as it may be to use drugs that appropriately affect surrogate end points, the therapist must beware. There are a number of examples in which drugs that alter surrogate end points enhance mortality (antiarrhythmics to decrease ventricular premature beats, MER 29 to reduce cholesterol levels, antitumor drugs used to manage nodular lymphomas). The therapist should try to obtain data on the overall effects of the drug on morbidity and mortality before embracing its use because it works on surrogate end points.*

Progesterone. The hyperventilation produced by progesterone has been known for many years. Progesterone appears to stimulate ventilation by increasing the sensitivity of the respiratory center to CO_2. Its role in the management of hypoventilation syndromes is questionable.

Acetazolamide. This carbonic anhydrase inhibitor induces metabolic acidosis and thereby stimulates ventilation. It has not proved useful in practice, and the metabolic imbalance it produces may be detrimental. The drug is useful in the prevention of acute mountain (high-altitude) sickness (Milledge, 1983).

Naloxone. Naloxone is a competitive opioid receptor antagonist. Its chemical value as a respiratory stimulant is to counter the respiratory depression caused by opioids. It is given as an IV bolus and, if effective, can be continued as an infusion. It is important to continue the naloxone infusion because the duration of respiratory depression induced by drugs such as methadone may be long compared with the half-life of naloxone.

Flumazenil. Flumazenil is a CNS benzodiazepine-receptor antagonist that can reverse the respiratory depression induced by overdoses of benzodiazepines. It is given by slow IV injection.

Protriptyline. Protriptyline has been used to treat sleep apnea, but the mechanism of its action is unclear. It may increase discharge of motor nerves in the upper airways and thus reduce the risk of hypotonia of the upper airways.

Oxygen

Oxygen therapy is important in correcting the acute and chronic hypoxemia of respiratory diseases. Hypoxemia usually is the result of impaired gas exchange in patients with pneumonia, exacerbations of chronic bronchitis, and/or left ventricular failure. Increasing the alveolar oxygen concentration by increasing inspired oxygen concentrations can relieve some of the problem. The concentration of oxygen given to patients should be carefully monitored to be sure that adequate oxygenation occurs at the lowest possible "doses" of oxygen thereby minimizing oxygen toxicity. *Principle: The principles of clinical pharmacology also apply to substances often not considered drugs (e.g., gases such as oxygen, salt, and water) when they are used in supraphysiologic quantities. Efficacy without risk may be difficult to achieve.*

Oxygen Delivery. Oxygen from cylinders or from domiciliary supplies may be delivered by a face mask that regulates the concentration of inspired oxygen based on the Venturi principle so that room air is entrained. Oxygen can be delivered at concentrations of 24%, 28%, and 32%. Above 32% a simple face mask is needed. Oxygen also may be delivered by nasal prongs that are not as reliable for delivery of a constant concentration but may be better tolerated by patients than a mask.

Adverse Effects. In patients with COPD who are hypercapnic, the respiratory sensibility to rising concentrations of CO_2 may be impaired. If so, the hypoxic contribution may be more important in determining respiratory drive than that ordinarily developed by hypercapnia. Relief of hypoxia with oxygen may therefore remove the last remaining drive to breathing, leading to underventilation and a further rise in PCO_2.

High concentrations of inspired oxygen (over 50%) may predispose to absorption atelectasis and also may directly damage type 1 pneumocytes and endothelial cells, resulting in a syndrome similar to adult respiratory distress syndrome (Massaro, 1980). Long-term exposure to high oxygen tension may lead to pulmonary fibrosis. It is therefore important to keep the inspired oxygen concentration below 50%.

Increasing inspired oxygen concentrations in premature neonates may result in retinal vascular damage with new vessel formation leading to retrolental fibroplasia. The result is permanent blindness. Therefore, arterial PO_2 should not be allowed to rise above 70 mm Hg (9 kPa) in infants who require supplemental oxygen.

Domiciliary Oxygen. Oxygen supplied at home may be used (usually for short periods) for the relief of breathlessness in patients with severe respiratory disease (Stretton, 1985). In view of the expense involved and the potential for subtle but important toxicity, assessment of whether the oxygen actually improves aspects of the disease should be made. Does use of the drug increase walking distance, allow the patient to accomplish new chores, lead to more exercise tolerance, and so forth?

Long-term oxygen also has been used to improve the prognosis of patients with COPD and severe hypoxemia (Petty, 1983). The cheapest form of supply for long-term oxygen therapy is an oxygen concentrator.

Supplemental O_2 should be used cautiously in patients with a history of documented or suspected CO_2 retention. Remember also that COPD is a dynamic process, and even though a patient has been free of serious hypercapnia in the past, an infectious insult or the natural course of the disease could worsen the situation. Every patient requiring supplemental O_2 for an acute exacerbation of pulmonary disease needs periodic estimations of blood-gas concentrations. Long-term therapy should not go unmonitored.

CLINICAL APPLICATIONS

Asthma

Despite a marked increase in treatments prescribed for asthma, the morbidity and even mortality caused by asthma appear to be increasing in industrialized countries. This may be related to inappropriate use of available medication or to a lack of availability of appropriate therapies. It is possible that virtually all deaths from asthma could be avoided by intelligent maintenance therapy and careful management of acute attacks.

Pathophysiology. Our understanding of asthma has changed markedly over the past few years. Asthma is now believed to be a chronic inflammatory disease of the airways. Even the clinically mildest of asthmatic patients have features of mucosal inflammation in the airways (Barnes, 1989b). Although in the past treatment was dominated by bronchodilators that relieve bronchoconstriction, it may be more efficacious to introduce anti-inflammatory treatment at an early stage of the disease (Barnes, 1989a). Asthma usually is easy to diagnose, yet often is underdiagnosed and undertreated because some patients do not have fully developed chronic bronchospasm. For example, they may simply present with a chronic cough.

The precise mechanisms involved in asthmatic inflammation are uncertain. Several inflammation cells appear to be involved, including mast cells, macrophages, T lymphocytes, and eosinophils. Eosinophilic "inflammation" is very characteristic of asthmatic airways, and indeed asthma may be considered as "chronic eosinophilic bronchitis." Several inflammatory mediators, including histamine, prostaglandins, leukotrienes, PAF, and bradykinin, as well as cytokines such as IL-3 and IL-5, are likely to be involved (Barnes et al.,

1988). Microvascular leak and edema of the airway wall also are important, as is hypersecretion of mucus, in addition to contraction of airway smooth muscle.

Principles of Management. The aim of management of asthma is to allow patients to lead as normal a life as possible. They should be able to participate in sports, have infrequent and mild exacerbations, and achieve control with minimal adverse effects of therapy.

General therapeutic measures include avoidance of allergens where this is practical. This is particularly important in occupational asthma. There are rather few categories of drug needed and available for the therapy of asthma (Fig. 7–6).

For patients with only occasional symptoms, an inhaled β_2-adrenergic agonist should be used when necessary. Oral bronchodilators are less satisfactory because of slower onset of action and adverse effects. Other types of patients with asthma present more difficult therapeutic challenges.

Chronic Asthma. For patients with more frequent symptoms (e.g., daily), some form of prophylactic treatment should be considered (Barnes, 1989d). Either low-dose inhaled steroids (for adults) or cromolyn sodium (for children) should be introduced in addition to an inhaled β_2-adrenergic agonist as required. If there is a convincing clinical history of intermittent wheezing, the use

of bronchodilators should not be abandoned on the basis of failure to respond to them on one occasion. Repeated tests of their efficacy may demonstrate that the patient's bronchi are labile and that long-term use of the bronchodilator is appropriate.

If satisfactory control is not achieved, then the dose of inhaled steroid should be increased. Inhaled doses of up to 2 mg (2000 μg) may be given before systemic effects or adrenocortical suppression begin to be seen. Inhaled steroids should be given four times daily until control is achieved; however, they may then be given twice daily if this regimen results in better compliance. When doses over 500 μg daily are needed, a spacer device should be used to reduce the risk of oropharyngeal adverse effects. If cromolyn is ineffective in children after 1 month of therapy, then low-dose inhaled steroids should be introduced. It may be useful to precede cromolyn treatment by inhalation of a sympathomimetic bronchodilator. This can prevent episodes of bronchospasm and might serve to improve distribution of the cromolyn.

Theophylline, given as a slow-release preparation, may be added as a third-line treatment. The dose must be carefully monitored so that therapeutic concentrations of drug in plasma are obtained.

Anticholinergic drugs have little value in the treatment of chronic asthma. Ketotifen and antihistamines do not provide any convincing benefit in the management of chronic asthma.

ASTHMA THERAPY

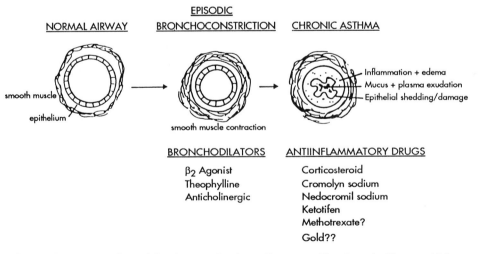

Fig. 7–6. Drugs currently used for therapy of asthma. Drugs are either *bronchodilators*, which act predominantly by relaxing airway smooth muscle, or *antiinflammatory drugs*, which suppress the chronic inflammation in the airway mucosa.

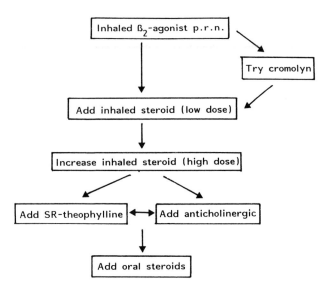

Fig. 7-7. Stepwise approach to therapy of asthma.

When asthma is more difficult to control, the use of oral steroids may be necessary. Prednisone or prednisolone are the drugs of choice. The lowest doses that control the symptoms should be used in order to avoid or at least minimize long-term complications of the corticosteroids. Oral steroids should be given as a single dose in the morning. Alternate-day dosing definitely reduces the incidence of adverse effects but almost always gives less satisfactory control. Some patients who have particular problems with oral steroids (e.g., osteoporosis in postmenopausal women) may be candidates for use of low-dose oral methotrexate (15 mg/week). The combination may spare (i.e., reduce) the dose of oral steroid that is required.

A stepwise approach to therapy is recommended (Fig. 7-7). The value of each step should be monitored by recording of peak airflow in the patient. The inflammation that underlies asthma is variable in its intensity; consequently, the doses of antiasthma treatments can be varied from time to time to match the intensity of the disease. The frequency of need to use β_2-adrenergic agonists by inhalation is a rough guide to the adequacy of control. If their use increases, then the amount of prophylactic treatment given should be increased.

Exacerbations of asthma should be treated with a short course of oral steroids (e.g., prednisone 30 mg daily for 2 weeks and then rapidly tapered off). Less severe exacerbations may be treated by doubling the dose of inhaled steroids. Patients with severe chronic asthma should be given a "crisis management plan" that clearly defines when they should initiate a course of oral steroids. The plan should use the measurement of peak flow at home as a quantitative indicator of severity as well as response to therapy. Such self-administration treatment has been shown to reduce hospital admissions and is acceptable to patients (Beasley et al., 1989).

Exercise-Induced Asthma. Exercise-induced asthma is a sign of poor control and usually responds to an increase in inhaled steroids. Inhalation of a β_2-adrenergic agonist or inhaled cromolyn 10 minutes prior to exercise usually prevents exercise-induced wheeze. Anticholinergics, theophylline, and oral β-adrenergic agonists are less satisfactory. In the future, long-acting β-adrenergic agonists may be suitable for prophylactic treatment of exercise-induced bronchoconstriction.

Nocturnal Asthma. Nocturnal wheezing also is a sign of poor control of asthma. It usually responds to inhaled steroids (Barnes, 1984; Dahl et al., 1989). If nocturnal symptoms persist, even after high-dose inhaled steroids, the addition of a slow-release theophylline preparation taken at night may be helpful (Barnes et al., 1982; Heins et al., 1988). Slow-release oral β-adrenergic agonists also may be useful in some of these patients. Again, long-acting inhaled β_2-adrenergic agonists may become the treatment of choice.

Severe Asthma. Occasionally, asthma can be difficult to control despite seemingly adequate doses of recommended medications (Barnes and Chung, 1989). The severity often is related to poor compliance to the prescriptions, which should be carefully checked. ***Principle: Reasons for and patterns of noncompliance are not straightforward, predictable, or necessarily con-***

sistent (see chapter 33). Simple direct questions may not be useful to detect the noncomplier. Whenever possible try to observe some effect in addition to efficacy of the drug to determine whether patients are taking the prescribed drugs. For example, β-adrenergic agonists and theophylline increase heart rates, and the latter may contribute to diuresis. Methotrexate reduces platelet and white cell counts, and so forth. If a patient is not responding to β-adrenergic agonists but the heart rate is elevated, there is evidence of compliance and inadequacy of the therapy. Try to carry through on this line of reasoning for as many therapeutic settings as possible.

A few patients have "brittle" asthma that is unpredictable. Some of these patients respond to subcutaneous β_2-adrenergic agonists (O'Driscoll et al., 1988). Others are relatively "steroid-resistant" even to high doses (Carmichael et al., 1981). These patients are difficult to manage, and methotrexate may be needed in combination with the steroids. A variant of steroid-resistant asthma is severe premenstrual asthma that may respond to parenteral progesterone (Beynon et al., 1988).

Asthma in Infants. Children under 2 years old may be difficult to manage simply because inhaled drugs are difficult to administer (another example of noncompliance) (Warner, 1988). Infants do not respond well to β-adrenergic agonists; in fact, anticholinergics are the most useful bronchodilators in such patients (Hodges et al., 1981). The anticholinergics may be delivered by MDI into a spacer device fitted with a face mask. For severe exacerbations, a course of oral steroids may be given in addition to nebulized ipratropium bromide. Preliminary evidence suggests that nebulized steroids also may be useful.

Asthma in Pregnancy. Asthma often improves during pregnancy, but some patients may deteriorate (Schatz et al., 1988). The principles of treatment are the same as for nonpregnant asthmatics (Chung and Barnes, 1987). Inhaled treatments should be used because inhaled β-adrenergic agonists, corticosteroids, and cromolyn are less likely to be absorbed. Oral medication should be avoided whenever possible. Oral steroids have been associated with cleft palate of the newborn when given in the first trimester of pregnancy. From the point of view of adverse effects on the fetus, most antiasthma medications appear to be relatively safe but have not been rigorously studied. There are very few registries of observations of drug effects on the fetus. If a drug-related event is only relatively severe, its relative risk is in the range of 2 or less, and its incidence is less than 1 : 10,000, we probably do not know about it (see chapters 29, 32, 34, and 41).

Severe Acute Asthma. Severe exacerbations of asthma usually respond to high doses of inhaled β-adrenergic agonists. Less severe episodes may be managed at home using a nebulizer or a spacer device. More severe episodes require admission to a hospital. Nebulized β_2-adrenergic agonists (e.g., albuterol 5 mg in 2 ml of saline nebulized over 10 minutes) is the initial treatment of choice and is more convenient to administer and as effective as IV β_2-adrenergic agonist (Williams et al., 1981). The nebulizer should be driven by oxygen to avoid the fall in Po_2 that may occur from the pulmonary vasodilation. If there is no response, the nebulization should be repeated within 20 minutes. Once response begins, the nebulization should be repeated every 3 to 4 hours.

Intravenous aminophylline is more difficult to use than adrenergic agents and may be associated with adverse effects. If the patient was taking a theophylline preparation at the time of exacerbation, the concentration of theophylline in plasma should be measured on admission. The loading dose of aminophylline should be reduced appropriately. Aminophylline should be used only if the patient fails to respond satisfactorily to a nebulized β_2-adrenergic agonist. That lack of response is rare.

Corticosteroids should be given to all patients who require hospitalization due to acute asthma. Intravenous hydrocortisone (200 mg 6 hourly) usually is given, but prednisolone 60 mg given orally is just as effective unless the patient is very ill (and therefore has impaired enteric absorption) (Harrison et al., 1986).

Although it has a slower onset of action, nebulized ipratropium bromide also is effective as a bronchodilator. But since there is a risk that it will produce paradoxical bronchoconstriction if used alone, it should be used in *addition* to a β_2-adrenergic agonist. A combination of a β_2-adrenergic agonist with ipratropium bromide (1 mg) often is used to spare the doses of the adrenergic agonist (Ward et al., 1981; Rebuck et al., 1987).

Careful monitoring is necessary in all patients who have been admitted to hospital because of acute severe asthma. The patients should be changed from nebulized bronchodilators to regular inhalers well before discharge from the hospital. They should be given a crisis management plan that clearly indicates when oral steroids should be introduced. Once again, the trigger to use the corticosteroids should be based on daily measurement of peak expiratory air flow.

COPD

Chronic obstructive pulmonary disease may be produced by chronic bronchitis that involves progressive obstruction of bronchi, and by emphysema that involves destruction of the lung parenchyma. Because these different disease processes share the same etiologic factors, they often occur together. The pharmacologic management of each type of dominant sign is essentially the same (Sackner, 1985).

Pathophysiology. Chronic bronchitis is characterized by an increase in mucus secretion and recognized as a chronic productive cough. Mucus hypersecretion resulting from chronic irritants such as cigarette smoke impairs mucociliary clearance. This in turn predisposes to infection and eventually can result in damage to and irreversible obstruction of the airways.

Emphysema is due to enzymatic destruction of lung parenchyma. The result is loss of the elastic recoil that normally keeps airways open, thus leading to narrowing of the airways. The enzyme responsible for this process is predominantly elastase that is derived from neutrophils and macrophages. This enzyme is normally counteracted by a number of serum protease inhibitors, such as α_1-antitrypsin and α_2-immunoglobulin (Flenley et al., 1986). Patients with an inherited deficiency of α_1-antitrypsin have a particularly severe form of emphysema.

Progressive airway obstruction leads to chronic hypoxemia that increases pulmonary vascular pressures via hypoxic vasoconstriction. The process eventually may lead to right ventricular failure (cor pulmonale). In patients with emphysema, destruction of the pulmonary vascular bed exacerbates the pulmonary vascular resistance. So does chronic hypoxemia in some patients, as it stimulates the release of erythropoietin, resulting in polycythemia. The rising blood viscosity contributes to pulmonary hypertension.

Goals of Treatment. The predominant aims of management are to treat exacerbations of infection promptly, to alleviate symptoms, and to prevent complications. Patients with mild symptoms should be encouraged to stop smoking, which can decrease the rate of progressive decline in lung function. Yearly vaccination for influenza is recommended, as is active immunization with polyvalent pneumococcal vaccine. Acute exacerbations associated with production of purulent sputum usually are due to *Hemophilus influenzae* or *Streptococcus pneumoniae*. These infections should be treated promptly with an appropriate antibiotic, such as amoxicillin or cotrimoxazole. The bronchial obstruction and plugging that is part of the pathogenesis of the disease allows ordinarily nonpathogenic bacterial to accumulate and cause serious infection. In such a setting normal flora can cause the disease, so that sputum culture may not be useful for deciding which antibiotic to use. Empirical data indicate that more expensive antibiotics such as oral cephalosporins rarely are necessary to manage acute infections in patients with COPD. Tetracycline may still play an important role in managing the disease.

Treatment with Bronchodilators. The degree of bronchodilation achievable in patients with COPD generally is considerably less than can be induced in patients with asthma. Inhaled β-adrenergic agonists and anticholinergics are the bronchodilators of choice. The only reversible element of bronchoconstriction in patients with COPD is cholinergic tone. The anticholinergics specifically antagonize the tone, and β-adrenergic agonists (that can overcome bronchoconstriction nonspecifically) are equally effective. Anticholinergics have been reported to be more effective in emphysematous patients (Gross and Skorodin, 1984b), but the reasons are not clear. Because obstruction of airflow often is very marked in patients with COPD (FEV$_1$ values can be less than 1 liter), only a very small proportion (less than 1% of the inhaled dose) enters the lung. For this reason, home nebulizers are a useful device for delivering large doses of these agents.

Theophylline is a relatively ineffective bronchodilator but increases the walking distance in patients with COPD (Taylor et al., 1985). This effect may be caused by deflation of the hyperinflated lungs, possibly through a selective action on peripheral airways (Chrystyn et al., 1988). Furthermore, theophylline may have an effect on respiratory muscles that increases ventilatory efficiency (Murciano et al., 1989). Smoking induces hepatic enzyme activity and thereby increases theophylline clearance; thus the dose of theophylline may need to be higher than usual in patients who continue to smoke.

Oxygen. Controlled administration of oxygen is needed to correct hypoxemia during acute exacerbations of COPD. In hypercapnic patients only low concentrations can be used until confidence can be gained that the oxygen will not depress respiratory drive. Home (domiciliary) oxygen, best supplied by an oxygen concentrator, also is indicated for patients with very severe COPD when hypoxemia limits daily activity. Some measure of objective improvement should be demonstrated, however, before this treatment is begun, and it must be monitored relatively frequently thereafter.

Mucolytics and Antitussives. Patients with chronic bronchitis generally have a chronic productive cough. The production of sputum usually decreases when the patient stops smoking. There is no evidence that currently available mucolytic drugs are of any benefit in clearing mucus. Antitussives are not indicated, because coughing is useful in clearing the respiratory tract. Furthermore, opioids may impair ventilatory drive and should be avoided.

Anti-inflammatory Drugs. There is no convincing evidence that corticosteroids, or any other anti-inflammatory treatment, are useful in the chronic management of patients with COPD. Indeed, if a patient improves while taking steroids, it is safe to assume that he or she is asthmatic and should be treated accordingly. A formal trial of steroids (prednisone 30 mg daily for 2 weeks) may be indicated when the diagnosis is uncertain. Peak expiratory flow should be measured to demonstrate an objective improvement associated with the therapy.

Drugs for Breathlessness. Bronchodilators should reduce breathlessness, as might the use of oxygen chronically. However, breathlessness may be extreme in a few patients. Drugs, such as dihydrocodeine or diazepam, may have some efficacy in reducing breathlessness, but they also depress ventilation. These drugs must be used with caution. *Principle: Drugs with poorly documented efficacy and well-documented toxicity should be used cautiously if at all. Caution in this regard means setting the lower limits of acceptable toxicity before starting therapy and assessing the effects of the drugs frequently.*

Cor Pulmonale. Pulmonary hypertension is a direct effect of alveolar hypoxia and chronic hypoxemia. If it persists, the destruction of the pulmonary vascular bed is progressive. In patients with emphysema, the process may lead to right ventricular failure, fluid retention, and peripheral edema.

Pulmonary hypertension may be reduced by long-term home oxygen therapy, although it may be necessary to take the oxygen for over 15 hours daily (Medical Research Council Working Party, 1981). Pulmonary hypertension also may be reduced by various vasodilators (e.g., prostacyclin, calcium-channel blockers, and hydralazine). None of these has a selective effect on the pulmonary circulation. The fall they produce in systemic vascular resistance, blood pressure, and cardiac output may outweigh any of their beneficial effects on the pulmonary circulation (Packer et al., 1982; Long and Rubin, 1987). Although the search for a selective pulmonary vasodilator has been long and continues, none is yet available.

If treatment becomes necessary, peripheral edema usually responds to diuretics, particularly if hypoxia can be relieved. Care should be taken with potassium-wasting diuretics, since they may exacerbate any hypokalemia induced by large doses of nebulized β-adrenergic agonists or use of corticosteroids. Potassium-sparing diuretics are preferable. Digoxin has not been demonstrated to have efficacy in patients with cor pulmonale, and patients with hypoxemia may be more prone to develop digoxin-induced arrhythmias. *Principle: Treatment of minor symptoms such as peripheral edema with drugs capable of causing major adverse effects (e.g., hypokalemia) may be counterproductive and even dangerous* (see chapter 11).

α_1-Protease Inhibitor Therapy. The gene for α_1-protease inhibitor (α_1PI, or α_1-antitrypsin) has been cloned, and human recombinant α_1PI has been synthesized. The recombinant product is now being tested in patients with homozygous α_1PI deficiency. Preliminary results suggest that when the protein is given by infusion each week, it can maintain concentrations of α_1PI in plasma that are required to neutralize lung elastase (Brantley et al., 1988). Site-directed mutagenesis also is being used to increase the stability of the protein (Brantley et al., 1989). Such treatment is available only to a few selected patients with α_1PI deficiency and is unlikely to be applicable to most patients with emphysema caused by smoking. *Principle: Drugs derived from the "new biology" are exciting to anticipate. New drugs may appear to be more attractive than old ones, mainly because of their promise* and *because the problems they will cause are not known. They may have unique properties never seen before. But as in all other settings of therapy, theoretical advantages of untested drugs must be proved. Even the relative value of α_1PI purified from pooled human serum versus the recombinant product must be tested to be understood.*

Respiratory Failure

Respiratory failure is defined by a low PaO_2 (less than 60 torr or 8 kPa) and/or a high PCO_2 (greater than 50 torr or 7 kPa). The causes include central depression of respiration (e.g., postoperatively from anesthesia, from drug overdose) or from a problem with gas exchange (e.g., COPD, asthma, left ventricular failure, adult respiratory distress syndrome). The two key steps in management are to provide adequate ventilation and to treat the underlying condition. Specific pharmacologic treatments have little role. Doxapram given by infusion is the most useful respiratory stimulant, but it must be used with great care. It is only truly useful when central depression of respiration is the major cause of disease.

Adult Respiratory Distress Syndrome. Adult respiratory distress syndrome (ARDS) is due to widespread leakage of fluid from pulmonary capillaries into alveoli, often related to neutrophil sequestration and activation. There are many causes (e.g., trauma, burn, sepsis, pancreatitis), and these should be treated vigorously and specifically. Oxygenation is the most important supportive treatment. There is little evidence that corticosteroids are effective, and they actually may increase the intensity and complications of infection (Bernard et al., 1987). If introduced early in the syndrome, methylprednisolone (500 mg IV 12 hourly) may help some patients. More specific therapy may arise from studies of pathogenesis, and evidence that tumor necrosis factor (TNF) is involved have prompted trials of anti-TNF antibodies or antagonists (Tracey et al., 1988). A methylxanthine, pentoxifylline, protects against experimental ARDS, although its mode of action is not certain (Welsch et al., 1988).

DRUG-INDUCED LUNG DISEASE

Over 40 drugs have now been implicated as causing a variety of lung diseases. Drugs may affect lung function by causing predictable pharmacologic effects (e.g., depression of ventilatory drive by opioids), by causing hypersensitivity (e.g., nitrofurantoin-induced pulmonary eosinophilia), or by causing a direct toxic effect (e.g, practolol- and paraquat-induced pulmonary fibrosis). Drugs may affect airways, pulmonary vasculature, or parenchyma.

Airway Disease and Asthma

Several drugs may lead to deterioration of asthmatic or other airway diseases by different mechanisms.

Sedatives. Any sedative (opiate, benzodiazepine) reduces ventilatory drive and should therefore be avoided in patients with COPD and with severe asthma.

β-Adrenergic Antagonists. β-Adrenergic antagonists should be avoided in patients with asthma. The mechanism by which β-adrenergic antagonists impair airway function is not yet certain. The actions appear to be mediated by blockade of β_2 receptors, but even "selective" β_1 blockers are potentially dangerous because their selectivity is modest. Even low doses of β-adrenergic blockers, such as timolol given as eye drops, can cause severe worsening of asthma (Shoene, 1981; Dunn et al., 1986), and fatalities continue to be reported. The effect is likely to be mediated via airway cholinergic nerves and may be very severe (Ind et al., 1989). Patients with COPD are less likely to be affected by β-adrenergic blockers, but some patients with COPD have an unrecognized component of asthma. Alternative treatments for hypertension and ischemic heart disease such as calcium-channel blockers are safe. Propafenone is a new antiarrhythmic agent that is structurally similar to propranolol and has been reported to increase bronchoconstriction in asthmatic patients (Hill et al., 1986).

Aspirin. A small proportion of asthmatics (3%–5%) develop worsening of their asthma on exposure to aspirin. These patients usually have late-onset asthma, rhinitis, and nasal polyps (Szczeklik, 1982; Stevenson, 1984). Other structurally unrelated NSAIDs also may cause similar effects in these patients, suggesting that cyclooxygenase inhibition underlies the phenomenon. Blocking the formation of bronchodilator prostaglandins (such as PGE-2) is one possible pathogenetic factor in such patients, but the explanation may be more complicated. Acetylsalicylic acid but not sodium salicylate can cause the syndrome, even though both are potent inhibitors of cyclooxygenase.

ACE Inhibitors. Angiotensin-converting enzyme (ACE) inhibitors such as captopril and enalapril may cause irritating nonproductive cough in 5% to 10% of patients (Fuller, 1989). Cough may occur in any patient and is no more frequent in patients with asthma, nor is there any convincing evidence that asthma gets worse with cough due to ACE inhibitors. The mechanism of the cough is unknown but may be caused by reduced degradation of peptides, such as bradykinin, in the lungs. The NSAIDs appear to be useful in inhibiting the cough (McEwan et al., 1990).

Pulmonary Vascular Disease

Oral contraceptives are associated with venous thrombosis and pulmonary thromboembolism that may result in pulmonary hypertension. Aminorex is an appetite-suppressant drug that was used in some European countries. It may lead to a severe form of pulmonary hypertension resembling primary pulmonary hypertension. Very rarely a similar syndrome has been reported in patients taking amphetamine-like agents, fenfluramine, or phenformin.

Parenchymal Disease

Several drugs may cause pulmonary shadowing, dyspnea, and crepitations, but little is known of the mechanisms involved. It is difficult to classify these effects (Cooper et al., 1986a and 1986b). Furthermore, some drugs appear to have variable effects in different patients, indicating differences in metabolism or tissue response to the drug. A further difficulty is encountered when there are only a few case reports of a particular drug effect; it may be difficult to know whether one is seeing a side effect of the drug itself or a rare manifestation of the disease being treated with the drug. For example, penicillamine is used in the treatment of severe rheumatoid arthritis and was implicated in causing obliterative bronchiolitis. However, it now seems more likely that this is a rare manifestation of rheumatoid disease (Geddes et al., 1977).

Pulmonary Infiltrates with Peripheral Eosinophilia. Pulmonary shadowing associated with blood eosinophilia has been associated with over 30 drugs. The most commonly associated drugs appear to be nitrofurantoin (Penn and Griffin, 1982), *p*-aminosalicylic acid, sulfonamides, penicillins, naproxen, carbamazepine, gold salts, and methotrexate. Symptoms usually develop within a few days of starting the drug and resolve when the drug is withdrawn.

Diffuse Fibrosis. Several drugs can cause interstitial alveolar infiltrates, thought to reflect immunologically mediated injury to alveolar cells, causing desquamation and later fibrosis. This is seen with cytotoxic and immunosuppressive drugs (especially bleomycin, busulphan, carmustine, methotrexate) (Cooper et al., 1986b), and also with the antiarrhythmic drug amiodorone (Liu et al., 1986). The mechanism of alveolar injury appears to depend on the generation of oxygen radicals. Nitrofurantoin and gold salts also may produce this picture, which probably results from hypersensitivity or immune-mediated reactions, because T-suppressor lymphocytes have been implicated.

Paraquat may induce an acute form of alveolar injury that often is fatal. Paraquat accumulates in lung tissue and generates oxygen radicals that produce the ARDS-like state. High concentrations of oxygen also lead to an ARDS-like picture (Massaro, 1980).

SLE-Like Syndrome. Several drugs induce a systemic lupus erythematosus–like syndrome that may involve the lungs with pleurisy and pleural effusions and occasionally lung fibrosis. Drugs most commonly implicated are hydralazine, procainamide, isoniazid, and sulfonamides. The syndrome usually regresses when the drug is withdrawn.

REFERENCES

Altounyan, R. E. C.: Review of clinical activity and mode of action of sodium cromoglycate. Clin. Allergy, 10:481–489, 1980.

Anderson, S. D.; Seale, J. P.; Rozea, P.; Bandler, L.; Theobald, G.; and Lindsay, D. A.: Inhaled and oral sulbutanol in exercise-induced asthma. Am. Rev. Respir. Dis., 114:493–498, 1976.

Appel, D.; Karrel, J. P.; and Sherman, M.: Epinephrine improves expiratory flow rates in patients with asthma who do not respond to inhaled metaproterenol sulfate. J. Allergy Clin. Immunol., 84:90–98, 1989.

Arvidsson, P.; Larsson, S.; Lofdahl, C. G.; Melander, B.; Wahlander, L.; and Svedmyr, N.: Formoterol, a new long-acting bronchodilator for inhalation. Eur. Resp. J., 2:325–330, 1989.

Aubier, M.; DeTroyer, A.; Sampson, M.; Macklem, P. T.; and Roussos, C.: Aminophylline improves diaphragmatic contractility. N. Engl. J. Med., 305:249–252, 1981.

Barclay, J.; Whiting, B.; Meredith, P. A.; and Addis, G. J.: Theophylline-salbutamol interaction: Bronchodilator response to salbutamol at maximally effective plasma theophylline concentrations. Br. J. Clin. Pharmacol., 11:203–208, 1981.

Barnes, P. J.: Effect of corticosteroids on airway hyperresponsiveness. Am. Rev. Respir. Dis., 141:S70–S76, 1990.

Barnes, P. J.: A new approach to asthma therapy. N. Engl. J. Med., 321:1517–1527, 1989a.

Barnes, P. J.: New concepts in the pathogenesis of bronchial hyperresponsiveness and asthma. J. Allergy Clin. Immunol., 83:1013–1026, 1989b.

Barnes, P. J.: Muscarinic receptor subtypes: Implications for lung disease. Thorax, 44:161–167, 1989c.

Barnes, P. J.: Chronic asthma. In, Current Therapy of Respiratory Disease, Vol 3 (Cherniak, R. M., ed.). B. Decker, Toronto, pp. 132–136, 1989d.

Barnes, P. J.: Airway pharmacology. In, Textbook of Respiratory Medicine (Murray, J. F.; and Nadel, J. A.; eds.). W. B. Saunders, Philadelphia, pp. 249–268, 1988.

Barnes, P. J.: Cholinergic control of airway smooth muscle. Am. Rev. Respir. Dis., 136:S42–S45, 1987a.

Barnes, P. J.: Using anticholinergics to best advantage. J. Respir. Dis., 8:84–95, 1987b.

Barnes, P. J.: Nocturnal asthma: Mechanisms and treatment. Br. Med. J., 288:1397–1398, 1984.

Barnes, P. J.; and Chung, K. F.: Difficult asthma. Br. Med. J., 299:695–698, 1989.

Barnes, P. J., and Pride, N. B.: Dose-response curves to inhaled beta-adrenoceptor agonists in normal and asthmatic subjects. Br. J. Clin. Pharmacol., 15:677–682, 1983.

Barnes, P. J.; Chung, K. F.; and Page, C. P.: Inflammatory mediators in asthma. Pharmacol. Rev., 40:49–84, 1988.

Barnes, P. J.; Greening, A. P.; Neville, L.; Timmers, J.; and Poole, G. W.: Single dose slow-release aminophylline at night prevents nocturnal asthma. Lancet, 1:299–301, 1982.

Baum, G. L.; and Wolinsky, E. (eds.): Textbook of Pulmonary Diseases. Little, Brown, Boston, 1989.

Beasley, R.; Cushley, M.; and Holgate, S. T.: A self management plan in the treatment of adult asthma. Thorax, 44:200–204, 1989.

Benatar, S. R.: Fatal asthma. N. Engl. J. Med., 314:423–429, 1986.

Bernard, G. R.; Luce, J. M.; and Sprung, C. L.: High dose corticosteroids in patients with adult respiratory distress syndrome. N. Engl. J. Med., 317:1565–1570, 1987.

Ber, stein, D. I.; Bernstein, I. L.; Bodenheimer, S. S.; and Pietrusro, R. G.: An open study of Auranofin in the treatment of steroid-dependent asthma. J. Allergy Clin. Immunol., 81:6–16, 1988.

Bernstein, I. L.: Cromolyn sodium in the treatment of asthma: Coming of age in the United States. J. Allergy Clin. Immunol., 76:381–388, 1985.

Beynon, H. L. C.; Garbett, N. D.; and Barnes, P. J.: Severe premenstrual exacerbations of asthma: Effect of intramuscular progesterone. Lancet, 2:370–372, 1988.

Boman, G.; Backer, U.; Larsson, S.; Melander, B.; and Wahlander, L. L.: Oral acetylcystine reduces exacerbation rate in chronic bronchitis: Report of a trial organized by the Swedish

Society for Pulmonary Diseases. Eur. J. Respir. Dis., 64:405–415, 1983.

Boschetto, P.; Roberts, N. M.; Rogers, D. F.; and Barnes, P. J.: Effect of anti-asthma drugs on microvascular leakage in guinea-pig airways. Am. Rev. Respir. Dis., 139:416–421, 1989.

Brantley, M.; Courtney, M.; and Crystal, R. G.: Repair of the secretion defect in the Z form of alpha-1-antitrypsin by addition of a second mutation. Science, 242:1700–1701, 1989.

Brantly, M.; Nukiwa, Y.; and Crystal, R. G.: Molecular basis of alpha-1-antitrypsin deficiency. Am. J. Med., 84:13–31, 1988.

Brattsand, R.: Glucocorticosteroids for inhalation. In, New Drugs for Asthma (Barnes, P. J., ed.). IBC Publications, London, pp. 117–130, 1989.

Brenner, M.; Berkowitz, R.; Marshall, N.; and Strunk, R. C.: Need for theophylline in severe steroid-requiring asthmatics. Clin. Allergy, 18(2):143–150, 1988.

British Thoracic Society Research Committee: Oral N-acetylcysteine and exacerbation rates in patients with chronic bronchitis and severe airway obstruction. Thorax, 40:832–835, 1985.

Carmichael, J.; Paterson, K.; Diaz, P.; Crompton, G. K.; Kay, A. B.; and Grant, I. W. B.: Corticosteroid resistance in chronic asthma. Br. Med. J., 282:1419–1422, 1981.

Carstairs, J. R.; Nimmo, A. J.; and Barnes, P. J.: Autoradiographic visualization of beta-adrenoceptor subtypes in human lung. Am. Rev. Respir. Dis., 132:541–547, 1985.

Chrystyn, H.; Mulley, B. A.; and Peake, M. D.: Dose response relation to oral theophylline in severe chronic obstructive airways disease. Br. Med. J., 297:1506–1510, 1988.

Chung, K. F.; and Barnes, P. J.: Prescribing in pregnancy. Treatment of asthma. Br. Med. J., 294:103–105, 1987.

Church, M. K.: Cromoglycate-like anti-allergic drugs. Drugs Today, 14:281–341, 1978.

Church, M. K.; and Gradidge, C. F.: Oxatomide: Inhibition and stimulation of histamine release from human lung and leucocytes in vitro. Agents Actions, 10:4–7, 1980.

Church, M. K.; and Hiroi, J.: Inhibition of IgE-dependent histamine release from human dispersed lung mast cells by antiallergic drugs and salbutamol. Br. J. Pharmacol., 90:421–429, 1987.

Cockcroft, D. W.; and Murdock, K. Y.: Comparative effects of inhaled salbutamol, sodium cromoglycate and beclomethasone diproprionate on allergen-induced early asthmatic responses, late asthmatic responses and increased bronchial responsiveness to histamine. J. Allergy Clin. Immunol., 79:734–740, 1987.

Cockcroft, D. W.; Murdock, K. Y.; Gore, B. P.; O'Byrne, P. M.; and Manning, P.: Theophylline does not inhibit allergen-induced increase in airway responsiveness to methacholine. J. Allergy Clin. Immunol., 83:913–920, 1989.

Coe, C. I.; and Barnes, P. J.: Reduction of nocturnal asthma by an inhaled anticholinergic drug. Chest, 90:485–488, 1986.

Collins, J. V.; Clarke, T. J. H.; Brown, D.; and Townsend, J.: The use of corticosteroids in the treatment of acute asthma. Q. J. Med., 44:259–273, 1975.

Cooper, J. A. D.; White, D. A.; and Matthay, R. A.: Drug-induced pulmonary disease: Part I. Cytotoxic drugs. Am. Rev. Respir. Dis., 133:321–340, 1986a.

Cooper, J. A. D.; White, D. A.; and Matthay, R. A.: Drug-induced pulmonary disease: Part II: Noncytotoxic drugs. Am. Rev. Respir. Dis., 133:488–505, 1986b.

Cox, J. S.: Disodium cromoglycate (FPL 670) ("Intal"): A specific inhibitor of reaginic antibody–antigen mechanisms. Nature, 216:1328–1329, 1967.

Coupe, M. O.; Guly, U.; Brown, E.; and Barnes, P. J.: Nebulised adrenaline in acute severe asthma: Comparison with salbutamol. Eur. J. Respir. Dis., 71:227–232, 1987.

Crystal, R. G.; Bitterman, P. B.; Rennard, S. I.; Hance, A. J.; and Keogh, B. A.: Interstitial lung diseases of unknown cause: Disorders characterized by chronic inflammation of the lower respiratory tract. N. Engl. J. Med., 310:154–166, 1984.

Cushley, M. J.; and Holgate, S. T.: Bronchodilator actions of xanthine derivatives administered by inhalation in asthma. Thorax, 40:176–179, 1985.

Cushley, M. J.; Tattersfield, A. E.; and Holgate, S. T.: Adenosine-induced bronchoconstriction in asthma: Antagonism by inhaled theophylline. Am. Rev. Respir. Dis., 129:380–384, 1984.

Dahl; R., and Johansson, S.-A.: Importance of duration of treatment with inhaled budesonide on the immediate and late bronchial reaction. Eur. J. Respir. Dis., 62:167–175, 1982.

Dahl, R.; Pedersen, B.; and Hagglof, B.: Nocturnal asthma: Effect of treatment with oral sustained-release terbutaline, inhaled budesonide and the two in combination. J. Allergy Clin. Immunol., 83:811–815, 1989.

Dajani, B. M.; Sliman, N. A.; Shubair, K. S.; and Hamzeh, Y. S.: Bronchospasm caused by intravenous hydrocortisone sodium succinate (Solu-Cortef) in aspirin-sensitive asthmatics. J. Allery Clin. Immunol., 68: 201–206, 1981.

Davis, A. O., and Lefkowitz, R. J.: Corticosteroid-induced differential regulation of beta-adrenergic receptors in circulating human polymorphonuclear leucocytes and mononuclear leucocytes. J. Clin. Endocrinol. Metab., 51:599–605, 1980.

Dixon, M.,; Jackson, D. M.; and Richards, I. M.: The effect of sodium cromoglycate on lung irritant receptors and left ventricular receptors in anaesthetised dog. Br. J. Pharmacol., 67:569–574, 1979.

Dunn, T. L.; Gerbert, M. J.; Shen, A. S.; Fernandez, E.; Iseman, M. D.; and Cherniak, R. M.: The effect of topical ophthalmic instillation of timolol and betaxolol on lung function in asthmatic subject. Am. Rev. Respir. Dis., 133:264–268, 1986.

Ellul-Micallef, R.: Glucocorticosteroids — The pharmacological basis of their therapeutic use in bronchial asthma. In, Asthma: Basic Mechanisms and Clinical Management (Barnes, P. J.; Rodger, I. W.; and Thomson, N. C.; eds.). Academic Press, London, pp. 653–692, 1988.

Ellul-Micallef, R.: Effect of terbutaline sulphate in chronic "allergic" cough. Br. Med. J., 287:940–943, 1983.

Ellul-Micallef, R.; and French, F. F.: Intravenous prednisolone in chronic bronchial asthma. Thorax, 30:312–315, 1975.

Erjefalt, I.; and Persson, C. G. A.: Anti-asthma drugs attenuate inflammatory leakage into airway lumen. Acta Physiol. Scand., 128:653–655, 1986.

Evans, R. M.: The steroid and thyroid hormone receptor superfamily. Science, 247:889–895, 1988.

Flenley, D. C.; Downing, I.; and Greening, A. P.: The pathogenesis of emphysema. Bull. Eur. Physiopathol. Respir., 22:245–252S, 1986.

Flower, R. J.: Lipocortin and the mechanism of action of the glucocorticoids. Br. J. Pharmacol., 94:987–1015, 1988.

Frith, P. A.; Jenner, B.; Dangerfield, R.; Atkinson, J.; and Drennan, C.: Oxitropium bromide. Dose response and time-response study of a new anticholinergic bronchodilator drug. Chest, 89:249–253, 1986.

Fuller, R. W.: Cough associated with angiotensin converting enzyme inhibitors. J. Hum. Hypert., 3:159–161, 1989.

Gambertoglio, J. G.; Amend, W. J. C.; and Benet, L. Z.: Pharmacokinetics and bioavailability of prednisone and prednisolone in healthy volunteers and patients: A review. J. Pharmacokinet. Biopharm., 8:1–52, 1980.

Geddes, D.; Corrin, B.; Bremerton, D. A.; Davies, R. J.; and Turner-Warwick, M.: Progressive airways obliteration in adults and its association with rheumatoid disease. Q. J. Med., 46:427–437, 1977.

Gonzalez, J. P.; and Brogden, R. N.: Nedocromil sodium. A preliminary review of its pharmacodynamic and pharmacokinetic properties and therapeutic efficacy in the treatment of reversible obstructive airways disease. Drugs, 34:560–577, 1987.

Gross, N. J.: Ipratropium bromide. N. Engl. J. Med., 319:486–494, 1988.

Gross, N. J.; and Skorodin, M. S.: Anticholinergic antimuscarinic bronchodilators. Am. Rev. Respir. Dis., 129:856–870, 1984a.

Gross, N. J.; and Skorodin, M. S.: Role of the parasympathetic system in airway obstruction due to emphysema. N. Engl. J. Med., 311:321–325, 1984b.

Haalboom, J. R. E.; Deenstra, A.; and Struyvenberg, A.: Hypokalaemia induced by inhalation of fenoterol. Lancet, 1: 1125–1127, 1985.

Harrison, B. D. W.; Hart, G. J.; Ali, N. J.; Stokes, T. C.; Vaughan, D. A.; and Robinson, A. A.: Need for intravenous hydrocortisone in addition to oral prednisolone in patients admitted to hospital with severe asthma without ventilatory failure. Lancet, 2:181–184, 1986.

Heins, M.; Kurtin, L.; Oellerich, M.; Maes, R.; and Sybrecht, G. W.: Nocturnal asthma: Slow-release terbutaline versus slow release theophylline therapy. Eur. Respir. J., 1:306–310, 1988.

Hill, M. R.; Gotz, V. P.; Harmann, E.; McLeod, I.; and Hendeles, L.: Evaluation of the asthmogeneity of propafenone, a new antiarrhythmic drug. Chest, 90:698–702, 1986.

Hodges, I. G. C.; Griggins, R. C.; Milner, A. D.; and Stoke, S.: Bronchodilator effect of inhaled ipratropium bromide in wheezing toddlers. Arch. Dis. Child., 56:729–732, 1981.

Holgate, S. T.; Baldwin, C. J.; and Tattersfield, A. E.: Beta-adrenergic agonist resistance in normal human airways. Lancet, 2:375–377, 1977.

Howard, P.: Almitrine bismesylate (Vectarican). Bull. Eur. Physiopathol. Respir., 20:99–103, 1984.

Howarth, P. H.; Durham, S. R.; Lee, T. H.; Kay, A. B.; Church, M. K.; and Holgate, S. T.: Influence of albuterol, cromolyn sodium and ipratropium bromide on the airway and circulating mediator responses to allergen bronchial provocation in asthma. Am. Rev. Respir. Dis., 132:986–922, 1985.

Hunt, C. E.; Inwood, R. J.; and Shannon, D. C.: Respiratory and non-respiratory effects of doxapram in congenital central hyperventilation syndrome. Am. Rev. Respir. Dis., 119:263–269, 1979.

Ind, P. W.; Dixon, C. M. S.; Fuller, R. W.; and Barnes, P. J.: Anticholinergic blockade of beta-blocker induced bronchoconstriction. Am. Rev. Respir. Dis., 139:1390–1394, 1989.

Irwin, R. S.; Corrao, W. M.; and Pratter, M. R.: Chronic persistent cough in the adult: The spectrum and frequency of causes and successful outcome of specific therapy. Am. Rev. Respir. Dis., 123:413–417, 1981.

Iversen, L. L.: Role of transmitter uptake mechanisms in synaptic neurotransmission. Br. J. Pharmacol., 41:571–591, 1971.

Kerrebijn, K. F.; von Essen-Zandvliet, E. E. M.; and Neijens, H. J.: Effect of long-term treatment with inhaled corticosteroids and beta-agonists on bronchial responsiveness in asthmatic children. J. Allergy Clin. Immunol., 79:653–659, 1987.

Konig, P.: Inhaled corticosteroids—Their present and future role in the management of asthma. J. Allergy Clin. Immunol., 82:297–306, 1988.

Kraan, J.; Koeter, G. H.; van der Mark, T. W.; Sluiter, H. J.; and de Vries, K.: Changes in bronchial hyperreactivity induced by 4 weeks of treatment with antiasthma drugs in patients with allergic asthma: A comparison between budesonide and terbutaline. J. Allergy Clin. Immunol., 76:628–636, 1985.

Long, W. A.; and Rubin, L. J.: Prostacyclin and PGE1 treatment of pulmonary hypertension. Am. Rev. Respir. Dis., 136:773–776, 1987.

Liu, L.-W. F.; Cohen, R. D.; Downar, E.; Butany, J. W.; Edelson, J. D.; and Rebuck, A. S.: Amiodorone pulmonary toxicity: Functional and ultrastructural evaluation. Thorax, 41:100–105, 1986.

Loftus, B. G.; and Price, J. F.: Long-term, placebo-controlled trial of ketotifen in the management of preschool children with asthma. J. Allergy Clin. Immunol., 79:350–355, 1987.

Maguire, W. G.; and Nair, S.: Ventilation and perfusion effects of inhaled alpha and beta agonists in asthma patients. Chest, 73:983–985, 1978.

Mann, J. S.; and George, C. F.: Anticholinergic drugs in the treatment of airways disease. Br. J. Dis. Chest, 79:209–228, 1985.

Martin, U.; and Baggliolini, M.: Dissociation between the anti-anaphylactic and antihistaminic action of ketotifen. Arch. Pharmacol., 316:186–189, 1981.

Massaro, F. L.: Oxygen toxicity. Am. J. Med., 69:117–126, 1980.

McEwan, J. R.; Choudry, N. B.; and Fuller, R. W.: The effect of sulindac on the abnormal cough reflex associated with dry cough. J. Appl. Physiol., in press, 1990.

McFadden, E. R.: Beta 2 receptor agonists—Metabolism and pharmacology. J. Allergy Clin. Immunol., 68:91–96, 1981.

Medical Research Council Working Party: Long-term domiciliary oxygen therapy in chronic hypoxic cor pulmonale complicating bronchitis and emphysema. Lancet, 1:681–686, 1981.

Meltzer, E. O.; Kemp, J. P.; Welch, M. J.; and Orgel, H. A.: Effect of dosing schedule on efficacy of beclomethasone diproprionate aerosol in chronic asthma. Am. Rev. Respir. Dis., 131:732–736, 1985.

Milledge, J. S.: Acute mountain sickness. Thorax, 38:641–645, 1983.

Minette, A.: Background of mucolytic treatments in chronic bronchitis. Eur. J. Respir. Dis., 64:401–404, 1983.

Morris, H. G.: Mechanisms of action and therapeutic role of corticosteroids in asthma. J. Allergy Clin. Immunol., 75:1–14, 1985.

Mullarkey, M. F.; Blumenstein, B. A.; Andrade, P.; Bailey, G. A.; Olason, I.; and Wetzel, C. E.: Methotrexate in the treatment of corticosteroid-dependent asthma. A double-blind crossover study. N. Engl. J. Med., 318:603–607, 1988.

Muranaka, M.; Mivamoto, T.; Shida, T.; Kabe, J.; Makinso, S.; Okumara, H.; Takeda, K.; Suzuki, S.; and Horiuchi, Y.: Gold salt in the treatment of bronchial asthma. Ann. Allergy, 40:132–137, 1978.

Murciano, D.; Auclaire, M. H.; Pariente, R.; and Aubier, M.: A randomized, controlled trial of theophylline in patients with severe chronic obstructive pulmonary disease. N. Engl. J. Med., 320:1521–1525, 1989.

Murray, J. F.; and Nadel, J. A. (eds.): Textbook of Respiratory Medicine. W. B. Saunders, Philadelphia, 1988.

Nadel, J. A.; Widdicombe, J. G.; and Peatfield, A. C.: Regulation of airway secretion, ion transport and water movement. In, Handbook of Physiology—The Respiratory System. American Physiology Society, Baltimore, pp. 419–445, 1985.

Nelson, H. S.: Adrenergic therapy of bronchial asthma. J. Allergy Clin. Immunol., 77:771–785, 1986.

Newcomb, R.; Thaskin, D. P.; Hu, K. K.; Conolly, M. E.; Lee, E.; and Dauphinee, B.: Rebound hyperresponsiveness to muscarinic stimulation after chronic therapy with an inhaled muscarinic antagonist. Am. Rev. Respir. Dis., 132:12–15, 1985.

Newhouse, M. T.; and Dolovich, M. B.: Control of asthma by aerosols. N. Engl. J. Med., 315:870–874, 1986.

Newman, S. P.; Pavia, D.; Moren, F.; Sheahan, N. F.; and Clarke, S. W.: Deposition of pressurised aerosols in the human respiratory tract. Thorax, 36:52–55, 1981.

O'Driscoll, B. R. C.; Ruffles, S. P.; Ayres, J. G.; and Cochrane, G. M.: Long term treatment of severe asthma with subcutaneous terbutaline. Br. J. Dis. Chest, 82:360–367, 1988.

Packer, M.; Greenberg, B.; Massie, B.; and Dash, H.: Deleterious effects of hydralazine in patients with primary pulmonary hypertension. N. Engl. J. Med., 306:1326–1331, 1982.

Patel, U. R.: Terfenadine in exercise-induced asthma. Br. Med. J., 288:1496–1497, 1984.

Pavia, D.; Bateman, J. R. M.; and Clarke, S. W.: Deposition and clearance of inhaled particles. Bull. Eur. Physiopathol. Respir., 16:335–366, 1980.

Pedersen, S.; Frost, L.; and Arnfred, T.: Errors in inhalation techniques and efficiency in inhaler use in asthmatic children. Allergy, 41:118–124, 1986.

Penn, R. G.; and Griffin, J. P.: Adverse reactions to nitrofurantoin in the United Kingdom, Sweden, and Holland. Br. Med. J., 284:1440–1442, 1982.

Persson, C. G. A.: Xanthines as airway anti-inflammatory drugs. J. Allergy Clin. Immunol., 81:615–617, 1988.

Persson, C. G. A.: Overview of effects of theophylline. J. Allergy Clin. Immunol., 78:780–787, 1986a.

Persson, C. G. A.: Development of safer xanthine drugs for the treatment of obstructive airways disease. J. Allergy Clin. Immunol., 78:817–824, 1986b.

Petty, T. L.: Selection criteria for long term oxygen therapy. Am. Rev. Respir. Dis., 127:397–398, 1983.

Petty, T. L.; Rollins, D. R.; Christopher, K.; Good, J. T.; and Oakley, R.: Cromolyn sodium is effective in adult chronic asthmatics. Am. Rev. Respir. Dis., 139:694–701, 1989.

Rachelefsky, G. S.; Wo, J.; Adelson, J.; Mickey, M. R.; Spector, S. L.; Katz, R. M.; Siegel, S. C.; and Rahr, A. S.: Behaviour abnormalities and poor school performance due to oral theophylline use. Pediatrics, 78:1133–1138, 1986.

Rafferty, P.; Beasley, R.; and Holgate, S. T.: Comparison of the efficacy of preservative free ipratropium bromide and Atrovent nebuliser solution. Thorax, 43:446–450, 1988.

Rafferty, P.; Beasley, R.; and Holgate, S. T.: The contribution of histamine to immediate bronchoconstriction provoked by inhaled allergen and adenosine 5′ monophosphate in atopic asthma. Am. Rev. Respir. Dis., 136:369–373, 1987.

Rebuck, A. S.; Chapman, K. R.; Abboud, R.; Pare, P. D.; Kreisman, H.; Wolkove, N.; and Vickerson, P.: Nebulized anticholinergic and sympathomimetic treatment of asthma and chronic obstructive airways disease in the emergency room. Am. J. Med., 82:59–64, 1987.

Reinberg, A.; Gervais, P.; Chaussade, M.; Fraboulet, G.; and Duburque, B.: Circadian changes in effectiveness of corticosteroids in eight patients with allergic asthma. J. Allergy Clin. Immunol., 71:425–433, 1983.

Rhoden, K. J.; Meldrum, L. A.; and Barnes, P. J.: Inhibition of cholinergic neurotransmission in human airways by beta2-adrenoceptors. J. Appl. Physiol., 65:700–705, 1988.

Richardson, P. S.; and Phipps, R. J.: The anatomy, physiology, pharmacology and pathology of tracheobronchial mucus secretion and the use of expectorants in human disease. Pharmacol. Ther., 3:441–479, 1978.

Rossing, T. H.; Fanta, C. H.; Goldstein, D. H.; Snapper, J. R.; and McFadden, E. R.: Emergency therapy of asthma: Comparison of acute effects of parenteral and inhaled sympathomimetic and infused aminophylline. Am. Rev. Respir. Dis., 122:365–371, 1980.

Sackner, M. A.: Recent advances in the management of obstructive airways disease. Chest, 88(suppl.):77S–170S, 1985.

Schatz, M.; Harden, K.; and Forsythe, A.: The course of asthma during pregnancy, post partum, and with successive pregnancies: A prospective analysis. J. Allergy Clin. Immunol., 81:509–517, 1988.

Schnack, C.; Podolsky, A.; Watzke, H.; Schernthaner, G.; and Burghuber, O. C.: Effects of somatostatin and oral potassium administration on terbutaline-induced hypokalemia. Am. Rev. Respir. Dis., 139:176–180, 1989.

Shenfield, G. M.: Combination bronchodilator therapy. Drugs, 24:414–439, 1982.

Shoene, R. B.; Martin, T. R.; Charan, N. B.; and French, C. L.: Timolol-induced bronchospasm in asthmatic bronchitis. J.A.M.A., 245:1460–1461, 1981.

Silver, P. J.; and Stull, J. T.: Phosphorylation of myosin light chain kinase and phosphorylase in tracheal smooth muscle in response to KCl and carbachol. Mol. Pharmacol., 25:267–274, 1984.

Sly, R. M.; and Kemp, J. P.: The use of antihistamines in patients with asthma. J. Allergy Clin. Immunol., 82:481–482, 1988.

Stephan, W. C.; Chick, T. W.; Avner, B. P.; and Jenne, J. W.: Tachyphylaxis to inhaled isoproterenol and the effect of methylprednisolone in dogs. J. Allergy Clin. Immunol., 65:105–109, 1980.

Stevenson, D. D.: Diagnosis, prevention and treatment of adverse reactions to aspirin and nonsteroidal anti-inflammatory drugs. J. Allergy Clin. Immunol., 74:617–622, 1984.

Stolley, P. D.: Asthma mortality: Why the United States was spared an epidemic of asthma deaths due to asthma. Am. Rev. Respir. Dis., 105:883–890, 1972.

Stradling, J. R.; Nicholl, C. G.; Cover, D.; Davies, E. C.; and Hughes, J. M. B.: The effects of oral almitrine on pattern and gas exchange in patients with chronic obstructive lung disease. Clin. Sci., 66:435–442, 1984.

Stradling, J. R.; Barnes, P.; and Pride, N. B.: The effects of almitrine on the ventilatory response to hypoxia and hypercapnia in normal subjects. Clin. Sci., 63:401–404, 1982.

Stretton, T. B.: Provision of long-term oxygen therapy. Thorax, 40:801–805, 1985.

Szczeklik, A.: Aspirin and asthma. Eur. J. Respir. Dis., 63: 376–379, 1982.

Tattersfield, A. E.: Tolerance to beta-agonists. Clin. Respir. Physiol., 21:1–5, 1985.

Taylor, D. R.; Buick, B.; Kinney, C.; Lowry, R. C.; and McDevitt, D. G.: The efficacy of orally administered theophylline, inhaled salbutamol, and a combination of the two as chronic therapy in the management of chronic bronchitis with reversible air-flow obstruction. Am. Rev. Respir. Dis., 131:747–751, 1985.

Taylor, D. R.; Duffin, D.; Kinney, C. D.; and McDevitt, D. G.: Investigation of diurnal changes in the disposition of theophylline. Br. J. Clin. Pharmacol., 16:413–416, 1983.

Thomson, N. C.: Nedocromil sodium: an overview. Resp. Med., 83:269–276, 1989.

Toogood, J. H.; Jennings, B.; and Baskerville, J. C.: Aerosol corticosteroids. In, Bronchial Asthma: Mechanisms and Therapeutics (Weiss, E. B.; Segal, M. S.; and Stein, M.; eds.). Little, Brown, Boston, pp. 698–713, 1985.

Toogood, J. H.; Baskerville, J.; Jennings, B.; Lefcoe, N. M.; and Johansson, S.-A.: Use of spacers to facilitate inhaled corticosteroid treatment of asthma. Am. Rev. Respir. Dis., 129:723–729, 1984.

Torphy, T. J.: Selective inhibitors of phosphodiesterase as bronchodilators. In, New Drugs for Asthma (Barnes, P. J., ed.). IBC Publications, London, pp. 66–77, 1989.

Torphy, T. J.; Freese, W. B.; Rinard, G. A.; Brunton, L. L.; and Mayer, S. E.: Cyclic nucleotide-dependent protein kinase in airway smooth muscle. J. Biol. Chem., 257:11609–11616, 1982.

Tracey, K. S.; Lowry, S. F.; and Cerami, A.: Cachectin/TNF-a in septic shock and septic adult respiratory distress syndrome. Am. Rev. Respir. Dis., 138:1377–1379, 1988.

Ullah, M. I.; Newman, G. B.; and Saunders, K. B.: Influence of age on response to ipratropium and salbutamol in asthma. Thorax, 36:523–529, 1981.

Ullman, A.; and Svedmyr, N.: Salmeterol, a new long acting inhaled β_2-adrenoceptor agonist: Comparison with salbutamol in adult asthmatic patients. Thorax, 43:674–678, 1988.

Vathenen, A. S.; Knox, A. J.; Higgins, B. G.; Britton, J. R.; and Tattersfield, A. E.: Rebound increase in bronchial responsiveness after treatment with inhaled terbutaline. Lancet, 1:554–558, 1988.

Vozeh, S.; Kewitz, G.; Perruchoud, A.; Tachan, M.; Kopp, C.; Heitz, M.; and Follath, F.: Theophylline serum concentration and therapeutic effect in severe acute bronchial obstruction: The optimal use of intravenously administered aminophylline. Am. Rev. Respir. Dis., 125(2):181–184, 1982.

Ward, M. J.; Fentem, P. H.; Roderick Smith, W. H.; and Davies, D.: Ipratropium bromide in acute asthma. Br. Med. J., 282:590–600, 1981.

Warren, J. B.; Cuss, F.; and Barnes, P. J.: Posture and theophylline kinetics. Br. J. Clin. Pharmacol., 19:707–709, 1985.

Warner, J. O.: The management of childhood asthma. In, Asthma: Basic Mechanisms and Clinical Management (Barnes, P. J.; Rodger, I. W.; and Thomson, N. C.; eds.). Academic Press, London, pp. 733–750, 1988.

Weinberger, M.: The pharmacology and therapeutic use of theophylline. J. Allergy Clin. Immunol., 73:525–540, 1984.

Weinberger, M.; and Hendeles, L.: Slow-release theophylline. Rationale and basis for product selection. N. Engl. J. Med., 308:760–764, 1983.

Welsch, C. H.; Lien, D.; Worthen, G. S.; and Weil, J. V.: Pentoxifylline decreases endotoxin-induced pulmonary neutrophil sequestration and extramuscular protein accumulation in the dog. Am. Rev. Respir. Dis., 138:1106–1114, 1988.

Williams, S.; Winner, S. J.; and Clark, T. J. H.: Comparison of inhaled and intravenous terbutaline in acute severe asthma. Thorax, 36:629–631, 1981.

Wilson, J. D.; Sutherland, D. C.; and Thomas, A. C.: Has the change to beta agonists combined with oral theophylline increased cases of fatal asthma. Lancet, 1:1235–1237, 1981.

Wong, S. C.; and Ward, J. W.: Analeptics. Pharmacol. Ther., 3:123–165, 1977.

Woolcock, A. J.; Yan, K.; and Salome, C. M.: Effect of ther-

apy on bronchial hyperresponsiveness in the long-term management of asthma. Clin. Allergy, 18:165–176, 1988.

Yukawa, T.; Kroegel, C.; Dent, G.; Chanez, P.; Ukena, D.; Chung, K. F.; and Barnes, P. J.: Effect of theophylline and adenosine on eosinophil function. Am. Rev. Respir. Dis., 140:327–333, 1989.

Zaagsma, J.; van der Heijden, P. J. C. M.; van der Schaar, M. W. G.; and Blank, C. M. C.: Comparison of functional β-adrenoceptor heterogeneity in central and peripheral airway smooth muscle of guinea pig and man. J. Recept. Res., 3:89–106, 1983.

8

Gastrointestinal Disorders

Gabriel Garcia

Many common symptoms relate to dysfunction or disease of the GI tract. Digestive diseases afflict 12% of all American adults and account for 16% of all absences from work. In a study of 25,000 illnesses in a group of Cleveland families, acute diarrheal illness was one of the most common illnesses reported, second only to the common cold (Dingle et al., 1964). Therefore, some of the most commonly used drugs are those directed at symptoms and diseases of the alimentary tract.

SPECIAL FEATURES OF THE CLINICAL PHARMACOLOGY OF THE DIGESTIVE TRACT

The therapy of diseases of the alimentary system presents a number of special challenges that arise from the several special characteristics of the digestive tract. The digestive tract is the usual route of administration for most drugs; they may have a direct action within the GI tract or upon its mucosal lining at relatively high concentrations. For example, salicylates and other NSAIDs may produce bleeding or erosive gastritis by a direct toxic effect on gastric mucosa.

A therapeutic benefit from certain drugs can be achieved without the drug's entering the circulation. Some drugs exert their action solely within the lumen of the GI tract. For example, the poorly absorbed antacids function only within the lumen of the stomach and duodenum to neutralize gastric acid. Some antibiotics or disaccharides such as lactulose, useful for their action on the GI flora, are poorly absorbed and exert their effects locally.

The presence of an enterohepatic cycle dependent on intestinal absorption, hepatic uptake, and biliary excretion may be exploited in the design of therapeutic regimens. Poisoning or overdoses with drugs that have an extensive enterohepatic circulation, such as theophylline, may be successfully treated with oral activated charcoal even after the initial dose has been completely absorbed (Park et al., 1986).

The GI tract harbors a rich microbial flora; some drugs require metabolism by bacteria to attain their full therapeutic activity. The action of sulfasalazine in the treatment of ulcerative colitis may depend upon the cleavage of its azo bond by bacteria of the lower bowel (Goldman and Peppercorn, 1975). Bacteria may lead to the production of toxic metabolites from otherwise safe drugs. If cyclamates represent a carcinogenic hazard (the magnitude of this risk is uncertain in humans), they may do so because of bacterial conversion of cyclamates to a known carcinogen. Bacterial enzymes are further complemented by metabolizing enzymes of the intestinal mucosa that may modify drug pharmacokinetics, as in the case of phenacetin (Pantuck et al., 1975).

Because the alimentary tract is the route of administration of most drugs, there are potentially many drug–drug and drug–food interactions that could influence the absorption and effectiveness of various therapeutic agents (see chapters 10 and 40). Examples of these include the adsorption of tetracycline by aluminum, calcium, or magnesium antacids; and the binding and inactivation of digitalis glycosides by the bile acid sequestrant cholestyramine (see chapter 40). Because food may have a marked effect on the rate of absorption of drugs and vitamins and upon their unwanted effects, it is very important to consider the impact of meals upon the rate of absorption and effectiveness of orally administered drugs.

The gut is one of the richest endocrine organs of the body, and endogenous control or exogenous manipulation of GI hormones may be critical in control of symptoms.

Finally, it is worth noting that the effectiveness of any therapeutic regimen that utilizes orally administered drugs may be influenced by disease and dysfunction of the GI tract. For example, patients with AIDS and candidal esophagitis frequently fail to respond to oral ketoconazole. The bioavailability of ketoconazole has been found to be reduced as a result of gastric achlorhydria, commonly seen in patients with AIDS. This effect can be reversed by concurrent administration of dilute hydrochloric acid (Lake-Bakaar et al., 1988; see chapter 24). Similarly, it is unsound to extrapolate expected drug effects from one population to another when the rates of coexisting diseases (parasitic infestations and diarrheal illnesses) are different in the population tested from those in the target population. *Principle: The effects of disease of one organ on the diagnosis and treatment of disease in another organ should make the "specialist" aware that focus on the disorders of a single organ system cannot be allowed to result in underappreciation of the complex relationships between organ systems.*

A general principle, shared with other organ systems, is that an understanding of the pathophysiology of a symptom or symptom complex in an individual patient usually will result in more selective and more effective therapy. For example, diarrhea as a symptom of enteric infection is more effectively and more definitively treated by specific therapy directed at the enteric pathogen than by nonspecific antidiarrheal agents. Sometimes therapy must be empirically directed at symptoms without a full understanding of their genesis; usually this practice is reserved for temporary control of symptoms during diagnostic evaluation or for those instances in which diagnostic analysis has failed to yield a full understanding of the cause of symptoms. *Principle: Continued use of drugs to control symptoms, without a comprehensive effort to understand the disease process that underlies these symptoms, is incomplete and dangerous medicine, delaying correct diagnosis and specific therapy.*

Some GI symptoms may be controlled or eliminated by withdrawal of an offending agent. Many drugs produce GI symptoms; when such drugs are withdrawn or decreased in dose, symptoms usually abate or disappear. Orally administered drugs often exert a direct toxic effect on the GI mucosa. Salicylates are believed to interfere with the integrity of the gastric epithelial membrane, allowing back diffusion of hydrogen ions. Neomycin causes malabsorption partly because of its direct toxicity on the small intestinal epithelium. Broad-spectrum antibiotics cause colitis by altering the bacterial flora of the gut.

Drug dependency is not as frequent in patients with GI disease as it is in patients with disease of other organ systems. However, the individual who abuses laxatives, in western man's common quest for a regular bowel movement, may so interrupt normal reflex function as to become functionally dependent on laxatives. Once again, the withdrawal of laxatives and appropriate changes in diet, with reeducation of and dependence upon GI reflex function, will result in a successful return to normal physiology. *Principle: In most societies addiction is not considered important unless the drug dominantly affects the CNS. Such an attitude is unrealistic. Furthermore, education of the patient during withdrawal may be the critical determinant of success of such withdrawal.*

Patients commonly attribute GI symptoms to specific foods. Although many of these cause-and-effect relationships fade under controlled scrutiny (Koch and Donaldson, 1964), others, such as diarrhea and distension after ingestion of milk by individuals with deficiency of intestinal lactase, have a firm basis in the pathophysiology of the GI system. In such patients the undigested lactose is fermented by colonic bacteria with generation of hydrogen gas and organic acids. Much more rarely, however, foods are the cause of intestinal disease rather than of intestinal symptoms; in these instances, there usually is a genetic predisposition (see chapter 32). An example is celiac sprue, in which the injury to the intestinal mucosa is caused by a genetically determined sensitivity to dietary gluten (wheat protein). Both the mucosal injury and the malabsorption syndrome are reversed by fastidious withdrawal of gluten from the diet. Far less common than celiac disease, but greatly overdiagnosed, is the problem of food allergy. Milk-protein allergy is the best studied and most clearly documented (Gryboski, 1985). Withdrawal of the offending protein, such as cow's milk, may result in dramatic clinical recovery and reversal of the morphologic abnormality of the intestinal mucosa.

When GI disease impairs digestive or absorptive function, resulting nutritional deficiencies are managed by replacement of missing factors or supplemental administration of deficient nutrients, or both (see chapter 10). Intuitively one might think that loss by disease or surgical resection of the acid- and pepsin-producing cells of the stomach might adversely affect digestion and could, therefore, call for replacement therapy. In practice, the peptic activity of the stomach is unnecessary for the individual eating a diet of cooked proteins. Such is not the case with disease or resection of the exocrine pancreas. Although the reserve is very great (90% of the pancreas must be destroyed before maldigestion occurs), such dysfunction can have very serious effects on intestinal digestion and nutrition. Under these circumstances, oral administration of pancreatic enzymes may improve the digestion and absorption of food (Graham, 1977).

Replacement therapy may also be required for restoration of nutrients lost because of malabsorption associated with GI disease. The patient with pernicious anemia, who lacks gastric intrinsic factor, requires vitamin B_{12} by injection. The patient with steatorrhea due to pancreatic or intestinal disease may well require supplemental replacement of vitamins by oral or parenteral routes (see chapter 10).

Gastrointestinal therapeutics may require interruption of normal or abnormal physiologic processes. Often a process that is qualitatively normal but quantitatively excessive can result in GI disease. Thus, peptic ulcer of the duodenum is associated with normal or excessive gastric acid secretion and may be treated by pharmacologic inhibition or neutralization of acid secretion. *Principle: Understanding the pathogenesis of a disease and the pharmacology of a drug clearly allows the imaginative and effective design of new uses for old drugs. The main challenge in therapy to most informed physicians is in construction of a new and logical hypothesis, in testing it with sound design, and in drawing valid conclusions related to the cause-and-effect relationship of drug–patient response* (see chapter 36).

Therapy is often directed at decreasing the functional stimulus to actively inflamed or diseased organs. An example of this principle is the effort to decrease the secretory responses of the pancreas in the presence of acute pancreatitis. By decreasing the flow of acid and food into the duodenum, one may decrease neural and hormonal stimuli to pancreatic secretion. In severe pancreatitis, this may require nasogastric suction; under milder conditions, small-volume feedings might minimize the pancreatic and gastric secretory response. Similarly, the inflamed small intestine or colon in Crohn disease or ulcerative colitis is "put at rest" to diminish diarrhea, abdominal pain, and cramping by decreasing dietary intake or, more drastically, by changing to an elemental diet resulting in a decreased residue and decreased stimulus to bowel function (see chapter 10). In the most symptomatic individuals, bowel rest is not achieved without placing the patient on a nothing-by-mouth regimen and substituting IV administration of fluids and medications. Total parenteral nutrition is used to prevent the worsening catabolic state associated with inadequate intake of calories and nitrogen when standard IV therapy is prolonged (see chapter 10).

In the absence of defined etiology or specific therapy, empiric therapy of proven utility should be used even if the mechanism of its benefit is not understood. This empiric approach to therapy is of particular importance in inflammatory diseases such as regional enteritis and ulcerative colitis; controlled clinical trials have shown the benefit of anti-inflammatory drugs such as corticosteroids and sulfasalazine although the pathophysiologic basis of this therapeutic benefit is not completely known. *Principle: When a drug whose pharmacology is reasonably understood is empirically found to have efficacy in a disease whose pathogenesis is poorly understood, the finding of efficacy ultimately may shed light on the mechanism of disease.*

DRUG-INDUCED GI DISORDERS

The GI tract is at risk of damage by direct contact with orally administered drugs as well as by their systemic effects. Drug-related erosive gastritis, ulcers, and diarrhea are common adverse effects of medications. The consequences can lead to serious complications or death. Because the offending agents are readily available and frequently used, it is important to discuss these adverse effects in detail.

Erosive Gastritis and Ulcers

Many medications cause erosions and ulcerations of the GI tract (alcohol, potassium chloride, corticosteroids, and aspirin). Nonsteroidal anti-inflammatory drugs are used by millions on a daily basis for long periods of time; they can cause both acute and chronic injury to the mucosa of the GI tract.

Endoscopic studies of acute drug injury, best characterized for aspirin, typically show the development of submucosal hemorrhage or active bleeding within 2 hours of ingestion of the drug. Acute drug-induced injury to the gastroduodenum can be diminished by enteric coating of the drug or by measures that decrease stomach content of acid (Lanza et al., 1980). Approximately 25% to 50% of patients who use NSAIDs on a regular basis will complain of dyspepsia; however, only rarely are GI symptoms severe enough to result in the inability to continue using the medications. Endoscopic studies have shown erosive gastritis in about 40% to 50% and ulcers of the stomach or duodenum in about 10% to 25% of chronic NSAID users. Unfortunately, the presence or absence of symptoms does not necessarily predict the findings at endoscopy (Graham and Smith, 1988). In addition, the drugs that cause the greatest degree of acute hemorrhagic gastritis are not the ones that necessarily lead to a higher rate of ulceration during chronic use; consequently, endoscopic measurements of acute drug injury do not accurately predict the differences in rates of ulcer formation from chronic use of different NSAIDs (Carson, 1987b).

Although sensitive endoscopic techniques to

evaluate the upper GI tract have described in detail the extent of acute and chronic mucosal injury caused by NSAIDs, the clinical significance of this injury is not as well delineated. In a case-control study that examined complications of ulcer disease (GI bleeding and death) in patients chronically using NSAIDs, the relative risk of developing GI bleeding 30 days after exposure to an NSAID was 1.5 (Carson, 1987b). There were dose–response and duration of exposure-response relationships noted between NSAID use and GI bleeding; however, the magnitude of the overall risk was small and suggests that only one of three bleeding ulcers in patients who use NSAIDs regularly may actually be caused by the drug. Data from prospectively followed groups of NSAID users will be necessary to corroborate this finding. Until such data are available, the clinician must be guided by complaints and findings that are independent of NSAID use in planning therapy for patients. *Principle: Few adverse effects of drugs cannot be caused by spontaneous disease. A major therapeutic error would be to attribute all adverse events to a drug that could cause them when the relative risks of such cause and effect are low and when the drug is vitally important to the patient's well-being.*

Prophylactic therapy with misoprostil, a synthetic prostaglandin E analog with antisecretory and cytoprotective properties, decreased the incidence of gastric ulcers in patients with osteoarthritis who were taking NSAIDs continually and had abdominal pain (Dajani, 1987; Silverstein et al., 1986). Ulcers were visualized in 21.7% of placebo recipients, and 4.2% and 0.7% of misoprostil-treated patients (100 or 200 μg four times daily, respectively) in three upper endoscopies over a 3-month period of surveillance. The effect on abdominal pain was not as clear-cut, as 30% of misoprostil-treated patients and 43% of placebo recipients still had abdominal pain during follow-up, despite healing of the ulcer. Diarrhea occured in 39% of patients receiving the higher dose of misoprostil but in only 13% of placebo-treated patients (Graham et al., 1988). If the serious GI complications of long-term use of NSAIDs are attributable only to their propensity to cause ulcers, then misoprostil should be widely used. However, the toxicity of long-term use of misoprostil and its ability to prevent ulcers over a long period of therapy with NSAIDs are yet to be determined. *Principle: Surrogate end points must be evaluated as carefully as any other drug effect. However, the physician must be careful to distinguish one type of end point from another when reading studies or treating patients.*

Diarrhea

Diarrhea can be defined as an abnormal increase in stool frequency, weight, or liquidity.

The former two are relatively straightforward to measure; the wet weight of stools is cumbersome to quantitate but likely to be the factor that most easily correlates with the patient's complaint. The average person eating three meals each day is likely to have 9000 ml of fluid traversing the duodenum, 1000 ml traversing the ileocecal valve, and 100 ml exiting as stool. Since the fluid balance of the gut must be exceedingly well controlled in order to have a normal water content in stools, minor changes in absorptive capacity of the bowel can likely play a major role in determining stool water content despite the ability of the bowel to adjust to changes in the delivery of abnormal quantities of fluid (Fine et al., 1989).

Diarrhea has many diverse causes but can be classified mechanistically into malabsorptive, maldigestive, or secretory processes; inflammatory states; and deranged intestinal motility (Fordtran, 1967). The differential diagnosis of diarrhea is lengthy and has been reviewed elsewhere (Fine et al., 1989). As with other GI symptoms, it is important to judge its severity and prognosis so that the need for treatment can be established, and to identify and specifically treat the underlying condition if possible and necessary.

Drug-induced diarrhea may be caused by any of the above mechanisms. Most commonly, diarrhea is caused by the use of laxatives or stool softeners. These may be poorly absorbed sugars such as lactulose and sorbitol that are fermented by intestinal bacteria in the colon or poorly absorbed salts of magnesium (sulfate, oxide, or hydroxide) or sodium (sulfate or citrate) ions. The diarrhea that ensues is characterized by a stool osmolality higher than that of plasma. Other commonly used laxatives (ricinoleic acid, phenolphthalein, dioctyl sodium sulfosuccinate, and senna) cause diarrhea characterized by its continuance even during fasting and a stool osmolality gap of less than 50 mOsm/kg (Binder, 1977).

The most serious drug-induced diarrheal state is antibiotic-related pseudomembranous colitis due to *Clostridium difficile*. Most patients with antibiotic-related diarrhea have a benign illness that begins during administration of the drug and lasts less than 1 week following discontinuation of the offending agent. A small percentage of patients will develop severe diarrhea with evidence of invasive colitis (fever, tenesmus, mucus, or bloody stools) that persists after the antibiotic is discontinued. Patients in this group are generally elderly and in the hospital or a skilled nursing facility, where their fecal flora is conditioned with antibiotics, and they acquire *C. difficile* as a nosocomial superinfection. The antibiotics most frequently implicated are ampicillin or amoxicillin, clindamycin, and cephalosporins (Bartlett, 1981). Laboratory studies may reveal hypoalbuminemia and fecal leukocytes, and flexible sigmoidoscopy demonstrates the characteristic 3- to 20-mm pseudomembranes bordered by normal or hyperemic colonic mucosa. Microbiologic studies reveal the presence of *C. difficile* toxin in the stool.

Therapy consists of discontinuing the implicated antibiotic, maintaining an adequate state of hydration and nutrition, and instituting enteric isolation procedures to limit person-to-person spread. Specific antibiotic therapy directed against *C. difficile* should be given to patients with signs and symptoms of moderate to severe colitis, or to those who fail to improve following nonspecific measures and discontinuation of antibiotics. Oral vancomycin and metronidazole appear to be equally efficacious; bacitracin may have equal activity, although it has not been as extensively studied. Parenteral metronidazole should be administered only to patients who cannot take oral medications. Therapy is generally accompanied by rapid defervescence and loss of diarrhea within 7 days; toxin generally is still present in the stool at the end of successful therapy. Relapses occur in 20% to 25% of patients treated with any of the three antibiotics and are heralded by recurrent symptoms within 7 days of the end of therapy. Relapses may be treated with another course of antibiotics if the seriousness of the colitis warrants specific treatment.

An alternative treatment for antibiotic-related pseudomembranous colitis involves administration of cholestyramine, which binds the toxin, leading to symptomatic improvement. However, this approach is not as efficacious as specific antibiotic therapy and should not be used in seriously ill patients. *Principle: Understanding the details of pharmacology of a drug and pathogenesis of a disease occasionally leads to otherwise nonobvious use of the drug in the disease with gratifying rewards for having considered the hypothesis.*

TREATMENT OF GI DISORDERS

Nausea and Vomiting

Vomiting is a complex clinical behavior that results in the evacuation of stomach contents and involves coordinated activity of the GI tract and the nervous system. It is frequently preceeded by nausea (an unpleasant sensation that has been felt by most people but is difficult to describe) and retching, or contractions of the diaphragm and chest wall against a closed glottis.

The neurophysiology of vomiting has been studied in detail in cats since the 1950s (Borison and Wang, 1953). Findings in studies of cats have generally been very relevant to humans. In brief, a vomiting center (VC), located in the dorsal portion of the lateral reticular formation of the medulla, coordinates the many organs involved in the intricate act of vomiting. The VC can be stimulated by a chemoreceptor trigger zone (CTZ) lo-

cated in the area postrema of the medulla on the floor of the fourth ventricle. The CTZ, in turn, is sensitive to chemical stimulation, including direct application of drugs such as apomorphine or toxins such as uremic plasma. Dopamine receptors in the CTZ likely play a role in the act of vomiting; dopamine agonists such as apomorphine or levodopa initiate vomiting, and dopamine antagonists such as metoclopramide or domperidone diminish vomiting (Jenner and Marsden, 1979). The VC can also be stimulated by afferent nerve stimuli originating in the gut and pharynx and probably other sites in the body; these stimuli are likely to travel via the vagus nerve.

Numerous conditions can cause nausea and vomiting, and most can be explained from these neurophysiologic relationships. Structural abnormalities of the GI tract may lead to nausea and vomiting by either of two general mechanisms: mechanical obstruction of a hollow viscus (such as congenital pyloric stenosis, achalasia, or Crohn disease of the small intestine) or by a nonobstructing lesion affecting any or all components of the wall of GI organs (such as an antral peptic ulcer, erosive gastritis, acute cholecystitis). Systemic conditions may have local or distant effects on the gut or on any neuromuscular component of the vomiting reflex: examples are drugs, diabetes mellitus (either through ketoacidosis or local effects on the innervation of the stomach leading to gastroparesis), uremia, pregnancy, adrenal insufficiency, or infiltration by mass lesions (tumors, amyloid) in critical areas of the nervous system or the intrinsic musculature of the stomach wall. Finally, psychiatric illness may manifest itself as predominantly a vomiting disorder, most vividly seen in bulimia. These conditions and others that can lead to nausea and vomiting have been discussed in detail (Malagelada and Camilleri, 1984; Hanson and McCallum, 1985).

The therapy of nausea and vomiting must first be directed at identifying the underlying condition that has precipitated the problem. Healing a pyloric channel ulcer with antisecretory therapy or the surgical removal of an acutely inflamed, calculous gallbladder is the appropriate therapy to manage the vomiting that frequently accompanies these disorders. However, there are many conditions accompanied by vomiting that have no specific treatment (e.g., viral gastroenteritis or hepatitis) or have vomiting as a predictable effect of therapy (e.g., cisplatin chemotherapy, total nodal radiation). In these cases, the vomiting must be managed without being able to address its cause directly.

Management of vomiting in situations where therapy is indicated must take into account the neurophysiologic correlates of vomiting as well as learned responses resulting from prior associations. This has been best studied in situations where vomiting is predictable and severe, such as that caused by the IV infusion of high doses of cisplatin during the therapy of various solid tumors. Even if there has been no prior experience with emetogenic chemotherapy, one must expect the patient to develop purely anticipatory nausea and vomiting. Such nausea and vomiting can be triggered by sights, odors, or any other memory associated with prior episodes of vomiting. These symptoms have been successfully treated with behavioral modification techniques or anxiolytic-amnesic agents such as lorazepam, or both (Laszlo et al., 1985).

Gastric distension can be avoided by beginning therapy following an overnight fast or, if there is an impediment to emptying the stomach, by evacuating its contents using a nasogastric tube. Maintaining adequate hydration is an important goal during potentially dehydrating therapy, and a large-bore IV line with adequate fluid replacement must be used. Prevention of nausea and vomiting, rather than rescue therapy, should be the goal of treatment (see chapter 23).

Drug therapy of vomiting is aimed at the interruption of the vomiting reflex at any and all levels. Phenothiazines such as prochlorperazine were first used for this purpose in the 1950s, and since that time agents with similar, substantial antidopaminergic effects have been employed. These include the butyrophenones such as droperidol and substituted benzamides such as metoclopramide (Wampler, 1983) (see chapter 13). Corticosteroids such as dexamethasone or methylprednisolone have been found to be useful, although the nature of their antiemetic action is unclear (Markman et al., 1984). Similarly, natural or synthetic cannabinoids have been employed in antiemetic therapy following the empiric observation of an antiemetic effect in habitual users who were undergoing chemotherapy. However, their mechanism of action is unknown, and their efficacy has not yet been adequately demonstrated in well-designed studies (Carey et al., 1983). Most recently, ondansetron, a selective inhibitor of serotonin S_3 receptors, was observed to prevent the vomiting induced by cisplatin in laboratory animals. This led to two controlled studies in patients with cancer undergoing cisplatin therapy. The studies showed the drug to be effective in preventing cisplatin-induced vomiting (Cubeddu et al., 1990; Marty et al., 1990). One of the studies also suggested that cisplatin treatment increased the release of serotonin from enterochromaffin cells, as measured by urinary excretion of 5-hydroxyindolacetic acid (Cubeddu et al., 1990), thus providing a possible mechanism for cisplatin-induced emesis and the beneficial effect of the drug.

Because single agents lack universal effectiveness in the prevention of vomiting, regimens using combinations of drugs are sensible and useful. The goal of combining drugs for this indication is the same as for any indication where combinations are used. The combination should result in a nausea-free patient, and minimize or abolish the potential adverse effects of the high doses of agents that would be necessary if they were used alone. One should choose combination therapy using agents whose efficacy is proved, modes of action are different, and potential toxicities are nonoverlapping. *Principle: Drug combinations can be useful when single agents fail to provide the desired efficacy or freedom from toxicity. Knowledge of the mode of action, pharmacology, and toxicity of drugs as single agents is useful in the rational planning of combination therapy. Drugs may have additive or even unique toxicities when used together, and the therapist must be alert to make observations that may not be predicted by studies on single agents.*

The information learned from drug studies in patients receiving highly emetogenic drugs is applicable to other clinical situations and should be used to plan therapy of patients who vomit for other reasons. For example, the routine care of patients with severe vomiting from an exacerbation of chronic pancreatitis should include nasogastric suction to empty the stomach, fluid and caloric support by the parenteral route, and prevention or treatment of nausea and vomiting as necessary to maintain patient comfort. This does not exclude therapy that may be specific to the underlying disease, such as surgery to drain pseudocysts or endoscopic sphincterotomy to remove a common bile duct stone. Therapy that is specific to the underlying disease should always be a part of the patient's management.

Peptic Ulcer Disease

Peptic ulcer disease is a heterogeneous group of illnesses whose hallmark is a mucosal defect in the stomach or duodenum that extends through the muscularis mucosa. It is a common disorder, with lifetime prevalences approaching 10% and point prevalences of 1% to 2% in American males (Grossman, 1980). Current thinking on the pathophysiology of peptic ulcer disease emphasizes the interplay between ulcerogenic factors (acid and pepsin) and the breakdown of normal mucosal defenses; the latter may be related to stress, smoking, alcohol or other drug use, or infection with the newly characterized *Helicobacter pylori* organism, the cause of antral gastritis, a condition nearly always present in patients with duodenal and gastric ulcers (Graham, 1989). Since acute mucosal breaks, such as those caused by endoscopic biopsies, heal rapidly in patients despite constant bathing by acid and pepsin, the interplay of aggressive and protective factors cannot be understated. Even in patients with gastrinomas, whose mucosal surfaces are constantly bathed with large amounts of pepsin and acid, peptic ulceration is an intermittent, albeit severe, condition with spontaneous exacerbations and remissions and multiple recurrences over the lifetime of affected individuals. Since there are now effective and safe methods to heal an acute peptic ulcer, the most important problem facing the therapist is not how to heal an ulcer, but how to prevent its recurrence and its complications.

Factors that are important in maintaining an intact mucosal barrier include the production of mucus and bicarbonate by surface epithelial cells with maintenance of a surface barrier to injury, and the ability to maintain adequate mucosal blood flow during and after a break in the surface defense mechanisms. Studies of rabbits administered antibodies against prostaglandins and NSAID-induced gastric erosions and ulcerations suggest that endogenous prostaglandins may play a critical role in protecting the integrity of the surface epithelium, although the ability of exogenous prostaglandins to reproduce these beneficial effects is at best partial. Endogenous sulfhydryl compounds, through their capacity to be free-radical scavengers, and epidermal growth factor may also contribute to mucosal resistance to injury (Soll, 1990).

Traditional therapy against peptic ulceration has been directed against the acid or ulcer-promoting factors. Therapies include the buffering of stomach acid with antacids, and use of agents that block parietal cell acid secretion. Antacids were the first drugs to be used in promoting healing of peptic ulcers. With time, the development of insoluble and nonabsorbable antacids such as aluminum hydroxide and magnesium trilisate allowed therapy without the systemic absorption of alkali seen with sodium bicarbonate and milk that had led to systemic alkalosis, hypercalcemia, and renal insufficiency. Their relative ease of administration and low cost made them very popular among patients with ulcers, but their high incidence of adverse effects (diarrhea, binding of coadministered drugs) and cumbersome regimens with up to seven daily doses made the search for alternate modes of therapy necessary (Lam, 1988). A combination of aluminum hydroxide and magnesium carbonate four times daily (acid-neutralizing capacity only 120 mmol/day) has been efficacious in healing doudenal ulcers, suggesting that antacids may heal duodenal ulcers by mechanisms in addition to their acid-buffering capabilities (Weberg et al., 1988).

Basic physiologic observations of the nature of the stimuli that lead the parietal cell to secrete acid led to therapies with anticholinergic agents and histamine H_2-receptor antagonists. Therapy with anticholinergic agents such as probanthine and atropine was attempted but essentially abandoned when it became clear that doses necessary to achieve enough acid reduction to heal ulcers also led to predictable adverse effects such as dry mouth, blurred vision, and urinary retention. Pirenzepine, a relatively M_1-selective antimuscarinic agent, may lead to enough reduction of acid secretion to promote ulcer healing without the high incidence of anticholinergic effects from inhibition of myocardial and smooth muscle function and salivary secretion (Feldman, 1984; Carmine and Brogden, 1985).

Histamine H_2-receptor antagonists were developed specifically for the treatment of duodenal ulcer disease. All are competitive inhibitors of the action of histamine at H_2 receptors; their structure is based on modifications of a molecule with the histamine imidazole ring structure (cimetidine), furan ring (ranitidine), and thiazole ring (famotidine and nizatidine). H_2-receptor antagonists became the drugs of choice in the healing of peptic ulcer because they are safe and are easy to administer once or twice daily in regimens that result in healing of 80% to 90% of peptic ulcers after 4 to 8 weeks of therapy. Drug-related adverse effects have been unusual. Antiandrogenic effects leading to gynecomastia and drug interactions secondary to cytochrome P450 enzyme inhibition have been attributed to cimetidine but not the others; presumably these are related to the imidazole ring structure and not to its H_2-receptor antagonism (McCarthy, 1983; Powell and Donn, 1983). Since lymphocytes and cardiac muscle have H_2 receptors, immune modulation and bradycardia seen with H_2 blockers is likely to be a generic adverse effect of this class of drugs, or perhaps in the future an alternate indication for using H_2 blockers (Siegel et al., 1982).

Prostaglandins such as misoprostil (see above) can lead to suppression of acid secretion and can lead to rates of ulcer healing comparable to those produced with the H_2 blockers. However, the need to administer these drugs two to four times daily and their diarrheogenic and uterotonic effects make them unlikely first-line drugs for the therapy of peptic ulcer disease (Sontag, 1986).

Omeprazole, a substituted benzimidazole that inhibits hydrogen-potassium ATPase, the proton pump of the parietal cell, can lead to sustained achlorhydria in humans by abolishing gastric acid secretion (McArthur et al., 1986). The result is an accelerated rate of ulcer healing in patients with peptic ulcer disease or severe erosive or ulcerative esophagitis (Archambult et al., 1988). Although this agent appears to offer distinct advantages over other antisecretory drugs because of its efficacy, the sustained achlorhydria it induces ma·

have as-yet-undetected adverse effects. Laboratory animals that are treated with relatively large doses of this agent have developed chronic elevations in serum gastrin concentrations and enterochromaffin cell hyperplasia, which is sometimes accompanied by malignant carcinoid tumors (Havu, 1986). Although carcinoid tumors have not been found in patients using the regimen currently recommended for healing ulcers or for patients with gastrinomas, these findings raise concerns that may limit the long-term usefulness of this drug (Maton et al., 1989).

Attempts to heal ulcers by methods that do not reduce gastric acid is a desirable goal in the rare patient intolerant to acid-reduction therapy or as adjunctive therapy. Cessation of smoking and ingestion of alcohol or NSAIDs is important. The capacity of prostaglandins to induce healing is not as great as that of antisecretory therapy (Brand et al., 1985). Prostaglandins appear to be useful in the prevention of NSAID-induced gastric ulcers; however, their superiority to antisecretory drugs in achieving this goal has not yet been tested.

Sucralfate (a sulfated disaccharide complex with aluminum hydroxide) acts by mechanisms other than the reduction of gastric acid production to promote ulcer healing. Sucralfate binds to the ulcer base, forms complexes with pepsin, and stimulates local production of bicarbonate and mucus; one or more of these mechanisms may be responsible for its mode of action. It is as effective as H_2 blockers in promotion of ulcer healing and maintains the gastric acid barrier to microorganisms during the healing process (Marks, 1987). This may be important in hospitalized patients at risk for extensive colonization of the stomach with bacteria, since such colonization may predispose patients to develop aspiration pneumonia. Adverse effects include constipation and nausea. The absorption of sucralfate from the GI tract has not been well studied; 0.5% to 2.2% of $[^{14}C]$ sucrose sulfate administered as sucralfate is excreted unchanged in the urine by normal subjects (Giesing et al., 1982). If a significant amount of aluminum is absorbed and deposited in tissues, resulting in chronic aluminum toxicity and the potential for encephalopathy, the usefulness of sucralfate may be limited to short-term therapy. To date, however, no cases of aluminum toxicity have been assessed in patients only on sucralfate therapy.

Bismuth compounds also have been shown to heal ulcers by unknown mechanisms. They bind to the ulcer base, inhibit pepsin activity, and lead to local prostaglandin synthesis. Their antimicrobial effect against *H. pylori* does not result in a predictable eradication of this organism to explain their promotion of ulcer healing. Therapy with tripotassium dicitrate bismuthate leads to fewer recurrent ulcers within the year following therapy when compared with H_2 antagonists (Miller and Faragher, 1986). This may be due to their bactericidal effect against *H. pylori*, or to systemic absorption and sustained release of bismuth from body stores following therapy. Although cases of bismuth encephalopathy have not been reported in patients treated with bismuth compounds for peptic ulcer disease, this potential adverse effect may limit the use of these agents to 4- to 8-week courses of therapy (Bradley et al., 1989).

Treatment of peptic ulcers must be guided by host factors, the location of the ulcer, and whether complications (perforation, penetration, gastric outlet obstruction, bleeding, or intractable pain) have occurred. Several simple, safe, and effective regimens are available to the therapist. Uncomplicated duodenal ulcers can heal with agents that effectively decrease nocturnal acid production without affecting daytime acid production; increasing the degree of acid suppression accelerates the healing process (Jones et al., 1987). A typical regimen would consist of cimetidine 800 mg once nightly; this has been shown to heal duodenal ulcers in 80% of patients after 4 weeks of treatment and in 95% of patients after 8 weeks. Similar results would be expected with ranitidine 300 mg or famotidine 40 mg nightly. The presence of continued pain or a complication would require establishing the presence of a persistent ulcer and a change in therapy to an agent and regimen that would lead to more profound acid suppression, such as omeprazole 20 to 40 mg daily, or change to a drug that works by a different mechanism, such as sucralfate 2 g twice daily (McFarland et al., 1990).

The healing of gastric ulcers by different drugs and regimens correlates best with total duration of treatment and poorly with the ability to suppress acid production over 24 hours (Howden et al., 1988). In order to achieve the healing rates of 90% or more seen with 8 weeks of antisecretory therapy in patients with duodenal ulcer, patients with gastric ulcer should be treated for 10 to 12 weeks. This may indicate that the pathogenesis of gastric ulcer may depend less on acid-peptic aggressive factors and more on local mucosal defenses. A typical regimen would be cimetidine 400 mg twice daily or ranitidine 150 mg twice daily. Patients with gastric ulcers should have documentation of complete healing of their ulcer in 10 to 12 weeks by gastroscopy and biopsy to exclude the small chance of a malignant ulcer. If an unhealed gastric ulcer is present, operative resection should be considered even when biopsies do not reveal malignant tissue, because of the possibility of gastric cancer.

Complications of peptic ulcers such as perforation, penetration, GI bleeding, gastric outlet obstruction, and intractable pain have in the past led to operative therapy of peptic ulcer disease. Because of the relatively morbid nature of surgery for peptic ulcer disease and its potential mortality even in otherwise healthy subjects, the advent of new drug therapies for peptic ulcer disease have led to attempts to manage nonemergent complications of ulcers without surgery. Whether this more conservative approach will ultimately benefit patients is yet to be proved.

A major dilemma in the care of patients with peptic ulcer disease is how to prevent recurrence of ulcers. About 90% of patients with duodenal ulcers that heal with antisecretory therapy will have a recurrent ulcer within a year; patients who heal with tripotassium dicitrate bismuthate recur 60% of the time (Miller and Faragher, 1986). Most recurrent ulcers are asymptomatic. Patients with a single episode of an uncomplicated ulcer should probably be observed without treatment and treated only if they have a symptomatic recurrence (Bardhan, 1988).

Patients in whom symptomatic ulcers frequently recur, or in whom a complication not requiring emergent surgery has occurred, should be considered candidates for prophylactic acid-suppressive therapy with an H_2 blocker, at half the usual dose required for healing, or sucralfate 1 g twice daily. This maintenance therapy can be expected to result in ulcer recurrence rates of less than 30% yearly (Bodemar and Walan, 1978). The appropiate length of prophylactic therapy is controversial. Elderly patients with serious coexisting illnesses should probably receive lifelong prophylactic therapy, since the potential for ulcer-related morbidity and mortality is greater in this group (Piper et al., 1975). Whether young patients without comorbid illnesses benefit from maintenance therapy is also unclear. A model proposed to evaluate the outcome of patients treated with intermittent versus maintenance therapy predicted that the point prevalence of ulcers at any time would be 16.5% in the intermittently treated group and 3% in the maintenance-therapy group and thus may result in patients intermittently treated being at greater risk for complications (Pounder, 1981). Failure of prophylactic therapy should signal the need for aggressive acid-reduction therapy and possibly surgery. The role of eradication of *H. pylori* infections in the prevention of ulcer recurrence is yet to be determined but may prove to be a critical step in the management of all patients with peptic ulcers.

Constipation

Constipation is generally perceived by people as an inability to have stools frequently; some complain of a sensation of incomplete evacuation of their rectum, or stools that are too firm, or too difficult to pass. These are common problems for which patients spend hundreds of millions of dollars for drugs in the United States every year. Most drugs are used to increase the frequency and water content of the stool. The frequency of bowel movements depends greatly on the diet, the use of drugs that may change (particularly decrease) GI motility or the water content of stools, the level of physical activity, and water intake. Ninety-nine percent of healthy adults in Britain have stools more than twice a week and no more than three times daily (Connell et al., 1965). However, people commonly perceive the absence of a daily bowel movement as a sign of illness because of accumulation of toxins. Numerous medications are used to achieve a once-a-day stool.

The physician who cares for a patient complaining of chronic constipation must first address whether the patient truly has a problem. If complaints suggest an underlying organic illness of the digestive tract (a sudden decrease in stool frequency or caliber, the presence of blood in the stool, or associated systemic complaints), then evaluation aimed at ruling out serious organic disease must be undertaken. Colonoscopy or a barium enema may be considered. If the patient complains of an inability to initiate a bowel movement, or if he or she has a sense of incomplete evacuation of the rectum, anorectal manometry and defecography may be useful diagnostic tests (Mahieu et al., 1984). If the patient complains of infrequent bowel movements, measurement of colonic transit time using radioopaque markers and anorectal manometry may be useful in determining the presence and segmental location causing the delayed transit (Wald, 1986).

The majority of patients who have chronic constipation do not have serious organic disease. Reeducation regarding "normal stool habits" and the benefits from increasing their physical activity, water intake, and amount of fiber in their diet may suffice. Patients should be encouraged to promptly respond to their urge to defecate. If necessary, a postprandial routine following breakfast or dinner should be established, to take advantage of the gastrocolic reflex. A careful search of the history of medications for those that may cause constipation should be performed. Nonessential drugs should be discontinued, and essential medications that can also alter GI mobility should be changed, if possible. The use of laxatives to treat patients with chronic constipation is generally reserved for those who fail to respond to simple nonpharmacologic measures.

Laxatives are generally classified into five categories: bulk-forming, emollients, lubricants, stimulants, and osmotic laxatives (Tedesco and

DiPiro, 1985). Preparations have been assigned to these categories on the basis of their presumed mechanism of action. For many drugs, the mechanism of action is poorly understood or current concepts differ from those presumed at the time the classification was constructed (Binder and Donowitz, 1975; Donowitz, 1979).

Bulk-Forming Agents. Bulk-forming agents are generally complex plant polysaccharides or cellulose derivatives that swell on contact with water. The most commonly used products contain powdered psyllium seed (Effersyllium, Hydrocil, Metamucil). The dose of the product needs to be adjusted so that the patient is ingesting a total of 15 g or more of dietary fiber daily; little may be required if the patients can increase the daily intake of fiber from foods. Softer, bulkier stools should be achieved within 24 to 48 hours. No systemic absorption of the drug is predicted, but systemic effects of high fiber intake occur. These can include lowering of serum lipid concentrations by drug binding of cholesterol excreted in the bile (Anderson and Gustafson, 1988). An adequate amount of water (8–16 oz of water per typical 4- to 6-g dose) should be simultaneously ingested; this will prevent the rare but predictable GI obstruction that can follow the use of these agents. If strictures of the GI tract are already present at the time the drug is started, bulk-forming agents may precipitate obstruction.

Emollient Laxatives. Emollient laxatives increase water secretion in the intestine and colon and act as surfactants to improve fecal mixing. Commonly used products include docusate sodium (Colace or Doxinate) or docusate calcium (Surfak). All these preparations are used in doses of 50 to 360 mg daily. Traditionally, these agents have been used in hospitalized patients following myocardial infarction or surgery, when straining at defecation should be avoided but activity and fluid intake may be restricted. They have little role in the management of chronic constipation, except when the patient is fluid-restricted or incapable of increasing his or her dietary fiber or activity.

Lubricants. Lubricants are mineral oil products (e.g., Haley's M-O). They coat the bowel and decrease colonic absorption of water, allowing easier passage of stool. Doses of 15 to 30 ml daily result in soft stools within hours. Because of the potential of aspirating the oil resulting in lipoid pneumonia in a patient who needs to be recumbent or less than normally active, the malabsorption of fat-soluble vitamins with chronic use, or the irritation of the perianal area and de-velopment of pruritus ani, these agents should not be used when potentially less toxic products are available and have not been tried.

Stimulant Laxatives. Stimulant laxatives are derivatives of anthraquinones (cascara sagrada, or "holy peel," senna) and dimethylethane (bisacodyl) that are felt to stimulate intestinal motility. More likely they work by increasing fluid secretion in the small intestine and colon. A bowel movement can be expected 6 to 8 hours after an oral dose or 15 to 60 minutes after the preparation is taken rectally. The drugs may damage the myenteric plexus and have a potential for causing serious acute (severe abdominal cramps, electrolyte and acid-base disorders, erythema multiforme) and chronic (melanosis coli, atonic colon) adverse effects (Smith, 1968). These agents are not recommended for chronic use, and even their short-term use can cause toxicity that exceeds that of the osmotic laxatives.

Osmotic Laxatives. Osmotic laxatives are poorly absorbed by the intestine and colon and result in net water movement into the GI tract along an osmotic gradient. They include ions of magnesium, sulfate, phosphate, and citrate; lactulose, and sorbitol. The onset of action generally is within 30 minutes to 3 hours after oral administration. These drugs have the capability of causing abdominal cramps, electrolyte and acid-base disorders, and volume depletion. Their use generally is limited to clinical settings when prompt evacuation of bowel contents is needed (e.g., following the use of activated charcoal or potassium-binding resins used in poisonings and hyperkalemia, or in preparation for GI endoscopy or surgery). These agents rarely may be required for patients with acute exacerbations of chronic constipation or acute constipation associated with a self-limited process (Koletzko et al., 1989). A balanced salt solution containing polyethylene glycol (Golytely, Colyte) works in a similar manner but causes little *net* water movement across the intestinal wall.

Diarrhea

Diarrhea generally is defined as the passing of watery stools or an increased frequency of relatively loose stools. Acute diarrhea is a common condition. It affects adults in developed countries once a year on the average. This illness is not likely to lead to consultation with a health care worker unless the patient is an infant or small child, or the illness is particularly severe. Chronic diarrhea, lasting longer than 3 weeks, is an uncommon condition. It requires a diagnostic workup that can be extensive and often requires a specialist. After illnesses that are managed with specific therapy have been identified and treated, the management of either acute or chronic diarrhea may be similar.

Acute diarrhea generally is regarded as an attempt by the GI tract to get rid of disease-causing microorganisms and toxins. This is felt to be adaptive, and therapy meant merely to decrease the number and volume of stools generally is not recommended. More likely, however, diarrhea provides an efficient way to disseminate and propagate the organisms that cause it and is an adaptive mechanism of the parasite, and not the host.

The mechanisms by which diarrhea occurs fall under four general categories: increased osmolality of intestinal contents, decreased fluid absorption, increased intestinal secretion, or abnormal intestinal motility. Any of these mechanisms may be responsible for diarrhea from any given cause. For example, loss of mature intestinal cells in villus tips due to an acute rotavirus infection is likely to lead to decreased mucosal absorptive surface, decreased fluid absorption, and a self-limited lactose intolerance and osmotic diarrhea with ingestion of milk (Starkey et al., 1986). *Escherichia coli* or *Vibrio cholera* infections cause diarrhea through an enterotoxin that causes net excretion of chloride by the enterocyte (Moss and Vaughan, 1989).

The ability of acute diarrhea to cause severe dehydration in children, leading to death in areas of the world where poverty and malnutrition are common, makes it an important worldwide health care problem. In industrialized countries, acute diarrhea is likely to be due to a viral agent (rotavirus, Norwalk virus, or similar viruses) and requires no specific treatment. Travelers to less developed nations are exposed to diarrheal illnesses not common in their native countries (cholera, enterotoxigenic *E. coli* infections, *Entamoeba histolytica*) and must be aware of the symptoms and correct management of these illnesses (see chapter 24). When diarrhea occurs in a traveler, is accompanied by signs of dysentery (temperature $\geq 103\,^\circ F$, systemic symptoms, bloody stools, or severe abdominal or rectal pain), or lasts longer than 14 days, one must consider a bacterial or protozoan cause. Further evaluation is necessary to determine whether specific antimicrobial therapy will be necessary.

For the vast majority of people with diarrhea who do not have an invasive infection and will have a self-limited condition, the goal of therapy is to maintain an adequate state of hydration. Simple measures such as avoiding substances that may increase intestinal secretion and motility (caffeinated beverages, ethanol, spicy foods, milk products) and adequate intake (2–3 liters or more per day) of fruit juices and noncarbonated beverages generally are sufficient.

Oral solutions of rehydration represent a major advance in the therapy of severe diarrhea. They take advantage of glucose-coupled sodium uptake and solvent drag in the small intestine. Both are processes that result in absorption of sodium and free water even in the face of bacterial toxin-induced secretory diarrhea (Field et al., 1989). When moderate or severe dehydration is already present and the potential for further dehydration is high (such as during cholera), a solution high in sodium is necessary in order to prevent hyponatremia. The World Health Organization has recommended an oral rehydration solution containing 90 mEq/l of sodium, 20 mEq/l of potassium, 80 mEq/l of chloride, 30 mEq/l of bicarbonate, and 20 g/l of glucose. For a less serious degree of dehydration or to prevent it from occurring, solutions containing 45 to 50 mEq/l of sodium are commercially available (Infalyte powder or Pedialyte liquid). If dehydration is very severe (greater than 10% of body weight loss) or if the diarrheal illness is accompanied by vomiting or inability to comply with oral fluid therapy, then IV fluids will be necessary.

If diarrhea is not accompanied by signs suggestive of an invasive infection, then symptomatic therapy with antidiarrheals should be considered. Two different classes of agents have been proved to be useful: opiates and NSAIDs. Adsorptive compounds such as kaolin or pectin have been used to treat diarrhea for centuries. They alter stool composition, turning loose stool into lumpy stool. They do not decrease stool volume or frequency and are not recommended (Ludan, 1988).

Opiates (diphenoxylate with atropine, loperamide, deodorized tincture of opium) decrease intestinal motility, increase mucosal absorption, and decrease fluid and electrolyte secretion. Presumably they act on intestinal μ opioid receptors (see chapter 25). Their net effect is to reduce stool volume and alleviate tenesmus and abdominal cramps. Loperamide (4 mg at the onset of diarrhea, and 2 mg after each bowel movement not to exceed 16 mg in 24 hours) is useful for treating "traveler's diarrhea" from multiple causes (DuPont et al., 1990). A theoretical advantage of this drug is that it crosses the blood–brain barrier poorly and is likely to have few CNS effects. Opiates are not recommended for children under 2 years of age because they can blunt alertness and interfere with oral rehydration therapy.

NSAIDs such as aspirin or indomethacin can decrease stool volume in the setting of acute infectious diarrhea but generally not to the degree that would make them clinically useful. Bismuth subsalicylate in large doses (30–60 ml every half hour for 8 doses following the onset of diarrhea) can decrease stool frequency and abdominal pain in mild to moderate acute self-limited diarrhea. However, this amount of salicylate may lead to toxic salicylate concentrations in the blood. It is not recommended for patients with renal failure or with concomitant use of other salicylates (see chapter 11). Loperamide is more effective for treating severe diarrhea (DuPont et al., 1990).

Specific antimicrobial treatment is currently recommended for symptomatic cases of diarrhea caused by *Shigella* spp., *Clostridium difficile*, *Salmonella typhi* with typhoid fever, *Giardia lamblia*, *Entamoeba histolytica*, and *Vibrio cholerae*. Certain patients with *E. coli* (enterohemorrhagic or enterotoxigenic *E. coli*, infants with enteropathogenic or enteroadherent *E. coli*), *Salmonella* infections without typhoid fever, or prolonged *Campylobacter jejuni* diarrhea may also benefit from specific antimicrobial treatment. Details of specific antimicrobial therapy change frequently and are best obtained from a frequently revised guide (Sanford, 1990) (see chapter 24). However, most bacterial causes of diarrhea can be treated effectively with ciprofloxacin 500 mg twice daily for 5 days. This empiric therapy may be used while awaiting the results of specific cultures (Goodman et al., 1990).

Therapy for chronic diarrhea generally is directed at the underlying disease. If the underlying disease cannot be identified or cured, then the general principles of management of acute diarrheal states are implemented. Other drugs may be considered to manage difficult cases of chronic diarrhea. Clonidine and lithium carbonate increase sodium chloride absorption in the gut; they have been used in chronic secretory diarrheas due to tumors elaborating vasoactive intestinal peptide (VIPomas) with limited success (O'Dorisio et al., 1989). Somatostatin or its analog octreotide decreases fluid and electrolyte secretion, decreases intestinal motility, and may decrease the release of a secretagogue from tumors such as VIPomas or nonmalignant tissue (Maton, 1989). Because of its reduction of release of growth hormone, somatostatin should not be used in children.

Acknowledgments—The author is indebted to Drs. Irwin H. Rosenberg and Charles S. Winams, whose section on gastrointestinal disorders in the prior edition of this textbook inspired and formed the framework for the current chapter.

REFERENCES

Anderson, J. W.; and Gustafson, N. J.: Hypocholesterolemic effects of oat and bean products. Am. J. Clin. Nutr., 48(3, suppl.):749–753, 1988.

Archambult, A. P.; Pare, P.; Bailey, R. J.; Navert, H.; Williams, C. N.; Freeman, H. J.; Baker, S. J.; Marcon, N. E.;

Hunt, R. H.; Sutherland, L.; Kepkay, D. L.; Saibil, F. G.; Hawken, K.; Farley, A.; Levesque, D.; Ferguson, J.; and Westin, J.-A.: Omeprazole (20 mg daily) versus cimetidine (1200 mg daily) in duodenal ulcer healing and pain relief. Gastroenterology, 94(5, pt. 1):1130–1134, 1988.

Bardhan, K. D.: Intermittent treatment of duodenal ulcer for long term medical management. Postgrad. Med. J., 64(suppl. 1):40–46, 1988.

Bartlett, J. G.: Antibiotic-associated pseudomembranous colitis. Hosp. Pract. (Off), 16(12):85–88, 1981.

Binder, H. J.: Pharmacology of laxatives. Annu. Rev. Pharmacol. Toxicol, 17:355–367, 1977.

Binder, H. J.; and Donowitz, M.: A new look at laxative action. Gastroenterology, 69(4):1001–1005, 1975.

Bodemar, G.; and Walan, A.: Maintenance treatment of recurrent peptic ulcer by cimetidine. Lancet, 1(8061):403–407, 1978.

Borison, H.; and Wang, S.: Physiology and pharmacology of vomiting. Pharmacol. Rev., 5:193–230, 1953.

Bradley, B.; Singleton, M.; and Po, A. L.: Bismuth toxicity—A reassessment. J. Clin. Pharmacol. Ther., 14(6):423–441, 1989.

Brand, D. L.; Roufail, W. M.; Thomson, A. B.; and Tapper, E. J.: Misoprostol, a synthetic PGE1 analog, in the treatment of duodenal ulcers. A multicenter double-blind study. Dig. Dis. Sci., 30(11, suppl.):147s–158s, 1985.

Carey, M. P.; Burish, T. G.; and Brenner, D. E.: Delta-9-tetrahydrocannabinol in cancer chemotherapy: Research problems and issues. Ann. Intern. Med., 99(1):106–114, 1983.

Carmine, A. A.; and Brogden, R. N.: Pirenzepine. A review of its pharmacodynamic and pharmacokinetic properties and therapeutic efficacy in peptic ulcer disease and other allied diseases. Drugs, 30(2):85–126, 1985.

Carson, J. L.; Strom, B. L.; Morse, M. L.; West, S. L.; Soper, K. A.; Stolley, P. D.; and Jones, J. K.: The relative gastrointestinal toxicity of the nonsteroidal anti-inflammatory drugs. Arch. Intern. Med., 147(6):1054–1059, 1987a.

Carson, J. L.; Strom, B. L.; Soper, K. A.; West, S. L.; and Morse, M. L.: The association of nonsteroidal anti-inflammatory drugs with upper gastrointestinal tract bleeding. Arch. Intern. Med., 147(1):85–88, 1987b.

Connell, A. M.; Hilton, C.; Irvine, G.; Lennard, J. J.; and Misiewicz, J. J.: Variation of bowel habit in two population samples. Br. Med. J., 5470:1095–1099, 1965.

Cubeddu, L. X.; Hoffmann, I. S.; Fuenmayor, N. T.; and Finn, A. L.: Efficacy of ondansetron (GR 38032F) and the role of serotonin in cisplatin-induced nausea and vomiting. N. Engl. J. Med., 322(12):810–816, 1990.

Dajani, E. Z.: Perspective on the gastric antisecretory effects of misoprostol in man. Prostaglandins, 33(suppl.):68–77, 1987.

Dingle, J.; Badger, G.; and Jordan, W.: Illness in the Home: A Study of 25,000 Illnesses in a Group of Cleveland Families. Press of Western Reserve University, Cleveland, 1964.

Donowitz, M.: Current concepts of laxative action: Mechanisms by which laxatives increase stool water. J. Clin. Gastroenterol., 1(1):77–84, 1979.

DuPont, H. L.; Flores, S. J.; Ericsson, C. D.; Mendiola, G. J.; DuPont, M. W.; Cruz, L. A.; and Mathewson, J. J.: Comparative efficacy of loperamide hydrochloride and bismuth subsalicylate in the management of acute diarrhea. Am. J. Med., 88(6A):15s–19s, 1990.

Feldman, M.: Inhibition of gastric acid secretion by selective and nonselective anticholinergics. Gastroenterology, 86(2):361–366, 1984.

Field, M.; Rao, M. C.; and Chang, E. B.: Intestinal electrolyte transport and diarrheal disease. N. Engl. J. Med., 321:800–806, 879–883, 1989.

Fine, K.; Krejs, G.; and Fordtran, J.: Diarrhea. Gastrointestinal Disease. Sleisenger, M. H. and Fordtran, J. S. (eds.). W. B. Saunders, Philadelphia, 1989.

Fordtran, J. S.: Speculations on the pathogenesis of diarrhea. Fed. Proc., 26(5):1405–1414, 1967.

Giesing, D.; Lanman, R.; and Runser, D.: Absorption of sucralfate in man. Gastroenterology, 82:1066, 1982.

Goldman, P.; and Peppercorn, M. A.: Drug therapy: Sulfasalazine. N. Engl. J. Med., 293(1):20–23, 1975.

Goodman, L. J.; Trenholme, G. M.; Kaplan, R. L.; Segreti, J.; Hines, D.; Petrak, R.; Nelson, J. A.; Mayer, K. W.; Landau, W.; and Parkhurst, G. W.: Empiric antimicrobial therapy of domestically acquired acute diarrhea in urban adults. Arch. Intern. Med., 150(3):541–546, 1990.

Graham, D. Y.: Enzyme replacement therapy of exocrine pancreatic insufficiency in man. Relation between in vitro enzyme activities and in vivo potency in commercial pancreatic extracts. N. Engl. J. Med., 296(23):1314–1317, 1977.

Graham, D. Y.; and Smith, J. L.: Gastroduodenal complications of chronic NSAID therapy. Am. J. Gasterenterol., 83(10):1081–1084, 1988.

Graham, D. Y.; Agrawal, N. M.; and Roth, S. H.: Prevention of NSAID-induced gastric ulcer with misoprostol: Multicentre, double-blind, placebo-controlled trial. Lancet, 2(8623): 1277–1280, 1988.

Graham, D. Y.: *Campylobacter pylori* and peptic ulcer disease. Gastroenterology, 96(2, Pt. 2, suppl.):615–625, 1989.

Grossman, M.: Peptic ulcer: Definition and epidemiology. In, The Genetics and Heterogeneity of Common Gastrointestinal Disorders (Rotter; Samloff; and Rimoin; eds.). Academic Press, New York, 1980.

Gryboski, J. D.: The role of allergy in diarrhea: Cow's milk protein allergy. Pediatr. Ann., 14(1):31–32, 1985.

Hanson, J. S.; and McCallum, R. W.: The diagnosis and management of nausea and vomiting: A review. Am. J. Gastroenterol., 80(3):210–218, 1985.

Havu, N.: Enterochromaffin-like cell carcinoids of gastric mucosa in rats after life-long inhibition of gastric secretion. Digestion, 35(suppl. 1):42–55, 1986.

Herting, R. L.; and Nissen, C. H.: Overview of misoprostol-clinical experience. Dig. Dis. Sci., 31(2, suppl.):47s–54s, 1986.

Howden, C. W.; Jones, D. B.; Peace, K. E.; Burget, D. W.; and Hunt, R. H.: The treatment of gastric ulcer with antisecretory drugs. Relationship of pharmacological effect to healing rates. Dig. Dis. Sci., 33(5):619–624, 1988.

Jenner, P.; and Marsden, C. D.: The substituted benzamides — A novel class of dopamine antagonists. Life Sci., 25(6):479–485, 1979.

Jones, D. B.; Howden, C. W.; Burget, D. W.; Kerr, G. D.; and Hunt, R. H.: Acid suppression in duodenal ulcer: A meta-analysis to define optimal dosing with antisecretory drugs. Gut, 28(9):1120–1127, 1987.

Koch, J.; and Donaldson, R.: A survey of food intolerances in hospitalized patients. N. Engl. J. Med., 271:657–660, 1964.

Koletzko, S.; Stringer, D. A.; Cleghorn, G. J.; and Durie, P. R.: Lavage treatment of distal intestinal obstruction syndrome in children with cystic fibrosis. Pediatrics, 83(5):727–733, 1989.

Lake-Bakaar, G.; Tom, W.; Lake, B. D.; Gupta, N.; Beidas, S.; Elsakr, M.; and Straus, E.: Gastropathy and ketoconazole malabsorption in the acquired immunodeficiency syndrome (AIDS). Ann. Intern. Med., 109(6):471–473, 1988.

Lam, S. K.: Antacids: the past, the present, and the future. Baillieres Clin. Gastroenterol., 2(3):641–654, 1988.

Lanza, F. L.; Royer, G. J.; and Nelson, R. S.: Endoscopic evaluation of the effects of aspirin, buffered aspirin, and enteric-coated aspirin on gastric and duodenal mucosa. N. Engl. J. Med., 303(3):136–138, 1980.

Laszlo, J.; Clark, R. A.; Hanson, D. C.; Tyson, L.; Crumpler, L.; and Gralla, R.: Lorazepam in cancer patients treated with cisplatin: A drug having antiemetic, amnesic, and anxiolytic effects. J. Clin. Oncol., 3(6):864–869, 1985.

Ludan, A. C.: Current management of acute diarrhoeas. Use and abuse of drug therapy. Drugs, 3(suppl. 4):18–25, 1988.

Mahieu, P.; Pringot, J.; and Bodart, P.: Defecography: I. Description of a new procedure and results in normal patients. Gastrointest. Radiol., 9(3):247–251, 1984.

Malagelada, J. R.; and Camilleri, M.: Unexplained vomiting:

A diagnostic challenge. Ann. Intern. Med., 101(2):211–218, 1984.

Markman, M.; Sheidler, V.; Ettinger, D. S.; Quaskey, S. A.; and Mellits, E. D.: Antiemetic efficacy of dexamethasone. Randomized, double-blind, crossover study with prochlorperazine in patients receiving cancer chemotherapy. N. Engl. J. Med., 311(9):549–552, 1984.

Marks, I. N.: The efficacy, safety and dosage of sucralfate in ulcer therapy. Scand. J. Gastroenterol., 140(suppl.):33–38, 1987.

Marty, M.; Pouillart, P.; Scholl, S.; Droz, J. P.; Azab, M.; Brion, N.; Pujade, L. E.; Paule, B.; Paes, D.; and Bons, J.: Comparison of the 5-hydroxytryptamine3 (serotonin) antagonist ondansetron (GR 38032F) with high-dose metoclopramide in the control of cisplatin-induced emesis. N. Engl. J. Med., 322(12):816–821, 1990.

Maton, P. N.: The use of the long-acting somatostatin analogue, octreotide acetate, in patients with islet cell tumors. Gastroenterol. Clin. North Am., 18(4):897–922, 1989.

Maton, P. N.; Vinayek, R.; Frucht, H.; McArthur, K. A.; Miller, L. S.; Saeed, Z. A.; Gardner, J. D.; and Jensen, R. T.: Long-term efficacy and safety of omeprazole in patients with Zollinger-Ellison syndrome: A prospective study. Gastroenterology, 97(4):827–836, 1989.

McArthur, K. E.; Jensen, R. T.; and Gardner, J. D.: Treatment of acid-peptic diseases by inhibition of gastric H^+,K^+-ATPase. Annu. Rev. Med., 37:97–105, 1986.

McCarthy, D. M.: Ranitidine or cimetidine. Ann. Intern. Med., 99(4):551–553, 1983.

McFarland, R. J.; Bateson, M. C.; Green, J. R.; O'Donoghue, D. P.; Dronfield, M. W.; Keeling, P. W.; Burke, G. J.; Dickinson, R. J.; Shreeve, D. R.; Peers, E. M.; and Richardson, P. D. I.: Omeprazole provides quicker symptom relief and duodenal ulcer healing than ranitidine. Gastroenterology, 98(2):278–283, 1990.

Miller, J. P.; and Faragher, E. B.: Relapse of duodenal ulcer: Does it matter which drug is used in initial treatment? (editorial). Br. Med. J. (Clin. Res.), 293(6555):1117–1118, 1986.

Moss, J.; and Vaughan, M.: Guanine nucleotide-binding proteins (G proteins) in activation of adenylyl cyclase: Lessons learned from cholera and "travelers' diarrhea." J. Lab. Clin. Med., 113(3):258–268, 1989.

O'Dorisio, T. M.; Mekhjian, H. S.; and Gaginella, T. S.: Medical therapy of VIPomas. Endocrinol. Metab. Clin. North Am., 18(2):545–556, 1989.

Pantuck, E. J.; Hsiao, K. C.; Kuntzman, R.; and Conney, A. H.: Intestinal metabolism of phenacetin in the rat: Effect of charcoal-broiled beef and rat chow. Science, 187(4178): 744–746, 1975.

Park, G. D.; Spector, R.; Goldberg, M. J.; and Johnson, G. F.: Expanded role of charcoal therapy in the poisoned and overdosed patient. Arch. Intern. Med., 146(5):969–973, 1986.

Piper, D. W.; Greig, M.; Coupland, G. A.; Hobbin, E.; and Shinners, J.: Factors relevant to the prognosis of chronic gastric ulcer. Gut, 16(9):714–718, 1975.

Pounder, R. E.: Model of medical treatment for duodenal ulcer. Lancet, 1(8210):29–30, 1981.

Powell, J. R.; and Donn, K. H.: The pharmacokinetic basis for H2-antagonist drug interactions: Concepts and implications. J. Clin. Gastroenterol., 5(suppl. 1):95–113, 1983.

Sanford, J.: Guide to Antimicrobial Therapy 1990. Antimicrobial Therapy, West Bethesda, 1990.

Siegel, J. N.; Schwartz, A.; Askenase, P. W.; and Gershon, R. K.: T-cell suppression and contrasuppression induced by histamine H2 and H1 receptor agonists, respectively. Proc. Natl. Acad. Sci. U.S.A., 79(16): 5052–5056, 1982.

Silverstein, F. E.; Kimmey, M. B.; Saunders, D. R.; and Levine, D. S.: Gastric protection by misoprostol against 1300 mg of aspirin. An endoscopic study. Dig. Dis. Sci., 31(2, suppl.):137s–141s, 1986.

Smith, B.: Effect of irritant purgatives on the myenteric plexus in man and the mouse. Gut, 9(2):139–143, 1968.

Soll, A. H.: Pathogenesis of peptic ulcer and implications for therapy. N. Engl. J. Med., 322(13):909–916, 1990.

Sontag, S. J.: Prostaglandins and acid peptic disease. Am. J. Gastroenterol., 81(11):1021–1028, 1986.

Starkey, W. G.; Collins, J.; Wallis, T. S.; Clarke, G. J.; Spencer, A. J.; Haddon, S. J.; Osborne, M. P.; Candy, D. C.; and Stephen, J.: Kinetics, tissue specificity and pathological changes in murine rotavirus infection of mice. J. Gen. Virol., 67(12):2625–2634, 1986.

Tedesco, F. J.; and DiPiro, J. T.: Laxative use in constipation. American College of Gastroenterology's Committee on FDA-Related Matters. Am. J. Gastroenterol., 80(4):303–309, 1985.

Wald, A.: Colonic transit and anorectal manometry in chronic idiopathic constipation. Arch. Intern. Med., 146(9):1713–1716, 1986.

Wampler, G.: The pharmacology and clinical effectiveness of phenothiazines and related drugs for managing chemotherapy-induced emesis. Drugs, 25(suppl. 1):35–51, 1983.

Weberg, R.; Aubert, E.; Dahlberg, O.; Dybdahl, J.; Ellekjaer, E.; Farup, P. G.; Hovdenak, N.; Lange, O.; Melsom, M.; Stallemo, A.; Vetvik, K. R.; and Berstad, A.: Low-dose antacids or cimetidine for duodenal ulcer? Gastroenterology, 95(6):1465–1469, 1988.

9

Treatment of Hepatic Disorders and the Influence of Liver Function on Drug Disposition

Gabriel Garcia

Chapter Outline

Withdrawal of Potentially Hepatotoxic
    Drugs, Dietary Components, or
    Environmental Agents
Drug-Induced Liver Disease
Removal of Offending Dietary Constituents
Avoidance of Certain Toxic Food
    Substances
Removal of "Toxic" Endogenous
    Substances
Replacement of Depleted Constituents:
    Role of Dietary Therapy
Temporizing

Prophylactic Therapy
Management of Complications of Advanced
    Liver Diseases
Portal Hypertension
Esophageal Variceal Hemorrhage
Ascites
Hepatic Encephalopathy
Specific Drug Therapy Aimed at an
    Underlying Disease
Gallstones
Viral Hepatitis
Alcoholic Liver Disease

A drug or a toxin will be the cause of disease in 50% or more of patients hospitalized for the management of liver disease, whether this be fulminant hepatic failure or complications of cirrhosis. This chapter discusses injury to the liver by drugs and environmental toxins and outlines principles of management of patients with drug-induced liver disease. Those few liver diseases that have specific drug therapy are also discussed; the rest of the chapter focuses on the management of the complications of advanced liver disease.

WITHDRAWAL OF POTENTIALLY HEPATOTOXIC DRUGS, DIETARY COMPONENTS, OR ENVIRONMENTAL AGENTS

Because many acute and chronic forms of liver injury may be caused by exposure of the patient to toxic substances, the physician must obtain a detailed history of drug use (both prescription and OTC pharmaceuticals), use of vitamins or hormones, or exposure to environmental or industrial toxins.

Drug-Induced Liver Disease

The liver's pivotal role in the processing of foreign substances also makes it susceptible to injury by those xenobiotics. Some chemical agents are predictable or intrinsic hepatotoxins: the injury they induce generally is dose-related, is seen above a threshold dose, and can be reproduced in experimental animals. These agents often produce tissue injury that results in metabolic defects and cell death or dysfunction. Examples of such direct hepatotoxins include the chlorinated hydrocarbons (e.g., carbon tetrachloride) and acetaminophen. Other agents may act indirectly, by interfering with a metabolic activity essential to cell function and survival.

Another group of chemical agents depend on idiosyncrasy in the host for their toxicity: their injury generally is not dose-related, is seen in only a few patients exposed to the drug (generally within 1–4 weeks after the onset of drug use), and may not be reproducible in other species. In certain cases, such as phenothiazine-induced hepatic injury, features of systemic hypersensitivity (fever, rash, eosinophilia, lymphocytosis, and lymphadenopathy) are present. In some cases, involvement of the immune system can be documented, confirming the presence of a true drug allergy. Liver biopsy obtained during the illness also may be typical of an allergic reaction, with eosinophilic and/or granulomatous infiltration and cellular necrosis.

With some drugs, liver injury depends on a metabolic idiosyncrasy that leads to accumulation of a metabolite that is capable either of inciting intrinsic liver damage or an allergic reaction. These reactions can occur over a much longer period of time than would be expected in a typical hypersensitivity reaction, and can result from genetic or acquired qualitative or quantitative differences in the handling of drugs. For example, patients with phenytoin-induced liver damage are unable to detoxify a potentially toxic metabolite, the arene oxide; this is related to decreased liver epoxide hydrolase activity in affected individuals (Spielberg et al., 1981).

Liver biopsy in drug-induced liver disease generally shows cytotoxic or cholestatic injury. Cytotoxic injury may be accompanied by necrosis or steatosis; cholestatic lesions may be exudative or bland. Less common types of injury include vascular (large or small hepatic vein occlusion, peliosis hepatitis, or other sinusoidal lesions), granulomatous, or neoplastic (benign and malignant) lesions. The purpose of a liver biopsy in patients with possible drug-induced liver injury is to establish the diagnosis, to suggest or establish another cause for the liver injury, and occasionally to stage the degree of liver injury.

Although the histologic pattern of the injury to the liver may be useful in determining the presence of drug-induced liver disease, one must remember that the liver has a limited repertoire of responses to injury, and the findings in the liver biopsy in patients with drug injuries may mimic other metabolic or infectious diseases. The histologic similarities between different conditions leading to liver disease may suggest a common pathway of injury.

For example, microvesicular fatty change is a characteristic histologic finding in patients with valproic acid–induced hepatic failure, Reye syndrome, and Jamaican vomiting disease, all conditions that are most commonly seen in children. Because a similar histologic picture has been seen in animals treated with 4-pentenoic acid, the hypothesis was put forth that a metabolite of the Ω-oxidation pathway may be responsible for hepatoxicity caused by these seemingly disparate drug and metabolic insults. Such a metabolite of valproic acid has been isolated, and administration of this metabolite to rats has led to microvesicular fatty change (Lewis et al., 1982). *Principle: The full spectrum of a drug's toxicity is not known when it is first used. Considerable experience with the drug in patients and careful observation are required to link an infrequent adverse response to a drug. Establishing a mechanism for an adverse response is even more difficult. However, once a mechanism is defined, it often can be retrospectively used to detect undiscovered reactions of an analogous nature.*

Reproduction of the clinical and biochemical signs of liver injury on rechallenge with the drug can be useful in allowing the therapist the certainty of the connection between the drug and the idiosyncratic drug reaction. This is most important clinically when no alternate therapy exists for a serious disorder. The therapist must weigh the potential benefit of greater diagnostic certainty by observing the response to rechallenge with the rare possibility that it may lead to a life-threatening injury.

The toxins or drugs that most commonly cause liver injury have changed over time as toxic or less effective agents have been removed from the workplace, the environment, and the pharmacy shelf. Predictably, new drugs and environmental agents have led to liver injury not suspected during the studies that determined their efficacy. Every time a drug is used, the therapist must be alert to the possibility of drug toxicity mimicking another disease and be aware of the relationships between drugs that predict similar toxicities. The reader is referred to a standard text of hepatotoxicity for an extensive list of drugs and chemicals that result in liver injury and for discussion of their clinical manifestations (Zimmerman, 1978).

Removal of Offending Dietary Constituents

Ordinary dietary constituents may occasionally produce liver injury or toxic side effects in a genetically susceptible individual. Treatment must then be directed at the removal of such substances from the diet. For example, removal of galactose-containing carbohydrates reverses jaundice, ascites, and hepatosplenomegaly in infants with galactosemia (Hsia and Walker, 1961). Removal of protein may reverse coma in a child with a urea cycle enzyme deficiency or in a cirrhotic patient with portal systemic encephalopathy. Reduction of carbohydrate ingestion improves fatty infiltration of the liver and hepatomegaly in patients who have a genetic susceptibility to carbohydrate-induced type IV hyperlipidemia, or in patients receiving total parenteral nutrition containing high concentrations of glucose.

Avoidance of Certain Toxic Food Substances

Naturally occurring organic compounds also have been associated with liver injury in man. The alkaloid senecio, found in certain herbal teas, produces hepatic vein occlusion. Aflatoxin is produced by a fungus, *Aspergillus flavus*, that grows on grains and nuts. In animals, prolonged consumption of aflatoxin may lead to cirrhosis or hepatoma. In humans, the level of aflatoxin in the diet has been found to be a cocarcinogen with hepatitis B infection in an epidemiologic study of hepatocellular carcinoma in rural China (Yeh et al., 1989). Mushrooms of the *Amanita* genus contain several toxins, of which α-amanitin and phalloidin can produce extensive hepatocellular necrosis that is frequently fatal (Welper and Opitz, 1972).

Removal of "Toxic" Endogenous Substances

Several endogenous substances (iron, copper, ammonia, bile acids, porphyrins) may accumulate as a result of disorders in intermediary metabolism or acquired liver injury. They may contribute further to liver injury and lead to other systemic effects. Therapy directed at removal of these substances often is beneficial, particularly if instituted during the precirrhotic phase of some of these illnesses. For example, D-penicillamine is used to remove copper in patients with Wilson disease (Scheinberg and Sternlieb, 1960; Sternlieb, 1980); phlebotomy is employed to reduce the body burden of iron in patients with idiopathic hemochromatosis (Bassett et al., 1980).

Replacement of Depleted Constituents: Role of Dietary Therapy

Although removal of hepatotoxic substances is critical in the therapy of some hepatic disorders, attention must also be directed to replenishing substances that are likely to become deficient in patients with hepatic disease. Three categories of deficiencies should be considered: (1) vitamins and minerals that are depleted because of dietary deficiencies, (2) vitamins and nutrients that are diminished as a result of impairment of the enterohepatic circulation, and (3) endogenous substances that become depleted as a result of impairment of hepatic function.

Patients with cholestatic liver disease are unable to excrete bile at a normal rate, and an intestinal luminal deficiency of bile salts results. Consequently, the absorption of fat-soluble vitamins as well as other lipid substances is impaired and deficiencies may develop. Malabsorption of vitamin K will lead to an impairment of the hepatic synthesis of vitamin K–dependent clotting factors. Similarly, vitamin A and D malabsorption may lead to the clinical syndromes typical of their deficiencies. In early stages of cholestasis, these deficiencies may be very difficult to detect.

Severe liver damage is almost always associated with impairment in the production of serum proteins that are synthesized in the liver. Intravenous administration of salt-poor albumin, plasma, or plasma fractions may be necessary to lessen these acquired deficiencies, especially in patients with clinically important bleeding who are deficient in hepatically generated clotting factors II, III, IX, and X.

TEMPORIZING

One of the most dramatic and imperfectly understood properties of the liver is its capacity to regenerate. After surgical removal of two thirds of the rat liver, the liver mass is restored within 7 to 10 days. A similar percentage of the human liver can be surgically removed, and sufficient regeneration can occur to support hepatic function at "normal" levels. The therapist must take advantage of this remarkable regenerative capability. There are many occasions when temporizing (i.e., making the deliberate decision not to treat with drugs) is the best therapeutic decision, allowing normal physiologic processes to reestablish homeostasis. *Principle: The decision not to treat is a therapeutic decision that often is medically wiser than offering a patient drugs. The decision not to give a drug has its own inherent potential efficacy and toxicity; like any other therapeutic maneuver, consideration of relative risks and benefits is necessary.*

The physician who waits and watches a patient with liver injury has an opportunity to observe the pattern of the disease and judge whether the liver injury will spontaneously resolve or whether it will become fulminant. This may require days or weeks of observation following acute viral or drug-induced hepatitis. Attention to the state of nutrition and hydration, and prompt identification and treatment of complications such as infection or electrolyte and acid–base disturbances, is key to the proper management of the patient. If fulminant hepatic failure develops (the presence of encephalopathy within 8 weeks of an acute liver injury in a patient without evidence of prior liver disease), the patient should be observed in an intensive care unit, and a determination should be made quickly whether the patient is a candidate for liver transplantation.

As a result of improved surgical and anesthetic techniques, better immunosuppressive regimens, and improved preservation of removed organs, liver transplantation is now a well-established therapeutic option for many patients whose liver disease has been complicated by liver failure. Five-year survival rates of >60% have been achieved in patients undergoing treatment for end-stage cirrhosis or fulminant hepatic failure. Absolute contraindications for liver transplantation include sepsis, malignancy outside the hepatobiliary tree, and active alcoholism (Starzl et al., 1989). *Principle: The use of devices and procedures as alternatives to drugs for the same indications is becoming a major responsibility of the therapist. However, it should be recognized that the requirements to put devices and procedures on the market are considerably less stringent than those that control marketing of a drug.*

Patients presenting with hyperbilirubinemia may have conditions causing either extrahepatic biliary obstruction or intrahepatic cholestasis. The therapist must choose between mechanical decompression of the biliary tract and careful observation based on the bedside evaluation and biliary-imaging studies. Patients in whom there is a high clinical suspicion of obstruction of the common bile duct and secondary cholangitis require prompt decompression (surgical or endoscopic) of the infected biliary tree and antibiotic therapy to treat and contain the bacterial infection. In the patient without clinical evidence of cholangitis, the choice to observe the patient during withdrawal of potentially hepatotoxic agents or identification of viral hepatitis will not expose patients with intrahepatic disease to unnecessary operative morbidity and mortality. Delay of an operative procedure until its need is established will not expose the patient to undue injury, because the development of secondary biliary cirrhosis takes weeks and may be surgically reversed after its onset (Bunton and Cameron, 1963).

PROPHYLACTIC THERAPY

Viral hepatitis often can be prevented or attenuated by postexposure prophylaxis with immune or hyperimmune serum. Other examples of prophylactic therapy in patients with liver disease include the diagnosis and treatment of asymptomatic patients who have hemochromatosis and Wilson disease. However, most prophylactic measures are not as specific as the measures that can be taken to manage or prevent the severe complications of these latter diseases. For instance, the avoidance of high doses of potent diuretics in patients with ascites who might otherwise develop renal insufficiency is a prudent, but nonspecific therapeutic decision. So too are the use of cleaning enemas and "nonabsorbable" antibiotics to prevent hepatic encephalopathy in a cirrhotic patient with GI bleeding, and the avoidance of surgery in the decompensated cirrhotic patient in whom the stress of anesthesia may precipitate irreversible hepatic failure. Prevention of GI hemorrhage with H_2-receptor antagonists in patients with severe liver failure is another example (MacDougall et al., 1977).

MANAGEMENT OF COMPLICATIONS OF ADVANCED LIVER DISEASES

Portal Hypertension

Portal hypertension is generally a consequence of the relationship between portal blow flow and the disruption of lobular and sinusoidal architecture that accompanies cirrhosis from any cause. Portal hypertension also may result from hypertension or obstruction at any level of the hepatic venous circulation, from thrombosis of the portal vein (presinusoidal causes) to obliteration or thrombosis of major or terminal hepatic veins (postsinusoidal causes). The major consequences of portal hypertension include (1) the development of a collateral circulation through the submucosa of the GI tract, the peritoneal surfaces, and the anterior abdominal wall, (2) an increase in lymphatic flow exiting through the thoracic duct, and (3) an increase in plasma volume and cardiac output with a loss of effective arterial tone.

As one would predict by Poiseuille's law, changes in portal pressure generally are caused by changes in vascular resistance or blood flow, because changes in the length of blood vessels or blood viscosity are not hemodynamically significant events in most clinical situations. A hyperdynamic state with a high blood flow and low vascular resistance in both the systemic and the portal circulation is the rule in patients with cirrhosis and portal hypertension. This is accompanied by increases in plasma volume and by both increased resistance and increased blood flow through the portal circulation as a result of expansion of collateral channels (Groszmann et al., 1988). Serious clinical manifestations that accompany these changes include hemorrhage from GI varices (predominantly esophageal, rarely hemorrhoidal), hepatic encephalopathy, and ascites.

Patients with chronic liver disease who develop symptoms and signs of portal hypertension must be considered candidates for liver transplantation if their underlying liver disease is amenable to this treatment modality. Since the 1-year mortality following the development of variceal hemorrhage, ascites, or hepatic encephalopathy varies from 20% to 80% in patients with chronic liver disease, one has the opportunity to improve both length and quality of life by a procedure whose overall 5-year survival is 50% to 70% (Starzl et al., 1989).

Esophageal Variceal Hemorrhage

Esophageal variceal hemorrhage is a dramatic, unpredictable clinical event in the natural history of cirrhosis that has a high mortality (20%–80% per episode of bleeding), and a 50% chance of recurrence within 6 months (Graham and Smith, 1981). Patients at high risk for bleeding generally have large varices, high portal pressures, and a variety of endoscopically described local signs (red wales, cherry-red spots, and varices-on-varices, collectively named *red color signs*; Beppu et al., 1981). Massive GI bleeding in patients with advanced liver disease usually stems from variceal bleeding, but other causes include gastritis, peptic ulcer disease, and Mallory-Weiss tears. Emergency upper endoscopy can differentiate among these causes, and an experienced therapeutic endoscopist can attempt local control of the hemorrhage through sclerotherapy, chemical coagulation, or thermal coagulation. Although the ultimate prognosis of patients following variceal hemorrhage is dictated by the seriousness of the underlying liver disease, attempts at medical management of variceal bleeding can reduce the need for massive blood transfusion and high-risk of surgery done under emergency conditions.

Medical management of patients with variceal bleeding should take place in an intensive care unit where the patient can be monitored closely. Attention to the hemodynamic status of the patient requires monitoring of urine output, central venous and arterial pressures, hematocrit, electrolytes, and acid-base status (see chapter 26). General supportive care of the patient is important to provide adequate oxygen-carrying capacity, platelets, and coagulation factors. The goal of transfusion therapy should be to reverse hypovolemia and to provide adequate oxygen-carrying capacity, because overexpansion of the blood volume may raise portal pressures and lead to continued bleeding.

More specific therapy of variceal bleeding is aimed at reduction of portal pressure. Both vasopressin and somatostatin decrease splanchnic blood flow, portal pressure, and collateral flow as measured by azygos vein flow. Vasopressin, or antidiuretic hormone, was isolated and chemically synthesized in 1954 (duVigneaud et al., 1954). Secretion of this hormone by the hypothalamus is induced by hyperosmolarity, volume depletion, emotional or physiologic stress, pharmacologic agents, and painful stimuli (Schrier, 1979). Its half-life in the circulation after secretion or IV administration is approximately 10 minutes; it is inactivated by peptidases in many tissues, but principally in the kidney (Rabkin et al., 1979). In addition to its renal antidiuretic effect, vasopressin causes constriction of vascular smooth muscle, and contraction of smooth muscle in the uterus and GI tract, leading to increased propulsive forces of both organs. Although therapy with a continuous infusion of IV vasopressin is generally accepted to be effective in stopping variceal bleeding, it has been difficult to prove in the acutely bleeding patient, because most such patients will cease to bleed spontaneously (Fogel et al., 1982). The intense vasospasm that can accompany the use of vasopressin can compromise blood flow in the coronary, cerebral, and mesenteric circulations, leading to ischemia and infarction. Attempts to reduce the systemic effects of vasopressin have included the simultaneous use of systemic vasodilators (nitroglycerin, nitroprusside) or the use of the triglycyl hormonogen of vasopressin-glypressin that causes fewer systemic effects (Gelman and Ernst, 1979; Groszmann, 1982; Freeman et al., 1982). Efficacy of this latter therapy is yet to be proved.

Somatostatin was first isolated as a polypeptide that inhibited the secretion of growth hormone by the pituitary gland (Brazeau et al., 1973). It is found in many tissues throughout the body but is most concentrated in the GI tract and pancreas (Arimura et al., 1975). The physiologic functions of somatostatin in the GI tract are yet to be defined; in general, it inhibits the secretion of GI hormones and pancreatic juice, and the motility of the GI tract. Infusion of somatostatin to normal volunteers and patients with cirrhosis leads to a reduction in mesenteric blood flow and portal pressures without significant hemodynamic effects on the systemic circulation (Bosch et al., 1981). The half-life of somatostatin is measured in minutes, and it must be administered IV. Octreotide, a cyclic octapeptide with similar biologic activity, can be administered subcutaneously and has a half-life of 1 to 2 hours. It is therefore easier to administer than the native molecule (O'Donnell and Heaton, 1988). Clinical trials have demonstrated that octreotide and vasopressin have equal efficacy in controlling variceal bleeding (Kravetz et al., 1984).

Sclerotherapy of esophageal varices requires injection of a sclerosing agent (polidocanol, tetradecylsulfate, sodium morrhuate, ethanol, or ethanolamine oleate) either into or next to the varices in the distal esophagus. Fibrosis of the mucosa and submucosa probably leads to progressive obliteration of the mucosal and submucosal vascular channels. Although sclerotherapy can be technically difficult at the time of active variceal bleeding, it leads to control of bleeding in the majority of the patients and has been shown to decrease length of hospitalization, units of blood transfused, and acute mortality from massive variceal bleeding (Infante et al., 1989).

When all medical treatments fail to control variceal bleeding, surgery to decompress the portal circulation or devascularize the distal esophagus will control bleeding. Shunt surgery has a high mortality and is often complicated by hepatic encephalopathy in patients with poor hepatic reserve. However, surgery leads to less recurrent bleeding than sclerotherapy and may be favored in patients with relatively good liver function (Cello et al., 1987). Esophageal transection is a simpler surgical technique that in experienced hands is as effective as shunt surgery in the control of active bleeding. However, higher rates of rebleeding may be expected (Huizinga, 1985).

Because the seriousness of the underlying liver disease affects both short-term and long-term survival following variceal bleeding, the physician can use well-established prognostic indicators to guide the management of patients with active variceal bleeding. Patients with acute variceal bleeding should be treated with variceal sclerotherapy until obliteration of distal esophageal varices is achieved. If rebleeding occurs, patients with adequate hepatic reserve should have surgery to control bleeding. The choice of operation should take into account the experience of the surgeon. The success of these surgical and endoscopic techniques is related to the expertise of the operator. *Principle: Therapeutic options that involve invasive techniques introduce a new variable in determining both efficacy and toxicity: the experience and skill of the physician himself or herself.*

Prophylactic therapy (therapy aimed at prevention of bleeding, either prior to or after the first bleeding episode) has been attempted with agents that reduce portal pressure (β-adrenergic blockers), sclerotherapy, and surgical shunts. The previously discussed guidelines have been used to classify patients into high- and low-risk groups for rebleeding. Studies using nonselective β-adrenergic blockers have had mixed, although generally positive, results, in both the prevention of the first bleed and the prevention of rebleeding. Unfortunately, it is difficult to predict which patients are most likely to experience a fall in portal pressure without invasive studies. In addition, the acute hemodynamic response to drug may not predict the long-term efficacy of treatment.

Both surgery and sclerotherapy appear to be too risky to be used in patients prior to their first bleed. This risk/benefit assessment might change if we were able to determine with more accuracy which 10% of patients with varices would bleed in any given year (Baker et al., 1959).

Ascites

The development of ascites, a collection of free fluid in the peritoneal cavity, is a common clinical feature of end-stage liver disease. A combination of avid renal sodium reabsorption and a decreased "effective" arterial volume leads to an increased extracellular fluid volume. Local peritoneal factors and increased hepatic production of lymph result in the accumulation of fluid within the peritoneal space. Hypoalbuminemia plays a role through Starling forces, but its magnitude is unclear. The formation of ascites in cirrhotic patients and the current hypotheses concerning the interplay between hormonal, hemodynamic, and neural mechanisms have been recently reviewed (Epstein, 1988).

Ascites can be associated with untoward clinical events. It is a source of significant discomfort, frequently leads to anorexia and vomiting in an already-malnourished patient, and may predispose to serious bacterial infections. For these reasons, massive ascites should always be treated. Therapy for lesser degrees of ascites should be individualized, as survival of the patient will depend on the seriousness of the underlying liver disease and not the presence or absence of ascites. Therapy with diuretics or paracentesis can lead to serious complications including encephalopathy, renal insufficiency, electrolyte disorders, and spontaneous bacterial peritonitis.

Important general measures for the management of ascites include withdrawal of potentially toxic agents (alcohol because of its direct toxic effects on the liver, and NSAIDs because of their tendency to cause fluid retention and reduce the glomerular filtration rate) and adherence to a nourishing, sodium-restricted diet. Spontaneous diuresis generally ensues in most patients with new-onset ascites that is not severe. Very severe sodium restriction (500 mg/day or less), although desirable, can make meals so unappetizing that caloric intake becomes compromised. The therapist should obtain a sample of the ascitic fluid for total granulocyte count and bacterial culture at the bedside, because spontaneous bacterial peritonitis can present without the usual signs and symptoms of inflammation and peritoneal irritation (Runyon et al., 1987, 1988). Granulocytic ascites should be treated presumptively for spontaneous bacterial peritonitis. Monitoring the patient's electrolytes and renal function is important. Hypokalemia, hyponatremia, and azotemia are particularly serious complications.

If the response to sodium restriction is inadequate, the therapist may proceed to other potential therapeutic modalities with greater efficacy and risk. Therapy with diuretics is discussed in other sections of this book (see chapter 11). When diuretics are used to treat cirrhotic ascites, it is important not to exceed the capacity for reabsorption of ascitic fluid by the systemic circulation (approximately 700–900 ml/day), because greater urinary losses may lead to severe contraction of plasma volume, which can induce hepatic encephalopathy or the hepatorenal syndrome (Shear et al., 1970). Regimens that lead to a modest natriuresis (spironolactone 100–400 mg daily and/or furosemide 20–240 mg daily) are best suited for diuresis of ascites, the goal being to produce a "gentle" diuresis. One should start with the lowest doses suggested, and increase until weight loss of 0.5 to 1.0 kg daily is achieved. Since mobilization of fluid from peripheral edema is more efficient than from the peritoneal cavity, the 0.5 to 1.0-kg/day guidelines may be exceeded as long as the patient has peripheral edema. One should not underestimate the toxicity of diuretic therapy; the physician should follow end points of efficacy (daily weight, physical exam) and toxicity (electrolytes and renal function tests) to guide therapy. *Principle: The rate of improvement may determine the likelihood of toxicity. Rapid success for the physician may lead to serious trouble for the patient.*

Large-volume paracentesis is a technique by which 4 to 6 liters of fluid a day are removed from the peritoneal cavity in patients with massive ascites. Intravenous administration of albumin generally is used to replace protein losses gram for gram (Ginès et al., 1987). One might have predicted that the length of hospitalization and the incidence of serious acid–base or electrolyte abnormalities might be reduced in patients treated by paracentesis when compared with diuretic therapy. A surprising finding, counter to traditional teaching, is that patients are less likely to develop azotemia and hypovolemia when therapeutic paracentesis is employed (Ginès et al., 1987). Unfortunately, paracentesis has led to a higher rate of spontaneous bacterial peritonitis, presumably because of dilution of opsonins through direct removal and replacement with albumin (Runyon, 1988). One may predict similar results with newer techniques that mechanically remove fluid such as ultrafiltration of ascites fluid. *Principle: The theoretical and intellectual appeal of a new treatment must be balanced against the well-established data concerning efficacy and toxicity of customary therapy. The eventual role of newer therapeutic modalities can become clear only as data accumulate concerning their true efficacy and toxicity.*

Return of ascites to the central venous circulation by reinfusion devices (extracorporeal or internal) has been proposed as treatment for massive ascites that would not result in protein losses. The best-studied technique is peritoneovenous shunting achieved using Le Veen or Denver shunts, in which a tube containing a one-way valve is tunneled under the skin to connect the peritoneal cavity with a vein of the central circulation. Studies of peritoneovenous shunts compared with therapeutic paracentesis show comparable patient survival. Both techniques induce more rapid diuresis than is generally achieved with diuretics alone; however, surgical mortality and serious morbidity (massive hemorrhage, infection, premature shunt closure) in patients with serious, end-stage liver disease is appreciable in the shunted groups (Stanley et al., 1989). Consider a trial of therapeutic paracentesis in patients truly refractory to diuretics, in whom ascites must be reduced prior to consideration of a peritoneovenous shunt.

Hepatic Encephalopathy

Hepatic encephalopathy is a syndrome that accompanies severe hepatic insufficiency; it is characterized by altered mental status. Abnormal concentrations or production of ammonia, amino acids, short-chain fatty acids, endogenous benzodiazepines, and false neurotransmitters have been implicated in the pathogenesis of this syndrome, but no specific abnormality appears to explain all the clinical manifestations. The diagnosis rests on finding symptoms and signs of a metabolic encephalopathy (impaired cognitive or motor function, asterixis, incontinence, or frank coma) in a patient with signs of serious liver disease or portal hypertension. Abnormal electroencephalograms and elevated serum ammonia and cerebrospinal glutamine concentrations are generally seen in patients with hepatic encephalopathy, and their presence helps support the diagnosis (Fraser and Arieff, 1985).

General therapeutic measures are important in the management of patients with hepatic encephalopathy. Endogenous or exogenous factors potentially precipitating encephalopathy must be sought and reversed. These can include nitrogen loads from azotemia or GI hemorrhage, hypokalemia, hyponatremia, alkalosis, dehydration, psychoactive drugs, dietary protein overload, and severe infections. Most patients dramatically improve after withdrawal of drugs or alcohol, and institution of simple support measures.

Preventive measures must be exercised in all patients with advanced liver disease. These include avoiding the use of psychoactive drugs, maintaining soft stools, and limiting protein intake if there is a history of protein intolerance.

Efficacy of treatment can best be monitored by careful staging of hepatic encephalopathy and coma. This must be performed frequently and regularly. For patients with lesser degrees of encephalopathy, standard tests of cognition and fine motor skills, as simple as asking the patient to sign his or her name or draw the face of a clock, can show dramatic differences over time as the severity of encephalopathy changes.

Specific drug therapy is aimed at reducing the absorption of ammonia from the colon. Drugs used for this purpose may be delivered orally or by enema. Neomycin, an antibiotic poorly absorbed from the GI tract, may work by decreasing colonic urease activity through quantitative reduction in bowel flora. A recommended dosage is 1 to 2 g daily in divided doses. Because of its low oral bioavailability, treatment with oral neomycin is rarely complicated by ototoxicity or nephrotoxicity. However, other antibiotics may be indicated in patients with renal insufficiency. Lactulose (or other sugars that are not readily absorbed by the small bowel) can reach the colon, where it is metabolized by bacteria to small organic acids. These result in acidification of the stool, which favors conversion of ammonia to ammonium ion and traps the latter in the colonic lumen. The organic acids also stimulate an osmotic catharsis that expels the trapped ammonium. The oral dose of lactulose is titrated to cause two or three soft stools a day. Patients must be observed for severe diarrhea during treatment with lactulose. The diarrhea itself may cause dehydration or hypernatremia and aggravate the encephalopathy (Conn et al., 1977).

The finding of abnormal plasma and cerebrospinal amino acid profiles in patients with hepatic encephalopathy, and interest in the false-neurotransmitter hypothesis, has led to the use of amino acid solutions enriched with branched-chain amino acids (BCAA). The purpose of such therapy is to alter the plasma amino acid profile to one with fewer aromatic amino acids, the potential precursors of false neurotransmitters. Merely removing protein or amino acids from the diet would not cause this change, because plasma amino acid concentrations depend primarily on endogenous production and metabolism. In a controlled study of BCAA solution versus neomycin in the therapy of patients with spontaneous encephalopathy, treatment with BCAA led to fewer deaths and better recovery from encephalopathy within a 14-day period of treatment (Cerra et al., 1985).

Nutritional support for the hospitalized patient with serious liver disease needs to be adjusted for the presence of encephalopathy. Patients without encephalopathy who require parenteral nutrition should be given relatively low concentrations of standard amino acid solutions, and the concentration should be increased as tolerated to deliver a total of 1 to 1.5 g of protein per kilogram of body weight daily. The presence of encephalopathy should lead to therapy with a BCAA-enriched formula until the patient recovers. Attempts to convert to standard amino acid formulas once the patient recovers are desirable. There is no evidence to show that prolonged therapy with BCAA is necessary as long as precipitating factors are identified and corrected (Blackburn and O'Keefe, 1989).

SPECIFIC DRUG THERAPY AIMED AT AN UNDERLYING DISEASE

Gallstones

Gallstone disease afflicts approximately 10% of the adult population of the United States (Ingelfinger, 1968). There are two distinct classes of gallstones: cholesterol stones and pigment stones. In western countries, 90% of the stones removed are either pure or mixed cholesterol stones. Cholesterol gallstones form in the gallbladder following a nucleation event that results in a nidus capable of supporting deposition and growth of cholesterol crystal. Several factors predispose patients to develop cholesterol gallstones. Bile may

become supersaturated because of biliary hypersecretion of cholesterol, or hyposecretion of bile salt or lecithin. An imbalance may develop between nucleation factors (such as gallbladder mucin) and antinucleating factors still to be characterized. Finally, impaired gallbladder function may lead to stasis and the development of biliary sludge (Holzbach, 1986). The prevalence of cholesterol gallstones increases with age and is heterogeneously distributed among racial and ethnic groups. Other risk factors include female sex, massive obesity, rapid weight loss (particularly in patients using lipid-lowering drugs), parity, ileal dysfunction, and cystic fibrosis.

Pigment stones may be brown or black (Soloway et al., 1977). Black pigment stones generally occur in patients with hereditary hemolytic disorders or other conditions that lead to decreased red blood cell survival. Brown pigment stones generally are seen in Asian women who are malnourished and have evidence of recurrent biliary tract infection.

The advent of real-time ultrasonography as a rapid and reliable screening test for the evaluation of abdominal pain and jaundice, coupled with progress in surgical and perioperative management of patients, has led to the frequent removal of diseased gallbladders containing gallstones. Approximately 500,000 cholecystectomies are performed yearly in the United States. Patients with asymptomatic gallstones will not have biliary complications frequently enough to risk the potential hazard of prophylactic surgery (Gracie and Ransohoff, 1982; Ransohoff et al., 1983). The same caution also applies to patients with diabetes mellitus or renal insufficiency who have asymptomatic gallstones, despite the fact that they may be at increased risk for serious morbidity or mortality should they require emergency surgery (Friedman et al., 1988).

Once symptomatic gallbladder disease develops, the potential for serious complications (acute gangrenous cholecystitis, ascending cholangitis, common bile duct obstruction, and pancreatitis) is frequent enough that specific therapy needs to be considered. Because of the safety and efficacy of cholecystectomy, it remains the treatment of choice for the vast majority of patients with symptomatic gallstones. In an otherwise healthy adult younger than 50 years of age, an elective cholecystectomy should be performed with less than 0.1% mortality (Jarvinen and Hasrbacka, 1980).

Interest in nonsurgical therapy for gallstone disease has been fueled by the small but finite number of deaths that occur each year from gallbladder surgery, by the fact that gallstone disease tends to occur with advancing age in patients with comorbid illnesses that make surgery more hazardous, and by the fact that we seem to understand its pathogenesis and a medical way to intercede. The recognition of the importance of bile supersaturation in the formation and growth of cholesterol gallstones has led to medical therapy specifically designed to change the physicochemical properties of bile. Both chenodeoxycholic acid (CDCA) and its 7β epimer ursodeoxycholic acid (UDCA), major bile acids of humans and bears, respectively, are effective in dissolving gallstones in selected patients (Schoenfield and Lachin, 1981; Roda et al., 1982).

Both CDCA and UDCA act by expanding the total bile acid pool and decreasing the secretion of biliary cholesterol, thereby decreasing the amount of time supersaturated bile is present in the gallbladder (Ward et al., 1984). Other bile acids such as cholic acid that fail to decrease the secretion of cholesterol into bile do not have a beneficial effect on bile lithogenicity or gallstone dissolution. CDCA also inhibits 3–hydroxy–3–methylglutaryl coenzyme A (HMG-CoA) reductase, the rate-limiting step in cholesterol biosynthesis; the same mechanism has been suggested but not proved for UDCA. CDCA inhibits the synthesis of other bile acids, whereas UDCA does not. UDCA forms a liquid-crystalline phase in the bile rather than a micellar phase.

The largest study of gallstone dissolution in the United States, the National Cooperative Gallstone Study, enrolled 916 adults who had radiolucent, not calcified gallstones discernible on an oral cholecystogram (OCG) (Schoenfield and Lachin, 1981). Patients were randomly allocated to receive 750 mg/day CDCA, 375 mg/day CDCA, or placebo for 2 years. Patients in the highest-dose group had 13.5% complete dissolution and 27% partial dissolution, using the presence of stones by OCG as the end point. When therapy was extended to 3 years, a total of 20% of patients treated with 750 mg/day of CDCA achieved total dissolution. Side effects of therapy included dose-related diarrhea that occurred in 40% of patients treated with 750 mg/day and was likely due to bile acid–induced colonic secretion of water and electrolytes. CDCA also increased the serum cholesterol concentration by 20 mg/dl, most of which was LDL cholesterol. The HDL cholesterol concentration was unchanged, and the triglyceride concentrations were mildly decreased. Minor elevations of aminotransferase concentrations were seen in 30% of patients receiving 750 mg/day, and clinically significant but reversible liver disease was seen in 3% of the group. Lithocholic acid, a product of intestinal bacterial 7α-hydroxylation of CDCA, has been implicated in this adverse effect. Analysis of the effect of treatment on bile lithogenicity has suggested that an optimum effect is not achieved until 15 mg/kg

CDCA daily is administered; at this dose one would expect more of the dose-related side effects than were seen at 750 mg/day.

When UDCA therapy is compared with CDCA therapy, the two drugs are equally efficacious at doses with equivalent effects on bile lithogenicity (Enrico et al., 1982; Erlinger et al., 1984; Fisher et al., 1985; Podda et al., 1989). UDCA is better tolerated by patients with essentially no diarrhea, hypercholesterolemia, or abnormal liver tests. Because of its relative lack of serious side effects, it can be used at its optimum dose of 10 mg/kg daily and ultimately may lead to more rapid and frequent dissolution. In study populations not optimally selected, the total gallstone dissolution rate is approximately 20% at 2 years. However, the range of gallstone dissolution seen in studies of UDCA has been wide and seems to be dependent on the characteristics of the study subjects. The best results (>50% total dissolution after 12–24 months of therapy) have been seen in women with small (<15 mm) floating stones in functioning gallbladders. Stones with a small calcific nidus or an incomplete rim of calcification also may be dissolved, albeit with less success. Patients on drugs or diets that promote cholesterol saturation of bile (estrogens, cholestyramine, or clofibrate, but not lovastatin) are less likely to respond.

Because medical dissolution of gallstones does not lead to removal of the diseased gallbladder, the issue of recurrence of the stones is important. About 50% of patients who have had successful dissolution of their gallstones with oral bile salt therapy have had recurrent gallstones within 5 years of discontinuation of oral bile salt therapy. Low doses of oral bile acids may not prevent recurrent gallstones. In 53 patients whose gallstones were dissolved during therapy with CDCA, subsequent therapy with either 375 mg/day of CDCA or placebo resulted in a recurrence rate of 27% during a 2- to 4.5-year follow-up period (Marks et al., 1984). Not all recurrent gallstones are symptomatic; thus whether patients whose gallstones are successfully dissolved will require lifelong therapy to prevent recurrent stones is an issue yet to be resolved. Attempts to modify other factors that contribute to stone formation such as modifying nucleating or antinucleating factors or improving gallbladder motility may play a future role in prevention of stone recurrence. ***Principle: The efficacy and toxicity seen during short-term drug therapy should not be extrapolated to chronic drug treatment without proof. Only drug trials designed to assess efficacy and toxicity during chronic administration will give an accurate answer.***

Other nonsurgical approaches to gallstone dissolution being evaluated at this time include extracorporeal shock wave lithotripsy (ESWL) and contact dissolution with the potent cholesterol-dissolving agent methyl *tert*-butyl ether (MTBE) delivered by needle puncture into the gallbladder. Because ESWL can fragment large stones into smaller (and potentially more easily dissolved) fragments, it may find its role in extending the usefulness of UDCA dissolution therapy to patients with large stones or stones that have calcified rims. However, ESWL may produce fragments that are small enough to exit the gallbladder and cause bile duct or pancreatic duct obstruction; 2% of patients in the largest published series had pancreatitis. ESWL can cause damage to other organs as well; 4% of patients had gross hematuria, presumably due to contusion of the right kidney (Sackmann et al., 1988).

Dissolution with MTBE is an attractive option because of the rapidity with which gallstone dissolution may be achieved following catheterization of the gallbladder. Potential adverse effects of MTBE are those related to small-bowel delivery and absorption of the drug (duodenitis, hemolysis, general anesthesia) or to the transhepatic gallbladder puncture (bleeding, bile peritonitis) (Allen et al., 1985; Thistle, 1987).

Current clinical studies suggest that patients with gallstone symptoms that are neither severe nor life-threatening should be considered for gallstone dissolution therapy if they are older than 50 years, have a high operative risk because of associated illnesses, and have clinical and radiologic features that predict a high rate of dissolution (one to three floating, radiolucent stones less than 1.5 cm in diameter in a functioning gallbladder). Therapy should be continued beyond the point of gallstone dissolution, and possibly indefinitely, in order to avoid the high rate of recurrence. It seems prudent to consider for further clinical investigation only those bile acids that increase cholesterol secretion into bile and that are not biotransformed into potentially toxic secondary bile acids. *Principle: Studies that prove the efficacy of a drug cannot encompass all the clinical indications nor the eventual regimen that will prove to be most useful. The therapist must use all the available basic and clinical data to decide the best use of the drug in individual patients and must be able to modify use of the drug based on experience and on further postmarketing testing of the drug.* Once gallstone disease is complicated by acute cholecystitis, common bile duct obstruction, pancreatitis, or ascending cholangitis, surgical measures are often necessary to provide adequate drainage of the biliary tree. This is generally performed by removal of the gallbladder and surgical exploration of the biliary tree. Endoscopic cholangiography, papillotomy, and extraction of stones from the common bile duct may play a more prominent role in the future in selected patients. Systemic antibiotics should be administered to patients with cholangitis in order to prevent or treat septicemia, and to help sterilize the biliary tree. Antibiotics are selected to provide coverage for the organisms that generally infect the biliary tract (gram-negative bacilli and anaerobes), taking into consideration the ability of the drug to be excreted into bile. Extended-spectrum penicillins and cephalosporins have been found to be clinically useful as single-agent therapy.

Viral Hepatitis

Identification of the agents responsible for acute and chronic viral hepatitis has led to a better understanding of the natural history of infection with different viruses. However, no agent has yet been proved to be safe and effective in eradicating the infection in any of the common types of viral hepatitis. Progress in viral hepatitis has been most successful in preventing it. Passive immunization with immune globulin is useful for individuals exposed to hepatitis A and B. Active immunization using hepatitis B vaccine is useful for individuals at high risk of acquiring hepatitis B.

General measures important in the care of patients with acute viral hepatitis include maintenance of adequate oral fluid intake and nutrition, and observation for the signs of fulminant viral hepatitis. These signs include altered mental status, the presence of ascites, or evidence of other signs of acute portal hypertension. If a patient is unable to keep himself or herself adequately nourished and hydrated, or if there are signs of hepatic failure, hospitalization is necessary for adequate patient management. Antiemetics may be useful in the management of nausea and vomiting and should be administered when adequate hydration does not relieve this complaint. Strict isolation is not necessary, even in cases of viral hepatitis A and E (which are transmitted by the oral–fecal route), unless the patient is incontinent and unable to properly dispose of his or her own urine and stool. However, frequent hand washing and the use of care and gloves when handling potentially infectious material (blood, stool, other body secretions) is mandatory.

The agent that causes outbreaks of water-borne or food-related fecal–orally transmitted viral hepatitis worldwide has been identified as the hepatitis A virus (HAV), a small RNA virus classified as enterovirus 72. This infection is not associated with a chronic carrier state; although the disease can be severe, it is only rarely fulminant. Reduced contamination of the water supply and improved sewage handling have resulted in fewer children being exposed to hepatitis A and a larger pool of adults not being immune. This loss of "herd immunity" leads to occasional outbreaks following the ingestion of contaminated food or water.

Clinically recognizable hepatitis A can be prevented in 80% to 90% of acutely exposed patients treated intramuscularly with 0.02 ml/kg of standard immune serum globulin (Stokes and Neefe, 1945). Controlled clinical trials have supported the use of immune serum globulin having an anti-HAV titer of at least 1:2000 within 2 weeks of a household exposure. This finding should be extended to situations in which the likelihood of acute exposure to hepatitis A is high. This includes exposures to infected children in day care centers, infected patients in institutions for the mentally retarded, and infectious food handlers. Similarly, prophylaxis is warranted for travelers to areas with an active hepatitis A epidemic. No vaccine is currently available (Balistreri, 1988).

A similar disease occurring in developing countries in Asia, Africa, and Central and South America is now known to be due to the as yet incompletely characterized hepatitis E virus (HEV). This disease is similar in its epidemiology to hepatitis A; however, it is absent from the United States except in imported cases, and it may cause fulminant hepatitis in pregnant, malnourished women. No specific treatment is available. Although serologic tests for this disease are still in the developmental stage, the prevalence of anti-HEV antibodies in blood samples from anicteric individuals living in areas where active HEV outbreaks are occurring is low. This suggests that there are relatively few anicteric cases and that immune globulin prepared from these sources may not be efficacious in preventing this disease (Ramalingaswami and Purcell, 1988).

Hepatitis B is endemic in Asia, equatorial Africa, and America. It leads to a chronic carrier rate of 5% to 10% of these populations, to serious chronic morbidity and mortality from end-stage liver disease, and to hepatocellular carcinoma. It is transmitted from mother to child by blood contamination at the time of birth, between people of any age through intimate contact, and by percutaneous exposure to infectious blood or blood products. Prevention of transmission following exposure in children of hepatitis B carrier mothers (Stevens et al., 1987), or in settings of high risk for transmission in sexually active homosexual men (Hadler et al., 1986), has been achieved with the use of hepatitis B immune globulin (HBIG; anti-HBs titer >1 : 100,000) and/or the hepatitis B vaccine. The currently recommended regimen for postexposure prophylaxis is 0.06 ml/kg HBIG intramuscularly (1 ml in neonates) followed by hepatitis B vaccine at 0, 1, and 6 months. Currently available hepatitis B vaccines are made from the small hepatitis B surface antigen (HBsAg) particles extracted from the plasma of chronic carriers of the virus, or manufactured in yeast by recombinant DNA techniques. Both vaccines stimulate antibody formation against a single determinant. About 5% to 10% of patients vaccinated do not develop significant titers of anti-HBs, and this appears to be a recessive trait (Alper et al., 1989) linked to the major histocompatibility complex (MHC). This nonresponsiveness may be circumvented by the inclusion in the vaccine of highly immunogenic epitopes from the large HBsAg molecule, present in very small numbers in hepatitis B carrier plasma, but able to be produced in large numbers in yeast by recombinant DNA techniques. *Principle: When a fundamental mechanism of drug resistance is revealed (e.g., MHC restriction) and the molecular means to circumvent it are discovered, look for the same concept to be explored for other drugs with other indications (vaccines).*

Treatment of established infections is supportive. Liver transplantation has been associated with a nearly universal recurrence of hepatitis B in the transplanted liver, which undergoes an accelerated progression to cirrhosis and liver failure. Hepatitis B can be complicated by simultaneous infection with the hepatitis D virus, a small RNA virus most closely related to viroids of plants. This virus is defective and requires simultaneous hepatitis B infection for infection and multiplication in most hosts. Hepatitis D infection is frequently associated with a rapidly progressive chronic active hepatitis or cirrhosis, or with a fulminant acute presentation. There are no known preventive measures or useful treatment (Rizzetto et al., 1988).

The hepatitis C virus, an RNA virus similar to flaviviruses, was isolated and characterized from the plasma of a chimpanzee infected with a plasma concentrate known to have transmitted non-A non-B hepatitis to humans. The development of a specific antibody test has enabled retrospective studies on previously banked blood and prospective studies on patients with previously uncharacterized chronic hepatitis classified as non-A non-B hepatitis. These studies establish the presence of antibodies to hepatitis C virus in over 90% of patients with posttransfusion hepatitis, and in at least 60% of patients with non-transfusion-associated chronic non-A non-B disease (Kuo et al., 1989). The use of globulin prophylaxis prior to blood transfusion has not been clearly shown to prevent posttransfusion hepatitis C (non-A non-B hepatitis) (Seeff et al., 1977). The reduction of posttransfusion hepatitis from 20% in the 1960s to the current estimated level of 1% to 2% has been achieved mainly by the use of volunteer blood and measures to screen volunteers for risks of parenterally transmitted viral disease through community educational programs and direct questioning at the time of donation. Testing of donated blood for the presence of hepatitis C virus is likely to lead to further decreases in the rate of posttransfusion hepatitis, since a worldwide sampling of healthy first-time blood donors revealed that 0.4% to 2.4% test positive in the currently available antibody test to hepatitis C virus.

In summary, hepatitis A and B are preventable diseases. All patients with viral hepatitis should receive supportive therapy, the intensity of which is related to their degree of liver failure. Although liver transplantation is a therapeutic option in the patient with viral hepatitis of any cause and liver failure, recurrent disease is common with hepatitis B and D and leads to early deaths from liver failure.

Alcoholic Liver Disease

Alcohol consumption greater than 80 g/day for 15 years or more has been associated with the development of clinically significant liver disease. The major pathologic manifestations of alcohol-induced liver injury are fatty liver, alcoholic hepatitis, and cirrhosis. Other less specific histologic findings include fibrosis, chronic active hepatitis, and hepatocellular carcinoma. The death rate from alcoholic liver disease in a given country is proportional to the consumption of ethanol. In individuals with alcoholic liver disease, prognosis deteriorates once severe clinical manifestations of the disease occur. Patients with alcoholic liver disease have at least a 35% death rate during the year following their first episode of jaundice, ascites, or hematemesis. Longer survival is seen in those who abstain from alcohol. Therefore, the most important treatment modality for patients with alcoholic liver disease is lifelong abstinence, and all other potential treatments must be considered adjunctive therapy.

Because ethanol metabolism mediated by alcohol dehydrogenase leads to production of acetaldehyde, the pathogenesis of alcohol-related liver injury generally has been attributed to direct or indirect effects of acetaldehyde. Recent work has focused on the role of an ethanol-inducible cytochrome P450IIE1 in ethanol metabolism and tolerance, and its ability to activate other potential hepatotoxins. Additional evidence suggests a role for acetaldehyde-protein adducts in the establishment of immune injury or in production of free radicals or lipid peroxidation (Lieber, 1988). However, the actual mechanism of hepatocellular injury is unknown, so recent trials have embarked on empiric therapy based on theoretical mechanisms of injury that may never be proved correct. Colchicine, steroid hormones, and propylthiouracil have all been evaluated for this indication.

Colchicine is a relatively safe drug when used over years of continual treatment. It is relatively inexpensive and has been shown to inhibit fibrogenesis in vitro. It was recently studied in Mexico City in a randomized, placebo-controlled trial of 100 patients with predominantly alcoholic cirrhosis (Kershenobich et al., 1988). Patients who received colchicine 1 mg daily had a median survival of 11 years; those randomized to placebo had a median survival of 3.5 years. Enhanced survival was accompanied by histologic improvement as determined by follow-up needle biopsies of the liver. Interpretation of the data from this study is made difficult by a high rates of noncompliance and dropout and by persistent use of alcohol in both groups. Also, a lower serum albumin concentration in the control group at baseline may indicate failure of randomization to balance treatment and placebo groups with respect to this important marker of the severity of liver disease.

Corticosteroids have been studied repeatedly in patients with alcoholic liver injury because of their potential effects on mediators of inflammation and fibrogenesis. Data supporting their use have been mixed; most recently, a randomized, placebo-controlled multicenter study of 263 patients showed no efficacy of prednisolone (Mendenhall et al., 1984). The same study suggested a long-term but no short-term benefit associated with use of oxandrolone, 80 mg daily for 1 month. Because of the possibility that failure to demonstrate efficacy was due to the presence of an overwhelming number of patients with a favorable clinical outcome in the studies to date, another multicenter, randomized, placebo-controlled study was designed to enroll and study only those patients predicted to have a high 30-day mortality because of the presence of high concentrations of serum bilirubin, markedly prolonged prothrombin time and/or the presence of spontaneous hepatic encephalopathy (Maddrey et al., 1986). The 30-day mortality was 2/35 in the treatment group versus 11/31 in the control group. Confirmation of these dramatic results in a similar group of patients at high risk of death and longer follow-up of the study cohort are both necessary.

The use of propylthiouracil (PTU) in patients with alcoholic hepatitis arises from the suggestion that a hypermetabolic state making the centrilobular area of the liver relatively susceptible to ischemic or toxic damage is fundamental to the pathogenesis of alcoholic liver disease and its characteristic early lesion of perivenular fibrosis. In hospitalized patients with mild to moderate alcoholic hepatitis, administration of propylthiouracil 300 mg/day did not result in decreased mortality (7/31 in the treatment group versus 7/36 in placebo recipients) or improved tests of liver function (Halle et al., 1982). However, in a randomized, placebo-controlled study of 310 outpatients with various degrees of alcoholic liver injury, a significant survival advantage was seen in the propylthiouracil treatment group over the placebo group, despite continued alcohol ingestion (Orrego et al., 1987). The high dropout rate in this study led to insufficient data for analysis of the effect on tests of liver function.

Until more definitive studies are conducted in patients with similar conditions, the therapist must make a decision for his or her patients based on inconclusive and conflicting data. One may consider the relatively safe and inexpensive therapy with colchicine in patients with chronic stable alcoholic cirrhosis as an adjunct to abstinence and await further data on steroids and antithyroid drugs. One may also identify a subgroup of patients who are likely to have a poor prognosis (such as those with acute severe alcoholic hepatitis with spontaneous hepatic encephalopathy) and choose to treat them with prednisolone because it is the drug with most promise in this setting.

Because the effects of these three drugs on tests of liver function or other predictors of success is still unclear, one is faced with the use of potentially harmful drugs without the ability to individualize drug dosage, minimize side effects, or monitor efficacy. *Principle: Physicians almost never have information adequate to optimize therapy. The clinician can gain some solace in knowing that more information is coming and that a number of answers will involve new indications for old drugs (e.g., colchicine, PTU, or corticosteroids for cirrhosis; aspirin for myocardial infarction). When experimental results are conflicting and final conclusions are unclear, choose the least toxic drug and monitor the patient carefully. Be prepared to change the therapeutic plan as new or confirmed data are published.*

Acknowledgment — The author is indebted to Drs. James L. Boyer and L. Frederick Fenster, whose section on hepatic disorders in the prior edition of this textbook inspired and formed the framework for the current chapter.

REFERENCES

Allen, M. J.; Borody, T. J.; Bugliosi, T. F.; May, G. R.; LaRusso, N. F.; and Thistle, J. L.: Rapid dissolution of gallstones by methyl *tert*-butyl ether. Preliminary observations. N. Engl. J. Med., 312(4):217–220, 1985.

Alper, C.; Kruskall, M.; Marcus-Bagley, D.; Craven, D.; Katz, A.; Brink, S.; Dienstag, J.; Awdeh, Z.; and Yunis, E.: Genetic prediction of nonresponse to hepatitis B vaccine. N. Engl. J. Med., 321(11):707–712, 1989.

Arimura, A.; Sato, H.; Dupont, A.; Nishi, N.; and Schally, A. V.: Somatostatin: Abundance of immunoreactive hormone in rat stomach and pancreas. Science, 189(4207):1007–1009, 1975.

Baker, C.; Smith, C.; and Lieberman, G.: The natural history of esophageal varices. Am. J. Med., 26:228–237, 1959.

Balistreri, W.: Viral hepatitis. Pediatr. Clin. North. Am., 35: 637–669, 1988.

Bassett, M. L.; Halliday, J. W.; and Powell, L. W.: Hemochro-

matosis — Newer concepts: Diagnosis and management. D.M., 26(4):1–44, 1980.

Beppu, K.; Inokuchi, K.; Koyanagi, N.; Nakayama, S.; Sakata, H.; Kitano, S.; and Kobayashi, M.: Prediction of variceal hemorrhage by esophageal endoscopy. Gastrointest. Endosc., 27(4):213–218, 1981.

Blackburn, G.; and O'Keefe, S.: Nutrition in liver failure. Gastroenterology, 97:1049–1051, 1989.

Bosch, J.; Kravetz, D.; and Rodes, J.: Effects of somatostatin on hepatic and systemic hemodynamics in patients with cirrhosis of the liver: Comparison with vasopressin. Gastroenterology, 80(3):518–525, 1981.

Brazeau, P.; Vale, W.; Burgus, R.; Ling, N.; Butcher, M.; Rivier, J.; and Guillemin, R.: Hypothalamic polypeptide that inhibits the secretion of immunoreactive pituitary growth hormone. Science, 179:77–79, 1973.

Bunton, G.; and Cameron, R.: Regeneration of liver after biliary cirrhosis. Ann. N.Y. Acad. Sci., 111:412–421, 1963.

Cello, J.; Grendell, J.; Crass, R.; Weber, T.; and Trunkey, D.: Endoscopic sclerotherapy versus portacaval shunt in patient with severe cirrhosis and acute variceal hemorrhage. N. Engl. J. Med., 316:11–15, 1987.

Cerra, F. B.; Cheung, N. K.; Fischer, J. E.; Kaplowitz, N.; Schiff, E. R.; Dienstag, J. L.; Bower, R. H.; Mabry, C. D.; Leevy, C. M.; and Kiernan, T.: Disease-specific amino acid infusion (F080) in hepatic encephalopathy: A prospective, randomized, double-blind, controlled trial. J. Parenter. Enter. Nutr., 9(3):288–295, 1985.

Conn, H. O.; Leevy, C. M.; Vlahcevic, Z. R.; Rodgers, J. B.; Maddrey, W. C.; Seeff, L.; and Levy, L. L.: Comparison of lactulose and neomycin in the treatment of chronic portalsystemic encephalopathy. A double blind controlled trial. Gastroenterology, 72(pt. 1):573–583, 1977.

duVigneaud, V.; Gish, D.; and Katsoyannis, P.: A synthetic preparation possessing biological properties associated with arginine vasopressin. J. Am. Chem. Soc., 76:4751–4752, 1954.

Enrico, R.; Bazzoli, F.; Labate, A.; Mazzella, G.; Roda, A.; Sama, C.; Festi, D.; Aldini, R.; Taroni, F.; and Barbara, L.: Ursodeoxycholic acid vs. chenodeoxycholic acid as cholesterol gallstone–dissolving agents: A comparative randomized study. Hepatology, 2(6):804–809, 1982.

Epstein, M.: The Kidney in Liver Disease. Elsevier-North Holland, New York, 1988.

Erlinger, S.; Le Go, A.; Husson, J.; and Fevery, J.: Franco-Belgian Cooperative Study of ursodeoxycholic acid in the medical dissolution of gallstones: A double-blind, randomized, dose–response study, and comparison with chenodeoxycholic acid. Hepatology, 4(2):308–314, 1984.

Fisher, M. M.; Roberts, E. A.; Rosen, I. E.; Shapero, T. F.; Sutherland, L. R.; Davies, R. S.; Bacchus, R.; and Lee, S. V.: The Sunnybrook Gallstone Study: A double-blind controlled trial of chenodeoxycholic acid for gallstone dissolution. Hepatology, 5(1):102–107, 1985.

Fogel, M. R.; Knauer, C. M.; Andres, L. L.; Mahal, A. S.; Stein, D. E.; Kemeny, M. J.; Rinki, M. M.; Walker, J. E.; Siegmund, D.; and Gregory, P. B.: Continuous intravenous vasopressin in active upper gastrointestinal bleeding. Ann. Intern. Med., 96(5):565–569, 1982.

Fraser, C. L.; and Arieff, A. I.: Hepatic encephalopathy. N. Engl. J. Med., 313(14):865–873, 1985.

Freeman, J. G.; Cobden, I.; Lishman, A. H.; and Record, C. O.: Controlled trial of terlipressin (Glypressin) versus vasopressin in the early treatment of oesophageal varices. Lancet, 2:66–68, 1982.

Friedman, L. S.; Roberts, M. S.; Brett, A. S.; and Marton, K. I.: Management of asymptomatic gallstones in the diabetic patient. A decision analysis. Ann. Intern. Med., 109(11):913–919, 1988.

Gelman, S.; and Ernst, E.: Nitroprusside prevents adverse hemodynamic effects of vasopressin. Arch. Surg., 113:1465–1471, 1979.

Ginès, P.; Tító, L.; Arroyo, V.; Planas, R.; Panés, J.; Viver, J.; Torres, M.; Humbert, P.; Rimola, A.; Llach, J.; Badalamenti, S.; Jiménez, W.; Gaya, J.; and Rodés, J.: Randomized comparative study of therapeutic paracentesis with and without intravenous albumin in cirrhosis. Gastroenterology, 94(6):1493–1502, 1988.

Ginèzs, P.; Arroyo, V.; Quintero, E.; Planas, R.; Bory, F.; Cabrera, J.; Rimola, A.; Viver, J.; Camps, J.; Jiménez, W.; Mastai, K.; Gaya, J.; and Rodés, J.: Comparison of paracentesis and diuretics in the treatment of cirrhotics with tense ascites. Results of a randomized study. Gastroenterology, 93(2):234–241, 1987.

Gracie, W.; and Ransohoff, D.: The natural history of silent gallstones: The innocent gallstone is not a myth. N. Engl. J. Med., 307(13):798–816, 1982.

Graham, D. Y.; and Smith, J. L.: The course of patients after variceal hemorrhage. Gastroenterology, 80(4):800–809, 1981.

Groszmann, R.; Blei, A.; and Atterbury, C.: Pathophysiology of portal hypertension. Liver: Biol. Pathobiol., 1147–1158, 1988.

Groszmann, R. J.; Kravetz, D.; Bosch, J.; Glickman, M.; Bruix, J.; Bredfeldt, J.; Cohn, H. O.; Rodes, J.; and Storer, E. H.: Nitroglycerin improves the hemodynamic response to vasopressin in portal hypertension. Hepatology, 2:757–762, 1982.

Hadler, S. C.; Francis, D. P.; Maynard, J. E.; Thompson, S. E.; Judson, F. N.; Echenberg, D. F.; Ostrow, D. G.; O'Malley, P. M.; Penley, K. A.; Altman, N. L.; Braff, E.; Shipman, G. F.; Coleman, P. J.; and Mandel, E. J.: Long-term immunogenicity and efficacy of hepatitis B vaccine in homosexual men. N. Engl. J. Med., 315(4):209–214, 1986.

Halle, P.; Pare, P.; Kaptein, E.; Kanel, G.; Redeker, A. G.; and Reynolds, T. B.: Double-blind, controlled trial of propylthiouracil in patients with severe acute alcoholic hepatitis. Gastroenterology, 82(5, pt. 1):925–931, 1982.

Holzbach, R.: Recent progress in understanding cholesterol crystal nucleation as a precursor to human gallstone formation. Hepatology, 6:1403–1446, 1986.

Hsia, D.; and Walker, F.: Variability in the clinical manifestations of galactosemia. J. Pediatr., 59:872–883, 1961.

Huizinga, W.: Esophageal transection versus injection sclerotherapy in the management of bleeding esophageal varices in patients at high risk. Surg. Gynecol. Obstet., 160:539–546, 1985.

Infante, R.; Esnaola, S.; and Villeneuve, J.: Role of endoscopic variceal sclerotherapy in the long-term management of variceal bleeding: A meta-analysis. Gastroenterology, 96(4):1087–1092, 1989.

Ingelfinger, F. J.: Digestive disease as a national problem: V. Gallstones. Gastroenterology, 55(1):102–104, 1968.

Jarvinen, H.; and Hasrbacka, J.: Early cholecystectomy for acute cholecystitis. A prospective randomized study. Ann. Surg., 191:501–505, 1980.

Kershenobich, D.; Vargas, F.; and Garcia-Tsao, G.: Colchicine in the treatment of cirrhosis of the liver. N. Engl. J. Med., 318:1709–1713, 1988.

Kravetz, D.; Bosch, J.; Teres, J.; Bruix, J.; Rimola, A.; and Rodes, J.: Comparison of intravenous somatostatin and vasopressin infusions in treatment of acute variceal hemorrhage. Hepatology, 4(3):442–446, 1984.

Kuo, G.; Choo, Q. L.; Alter, H. J.; Gitnick, G. L.; Redeker, A. G.; Purcell, R. H.; Miyamura, T.; Dienstag, J. L.; Alter, M. J.; Stevens, C. E; Tegtmeier, G. E.; Fonino, F.; Colombo, M.; Lee, W.-S.; Koo, C.; Berger, K.; Shuster, J. R.; Overby, L. R.; Bradley, D. W.; and Houghton, M.: An assay for circulating antibodies to a major etiologic virus of human non-A, non-B hepatitis. Science, 244(4902):362–364, 1989.

Lewis, J. H.; Zimmerman, H. J.; Garrett, C. T.; and Rosenberg, E.: Valproate-induced hepatic steatogenesis in rats. Hepatology, 2(6):870–873, 1982.

Lieber, C.: Metabolic effects of ethanol and its interaction with other drugs, hepatotoxic agents, vitamins, and carcinogens: A 1988 update. Semin. Liver Dis., 8(1):47–67, 1988.

MacDougall, B.; Bailey, R.; and Williams, R.: H_2 receptor antagonists and antacids in the prevention of acute gastrointestinal hemorrhage in fulminant hepatic failure, two controlled trials. Lancet, 1:617–619, 1977.

Maddrey, W.; Carithers, R. Jr.; Combes, B.; Diehl, A. M.;

Shaw, E.; and Fallon, H. J.: Prednisolone therapy in patients with severe alcoholic hepatitis: Results of multi-center trial. Hepatology, 6:1202, 1986.

Marks, J.; Lan, S.; and the National Cooperative Gallstone Study Committee: Low dose chenodiol for the prevention of gallstone recurrence following dissolution therapy: The National Cooperative Gallstone Study. Ann. Intern. Med., 100:376–381, 1984.

Mendenhall, C.; Anderson, S.; and Garcia-Pont, P.: Short-term and long-term survival in patients with alcoholic hepatitis treated with oxandrolone and prednisolone. N. Engl. J. Med., 311:1464–1469, 1984.

O'Donnell, L.; and Heaton, K.: Recurrence and re-recurrence of gall stones after medical dissolution: A longterm follow-up. Gut, 29:655–658, 1988.

Orrego, H.; Blake, J.; Blendis, L.; Compton, K. V.; and Isreal, Y.: Long-term treatment of alcoholic liver disease with propylthiouracil. N. Engl. J. Med., 317:1421–1427, 1987.

Podda, M.; Zuin, M.; Battezzati, P. M.; Ghezzi, C.; de Fazio, C.; and Dioguardi, M. L.: Efficacy and safety of a combination of chenodeoxycholic acid and ursodeoxycholic acid for gallstone dissolution: A comparison with ursodeoxycholic acid alone. Gastroenterology, 96(1):222–229, 1989.

Rabkin, R.; Share, L.; Payne, P.; Young, J.; and Crofton, J.: The handling of immunoreactive vasopressin by the isolated perfused rat kidney. J. Clin. Invest., 63:6–13, 1979.

Ramalingaswami, V.; and Purcell, R.: Waterborne non-A, non-B hepatitis. Lancet, 1:571–573, 1988.

Ransohoff, D.; Gracie, W.; Wolfenson, L.; and Neuhauser, D.: Prophylactic cholecystectomy or expectant management for silent gallstones. Ann. Intern. Med., 99:199–204, 1983.

Rizzetto, M.; Bonino, F.; and Verme, G.: Hepatitis delta virus infection of the liver: Progress in virology, pathobiology, and diagnosis. Semin. Liver Dis., 8(4):350–356, 1988.

Roda, E.; Bazzoli, F.; Labate, A.; Mazzela, G.; Roda, A.; Sama, C.; Festi, D.; Aldini, R.; Taroni, F.; and Barbara, L.: Ursodeoxycholic acid vs. chenodeoxzycholic acid as cholesterol gallstone–dissolving agents: A comparative randomized study. Hepatology, 2:804–810, 1982.

Runyon, B.: Patients with deficient ascitic fluid opsonic activity are predisposed to spontaneous bacterial peritonitis. Hepatology, 8:632–635, 1988.

Runyon, B.; Umland, E.; and Merlin, T.: Inoculation of blood culture bottles with ascitic fluid; improved detection of spontaneous bacterial peritonitis. Arch. Intern. Med., 147:73–75, 1987.

Runyon, B. A.; Canawati, H. N.; and Akriviadis, E. A.: Optimization of ascitic fluid culture technique. Gastroenterology, 95(5):1351–1355, 1988.

Sackmann, M.; Delius, M.; Sauerbruch, T.; Holl, J.; Weber, W.; Ippisch, E.; Hagelauer, U.; Wess, O.; Hepp, W.; Brendel, W.; and Paumgartner, G.: Shock-wave lithotripsy of gallbladder stones. The first 175 patients. N. Engl. J. Med., 318(7):393–397, 1988.

Scheinberg, I. H.; and Sternlieb, I.: The long-term management of hepatolenticular degeneration. Am. J. Med., 29:316–333, 1960.

Schoenfield, L.; Lachin, J.; and the Steering Committee, National Cooperative Gallstone Study: A controlled trial of the efficacy and safety of chenodeoxycholic acid as cholesterol gallstone–dissolving agents: A comparative randomized study. Ann. Intern. Med., 95:257–282, 1981.

Schrier, R.: Osmotic and nonosmotic control of vasopressin release. Am. J. Physiol., 236:F321–F332, 1979.

Seeff, L. B.; Zimmerman, H. J.; Wright, E. C.; Finkelstein, J. D.; Garcia, P. P.; Greenlee, H. B.; Dietz, A. A.; Leevy, C. M.; Tamburro, C. H.; Schiff, E. R.; Schimmel, E. M.; Zemel, R.; Zimmon, D. S.; and McCollum, R. W.: A randomized, double blind controlled trial of the efficacy of immune serum globulin for the prevention of post-transfusion hepatitis. A Veterans Administration cooperative study. Gastroenterology, 72(1):111–121, 1977.

Shear, L.; Ching, S.; and Gabuzda, G. J.: Compartmentalization of ascites and edema in patients with hepatic cirrhosis. N. Engl. J. Med., 282(25):1391–1396, 1970.

Soloway, R.; Trotman, B.; and Ostrow, J.: Pigment gallstones. Gastroenterology, 72:167–182, 1977.

Spielberg, S. P.; Gordon, G. B.; Blake, D. A.; Goldstein, D. A.; and Herlong, H. F.: Predisposition to phenytoin hepatotoxicity assessed in vitro. N. Engl. J. Med., 305(13):722–727, 1981.

Stanley, M. M.; Ochi, S.; Lee, K. K.; Nemchausky, B. A.; Greenlee, H. B.; Allen, J. I.; Allen, M. J.; Baum, R. A.; Gadacz, T. R.; Camara, D. S.; Caruana, J. A.; Schiff, E. R.; Livingstone, A. S.; Samanta, A. K.; Najem, A. Z.; Glick, M. E.; Juler, G. L.; Adham, N.; Baker, J. D.; Cain, G. D.; Jordan, P. H.; Wolf, D. L.; Iulenwider, J. T.; and James, K. E.: Peritoneovenous shunting as compared with medical treatment in patients with alcoholic cirrhosis and massive ascites. Veterans Administration Cooperative Study on Treatment of Alcoholic Cirrhosis with Ascites. N. Engl. J. Med., 321(24):1632–1638, 1989.

Starzl, T.; Demetris, A.; and Van Thiel, D.: Liver transplantation (first of two parts). N. Engl. J. Med., 321:1013–1022, 1989.

Sternlieb, I.: Copper and the liver. Gastroenterology, 78:1615–1628, 1980.

Stevens, C. E.; Taylor, P. E.; Tong, M. J.; Toy, P. T.; Vyas, G. N.; Nair, P. V.; Weissman, J. Y.; and Krugman, S.: Yeast-recombinant hepatitis B vaccine. Efficacy with hepatitis B immune globulin in prevention of perinatal hepatitis B virus transmission. J.A.M.A., 257(19):2612–2616, 1987.

Stokes, J. Jr.; and Neefe, J.: The prevention and attenuation of infectious hepatitis by gamma globulin. J.A.M.A., 127: 44–45, 1945.

Thistle, J.: Direct contact dissolution of gallstones. Semin. Liver Dis., 7:311–316, 1987.

Ward, A.; Brogden, R.; Heel, R.; Speight, T. M.; and Avery, S. S.: Ursodeoxycholic acid — A review of its pharmacological properties and therapeutic efficacy. Drugs, 27(2):95–131, 1984.

Welper, W.; and Opitz, K.: Histologic changes in the liver biopsy in *Amanita phalloides* intoxication. Hum. Pathol., 3: 249–254, 1972.

Yeh, F.; Yu, M.; Mo, C.; Luo, S.; Tong, M.; and Henderson, B.: Hepatitis B virus, aflatoxins, and hepatocellular carcinoma in southern Guangxi, China. Cancer Res., 49(9):2506–2509, 1989.

Zimmerman, H.: Hepatotoxicity: The Adverse Effects of Drugs and Other Chemicals on the Liver. Appleton-Century-Crofts, New York, 1978.

10

Nutrition

Irwin H. Rosenberg and Elliot M. Berry

There are many therapeutic modalities available to the practicing physician. Some patients require drug medication, some require the application of a device, and others may benefit from physiotherapy—but all require adequate nutrition. Some 50% of patients hospitalized for surgery show some signs of undernutrition (Butterworth and Blackburn, 1975). That an even greater proportion are undernourished at discharge is testimony to the requirement for greater attention to the nutritional management of the hospitalized patient. By contrast, in the outpatient setting a considerable proportion of the population suffers from overnutrition or obesity. Correct nutritional management deserves high priority in both inpatient and ambulatory settings. Nutritional problems may be more acute in surgery, where patients spend long periods of time on IV therapy with low calorie intakes. In the past decade, the management of the severely ill patient has been altered radically by the advent of total parenteral nutrition (TPN). Diet therapy is an integral part of the management of heart disease, hypertension, liver, GI, and renal disease, endocrine-metabolic problems such as diabetes mellitus and the hyperlipidemias, and also as an adjunct to cancer therapy. The list is not comprehensive, but it emphasizes the variety of diseases affected by the state of nutrition. Yet, despite this, insufficient attention is given to the nutritional aspects of patient management. *Principle: It would be limiting for a doctor to have no tools to interdict disease; worse would be to misuse or neglect to use those that could work; and most inappropriate would be to use a tool so that harm were the only noticeable effect. Nutrition therapy should not be any more neglected than drug therapy.*

Good medical practice requires that every patient—whether in the hospital or in the clinic—be given a nutritional plan. Such a plan will take into account the nutritional status of the patient, the nature of his or her disease, and the social circumstances concerning food availability and cooking. In many ways formulating a nutritional plan is like prescribing a drug; it requires attention to detail and a knowledge of metabolism and pathophysiology, as well as the lifestyle of the patient. It also requires setting clear-cut objectives that can be followed to assess the adequacy of the "prescription."

In this chapter we consider the pathophysiologic concepts underlying nutritional status in health and disease, the interactions between diet, medication, and disease, and the basis for a quantitative approach to the nutritional management of the patient.

NUTRITIONAL REQUIREMENTS IN HEALTH AND DISEASE

Caloric Requirements

A comprehensive nutritional plan must begin with an estimation of individual nutritional requirements of the patient. The patient's caloric requirements are determined by the basal metabolic rate (BMR), activity level, and disease severity. In practice the BMR and the resting energy expenditure (REE) differ by less than 10%, and therefore the terms may be used interchangeably. The REE accounts for approximately two thirds of the total energy requirements and is affected by body build (in particular lean body mass), age, sex, and habitus. Convenient formulas for calculating the REE are shown in Table 10–1. Note that the REE declines approximately 2% per decade over the age of 45 years. The REE also includes the energy requirements for absorbing, digesting, and processing nutrients, the so-called diet-induced thermogenesis (DIT). In hypermetabolic patients, DIT is less marked because heat production is already elevated. In calculating additional energy requirements for such patients, the DIT should be estimated at no more than 5% of total energy requirements.

Energy for Activity. The energy of physical activity is about one third of the total expenditure and can vary from 2 to 12 kcal/min. This factor is more important in calculating energy requirements for active, ambulatory patients. If the proportion of time spent in exercise is unknown, then it is possible to use activity factors as a multiple of the REE; these have been converted to energy expenditure in kilocalories per kilogram per day (Table 10–2). For example, the caloric requirements of a 70-kg man on a moderate work schedule can be calculated from the table at 70 kg × 41 kcal/kg per day = 2870 kcal/day. For a 58-kg woman on a light routine, the calculation would be 58 kg × 35 kcal/kg per day = 2030 kcal/day.

Activity level declines over the age of 45 by about 200 kcal/day and reaches 500 kcal/day less for persons over the age of 70 years.

Additional Energy Requirements of Illness. Heat production increases with fever and inflammation. However, in the patient with inflammation, as oxygen consumption increases, DIT decreases, and the energy of activity declines owing to immobility. For these reasons, the daily energy requirement of ill persons is usually only slightly greater than the requirement of the healthy. Indeed, the energy requirement for most patients, even during severe illness, rarely exceeds 3000 kcal/day. The earlier estimates of massively increased calorie requirements in patients with sepsis have not been substantiated. *Principle: While clinical cliches can be attractive and seem by their age and nature to ring true, be certain that they are based on fact before using them. How efficacious is it to "feed a fever"?*

Malabsorption is another cause of altered energy balance. The most accurate way to assess calorie loss due to malabsorption would be calorimetry of the feces. A more practical way is to multiply the daily fat excretion in grams by a factor of 9 kcal/g (the caloric value for fat). To estimate the total fecal energy loss, this value should be then multiplied by 2.5, assuming average dietary composition and equivalent malabsorption of fat, carbohydrate, and protein. Thus, in summary, the total energy equivalent lost in the feces per day = fecal fat (g/day) × 9 kcal/g × 2.5.

Caloric requirements may be estimated for different patients according to the severity of disease, as well for the extra needs during pregnancy and lactation using the factors in Table 10–3.

Protein Requirements

Calculation of the total caloric requirements alone is not sufficient for optimal patient care. Attention must be given to the quality of the diet, in particular the protein content. Unlike the storage of triglycerides and glycogen, the storage of proteins (or amino acids) in the body for utilization in times of need does not occur. Every protein serves a structural or metabolic function, and when excess protein is ingested, the amino acids are deaminated and the nonnitrogenous portion of the molecule serves as a source of calories for storage as glycogen or fat.

In conditions of malnutrition or acute starvation, several tissues including the brain can utilize only glycolytic pathways to obtain energy. Since the conversion of fatty acids to carbohydrate is inadequate in humans, such glucose-requiring tissues must utilize either glucose or substrates that can be converted to glucose. During prolonged

Table 10–1.   EQUATIONS FOR PREDICTING RESTING ENERGY EXPENDITURE FROM BODY WEIGHT*

AGE RANGE (YEARS)	EQUATION TO DERIVE REE IN KCAL/DAY
Males	
0–3	(60.9 × wt) − 54
3–10	(22.7 × wt) + 495
10–18	(17.5 × wt) + 651
18–30	(15.3 × wt) + 679
30–60	(11.6 × wt) + 879
>60	(13.5 × wt) + 487
Females	
0–3	(61.0 × wt) − 51
3–10	(22.5 × wt) + 499
10–18	(12.2 × wt) + 746
18–30	(14.7 × wt) + 496
30–60	(8.7 × wt) + 829
>60	(10.5 × wt) + 596

* Modified from WHO (1985). These equations were derived from BMR data.

Table 10-2. FACTORS FOR ESTIMATING DAILY ENERGY ALLOWANCES AT VARIOUS LEVELS OF *PHYSICAL ACTIVITY* FOR MEN AND WOMEN (AGES 19-50)

KCAL/MIN	ACTIVITY FACTOR ($\times$ REE)	ENERGY EXPENDITURE EXAMPLE (KCAL/KG PER DAY)	
Resting (REE)			
Men 1.0	1.0	24	Sleeping
Women 1.0	1.0	23	Reclining
Very Light			
Men <2.5	1.3	31	Clerical
Women 2.0	1.3	30	Driving
Light			
Men 2.5-5.0	1.6	38	Housework, child care
Women 2.0-4.0	1.5	35	Golf, strolling
Moderate			
Men 5.0-7.5	1.7	41	Carrying a load
Women 4.0-6.0	1.6	37	Walking 4 mph
Heavy			
Men 7.5-12.0	2.1	50	Running
Women 6.0-10.0	1.9	44	Walking uphill with load

Table 10-3. CALORIC AND PROTEIN REQUIREMENTS UNDER VARIOUS CIRCUMSTANCES*†

	CALORIES (KCAL/KG PER DAY)	PROTEIN (G/KG PER DAY)	COMMENT
Normal adult	25	0.8	
Mild stress	30	1.0	Uncomplicated surgery, vigorous exercise
Moderate stress	35	1.2	Sepsis, trauma
Severe stress	40	1.4	40% surface burn
Pregnancy	30	1.0	Additional 300 kcal/day
Lactation	35	1.2	Additional 500 kcal/day and 15 g protein/day

* Requirements for infants and children vary considerably with age, and reference tables (RDA) should be consulted.

† The use of doubly labeled water in the future is likely to revolutionize the measurement of energy expenditure in free-living subjects and patients alike.

starvation, ketone bodies increasingly become a source of energy. Amino acids derived primarily from skeletal muscle constitute the major endogenous source of carbon for production of glucose for this purpose. Since there is no storage form of protein, a fasting individual sustains a constant daily loss of functionally or structurally significant protein. Thus, the maintenance of adequate protein balance is a major consideration when planning nutritional rehabilitation.

On a diet adequate in calories but free of protein, the minimal nitrogen loss from a 70-kg person approximates 1.9 to 3.1 g/day in urine, 0.7 to 2.5 g/day in stool, and 0.3 g/day from the skin. This obligatory nitrogen loss from the body has been extensively studied under metabolic conditions, and the values calculated have been in close agreement at an average of 53 (41-69) mg of nitrogen per kilogram per day. The equivalent protein loss may be calculated by multiplying the nitrogen loss by 6.25, which for a 70-kg man comes to 23 g/day, or about 0.33 g/kg body

weight. The lean body mass is about 16% to 20% protein; thus this loss corresponds to a daily loss of about 130 g of lean body mass. In order to accommodate for differences in the biologic quality of dietary protein and for the inefficiency of its utilization, the recommended daily protein allowance for adults is raised to 0.8 g/kg for both sexes. Vigorous exercise in normal people or the stress of illness may increase this requirement to 1.0 g/kg of body weight or higher (Table 10-3). A convenient and practical way of approximating nitrogen balance is to use the following approximate formula, where UUN is urinary urea nitrogen and the units are in grams per 24 hours:

Nitrogen balance =

$$\frac{\text{protein intake}}{6.25} - (\text{UUN} + 4)$$

On a diet of 0.8 g/kg per day in a 70-kg person, a UUN of less than 9 g per 24 hours is normal;

above 9 g per 24 hours represents negative nitrogen balance, and values above 12 g indicate severe catabolism of protein and metabolic stress. Dependence on the UUN may result in erroneous underestimation of the severity of negative nitrogen balance if major protein losses occur from other body sites such as from the GI tract or urine, or from the skin in severe burns.

Vitamin and Mineral Requirements

The current consensus for estimation of vitamin and mineral requirements is that of the recommended dietary allowances (RDAs) of the National Research Council, National Academy of Sciences (Table 10-4).

The RDAs are defined as "the levels of intake of essential nutrients considered, in the judgment of the Committee on Dietary Allowances of the Food and Nutrition Board on the basis of available scientific knowledge, to be adequate to meet the known nutritional needs of practically all healthy persons." The RDAs are not requirements for an individual, but recommendations for the daily amounts of nutrients to be consumed over a period of time to protect members of that population. With exception of the allowances for energy,

Table 10-4. RECOMMENDED VITAMIN AND MINERAL INTAKES FOR HEALTHY ADULTS (OVER 25 YEARS)*

	RANGE OF ADULT DIETARY ALLOWANCE
Vitamin A (μg retinol equivalent)	800–1000
Vitamin D (μg)	5.0–7.5
Vitamin E (mg α-tocopherol equivalents)	8–10
Vitamin C (mg)	60
Thiamine (mg)	1.0–1.5
Riboflavin (mg)	1.2–1.7
Niacin (mg niacin equivalent)	13–19
Vitamin B_6 (mg)	1.6–2.0
Folacin (μg)	180–200
Vitamin B_{12} (μg)	2.0
Calcium (mg)	800–1200
Phosphorus (mg)	800
Magnesium (mg)	280–350
Iron (mg)	10–15
Zinc (mg)	12–15
Iodine (μg)	150
Copper (mg)*	2.0–3.0
Manganese (mg)*	2.0–5.0
Fluoride (mg)*	1.5–4.0
Chromium (μg)*	50–200
Selenium (μg)*	55–70
Molybdenum (μg)*	75–250

* Estimated safe and adequate daily dietary intakes. From the National Research Council Recommended Dietary Allowances. National Academy of Sciences, Washington, D.C., 1989.

RDAs are estimated to exceed the requirements of most individuals to ensure that the needs of nearly all members of a population will be met. In this country, RDAs are usually set approximately 2 standard deviations (SDs) above the mean requirement and will therefore meet the needs of 97% of the population. Allowances are established for a wide range of age, weight, and sex groups and for pregnancy and lactation. The RDAs have not been set for all recognized essential nutrients. In the 10th edition of *Recommended Dietary Allowances*, issued in 1989, RDAs were set for 11 of the 13 known vitamins. Because of the lack of information on which to base allowances, the RDA committee established ranges of estimated safe and adequate daily dietary intakes for pantothenic acid and biotin. *Principle: The recommended allowances of nutrients and vitamins are almost equivalent to "doses of prescription drugs." In each case they can only be used as guidelines for the average person and in no way can substitute for careful individualization.*

Since the RDAs are established for healthy people, they do not cover special needs of persons with specific clinical problems, such as premature birth, inherited metabolic disorders, or infections; persons with specific catabolic states, including those who are attempting weight reduction; or those with chronic diseases or on drug therapy, all of which may alter requirements for given vitamins as discussed later.

PATHOGENESIS OF NUTRITIONAL DEFICIENCY

This section gives examples of the different mechanisms that may be involved in the pathogenesis of nutritional deficiency, especially of vitamins, minerals, or trace metals.

Decreased Dietary Intake

Insufficient intake of nutrients may result from anorexia, nausea and vomiting, or postprandial pain as in patients with peptic ulcer disease. Nutritional deficiency may also be iatrogenic and result from the highly restrictive diets that are often prescribed without sufficient attention to their nutritional value. In such cases, replacement therapy need only be directed at provision of those nutrients whose intake fails to meet the recommended dietary requirements.

Malabsorption

Disease of the pancreas, biliary tract, or small intestine may be associated with deficiencies of vitamins and minerals as well as malabsorption of fat, carbohydrate, and protein. In regard to vitamin malabsorption, the separation of vitamins into fat-soluble (A, D, E, K) and water-soluble (thiamine, riboflavin, niacin, pyridoxine, pantothenic acid, folate, vitamin B_{12}, and vitamin C) vitamins has some pragmatic clinical value. Deficiencies of the fat-soluble vitamins are most likely to occur when there is severe malabsorption of fat (steatorrhea). Deficiencies of water-soluble vitamins more closely reflect malabsorption of water-soluble macronutrients such as sugars and amino acids. Deficiencies usually are multiple and should be treated by multivitamin-mineral preparations.

Increased Loss

In addition to increased loss of nutrients by malabsorption, GI disease may be complicated by fecal nutrient loss caused by increased mucosal permeability as in protein-losing enteropathy. Severe diarrhea may lead to depletion of electrolytes such as potassium and magnesium and theoretically some water-soluble vitamins. Other sources of protein and electrolyte depletion are renal disease (e.g., nephrotic syndrome) and large-area burns.

Defective Utilization

Since most vitamins are ingested in a form that is not identical to their functional coenzyme state, they must undergo metabolic transformation in the intestinal mucosa or elsewhere. A defect in this transformation would have the same clinical effect as inadequate intake or malabsorption. An example of this phenomenon is the impaired final hydroxylation of vitamin D during severe renal disease that contributes to osteodystrophy (see chapter 11). A defect in the initial hepatic hydroxylation of vitamin D has been proposed as a factor in the bone disease associated with primary biliary cirrhosis. Some drugs may interfere with vitamin metabolism. Oral contraceptives interfere with pyridoxine; azulfidine, methotrexate, and alcohol interfere with folate.

Increased Requirement

Increased turnover of mucosal cells in celiac sprue and in ulcerative colitis, along with the increased demand for mobilization of inflammatory cells in those conditions, may contribute to the depletion of key nutrients such as folic acid that are required for cellular proliferation.

Drugs may influence all the above mechanisms. These aspects are dealt with separately below.

DEVELOPMENTAL STAGES OF NUTRIENT DEFICIENCY

Table 10-5 reviews the typical sequence of events in the evolution of vitamin deficiency and

Table 10-5.   STAGES OF VITAMIN DEFICIENCY

SUBCLINICAL DEFICIENCY	CLINICAL DEFICIENCY
Lowered plasma concentrations	Functional impairment
Lowered cell content	On challenge
Decreased apoenzyme activity	Spontaneous
Response to coenzyme addition	Tissue organ changes
Altered response to challenge	Reversible
	Irreversible

proposes a reasonable separation between subclinical and clinical deficiency states. The concept of subclinical deficiency is useful for describing stages of true vitamin depletion that precede symptoms and signs of clinical deficiency. One must recognize that deficiency states proceed through a temporal sequence with considerable individual variability (according to subject and nutrient) in the duration of each stage.

Although there are exceptions, the first step in depletion usually is a fall in circulating levels of the vitamin or its coenzyme state. This is followed by decreased urinary excretion, and finally by diminished concentration of the vitamin in tissue. This last stage is best demonstrated by a fall in vitamin content of circulating blood cells. Tissue depletion is accompanied by diminished coenzyme function or fat-soluble synthetic function, and these disturbances lead to functional abnormalities in vitamin-dependent metabolic pathways. At this stage of functional disturbance, symptoms of deficiency are most likely to be noted, although their manifestations may be very subtle. At more advanced stages of deficiency, visible signs appear, including changes in the skin and mucous membranes that represent pathologic manifestations of functional abnormalities. *Principle: The detection of nutritional deficiencies is equivalent to detection of most diseases. The earlier the abnormality, the more readily therapy will work to lower morbidity.*

FORMULATING A PLAN FOR NUTRITIONAL CARE

The components of a nutrition care plan are (1) assessing nutritional status, (2) setting nutritional goals, (3) implementing a nutritional plan and monitoring nutritional status. Assessment summarizes individual nutritional problems and needs based on history, physical examination, and relevant laboratory tests. The goals of the nutritional treatment are then set at the planning stage, and the diet prescription and appropriate patient education implemented. Since most dietary interventions involve a change in habits and behavior, the best plans will only be of use if compliance is carefully monitored by regular follow-up. *Principle: Nutrients may be thought of like drugs. Diagnosis directs the need to use them and the strategy for their use. Evaluation of efficacy and toxicity is needed in precisely the same way as for prescribing any other drug.*

Nutritional Assessment

The assessment of the nutritional status of a patient involves two components: the regular dietary intake (a modified diet history) and the level of nutrition, the latter of which reflects the interaction of diet and disease. The diet may have contributed to the disease, or the disease may cause additional dietary requirements.

Dietary Assessment. There are two levels of dietary assessment, qualitative and quantitative. Qualitative assessment involves a history of what the patient usually eats and what he or she avoids, recent weight changes, whether the patient is following a special diet, and if supplements or vitamins are taken (Table 10-6). Problems in eating (chewing, swallowing) and bowel function should also be noted. A balanced diet comprises choices from the major food categories — milk and eggs, fish and meat, cereals, and fruits and vegetables — as well as an adequate intake of fluid — at least five glasses a day.

Current recommendations for a healthful diet suggest four or more daily servings of breads, cereals, or legumes; four or more servings of fruits and vegetables; and two servings of poultry, meat, or fish. If the semiqualitative assessment suggests that there may be problems in nutrition, a detailed quantitation may be needed. This is usually done by a qualified dietician who utilizes methods such as 24-hour recalls and questionnaires regarding the frequency of food intake. Standard food composition tables are currently widely available as the data base for computer programs that can be used to establish the level of each nutrient and vitamin.

When considering the assessment of nutritional status, do not overlook the history and the physical examination by moving too quickly to more quantitative, biochemical, or microbiologic assays. As it is in other areas of therapeutics, a carefully performed history may be the most valuable means of screening for patients at particular risk as well as for identifying symptoms that suggest nutritional deficiency. The physical examination can often establish the severity of the problem and some of the pathogenic factors. The laboratory can help to confirm clinical suspicions but also may identify nutritional depletion at stages earlier than those represented by symptoms and physical findings.

Clinical History. Recent or prolonged changes in body weight in adults or changes of the velocity of growth in children are important risk factors for vitamin depletion. The past medical and surgical history may reveal diseases or conditions that place the individual at special risk for nutrition depletion. These factors are summarized in Table 10-6. This information raises the concern that there might be a problem in nutrition and helps focus the physical examination to find further clues of nutritional disease.

Physical Examination. The physical examination may identify signs of deficiency. Table 10-7 details the physical findings associated with a deficiency of nutrients. Like the historical data, however, many physical signs are nonspecific and require further confirmation from quantitative dietary or laboratory analysis. An example of such nonspecificity is skin pallor suggestive of anemia that may raise the possibility of inadequate iron, folic acid, or vitamin B_{12}. But there are many other nonnutritional causes of anemia. Similarly, changes in the skin or mucous membranes compatible with vitamin deficiency are rarely pathognomonic but rather help to identify elements in the differential diagnosis than can direct a more specific selection of laboratory diagnostic studies.

The overall nutritional assessment of a patient may be determined at the bedside without the need for sophisticated equipment or expensive laboratory tests. Weight and height are both important. Also, the body mass index (BMI) should

---

Table 10-6. FINDINGS IN THE MEDICAL HISTORY SUGGESTING INCREASED RISK OF NUTRIENT DEFICIENCY

Recent weight loss
Restricted dietary intake (limited variety)
  Drastic weight-loss program, liquid diet
  Fad diets
  Food avoidances
  Eating disorder — anorexia, bulimia
Problems with eating, chewing, swallowing
Previous GI surgery (e.g., partial gastrectomy, bowel resection)
Increased losses due to GI disorders such as malabsorption and diarrhea
Systemic disease interfering with appetite or eating (chronic lung, liver, heart and renal disease, abdominal angina, cancer)
Excessive alcohol use
Medications that might interfere with vitamin or nutrient metabolism
Psychosocial situation
  Depression, cognitive impairment
  Isolation, economic difficulties

Table 10-7. SIGNS CAUSED BY NUTRITIONAL DEFICIENCIES*

NUTRIENT	PHYSICAL SIGNS OF DEFICIENCY
Calories (energy)	Weight loss, loss of subcutaneous fat, muscle wasting, growth retardation
Protein	Muscle wasting, edema, skin and hair changes, dyspigmentation, hepatomegaly
Essential fatty acid	Scaly, eczematoid skin rash on face and extremities, hepatomegaly
Calcium	Tetany, convulsions, growth failure
Phosphorus	Weakness, osteomalacia
Magnesium	Weakness, tremor, tetany
Iron	Pallor, anemia, weakness, lingual atrophy, koilonychia
Zinc	Hypogeusia, acrodermatitis, slow wound healing, growth failure, hypogonadism, delayed puberty
Copper	Bone marrow suppression
Chromium	Glucose intolerance
Thiamine	Beriberi, muscle weakness, hypesthesia, tachycardia, heart failure
Riboflavin	Angular stomatitis, cheilosis, corneal vascularization, dermatoses
Niacin	Pellagra, glossitis, dermatosis, dementia, diarrhea
Vitamin B_6	Nasolabial seborrhea, peripheral neuropathy
Biotin	Organic aciduria
Folic acid	Macrocytosis, megaloblastic anemia, glossitis
Vitamin B_{12}	Megaloblastic anemia, paresthesias, mental changes, combined system degeneration
Vitamin A	Xerophthalmia, hyperkeratosis of skin
Vitamin D	Rickets and growth failure in children; osteomalacia in adults
Vitamin K	Bleeding, ecchymoses
Vitamin E	Cerebellar ataxia, areflexia

* Modified from Alpers et al. (1987).

be calculated. This is the ratio of the weight (in kilograms) to the square of the height (in meters^2), which standardizes body weight in relation to build. The range of normal values for the BMI varies with age as shown in Table 10–8, which is derived from age-specific mortality rates. If the BMI is below the lowest value appropriate for the patient's age, then the patient is probably undernourished. Subjects with a BMI above 27 are usually overweight, and those with a BMI above 30 are definitely obese. If the ratio is over 40 then the condition is called morbid obesity. All subjects with a BMI over 30, and especially those

Table 10-8. DESIRABLE BMI RANGE IN RELATION TO AGE*

AGE GROUP (YEARS)	BMI (KG/M^2)
19–24	19–24
25–34	20–25
35–44	21–26
45–54	22–27
55–64	23–28
65 +	24–29

* Modified from Bray (1976).

with an abdominal distribution of obesity—where the waist/hip ratio is greater than 1.0 in men or 0.8 in women—are at risk from the sequelae of obesity, in particular the metabolic complications such as non-insulin-dependent diabetes, hyperlipidemia, and cardiovascular disease (Kissebah et al., 1989). Again these figures represent averages and must be considered as a guide together with a weight history, which should include documentation of the dates of the highest and lowest weights. A patient with a reduced body weight and BMI over a decade is clearly in a different category from one who has lost 10 kg in the past 6 months. Clues to such weight loss may be seen from impressions on belt holes or a history of changing requirements in dress sizes. Laboratory indices for determining levels of energy-protein undernutrition may be found in Table 10–9.

The Nutritional Prescription

Based on clinical and laboratory assessment, a plan for care is devised to maintain status or correct deficiencies. The approach must be quantitative, and the route of administration of the diet must be specified.

Table 10–9.   QUANTITATIVE VALUES COMMONLY USED TO STRATIFY CALORIE-PROTEIN NUTRITIONAL STATUS

METHOD OF ASSESSMENT	MODERATELY MALNOURISHED	SEVERELY MALNOURISHED
% ideal weight	60–80	<60
Creatinine height index Actual 24-h urine creatinine × 100 Ideal 24-h urine creatinine for height and sex	60–80	<60
Serum albumin	2.1–3.0 g/dl (21–30 g/l)	<2.1
Serum transferrin	100–150 mg/dl (1–1.5 g/l)	<100
Total lymphocyte count	800–1200/mm^3 (0.8–1.2 × 10^9/l)	<800
Delayed hypersensitivity index*	1†	0†

* Delayed hypersensitivity index quantitates the amount of induration elicited by skin testing with a common antigen such as *Candida, Trichophyton*, or mumps virus.
† Induration graded in cm: 0 < 0.05, 1 = 0.5, 2 = 1.0.

Therapeutic Diets. The following discussion highlights the main types of diets. As with any treatment, the physician should learn their approximate compositions and the indications for their use.

When feasible, protein-calorie malnutrition is treated by diet. The calculation of the energy cost of weight gain is not straightforward since it depends on the composition of the tissue laid down. The caloric cost to synthesize 1 g of lean body mass (LBM) containing 16 to 20% protein is about 2 kcal, while that to synthesize adipose triglyceride is about 9 kcal/g. The overall caloric cost will be different when a patient is gaining weight reversing a state of malnutrition (increase mainly in LBM), versus going from overweight to obese, when fat is the predominant tissue synthesized.

There are a number of diseases for which a specific diet is the definitive intervention. For example, a gluten-free diet will treat celiac disease and also dermatitis herpetiformis. Patients with malabsorption of lactose respond to a lactose-free or low-lactose diet. Yogurt is the one lactose-containing food that may be well tolerated by lactose-intolerant persons, because fermentation of the lactose by yogurt bacteria occurs in the small-intestinal lumen. Such tolerance must be titrated by a trial (i.e., dose-response) basis. The lactose content of yogurt often is lower than that in equivalent amounts of milk, 7 to 8 g versus 12 g per cup. Most cheeses contain only 0.5 to 1 g of lactose per ounce. Since most patients with lactose intolerance can ingest 3 g of lactose with no ill effects, a few ounces of cheese are generally well tolerated. All deserts and sauces made with milk, cream, cheese, or milk chocolate are avoided in a low-lactose diet. Sorbets, ices, and oleomargarines usually are not made from milk products and therefore do not contain lactose.

Weight Reduction Diets. While hospitalized patients often present problems of undernutrition, the commonest nutritional disorder seen in the outpatient department in the western world is overnutrition and obesity. The first line of treatment in the management of hypertension, non-insulin-dependent diabetes, and hyperlipidemias is weight control. The economics of changes in body weight are in strict accordance with the first law of thermodynamics. That is, weight gain occurs when energy input exceeds output, and weight loss occurs under reverse conditions.

Calculating the estimated rate of weight loss is instructive. The caloric value of 1 kg of stored adipose tissue including water and supporting elements is approximately 7000 kcal. If a person changes his or her dietary intake from 2000 kcal/day to half that amount, the negative balance of 1000 kcal/day or 7000 kcal/week results. This means that the maximum weight loss that may be expected is 1 kg/week or 2.2 lb/week. Any loss over this amount is not tissue but water (due to changes in sodium intake and consequent diuresis) and occurs early in the diet (a useful boost to compliance). In practice, the rate of weight loss decreases over time to a more frustrating 0.5 kg per week. This is because various compensatory mechanisms are activated in response to diminished intake of food. They include a reduction in REE and thyroid hormone secretion (low T3, increase in rT3).

Any potential dieter should be given realistic goals. Emphasis should be on the long-term aim: a steady loss over 6 months of up to 20 to 35 lb (10–16 kg). The number of diet books and weight-loss plans available on the market testifies to the absence of a definitive solution to the problem of obesity. More gullible members of the public want something (weight loss) for nothing (no exertion). But dieting alone is not enough to lose and keep off substantial weight.

Any program for weight loss that does not include behavioral modification and a regular exercise routine is doomed to failure. Exercise means maintaining about 75% of the target heart rate (where the target is 220 – age) for at least 20 minutes, three times a week (Segal and Pi-Sunyer, 1989). Advice to the overworked, sedentary, fast-food-eating patient is to begin walking for 30 minutes at a time and then gradually increase the intensity of the exercise program.

Weight reduction is a key subject of diet therapy because obesity is a major source of morbidity in the general population and weight reduction is a mainstay in the management of heart disease, hypertension, hyperlipidemia, and non-insulin-dependent diabetes mellitus. If defined as more than 20% above the desirable body weight (which corresponds to a BMI of roughly 27.5), then obesity affects over 35 million Americans (Kissebah et al., 1989). Approximately 80% of patients with non-insulin-dependent diabetes are obese, and hypertension is twice as prevalent in the obese as in the population with normal weight (National Research Council, 1989). Thus, every physician should know how to prescribe and supervise the effects of a weight-reducing diet. Such diets usually contain about 1000 kcal per day for women or 1200 kcal per day for men. The quantity of the calories is more important than the quality. Since on a weight-for-weight basis the caloric value of fat is 2.25 times that of carbohydrate and proteins, and since dietary calories are more efficiently connected to body fat, reduction in the amount of fat consumed is a major goal in revamping a patient's diet.

The problem of maintaining a new lower body weight usually receives too little attention, possibly because it is so difficult. Maintaining a new low body weight may be even harder than losing weight in the first place. The appropriate recommendation for "success" may be summarized as "once the need for dietary control, always the need."

Low-Salt Diets. Low-salt diets are used as adjunctive measures in the management of hypertension and edematous states associated with heart or liver failure. The principal source of sodium in the diet is salt that is added to food during its preparation and preservation, and at the table before eating. Other sodium-containing chemicals are found in leavening agents (baking powder, soda), disodium phosphate (used in some cereals and cheeses), monosodium glutamate (flavor), sodium alginate (some ice creams and chocolate milks), sodium hydroxide (food processing), sodium benzoate (preservative), sodium propionate (inhibitor of molds), and sodium sulfite (a bleach for certain fruits and a preservative). With such varied sources of ingestible salt, the careful patient becomes familiar with techniques for detecting subtle sources of salt by reading food labels. Each molecule of salt is approximately 40% sodium, and thus, as a rule of thumb, 1 teaspoon of salt (5 g) contains approximately 2000 mg or 90 mEq of sodium. Three levels of sodium restriction have been established by convention. Mild sodium restriction ("no added salt") usually means 2400 to 4500 mg (100–200 mEq) of sodium used daily. With this diet, some may be added during cooking, but none is added to the meal. All salty foods and snacks are forbidden.

Moderate sodium restriction usually means 1000 to 2000 mg (45–90 mEq) of sodium used daily. At this level of restriction, salt is added sparingly in food preparation, and the daily allowance is a quarter of a teaspoon (1200 mg) in carefully selected food items. A slice of bread, for example, contains 150 mg of sodium.

Severe sodium restriction usually means 500 to 1000 mg (20–45 mEq) of sodium used daily. If, for example, edema persists despite moderate restriction plus diuretics, then the sodium intake may be lowered further by providing the patient with distilled rather than tap water.

Moderate restriction of dietary sodium may help reduce elevated blood pressure, but the response of an individual patient to such restriction is unpredictable (Bittle et al., 1985).

A major problem of compliance to a low-salt diet is lack of palatability. Although salt substitutes that contain potassium chloride are available, they are rather bitter and have not been widely accepted. A better approach that aids compliance is to encourage the generous use of spices that usually contain negligible (0.05%–0.1%) amounts of salt. Celery and parsley spices are excluded from that list. In heart failure, special attention must be given not only to the sodium in the diet, but also to dietary potassium that can counter the toxicity of diuretics (see chapter 11). Drugs, too, may contain sodium or potassium (see Table 10–10). For example, aqueous penicillin G is available as either the sodium or potassium salt. *Principle: The form of a chemical entity and the excipients used in the product may be important nuances in the ultimate effects of a drug.*

Diets in Diabetes. Diet and weight control along with insulin are the cornerstones of the therapy of non-insulin-dependent diabetes mellitus if good glycemic control is to be achieved.

**Table 10–10.   SODIUM AND POTASSIUM CONTENTS
OF SOME COMMON MEDICATIONS***

Sodium content of oral medications		
Alka-Seltzer, antacid	296	mg/tab
Alka-Seltzer, pain reliever	551	mg/tab
Alka-Seltzer Plus	482	mg/tab
Alevaire	80	mg/5 ml
Di-Gel	10.6	mg/tab
Di-Gel, liquid	8.5	mg/5 ml
Dristan Cough Formula	58	mg/5 ml
Fleet Phospho-Soda	550	mg/5 ml
Phosphagel	12.5	mg/5 ml
Rolaids	53	mg/tab
Sodium Salicylate, tablet	49	mg/5 gr
Titralac liquid	11	mg/5 ml
Vicks Cough Syrup	41	mg/5 ml
Formula 44D Decongestant Cough mixture	51	mg/5 ml
Neutra-Phos	164	mg/capsule
Sodium content of parenteral medications		
Azlocillin	49.9	mg/g
Cefoxitin	52.9	mg/g
Mezlocillin	42.6	mg/g
Penicillin G Potassium	12.2	mg/g
Penicillin G Sodium	62.6	mg/g
Piperacillin	45.5	mg/g
Ticarcillin	119.6–149.5	mg/g
Potassium content of oral and parenteral medications		
Mysteclin F	21	mg/5 ml
Neutra-Phos	278	mg/capsule
Neutra-Phos-K	556	mg/capsule
Penicillin G Potassium	66.3	mg/million units
Pfizerpen VK	1.7	mg/250 mg

* Modified from Roe (1989).

The quantity of food is far more important than either its quality or the timing of meals taken by the diabetic patient who does not need exogenous insulin (National Institutes of Health, 1986). In contrast, for those patients who need insulin, the timing of both the insulin doses and meals as well as their caloric content is crucial to good care (see chapter 16). Recent work also suggests that low-protein diets may delay the progression of diabetic and other nephropathy (Ciavarella et al., 1987). This work remains to be substantiated and is the subject of a multicenter trial sponsored by the National Institutes of Health (see chapters 11 and 16). *Principle: The full value and risks of any therapy, particularly when they are not anticipated by known pharmacologic profiles, take considerable time to reveal themselves. The therapist must maintain a systematic update on any therapy he or she uses.*

Diet in Hyperlipidemia. The first step in the management of the hyperlipidemia is dietary (see chapter 15). The aim is to control both the cholesterol content and the types of fatty acids ingested. Initially (step 1) the diet is chosen to facilitate achieving ideal body weight. In this period an intake of saturated fat that accounts for less than 10% of calories, total fat that accounts for less than 30% of calories, and dietary cholesterol that is less than 300 mg/day is suggested. Remember, one egg yolk contains about 260 mg of cholesterol; a 3-oz (90-g) piece of meat, fish, or poultry has 60 to 90 mg of cholesterol; but a similar portion of liver contains 390 mg of cholesterol.

A comparison of this so-called prudent diet with the average American menu is shown in Table 10–11. Table 10–12 offers an outline of the food that can be used for a low-fat diet. On a 2000-kcal total intake, if fat is approximately 30% of the calories, the daily fat intake is about 65 g. When treating hypertriglyceridemia, restriction of carbohydrates and sucrose is advisable as it may decrease the hepatic synthesis of very-low-density lipoproteins (Ahrens, 1986).

Fiber. Commonly, prescriptions for diets specify an increase or decrease in "residue," or fiber (see summary in National Research Council, 1989, and chapter 8). "Fiber" is a heterogeneous group of substances with many different

**Table 10-11.   COMPARISON BETWEEN THE AVERAGE AMERICAN DIET AND
THE STEP-1 CHOLESTEROL-LOWERING DIET**

	AVERAGE AMERICAN DIET	CHOLESTEROL-LOWERING
Total fat	35–40% total calories	<30% total calories
Saturated	15–20% total calories	<10% total calories
Monounsaturated	14–16% total calories	10–15% total calories
Polyunsaturated	7% total calories	up to 10% total calories
Protein	16% total calories	up to 20% total calories
Carbohydrate	47% total calories	50–60% total calories
Cholesterol	350–450 mg/d	<300 mg/d
Total calories	"Excessive"	To achieve and maintain desirable weight

Table 10-12.   OUTLINE OF A LOW-FAT DIET

FAT INTAKE (G/DAY)	APPROPRIATE FOODS
40	Vegetables, fruits, breads, cereals with skim milk, two 3-oz servings of lean meat, one egg, 1 tsp. margarine
60	In addition to the above foods: 2 cups of 2% milk, or 1 more ounce of meat with each serving, or one egg, or 4 tsp. of margarine or oil
75	In addition to foods allowed on a 60-g diet: whole milk instead of 2%, or two slices of bacon, or 4 oz of ice cream, or two servings of lean meat—6 oz each

properties. Table 10-13 shows the approximate fiber content of common foods. Fiber in the diet may be either insoluble (e.g., lignin and cellulose) or soluble (e.g., pectin and gums). The former is found in vegetables and cereals and increases fecal bulk, thereby decreasing intestinal transit

**Table 10-13.   FIBER CONTENT OF
COMMONLY USED FOODS**

APPROXIMATE CONTENT OF DIETARY FIBER (G/SERVING)	REPRESENTATIVE FOODS
5	Bran-containing cereals, stewed prunes, grapes, baked beans, raspberries
4	Peas, broccoli, pears, apples, potato skins, canned fruit, fruit pies
2	Citrus fruits, root vegetables, peanut butter, strawberries, cherries, wheat and corn cereals
1	Melons, white bread, salad vegetables, popcorn, rice cereals
<0.2	Milk, egg, meat, sugar, fats, strained juices

time. Soluble fiber is found in citrus fruit, legumes, oats, and barley. It delays gastric emptying and slows absorption of glucose; it may also lower serum cholesterol concentrations by increasing fecal losses of steroids. The amount of "roughage," or fiber, in the diet plays an important role in the treatment of inflammatory bowel disease and may also influence the progression of diverticulosis in some patients (LSRO, 1987). As more information is obtained, recommendations will be established for which specific type of fiber is indicated to treat or prevent a given disease.

At present there are no clear-cut guidelines for ingestion of fiber; although the National Cancer Institute recommends a daily fiber intake of between 20 and 30 g, such an intake should be achieved by the consumption of natural foods rather than by adding fiber concentrates to the diet (RDA, 1989).

Restriction of Protein. The management of acute and chronic renal failure depends on correct counseling with regard to dietary protein and fluid and electrolyte balance (see chapter 11). Restriction of protein (0.6 g/kg per day) is advised when the creatinine clearance is below 20 ml/min and there is no nephrotic component to the disease. In the nephrotic syndrome, protein losses may be over 20 g/day. Dialysis, whether peritoneal dialysis or hemodialysis, causes loss of protein at a rate of about 1 g/h. This must be compensated for by suitable allowances in the diet. When protein restriction is commenced, at least 75% of the protein should be of high biologic value containing the essential amino acids. The body may then use the extra nitrogen to synthesize the nonessential amino acids and thus reduce the burden of urea that must be excreted. Proteins of high biologic value are contained in eggs, meat, fish, poultry, and milk products. The protein of cereals, fruits, and vegetables lacks essential amino acids and for this reason is considered of low biologic value.

Vitamin Therapy and Supplements. The major indications for the use of vitamins in medical management are (1) the prevention of vitamin deficiency and (2) the treatment of specific or multiple deficiencies. Rarely, vitamins are used in high doses in the treatment of uncommon genetic disorders that impair the absorption or utilization of a specific vitamin. The doses and routes of administration differ depending on the indication for vitamin or mineral use.

For the great majority of healthy individuals, maintenance of normal vitamin and mineral status or prevention of deficiency is accomplished by attention to a diet that uses a variety of food sources and meets usual caloric requirements. There are, however, circumstances under which vitamin and/or mineral supplementation should be recommended even for healthy individuals. At the extremes of age (infants or the elderly), diets may not be adequate to meet special nutritional requirements, and supplements are commonly recommended. Iron supplements are needed to meet the needs of some women of childbearing age. Those who are on special restricted diets for weight loss or other reasons (for example, strict vegetarians avoiding all animal products), or persons with multiple food allergies, benefit from vitamin and mineral supplements. Under these circumstances, supplementation should always take the form of multiple vitamins, since individual deficiencies are uncommon in the setting of restricted diets. There is rarely a need for doses of vitamins or minerals beyond 100% of the RDA (Table 10–14), and such formulations of multiple vitamins are readily available over the counter.

For those that at special risk of vitamin or mineral deficiency because of increased requirements (e.g., pregnancy), special habits (e.g., excessive alcohol use), or disease (e.g., malabsorption or diabetes), higher doses of multiple vitamins are needed to prevent or reverse deficiency. Multivitamin-mineral preparations for pregnancy ordinarily contain higher doses of certain vitamins and minerals such as folate and iron because of the special increased requirements. Patients who drink alcohol excessively and those with malabsorption may require therapeutic doses of vitamins (5–10 times preventive doses) to overcome excessive losses (Council on Scientific Affairs, 1987). In clinical settings where vitamin deficiency is manifest, usually because of disease or trauma or surgery that has prevented adequate intake and utilization of vitamins, vitamins are needed in higher doses to reverse the deficiency state. In such therapeutic situations, vitamin doses are commonly five to ten times the RDA or daily requirement so that repletion and restitution of normal metabolic pathways will be achieved as quickly as possible. Usually vitamins and minerals are administered by mouth, but for those who cannot take oral medication, parenteral routes of medication may be used. The patient with pernicious anemia or who has had extensive gastric or distal small-bowel surgery presents a special instance in the treatment and prevention of vitamin B_{12} deficiency, and under such clinical circumstances, parenteral vitamin B_{12} therapy is mandatory.

Some individuals may express a genetic defect in the absorption, transport, or metabolism of a given vitamin and thus present with a nutritional deficiency disease despite the usual dietary intakes of the vitamin. These rare genetic syndromes that usually are discovered in early infancy are called vitamin *dependency* syndromes to distinguish them from vitamin *deficiency* syndromes. Substantial improvement of vitamin-dependent metabolic pathways in some of these patients can be

Table 10–14. RDA RANGES OF VITAMINS FOR PREVENTION AND TREATMENT OF DEFICIENCIES, AND DOSES FOR PATIENTS WITH SPECIAL NEEDS

VITAMIN	PREVENTION OF VITAMIN DEFICIENCY	TREATMENT OF VITAMIN DEFICIENCY	TREATMENT OF GENETIC VITAMIN-DEPENDENCY SYNDROMES
Vitamin A (μg)	800–1000	4000–10,000	1250–5000
Vitamin D (μg)	5	50–250	
Vitamin E (μg)	8–10	100–800	
Vitamin K (μg)	65–80	1000 (IM)	
Ascorbic acid (mg)	60	500	
Thiamine (mg)	1.1–1.5	5–25	25–500
Riboflavin (mg)	1.3–1.7	5–25	
Niacin (mg)	15–19	25–50	50–250
Vitamin B_6 (mg)	1.6–2.0	5–25	
Pantothenic acid (mg)	4–7	5–20	
Biotin (μg)	30–100	150–300	10
Folic acid (μg)	180–200	1000	
Pyridoxine (mg)	2	5–25	10
Vitamin B_{12} (μg)	2	1000 (IM) per month	1–40

achieved with very high doses of the relevant vitamin. To achieve normal function, doses as high as 1000 times the usual requirement may be needed (Council on Scientific Affairs, 1987). *Only in these rare circumstances are such high doses indicated!* There are claims for so-called megadoses of vitamins that are neither based on sound therapeutic principles nor safe. Vitamins, like all other therapeutic substances, have their proper dose range for appropriate indications, as noted above and in Table 10–14. This is true of water-soluble and fat-soluble vitamins. There are doses that are safe and adequate and doses that are potentially toxic. The difference between a preventive or therapeutic dose and a toxic dose is highly variable among nutrients: toxic/therapeutic dose ratios for vitamins may vary from 10- to 300-fold. One of the physician's responsibilities with respect to using vitamins is to see that self-administered vitamins are taken in safe dosages as supplements, not in so-called megadoses that provide no added benefit and risk toxic accumulations. Toxicity syndromes for vitamin A, vitamin D, niacin, and iron have been associated with chronic disease or death (Roe, 1989).

Some examples of the use of vitamins may be instructive.

Case Histories

A 95-lb woman, aged 75, who is not very active has a caloric requirement of only 1000 calories. The small amount of food required to meet this caloric need may not contain adequate amounts of vitamins and minerals to meet the usual, or the extra, needs of the elderly. A multivitamin-mineral preparation that contains 100% of the RDA for all vitamins along with some zinc, chromium, and magnesium would be a prudent recommendation for the prevention of vitamin and mineral deficiency.

A middle-aged male presents to a physician with early findings of liver disease. The patient has been obtaining in excess of 50% of his calories from alcohol for some years and presents with folate deficiency anemia and some peripheral neuropathy suggestive of multiple B-vitamin deficiencies. This patient should be treated with multivitamin therapy containing 5 to 10 times the requirement of the B vitamins with a dose of folic acid of at least 1 mg/day. Multivitamin-mineral preparations containing higher doses of iron are not indicated under these circumstances because of the tendency of alcoholics to have increased total body iron. Also, high doses of vitamin A may exacerbate the hepatotoxic effects of alcohol.

Principle: Not all vitamin and mineral preparations are the same. Select the dose and nutrient content that are appropriate for the specific indication for use.

In general, a range of doses is recommended depending on the clinical situation. The range extends from a minimum effective dose to an upper dose beyond which no greater benefit is achieved and the benefit-to-risk ratio diminishes. The minimum effective dose for prevention of nutritional deficiency is based on studies in humans of all ages and both sexes and is approximately the RDA for that nutrient. The minimum effective dose for treatment is based, when possible, upon successful quantitative therapeutic studies on patients with vitamin and/or mineral deficiencies, as well as known dangers of higher doses and the likelihood of toxicity. Studies on treating deficiencies have arbitrarily used doses of vitamins or minerals that are 5 to 10 times the doses needed to prevent deficiency. The rationale for this is based on observations that the higher doses more quickly replenish depleted stores.

INTENSIVE NUTRITIONAL THERAPY

Most problems relating to nutritional support in hospital patients arise from the difficulty in meeting calorie and protein requirements. Vitamins and minerals usually are more easily replaced because required doses are manageable and relatively small. Calorie and nitrogen sources, on the other hand, require larger volumes just to meet daily requirements, and even more to restore altered nutritional status to normal. Therefore, emphasis in this discussion is placed on choosing the most convenient yet effective means of providing these macronutrients.

The therapist needs to develop a rational approach to the selection and management of patients who need these forms of nutritional therapy. Consider the answer to the following questions in selecting patients for intensive nutritional support:

1. What is the current protein-calorie nutritional status of the patient?
2. How severe is the current negative nitrogen and calorie balance?
3. What is the anticipated duration of negative balance?
4. Is the intestinal tract available and adequate for digestion and absorption?
5. What options are available for protein-calorie therapy?

Use of Commercially Available Supplements

The protein and calorie content of the patient's usual diet can be bolstered by the use of commercially available supplements. Calorie supplements can be largely nonprotein (carbohydrates or fats), protein, or both. Products designed as supplements should not be used as the sole dietary constituent unless they are nutritionally complete, that is, unless the regimen meets daily requirements for vitamins and minerals. Many of the supplements have features that make them especially useful in certain disorders; for example, lactose-free products contain less than 1 g of the disaccharide per 1000 kcal and are useful for those who do not tolerate this disaccharide. The carbohydrate sources are usually sucrose, glucose oligosaccharides, and corn syrup solids. A few supplements are blended formulas containing some fibrous animal or vegetable products. However, most commercially available supplements are devoid of indigestible fiber and are consequently low in residue. Supplements that are also low in fat content provide substrate that is least conducive to colonic bacterial growth. Low-residue supplements are particularly useful for hospitalized patients in whom decreased ileal effluent is desired (e.g., because of bowel disease, or while the patient is undergoing preparation for radiologic or endoscopic procedures). Commercial supplements with increased fiber content have recently become available and may be advantageous for some patients requiring long-term use of liquid formula products. The features of several commonly used nutritional supplements are summarized in Table 10–15.

Medium-chain triglyceride (MCT) oil is a distilled derivative of coconut oil and can be an important calorie supplement. Triglycerides with fatty acid moieties of 8- and 10-carbon chain length compose over 95% of the oil. They are absorbed even in the presence of minimal amounts of pancreatic enzymes and in the absence of bile salts, and the medium-chain fatty acids appear directly in the portal blood. Although this oil can act as a valuable calorie supplement in patients with malabsorption of fat of any cause, only 400 cal/day (60 ml/day) can be effectively used because higher doses are likely to cause diarrhea.

Differences in the metabolism of the various sources of calories used in enteral diets have been of recent interest, particularly in patients with pulmonary disease. When carbohydrates are completely metabolized in the presence of oxygen to CO_2 and H_2O, one molecule of CO_2 is produced for each molecule of oxygen consumed, and the resultant respiratory quotient (RQ) is 1.0. The RQ for fats is 0.7, less CO_2 being produced in relation to oxygen consumed. Taking into account the different caloric values of fats and carbohydrates, one can see that these ratios indicate that provision of an isocaloric diet with higher fat content would be accompanied by less production of CO_2 than if the calories were supplied in the form of carbohydrates. The reduced production of CO_2 theoretically might be advantageous to patients with severe pulmonary disease and CO_2 retention. Precipitation of respiratory failure and difficulties with weaning patients from ventilatory support have been attributed to high-carbohydrate parenteral feeding. Possibly the CO_2 production accompanying overfeeding in general has been a factor in precipitating narcosis to the CO_2 ventilatory drive (Askanazi et al., 1980) (see chapter 7). Differing energy sources will affect CO_2 production and minute ventilation. Comparisons of the calculated RQ of various commercially available products indicate that the traditional elemental

Table 10–15. CHARACTERISTICS OF ENTERAL SUPPLEMENTS FOR SPECIAL USE

PRODUCT	KCAL/ 1000 ML	PROTEIN (G/L)	CHO† (G/L)	FAT (G/L)	OSMOLALITY (MOSM/ KG H_2O)	COMMENTS†
Hepatic Aide II	1200	44	168	36	560	↑BCAA, ↓AAA and methionine; negligible electrolytes; vitamin- and mineral-free
Travasorb hepatic	1110	26	194	13	600	↑BCAA, ↓AAA; contains electrolytes, vitamins and minerals
Amin Aid	2000	19	366	46	700	EAA and histidine; high calorie/nitrogen ratio; negligible electrolytes; vitamin- and mineral-free
Travasorb Renal	1350	22	274	18	590	60% EAA, 40% NEAA; contains water-soluble vitamins; negligible electrolytes; mineral- and fat-soluble-vitamin-free

* When prepared in standard dilution.
† BCAA = branched chain amino acids; AAA = aromatic amino acids; EAA = essential amino acids; NEAA = nonessential amino acids; CHO = carbohydrate.

diets have higher values than other chemically defined diets, reflecting the higher carbohydrate content of the elemental feedings. Products are being designed that contain more fat and have lower RQ values than standard formulations (e.g., Pulmocare, 0.80, versus Ensure Plus, 0.87). *Principle: Clinicians must consider all maneuvers from behavioral modification to nutrition to application of drugs, devices, and procedures as potentially therapeutic. Even nutritional supplements have specific indications and contraindications.*

Modified defined-formula diets are available for patients with renal failure and/or liver disease (Table 10–16). Formulas for treating patients with uremia contain essential amino acids and histidine as the nitrogen sources. In principle, the nonessential amino acids will be formed endogenously, possibly by utilizing retained nitrogen. As a nutritional supplement to a low-protein diet, essential amino acids will reduce the BUN/creatinine ratio and can assist in prolonging the predialysis period without endangering the life expectancy of the patients (Alvestrand et al., 1980).

Formulas for patients with liver failure contain a high proportion of branched-chain amino acids (valine, leucine, and isoleucine) and arginine and reduced amounts of aromatic amino acids and methionine (see chapter 9). This modification was developed from the observation of a relative increase in plasma concentrations of certain aromatic amino acids and methionine in patients with liver insufficiency and portosystemic enceph-

alopathy. Modest improvement in objective and subjective parameters of encephalopathy has been demonstrated with the use of branched-chain amino acids themselves or as α-keto analogs in supplemental form to a protein-restricted diet (Fischer et al., 1973).

These specialized formulas may contain no vitamins and minimal electrolytes; depending on the clinical situation, supplementation will be necessary if no other diet is used. The full extent of the clinical application of these diets and similar commercial products awaits further study.

Tube Feeding at Home

Long-term enteral feeding is accomplished either through a transnasal feeding tube or through a gastrostomy or jejunostomy. Simplified methods of gastrostomy may be utilized even for patients with relatively short courses of planned nutritional support, such as during radiation therapy or following radical head and neck surgery. However, use of a transnasal feeding tube certainly is more cost-effective if the patient can tolerate the appearance and psychological and technical aspects of this approach. It is feasible to continue enteral feeding in a patient's home. The technique is considerably cheaper (one tenth to one twentieth the cost) than comparable support with parenteral nutrition. In addition, serious complications are much less frequent with the enteral technique.

Patients have been treated for months without

Table 10–16. CHARACTERISTICS OF REPRESENTATIVE NUTRITIONALLY COMPLETE ENTERAL FORMULAS

PRODUCT	KCAL/L*	PROTEIN (G/L)	CHO (G/L)†	FAT (G/L)	OSMOLALITY (MOSM/KG)	COMMENTS
Meritene	960	58	110	32	505	Milk-based
Sustacal	1000	61	140	23	620	Lactose-free
Ensure	1060	37	145	37	470	Lactose-free
Complete	1070	43	128	43	405	Blenderized food
Isocal	1060	34	133	44	300	Tube feeding only
Osmolite	1060	37	145	38	300	Tube feeding only
Ensure Plus	1500	55	200	53	690	Higher cal., protein
Sustacal HC	1500	61	190	58	650	Higher cal., protein
Pulmocare	1500	63	106	92	490	Lower CHO
Isocal HCN	2000	75	200	102	690	Highest cal. density
Magnacal	2000	70	250	80	590	Highest cal. density
Criticare HN	1060	38	220	5	650	Low-fat, low-residue
Vital HN	1000	42	185	11	500	Low-fat, low-residue
Vivonex T.E.N.	1000	38	206	3	630	Low-fat, low-residue
Travasorb MCT	1000	49	123	33	312	Contains MCT
Enrich	1100	40	162	37	480	Fiber-containing
Jevity	1060	44	152	37	310	Fiber-containing

* When prepared in standard solution.
† CHO = carbohydrate.

detrimental changes in laboratory profile. They do gradually develop zinc deficiency and other micronutrient deficiencies. *Principle: When an event occurs slowly and is subtle until grossly evident, the therapist may have difficulty recognizing the problem. Anticipation and prevention become more important.*

Complications of Tube Feeding. Complications of the nasogastric and nasoenteral tube feeding techniques are infrequent. Nasal and oropharyngeal irritation are less common when small-caliber, soft, flexible nasogastric or naso-duodenal tubes are used. Gastrointestinal distress is more frequent when the feeding is directly into the small bowel as opposed to the intragastric feeding. The irritation can usually be improved by reducing the infusion rate or temporarily diluting the formula. Diarrhea can result from infusion that is too rapid, from infusion that is hyperosmolar, from concomitant use of antibiotics, or from malabsorption of fats due to underlying GI disease. Appropriate modification of the feeding protocol usually will result in a decrease in stool output. Occasionally codeine sulfate or drops of deodorized tincture of opium may be used to stop the diarrhea.

Rare complications include inadvertent IV administration of the diet and precipitation of the syndrome of intestinal pseudoobstruction (Stellato et al., 1984). Perforation of a bronchus or penetration into the lung parenchyma with passage of the feeding tube into the pleural space can occur especially if a stylet is used to place a transnasal feeding tube (Miller et al., 1985).

Tracheobronchial aspiration and aspiration pneumonia are serious complications of forced enteral feeding. Passage of the tube into the distal duodenum, preferably beyond the ligament of Treitz, should reduce this likelihood. However, even a feeding jejunostomy may not eliminate the chances of tracheobronchial aspiration. Patients receiving continuous enteral infusions should have their heads elevated 30 degrees from the horizontal at all times, and those receiving intermittent bolus feeding should remain in a tilted or upright position for at least 2 hours after each feeding.

Forced feeding with defined-formula diets can result in significant electrolyte abnormalities. Careful monitoring in the first 1 to 2 weeks of therapy, similar to monitoring total parenteral nutrition therapy, is important. A syndrome of hyperosmotic, nonketotic dehydration has occurred as a result of inadequate supplementation with water (Walike, 1969). Patients with this syndrome appear lethargic, dehydrated, and occasionally febrile and respond to rehydration with hypotonic fluids.

Parenteral Nutrition

The general indications for parenteral nutrition are to correct severe nutritional depletion in patients unable to maintain adequate oral intake and to meet nutritional needs during periods without any enteral intake (Butterworth and Blackburn, 1975). Considering the frequency with which nothing-by-mouth regimens or nasogastric suction is used in the management of severe GI disorders and the likelihood that such patients suffer from nutritional depletion on presentation, it is not surprising that patients with GI disorders have been among those most commonly treated with total parenteral nutrition.

Techniques in Parenteral Nutrition. Parenteral nutrition refers to the IV administration of carbohydrates, proteins (as amino acids), and fats in amounts capable of maintaining or restoring protein and energy needs. The term *total parenteral nutrition* (TPN) needs qualification. Many patients selected for protein-calorie therapy may require total support without any other sources of calories or proteins. However, in the absence of clinical indications for complete bowel rest or nasogastric or nasoenteric suction, parenteral nutrition therapy can be used to *supplement oral intake* that by itself cannot meet nutritional goals. Partial or supplemental nutritional support often is administered by peripheral vein. This is possible because the contribution of IV nutrition to total calorie requirement is low enough to permit the use of mildly hypertonic solutions. These solutions can be safely infused into peripheral veins. Central IV lines can be used for both partial and total nutrition support via the IV route. The physician should establish the nutritional goal for the patient (as described earlier in this chapter) and then select the therapeutic technique best suited to meet these goals. Combined calorie and protein support is generally required for patients who need intensive nutrition support by vein. "Protein-sparing" therapy that employs IV amino acids in hypocaloric regimens has little application in the management of patients with GI disease.

Total nutritional support can be provided in some patients via peripheral vein for limited periods of time if the hypertonicity of the solutions is limited. Carbohydrate as dextrose solutions in concentrations of up to 30% can be used when the administration is into a large central vein, such as the superior vena cava (SVC). Concentrations above 10% dextrose are very hypertonic (>500 mOsm/l) and too corrosive to use in smaller peripheral veins. Lipid emulsions in concentrations of 10% to 20% by volume have the advantage of delivering a highly concentrated source of calories in an isotonic solution. With the use of such emulsions, it is possible to administer close to 2000 kcal/day by peripheral vein, employing 2.5 liters of 10% dextrose with appropriate amino acids and 1000 ml of a 10% lipid emulsion. When more calories are provided as lipids, intakes above 2500 kcal/day can be accomplished. But lipid sources should not supply more than 60% to 70% of the daily nonprotein calories (Skeie et al., 1988). Nutritional support via peripheral veins is most attractive for younger patients whose peripheral veins offer a continuing reliable conduit and when caloric requirements can be met relatively easily. Such therapy is usually employed for short periods (less than 2 weeks). Nutrition support therapy by peripheral veins also is attractive when the patient continues to eat and the total caloric requirement can be met by a combination of ingested food or formula plus IV nutrition.

Parenteral nutrition by central vein is normally provided through a catheter passed via the subclavian vein into the SVC. To keep complications to a minimum and to maximize therapeutic effectiveness, this technically demanding approach is best executed by an experienced group consisting of a physician or surgeon trained in nutritional decision making and management in addition to catheter placement, a nurse trained in catheter care and patient monitoring, a pharmacist responsible for preparation and monitoring of the IV solutions, and a clinical nutritionist who can aid in establishing initial goals and in monitoring signs of nutritional progress.

A detailed description of catheter insertion and care, preparation of parenteral nutritional solutions, and details of patient monitoring are beyond the scope of this text. Many publications offer detailed guidance on these matters (Alpers et al., 1987). Fundamental principles in the formulation of a prescription for IV nutritional therapy include the following.

Setting calorie and protein goals utilizing sound nutritional principles have been described in this chapter. In some centers the caloric goals are based on achieving or maintaining ideal body weight based on insurance company actuarial statistics. Weights listed in such tables are those associated with lowest mortality. In some patients the usual body weight may be a more useful basis for judging the caloric requirements, particularly when that weight has been the patient's standard for a long period of good health. The daily requirement for most patients with no more than moderate metabolic stress is 30 to 35 kcal/kg for maintenance of weight and 40 kcal/kg for weight gain at a modest rate.

One gram of protein per kilogram of ideal body weight (or usual body weight) per day is usually ample to maintain or promote positive nitrogen balance. Patients with active disease resulting in loss of protein into the GI tract or through fistulas often require as much as 1.5 g of protein per kilogram per day.

Choosing Among Sources of Calories. Two sources of nonprotein calories are commercially available: dextrose solutions and lipid emulsions. Both can provide energy through oxidation, and both are capable of sparing body protein by providing calories that inhibit breakdown of protein for gluconeogenesis. Maximal suppression of gluconeogenesis occurs when infusions of glucose approach 400 g, or about 1600 kcal/day. There appears to be a limit to the capacity to derive energy from infused glucose. The limits of the nitrogen-sparing effects of glucose infusion are observed at about 35 kcal/kg per day. Above this dose, one can expect increased synthesis of fat from glucose and deposition of fat in the liver. Before the widespread use of lipid emulsions, hepatomegaly, right upper quadrant pain, and abnormalities in liver function were common complications of intensive nutrition support with hypertonic dextrose and amino acid solutions. Lipid emulsions not only provide a high-energy source of calories (9 kcal/g of fat) but also provide a source of essential fatty acids (EFAs). Thus deficiency of EFAs is prevented. Intravenous lipid emulsions are a suitable source of nonprotein calories that contribute to conservation of body protein.

Recent clinical studies have confirmed that the most effective approach to providing energy is the combination of carbohydrate and fat. A regimen in which the calorie source was glucose alone compared with one in which calories were derived nearly equally from fat and glucose resulted in similar weight gain, but repletion of protein was achieved only in the combined regimen (MacFie et al., 1981). Thus, a regimen by which calories are supplied in the form of both dextrose and lipid (with fat providing 30% or more of total calories) appears to be most effective.

Patients who have difficulty clearing these IV lipid particles that are metabolized almost identically to chylomicrons must be given these supplements with great care to avoid persistent lipidemia and complications such as pancreatitis.

Essential Fatty Acids. Small quantities of EFAs must be ingested in order to maintain health. Deficiency of the *n*-6 fatty acid linoleic acid [18:2 (carbon chain length: double bonds)] is associated with scaly skin, hair loss, and impaired wound healing and has been described in patients receiving IV fluids without any fat supplements (Richardson and Sgoutas, 1975).

Under normal circumstances linoleic acid may be desaturated and elongated to form arachidonic acid (20:4), which is a precursor of eicosanoids. Arachidonic acid is also considered essential, but only when linoleic acid deficiency exists. The third fatty acid traditionally classified as being essential is the n-3 polyunsaturated α-linolenic acid (18:3), which is a precursor of eicosapentaenoic acid (EPA)(20:5) and docosahexaenoic acid (DHA)(22:6). These fatty acids, in addition to the roles in eicosanoid formation, are essential constituents of the retina and brain membranes (RDAs, 1989).

Deficiency of EFAs has been observed only in patients with medical problems affecting fat intake or absorption (e.g., cystic fibrosis and biliary atresia); there are no RDAs for these fatty acids (RDAs, 1989). Linoleic acid at levels of 1% to 2% of total calories is sufficient to prevent the biochemical and clinical evidence of EFA deficiency (Holman, 1970).

The National Research Council (1989) recommended that the average intake of n-6 fatty acids remain at about 7% of total calories and not exceed 10%. The reason for this is that while EFAs may affect platelet function, inflammatory responses, and blood triglyceride levels to a variable extent after acute supplementation, little is known concerning the long-term consequences of higher intakes (Leaf and Weber, 1988).

Lipid emusions for IV use are derived from soybean oil, safflower oil, or both and contain nearly 50% of fatty acids as linoleic (18:2) and 4% to 8% as linolenic acid (18:3). While the requirement for EFAs can be met by weekly provision of 500 ml of a 10% lipid emulsion or 250 ml of a 20% emulsion, it is normally recommended that more than 20% of total daily nonprotein calories be provided as lipid.

Protein Source. Infusion of a commercial mixture of essential and nonessential amino acids, in a ratio of about 1 : 4, in the presence of adequate calories, can meet needs for protein balance (Peters and Fischer, 1980). The optimal calorie/nitrogen ratio appears to be about 160 : 1 cal/g. At a ratio of 100 : 1, weight loss and negative nitrogen balance have been observed.

Fluids. The 70-kg adult normally requires about 30 ml of water per kilogram of body weight per day, or about 1 ml of fluid per kilocalorie per day. The increased fluid and electrolyte requirements of patients with fever, diarrhea, short-bowel syndrome, or extensive drainage from fistula must be provided. In patients with limitations of fluid intake imposed by cardiac failure or cirrhosis, total fluid volume will be an important factor in selecting solutions and the rate of infusion.

Vitamins, Minerals, and Trace Elements. Vitamins and minerals should be added to parenteral alimentation solutions in amounts designed to meet daily requirements of patients with disease (Table 10–17). Because these doses are several times the recommended dietary dose, they may be slightly higher than needed in some patients. Research on IV vitamin requirements is needed. Still, the usual values appear to have served well in view of the successful support of patients on home TPN for more than 10 years. Experience with home TPN has reemphasized the necessity for certain vitamins and trace elements in human nutrition. Deficiency syndromes of biotin, selenium, zinc, or copper have been reported when any of these materials has been excluded from parenteral solutions. This experience reinforces the need to include all essential nutrients in parenteral solutions, particularly when prolonged IV therapy is planned (Solomons et al., 1976; Mock et al., 1981; Johnson et al., 1981).

Special problems exist in meeting iron requirements. Iron salts are generally incompatible with the usual IV solutions, and iron needs are therefore met by intermittent parenteral infusions or injections. Since there is no need to absorb dietary calcium from the gut, the IV requirements for vitamin D are uncertain. About 150 to 200 mEq of chloride and 90 to 120 mEq of sodium are required per day. Patients with fistulas of the GI tract or those with gastroduodenal drainage may require up to twice that amount.

Some patients require large amounts of phosphate, potassium, and magnesium. These electrolytes are incorporated into cells during nutritional repletion, and their omission contributes to the nutritional refeeding syndrome. Calcium intake is designed to meet or exceed calcium excretion in urine and stool as predicted from studies of calcium balance. Adequate zinc is required for nutritional restitution, for positive nitrogen balance, and for wound healing. The requirements of zinc may be two or three times normal in patients with diarrhea and GI fistulas.

Home Parenteral Nutrition. The development of techniques for home TPN has revolutionized the management of patients whose nutritional disability is of long duration or permanent. Such regimens require intensive training of the patient and family and vigorously organized follow-up. Financial savings are substantial compared with TPN in hospital, and home TPN with infusion overnight permits return to a reasonably normal daytime routine and aids in social adjustment. The details of management differ somewhat, but the principles are constant. With experience now spanning more than 15 years, TPN at home is increasingly used, progressively safer, and capable

Table 10-17. TYPICAL DAILY TPN PRESCRIPTION FOR ADULT PATIENTS

Calories: 30–40 kcal/kg of IBW*		Lipid: 1/3 nonprotein calories	
Protein: 1.0–1.5 gm/kg of IBW		Dextrose: 2/3 nonprotein calories	
Electrolytes and Minerals (mEq)		*Vitamins*	
Sodium	90–120	A (IU)	3300
Potassium	90–150	C (mg)	100
Calcium	12–16	D (IU)	200
Magnesium	150–200	E (IU)	10
Chloride	12–16	K (mg)‡	—
Acetate	20–30	Thiamine, B_1 (mg)	3
Phosphorus (mmol)	20–40	Riboflavin, B_2 (mg)	3.6
Sulfate	12–16	Pyridoxine, B_6 (mg)	4
Trace Elements		Niacinamide (mg)	40
Zinc (mg)	3–9	B_{12} (μg)	5
Copper (mg)	1–1.6	Pantothenate (mg)	15
Manganese (mg)	0.5	Biotin (μg)	60
Chromium (μg)	10–15	Folic acid (μg)	60
Selenium (μg)	40		
Molybdenum (μg)	20		
Iron (mg)	2–3†		

* IBW = ideal body weight.
† Doses greater than 5 mg/day have been associated with anaphylactoid or other types of adverse reactions.
‡ Vitamin K is added to the TPN or administered IM 5 mg/week.

of achieving both nutritional and social rehabilitation in a majority of patients so treated.

The patients in whom TPN has been employed at home represent a difficult challenge. Increased survival after massive intestinal resection is directly related to this mode of support. Home TPN has transformed the outcome of severe radiation enteritis and pseudoobstruction, and some promising results have been reported in the subacute treatment of patients with Crohn disease at home rather than in the hospital (Kushner et al., 1986).

DRUGS THAT AFFECT NUTRITIONAL STATUS

Many medications have effects on energy and protein homeostasis. An obvious example is thyroid hormone therapy. Overmedication with thyroxine increases metabolic rate and leads to weight loss not only of fat but also of LBM (see chapter 14). This latter action precludes the use of thyroid pills as a treatment for obesity. Treatment with corticosteroids other than for replacement therapy leads to weight gain despite progressive negative nitrogen balance. This accounts for the clinical picture of osteoporosis, poor wound healing, and redistribution of body fat seen in patients who take corticosteroids for a prolonged period. Patients who require long-term, high-dose corticosteroids, as during the treatment of asthma or pemphigus, are told to increase the protein content of their diet—although the value of this logical precaution has yet to be properly documented. In children, prolonged use of corticosteroids may retard growth. For this reason, ACTH may be preferable. Many other medications may influence appetite and satiety and thus indirectly alter energy balance.

Drugs That Increase Appetite

Cyproheptadine hydrochloride (Periactin) may cause weight gain in debilitated children and adults. It probably acts as a serotonin antagonist to stimulate appetite. When eating is associated with physical pain or mental anguish, as in anorexia nervosa, the drug is not effective. Psychotropic drugs such as phenothiazines, and the tricyclic antidepressants, promote appetite when administered chronically, and benzodiazepines increase food intake in both healthy and sick persons. If tranquilizers are given to geriatric patients in whom there may be decreased drug metabolism, then excessive somnolence can occur, leading to the opposite effect—disinterest and a decreased food intake.

Drugs That Decrease Food Intake

Amphetamines and related drugs such as fenfluramine, a trifluoromethyl-substituted amphetamine, have long been used in the treatment of obesity. Their effects probably are due to their actions on the catecholaminergic or serotonergic pathways. While these drugs may have a place in the initial treatment of obesity (for a period of 3 months), they should not be used indefinitely because of their adverse effects and because they provide an inadequate substitute for the necessary diet, exercise, and behavior changes. Patients should be instructed that such medications help compliance but should not be used instead of proper diet therapy.

Drug–Nutrient Interactions

There is a reciprocal relationship between drug therapy and nutrients (Robinson et al., 1986; Roe, 1989; Tatro, 1990). Drugs may influence the intake, absorption, and metabolism of foods, and foods can affect drug absorption, metabolism, and excretion. Patients at increased risk include the very young and the elderly, the former because of the narrow range between therapy and toxicity and the latter because the elderly are often on continual long-term medication and may also have a borderline-adequate diet (Morley, 1988). About 16% of U.S. citizens older than 60 years ingest fewer than 1000 calories per day (Abraham et al., 1977). Table 10–18 lists the drugs that most commonly cause nutritional depletion.

Effects of Drugs on the Availability of Nutrients.   Primary drug-induced malabsorption is due to direct effects on luminal events or on the intestinal mucosa. Mineral oil and cholestyramine are examples of the former, and methotrexate and colchicine of the latter mechanism. Secondary malabsorption occurs when a drug interferes with the absorption, disposition, or metabolism of one nutrient that in turn leads to malabsorption and deficiency of a second nutrient. Phenytoin (diphenylhydantoin) suppresses absorption and metabolism of vitamin D, thereby leading to malabsorption of calcium and eventually to osteomalacia. Methotrexate, in addition to causing mucosal damage, also impairs the utilization of folate.

Drugs Affecting Mineral Metabolism.   Any drug that affects renal function, salt and water balance, or mineralocorticoid activity may be expected to alter the serum concentrations of sodium, potassium, magnesium, and calcium (see chapter 11). Diuretics are perhaps the best examples of drugs that affect serum electrolyte concentrations, in particular potassium concentrations. Aldosterone antagonists cause the opposite effect, hyperkalemia. Sodium concentrations are altered by diuretics and drugs that affect antidiuretic hormone secretion. Calcium concentrations are also affected by diuretics (see chapter 11).

Drugs That Antagonize Vitamins.   Methotrexate, pyrimethamine, triamterene, and trimethoprim are all antagonists of folic acid. Isoniazid, hydralazine, cycloserine, and levodopa interact with vitamin B_6, nitrous oxide with vitamin B_{12},

and coumarin anticoagulants with vitamin K. Recognition of such effects makes it possible to devise replacement therapy and decrease some adverse effects.

EFFECTS OF FOOD ON DRUG BIOAVAILABILITY

Food in the GI tract may influence the absorption of certain drugs and thereby dictate the optimal times for taking a dose. For example, penicillin G is inactivated by gastric acid and thus should be given on an empty stomach. For all practical purposes an "empty stomach" occurs either 1 hour or more before or at least 3 hours after a meal. Most other oral penicillins also should be taken on an empty stomach since food affects absorption in a variable and unpredictable way. Amoxicillin is a notable exception, since blood concentrations are independent of meals. Tetracycline bioavailability is also altered by food: the calcium in milk and dairy products can form poorly absorbed chelates with tetracyclines, which should therefore be taken before meals.

Cholestyramine is a classic example of a drug that frequently interacts with nutrients and other drugs in the GI tract. Cholestyramine is an anion-exchange resin used for the treatment of hyperlipidemia and also primary biliary cirrhosis (see chapter 15). If used in doses over 24 g/day, it impedes absorption of fat and causes steatorrhea. Cholestyramine also binds with other drugs and thus prevents their absorption. The list of drugs whose absorption is impaired is long and includes thyroid hormone, digoxin, coumarin-derived anticoagulants, fat-soluble vitamins, folic acid, thiazide diuretics, amiodarone, and some β blockers.

The major adverse effect of cholestyramine, however, is constipation. This serves as a general reminder that the most common drug–nutrition interaction is the effect of many drugs on GI function, including appetite, presence of nausea and vomiting, and alteration in bowel habits, whether constipation or diarrhea. Nausea and vomiting are problems with chemotherapeutic agents and an important determinant of compliance with cancer treatment.

Probably one of the most important clinically relevant interactions of food with drugs is the potentiation of the pressor effects of tyramine by monoamine oxidase (MAO) inhibitors (see chapter 2). Patients taking these medications may experience marked elevation of blood pressure, hypertensive crisis, and/or hemorrhagic strokes if foods with a high tyramine content are consumed concurrently or up to 4 weeks after cessation of the therapy. Tyramine and other amines capable of elevating blood pressure may be found in aged, overripe, and fermented foods and drinks. Red

**Table 10–18. COMMON DRUGS AND DRUG CLASSES THAT MAY CAUSE
NUTRITIONAL DEPLETION AND DEFICIENCY**

DRUG CLASS	DRUG	DEFICIENCY
Antacids	Sodium bicarbonate, aluminum hydroxide	Folate, phosphate, calcium, copper
Anticonvulsants	Phenytoin, phenobarbital, primidone Valproic acid	Vitamins D and K Carnitine
Antibiotics	Tetracycline Gentamicin Neomycin	Calcium Potassium, magnesium Fat, nitrogen
Antibacterial agents	Boric acid Trimethoprim Isoniazid	Riboflavin Folate Vitamin B_6, niacin, vitamin D
Antimalarials	Pyrimethamine	Folate
Anti-inflammatory agents	Sulfasalazine Aspirin Colchicine	Folate Vitamin C, folate, iron Fat, vitamin B_{12}
Anticancer drugs	Methotrexate Cisplatin	Folate, calcium Magnesium
Anticoagulants	Warfarin	Vitamin K
Antihypertensive agents	Hydralazine	Vitamin B_6
Diuretics	Thiazides Furosemide Triamterene	Potassium, magnesium Potassium, calcium, magnesium Folate
H_2-receptor antagonists	Cimetidine Ranitidine	Vitamin B_{12}
Hypocholesterolemic agents	Cholestyramine Colestipol	Fat Vitamin K, vitamin A, folate, vitamin B_{12}
Laxatives	Mineral oil Phenolphthalein Senna	Carotene, retinol, vitamins D, K Potassium, fat, calcium Fat, calcium
Oral contraceptives	Estrogens/progestagens	Vitamin B_6, folate, vitamin C
Tranquilizers	Chlorpromazine	Riboflavin

wines (in particular chianti), some imported beers, yeast extracts, broad beans, chicken or beef liver, caviar, pickled herring, fermented sausage (e.g., bologna, pepperoni, salami, summer sausage), overripe avocados, and various cheeses (e.g., Boursault, Brie, Camembert, cheddar, Emmenthaler, Gruyère, mozzarella, Parmesan, Romano, Roquefort, and Stilton). Providing a list of these contraindicated foods may even serve as a spur to recovery in patients receiving MAO inhibitors (see chapter 13).

Another possible drug-nutrient interaction is the influence of the composition of a meal—in particular the balance between carbohydrates and proteins—on absorption of levodopa across the blood–brain barrier (see chapter 12). Levodopa shares the same carrier as the large neutral amino acids (LNAA—valine, leucine, isoleucine, tyrosine, and tryptophan). Therefore, any dietary manipulation affecting the circulating levels of these amino acids, and thereby the levodopa/LNAA ratio, may conceivably modulate the biologic and clinical effects of levodopa. The nature of the carrier competition is not clearly understood, but some Parkinson patients show marked "on–off" switches (corresponding to over- and undermedication) in their clinical condition in relation to their diet. Another interaction of interest is levodopa with pyridoxine. Pyridoxine may inhibit the therapeutic efficacy of levodopa by stimulating peripheral conversion of levodopa to dopamine so that less is available for this conversion in the brain. Therefore, high-dose vitamin B_6 supplementation should be avoided in patients with Parkinson disease.

Nutrients also may influence the excretion of

certain drugs. Citrus fruits and low-protein diets lead to increased urinary pH, and this leads to increased renal reabsorption of quinidine, which may in turn cause drug toxicity. On the other hand, alkalinization of the urine increases the excretion of nitrofurantoin, which thereby increases the effectiveness of this antibiotic used for infections of the urinary tract. Alkaline diuresis may be used to increase the rate of excretion of some anionic drugs such as phenobarbital and salicylate.

A high-protein diet leads to the converse — an acidic urine. Lower urine pH increases the rate of excretion of cationic drugs such as amitriptyline. High-protein diets also may influence the metabolism of theophylline. Lithium toxicity may follow concurrent treatment with a sodium-free diet, since under such circumstances renal reabsorption is enhanced. *Principle: There are so many ways for diet to influence the outcome of disease or therapy that it must always be considered as part of a therapeutic regimen. Reconsider diet when drugs are not performing as expected.*

REFERENCES

Abraham, S.; Carroll, M. D.; and Dresser, C. M.: Dietary Intake of Persons 1–74 Years of Age in the United States. Advance Data from Vital and Health Statistics No. 6. DHEW Publication No. (HRA) 77-1647. U.S. Department of Health, Education and Welfare. Health Resources Administration, Public Health Service, Rockville, Md., 1977.

Ahrens, E. J.: Carbohydrates, plasma triglycerides and coronary heart disease. Nutr. Rev., 44:60–64, 1986.

Alpers, D. H.; Clouse, R. E.; and Stenson, W. K.: Manual of Clinical Therapeutics, 2nd ed. Little, Brown, Boston, 1987.

Alvestrand, A.; Ahlberg, M.; Furst, P.; and Bergstrom, J.: Clinical experience with amino acid and keto acid diets. Am. J. Clin. Nutr., 33:1654–1666, 1980.

Askanazi, J.; Elwyn, D. H.; Silverberg, P. A.; Rosenbaum, S. H.; and Kinney, J. M.: Respiratory distress secondary to a high carbohydrate load: A case report. Surgery, 87:596–598, 1980.

Bittle, C. C. Jr.; Molina, D. J.; and Bartter, F. C.: Salt sensitivity in essential hypertension as determined by the Cosinor method. Hypertension, 7:989–994, 1985.

Bray, G. A.: The Obese Patient: Major Problems in Internal Medicine. W. B. Saunders, Philadelphia, 1976.

Butterworth, C. E.; and Blackburn, G. L.: Hospital malnutrition and how to assess the nutritional status of a patient. Nutr. Today, 10:8–18, 1975.

Ciavarella, A.; DiMizio, G.; Stefoni, S.; Borgnino, L. C.; and Vannini, P.: Reduced albuminuria after dietary protein restriction in insulin-dependent diabetic patients with clinical nephropathy. Diabetes Care, 10:407–413, 1987.

Council on Scientific Affairs: Vitamin preparations as dietary supplements and as therapeutic agents. J.A.M.A., 257:1929–1936, 1987.

Fischer, J. E.; Yoshimura, N.; Aguirre, A. L.; James, J. H.; Cummings, M. G.; Abel, R. M.; and Deindoerfer, F: Plasma amino acids in patients with hepatic encephalopathy: Effects of amino acid infusions. Am. J. Surg., 127:40–47, 1973.

Holman, R. T.: Biological activities of and requirements for polyunsaturated acids. In, Progress in the Chemistry of Fat and Other Lipids, Vol. 9. Pergamon Press, New York, N.Y., pp. 607–682, 1970.

Johnson, R. A.; Baker, S. S.; Fallon, J. T.; Maynard, E. P.; Ruskin, J. B.; Wen Z.; Keyou, G.; and Cohen, H. J.: An accidental case of cardiomyopathy and selenium deficiency. N. Engl. J. Med., 304:1210–1212, 1981.

Kissebah, A. H.; Freeman, D. S.; and Peiris, A. N.: Health risks of obesity. Med. Clin. North Am., 73:111–138, 1989.

Kushner, R. F.; Shapir, J.; and Sitrin, M. D.: Endoscopic, radiographic and clinical response to prolonged bowel rest and home parenteral nutrition in Crohn's disease. J.P.E.N., 10:568–577, 1986.

Leaf, A.; and Weber, P. C.: Cardiovascular effects of *n*-3 fatty acids. N. Engl. J. Med., 318:549–557, 1988.

LSRO (Life Sciences Research Office): Physiological Effects and Health Consequences of Dietary Fiber. Federation of American Societies for Experimental Biology, Bethesda, Md., 1987.

MacFie, J.; Smith, R. C.; and Hill, G. L.: Glucose or fat as a non-protein energy source? A controlled clinical trial in gastrointestinal patients requiring intravenous nutrition. Gastroenterology, 80:103–107, 1981.

Miller, K. S.; Tomlinson, J. R.; and Sahn, S. A.: Pleuropulmonary complications of enteral tube feedings. Two reports, review of the literature, and recommendations. Chest, 88: 230–233, 1985.

Mock, D. M.; Delorimer, A. A.; Liebman, W. M.; Sweetman, L.; and Baker, H.: Biotin deficiency: An unusual complication of parenteral alimentation. N. Engl. J. Med., 304:820–822, 1981.

Morley, J. E.: Moderator, nutrition in the elderly. Ann. Intern. Med., 109:890–904, 1988.

National Institutes of Health: Diet and Exercise in Non-Insulin Dependent Diabetes Mellitus. Vol. 6, National Institutes of Health Consensus Development Conference Statement. National Institute of Arthritis, Diabetes and Digestive and Kidney Diseases and the Office of Medical Applications of Research. U.S. Department of Health and Human Services, Bethesda, Md., 1986.

National Research Council (U.S.) Committee on Diet and Health: Diet and health: Implications for reducing chronic disease risk. National Academy Press, Washington, D.C., 1989.

Peters, C.; and Fischer, J. E.: Studies on calorie to nitrogen ratio for total parenteral nutrition. In, Davis, L. (ed.): Chicago, IL, Surg. Gynecol. Obstet., 151:1–8, 1980.

Recommended Dietary Allowances, 10th ed. National Academy of Sciences, Washington, D.C., 1989.

Richardson, T. J.; and Sgoutas, D.: Essential fatty acid deficiency in four adult patients during total parenteral nutrition. Am. J. Clin. Nutr., 28:258–263, 1975.

Robinson, C. H.; Lawler, M. R.; Chenoweth, W. L.; and Garwick, A. E. (eds.): Normal and Therapeutic Nutrition, 17th ed. Macmillan, New York, 1986.

Roe, D. A.: Diet and Drug Interactions. Van Nostrand Reinhold, New York, 1989.

Segal, K. R.; and Pi-Sunyer, F. X.: Exercise and obesity. Med. Clin. North Am., 73:217–236, 1989.

Skeie, B.; Askanazi, J.; Rothkopf, M. M.; Rosenbaum, S. H.; Kvetan, V.; and Thomashow, B.: Intravenous fat emulsions and lung function: A review. Crit. Care Med., 16:1883–1894, 1988.

Solomons, N. W.; Layden, T. J.; Rosenberg. I. H.; Vo-Khactu, K.; and Sandstead, H. H.: Plasma trace metals during total parenteral alimentation. Gastroenterology, 70:1022–1025, 1976.

Stellato, T. A.; Danziger, L. H.; Nearman, H. S.; and Creger, R. J.: Inadvertent intravenous administration of enteral diet. J.P.E.N., 8:453–459, 1984.

Tatro, D. S. (ed.): Drug Interaction Facts. J. B. Lippincott Co., St. Louis, Mo., 1990.

Walike, J. W.: Tube feeding syndrome in head and neck surgery. Arch. Otolaryngol., 29:533–536, 1969.

WHO (World Health Organization): Energy and Protein Requirements. Report of a Joint FAO/WHO/UNU Expert Consultation. Technical Report Series 724. World Health Organization, Geneva, p. 206, 1985.

11

Treatment of Renal Disorders and the Influence of Renal Function on Drug Disposition

D. Craig Brater

PHARMACOTHERAPY OF COMMON RENAL DISORDERS

Acute Renal Failure

Pathophysiology. Acute renal failure (ARF) is a syndrome in which a rapid decline in renal function occurs and is reflected in increases in concentrations of blood urea nitrogen (BUN) and especially creatinine in serum. Acute renal failure can occur on the background of normal renal function or may be superimposed on chronic renal insufficiency (CRI). In addition, factitious increases in BUN and/or creatinine concentrations can occur. For example, excess tissue catabolism or antianabolic agents like the tetracyclines can cause increases in BUN concentrations (Shils, 1963). Drugs such as cimetidine that block the secretory component of creatinine elimination can increase serum concentrations of creatinine (McKinney et al., 1981). In these settings no actual decline in renal function has occurred. Thus, when faced with a patient with the presumptive diagnosis of ARF, one must first determine whether the change in observed measurements of renal function actually represents a decline in renal function.

When a patient is seen for the first time, determining whether the patient has ARF or CRI is sometimes difficult. Anemia, osteodystrophy, neuropathy, and shrunken kidneys are more con-sistent with CRI. Hyperphosphatemia and hypocalcemia can develop quickly during ARF and are less helpful clues. Differentiating ARF superimposed upon CRI also can be difficult, since renal function in most patients with CRI declines progressively over time. Thus, it is sometimes enigmatic whether a patient manifests the natural progression of his or her disease or, alternatively, whether an acute and possible remedial insult has occurred. A graph of creatinine clearance (or less accurately the reciprocal of serum creatinine concentrations) against time usually reveals a linear deterioration in renal function (Mitch et al., 1976; Jones et al., 1979). A negative deviation from such a plot indicates a new insult and serves as presumptive evidence of ARF until proved otherwise.

Once a diagnosis of ARF is established, its pathogenesis must be determined so that a rational therapeutic strategy can be developed. To facilitate diagnosis, ARF can be classified according to Table 11–1. Both noninvasive and invasive tests can be utilized to formulate a specific diagnosis (Harrington and Cohen, 1975; Miller et al., 1978). For example, assessment of the urinary sediment can be helpful: red blood cell casts and proteinuria focus one's attention on glomerulonephritis or vasculitis; calcium oxalate or urate crystals raise the possibility of urinary tract calculi causing obstruction; granular casts implicate a

Table 11–1. CLASSIFICATION OF TYPES OF ACUTE RENAL FAILURE

Renovascular — Acute obstruction of renal arterial supply (bilateral) or renal vein thrombosis

Prerenal azotemia — Functional renal hypoperfusion due to diminished actual or effective circulating volume such as volume depletion, congestive heart failure, hepatorenal syndrome, etc.

Acute glomerulonephritis or vasculitis

Acute tubular necrosis — either oliguric (urinary volume < 20 ml/h) or nonoliguric (> 20 ml/h)

Nephrotoxic acute renal failure

Acute interstitial nephritis

Postrenal (obstructive) azotemia

nephrotoxic insult; and eosinophiluria raises the specter of interstitial nephritis. Since in prerenal azotemia the kidney behaves as if volume depletion were present, urinary sodium excretion is low (fractional excretion of sodium < 1%) and the urine is concentrated so that its specific gravity or osmolality is high (> 500 mOsm/kg). Moreover, the BUN concentration rises disproportionally to the creatinine concentration. In contrast, when tubular function is impaired, as with acute tubular necrosis (ATN) or interstitial nephritis, sodium reabsorption is diminished so that fractional excretion of sodium is increased; in addition, both urinary dilution and concentration are impaired so that isosthenuria occurs.

If noninvasive assessment and other clinical clues (e.g., exposure to drugs, vascular surgical procedures, presence of decompensated cardiac or hepatic disease, etc.) do not allow a firm diagnosis, invasive studies such as arteriography, renal biopsy, or retrograde pyelography may be indicated. Fortunately, such procedures often can be avoided.

Clinical Pharmacology of Drugs Used in Acute Renal Failure. Obstruction of the renal arteries is not amenable to drug therapy. However, it often is associated with elevated blood pressure that can further damage the kidney. Hypertension should be controlled as discussed in chapter 2. In this setting, however, use of angiotensin-converting enzyme (ACE) inhibitors can further impair renal function. When both kidneys are tightly obstructed or when renal perfusion is severely diminished, as may occur in end-stage heart failure, residual glomerular filtration becomes dependent upon efferent arteriolar constriction from intrarenal production of angiotensin II. Inhibition of converting enzyme can thereby result in a precipitous fall in renal function (Keane et al., 1989).

Treatment of prerenal azotemia depends upon the underlying disorder. Volume repletion quickly restores renal function in depleted patients. In contrast, treatment of conditions such as severe

heart failure or hepatorenal syndrome may not fully restore renal perfusion to normal and patients may remain with some degree of prerenal azotemia. In fact, the degree of prerenal azotemia can sometimes be used as a helpful guide to therapy. For example, a patient with severe decompensated heart failure might present with a markedly elevated BUN/creatinine ratio. With therapy and diuresis, this ratio should diminish, although it may not return to normal. With further diuresis, the ratio might begin to escalate again, indicating overly vigorous diuresis and the onset of iatrogenic relative volume depletion, not worsening heart failure. In some patients this may even occur despite the persistence of peripheral edema. A proper response to this scenario would be a decrease in the dose of diuretic and/or liberalized sodium intake.

Glomerulonephritides and vasculitides are treated with immunosuppressive agents that are discussed elsewhere (see chapters 19 and 20). Since the precise etiology of these syndromes is unknown, such therapy is empiric and should be guided by well-controlled clinical trials.

Acute tubular necrosis represents a syndrome wherein an insult to the kidney (usually ischemic) has progressed to a stage of cell death. Before this stage occurs, renal dysfunction is readily reversible by ameliorating the original insult. For example, if renal ischemia has occurred because of hypotension during a surgical procedure or due to NSAID-induced vasoconstriction (see the section on adverse effects of drugs on renal function), prompt restoration of blood pressure or stopping the offending NSAID can restore renal perfusion before an ischemic insult to tubular cells occurs.

Once ATN is manifest, it is generally characterized by poor reabsorption of sodium and inability to concentrate or dilute the urine. Thus, as noted previously, the fractional excretion of sodium (FE_{Na}) is elevated (> 1%) and urine is isosthenuric (Miller et al., 1978). FE_{Na} (in percent) is calculated as follows:

$$FE_{Na} = \left(\frac{\text{clearance of Na}^+}{\text{GFR}} \right) \times 100\%$$

$$= \left(\frac{U_{Na}V}{S_{Na}} \Big/ \frac{U_{Cr}V}{S_{Cr}} \right) \times 100\%$$

where U is urinary concentration of either Na^+ or creatinine (Cr), S is concentration in serum, GFR is glomerular filtration rate, and V is urinary flow rate. The V cancels, leaving:

$$FE_{Na} = \left(\frac{U_{Na}}{S_{Na}} \Big/ \frac{U_{Cr}}{S_{Cr}} \right) \times 100\%$$

Another parameter for diagnosing causes of ARF is the so-called renal failure index (RFI):

$$\text{RFI} = U_{\text{Na}} \left/ \frac{U_{\text{Cr}}}{S_{\text{Cr}}} \right.$$

An RFI <1 mEq/l indicates prerenal azotemia, and a value >1 mEq/l indicates ATN.

Note that the indices described above are not absolute in a diagnostic sense. Thus, patients, particularly those with underlying disorders characterized by sodium avidity, may have ATN but $FE_{\text{Na}} < 1\%$ even though their urine volume is substantial (Diamond and Yoburn, 1982).

Patients with ATN usually are subdivided into those with oliguria (urine output <20 ml/h) and those who are nonoliguric. Nonoliguric renal failure appears to be less severe than does oliguric in that patients have fewer complications, require less dialysis, and have lower mortality rates (Anderson et al., 1977; McMurray et al., 1978; Minuth et al., 1976). These observations have provoked controversy as to whether patients with oliguric ARF should be treated with the objective of converting them to a nonoliguric state.

Treatment of ATN has focused on use of either mannitol, as an osmotic diuretic, or loop diuretics. In animal models of ARF, prophylactic treatment with mannitol or loop diuretics can prevent the development of ARF (Stein et al., 1978). The mechanism by which mannitol affords this protection is unclear. By blocking reabsorptive pumps, loop diuretics decrease metabolic demands of the medullary segment of the thick limb of the loop of Henle. This area is in tenuous oxygen balance and thereby exquisitely sensitive to ischemic insults. When this nephron segment is put "at rest," an ischemic insult is better tolerated (Brezis et al., 1984).

Though no studies have directly addressed the question, it seems plausible that prophylactic use of osmotic or loop diuretics is a reasonable strategy in patients about to undergo a surgical procedure with a substantial risk of an ischemic renal insult.

Whether mannitol or loop diuretics are efficacious after an insult has occurred is vigorously debated. Mannitol is a poor choice of drug in a patient with renal insufficiency; we recommend that it not be used. Mannitol depends upon the kidney for excretion. Its pharmacokinetics in patients with normal as contrasted to end-stage renal disease (and presumably ARF) are presented in Table 11–2 (Cloyd et al., 1986). In patients with normal renal function, 80% of an IV dose is excreted unchanged in the urine. Mannitol is freely filtered at the glomerulus and on entering the tubular fluid exerts its osmotic effect throughout the length of the nephron to blunt solute re-

Table 11–2. PHARMACOKINETICS OF MANNITOL

	NORMAL RENAL FUNCTION	END-STAGE RENAL DISEASE
Volume of distribution (l/kg)	0.5	—
Clearance (ml/min per kg)	7	0.03
Half-life (h)	1.2	36

absorption. This effect is most pronounced in the proximal tubule and the thick ascending limb of the loop of Henle. Because of mannitol's dependence on renal excretion, it is predictably retained in patients with decreased renal function.

Thus, if mannitol does not improve renal function in a patient with ARF, it persists in plasma, where its osmotic effect can cause intravascular volume expansion sufficient to precipitate heart failure; in addition, severe hyponatremia can occur (Warren and Blantz, 1981; Borges et al., 1982). In this setting, its pharmacodynamics as an osmotic agent in the systemic circulation are deleterious. In contrast, in patients with cerebral edema, the systemic osmotic effect is beneficial. Thus, the benefit–risk assessment for the drug is dependent upon the clinical indication and the patient's renal status. A tenuous potential beneficial effect in ARF seems outweighed by substantial risks, arguing that mannitol's use in patients with ARF is only of historical interest.

If mannitol is administered to a patient with renal insufficiency and adverse effects occur, it is eliminated so slowly (Table 11–2) (half-life = 6 h) that hemodialysis may be necessary to hasten its removal.

The utility of loop diuretics in patients with ARF is debated. Some investigators argue that they may help improve prognosis by converting the patient from the oliguric to the nonoliguric state (Beaufils et al., 1972; Cantarovich et al., 1973). On the other hand, other studies have demonstrated no benefit, or at best a need for a diminished number of dialysis sessions (Epstein et al., 1975; Minuth et al., 1976; Graziani et al., 1984). In addition, use of loop diuretics in patients with ARF also has been associated with ototoxicity, so their administration entails some risk, albeit not as grave as with mannitol (Nierenberg, 1980). In the absence of convincing data, it seems illogical to use diuretics for most patients with ARF.

Chronic Renal Insufficiency

Pathophysiology. Chronic renal insufficiency can result from many disorders such as hypertension, diabetes mellitus, polycystic kidney disease, collagen-vascular diseases, and so forth. Once a decline in renal function occurs by way of any insult, inexorable progression of renal dysfunction usually occurs. No matter what the etiology, end-stage kidneys all show interstitial fibrosis and glomerulosclerosis, raising the hypothesis that a single mechanism accounts for the progressive deterioration of renal function. The considerable efforts that have focused on a possible unifying mechanism of continuing renal injury have led to the hypothesis that the final common pathway of the process occurs by glomerular hyperfiltration as illustrated in Fig. 11-1 (Brenner, 1983; Zeller, 1987; Keane et al., 1989). Simplistically, once a renal insult has occurred, remnant nephrons must work harder. They suffer increased glomerular pressures and glomerular hyperfiltration. Hyperfiltration is associated with a loss in glomerular permselectivity that results in protein filtration, and possible direct tissue injury. Both these effects cause glomerular mesangial injury and stimulation, the culmination of which is glomerulosclerosis. Interestingly, early diabetes mellitus is characterized by glomerular hyperfiltration even when the nephron mass is normal (Reddi and Camerini-Davalos, 1990). Animal models of various types of renal injury have documented many elements of this hypothesis (Keane et al., 1989). On the other hand, not all data are consistent with this model (Klahr et al., 1988).

The hyperfiltration hypothesis has led to a number of potential therapeutic interventions to arrest the progression of renal disease over and above vigorous treatment of the primary disease (e.g., hypertension, diabetes mellitus). The observation that dietary protein in experimental animals caused glomerular hyperfiltration has led to

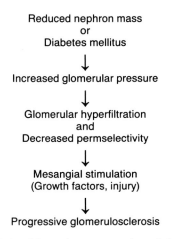

Fig. 11-1. Schematic representation of the glomerular hyperfiltration hypothesis of progressive renal dysfunction.

studies indicating that diminished protein intake (usually 0.4 g of protein per kilogram body weight per day) slows the rate of progression of renal disease (Rosman et al., 1984; Zeller, 1987; Ihle et al., 1989; Keane et al., 1989). In some patients this benefit is outweighed by protein-calorie malnutrition; the degree of protein restriction must be tailored to individual patients.

Experimental studies also have shown that ACE inhibitors diminish glomerular hyperfiltration by ameliorating the intrarenal effects of angiotensin II (Brenner, 1983; Keane et al., 1989). These drugs reverse or arrest albuminuria in normotensive diabetic patients, and they are currently being studied clinically to determine their ability to curtail progression of renal disease (Marre et al., 1988; Parving et al., 1989). In the absence of data confirming their utility, it seems unreasonable to use these agents as a preventive. On the other hand, if a patient with renal insufficiency or diabetes mellitus requires treatment of systemic hypertension, a converting enzyme inhibitor is a logical first choice. This is particularly true since lowering the systemic blood pressure per se is not tantamount to decreasing glomerular hyperfiltration. Other antihypertensives such as diuretics and vasodilators may, in fact, increase glomerular pressure, if not leave it unabated. For calcium-channel antagonists, data are conflicting (Keane et al., 1989).

The diminished renal function in patients with CRI results in a number of conditions often requiring pharmacologic therapy. Loss of nephron mass affects solute homeostasis. Even though patients with CRI have an obligate sodium loss of 20 to 30 mEq/day (Danovitch et al., 1977), compromised ability to excrete amounts of sodium commonly ingested usually results in a need for diuretics to enhance sodium excretion.

Diminished ability to excrete phosphate causes its elevation in plasma with a reciprocal lowering of calcium concentrations, which in turn stimulates release of parathyroid hormone. Ordinarily, parathyroid hormone, among other effects, stimulates 1-hydroxylation of $25[OH]-D_3$ by the kidney, which restores concentrations of calcium toward normal. However, the diminished nephron mass results in decreased capacity to synthesize $1,25[OH]_2-D_3$ such that pharmacologic replacement may be needed (Cushner and Adams, 1986; Feinfeld and Sherwood, 1988).

Correction of the serum calcium concentration without lowering the phosphate concentration may cause precipitation of calcium phosphate in soft tissue. Thus, treatment of hyperphosphatemia is important. Historically, aluminum-containing antacids have been used to irreversibly bind dietary phosphate in the gut precluding its absorption. Aluminum was preferred because of the assumption that it was not absorbed and was thereby innocuous. In contrast, calcium-containing antacids could result in hypercalcemia from absorbed calcium, and magnesium-containing antacids could cause hypermagnesemia with neurologic sequelae (Randall et al., 1964). More recent data have documented considerable accumulation of aluminum in patients with CRI, particularly those treated by chronic dialysis (Cushner and Adams, 1986; Molitoris et al., 1989). Accumulated aluminum has been implicated as a cause of dialysis dementia and as causal or contributory to renal osteodystrophy (Cushner and Adams, 1986; Feinfeld and Sherwood, 1988; Molitoris et al., 1989). Moreover, absorption of aluminum is enhanced by citrate (Molitoris et al., 1989). Unfortunately, citrate-containing preparations have been frequently used to treat the metabolic acidosis of CRI.

Diminished renal function is also associated with a decrease in the kidney's ability to synthesize erythropoietin, accounting for the anemia of patients with CRI (Fried, 1973; Erslev, 1975). Until recently, androgenic steroids and transfusion were the only therapeutic modalities available. The gene for erythropoietin has been cloned and expressed in bacteria, so that pharmacologic doses of human erythropoietin now are available (Groopman et al., 1989). Replacement of this hormone has been proved to normalize red cell mass in patients with CRI, to reverse the iron overload that occurs in many transfusion-dependent patients, and to improve their quality of life (Eschbach et al., 1989a, 1989b).

All patients with CRI become hyperuricemic but are rarely symptomatic from it (gout). Uric acid normally is freely filtered at the glomerulus, after which it is quantitatively reabsorbed by the proximal tubule and then secreted back into the lumen of the nephron, again by the proximal tubule. Diminished GFR from any cause results in elevated uric acid concentrations with the potential risk of gout, urolithiasis, and urate nephropathy. An extensive literature now documents that the risks of asymptomatic hyperuricemia, either de novo, secondary to diuretics, or due to CRI, are negligible (Berger and Yu, 1975; Emmerson and Row, 1975; Fessel, 1979; Yu et al., 1979; Foley and Weinman, 1984; Langford et al., 1987). Rare patients develop gout: 15 episodes over 5 years in 3693 patients with thiazide-induced hyperuricemia (Langford et al., 1987). The risk of urolithiasis is negligible: 1 stone in about 300 patients with hyperuricemia compared with 1 stone in about 850 normouricemic patients (Fessel, 1979); and urate nephropathy is so unusual that some experts question its existence as a distinct clinical entity (Foley and Weinman, 1984). Thus, hyperuricemia in patients with CRI should only be treated if patients are symptomatic, that is, with attacks of gout or with uric acid nephrolithiasis.

Many other associated conditions require treatment in patients with CRI, and doing so is usually made more complicated by the compromised renal function. For example, diabetes mellitus and hypertension frequently cause CRI in the first place. Their control is paramount in patients with diminished renal function in order to preserve residual renal function as much as possible. Many of the drugs used to treat hypertension and other diagnoses have altered disposition and/or pharmacodynamics in patients with CRI, and dosing strategies must be altered. This aspect of therapy is subsequently discussed in detail. *Principle: The number of different factors that influence renal function illustrates the biologic sophistication of the organ and the difficulty presented to the therapist in interpreting drug- or disease-induced changes. Nevertheless, such interpretations must be made if one is to judge when an intervention is required and how to assess the effect of intervention. The major difficulties include the following: (1) disease- or drug-induced changes may be subtly evident because mechanisms for homeostasis are complex and to some extent "fail-safe," but (2) some diseases of other organs are likely to be confused with diseases that can be caused by the kidney (e.g., hypercalcemia), and thus "what to treat, sign or pathogenesis, may be easily forgotten," and (3) some drugs used for therapy of diseases not related to the kidney may modulate renal function (e.g., indomethacin for treatment of inflammatory disease). The challenges for proper responses by the therapist are great and clinically important.*

Clinical Pharmacology of Drugs Used in Chronic Renal Insufficiency. Pharmacotherapy in patients with CRI is aimed at preserving renal function and at treating disorders that arise from the loss of nephron mass itself. Preservation of renal function first entails treatment of primary diseases such as hypertension or diabetes mellitus that can cause further decrements in renal function if they are not controlled. The pharmacology and clinical pharmacokinetics of drugs used in these disorders are discussed in chapters 2 and 16, respectively. Other primary causes of CRI such as polycystic kidney disease are untreatable, though complications such as infection, which hastens renal deterioration, can be treated.

Other than treating primary diseases with adverse effects on renal function, another therapeutic goal is arrest of progressive renal deterioration. As discussed previously, glomerular hypertension may represent a final common pathway for the persistent decrement in renal function that occurs in most patients with CRI (Fig. 11-1), though some experts feel this explanation to be too simplistic and that multifactorial factors that differ among diseases are etiologic (Brenner, 1983; Klahr et al., 1988). Despite this debate, data support limiting protein intake to 0.4 g/kg body weight per day if nutritional status can be maintained (Rosman et al., 1984; Zeller, 1987; Ihle et al., 1989; Keane et al., 1989). In addition, data in animals are sufficient to recommend preferential use of ACE inhibitors to treat hypertension in patients with CRI (Keane et al., 1989). The clinical pharmacology of these drugs is discussed in chapter 2.

Strategies for maintaining calcium and phosphate homeostasis have changed recently. The heretofore universal use of aluminum-containing antacids to bind phosphate in the gut has for the most part been abandoned in order to avoid aluminum toxicity (Cushner and Adams, 1986). Similarly, calcium citrate is no longer favored as a phosphate binder and calcium replacement, since citrate increases aluminum absorption (Molitoris et al., 1989). Instead, calcium carbonate or calcium acetate should be used to bind phosphate and simultaneously supplement calcium (Sheikh et al., 1989). If hyperphosphatemia is not controlled, judicious use of aluminum-containing antacids can be employed if ingested with meals. If plasma phosphate is normal but calcium remains depressed, $1,25[OH]_2-D_3$ is used to restore calcium homeostasis and thereby reverse secondary hyperparathyroidism (Cushner and Adams, 1986; Feinfeld and Sherwood, 1988).

Reversal of erythropoietin deficiency is now possible through use of the genetically engineered human hormone. In virtually all patients, including those treated with chronic dialysis, red cell mass can be restored to normal within 12 weeks. Lack of response implies another disorder such as blood loss, myelofibrosis, and so forth. Although many patients who receive erythropoietin are iron-overloaded because of repeated blood transfusions, the increased iron needs for new red blood cell propagation results in iron deficiency in over 40% of patients; thus many, if not most, patients require iron supplements. The increased blood volume that occurs also results in hypertension or worsened hypertension in about one third of patients. Initial concerns of an increased rate of clotting of vascular access has been disproved (Eschbach et al., 1989a, 1989b). The improved patient well-being and quality of life far outweigh the deleterious effects of erythropoietin, and its availability represents a major advance in therapy of CRI and an excellent example of the utility and potential of extrapolation of molecular biology to clinical medicine.

Treatment of symptomatic hyperuricemia entails either decreasing the rate of synthesis of uric acid or increasing its excretion. The latter is not a therapeutic option in patients with CRI since uricosuric agents are ineffective because of the decreased renal function. Thus, allopurinol is used, but at decreased doses to avoid accumulation of its potentially toxic active metabolite, oxipurinol.

Allopurinol and its metabolite oxipurinol decrease production of uric acid by inhibiting xanthine oxidase. Allopurinol itself has a bioavailability of about 65%. It is eliminated quickly with a half-life of about 1.5 hours. With chronic dosing, oxipurinol accumulates, since its half-life is 15 to 30 hours, accounting for the satisfactory response to once-daily dosing. This observation also confirms that the majority of the hypouricemic effect with chronic dosing is due to the metabolite rather than the parent drug (Murrell and Rapeport, 1986). In contrast to allopurinol, which is metabolized in the liver, oxipurinol is excreted in the urine. Thus, patients with CRI accumulate oxipurinol, which has a half-life in patients with severe CRI of about 1 week (Elion et al., 1968; Murrell and Rapeport, 1986). If the dose of allopurinol is not decreased to about one third of normal or less in such patients, severe oxipurinol toxicity, which manifests as a systemic vasculitis, can occur (Young et al., 1974).

Most patients with CRI require treatment with diuretics at some point during the course of their disease either as antihypertensive agents or to reverse sodium accumulation. The pharmacology of diuretic agents will be subsequently discussed in the section on fluid and electrolytes. Since diuretics used in patients with CRI are for the most part restricted to loop diuretics, their use will be discussed here.

The diminished filtered sodium in patients with CRI often makes diuretic therapy vexing because even highly efficacious loop diuretics are limited in their effects. As a consequence, patients can easily ingest sufficient sodium to overcome any drug-induced diuresis, making dietary restriction of sodium a mainstay of therapy in patients with CRI, just as it is in some edematous disorders.

The loop diuretics bumetanide, ethacrynic acid, and furosemide all must reach the lumen of the nephron to exert an effect (Odlind and Beermann, 1980; Odlind et al., 1983). Renal clearance of these diuretics decreases in parallel with the diminished renal perfusion of CRI, so that less drug reaches the site of action. For example, in patients with severe renal insufficiency, only one fifth as much furosemide reaches the urine as after administration of the same dose to a patient with normal renal function (Brater et al., 1986; Voelker et al., 1987). With bumetanide, the comparable value is one tenth (Voelker et al., 1987).

Similar data have not been published with ethacrynic acid, a diuretic little used except in patients with allergic reactions to furosemide or bumetanide. *These findings suggest that a 5-fold higher dose of furosemide and a 10-fold higher dose of bumetanide would be needed in a patient with severe renal insufficiency compared with a patient with normal renal function* (Voelker et al., 1987; Brater, 1988).

Recent studies have documented that residual nephrons respond normally to amounts of loop diuretic reaching them with a maximal fractional excretion of sodium of about 20% (Brater et al., 1986; Voelker et al., 1987). In a patient with normal GFR, this level of response amounts to a maximal sodium excretion rate of about 3 mEq/min that constitutes a substantial natriuresis even if sustained over only a short period of time. In contrast, a patient with CRI having a GFR one tenth of normal would have a maximal sodium excretion rate of only about 0.3 mEq/min. Even if sustained over several hours, this magnitude of response may be inadequate in many patients, mandating ancillary measures for removing sodium, such as dialysis. If a therapeutic trial is possible, occasional patients with CRI respond to a combination of loop and thiazide diuretics. The rationale for such therapy will be discussed in the section on fluid and electrolytes.

Recent data have shown that maximal doses of loop diuretics in patients with severe CRI (GFR < 15 ml/min) are 8 to 10 mg of oral or IV bumetanide and 200 mg of IV or 400 mg of oral furosemide (Brater et al., 1986; Voelker et al., 1987). Higher doses add no increment of efficacy and simply risk toxicity. Though the therapeutic margin of loop diuretics is large, ototoxicity that usually is reversible can occur. Ototoxicity usually has been reported with large doses given to patients with renal insufficiency particularly if they were concomitantly treated with other ototoxic drugs such as aminoglycoside antibiotics (Sheffield and Turner, 1971; Cooperman and Rubin, 1973; Gallagher and Jones, 1979).

The pharmacokinetics of loop diuretics are listed in Table 11-3 (Hammarlund-Udenaes and Benet, 1989; Brater, 1990). No data are available for ethacrynic acid, but as noted above, it is little used. Bumetanide and furosemide are considered to be essentially equivalent in terms of their pharmacologic effects. They differ, however, in their disposition and the influence of disease thereon. On average, about half of an oral dose of furosemide is absorbed; switching from IV to oral dosing requires doubling the dose. In contrast, bumetanide is essentially completely absorbed; IV and oral doses are identical.

Both bumetanide and furosemide are highly protein-bound (>90%), accounting for the small volumes of distribution listed in Table 11-3. Distribution volume is not appreciably changed in the diseases in which it has been assessed. These two loop diuretics differ considerably in their metabolism. In healthy subjects, about half of an IV dose reaches the urine and accounts for the diuretic effect. The remaining 50% of bumetanide is metabolized by the cytochrome P450 mixed-function oxidase system, whereas the remaining half of furosemide is conjugated with glucuronide (Brater, 1990). In patients with severe renal insufficiency, nonrenal as well as renal pathways for furosemide's elimination are impaired, causing an overall clearance of one third normal that more than doubles the elimination half-life. In contrast, bumetanide in patients with severe CRI still retains its nonrenal elimination pathways such that overall clearance is less depressed (two thirds normal) and the half-life of elimination is unchanged. Thus in CRI, furosemide persists in plasma and similarly in urine longer than does bumetanide. Whether this is clinically important is unknown.

The differing routes of nonrenal elimination of bumetanide and furosemide also result in a different pattern of the effect of liver disease on their disposition (Table 11-3). Thus, for bumetanide, cirrhosis results in diminished nonrenal clearance and a substantial fall in overall clearance with a doubling of the elimination half-life. In contrast, with furosemide, hepatic dysfunction results in only slight decreases in overall clearance and negligible effects on half-life. As such, in contrast to patients with CRI, in cirrhosis, bumetanide persists in plasma and urine longer than does furosemide.

The disposition of bumetanide has not been well studied in patients with heart failure but likely differs little from its disposition in healthy subjects unless considerable congestive hepatopathy prevails. This could cause a decrease in metabolism of the drug.

Changes in disposition of furosemide in patients with heart failure are explained by moderate decreases in renal function that occur in many such patients (Brater et al., 1982). These changes on average dictate a twofold increase in doses needed in patients with heart failure.

Studies with both bumetanide and furosemide in patients with heart failure have shown a delay in absorption though the total quantity of diuretic absorbed (i.e., bioavailability) is unaltered (Brater et al., 1984; Vasko et al., 1985). Moreover, patients in the decompensated state show a greater delay of absorption than when they have been treated to a stable clinical condition (Vasko et al., 1985). The clinical importance of these ob-

Table 11–3. **PHARMACOKINETICS OF LOOP DIURETICS**

	HEALTHY VOLUNTEERS	END-STAGE RENAL DISEASE	CIRRHOSIS	CONGESTIVE HEART FAILURE
Bumetanide				
Bioavailability (%)	80	80	95	—
Volume of distribution (l/kg)	0.17	0.23	0.09	—
Clearance (ml/min per kg)	2.6	1.6	0.6	—
Half-life (h)	1.2	1.5	2.3	1.8
Fraction of IV dose excreted in urine unchanged (%)	65	5	70	—
Furosemide				
Bioavailability (%)	50	45	60	50
Volume of distribution (l/kg)	0.16	0.12	0.16	0.16
Clearance (ml/min per kg)	2.2	0.8	1.7	1.6
Half-life (h)	1.0	2.5	1.2	1.4
Fraction of IV dose excreted in urine unchanged (%)	60	10	55	60

servations is that patients with decompensated heart failure absorb loop diuretics so slowly that they often require treatment by IV dosing.

Urinary Tract Infections

Pathophysiology. Urinary tract infections (UTIs) encompass infections from the urethra to the kidney itself. In addition, vaginitis often can present with symptoms consistent with a UTI, though it often can be distinguished from a true UTI by superficial burning that occurs after urination as opposed to true dysuria.

Therapeutic strategies in patients with a UTI are dictated by whether the patient is male or female, whether the infection is symptomatic, and whether the infection is in the lower or upper urinary tract. Infection of the male urinary tract implies an underlying pathologic condition, either anatomic or a set of host factors increasing susceptibility to infection. In contrast, UTI is frequent in women, with 10% to 20% of all women suffering a UTI during their life (Johnson and Stamm, 1989). A search for an underlying pathologic condition in women with UTI is indicated only when infections recur; three or more infections in a woman during one year warrant further investigation (Komaroff, 1984).

Asymptomatic bacteriuria is frequent, particularly in elderly patients, affecting up to 20% of women and 10% of men over 65 years of age (Boscia et al., 1987). There is no evidence that asymptomatic bacteriuria leads to progressive renal insufficiency or other complications; thus, it need not be treated (Boscia et al., 1987). If symptoms occur, treatment is, however, indicated. The exception to this general rule is pregnancy, wherein even asymptomatic bacteriuria (which occurs frequently) should be treated, accounting

for the rationale for screening urinalyses throughout pregnancy (Komaroff, 1986).

When a patient's UTI presents, it is important to distinguish upper (pyelonephritis) from lower (cystitis) tract infection. Table 11–4 offers clinical signs and symptoms that can help differentiate upper from lower UTI (Johnson and Stamm, 1989). However, up to one third of patients with the characteristic presentation of cystitis have concomitant upper tract infection. If a patient is treated for cystitis and treatment failure occurs or relapse with the same organism occurs within 2 weeks of the completion of therapy, upper tract infection should be assumed (Komaroff, 1984).

Clinical Pharmacologic Considerations in Treating UTIs. Traditional dictum is that treatment of any UTI requires antecedent cultures and

Table 11–4. **SIGNS AND SYMPTOMS TO DIFFERENTIATE UPPER FROM LOWER URINARY TRACT INFECTION**

Upper Tract
  Localized flank, low back, or abdominal pain
  Systemic signs and symptoms:

Fever	Nausea
Rigors	Vomiting
Sweats	Malaise
Headache	Prostration

Lower Tract
  Dysuria
  Frequency
  Nocturia
  Urgency
  Frequent small voidings
  Incontinence
  Suprapubic tenderness—occurs in only about 10% of patients but is specific for cystitis

Adapted from Johnson and Stamm (1989).

sensitivity testing. However, patients with signs and symptoms suggesting lower tract disease and pyuria (two to five white blood cells per high-power field) in an adequate, spun specimen can be treated cost-effectively without the guidance of a urine culture (Komaroff, 1986; Johnson and Stamm, 1989). Moreover, microscopic hematuria and particularly bacteriuria in the presence of typical symptoms of cystitis are highly specific though not as sensitive as pyuria (Johnson and Stamm, 1989).

If cultures of urine are obtained in a patient with signs and symptoms of a UTI, the usual cut-off value of 10^4 bacterial colonies per milliliter is too rigid, and 10^2 colonies per milliliter should be considered confirmatory of infection (Johnson and Stamm, 1989).

Adequate treatment of uncomplicated cystitis can be accomplished with a variety of drugs and a variety of regimens. Therapy for 1 day, for 3 days, and for a complete 7- to 10-day course has been assessed. One day of therapy is effective and inexpensive and entails fewer side effects than longer courses of treatment. If a 1-day regimen is utilized, trimethoprim alone is as effective as trimethoprim plus sulfamethoxazole and has fewer adverse effects. In addition, fewer relapses occur with these two drugs compared with ampicillin, amoxicillin, or an oral cephalosporin (Johnson and Stamm, 1989). Three days of therapy with trimethoprim, trimethoprim plus sulfamethoxazole, amoxicillin, or doxycycline has the same efficacy as a 10-day course of treatment but has as low an incidence of adverse effects as a 1-day course and is intermediate in expense. It likely represents the best regimen for most patients (Johnson and Stamm, 1989).

Upper tract infections and those with a greater likelihood of resistant pathogens (Table 11-5) require more aggressive therapy and guidance by culture and sensitivity testing. Intravenous antibiotic therapy is sometimes necessary, with the choice of antibiotics dependent upon local sensitivity patterns, aspects of patient history that might indicate the infecting organism, and sever-

Table 11-5. PATIENT FACTORS INDICATING THE LIKELIHOOD OF UTI WITH RESISTANT PATHOGENS

Hospital-acquired
Pregnancy
Indwelling bladder catheter
Recent urinary tract instrumentation
Urinary tract anatomic abnormality
Urinary tract stone
Recent antibiotic use
Diabetes mellitus
Immune compromise

Adapted from Johnson and Stamm (1989).

Table 11-6. FACTORS THAT PREDISPOSE TO FORMATION OF URINARY TRACT STONES

Enhanced Precipitation from Urine
Increased excretion of the precipitant (e.g., hypercalciuria, hyperuricosuria, hyperoxaluria, cystinuria)
Decreased saturability of the urine
Urine pH decreasing solubility (e.g., RTA)
Low urine volume
Decrease in Inhibitors of Crystalization
Hypocitraturia
Decreased urinary pyrophosphate
Deficits in other inhibitors?

ity of illness (see chapter 24 for discussion of specific antibiotics). Once culture results identify the infecting organism, oral drug dosing can commence with treatment for 14 days. If relapse occurs, a 6-week course of therapy should be employed. If the patient has not improved within 3 days of therapy, a complication such as nephrolithiasis, obstruction, or abscess must be considered (Johnson and Stamm, 1989).

Some patients have recurrent UTIs. If infections occur three or more times per year, prophylactic therapy is cost-effective (Stamm et al., 1980, 1981). Any of a variety of agents are effective, and therapy is guided by results of urine cultures. Treatment should last for 6 months; if symptomatic recurrences continue, prophylactic therapy may need to be indefinite (Ronald and Harding, 1981; Stamm et al., 1980, 1981).

Chlamydial infection is worthy of specific comment (Schachter, 1978). This common pathogen should be particularly suspected in women with a stuttering and prolonged onset of dysuria and other lower urinary tract symptoms. Both the patient and his or her sexual partner should be treated with a 7-day course of either erythromycin or tetracycline (Komaroff, 1986).

Urinary Tract Stones

Pathophysiology. Urinary tract stones can be formed from many constituents in urine including calcium, uric acid, cystine, oxalate, and even some drugs and metabolites of drugs excreted in the urine such as triamterene and oxipurinol (Landgrebe et al., 1975; Ettinger, 1985). Formation of a stone requires a nidus and supersaturated urine, both of which combine to produce precipitation, followed by crystal growth and aggregation or agglomeration. Growth of the crystal and aggregation may be the most important elements, since a simple precipitate still can be excreted in the urine.

A predilection to formation of a stone can occur by several general mechanisms (Table 11-6). Increased excretion of the precipitant can occur from a variety of disorders. For example, hypercalciuria can occur from hyperparathyroidism or other primary disorders or can be idiopathic, which in turn has been classified as either absorptive or renal (Pak et al., 1974a; Pak, 1979). Similar examples can be enumerated for causes of hyperuricosuria, hyperoxaluria, and cystinuria (Coe and Favus, 1986). *Principle: Making a specific diagnosis (the basis of the hyperexcretion) is required to target therapy specifically toward the pathogenesis of the underlying disorder.*

An increase in the likelihood of precipitation from supersaturated urine can occur through simply physical factors such as urinary pH and volume. A low urine volume can increase saturation beyond the point of solubility. A corollary of this principle is that increased fluid intake is a reasonable prescription for any patient with nephrolithiasis, no matter what the cause (Pak et al., 1980b). The solubility of many of the causal factors of renal stones is influenced by pH. As such, an alkaline urine greatly increases the solubility of uric acid and cystine and is a therapeutic goal in patients suffering these types of stones (Pak, 1985). On the other hand, the persistently alkaline urine of renal tubular acidosis (RTA) diminishes the solubility of calcium salts and can cause not only nephrolithiasis, but also nephrocalcinosis.

Clearly, the urine contains inhibitors of crystalization. Pyrophosphate and citrate serve this function, but other as-yet-unidentified inhibitors also are likely to be present (Pak, 1985; Coe and Favus, 1986). Phosphate, diphosphonates, and synthetic analogs of pyrophosphate can be given to humans, but the effects of the latter two on bone mineralization preclude their use to replenish urinary inhibitory activity. In contrast, some stone disorders are characterized by hypocitraturia that can be corrected by administration of alkali (e.g., sodium or potassium bicarbonate) or citrate-containing salts (Pak and Fuller, 1986; Kok et al., 1990).

Clinical Pharmacology in the Treatment of Stones in the Urinary Tract. The treatment employed requires a diagnosis of the cause of the formation of the stone. The first step is to analyze the stone itself. From 40% to 75% of stones will prove to be due to hypercalciuria (Pak, 1985). Another 5% to 25% will be accounted for by hyperuricosuria (Coe and Favus, 1986). Other causes of stone formation are uncommon. If hyperexcretion of a substance that causes stone is found, further workup entails identification of pathogenesis. For example, if hypercalciuria is found, assessment for hyperparathyroidism or for the different forms of idiopathic hypercalciuria should ensue. Relatively simple methods for such assessment have been described. They are feasible for most patients in an outpatient setting

and do not require complex or expensive analytical techniques (Pak et al., 1975, 1980a).

Once the cause of the stone formation is established, one must decide whether to treat. Since the median time to recurrence of untreated calcium-containing stones is about 7 years (Coe et al., 1977) and since drug treatment entails potential adverse effects, it is reasonable to defer drug treatment until more than one episode occurs (Uribarri et al., 1989). Moreover, this admonition means that metabolic evaluation to determine causality can be deferred until more than one episode occurs. Conservative measures such as increasing fluid intake and decreasing calcium and urate intake should be recommended to delay (if not prevent) recurrence as long as possible.

If treatment is necessary, the therapeutic regimen is based on the cause of the pathogenesis of the stone as summarized in Table 11-7. Hyperparathyroidism usually is remedied surgically. The incidence of the diagnosis of hyperparathyroidism has considerably increased with the routine measurement of serum calcium concentrations made possible by the autoanalyzers and by the availability of accurate radioimmunoassays for determining the circulating concentration of parathyroid hormone (Bilezikian, 1982; Mallette, 1987). It appears that asymptomatic patients without bone, ulcer, or stone disease can be followed conservatively; however, the occurrence of a stone is an indication for surgical correction (Bilezikian, 1982; Mallette, 1987).

Most hypercalciuria is idiopathic, making this diagnosis the most common in patients with nephrolithiasis. Thiazide diuretics are effective for both absorptive and renal hypercalciurias. Some experts recommend these diuretics for both forms of this disorder (Coe and Favus, 1986). Others

Table 11-7. TREATMENT OF URINARY TRACT STONES

CAUSE	TREATMENT
Hypercalciuria	
Hyperparathyroidism	Parathyroidectomy
Idiopathic	
Absorptive	Sodium cellulose phosphate
Renal	Thiazide diuretics
Hyperuricosuria	Allopurinol
	Alkali
Distal renal tubular acidosis	Alkali
Hyperoxaluria	
Metabolic	Pyridoxine
Enteric	Chloestyramine
Cystinuria	D-Penicillamine
	Mercaptopropionylglycine
Normocalciuric idiopathic	Phosphate

argue that more specifically directed therapy is appropriate. They use sodium cellulose phosphate to retard absorption of calcium in patients with the absorptive form of this disorder (Pak et al., 1974b). Thiazides are then reserved for patients with renal hypercalciuria. If sodium cellulose phosphate is used, substantial negative calcium balance that may adversely affect bone metabolism can occur; patients should be monitored for such an adverse effect.

It seems somewhat paradoxical that diuretics are used to decrease excretion of calcium. Acute administration of loop and thiazide diuretics causes an increase in calcium excretion that parallels the increased sodium excretion. Chronic use of thiazide diuretics, however, causes mild volume depletion that, in turn, stimulates proximal and distal tubular reabsorption of solute, including calcium (Brickman et al., 1972; Breslau et al., 1976). The net result is decreased excretion of calcium in urine with amelioration of stone formation. Interestingly, it appears that this therapy results in a net positive calcium balance and increased bone density that appear protective against hip fracture in elderly patients (LaCroix et al., 1990). *Principle: Once one is on the trail of a fundamental undiscovered mechanism of action of a drug, it pays to follow up on all its implications.*

Though uric acid stones are less common than are calcium-containing stones, calcium stones in the setting of hyperuricosuria responds to measures that decrease urinary excretion of uric acid, such as dietary restriction of purine or the use of allopurinol (Coe and Raisen, 1973; Coe, 1978; Ettinger et al., 1986). The mechanism by which decreases in uric acid excretion diminish formation of calcium stones depends upon the fact that the precipitated uric acid serves as a nidus for stone formation. Since even normal excretion of calcium results in a supersaturated urine, a nidus of uric acid allows epitaxial crystal growth with calcium salts (usually oxalate).

Treatment of hyperuricosuria with allopurinol depends mainly upon the activity of its active metabolite, oxipurinol. Both compounds lower uric acid formation by inhibiting xanthine oxidase, the enzyme that converts hypoxanthine to xanthine and also xanthine to uric acid. With chronic therapy, oxipurinol (with a half-life of 15 to 30 hours) accumulates in excess of allopurinol (half-life of 1.5 hours) and accounts for the majority of inhibition of xanthine oxidase. Oxipurinol depends on renal function for elimination (e.g., in patients with end-stage renal disease, its half-life is about 1 week). It can accumulate to toxic concentrations in patients with renal insufficiency unless doses are diminished in relationship to the level of renal function. Oxipurinol toxicity resembles a hypersensitivity reaction with skin rash, fever, hepati-

tis, nephritis, and eosinophilia (Young et al., 1974; Al-Kawas et al., 1981).

Stones in patients with distal renal tubular acidosis usually are calcium phosphate, and their formation is a result of not only increased calcium and phosphate excretion but also the additional pathogenetic factors of alkaline pH and hypocitraturia (Coe and Favus, 1986). Since the urine is already alkaline, treatment with alkali seems paradoxical; however, so doing increases urinary citrate that acts as an inhibitor of stone formation.

Hyperoxaluria can generally be classified as metabolic or enteric, each of which has a variety of causes. The former is rare, and the latter usually is associated with inflammatory bowel disease, intestinal bypass surgery, or malabsorption syndromes. Metabolic hyperoxaluria is treated with pyridoxine. Enteric hyperoxaluria is treated with restriction of dietary fat or replacement of pancreatic enzymes if there is associated steatorrhea, restriction of dietary oxalate, or use of oral calcium carbonate supplements and/or cholestyramine. Calcium supplements increase enteric calcium that binds with enteric oxalate to prevent its absorption. The binding of bile acids by cholestyramine diminishes saponification of dietary fats that bind calcium in the proximal intestine. Thus, more calcium becomes available for binding with oxalate.

Cystinuria is a rare metabolic disorder that is occasionally associated with stone formation. Therapy consists of increasing fluid intake to dilute the urine and ingesting large doses of alkali to alkalinize the urine. The latter is only marginally beneficial since cystine's solubility does not appreciably increase until the urine pH exceeds 7.5, a value close to the maximum physiologic pH of about 8.0. If these conservative maneuvers fail, either D-penicillamine or mercaptopropionylglycine can be used. The efficacy of these drugs depends upon disulfide exchange. Cystine is the disulfide of cysteine. Treatment with D-penicillamine that contains a free thiol group results in a mixed disulfide, D-penicillamine-S-S-cysteine, which is more soluble than is cystine (Crawhall and Watts, 1968; Broadus and Thier, 1979).

D-Penicillamine is used as a last resort in patients with cystinuria because of its adverse effects, particularly nephrotoxicity, which usually first manifests as proteinuria from membranous glomerulonephritis (Hall et al., 1988). Other common adverse effects include rash, loss of taste, stomatitis, thrombocytopenia, and leukopenia (Stein et al., 1980; Steen et al., 1986). Up to 50% of patients will have an adverse effect, and up to one third will have to discontinue the drug. Clinical experience with mercaptopropionylglycine is insufficient to know its benefit-to-risk profile.

Some patients with nephrolithiasis have no

identifiable metabolic abnormality. They are classified as normocalciuric idiopathic stone formers. These patients can be treated with inorganic phosphate that also is effective in patients with hypercalciuria (Ettinger and Kolb, 1973). However, even phosphate likely entails more risks than using alkali to increase urinary citrate, which seems the logical first approach to therapy in these patients.

Fluid and Electrolyte Disorders

Pathophysiology. A number of diseases and drugs themselves cause abnormalities in fluid and electrolyte status. Understanding the physiology of renal regulation of electrolyte and volume homeostasis is necessary to correct abnormalities thereof.

Volume and Osmolality. Total body fluid volume is determined by body sodium content and is independent of sodium concentration. Thus, a patient can be volume-expanded yet be hyponatremic. A good example is a patient with severe congestive heart failure. The serum sodium *concentration* is an index of osmolality. As such the patient described above with hyponatremia would be hypoosmolar unless solutes other than sodium were circulating in plasma (e.g., elevated blood glucose concentration). Osmolality, in turn, is determined by free-water homeostasis. A patient with severe CHF and hyponatremia thereby has a diminished concentration of sodium in serum because of free-water retention that is independent of overall sodium and volume homeostasis.

Figure 11–2 depicts a schematized renal tubule that highlights the major components of regulation of sodium and water and thus the control of volume and osmolality. In addition to these tubular functions, regulation is also facilitated by humoral and hemodynamic components. For example, volume depletion increases circulating catecholamine concentration and activates the systemic and intrarenal renin-angiotensin systems. Proximal tubular receptors to norepinephrine and to angiotensin II stimulate sodium reabsorption (Schuster et al., 1984; DiBona, 1985; Douglas, 1987; Nord et al., 1987). Effects of these autacoids on renal hemodynamics also enhance sodium reabsorption. Conversely, volume expansion activates atrial stretch receptors that release atrial natriuretic peptide, causing an increased GFR and filtered sodium with resulting increased sodium excretion (Ballermann and Brenner, 1985; de Bold, 1985; Trippodo et al., 1987).

Isosmotic reabsorption of 60% to 70% of ions and water occurs in the proximal tubule. Sodium and water reabsorption passively follow the active transport of organic solute. In addition, sodium is actively reabsorbed (Windhager and Giebisch, 1976; Cogan, 1982; Rector, 1983). Normally,

more than 85% of filtered bicarbonate is reabsorbed as sodium bicarbonate. High permeability to water in the proximal tubule allows the passive reabsorption of water with sodium.

In the thick loop of Henle, reabsorption of 20% to 30% of the filtered sodium as sodium chloride occurs via active transport of two Cl^- ions coupled to one Na^+ and one K^+ ion (Greger, 1985). Saturation of this transport system cannot be demonstrated under physiologic conditions (Burg, 1976). This means that increased rejection of solute from the proximal nephron can be reclaimed at the loop of Henle and the contribution of the loop to overall sodium reabsorption can increase dramatically.

The thick ascending limb of the loop of Henle is impermeable to water. Solute reabsorption from a segment of the nephron that is impermeable to water ultimately leaves in the tubule fluid that is hypotonic to plasma. This hypotonic fluid consists of two hypothetical volumes, one isosmotic with plasma and the other free of osmotic activity (solute-free water or *free water*). Therefore, production of free water occurs in the ascending limb of the loop of Henle. In the cortical segment of the limb, fluid actually becomes hypotonic; consequently this segment also is referred to as the *diluting* segment. Production of dilute urine depends upon the delivery of sodium chloride to that site (i.e., if less sodium is delivered to the diluting site, less dilution can occur), active transport of solute, and the tubule's impermeability to water. The tubular fluid in the early distal region remains hypotonic, and if there is no stimulus for conservation of water, this dilute fluid will be excreted in the urine, thereby providing a mechanism for excretion of free water. Considered in another way, this capacity to excrete a dilute urine provides the body's defense against hypoosmolality. For example, ingestion of distilled water would cause hyponatremia and hypoosmolality unless the kidney could excrete the water load. Conversely, impaired ability to excrete a water load caused by drugs (see the section on adverse effects of drugs on renal function) or disease states can result in a hypoosmolar state and hyponatremia.

The thick ascending limb of the loop of Henle also contributes to the ability to concentrate the urine. The active reabsorption of solute coupled with passive transport of urea at this segment allows the development of a hypertonic medullary interstitium (Jamison et al., 1967; Jamison, 1968; Kokko and Rector, 1972; Berliner, 1976). This hypertonic interstitium provides the osmotic driving force for water reabsorption when the kidney needs to conserve water. Any interruption of this capacity, then, impairs a patient's ability to conserve water and subjects him or her to the risk of a hyperosmolar state and hypernatremia.

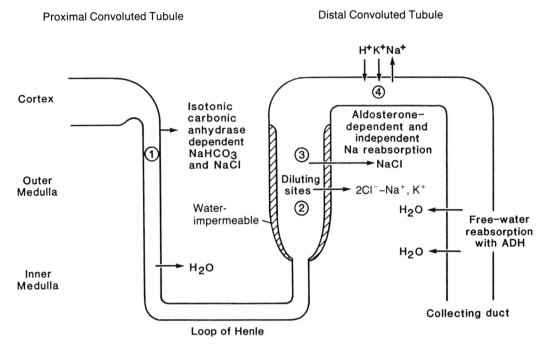

Fig. 11-2. Diagram of a nephron indicating functional areas involved in regulation of salt and water homeostasis. Circled numbers represent sites of action of diuretics (see Table 11-8).

In the distal tubule (including the collecting duct) reabsorption of the remaining 5% of filtrate occurs. At this segment, reabsorption of sodium enhances secretion of potassium and hydrogen and is partly dependent for this action on aldosterone (Knochel, 1973; Marver and Kokko, 1983). The presence of aldosterone-dependent and -independent sodium reabsorptive mechanisms accounts for two specific pharmacologic interventions at this site.

In this segment of the nephron, sodium and potassium move in opposite directions, whereas in all more proximal nephron sites, sodium and potassium movement is parallel. Therefore, anything that decreases sodium reabsorption at more proximal sites also decreases potassium reabsorption and can lead to potassium depletion. In contrast, a decrease in reabsorption of sodium at the distal tubule results in retention of potassium.

The tubule's permeability to water in the collecting duct is increased by antidiuretic hormone (ADH) that is secreted by the pituitary in response to both osmotic and nonosmotic stimuli (Schrier and Berl, 1975; Hays, 1976; Schrier et al., 1979; Schrier and Bichet, 1981). An increase in serum osmolality causes increased ADH release with retention of free water by the kidney in order to correct the hyperosmolar state. In addition, activation of the sympathetic nervous system also stimulates ADH release even during hypoosmolar

states. This pathophysiology accounts for the free-water retention and hyponatremia that occurs in patients with heart failure, liver disease, and other disorders.

As noted previously, release of ADH must be coupled with an osmotic driving force for free-water reabsorption to occur. In other words, a hypertonic medullary interstitium is necessary to achieve maximal concentration of urine in response to ADH (Berliner and Bennett, 1967).

Overall, then, two interdependent regulatory systems are responsible for the normalization of volume and osmolality: (1) extracellular fluid volume is primarily regulated by the retention or excretion of sodium, and (2) total solute concentration (i.e., osmolality) is regulated by variation in the water intake and by the renal excretion of water modulated by ADH. In general, the balanced intake and excretion of sodium maintain extracellular fluid volume. Increased sodium intake sufficient to expand extracellular fluid and vascular volume leads to increased glomerular filtration, decreased aldosterone secretion, and operation of physical and humoral factors that result in natriuresis. Sodium loss is self-limited by a reversal of these processes.

Potassium Homeostasis. More than 90% of the potassium filtered at the glomerulus is reabsorbed in the proximal tubule. At the distal tubule, both reabsorption and secretion of potassium occur. In the presence of mineralocorticoids such as aldosterone that stimulate distal sodium reabsorption, potassium is secreted. In addition, reabsorption of sodium leaves behind nonreabsorbable anions that make the lumen electronegative, facilitating excretion of potassium. Impaired secretion of potassium and its retention may occur if delivery of sodium to the distal tubule is reduced by any of a number of mechanisms. Reduction in mineralocorticoid concentration also enhances retention of potassium. Decreased production of aldosterone most often occurs in patients with mild renal disease due to diabetes mellitus. In these patients, effects on the juxtaglomerular apparatus result in hyporeninemia and secondary hypoaldosteronemia (Schambelan et al., 1972; Schambelan, 1973). This syndrome also can be caused by drugs that decrease aldosterone secretion such as NSAIDs and ACE inhibitors.

Hyperkalemia may occur in patients who have an impaired ability to excrete potassium, such as those with renal insufficiency, or who have systemic acidemia that causes potassium to shift extracellularly. In addition, hemolysis and any type of tissue necrosis result in release of potassium to the extracellular space. Commercially available premixed electrolyte solutions, salt substitutes, and low-sodium products prepared with potassium, such as potassium penicillin G, are sources of excess potassium that should be avoided in patients with impaired ability to excrete potassium.

Depletion of potassium occurs in primary or secondary adrenocortical overactivity, with use of diuretics that inhibit sodium reabsorption proximal to sites at which sodium and potassium exchange, and during both acidosis and alkalosis of any cause. Note that depletion of potassium may occur while the serum potassium concentration is maintained (Moore et al., 1953; Maffly and Edelman, 1961; Croxson et al., 1972). The clinician should be aware of the signs of potassium depletion in the setting of normal serum concentrations including alkalosis, especially in the presence of an acid urine, hypochloremia, and hyponatremia (in the absence of obvious sodium depletion and/or fluid overload) (Edelman et al., 1958).

Calcium Homeostasis. Control of concentrations of calcium in plasma depends upon the interaction between parathyroid hormone and vitamin D. These hormones exert their effects on bone, the intestinal epithelium, and the kidney to maintain calcium homeostasis (Habener and Potts, 1978; Agus et al., 1982; Reichel et al., 1989). Vitamin D_3 is either ingested in the diet or synthesized by the skin on exposure to sunlight. The liver then converts vitamin D_3 to 25[OH]-D_3 that in turn is further hydroxylated by the kidney to form 1,25[OH]$_2$-D_3. This final product modu-

lates the effects of parathyroid hormone on bone, increases intestinal absorption of calcium, and increases renal reabsorption of calcium. Parathyroid hormone is released when serum calcium concentrations diminish. The hormone induces release of calcium from bone, stimulates 1-hydroxylation of 25[OH]-D_3 by the kidney, and promotes renal reabsorption of calcium. Thus, the effects of parathyroid hormone and vitamin D_3 in concert preserve calcium homeostasis by their effects on multiple organs. Drugs affect calcium homeostasis in two ways. They can cause disorders of calcium homeostasis, as will be discussed in the section on adverse effects of drugs on renal function, and they are used to treat abnormalities of concentration of calcium in serum concentration as discussed below.

In the kidney, handling of calcium generally parallels that of sodium (Agus et al., 1982). Thus calcium that is not bound to albumin is freely filtered at the glomerulus, after which it undergoes reabsorption throughout the length of the nephron. Inhibition of reabsorption of sodium at a particular nephron site also results in less reabsorption of calcium; the converse also is true.

When the calcium homeostasis of a patient is evaluated, the usual value reported from the laboratory is the total concentration of calcium in serum. That concentration includes the unbound calcium plus the majority of calcium in serum that is bound to albumin. Changes in the concentration of albumin can affect total concentrations of calcium in serum without affecting the physiologically relevant unbound (also referred to as *ionized* or *free*) concentration. In settings of abnormal concentrations of albumin in serum the measured total concentration of calcium in serum can be "normalized" by adding 0.8 mg/100 ml to the calcium concentration for every 1 g/100 ml that the serum albumin is below a "normal" value of 4 g/100 ml.

Acid–Base Balance. The body's extracellular fluid environment is maintained relatively constant at approximately pH 7.4; intracellular fluid generally is more acidic.

Cell metabolism releases large quantities of CO_2 and hydrogen ion. The hydrogen ion is fixed by combination with bases and eliminated, so that release, fixation, and excretion are constant at steady state. If bicarbonate is inappropriately lost by excretion into the urine, retention of hydrogen ion and acidemia result. Conversely, administration of bicarbonate reduces the concentration of hydrogen ion and results in alkalemia.

Most acid is excreted as CO_2 by the lungs. However, the kidney must eliminate 1 to 2 mEq of hydrogen ion per kilogram per day to maintain acid–base balance. Removal of this excess hydrogen ion is accomplished by the secretion of hydrogen ion into the urine. To acidify the urine, three processes must operate effectively: (1) reabsorption of bicarbonate, (2) formation of titratable acid, and (3) production of ammonia. The buffering of acid excretion by phosphate and ammonia allows a greater capacity for elimination of hydrogen ion. Without these buffers, a urinary pH would soon be reached that would preclude further secretion of H^+ ions by tubular cells.

The tubular secretion of hydrogen ion results in removal of luminal bicarbonate so that bicarbonate is reabsorbed; further hydrogen ion secretion acidifies the urine. Most hydrogen is secreted in the proximal nephron in exchange for sodium, and the process serves to reclaim most of the filtered bicarbonate. Reabsorption of bicarbonate is facilitated by carbonic anhydrase.

Acidemia and alkalemia occur when exogenous administration or production of endogenous acid or alkali exceeds removal by metabolism and/or excretion. The metabolic acidosis of uncontrolled diabetes mellitus provides a good example. In this condition, breakdown of fat occurs so rapidly that acetoacetic acid and β-hydroxybutyric acid accumulate. The accumulation of ketoacids exceeds the normal buffering and excretory mechanisms responsible for acid–base regulation — diabetic acidemia ensues. If insulin is administered, ketoacid production decreases and acid–base balance is restored.

Metabolic acidosis may result from either production or administration of acid at a rate faster than can be excreted by the normal kidney, from selective loss of base, or from the inability of a diseased kidney to excrete normal amounts of acid. Loss of base usually occurs via GI losses such as during diarrhea or is due to failure of the kidney to reabsorb bicarbonate, in which case the acidosis is accompanied by an inappropriately alkaline urine. This defect may be the result of a primary abnormality in reabsorption of bicarbonate in the proximal tubule or of a defect in the ability to maintain a hydrogen ion gradient in the distal tubule (Morris et al., 1972). In addition, drugs such as carbonic anhydrase inhibitors can cause excessive loss of bicarbonate. Lastly, hyporeninemic-hypoaldosteronism or similar pathophysiologic syndromes caused by NSAIDs or ACE inhibitors diminish the hydrogen secretory ability of the distal tubule causing a metabolic acidosis (Perez et al., 1974; Sebastian et al., 1977; Tan et al., 1979; Warren and O'Connor, 1980).

Generation of a metabolic alkalosis occurs when acid is lost or bicarbonate is gained in excess of endogenous production of acid. Acid loss can occur due to vomiting, nasogastric suctioning, or by the kidney during potassium depletion or states of mineralocorticoid excess. With each millimole of acid lost, a millimole of bicarbonate is generated systemically. Bicarbonate also can be gained by exogenous administration.

Maintenance of a metabolic alkalosis occurs during depletions of volume, potassium, or chloride, or during elevations of P_{CO_2} or mineralocorticoid concentration (Coe, 1977; Jacobson and Seldin, 1983; Sabatini and Kurtzman, 1984). Persistence of any of these conditions maintains a metabolic alkalosis, and successful therapy requires reversal of all the contributing factors in a given patient.

There is an expected degree of respiratory compensation for each metabolic disturbance in acid–base status (Elkinton, 1965; Winters, 1965). For example, in a simple metabolic acidemia, each decrement in the serum bicarbonate concentration is accompanied by a predictable reduction in the arterial blood P_{CO_2}. When the response to metabolic acidemia results in a greater- or lesser-than-predicted change in P_{CO_2} the presence of a separate, independent respiratory acid–base disorder should be suspected. The physician can recognize the presence of mixed acid–base disturbances because of the predictable compensatory responses; by defining the separate components of the mixed disturbance, he or she can design a more comprehensive therapeutic program.

Clinical Pharmacology of Drugs Used in Fluid and Electrolyte Disorders

Abnormalities of Volume and Osmolality. Hypovolemia is readily treated by administering appropriate fluids whether by blood replacement, isotonic saline, or more dilute saline solutions as dictated by the individual patient's needs. Increased total body sodium is treated with diuretics.

USE OF DIURETICS. The rational use of diuretics requires an understanding of the pathogenesis of the entity being treated, the mechanisms by which the kidney handles sodium and water (Fig. 11–2), and the pharmacology of the diuretics. Such knowledge is the basis for establishing rational end points for efficacy and toxicity during diuretic therapy. The diuretics are one of the most important groups of pharmacologic agents acting directly on the kidney. As discussed above, although they are given to produce negative sodium balance, they also affect tonicity, acid–base regulation, potassium balance, calcium homeostasis, and so forth. In addition, understanding their diverse nondiuretic effects allows their rational use in nonedematous disorders (see below).

Studies on the mechanisms of formation of edema have shown that whatever the primary disturbance, the result is increased renal retention of sodium, which leads to an increase in total exchangeable sodium. Decreased renal excretion of sodium in some instances may be primarily due to reduced GFR and thereby be due to renal dysfunction per se. More commonly, the kidney is not diseased but is responding to signals (many or most of which are unknown) stimulated by diseases of other organ systems. These signals affect the regulation of tubular function causing enhanced reabsorption of sodium (Frazier and Yager, 1973; Klahr and Slatopolsky, 1973).

The net loss of sodium from body fluids caused by a diuretic contracts the extracellular fluid space. Since the sodium excreted by the kidney immediately derives from the intravascular space, rational goals of therapy entail clinical assessment of the patient's vascular volume. For example, a patient in CHF with an increased intravascular volume predictably tolerates a rapid diuresis more readily than does a patient with a normal or decreased intravascular volume as occurs in patients with nephrotic syndrome or cirrhosis. The maximum rate to mobilize ascitic or pleural fluid safely is approximately 1 l/day (Shear et al., 1970). Consequently, when reduction of intravascular volume would be potentially harmful, diuretic-induced weight loss should be limited to 1 kg/day. Patients with peripheral edema and those with expanded intravascular volumes can withstand even more rapid mobilization of fluid.

Just as sodium and water are handled differently along the length of the tubule (Fig. 11–2), diuretics act by different mechanisms and at different sites along the nephron (Table 11–8). In addition, as indicated in this table, routes of access of diuretics to their site(s) of action differ. All diuretics except spironolactone must reach the lumen of the nephron to inhibit sodium reabsorption. Osmotic diuretics are filtered at the glomerulus and reach this site by that mechanism. In contrast, the remaining diuretics depend upon secretion to reach the urine. The carbonic anhydrase inhibitors, loop diuretics, and thiazides are acidic drugs and are secreted through the organic

acid secretory system of the proximal tubule (Odlind and Beermann, 1980; Odlind et al., 1983). In contrast, amiloride and triamterene are secreted by the organic base secretory system (Kau, 1978; Besseghir and Rennick, 1981). Since the majority of diuretics must reach the tubular lumen to cause their effects, it follows that any impairment of delivery of diuretic to this site will result in diminished response.

Understanding the overall response to a diuretic is facilitated by a few simple principles. First, when a diuretic interferes with the reabsorption of sodium at any site in the tubule, it results in inhibition of other renal functions related to reabsorption of sodium at that site (e.g., calcium reabsorption) and to an enhanced effect of reabsorption of sodium at all more distal tubular sites (e.g., exchange with potassium). Thus, interference with reabsorption of sodium in the proximal tubule leads to increased delivery of sodium chloride to the ascending limb of the loop of Henle and the distal tubule. This facilitates the creation and reabsorption of free water and increases potassium loss, respectively. Similarly, interference with reabsorption of sodium chloride in the ascending limb of the loop of Henle interferes with the ability to create or reabsorb free water but continues to potentiate excretion of potassium. Finally, interference with sodium reabsorption at the distal nephron and the collecting duct reduces excretion of potassium. A second consideration is that diuretics act only if sodium reaches their site of action. Thus, more distally acting diuretics lose their effectiveness if proximal sodium reabsorption is increased, as occurs in a number of edema-forming states. Finally, diuretics acting at different sites or at the same site by different mechanisms may be additive or synergistic in their effects, and the increased effect of combining drugs can be used to great clinical advantage.

Table 11–8. **ROUTES OF ACCESS TO, SITES OF ACTION OF, AND EFFICACY OF DIURETICS**

DIURETIC	ROUTE OF ACCESS	SITE OF ACTION*	RELATIVE EFFICACY
Carbonic anhydrase inhibitors	Organic acid secretion	Proximal tubule (1)	2
Osmotic diuretics	Glomerular filtration	Proximal tubule and thick ascending limb of loop of Henle (1, 2, 3)	6
Loop diuretics	Organic acid secretion	Thick ascending limb of loop of Henle (2)	10–15
Thiazide diuretics	Organic acid secretion	Proximal tubule (clinically negligible) and distal tubule (3)	4
Potassium-Retaining Diuretics			1
Amiloride	Organic base secretion	Distal tubule and collecting duct (4)	
Spironolactone	Peritubular circulation	Distal tubule and collecting duct (4)	
Triamterene	Organic base secretion	Distal tubule and collecting duct (4)	

* Numbers in parentheses refer to the site of action shown schematically in Fig. 11–2.

CARBONIC ANHYDRASE INHIBITORS. The first orally effective diuretic was acetazolamide. Its synthesis was stimulated by the observation that sulfanilamide, a sulfonamide antibiotic, caused a diuresis of sodium bicarbonate and a metabolic acidosis. Studies showed that the mechanism of this effect is inhibition of carbonic anhydrase. Acetazolamide was then developed by synthesizing derivatives of sulfanilamide.

Currently, acetazolamide is rarely used as a diuretic. It has been supplanted by more efficacious agents with fewer adverse effects. It might seem to be surprising that other agents are more efficacious, since 60% or more of filtered sodium is reabsorbed in the proximal tubule that is the site of action of acetazolamide. One could speculate that acetazolamide would cause more sodium excretion than any other diuretic. However, only a fraction of proximal tubular reabsorption of sodium is as $NaHCO_3$ and thereby linked to carbonic anhydrase. In addition, much of the sodium rejected from the proximal tubule under the influence of acetazolamide is reabsorbed at more distal nephron sites, particularly the thick ascending limb of the loop of Henle. The net effect is that acetazolamide is a relatively weak diuretic (see Table 11–8 for relative efficacy compared to other diuretics).

Acetazolamide occasionally is used as a diuretic in the few patients with severe edematous disorders who are poorly responsive or refractory to large doses of potent loop diuretics (Table 11–9). Some of these patients, particularly those with heart failure, have increased proximal tubular reabsorption of sodium. Thus, the loop diuretic is limited in its efficacy because less sodium is being delivered to the loop. Coadministration of acetazolamide in this setting can cause a clinically important diuresis when such was unobtainable with maximally tolerated doses of loop diuretics. This additive effect is predictable based on known renal physiology and the separate tubular sites of action of diuretics. *Principle: In general, drugs that produce similar effects by different mechanisms are good candidates to maximize effects that are insufficient when only one is used.*

Most diuretics also are used for their pharmacologic effects unrelated to sodium reabsorption (Martinez-Maldonado et al., 1973) (Table 11–9). Since carbonic anhydrase is important for intraocular fluid formation, inhibitors of this enzyme decrease intraocular pressure and are therefore used to treat glaucoma. Acetazolamide itself is little used for this purpose, since derivatives such as methazolamide have been developed that affect ocular carbonic anhydrase but have little systemic or renal effect. Acetazolamide itself is now mainly of historical interest.

OSMOTIC DIURETICS. The most common setting of osmotic diuresis is a disease rather than therapy, namely, that caused by renal excretion of glucose that occurs in uncontrolled diabetes mellitus. As diuretics per se, osmotic agents (mannitol) have been used in patients with acute renal failure but as has been discussed previously in this chapter, it seems that the risks of this therapy outweigh any potential benefit.

On the other hand, because the osmotic effect of mannitol is highly effective in short-term treatment of cerebral edema, it is used widely in neurosurgical procedures and for patients with head trauma (Table 11–9). This use may be associated with a pronounced diuresis and even unwanted hypotension. Scrupulous attention is therefore paid to the patient's vital signs to make certain that too much volume depletion is avoided.

LOOP DIURETICS. Loop diuretics are the most effective diuretics available (Table 11–8). For this reason and because they are often effective when other diuretics are not, they also are called *high-ceiling* diuretics. Their site of action is the thick ascending limb of the loop of Henle, where they block the $2Cl^- - Na^+, K^+$ reabsorption pump (Fig. 11–2). This segment normally reabsorbs 20% to

Table 11–9. THERAPEUTIC USES OF DIURETIC AGENTS

	USES	
TYPE	DIURETIC*	"NONDIURETIC"
Carbonic anhydrase inhibitors	With loop diuretics in patients with resistance to diuretics	Glaucoma, metabolic alkalosis, altitude sickness
Osmotic agents	Acute renal failure	Cerebral edema
Loop diuretics	Edematous disorders, acute renal failure, hypertension in patients with Cl_{creat} 40 ml/min or in those with extensive fluid retention	Hypercalcemia, hyponatremia, renal tubular acidosis
Thiazide diuretics	Edematous disorders	Hypertension, hypercalciuria, diabetes insipidus
Potassium-retaining diuretics	Edematous disorders (particularly primary or secondary hyperaldosteronism; e.g., cirrhosis)	Potassium and/or magnesium loss

* Cl_{creat} = creatinine clearance.

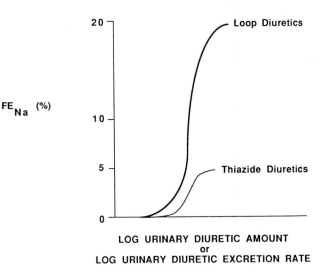

FE_{Na} (%)

20

10

5

0

Loop Diuretics

Thiazide Diuretics

LOG URINARY DIURETIC AMOUNT
or
LOG URINARY DIURETIC EXCRETION RATE

Fig. 11–3. Schematized "dose"–response relationship for loop and thiazide diuretics.

30% of filtered sodium. Since the loop diuretics are able to block virtually all reabsorption of the ion at this site, and since only small amounts of sodium can be reclaimed at more distal nephron sites, these agents cause excretion of up to 20% of the sodium that is filtered at the glomerulus. If response to a loop diuretic is assessed relative to the amount of diuretic reaching the site of action within the tubular lumen (reflected by amounts in the urine), a classic pharmacologic concentration–response curve results. The upper plateau of the response curve represents the reabsorptive capacity of the thick ascending limb of the loop of Henle (Fig. 11–3). The figure schematically illustrates this relationship and contrasts the efficacy of a loop diuretic with the lesser response that occurs to a thiazide diuretic.

Many patients require loop diuretics to control edema, particularly those patients with severe heart failure, severe cirrhosis, nephrotic syndrome, and renal insufficiency. If creatinine clearance is less than about 40 ml/min, other diuretics are unlikely to be effective and loop diuretics usually are needed. Patients may require large doses of these drugs, but the magnitude of their effect demands that small doses be tried first, followed by upward titration adjusting to the clinical response. Thus, 40 mg of furosemide or the equivalent dose of either bumetanide or ethacrynic acid is given first. If inadequate, the dose can be sequentially doubled until a response ensues or until a maximum tolerated dose is reached. The maximum single dose that should be tried differs for different clinical conditions (Table 11–10). Nothing is gained by administering larger doses than those listed, and toxicity, which is usually auditory, may occur.

The loop diuretics are intense but short-acting in their effects, so that diuresis after a given dose lasts only several hours. Once an effective dose is found, it may need to be administered several times a day. The frequency of administration is determined for each individual and depends on the amount of cumulative excretion of sodium that is needed and the amount of sodium restriction that the patient will tolerate. For example, if the goal is to cause a *net* loss of 200 mEq of sodium and each dose of diuretic effects 100 mEq of excretion, twice-daily dosing would be sufficient if the patient ingested no sodium. If the patient ingests 100 mEq of sodium, then dosing three times a day is necessary.

Other renal effects of loop diuretics are useful for treating hypercalcemia, hyponatremia, and occasionally renal tubular acidosis (Table 11–9). The major site of reabsorption of calcium is the thick ascending limb of the loop of Henle (Agus et al., 1982). Thus, by inhibiting solute reabsorption at this segment of the nephron, loop diuretics increase excretion of calcium and are effective adjunctive therapy of hypercalcemia. Most patients with hypercalcemia are volume-depleted, so the first step of therapy is replacement of volume with saline. The saline diuresis in and of itself will increase excretion of calcium and is sufficient for many patients. If additional therapy is needed, loop diuretics plus replacement of fluid losses sufficient to prevent volume depletion can be helpful. *Principle: The physician can make use of valuable interactions between drugs, water, and electrolytes.*

By increasing delivery of solute to the diluting segment, loop diuretics increase free-water formation; in other words, they cause excretion of water in excess of sodium (Schrier et al., 1973). As such, if patients who are hyponatremic also

Table 11–10.   MAXIMUM SINGLE DOSES OF LOOP DIURETICS*

	DOSE (MG)			
	FUROSEMIDE		BUMETANIDE	ETHACRYNIC ACID
CLINICAL CONDITION†	IV	P.O.	IV & P.O.	IV & P.O.
Renal Insufficiency				
20 < Cl_{creat} < 50	80	160	2	100
Cl_{creat} < 20	200	400	8–10	250
Nephrotic syndrome	120	240	4	150
Cirrhosis	40	80	1	50
Congestive heart failure	120	240	4	150

* See Brater (1988, 1990) for documentation of the derivation of the maximum single doses.

† Cl_{creat} = creatinine clearance.

have loop diuretic–induced volume losses replaced with iso- or hypertonic saline, there will be a net gain of sodium relative to water. This sequence causes the concentration of sodium in serum to increase (Hantman et al., 1973). This strategy is only rarely used, particularly since overly rapid correction of chronic hyponatremia can be deleterious (Berl, 1990).

In some patients with distal renal tubular acidosis who are unable to maintain an adequate systemic pH with conventional therapy, loop diuretics allow excretion of an acid urine and facilitate correction of the metabolic acidosis (Rastogi et al., 1984).

Both the effects on urinary acidification and formation of free water are not primary uses of loop diuretics, but they illustrate that knowledge of a drug's pharmacology can be coupled with known pathophysiology to allow its logical use for otherwise nonobvious indications (Table 11-9).

THIAZIDE DIURETICS.   After discovery of the carbonic anhydrase inhibitors, it was deemed desirable to find a diuretic that would cause a diuresis of sodium chloride. Systematic study of the diuretic effects of chemical modifications of compounds having carbonic anhydrase inhibitory activity resulted in the discovery of chlorothiazide. Additional derivatives have resulted in the large group of thiazide diuretics.

Thiazide diuretics block electroneutral reabsorption of NaCl at the distal convoluted tubule, connecting tubule, and early collecting duct, causing diuresis of the salt (Shumizu et al., 1988; Stokes, 1989). These segments are collectively referred to as the distal tubule. At suprapharmacologic concentrations, all thiazides inhibit carbonic anhydrase. However, in clinically used doses, any such effect at the proximal tubule is negligible. The enhanced distal delivery of Na^+ caused by thiazides predictably facilitates secretion of potassium; these drugs deplete potassium. Because the distal tubule reabsorbs only about 5% of filtered

sodium, the maximal effect of thiazides is much less than is that of loop diuretics (Table 11-8) (Fig. 11-3). However, these drugs are still adequate for many patients with mild edematous disorders unless patients have concomitant renal dysfunction. In such cases, limited filtration of sodium and delivery of thiazides into the tubular lumen compromise efficacy. Thus loop diuretics may be required.

Thiazide diuretics have shallow dose–response curves (Fig. 11-3), but all have the same efficacy; that is, the maximal response to each is the same. These drugs differ from each other only in terms of cost and their duration of action (Table 11-11). *Principle: The relative potencies of drugs that produce equivalent efficacy and toxicity should have little importance to the wise therapist.*

Historically, the greatest use of thiazide diuretics has been as antihypertensive agents (see chapter 2). In patients with hypertension, initial doses of a thiazide are associated with diuresis-induced decreases in blood volume and consequent lowering of blood pressure. This decrease in blood vol-

Table 11-11.   DURATION OF ACTION OF THIAZIDE DIURETICS

DIURETIC	DURATION OF ACTION
Short-Acting	Up to 12 hours
Chlorothiazide	
Hydrochlorothiazide	
Intermediate-Acting	12 to 24 hours
Bendroflumethiazide	
Benzthiazide	
Cyclothiazide	
Hydroflumethiazide	
Metolazone	
Quinethazone	
Trichloromethiazide	
Long-Acting	>24 hours
Chlorthalidone	
Indapamide	
Methyclothiazide	
Polythiazide	

ume, however, triggers homeostatic reflexes such as the renin-angiotensin-aldosterone and sympathetic nervous system responses that cause renal sodium retention and restoration of blood volume. However, the antihypertensive effect persists. Chronic use of these agents results in diminished peripheral vascular resistance by unknown mechanisms.

The homeostatic reflexes that restore blood volume when thiazides are used to treat hypertension can be helpful in treating hypercalciuria and diabetes insipidus (Table 11-9). As discussed previously, some patients with nephrolithiasis have idiopathically increased urinary excretion of calcium (Pak, 1979). Increased reabsorption of solute, including calcium, proximal to sites at which the thiazides act, plus increased distal reabsorption, results in diminished excretion of calcium and amelioration of formation of renal stones (Brickman et al., 1972; Breslau et al., 1976). This effect also will cause slight increases in concentration of calcium in serum. Thus, while loop diuretics can be used to lower the serum calcium concentration, thiazide diuretics can increase it. Importantly, these effects are predictable based on the pharmacology of the drugs and the physiology of calcium homeostasis. *Principle: Fully defining the mechanisms of action of drugs often leads to new understanding of the pathogenesis of disease and new indications for the drugs.*

Similarly, the increased proximal tubular reabsorption of solute that occurs with chronic administration of thiazide can affect the concentrations of other cations. Since the major component of lithium reabsorption occurs at the proximal tubule, use of thiazides predictably increases reabsorption of lithium. Thiazides can cause accumulation of lithium to potentially toxic concentrations. As a consequence, patients concomitantly treated with thiazides and lithium should be given lower-than-usual doses of lithium and the dosing regimen should be guided by measuring the concentration of lithium in serum.

The increased proximal reabsorption of solute with chronic use of thiazide also is accompanied by increased reabsorption of water. In addition, the distal site at which thiazides act is responsible for generating a dilute urine. As a consequence, thiazide diuretics impair the ability to maximally dilute the urine. On the one hand, this effect predisposes to hyponatremia if patients treated with thiazides ingest large amounts of hypotonic fluids (Friedman et al., 1989). On the other hand, thiazides can be useful therapy in diabetes insipidus (Table 11-9). Patients with central diabetes insipidus are plagued by a maximally dilute urine that can result in urine volumes of up to 20 l/day. Thiazides in such patients often can diminish urinary output to about 10 l/day, a nontrivial decrease that improves the quality of these patients' lives. Thus, a diuretic agent actually can be used to diminish the volume of urine! The paradoxical effect makes sense once understanding of the site of action and pharmacology of the drug is coupled with understanding of the pathophysiology of central diabetes insipidus. *Principle: The rewards of thinking about mechanisms of drug and disease can yield very satisfying results that would not occur if one classified drugs simply by their rubric mechanisms of action.*

The mechanisms of other effects of thiazides are poorly understood. Disruption of glucose homeostasis is a good example. In patients with borderline control of blood glucose concentrations, institution of thiazides may cause significant hyperglycemia. Some have attributed this adverse effect to depletion of potassium or to reduced secretion of insulin; there is little support for these hypotheses.

Thiazide diuretics also cause a worrisome increase in low-density lipoprotein (LDL) and a slight decrease in high-density lipoprotein (HDL) cholesterol. These effects could be associated with increased cardiac risk. Though the effect is rather small (about a 10% increase in LDL), it is persistent and over time may be sufficient to cause adverse effects in patients. One example might be a young patient with mild essential hypertension (Ames, 1986). This adverse effect of thiazides has caused reassessment of their role as primary therapy for hypertension (see also chapter 2). The mechanism of this effect is unknown.

POTASSIUM-RETAINING DIURETICS. In the distal nephron and collecting duct, sodium exchanges with K^+ and H^+. The exchange process is blocked by amiloride and triamterene (Frelin et al., 1987). Sodium reabsorption at these nephron segments also is stimulated by aldosterone. Cells responsive to aldosterone contain cytoplasmic receptors that bind mineralocorticoids. Receptor binding results in translocation of the hormone-receptor complex to the nucleus, where synthesis of mRNA presumably coding for a protein of Na^+ pumps is stimulated (Corvol et al., 1981). This entire sequence of events can be inhibited by spironolactone, which blocks the receptor for aldosterone.

Thus, there are two different mechanisms by which this class of drugs blocks Na^+ reabsorption. That for amiloride and triamterene is independent of aldosterone, while that for spironolactone can only antagonize the effects of aldosterone. This latter mechanism of action provides the rationale for specifically using spironolactone in patients with primary or secondary hyperaldosteronism. The dose of spironolactone needed will be dependent upon the endogenous level of mineralocorticoid in each individual patient. Thus, each patient must undergo titration until an effective dose is reached. The appropriate dose can be gauged by monitoring urinary electrolyte concentrations. A pharmacologic effect has been reached when a urine characterized by low amounts of Na^+ and high amounts of K^+ reverses to one in which Na^+ is in excess of K^+. Since the mechanism of action of spironolactone involves blockade of protein synthesis, the duration of effect of spironolactone is one or more days and the plateau of effect is not reached until 3 or 4 days of therapy. Therefore, in titrating the drug, doses should not be increased more frequently than every 3 or 4 days.

The actions of amiloride and triamterene contrast with those of spironolactone. Mineralocorticoid is not needed for them to work, and they are shorter-acting, making dosage adjustments possible on a daily basis if necessary. These agents are preferable to spironolactone if a potassium-retaining diuretic is needed in a patient without excess mineralocorticoid.

Since only a small amount of sodium is reabsorbed at the site of action of these agents, they produce only weak natriuresis and diuresis in most patients (excluding those with mineralocorticoid excess) (Table 11-8). Their use, then, is to correct or prevent potassium and/or magnesium deficiency (Table 11-9).

Potassium-retaining diuretics are most frequently used in combination with thiazide diuretics. Preparations often contain fixed doses of each drug. The rationale for these preparations is that the potassium-retaining agents offset the potassium-wasting effects of the thiazides. Thereby the combination maintains potassium and magnesium homeostasis. As such, the combination is presumed to have a neutral effect on potassium and magnesium excretion while maintaining the efficacious diuretic or antihypertensive effects. This rationale for combination products is, however, flawed. Since only about 5% of patients receiving thiazide diuretics become potassium-depleted, the remaining 95% of patients do not require additional therapy with potassium-retaining diuretics. Secondly, potassium-retaining diuretics may produce hyperkalemia in about 5% of patients, an effect that may be more dangerous than depletion of potassium. Thirdly, patients with a true need for potassium-retaining diuretics often require amounts that are not available in fixed-combination preparations. Thus, when used, each of these drugs should be individually titrated to the desired effect. *Principle: There is nothing inherently advantageous or disadvantageous about fixed-dose combination products. They may be tested in the usual clinical settings where their components are or can be given separately for relative rates of efficacy and toxicity.*

Then the decision about their general utility can follow. In comparisons of fixed-dose products with their separate entities, relative price for a given effect should also be considered.

The most rational use of potassium-sparing diuretics is in patients who have actually become hypokalemic or hypomagnesemic rather than as prophylaxis for such imbalance. These drugs are more effective at attaining and maintaining homeostasis of these cations than is exogenous supplements of the ions.

Blockade of H^+ exchange for Na^+ by these drugs causes renal tubular acidosis, type IV (Hulter et al., 1980). Patients with mild renal insufficiency or with diabetes mellitus may be particularly susceptible. Other adverse effects of potassium-retaining diuretics are not extensions of their pharmacologic effects. Rarely, the metabolite of triamterene can precipitate in concentrated urine (Ettinger, 1985). High doses of spironolactone have antiandrogenic effects that can cause gynecomastia (Ochs et al., 1978). This rarely occurs while using conventional doses.

COMBINATIONS OF DIURETICS. The rationale for combining potassium-retaining and other diuretics has been discussed.

Other combinations of diuretics are used to obtain additive or even synergistic natriuretic effects in patients who respond poorly to single agents. Such patients invariably have severe disease, for example, end-stage heart failure, severe renal insufficiency, severe cirrhosis with persistent ascites, and so forth. In spite of receiving maximal doses of loop diuretics, the sodium excretion in these patients is inadequate. By blocking additional sites in the nephron, a greater response often can be achieved. The most useful combination of agents for this purpose is that of a loop plus a thiazide diuretic. Response to a loop diuretic alone can be considerably blunted by increased reabsorption of sodium at sites distal to the thick ascending limb. In fact chronic dosing of loop diuretics appears to cause hypertrophy of distal tubule cells with an enhanced capacity to reabsorb sodium (Kaissling and Stanton, 1988; Stanton and Kaissling, 1988; Ellison et al., 1989; Loon et al., 1989). Blocking reclamation of sodium at these distal sites with thiazide diuretics can often increase response to a clinically important degree and can occasionally result in a pronounced diuresis in patients with minimal or no response to a loop diuretic alone. This effect is schematically shown in Fig. 11-4. Patients should be carefully monitored for volume and potassium status when such combinations are used.

Some patients, particularly those with severe heart failure, have increased proximal tubular reabsorption of sodium that blunts response to more distally acting agents. Addition of an agent

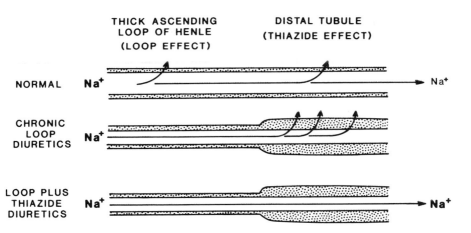

Fig. 11–4.   Schematic illustration of the synergy between loop and thiazide diuretics. Chronic therapy with loop diuretics causes hypertrophy at the distal tubule with enhanced reabsorption of sodium. Inhibition of this site by thiazide diuretics amplifies the effects of the loop diuretic.

with proximal effects such as acetazolamide can be a helpful adjunct to therapy in some of these patients. It is best to try combinations of thiazides and loop diuretics first and reserve addition of acetazolamide for those still unresponsive. Fortunately, such patients are rarely encountered.

Treatment of Disorders of Osmolality (Hyper- and Hyponatremia).   Treatment of hyper- or hyponatremia is dictated by its pathogenesis. The first step in therapy is to decipher the genesis of the disorder (Narins et al., 1982).

Hypernatremia may be caused by loss of free water, as in diabetes insipidus of central or nephrogenic origin. The former can be treated with the vasopressin analog 1-deamino-δ-D-arginine vasopressin (DDAVP) (Robinson, 1976); thiazide diuretics also may be helpful. As discussed previously, elderly persons have decreased thirst relative to the degree of tonicity and are subject to hypernatremia that has considerable morbidity (Phillips et al., 1984; Snyder et al., 1987). On the other hand, hypernatremia may primarily occur from sodium excess that includes such iatrogenic causes as parenteral administration of hypertonic sodium, mistaken feeding of high-sodium-containing formulas to infants, and so forth (Snyder et al., 1987). In addition, a number of drugs can cause hypernatremia.

Hyponatremia has many causes that dictate disparate treatments (Narins et al., 1982). Some patients present with acute, symptomatic hyponatremia that often is iatrogenic, for example, caused by receipt of large volumes of hypotonic parenteral fluids postoperatively. Whether and how fast hyponatremia should be corrected is a vigorously debated issue (Berl, 1990). Rapid correction of the concentration of sodium in serum (within hours) by administration of hypertonic saline with or without loop diuretics seems appropriate for most causes of severe hyponatremia. In contrast, patients with insidious onset of asymptomatic hyponatremia should be slowly corrected. Rapid reversal in such patients apparently can cause osmotic disequilibrium of the CNS with considerable morbidity and mortality. In this circumstance, the serum concentration of sodium should be corrected no more rapidly than 2.5 mEq/l per hour. Total correction should not exceed 20 mEq/l per day (Berl, 1990).

Patients with chronic hyponatremia may not need treatment with other than fluid restriction to 500 ml/day. If chronic therapy is needed, demeclocycline or lithium can be used, taking advantage of the nephrogenic diabetes insipidus that both these drugs can cause (Forrest et al., 1978). Of these drugs, demeclocycline usually is preferable because of its relatively safe profile.

Potassium Abnormalities.   Hyperkalemia can be treated acutely by maneuvers that shift the ion into cells. Administration of bicarbonate usually is the first therapeutic step, since alkalemia drives potassium intracellularly. If the patient cannot be given bicarbonate or if it is ineffective, glucose plus insulin causes glucose and potassium entry into cells. Treatment of chronic hyperkalemia entails use of sodium polystyrene sulfonate, an ion-exchange resin that prevents absorption of potassium by binding it in the gut.

Treatment of hypokalemia is confounded by the fact that concentrations of potassium in serum poorly reflect the state of intracellular potassium stores. For example, at normal systemic pH, reduction of the serum potassium concentration to less than 3 mEq/l reflects a deficit of 400 mEq or more of total body potassium (Scribner and Burnell, 1959). As the serum potassium concentration falls further, total body potassium deficits rise exponentially. A correlation between the concentration of potassium in serum with pH indicates that about an 0.5 to 1.0 mEq/l rise in potassium concentration will occur for each fall of 0.1 pH unit in arterial blood. Such estimates of potassium requirements represent averages and are applicable only as guidelines to individual cases. Less potassium should be replaced than the estimated deficit and at the same time that the causative abnormalities in pH are being corrected. Careful monitoring of the effects of therapy is required.

Since the physiologic effect of potassium is reflected in important and easily measured functions, the efficacy and safety of rapid replacement may be followed by observing changes in the electrocardiogram. This indicator of intracellular concentration may be more useful to measure than its serum concentration. Both measures of potassium should be used.

Use of potassium-retaining diuretics to maintain potassium homeostasis was previously discussed.

Calcium Abnormalities. Most hypercalcemic patients are volume-depleted. The mainstay of their therapy is restoration of normal intravascular volume. Acute therapy of hypercalcemia relies on the parallel reabsorption of sodium and calcium by the nephron. Thus, decreased reabsorption of sodium results in increased excretion of calcium. Parenteral administration of saline often is sufficient to cause calciuresis. If not, loop diuretics can be used, but scrupulous attention must be paid to preventing contraction of volume.

Chronic treatment of hypercalcemia depends on the cause. For example, hyperparathyroidism is usually treated surgically, that associated with sarcoid responds to steroids, and so forth. The most vexing form of hypercalcemia to treat is that caused by malignancy. There the hypercalcemia may be due to destruction of bone, to synthesis of bone-resorbing prostaglandins, or to synthesis of other bone-resorbing factors like transforming growth factor α, lymphotoxin, or, intriguingly, synthesis of a parathyroid hormone–like peptide by the tumor (Seyberth et al., 1975; Horiuchi et al., 1987; Broadus et al., 1988; Mundy, 1988). Other than using indomethacin in patients with the rare tumors that produce prostaglandin-mediated hypercalcemia, only nonspecific therapy is available. Oral phosphate, mithramycin, glucocorticoids, and diphosphonates can be employed (Mundy et al., 1983). Glucocorticoids often are ineffective. Since administration of phosphate orally is simple, it is often tried first. Later either mithramycin or diphosphonates can be used.

Hypocalcemia, if not simply factitious due to hypoalbuminemia, can be treated with calcium supplements given orally with or without vitamin D analogs. Of the latter, $1,25[OH]_2$–D_3 has the shortest duration of action, that is advantageous if patients become hypercalcemic. On the other hand, it is expensive. Other preparations such as dihydrotachysterol are less expensive, but their effects persist for a long time. Which agent to use must be tailored to the individual patient.

Acid–Base Abnormalities. Treatment of metabolic acidemia requires defining and treating the underlying disease (i.e., treatment of diabetic acidosis, correction of poor tissue perfusion, removal of acidifying drugs, etc.). If one needs to treat the acidemia, the bicarbonate deficit must be calculated. Then one must remember that usually approximately one half the acid load is buffered intracellularly and one half extracellularly (Swan and Pitts, 1955). In severe acidemia, bicarbonate replacement to restore intra- and extracellular pH is greater than would be calculated on the assumption that only one half the acid load is buffered in the cell (Garella et al., 1973). The objective of therapy with bicarbonate is to restore buffering capacity. Replacement should be slow and cautious since improvement in the patient's clinical condition will recruit endogenous mechanisms for correcting the abnormality. As such, a calculated replacement may prove excessive, resulting in alkalemia.

Alkalemia, hypokalemia, or changes in ionized calcium may occur with bicarbonate therapy and complicate the disease state. As metabolic acidemia develops, potassium leaves cells and is excreted by the kidney. Depletion of total exchangeable potassium may be masked by an apparently normal or even mildly elevated concentration of potassium in serum caused by the acidemia. Abrupt correction of the acidemia may move potassium back into cells, resulting in hypokalemia with its attendant effects on muscular, neuromuscular, and cardiac functions.

Metabolic alkalosis can be subdivided into that which is saline-responsive (where urinary chloride excretion is < 10 mEq/day) as opposed to saline-unresponsive (where urinary chloride excretion is > 10 mEq/day) (Parker et al., 1980; Narins et al., 1982). There are multiple causes of each of these entities, but the former responds to treatment with saline alone; the latter requires therapy of the primary abnormality, replacement of chloride deficits, and concomitant replacement of potassium losses.

ADVERSE EFFECTS OF DRUGS ON RENAL FUNCTION

Drugs can adversely affect renal function in a variety of ways. In doing so the adverse effects can mimic almost any renal disease. Thus, whenever a patient presents with a renal disorder, adverse drug reactions should be considered in the differential diagnosis. If a renal syndrome is not appropriately attributed to an offending drug, therapy with that drug will continue while additional misdirected treatment is aimed at some other cause. The patient is likely to worsen and potentially incur an irreversible insult.

The manner in which drugs adversely affect renal function can be categorized (Table 11–12). Examples of each type of effect will be briefly discussed. An exhaustive listing of drugs and their effects on the kidney is beyond the scope of this chapter.

Factitious Increases in Creatinine

As indicated in the section on acute renal failure, factitious increases in BUN and creatinine concentrations can occur that could lead to an erroneous diagnosis of an adverse effect on the kidney. For example, the catabolic effect of glucocorticoids and the antianabolic effect of tetracyclines can elevate the BUN concentration (Shils, 1963). Other drugs such as cimetidine can block the secretory component of creatinine elimination, causing its concentration in plasma to increase in patients who already have renal dysfunction (McKinney et al., 1981). The secretory component of creatinine's elimination entails only about 15% of its overall excretion in subjects with normal renal function. Thus, competition for secretion is quantitatively unimportant, and an effect of cimetidine on this component of excretion would not be clinically noticeable in a normal person. In contrast, as renal function declines, the secretory component becomes noticeable and interference with that secretion can cause a readily detectable increase in creatinine concentrations. Clinicians should be aware of this pitfall.

Decreased Renal Perfusion

Renal perfusion can be impaired by a number of drugs. Any adverse reaction sufficient to cause

Table 11–12. TYPES OF ADVERSE EFFECTS OF DRUGS ON RENAL FUNCTION AND THEIR PROTOTYPES

Factitious (glucocorticoids, tetracyclines, cimetidine)
Hemodynamic (ACE inhibitors, NSAIDs, cyclosporine)
Glomerular
  "Toxic" (NSAIDs, gold, penicillamine)
  Immunologic (sulfonamide vasculitides, drug-induced lupus, organic solvents)
Interstitial
  "Toxic" (cyclosporine, analgesics, heavy metals)
  Immunologic (penicillins, sulfonamide derivatives)
Collecting system (sulfonamides, oxipurinol, triamterene, increased uric acid excretion)
Renal tubular

systemic hypotension or reduce cardiac output can diminish renal perfusion. Such an effect may result in prerenal azotemia or, if extreme, can result in acute renal failure. Common examples of adverse hemodynamic effects of drugs are observed with ACE inhibitors, NSAIDs, and cyclosporine.

During states of already severely compromised renal blood flow, maintenance of glomerular filtration depends upon intrarenal generation of angiotensin II (AII), which constricts the glomerular efferent arteriole. Inhibition of AII formation with any ACE inhibitor in this setting will result in prompt decrements in GFR manifested as acute oliguric renal failure (Keane et al., 1989). This syndrome occurs most often in patients with severe bilateral renal artery stenosis, in those with severe stenosis of a solitary functioning kidney, or in patients with profoundly low cardiac output. In fact, in the absence of severe cardiac disease, acute renal failure from an ACE inhibitor should prompt an evaluation of the patient for renal artery stenosis.

One of the several renal effects of NSAIDs is acute ischemic renal failure. In clinical conditions of diminished actual or effective circulating volume, renal perfusion becomes dependent upon local synthesis of vasodilating prostaglandins (PGs). Prostacyclin is synthesized by the renal vascular endothelium. In such settings, inhibition of renal PGs by NSAIDs allows unopposed vasoconstriction by circulating catecholamines and AII. The constrictor can cause acute and sometimes profound decreases in renal perfusion. Patients susceptible to this effect include those who are volume-depleted, whether by disease or diuretics, and those with CHF, cirrhosis, or renal insufficiency (including nephrotic syndrome) (Dunn and Zambraski, 1980; Levenson et al., 1982). When such patients are to receive an NSAID, their renal function should be assessed within several days of commencing therapy in order to detect an adverse effect while it is reversible.

Cyclosporine is extensively used in organ transplantation and now in diseases of abnormal immune expression. It has multiple effects on the kidney, one of which is to cause renal vasoconstriction (Myers, 1986; Kahan, 1989). The mechanism of this effect is unknown, but it may cause the hypertension that is frequently associated with cyclosporine's use (Porter et al., 1990). The hypertension responds to both calcium antagonists and ACE inhibitors. Whether this vasoconstrictive effect of cyclosporine is the mechanism of the progressive decline in renal function that occurs with chronic use of this agent is unclear.

Glomerular Injury

Drugs can affect the glomerulus either by a "toxic" effect (meaning the mechanism is not known) or by causing glomerulonephritis. A toxic effect includes not only hemodynamically mediated decrements in GFR discussed above but also drug-induced nephrotic syndrome that does not appear to have an immunologic basis. Chronic use (months or years of therapy) of NSAIDs can rarely result in nephrotic syndrome that is unusual histologically in that glomeruli appear benign in contrast to a marked interstitial nephritis (Clive and Stoff, 1984; Carmichael and Shankel, 1985). Thus, this syndrome represents the paradox of a primarily interstitial disease that becomes clinically manifest because of what appears to be a secondary glomerulopathy.

Gold salts and penicillamine commonly cause proteinuria, the mechanism of which is unknown (Katz et al., 1984; Hall et al., 1987, 1988). Patients receiving these drugs need regular monitoring for urinary protein in order to detect an adverse effect early when it can be reversed by discontinuing the offending drug.

Other drugs cause glomerulonephritis. The vasculitides that rarely occur with sulfonamide antibiotics can include a glomerular component. Several drugs including procainamide, hydralazine, isoniazid, and phenytoin can cause a systemic lupus erythematosus syndrome (Hess, 1988). Presumably, the development of antibodies to these drugs is causal (Hahn et al., 1972; Wilson, 1980; Totoritis et al., 1988). In contrast to spontaneously occurring lupus, the drug-induced syndrome usually does not manifest glomerulonephritis. The reasons for this difference are unknown.

Organic solvents, including gasoline, cause renal tubular injury (see below). They have also been implicated in antiglomerular basement membrane antibody–mediated glomerulonephritis including an association with pulmonary involvement (i.e., Goodpasture syndrome) (Cullen et al., 1990).

Interstitial Injury

Interstitial nephritis can be caused by a number of drugs. The NSAIDs can produce an interstitial inflammatory infiltrate. Cyclosporine also causes an interstitial reaction that may be the mechanism by which its use over time results in declines in renal function in many patients (Myers et al., 1984; Berg et al., 1986; Palestine et al., 1986).

The entity of analgesic nephropathy is likely different from the interstitial nephritis caused by NSAIDs noted above. Analgesic nephropathy has an interstitial component, but this may be secondary rather than primary scarring. The hallmark of analgesic nephropathy is papillary necrosis. The mechanism of the progression from this lesion to end-stage renal disease is unknown. Development of analgesic nephropathy requires years of persistent ingestion of the analgesic. The reasons for

distinct geographic distribution (e.g., Scandinavia, Switzerland, Australia, and the southeastern United States) are unknown. Likewise, the offending agent(s) is unclear (Kincaid-Smith, 1980; Dubach et al., 1983; Buckalew and Schey, 1986). Originally phenacetin was presumed to be a major cause of analgesic nephropathy. However, removal of phenacetin from the market in countries with a high prevalence of this syndrome has not decreased its frequency (Buckalew and Schey, 1986). ***Principle: If a drug is banned for the wrong reason, its therapeutic value is unjustly lost and lost forever*** (Melmon, 1989). Many investigators now feel that the salicylate component is incriminated or that causality is related to combination products somehow having an additive or synergistic toxic effect on the kidney (Dubach et al., 1983). Whether currently marketed nonsalicylate NSAIDs will cause this syndrome is unknown. Interestingly, case reports of NSAID-induced papillary necrosis have appeared (Clive and Stoff, 1984). Whether analgesic nephropathy from chronic use of these compounds will become manifest in future years is unknown but worrisome, particularly because these drugs are available over the counter in the United States.

Heavy metals, particularly lead, cause intestinal nephropathy (Batuman et al., 1981). Exposure usually occurs through occupational sources and has been implicated in causing "saturnine" gout and hypertension (Cullen et al., 1990).

Immunologically mediated interstitial nephritis has been described with penicillins and other drugs (Neilson, 1989). In some cases, drug-induced development of antibodies to renal tubular basement membranes has been documented (Border et al., 1974; Bergstein and Litman, 1975). Histologically, this lesion reveals an inflammatory infiltrate with many eosinophils; in fact, systemic eosinophilia and eosinophiluria may aid the diagnosis. Finding eosinophils in the urine is highly specific for this disorder but is not sensitive since many false negatives occur. Patients usually manifest this syndrome after days, weeks, or even longer duration of therapy. Renal function declines in the absence of other causes. Stopping the medication usually results in prompt resolution. Administration of a structurally dissimilar drug usually is safe. For example, patients suffering interstitial nephritis from furosemide can be successfully managed with ethacrynic acid. In contrast, substituting bumetanide for the structurally similar furosemide would not be wise.

Damage to the Collecting System

Just as minerals can precipitate in the urinary collecting system, some drugs also can crystallize and serve as the nidus for stone formation. The risk of this effect is greatest if urine flow is low and drugs attain high concentrations in the urine. Sulfonamide diuretics are classic examples of this phenomenon. In fact, this property precluded use of some of them. This risk also historically led to the use of preparations containing several different sulfonamide antibiotics since they had additive antibacterial effects but did not entail an additive risk of precipitation in urine. Thus, with a combination of sulfonamides, the efficacy of a large dose of a single agent could be attained but each component would not reach sufficient concentrations in urine to precipitate. Thus, this simple strategy improved the benefit-to-risk ratio.

Oxipurinol, the active metabolite of allopurinol, and triamterene have rarely been found as renal stones in patients (Landgrebe et al., 1975; Ettinger, 1985). If a patient with no history of nephrolithiasis develops renal colic while taking one of these drugs, one should suspect stones generated from the drug.

Drugs can increase excretion of uric acid by several mechanisms sufficient to cause precipitation and uropathy from urates. For example, suprofen, a NSAID with uricosuric properties, caused sufficient acute uropathy to be removed from the market (Hart et al., 1987). By a different mechanism, rapid necrosis of malignancies (particularly hematologic) can cause a sudden increase in the production and excretion of uric acid resulting in acute renal failure (Beck, 1981). Pretreatment of such patients with allopurinol inhibits formation of uric acid and prevents the syndrome.

Effects on Renal Tubules

Effects of drugs on renal tubular function can result in alterations in fluid and electrolyte homeostasis. As shown in Table 11–13, virtually any fluid and electrolyte disorder can be caused by drugs (Brater, 1985). Space does not permit discussion of the mechanisms for the effects listed. Nevertheless clinicians should consider a drug-induced cause for any electrolyte disorder encountered in a patient.

EFFECTS OF RENAL IMPAIRMENT ON DRUG DISPOSITION

Well over 100 drugs are eliminated by the kidney. Many others are metabolized or conjugated, usually in the liver, and the polar metabolites are excreted by the kidney. Renal impairment results in the accumulation of exogenously administered drugs and their polar metabolites. To compensate for such accumulation, doses of affected drugs must be adjusted to attain concentrations similar to those obtained in patients with normal renal function.

The pharmacologic and biochemical characteristics of a drug sometimes allow prediction of whether renal dysfunction is likely to affect their disposition (Table 11–14) (Brater, 1989). If a drug has a wide therapeutic margin, accumulation has little if any consequence and dose adjustment is less critical. Penicillin derivatives and many cephalosporins are examples of this type of drug. Though toxic accumulation of these drugs can occur, it is usually only with massive (and often inappropriate) doses in patients with compromised excretion.

Drugs can bind to plasma proteins, the most important of which are albumin and α_1 acid glycoprotein (Jusko and Gretch, 1976; Vallner, 1977). Acidic compounds predominantly bind to albumin, whereas basic compounds bind to α_1 acid glycoprotein. Patients with renal insufficiency accumulate endogenous organic acids that normally are excreted by the kidney. These compounds are able to displace acidic drugs from albumin's binding sites (Reidenberg and Drayer, 1984). The clinical importance of this effect depends upon the degree of binding of the drug. For drugs bound less than 90%, the magnitude of effect is so small as to be irrelevant. In contrast, drugs bound >90% may be importantly affected by changes in protein binding.

The extent of protein binding also predicts the potential for removal of the drug by dialysis. Substantial binding means that only small amounts of drug are free in plasma. Only the free fraction can be removed by dialysis. Only negligible amounts of drugs that are more than 90% bound to plasma proteins are removed by dialytic procedures (excepting hemoperfusion).

Knowing the amount of a drug or active metabolite that is excreted in the urine allows one to predict the potential for clinically important accumulation of drug or metabolite in patients with renal insufficiency. Unless the drug has a wide therapeutic margin, if 40% or more is excreted unchanged in urine, adjustment of the dose will be needed in patients with renal insufficiency.

The drug's volume of distribution also can help predict its removal by hemodialysis. Drugs with volumes of distribution on the order of total body water or less (i.e., ≤ 0.7 l/kg) are likely restricted to the extracellular space and are accessible to dialysis. A large volume of distribution implies that the majority of drug is not dialyzable. Thus, a drug with a small volume of distribution and low protein binding (e.g., aminoglycoside antibiotics) would be predicted to be substantially removed by dialytic procedures and likely require supplemental dosing after dialysis. In contrast, even though a drug with a large volume of distribution may pass through a dialysis membrane, so little of it is in the plasma relative to overall body

Table 11–13. **EXAMPLES OF FLUID AND ELECTROLYTE DISORDERS CAUSED BY DRUGS**

DISORDER	DRUG	MECHANISM
Hypernatremia	Osmotic cathartics (e.g., lactulose)	Intestinal water loss
	Povidone-iodine	Cutaneous water loss
	Lithium Demeclocycline Vinblastine	Decreased renal response to ADH
Hyponatremia	Thiazide diuretics Amiloride	Decreased function of "diluting segment"
	Chlorpropamide Cyclophosphamide	Increased response to ADH
	Cisplatin Carboplatinum Antidepressants	Unknown
Hyperkalemia	Cardiac glycosides Succinycholine Arginine hydrochloride	Shift from intracellular stores
	Potassium salts	Increased intake
	β-Adrenergic antagonists NSAIDs ACE inhibitors Heparin Cyclosporine	Hyporenin and/or hypoaldosterone
	Potassium-retaining diuretics	Decreased potassium secretion
Hypokalemia	Glucose Insulin β_2-Adrenergic agonists Theophylline Laxatives	Distribution into cells
	Carbonic anhydrase inhibitors Osmotic diuretics Loop diuretics Thiazide diuretics	Decreased tubular reabsorption
	Carbenoxolone True licorice	Increased mineralocorticoid effect
	Penicillins	Increased secretion due to nonreabsorbable anion
Metabolic acidosis Increased anion gap	Biguanides	Lactic acidosis
	Ethanol Papaverine Nalidixic acid Nitroprusside Iron Salicylates Paraldehyde Methanol Ethylene glycol Toluene	Unmeasured anions
Normal anion gap	Laxatives Cholestyramine	Gastrointestinal HCO_3^- loss
	Carbonic anhydrase inhibitors	Renal HCO_3^- loss
	Toluene Amphotericin B Lithium NSAIDs Potassium-retaining diuretics	Decreased H^+ secretion
	NH_4Cl Arginine Lysine Histidine	Exogenous acid

(continued)

Table 11–13.   *(CONTINUED)*

DISORDER	DRUG	MECHANISM
Metabolic alkalosis	Potassium-losing diuretics	Renal K^+ loss
	Tolazoline Drug-induced vomiting	Gastrointestinal H^+ loss
Hypercalcemia	Milk plus soluble alkali Vitamin D	Increased gastrointestinal CA^{2+} absorption
	Vitamin D Vitamin A Tamoxifen	Increased mobilization from bone
	Thiazide diuretics	Decreased renal excretion
Hypocalcemia	Anticonvulsants Glutethimide	Increased degradation of endogenous vitamin D
	Mithramycin Calcitonin	Decreased mobilization from bone
	EDTA Phosphate	Physicochemical complexing
Hypermagnesemia	Mg^{2+} salts	Increased intake
Hypomagnesemia	Laxatives	Decreased GI absorption
	Potassium-losing diuretics Aminoglycoside antibiotics Cisplatin Amphotericin	Increased renal loss
Hyperphosphatemia	Drug-induced rhabdomyolysis	Tissue release
Hypophosphatemia	Glucose Insulin	Distribution into cells
	Aluminum- and magnesium- containing antacids	Decreased GI absorption

stores that the total amount removed is negligible.

Data describing the amount of drug removed by a dialytic procedure can be used to help predict likely need for adjustment of dose. If no drug is removed by dialysis, then the only dose adjustment needed is that for the patient's endogenous level of renal function (presumably end stage). In contrast, if more than 30% of a dose of a drug is removed by a dialytic procedure, supplemental dosing to replace the amount removed may be necessary. In addition, dialysis, particularly hemodialysis or hemoperfusion, occasionally is considered for therapeutic intervention in settings of

**Table 11–14.   CHARACTERISTICS OF A DRUG THAT PREDICT
IMPORTANT EFFECTS OF RENAL COMPROMISE**

CHARACTERISTICS	IMPLICATIONS
Therapeutic margin	If the drug has a wide therapeutic margin, its accumulation poses negligible risk.
Protein binding	A high degree of binding (>90%) to albumin makes displacement likely; a high degree of binding to either albumin or α_1 acid glycoprotein means little drug is available for removal by dialysis.
Amount of drug excreted in the urine unchanged	If 40% or more of a drug is excreted in the urine unchanged, it is highly likely to accumulate in patients with renal insufficiency.
Active metabolites are excreted in the urine	The metabolites can accumulate with attendant effects.
Volume of distribution	A small volume of distribution (that of total body water or less; i.e., ≤ 0.7 l/kg) means the drug may be accessible for removal by dialysis *if* it is *not* highly protein-bound; a large volume of distribution means little if any removal by dialysis.
Dialyzability	Removal of more than 30% of a drug by a dialytic procedure means supplemental dosing may be necessary; in overdose settings, an increment in endogenous clearance of more than 30% indicates that dialysis may be useful therapeutically.

overdose. For such adjuncts to be helpful, the dialytic procedure should increase endogenous clearance of the poison by 30% or more. For increments less than this value, the risks of the procedure likely outweigh any benefits.

The foregoing discussion implies that one can make reasonable predictions as to the need for adjusting therapy even for drugs that have not been explicitly studied in patients with renal insufficiency. Though lack of quantitative guidelines makes dose adjustments tentative, a worse problem is ignoring the need to do so. When no information about a particular drug is available, consider using a drug of the same class but with no dependence on the kidney for elimination. For example, rather than using a modified dose of atenolol as a selective β-adrenergic antagonist in a patient with renal insufficiency, one could administer metoprolol, which is eliminated by the liver and needs no dose adjustment in patients with renal insufficiency (Brater, 1989). The converse would apply to patients with liver disease.

Effects of Renal Function on Pharmacokinetic Variables

Absorption. No primary influences of the kidney on drug absorption have been identified. The potential exists for a number of secondary influences. For example, dehydration from salt wasting might affect perfusion to and absorption from intramuscular or intestinal sites. Potassium depletion might significantly affect GI motility and thereby change the degree and/or rate of absorption of a drug. The clinician should be aware of the potential for a variety of changes in absorption kinetics and prospectively derive therapeutic and toxic end points to follow in each patient.

Distribution. The kidney may affect distribution of a drug by several mechanisms. Changes in acid–base balance may affect the amount of ionized relative to nonionized drug. A pH favoring the nonionized form of a weak acid or base can facilitate its distribution out of plasma and into tissues. For example, with salicylate, a more acidic systemic pH increases the relative amount of nonionized salicylate and increases the amount reaching the CNS. The larger the amount in the CNS, the greater the chances of toxicity (Hill, 1971, 1973). Presumably, the acidemia of uremia would enhance distribution of salicylate toward the CNS.

Protein binding is another major determinant of a drug's distribution. Diminished binding of acidic drugs frequently occurs in patients with renal insufficiency, because accumulated endogenous organic acids displace exogenously administered xenobiotics (Reidenberg and Drayer, 1984). This decreased binding increases the percentage of free (unbound) drug in plasma. A popular misconception is that such an effect results in increased *concentrations* of unbound, pharmacologically active drug, causing an enhanced effect, including toxicity. In the majority of instances, however, there is no increase in concentration of unbound drug and therefore no changes in response unless it is caused by pharmacodynamic factors (Klotz, 1976; Greenblatt et al., 1982; MacKichan, 1989). Consider an example of phenytoin. Reductions in protein binding of phenytoin during uremia or in the patient with hypoalbuminemia of nephrotic syndrome can lead to misinterpretation of its concentrations in serum. In both clinical conditions, protein binding of phenytoin is decreased; unbound concentrations are unchanged though total concentrations are diminished. When concentrations of phenytoin in plasma are obtained, the clinical laboratory measures only its total concentration. This could be misinterpreted as being too low even though unbound concentrations are usual and "therapeutic." If the clinician is misled and increases the dose of phenytoin in an attempt to attain a total concentration in the usual therapeutic range, an increase in the unbound concentration of phenytoin could result in toxicity. This problem could be avoided by measuring unbound concentrations (see chapter 37). Alternatively, one must redefine the therapeutic range of the drug in uremic and hypoalbuminemic patients. The therapeutic range for this drug in terms of its total concentration in plasma is about one half to two thirds of the value obtained in normal patients.

Displacement of drug from albumin binding sites in patients with renal insufficiency has been misinterpreted (Klotz, 1976; Greenblatt et al., 1982; MacKichan, 1989). It is mistakenly cited as a mechanism for altered response to drugs in patients with renal disease. However, since unbound concentrations of drug may not change, this mechanism cannot explain altered response to drugs in many, if not most, uremic patients. It also follows that protein binding usually does not mandate a change in drug dosing. Clinicians should avoid false conclusions regarding drug disposition from what may be incomplete data in the medical literature, namely, studies of highly bound drugs that quantify only total and not unbound concentrations.

Digoxin represents a drug for which volume of distribution (V_d) decreases as renal function diminishes (Sheiner et al., 1977):

$$V_d \text{ (in l/kg)} = 3.84 + 0.0446\, Cl_{\text{creat}} \text{ (in ml/min)}$$

where Cl_{creat} is creatinine clearance.

The mechanism of this effect is unknown, but the magnitude is sufficient to require adjustment of dose. Since volume of distribution influences the loading dose of a drug (as opposed to the maintenance dose), this effect is important only in patients to whom a loading dose of digoxin is administered. As such, the loading dose of digoxin for a patient with end-stage renal disease should be approximately one half that of a patient with normal renal function.

Metabolism. The kidney metabolizes numerous drugs, but its quantitative contribution to overall elimination of drugs is for the most part unknown (Anders, 1980). The proximal tubule has high levels of glucuronyl transferase and sulfotransferase (Besseghir and Roch-Ramel, 1987). Renal glucuronidation may be substantial; for example, approximately 20% of an IV dose of furosemide and 50% of a dose of morphine may be glucuronidated by the kidney itself (Smith et al., 1980; Jacqz et al., 1986).

The proximal tubule also contains mixed-function cytochrome P450 oxidases, but in lower amounts than in the liver. There are no data that allow conclusions about the quantitative importance of this potential pathway for drug metabolism (Anders, 1980; Besseghir and Roch-Ramel, 1987).

The kidney metabolizes proteins, in particular insulin. In patients with normal renal function, up to 50% of insulin's elimination occurs via metabolism by the kidney. This component of overall elimination diminishes in patients with renal insufficiency and partially accounts for the decreased insulin requirement as a patient's renal function deteriorates (Rabkin et al., 1970).

In addition to actual metabolism by the kidney, the kidney excretes many drug metabolites that are formed in the liver. Renal insufficiency does not necessarily mean that metabolites of drugs will accumulate since other excretory pathways such as biliary excretion exist. Many drug metabolites have no pharmacologic effects, but some do (Drayer, 1976; Verbeeck et al., 1981). Sometimes the active metabolites exert pharmacologic effects similar to those of the parent compound (e.g., primidone). Others account for all the pharmacologic activity of the parent (e.g., enalapril). In additional examples, the metabolite has a different pharmacologic profile from that of the parent drug. For example, normeperidine excites the CNS and can cause seizures, in contrast to the sedating and analgesic effects of meperidine (Szeto et al., 1977). In order to safely use drugs in patients with renal insufficiency, one must not only know the pharmacologic profile of the parent drug, but also its metabolite(s). In patients with renal disease, one should avoid using drugs that form active metabolites.

Excretion

Filtration. The integrity of the glomerulus, the size and charge of the molecule to be filtered, and the extent of protein binding determine the amount of a drug that is filtered. Highly protein-bound drugs are not appreciably filtered since only the unbound (free) drug is able to pass through the glomerulus. Protein binding, however, does not preclude substantial elimination by the kidney, since postglomerular secretory sites can efficiently excrete many drugs (see below).

The glomerulus offers no barrier to filtration of most drugs that are free in plasma. Exceptions include larger proteins and dextran. Dextran is administered as a mixture of several molecules and is a good example of the relationship between molecular size and glomerular filtration. Thus, dextran 1 (molecular weight 1000) is freely filtered and eliminated rapidly by the kidney with a half-life of elimination of about 2 hours. In contrast, dextran 70 (average molecular weight 70,000) is too big to be filtered and is eliminated slowly by metabolism. It is detectable in plasma for 4 to 6 weeks (Klotz and Kroemer, 1987). Dextran 40 is a mixture of both high- and low-molecular-weight forms so that the smaller dextrans are freely filtered and eliminated quickly with selective retention of the larger components (Data and Nies, 1974).

The status of the glomerulus is reflected by its rate of filtration and its integrity as a sieve. In the nephrotic syndrome this integrity is compromised, with loss of protein in the urine. One might predict that highly protein-bound drugs could be carried out with the protein into the urine, significantly increasing their excretion rate. This phenomenon has been investigated for phenytoin and clofibrate, both of which are highly bound to albumin. Their excretion is increased in patients with the nephrotic syndrome. However, there also is a concomitant decrease in protein binding of the two drugs with no change in the clinically important amount of free drug in the serum (Gugler et al., 1975).

The clinical significance of decrements in glomerular filtration rate on drug kinetics is widely known. This effect is important for many drugs, including cardiovascular agents (digoxin, procainamide, and various antihypertensives), antibiotics (aminoglycosides, macrolides, sulfas and their nonantibiotic derivatives), diuretics, and so forth. The scope of agents is so broad that the clinician should consult the literature on the drugs that might be used in uremic patients.

Frequently updated compilations of data on

elimination of individual drugs in patients with renal insufficiency are readily available and should be part of every clinician's resources (Bennett et al., 1987; Brater, 1989). Despite the accessibility of guidelines, clinicians should also be aware that such information is not available for all drugs. There simply is no way to circumvent understanding the pharmacology of the agents needed so that clinical end points of efficacy and toxicity, and concentrations of drug in serum (if feasible), can be followed as determinants of dosing and dosing intervals.

Secretion. At the pars recta, or straight segment of the proximal tubule, active secretion of organic acids and bases into the tubular lumen occurs. There appear to be two pathways, one for acids and one for bases, each of which is nonspecific in that a variety of acids can compete with each other for transport, as can a variety of bases (Table 11–15). There are a number of clinically important interactions in these two groups. Probenecid significantly prolongs the half-life of the penicillins. This fact is clinically utilized for the treatment of gonorrhea, in which the coadministration of the two drugs allows therapeutic concentrations of penicillin to be maintained in plasma for longer periods of time. This interaction results in increased efficacy of the penicillin. In contrast, inadvertent administration of probenecid, salicylates or other NSAIDs with methotrexate has resulted in severe methotrexate toxicity, including death (Aherne et al., 1978; Thyss et al., 1986). Similarly, histamine H₂ antagonists

Table 11–15. EXAMPLES OF ORGANIC ACIDS AND BASES SECRETED BY THE KIDNEY

Acids
  Cephalosporins (most)
  Loop diuretics
  Methotrexate
  NSAIDs (including salicylate)
  para-Aminohippurate (PAH)*
  Penicillins (most)
  Probenecid
  Sulfonamides (most)
  Thiazide diuretics
Bases
  Amiloride
  Choline
  Ephedrine and pseudoephedrine
  Histamine H₂ antagonists (cimetidine, famotidine, nizatidine, ranitidine)
  Mepiperphenidol*
  Morphine
  N-Methylnicotinamide (NMN)*
  Procainamide and *N*-acetylprocainamide
  Quinine
  Tetraethylammonium (TEA)*
  Triamterene

* Substrates used as prototypes in experimental settings.

Table 11–16. EXAMPLES OF DRUGS WHOSE ELIMINATION IS URINARY pH–DEPENDENT

Weak Acids (increased excretion in alkaline urine)
  Chlorpropamide
  Methotrexate
  Phenobarbital
  Salicylates
  Sulfonamide derivatives
  Trimethoprim
Weak Bases (increased excretion in acidic urine)
  Amphetamine
  Ephedrine
  Mexiletine
  Pseudoephedrine
  Quinine
  Tocainide

can compete with procainamide and *N*-acetylprocainamide for secretion, potentially causing accumulation to toxic concentrations (Somogyi et al., 1983; Christian et al., 1984; Somogyi and Bochner, 1984). When patients need concomitant administration of the drugs listed in Table 11–15, one should be alert to possible drug interactions. For drugs with narrow therapeutic indices, alternative drugs may be sought, or careful plans for dose adjustment should be made.

Digoxin is not only filtered at the glomerulus, but a clinically important component also is secreted in the distal nephron (Koren, 1987). The mechanism of this secretion is unknown. Quinidine, verapamil, diltiazem, flecanide, amiodarone, and spironolactone can block digoxin's secretion and thereby cause increases in its concentration in serum (Koren, 1987). This interaction is greatest with quinidine, which causes the serum digoxin concentration to double in at least 90% of patients (Bigger and Leahey, 1982). The magnitude and clinical implications of the interaction are much more variable with the other drugs noted above. Individual patients need close monitoring when these possible inhibitors of digoxin secretion are coadministered.

Reabsorption. Reabsorption from the tubular lumen back into the systemic circulation occurs with a number of drugs (Table 11–16). Clinically important modulators of this transport process are urine flow rate and pH. High rates of urine formation decrease the concentration of a drug in the distal tubule and decrease the time for the agent to diffuse from the lumen. Increased renal clearance results. This process occurs to a significant extent with phenobarbital, but the effect has not been investigated for clinical importance during the use of other drugs.

A number of drugs demonstrate urine pH–dependent kinetics that follows the principle of passive nonionic diffusion. For both weak acids and weak bases, the nonionized form of the drug is more readily reabsorbed across the lipid cell membrane than the ionized form. The pK_a of the drug and the pH of the urine determine the relative amounts of ionized versus nonionized component, as illustrated in Fig. 11–5 (Milne et al., 1958; Mudge et al., 1975).

This effect is clinically important with a number of agents. Salicylate is a weak acid, and alkalinization of the urine increases its rate of excretion. This fact is clinically used to advantage in cases of salicylate overdose, in which bicarbonate diuresis significantly increases clearance. Though phenobarbital is a weak acid, its excretion is less pH- and more flow-dependent. Though a number of sulfa antibiotics are weak

Weak Acids

$$HA \rightarrow H^+ + A^-$$

$$K_a = \frac{(H^+)\,(A^-)}{(HA)}$$

$$-\log K_a = pK_a = -\log(H^+) - \log \frac{(A^-)}{(HA)}$$

or

$$pK_a = pH - \log \frac{(A^-)}{(HA)}$$

or

$$pH - pK_a = \log \frac{(A^-)}{(HA)} = \log \frac{\text{(ionized drug)}}{\text{(nonionized drug)}}$$

Therefore, for a weak acid, as pH increases, the concentration of ionized drug increases.

Weak Bases

$$BH^+ \rightarrow B + H^+$$

$$K_a = \frac{(B)\,(H^+)}{(BH^+)}$$

$$-\log K_a = pK_a = -\log (H^+) - \log \frac{(B)}{(BH^+)}$$

or

$$pK_a = pH - \log \frac{(B)}{(BH^+)}$$

or

$$ph - pK_a = \log \frac{(B)}{(BH^+)} = \log \frac{\text{(nonionized drug)}}{\text{(ionized drug)}}$$

Therefore, for a weak base, as pH increases, the concentration of nonionized drug increases.

Fig. 11–5. Relationship between pH and the ionization of weak acids and bases.

acids with pH-dependent kinetics, the increment in their renal clearance caused by changes in urine pH is not significant when compared with overall clearance.

Weak bases similarly follow pH-dependent kinetics. Excretion of amphetamine is highly dependent on urine pH (Beckett and Rowland, 1965). At alkaline pH, only 2.7% of the drug is excreted in 16 hours while 57% is eliminated during the same period at acidic pH. Unfortunately, addicts may be more aware of this phenomenon than clinicians in that they regularly take baking soda before and during their abuse of amphetamine to prolong the "high." Ephedrine and pseudoephedrine also have significantly decreased renal clearance at alkaline urine pH. Children with renal tubular acidosis and persistently alkaline urine have developed severe pseudoephedrine toxicity due to accumulation of the drug when they are given "normal" doses (Brater et al., 1980).

It should be apparent that clinicians need to be aware of the influence of pH on drug disposition. As such, they should be alert to a patient's urinary pH, a clinical parameter that is often obtained but too little heeded.

Dialysis. Just as dialytic procedures are used to remove accumulated endogenous end products of metabolism, they also can remove drugs. The amount removed can be sufficient so that supplemental dosing is required. In poisoning, dialysis may speed the elimination of the toxin(s).

As noted previously, several characteristics of drug disposition can help predict removal of a drug by dialysis. Intuitively, a high degree of protein binding restricts the concentration of unbound (free) and therefore dialyzable drug. Similarly, a large volume of distribution means that only a small portion of the total body burden of drug is in plasma and accessible to dialytic removal. These considerations apply not only to conventional hemodialysis, but also to the newer techniques of continuous AV hemofiltration (CAVH) and continuous venovenous hemofiltration (CVVH). For these latter two techniques, ultrafiltration through the dialysis membrane is the sole mode of elimination and dialytic removal is equal to the unbound fraction times the ultrafiltration rate. This value can be used to estimate whether supplementary drug dosing needs to be given and, if so, the amount. For conventional hemodialysis, updated reference sources should be kept accessible so that the need for supplemental dosing can be determined in individual patients (Bennett et al., 1987; Brater, 1989).

Hemoperfusion techniques allow removal of substantially greater amounts of some drugs than can be accomplished with other dialysis or ultrafiltration methods. In fact, these methods are so efficient that all drug entering the dialysis

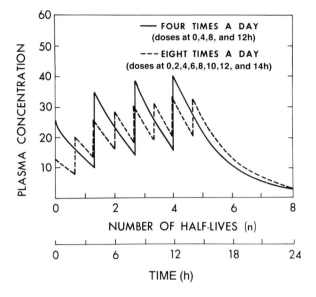

Fig. 11-6. Serum concentration of a drug related to dosing interval. The same total amount of drug is administered in both examples. Half as much drug is administered twice as frequently in the regimen depicted by the broken line compared with that depicted by the solid line.

cartridge is removed (Rosenbaum et al., 1976; Winchester and Gelfand, 1978). However efficient this removal of drug from blood may be, it still may not remove a clinically important amount of drug from the body. For example, if only a minor percentage of the total amount of drug in the body is circulating in plasma, even if hemoperfusion removes all the circulating drug, most of it is still left in body reservoirs inaccessible to the dialyzer yet still in equilibrium with the plasma. As soon as dialysis is stopped, these reservoirs serve to refill the circulating compartment such that decrements in circulating concentrations of drug caused by hemoperfusion are only transient. This phenomenon accounts for the lack of efficacy of hemoperfusion in treating poisoning with highly lipid-soluble sedative-hypnotics having large volumes of distribution (e.g., glutethimide and methaqualone).

Interestingly, most drugs are negligibly removed by peritoneal dialysis. This finding is in contrast to the substantial absorption of many drugs from the peritoneal space (Somani et al., 1982). The mechanism for this unidirectional peritoneal transport is unknown.

Dosing Regimens

In patients with renal disorders, the clinician often needs to decrease the amount of drug administered to prevent its accumulation and toxicity. Perturbations of any of the pathways of renal handling of drugs may necessitate alterations in dosage regimens. With a number of drugs, such as the aminoglycoside antibiotics and digoxin, various experimentally validated guidelines to therapy exist. These suffice only as first approximations, and the clinician cannot assume that the predicted concentrations of drug in serum derived from a nomogram or formula will be attained in a specific patient. When possible, patients should be monitored for serum concentrations of drugs with a narrow therapeutic margin. In addition, however, disease states may alter not only the relation between dose and serum concentration attained but also between concentration and effect. Determination of the concentration of drugs in serum is useful and beneficial, but is not a substitute for and must be supplemented with clinical end points of efficacy and toxicity for each drug administered.

There are two general approaches to decreasing the total amount of administered drug: maintaining the same dose as in patients with normal renal function and giving it at wider intervals (variable-interval regimen) or administering smaller doses at the same dosing interval (variable-dosage regimen). Most reports emphasize the approach using variable intervals. This may not be ideal for all drugs. If the goal is a regimen that provides constant concentrations in plasma within a certain range, the most effective method of maintaining that level is with an IV infusion. This approach often is not practical in clinical settings and in its stead multiple, intermittent administration of the drug is recommended. Obviously, small amounts of a drug given at closely spaced intervals more nearly approximates a continuous infusion than does administration of large amounts of the drug at widely spaced time intervals (the total amount of drug administered being the same). Figure 11-6 illustrates this concept.

Frequent dosing provides less variation in zenith and nadir concentrations of drug. If the range of effective concentrations of the drug is large, the efficacy of the two methods may not differ. However, if the therapeutic range is small, wide swings from peak to trough may result in periods during which concentrations of drug are subtherapeutic and other periods when they are toxic. Monitoring concentrations and clinical signs of pharmacologic effect in serum 1 hour after administration of a drug and just before administration of the next dose should enable the clinician to ascertain the appropriateness of the dosing regimen. *Principle: The kidney is a major organ that determines drug kinetics and is a major site of drug action. Renal function must be considered in the development of most therapeutic strategies.*

REFERENCES

Agus, Z. S.; Wasserstein, A.; and Goldfarb, S.: Disorders of calcium and magnesium homeostasis. Am. J. Med., 72:473–488, 1982.

Aherne, G. W.; Piall, E.; Marks, V.; Mould, G.; and White, W. F.: Prolongation and enhancement of serum methotrexate concentrations by probenecid. Br. Med. J., 1:1097–1099, 1978.

Al-Kawas, F. H.; Seeff, L. B.; Berendson, R. A.; Zimmerman, H. J.; and Ishak, K. G.: Allopurinol hepatotoxicity. Report of two cases and review of the literature. Ann. Intern. Med., 95:588–590, 1981.

Ames, R. P.: The effects of antihypertensive drugs on serum lipids and lipoproteins. I. Diuretics. Drugs, 32:260–278, 1986.

Anders, M. W.: Metabolism of drugs by the kidney. Kidney Int., 18:636–647, 1980.

Anderson, R. J.; Linas, S. L.; Berns, A. S.; Henrich, W. L.; Miller, T. R.; Gabow, P. A.; and Schrier, R. W.: Nonoliguric acute renal failure. N. Engl. J. Med., 296:1134–1138, 1977.

Ballermann, B. J.; and Brenner, B. M.: Biologically active atrial peptides. J. Clin. Invest., 76:2041–2048, 1985.

Batuman, V.; Maesaka J. K.; Haddad, B.; Tepper, E.; Landy, E.; and Wedeen, R. P.: The role of lead in gout nephropathy. N. Engl. J. Med., 304:520–523, 1981.

Beaufils, F.; deMuttenaere, S.; Rohan, J.; and Chapman, A.: Effects du furosemide chez les malades en insuffisance renale aigue. Nouv. Presse Med., 16:1073–1078, 1972.

Beck, L. H.: Clinical disorders of uric acid metabolism. Med. Clin. North Am., 65:401–411, 1981.

Beckett, A. H.; and Rowland, M.: Urinary excretion kinetics of amphetamine in man. J. Pharm. Pharmacol., 17:628–639, 1965.

Bennett, W. M.; Aronoff, G. R.; Golper, T. A.; Morrison, G.; Singer, I.; and Brater, D. C.: Drug Prescribing in Renal Failure. Dosing Guidelines for Adults. American College of Physicians, Philadelphia, 1987.

Berg, K. J.; Førre, Ø.; Bjerkhoel, F.; Amundsen, E.; Djøseland, O.; Rugstad, H. E.; and Westre, B.: Side effects of cyclosporin A treatment in patients with rheumatoid arthritis. Kidney Int., 29:1180–1087, 1986.

Berger, L.; and Yu, T. F.: Renal function in gout: IV. An analysis of 524 gouty subjects including long-term follow-up studies. Am. J. Med., 59:605–613, 1975.

Bergstein, J.; and Litman, N.: Interstitial nephritis with antitubular-basement-membrane antibody. N. Engl. J. Med., 292:875–878, 1975.

Berl, T.: Treating hyponatremia: Damned if we do and damned if we don't. Kidney Int., 37:1006–1018, 1990.

Berliner, R. W.: The concentrating mechanism in the renal medulla. Kidney Int., 9:214–222, 1976.

Berliner, R. W.; and Bennett, C. M.: Concentration of urine in the mammalian kidney. Am. J. Med., 42:777–789, 1967.

Besseghir, K.; and Rennick, B.: Renal tubule transport and electrolyte effects of amiloride in the chicken. J. Pharmacol. Exp. Ther., 219:435–441, 1981.

Besseghir, K.; and Roch-Ramel, F.: Renal excretion of drugs and other xenobiotics. Renal Physiol., 10:221–241, 1987.

Bigger, J. T.; and Leahey, E. B.: Quinidine and digoxin. An important interaction. Drugs, 24:229–239, 1982.

Bilezikian, J. P.: The medical management of primary hyperparathyroidism. Ann. Intern. Med., 96:198–202, 1982.

Border, W. A.; Lehman, D. H.; Egan, J. D.; Sass, H. J.; Glode, J. E.; and Wilson, C. B.: Antitubular basement-membrane antibodies in methicillin-associated interstitial nephritis. N. Engl. J. Med., 291:381–384, 1974.

Borges, H. F.; Hocks, J.; and Kjellstrand, C. M.: Mannitol intoxication in patients with renal failure. Arch. Intern. Med., 142:63–66, 1982.

Boscia, J. A.; Abrutyn, E.; and Kaye, D.: Asymptomatic bacteriuria in elderly persons: Treat or do not treat? Ann. Intern. Med., 106:764–766, 1987.

Brater, D. C.: Diuretics. In, Rational Therapeutics. A Clinical Pharmacologic Guide for the Health Professional (Williams, R. L.; Brater, D. C.; and Mordenti, J.; eds.). Marcel Dekker, New York, pp. 269–315, 1990.

Brater, D. C.: Pocket Manual of Drug Use in Clinical Medicine, 4th ed. B. C. Decker, Toronto, 1989.

Brater, D. C.: Use of diuretics in chronic renal insufficiency and nephrotic syndrome. Semin. Nephrol., 8:333–341, 1988.

Brater, D. C.: Drug induced electrolyte disorders. In, Clinical Aspects of Fluid and Electrolyte Disorders (Tannen, R. L.; and Kokko, J. P.; eds.). W. B. Saunders, Philadelphia, pp. 760–787, 1985.

Brater, D. C.; Anderson, S. A.; and Brown-Cartwright, D.: Response to furosemide in chronic renal insufficiency: Rationale for limited doses. Clin. Pharmacol. Ther., 40:134–139, 1986.

Brater, D. C.; Day, B.; Burdette, A.; and Anderson, S.: Bumetanide and furosemide in heart failure. Kidney Int., 26:183–189, 1984.

Brater, D. C.; Seiwell, R.; Anderson, S.; Burdette, A.; Dehmer, G. J.; and Chennavasin, P.: Absorption and disposition of furosemide in congestive heart failure. Kidney Int., 22:171–176, 1982.

Brater, D. C.; Kaojarern, S.; Benet, L. Z.; Lin, E. T.; Lockwood, T.; Morris, R. C.; McSherry, E. J.; and Melmon, K. L.: Renal excretion of pseudoephedrine. Clin. Pharmacol. Ther., 28:690–694, 1980.

Brenner, B. M.: Hemodynamically mediated glomerular injury and the progressive nature of kidney disease. Kidney Int., 23: 647–655, 1983.

Breslau, N.; Moses, A. M.; and Wiener, I. M.: The role of volume expansion in the hypocalciuric action of chlorothiazide. Kidney Int., 10:164–170, 1976.

Brezis, M.; Rosen, S.; Silva, P.; and Epstein, F. H.: Renal ischemia: A new perspective. Kidney Int., 26:375–383, 1984.

Brickman, A. S.; Massry, S. G.; and Coburn, J. W.: Changes in serum and urinary calcium during treatment with hydrochlorothiazide: Studies on mechanisms. J. Clin. Invest., 51: 945–954, 1972.

Broadus, A. E.; and Thier, S. O.: Metabolic basis of renal-stone disease. N. Engl. J. Med., 300:839–845, 1979.

Broadus, A. E.; Mangin, M.; Ikeda, K.; Insogna, K. L.; Weir, E. C.; Burtis, W. J.; and Stewart, A. F.: Humoral hypercalcemia of cancer. Identification of a novel parathyroid hormone-like peptide. N. Engl. J. Med., 319:556–563, 1988.

Buckalew, V. M.; and Schey, H. M.: Renal disease from habitual antipyretic analgesic consumption: An assessment of the epidemiologic evidence. Medicine, 11:291–303, 1986.

Burg, M. B.: Tubular chloride transport and the mode of action of some diuretics. Kidney Int., 9:189–197, 1976.

Cantarovich, F.; Galli, C.; Benedetti, L.; Chena, C.; Castro, L.; Correa, C.; Perez-Loredo, J.; Fernandez, J. C.; Locatelli, A.; and Tizado, J.: High dose furosemide in established acute renal failure. Br. Med. J., 4:449–450, 1973.

Carmichael, J.; and Shankel S. W.: Effects of nonsteroidal anti-inflammatory drugs on prostaglandins and renal function. Am. J. Med., 78:992–1000, 1985.

Christian, C. D.; Meredith, C. G.; and Speeg, K. V.: Cimetidine inhibits renal procainamide clearance. Clin. Pharmacol. Ther., 36:221–227, 1984.

Clive, D. M.; and Stoff, J. S.: Renal syndromes associated with nonsteroidal antiinflammatory drugs. N. Engl. J. Med., 310: 563–572, 1984.

Cloyd, J. C.; Snyder, B. D.; Cleeremans, B.; and Bundlie, S. R.: Mannitol pharmacokinetics and serum osmolality in dogs and humans. J. Pharmacol. Exp. Ther., 236:301–306, 1986.

Coe, F. L.: Calcium-uric acid nephrolithiasis. Arch. Intern. Med., 138:1090–1093, 1978.

Coe, F. L.: Metabolic alkalosis. J.A.M.A., 238:2288–2290, 1977.

Coe, F. L.; and Favus, M. J.: Disorders of stone formation in the kidney. (Brenner, B. M.; and Rector, F. C.; eds.). W. B. Saunders, Philadelphia, pp. 1403–1442, 1986.

Coe, F. L.; and Raisen, L.: Allopurinol treatment of uric-acid disorders in calcium-stone formers. Lancet, 1:129–131, 1973.

Coe, F. L.; Keck, J.; and Norton, E. R.: The natural history of calcium urolithiasis. J.A.M.A., 238:1519–1523, 1977.

Cogan, M. G.: Disorders of proximal nephron function. Am. J. Med., 72:275–288, 1982.

Cooperman, L. B.; and Rubin, I. L.: Toxicity of ethacrynic acid and furosemide. Am. Heart J., 85:831–834, 1973.

Corvol, P.; Claire, M.; Oblin, M. E.; Geering, K.; and Rossier, B.: Mechanism of the antimineralocorticoid effects of spirolactones. Kidney Int., 20:1–6, 1981.

Crawhall, J. C.; and Watts, R. W. E.: Cystinuria. Am. J. Med., 45:736–755, 1968.

Croxson, M. S.; Neutze, J. M.; and John, M. B.: Exchangeable potassium in heart disease: Long-term effects of potassium supplements and amiloride. Am. Heart J., 84:53–60, 1972.

Cullen, M. R.; Cherniack, M. G.; and Rosenstock, L.: Occupational medicine. N. Engl. J. Med., 322:594–601, 1990.

Cushner, H. M.; and Adams, N. D.: Review: Renal osteodystrophy—pathogenesis and treatment. Am. J. Med. Sci., 4: 264–275, 1986.

Danovitch, G. M.; Bourgoignie, J.; and Bricker, N. S.: Reversibility of the "salt-losing" tendency of chronic renal failure. N. Engl. J. Med., 296:14–19, 1977.

Data, J. L.; and Nies, A. S.: Dextran 40. Ann. Intern. Med., 81:500–504, 1974.

de Bold, A. J.: Atrial natriuretic factor: A hormone produced by the heart. Science, 230:767–770, 1985.

Diamond, J. R.; and Yoburn, D. C.: Nonoliguric acute renal failure associated with a low fractional excretion of sodium. Ann. Intern. Med., 96:597–600, 1982.

DiBona, G. F.: Neural regulation of renal tubular sodium reabsorption and renin secretion. Fed. Proc., 44:2816–2822, 1985.

Douglas, J. G.: Angiotensin receptor subtypes of kidney cortex. Am. J. Physiol., 253:F1–F7, 1987.

Drayer, D. E.: Pharmacologically active drug metabolites: Therapeutic and toxic activities, plasma and urine data in man, accumulation in renal failure. Clin. Pharmacokinet., 1: 426–443, 1976.

Dubach, U. C.; Rosner, B.; and Pfister, E.: Epidemiologic study of abuse of analgesics containing phenacetin. N. Engl. J. Med., 308:357–362, 1983.

Dunn, M. J.; and Zambraski, E. J.: Renal effects of drugs that inhibit prostaglandin synthesis. Kidney Int., 18:609–622, 1980.

Edelman, I. S.; Leibman, J.; O'Meara, M. P.; and Birkenfeld, L. W.: Interrelations between serum sodium concentration, serum osmolarity and total exchangeable sodium, total exchangeable potassium and total body water. J. Clin. Invest., 37:1236–1256, 1958.

Elion, G. B.; Yu, T. F.; Gutman, A. B.; and Hitchings, G. H.: Renal clearance of oxipurinol, the chief metabolite of allopurinol. Am. J. Med., 45:69–76, 1968.

Elkinton, J. R.: Acid-base disorders and the clinician. Ann. Intern. Med., 63:893–899, 1965.

Ellison, D. H.; Velazquez, H.; and Wright, F. S.: Adaptation of the distal convoluted tubule of the rat. Structural and functional effects of dietary salt intake and chronic diuretic infusion. J. Clin. Invest., 83:113–126, 1989.

Emmerson, B. T.; and Row, P. G.: An evaluation of the pathogenesis of the gouty kidney. Kidney Int., 8:65–71, 1975.

Epstein, M.; Schneider, N. S.; and Befeler, B.: Effect of intrarenal furosemide on renal function and intrarenal hemodynamics in acute renal failure. Am. J. Med., 58:510–515, 1975.

Erslev, A. J.: Biogenesis of erythropoietin. Am. J. Med. 58: 25–30, 1975.

Eschbach, J. W.; Abdulhadi, M. H.; Browne, J. K.; Delano, B. G.; Downing, M. R.; Egrie, J. C.; Evans, R. W.; Friedman, E. A.; Graber, S. E.; Haley, N. R.; Korbet, S.; Krantz, S. B.; Lundin, A. P.; Nissenson, A. R.; Ogden, D. A.; Paganini, E. P.; Rader, B.; Rutsky, E. A.; Stivelman, J.; Stone, W. J.; Teschan, P.; Van Stone, J. C.; Van Wyck, D. B.; Zuckerman, K.; and Adamson, J. W.: Recombinant human erythropoietin in anemic patients with end-stage renal disease. Results of a phase III multicenter clinical trial. Ann. Intern. Med., 111:992–1000, 1989a.

Eschbach, J. W.; Kelly, M. R.; Haley, N. R.; Abels, R. I.; and Adamson, J. W.: Treatment of the anemia of progressive renal failure with recombinant human erythropoietin. N. Engl. J. Med., 321:158–163, 1989b.

Ettinger, B.: Excretion of triamterene and its metabolite in triamterene stone patients. J. Clin. Pharmacol., 25:365–368, 1985.

Ettinger, B.; and Kolb, F. O.: Inorganic phosphate treatment of nephrolithiasis. Am. J. Med., 55:32–37, 1973.

Ettinger, B.; Tang, A.; Citron, J. T.; Livermore, B.; and Williams, T.: Randomized trial of allopurinol in the prevention of calcium oxalate calculi. N. Engl. J. Med., 315:1386–1389, 1986.

Feinfeld, D. A.; and Sherwood, L. M.: Parathyroid hormone and 1,25(OH)$_2$D$_3$ in chronic renal failure. Kidney Int., 33: 1049–1058, 1988.

Fessel, W. J.: Renal outcomes of gout and hyperuricemia. Am. J. Med., 67:74–82, 1979.

Foley, R. J.; and Weinman, E. J.: Review: Urate nephropathy. Am. J. Med. Sci., 288:208–211, 1984.

Forrest, J. N.; Cox, M.; Hong, C.; Morrison, G.; Bia, M.; and Singer, I.: Superiority of demeclocycline over lithium in the treatment of chronic syndrome of inappropriate secretion of antidiuretic hormone. N. Engl. J. Med., 298:173–177, 1978.

Frazier, H. S.; and Yager, H.: The clinical use of diuretics. N. Engl. J. Med., 288:246–249, 455–459, 1973.

Frelin, C.; Vigne, P.; Barbry, P.; and Lazdunski, M.: Molecular properties of amiloride action and of its Na$^+$ transporting targets. Kidney Int., 32:785–793, 1987.

Fried, W.: Erythropoietin. Arch. Intern. Med., 131:929–938, 1973.

Friedman, E.; Shadel, M.; Halkin, H.; and Zarfel, Z.: Thiazide-induced hyponatremia. Reproducibility by single dose rechallenge and an analysis of pathogenesis. Ann. Intern. Med., 110:24–30, 1989.

Gallagher, K. L.; and Jones, J. K.: Furosemide-induced ototoxicity. Ann. Intern. Med., 91:744–745, 1979.

Garella, S.; Dana, C. L.; and Chazan, J. A.: Severity of metabolic acidosis as a determinant of bicarbonate requirements. N. Engl. J. Med., 289:121–126, 1973.

Graziani, G.; Cantaluppi, A.; Casati, S.; Citterio, A.; Scalamogna, A.; Aroldi, A.; Silenzio, R.; Brancaccio, D.; and Ponticelli, C.: Dopamine and furosemide in oliguric acute renal failure. Nephron, 37:39–42, 1984.

Greenblatt, D. J.; Sellers, E. M.; and Koch-Wester, J.: Importance of protein binding for the interpretation of serum or plasma drug concentrations. J. Clin. Pharmacol., 22:259–263, 1982.

Greger, R.: Ion transport mechanisms in thick ascending limb of Henle's loop of mammalian nephron. Physiol. Rev., 65: 760–797, 1985.

Groopman, J. E.; Molina, J. M.; and Scadden, D. T.: Hematopoietic growth factors. Biology and clinical applications. N. Engl. J. Med., 321:1449–1459, 1989.

Gugler, R.; Shoeman, D. W.; Huffman, D. H.; Cohlmia, J. B.; and Azarnoff, D. L.: Pharmacokinetics of drugs in patients with the nephrotic syndrome. J. Clin. Invest., 55: 1182–1184, 1975.

Habener, J. F.; and Potts, J. T.: Biosynthesis of parathyroid hormone. N. Engl. J. Med., 299:580–585; and 635–644, 1978.

Hahn, B. H.; Sharp, G. C.; Irvin, W. S.; Kantor, O. S.; Gardner, C. A.; Bagby, M. K.; Perry, H. M. Jr.; and Osterland, C. K.: Immune responses to hydralazine and nuclear antigens in hydralazine-induced lupus erythematosus. Ann. Intern. Med., 76:365–374, 1972.

Hall, C. L.; Jawad, S.; Harrison, P. R.; MacKenzie, J. C.; Bacon, P. A.; Klouda, P. T.; and MacIver, A. G.: Natural course of penicillamine nephropathy: A long term study of 33 patients. Br. Med. J., 296:1083–1086, 1988.

Hall, C. L.; Fothergill, N. J.; Blackwell, M. M.; Harrison, P. R.; MacKenzie, J. C.; and MacIver, A. G.: The natural course of gold nephropathy: Long term study of 21 patients. Br. Med. J., 295:745–748, 1987.

Hammarlund-Udenaes, M.; and Benet, L. Z.: Furosemide pharmacokinetics and pharmacodynamics in health and disease—An update. J. Pharmacokinet. Biopharm., 17:1–46, 1989.

Hantman, D.; Rossier, B.; Zohlman, R.; and Schrier, R.: Rapid correction of hyponatremia in the syndrome of inappropriate secretion of antidiuretic hormone: An alternative treatment to hypertonic saline. Ann. Intern. Med., 78:870–875, 1973.

Harrington, J. T.; and Cohen, J. J.: Acute oliguria. N. Engl. J. Med., 292:89–91, 1975.

Hart, D.; Ward, M.; and Lifschitz, M. D.: Suprofen-related nephrotoxicity. Ann. Intern. Med., 106:235–238, 1987.

Hays, R. M.: Antidiuretic hormone. N. Engl. J. Med., 295: 659–665, 1976.

Hess, E.: Drug-related lupus. N. Engl. J. Med., 318:1460–1462, 1988.

Hill, J. B.: Salicylate intoxication. N. Engl. J. Med., 288:1110–1113, 1973.

Hill, J. B.: Experimental salicylate poisoning: Observations on the effects of altering blood pH on tissue and plasma salicylate concentrations. Pediatrics, 47:658–665, 1971.

Horiuchi, N.; Caulfield, M. P.; Fisher, J. E.; Goldman, M. E.; McKee, R. L.; Reagen, J. E.; Levy, J. J.; Nutt, R. F.; Rodan, S. B.; Schofield, T. L.; Clemens, T. L.; and Rosenblatt, M.: Similarity of synthetic peptide from human tumor to parathyroid hormone in vivo and in vitro. Science, 238:1566–1570, 1987.

Hulter, H. N.; Licht, J. H.; Glynn, R. D.; and Sebastian, A.: Pathophysiology of chronic renal tubular acidosis induced by administration of amiloride. J. Lab. Clin. Med., 95:637–653, 1980.

Ihle, B. U.; Becker, G. J.; Whitworth, J. A.; Charlwood, R. A.; and Kincaid-Smith, P. S.: The effect of protein restriction on the progression of renal insufficiency. N. Engl. J. Med., 321:1773–1777, 1989.

Jacobson, H. R.; and Seldin, D. W.: On the generation, maintenance, and correction of metabolic alkalosis. Am. J. Physiol., 245:F425–F432, 1983.

Jacqz, E.; Ward, S.; Johnson, R.; Schenker, S.; Gerkens, J.; and Branch, R. A.: Extrahepatic glucuronidation of morphine in the dog. Drug Metab. Disp., 14:627–630, 1986.

Jamison, R. L.: Micropuncture study of segments of thin limb of Henle in the rat. Am. J. Physiol., 215:236–242, 1968.

Jamison, R. L.; Bennett, C. M.; and Berliner, R. W.: Countercurrent multiplication by the thin loops of Henle. Am. J. Physiol., 212:357–366, 1967.

Johnson, J. R.; and Stamm, W. E.: Urinary tract infections in women: Diagnosis and treatment. Ann. Intern. Med., 111: 906–917, 1989.

Jones, R. H.; Hayakawa, H.; Mackay, J. D.; Parsons, V.; and Watkins, P. J.: Progression of diabetic nephropathy. Lancet, 1:1105–1106, 1979.

Jusko, W. J.; and Gretch, M.: Plasma and tissue protein binding of drugs in pharmacokinetics. Drug Metab. Rev., 5:43–140, 1976.

Kahan, B. D.: Cyclosporine. N. Engl. J. Med., 321:1725–1738, 1989.

Kaissling, B.; and Stanton, B. A.: Adaptation of distal tubule and collecting duct to increased sodium delivery: I. Ultrastructure. Am. J. Physiol., 255:F1256–F1268, 1988.

Katz, W. A.; Blodgett, R. C.; and Pietrusko, R. G.: Proteinuria in gold-treated rheumatoid arthritis. Ann. Intern. Med., 101: 176–179, 1984.

Kau, S. T.: Handling of triamterene by the isolated perfused rat kidney. J. Pharmacol. Exp. Ther., 206:701–709, 1978.

Keane, W. F.; Anderson, S.; Aurell, M.; deZeeuw, D.; Narins, R. G.; and Povar, G.: Angiotensin converting enzyme inhibitors and progressive renal insufficiency. Ann. Intern. Med., 111:503–516, 1989.

Kincaid-Smith, P.: Analgesic abuse and the kidney. Kidney Int., 17:250–260, 1980.

Klahr, S.; and Slatopolsky, E.: Renal regulation of sodium excretion. Function in health and in edema-forming states. Arch. Intern. Med., 131:780–791, 1973.

Klahr, S.; Schriener, G.; and Ichikawa, I.: The progression of renal disease. N. Engl. J. Med., 318:1657–1666, 1988.

Klotz, U.: Pathophysiological and disease-induced changes in drug distribution volume: Pharmacokinetic implications. Clin. Pharmacokinet., 1:204–218, 1976.

Klotz, U.; and Kroemer, H.: Clinical pharmacokinetic considerations in the use of plasma expanders. Clin. Pharmacokinet., 12:123–135, 1987.

Knochel, J. P.: The role of aldosterone in renal physiology. Arch. Intern. Med., 131:876–884, 1973.

Kok, D. J.; Papapoulos, S. E.; and Bijvoet, O. L. M.: Crystal agglomeration is a major element in calcium oxalate urinary stone formation. Kidney Int., 37:51–56, 1990.

Kokko, J. P.; and Rector, F. C. Jr.: Countercurrent multiplication system without active transport in inner medulla. Kidney Int., 2:214–223, 1972.

Komaroff, A. L.: Urinalysis and urine culture in women with dysuria. Ann. Intern. Med., 104:212–218, 1986.

Komaroff, A. L.: Acute dysuria in women. N. Engl. J. Med., 310:368–375, 1984.

Koren, G.: Clinical pharmacokinetic significance of the renal tubular secretion of digoxin. Clin. Pharmacokinet., 13:334–343, 1987.

LaCroix, A. Z.; Wienpahl, J.; White, L. R.; Wallace, R. B.; Scherr, P. A.; George, L. K.; Cornoni-Huntley, J.; and Ostfeld, A. M.: Thiazide diuretic agents and the incidence of hip fracture. N. Engl. J. Med., 322:286–290, 1990.

Landgrebe, A. R.; Nyhan, W. L.; and Coleman, M.: Urinary-tract stones resulting from the excretion of oxypurinol. N. Engl. J. Med., 292:626–627, 1975.

Langford, H. G.; Blaufox, M. D.; Borhani, N. O.; Curb, J. D.; Molteni, A.; Schneider, K. A.; and Pressel, S.: Is thiazide-produced uric acid elevation harmful? Analysis of data from the hypertension detection and follow-up program. Arch. Intern. Med., 147:645–649, 1987.

Levenson, D. J.; Simmons, C. E. Jr.; and Brenner, B. M.: Arachidonic acid metabolism, prostaglandins and the kidney. Am. J. Med., 72:354–374, 1982.

Loon, N. R.; Wilcox, C. S.; and Unwin, R. J.: Mechanism of impaired natriuretic response to furosemide during prolonged therapy. Kidney Int., 36:682–689, 1989.

MacKichan, J. J.: Protein binding drug displacement interactions. Fact or fiction? Clin. Pharmacokinet., 16:65–73, 1989.

Maffly, R. H.; and Edelman, I. S.: The role of sodium, potassium and water in the hypo-osmotic states of heart failure. Prog. Cardiovasc. Dis., 4:88–104, 1961.

Mallette, L. E.: Review: Primary hyperparathyroidism, an update: Incidence, etiology, diagnosis, and treatment. Am. J. Med. Sci., 293:239–249, 1987.

Marre, M.; Chatellier, G.; Leblanc, H.; Guyene, T. T.; Menard, J.; and Passa, P.: Prevention of diabetic nephropathy with enalapril in normotensive diabetics with microalbuminuria. Br. Med. J., 297:1092–1095, 1988.

Martinez-Maldonado, M.; Eknoyan, G.; and Suki, W. N.: Diuretics in nonedematous states. Physiological basis for the clinical use. Arch. Intern. Med., 131:797–808, 1973.

Marver, D.; and Kokko, J. P.: Renal target sites and the mechanism of action of aldosterone. Min. Elect. Metab., 9:1–18, 1983.

McKinney, T. D.; Myers, P.; and Speeg, K. V.: Cimetidine secretion by rabbit renal tubules in vitro. Am. J. Physiol., 241:F69–F76, 1981.

McMurray, S. D.; Luft, F. C.; Maxwell, D. R.; Hamburger, R. J.; Futty, D.; Szwed, J. J.; Lavelle, K. J.; and Kleit, S. A.: Prevailing patterns and predictor variables in patients with acute tubular necrosis. Arch. Intern. Med., 138:950–955, 1978.

Melmon, K. L.: Adverse effects of drug banning. J. Clin. Epidemiol., 42(9):921–923, 1989.

Miller, T. R.; Anderson, R. J.; Linas, S. L.; Henrich, W. L.; Berns, A. S.; Gabow, P. A.; and Schrier, R. W.: Urinary diagnostic indices in acute renal failure. A prospective study. Ann. Intern. Med., 89:47–50, 1978.

Milne, M. D.; Scribner, B. H.; and Crawford, M. A.: Non-ionic diffusion and the excretion of weak acids and bases. Am. J. Med., 24:709–729, 1958.

Minuth, A. N.; Terrell, J. B.; and Suki, W. N.: Acute renal failure: A study of the course and prognosis of 104 patients and of the role of furosemide. Am. J. Med. Sci., 271:317–324, 1976.

Mitch, W. E.; Walser, M.; Buffington, G. A.; and Lemann, J.: A simple method of estimating progression of chronic renal failure. Lancet, 2:1326–1328, 1976.

Molitoris, B. A.; Froment, D. H.; Mackenzie, T. A.; Huffer, W. H.; and Alfrey, A. C.: Citrate: A major factor in the toxicity of orally administered aluminum compounds. Kidney Int., 36:949–953, 1989.

Moore, F. D.; Edelman, I. S.; Olney, J. M.; James, A. H.; Brooks, L.; and Wilson, G. M.: Body sodium and potassium: III. Inter-related trends in alimentary, renal and cardiovascular disease; lack of correlation between body stores and plasma concentration. Metabolism, 3:334–350, 1953.

Morris, R. C.; Sebastian, A.; and McSherry, E.: Renal acidosis. Kidney Int., 1:322–340, 1972.

Mudge, G. H.; Silva, P.; and Stibitz, G. R.: Renal excretion by non-ionic diffusion (the nature of the disequilibrium). Med. Clin. North Am., 59:681–698, 1975.

Mundy, G. R.: Hypercalcemia of malignancy revisited. J. Clin. Invest., 82:1–6, 1988.

Mundy, G. R.; Wilkinson, R.; and Heath, D. A.: Comparative study of available medical therapy for hypercalcemia of malignancy. Am. J. Med., 74:421–432, 1983.

Murrell, G. A. C.; and Rapeport, W. G.: Clinical pharmacokinetics of allopurinol. Clin. Pharmacokinet., 11:343–353, 1986.

Myers, B. D.: Cyclosporine nephrotoxicity. Kidney Int., 30:964–974, 1986.

Myers, B. D.; Ross, J.; Newton, L.; Luetscher, J.; and Perlroth, M.: Cyclosporine-associated chronic nephropathy. N. Engl. J. Med., 311:699–705, 1984.

Narins, R. G.; Jones, E. R.; Stom, M. C.; Rudnick, M. R.; and Bastl, C. P.: Diagnostic strategies in disorders of fluid, electrolyte and acid-base homeostasis. Am. J. Med., 72:496–520, 1982.

Neilson, E. G.: Pathogenesis and therapy of interstitial nephritis. Kidney Int., 35:1257–1270, 1989.

Nierenberg, D. W.: Furosemide and ethacrynic acid in acute tubular necrosis. West. J. Med., 133:163–170, 1980.

Nord, E. P.; Howard, M. J.; Hafezi, A.; Moradeshagi, P.; Vaystub, S.; and Insel, P. A.: Alpha$_2$ adrenergic agonists stimulate Na$^+$-H$^+$ antiport activity in the rabbit renal proximal tubule. J. Clin. Invest., 80:1755–1762, 1987.

Ochs, H. R.; Greenblatt, D. J.; Bodem, G.; and Smith, T. W.: Spironolactone. Am. Heart J., 96:389–400, 1978.

Odlind, B.; and Beermann, B.: Renal tubular secretion and effects of furosemide. Clin. Pharmacol. Ther., 27:784–790, 1980.

Odlind, B.; Beermann, B.; and Lindstrom, B.: Coupling between renal tubular secretion and effect of bumetanide. Clin. Pharmacol. Ther., 34:805–809, 1983.

Pak, C. Y. C.: Pathophysiology of calcium nephrolithiasis. In, The Kidney: Physiology and Pathophysiology (Seldin, D. W.; and Giebisch, G.; eds.). Raven Press, New York, pp. 1365–1379, 1985.

Pak, C. Y. C.: Physiological basis for absorptive and renal hypercalciurias. Am. J. Physiol., 237:F415–F423, 1979.

Pak, C. Y. C.; and Fuller, C.: Idiopathic hypocitraturic calcium-oxalate nephrolithiasis successfully treated with potassium citrate. Ann. Intern. Med., 104:33–37, 1986.

Pak, C. Y. C.; Britton, F.; Peterson, R.; Ward, D.; Northcutt, C.; Breslau, N. A.; McGuire, J.; Sakhaee, K.; Bush, S.; Nicar, M.; Norman, D.; and Peters, P.: Ambulatory evaluation of nephrolithiasis: Classification, clinical presentation, and diagnostic criteria. Am. J. Med., 69:19–30, 1980a.

Pak, C. Y. C.; Sakhaee, K.; Crowther, C.; and Brinkley, L.: Evidence justifying a high fluid intake in treatment of nephrolithiasis. Ann. Intern. Med., 93:36–39, 1980b.

Pak, C. Y. C.; Kaplan, R.; Bone, H.; Townsend, J.; and Waters, O.: A simple test for the diagnosis of absorptive, resorptive and renal hypercalciurias. N. Engl. J. Med., 292:497–500, 1975.

Pak, C. Y. C.; Ohata, M.; Lawrence, E. C.; and Snyder, W.: The hypercalciurias. Causes, parathyroid functions, and diagnostic criteria. J. Clin. Invest., 54:387–400, 1974a.

Pak, C. Y. C.; Delea, C. S.; and Bartter, F. C.: Successful treatment of recurrent nephrolithiasis (calcium stones) with cellulose phosphate. N. Engl. J. Med., 290:175–180, 1974b.

Palestine, A. G.; Austin, H. A.; Balow, J. E.; Antonovych, T. T.; Sabnis, S. G.; Preuss, H. G.; and Nussenblatt, R. B.: Renal histopathologic alterations in patients treated with cyclosporine for uveitis. N. Engl. J. Med., 314:1293–1298, 1986.

Parker, M. S.; Oster, J. R.; Perez, G. O.; and Taylor, A. L.: Chronic hypokalemia and alkalosis. Approach to diagnosis. Arch. Intern. Med., 140:1336–1337, 1980.

Parving, H. H.; Hommel, E.; Nielsen, M. D.; and Giese, J.: Effect of captopril on blood pressure and kidney function in normotensive insulin dependent diabetics with nephropathy. Br. Med. J., 299:533–536, 1989.

Perez, G. O.; Oster, J. R.; and Vaamonde, C. A.: Renal acidosis and renal potassium handling in selective hypoaldosteronism. Am. J. Med., 57:809–816, 1974.

Phillips, P. A.; Rolls, B. J.; Ledingham, J. G. G.; Forsling, M. L.; Morton J. J.; Crowe, M. J.; and Wollner, L.: Reduced thirst after water deprivation in healthy elderly men. N. Engl. J. Med., 311:753–759, 1984.

Porter, G. A.; Bennett, W. M.; and Sheps, S. G.: Cyclosporine-associated hypertension. Arch. Intern. Med., 150:280–283, 1990.

Rabkin, R.; Simon, N. M.; Steiner, S.; and Colwell, J. A.: Effect of renal disease on renal uptake and excretion of insulin in man. N. Engl. J. Med., 282:182–187, 1970.

Randall, R. E.; Cohen, M. D.; Spray, C. C.; and Rossmeisl, E. C.: Hypermagnesemia in renal failure. Etiology and toxic manifestations. Ann. Intern. Med., 61:73–88, 1964.

Rastogi, S. P.; Crawford, C.; Wheeler, R.; Flanigan, W.; and Arruda, J. A. L.: Effect of furosemide on urinary acidification in distal renal tubular acidosis. J. Lab. Clin. Med., 104:271–282, 1984.

Rector, F. C.: Sodium, bicarbonate, and chloride absorption by the proximal tubule. Am. J. Physiol., 244:F461–F471, 1983.

Reddi, A. S.; and Camerini-Davalos R. A.: Diabetic nephropathy. Arch. Intern. Med., 150:31–43, 1990.

Reichel, H.; Koeffler, H. P.; and Norman, A. W.: The role of the vitamin D endocrine system in health and disease. N. Engl. J. Med., 320:980–991, 1989.

Reidenberg, M. M.; and Drayer, D. E.: Alteration of drug-protein binding in renal disease. Clin. Pharmacokinet., 9(suppl. 1):18–26, 1984.

Robinson, A. G.: DDAVP in the treatment of central diabetes insipidus. N. Engl. J. Med., 294:507–511, 1976.

Ronald, A. R.; and Harding, G. K. M.: Urinary infection prophylaxis in women. Ann. Intern. Med., 94:268–270, 1981.

Rosenbaum, J. L.; Kramer, M. S.; and Raja, R.: Resin hemoperfusion for acute drug intoxication. Arch. Intern. Med., 136:263–266, 1976.

Rosman, J. B.; Meijer, S.; Sluiter, W. J.; Ter Wee, P. M.; Piers-Becht, T. P. M.; and Donker, A. J. M.: Prospective randomised trial of early dietary protein restriction in chronic renal failure. Lancet, 2:1291–1295, 1984.

Sabatini, S.; and Kurtzman, N. A.: The maintenance of metabolic alkalosis: Factors which decrease bicarbonate excretion. Kidney Int., 25:357–361, 1984.

Schachter, J.: Chlamydial infections. N. Engl. J. Med., 298: 428–434; 490–495; and 540–547, 1978.

Schambelan, M.: Isolated hypoaldosteronism. West. J. Med., 118:33–38, 1973.

Schambelan, M.; Stockigt, J. R.; and Biglieri, E. G.: Isolated hypoaldosteronism in adults. A renin-deficiency syndrome. N. Engl. J. Med., 287:573–578, 1972.

Schrier, R. W.; and Berl, T.: Nonosmolar factors affecting renal water excretion. N. Engl. J. Med., 292:81–88; 141–145, 1975.

Schrier, R. W.; and Bichet, D. G.: Osmotic and nonosmotic control of vasopressin release and the pathogenesis of impaired water excretion in adrenal, thyroid, and edematous disorders. J. Lab. Clin. Med., 98:1–15, 1981.

Schrier, R. W.; Berl, T.; and Anderson, R. J.: Osmotic and nonosmotic control of vasopressin release. Am. J. Physiol., 236:F321–F332, 1979.

Schrier, R. W.; Lehman, D.; Zacherle, B.; and Earley, L. E.: Effect of furosemide on free water excretion in edematous patients with hyponatremia. Kidney Int., 3:30–34, 1973.

Schuster, V. L.; Kokko, J. P.; and Jacobson, H. R.: Angiotensin II directly stimulates sodium transport in rabbit proximal convoluted tubules. J. Clin. Invest., 73:507–515, 1984.

Scribner, B. H.; and Burnell, J. M.: Interpretation of serum potassium concentration. Metabolism, 5:468–479, 1959.

Sebastian, A.; Schambelan, M.; Lindenfeld, S.; and Morris, R. C.: Amelioration of metabolic acidosis with fludrocortisone therapy in hyporeninemic hypoaldosteronism. N. Engl. J. Med., 297:576–583, 1977.

Seyberth, H. W.; Segre, G. V.; Morgan, J. L.; Sweetman, B. J.; Potts, J. T.; and Oates, J. A.: Prostaglandins as mediators of hypercalcemia associated with certain types of cancer. N. Engl. J. Med., 293:1278–1283, 1975.

Shear, L.; Ching, S.; and Gabuzda, G. J.: Compartmentalization of ascites and edema in patients with hepatic cirrhosis. N. Engl. J. Med., 282:1391–1396, 1970.

Sheffield, P. A.; and Turner, J. S.: Ototoxic drugs: A review of clinical aspects, histopathologic changes and mechanisms of action. South Med. J., 64:359–363, 1971.

Sheikh, M. S.; Maguire, J. A.; Emmett, M.; Santa Ana, C. A.; Nicar, M. J.; Schiller, L. R.; and Fordtran, J. S.: Reduction of dietary phosphorus absorption by phosphorus binders. A theoretical, in vitro, and in vivo study. J. Clin. Invest., 83: 66–73, 1989.

Sheiner, L. B.; Rosenberg, B. G.; and Marathe, V. V.: Estimation of population characteristics of pharmacokinetic parameters from routine clinical data. J. Pharmacokinet. Biopharm., 5:445–479, 1977.

Shils, M. E.: Renal disease and the metabolic effects of tetracycline. Ann. Intern. Med., 58:389–408, 1963.

Shumizu, T.; Yoshitomi, K.; Nakamura, M.; and Imai, M.: Site and mechanism of action of trichlormethiazide in rabbit distal nephron segments perfused in vitro. J. Clin. Invest., 82:721–730, 1988.

Smith, D. E.; Lin, E. T.; and Benet, L. Z.: Absorption and disposition of furosemide in healthy volunteers, measured with a metabolite-specific assay. Drug Metab. Disp., 8:337–342, 1980.

Snyder, N. A.; Feigal, D. W.; and Arieff, A. I.: Hypernatremia in elderly patients. A heterogenous, morbid, and iatrogenic entity. Ann. Intern. Med., 107:309–319, 1987.

Somani, P.; Shapiro, R. S.; Stockard, H.; and Higgins, J. T.: Unidirectional absorption of gentamicin from the peritoneum during continuous ambulatory peritoneal dialysis. Clin. Pharmacol. Ther., 32:113–121, 1982.

Somogyi, A.; and Bochner, F.: Dose and concentration dependent effect of ranitidine on procainamide disposition and renal clearance in man. Br. J. Clin. Pharmacol., 18:175–181, 1984.

Somogyi, A.; McLean, A.; and Heinzow, B.: Cimetidine-procainamide pharmacokinetic interaction in man: Evidence of competition for tubular secretion of basic drugs. Eur. J. Clin. Pharmacol., 25:339–345, 1983.

Stamm, W. E.; McKevitt, M.; Counts, G. W.; Wagner, K. F.; Turck, M.; and Holmes, K. K.: Is antimicrobial prophylaxis of urinary tract infections cost effective? Ann. Intern. Med., 94:251–255, 1981.

Stamm, W. E.; Counts, G. W.; Wagner, K. F.; Martin, D.; Gregory, D., McKevitt, M.; Turck, M.; and Holmes, K. K.: Antimicrobial prophylaxis of recurrent urinary tract infections. A double-blind, placebo-controlled trial. Ann. Intern. Med., 92:770–775, 1980.

Stanton, B. A.; and Kaissling, B.: Adaptation of distal tubule and collecting duct to increased Na delivery: II. Na^+ and K^+ transport. Am. J. Physiol., 255:F1269–F1275, 1988.

Steen, V. D.; Blair, S.; and Medsger, T. A.: The toxicity of D-penicillamine in systemic sclerosis. Ann. Intern. Med., 104: 699–705, 1986.

Stein, H. B.; Patterson, A. C.; Offer, R. C.; Atkins, C. J.; Teufel, A.; and Robinson, H. S.: Adverse effects of D-penicillamine in rheumatoid arthritis. Ann. Intern. Med., 92:24–29, 1980.

Stein, J. H.; Lifschitz, M. D.; and Barnes, L. D.: Current concepts on the pathophysiology of acute renal failure. Am. J. Physiol., 234:F171–F181, 1978.

Stokes, J. B.: Electroneutral NaCl transport in the distal tubule. Kidney Int., 36:427–433, 1989.

Swan, R. C.; and Pitts, R. F.: Neutralization of infused acid by nephrectomized dogs. J. Clin. Invest., 34:205–212, 1955.

Szeto, H. H.; Inturrisi, C. E.; Houde, R.; Saal, S.; Cheigh, J.; and Reidenberg, M. M.: Accumulation of normeperidine, an active metabolite of meperidine, in patients with renal failure or cancer. Ann. Intern. Med., 86:738–741, 1977.

Tan, S. Y.; Shapiro, R.; Franco, R.; Stockard, H.; and Mulrow, P. J.: Indomethacin-induced prostaglandin inhibition with hyperkalemia. A reversible cause of hyporeninemic hypoaldosteronism. Ann. Intern. Med., 90:783–785, 1979.

Thyss, A.; Kubar, J.; Milano, G.; Namer, M.; and Schneider, M.: Clinical and pharmacokinetic evidence of a life-threatening interaction between methotrexate and ketoprofen. Lancet, 1:256–258, 1986.

Totoritis, M. C.; Tan, E. M.; McNally, E. M.; and Rubin, R. L.: Association of antibody to histone complex H2A-H2B with symptomatic procainamide-induced lupus. N. Engl. J. Med., 318:1431–1436, 1988.

Trippodo, N. C.; Cole, F. E.; Macphee, A. A.; and Pegram, B. L.: Biologic mechanisms of atrial natriuretic factor. J. Lab. Clin. Med., 109:112–119, 1987.

Uribarri, J.; Oh, M. S.; and Carroll, H. J.: The first kidney stone. Ann. Intern. Med., 111:1006–1009, 1989.

Vallner, J. J.: Binding of drugs by albumin and plasma protein. J. Pharm. Sci., 66:447–465, 1977.

Vasko, M. R.; Brown-Cartwright, D.; Knochel, J. P.; Nixon, J. V.; and Brater, D. C.: Furosemide absorption altered in decompensated congestive heart failure. Ann. Intern. Med., 102:314–318, 1985.

Verbeeck, R. K.; Branch, R. A.; and Wilkinson, G. R.: Drug metabolites in renal failure: Pharmacokinetic and clinical implications. Clin. Pharmacokinet., 6:329–345, 1981.

Voelker, J. R.; Cartwright-Brown, D.; Anderson, S.; Leinfelder, J.; Sica, D. A.; Kokko, J. P.; and Brater, D. C.: Comparison of loop diuretics in patients with chronic renal insufficiency. Kidney Int., 32:572–578, 1987.

Warren, S. E.; and Blantz, R. C.: Mannitol. Arch. Intern. Med., 141:493–497, 1981.

Warren, S. E.; and O'Connor, D. T.: Hyperkalemia resulting from captopril administration. J.A.M.A., 244:2551–2552, 1980.

Wilson, J. D.: Antinuclear antibodies and cardiovascular drugs. Drugs, 19:292–305, 1980.

Winchester, J. F.; and Gelfand, M. C.: Hemoperfusion in drug intoxication: Clinical and laboratory aspects. Drug Metab. Rev., 8:69–104, 1978.

Windhager, E. E.; and Giebisch, G.: Proximal sodium and fluid transport. Kidney Int., 9:121–133, 1976.

Winters, R. W.: Terminology of acid–base disorders. Ann. Intern. Med., 63:873–884, 1965.

Young, J. L.; Boswell, R. B.; and Nies, A. S.: Severe allopurinol hypersensitivity. Association with thiazides and prior renal compromise. Arch. Intern. Med., 134:553–558, 1974.

Yu, T. F.; Berger, L.; Dorph D. J.; and Smith, H.: Renal function in gout: V. Factors influencing the renal hemodynamics. Am. J. Med., 67:766–771, 1979.

Zeller, K. R.: Review: Effects of dietary protein and phosphorus restriction on the progression of chronic renal failure. Am. J. Med. Sci., 294:328–340, 1987.

12

Neurologic Disorders

Gregory W. Albers and Stephen J. Peroutka

Chapter Outline

Headache
  Muscle Contraction, or Tension, Headache
  Treatment of Acute Migraine
  Prophylaxis of Migraine
Epilepsy
  Classification of Seizures and Epileptic
    Syndromes
  Antiepileptic Drugs
  Optimal Use of Antiepileptic Drugs
Cerebral Vascular Disease
  Clinical Aspects of Stroke
  Management of Acute Stroke
  Prophylactic Treatments for Stroke
Parkinsonism

Clinical Aspects of Parkinsonism
Treatment of Parkinson Disease
Side Effects of Antiparkinsonian
  Medications
New Treatment Strategies
Drug-Induced Neurologic Disorders
  Cerebral Cortex
  Headache
  Cranial Nerve Disorders
  Involuntary Movement Disorders
  Peripheral Neuropathies
  Inhibition of Neuromuscular Transmission
  Autonomic Nervous System

HEADACHE

Headache is probably the most common human ailment. It is also the most common complaint of patients evaluated by neurologists (Kurtzke et al., 1986). Although headache can be caused by a large variety of conditions (Table 12–1), muscle contraction (or tension) headache and migraine are the most common causes. Muscle contraction headache afflicts as many as 80% of people per year with relatively low morbidity, while migraine afflicts approximately 10% to 20% of the population and is associated with appreciable morbidity. It is estimated that approximately 64 million workdays are lost in the United States each year due to migraine. Since the pathophysiology and treatment of these two types of headache differ, it is imperative that physicians

Table 12–1. COMMON CAUSES OF HEADACHE

Muscle contraction, or tension, headache
Migraine
Cervical spine disease
Sinusitis
Pseudotumor cerebri
Cluster headache
Intracranial mass
Cerebrovascular disorders
Trigeminal neuralgia
Temporal arteritis
Meningitis or encephalitis

easily distinguish them. Rational treatment of headache is based upon first making an accurate diagnosis of the type of headache presented by the patient.

Muscle Contraction, or Tension, Headache

Many patients who claim to have migraine may in fact suffer from *muscle contraction*, or *tension, headaches*. These terms are synonymous and are used to define headaches that are described by the patient as a "constant, dull, pressure sensation" around the head or neck region. These patients may state that they are "never headache-free." They rarely complain of a throbbing pain or associated nausea, symptoms that are more suggestive of a migraine headache. However, muscle contraction, or tension, headaches may be coincident with migraine (a condition designated as *mixed headache syndrome*).

The appropriate treatment program for patients with muscle contraction headaches extends far beyond the scope of this chapter. An attempt should be made to identify contributing sources of stress or depression. In addition, relaxation therapy (ranging from simple exercise to formal biofeedback techniques) is recommended. Finally, pharmacologic therapies can be useful and may be divided into two major categories: simple analgesics such as aspirin or acetaminophen, and combination analgesics containing additional agents such as caffeine and/or a small amount of a barbiturate (Table 12–2).

Available combination preparations include Axotal, Fiorinal, and Phrenilin, all of which are indicated for the treatment of muscle contraction headaches. *Principle: Narcotics are never indicated for treatment of muscle contraction headaches. The recurrent and/or nearly constant pattern of the disorder makes their addictive potential extremely high.* Indeed, caution should be exercised in the use of medications containing low-dose barbiturates (e.g., butalbital) because these agents are also addictive. Finally, there is no known justification for the determination of plasma concentrations of these agents in this clinical setting.

Treatment of Acute Migraine

Migraine is a specific neurologic syndrome that has a wide variety of manifestations (Lance and Anthony, 1966; Olesen, 1978; Dalessio, 1980). At the most basic level, migraine can be defined as a throbbing headache (usually unilateral) with associated nausea. A premonitory phase may begin up to 24 hours before the headache and often consists of changes in mood or appetite. The headache itself is often accompanied by photophobia, hyperacusis, polyuria, or diarrhea. An acute migraine attack can last from hours to days and is followed by prolonged pain-free intervals. The headache frequency is extremely variable but usually ranges from several per year to several per month.

A commonly used classification system for migraine is summarized in Table 12–3. A *classic* migraine begins with neurologic symptoms that constitute the aura, or prodrome, of the headache. Visual distortions are the most common complaint of patients and usually consist of blurred vision, scintillating scotomata (a blind spot with shimmering edges), or fortification spectra (zigzag lines). These symptoms evolve over the course of 15 to 20 minutes. A severe, throbbing pain then begins on the side of the head contralateral to the visual distortions. In 70% to 80% of patients, the pain is unilateral; in most patients, the headache tends to recur on the same

Table 12–3. CLASSIFICATION OF MIGRAINE

TYPES OF MIGRAINE	SYMPTOMS
Common	Unilateral (80%) throbbing headache with associated nausea
Classic	Same as common migraine but preceded by a visual aura, or prodrome
Complicated	
Hemiplegic	Sudden onset of hemiparesis followed by a contralateral throbbing headache
Ophthalmoplegic	Unilateral eye pain and ipsilateral ophthalmoplegia
Basilar Artery	Visual aura with alterations in consciousness prior to headache

side of the head. Nausea is frequently present, and the patient may occasionally vomit.

A *common* migraine is identical to the above except that it lacks the aura, or *prodrome*, phase of the headache. If the patient has focal neurologic deficits other than visual distortions, the migraine is designated *complicated*.

Although attacks are associated with disordered vasoconstriction and later vasodilation of cerebral vessels, the detailed pathophysiology of acute migraine attacks is not entirely clear. The cause of this abnormal cerebrovascular motor activity may be related to the elevated blood concentrations of norepinephrine, histamine, or serotonin, which have been observed during attacks. In addition, attacks are associated with increased platelet aggregability. Whether these observations represent cause or effect of the attack is not clear. However, it is likely that the portion of the acute attack manifested by pain may be related to excessive pulsation of (extracranial) arteries. Some, but not all, patients suffering such acute attacks can discern activities that can trigger these attacks. The present lack of understanding of the pathophysiology of these attacks makes therapeutic management less than optimal. Management is directed at preventing initial vasoconstriction, antagonizing the effects of serotonin, combating

Table 12–2. DRUGS USEFUL IN THE MANAGEMENT OF MUSCLE CONTRACTION (TENSION) HEADACHE

DRUG(S)	TRADE NAME	DOSAGE
Aspirin	(many)	650 mg q4h
Acetaminophen	(many)	650 mg q4h
Aspirin, butalbital	Axotal	One tablet q4h (maximum six tablets)
Aspirin, caffeine, butalbital	Fiorinal	One or two tablets q4h (maximum six tablets)
Acetaminophen, butalbital	Phrenilin	One or two tablets q4h (maximum six tablets)

later vasodilation, treating associated nausea, and encouraging rest by administering sedatives.

The primary treatment for an acute migraine attack is nonopioid analgesics. For patients who are unresponsive to these analgesics and behavioral measures, other more effective but also more potentially toxic pharmacologic options such as ergots and antiemetics are available. The use of opioid (narcotic) analgesics should be limited to severe cases in which other measures have proved inadequate.

Analgesics. Nearly all migraine attacks can be treated satisfactorily with symptomatic measures (Table 12–4). At the first onset of symptoms, mild analgesics such as aspirin or acetaminophen should be taken. Aspirin has been used for over 90 years and remains the drug used most frequently to abort an acute attack. The NSAIDs are also effective pain relievers and differ from aspirin primarily in cost to the patient. Such analgesics should be taken at the first sign of the onset of an acute attack and then every 4 hours until the headache is completely relieved. Mild analgesics are most effective if taken very early in the course of the headache. These drugs are rarely able to completely relieve the pain associated with moderate-to-severe migraine attacks.

A number of stronger nonnarcotic analgesics have been developed. Most are combination products containing aspirin or acetaminophen with a sedative such as butalbital. A few also contain mild vasoconstrictors such as isometheptene, a sympathomimetic amine that has been reported to reduce carotid blood flow in anesthetized cats

(Spierings and Saxena, 1980). Two of these commercial products (Midrin and Migralam) have been officially indicated for use in migraine. By contrast Axotal, Fiorinal, and Phrenilin are similar compounds officially indicated for muscle contraction headaches that can be used to treat relatively mild migraines. *Principle: Although combination products may appear to be more attractive than medications containing only one ingredient, they are not necessarily more effective. Each component must be present in an amount sufficient to cause its intended pharmacologic effect. Often multiple components may fail to contribute to overall efficacy, but may contribute to overall adverse effects.* In general, these combination products should be used only after a simple analgesic has been found to be insufficient for a patient with migraine.

Ergots. A large proportion of migraine patients respond to mild analgesics, antiemetics, and sleep. While ergots are more effective, their increased toxicity suggests they should be reserved for use in patients whose migraine is severe and likely to be refractory to measures described above. For refractory patients, ergot preparations have been recommended since the 1920s. These drugs have potent vasoconstrictor effects and interact with a number of neurotransmitter receptors (McCarthy and Peroutka, 1989). The use of ergots for acute migraine attacks should be restricted to patients having infrequent but severe migraine. Ergot preparations can be taken orally, sublingually, rectally, IM, IV, or via inhalers.

The patient with a severe migraine should be

Table 12–4. NONOPIOID DRUGS USED TO TREAT ACUTE MIGRAINE

DRUG	TRADE NAME(S)	DOSAGE
Aspirin	(many)	650 mg q4h
Acetaminophen	(many)	650 mg q4h
Acetaminophen, isometheptene, dichloralphenazone	Midrin	Two capsules at onset followed by one capsule q1h (maximum five capsules)
Acetaminophen, caffeine, isometheptene	Migralam	Two capsules at onset followed by one capsule q1h (maximum five capsules)
Aspirin, butalbital	Axotal*	One tablet q4h (maximum six tablets)
Aspirin, caffeine, butalbital	Fiorinal*	One or two tablets q4h (maximum six tablets)
Acetaminophen, butalbital	Phrenilin*	One or two tablets q4h (six capsules maximum)
Ergotamine, caffeine	Wigraine; Cafergot	Two tablets at onset then one tablet q$\frac{1}{2}$h (maximum 6 per day, 10 per week)
Ergotamine, caffeine, belladonna, pentobarbital	Cafergot P-B; Wigraine P-B	One suppository at onset then 1 hour later (maximum two per day or five per week)
Ergotamine	Ergostat; Ergomar	One sublingual tablet at onset and q$\frac{1}{2}$h (maximum three per day, five per week)
Ergotamine	Medihaler-Ergotamine	Single inhalation at onset followed by q5min (maximum 6 per day; 15 per week)
Dihydroergotamine	D.H.E. 45	1 ml IM or IV at onset and q1h (maximum 3 ml per day, 6 ml per week)

* Not specifically indicated by FDA for migraine.

advised to take ergot preparations as soon as possible after the onset of a headache. Gastrointestinal absorption of ergots is erratic; this fact may explain the large variation in patient response to these drugs (Fozard, 1986). Coadministration of caffeine has been reported to increase intestinal absorption of ergots, which provides a rationale for the use of combination pills containing caffeine (Ala-Hurula, 1982). Various preparations of ergots are available, most of which contain additional ingredients such as caffeine and/or barbiturate derivatives (see Table 12–4). *Principle: Understanding the multiple mechanisms by which drug interactions occur enables finding optimal strategies for the use of those drugs.*

With ergotamine preparations, a dose of 1 to 2 mg should be taken at the onset of the headache, followed by up to four additional 1-mg tablets taken 30 minutes apart. No more than 10 mg/week of ergotamine should be taken. Ergotamine has a relatively long biologic half-life, and administration of greater than 1 mg/day may cause peripheral vasospasm and, rarely, gangrene (Peatfield et al., 1986). The manifestations of ergotism should be evaluated in patients receiving long-term therapy.

Ergotamine preparations are contraindicated in pregnant women and patients with peripheral vascular disease, angina, and hypertension. It has been recommended that ergots be avoided in patients with complicated migraine due to fears that drug-induced vasoconstriction may lead to cerebral infarctions. Data concerning this issue are lacking. Nausea and vomiting are probably the most common side effects of ergots, as well as common presenting complaints of the disease itself. *Principle: When a disease and its therapy cause similar symptoms, it becomes increasingly difficult to distinguish undertreatment from drug toxicity.*

The use of IV ergots has been recommended for the treatment of severe or refractory migraine. In a study of acute migraine patients, the use of 0.75 mg IV dihydroergotamine (D.H.E. 45) (Fig. 12–1) was found to be safe and effective (Callaham and Raskin, 1986). This regimen also significantly decreased the need for narcotics. Raskin (1986) has also reported that 49 of 55 patients were headache-free within 48 hours after receiving 0.5 mg of dihydroergotamine and 10 mg of metoclopramide (Reglan) every 8 hours.

These results demonstrating the efficacy of IV dihydroergotamine in patients with severe, refractory migraine may enable physicians to avoid administering opioids to such patients. Given the recurrent nature of the disease, such recurrent use of opioids carries a high risk of causing dependence, as discussed below. *Principle: When two drugs are comparably effective, the choice of* *drug is often dictated by comparison of the toxicity profiles of the two drugs.*

Sumatriptan. Recently, sumatriptan (formerly called GR 43175) (Fig. 12–1) has been reported to be extremely effective in the treatment of acute migraine. Although its mechanism of action was initially unclear, it has been suggested that sumatriptan may selectively stimulate a subpopulation of 5-HT (5-hydroxytryptamine, serotonin) receptors (Humphrey et al., 1988; McCarthy and Peroutka, 1989). Indeed, the hypothesis to be tested is that the ability of sumatriptan to stimulate 5-HT_{1D} receptors might account for its antimigraine efficacy (McCarthy and Peroutka, 1989).

In one study, sumatriptan 2 mg IV completely abolished migraine symptoms in 71% of 24 migraine attacks and significantly reduced headache symptoms in the remaining patients (Doenicke et al., 1988). Only minor side effects (transient pressure in the head, feeling of warmth or tingling) were observed. Sumatriptan is now in phase III trials, and it continues to show great promise as therapy for acute migraine, with minimal side effects.

Antiemetics. Antiemetics are an important yet infrequently used drug class in the treatment of acute migraine (Peatfield et al., 1986). As many as 90% of migraine patients complain of nausea and/or vomiting with the headache (Olesen, 1978). Treatment with antiemetic medications such as prochlorperazine, promethazine, or metoclopramide can help relieve the nausea associated with acute migraine. Each of these agents is known to block dopamine D_2 receptors, a pharmacologic property that theoretically accounts for their antiemetic effects (Hamik and Peroutka, 1989). Metoclopramide is unique among currently available antiemetic agents in that it possesses both dopamine D_2 and 5-HT_3 receptor antagonist properties at equimolar concentrations (Hamik and Peroutka, 1989).

In addition, gastric absorption is altered during a migraine attack. Metoclopramide appears to have specific gastrokinetic properties that correct this disturbance of absorption (Volans, 1975). These properties may be particularly important when oral ergots are used. Therefore, the use of metoclopramide appears to be warranted for both the symptomatic treatment of the nausea associated with migraine and for its ability to increase GI motility and gastric emptying (Volans, 1975; Hakkarainen and Allonen, 1982).

Other Agents. Other medications have been recommended for treatment of acute migraine attacks. Unfortunately, many patients are routinely

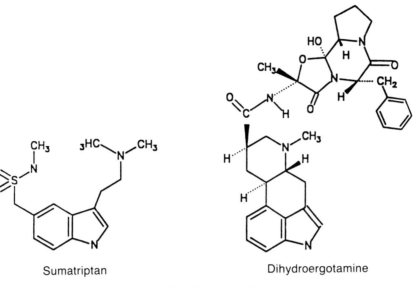

Sumatriptan   Dihydroergotamine

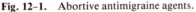

Fig. 12–1. Abortive antimigraine agents.

treated with potent narcotics, despite the fact that such potentially addicting drugs have no effect on the underlying migraine process. Therefore, the use of narcotics such as meperidine should be limited to patients with severe acute migraine attacks refractory to all other measures. Long-term use of narcotics to treat migraine is never indicated. Finally, it appears to be useful to have the patient enter a dark and quiet room. Patients should attempt to sleep, because they often awaken without a headache (Wilkinson, 1983, 1988).

Prophylaxis of Migraine

A small proportion of migraine patients have frequent headache attacks. A general consensus among neurologists is to prophylactically treat patients having three or more migraines per month (Peatfield et al., 1986). This section discusses the medications that have demonstrated efficacy in the prophylactic treatment of migraine (see Table 12–5). However, none of the following agents is effective in more than 60% to 70% of patients (Peatfield et al., 1986). Therefore, none of the agents has been established as the "drug of first choice" for migraine prophylaxis. *Principle: The selection of the first agent tried in any given patient with migraine depends more on the contraindications and side effects than on clinically substantiated differences in expected efficacy.* Because migraine is a sporadically recurrent disorder, a medication trial period of at least 4 to 6 weeks is generally considered necessary to evaluate drug efficacy.

Unfortunately, plasma concentrations of these

Table 12–5. DRUGS USEFUL FOR MIGRAINE PROPHYLAXIS

DRUG	TRADE NAME	DOSAGE
β-Adrenergic Receptor Antagonists		
Propranolol	Inderal	80–320 mg qd
Atenolol	Tenormin*	50–100 mg qd
Nadolol	Corgard*	40–80 mg qd
Metoprolol	Lopressor*	100–450 mg qd
Timolol	Blocadren*	20–60 mg qd
Antidepressants		
Amitriptyline	Elavil*	50–150 mg qd
Phenelzine	Nardil*	15 mg t.i.d.
Isocarboxazid	Marplan*	10 mg q.i.d.
Calcium-Channel Blockers		
Diltiazem	Cardizem*	180–240 mg qd
Nifedipine	Procardia*	10–40 mg t.i.d.
Verapamil	Isoptin*; Calan*	80–120 mg t.i.d.
Serotonergic-Receptor Antagonists		
Methysergide	Sansert	4–8 mg qd
Cyproheptadine	Periactin*	4–16 mg qd
Ergots		
Ergonovine	Ergotrate*	0.2 mg t.i.d.

* Not specifically approved by the FDA for this indication.

drugs are of no known therapeutic benefit. Therefore, the physician must depend on patient self-reports to assess whether the therapy is successful. Clearly, the lack of objective diagnostic and/or therapeutic tests in migraine has severely hindered clinical pharmacologic studies of this disorder.

Ideally, the physician and patient will be able to identify an agent that leads to an appreciable decrease in the frequency, intensity, or duration of the migraine attacks. Once the patient and physician believe that a particular prophylactic medication is efficacious, then the drug should be continued for a period of at least 6 months. In the opinion of the authors, an attempt should then be made to discontinue the treatment because of the high incidence of complete remission in migraine. If a rebound of headache occurs after the discontinuation of a successful prophylactic therapy, then the medication regimen should be reinstituted for at least another 6-month period. *Principle: Determining the efficacy of a prophylactic agent depends on the natural course of the disease. If the disease is not chronically and constantly signaling its presence, "cure" by a prophylactic will take several ordinary cycles of the disease for evaluation. Failure to recognize the time requirements may keep a patient on long-term administration of a useless drug or cause discontinuation of a partially useful one.*

β-Adrenergic Receptor Antagonists. In the late 1960s, a serendipitous observation in patients with exertional angina suggested that propranolol (Fig. 12-2) is able to prevent frequent migraine attacks (Raskin, 1986; Wykes, 1968). A review of multiple clinical studies shows that 50% to 70% of patients derive some benefit from prophylactic propranolol therapy (Peatfield et al., 1986). Approximately one third of such patients report greater than 50% reduction in the number of attacks with treatment. A dose of 40 mg twice a day is usually begun; doses as great as 320 mg/day should be given for at least 4 to 6 weeks before deciding that the patient is nonresponsive to therapy.

A variety of other β-adrenergic receptor antagonists have been used to prevent migraine (Weerasuriya et al., 1982). Atenolol, metoprolol, nadolol, and timolol appear to be as effective as propranolol for migraine prophylaxis. More variable results have been obtained with pindolol. By contrast, a number of other β-adrenergic receptor antagonists (e.g., acebutolol, oxprenolol, alprenolol) do not appear to be effective for migraine therapy (Weerasuriya et al., 1982; Peatfield et al., 1986). *Principle: The full effects of a marketed drug cannot be known until it is in the field. Propranolol's uses have broadened greatly from its original indications. Obviously, detection of an effect such as that described here requires a clinican with a low barrier for accepting what he or she sees as a drug effect (even when the effect has not been described by someone else) (Melmon, 1984). Generally, the barriers to making the first observation of an unanticipated drug effect are high.*

The pharmacologic basis for the effectiveness of certain β-adrenergic receptor antagonists in migraine is not known. However, no single pharmacologic property of this class of drugs can explain their apparent clinical efficacy (Fozard, 1982). Antimigraine effects of these drugs do not correlate with their potency at blocking β-adrenergic receptors, because not all β-adrenergic receptor antagonists are effective migraine agents. The ability of certain β-adrenergic agents to modulate serotonergic systems has also been suggested to be the basis of their antimigraine efficacy (Raskin, 1981; Fozard, 1982; McCarthy and Peroutka, 1989). Alternatively, it has been suggested that only pure β-adrenergic receptor antagonists are effective agents for migraine prophylaxis (Weerasuriya et al., 1982; Fanchamps, 1985). Drugs that display "intrinsic sympathomimetic activity" (i.e., partial agonist activity) at the β-adrenergic receptor may be less effective migraine prophylactic agents. *Principle: Trying to describe all of a drug's effects by the rubric of its mechanism of action (e.g., β-adrenergic receptor antagonist) may unduly restrict curiosity about the mechanisms of drug effects and narrow the pharmacologic and therapeutic profile of a chemical entity.*

Adverse effects of β-adrenergic receptor antagonists are seldom severe in otherwise healthy patients. However, these drugs are contraindicated in patients with asthma, sinus bradycardia, congestive heart failure, and diabetes mellitus (see chapters 3, 6, 16). Common side effects include lethargy, GI upset, and orthostatic hypotension. However, these side effects rarely necessitate discontinuation of the drug.

Amitriptyline. The tricyclic antidepressant amitriptyline (Fig. 12-2) is an effective prophylactic agent in migraine, independent of its antidepressant actions (Gomersall and Stuart, 1973; Couch et al., 1976; Couch and Hassanein, 1979). Amitriptyline is a potent blocker of serotonin and norepinephrine uptake and is also an antagonist of multiple neurotransmitter receptors. However, its mechanism of action in migraine prophylaxis remains unknown. Amitriptyline is not officially indicated for the treatment of migraine despite its widespread clinical use for this disorder.

Amitriptyline is commonly used to treat patients with "mixed" headaches (i.e., patients having symptoms of both migraine and muscle contraction headaches). Patients are typically started on a 25- or 50-mg dose at bedtime, and the dose may be gradually increased to from 150 to 200 mg/day. A significant proportion of patients complain of excessive sedation caused by the drug. If this problem occurs, the dose should be halved. A 4- to 6-week trial is recommended before the drug is considered ineffective. Side effects are usually related to the anticholinergic

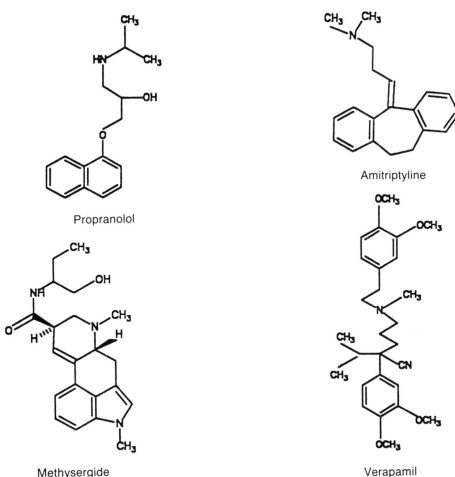

Fig. 12–2. Prophylactic antimigraine agents.

properties of the drug (i.e., dry mouth, dizziness, blurred vision, urinary retention) and are discussed in chapter 13. Its ability to predispose to cardiac arrhythmias, and its relative contraindication in patients with heart disease, are widely believed but not firmly proved.

Methysergide. Serotonergic-receptor antagonists such as methysergide (Fig. 12–2) represent the first class of drugs to be shown effective in migraine prophylaxis (Lance, 1970, 1981). In 1959, Sicuteri reported that chronic methysergide therapy decreased migraine frequency (Sicuteri, 1959). Methysergide is an ergot derivative that has complex effects on serotonergic and other neurotransmitter systems. Methysergide has been shown to be effective in 60% to 80% of migraine patients and should be given for at least a 3- to 6-week trial (Lance, 1970). Common side effects include nausea, vomiting, and diarrhea. The oral

bioavailability of methysergide has been reported to be only 13%, reflecting its considerable first-pass effect and suggesting that a metabolite such as methylergometrine may be the active therapeutic agent (Tfelt-Hansen et al., 1985).

Unfortunately, as clinical experience with methysergide increased during the 1960s, a small number of patients developed retroperitoneal fibrosis and fibrotic processes involving the aorta, heart, and lungs. The onset of these side effects was delayed 7 to 79 months into methysergide therapy (Graham, 1979). It has been recommended that methysergide be administered for a maximal period of 4 consecutive months; the patient should then discontinue the medication for at least 2 weeks in order to minimize the risk of fibrotic complications (Graham, 1979). The efficacy of this approach has not been documented clinically. Because of continued concerns of potential fibrotic side effects, the use of methysergide for migraine prophylaxis has progressively diminished during the past decade. Although other serotonin-receptor antagonists such as pizotifen have also been reported to be effective for migraine prophylaxis, cyproheptadine is the only other serotonergic agent currently available in the United States. *Principle: The most effective drug in a given situation may not be the agent of choice. Efficacy and toxicity are not absolute values, but are relative values with respect to the severity of the disease process and each other. Similarly, drug indications and contraindications usually are relative.*

Calcium-Channel Blockers. Calcium-channel blockers represent a potentially novel class of antimigraine agents (Peroutka, 1983; Greenberg, 1986). These drugs block the entrance of extracellular calcium into vascular smooth muscle cells and thereby prevent vasoconstriction. In fact, no known endogenous vasoactive agent can contract intracranial blood vessels in the presence of an adequate concentration of a calcium-channel antagonist drug such as verapamil (Fig. 12–2) (Peroutka, 1983). Although generally considered a single-drug class, the calcium-channel blockers are a structurally diverse group of agents. At least three classes of calcium-channel blockers have been described. All agents share the ability to prevent contractions of vascular smooth muscle.

Since 1981 several clinical trials have reported that calcium-channel blockers are effective for migraine prophylaxis (Schuler et al., 1987; Jonsdottir et al., 1988). Flunarizine, a relatively weak calcium-channel antagonist, has been studied extensively (Amery, 1983). The drug was found to be safe and effective for the treatment of both classic and common migraine. In addition, a number of recent case reports and studies have documented the effectiveness of diltiazem, verapamil, nifedipine, and nimodipine in the prophylactic treatment of migraine. These drugs appear to decrease both the frequency and severity of classic and common migraine. At present, none of these agents have been specifically approved by the FDA for use in migraine prophylaxis. Moreover, recent studies have questioned the effectiveness of calcium-channel blockers in migraine and have reported a high incidence of side effects in migraine patients (Albers et al., 1989b; McArthur et al., 1989). Side effects can be expected to develop in 20% to 60% of the patients but are usually mild and consist of constipation and mild orthostatic hypotension (Albers et al., 1989b). These drugs are relatively contraindicated in pregnant women because of available data suggesting fetal toxicity in animals and the absence of sufficient data in humans to allow firm conclusions.

Other Agents. Other medications have been reported to be effective for migraine prophylaxis. Chlorpromazine (see chapter 13), a phenothiazine with antiemetic properties, has been recommended as a first-line drug for migraine prophylaxis (Caviness and O'Brien, 1980). The NSAID naproxen, and monoamine oxidase (MAO) inhibitors such as phenelzine and isocarboxazid, have been reported to be effective for migraine prophylaxis (Ziegler and Ellis, 1985; Peatfield et al., 1986). The MAO inhibitors may be effective because of their ability to increase concentrations of endogenous serotonin. However, their side effects include orthostatic hypotension, insomnia, and nausea. Narcotics are definitely contraindicated for migraine prophylaxis because of their lack of efficacy and their potential for causing tolerance, dependence, and addiction. *Principle: When a variety of drugs with numerous mechanisms of action appear to be useful but not definitive in managing a disease, at least two points should be considered: (1) the drugs may be doing very little but the characteristics of the disease make it difficult to negate apparent efficacy, or (2) the drugs may be working at different points of pathogenesis of disease and might be combined for additive efficacy* (see hypertension, chapter 2).

EPILEPSY

Epilepsy is a general term for a group of disorders characterized by recurrent seizures. A seizure is defined as a sudden, transient disturbance in cognitive, motor, sensory, or autonomic function that is accompanied by an abnormal, excessive electrical discharge in the brain. Convulsive seizures that involve involuntary muscle contractions are more common than nonconvulsive seizures. Seizures may be primary (idiopathic), or a secondary manifestation of a variety of pathologic conditions, many of which require specific management.

Major causes of epilepsy include trauma, vascular disorders, tumors, toxic or metabolic disturbances, and infections (see Table 12–6). However, many epileptic patients have no identifiable pathologic brain lesion, and these patients are generally thought to have a genetic predisposition toward seizures. Therefore, in considering treatment for a patient with epilepsy, identification of the underlying cause is crucial in order to identify the primary target for therapy. *Principle: Rational treatment of a syndrome that may be caused by a variety of underlying conditions requires that the therapist first determine the underlying disease causing the syndrome. Successfully treating a syndrome while ignoring feasible treatment of its cause does not represent optimal therapeutics.*

Table 12-6. COMMON CAUSES OF EPILEPSY

Head injury
Infarct
Hemorrhage
Vascular malformations
Primary brain tumors
Metastatic tumors
Toxic or metabolic processes
Alcohol or drugs
Electrolyte disturbances
Meningitis
Encephalitis
Idiopathic or inherited factors

Classification of Seizures and Epileptic Syndromes

Specific types of epilepsy respond differentially to individual agents; thus, it is important to make a definitive diagnosis in order to choose a medication most likely to be effective. For example, valproic acid is more effective for generalized seizures than for partial seizures. Ethosuximide is effective for treatment for typical absence seizures but ineffective for other seizure types. For each seizure or epilepsy type, there are usually several medications from which to choose. Therefore, the side effects of the different agents will influence the choice of a final medication. *Principle: When several medications of equal efficacy are available, other features such as side effects and dosing schedules should be considered.*

Classification of Seizures. Seizures have been classified in a variety of ways. Currently, the International League Against Epilepsy classifies seizures into two general categories: partial (focal) or generalized (Commission on Classification and Terminology of the International League Against Epilepsy, 1981) (Table 12-7). Partial seizures arise from a specific abnormal location in the brain—usually an area damaged by a known pathologic condition (e.g., trauma, tumor, infarct, or hemorrhage). Electroencephalography

Table 12-7. CLASSIFICATION OF SEIZURES

Partial (Focal, Local) Seizures
  Simple partial (no impairment of consciousness)
  Complex partial (consciousness impaired)
  Secondarily generalized
Generalized Seizures
  Tonic-clonic
  Absence
  Atypical absence
  Myoclonic
  Atonic
  Clonic
  Tonic

(EEG) of patients with partial seizures often reveals a localized abnormality overlying the seizure focus. Partial seizures may be classified as either simple or complex. In simple partial seizures, consciousness is preserved during the entire event. For example, a seizure consisting only of clonic contractions of the arm without disturbance of consciousness would be classified as a simple partial motor seizure.

The defining feature of complex partial seizures is impaired consciousness during the ictal event. These seizures arise most commonly from the temporal lobe and are often associated with unusual symptoms such as hallucinations and "psychic phenomena." Both simple and complex partial seizures may spread to involve both hemispheres of the brain and become "secondarily generalized" with convulsions of all extremities and loss of consciousness.

In generalized seizures, epileptic activity is initiated simultaneously in both hemispheres. Generally, consciousness is lost or impaired and motor manifestations are bilateral. Frequently, no pathologic process is discovered in patients with generalized seizures, suggesting a hereditary cause. Electroencephalographic abnormalities are typically bilateral and generalized. A variety of subtypes of generalized seizures occur, ranging from absence seizures (manifested by only brief impairment of consciousness) to generalized tonic-clonic seizures (with convulsions and loss of consciousness). These different seizure types are outlined in Table 12-7.

Classification of Epileptic Syndromes. In addition to determining what type of seizures a patient has had, it is important to investigate the underlying cause of the seizures. More effective therapeutic decisions can be made if the cause is identified. The term *epileptic syndrome* refers to the classification of an epileptic disorder on the basis of important factors such as seizure types, age of onset, EEG findings, and prognosis (Commission on Classification and Terminology of the International League Against Epilepsy, 1989). Recognition of different epileptic syndromes is particularly important for patients with idiopathic or hereditary forms of epilepsy. For example, juvenile myoclonic epilepsy is an inherited disorder in which patients typically develop generalized tonic-clonic and myoclonic seizures during adolescence (Delgado-Escueta and Enrile-Bascal, 1984). This syndrome has a characteristic EEG pattern and responds poorly to treatment with phenytoin. Valproic acid is the most effective anticonvulsant for these patients and usually must be continued long term because of a high relapse rate after withdrawal. *Principle: Empirical observations that match disease patterns with their re-*

sponses to specific drugs often must be used in therapeutic decisions. Although therapists would like to know the pathogenesis of all diseases and mechanisms of action of all drugs, we are nowhere close to that level of sophistication. The evaluation of suggestions made on empirical data is equivalent to the evaluation of any other experimental data.

Antiepileptic Drugs

Some secondary seizures respond to correction of the underlying process (e.g., corrections of hypoglycemia, reduction of fever), but in most situations antiepileptic medications are used as the primary treatment option for managing epilepsy. In unusual, refractory cases, other options such as surgery may be appropriate. The primary goal of treatment is to control seizures while minimizing drug-related side effects and patient inconvenience. Usually, both goals can be accomplished by choosing a single antiepileptic drug and carefully escalating the dose to obtain seizure control. If significant toxicity is encountered, the dose may need to be reduced and subsequently increased more slowly, or an alternative medication may be necessary.

Over the past several years, it has become clear that, whenever possible, epilepsy should be treated with one medication (*monotherapy*) rather than with multiple medications (*polytherapy*). Patients receiving monotherapy tend to experience fewer side effects, fewer drug interactions, lower medication costs, and usually better compliance (Wilder and Rangel, 1988). In addition, numerous studies have shown that the majority of patients actually have better seizure control with monotherapy than with polytherapy (Wilder, 1987). If it becomes clear that the patient cannot be controlled by a single drug, then combination therapy can be instituted. When choosing a drug combination, it is useful to begin by selecting agents that have different mechanisms of action (see below). *Principle: For many diseases, monotherapy is preferable if satisfactory end points for efficacy can be achieved.*

Although a large variety of anticonvulsants are available for clinical use, the majority of patients with epilepsy can be well controlled by using one of the medications shown in Table 12–8.

Mechanism of Action of Antiepileptic Drugs.

The mechanism of action of anticonvulsant drugs is a complex and incompletely understood topic that is beyond the scope of this chapter. These medications produce a wide array of complex neurophysiologic and neurochemical effects. The relationship between these effects and their anticonvulsant properties is often not clear.

Table 12–8. COMMONLY PRESCRIBED ANTIEPILEPTIC DRUGS

DRUG	TRADE NAME	DOSAGE
Phenytoin	Dilantin	300–400 mg qd
Carbamazepine	Tegretol	200–400 mg t.i.d.
Phenobarbital	—	90–120 mg qd
Valproic acid	Depakote	250–500 mg t.i.d.
Ethosuximide	Zarontin	250–500 mg t.i.d.
Clonazepam	Klonopin	1–5 mg t.i.d.

Major mechanisms of action appear to relate to modification of ionic conductances in neuronal membranes, particularly those of sodium and calcium (Ferrendelli, 1987). Phenytoin and carbamazepine appear to have many similarities in their mechanisms of action. Both inhibit sustained, high-frequency, repetitive neuronal firing (Macdonald and McLean, 1986). Barbiturates, benzodiazepines, and valproic acid all influence gamma-aminobutyric acid (GABA)-mediated synaptic inhibition (Macdonald and McLean, 1986). Ethosuximide appears to inhibit thalamic low-threshold calcium current, which may influence rhythmic thalamic activity (Coulter et al., 1989).

Phenytoin. Phenytoin is the most thoroughly studied anticonvulsant drug in our therapeutic arsenal. It was first synthesized in 1908, but its anticonvulsant properties were not noted until many years later. In contrast to previous experience with phenobarbital, phenytoin demonstrated antiseizure efficacy with minimal sedation. The concept that antiseizure and sedative effects of a drug were not invariably linked represented a significant advance in therapy and appreciation of pathogenesis of the disease. Many compounds containing the heterocyclic hydantoin ring are anticonvulsants (see Fig. 12–3). Of these, phenytoin is the most widely used.

Phenytoin is effective for partial seizures and for most generalized tonic-clonic seizures. Phenytoin is usually administered orally. Oral bioavailability varies significantly between individuals and is altered by a variety of factors including pregnancy, concomitant antacids, manufacturer, liquid versus solid preparation, rapid- versus sustained-release formulation, and so forth. Therefore, patients should not be switched between different formulations.

The IV formulation is delivered with a saline solution because it may precipitate in 5% glucose. The rate of infusion should not exceed 50 mg/min, because both the drug and its vehicle are capable of inducing hypotension if administered too quickly. Phenytoin is approximately 90% protein-bound and is metabolized in the liver to a parahydroxylated metabolite by the cytochrome

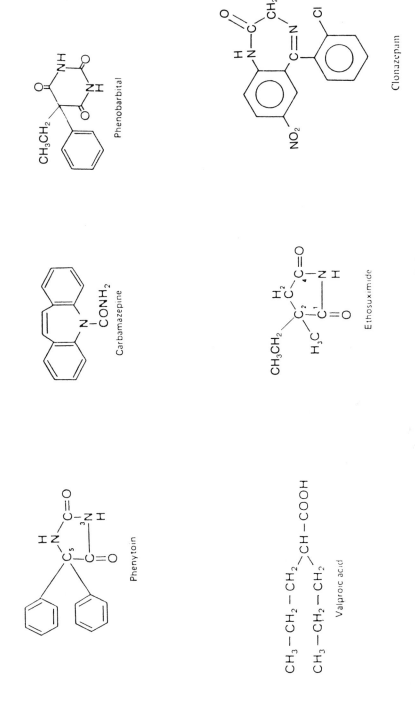

Fig. 12–3. Anticonvulsant agents.

Phenobarbital

Clonazepam

Carbamazepine

Ethosuximide

Phenytoin

Valproic acid

p450 system (Kutt and Verebely, 1970). Less than 5% is excreted unchanged in the urine. In patients with advanced renal failure, protein binding is decreased, leading to higher free fractions (% unbound) of phenytoin. Therefore, lower total serum concentrations are acceptable, and even desirable, in uremic patients because the free concentration of the drug is greater than in patients with normal renal function (see chapter 11).

The pharmacokinetics of phenytoin are different from those of other commonly used anticonvulsants and must be understood in order to achieve proper plasma concentrations. Phenytoin clearance becomes nonlinear (i.e., its rate of metabolism becomes constant) at serum concentrations in the low therapeutic range (approximately 10 mg/l) (Richens, 1975). Therefore, above this serum concentration, small increases in dose may lead to large increases in serum concentration. Because of this, intoxication with phenytoin is more common than with the other anticonvulsants. Significant toxicity can usually be avoided by increasing the dose in small increments once the low therapeutic range is reached and waiting for 2 weeks to evaluate the full effects of that dosage change. *Principle: Understanding a drug's detailed pharmacokinetics, especially when they are atypical, is essential in order to prescribe the drug rationally.*

Excessive serum concentrations of phenytoin produce a variety of unwanted effects, including ataxia, dizziness, diplopia, nausea, and drowsiness. Horizontal nystagmus on lateral gaze is often seen even when plasma concentrations are in the therapeutic range (10–20 mg/l). Chronic use of phenytoin may produce a variety of adverse effects including gingival hyperplasia, hirsutism, nausea, and coarsening of facial features. Chronic metabolic effects can include folate deficiency and effects on vitamin D and calcium metabolism. Other concerns during chronic therapy with phenytoin include an association with cerebellar atrophy and a rare association with lymphoma or "pseudolymphoma" and bone marrow depression (Reynolds, 1975). Some of the many reported drug interactions that can occur when phenytoin is prescribed will be described later in this chapter.

Carbamazepine. While carbamazepine was approved in the early 1960s for the treatment of trigeminal neuralgia, it is better known as an excellent antiseizure medication. Carbamazepine is a tricyclic dibenzepine derivative similar in structure to the tricyclic antidepressants. Like phenytoin, carbamazepine is most effective for partial and generalized tonic-clonic seizures.

Because of its poor water solubility, parenteral formulations of carbamazepine are not available.

Solubility can be improved by taking the drug with meals. While absorption following an oral dose is prompt, oral bioavailability is variable (average 70%). Peak plasma levels are typically achieved 4 to 6 hours after an oral dose. Carbamazepine is less strongly bound to plasma proteins than phenytoin (approximately 75% bound) and is primarily metabolized by the liver. Less than 1% of a dose is excreted unchanged in the urine. The main metabolite is carbamazepine 10,11-epoxide, which may contribute to carbamazepine-related adverse effects. Other anticonvulsants that influence liver enzymes may lead to an increased epoxide/carbamazepine ratio (Altafullah et al., 1989). Therefore, higher concentrations of carbamazepine may be better tolerated in patients being treated with monotherapy. Because drowsiness and nausea are usually most significant during peak serum concentrations, it is often beneficial to give the largest carbamazepine dose at bedtime. A controlled-release formulation of carbamazepine that produces less rapid charges in serum concentrations is being evaluated (Larkin et al., 1989).

When prescribing carbamazepine, the physician must be aware of its tendency to induce its own metabolism (time-dependent kinetics) (Patel et al., 1978). During the first few weeks of therapy, the metabolism of carbamazepine increases significantly, resulting in up to a 50% reduction in carbamazepine half-life. Therefore, patients who are "stabilized" in the therapeutic range during the first week or two of treatment often have subtherapeutic plasma concentrations by week 4. Measurement of serum levels and appropriate dose adjustments are usually required during the first few months of treatment.

Advantages of carbamazepine include its minimal effects on cognitive function (Trimble, 1987) and the absence of gingival hyperplasia and hirsutism. Disadvantages of this drug include the lack of a parenteral formulation, and its short half-life that necessitates at least twice-a-day dosing. There has been significant concern about serious bone marrow toxicity associated with carbamazepine. However, a careful review of reported carbamazepine-associated hematologic abnormalities indicated that the incidence of fatal aplastic anemia or agranulocytosis in patients receiving carbamazepine is only 2.2/million patients (Pellock, 1987). This rate of hematologic fatalities appears to be considerably less that of many other commonly used medications such as phenothiazines, which have been found to have an incidence of agranulocytosis of 1/1300 (Vincent, 1986). The risk of significant bone marrow toxicity from phenytoin and most other anticonvulsants is not well established.

Carbamazepine dose-related adverse effects in-

clude drowsiness, nausea, dizziness, ataxia, diplopia, and blurred vision. Hyponatremia and decreased plasma osmolality are an occasional side
effect of carbamazepine, particularly when high
doses are used in elderly individuals. This effect
appears to be mediated by excessive secretion of
antidiuretic hormone and can usually be managed
by mild water restriction or dose reduction. If
necessary, the addition of phenytoin or demeclocycline is also effective (Ringel and Brick, 1986).
Carbamazepine may exacerbate certain seizure
types including atonic, myoclonic, and atypical
absence seizures (Pellock, 1987).

Other uses for this drug include treatment of
chronic pain syndromes and treatment of pain
associated with trigeminal neuralgia.

Phenobarbital. Phenobarbital has been used
as an anticonvulsant since the early 1900s and is
still widely used despite its high incidence of sedative and behavioral side effects. Phenobarbital is
effective for partial and generalized tonic-clonic
seizures.

Phenobarbital is well absorbed whether it is
administered orally, IM, or IV. However, peak
serum levels may not be obtained for 18 hours
after oral administration of large doses. Phenobarbital is less bound to plasma proteins (about
50% bound) than most other anticonvulsants, so
alterations in serum protein binding do not significantly interfere with its distribution or therapeutic effects. Its half-life (70–100 hours) is longer
than that of other anticonvulsants, which allows
once daily dosing and affords prolonged protection for patients with poor compliance. However,
because of the long half-life, steady state may not
be reached for several weeks after dose adjustment.

Phenobarbital is predominantly cleared by hepatic metabolism; conjugated metabolites are excreted by the kidney. Only about 25% of the drug
is excreted unchanged in the urine. However, the
renal clearance of phenobarbital is altered by
changes in urinary pH. As urinary pH increases,
phenobarbital (a weak acid) becomes more highly
ionized and is less well reabsorbed from the kidney. Therefore, alkalinization of the urine increases renal excretion and can be used to treat
phenobarbital overdose.

Extensive clinical experience has shown phenobarbital to be a safe medication with few serious
adverse effects. The most frequent side effect is
a morbilliform rash that often resolves without
discontinuation of the medication. Severe dermatologic reactions, bone marrow depression, or
hepatitis rarely may occur. The most common
reasons for discontinuation of the medication are
sedation in adults and a variety of adverse cognitive effects in children, including hyperactivity

and impaired performance on neuropsychological
tests (Trimble, 1987).

Valproic Acid. Valproic acid is a branched-
chain carboxylic acid that was originally used as a
solvent. The anticonvulsant properties of valproic
acid were discovered serendipitously in the early
1960s when it was being used as a solvent for other
potential anticonvulsant compounds. Valproic
acid is very effective for virtually all types of
generalized seizures including generalized tonic-
clonic, absence, and myoclonic seizures. Recently, its effectiveness has also been documented
in patients with partial seizures—particularly *secondarily generalized* seizures (Penry and Dean,
1988).

As with carbamazepine, no parenteral formulation of valproic acid is available. Valproic acid
is most commonly administered orally as an
enteric-coated compound with sodium valproate
to provide good GI tolerance (Wilder, 1983). This
formulation is well tolerated; however, its absorption may be significantly delayed if taken with
food (Fischer, 1988). Although frequent dosing is
often recommended because of the short serum
half-life, recent studies have indicated that adequate seizure control can be achieved with dosing
every 12 or even every 24 hours (Covanis and
Jeavons, 1980; Gjerloff, 1984). *Principle: The
half-life of a drug in serum may not correlate with
the drug's pharmacodynamic half-life.* Valproic
acid has a small volume of distribution and is
highly bound to plasma proteins (about 90%
bound). At high serum concentrations of valproic
acid, protein binding sites become saturated and
free–valproic acid concentrations increase out of
proportion to the total serum concentrations.

The primary concern surrounding valproic acid
has been the occurrence of fatal hepatic toxicity
associated with the drug. Recent studies by Dreifuss and co-workers have indicated that high-risk
groups for valproic acid–associated hepatic toxicity can be identified in advance (Dreifuss, 1987;
Dreifuss et al., 1989). Patients younger than 2
years of age who are taking multiple anticonvulsants constitute the highest-risk group. Conversely, adults receiving valproate monotherapy
appear to be at minimal risk. The increased risk
associated with polytherapy appears to be related
to an increased production of hepatotoxic metabolites of valproic acid when other liver enzyme-
inducing anticonvulsants are also being used.
Since the recognition of these patient groups at
different risk, the incidence of valproate-related
hepatic fatalities has decreased significantly despite an overall increase in valproic acid usage
(Dreifuss et al., 1989).

Other valproic acid–related side effects include
nausea, tremor, weight gain, and alopecia. Val-

proic acid is highly protein-bound at therapeutic concentrations and has an inhibitory effect on hepatic drug-metabolizing enzymes. These factors lead to a number of drug interactions (see below). Advantages of valproic acid include minimal sedative effects and little evidence of adverse cognitive effects (Vining, 1987).

Ethosuximide. Ethosuximide is the most common succinimide derivative used as an anticonvulsant. It is the product of a deliberate search to find less toxic alternatives for treatment of clinical absence seizures. Ethosuximide is effective only for seizures of this type.

After slow and variable absorption, the drug is not appreciably bound to plasma proteins. About 20% of the drug is eliminated unchanged in the urine; the rest of it undergoes hepatic biotransformation. The drug has a relatively long half-life of elimination (about 60 hours) but usually is given in divided dosage to avoid gastric irritation. Toxicity is usually mild, with gastric distress being the most common side effect. This can generally be avoided by starting therapy at a low dose and then gradually increasing the dose until therapeutic concentrations are achieved. Drug interactions are rarely a problem.

Benzodiazepines. Diazepam, clonazepam, and lorazepam are the most commonly used benzodiazepines for controlling seizures. Diazepam and lorazepam are available in IV formulations and are rapidly distributed to the CNS. These medications frequently are used for acute treatment of status epilepticus. When used in this setting, both drugs are given rapidly via the IV route as a loading dose. The most important acute toxicity is respiratory depression. The antiseizure effects last only 15 to 60 minutes because of rapid redistribution of the drug. The half-life of elimination is much longer for both drugs. Because of this kinetic profile and the ability of sustained concentrations in plasma to produce daytime somnolence, these drugs have not been drugs of choice for chronic control of seizures. *Principle: Both the pharmacokinetic and the pharmacodynamic properties of a drug help determine how the drug can be used to maximize efficacy and minimize toxicity.*

Oral clonazepam is often effective for generalized seizures, particularly myoclonic seizures (Nanda, 1977). Use of this agent is often limited by side effects, primarily sedation. The clinical pharmacology and pharmacokinetics of the benzodiazepines are discussed in chapters 13 and 27.

Optimal Use of Antiepileptic Drugs

Antiepileptic drugs exhibit a number of complex drug interactions that are often clinically important. In addition, they typically have a narrow therapeutic index. Therefore, optimal use of these agents requires a detailed understanding of their pharmacologic properties.

Antiepileptic Drug Interactions. Although anticonvulsants are involved in numerous complex drug interactions, many of these can be predicted by understanding how these agents influence hepatic drug-metabolizing enzymes. In general, phenobarbital, phenytoin, and carbamazepine induce liver enzyme activity, while valproic acid inhibits liver enzymes. Therefore, valproic acid tends to slow metabolism of other drugs, leading to higher serum concentrations. For example, if a patient currently taking phenobarbital adds valproic acid, the phenobarbital concentration is likely to increase, often to the point of toxicity (Bourgeois, 1988). Therefore, it is usually necessary to reduce the phenobarbital dose, often by as much as 50%, when valproic acid is added.

Conversely, because of their enzyme-inducing effects, phenobarbital, carbamazepine, or phenytoin often reduce the plasma concentrations of other anticonvulsant drugs. For example, enzyme-inducing anticonvulsants may increase the metabolism of estrogens in birth control pills and lead to contraceptive failure (Mattson, 1986).

Other medications can also alter anticonvulsant-drug metabolism. For example, erythromycin, propoxyphene, cimetidine, and isoniazid can all inhibit hepatic metabolism of carbamazepine, leading to increased plasma concentrations and toxicity (Pippenger, 1987).

Other types of drug interactions also occur with antiepileptic drugs. Since most anticonvulsants are highly protein-bound, they can displace other protein-bound drugs. Valproic acid can displace carbamazepine or phenytoin from plasma proteins, leading to transient elevations in free-drug concentrations that may cause toxicity. Sometimes this problem can be avoided by scheduling drug-dosing times so that levels of highly protein-bound agents do not peak simultaneously. Other protein-bound drugs such as aspirin can displace anticonvulsants from protein binding sites and produce toxicity (Paxton, 1980; Goulden et al., 1987). The interactions mentioned above are among those most likely to occur and to be clinically significant. Additional interactions have been reported that occur only occasionally, or that produce minimal clinical impact. Some interactions occur in only a small percentage of patients. *Principle: Knowledge of drug–drug interactions helps the prescriber maximize the chances of a successful course of therapy. However, a known interaction will not necessarily occur in all patients receiving both agents, nor is it certain that an interaction will not occur if it has not been previously reported. Also, by modifying drug doses, it may be possible to avoid adverse effects from kinetic interactions* (also see chapters 38 and 40).

Initiation of Treatment. Not all patients who have seizures require treatment with antiepileptic medications. The decision to initiate antiepileptic therapy is based on a variety of factors including the type of seizure, underlying cause and precipitating factors, and social and environmental factors. If a "reversible" cause such as a toxic or metabolic disturbance (e.g., hypoglycemia) is identified, it may be corrected and antiepileptic therapy averted. Even if no cause for the seizure is discovered, the physician may elect to withhold antiepileptic therapy. For example, a patient with a single generalized tonic-clonic seizure and a normal neurologic evaluation is generally felt to have less than a 50% chance of having a second seizure (Hauser et al., 1982). In this specific situation, there is no reliable evidence that anticonvulsant therapy alters the risk of recurrence; therefore, the side effects and inconvenience associated with long-term antiepileptic therapy may not be justifiable. However, if the patient must operate a motor vehicle or dangerous machinery, then potential benefits of treatment may outweigh potential risks.

If the decision is made to initiate therapy, pharmacologic features of the agent chosen must be considered from the onset. When anticonvulsants are administered during an urgent or emergency situation with the patient actively seizing, an IV loading dose of diazepam or lorazepam is required to achieve prompt effect. The 15 to 60 minutes of control that this produces allows the physician to initiate the more gradual process of loading the patient with a longer-acting and less promptly effective drug such as phenytoin or phenobarbital.

Phenytoin can be loaded either IV or orally and is usually well tolerated. The typical loading dose required for an adult is 18 mg/kg. The rate of administration should not exceed 50 mg/min because of the risk of hypotension or cardiac arrhythmias (Cranford et al., 1978). Phenobarbital loading can be accomplished orally, IM, or IV; however, significant sedation will result. Loading doses of carbamazepine and valproic acid usually are not well tolerated because of GI and other side effects, making them poor choices in urgent situations. Initiation of therapy with these agents usually must be done slowly and occasionally requires several weeks of gradual dose escalation to achieve therapeutic effects without encountering significant adverse effects.

Target Concentrations. Obtaining plasma anticonvulsant concentrations is often very helpful when managing epileptic patients. The timing of the concentration in relation to dose is important, especially for drugs with short half-lives. Random concentrations are often misleading and can lead to therapeutic errors (Troupin, 1984). Trough concentrations are ideal and are usually most conveniently obtained prior to the morning dose.

Many misconceptions exist regarding how to interpret anticonvulsant concentrations. The therapeutic range represents a guide but should not be taken as an absolute when dealing with individual patients. Many patients will obtain complete seizure control without side effects at serum concentrations significantly above the upper limit of the "therapeutic range" (Lesser et al., 1984). Similarly, "subtherapeutic" concentrations may provide adequate seizure control for other patients.

In general, serum concentrations of drugs should not be measured until the patient has reached the steady state. If the concentrations are measured prior to this, results must be interpreted with caution, and a follow-up concentration should be obtained after reaching the steady state. Serum concentrations may be particularly helpful immediately following a seizure to help document compliance and to facilitate decisions about dose changes. Plasma concentrations are also useful when a patient complains of a potentially dose-related side effect.

The discussion above has appropriately focused on the pharmacokinetic and pharmacodynamic properties of antiseizure drugs that help determine how they can be optimally prescribed. However, it is important not to lose sight of another point. *Principle: In the management of the patient with epilepsy, the physician's responsibility is far from over after he or she gives the patient an appropriate drug. The drug must be used in a way that maximizes the chances for success and minimizes the chances for toxicity or an unexpected drug interaction. The physician must help educate the patient with respect to behaviors that might lessen control of the seizures, including poor compliance. This approach to the alliance with the patient is equally important in treating patients with epilepsy, hypertension, angina, and so forth.*

CEREBRAL VASCULAR DISEASE

Cerebral vascular disease is a major cause of death and disability throughout the world. It is the third most common cause of death in the United States. The major consequence of cerebrovascular disease is stroke.

Clinical Aspects of Stroke

To ensure optimal clinical management of an acute stroke, the underlying pathophysiologic process must be understood. The term *stroke* refers to the neurologic damage resulting from an acute impairment of cerebral blood flow caused by vascular occlusion or hemorrhage. The most common modes of vascular occlusion are thrombosis and embolism. Stroke is a heterogeneous disease with numerous causes and a wide spectrum of clinical outcomes. In stroke caused by vascular occlusion, brain tissue is infarcted as a result of local ischemia. In cerebral hemorrhage, damage results both from ischemia and the adverse effects of intracerebral blood.

Cerebrovascular Terminology. Cerebrovascular terminology can be confusing. The term *cerebral vascular accident* (CVA) is an imprecise term that is frequently used as a synonym for stroke. A transient ischemic attack (TIA) is defined as a brief, reversible episode of neurologic dysfunction caused by transient cerebral ischemia. Most TIAs last less than 1 hour and leave the patient without residual neurologic deficit. However, TIAs are an important warning sign, indicating a high risk for subsequent stroke. Patients who experience a TIA have a subsequent stroke risk of about 5%/year (Barnett, 1980).

Stroke in evolution implies acute, progressive neurologic deterioration from a stroke. Although a number of factors can contribute to poststroke deterioration, the term *stroke in evolution* generally implies progressive, ongoing, vascular occlusion. A *lacune* is a tiny infarct (usually less than 5 mm) typically located deep within the brain and usually attributed to atheromatous occlusion of deep penetrating branches (Fisher, 1969).

Risk Factors. Hypertension is by far the most important and most treatable risk factor for stroke. Other major risk factors include heart disease, diabetes mellitus, smoking, and oral contraceptive use. Cardiac diseases that may cause embolic stroke include chronic or intermittent arrhythmias, acute myocardial infarction (MI), cardiomyopathy, valvular heart disease, and endocarditis.

Clinical Presentation. Classically, the clinical presentation of an acute stroke is that of an abrupt onset of a focal neurologic deficit. Because vascular occlusion or hemorrhage generally produces an immediate deficit, the hallmark of stroke is the acute onset of the disability. The particular clinical features of the neurologic deficit depend upon the location of the vascular lesion. For example, an embolus from the heart may lodge in the left middle cerebral artery and present with language dysfunction and sensory or motor loss on the right side of the body. Alternatively, an atherosclerotic occlusion of the poste-

rior cerebral artery will cause a stroke in the occipital lobe and produce partial visual loss.

Diagnostic Evaluation. The most common cause of stroke is arterial obstruction secondary to atherosclerosis. However, a number of diverse pathologic entities may cause stroke. Many of these conditions are listed in Table 12–9. Because of the wide range of causative factors and associated conditions, it is important to establish the cause of a stroke prior to making treatment decisions. Because some of the primary conditions leading to stroke require specific therapy in and of themselves (e.g., antibiotics for endocarditis), rational treatment demands that diagnosis of underlying conditions be made if at all possible.

One of the first steps in evaluating a stroke patient is to image the brain with computed tomography (CT) or magnetic resonance imaging (MRI). These studies are extremely useful for clarifying the location of the stroke and determining whether or not it is hemorrhagic. Subsequently, stenotic or ulcerated vascular lesions that may lead to stroke can be visualized by carotid ultrasound or cerebral angiography. Sometimes these lesions may be surgically correctable. In addition, blood tests can help document coagulation disorders or systemic illnesses that can predispose to stroke. Echocardiography can be used to visualize a potential cardiac source of embolic material.

Management of Acute Stroke

Therapy for stroke can be divided into preventive measures and acute interventions. Attempts to develop effective therapies for acute stroke have typically focused on increasing blood flow to the ischemic area or on improving the intrinsic ability of brain parenchyma to withstand ische-

Table 12–9. COMMON CAUSES OF STROKE

Vascular Occlusion
  Atherosclerosis
  Vasculitis
  Drugs (oral contraceptives, cocaine)
  Hypercoagulable states
  Arterial dissection
Embolism
  Ulcerative carotid lesions
  Atrial fibrillation
  Acute myocardial infarction
  Ventricular aneurysm
  Rheumatic heart disease
  Prosthetic cardiac valves
Hemorrhage
  Aneurysm
  Arteriovenous malformation
  Hypertension

mia. Numerous therapeutic agents have been tested in the setting of acute stroke, but none has been shown to be clearly beneficial. *Principle: The frustration of not being able to "do anything" to treat a disease should not result in the irrational prescribing just to "do something." When efficacy cannot be expected, only toxicity can.*

Previous Unsuccessful Drug Trials. Barbiturates have been shown to improve neuronal tolerance to ischemia in various animal models of stroke. Unfortunately, clinical trials with barbiturates have been discouraging (Yatsu, 1983). One recent study demonstrated fewer neuropsychological complications in patients undergoing cardiac bypass surgery who were treated with high doses of barbiturates during the operation (Nussmeier et al., 1986). Neuropsychological dysfunction following bypass surgery is common and appears to be related to cerebral ischemia secondary to bypass-related embolization.

It was thought that corticosteroids might reduce morbidity from stroke by a variety of mechanisms, including reducing edema, inhibiting lysosomal enzymes, or reducing the production of free radicals (Hass et al., 1989). However, several randomized clinical trials have failed to reveal any clinical benefit of corticosteroids. In fact, some studies suggest that stroke patients treated with steroids had worse outcomes (Hass et al., 1989).

Increases in cerebral blood flow can be achieved by lowering the hematocrit and blood viscosity through hemodilution. A variety of therapeutic agents and techniques can produce hemodilution, including infusions of low-molecular-weight dextran or hetastarch (see chapter 26). Multicenter trials with these techniques have been performed, but the results have so far been unimpressive.

New Treatment Strategies for Stroke. Despite the poor results obtained in trials of previous agents, effective therapeutic drugs may soon be available. Several new classes of potentially neuroprotective agents, including *N*-methyl-D-aspartate antagonists, have shown promising results in animal models of stroke (Albers et al., 1989a). Furthermore, calcium-channel blockers potentially offer both improved perfusion to ischemic areas and direct neuroprotective effects. Encouraging results from clinical trials using nimodipine have already been reported (Gelmers et al., 1988). In addition, fibrinolytic agents that are capable of reopening recently thrombosed vessels are currently under clinical investigation (Hass et al., 1989). However, fibrinolytic therapy may prove to be less effective in cerebral thrombosis than in cardiac thrombosis because of the increased risk of brain hemorrhage.

Prophylactic Treatments for Stroke

Although pharmacologic options for treatment of acute stroke are limited, several drugs have proven ability to reduce the risk of stroke in selected patient populations.

Anticoagulation. For patients with certain cardiac disorders, anticoagulant therapy can reduce risk of stroke. The subgroups of cardiac patients that benefit from anticoagulation are not firmly established, but it appears that cardiac conditions that carry a 5%/year or greater risk of embolization are likely to benefit from anticoagulant therapy. These subgroups include atrial fibrillation associated with any of the following conditions: previous embolization, valvular disease (either rheumatic or prosthetic), congestive heart failure, recent MI, sick sinus syndrome, cardiomyopathy, or thyrotoxicosis (Halperin and Hart, 1988; Dunn et al., 1989; Stein et al., 1989; Stratton, 1989; Petersen, 1990). Benefit of anticoagulation in patients with nonvalvular atrial fibrillation has also been demonstrated in two large prospective randomized trials (Petersen et al., 1989; Stroke Prevention in Atrial Fibrillation Study Group Investigators, 1990). Anticoagulation may *not* be indicated in patients with lone atrial fibrillation who are younger than 60 years of age (Kopecky et al., 1987; Cerebral Embolism Task Force, 1989), but results may depend upon the degree of anticoagulation obtained. Other cardiac conditions in which anticoagulation appears to be indicated include recent anterior MI (especially if a new left ventricular thrombus is detected), rheumatic mitral valve disease with an enlarged left atrium, mechanical prosthetic valves, and cardiomyopathy (Cerebral Embolism Task Force, 1989). In addition, anticoagulation is recommended for secondary prevention of stroke in some subgroups of patients who present with a cardioembolic stroke (Yatsu et al., 1988). Several large, randomized clinical trials are in progress to help clarify the role of prophylactic anticoagulation in patients with previous cardioembolic stroke. Oral anticoagulation with warfarin (Coumadin) reduces stroke risk by about 60% in patients with cardioembolic sources (Cerebral Embolism Task Force, 1989). However, the decision to anticoagulate such patients is difficult because of the risk of hemorrhage. Over the last decade, it has become evident that the risk/benefit ratio may be improved by targeting less intense levels of anticoagulation than were previously employed. *Principle: Choosing an optimal target for drug therapy is also important when the end point is a physiologic effect rather than a concentration of drug in plasma (a surrogate end point).*

The mechanism of action of warfarin involves inhibition of the hepatic synthesis of vitamin K–dependent clotting factors. The prothrombin time (PT) is the most common method of monitoring the intensity of oral anticoagulant therapy. This laboratory test can quantify the reduction in circulating vitamin K–dependent coagulation factors. Reduction in vitamin K–dependent factors by warfarin leads to a prolongation of the PT. There has been controversy concerning the optimal intensity of anticoagulation. In the laboratory, the PT test is performed by adding calcium and a thromboplastin to citrated plasma. The more responsive the thromboplastin, the larger the prolongation of the PT ratio by warfarin. In the l950s, the recommended therapeutic range for oral anticoagulation was established to be prolongation of the PT by a factor of 2.0 to 2.5. This recommendation was based on the use of a more responsive thromboplastin than is used today in most North American laboratories. But when less responsive thromboplastins began to be employed, the recommended range for anticoagulation intensity was not adjusted accordingly (Hirsh et al., 1989). This oversight has led to significant overanticoagulation of patients and an increased incidence of bleeding complications from oral anticoagulant therapy. Numerous recent studies have shown that a less intense level of anticoagulation (PT ratio of 1.2–1.5) provides equivalent protection from embolic stroke with significantly less risk of hemorrhage (Hirsh et al., 1989). *Principle: Excessive drug effect frequently increases side effects without increasing therapeutic efficacy.*

The role of anticoagulants for stroke prevention in patients with previous TIAs has been controversial. It has been suggested that anticoagulants may be effective in patients with stenotic lesions of large blood vessels where slow flow is likely to produce thrombus formation (Caplan, 1986). However, a recent meta-analysis of studies evaluating the role of anticoagulation in patients with TIAs failed to establish any benefit of anticoagulation in stroke prophylaxis (Jonas, 1988). Unfortunately, the majority of these studies do not meet currently accepted criteria for adequate clinical trials, leaving the role of anticoagulants in this setting unresolved. Since both platelets and clotting factors are involved in thrombosis, ongoing studies are evaluating the efficacy of combined therapy with low-intensity anticoagulation and antiplatelet agents.

Antiplatelet Agents. A number of large, well-controlled studies have examined the role of antiplatelet agents in reducing stroke incidence in patients with previous TIAs or minor stroke.

Antiplatelet agents may reduce the formation of platelet aggregates, thereby decreasing the risk of vascular occlusion. Irregular vascular surfaces such as ulcerated carotid plaques are thought to be particularly likely to induce platelet aggregation. Platelet aggregates may also embolize distally and contribute to vessel occlusion.

Aspirin is the best-studied antiplatelet agent for stroke prevention. Substantial evidence exists that aspirin therapy reduces stroke risk by about 25% (Sherman et al., 1989). The major antithrombotic effects of aspirin are thought to be mediated by its irreversible inhibition of the enzyme cyclooxygenase. In platelets, cyclooxygenase is responsible for converting arachidonic acid to thromboxane A_2, and in vascular endothelium cyclooxygenase leads to the production of prostacyclin. Prostacyclin prevents platelet aggregation and causes vasodilation, and thromboxane A_2 induces platelet aggregation and vasoconstriction.

The optimal dose of aspirin for stroke prophylaxis has been a matter of disagreement. Some in vitro studies have shown that low doses of aspirin (approximately 40 mg/day) may inhibit thromboxane A_2 synthesis without significantly altering prostacyclin production (Hirsh et al., 1989). This observation suggests that low doses of aspirin may be more effective than high doses. However, most clinical trials have been performed with higher doses of aspirin (as much as 1300 mg/day). Currently, there is no clinical evidence that low-dose aspirin is either more or less effective than high-dose aspirin. However, since low doses (80–325 mg/day) produce fewer GI side effects, they are currently preferred by most clinicians (Sherman et al., 1989). *Principle: It is not always true that if a low plasma concentration (or dose) of a drug is good, a higher concentration (or dose) is better. Higher doses may be associated with increased toxicity, and in some situations, decreased efficacy.*

Ticlopidine is a recently developed antiplatelet agent that has been evaluated in two large stroke-prevention trials. In one study, ticlopidine was found to be superior to aspirin for stroke prevention in patients with a history of TIA. Ticlopidine produced a 21% reduction in stroke risk at 3 years compared with aspirin (Hass et al., 1989). Another study demonstrated that patients with a recent history of stroke who took ticlopidine had an approximately 30% reduction in subsequent stroke compared with patients who received a placebo (Gent et al., 1989).

Ticlopidine's antiplatelet effects differ from those of aspirin in that it does not inhibit platelet aggregation induced by arachidonic acid, but it does inhibit aggregation induced by platelet-activating factor or adenosine diphosphate (Uchiyama et al., 1989). These pharmacologic differences provide a rationale for combined treatment with aspirin and ticlopidine.

Although ticlopidine may be more effective than aspirin for stroke prevention, its use may be limited to high-risk patients and aspirin-intolerant patients because of adverse effects. Significant neutropenia occurs in up to 1% of patients, necessitating routine hematologic monitoring. Severe skin rash and diarrhea occur in about 2% of patients. *Principle: When considering prescribing a newly marketed drug, remember two facts: (1) the adverse effects that are discovered during drug development and clinical testing may be more common or more severe during routine clinical use and (2) adverse effects that appear after chronic administration, even if severe, may be recognized only during postmarketing surveillance* (also see chapters 34 and 39).

Dipyridamole (Persantine) is another antiplatelet agent that has been tested in stroke-prevention trials. Its mechanism of action appears to involve inhibition of cyclic AMP phosphodiesterase. There is no clear evidence that dipyridamole, whether used alone or in combination with aspirin, is effective for prevention of stroke in patients with previous TIAs or minor stroke (Bousser et al., 1983; The American-Canadian Co-operative Study Group, 1985). Dipyridamole may help reduce stroke risk in patients with mechanical heart valves (Sullivan et al., 1969; Chesebro et al., 1983).

In summary, aspirin continues to be the primary pharmacologic therapy used to help prevent stroke. Anticoagulation with warfarin is appropriate for stroke prophylaxis in patients with specific cardiac disorders. The role of combined therapy using low-dose anticoagulants and antiplatelet agents is under investigation.

PARKINSONISM

In 1817, Sir James Parkinson wrote the classic paper describing "paralysis agitans" or Parkinson syndrome. The onset of the syndrome usually occurs between 40 and 70 years of age with peak age of onset in the 60th year. Only 1% of cases begin in patients younger than 30 years of age. Parkinson disease occurs in all countries, among all ethnic groups and all socioeconomic classes. The disease afflicts approximately 1 million patients in the United States, or about 1% of the population over the age of 50 years.

Clinical Aspects of Parkinsonism

Parkinsonism refers to a clinical condition that results from dysfunction of the nigrostriatal dopaminergic system due to degenerative, destructive, or pharmacologic processes. Parkinson disease is only one of a diverse group of disorders that causes parkinsonism. Therefore, diagnostic considerations are important prior to making treatment decisions.

Clinical Signs. The classic clinical triad of parkinsonism includes tremor, rigidity, and bradykinesia. Tremor is the most common and often earliest symptom of parkinsonism. The tremor is a coarse 3 to 4 per second "pill rolling" tremor usually involving the thumb and fingers, but it may also involve the jaw, tongue, eyelids, or foot. The tremor typically occurs at rest, and volitional movements usually dampen the tremor momentarily. Although it rarely produces a serious disability, tremor is often the most bothersome symptom to the patient. The tremor increases with stress but disappears during sleep. Electromyography reveals alternating bursts of activity in agonist and antagonist muscles during the tremor.

Patients also exhibit a "lead pipe" rigidity, which is characterized by resistance to passive flexion and extension movements. This rigidity, coupled with the resting tremor, produces the classic "cogwheel" phenomenon (i.e., moves "like a ratchet") that is felt when the patient's extremities are passively moved. The rigidity is usually increased with simultaneous movement of the opposite limb.

The third clinical hallmark of parkinsonism is the bradykinesia that underlies the characteristic paucity of movements. Repetitive movements become increasingly hampered. Patients typically exhibit psychomotor retardation, sitting nearly motionless. In addition, patients often develop a characteristic hand posture that includes straightening of the fingers with adduction and some flexure at the metacarpal–phalangeal joint. Facial expression is blunted, producing "masked" facies. The gait gradually deteriorates, with decreased arm swing as a first sign. Eventually, the gait becomes progressively stooped, with a flexed posture, shuffling steps, and festination. Small steps are taken as the patient leans forward and tries to maintain his or her center of balance.

Differential Diagnosis. The differential diagnosis of parkinsonism is quite large and is summarized in Table 12–10. Parkinson disease, also known as paralysis agitans, is the prototypic form of parkinsonism. This idiopathic disorder results from degeneration of dopamine-containing neurons in the substantia nigra. Unfortunately, the most common cause of parkinsonism is actually iatrogenic: medications that interfere with dopaminergic function.

**Table 12-10. DIFFERENTIAL DIAGNOSIS
OF PARKINSONISM**

Parkinson disease
Drug-induced (neuroleptic)
Postencephalitic (encephalitis lethargica)
Toxins (manganese)
MPTP*
Metabolic (hypoparathyroidism)
Multiple cerebral infarcts
Posthypoxic
Other degenerative neurologic conditions
Progressive supernuclear palsy
Juvenile Huntington chorea
Multiple system atrophies

* MPTP = 1-methyl-4-phenyl-1,2,3,6-tetrahydropyridine.

Neuroleptics such as chlorpromazine and haloperidol, and metoclopramide cause signs of parkinsonism based on their pharmacologic ability to block dopamine receptors. *Principle: The neuroleptic-induced symptoms of a slight "masked" facies, stiffness of the trunk and limbs, lack of arm swing, tremor of the hands, and mumbling speech are often mistaken as Parkinson disease.* Other drugs such as reserpine and α-methyldopa can cause parkinsonism by interfering with dopamine metabolism.

Shortly after World War I (1919–1926), an outbreak of viral encephalitis occurred worldwide (called von Economo encephalitis or encephalitis lethargica) and left its victims with parkinsonism. The interval between infection and development of parkinsonism varied from months to years. Patients suffered from a classic parkinsonian illness accompanied by a variety of additional symptoms including oculogyric crises, convergence paresis, bizarre movements and postures, tics, and psychopathic behavior. No new cases of this specific form of encephalitis have been recorded since 1930. However, it is likely that rare cases of other forms of viral postencephalitic parkinsonism still occur.

Toxins such as manganese and carbon monoxide may sometime cause a parkinsonian syndrome. There is also a Parkinson-dementia syndrome in Guam that appears to be the result of a dietary neurotoxin. Recently, the drug 1-methyl-4-phenyl-1,2,3,6-tetrahydropyridine (MPTP) has been discovered to cause parkinsonism (Calne et al., 1984; Ballard et al., 1985). Chemically, MPTP is a synthetic derivative of meperidine or "street heroin," and was inadvertently synthesized by drug abusers in northern California. It directly destroys dopamine-containing neurons in the substantia nigra and was found to cause irreversible parkinsonian symptoms in young drug abusers in the San Jose area in the summer of 1982. Neurotoxicity is dependent upon the oxidation of MPTP to MPP^+. This conversion is catalyzed by monoamine oxidase B (MAO-B). MPP^+ is then selectively taken up by the dopamine-uptake system and subsequently destroys dopaminergic cells. These findings have led to the development of various animal models of Parkinson disease, which have been used to evaluate novel therapeutic alternatives (see below). *Principle: By causing disease, drugs or xenobiotics may tell us much about pathophysiology, or allow new models of disease to be developed with which to evaluate new therapeutic agents. The discovery of unexpected toxicity of drugs or chemicals may prove useful to the prepared observer.*

Other degenerative neurologic syndromes may present with a parkinsonism-like clinical picture. Such disorders include Shy-Drager syndrome, progressive supranuclear palsy, striatonigral degeneration, olivopontocerebellar degeneration, calcification of the basal ganglia, Alzheimer disease, Huntington chorea (in patients under the age of 20), and Wilson disease (in patients under the age of 40).

Treatment of Parkinson Disease

Principle: The primary treatment strategy for Parkinson disease has focused on restoring the normal balance between dopaminergic and cholinergic neurotransmission within the CNS. This can be achieved, at present, by use of three major classes of pharmacologic agents: anticholinergic drugs, dopamine precursors, and dopamine agonists. The therapeutic options for patients with parkinson disease and other treatable parkinsonian syndromes are summarized in Table 12-11.

Anticholinergic Drugs. Anticholinergic agents have been used for the treatment of parkinsonism since the early 20th century and until the late

**Table 12-11. DRUGS USED TO
TREAT PARKINSONISM**

DRUG	TRADE NAME	DOSE
Anticholinergics		
Benztropine	Cogentin	1–4 mg b.i.d.
Trihexyphenidyl	Artane	5–10 mg t.i.d.
Biperiden	Akineton	2–12 mg t.i.d.
Amantadine	Symmetrel	100 mg b.i.d.
Dopamine Precursors		
Levodopa/ carbidopa	Sinemet	25 mg/100 mg t.i.d.
Levodopa	Larodopa	1500 mg t.i.d.
Dopamine Agonists		
Bromocriptine	Parlodel	5–15 mg t.i.d.
Pergolide	Permax	2–4 mg qd
MAO-B Inhibitor		
Deprenyl (selegiline)	Eldepryl	5 mg b.i.d.

1960s were the only therapeutic agents available. The recent introduction of more effective therapies has limited the indications for anticholinergics in the treatment of parkinsonism. At present, anticholinergics might be considered the drugs of first choice for patients presenting with tremor and/or the earliest stages of parkinsonism (Lang, 1984; Kurlan, 1987). In addition, they are frequently used to counteract parkinsonian symptoms induced by neuroleptic drugs.

The efficacy of anticholinergics in parkinsonism probably results from their ability to antagonize the secondary hypercholinergic state caused by the loss of inhibitory dopaminergic neurons. Since sialorrhea is a common problem in parkinsonism, the usual anticholinergic "side effect" of dry mouth due to inhibition of salivary secretions is actually an advantageous effect of anticholinergics in the treatment of parkinsonism. Other anticholinergic side effects such as mental confusion and urinary retention are more difficult. The drugs are usually given on a b.i.d. or t.i.d. schedule. Available agents include trihexyphenidyl, benztropine, and biperiden. There are no significant pharmacologic differences between these agents.

Amantadine. Amantadine, which was introduced initially as an antiviral agent, unexpectedly was found to have antiparkinsonian properties in the late 1960s (Schwab et al., 1972). Amantadine has been reported to induce the release of dopamine. As a result, amantadine is sometimes used as an adjunctive therapeutic agent in parkinsonian patients since it may enhance the effects of levodopa (see below). Amantadine is rapidly absorbed from the GI tract and is excreted unchanged in the urine. Side effects, if present, are usually mild and include mental confusion, hallucinations, and nightmares. The usual dose is 100 mg b.i.d.

Dopamine Precursors. A major breakthrough in the pharmacotherapy of parkinsonism occurred in the 1960s, with the introduction of levodopa (L-dopa or L-3,4-dihydroxyphenylalanine). Levodopa is unquestionably the most effective agent for the treatment of Parkinson disease. The theoretical basis for the administration of dopamine precursors was the observation that striatal dopamine is depleted in patients suffering with parkinson disease. This depletion is caused by the death of dopamine-containing neurons in the substantia nigra. Levodopa crosses the blood–brain barrier and is metabolized to dopamine by the cytoplasmic enzyme dopa decarboxylase. The use of levodopa has been documented to both increase the quality of life and prolong the average life span of patients with parkinsonism (Fahn and Bressman, 1984; Muenter, 1984; Yahr, 1984).

The use of levodopa is associated with a high incidence of nausea and vomiting, which apparently result from the peripheral conversion of levodopa to dopamine. Levodopa is rapidly absorbed from the small bowel via an active transport system for aromatic amino acids. Peak plasma concentrations are achieved in 0.5 to 2 hours, and the plasma half-life is short (approximately 1–3 hours).

As much as 95% of the absorbed levodopa is rapidly decarboxylated in the periphery to form dopamine. Dopamine itself cannot cross the blood–brain barrier. As a result, less than 1% of orally absorbed levodopa is thought to reach the CNS. In order to achieve higher brain concentrations of levodopa and of dopamine, and to lessen the side effects associated with high peripheral concentrations of dopamine, combination medications have been developed that include both levodopa and a dopamine decarboxylase inhibitor such as carbidopa (Sinemet). This decarboxylase inhibitor does not cross the blood–brain barrier. Therefore, the enzymatic conversion of levodopa to dopamine catalyzed by dopa decarboxylase is inhibited only in the periphery, while enzymatic conversion in the CNS is not impeded. In effect, the combination of levodopa and carbidopa prevents the rapid conversion of levodopa to dopamine in the blood but promotes increased brain concentrations of dopamine using a much lower dose of levodopa. Nonetheless, side effects are still observed with the combination medications and include psychiatric symptoms, nausea, and/or involuntary movements (e.g., dyskinesias and/or choreoathetosis) (Jankovic, 1982). *Principle: A drug's selectivity of action, and even its therapeutic index, may be modulated by using knowledge of the drug's metabolic pathways to design specific inhibitors of biotransformation reactions. Such exploitation of a drug's biotransformation is yet another way in which knowledge of a drug's pharmacokinetic properties is essential to the practice of rational therapeutics. Consider additional examples of this principle, for example, allopurinol and 6-mercaptopurine or azathioprine.*

Direct-Acting Dopamine-Receptor Agonists. A number of ergoline derivatives have been developed that share the ability to directly stimulate postsynaptic dopamine receptors (Calne et al., 1984). Drugs such as bromocriptine and pergolide became available in the United States in the 1980s, and lisuride is available in other countries. These agents, which are readily absorbed and reach peak plasma concentrations in 1 to 2 hours, are used most commonly as adjunctive agents to levodopa-containing compounds. The dosage schedule for bromocriptine is t.i.d. whereas pergolide can be given once a day. The side-effect profile of these drugs is similar to that of levodopa and includes nausea, vomiting, and orthostatic hypotension.

Monoamine Oxidase B Inhibitors. The discovery of MPTP-induced parkinsonism provided an animal model useful for evaluating new treatment strategies for parkinson disease. One hypothesis is that neurotoxic compounds similar to MPTP may occur in the environment. Since activation of MPTP is dependent on the enzyme MAO-B, it is hoped that inhibitors of this enzyme might prevent the progression of Parkinson disease.

In 1989, two studies were completed that had been designed to determine whether treatment with deprenyl (selegiline) would increase the period of time between onset of parkinsonism and need for treatment with levodopa (Tetrud and Langston, 1989; Parkinson Study Group, 1989). The data indicated that the use of deprenyl (Eldepryl) delayed the onset of disability in patients with early, untreated disease. The investigators have suggested three possible interpretations of their data:

1. Deprenyl may have had a subtle but significant effect on the symptoms of parkinsonism. For example, other investigators have demonstrated that metabolism of (−)deprenyl to amphetamine and methamphetamine may be responsible for some of the therapeutic effects of the drug (Karoum et al., 1982).

2. Deprenyl may have intrinsic antidepressant properties or may have produced a more general sense of "well-being" in the study patients (Parkinson Study Group, 1989).

3. Deprenyl may have delayed the progression of parkinsonism, theoretically as a result of its inhibition of MAO-B. The authors conclude that "nothing in our data is inconsistent with this interpretation."

Studies of longer duration, as well as more objective clinical and pathologic data, are needed before the relative importance of each of these three possibilities can be determined. The appropriate clinical role of deprenyl in parkinsonism can be expected to be a major area of research activity in the years ahead.

Other Agents. Dopamine-uptake inhibitors such as mazindol are effective in preventing MPTP toxicity in animals, potentially offering another therapeutic option. Antioxidants such as vitamin E are able to prevent the neuronal damage induced by free radicals, compounds that are known to be created by MPTP administration. Clinical trials with vitamin E have already been initiated in patients with Parkinson disease.

Side Effects of Antiparkinsonian Medications

Dyskinesias. A variety of unusual side effects are associated with antiparkinsonian medications. Dyskinesias, which usually consist of choreiform movements of the head, limbs, and trunk, frequently occur as a result of increased synaptic dopamine concentration. Dyskinesias typically accompany peak levodopa concentrations and usually improve if the dose is reduced. By contrast, dystonias tend to occur more frequently when levodopa concentrations fall.

End-of-Dose or Wearing-off Effect. Frequently the most challenging problem encountered in the management of Parkinson disease is the *wearing-off* effect known as *end-of-dose failure*. This problem typically occurs after many years of antiparkinsonian therapy. Strategies to deal with this problem include decreasing the time between doses, use of sustained-release levodopa, the addition of dopamine agonists, or increasing the amount of carbidopa (Jankovic and Marsden, 1988).

On–Off Phenomenon. A less common and less predictable side effect of levodopa medication is the on–off phenomenon (Nutt et al., 1984; Nutt, 1987). In this condition, patients abruptly develop improvement or exacerbation of their symptoms in a manner that appears unrelated to their daily dose of levodopa. This phenomenon presents therapeutic problems that can be dealt with by dividing the total daily dose into smaller portions administered more frequently or combining direct agonists or anticholinergic drugs in a different ratio. Recently, a number of studies have demonstrated that fluctuations in serum concentrations of dietary amino acids are the likely pathophysiologic basis for the on–off phenomenon (Eriksson et al., 1988; Carter et al., 1989). Indeed, reducing the amount of dietary protein improves the effectiveness of levodopa therapy (Tsui et al., 1989; Carter et al., 1989). Future data may yield an "optimized" dietary plan for certain parkinsonian patients who suffer clinically as a result of the on–off phenomenon. *Principle: Interactions between dietary components and drugs are frequent and can alter a drug's efficacy or toxicity. Such drug–nutrient interactions are becoming recognized more frequently* (see chapters 10, 39, and 40).

New Treatment Strategies

In the mid-20th century, investigators developed surgical therapies that involved stereotaxic placement of destructive lesions in the central nuclei of the globus pallidus or ventral thalamus contralateral to the side of the body chiefly affected. This technique was used in refractory asymmetric disease and had only limited success.

More recently, a new surgical approach has been developed, involving autologous transplantation of adrenal tissue to the basal ganglia (Backlund et al., 1985). Although initial clinical reports were strikingly positive (Madrazo et al., 1987), more recent data suggest a much less significant beneficial effect of the procedure (Allen et al., 1989). Future studies are needed to determine what, if any, role this procedure will play in the management of parkinsonism.

DRUG-INDUCED NEUROLOGIC DISORDERS

Many drugs produce adverse reactions that lead to altered function of the nervous system. Since the nervous system is complex, the list of possible adverse drug effects expressed in the nervous system is large. In this section, many of the more common drug-induced neurologic adverse reactions and the agents that cause them are summarized. The list is not exhaustive. Detailed reviews of this subject, with extensive references, are included in Lane and Routledge (1983) and Blain and Stewart-Wynne (1985).

Cerebral Cortex

Seizures. Increased frequency of seizures can occur in patients with underlying seizure disorders, or seizures can occur de novo in otherwise healthy patients. Many of the penicillins and related drugs such as imipenem can cause seizures when high plasma concentrations of drug occur. Such toxic concentrations are especially likely to occur in patients with abnormal renal function (see chapter 11). Isoniazid, phenothiazines, theophylline, lithium, cocaine, and lidocaine also can cause seizures. Sulfonylureas cause seizures by producing hypoglycemia. Normeperidine, a toxic metabolite of meperidine, can accumulate in certain patients (particularly those with renal compromise receiving high doses) and result in myoclonus or seizures.

Stroke. Oral contraceptives can lead to a hypercoagulable state that results in cerebral venous thrombosis. Smokers and women who have underlying migraine appear to be at higher risk of this complication. Nifedipine has been reported to cause acute stroke, possibly by lowering blood pressure too quickly. Patients receiving β blockers or MAO inhibitors can experience hypertensive crises precipitated by the administration of epinephrine or indirectly acting sympathomimetics, respectively, thereby leading to acute cerebral hemorrhage or subarachnoid hemorrhage. Hypertensive crisis with secondary stroke can result from sudden loss of control of hypertension. The abrupt withdrawal of a drug such as clonidine or propranolol ("rebound" hypertension), or the addition of a tricyclic antidepressant to a patient dependent on guanethidine, can set in motion an adverse sequence of events beginning with an acute hypertensive crisis. Cocaine and other sympathomimetic agents have also been reported to cause nonhemorrhagic stroke.

Cognitive Impairment. A number of drugs cause dementia, obtundation, or in extreme cases, coma. The variety is striking and includes drugs under the rubric of antihistamines, sedative-hypnotics, opioids, phenothiazines, tricyclic antidepressants, and anticonvulsant drugs. It is well known that salicylate intoxication can lead to delirium and coma, but less well appreciated that β blockers and methyldopa also cause sedation and obtundation. Hypoglycemic agents and diuretics can contribute to changes in the CNS by causing hypoglycemia and hyponatremia, respectively. One recent review concluded that drugs causing cognitive impairment are an important source of excess morbidity in elderly patients, especially those with preexisting, underlying dementia (Larson et al., 1987).

Syncope. Sudden loss of consciousness is an uncommon adverse drug effect. Drugs causing volume depletion or venodilation such as diuretics and nitrates can exacerbate orthostatic hypotension, thereby contributing to syncope. β-Adrenergic receptor antagonists and calcium-entry blockers can increase AV block and produce bradyarrhythmias, especially when they are used simultaneously. An increasing number of antiarrhythmic agents including digoxin, quinidine, and some of the type IC drugs have been recognized as being proarrhythmic agents (see chapter 6). Any of the drug-induced arrhythmias, but particularly supraventricular and ventricular arrhythmias, can lead to syncope.

Headache

Headaches caused by drugs may be associated with excessive vasodilation, or increased intracranial pressure. Vasodilating drugs such as nitrates, nifedipine, or hydralazine commonly cause headaches. In a similar fashion, withdrawal of drugs that have vasoconstrictive properties such as ergotamine, amphetamines, or caffeine can cause headache by allowing rebound vasodilation. The mechanism of production of headache by withdrawal from benzodiazepines is not clear.

Drugs can increase intracranial pressure without mass effect, a condition known as pseudotumor cerebri. Retinol (vitamin A), tetracycline, and lithium all produce headache by this mechanism.

Some drugs can cause headache by initiating a noninfectious aseptic meningitis. Several of the NSAIDs including sulindac, ibuprofen, and tolmetin have been reported to cause this syndrome.

Cranial Nerve Disorders

While any of the cranial nerves or the retina can be damaged or affected by drugs, the most common problems are associated with the second and eighth cranial nerves. Prolonged therapy with chloroquine can lead to a serious retinopathy in 2% to 17% of patients. Although reversible in its early stages, it may become irreversible if the drug is continued. Thioridazine (Mellaril) causes a similar process, but it tends to develop more rapidly and fortunately usually is reversible if it is detected quickly. Recognition of this syndrome has led to recommendations that the daily dose of thioridazine should not exceed 800 mg. Optic neuritis occasionally can be caused by antituberculous antibiotics. Other drugs causing toxicity to the optic nerve are discussed in an excellent review (Lane and Routledge, 1983).

Drug-induced problems of either the auditory or vestibular branches of the eighth cranial nerve are common. Many drugs can cause vestibulotoxicity, cochleotoxicity, or both. The most common offenders are the aminoglycoside antibiotics, polymyxin, and loop diuretics (especially ethacrynic acid). Toxicity associated with aminoglycosides may be subtle and irreversible, since high-frequency hearing loss and vestibular toxicity can be easy to miss unless it is rigorously evaluated. Deafness caused by ethacrynic acid usually is reversible and usually avoidable if the drug is not administered rapidly IV. Aspirin, quinine, and quinidine can cause dose-related tinnitus that can progress to deafness if it is not recognized and treated.

Involuntary Movement Disorders

Drugs can cause a variety of abnormal, involuntary movement disorders. These syndromes range from trivial to life-threatening, asymptomatic to painful, and acute to chronic. While many are reversible or treatable, several may leave permanent residue even if the offending drug is discontinued.

Tremor. Tremor is perhaps the least serious of the drug-induced involuntary movement disorders. The most common cause of drug-related tremor probably is withdrawal from ethanol or benzodiazepines. Sympathomimetics such as β-receptor agonists commonly cause tremor that may be improved by switching from oral therapy to inhalational therapy. Tricyclic antidepressants, lithium, and caffeine also cause tremors. As already has been discussed, tremor may present as a manifestation of drug-induced parkinsonism. Asterixis and myoclonus are movement disorders closely related to tremor and are well-known toxic reactions to several of the anticonvulsant drugs (Lane and Routledge, 1983).

Acute Dystonic Reactions. So-called extrapyramidal movement disorders include acute dystonic reactions as well as akathisia, parkinsonism, and tardive dyskinesia. All are associated with the use of neuroleptic agents or other drugs, such as metoclopramide, that act as dopaminergic-receptor antagonists. Acute dystonic reactions usually occur in younger patients early in the course of therapy. They present with frightening and at times painful contractions of muscles of the eyes (blepharospasm, oculogyric crisis), face (trismus), neck (torticollis), trunk (opisthotonos), or body. A physician unfamiliar with this common adverse reaction may mistakenly conclude that the patient is suffering from hysteria, a seizure disorder, or even tetany. Spasm of laryngeal muscles not only can be frightening but also life-threatening. These acute dystonias respond to discontinuation of the drug. Clinical experience suggests that treatment with diphenhydramine or anticholinergic drugs such as benztropine is useful. In young adults at high risk, some psychiatrists routinely administer benztropine prophylactically with new prescriptions of neuroleptic drugs.

Akathisia. This is another extrapyramidal reaction that usually occurs early during the course of treatment with a neuroleptic agent. It is characterized by extreme nervousness and the inability to sit still. The patient moves about and fidgets uncontrollably. Unfortunately, there seems to be little effective treatment for akathisia other than lowering the dose of the neuroleptic agent.

Parkinsonism. As discussed in chapter 13, drug-induced parkinsonism presents in a similar fashion to Parkinson disease. Drug induction of the disease may account for about half of all elderly patients presenting with new manifestations of parkinsonism (Stephen and Williamson, 1984). Drug-induced parkinsonism probably is the most common drug-induced movement disorder. It occurs to a mild degree in many patients receiving phenothiazines. Bradykinesia, rigidity, tremor, paucity of movement, and psychomotor retardation are similar in both the spontaneous and the drug-induced diseases. Antidopaminergic drugs such as neuroleptics and metoclopramide are responsible for most cases, although reserpine and methyldopa also have been reported as causative agents. Drug-induced parkinsonism responds to reduction or elimination of the antidopaminergic drug. If the dose cannot be reduced (as in treatment of a psychotic patient), then symptoms may be relieved by the addition of an anticholinergic drug such as benztropine. The decision to treat an adverse effect of a drug with another drug is a serious decision implying that the indication of the first drug is irrefutable and that there are no other drugs useful for the same indication. In many patients, the offending neuroleptic agent may be discontinued, particularly if it was originally prescribed for an unclear or improper indication. Elderly patients, especially those in nursing homes, appear to receive excessive prescriptions for neuroleptic agents used to control minimally disturbed behavior, or as hypnotic agents when safer alternatives are available.

Tardive Dyskinesia. After years of therapy with neuroleptic agents, some patients develop a progressive and disabling pattern of gross movements of the tongue, mouth, face, and body characteristic of tardive dyskinesia. This disorder is especially troubling since reducing the dose of the offending drug may make the disorder worse, and the problem may become irreversible. In addition, it is unclear that any treatment results in improvement in most patients. Therefore, patients begun on neuroleptic agents must be informed of this risk of long-term treatment. In addition, this toxic class of drugs should not be used for trivial indications, or when safer alternatives are available.

Neuroleptic Malignant Syndrome. The most dangerous disorder associated with use of neuroleptic agents is the neuroleptic malignant syndrome. It occurs in about 1% of patients exposed to these agents. The syndrome usually consists of the sudden onset of high fevers, rigidity, altered mental status (coma, mutism, catatonia), and autonomic instability (Rosenberg and Green, 1989; Rosebush and Stewart, 1989). Respiratory distress and renal compromise may occur, and the creatine phosphokinase (CPK) level is elevated in most patients as well. Optimal treatment includes general supportive measures, discontinuing the offending agent, and administering a dopaminergic-receptor agonist (e.g., bromocriptine), or a muscle relaxant (e.g., dantrolene). The latter two drugs can create their own problems and the data suggesting their efficacy in these settings are limited. Although more difficult to recognize, less severe and gradually developing forms of the syn-

drome also occur; fever may be lacking in such presentations.

Peripheral Neuropathies

Peripheral neuropathies may present as mixed sensorimotor neuropathies, predominantly sensory neuropathies, or predominantly motor neuropathies. Several drugs can cause each and all of these presentations. Antibacterial and antineoplastic agents are particularly noted in these neuropathic syndromes (Snavely and Hodges, 1984; Weiss et al., 1974).

Mixed Sensorimotor Neuropathy. A distal, mixed neuropathy probably is the most common type of drug-induced peripheral neuropathy. As in other peripheral neuropathies of a mixed nature, patients may note a symmetric distal loss of sensation, greater in the feet, with painful dysesthesia. The distribution may be of the *stocking-glove* type; deep tendon reflexes are often diminished. Some of the more commonly used agents that cause this type of peripheral neuropathy include ethanol, chlorambucil, ethambutol, gold, isoniazid (preventable by administering vitamin B_6), nitrofurantoin, penicillamine, phenytoin, vinblastine, and vincristine. Possible mechanisms for this adverse effect, as well as a more comprehensive list with references, have been discussed in Blain and Stewart-Wynne (1985).

Sensory Neuropathy. Most of the drugs causing a mixed neuropathy can present as a predominantly sensory neuropathy. Other drugs that cause a predominantly sensory type of peripheral neuropathy include ergotamine (see earlier discussion of ergots for migraine), propylthiouracil, nalidixic acid, and streptomycin.

Motor Neuropathy. A few drugs may cause a predominantly motor peripheral neuropathy. They include the sulfonamides, nitrofurantoin, amitriptyline, dapsone, and gold.

Inhibition of Neuromuscular Transmission

A variety of drugs cause motor weakness or even paralysis by interfering with normal function of the neuromuscular junction. Drugs such as succinylcholine or pancuronium are administered to cause such effects, and these direct pharmacologic actions would not be termed adverse reactions. Unintended curarelike effects have been observed when using the aminoglycosides and polymixin. Chloroquin also has been reported to have such effects. In patients with underlying neuromuscular problems such as myasthenia gravis, even drugs with weak curarelike effects such as quinine, quinidine, and procainamide may have clinically important adverse effects.

Even the syndrome of myasthenia gravis can be mimicked by the drug penicillamine, which in addition to many other adverse autoimmune effects has been reported to stimulate the development of autoantibodies directed against nicotinic acetylcholine receptors.

Autonomic Nervous System

Drugs that produce known pharmacologic effects upon the sympathetic or parasympathetic nervous system are commonly used with that intent. It is surprising how many other drugs with different indications produce unintended and undesired effects upon the antonomic nervous system.

For example, many classes of drugs produce unintended antagonism at muscarinic receptors located throughout the body. Elderly patients may be at greater risk for such effects, which can include dry mouth, visual problems, delirium, heat stroke, ileus, constipation, tachycardia, loss of detrusor tone, and acute urinary retention (especially in elderly men with enlarged prostates). In an extreme situation, patients can exhibit many of the anticholinergic effects summarized in the saying, "Mad as a hatter, blind as a bat, dry as a bone, hot as a pistol, and red as a beet."

The phenothiazines, tricyclic antidepressants, antiemetics, and antihistamines are perhaps the largest drug classes that have undesired anticholinergic properties. However, other classes of drugs may be prescribed by physicians without their realizing that a primary action is an antimuscarinic effect. Antiparkinsonian drugs (e.g., benztropine), mydriatics (e.g., tropicamide), drugs used for ulcer disease (e.g., propantheline), preanesthetics (e.g., scopolamine), bronchodilators (e.g., ipratropium), and antispasmodics and antidiarrheals (e.g., belladonna tincture) all contain anticholinergic drugs. The magnitude of this problem has been well described (Peters, 1989).

In summary, a large number of drugs can produce undesired toxicity at many sites within the central and peripheral nervous system, involving motor, sensory, and autonomic functioning. Adverse drug reactions should be kept in the differential diagnosis in patients presenting with neurologic problems.

REFERENCES

Ala-Hurula, V.: Correlation between pharmacokinetics and clinical effects of ergotamine in patients suffering from migraine. Eur. J. Clin. Pharmacol., 21:397–402, 1982.

Albers, G. W.; Goldberg, M. P.; and Choi, D. W.: N-methyl-D-aspartate antagonists: Ready for clinical trial in brain ischemia. Ann. Neurol., 25:398–403, 1989a.

Albers, G. W.; Simon, L. T.; Hamik, A.; and Peroutka, S. J.:

Nifedipine versus propranolol for the initial prophylaxis of migraine. Headache, 29:215–218, 1989b.

Allen, G. S.; Burns, R. S.; Tulipan, N. B.; and Parker, R. A.: Adrenal medullary transplantation to the caudate nucleus in Parkinson's disease. Arch. Neurol., 46:487–491, 1989.

Altafullah, I.; Talwar, D.; Loewenson, R.; Olson, K.; and Lockman, L. A.: Factors influencing serum levels of carbamazepine and carbamazepine-10,11-epoxide in children. Epilepsy Res., 4:72–80, 1989.

The American-Canadian Co-Operative Study Group: Persantine aspirin trial in cerebral ischemia: Part II. Endpoint results. Stroke, 16:406–415, 1985.

Amery, W. K.: Flunarizine, a calcium channel blocker: A new prophylactic drug in migraine. Headache, 23:70–74, 1983.

Backlund, E. O.; Granberg, P. O.; Hamberger, B.; Knutsson, E.; Martensson, A.; Sedvall, G.; Seiger, A.; and Olson, L.: Transplantation of adrenal medullary tissue to striatum in parkinsonism. J. Neurosurg., 62:169–173, 1985.

Ballard, P. A.; Tetrud, J. W.; and Langston, J. W.: Permanent human parkinsonism due to 1-methyl-4-phenyl-1,2,3,6-tetrahydropyridine (MPTP): Seven cases. Neurology, 35:949–956, 1985.

Barnett, H. J. M.: Progress towards stroke prevention: The Robert Wartenberg lecture. Neurology, 30:1212–1225, 1980.

Blain, P. G.; and Stewart-Wynne, E.: Neurological disorders. In, Textbook of Adverse Drug Reactions, 3rd ed. (Davies, D. M., ed.). Oxford University Press, New York, pp. 494–514, 1985.

Bourgeois, B. F. D.: Pharmacologic interactions between valproate and other drugs. Am. J. Med., 84:29–33, 1988.

Bousser, M. D.; Eschwege, E.; and Haguenau, M.: "AICLA" controlled trial of aspirin and dipyridamole in the secondary prevention of athero-thrombotic cerebral ischemia. Stroke, 14:5–14, 1983.

Callaham, M.; and Raskin, N.: A controlled study of dihydroergotamine in the treatment of acute migraine headache. Headache, 26:168–171, 1986.

Calne, D. B.; Burton, K.; and Beckman, J.: Dopamine agonists in Parkinson's disease. Can. J. Neurol. Sci., 11:221–224, 1984.

Caplan, L. R.: Anticoagulation for cerebral ischemia. Clin. Neuropharmacol. 9:399–414, 1986.

Carter, J. H.; Nutt, J. G.; Woodward, W. R.; Hatcher, L. F.; and Trotman, T. L.: Amount and distribution of dietary protein affects clinical response to levodopa in Parkinson's disease. Neurology, 39:552–556, 1989.

Caviness, V. S.; and O'Brien, P.: Headache. N. Engl. J. Med., 302:446–450, 1980.

Cerebral Embolism Task Force: Cardiogenic brain embolism. Arch. Neurol., 46:727–743, 1989.

Chesebro, J. H.; Fuster, V.; Elveback, L. R.; McGoon, D. C.; Pluth, J. R.; Puga, F. J.; Wallace, R. B.; Danielson, G. K.; Orszulak, T. A.; Piehler, J. M.; and Schaff, H. V.: Trial of combined warfarin plus dipyridamole or aspirin therapy in prosthetic heart valve replacement: Danger of aspirin compared with dipyridamole. Am. J. Cardiol., 51:1537–1541, 1983.

Commission on Classification and Terminology of the International League Against Epilepsy: Proposal for revised classification of epilepsies and epileptic syndromes. Epilepsia, 30:389–399, 1989.

Commission on Classification and Terminology of the International League Against Epilepsy: Proposal for revised clinical and electroencephalographic classification of epileptic seizures. Epilepsia, 22:489–501, 1981.

Couch, J. R.; and Hassanein, R. S.: Amitriptyline in migraine prophylaxis. Arch. Neurology, 36:695–699, 1979.

Couch, J. R.; Ziegler, D. K.; and Hassanein, R.: Amitriptyline in the prophylaxis of migraine. Neurology, 26:121–127, 1976.

Coulter, D. A.; Huguenard, J. R.; and Prince, D. A.: Characterization of ethosuximide reduction of low-threshold calcium current in thalamic neurons. Ann. Neurol., 6:582–590, 1989.

Covanis, A.; and Jeavons, P. M.: Once daily sodium valproate in the treatment of epilepsy. Dev. Med. Child. Neurol., 22: 202–204, 1980.

Cranford, R. E.; Leppik, I. E.; and Patrick, B.: Intravenous phenytoin: Clinical and pharmacokinetic aspects. Neurology, 28:874–876, 1978.

Dalessio, D. J.: Wolff's Headache and Other Head Pain, 4th ed. Oxford University Press, New York, 1980.

Delgado-Escueta, A. V.; and Enrile-Bascal, F. E.: Juvenile myoclonic epilepsy of Janz. Neurology, 34:285–294, 1984.

Doenicke, A.; Brand, J.; and Perrin, V. L.: Possible benefit of GR 43175, a novel 5-HT₁ like receptor agonist, for the acute treatment of severe migraine. Lancet, 1:1309–1311, 1988.

Dreifuss, F. E.: Valproic acid hepatic fatalities: A retrospective review. Neurology, 37:379–385, 1987.

Dreifuss, F. E.; Langer, D. H.; Moline, K. A.; and Maxwell, J. E.: Valproic acid hepatic fatalities: II. US experience since 1984. Neurology, 39:201–207, 1989.

Dunn, M.; Alexander, J.; de Silva, R.; and Hildner, F.: Antithrombotic therapy in atrial fibrillation. Chest, 95:118S–125S, 1989.

Eriksson, T.; Granerus, A.-K.; Linde, A.; and Carlsson, A.: "On-off" phenomenon in Parkinson's disease: Relationship between dopa and other large neutral amino acids in plasma. Neurology, 38:1245–1248, 1988.

Fahn, S.; and Bressman, S. B.: Should levodopa therapy for Parkinsonism be started early or late? Evidence against early treatment. Can. J. Neurol. Sci., 11:200–206, 1984.

Fanchamps, A.: Why do not all beta-blockers prevent migraine? Headache, 25:61–62, 1985.

Ferrendelli, J. A.: Pharmacology of antiepileptic drugs. Epilepsia, 28:S14–S16, 1987.

Fischer, J. H.: Effect of food on the serum concentration profile of enteric-coated valproic acid. Neurology, 38:1319–1322, 1988.

Fisher, C. M.: The arterial lesions underlying lacunes. Acta Neuropathol., 12:1–15, 1969.

Fozard, J. R.: Migraine—A critique of therapy. In, The Modern Approach to Headache (Rose, F. C., ed.). Oxford University Press, Oxford, U.K., 1986.

Fozard, J. R.: Basic mechanisms of antimigraine drugs. Adv. Neurol., 33:295–307, 1982.

Gelmers, H. J.; Gorter, K.; Weerdt, D.; and Wiezer, H. J.: A controlled trial of nimodipine in acute ischemic stroke. N. Engl. J. Med., 318:203–207, 1988.

Gent, M.; Blakely, J. A.; and Easton, J. D.: The Canadian American Ticlopidine Study (CATS) in thromboembolic stroke. Lancet, 1:1215–1220, 1989.

Gjerloff, I.: Monodose versus three daily doses of sodium valproate: A controlled trial. Acta. Neurol. Scand., 69:120–124, 1984.

Gomersall, J. D.; and Stuart, A.: Amitriptyline in migraine prophylaxis. J. Neurol. Neurosurg. Psychiatry, 36:684–690, 1973.

Goulden, K. J.; Dooley, J. M.; Camfield, P. R.; and Fraser, A. D.: Clinical valproate toxicity induced by acetylsalicylic acid. Neurology, 37:1392–1394, 1987.

Graham, J. R.: Migraine headache: Diagnosis and management. Headache, 19:133–141, 1979.

Greenberg, D. A.: Calcium channel antagonists and the treatment of migraine. Clin. Neuropharmacol., 9:311–328, 1986.

Hakkarainen, H.; and Allonen, H.: Ergotamine vs. metoclopramide vs. their combination in acute migraine attacks. Headache, 22:10–12, 1982.

Halperin, J. L.; and Hart, R. G.: Atrial fibrillation and stroke: New ideas, persisting dilemmas. Stroke, 19:937–941, 1988.

Hamik, A.; and Peroutka, S. J.: Differential interactions of traditional and novel antiemetics with dopamine D₂ and 5-hydroxytryptamine₃ receptors. Cancer Chemother. Pharmacol., 24:307–310, 1989.

Hass, W. K.; Easton, J. D.; Adams, H. P. Jr.; Pryse-Phillips, W.; Molony, B. A.; Anderson, S.; and Kamm, B.: A randomized trial comparing ticlopidine hydrochloride with aspirin for the prevention of stroke in high-risk patients. N. Engl. J. Med., 321:501–507, 1989.

Hauser, W. A.; Anderson, V. E.; Loewenson, R. B.; and McRoberts, S. M.: Seizure recurrence after a first unprovoked seizure. N. Engl. J. Med., 307:522–528, 1982.

Hirsh, J.; Poller, L.; Deykin, D.; Levine, M.; and Dalen, J. E.: Optimal therapeutic range for oral anticoagulants. Chest, 95:5S–10S, 1989.

Humphrey, P. P. A.; Feniuk, W.; and Perren, M. J.: GR 43175, a selective agonist for the 5-HT₁-like receptor in dog isolated saphenous vein. Br. J. Pharmacol., 94:1123–1132, 1988.

Jankovic, J.: Management of motor side effects of chronic levodopa therapy. Clin. Neurol., 5:S19–S28, 1982.

Jankovic, J.; and Marsden, C. D.: Therapeutic strategies in Parkinson's disease. In, Parkinson's Disease and Movement Disorders (Jankovic, J.; and Tolosa, E.; eds.). Urban and Schwarzenberg, Baltimore, pp. 95–119, 1988.

Jonas, S.: Anticoagulant therapy in cerebrovascular disease: Review and meta-analysis. Stroke, 19:1043–1048, 1988.

Jonsdottir, M.; Meyer, J. S.; and Rogers, R. L.: The role of calcium channel blocking agents in the prevention of migraine. Drug. Intell. Clin. Pharm., 22:187–191, 1988.

Karoum, F.; Chuang, L.-W.; Eisler, T.; Calne, D. B.; Liebowitz, M. R.; Quitkin, F. M.; Klein, D. F.; and Wyatt, R. J.: Metabolism of (−)deprenyl to amphetamine and methamphetamine may be responsible for deprenyl's therapeutic benefit: A biochemical assessment. Neurology, 32:503–509, 1982.

Kopecky, S. L.; Gerah, B. J.; McGoon, M. D.; Whisnant, J. P.; Holmes, D. R.; Ilstrup, D. M.; and Frye, R. L.: The natural history of lone atrial fibrillation. N. Engl. J. Med., 317:669–674, 1987.

Kurlan, R.: Practical therapy of Parkinson's disease. Semin. Neurol., 7:160–166, 1987.

Kurtzke, J. F.; Bennett, D. R.; Berg, B. O.; Beringer, G. B.; Goldstein, D. O.; and Vates, T. S.: On national needs for neurologists in the United States. Neurology, 36:383–388, 1986.

Kutt, H.; and Verebely, K.: Metabolism of diphenylhydantoin by rat liver microsomes: I. Characteristics of the reaction. Biochem. Pharmacol., 19:675–683, 1970.

Lance, J. W.: Headache. Ann. Neurol., 10:1–10, 1981.

Lance, J. W.: Comparative trial of serotonin antagonists in the management of migraine. Br. Med. J., 2:327–330, 1970.

Lance, J. W.; and Anthony, M.: Some clinical aspects of migraine. Arch. Neurol., 15:356–361, 1966.

Lane, R. J. M.; and Routledge, P. A.: Drug-induced neurological disorders. Drugs, 26:124–147, 1983.

Lang, A. E.: Treatments of Parkinson's disease with agents other than levodopa and dopamine agonists: Controversies and new approaches. Can. J. Neurol. Sci., 11:210–220, 1984.

Larkin, J. G.; McLellan, A.; Munday, A.; Sutherland, M.; Butler, E.; and Brodie, M. J.: A double-blind comparison of conventional and controlled-release carbamazepine in healthy subjects. Br. J. Clin. Pharmacol., 27:313–322, 1989.

Larson, E. B.; Kukull, W. A.; Buchner, D.; and Reifler, B. V.: Adverse drug reactions associated with global cognitive impairment in elderly persons. Ann. Int. Med., 107:169–173, 1987.

Lesser, R. P.; Pippenger, C. E.; Luders, H.; and Dinner, D. S.: High-dose monotherapy in treatment of intractable seizures. Neurology, 34:707–711, 1984.

Macdonald, R. L.; and McLean, M. J.: Anticonvulsant drugs: Mechanisms of action. Adv. Neurol., 44:713–736, 1986.

Madrazo, I.; Drucker-Colin, R.; Diaz, V.; Martinez-Mata, J.; Torres, C.; and Begerril, J. J.: Open microsurgical autograft of adrenal medulla to the right caudate nucleus in two patients with intractable Parkinson's disease. N. Engl. J. Med., 316:831–834, 1987.

McArthur, J. C.; Marek, K.; Pestronk, A.; McArthur, J.; and Peroutka, S. J.: Nifedipine in the prophylaxis of classic migraine: A cross-over, double-masked, placebo-controlled study of headache frequency and side effects. Neurology, 39: 284–286, 1989.

McCarthy, B. G.; and Peroutka, S. J.: Comparative neuropharmacology of dihydroergotamine and sumatriptan (GR 43175). Headache, 29:420–422, 1989.

Mattson, R.: Use of oral contraceptives by women with epilepsy. J.A.M.A., 256:238–240, 1986.

Muenter, M. D.: Should levodopa therapy be started early or late? Can. J. Neurol. Sci., 11:195–199, 1984.

Melmon, K. L.: Will the sighted physician see? Pharos, 47:2–6, 1984.

Nanda, R. N.: Treatment of epilepsy with clonazepam and its effect on other anticonvulsants. J. Neurol. Neurosurg. Psychiatry, 40:538–543, 1977.

Nussmeier, N. A.; Arlund, C.; and Slogoff, S.: Neuropsychiatric complications after cardiopulmonary bypass: Cerebral protection by a barbiturate. Anesthesiology, 64:165–170, 1986.

Nutt, J. G.: On-off phenomenon: Relation to levodopa pharmacokinetics and pharmacodynamics. Ann. Neurol., 22:535–540, 1987.

Nutt, J. G.; Woodward, W. R.; Hammerstad, J. P.; Carter, J. H.; and Anderson, J. L.: The "on-off" phenomenon in Parkinson's disease. N. Engl. J. Med., 310:483–488, 1984.

Olesen, J.: Some clinical features of the acute migraine attack. An analysis of 750 patients. Headache, 18:268–271, 1978.

Parkinson Study Group. Effect of deprenyl on the progression of disability in early Parkinson's disease. N. Engl. J. Med., 321:1364–1371, 1989.

Patel, I. H.; Levy, R. H.; and Trager, W. F.: Pharmacokinetics of carbamazepine-10,11-epoxide before and after autoinduction in the rhesus monkey. J. Pharmacol. Exp. Ther., 206:607–613, 1978.

Paxton, J. W.: Effects of aspirin on salivary and serum phenytoin kinetics in healthy subjects. Clin. Pharmacol. Ther., 27:170–178, 1980.

Peatfield, R.; Fozard, J. R.; and Rose, F. C.: Migraine: Current concepts of pathogenesis and treatment. In, Handbook of Clinical Neurology (Vinken, P. J.; and Bruyn, G. W.; eds.). Vol. 4. Elsevier, New York, 173–216, 1986.

Pellock, J. M.: Carbamazepine side effects in children and adults. Epilepsia, 28:S64–S70, 1987.

Penry, J. K.; and Dean, J. C.: Valproate monotherapy in partial seizures. Am. J. Med., 84:14–16, 1988.

Peroutka, S. J.: The pharmacology of calcium channel antagonists: A novel class of anti-migraine agents? Headache, 23:278–283, 1983.

Peters, N. L.: Snipping the thread of life. Arch. Intern. Med., 149:2414–2420, 1989.

Petersen, P.: Thromboembolic complications in atrial fibrillation. Stroke, 21:4–13, 1990.

Petersen, P.; Godtfredsen, J.; and Boysen, G.: Placebo-controlled, randomized trial of warfarin and aspirin for prevention of thromboembolic complications in chronic atrial fibrillation. Lancet, 1:175–178, 1989.

Pippenger, C. E.: Clinically significant carbamazepine drug interactions: An overview. Epilepsia, 28:S71–S76, 1987.

Raskin, N.: Repetitive intravenous dihydroergotamine as therapy for intractable migraine. Neurology, 36:995–997, 1986.

Raskin, N. H.: Pharmacology of migraine. Ann. Rev. Pharmacol. Toxicol., 21:463–478, 1981.

Reynolds, E. H.: Chronic epileptic toxicity; A review. Epilepsia, 16:319–352, 1975.

Richens, A.: A study of the pharmacokinetics of phenytoin (diphenylhydantoin) in epileptic patients and the development of a nomogram for making dose increments. Epilepsia, 16:627–634, 1975.

Ringel, R. A.; and Brick J. F.: Perspective on carbamazepine induced water intoxication: Reversal by demeclocycline. Neurology, 36:1506–1507, 1986.

Rosebush, P.; and Stewart, T.: A prospective analysis of 24 episodes of neuroleptic malignant syndrome. Am. J. Psychiatry, 146:717–725, 1989.

Rosenberg, M. R.; and Green, M.: Neuroleptic malignant syndrome. Arch. Intern. Med., 149:1927–1931, 1989.

Schwab, R. S.; Poskanzer, D. C.; England, A. C.; and Young, R. R.: Amantadine in Parkinson's disease: Review of more than two years' experience. J.A.M.A., 222:792–795, 1972.

Schuler, M. E.; Goldman, M. P.; and Munger, M. A.: Efficacy, side effects and tolerance compared during headache treatment with three different calcium blockers. Headache, 27:364–369, 1987.

Sherman, D. G.; Dyken, M. L.; Fisher, M.; Harrison, M. J. G.; and Hart, R. G.: Antithrombotic therapy for cerebrovascular disorders. Chest, 95:140S–155S, 1989.

Sicuteri, F.: Prophylatic and therapeutic properties of 1-methyl-lysergic acid butanolamide in migraine. Int. Arch. Allergy, 15:300–307, 1959.

Snavely, S. R.; and Hodges, G. R.: The neurotoxicity of antibacterial agents. Ann. Intern. Med., 101:92–104, 1984.

Spierings, E. L. H.; and Saxena, P. R.: Effect of isometheptene on the distribution and shunting of 15μM microspheres throughout the cephalic circulation of the cat. Headache, 20:103–106, 1980.

Stein, B.; Fuster, V.; Halperin, J. L.; and Chesebro, J. H.: Antithrombotic therapy in cardiac disease: An emerging approach based on pathogenesis and risk. Circulation, 80:1501–1513, 1989.

Stephen, P. J.; and Williamson, J.: Drug-induced parkinsonism in the elderly. Lancet, 2(8411):1082–1083, 1984.

Stratton, J. R.: Common causes of cardiac emboli – Left ventricular thrombi and atrial fibrillation. West. J. Med., 151:172–179, 1989.

Stroke Prevention in Atrial Fibrillation Study Group Investigators: Preliminary report of the stroke prevention in atrial fibrillation study. N. Engl. J. Med., 322:863–868, 1990.

Sullivan, J. M.; Harken, D. E.; and Gorlin, R.: Effect of dipyridamole on the incidence of arterial emboli after cardiac valve replacement. Circulation, 39 (5)suppl:149–153, 1969.

Tetrud, J. W.; and Langston, J. W.: The effect of deprenyl (selegiline) on the natural history of Parkinson's disease. Science, 245:519–522, 1989.

Tfelt-Hansen, P.; Bredberg, U.; Eyjolfsdottir, G. S.; Paalzow, L.; and Tfelt-Hansen, V.: Kinetics of methysergide and its main metabolite, methylergometrine, in man. Cephalagia, 5S3:54–55, 1985.

Trimble, M. R.: Anticonvulsant drugs and cognitive function: A review of the literature. Epilepsia, 28:S37–S45, 1987.

Troupin, A. S.: Diagnostic decision. The measurement of anticonvulsant agent levels. Ann. Intern Med., 100:854–858, 1984.

Tsui, J. K.; Ross, S.; Poulin, K.; Douglas, J.; Postnikoff, D.; Calne, S.; Woodward, W.; and Calne, D. B.: The effect of dietary protein on the efficacy of L-dopa: A double-blind study. Neurology, 39:549–552, 1989.

Uchiyama, S.; Sone, R.; Nagayama, T.; Shibagaki, Y.; Kobayashi, I.; Maruyama, S.; and Kusakabe, K.: Combination therapy with low-dose aspirin and ticlopidine in cerebral ischemia. Stroke, 20:1643–1647, 1989.

Vincent, P. C.: Drug-induced aplastic anemia and agranulocytosis: Incidence and mechanisms. Drugs, 31:52–63, 1986.

Vining, E. P. G.: Cognitive dysfunction associated with antiepileptic drug therapy. Epilepsia, 28:S18–S22, 1987.

Volans, G. N.: The effect of metoclopramide on the absorption of effervescent aspirin in migraine. Br. J. Clin. Pharmacol., 2:57–63, 1975.

Weerasuriya, K.; Patel, L.; and Turner, P.: β-adrenoceptor blockade and migraine. Cephalalgia, 3:33–45, 1982.

Weiss, H. D.; Walker, M. D.; and Wiernick, P. H.: Neurotoxicity of commonly used antineoplastic agents. N. Engl. J. Med., 291:75–81, 127–133, 1974.

Wilder, B. J.: Treatment considerations in anticonvulsant monotherapy. Epilepsia, 28:S1–S7, 1987.

Wilder, B. J.: Gastrointestinal tolerance of divalproex sodium. Neurology, 33:808–811, 1983.

Wilder, B. J.; and Rangel, R. J.: Review of valproate monotherapy in the treatment of generalized tonic-clonic seizures. Am. J. Med., 84:7–13, 1988.

Wilkinson, M.: Treatment of migraine. Headache, 28:659–661, 1988.

Wilkinson, M.: Treatment of the acute migraine attack – Current status. Cephalalgia, 3:61–67, 1983.

Wykes, P.: The treatment of angina pectoris with coexistent migraine. Practitioner, 200:700–704, 1968.

Yahr, M. D.: Limitations of long-term use of antiParkinson drugs. Can. J. Neurol. Sci., 11:191–194, 1984.

Yatsu, F. M.: Pharmacologic protection against ischemic brain damage. Neurol. Clin., 1:37–53, 1983.

Yatsu, F. M.; Hart, R. G.; Mohr, J. P.; and Grotta, J. C.: Anticoagulation of embolic strokes of cardiac origin: An update. Neurology, 38:314–316, 1988.

Ziegler, D. K.; and Ellis, D. J.: Naproxen in prophylaxis of migraine. Arch. Neurol., 42:582–584, 1985.

13

Psychiatric Disorders

Leo E. Hollister

GENERAL PROBLEMS OF PSYCHIATRIC DIAGNOSIS AND NOSOLOGY

Diagnosis of psychiatric disorders remains the most clinically based system in medicine. Unlike other medical disciplines, which enjoy an abundance of diagnostic tools or eventually the priceless feedback from the autopsy room, psychiatry has few tests that validate diagnoses. Not surprisingly, expert opinion may vary considerably about the most appropriate diagnosis for any particular patient.

Sources of data are limited and highly subjective. We must rely on what patients tell us (sometimes not very reliably), what others tell us about the patient (possibly a bit better), and clinical observation of the patient's behavior. From these, we draw inferences about the diagnosis. Psychological testing usually confirms the clinical diagnosis but in difficult situations is often couched in such vague and comprehensive terms as to rival horoscopes. No specific electroencephalographic (EEG) patterns have been adduced for most psychiatric disorders; abnormalities usually lead to investigations of organic causes. A similar situation applies in the case of brain scans, where an abundance of minor abnormalities of unknown significance have been reported in patients with various diagnoses. Whether these are the cause or the result of the disorder is uncertain, but in any case their sensitivity and specificity have been remarkably low. The ability to measure regional cerebral blood flow and metabolism, or to image the distributions of various neurotransmitter receptors, may ultimately provide a totally new way of categorizing psychiatric disorders; at present, none of the reported abnormalities have been well established.

To compensate for these deficiencies, increasing efforts have been made to define psychiatric diagnoses in terms of presenting symptoms and signs, the natural history of the disorder, and various exclusionary criteria. The *Diagnostic and Statistical Manual* of the American Psychiatric Association (DSM) is being revised for a fourth edition. As desirable as a more precise definition of terms may be, one should recognize the defects of such a system. First, the definitions represent only the prevailing opinions of a group of experts at some period of time and are amenable to constant change. Second, definitions expounded by one group (DSM) may not be congruent with those of another, say the International Classification of Disease (ICD). Third, a variety of so-called research diagnostic criteria have been proposed for defining diagnoses. Many of these do not agree either with DSM or ICD criteria, or, for that matter, with each other (Overall and Hollister, 1979). Fourth, renaming an old disorder somehow carries the magical implication that by so doing one gains more insight into its cause and treatment. Today's fashionable diagnosis of panic disorder was called an acute anxiety attack 25 years ago. Fifth, old rubrics may be discarded (homosexuality and neurosis) while new ones may be added (late luteal phase dysphoria, a fancy name for premenstrual tension).

Considering these difficulties, psychiatrists do much better than might be expected. It is still possible to form a working diagnosis and try what might be construed as the best treatments for it. When diagnosis is less certain, it becomes possible to entertain a number of possibilities, in order of presumed certitude, and successively try a number of different treatments. Thus, it should not be surprising that some patients initially diagnosed as having generalized anxiety disorder may ultimately respond to an antidepressant, or someone initially thought to be schizophrenic might respond best to a drug useful for treating mania. Whether such examples reflect uncertainty of diagnosis, or the nonspecificity of action of the various drugs, or both, is still undetermined.

Anxiety Disorders

Prevalence. Surveys of the frequency of anxiety disorders have led to variable rates of prevalence. The most comprehensive and recent was the Epidemiologic Catchment Area (ECA) Survey sponsored by the National Institute of Mental Health. The 6-month prevalence of anxiety disorders ranged from 6.6% to 14.9% with lifetime prevalence rates varying between 10.4% and 25.1% (Myers et al., 1984; Robins et al., 1984). Anxiety disorders were the most frequent of all psychiatric disorders during any 6-month period (and quite likely one of the most frequent of all medical problems). The lifetime prevalence of substance abuse disorders was slightly higher. Even if these estimates are flawed, they indicate that anxiety is very common in the general population. No wonder that drugs for treating anxiety have found such a ready market.

Fear, panic, and anxiety have many qualitative similarities; the big differences are in the severity of clinical manifestations and the natural course (Table 13–1). In a sense, fear-anxiety may be considered one of the body's major defense mechanisms, and like so many others, operate through redundant mechanisms.

Possible Mechanisms of Anxiety Disorder

1. **Sympathomimetic Model.** Physiologic changes associated with fear-anxiety resemble those associated with stimulation of the sympathetic nervous system. Walter Cannon interpreted these as indicating that the organism is prepared for "fight or flight," implying the defensive function of fear-anxiety. Sympathomimetic compounds, such as epinephrine, often induce a sensation of anxiety, although the psychological changes may be less a model than the physiologic changes. The use of drugs that block the sympathetic nervous systems, such as β-adrenoreceptor blocking drugs, alleviate some aspects of fear-anxiety (Ananth and Lin, 1986).

2. **Locus Ceruleus, α_2-Adrenoreceptor Model.** The locus ceruleus, a blue streak of cells at the base of the fourth ventricle, is the origin of most of the norepinephrine innervation of the brain. Electrical stimulation of this area in animals mimics anxiety, but lesions prevent fearful behavior. α_2 Adrenoreceptors on the cell bodies act as autoreceptors. Drugs that act as α_2 antagonists, such as yohimbine and piperoxan, increase the firing of these cells and elicit some symptoms of anxiety. Drugs that act as α_2 agonists, such as clonidine, decrease firing and alleviate anxiety. Locus ceruleus cells also have inputs from other neurotransmitters, including serotonin, acetylcholine, γ-aminobutyric acid (GABA), and several neuropeptides (Charney and Heninger, 1986). Nonethe-

Table 13–1. **CLINICAL DIFFERENCES BETWEEN FEAR, PANIC, AND ANXIETY**

	ONSET	DURATION OF SIGNS OR SYMPTOMS	SEVERITY OF MANIFESTATION	PRECIPITANT	COURSE	OTHER PSYCHIATRIC DISORDERS
Fear	Sudden, un-anticipated	Brief, termi-nated by resolution of threat	Very severe	External, recognized	Single epi-sode, self-limiting	None
Panic	Sudden, un-anticipated	Brief, sponta-neous sub-sidence	Moderate to severe	Unknown, un-recognized	Repeated epi-sodes with remission	Other anxiety disorders, depression
Anxiety	Insidious, may be an-ticipated	Long-lived	Mild to mod-erate	Unknown, un-recognized	Chronic with varying re-mission	Other anxiety disorders, depression

less, the role of the locus ceruleus in mediating fear-anxiety in humans is still uncertain.

3. **GABA-Benzodiazepine-Receptor Model.** The discovery of a macromolecular complex with binding sites for GABA, benzodiazepines, barbiturates, and other sedative-hypnotics and some convulsants, such as picrotoxin, has stimulated much speculation about its physiologic functions (Martin, 1987). This complex regulates an ion channel for chloride ions, whose entry into the cell hyperpolarizes it. GABA-benzodiazepine-binding sites are selectively distributed in the human brain and occur in animals far down the phylogenetic line. This complex has the peculiar property of accommodating three confirmations: agonist, antagonist, and inverse agonist (Costa, 1988). The latter has been especially provocative, as the action may often mimic the effects of fear-anxiety. Whether or not endogenous inverse agonists exist is still under investigation. One might speculate that the major function of this complex would be to serve as a fear-anxiety mechanism, activated by endogenous inverse agonists. Persons with anxiety disorders might have an exaggerated mechanism that makes them more prone to become anxious than the general run of people. *Principle: It is tempting to assume that when a drug alleviates a manifestation its mechanisms of action provide clues to the origin of the manifestation. Deductions about pathogenesis based on the action of drugs must always be considered shaky.*

4. **Other Neurotransmitters.** The introduction of a new class of drugs for treating anxiety, exemplified by buspirone, renewed interest into possible serotonergic mechanisms of anxiety. Buspirone apparently exerts its major action by blocking serotonin receptors of the 5-HT$_{1A}$ type (Palmer, 1988). Unfortunately, increasing serotonin activity has not provided very good models of anxiety, and questions remain about the efficacy of buspirone. The principle stated above still applies.

Problems from the Broadened Concept of Anxiety Disorders. Formerly, virtually all anxiety disorders were encompassed by the term *anxiety neurosis.* However, the most recent classification of these disorders has broadened the concept. Most people would have no difficulty reconciling panic disorder in the group; some would insist that it always was included. The various phobias may deserve a place (the root of *phobia* is the Greek word for fear). But should obsessive-compulsive disorder be included? Recent work suggests that its pathogenesis might be considerably different from that of other forms of fear-anxiety (Rapoport, 1988). Thus, to the extent that the concept of anxiety disorders is broadened, so will be the potential pathogenetic mechanisms.

Sleep Disorders

Prevalence. Difficulty in initiating or maintaining sleep is a common complaint. During the course of a year, 35% of adults surveyed complained of insomnia and half of them thought it to be serious. Probably no more than 15% were treated, either with drugs or other means (Consensus Development Conference, 1984a). Considering the large number of persons involved, even a small percentage being treated with drugs represents a sizable use.

Biology of Sleep. The functions of sleep are unknown. No one ever dies from lack of it, yet few people can postpone it for much more than a few days. Sleep–wake rhythms are locked into the diurnal cycle, although when free-running, the rhythms do not always follow a 24-hour periodicity (Moore-Ede et al., 1983).

Sleep is a complex, nonhomogeneous state. Rapid eye movement (REM) sleep occurs periodically during the night (about 20% of total sleep time) and is often associated with dreaming. The remainder of sleep is non-REM sleep, which is arbitrarily divided into four stages based on slowing of waves on the EEG. Even a normal night of sleep may be punctuated by brief awakenings.

Serotonin seems to be involved in induction of non-REM sleep and acetylcholine in REM sleep, but the exact role of either of these, or other neurotransmitters, is not known. Peptides have been isolated from brain that appear to induce sleep and that accumulate with sleep deprivation (Krueger et al., 1986), which is the most important determinant of sleep.

Classification of Sleep Disorders. A number of classification systems have been proposed or are under revision. Two broad categories have been mentioned, the dyssomnias and the parasomnias. Dyssomnias include insomnia, hypersomnia, and disorders of the sleep–wake cycle. Parasomnias include aberrations of sleep, such as nightmares, sleep terror, and sleepwalking.

Insomnia is the most frequent complaint about sleep; either the patient does not sleep long enough or does not feel rested. The clinical diagnosis of insomnia is justified when inadequate sleep occurs several times a week for at least 1 month. When it is more than 3 months in duration, insomnia is said to be chronic.

Diagnosis relies heavily on the history, including one taken from a bed partner. Physical examination may reveal sources of pain that might interfere with sleep. Ordinary laboratory workup is usually noncontributory. Sleep laboratory studies need be done only rarely; they are expensive. About 35% of insomnia is thought to be associated with other psychiatric disorders, mainly anxiety and depression. An undetermined amount is due to drug taking, either social drugs such as alcohol or caffeine or a variety of medications with stimulant properties.

Sleep apnea and periodic movements of sleep are unusual causes of insomnia. Both may be suspected on the basis of testimony from a bed partner. Sleep apnea may cause hundreds of minor awakenings through the night. Even though patients may not be fully aware of being awake, they feel excessively fatigued the following day. The bed partner may describe periods in which the patient snores loudly followed by rapid breathing and then a period of quiet with barely noticeable respiration. Two types are recognized. Obstructive apnea is due to excessive laxity of the soft palate, which may fall back and occlude the airway. Surgical revision of the palate or placement of a permanent tracheostomy are the proper treatments for this cause. Central apnea is due to a lack of adequate respiratory drive. After a period of apnea in which the CO_2 tension increases, breathing resumes with a start followed by a brief period of hyperventilation. Drugs that stimulate respiration, such as almitrine, have been used suc-

cessfully in such patients. Sleep apneas are more frequent in elderly patients and those who are obese. Generally, any drug that may depress respiratory drive, which would include the benzodiazepines, should be avoided in such patients. The diagnosis may be suspected on clinical grounds: daytime sleepiness or napping; snoring or uneven respirations as noted by a bed partner; headaches and hypertension; or marked obesity. Sleep laboratory studies are usually definitive.

Periodic movements of sleep occur throughout the night. Restless legs disturb sleep not so much by causing awakenings but by reducing the depth of sleep. This diagnosis, too, may be suspected from the testimony of a bed partner. Sleep laboratory studies establish the diagnosis. Although clonazepam has been specifically recommended as treatment, quite likely any benzodiazepine would suffice. In this case, regular use of the drug may be justified.

Sleepwalking, sleep terrors, and enuresis occur during slow wave sleep. Enuresis has been satisfactorily treated with tricyclic antidepressants. The other conditions may respond to drugs that tend to eliminate or reduce slow wave sleep, which would include most benzodiazepines.

Many larger medical centers have a sleep laboratory. The normal architecture of sleep has been well described so that patients with sleep problems may be compared with the norm to determine the nature of the disturbance. Some patients are found to have a normal amount of sleep and normal sleep architecture despite a subjective complaint of poor sleep. The effects of drugs on the architecture of sleep can also be studied in sleep laboratories. In general, most hypnotic drugs reduce the amount of REM and slow-wave sleep and increase total sleep time.

Depressive Disorders

Prevalence. Serious depressive disorders should be referred for psychiatric care, as the morbidity is great and mortality, by suicide, is appreciable. Many depressed patients are seen by general physicians. A host of complaints mask the true disorder. Patients with many vague, unexplainable symptoms, affecting multiple organ systems, as well as those considered to be "crocks" with visits to many clinics, should be suspected of being depressed.

An epidemiologic survey in three communities found major depression to vary over a 6-month period from 2.2% to 3.5%, with minor depression (dysthymia) ranging between 2.1% and 3.8%. The lifetime prevalence of each was estimated as between 3.7% and 6.7%, and 2.1% and 3.8%, respectively (Myers et al., 1984; Robins et al., 1984). These estimates are somewhat less than

previous ones but still indicate a fairly high prevalence.

Etiologic Considerations

1. **Heterogeneity.** Depressions may have two
major bases, one psychologic and the other
genetic-biochemical. Psychologically, most depressions involve a feeling of loss. Anger engendered by the loss may be directed inward, with
feelings of worthlessness and guilt, or outward,
with expressions of hostility. Some psychological
treatments are directed at helping patients express
this repressed rage.

The depression evoked by reserpine suggested
that depression may have a biochemical basis.
Reserpine reduces stores of biogenic amines and
produces depression. Therefore, depression is
thought to be associated with reduced biogenic
amines. This simple syllogism was the basis for
the amine hypothesis of depression. *Principle.
Unwanted effects of drugs may sometimes provide clues to the pathogenesis of naturally occurring disorders. Another example would be the
Parkinson syndrome induced by some antipsychotic drugs.*

These two mechanisms also suggest the possibility of interaction. Patients with a genetic predisposition for depression may develop clinical
manifestations only when experiencing psychological stress. The biochemical basis may be a necessary but not sufficient condition for the phenotypic expression of depression.

2. **Amine Hypothesis.** The idea that deficient
biogenic amines may be related to depression was
given additional support by the action of antidepressant drugs (Green, 1987). Tricyclic antidepressants, as well as some of the "second-
generation" drugs, inhibit the uptake of these
amines, especially serotonin and norepinephrine.
Monoamine oxidase (MAO) inhibitors block their
catabolism. Sympathomimetics also increase the
availability of catecholamines at synapses. Thus,
all three possible treatments, in differing ways,
increase available neurotransmitter. The secondary effect of such increase is a compensatory decrease, or *down-regulation*, of postsynaptic receptors (Byerley et al., 1988). Nonetheless, direct
proof of the amine hypothesis has been difficult,
and, despite its heuristic value, it is still a hypothesis.

3. **Other Possibilities.** Many basic bodily
rhythms involving hunger, sleep, sexual desire,
and motor activity are altered in depression. This
has suggested that depression might be caused by
alteration of diurnal rhythms. Attempts have
been made to treat depression by advancing the
phase of sleep–wake cycles with variable success.

The fact that some patients seem to experience
depression associated with seasonal changes also
suggests some disturbance of bodily rhythms.
Winter depression is more common than summer
depression. It is believed to be due to more darkness during the winter months and has been
treated with exposure to bright light.

Biologic Correlates of Depression. Several biologic abnormalities have been associated to varying degrees with depression and have kindled
hope for a diagnostic test. The one most widely
studied has been nonsuppression of cortisol concentrations by dexamethasone. This escape from
suppression by the exogenous corticosteroid occurs in only about 50% of depressed patients, so
its sensitivity is low. It was first thought to be
highly specific, but more experience has shown
similar nonsuppression in manic, alcoholic, and
Alzheimer disease patients (Nierenberg and
Feinstein, 1988).

A blunted response of thyrotropin (TSH) to
thyrotropin-releasing hormone (TRH) has been
repeatedly found in 25% to 35% of depressed
patients. The development of increasingly sensitive assays for TSH may determine whether such
responses indicate subclinical hyperthyroidism.
On the other hand, patients who show an exaggerated response, which might be interpreted as
"subsubclinical hypothyroidism," have been said
to need supplements of liothyronine. Thyroid
function in depression is far from settled.

In about 80% of depressed patients studied in
the sleep laboratory, the first epoch of REM sleep
occurs in less than 60 minutes, as contrasted with
the usual time of about 90 minutes. This reduced
latency of REM sleep may be related to the disturbed diurnal rhythms mentioned above.

The excretion of a metabolite of norepinephrine, 3-methoxy-4-hydroxyphenylethylene glycol
(MHPG), has been said to be both "low" and
"high" in depressed patients. Those with low values are said to require drugs that block uptake
of norepinephrine while those with high rates of
excretion require drugs that block uptake of serotonin. Unfortunately, the range of such excretion
in normal persons covers the entire range reported
in depressed patients (Hollister et al., 1978).

Clinical Classification; Diagnosis. The nosol-
ogy of depression has been characterized by a variety of names that seem to change constantly.
Currently both *unipolar* (formerly *endogenous*)
and *bipolar* (formerly *manic-depressive*) depressions are lumped into the category *major affective
disorder*, the type being specified. Minor variants
of each are called *dysthymia* and *cyclothymic disorder*, respectively.

A depressed mood is less often the patient's
chief complaint than are somatic symptoms.

Thus, many depressed patients are first seen by general physicians rather than psychiatrists. Depression and anxiety are inextricable, leading often to the misdiagnosis of one of the anxiety disorders. Somatic complaints, besides those due to disturbed bodily rhythms, may affect multiple organ systems. Guilt is almost unique to depression. Depressed mood is, of course, the major diagnostic manifestation. Until the advent of AIDS, depression was well on its way to supplant syphilis and tuberculosis as the "great imitator."

Manic-Depressive Disorder

Nature and Prevalence. An elevated, expansive, or irritable mood is the primary characteristic of mania. Such elevations of mood may on other occasions be replaced by depressed mood, although the sequences between mania and depression may vary from one patient to another. The older name *manic-depressive disorder* was much more descriptive than the recent term, *bipolar mood disorder*. The diagnosis is established by the presence of a manic episode.

This affliction occurs in slightly less than 1% of the general population. Onset may be at any age but is most common in the third decade of life. Episodes are almost always recurrent with considerable morbidity and an appreciable mortality. In some patients, episodes assume a crescendo pattern with increased frequency and shorter symptom-free intervals. This pattern, as well as the response of some patients to anticonvulsants, has led to the *kindling* hypothesis (induction of seizures by repeated subthreshold stimuli). However, it has been impossible to prove this mechanism for the disorder (Post, 1987).

Possible Mechanism of Manic-Depressive Disorder. Because the disorder tends to run in families, a number of investigations have attempted to identify a genetic locus. Genetic linkage studies have reported an association with the X chromosome as well as two loci on chromosome 11 (Mendelwiez et al., 1987; Baron et al., 1987; Egeland et al., 1987). However, other studies have failed to identify a genetic marker. Thus, the issue is unresolved, or perhaps begged by assuming that the disorder may be heterogeneous.

A number of neurotransmitters have been implicated in mania, but none is paramount. Neuroleptics, which block dopamine receptors, are usually somewhat effective, pointing to involvement of dopamine. As mania has been induced by tricyclic antidepressants, which increase noradrenergic or serotonergic activity, these transmitters may also be involved. Increasing cholinergic activity has also been found to alleviate mania. A variety of disturbances of circadian rhythms have been

noted, but whether these are primary or secondary to the disorder remains uncertain.

Because of the more serious import and prognosis of manic disorder, it is likely that such patients should be referred to a biologically minded psychiatrist for management. Many episodes require hospitalization; even during periods of remission, patients require close clinical monitoring.

Schizophrenia

Nature and Prevalence. Modern concepts of schizophrenia were developed at the beginning of this century. Kraepelin (1905) considered significant hallmarks of the disorder to be negativisms, mannerisms, stereotypes, disturbances of volition, disruption of judgment, discrepancy between mood and the general reaction, peculiar attention and thinking disorders, and a deterioration of a differentiation between the real and the unreal. In more vernacular terms, patients appear to be crazy. Whether schizophrenia is a single disorder with multiple degrees of severity and manifestations, or whether it is a syndrome whose clinical manifestations represent a number of disorders of differing pathogenesis, remains unclear. Bleuler (1950) subscribed to the notion that schizophrenia is a syndrome, that is, a "group of schizophrenias."

Various subclassifications have been proposed: *paranoid, catatonic, disorganized, undifferentiated*, and *residual* are terms still used. Most clinicians try to make distinctions mainly between paranoid versus nonparanoid or undifferentiated types. Although not all patients suffer a chronic, deteriorating course, one makes the diagnosis with some trepidation because of the generally poor prognosis.

A more recent classification has proposed *organic* and *functional* types. The organic type is manifested by atrophy of various portions of the brain as shown by imaging techniques and is associated with a preponderance of negative symptoms (affective flattening and poverty of speech) and a poor response to drug therapy. The functional type is construed as representing some functional disorder of dopaminergic neurotransmission. It is manifested by positive symptoms (delusions, hallucinations, and thought disorder) but responds in varying degrees to antipsychotic drugs (Crow, 1980).

The 6-month prevalence rate for schizophrenia in three urban U.S. samples ranged from 0.6% to 1.1% for schizophrenia and from 0.1% to 0.2% for schizophreniform disorders (Myers et al., 1984). Lifetime prevalence rates were 1.0% to 1.9% and 0.1% to 0.3%, respectively (Robins et al., 1984). Such estimates are close to those made earlier, which suggested that about 1% to 2% of the population is susceptible to developing a schizophrenia-like psychosis at some time in their lives.

The burden of schizophrenia far outweighs its prevalence. The disorder tends to occur early in life and may last an entire lifetime. The cost in economic terms of supporting and treating patients is huge. The cost in personal tragedy, not only for the affected person but also for friends and family, is incalculable.

Possible Pathogenesis. The postulated mechanisms for producing schizophrenia have been numerous, as is usually the case in conditions that are poorly understood. The wide ranges of postulated disorders are summarized in Table 13-2. None has been proved or conclusively disproved.

The dopaminergic hypothesis, which postulates that for one reason or another dopaminergic activity is increased in the mesolimbic system of the brain, is the bedrock on which drug therapy is founded (McKenna, 1987). Evidence has been circumstantial: schizophrenia-like disorders have followed use of drugs that work through dopaminergic mechanisms (amphetamine psychosis); all effective antipsychotic drugs seem to act by blocking postsynaptic dopamine receptors; schizophrenia may be aggravated by dopamine precursors, such as levodopa, by dopamine releasers, such as amphetamines, and by dopamine-receptor agonists, such as apomorphine. Direct links to a

Table 13-2. SOME POSTULATED MECHANISMS FOR SCHIZOPHRENIA

Dopaminergic overactivity
  ? Increased dopamine receptors found at postmortem and demonstrated in vivo with PET scans
  Improvement with dopamine-receptor blocking drugs
Other catecholamine abnormalities
  ? β-Phenethylamine increased in CSF
  ? Improvement with β-adrenoreceptor blocking drugs
Indolealkylamine abnormalities
  Improvement with serotonin-receptor blocking drugs
Genetic factors
  Concordance rate in 50% of identical twins
  Concordance in 20% of first-degree relatives
Viral disease
  Season of birth, increased during winter
  ? Viral particles in CSF, cells of brain
Autoimmune disorders
  ? Antibrain antibodies
Structural and metabolic abnormalities
  Variable brain atrophy on CT and MRI scans
  Variable decrease in brain metabolism on PET scans
Environment
  Stress and emotional factors
  Parental influences

dopaminergic abnormality have been more difficult to establish (Reynolds, 1989). A search still continues for other possible mechanisms of drug action that may elucidate the problem of the biochemical pathogenesis of schizophrenia. This approach has been greatly stimulated by the well-established efficacy of clozapine, an atypical antipsychotic. This drug has only weak dopamine-receptor blocking activity but has a broader spectrum of effects on other receptor systems. Thus, the spectrum of pharmacologic actions may be more important than is an action on any single neurotransmitter or receptor system.

Unsolved Problems. An appraisal of the major public health problems in the United States at midcentury listed schizophrenia along with alcoholism, hypertension, arteriosclerosis, and cancer. It is rather disappointing that 4 decades later so little progress has been made in understanding the cause of schizophrenia and in advancing its treatment. Although in the 1950s one out of every four hospital beds was occupied by a schizophrenic patient, that problem has been solved: by turning psychiatric patients loose in the community, the numbers still hospitalized have decreased by 80% to 90%.

One of the great hopes is that molecular genetic approaches may identify a gene or genes associated with schizophrenia and that by finding ways to counter the gene product treat the disorder more rationally. Thus far, attempts to establish genetic linkages have been controversial. Part of the problem has been the difficulty in finding strongly affected families, both due to the comparative rarity of the condition and the disruption and dispersal of such families caused by the illness.

Childhood and Adolescent Disorders

Nature and Prevalence. Diagnosis of psychiatric disorders in children and adolescents is complicated by the fact that one is dealing with a developing person. Furthermore, the manifestations of such disorders in these age groups may be somewhat different from those of adult disorders. Finally, clinicians are much less keen about using definitive diagnostic terms in young persons because the mere fact of labeling may affect the future development of the person.

Because of these difficulties, no precise estimates of the prevalence of childhood disorders have been made. Although a surprising number of children and adolescents are hospitalized in psychiatric institutions at any given point in time, it is difficult to tell how many of them have true psychiatric disorders as opposed to problems in living. The best data probably pertain to the various forms of mental retardation, which are most clearly diagnosable even though the cause of the majority of instances remains obscure.

Disorders in Common with Adults. So far as one can tell, most of the common psychiatric disorders of adults can also be found in children and adolescents. Thus, one can make a diagnosis of anxiety disorders, depression, mania, and schizophrenia. However, these diagnoses are made far less commonly in children for reasons mentioned above. Anxiety in childhood may be manifested by a variety of behaviors, possibly labeled initially with the rather nonspecific term *conduct disorder*. Depression is more apparent in adolescence, being manifested tragically by the fact that suicide is a major cause of death in this age group. Schizophrenia characteristically tends to become evident in late adolescence and early adult life; earlier on, it may be mistaken for anxiety disorders. Mania may occur in children but is more likely first to be misdiagnosed as attention deficit/hyperactivity disorder (ADHD).

Disorders Peculiar to Children and Adolescents. Attention deficit/hyperactivity disorder usually becomes evident in the early school years. The pathogenesis is uncertain, but it is highly amenable to treatment. *Principle: One does not have to understand the cause of a disorder to treat it effectively.* Longer-term follow-up studies indicate that it may persist during adult life. Autism used to be considered to be a form of childhood schizophrenia but is now considered to be entirely separate. It may or may not be associated with mental retardation. A variety of other conditions have also been described. Conduct disorder is a diagnosis made frequently (about 4% of boys), but its boundaries are not clear; it may often be a "wastebasket" diagnosis. Enuresis is mainly found in children and declines with advancing years. Anorexia and bulimia are most likely to become evident during adolescence. Tourette syndrome, the "barking tic," usually first becomes recognized in adolescence. Narcolepsy can be recognized in adolescents, although its diagnosis may be deferred until adult life.

Unsolved Problems. One normally has some reluctance to start drug therapy early in life. Thus, systematic experience with the advantages and disadvantages of drug therapy in children and adolescents is not nearly as well developed as it is in adults. The use of drugs for treating some disorders, such as attention deficit, or hyperactivity syndrome, and enuresis, is well established. For many other disorders there is insufficient experience to determine the risk/benefit ratios. Fortunately, the successes of drug therapy in children

have engendered a more liberal attitude about such treatment and should expand the presently deficient knowledge.

Disorders in Old Age

Nature and Prevalence. Projections of an increasing population of aged persons in developed countries have been interpreted by some as indicating an impending "silent epidemic" of Alzheimer disease. This disease, also sometimes called *primary degenerative dementia* or *senile dementia of the Alzheimer type*, has become a major focus of inquiry, into both its causes and its treatment. Some evidence suggests that the disease may be heterogeneous. Early-onset forms (age below 58 years) are known to occur and seem to follow an autosomal-dominant mode of transmission. Later-onset forms, which may affect 10% of the population over 85 years of age, may be blamed on both a genetic predisposition and environmental influences (Davies, 1986). The progression of the disease may also vary from rapid to slow. The association of Alzheimer neuropathologic changes with Down syndrome has pointed a finger of suspicion at chromosome 21, which is triplicated in Down syndrome. This chromosome seems to be the locus of the β-amyloid gene, and amyloid deposits are a prominent part of the neuropathologic lesions, but whether the Alzheimer gene is located on this chromosome is unknown.

The only secure diagnosis of Alzheimer disease is neuropathologic, which hardly suffices for the clinician. Error rates for the clinical diagnosis of probable Alzheimer disease have varied from 5% to 25%, depending on the series. A great number of potentially reversible causes of dementias of old age have been reported, which creates a problem in determining how much medical workup is required. In general, most reversible causes are found in younger patients; an insidious onset of dementia in older patients is almost always due to Alzheimer disease. The two psychiatric states most likely to be confused are delirium and depression. Delirium is almost always associated with concurrent drugs or concomitant medical illness (Francis et al., 1990). Depression may create a pseudodementia, but close inquiry into cognitive functions shows a disparity between the degree of social withdrawal and the cognitive impairment.

Other Psychiatric Disorders of Old Age. Multiinfarct dementia may occur after a succession of small strokes that do not present with customary major neurologic impairments. Mental disturbances may be episodic with declines following each episode of infarct; these may be temporary or become stable until the next episode. As Alzheimer disease and cerebral arteriosclerosis often occur together in the same patient, the determination of which predominates may not always be clear, but imaging studies may help.

Some elderly patients with little history of prior psychiatric disorder develop a paranoid state. If other signs of schizophrenia are present, one may be dealing with a late-onset form of paranoid schizophrenia, so-called paraphrenia. On the other hand, one may be dealing with an affective disorder if mood changes predominate.

Elderly patients may also become highly hypochondriacal, becoming so obsessed with some bodily function as to appear somewhat psychotic. Usually, however, this problem is not difficult to recognize, although it may be difficult to treat.

Unsolved Problems. An extensive search for peripheral biologic markers of Alzheimer disease has not yet established any as clinically useful. Present investigations focus around peripheral deposits of amyloid around small blood vessels, such as might be examined by a skin biopsy, or the presence of a unique protein in the cerebrospinal fluid. As it is unlikely that any treatment possible in the near term could reverse the pathologic lesions of well-established Alzheimer disease, earlier detection might allow a potential treatment to show a greater effect. Ultimately, we should like to know better the pathogenetic mechanisms by which the degeneration of neurons and neurites occurs.

DRUG THERAPY OF PSYCHIATRIC DISORDERS

Overview of Current Drug Therapy

Discovery. It is somewhat paradoxical that serendipity has played a significant role in the drug treatment of psychiatric disorders. Reserpine was noted to have unusual sedative effects while being used for treating hypertensives, resurrecting the empirical observation of ayurvedic medicine that the drug is useful for "manic" states. Chlorpromazine was initially synthesized for potentiation of analgesics; it was first used clinically in a "lytic cocktail" for anesthesia. Again, its unusual mental effects led to its employment in treatment of schizophrenia. Iproniazid had an elating effect in patients treated for pulmonary tuberculosis, yet its potential use as an antidepressant was almost lost. As iproniazid had been rapidly replaced by isoniazid for treating pulmonary tuberculosis, a number of studies used the latter drug for treating treating depression, with negative results. Only when it was discovered that iproniazid, but not isoniazid, inhibits the enzyme MAO was the full potential of the

group of MAO inhibitors realized. Imipramine was synthesized to be an antipsychotic, the ring structure having been modified to a 6-7-6 configuration to differ from the 6-6-6 configuration of chlorpromazine. Clinical observation indicated that it has little value as an antipsychotic but that it alleviates depressive symptoms. Synthesis of benzodiazepines defied the chemical prediction for the reaction; this previously unknown type of compound was found to be sedative and quickly moved into clinical practice. Lithium urate was used in an experiment to determine how uric acid might modify the toxic effects in rats of urea in the urine of patients with mania. Somewhat surprisingly, lithium urate, as well as lithium carbonate, had a calming action in the animals that suggested use of the latter compound in manic patients. The rationale may have been wrong, but good observation made the discovery. *Principle: Pasteur's injunction that "chance favors the prepared mind" has been shown repeatedly to be true in the discovery of psychotherapeutic drugs.*

Multiple Drugs. As each new class of drugs was discovered, many chemical homologs were synthesized. Therapeutic effects were similar, but sometimes potency was increased or a modified array of side effects was achieved. Probably more than 100 phenothiazines with antipsychotic effects are known throughout the world. The pharmacologic properties of the original member, chlorpromazine, led to a battery of screening tests that discovered new chemicals but old drugs. A minor modification of the side chain of phenothiazines resulted in the thioxanthene group. Haloperidol, the first of a variety of butyrophenones, was somewhat atypical, not only in being highly potent but also in having a more specific spectrum of pharmacologic actions. The truly atypical antipsychotic drug clozapine was one of several compounds with a somewhat different chemical structure that still fulfilled requirements of screening tests for antipsychotic drugs.

A similar multiplication occurred among other classes of drugs. The number of tricyclic antidepressants or related compounds increased dramatically. Most were discovered because they blocked uptake of aminergic neurotransmitters, such as norepinephrine or serotonin. Another approach sought compounds with specific blocking action on the uptake of serotonin; the result was the increasing group of such drugs, exemplified by fluoxetine. Bupropion, which might be considered an attenuated amphetamine, has raised the question of a role for dopamine in depression.

Nowhere has the multiplicity of homologs been more evident than in the class of benzodiazepines. Just when one thinks that no more can possibly be found that are different, a drug such as midazolam, which is ultrashort-acting and water-soluble, appears on the scene. Whether the benzodiazepine era is at an end, to be supplanted by drugs of the buspirone type, remains to be seen. Buspirone, which has a structure resembling that of a butyrophenone, was synthesized as a potential antipsychotic. After it failed that use, its antianxiety effects were discovered.

Lithium remains the basic drug for treating mania, but carbamazepine is now considered to be a suitable alternative. The latter drug was discovered on the simplistic notion that because both mania and seizures are episodic, an anticonvulsant drug might have antimanic action. This concept has been incorporated into the kindling hypothesis of mania. A variety of other anticonvulsant drugs are currently under investigation.

These developments have had the consequence that clinicians now have an abundance of drugs from which to choose for treating various psychiatric disorders. The advantages of having such a wide choice are several: (1) patients may respond to one drug better than to another; the clinician can successively try drugs to determine which best meets the patient's need; unfortunately, there is no way to predict in advance which drug may be best for a given patient; and (2) some patients are better able to tolerate the side effects of one drug than another, even though both drugs may be equally effective. This wide choice allows attempts not only to find the most effective drug for an individual patient but also to identify the one best tolerated. A disadvantage is that physicians may be overwhelmed by the sheer number of these drugs; it is difficult even for those of us in the field to remember the generic and trade names, the doses, and the dosage forms of so many compounds. *Principle: Whenever there is an abundance of drugs for treating an illness, it is better to learn to use a few well than to attempt to use them all at the risk of doing so poorly.*

Limitations of Current Drugs. No therapeutic area has ideal drugs; psychiatric disorders are no exception. Antipsychotic drugs have revolutionized the treatment of psychotic persons, perhaps too much so. The reduction of the number of state hospital beds during the 1960s had a consequence recognized during the 1980s of producing a plethora of homeless mentally ill persons on the streets of our major cities. Even under the best conditions, antipsychotic drugs benefit only 60% to 65% of patients, and remissions are far from complete. Not only that, but the specter of the neurologic complication tardive dyskinesia is ever-present and has rapidly become a major source of litigation. Clozapine may be able to salvage some patients who have been refractory to the conventional antipsychotics, but it has the

major disadvantage of a life-threatening complication, agranulocytosis. As currently marketed, with mandatory expensive laboratory monitoring to protect against this complication, it seems likely that only a small fraction of patients who might potentially benefit from the drug will obtain it.

Antidepressants, too, are effective in only 65% to 70% of patients and seldom lead to complete recovery. The efficacy of these drugs in large groups of patients is roughly equivalent, with no substantial increase during the past 30 years. All have major side effects that limit their acceptance by patients; noncompliance with treatment is the major cause for relapse. Many antidepressants are potentially lethal in overdose, a consideration of importance for depressed patients.

It is generally agreed that benzodiazepines are effective for alleviating anxiety, but spontaneous fluctuations in this disorder have often led to relatively few demonstrable differences from placebo in comparative studies. The problems of dependence when these drugs are abused was recognized early in their use, but the new concept of *therapeutic-dose dependence* has put some desirable limitations on the amount of exposure to these drugs. Buspirone may mitigate this problem, but the lack of overt sedation, rather than being an advantage, seems to be a disadvantage for patients who have sleep problems.

Lithium has been relatively safe but also is not effective in all patients. Carbamazepine is no more effective overall but may help patients unresponsive to lithium. As keeping patients on medication is a most difficult problem with manic patients, the fact that neither of these drugs is available in any long-acting IM preparation limits their utility.

The number of available psychotherapeutic drugs has increased markedly during the past 35 years. However, increased efficacy has been difficult to attain, and reduced side effects have been limited to a relatively few. The ideal drug still remains elusive.

ANTIANXIETY DRUGS

Types

To date, seven different classes of drugs have been used for treating anxiety. The classic *sedative-hypnotic* type includes old drugs, such as phenobarbital and meprobamate, as well as the increasing number of benzodiazepines. A group that might be called *sedative-autonomic*, because of that combination of pharmacologic properties, includes sedative antihistamines as well as antipsychotics and tricyclic antidepressants used in small doses. Finally, a new class, which might be termed *nonsedating anxiolytics*, is exemplified by buspirone and its congeners. Some of the chemical structures of representatives of these classes are shown in Fig. 13–1.

Pharmacodynamics

The discovery of the GABA-benzodiazepine-receptor complex has provided a new basis for the understanding of the mode of action of these drugs as well as others in the sedative-hypnotic group. The complex, a tetramer or pentamer, surrounds a channel for the passage of chloride ions. Binding of GABA opens the chloride channel and allows chloride ions to hyperpolarize the cell, reducing the likelihood of its firing (Fig. 13–2). Benzodiazepines, which bind at a different locus on the complex, merely facilitate the physiologic action of GABA (Tallman et al., 1980). Although other potential mechanisms of action have been described for the benzodiazepines, either as a group or for individual drugs, this mechanism seems to be the most pertinent to their usual therapeutic uses. It is possible that barbiturates and other conventional sedative-hypnotics operate through a similar mechanism.

Buspirone represents a novel drug, both chemically and pharmacologically. Its structure is reminiscent of a butyrophenone, and its first clinical application was as an antipsychotic. It has neither overt sedative, hypnotic, nor autonomic actions. Its major proposed mechanism of action is by blocking 5-HT$_{1A}$ receptors; it also has weak dopamine D$_2$-receptor blocking action (Taylor, 1988). Because of its lack of sedative effects, it has not been abused, and withdrawal reactions are unknown. Most patients who have been treated with benzodiazepines prefer them, which has limited the use of buspirone.

Pharmacokinetics and Metabolism

Although various benzodiazepines are promoted for differing uses (sedative, hypnotic, antipanic, antidepressant, muscle relaxant, anticonvulsant, anesthetic), much of the selectivity is based on commercial considerations. Although a few pharmacodynamic differences have been reported, especially for alprazolam, clonazepam, and lorazepam, these are neither terribly compelling nor of any demonstrated clinical significance.

Pharmacokinetic differences are more pronounced (Greenblatt and Shader, 1985). Benzodiazepines can be classified, on the basis of plasma half-life, as very short acting (midazolam), short-acting (triazolam), intermediate-acting (alprazolam), long-acting (diazepam), and very long acting (flurazepam). These differences in plasma half-life do not always accurately define the clinical span of action of these drugs, but can be used

as guides. Table 13–3 summarizes pharmacokinetic characteristics of various antianxiety drugs.

Differences in metabolism have dubious clinical importance. Drugs that require only glucuronide formation (oxazepam, lorazepam) are said to be safer in patients whose drug-metabolizing capacity may be diminished, such as the elderly or those with liver damage. On the other hand, a traditional way of handling these situations might be to use a slightly smaller dose and to increase the dosing interval. Many of these drugs have active metabolites, nordiazepam being the major one for diazepam, chlordiazepoxide, clorazepate, prazepam, and halazepam. In fact, the latter three drugs are best considered as prodrugs for nordiazepam. When diazepam is given chronically, its active metabolite, nordiazepam, becomes more prevalent than the parent drug. As nordiazepam has a rather long half-life, while the half-life of diazepam is rather brief, the net result is that diazepam becomes a long-acting drug, even though its half-life is relatively short. This example indicates why determination of half-life alone is not always a good indicator of duration of action.

Pharmaceutical preparations may influence the uses of these drugs. Midazolam is water-soluble and is easily administered IV. Combined with its short duration of action, this property allows its exploitation as an IV anesthetic. Some drugs (diazepam, chlordiazepoxide), because of the diluent required, are not highly available when given IM. On the other hand, lorazepam is both well tolerated and highly available when given by that route.

Buspirone has a rather short half-life. Consequently, several divided doses each day are recommended. Whether this dosage schedule is really required has not been tested.

Therapeutic Indications

The extended concept of anxiety disorders has widened the scope of drugs useful in treating them. For most, antianxiety drugs will be the main treatment.

Generalized Anxiety Disorder. Formerly, virtually all anxiety was included under this diagnosis. Since the current fad for panic disorder, even the existence of generalized anxiety disorder has been questioned; it was not included as a possible diagnosis in the ECA Survey. General physicians will probably recognize this diagnosis more often and will tend to use either benzodiazepines or buspirone to treat it. Uniformly, it is found that patients who have previously been treated with benzodiazepines do not readily accept buspirone.

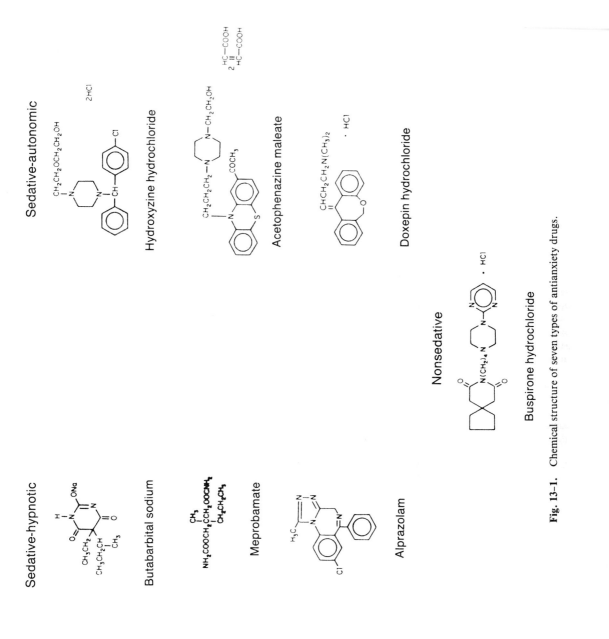

Fig. 13–1. Chemical structure of seven types of antianxiety drugs.

349

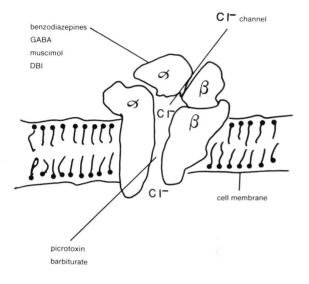

Fig. 13-2. Schematic representation of benzodiazepine-GABA-Cl⁻-channel macromolecular complex, tetrameric structure of two different proteins. Binding of benzodiazepines, comparable to that of GABA, opens the ion channel. Entry of Cl⁻ hyperpolarizes the cell. DBI = diazepam binding inhibitor.

On the other hand, patients being newly treated might find buspirone more acceptable (Olajida and Lader, 1987).

If a benzodiazepine is to be used, the physician should choose whichever one the patient previously found to be effective. Other than that guideline, there is little reason to choose among those indicated for anxiety. The principles outlined above should be followed.

Panic Disorder. *Panic* is the name that has been given to acute anxiety attacks that border on fear. It has existed under a variety of names over the past century, most recently as "neurocirculatory asthenia." The attacks can be quite frightening as well as embarrassing. Thus, some patients develop a secondary agoraphobia. Imipramine was found in the mid-1960s to be useful in treating this disorder. Later phenelzine, an MAO inhibitor, was also found to be effective. Alprazolam has been extensively studied as a treatment, and it is effective (treatment response about 65%–70% versus 30%–35% for placebo). The doses used have been quite high, sometimes enough to place the patient at risk of dependence. Weaning patients away from this drug is not easy, and relapse of panic attacks is frequent (Fyer et al., 1987). It now appears that an antipanic action is not unique to alprazolam but may be shown with other benzodiazepines, such as lorazepam and clonazepam, given in equivalent doses. While it might have been expected that a benzodiazepine would be effective in this manifestation of acute anxiety, just why the other drugs, such as tricyclics and MAO inhibitors, with markedly different mechanisms of action, are equally effective is unknown.

Agoraphobia. Fear of public places is the most common phobia. Previously, agoraphobia was considered to be of psychological origin. Now it is more often considered to be secondary to acute anxiety. The same drugs mentioned for treating panic disorder may be useful, as well as behavioral techniques aimed at desensitizing the fear.

Social Phobias. Fear of scrutiny by others is often associated with generalized anxiety disorder, which might be treated as indicated above. Or one may choose to use benzodiazepines in an ad hoc manner for situations that are likely to provoke this phobia.

Specific Phobias. Fear of specific stimuli, such as snakes, dogs, and others, is effectively treated with behavioral techniques.

Obsessive-Compulsive Disorder. Intrusive thoughts or a compelling urge to repeat meaningless rituals can be highly disabling. Whether this diagnosis belongs under the anxiety rubric may be questioned. It is currently believed to represent some sort of dysfunction of the basal ganglia. Usual antianxiety drugs have been of little help. A tricyclic antidepressant, clomipramine, has demonstrated efficacy. Because this drug works primarily through serotonin, it now is believed that this neurotransmitter plays some role (Rapoport, 1988). Other specific serotonin-uptake inhibitors, such as fluoxetine, have also been helpful.

Other Indications. Use of benzodiazepines as hypnotics is discussed separately. Other indica-

Table 13-3. PHARMACOKINETIC PARAMETERS AND DOSES OF COMMONLY USED ANTIANXIETY DRUGS

DRUG	$T_{1/2b}$ (H)	V_D (L/KG)	PROTEIN BINDING (%)	ACTIVE METABOLITES	$T_{1/2b}$ (H)	THERAPEUTIC CONCENTRATION (NG/ML)	DOSE (MG/DAY)
Very Short Acting							
Buspirone (Buspar)	2.5–3.0			1-Pyrimadylpiperazine (1-PP)			5–40
Short Acting							
Alprazolam (Xanax)	6–20	0.7–0.8	85	None			0.75–4
Lorazepam (Ativan)	9–22	0.7–1.0	86	None			2–6
Oxazepam (Serax)	6–24	0.6–1.6					30–180
Intermediate Acting							
Chlordiazepoxide (Librium)	10–29	0.3–0.6	93	Nordiazepam Desmoxepam Desoxydemoxepam	10–18 28–63 39–61		15–100
Clonazepam (Klonopin)	19–42						1–3
Diazepam (Valium)	14–61	0.7–2.6	98	Nordiazepam	36–200	400–1200	4–40
Halazepam (Paxipam)	9–28	0.1–1.3	98	Nordiazepam	36–200		20–160
Long Acting							
Clorazepate (Tranxene)		1.0–1.3	98	Nordiazepam	36–200	430	15–60
Prazepam (Centrax)		1.0–1.3	98	Nordiazepam	36–200	430	15–30

tions, which may be more familiar to the general physician than to psychiatrists, are mentioned here.

1. **Somatoform Disorders.** This is a new name for what were formerly called "psychophysiologic reactions," or what most general physicians recognized as "functional" disorders. Although these are common in the general practice of medicine, they were virtually missed in the ECA Survey. As most prescribing of benzodiazepines is done by nonpsychiatrists, it would follow that much of this use is for disorders of this type.

2. **Muscle Spasm.** Whether drugs can relieve muscle spasm by a central action other than sedation has always been questioned. The GABAergic action of benzodiazepines provides some rationale for their use, as GABA decreases the firing of motor neurons in the spinal cord via presynaptic inhibition.

3. **Alcohol Withdrawal.** Benzodiazepines are cross-tolerant with alcohol as well as being effective anticonvulsants. They have now replaced older sedatives for alleviating alcohol withdrawal. Although other types of drugs, such as clonidine or carbamazepine, have been effective, it still makes more sense to use benzodiazepines.

4. **Uncontrolled Seizures.** Intravenously administered benzodiazepines afford prompt relief with less respiratory depression than other sedatives. Because of their brief duration of effect, they must be followed with loading doses of phenytoin. Diazepam used to be the preferred drug for this indication, but lorazepam and midazolam are better tolerated when given by vein.

5. **Intravenous Anesthetic.** A short-acting IV anesthetic is useful for induction of general anesthesia, and for endoscopies, reduction of minor fractures, electric cardioversion, or dental surgery. Lorazepam and midazolam are now the preferred agents.

6. **Control of Agitation in Psychotic Patients.** The combination of a sedative-hypnotic drug with an antipsychotic has long been used for this purpose. Either IM lorazepam or sodium phenobarbital may be used (Garza-Trevino et al., 1989).

Principles of Use

Because of their controversial nature, benzodiazepines should be used prudently. Increasingly, malpractice actions are based on claims that a patient was made dependent on these drugs by his or her physician. The following principles should permit effective but safe use of these drugs:

1. The decision to use these drugs should be based on the degree of discomfort or disability that patients experience. Both can be consider-

able. As in any other branch of medicine, it is well to establish a working diagnosis and to document it in the patient's records. Patients should share in the decision to begin treatment.

2. Just because drug treatment is being started does not rule out the effective use of nonpharmacologic treatments. Some sort of psychotherapy might be indicated. Environmental manipulation to reduce stressors is often overlooked. Many patients find that a period of exercise during the day or meditation in the evening allays their symptoms. No evidence suggests that drugs interfere in any way with these treatment approaches.

3. The physician should propose to the patients that treatment courses will likely be brief and interrupted, allowing them to regain control of their lives and only treating episodes of anxiety. Usually a course of 2 to 3 weeks of treatment should provide near-maximal relief of symptoms. It is much easier at that time to get the patient to accept a period without drugs than after they have been treated for 6 months.

4. Extensive pharmacokinetic studies have shown that both maximal and steady-state plasma concentrations following chronic doses vary widely between individuals given the same dose. Doses should be titrated on the basis of the clinical effects the patient experiences and not chosen arbitrarily from the *Physicians' Desk Reference*. Nor do doses need to be divided equally throughout the day. A more sensible schedule might be to give the major dose at night, essentially as a hypnotic, with as-needed daytime doses in fractional amounts. The range of daily doses of various antianxiety drugs is shown in Table 13–3.

5. The response to treatment should be monitored carefully. Failure to respond may signify a misdiagnosis. Anxiety is a ubiquitous symptom and is quite often found in patients with depression or in the early stages of schizophrenia. Always consider other possibilities when symptoms remain unabated.

6. Patients should be warned that until their responses to the drug and dose are known, they should avoid potentially dangerous activities, especially close to the time of taking the drug. They may also have less tolerance for alcohol or other CNS depressants. Most of all, if they have been taking the drug for more than a few weeks, they should never stop it abruptly lest they experience a withdrawal reaction.

7. Benzodiazepines should be avoided in patients with any indication of alcohol or drug abuse. Other drugs of the sedative-autonomic type or buspirone would be better choices, as these are not abused. Limit amounts prescribed to those compatible with the planned dosage so that abuse becomes impossible.

Controversies about Use of Benzodiazepines

For most of the past 30 years, one or another benzodiazepine has been close to the top in number of prescriptions. Diazepam long was the most prescribed drug in the United States. Recently, its popularity has diminished, so that alprazolam and lorazepam are more popular. The almost exponential increase in use of these drugs since the introduction of diazepam in 1963 raised some concerns. However, two surveys sponsored by the National Institute of Mental Health have come up with somewhat reassuring findings. First, use is not widespread, with only about 15% of the adult population using these drugs at least once during a year and only 6% using them more or less chronically for 1 month or more. These patterns were right in the middle of the range of such use among nine countries of western Europe. Second, the pattern of use followed a medical model. The drugs were prescribed for older patients with high levels of psychic distress (and often concurrent physical illnesses) who seemed to derive considerable benefit from them. No evidence suggested that physicians prescribed them in a casual manner for trivial complaints (Mellinger et al., 1978). Third, the total use of these drugs has declined during the past decade, not so much in the number of people using them as in the amounts used.

Nonetheless, opinions vary widely, and sometimes sharply, about use of these drugs. Some physicians, mainly those in the substance abuse field, find no justification at all for their use, leaving many patients not being treated who might benefit. Each physician has to decide individually what course to follow. *Principle: Controversies are common in therapeutics. Clinical decisions must often be made on the basis of conflicting or imperfect data. Many times decisions are based more on the philosophical bent of the physician than on the evidence at hand.*

Adverse Effects of Benzodiazepines

After almost 30 years of extensive use, benzodiazepines have proved to be remarkably safe. Toxicity involving any of the major organ systems is rare. Virtually all problems have been related to the action on the CNS.

Oversedation. Most patients recognize when they are oversedated and spontaneously reduce the dose. Tolerance develops to this effect over time, so that the same dose that produced overt sedation initially may not after chronic use.

Dependence. Both physical and psychic dependence may occur with chronic use of benzodiazepines. Two types of physical dependence have been recognized. *Classic* dependence occurs in the context of taking excessive doses in an abusive pattern. The great majority of these instances have occurred in patients with other substance abuse problems. The manifestations of withdrawal have been those described for dependence of the alcohol-barbiturate type (Hollister et al., 1961). *Therapeutic-dose* dependence occurs in the context of therapeutic doses taken for rather long periods of time. The product of dose × time seems to determine its occurrence. Manifestations of withdrawal may be subtle and are easily confused with the symptoms being treated (Ladewig, 1984). They are usually qualitatively similar to those of classic dependence. Claims have been made of a protracted-abstinence syndrome, but these are difficult to evaluate. In any case, this type of dependence can be avoided if treatment is interrupted and withdrawal is accomplished gradually. In those patients who require continued treatment to maintain well-being, one may accept the risk of dependence rather than give up therapeutic gains.

Aggravation of Depression. Although benzodiazepines have been used with some success in treating minor depressions, occasional patients experience feelings of depression that are quickly relieved when the drug is discontinued. Some of these patients very likely are prone to become depressed, or may even have been depressed when the drug was prescribed. At the moment, no pharmacologic property of the benzodiazepines would suggest that they are intrinsically "depressogenic."

Release of Hostility. Drugs with disinhibiting effects may release underlying personality characteristics. Although benzodiazepines can do this, the most notable drug in this regard is alcohol.

Other Effects. Probably all benzodiazepines have some degree of amnesic effect. Amnesia could be an advantage when they are used as anesthetic agents. Triazolam has been most troublesome in this respect, although such instances are rare. Alprazolam has provoked mania, which has been adduced as evidence for an antidepressant effect. As the drug is widely used in depressed patients, it seems more likely that patients with manic-depressive disorder may have been erroneously treated with this drug. Hip fractures, especially in the elderly, are increased in patients taking sedatives of any type. Dysmorphogenesis remains an unresolved issue. One would have thought that if it were a major risk it would have become evident by now.

Buspirone. This new drug seems to have relatively few side effects, but experience is still being developed. Some patients have experienced anxiety, restlessness, insomnia, and maniclike symptoms. Digestive complaints are also more common with this drug.

Overdoses. Overdoses of benzodiazepines are remarkably safe. Supportive treatment usually suffices. Respiratory support is rarely needed unless other depressants, such as alcohol, have been ingested. If clinically desired, all the sedative effects can be reversed by a specific benzodiazepine antagonist, flumazenil.

HYPNOTICS

For practical purposes all hypnotic drugs other than benzodiazepines might be considered obsolete. Sedative antihistamines are often found in OTC sleep remedies but are seldom prescribed. Only three benzodiazepines have been marketed specifically as hypnotics, but because all benzodiazepines share many common properties, virtually any may be used as such. Chemical structures of the three, flurazepam, temazepam, and triazolam, are shown in Fig. 13–3.

Pharmacodynamics

Presumably the same mechanism of action accounts for the hypnotic effects as it does for the antianxiety effects. Benzodiazepine-receptor antagonists effectively counter the hypnotic action. A number of hypnotics under clinical investiga-

tion, such as zopiclone and suriclone, are not benzodiazepines but apparently also work through the GABA-benzodiazepine-receptor complex.

The GABA-benzodiazepine complex is not the only mechanism by which sleep may be induced. Blockade of histamine 1 receptors is known to produce sleepiness, which explains the use of such drugs as hypnotics. Blockade of α_1-adrenoreceptors also helps sleep. Sleepiness is also induced by melatonin, the secretion of which is induced by darkness. It would be surprising if such an important function as sleep did not have redundant mechanisms for its induction.

Pharmacokinetics

Paradoxically, the three benzodiazepines marketed as hypnotics virtually span the range of plasma half-lives (Table 13–4). Triazolam is short-acting, with a plasma half-life measured in a few hours, while flurazepam, via its active metabolite desalkylflurazepam, has a half-life measured in days. Temazepam has a half-life that is intermediate. Following single doses of each drug, differences are not especially apparent. Triazolam has been said to produce rebound insomnia or anxiety even within a single night, but this contention is controversial (Bixler et al., 1985). On the other hand, the long half-life of flurazepam opens the possibility of cumulative oversedation if doses are too high and the drug is taken chronically. Once again, the clinical importance

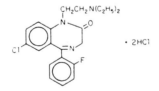

Flurazepam hydrochloride

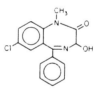

Temazepam

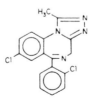

Triazolam

Fig. 13–3. Structures of three benzodiazepines promoted for use as hypnotics

Table 13–4. PHARMACOKINETIC PARAMETERS OF THREE BENZODIAZEPINE HYPNOTICS

	C_{max} (H)	PROTEIN BINDING (%)	ACTIVE METABOLITE	HALF-LIFE (H)
Flurazepam*	1–3	96	Desalkyl	40–114
Temazepam	2–3	96	None	9.5–12.4
Triazolam	0.7–2	80	None	1.3–3.9

*Data pertain to desalkylflurazepam.

of pharmacokinetic differences seems not to be of major consequence.

Therapeutic Indications

Treatment of sleep disorders should logically follow a diagnosis (Consensus Development Conference, 1984a). Unfortunately, the majority of cases of insomnia do not fit usual diagnoses. The major consideration is not to miss an underlying psychiatric disorder, physical cause, or insomnia due to drugs. Most cases of insomnia must be considered to be "primary," that is, of unknown cause. It is possible that persistent insomnia may herald the later appearance of depression. If so, early recognition and treatment might conceivably prevent future psychiatric disorders (Ford and Kamerow, 1989).

Transient sleep disturbances are ideal for drug treatment. These include sleeping in strange quarters, or moving through several time zones, or sleeping at a different time of day because of altered work schedules. Accommodation occurs quickly, and drugs may be needed for only a few days. A bigger problem is recurrent insomnia with no obvious cause. In this case, the possibility exists that drugs may be overused. Nonetheless, the greatest use of hypnotics is probably in patients with so-called primary insomnia.

The major contraindication to use of hypnotics is in patients with sleep apnea, in whom depression of respiration during sleep may lead to a fatal outcome. These drugs should also be used with great care in alcoholics, for the combination of high levels of blood alcohol and large doses of benzodiazepines could lead to unintentional suicide.

Principles of Use

Choice of Drug. Assuming that benzodiazepines will be used, how should one choose among them? The best criterion for making a choice is the preference of the patient. Triazolam is the current favorite, possibly because its short plasma half-life may minimize daytime hangover. Flurazepam has been used the longest; its long half-life might provide an advantage when some degree of daytime sedation is required for attendant anxiety. Temazepam has a half-life similar to that of

lorazepam. Diazepam, when given in single doses, is a relatively short acting drug, as its action is terminated largely by redistribution. Thus, almost any benzodiazepine used for treating anxiety might be equally suitable for treating insomnia. One should avoid at all costs the ridiculous situation of using one benzodiazepine for anxiety and a second benzodiazepine as a hypnotic.

A liquid preparation would be ideal for a hypnotic as one would like to obtain a prompt effect. None of these drugs is available in this form. Taking an adequate amount of fluid hastens disintegration of the tablet or capsule. Remaining upright for a while after taking the dose also facilitates absorption.

Dose. The proper dose is one that facilitates, rather than enforces, sleep. Therefore, one should start out with a small dose and increase it only as needed. For drugs that come as capsules, such as flurazepam and temazepam, one is limited to the dose contained in each capsule. A scored tablet, like triazolam, permits one to reduce the dose unit by cracking the tablet. For many persons, a dose of 0.125 mg of triazolam (half a 0.25-mg tablet) is sufficient. Maximum doses have been proposed for hypnotics: 0.5 mg for triazolam and 60 mg for either temazepam or flurazepam.

Frequency of Use. One wishes to avoid nightly use of hypnotics whenever possible. Prolonged, unremitting use of these drugs may induce withdrawal insomnia on discontinuation. Patients should be advised to use these drugs only occasionally. A reasonable system might propose a maximum use of only 1 night of every 3. The first dose would be taken because of a distressing complaint of insomnia. After a good night of sleep, no drug would be taken the second night. If patients had trouble sleeping the second night, they could be reassured that the sleep deprivation would make sleep come more easily on the third night. One might also consider, especially if the onset of sleep was delayed the second night, that they might have overslept the night before because of too large a dose of hypnotic. Should they not sleep well on the third night, they would be permitted to take another dose of hypnotic on the fourth night. Using such a pattern of hypnotic use should avoid habituation and is more consistent with what is known of the physiology of sleep. *Principle: The concept of sleep deprivation as the driving force for sleep explains several phenomena. First, even if hypnotics were not available, people with insomnia would eventually sleep. Second, oversleeping, by reducing the degree of deprivation, may be followed by insomnia.* These constructs are important in educating insomniac patients about the physiology of sleep.

Adverse Effects

Dependence. Although a few instances of dependence on benzodiazepines have been attributed to their use as hypnotics, closer inspection reveals that almost all involved gross misuse of the drugs. Small doses and infrequent administration (even when a single dose is taken each night) protect against dependence. Psychic dependence may be found among patients who feel that they simply must take a hypnotic every night.

Rebound Anxiety and Insomnia. These symptoms have been reported from use of short-acting hypnotics, mainly triazolam. However, others deny their existence. One could make a case that any insomnia the night following use of a hypnotic may simply reflect some degree of "oversleeping," with a subsequent reduced drive for sleep.

Oversedation. Too large a dose of hypnotic might result in daytime lethargy simply due to hangover effects. Accumulation of long-acting drugs, such as flurazepam, might result in mild intoxication.

Respiratory Depression. One of the great advantages of benzodiazepines has been less respiratory depression than from older hypnotics. Depression of respiration is a common precipitant of respiratory failure in patients with chronic obstructive pulmonary disease. Nonetheless, small doses of triazolam were well tolerated so long as patients did not have hypoxemia or carbon dioxide retention during the waking state (Timms et al., 1988).

Amnesia. Despite the failed memory of patients up to 36 hours following the dose, anterograde amnesia rarely follows use of triazolam. Whether amnesia is made more likely by a large dose or concomitant alcohol ingestion is uncertain.

Suicide. Because insomnia may be a symptom of more severe psychiatric illness, mainly depression, patients may attempt suicide with their hypnotics. Benzodiazepines are much safer than barbiturates and other drugs; it is virtually impossible to commit suicide with their use alone.

Nondrug Treatments

The effects of a warm bath, a massage, or relief of sexual tension for promoting sleep are well known. Bedtime rituals may provide a conditioning aspect for promoting sleep. Exercise during the day, enough to produce a moderate degree of fatigue, is helpful. Preferably it should not occur too close to the time of retiring. A patient who customarily awakens too early in the morning might well be advised to delay his or her bedtime. It must always be remembered that the primary drive for sleep comes from being sleep-deprived. Someone who has overslept the night before may find it difficult to court sleep the following night.

ANTIDEPRESSANTS

Not all patients with depression need drug therapy. Many patients become depressed as a reaction to temporary adverse circumstances. The *reactive* depressions usually subside with time; only when the depression is out of proportion to the problem or when it persists beyond resolution of the problem need drug therapy be considered.

Psychotherapy may be useful for all types of depression. Several specific types have been devised for treating depression, the cognitive-behavioral type being most widely used. Severely depressed patients may not be able to benefit from such treatment until after some alleviation of depression by drug therapy.

Drug therapy has been most effective for patients with *endogenous* depression. Such patients are characterized by having the disturbances of bodily rhythms mentioned earlier. They tend to have repeated episodes of depression throughout life; a family history of depression also supports the diagnosis. Often these depressions are autonomous, in that they may be precipitated, sometimes abruptly, without any evident psychosocial stressor.

Several different classes of drugs have been used as antidepressants and new ones are constantly being added. Drug therapy alleviates depression in only about 60% to 65% of patients, and many of the drugs used have significant drawbacks. New drugs are needed.

Tricyclics

Pharmacology. Promazine, like other phenothiazine derivatives, has a 6-6-6 three-ring structure, each ring having six members. A minor modification of this tricyclic structure to 6-7-6 was thought to preserve its antipsychotic action.

Quite unexpectedly, the first clinical study indicated that this new drug, imipramine, was not very effective as an antipsychotic but relieved depression in affected schizophrenics. Subsequently, its antidepressant action was confirmed in depressed patients. ***Principle: Minor alterations in chemical structure may cause profound changes in the pharmacology and clinical indications of a drug.***

Structures of the various members of this group are shown in Fig. 13–4. Both imipramine and amitriptyline have active monodemethylated side-chain metabolites, desipramine and nortriptyline, respectively, which have been marketed as separate entities. Doxepin and protriptyline differ from the other tricyclics only in minor modifications of the tricyclic ring structure. Clomipramine differs from imipramine only in having a chlorine atom at the 3 position of the tricyclic moiety.

Tricyclics are rather nonspecific in their pharmacologic actions. The principal action, by which the antidepressant effects are thought to be mediated, is their ability to block uptake of biogenic amine neurotransmitters. Amitriptyline and imipramine, by virtue of their active metabolites, have a mixed action in blocking uptake of both serotonin and norepinephrine. Only desipramine is specific for blocking uptake of norepinephrine. To the extent that the action of this neurotransmitter is increased, mild sympathomimetic effects may appear. Sedation may be due to a combination of antihistaminic and α_1-adrenoreceptor blocking actions. Anticholinergic action produces numerous side effects, such as dry mouth, blurred vision, urinary hesitancy, and constipation. α_1-Adrenoreceptor blockade also contributes to orthostatic hypotension. Most tricyclics are membrane-active local anesthetics, which may contribute to both an antiarrhythmic and an arrhythmogenic potential. Slight variations occur in this spectrum of pharmacologic actions among various tricyclics (Table 13–5).

Although reuptake of released neurotransmitters can be blocked by the very first doses of these drugs, the subsequent down-regulation of receptors may take longer. This delay in the ultimate consequence of these drugs has been adduced as an explanation for delays in clinical response (Sulser, 1987). Clinical response has been said to be delayed for at least 2 to 3 weeks; according to

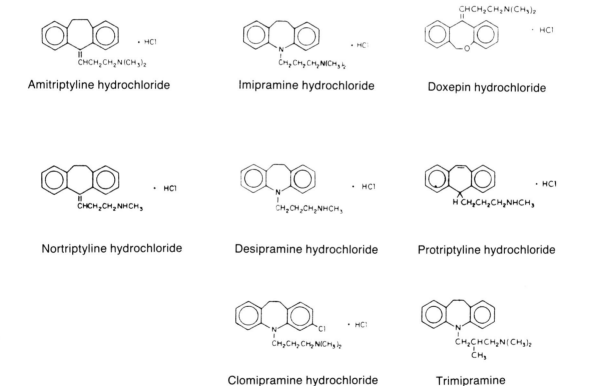

Fig. 13–4. Structures of various tricyclic antidepressants. Minor chemical modifications create changes in the spectrum of pharmacologic actions.

Table 13-5. EFFECTS OF VARIOUS ANTIDEPRESSANTS ON DIFFERENT RECEPTORS*

	β-ADRENERGIC† STIMULATION	SEROTONIN 2 RECEPTOR† STIMULATION	α₁-ADRENERGIC BLOCKADE	α₂-ADRENERGIC BLOCKADE	MUSCARINIC BLOCKADE	DOPAMINE 2 BLOCKADE	HISTAMINE 1 BLOCKADE
Tricyclics							
Imipramine	++	++	+++	+	++	+	++
Desipramine	+++	0	++	±	+	+	+
Amitriptyline	++	+++	+++	++	+++	+	+++
Nortriptyline	++	++	+++	+	+	+	++
Doxepin	++	++	+++	++	++	+	++++
Second-Generation							
Amoxapine	++	++	+++	±	+	++	++
Maprotiline	+++	+	+++	±	+	+	+++
Trazodone	±	++	++++	++	0	+	++
Fluoxetine	±	+++	±	±	±	0	±
Buproprion	±	±	±	0	0	?†	±

* Data obtained from a variety of sources as well as clinical estimates of side effects.
† β-Adrenoreceptor (norepinephrine) and serotonin 2 receptor are stimulated because of uptake inhibition; all others represent blockade of receptors.

some clinicians, a fair trial of these drugs should last 6 to 12 weeks, some responses being delayed that long. On the other hand, new evidence indicates that both the down-regulation of receptors and clinical response may occur much more quickly than formerly believed. When these drugs have been given intensively, either with large initial oral doses or following parenterally administered loading doses, clinical responses may occur within a few days. Thus, the relative contributions of pharmacodynamics and pharmacokinetics to the rate of clinical response to these drugs are still uncertain.

Pharmacokinetics. Most tricyclics have a widely variable and incomplete bioavailability because of extensive first-pass metabolism. They tend to be highly protein-bound, with large volumes of distribution. Plasma half-lives are variable and tend to be long, averaging about 24 hours (Table 13–6). Because the steady-state plasma concentrations of these drugs are not well correlated with dose, monitoring of plasma concentrations has been recommended.

Therapeutic ranges of plasma concentrations have been proposed for many of these drugs. Their reliability has been clouded by the fact that many studies have failed to demonstrate a therapeutic range and that active metabolites often have not been accounted for. Whether routine monitoring should be done is controversial and has not yet been shown to be cost-effective (Hollister et al., 1980). Most clinicians believe that the primary indication for monitoring is the failure of a patient to respond to what are adequate doses for most patients. Either the dose may be too low for that particular patient or compliance may be an issue.

Indications. The two approved indications for tricyclics are treatment of depressive symptoms, mainly those from endogenous depressions, and treatment of enuresis in children over the age of 6 years. Whether the action of these drugs in ameliorating enuresis is due to the sedative and anticholinergic effects or their actions on the architecture of sleep (reducing the sleep stage in which enuresis occurs) is uncertain. Action against enuresis does not seem to be related to the action that mediates the antidepressant effects.

Many other clinical uses have been found for these drugs over the years: relief of chronic pain states; reduction of bulimic episodes; management of narcolepsy; control of panic attacks, school phobias, and attention deficit disorder; and prophylaxis of migraine. The benefit of these drugs in these unrelated disorders does not appear to be due to their antidepressant action. Thus, the nonspecificity of action of tricyclics, which is troublesome for treating depression, becomes an advantage for extending their clinical uses. *Principle: Generic names of drug classes such as anti-depressant may not do justice to the versatility of their clinical uses. Neither do they signify that the mechanisms of action for these other uses are the same as for the generic indication.*

Clinical Use. Because of unpleasant side effects of tricyclics, including orthostatic hypotension, the custom has been to start treatment with small oral doses and augment them until a dose likely to be therapeutic (say 150 mg/day) is reached. Even the latter dose may be inadequate for some patients, so that doses up to 300 mg/day or more have been used. Thus, an exceptionally wide range of doses, from 30 to 75 mg/day in older frail women to 300 mg/day or more in robust young persons, can be used.

The duration of treatment before one sees a therapeutic result varies from days to weeks. Many physicians feel that if the patient has not shown an appreciable improvement by the third

Table 13–6. PHARMACOKINETIC PARAMETERS OF SOME ANTIDEPRESSANTS

	BIOAVAIL-ABILITY (%)	PROTEIN BINDING (%)	$T_{1/2B}$ (H)	METABOLITES	V_D (L/KG)	THERAPEUTIC CONCENTRATIONS (NG/ML)
Tricyclics						
Imipramine	29–77	88–93	6–20	Desipramine	20–30	>180 total
Desipramine	–	70–90	14–30	2-Hydroxy	22	145
Amitriptyline	31–61	82–96	19–31	Nortriptyline	15	>200 total
Nortriptyline	46–79	93	18–28	10-Hydroxy	21–57	50–1550
Doxepin	13–45	–	8–24	Desmethyl	9–33	–
Second-Generation						
Amoxapine	–	–	–	9-Hydroxy	–	200–400
Maprotiline	66–75	89	21–40	Desmethyl	52	200–300
Trazodone	–	73	8	*m*-Chlorphenylpiperazine	–	–
Fluoxetine	? 72	94	24–96	Norfluoxetine	20–45	–
Buproprion	–	85	11–14	? Active metabolites	–	25–100

week of treatment, other treatments should be considered. Exceptions do occur, however, and opinions differ as to what constitutes an adequate duration of treatment to conclude that the drug is not effective.

Because depression is a recurrent illness, maintenance and prophylactic treatment may be required in those patients who have had previous episodes. Maintenance treatment refers to continuation of drug until the depressive episode has definitely ended and is usually 3 to 4 months after a remission has been attained. Prophylactic treatment refers to very long term treatment, measured in years, with the goal of preventing future episodes of depression. Whether full therapeutic doses are needed either for maintenance or prophylactic treatment is still not settled.

Adverse Effects. Most common unwanted effects are minor but may lead to noncompliance. Sedative effects are usually well tolerated; they are greatest with amitriptyline and doxepin and least with protriptyline. Tremor is common, but propranolol may help. Anticholinergic effects include dry mouth, blurred vision, urinary hesitancy, and constipation. Palpitations, tachycardia, and orthostatic hypotension may occur early in treatment. Cardiac arrhythmias and abnormal ECGs are uncommon. Any delay in cardiac conduction represents a contraindication. Confusional states are common in older patients and are drug- and dose-related. Desipramine seems less likely than the others to produce this adverse reaction. Weight gain is frequent and is probably due to a central action rather than simply improved mood. Seizures are rare. Skin rashes and other allergic reactions are also uncommon.

Drug Interactions, Overdose. Pharmacodynamic drug interactions are generally predictable. Additive sedative and anticholinergic effects are noted when other drugs with similar actions are used concomitantly. Other membrane-active drugs such as thioridazine may produce additive arrhythmogenic effects. Reversal of the antihypertensive action of guanethidine often produces a dangerous overshoot of blood pressure. This drug, as well as methyldopa and clonidine, enters the nerve ending by the same amine pump blocked by tricyclics; thus the antihypertensive action is blocked. Pharmacokinetic interactions have generally been of little clinical import.

Overdoses of tricyclics are characterized by coma, convulsions, hypotension and abnormalities of cardiac conduction and rhythm. Ventricular arrhythmias are potentially life-threatening. Correction of metabolic acidosis, and administration of antiarrhythmics such as lidocaine, propranolol, and phenytoin should be used for pre-

vention and treatment. Removal of the drug by activated charcoal should be attempted because absorption in overdose situations may be quite slow.

MAO Inhibitors

When patients with pulmonary tuberculosis were first treated with iproniazid, they became euphoric. Shortly afterward, liver toxicity caused iproniazid to be replaced by isoniazid. The latter drug was used to exploit the euphoriant action in depressives but to no avail. It was only after iproniazid was found to be a potent inhibitor of the enzyme MAO and isoniazid a very weak inhibitor that it became apparent that enzyme inhibition was the key factor in any antidepressive action.

Pharmacology. The enzyme MAO works presynaptically to catabolize monoamine neurotransmitters (dopamine, norepinephrine, serotonin). Blocking this enzyme presumably allows more neurotransmitter to accumulate and become available for release at the synapse. Increased neurotransmitter at synapses leads to downregulation of postsynaptic receptors, the same end point attained with tricyclics (Pare, 1985).

These drugs may be either hydrazides (presence of a $-C-N-N-$ configuration) or nonhydrazides (Fig. 13–5). Phenelzine is now the most widely used, largely by default, as early fears of complications from use of these drugs curtailed their promotion. Tranylcypromine resembles dextroamphetamine in structure and retains some sympathomimetic action.

Two selective MAO inhibitors are under clinical investigation. Deprenyl (selegilene) inhibits MAO-B, a type of MAO that does not much degrade either serotonin or norepinephrine (Mann et al., 1989). Clorgiline is more specific for these two neurotransmitters. Whether selective MAO inhibition will confer clinical advantages is still uncertain. Selectivity of action may be lost with higher doses of each agent.

Although reversible MAO inhibitors are in the process of development, most currently available MAO inhibitors are irreversible. Thus, traditional pharmacokinetic studies of this class of drugs is meaningless. Inhibition of the enzyme can be measured in platelets to obtain an idea of the onset and persistence of inhibition. Inhibition is attained slowly and lost slowly, taking approximately 2 weeks in either direction. Studies of phenelzine indicate that a dose of 1 mg/kg per day is usually enough to attain the 88% inhibition of the enzyme required for clinical antidepressant action (Robinson et al., 1978). Measuring platelet MAO activity is too difficult to apply clini-

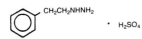

Phenelzine sulfate

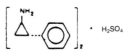

Tranylcypromine sulfate

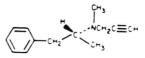

Clorgiline

Selegiline

Fig. 13–5. Structures of various types of MAO inhibitors. Phenelzine, with a C—N—N configuration, is a hydrazide. Tranylcypromine has a cyclopropyl side chain rather than the isopropyl side chain of the amphetamines.

cally, so no monitoring of dose is used with these drugs.

Pharmacodynamics. The slow rate of inhibition and regeneration of the enzyme has several important clinical consequences. First, response to treatment may be delayed by 2 weeks pending full inhibition of the enzyme. Second, full doses of these drugs should be used to begin treatment. Third, interacting drugs should be avoided until the enzyme is fully regenerated.

Indications. These drugs are mainly used for treating depression; they have also been used to treat panic-anxiety and phobias. Although lack of success with them early on suggested that they were not especially effective for endogenous depressions, they are effective if doses are sufficient. They have also been used with success in atypical depressions characterized by somatic complaints, anxiety, and phobias. Although some MAO inhibitors, such as pargyline, were used as antihypertensives, orthostatic lowering of blood pressure is not the most desirable method of control. They were also used briefly as antianginal drugs. Both of these uses have now been superseded.

Some patients have been found who are responsive to MAO inhibitors and no other antidepressants. Such a history should be reason to use these drugs first in subsequent episodes of depression. Ordinarily, they might be thought of as second-line drugs to follow a failed trial of tricyclics.

Clinical Use. A dose of 1 mg/kg per day of phenelzine is recommended. As the tablets are in 15 mg dose units, it is necessary to round off the calculated dose to the next 15 mg. Such a dose may be given right from the start of treatment, as it will take about 2 weeks for full inhibition of the enzyme. Some degree of orthostasis is probably

desirable to demonstrate that the drug is being given in adequate doses; this pharmacologic criterion is probably better than any laboratory measurement.

Tranylcypromine has some sympathomimetic action. Thus, dosage is usually small in the beginning with gradual increments until some sign, such as orthostasis or clinical improvement, suggests that a therapeutic dose has been reached. For a while, 30 mg/day was considered to be the maximum daily dose, but a few patients have been reported to respond to very large doses, such as 120 mg/day or more (Guze et al., 1987).

Duration of treatment should be at least 3 to 4 weeks to determine efficacy. If the drug is effective, the same considerations apply to continuation and prophylactic treatment as with tricyclics.

Adverse Reactions, Interactions, Overdoses. Common side effects of MAOs include dizziness, weakness and fatigue, orthostatic hypotension, constipation, neuromuscular irritability, and delayed ejaculation or anorgasmia. Major concern is possible interactions of these drugs with other drugs and with tyramine-containing foods. Excessive sedation to the point of coma has been experienced by patients concurrently taking opioids, anesthetics, and sedatives. Severe hypertensive crises have resulted when sympathomimetic drugs that act by releasing norepinephrine are used during MAO inhibition. Tyramine-containing foods, which include fermented products such as hard cheeses, dry sausage, pickled herring, and some beers or wines, may provoke severe hypertension leading to subarachnoid or intracerebral hemorrhage. It is obligatory that patients be given a list of foods and drugs most likely to cause these serious interactions, although the dangers are less than formerly believed (Folks, 1983).

Overdoses of MAO inhibitors are unusual. Agitation, delirium, and neuromuscular excitability are followed by obtunded consciousness, seizures, shock, and hyperthermia. Supportive treatment is generally adequate, although sedatives with α_1-adrenergic blocking action, such as chlorpromazine, may be useful.

Principles of treatment are similar to those for tricyclics.

Second-Generation Antidepressants

During the past decade a number of new heterocyclic antidepressants have been introduced. Most often they have been referred to as *second-generation* antidepressants (Coccaro and Siever, 1985). The major claims made for these drugs are that they have a more rapid onset of action, have fewer side effects, and are safer when taken in overdose. Such claims have not been fully justified. No claim has been made for greater overall efficacy.

Amoxapine. A demethylated metabolite of the antipsychotic loxapine, this was the first of the new drugs (Jue et al., 1982). A more rapid onset of action is extremely difficult to demonstrate and has not been convincingly demonstrated for this drug or any other of the second-generation group. Amoxapine has as many, and possibly more, side effects than tricyclics. In addition to having their spectrum of unwanted effects, amoxapine retains some of the unwanted effects of antipsychotics. Overdoses are characterized by severe neurotoxicity, which is just as dangerous as the cardiotoxicity of tricyclics.

Maprotiline. This drug came to the United States after a decade of use in Europe. It specifically blocks uptake of norepinephrine, as does desipramine, a drug to which it has some structural resemblance. Its major disadvantage is a predilection to cause seizures, which are dose-related (Barbaccia et al., 1986).

Trazodone. This phenylpiperazine derivative has a mixture of pharmacologic actions that are difficult to interpret. At some doses it acts as a serotonin antagonist and at others it blocks serotonin uptake or acts as a direct serotonin agonist. Trazodone also has antagonistic effects on both α_1 and α_2 adrenoreceptors. Clinically, sedation is most prominent and antidepressant effects have been more difficult to prove than with other drugs (Feighner and Boyer, 1988). It has been remarkably safe in overdoses.

Fluoxetine. Fluoxetine is the first specific serotonin-uptake inhibitor and should prove to be a useful pharmacologic tool. It has virtually no action on other neurotransmitter or receptor

systems, thus producing many fewer side effects than tricyclics (Sommi et al., 1987). The drug is characterized by having a very long plasma half-life and by inducing many pharmacokinetic interactions with other drugs. Its role in treatment requires a more extensive experience to evaluate. Such should be rapidly forthcoming, as the drug has been exceedingly popular.

Buproprion. This drug may be considered a "tamed" amphetamine, which it structurally resembles. It seems to work through a dopaminergic mechanism (Soroko et al., 1977). Dose-related seizures caused it to be temporarily removed from the market; with the lower doses now used, that risk is acceptable. The range of its clinical utility still remains to be determined by a more extensive experience.

Sympathomimetics and Lithium

Amphetamines have never been accepted as true antidepressants, yet a few patients do quite well with them. They may act by increasing release of norepinephrine and dopamine, as well as inhibiting their uptake and mimicking directly their action on receptors. Dextroamphetamine has been used concurrently with tricyclics to hasten clinical response; a good early response is said to augur a good ultimate response to the tricyclic.

Most authorities do not see much value of lithium as an antidepressant per se. It has been used to increase responsivity to tricyclics and for the prophylaxis of recurrent depression.

Principles of Use

Treatment of depression should be considered urgent. The most rapid recovery possible is desirable, as morbidity is great and mortality a possible outcome.

Indications. As mentioned, not all patients who appear depressed require drug treatment. Depression is considered to be a heterogeneous disorder. The more endogenous the depression, the more likely treatment with drugs will be effective. Even so, treatment-resistant patients may account for as many as one third of treated patients. Severely depressed patients with a risk of suicide are best treated with electroconvulsive therapy (ECT), which may be given concurrently with antidepressants. Psychotherapy is less effective than drug therapy for reducing acute symptoms of depression but may have more favorable long-term effects in improving social outcome and preventing recurrences.

Choice of Drugs. Tricyclics are still be a reasonable first-choice drug for many patients. A tremendous amount of clinical experience has delineated rather well their potential uses and disadvantages. Although occasional patients who do not respond to one tricyclic may respond to another, if a patient has failed to respond to an adequate dose and duration of treatment with a tricyclic, it may be well to consider other drug classes. Whether to try next the MAO inhibitors or one of the second-generation drugs is a matter of clinical judgment. Some patients have been specifically responsive to MAO inhibitors. They have generally been characterized as "atypical" depressions, that is with much anxiety, somatic complaints, phobias and "reversed" vegetative symptoms (hypersomnia, overeating, agitation). Among the second-generation drugs, only fluoxetine, buproprion, and trazodone are different enough from tricyclics to merit consideration.

Doses. Inadequate doses have been adduced as a major reason for treatment failures. Because doses do not always correlate well with plasma concentrations of drug, the latter may be more indicative of adequate treatment. Doses and the ranges of therapeutic plasma concentrations of various antidepressants are shown in Table 13–6. Whether doses should be more conservative in older patients has been disputed; most clinicians would tend to use smaller doses in the elderly.

Adverse Effects. Patients should be reassured that side effects represent normal actions of the drug and herald therapeutic benefits. Encouragement helps avoid premature termination of treatment or noncompliance.

Duration of Treatment. What constitutes a suitable therapeutic trial of antidepressant treatment is still debated. Some would feel that failure to respond after 3 weeks of treatment might be an indication that not all is going well, while others have recommended a course as long as 4 to 6 months. The old clinical axiom that the longer it takes for a drug to work, the more likely the response is nonspecific seems applicable here. How long to treat is determined in large part by how disabled the patient is.

Maintenance Treatment. Most episodes of depression have a finite length and then subside spontaneously. Because it is often uncertain when during an episode the patient was first treated, a general feeling exists that treatment should continue for as long as 4 months past remission to prevent relapse. Longer-term treatment may be considered to prevent recurrences of new episodes; such treatment may last for years and often uses doses smaller than those used for therapy.

Special Problems

Monitoring. Monitoring plasma concentrations of these drugs has been thought to be useful in determining whether the patient is being treated properly. Therapeutic ranges have not been clearly defined for many of these drugs, however. The most reasonable indication for measuring plasma concentrations might be in patients who have been treated with what would appear to be an adequate dose but who have failed to respond. A low concentration might signify noncompliance. Levels in the low therapeutic range might encourage one to increase doses to explore a higher range. An excessively high level might account for many side effects; reduction in dose might lead to a better result. Compliance during treatment has been a constant problem. In the case of some of the earlier classes of drugs, such as tricyclics, it was largely due to unwanted adverse effects. With some of the newer antidepressants, which are rather expensive, it may simply be lack of money.

The possibility of overdosing with these drugs in a suicidal attempt should be kept in mind. If there is any risk, let another family member or friend mind the supplies of medication; 100 25-mg dose units of most tricyclics can be a lethal weapon.

Combinations. Antidepressants may be safely, and sometimes effectively, combined with other psychotherapeutic drugs. Antipsychotics may be used concurrently when psychotic symptoms are present. Antianxiety drugs have been used early in therapy to assist sleep and reduce anxiety. Lithium and carbamazepine have been used as adjuncts when patients have failed to respond. There is no present justification for combining two antidepressants.

MOOD STABILIZERS

Although it is tempting to term all drugs used for treating mania *antimanic*, most are not especially effective for acute mania. Antipsychotics are more effective for such symptoms. Rather, drugs specific for mania might be construed as *mood stabilizers*, affecting the cycles of both mania and depression. Several drugs have been used with some success.

Lithium

Pharmacology. Lithium was discovered for all the wrong reasons. It was used in animals as lithium urate, the urate being thought to counter a nonexistent toxic substance in the urine. It turned out that the lithium component had a calming effect in the animals. When the first trial in humans with lithium carbonate was undertaken, an amazingly fortunate choice of dose, 600 mg three times daily, confirmed its efficacy (Amdisen, 1987).

The mode of action of lithium remains unclear. Three major lines of inquiry have suggested possible mechanisms. First, lithium may enter cells through the sodium-transport system and presumably stabilize cell membranes. Second, lithium may alter the effect of various neurotransmitters, such as dopamine, serotonin, and norepinephrine. Third, and currently most favored, is its effect on the inositol triphosphate, diacylglycerol second-messenger system. Lithium blocks conversion of inositol diphosphate to inositol phosphate, an essential step in the normal recycling of membrane phosphoinositides (Wood and Goodwin, 1987). This action ultimately leads to a depletion of both second messengers.

Pharmacokinetics. Lithium is a cation and has very simple kinetics, as outlined in Table 13–7. Two methods have been used to predict the proper loading dose to attain therapeutic serum levels. One uses a 24-hour determination of lithium concentration following a test dose (both the size of the test doses and the frequencies of obtaining levels have been varied) to make a prediction. The other, which is far simpler, is based on body weight. A dose of 0.5 mEq/kg (one 300-mg dose unit = 8 mEq) is adequate to produce initial concentrations in the therapeutic range (Stokes et al., 1976).

Monitoring of serum lithium concentrations is considered to be mandatory, as the therapeutic margins of this drug are small. Generally a range of 0.5 to 1.4 mEq/l has been recommended for acute treatment.

Because lithium must enter the cell to act, its onset of action is often slow, so that it may be a week or so before therapeutic effects are noted. Similarly, it may take a while for relapse to occur following its discontinuation. In severely manic patients, it is often necessary to initiate treatment with antipsychotics, alone or combined with sedative-hypnotics, to control agitated behavior.

Indications. The principal indication for lithium is for management of manic-depressive disor-

der. The drug is more effective against the manic than against depressive symptoms. Its major value has been its ability to prevent subsequent recurrent episodes of both mania and depression. Although it has been reported to be useful in unipolar depressions (that is without mania), tricyclics and other antidepressants are preferred. In schizoaffective disorders, lithium may be combined with antipsychotics to good effect. Its addition to antipsychotics in treatment-resistant schizophrenia or antidepressants in treatment-resistant depressions has been helpful. Its use in treating alcoholism has been controversial. Some feel that lithium is ineffective in the absence of a concurrent affective disorder, while others think it may curb drinking in the absence of clinically apparent affective disorder. Reports of efficacy in aggressive and violent patients (usually prisoners) suggest an interesting possible indication.

Doses and Duration of Treatment. If doses are related to body weight, extremes of 600 to 2400 mg/day may be considered. The majority of patients do well with doses of 1500 to 1800 mg/day. More important is monitoring of serum levels to keep patients within the therapeutic range. The first determination may be done 1 week after starting treatment with a fixed dose, when the patient presumably has reached a steady state. A simple arithmetic adjustment of dose can be made to fine-tune the therapeutic concentration. Once that is attained, measurement of levels is needed only because of signs of toxicity or changes in the status of the patient (an intercurrent illness, starting another medication).

Treatment of an acute manic episode is measured in weeks or months; prophylaxis against recurrent episodes is measured in months or years. Usually, two or more episodes during the span of a single year is considered an indication for prophylactic treatment. Serum concentrations during this phase of treatment may be lower than those during acute treatment (Consensus Development Conference, 1984b).

Drug Interactions. Thiazide diuretics decrease renal clearance of lithium by about 25%, so that doses need to be reduced; furosemide apparently

Table 13–7.   PHARMACOKINETIC PARAMETERS OF LITHIUM AND CARBAMAZEPINE

	BIOAVAIL-ABILITY (%)	PROTEIN BINDING (%)	V_D (L/KG)	$T_{1/2}$ (H)	METABOLITE	RENAL EXCRETION	THERAPEUTIC LEVELS
Lithium	100	0	0.7	20	None	20% of creatinine clearance	0.5–1.4 mEq/l
Carbamazepine	—	70–80	1.2	31–35	10,11-Epoxide	None	4–12 µg/ml

does not have such an action. A similar reduction in renal clearance has followed use of several newer NSAIDs; aspirin and ibuprofen do not do this.

Adverse Effects. Tremor is relatively frequent with therapeutic doses and is of little consequence. Other neurologic abnormalities, such as ataxia, dysarthria, neuromuscular irritability, and choreoathetosis, may herald toxicity. Appearance of any new neurologic or psychiatric symptoms during treatment is reason to stop the drug and assess serum concentrations. Gastrointestinal symptoms, such as anorexia, nausea, or vomiting may also herald toxicity, but diarrhea is common even at therapeutic concentrations.

Because lithium blocks adenylate cyclase in the distal nephron, the action of antidiuretic hormone is blocked. Mild symptoms are merely those of increased water turnover, but when excretion reaches 3 l/day or more, the patient is presumed to have nephrogenic diabetes insipidus. Amiloride is acceptable treatment (Battle et al., 1985). Chronic interstital nephritis has been reported but is controversial.

Thyroid functional impairment is thought to be common but rarely is of clinical significance. About 10% to 20% of patients develop a mild goiter during long-term treatment, with clinical hypothyroidism in a smaller number. Thyroid replacement treats both goiter and hypothyroidism (Maarbjerg et al., 1987).

Dysmorphogenesis characterized mainly by an increase in cardiac malformations has been associated with lithium treatment. Thus, it is contraindicated during pregnancy or, if the fetus has been inadvertently exposed, the woman should be counseled about possible choices. Lithium excretion decreases after parturition and postpartum toxicity has occurred. The ion readily enters the breast milk and can contribute to lethargy and poor reflexes in the neonate.

Other adverse effects of lithium that are frequent but of little concern are edema, acneiform eruptions, and leukocytosis. The latter is due to a direct effect on leukopoiesis and not simply recruitment from the marginal pool. Lithium has actually been employed as a treatment for drug-induced and other forms of granulocytopenia. Abnormal T waves are seen in the ECG, but exacerbations of the sick sinus syndrome are more serious; this condition would also constitute a contraindication to use of the drug.

Overdoses. Many overdoses are iatrogenic and occur during therapy with the drug. Intentional overdoses are life-threatening and may produce permanent neurologic residua (Sansone and Ziegler, 1985). Both peritoneal and hemodialysis are useful for eliminating the small lithium ion. Serum concentrations should be reduced to well below the therapeutic range before dialysis is stopped (Simard et al., 1989).

Carbamazepine

Carbamazepine was first used to treat manic-depressive disorder in 1971, based on a hypothesized similarity between the rhythmic mood alterations of manic-depressive disorder and epileptiform discharges. Although the reasoning was probably wrong, the drug has been proved effective in several blind studies. It is now considered to be equivalent to lithium and a suitable alternative to that drug.

Pharmacodynamics. Like lithium, carbamazepine has a multitude of pharmacologic actions, which vary on the basis of acute versus chronic administration (Post et al., 1987; Elphick, 1988).

Carbamazepine interacts with sodium channels, dampening the influx of sodium ions into neurons. Because this action would have a stabilizing effect on synaptic transmission, this may be the basis of carbamazepine's efficacy as an anticonvulsant and in the treatment of trigeminal neuralgia. As one would expect in any tricyclic, carbamazepine blocks the reuptake of norepinephrine, although it has only 25% the activity of imipramine. This action may contribute to its efficacy as an anticonvulsant, as the destruction of norepinephrine neurons blocks the anticonvulsant effects of carbamazepine. Moreover, this action may well explain its antidepressant effects in both bipolar and unipolar depression.

Carbamazepine enhances the release and blocks the reuptake of dopamine. It does not bind to or block postsynaptic dopamine receptors, but the presynaptic effect on dopamine is linked to the fact that, in animals, carbamazepine is capable of blocking neuroleptic-induced dopamine-receptor increases.

Carbamazepine is a competitive adenosine antagonist. However, whether this pharmacologic action is related to efficacy in manic-depressive illness awaits elucidation of adenosine's functions as a neurotransmitter.

Pharmacokinetics. The absorption of carbamazepine from the GI tract is slow. The attainment of peak serum concentrations can be highly variable (2–12 hours); the drug's half-life is relatively long (31–35 hours). Protein binding is approximately 70% to 80%. Achieving stable therapeutic serum concentrations of carbamazepine can be complicated by the fact that the drug can increase its own metabolism by hepatic enzymes. Thus, it may take several days to select a daily dose that maintains therapeutic serum concentrations ($4–12$ μg/ml). The relationship between dose and plasma concentrations is poor. Pharmacokinetic parameters are summarized in Table 13–7.

Metabolism of carbamazepine occurs as oxidation, first to a 10,11-epoxide metabolite and then to the 10,11-dihydroxide. One third of the 10,11-dihydroxide is then conjugated as the glucuronide and eliminated, while two thirds is eliminated in the free form. The drug is excreted in both the urine and feces. It should be noted that the 10,11-epoxide has potent anticonvulsant activity.

Indications. The primary indication for carbamazepine has been seizures. It is also useful for treating trigeminal neuralgia. The fact that lithium and carbamazepine have similar overall rates of efficacy in manic-depressive patients should not be construed to mean that they are interchangeable in individual patients. The clinical profile of the patient who benefits from carbamazepine may differ from that of a lithium responder. It makes good clinical sense that patients who are lithium failures should be tried on carbamazepine. In some cases of mania, concurrent administration of carbamazepine and lithium may be superior to treatment with either agent alone.

Doses. Clinical use of carbamazepine for manic-depressive illness follows similar guidelines as when it is used for epilepsy. One should begin carbamazepine treatment with a dosage schedule of 200 mg until a daily dose of 600 to 800 mg/day is achieved. Serum levels should be assessed 5 to 6 days after this dose has been reached, and additional dose increments can be performed as required. Most patients require a dose of no more than 1200 mg/day. As noted above, carbamazepine may induce its own metabolism; thus, the daily dose may require further adjustment for several days. In the treatment of manic-depressive disorder, it has been difficult to show correlations between serum concentrations and the degree of the clinical antimanic response. Some experts recommend that the daily dose of carbamazepine should be increased without regard to serum concentrations until intolerable side effects are encountered or until the dose reaches 1200 mg/day.

Duration of Treatment. As with lithium, patients who have responded to carbamazepine but who are thought to require prophylactic treatment may be continued on carbamazepine for months or even years (Kishimoto et al., 1983). For patients who do not seem to need long-term treatment, the drug can be gradually discontinued after remission has been maintained for 3 to 4 months.

Interactions. Clinically significant interactions between carbamazepine and other drugs are few. The one of greatest concern is a pharmacodynamic interaction, in which the combination of carbamazepine with lithium increases neurotoxicity.

Adverse Effects. Approximately one third of patients treated with carbamazepine experience side effects. The most commonly encountered side effects are related to the CNS, namely, sedation, nausea, weakness, ataxia, diplopia, and mild nystagmus. These side effects are dose-dependent and may be avoided by a dose reduction. Subtle interference with a variety of cognitive processes, such as memory or attention, may also occur, even when clear-cut sedation is absent.

Carbamazepine is known to produce leukopenia. In many cases this side effect is of a mild degree and spontaneously reversible and should not constitute an absolute contraindication for further therapy. In other cases, leukopenia may be irreversible and life-threatening. The drug should be immediately discontinued in these cases. Since leukopenia usually occurs early in treatment, a reasonable precaution is to obtain weekly leukocyte counts for the first 4 weeks of treatment and to discontinue treatment if a steadily progressive decrease in the leukocyte count occurs, or if the leukocyte count falls below 4000 per cubic millimeter on any occasion.

Overdoses. Carbamazepine overdose is potentially life-threatening. The initial symptoms are drowsiness and ataxia, associated with plasma concentrations of 11 to 15 μg/ml. As plasma concentrations rise to $15–25$ μg/ml, combativeness, hallucinations, and choreiform movements may follow. Concentrations above 25 μg/ml are associated with severe disturbance of consciousness, often coma. Coma usually lasts less than 24 hours. Although neurotoxic effects predominate, cardiotoxicity may include prolonged conduction and repolarization times. Cardiopulmonary arrest is a potential cause of death.

The kinetics of the drug change during massive overdose. Half-life is prolonged, and the epoxide metabolite increases, presumably contributing to toxicity. The usual methods are used in trying to rid the body of drug, including repeated oral gastric lavage followed by charcoal administration. Use of cathartics may spread the drug through the GI tract and defeat the purposes of lavage. Although the drug has a large volume of distribution, charcoal hemoperfusion may be considered. Supportive measures should include close cardiac monitoring and management of electrolyte abnormalities. Seizures may be treated with diazepam or phenytoin. In short, many of the same princi-

ated with hallucinogen use is easily accomplished by giving a large dose of benzodiazepines and permitting the subject to sleep through the effects of the hallucinogen.

REFERENCES

Addonizio, G.; Susman, V. L.; and Roth, S. D.: Neuroleptic malignant syndrome: Review and analysis of 115 cases. Biol. Psychiatry, 22:1004–1020, 1987.

Amdisen, A.: The history of lithium. Biol. Psychiatry, 22:522–524, 1987.

Ananth, J.; and Lin, K. M.: Propranolol in psychiatry: Therapeutic uses and side effects. Neuropsychobiology, 15:20–27, 1986.

Arana, G. W.; Goff, D. C.; Baldessarini, R. J.; and Keepers, G. A.: Efficacy of anticholinergic prophylaxis for neuroleptic-induced dystonia. Am. J. Psychiatry, 145:993–996, 1988.

Barbaccia, M. L.; Ravizza, L.; and Costa, E.: Maprotiline: An antidepressant with an unusual pharmacological profile. J. Pharmacol. Exp. Ther., 236:307–312, 1986.

Baron, M.; Risch, N.; Hamburger, R.; Mandel, B.; Kushner, S.; Newman, M.; Drumer, D.; and Belmaker, R. H.: Genetic linkage between X-chromosome markers and bipolar affective illness. Nature, 326:289–292, 1987.

Battle, D. C.; von Riotte, A. B.; Gaviril, M.; and Grupp, M.: Amelioration of polyuria by amiloride in patients receiving long-term lithium therapy. N. Engl. J. Med., 312:408–414, 1985.

Bixler, E. O.; Kales, J. D.; Kales, A.; Jacoby, J. A.; and Soldatos, C. R.: Rebound insomnia and elimination half-life: Assessment of individual subject response. J. Clin. Pharmacol., 25:115–124, 1985.

Bleuler, E.: Dementia Praecox or the Group of Schizophrenics. International Universities Press, New York, 1950.

Byerley, W. F.; McConnell, E. J.; McCabe, R. T.; Dawson, T. M.; Grosser, B. I.; and Wamsley, J. K.: Decreased beta-adrenergic receptors in rat brain after chronic administration of the selective serotonin uptake inhibitor, fluoxetine. Psychopharmacology, 94:141–143, 1988.

Campbell, M.: Fenfluramine treatment of autism. J. Child. Psychol. Psychiatry, 29:1–10, 1988.

Campbell, M.; Small, A. M.; Green, W. H.; Jennings, S. J.; Perry, R.; Bennett, W. G.; and Anderson, L.: Behavioral efficacy of haloperidol and lithium carbonate. A comparison in hospitalized aggressive children with conduct disorder. Arch. Gen. Psychiatry, 41:650–656, 1984.

Charney, D. S.; and Heninger, G. R.: Abnormal regulation of noradrenergic function in panic disorders. Arch. Gen. Psychiatry, 43:1042–1054, 1986.

Coccaro, E. F.; and Siever, L. J.: Second generation antidepressants: A comparative review. J. Clin. Psychopharmacol., 25: 241–260, 1985.

Consensus Development Conference: Drugs and insomnia. The use of medications to promote sleep. J.A.M.A., 251:2410–2414, 1984a.

Consensus Development Conference: Mood Disorder: Pharmacologic Prevention of Recurrences. Vol. 5, No. 4. National Institutes of Health, Bethesda, Md., 1984b.

Costa, E.: Polytypic signaling at GABAergic synapses. Life Sci., 42:1407–1017, 1988.

Crow, J. J.: Molecular pathology of schizophrenia. More than one disease process? Br. Med. J., 280:66–68, 1980.

Danielson, D. A.; Porter, J. B.; Lawson, D. H.; Soubrie, C.; and Jick, H.: Drug-associated psychiatric disturbances in medical inpatients. Psychopharmacology, 74:105–108, 1981.

Davies, P.: The genetics of Alzheimer's disease: A review and a discussion of the implications. Neurobiol. Aging, 7:459–465, 1986.

Davis, K. L.: Psychological effects of nonpsychiatric drugs. In, Psychopharmacology: From Theory to Practice (Barchas, J. D.; Berger, P. A.; Ciarnillo, R. D.; Elliott, G. R.; eds.). Oxford University Press, New York, pp. 469–480, 1977.

Egeland, J. A.; Gerhard, D. S.; Pauls, D. L.; Sussex, J. N.; Kidd, K. K.; Allen, C. R.; Hostetler, A. M.; and Hoosman, D. E.: Bipolar affective disorders linked to DNA markers on chromosome 11. Nature, 325:783–787, 1987.

Elphick, M.: The clinical uses and pharmacology of carbamazepine in psychiatry. Int. Clin. Psychopharmacol., 3:185–203, 1988.

Farde, L.; Wiesel, F. A.; Halldin, C.; and Sedvall, G.: Central D2-dopamine receptor occupancy in schizophrenic patients treated with antipsychotic drugs. Arch. Gen. Psychiatry, 45: 71–76, 1988.

Feighner, J. P.; and Boyer, W. R.: Overview of controlled trials of trazodone in clinical expression. Psychopharmacology, 95: S50–S53, 1988.

Flament, M. F.; Rapoport, J. L.; Berg, C. J.; Sceery, W.; Kilts, C.; Melstrom, B.; and Linnoila, M.: Clomipramine treatment of childhood obsessive-compulsive disorder. Arch. Gen. Psychiatry, 42:977–983, 1985.

Folks, D. G.: Monoamine oxidase inhibitors: Reappraisal of dietary considerations. J. Clin. Psychopharmacol., 3:249–252, 1983.

Ford, D. E.; and Kamerow, D. B.: Epidemiologic study of sleep disturbances and psychiatric disorders. An opportunity for prevention? J.A.M.A., 262:1479–1484, 1989.

Francis, J.; Martin, D.; and Kapoor, W. N.: A prospective study of delirium in hospitalized elderly. J.A.M.A., 263:1097–1101, 1990.

Fyer, A. J.; Liebowitz, M. R.; Gorman, J. G.; Campeas, R.; Levin, A.; Davies, S. O.; Goetz, D.; and Klein, D. F.: Discontinuation of alprazolam treatment in panic patients. Am. J. Psychiatry, 144:303–308, 1987.

Garland, B. J.; Wilder, D. E.; and Copeland, J.: Concepts of depression in the elderly: Signposts to future mental health needs. In, Aging 2000: Our Health Care Destiny (Gaitz, C. M.; and Samorajski, T.; eds.). Springer-Verlag, New York, pp. 443–451, 1985.

Garza-Trevino, E.; Hollister, L. E.; Overall, J. E.; and Alexander, W. F.: Efficacy of combination of intramuscular antipsychotics and sedative-hypnotics for control of psychotic agitation. Am. J. Psychiatry, 146:1598–1601, 1989.

Gittelman-Klein, R.; and Klein, D. F.: School phobia: Diagnostic considerations in the light of imipramine effects. J. Nerv. Ment. Dis., 166:199–215, 1973.

Golinko, B. E.: Side effects of dextroamphetamine and methylphenidate in hyperactive children—a brief review. Prog. Neuropsychopharmacol. Biol. Psychiatry, 8:1–8, 1984.

Greden, J. F.; Fontaine, P.; Lubetsky, M.; and Chamberlin, K.: Anxiety and depression associated with caffeinism among psychiatric patients. Am. J. Psychiatry, 135:963–966, 1978.

Green, A. R.: Evolving concepts on the interactions between antidepressant treatments and monoamine neurotransmitters. Neuropharmacology, 26:815–822, 1987.

Greenblatt, D. J.; and Shader, R. I.: Clinical pharmacokinetics of the benzodiazepines. In, The Benzodiazepines: Current Standards for Medical Practice (Smith, D. E.; and Wesson, D. R.; eds.). MTP Press, Lancaster, U.K., pp. 43–50, 1985.

Guze, B. H.; Baxter, L. R. Jr.; and Rego, J.: Refractory depression treated with high doses of monoamine oxidase inhibitor. J. Clin. Psychiatry, 48:31–32, 1987.

Hollister, L. E.: Drug-induced psychiatric disorders and their management. Med. Toxicol., 1:428–448, 1986.

Hollister, L. E.: Alzheimer's disease. Is it worth treating? Drugs, 29:483–488, 1985.

Hollister, L. E.; Pfefferbaum, A.; and Davis, K. L.: Monitoring nortriptyline plasma concentrations. Am. J. Psychiatry, 137: 485–486, 1980.

Hollister, L. E.; Davis, K. L.; Overall, J. E.; and Anderson, T.: Excretion of MHPG in normal subjects. Implications for biological classification of affective disorders. Arch. Gen. Psychiatry, 35:1410–1415, 1978.

Hollister, L. E.; Motzenbecker, F. P.; and Degan, R. O.: Withdrawal reactions from chlordiazepoxide ("Librium"). Psychopharmacology, 2:63–68, 1961.

Johnson, D. A. W.: Drug-induced psychiatric disorders. Drugs, 22:57–69, 1981.

Judd, B. W.; Meyer, J. S.; Rogers, R. L.; Gandhi, S.; Tanahashi,

N.; Mortel, K. F.; and Tawaklna, T.: Cognitive performance correlates with cerebrovascular impairments in multi-infarct dementia. J. Am. Geriatr. Soc., 34:355–360, 1986.

Jue, S. G.; Dawson, G. W.; and Brogden, R. N.: Amoxapine: A review of its pharmacology and efficacy in depressed states. Drugs, 24:1–23, 1982.

Kane, J.; Honigfeld, G.; Singer, J.; and Meltzer, H.: Clozapine for the treatment-resistant schizophrenic. A double-blind comparison with chlorpromazine. Arch. Gen. Psychiatry, 45(9): 789–760, 1988.

Kishimoto, A.; Ogura, C.; Hazama, H.; and Inoue, K.: Longterm prophylactic effects of carbamazepine in affective disorder. Br. J. Psychiatry, 143:327–331, 1983.

Kraepelin, F.: Lectures on Clinical Psychiatry. New York, William Wood, 1905.

Krueger, J. M.; Karaszewski, J. W.; Davenne, D.; and Shosham, S.: Somnogenic muramyl peptides. Fed. Proc., 45:2552–2555, 1986.

Ladewig, D.: Dependence liability of the benzodiazepines. Drug Alcohol Depend., 13:139–149, 1984.

Maarbjerg, K.; Vestergaard, P.; and Schou, M.: Changes in serum thyroxine (T_4) and serum thyroid-stimulating hormone (TSH) during prolonged lithium treatment. Acta. Psychiatr. Scand., 75:217–221, 1987.

Mann, J. J.; Aarons, S. F.; Wilner, P. J.; Kelly, J. G.; Sweeney, J. A.; Pearlstein, T.; Frances, A. J.; Kocsis, J. H.; and Brown, R. P.: A controlled study of the antidepressant efficacy of (–) deprenyl. A selective monoamine oxidase inhibitor. Arch. Gen. Psychiatry, 46, 45–50, 1989.

Martin, I. L.: The benzodiazepines and their receptors: 25 years of progress. Neuropharmacology, 26:957–970, 1987.

McKenna, P. J.: Pathology, phenomenology and the dopamine hypothesis of schizophrenia. Br. J. Psychiatry, 151:288–301, 1987.

Mellinger, G. D.; Balter, M. B.; Manheimer, D. I.; Cisin, I.; and Parry, H. S.: Psychic distress, life crisis, and use of psychotherapeutic medications. National household survey. Arch. Gen. Psychiatry, 35:1045–1052, 1978.

Mendlewiez, J.; Simon, P.; Sevy, S.; Charon, F.; Brocas, H.; Legros, S.; and Vassert, G.: Polymorphic DNA marker on X-chromosome and manic-depression. Lancet, 1:1230–1234, 1987.

Moore-Ede, M. C.; Czeisler, C. A.; and Richardson, G. S.: Circadian timekeeping in health and disease. N. Engl. J. Med., 309:469–536, 1983.

Myers, J. K.; Weissman, M. M.; Tischler, G. L.; Holzer, C. E. III; Leaf, P. J.; Orvaschel, H.; Anthony, J. C.; Boyd, J. H.; Bulke, J. D. Jr.; Kramer, M.; and Stoltzman, R.: Six-month prevalence of psychiatric disorders in three communities: 1980 to 1982. Arch. Gen. Psychiatry, 41:959–967, 1984.

Nierenberg, A. A.; and Feinstein, A. R.: How to evaluate a diagnostic test. Lessons from the rise and fall of dexamethasone suppression test. J.A.M.A., 259:1699–1702, 1988.

Olajida, D.; and Lader, M.: A comparison of buspirone, diazepam, and placebo in patients with chronic anxiety states. J. Clin. Psychopharmacol., 7:148–152, 1987.

Overall, J. E.; and Hollister, L. E.: Comparative evaluation of research diagnostic criteria for schizophrenia. Arch. Gen. Psychiatry, 36:1198–1205, 1979.

Palmer, D. P.: Buspirone, a new approach to the treatment of anxiety. Fed. Am. Soc. Exp. Biol. J., 2:2445–2452, 1988.

Pare, C. M. P.: The present status of monoamine oxidase inhibitors. Br. J. Psychiatry, 146:576–584, 1985.

Post, R. M.: Mechanisms of action of carbamazepine and related anticonvulsants in affective illness. In, Psychopharmacology: The Third Generation of Progress (Meltzer, H. Y., ed.). Raven Press, New York, pp. 567–576, 1987.

Post, R. M.; Uhde, T. W.; By-Byrne, R.; and Joffe, R. T.: Correlates of antimanic response to carbamazepine. Psychiatry Res., 21:71–83, 1987.

Preskorn, S. H.; Weller, E. B.; and Weller, R. A.: Depression in children: Relationship between plasma imipramine levels and response. Psychopharmacology, 43:450–453, 1982.

Rapoport, J. L.: The neurobiology of obsessive-compulsive disorder. J.A.M.A., 260:2888–2890, 1988.

Reynolds, G. P.: Beyond the dopamine hypothesis. The neurochemical pathology of schizophrenia. Br. J. Psychiatry, 155: 304–316, 1989.

Robins, L. N.; Helzer, J. E.; Weissman, M. M.; Orvaschel, H.; Gruenberg, E.; Burke, J. D. Jr.; and Regier, D. A.: Lifetime prevalence of specific psychiatric disorders in three sites. Arch. Gen. Psychiatry, 41:949–958, 1984.

Robinson, D. S.; Nies, A.; Ravaris, C. L.; Ives, J. O.; and Bartlett, H. D.: Clinical pharmacology of phenelzine. Arch. Gen. Psychiatry, 35:629–635, 1978.

Sansome, M. E.; and Ziegler, D. K.: Lithium toxicity: A review of neurologic complications. Clin. Neuropharmacol., 8:242–248, 1985.

Schentag, J. J.; Cerra, F. B.; Calleri, G.; DeGlopper, E.; Rose, J. Q.; and Bernhard, H.: Pharmacokinetic and clinical studies in patients with cimetidine-associated confusion. Lancet, 1: 177–181, 1979.

Shaarawy, M.; Fayad, M.; and Abdel-Azim, S.: Serotonin metabolism and depression in oral contraceptive users. Contraception, 26:193–196, 1982.

Simard, M.; Gumbiner, B.; Lee, A.; Lewis, H.; and Norman, D.: Lithium carbonate intoxication. A case report and review of the literature. Arch. Intern. Med., 149:36–46, 1989.

Simpson, G. M.; Pi, E. H.; and Stramek, J. J.: An update on tardive dyskinesia. Hosp. Community Psychiatry, 37:362–369, 1986.

Sommi, R. W.; Crismon, M. L.; and Bowden, C. L.: Fluoxetine: A serotonin-specific second-generation antidepressant. Pharmacotherapy, 7:1–15, 1987.

Soroko, F. E.; Mehta, N. B.; Maxwell, R. A.; Ferris, R. M.; and Schroeder, D. H.: Buproprion hydrochloride. A novel antidepressant agent. J. Pharm. Pharmacol., 29:767–770, 1977.

Sovner, R.; and Hurley, A.: The management of chronic behavior disorders in mentally retarded adults with lithium. J. Nerv. Ment. Dis., 169:191–195, 1981.

Stokes, P. E.; Kocsis, J. H.; and Arcuni, O. J.: Relationship of lithium chloride dose to treatment response in acute mania. Arch. Gen. Psychiatry, 33:1080–1084, 1976.

Sulser, F.: Serotonin-norepinephrine receptor interactions in the brain: Implications for the pharmacology and pathophysiology of affective disorders. J. Clin. Psychiatry, 48(suppl.):12–18, 1987.

Tallman, J. F.; Paul, S. M.; Skolnick, P.; and Gallagher, D. W.: Receptors for the age of anxiety: Pharmacology of the benzodiazepines. Science, 207:274–281, 1980.

Taylor, D. P.: Buspirone, a new approach to the treatment of anxiety. FASEB J., 2:2445–2452, 1988.

Thompson, T. L.; Moran, M. G.; and Nies, A. S.: Psychotropic drug use in the elderly. N. Engl. J. Med., 308:134–138, 194–199, 1983.

Timms, R. M.; Dawson, A.; Hajdukovic, R. M.; and Mitler, M. M.: Effect of triazolam on sleep and arterial oxygen saturation in patients with chronic obstructive pulmonary disease. Arch. Intern. Med., 149:2159–2163, 1988.

Walsh, B. T.; Stewart, J. W.; Roose, S. P.; Gladis, M.; and Glassman, A. H.: Treatment of bulimia with phenelzine. A double-blind, placebo-controlled study. Arch. Gen. Psychiatry, 41:1105–1109, 1984.

Wood, A. J.; and Goodwin, G. M.: A review of the biochemical and neuropharmacological actions of lithium. Psychol. Med., 17:579–600, 1987.

Youngerman, J.; and Canino, I.: Lithium carbonate use in children and adolescents. Arch. Gen. Psychiatry, 35:216–224, 1978.

14

Treatment of Endocrine Disorders: The Thyroid

Douglas S. Ross

Chapter Outline

Thyroid Physiology
Effects of Drugs and Illness on Thyroid
    Function Tests
Treatment of Thyroid Disorders
    Hypothyroidism
    Myxedema Coma
    Goiter: Thyroid Hormone Suppressive
      Therapy
    Hyperthyroidism

Thyroid Storm
Hyperthyroidism in Pregnancy
Prevention of Neonatal Graves Disease
Ophthalmopathy
Pretibial Myxedema
Subacute, Painless, and Postpartum
    Thyroiditis
Thyroid Cancer

THYROID PHYSIOLOGY

The major function of the thyroid gland is to synthesize thyroid hormone, store it in the colloid space, and release it into the circulation. The thyroid gland is regulated by its pituitary tropic hormone, thyrotropin [thyroid-stimulating hormone (TSH)]. TSH stimulates thyroid hormone synthesis and release; thyroid hormones in turn exert negative feedback control and inhibit the synthesis and release of pituitary TSH (Larsen, 1982). A third level of control involves hypothalamic TRH (thyrotropin-releasing hormone) that stimulates the release of TSH and is itself inhibited by the thyroid hormones. This complex regulatory system provides fairly constant levels of thyroid hormone in blood throughout the day (Fig. 14–1).

The thyroid synthesizes two hormonally active iodinated compounds, thyroxine (T_4) and triiodothyronine (T_3). Both compounds are synthesized within the structure of a large glycoprotein, thyroglobulin. Synthesis involves trapping circulating iodine against a concentration gradient, organifying the trapped iodine to tyrosyl residues on thyroglobulin via a specific microsomal thyroid peroxidase, and coupling mono- and diiodotyrosine residues to form the iodothyronines (DeGroot and Niepomniszcze, 1977). The thyroglobulin is stored within the colloid space surrounded by thyroid follicular cells. When the thyroid is stimulated to release hormone, colloid droplets are taken up into the follicular cells and merged with lysozymes. Following proteolysis, T_4 and T_3 are released into the circulation.

TSH stimulates all the stages of thyroid hormone synthesis and release. Several drugs can inhibit certain stages. Perchlorate and thiocyanate act as competitive inhibitors of the trapping of circulatory iodine. Because of their rapid excretion from the body and their toxic effects, which include aplastic anemia, they are not commonly useful as antithyroid drugs. The thiourea derivatives propylthiouracil and methimazole block organification and coupling and have been extremely useful in the management of hyperthyroidism (see below). Lithium inhibits the release of thyroid hormone. This may be an important adverse effect of the drug when it is used for CNS effects. *Principle: Even if drugs are efficacious, they may be impractical, and the choice between agents may be independent of their proven useful pharmacologic effects.*

Iodine itself plays an important role in the regulation of thyroid hormone synthesis and release, a phenomenon called autoregulation. Increased supply of iodide as a substrate for thyroid hormone can result in increased synthesis, especially when a patient lives in areas where iodine deficiency is common (endemic goiter), or in glands that have developed abnormal tissue that becomes autonomous of the usual regulatory mechanisms. Occasionally, iodide given to people with autonomous glands causes sufficient excessive synthesis of thyroid hormone to result in hyperthyroidism [Jod-Basedow phenomenon, or iodine-induced

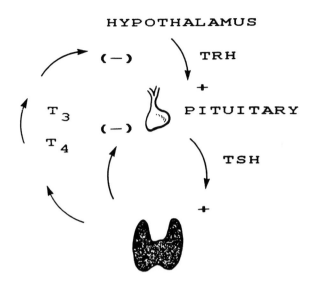

HYPOTHALAMUS

TRH

PITUITARY

TSH

THYROID

Fig. 14-1. The hypothalamic–pituitary–thyroid axis.

hyperthyroidism (Fradkin and Wolff, 1983)]. In contrast, normal thyroid glands respond to excessive iodine by reducing trapping, organification, coupling, and release of thyroid hormone. Trapping resumes when intrathyroidal iodine concentrations become subnormal. The inhibitory effects of iodine on its own organification to thyroglobulin are called the Wolff-Chaikoff effect (Wolff and Chaikoff, 1948). Normally, the thyroid escapes from this blockade of organification, but patients with underlying autoimmune thyroid disease, who may already have a mild acquired block in organification, may fail to escape from the Wolff-Chaikoff effect. Occasionally, patients with lymphocytic thyroiditis who are given iodide may become hypothyroid and develop goiters. Thus the effects of iodine on the thyroid are highly dependent upon the underlying state of the gland (Silva, 1985). Understanding this is essential before using iodine as a pharmacologic agent. For example, iodide given to a patient with hyperthyroidism due to an adenoma may make the hyperthyroidism worse despite some inhibition of hormone release. Iodide given to a patient with recurrent mild Graves disease following radioiodine ablation may be sufficient to control hyperthyroidism by blocking organification and release of hormone. Iodide can be used in thyroid storm to block release, but only after thionamides have been given to prevent the iodine from becoming organified and utilized as substrate for de novo synthesis. *Principle: The effects of a given pharmacologic agent often are dependent upon the mechanisms and extent of the underlying process that the agent is intended to alter. The result*

of therapy differs depending upon the specific pathophysiology and the degree of distortion of physiology.

Once secreted into the blood, T_4 and T_3 are avidly bound to three different serum proteins, thyroxine-binding globulin (TBG), thyroxine-binding prealbumin (TBPA), and albumin (Oppenheimer, 1968). The large bound pools are in equilibrium with considerably smaller free circulating fractions; for example, only 0.03% of T_4 circulates unbound in plasma. Only unbound hormone is immediately available for uptake into tissues, so the majority of thyroid hormone is present within an extracellular protein-bound pool that is in equilibrium with the biologically active free-hormone pool. The slightly less avid binding of T_3 to these proteins accounts in part for its more rapid turnover. Drugs and diseases that alter the serum concentrations of these binding proteins may have major effects on total hormone concentrations in serum and minimal effect on the availability of unbound hormone for organ utilization.

The thyroid is the only tissue that synthesizes T_4. In contrast, most tissues in the body have a specific 5'-monodeiodinase that converts T_4 to T_3 (Schimmel and Utiger, 1977). Only 10% to 15% of T_3 is actually synthesized in the thyroid gland. One may view T_4 as a prohormone that is first deiodinated to T_3 before it combines with its specific nuclear hormonal receptor. The T_4 itself may have about 10% of the intrinsic activity of T_3. When thyroid hormone interacts with its nuclear receptor, it alters the transcription rates of many genes in various tissues that are involved in basic metabolic processes including growth and development. Several drugs and diseases (discussed below) can alter thyroid function by directly inhibiting the deiodination of T_4 to T_3.

Iodine metabolism seems to be reasonably straightforward. Most of the ingested iodides are absorbed from the GI tract. Iodide may also enter the circulation from the deiodination of the thyroid hormones, or the "leak" of some iodide from the thyroid gland. Iodide is rapidly cleared from the circulation by the thyroid gland and the kidneys. Since the renal tubules passively reabsorb iodide, clearance is dependent upon the glomerular filtration rate. The recommended daily allowance of iodine is 150 μg. In the United States, iodine deficiency has been obliterated by the iodination of salt and the presence of iodinated compounds in bread. In this setting, iodide intake is about 500 to 800 μg daily.

The metabolism of the thyroid hormones is still not fully understood. The major pathway involves the repetitive deiodination of thyroid hormone into inactive metabolites (Engler and Burger, 1984). Deamination, decarboxylation, ether-link cleavage, and conjugation into glucuronide or sulfate derivatives are less important pathways. Excretion of glucuronide derivatives into bile results in a minor enterohepatic circulation.

EFFECTS OF DRUGS AND ILLNESS ON THYROID FUNCTION TESTS

The assessment of thyroid function has become more precise with the use of newer, more sensitive TSH assays that can detect subnormal TSH concentrations in patients with subclinical or overt hyperthyroidism (Ehrmann and Sarne, 1989). A log–linear negative-feedback relationship exists between changes in TSH and free-T_4 concentrations; consequently, measurement of serum TSH concentrations, in the absence of pituitary disease, provides the most sensitive and specific evaluation of thyroid function. An elevated concentration of TSH signifies hypothyroidism, while a subnormal TSH concentration indicates subclinical or overt hyperthyroidism. The degree of hyperthyroidism can be assessed by direct measurement of the thyroid hormones. There are fortunately very few diseases or drugs that can affect measurement of TSH. Clearly, in the presence of hypothalamic or pituitary disease, one cannot rely upon TSH measurements as an assessment of thyroid function; instead the direct measurement of the thyroid hormones is used. Seriously ill patients (nonthyroidal illness) may exhibit reduced pituitary production of TSH, but rarely to the concentration seen in hyperthyroid patients (Spencer et al., 1990). During recovery from nonthyroidal illness, there may be a transient increase in concentrations of TSH in serum above the normal range (Hamblin et al., 1986). Dopamine infused IV reduces TSH concentrations; hypothyroid patients with elevated TSH concentrations may have values reduced into the normal range with administration of dopamine. Metoclopramide and domperidone may cause transient elevations in serum TSH concentrations. Glucocorticoids may decrease serum concentrations of TSH, but the magnitude of these changes is small and does not overlap with values seen in hyperthyroid patients [when an appropriately sensitive TSH assay is used (Spencer et al., 1990)].

Thyroid function may also be assessed by the direct measurement of serum total-T_4 concentrations and a test to estimate free-hormone concentrations (Kaplan, 1985). Total T_4 is readily measured by radioimmunoassay. The most commonly used method of estimating free hormone is calculation of the free-T_4 index. This involves measurement of the thyroid hormone–binding index (THBI), formerly called the T_3 resin uptake test (T_3R). In this assay, the inverse of available binding sites on thyroid hormone–binding proteins is assessed by allowing labeled T_3 first to interact with binding proteins in vitro; then the remaining tracer is bound to the resin. The free-T_4 index is the total T_4 multiplied by the THBI. In states of excess of binding protein, most of the labeled T_3 added in vitro interacts with the increased binding proteins, and little is available to interact with the resin. The THBI is therefore subnormal, while the total T_4 is high because of increased T_4 binding to the excess binding proteins. The high T_4 multiplied by the low THBI results in a normal free-T_4 index. Similarly, states of low binding proteins are associated with a low T_4, a high THBI, and normal free-T_4 index. However, it is possible to estimate the free-T_4 fraction by nonequilibrium radioimmunoassays or methods similar to dialysis that calculate the free-hormone fraction.

Unlike TSH measurements, T_4 and free-T_4 measurements can be influenced by a number of disease states and drugs (Kaplan, 1985; Ehrmann and Sarne, 1989; Spencer et al., 1990). Estrogens, tamoxifen, 5-fluorouracil, perphenazine, clofibrate, narcotics, acute hepatitis, and acute intermittent porphyria may increase serum TBG concentrations and cause an elevated total-T_4 concentration. Hereditary TBG excess, a familial abnormal albumin or TBPA, and immunoglobulins that bind T_4 also may cause hyperthyroxinemia. Use of amphetamine is occasionally associated with high T_4 concentrations in serum. Several drugs—amiodarone, ipodate, iopanoic acid, and high doses of propranolol—inhibit T_4-to-T_3 conversion and block hepatic uptake of serum T_4, resulting in hyperthyroxinemia.

Other drugs and disease states reduce total concentrations of T_4 in serum (Kaplan, 1985). Androgens, glucocorticoids, L-asparaginase, danazol, colestipol-niacin therapy, severe illness, malnutrition, acromegaly, Cushing syndrome, and the nephrotic syndrome may decrease TBG concentrations. Phenytoin, and to a lesser extent barbiturates, may accelerate nondeiodinative metabolism of T_4 and may also slowly displace T_4 from serum proteins, resulting in hypothyroxinemia over time. High concentrations of salicylates, fenclofenac, furosemide, mitotane, and phenylbutazone in plasma also may displace T_4 from serum binding proteins. In addition, the higher serum concentrations of free fatty acids in the serum of severely ill patients may displace T_4 from plasma binding proteins. This effect may be exacerbated by low concentrations of albumin in serum that would normally buffer serum free fatty acids in these patients. *Principle: The use of a laboratory test for the detection of disease or the determination of drug dosage requires a thorough knowledge of the factors that can alter the results of the specific test. The test must also be coordinated with signs, symptoms, or other tests that verify the deficiency or excesses of hormone predicted by the test used for diagnosis or monitoring of the effects of therapy.*

Because of these multiple effects of drugs and nonthyroidal illness on serum T_4 concentrations, measurement of serum TSH concentrations in a sensitive assay generally provides the most accurate assessment of thyroid function in the absence of pituitary or hypothalamic disease (de los Santos et al., 1989). There is some evidence that patients with severe nonthyroidal illness may have abnormalities in hypothalamic-pituitary-thyroid function that may result in partial reduction of the concentrations of TSH (Hamblin et al., 1986). However, treatment of these patients with thyroid hormone does not appear to be beneficial (Brent and Hershman, 1986) and may in fact exacerbate their catabolic state. Such patients are usually regarded as euthyroid.

TREATMENT OF THYROID DISORDERS

Hypothyroidism

Hypothyroidism is a common disorder. In the United States, the most common cause of hypothyroidism is the autoimmune destruction of thyroid parenchyma accompanied by lymphocytic infiltration—chronic lymphocytic (Hashimoto) thyroiditis. A second potential autoimmune mechanism is related to the presence and effect of TSH-receptor blocking antibodies (Endo et al., 1978). Hypothyroidism is commonly a consequence of the treatment of hyperthyroidism by surgical removal of the thyroid gland or radioiodine ablation of thyroid tissue. Thyroidectomy for benign or malignant goitrous disease, congenital absence of the thyroid, or defects in thyroid hormone synthesis may result in hypothyroidism. Goitrogens, such as lithium and excessive iodine, as well as the recovery phases of painless and subacute thyroiditis, may be associated with transient hypothyroidism. Worldwide, iodine deficiency is an important cause of hypothyroidism, although iodine deficiency is rarely found in countries having iodized salt and iodinated compounds in bread. Hypothyroidism may also be caused by pituitary or hypothalamic disease—so-called secondary and central hypothyroidism, respectively.

Hypothyroidism is readily treated by ingestion of thyroid hormone. Nineteenth century prescriptions for the treatment of hypothyroidism included pan-fried sheep thyroid glands, desiccated thyroid, thyroid extract, or purified thyroglobulin. The latter preparations made the treatment of hypothyroidism palatable and effective, but these preparations always raise concern regarding the correct dosage. Preparations of synthetic thyroid hormone provide optimal replacement therapy. Table 14–1 lists the thyroid preparations currently available in the United States.

Levothyroxine. Levothyroxine is synthetically prepared and marketed as the monosodium salt, available as a soluble lyophilized powder for injection, or in tablet form for oral ingestion. Levothyroxine currently is considered the drug of choice for chronic replacement of thyroid hormone. While its absorption from the GI tract is variable and different commercial formulations may have slight differences in bioavailability, approximately 65% to 100% of the administered dose (average 81%) is absorbed (Fish et al., 1987). Absorption is reduced in disease states known to cause generalized malabsorption, and some thyroxine undergoes enterohepatic circulation. Because occasional generic preparations of levothyroxine have been found to contain significantly less hormone than stated (Stoffer and Szpunar, 1980), and because of potential variability in bioavailability, precise titration of dosage and maintenance therapy are best accomplished by continued use of the same commercial preparation in any given patient.

The average replacement dose of levothyroxine is 1.64 μg/kg (or 0.112 mg daily) (Fish et al., 1987). Because of its binding to serum proteins, levothyroxine has a clearance rate of only 0.0132 l/day per kilogram and a plasma half-life of 6 to 7 days. As a result, its onset of action is slow, and its duration of action is prolonged. Thyroxine is frequently viewed as a prohormone; about 25% of the administered dose is converted to T_3 by specific 5'-deiodinases present in most peripheral

Table 14–1. THYROID HORMONE PREPARATIONS

GENERIC NAMES	TRADE NAMES	APPROXIMATE EQUIVALENT DOSE	PREPARATIONS	COMMENTS
Levothyroxine (T_4)	Levothroid Levoxine Synthroid	100 μg	25-, 50-, 75-, 100-, 112-, 125-, 150-, 175-, 200-, 300-μg tablets	Drug of choice for chronic therapy.
Liothyronine (T_3)	Cytomel	25 μg	5-, 25-, 50-μg tablets	Short half-life in plasma. Used in patients with thyroid cancer in preparation for radioiodine scanning.
Liotrix	Thyrolar	1 unit	1 unit = T_4 50 μg plus T_3 12.5 μg	Fails to mimic physiologic serum T_4/T_3 ratio.
	Euthyroid		1 unit = T_4 60 μg plus T_3 15 μg 1/4, 1/2, 2, 3 units	
Thyroglobulin (pork)	Proloid	65 mg	32, 65, 100, 130, 200 mg	Contains approximately 36 μg of T_4 and 12 μg of T_3/65 mg.
Thyroid USP (pork or beef)	Armour Thyroid S-P-T Thyrar	60–65 mg	15-, 30-, 60-, 65-, 90-, 120-, 130-, 180-, 240-, 300-mg tablets	Contains approximately 38 μg of T_4 and 9 μg of T_3/65 mg.
	Thyroid Strong	40 mg	32.5, 65, 130, 200 mg	Contains approximately 50% more hormone than thyroid USP.

organs (Fig. 14–2). In most models of thyroid hormone action, T_3 is 10 times more potent than T_4. Hence, most of the biologic effects of levothyroxine therapy are mediated by its conversion to T_3.

Levothyroxine replacement therapy reverses all the clinical manifestations of hypothyroidism. Until recently titration of therapy was primarily accomplished by directly measuring concentrations of T_4 in serum. Measurements of T_4 are significantly affected by many factors that alter either the interaction of T_4 with its binding proteins or the actual level of binding proteins. Estimated measurements of unbound (free) T_4 concentrations are more accurate. Patients taking levothyroxine have higher serum T_4 concentrations than euthyroid patients on no medication (11.3 $\pm$ 1.5

vs. 8.7 $\pm$ 1.1 μg/dl; Fish et al., 1987). However, with the availability of measurements of TSH that can detect values below the normal euthyroid range, precise titration of levothyroxine therapy is best accomplished by monitoring concentrations of TSH in serum (Carr et al., 1988). Underreplacement is characterized by elevated serum TSH concentrations, and excessive replacement therapy results in suppression of serum TSH concentrations below the normal range. *Principle: The most useful surrogate end point to measure in a complicated feedback cycle of control is the first "driving hormone" affected by functional concentrations of the end product.*

Initial treatment of hypothyroidism is guided by both clinical judgment and pharmacologic principles. The long plasma half-life of T_4 results

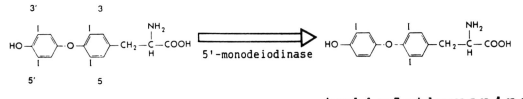

Fig. 14–2. Thyroxine is converted to T_3 by removal of the 5'-iodine by specific deiodinases present in most organs.

in a 3-week or longer delay before the full biologic effects of initial therapy or adjustments in therapy are realized (chapters 1, 37, and 38). Generally, adjustment and titration of dosages of T_4 are done at 4- to 6-week intervals (Sawin, 1985). Hypothyroidism may itself decrease the clearance of levothyroxine. As levothyroxine treatment is initiated, its clearance may increase as hypothyroidism resolves, so that plasma T_4 concentrations frequently do not vary linearly with increased dosage. *Principle: The effects of a pharmacologic agent on one or more organ systems may alter its own distribution or clearance* (see chapters 9, 11, and 37).

Patients are generally not started on full anticipated replacement doses, since it is feared that underlying heart disease in the form of angina, arrhythmia, or congestive heart failure may be exacerbated with too rapid restoration of euthyroidism. Patients started on levothyroxine may develop cardiac symptoms for the first time, presumably because their hypothyroidism had masked clinical symptoms. The factual basis for reducing the early loads of thyroid are largely anecdotal. Logic and caution simply must carry the day. Initial dosage therefore depends upon knowing whether underlying cardiac disease is likely, the age of the patient, and the severity of the hypothyroidism. A patient with angina, or an elderly patient, should be started with 0.025 mg of levothyroxine and the dosage increased by 0.025-mg increments every 4 to 8 weeks as tolerated until adequate replacement therapy is achieved. In some patients, the exacerbation or appearance of angina may limit therapy to less than full replacement. Patients without apparent or likely heart disease may be started with 0.050 mg of levothyroxine and the dosage can be increased by 0.025- to 0.050-mg increments every 4 to 6 weeks. Younger (less than 50 years), healthy patients may be started on 0.075 to 0.100 mg depending upon age and body weight. Levothyroxine crosses the placenta poorly and is safe for treating the pregnant woman (Fisher et al., 1964). Pregnancy changes T_4 distribution primarily because T_4-binding globulin is nearly doubled, increasing the size of the serum pool; however, there is no change in concentrations of the free hormone (Mulaisho and Utiger, 1977). Requirements of levothyroxine may increase during pregnancy (Pekonen et al., 1984). Treatment of hypothyroidism during pregnancy is essential since pregnancies complicated by hypothyroidism are associated with increased spontaneous abortions, still-births, and possibly fetal malformations (Davis et al., 1988).

Adrenal insufficiency can be precipitated by replacement of thyroid hormone in patients with secondary (pituitary) hypothyroidism, and/or with coexistent adrenal disease. Hypothyroidism prolongs the clearance of glucocorticoids. When secondary hypothyroidism is diagnosed, assessment of the pituitary–adrenal axis and, if indicated, appropriate glucocorticoid replacement are mandatory before initiating levothyroxine therapy. Patients with known adrenal insufficiency may require an increase in steroid dosage during the initiation of levothyroxine therapy. *Principle: When drug effects can modulate or be modulated by more than the target effect, all factors that contribute to efficacy or toxicity must be monitored and stabilized as a part of the target effects you seek.*

Several drugs can affect levothyroxine therapy. Cholestyramine interferes with the absorption of levothyroxine (Northcutt et al., 1969). These preparations should be administered as far apart as possible, at least 4 hours (see chapters 39 and 40). Phenytoin and phenobarbital have multiple effects on the pituitary–thyroid axis, including increased hepatic metabolism of levothyroxine by increasing metabolic cleavage of the ether linkage rather than the deiodinative pathways. Correction of hypothyroidism may have effects on the clearance and blood concentrations of other medications. Requirements for sedatives, narcotics, and digoxin commonly increase as hypothyroidism is treated. In contrast, correction of hypothyroidism may potentiate the effects of warfarin by increasing the catabolism of vitamin K–dependent clotting factors. Hypothyroidism may also ameliorate diabetes mellitus, and correction of hypothyroidism may necessitate an increase in the dose of insulin or hypoglycemic agents. *Principle: Do not be so focused on a specific outcome of drug therapy that you are slow to appreciate or respond to concomitant effects of the therapy that will also require intervention.*

Toxicity of levothyroxine is limited to overdosage and is manifest as hyperthyroidism. Since many of the biologic effects of levothyroxine are delayed, clinical features of hyperthyroidism may not become apparent until several days after the overdose. Management of acute overdosage includes gastric lavage and the use of charcoal, β-adrenergic receptor antagonists, and agents that block conversion of T_4 to T_3, for example, ipodate. There have been descriptions of occasional allergic reactions to the inert ingredients in levothyroxine preparations, especially to tartrazine (FD&C yellow dye No. 5), which is present in several of the formulations. Some manufacturers are eliminating tartrazine from their products. When allergies to dyes are suspected, patients can be treated with the uncolored 0.050-mg tablets.

Liothyronine. Liothyronine is synthetically prepared and available as the sodium salt of T_3

appropriate for oral administration. It differs from levothyroxine by the removal of the 5'-iodine and is three to four times more potent than levothyroxine. Greater than 90% is absorbed from the GI tract (Hays, 1970). It is less avidly bound to TBG and has a considerably shorter plasma half-life (approximately 1 day) than levothyroxine. As a result, patients taking liothyronine may have serum T_3 concentrations that exceed three times the normal range shortly after ingesting the hormone, and then drop to normal values after 12 to 24 hours (Surks et al., 1972). Possibly these large swings in hormone concentration are experienced by the patient, and there is concern that periods of hypertriiodothyronemia could have significant cardiovascular sequelae. In contrast, both serum T_4 and T_3 concentrations are relatively stable following daily levothyroxine therapy. As a result, liothyronine is *not* recommended for replacement therapy in hypothyroidism. Replacement doses have not been adequately assessed, but in general approximately 37.5 to 75 μg/day in two or three divided doses should be used.

There are three indications for the use of liothyronine. The most common use is in preparing patients with thyroid cancer for radioiodine scanning or treatment. This allows for the rapid withdrawal of thyroid hormone. Occasionally it is used to treat myxedema coma (see below). Formerly it was used to perform a *T_3-suppression test*. Liothyronine, 25 μg three times a day for 10 days, suppresses the radioiodine uptake in a normal gland but not in autonomous thyroid tissue or in the presence of thyroid-stimulating immunoglobulins. Many physicians now administer levothyroxine for approximately 4 weeks before getting a radioiodine suppression scan, rather than using a traditional T_3-suppression test.

Liotrix. Liotrix is a combination preparation of synthetic levothyroxine and liothyronine in a ratio of 4 : 1. The original intent in preparing this combination was to mimic serum concentrations of T_4 and T_3. Subsequent to its introduction, we learned that 80% to 85% of serum T_3 originates from deiodination of T_4 (Schimmel and Utiger, 1977). Therefore, liotrix fails to mimic the physiologic concentration in plasma. In addition, the short plasma half-life of liothyronine results in wide swings in concentrations of T_3 in serum. As a result, liotrix is not recommended for replacement therapy. *Principle: Theoretical advantages are not sufficient to choose and use a marketed drug. Proven value is the most important criterion for such use.*

Thyroid Extract and Thyroglobulin. Several preparations of thyroid hormone are available that are derived from hog and beef thyroid glands. Until recently, these preparations met USP standards if they contained 0.17% to 0.23% iodine and were free from inorganic or nonthyroidal iodinated compounds. One preparation, thyroid strong, is standardized to contain 0.3% iodine and is therefore 50% more potent than thyroid USP. While some manufacturers have performed *bioassays* of their products, studies have shown excessive variability in the T_4 and T_3 content of these preparations. Recent USP standards specify 38 μg of levothyroxine and 9 μg of liothyronine per 65 mg of thyroid USP, but assay and standardization of these preparations are difficult. Thyroglobulin is an extract of hog thyroid that under current USP standardization should contain 36 μg of levothyroxine and 12 μg of liothyronine per 65 mg of thyroglobulin. *Principle: Drugs that are simply extracts of tissues must be standardized by biologic and NOT chemical assays to be consistently reliable.*

These preparations are no longer recommended for the treatment of hypothyroidism since synthetic levothyroxine preparations are a superior alternative. Variable potency can be clinically apparent to patients. The liothyronine content results in variable serum concentrations of T_3 that may cause clinical symptoms or aggravate cardiovascular conditions. Additionally, monitoring therapy with these preparations can be confusing, since serum T_4 concentrations tend to be lower than those in nontreated euthyroid patients and serum T_3 concentrations tend to be higher than normal. Occasional patients develop hypersensitivity to various components in the pork or beef preparations.

Myxedema Coma

Myxedema coma or life-threatening severe hypothyroidism is not commonly encountered in clinical practice but is associated with an extremely high mortality. Effective treatment requires attention to adequate ventilation to correct CO_2 retention and hypoxia; reversal of hypothermia; correction of fluid and electrolyte abnormalities, especially water intoxication; and treatment of infection and underlying disease processes. Glucocorticoid replacement therapy is also appropriate until the pituitary–adrenal axis is assessed.

Because of the high mortality, rapid correction of the hypothyroidism has generally been felt to be appropriate. An initial loading dose of 0.3 to 0.5 mg of levothyroxine, followed by 0.050 mg a day, has been recommended (Holvey et al., 1964). Others have argued that conversion of levothyroxine to T_3 may be delayed, and that initial therapy should start with liothyronine 20 to 40 μg every 6 to 8 hours. Metabolic parameters do normalize more rapidly when liothyronine instead of levothyroxine is given to hypothyroid (noncomatose) patients (Ladenson et al., 1983). However, there is no commercial preparation of liothyronine for IV use. Hospital pharmacies can prepare their own by dissolving the powder in dilute NaOH, diluting further in saline containing 1% albumin, and sterilizing via Millipore filtration. There is no evidence yet that the morbidity of myxedema coma is reduced by initiating therapy with liothyronine.

Goiter: Thyroid Hormone Suppressive Therapy

Thyroid hormone may also be administered to previously euthyroid or hypothyroid patients for the purpose of suppressing serum TSH to subnormal concentrations with the aim of shrinking and/or preventing growth of goitrous or abnormal thyroid tissue. Patients with goitrous Hashimoto thyroiditis, multinodular goiters, endemic goiters, or benign solitary nodules (follicular or colloid adenomas); patients with a history of radiation treatment to the head or neck region; and patients who have had surgery for benign or cancerous growths of the thyroid may require thyroid hormone preparations for suppression of their pituitary–thyroid axis. Levothyroxine is the preparation of choice for the reasons outlined above. Patients taking truly suppressive doses of levothyroxine can be said to have subclinical hyperthyroidism. Such therapy may be associated with minor changes in hepatic enzyme activity, serum proteins, the systolic time interval, or bone density (Ross, 1988). Accordingly, suppressive therapy should be administered in the smallest possible doses that achieve suppression of TSH. Recently, more sensitive assays of TSH have demonstrated that TSH concentrations may be reduced only slightly to just below the normal range, or more profoundly to more than 10-fold below the lower limit of the normal range. The desired degree of TSH suppression may vary depending upon the indication (e.g., cancer vs. benign nodule). Studies in progress utilizing sensitive TSH assays will eventually determine guidelines for the optimal use of thyroid hormone suppressive therapy. *Principle: Subtle long-term side effects of drugs may be considered trivial when treating potentially life-threatening disease, but these minimal toxicities may impact on the long-term risk/benefit ratio when treatment of benign and chronic disease is contemplated.*

Hyperthyroidism

Hyperthyroidism can present as a dramatic illness, with significant weight loss, tremulousness, palpitations and arrhythmias, emotional lability, sweating and heat intolerance, and hyperdefecation. If untreated, hyperthyroidism may lead to thyroid storm, hemodynamic instability, hyperpyrexia, and death. The cause of hyperthyroidism must be determined in order to decide on the most appropriate therapy. Hyperthyroidism is most frequently due either to Graves disease or to toxic adenoma(s) that may occur as a solitary adenoma or as autonomous tissue within a multinodular goiter. In these instances, hyperthyroidism occurs as a consequence of synthesis of excess thyroid hormone. In Graves disease, specific immunoglobulins referred to as thyroid-stimulating immunoglobulins (TSIs) activate the TSH receptor. In toxic adenomas, the thyroid follicular cells become partially autonomous of TSH regulation and produce excessive thyroid hormone. Treatment is directed at interfering with thyroid hormone synthesis with the use of thionamides, or destroying thyroid tissue with radioiodine ablation or surgical excision.

One must recognize that not all hyperthyroidism is the result of excessive synthesis of thyroid hormones. In subacute (granulomatous), painless (lymphocytic), and post-partum (lymphocytic) thyroiditis, hyperthyroidism results from excess release of preformed thyroid hormone from an inflamed gland; synthesis of new hormone has already stopped because of the inflammation and disruption of normal follicular cell function and TSH suppression. Consequently in these patients, the use of thionamides is not beneficial. Factitious ingestion of thyroid hormone is another cause of hyperthyroidism that does not respond to therapies aimed at suppressing thyroid hormone synthesis.

Therefore, it is essential to determine the cause of the hyperthyroidism prior to starting therapy. Usually the 24-hour radioiodine uptake should be measured to document the increased synthetic activity (ongoing organification of iodine) prior to the administration of drugs that block organification or destroy the thyroid (e.g., radioiodine). *Principle: In the treatment of a syndrome that may be caused by several different diseases, appropriate therapy may depend critically on an exact diagnosis. On the other hand, in some syndromes (e.g., essential hypertension), appropriate therapy may be chosen relatively independently of an understanding of the mechanisms involved.*

Antithyroid Drugs. The goitrogenic effect of thiocyanates in humans was occasionally noted in studies using thiocyanates to treat hypertension (Barker et al., 1941). Animal studies of related compounds led to the appreciation of the therapeutic potential of thioureylene derivatives. Studies of the antibiotic sulfaguanidine on mouse intestinal flora found that the animals all had markedly hypertrophied thyroid glands (MacKenzie et al., 1941). Another study of taste preferences in rats using phenylthiocarbamide also demonstrated thyroid hypertrophy (Richter and Clisby, 1942). This led two groups of investigators in 1943 to systematically study these and related compounds; they concluded that their mechanism of action was an inhibition of thyroid hormone synthesis (MacKenzie and MacKenzie, 1943; Astwood et al., 1943). Additional studies led to the introduction of the two antithyroid drugs available in the United States: 6-propylthiouracil (PTU) and 1-methylmercaptoimidazole (methimazole) (Fig.14-3). These drugs are actively concentrated into thyroid tissue, where their major mechanism of action is inhibition of iodide organification to tyrosine residues on thyroglobulin, as well as inhibition of the coupling reaction between iodotyrosines. The drugs are themselves iodinated, and it is thought that they compete for oxidized iodine with thyroglobulin. They may also bind to thyroglobulin and have effects on thyroglobulin synthesis (Cooper, 1984).

The two drugs differ in some important respects. PTU is less soluble in aqueous solutions and is heavily protein-bound. As a result it crosses the placenta only a fourth as well as methimazole (Marchant et al., 1977) and is concentrated in breast milk only one tenth as well (Kampmann et al., 1980). Methimazole has a serum half-life of 4 to 6 hours, longer than the 75 minutes for PTU (Cooper et al., 1982, 1984). While both drugs are rapidly absorbed and reach peak concentrations in plasma in 1 to 2 hours, their mechanism of action requires high sustained intrathyroidal concentrations. Because of active transport into the thyroid, the thyroid/blood ratio is as high as 100 : 1 (Aungst et al., 1979). Since methimazole remains concentrated within the thyroid for 20 hours (Jansson et al., 1983) and has a duration of action as long as 40 hours, single-day dosage is effective despite the short plasma half-life. PTU is felt to have a shorter intrathyroidal residence (Cooper, 1984).

Clinicians have generally observed that methimazole is 10 times more potent than PTU (Cooper, 1984). The dosage and choice of antithyroid drug have been based on physician preference. However, a careful analysis would suggest that methimazole controls hyperthyroidism more easily, and is associated with less toxicity (Cooper,

1986). The appreciation of the pharmacokinetics of methimazole has led to clinical studies documenting its effectiveness when administered as a single daily dose (Bouma, 1980); the effectiveness of single-dose therapy with PTU is controversial (Cooper, 1984). In the United States, patients are usually started on methimazole 30 mg in single or divided doses, or PTU 300 mg in divided doses, usually three times a day. While this provides rapid inhibition of synthesis of thyroid hormone, one should note that these drugs do not inhibit release of stored thyroid hormones. Euthyroidism is therefore delayed until the extensive stores of thyroid hormone in the colloid are exhausted. Then doses of thionamide are frequently reduced to "maintenance concentrations," frequently one third or less of the starting dose. Recent studies have demonstrated that these lower maintenance doses can be used initially, and the duration of time to achieve euthyroidism is the same as with traditional higher doses (Mashio et al., 1988). The dosage of thionamide may need to be reduced to allow some thyroid hormone synthesis to occur; otherwise the patient may become hypothyroid. Some physicians continue relatively high doses of the antithyroid drugs and add levothyroxine to treat the hypothyroidism. The disadvantage to this approach is that it confounds attempts to determine whether the patient may still require active therapy.

One clear advantage of methimazole is its longer duration of action. This allows its use as a single daily dose (Bouma and Kammer, 1980). While many physicians still prefer to begin with split doses, possibly to minimize the GI side effects, one is usually able to taper the dose to 5 to 15 mg once in the morning. Patients taking PTU initially require multiple dosing, and many patients on maintenance therapy escape from the organification blockade if PTU is given only once daily. These differences between methimazole and PTU are listed in Table 14-2.

Before starting antithyroid drugs, it is essential to understand the anticipated end point of therapy. Patients with Graves disease may be given antithyroid drugs for a fixed period, frequently 1 or 2 years, in the hope that the disease will go into remission. Remission occurs in 20% to 40% of patients treated with antithyroid drugs. Remission is more likely in females, patients with mild hyperthyroidism and small glands, patients whose

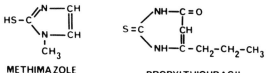

METHIMAZOLE   **PROPYLTHIOURACIL**

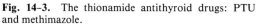

Fig. 14–3. The thionamide antithyroid drugs: PTU and methimazole.

Table 14-2. COMPARISON OF THE ANTITHYROID DRUGS

	PTU	METHIMAZOLE (TAPEZOLE)
Preparations	50-mg tablets	5-, 10-mg tablets
Pharmacology	Serum $t_{1/2}$ = 75 min	Serum $t_{1/2}$ = 4–6 h Intrathyroidal $t_{1/2}$ = 20+ h 10 times as potent
	Highly protein-bound	Not protein-bound Crosses placenta Concentrates in breast milk
	Inhibits T_4-to-T_3 conversion	
Initial dosage	100–150 mg q6–8h	10 mg q8h or 15–30 mg once daily
Toxicity	Rash, fever, athralgias, nausea Agranulocytosis 0.5% Hepatocellular necrosis	Rash, fever, athralgias, nausea Agranulocytosis less common if dose < 30 mg daily Cholestatic jaundice Congenital scalp defect

PTU = 6-propylthiouracil.

glands shrink rapidly after the onset of therapy, and patients with positive antithyroid antibodies (Greer et al., 1977; Takaichi et al., 1989). There is controversial evidence that the antithyroid drugs themselves are immunomodulatory and may make remissions more likely (Ratanachaiyavong and McGregor, 1985). In contrast to patients with Graves hyperthyroidism, patients with toxic adenoma(s) are not likely to have spontaneous remission of their disease, and these patients are treated with a short course of antithyroid drugs to render them euthyroid prior to the administration of radioiodine or surgery. Similarly, some patients with Graves disease who have opted for ablative therapy are first treated with a short course of antithyroid drugs to deplete thyroid hormone stores prior to radioiodine treatment, or to render them euthyroid prior to surgery.

During pregnancy, maternal hyperthyroidism is best treated with PTU since placental transfer is less than that of methimazole, and the chances of fetal hypothyroidism and goiter are decreased (Marchant et al., 1977). Additionally, methimazole may cause a rare scalp defect, aplasia cutis (Milham and Elledge, 1972). Pregnant women taking PTU need frequent assessment of thyroid function tests to avoid inadequate treatment or overtreatment. It is important to consider that serum T_4 concentrations are normally elevated in pregnancy because of increased thyroxine-binding globulin (Mulaisho and Utiger, 1977). Free-T_4 and sensitive TSH measurements are useful end points to follow.

Both antithyroid drugs have significant and overlapping toxicity, although the more serious toxicities may be associated with PTU. Rash, urticaria, fever, arthralgias, and arthritis occur in up to 5% of patients. Mild leukopenia is seen in some patients, although many patients with Graves disease have antineutrophilic antibodies

(Weitzman et al., 1985). Agranulocytosis is a serious complication of therapy, occurring in about 0.5% of patients. In retrospective analysis (Cooper et al., 1983), agranulocytosis was more likely to occur in older patients. Patients taking higher doses of methimazole (> 40 mg) were more likely to have agranulocytosis than patients taking a lower dose. The incidence was independent of dose with PTU. Therefore, treatment with doses of methimazole under 30 mg has been recommended, since the incidence of agranulocytosis was lowest with this regimen. Patients should be warned to discontinue use of these drugs and obtain a white cell count at the first sign of fever or infection; once agranulocytosis has been excluded, therapy with the drug can be resumed. Hepatocellular necrosis is a rare side effect seen with PTU therapy; methimazole may be associated with cholestatic jaundice. For patients who have a minor reaction to one antithyroid drug, the other drug can be substituted, although cross-sensitivity may be seen in up to 50% of cases (Jackson, 1975).

Radioiodine. The majority of patients with hyperthyroidism in the United States eventually receive radioiodine ablation of their thyroid glands. The ^{131}I is administered as an oral solution of sodium iodide. The isotope is concentrated and organified into active thyroid tissue, and the β emissions cause extensive tissue damage that will result in effective ablation of the gland after 6 to 18 weeks or longer (Graham and Burman, 1986). Currently there are two general approaches to ablative therapy. Most physicians recognize permanent hypothyroidism as the expected outcome of radioiodine treatment and treat with doses designed to administer 100 to 160 μCi/g of thyroid tissue; on average this is a total dose of 5 to 15 mCi. The dose delivered to the thyroid is usually between 5000 and 20,000 rad; however, the penetration of the β emissions is limited to only a few centimeters, so other tissues receive little exposure. Using these doses, 60% to 70% of patients are rendered hypothyroid within 6 to 12 months (Ross et al., 1983). About 10% remain hyperthyroid and require a second dose. Those patients who become euthyroid are at more risk for late recurrent hyperthyroidism, and 2% to 5% of treated euthyroid patients per year ultimately become hypothyroid. For those patients and physicians who feel that permanent hypothyroidism should be avoided, a compensated low-dose treatment program, usually requiring several smaller doses of radioiodine, can reduce the incidence of hypothyroidism (Sridama et al., 1984). However, this considerably delays the resolution of hyperthyroidism and its potential adverse long-term effects on other organ systems, especially bone (Smith et al., 1973).

Younger patients without cardiovascular disease may be given radioiodine as primary therapy. Older patients and patients with underlying medical illnesses are usually pretreated with antithyroid drugs to deplete thyroid hormone stores. This strategy prevents symptomatic exacerbation of hyperthyroid symptoms that may occasionally be seen when the radioiodine induces thyroiditis, with leakage of preformed hormone from the gland into the blood. Antithyroid drugs are stopped at least a few days before therapy so that organification of the isotope into thyroglobulin can proceed. Thionamides are restarted a few days after therapy to prevent new hormone synthesis while destruction of follicular cells proceeds.

Despite theoretic concerns about carcinogenicity, several studies of large numbers of patients followed for up to 15 to 20 years have failed to demonstrate an increased risk of cancer following radioiodine treatment of hyperthyroidism (Graham and Burman, 1986), including one prospective study of 36,000 patients that failed to detect an increased incidence of leukemia (Saenger et al., 1968). There is also no evidence that radioiodine is teratogenic to the unfertilized eggs stored in the ovary. Ovarian exposures are minimal, and similar to those of many diagnostic radiographic procedures such as a barium enema. Radioiodine is contraindicated in pregnancy, however, since, especially after the tenth week, destruction of fetal thyroid tissue would result. *Principle: The physician must be prepared to assess the long-range effects of therapy as well as the initial results. Data on prolonged and subtle effects of therapy are much more difficult to record than cause-and-effect events. However, such data may be most critical in establishing a risk/ benefit ratio for the therapy and, therefore, in establishing a logical choice between modes with differing acute effects.*

Surgery. Surgery is a reasonable alternative to radioiodine ablation in those patients who refuse radioiodine therapy, and in patients who have an extremely large gland or cosmetically large toxic adenoma (most diffuse glands and toxic adenoma shrink after radioiodine, but in very large glands the final appearance may not be optimal). The risks peculiar to thyroid surgery include damage to the recurrent laryngeal nerves and damage to the parathyroid glands. Surgeons, like radiotherapists, can remove nearly the entire gland, which results in hypothyroidism, or leave a remnant. Surgical remnants may reduce the incidence of postoperative hypothyroidism, but they also may grow and result in recurrent hyperthyroidism (Jortso et al., 1987). Since the risks of surgery are increased in untreated hyperthyroid patients, ideally patients are treated with antithyroid drugs to attain euthyroidism prior to surgery. Recently, the use of β-adrenergic antagonists and iodide alone have been successfully used in patients who are unable to take antithyroid drugs preoperatively (Feek et al., 1980).

β-Adrenergic Blocking Agents. Many of the manifestations of hyperthyroidism are mediated through increased effects of catecholamines on β-adrenergic receptors; in part this may be due to thyroid hormone–induced increased expression of β receptors (Bilezekian and Loeb, 1983). β-Adrenergic receptor blockade provides some relief from anxiety, palpitations, tremor, and heat intolerance without changing thyroid hormone levels (Grossman et al., 1971). Propranolol (Wiersinga and Touber, 1977) decreases serum T_3 concentrations by 15% to 20% by inhibiting T_4-to-T_3 conversion; the other β-adrenergic antagonists have little or no effect. While in vitro data demonstrate that all the β-adrenergic antagonists can block the hepatic monodeiodinase, inhibition occurs only at concentrations significantly higher than those usually obtained in plasma. Propranolol may be effective in vivo because of its lipid solubility and possible concentration in hepatic tissue (Shulkin et al., 1984). Despite this theoretical advantage, many patients find once-daily agents to be more convenient. Symptomatic hyperthyroid patients without a contraindication should be offered β-adrenergic blocking agents. When indicated because of coexisting medical conditions, β_1-selective agents can be employed.

Alternative Modalities: Iodide, Ipodate, Lithium, Perchlorate. While antithyroid drugs, radioiodine, and surgery are the traditional approaches to the treatment of conventional hyperthyroidism, several other drugs may occasionally be useful. Iodides themselves inhibit release of thyroid hormone and in patients with Graves disease inhibit organification. Burnt-sponge extract, one of the earliest treatments of hyperthyroidism, was replaced in the 19th century with specific iodide-containing elixirs, Lugol's solution (5% iodine and 10% potassium iodide; approximately 6.3 mg of iodine per drop) and saturated solution of potassium iodide (SSKI; approximately 38 mg of iodine per drop). Iodides are rarely useful as monotherapy to control hyperthyroidism; however, they may be useful adjunctive therapy following administration of radioiodine. If iodide therapy is started a week after radioiodine therapy, patients achieve euthyroidism more rapidly; however, subsequent follow-up may be prolonged because of the need to then taper the iodides (Ross et al., 1983). In patients who remain slightly hyperthyroid several months following radioiodine therapy for Graves disease, iodides alone may be sufficient to control the hyperthyroidism, since the "damaged" gland is more susceptible to the inhibitory effects of iodide.

It must be emphasized that the iodide may ameliorate hyperthyroidism by causing a persistent block in organification in patients with Graves hyperthyroidism, while patients with toxic adenoma frequently become worse with the use of iodide that then simply provides additional substrate for synthesis of hormone. Iodides are also used for 10 days prior to thyroid surgery for Graves disease to decrease the vascularity of the gland. Iodides occasionally cause sialadenitis, fever, urticaria, or a dose-dependent acneiform rash. Many commercial iodide preparations contain sodium bisulfite that may be the cause of allergic reactions.

Lithium may also block release of thyroid hormone, but its CNS and cardiovascular toxicity make it a poor choice for therapy.

Ipodate, a radiocontrast agent, both is rich in iodine and blocks conversion of T_4 to T_3. Rarely, this agent alone may be sufficient to control patients with Graves hyperthyroidism (Shen et al., 1985). The drug may also be useful in overcoming the effects of levothyroxine overdosage by blocking conversion of the latter into the more active hormone. Finally, the drug is used as adjunctive therapy for treating thyroid storm.

Perchlorate is not available in the United States as an antithyroid drug because of the high incidence of bone marrow toxicity. However, recently it has been used in combination with thionamides in hyperthyroid patients who develop iodine-induced hyperthyroidism due to amiodarone therapy (Martino et al., 1986). Amiodarone, a cardiac antiarrhythmic agent, contains 75 mg of iodine per tablet and is an increasingly common cause of iodine-induced thyroid dysfunction

(chapter 6). *Principle: The cross-system effects of drugs usually used by specialists are often subtle and easily missed by the physician interested dominantly if not exclusively in a single organ system.*

Thyroid Storm

Thyroid storm is rarely seen in modern practice since most hyperthyroid patients consult a physician before they become severely ill. Appropriate treatment usually is rapidly instituted. Like patients with myxedema coma, patients with thyroid storm frequently have a precipitating illness such as a severe infection. Treatment of the precipitating illness, hyperthermia, arrhythmias, and agitation is as important as treating the hyperthyroidism. Antithyroid drugs should be started as soon as possible (Robbins, 1988). PTU is preferred by some physicians because it also blocks conversion of T_4 to T_3. Because of its shorter half-life, PTU should be administered every 4 to 6 hours in severely hyperthyroid hospitalized patients. Methimazole may be used and has the advantage of a longer duration of action. Both drugs can be given rectally if the patient cannot take medication by mouth. Iodides are given to block thyroid hormone release; 750 mg to 1 g of sodium iodide per day IV, or 10 drops of SSKI three times daily provides more than enough iodide. Minimal or optimal doses are unknown. Administration should be delayed for at least 1 hour or longer after initiation of thionamide therapy to accomplish adequate blockade of organification; otherwise, the iodide may provide substrate for additional hormone synthesis. Another approach is to give ipodate with methimazole, since ipodate is a more powerful blocker of T_4-to-T_3 conversion than PTU and is also rich in iodine. β-Adrenergic blocking agents can be added to control sympathetic overactivity and may be useful in reducing heart rate and controlling arrhythmias. However, their use should be carefully monitored if congestive heart failure is present (Ikram, 1977). Propranolol is the agent commonly used since it is available for IV administration. Glucocorticoids are frequently given and have many theoretical benefits that have not actually been demonstrated in this setting. They inhibit T_4-to-T_3 conversion, ameliorate the underlying autoimmune disease, and treat possible relative adrenal insufficiency. Plasmapheresis may be used to remove thyroid hormone in cases that fail to respond rapidly to the usual measures. *Principle: Careful consideration allows choice of a nonconflicting sequence of drugs when it is likely that more than one drug will be necessary to manage a disease state.*

Hyperthyroidism in Pregnancy

The major therapy for a pregnant hyperthyroid patient involves PTU. Methimazole is relatively contraindicated because it can cause a rare fetal scalp defect, aplasia cutis. Radioiodine is harmful to the fetal thyroid. Iodides may cause fetal goiter and consequently impose a risk of asphyxiation at delivery. Surgery occasionally becomes necessary in the patient who cannot take PTU. The goals of therapy are essentially similar to those in the nonpregnant patient; however, therapy must be closely monitored to avoid overtreatment, which is associated with fetal hypothyroidism and fetal goiter. Since levothyroxine crosses the placenta poorly (Fisher et al., 1964), it should not be given to hyperthyroid pregnant women taking antithyroid drugs with the intent of preventing fetal hypothyroidism. If elevations of serum TSH concentrations occur, the dose of the antithyroid drug should be reduced to the lowest dose necessary to control the hyperthyroidism.

Prevention of Neonatal Graves Disease

Following radioiodine ablation or surgery, a woman may be taking levothyroxine for hypothyroidism but still may have a high titer of serum TSI. Some TSI, especially if present in high titers, has been shown to cross the placenta and cause fetal and neonatal hyperthyroidism. Pregnant women with a past history of ablative therapy for Graves disease have a 1% risk of having a child with neonatal Graves disease. If fetal hyperthyroidism is suspected because of high fetal heart rate, advanced ultrasonographic age compared with expected age based on the last menstrual period, craniosynostosis or fetal goiter on ultrasound examination, and/or high maternal TSI titers (>500%), one can consider PTU therapy during pregnancy to treat the fetus in utero (Zakarija and McKenzie, 1983).

Ophthalmopathy

Most patients with Graves disease, and some patients with Hashimoto thyroiditis, demonstrate an infiltration and inflammation of the retroorbital muscles and surrounding tissues with resultant proptosis and lid retraction (Jacobson and Gorman, 1984). Fortunately for most patients, the ophthalmopathy is not severe and can be treated conservatively. Local lubricants such as methylcellulose solutions, elevation of the head, and taping the eyelids closed at night are useful. In more severe cases, corneal ulceration, diplopia, and traction or compression of the optic nerve with loss of vision can occur. High-dose glucocorticoids (60–120 mg of prednisone daily) for prolonged periods may reduce orbital inflammation. When vision is threatened, external radiation therapy to the inflamed orbital tissues and/or decompressive surgery with removal of a portion of the bony structure of the orbit may be indicated. Corrective surgery on eye muscles, use of prisms,

and cosmetic surgery on eyelids and suborbital soft tissues may be required to restore function and appearance toward normal. *Principle: When possible therapies are diverse and clinical data are conflicting, the therapist must look for strengths and weaknesses in the data in order to make his or her own decision: (1) The conclusions related to results or to comparisons of results may be invalid by virtue of patient selection or improper design (see chapter 1). (2) The drugs may all be relatively ineffective (particularly with a disease whose natural history is either unknown or notoriously variable) or may not have been used in a manner that can establish their effect. (3) The pathogenesis of the disease may be so poorly understood that all therapy must be considered palliative, and heroic doses or irreversible measures should be approached with caution. (4) If alternative 3 applies (as with exophthalmos and perhaps with pretibial myxedema), the physician can recognize that his or her therapy is empirical and palliative, and use the therapy but remain open to valid studies suggesting unconventional approaches. If the disease is uncommon, the patient may be referred to therapists skilled in the special care of such patients. Often a carefully selected referral may be a valuable therapeutic maneuver.*

Pretibial Myxedema

Rarely, patients with Graves disease develop a violaceous, elevated, pruritic induration, most commonly over the pretibial area, due to the infiltration of mucopolysaccharides; this is termed *pretibial myxedema*. This unusual complication of Graves disease is felt to be autoimmune and responds poorly to therapy. Fluorinated glucocorticoid creams under occlusive dressings have been reported to be useful in some patients (Kriss et al., 1967).

Subacute, Painless, and Postpartum Thyroiditis

Subacute (granulomatous) thyroiditis is a dramatic painful inflammation of the thyroid gland that is frequently associated with a preceding upper respiratory illness, fever, malaise, and changes in Coxsackie or mumps viral titers (Volpe, 1979). Hyperthyroidism occurs because of the release of preformed hormone from the inflamed gland. The disease is usually self-limited, lasting for 1 to several months. The hyperthyroid phase is usually followed by a hypothyroid phase after the thyroid hormone stores are depleted and prior to recovery of synthetic function of the thyroid. Ultimately, recovery is usually complete. *The physician must realize that antithyroid drugs are not efficacious in treating this hyperthyroidism*, since the hyperthyroidism is not due to ongoing synthesis of hormone, but rather to the leakage of previously synthesized and stored hormone. β-Adrenergic antagonists are the mainstay of therapy. The neck pain is frequently the major complaint. Salicylates or NSAIDs are frequently sufficient to manage pain. Because the response to glucocorticoid therapy is rapid and dramatic, many physicians are quick to initiate prednisone therapy at doses that range from 20 to 60 mg daily (Volpe, 1979). However, once glucocorticoid therapy is started, attempts to taper it may result in recurrent symptoms and a prolonged course of glucocorticoid therapy. Many physicians therefore reserve the use of corticosteroids for the most severe cases.

Painless (lymphocytic) thyroiditis that frequently occurs in the postpartum period is an autoimmune disorder related to the other autoimmune thyroid diseases (Nikolai et al., 1982). Painless lymphocytic inflammation of the gland results in leakage of preformed hormone and a course of spontaneously resolving hyperthyroidism that is similar to that seen in subacute thyroiditis. The radioiodine uptake should be measured in these patients to confirm the diagnosis. While patients with Graves disease or toxic adenoma have an elevated radioiodine uptake, patients with painless (or subacute) thyroiditis have a suppressed uptake that is almost always less than 1%. Since the hyperthyroidism is not due to ongoing synthesis of new hormone, antithyroid drugs and radioiodine are not efficacious, and β-adrenergic antagonists are used to treat symptomatic patients. *Principle: Whenever possible, a proper diagnosis should be established before therapy is started. This requirement prevents the toxicity that will be the dominant effect of an improperly chosen drug.*

Thyroid Cancer

The treatment of papillary and follicular cancer of the thyroid is extremely controversial and may differ substantially in different centers. Papillary cancer of the thyroid accounts for about 70% of all thyroid cancer in the United States, and some cases are secondary to a prior history of head or neck irradiation for unrelated disorders. For the majority of patients, it is a rather indolent tumor associated with a good prognosis. Patients under the age of 40 to 50 years who have intrathyroidal lesions (even with cervical lymph node metastases) have recurrence and mortality rates of less than 3% to 10% and less than 1% to 5%, respectively (McConahey et al., 1986; Vickery et al., 1987). However, older patients with extrathyroidal spread or distant metastases at the time of presentation have 10-year mortality rates of 20% and 65%, respectively. Initial treatment is surgery, but the extent of initial surgery is controversial. Some centers recommend hemithyroidectomy for low-risk young patients with intrathy-

roidal lesions to avoid surgical complications such as recurrent laryngeal nerve injury or hypoparathyroidism (Hay et al., 1987), while other centers recommend total thyroidectomy for all patients to facilitate follow-up with radioiodine scanning and serum thyroglobulin measurements.

Papillary cancer may spread though lymphatic channels to lung, bone, or other organs. Follicular cancer, which accounts for 10% to 15% of thyroid cancer in the United States, spreads via hematogenous routes, occurs in somewhat older patients, and is associated with a slightly worse prognosis. However, young patients with minimally invasive disease generally have 10-year mortality rates of only 3% to 5%. Thyroid cancer is primarily a surgical disease, and aggressive surgical approaches are appropriate for patients with locally invasive disease. Thyroid hormone suppressive therapy (see above) is critical for all postsurgical patients since growth of any remaining differentiated thyroid cancer may be partially stimulated by TSH. Radioiodine is a uniquely effective antitumor therapy for patients with differentiated thyroid cancer (Hurley and Becker, 1983). In the presence of an elevated TSH concentration, large doses of administered radioiodine will be concentrated in functioning tumor recurrences and metastases and can be calculated to deliver local radiation doses of 3000 to 20,000 rads. Frequently, following primary surgery, normal thyroid remnants are first ablated with radioiodine. Subsequent total body scanning with radioiodine tracer identifies persistent, recurrent, and metastatic disease. Therapeutic doses may range from 30 to 200 mCi or more. Dosimetry is influenced by the uptake in the remnant or metastases, and the calculated dose to other organs. Complications of therapy include radiation thyroiditis in remnants, pain in metastases, rare nausea or vomiting, sialoadenitis, transient bone marrow suppression, and transient azoospermia. With repetitive high doses, long-term complications include pulmonary fibrosis in patients with extensive lung metastases, permanent bone marrow suppression, leukemia, permanent azoospermia, rare ovarian failure, and a slight increased incidence of bladder cancer (Edmonds and Smith, 1986).

Recurrent disease is frequently approached surgically. About one third of metastases or recurrences are nonfunctional, that is, fail to accumulate radioiodine. In these patients and patients with rapidly growing tumor, if a surgical approach is impossible, external radiotherapy may be utilized to reduce the growth rate and delay local complications from invasive disease (Tubiana et al., 1985). Chemotherapy has had a limited role in the treatment of differentiated thyroid cancer, primarily because the disease responds well to other modalities (Ahuja and Ernst, 1987). In several clinical series, adriamycin has occasionally produced reductions in tumor mass and prolonged survival in patients with nonfunctional metastases. Adriamycin combined with cisplatin is associated with a higher response rate, but combined therapy is also associated with increased toxicity.

There are several less common forms of thyroid cancer. Anaplastic thyroid cancer generally responds poorly to all therapeutic modalities. External radiation therapy may give short-term palliation, but most patients die within 6 to 12 months. Medullary cancer of the thyroid originates in the parafollicular cells and is frequently familial or a component of the multiple endocrine neoplasia II syndrome. Surgery is the primary therapy for the initial and recurrent disease. Thyroid lymphoma is responsive to external radiation therapy, and chemotherapy is utilized in patients with higher-stage or aggressive histologic findings.

REFERENCES

Ahuja, S.; and Ernst, H.: Chemotherapy of thyroid carcinoma. J. Endocrinol. Invest., 10:303–310, 1987.

Astwood, E. B.; Sullivan, J.; Bissell, A.; and Tyslowitz, R.: Action of certain sulfonamides and thiourea upon the function of the thyroid gland of the rat. Endocrinology, 32:210–225, 1943.

Aungst, B. J.; Vesell, E. S.; and Shapiro, J. R.: Unusual characteristics of the dose-dependent uptake of propylthiouracil by thyroid gland in vivo: Effects of thyrotropin, iodide, or phenobarbital pretreatment. Biochem. Pharmacol., 28:1479–1484, 1979.

Barker, M. H.; Lindberg, H. A.; and Wald, M. H.: Further experiments with thiocyanates. J.A.M.A., 117:1591–1594, 1941.

Bilezekian, J. P.; and Loeb, J. N.: The influence of hyperthyroidism and hypothyroidism on α- and β-adrenergic receptor systems and adrenergic responsiveness. Endocr. Rev., 4:378–388, 1983.

Bouma, D. J.; and Kammer, H.: Single daily dose methimazole treatment of hyperthyroidism. West. J. Med., 132:13–15, 1980.

Brent, G. A.; and Hershman, J. M.: Thyroxine therapy in patients with severe nonthyroidal illness and low serum thyroxine concentrations. J. Clin. Endocrinol. Metab., 63:1–8, 1986.

Carr, D.; McLeod, D. T.; Parry, G.; and Thornes, H. M.: Fine adjustment of thyroxine replacement dosage: Comparison of the thyrotropin releasing hormone test using a sensitive thyrotropin assay with measurement of free hormones and clinical assessment. Clin. Endocrinol., 28:325–333, 1988.

Cooper, D. S.: Which anti-thyroid drug? Am. J. Med., 80:1165–1168, 1986.

Cooper, D. S.: Antithyroid drugs. N. Engl. J. Med., 311:1353–1362, 1984.

Cooper, D. S.; Bode, H. H.; Nath, B.; Saxe V.; Maloof, F.; and Ridgway, E. C.: Methimazole pharmacology in man: Studies using a newly developed radioimmunoassay for methimazole. J. Clin. Endocrinol. Metab., 58:473–479, 1984.

Cooper, D. S.; Goldminz, D.; Levin, A. A.; Ladenson, P. W.; Daniels, G. H.; Molitch, M. E.; and Ridgway, E. C.: Agranulocytosis associated with antithyroid drugs: Effects of patient age and drug dose. Ann. Intern. Med., 98:26–29, 1983.

Cooper, D. S.; Saxe, V. C.; Meskell, M.; Maloof, F.; and Ridgway, E. C.: Acute effects of propylthiouracil (PTU) on thyroidal iodide organificaton and peripheral iodothyronine deiodination: Correlation with serum PTU levels measured by radioimmunoassay. J. Clin. Endocrinol. Metab., 54:101–107, 1982.

Davis, L. E.; Leveno, K. J.; and Cunnigham, F. G.: Hypothy-roidism complicating pregnancy. Obstet. Gynecol., 72:108–112, 1988.

DeGroot, L. J.; and Niepomniszcze, H.: Biosynthesis of thyroid hormone: Basic and clinical aspects. Metabolism, 26:665–718, 1977.

Edmonds, C. J.; and Smith, J.: The long-term hazards of the treatment of thyroid cancer with radioiodine. Br. J. Radiol., 59:45–51, 1986.

Ehrmann, D. A.; and Sarne, D. H.: Serum thyrotropin and the assessment of thyroid status. Ann. Intern. Med., 110:179–181, 1989.

Endo, K.; Kasagi, K.; Konishi, J.; Ikekubo, K.; Okuno, T.; Takeda, Y.; Mori, T.; and Torizuka, K.: Detection and properties of TSH-binding inhibitor immunoglobulins in patients with Graves' disease and Hashimoto's thyroiditis. J. Clin. Endocrinol. Metab., 46:734–739, 1978.

Engler, D.; and Burger, A. G.: The deiodination of the iodothyronines and of their derivatives in man. Endocr. Rev., 5:151–184, 1984.

Feek, C. M.; Sawers, S. A.; Irvine, W. J.; Beckett, G. J.; Ratcliffe, W. A.; and Toft, A. D.: Combination of potassium iodide and propranolol in preparation of patients with Graves' disease for thyroid surgery. N. Engl. J. Med., 302:883–885, 1980.

Fish, L. H.; Schwartz, H. L.; Cavanaugh, J.; Steffes, M. W.; Bantle, J. P.; and Oppenheimer, J. H.: Replacement dose, metabolism, and bioavailability of levothyroxine in the treatment of hypothyroidism. Role of triiodothyronine in pituitary feedback in humans. N. Engl. J. Med., 316:764–770, 1987.

Fisher, D. A.; Lehman, H.; and Lackey, C.: Placental transport of thyroxine. J. Clin. Endocrinol. Metab., 24:393–400, 1964.

Fradkin, J. E.; and Wolff, J.: Iodine induced thyrotoxicosis. Medicine, 62:1–20, 1983.

Graham, G. D.; and Burman, K. D.: Radioiodine treatment of Graves' disease. An assessment of its potential risks. Ann. Intern. Med., 105:900–905, 1986.

Greer, M. A.; Kammer, H.; and Bouma, D. J.: Short-term antithyroid drug therapy for the thyrotoxicosis of Graves disease. N. Engl. J. Med., 297:173–176, 1977.

Grossman, W.; Robin, N. I.; Johnson, L. W.; Brooks, H.; Selenhow, H. A.; and Dexter, L.: Effects of beta blockade on the peripheral manifestations of thyrotoxicosis. Ann. Intern. Med., 74:875–879, 1971.

Hamblin, P. S.; Dyer, S. A.; Mohr, V. S.; LeGrand, B. A.; Lim, C. F.; Tuxen, D. V.; Topliss, D. J.; and Stockigt, J. R.: Relationships between thyrotropin and thyroxine changes during recovery from severe thyrohypoxinemia of illness. J. Clin. Endocrinol. Metab., 62:717–722, 1986.

Hay, I. D.; Grant, C. S.; Taylor, W. F.; and McConahey, W. M.: Ipsilateral lobectomy versus bilateral lobar resection in papillary thyroid carcinoma: A retrospective analysis of surgical outcome using a novel scoring system. Surgery, 102:1088–1095, 1987.

Hays, M. T.: Absorption of triiodothyronine in man. J. Clin. Endocrinol. Metab., 30:675, 1970.

Holvey, D. N.; Goodner, C. J.; Nicoloff, J. T.; and Dowling, T. J.: Treatment of myxedema coma with intravenous thyroxine. Arch. Intern. Med., 113:89–96, 1964.

Hurley, J.; and Becker, D. V.: The use of radioiodine in the management of thyroid cancer. In, Nuclear Medicine Annual 1983 (Freeman, L. M.; and Weissmann, H. S., eds.). Raven Press, New York, pp. 329–384, 1983.

Ikram, H.: Hemodynamic effects of beta-adrenergic blockade in hyperthyroid patients with and without heart failure. Br. Med. J., 1:1505–1507, 1977.

Jackson, I. M. D.: Management of thyrotoxicosis. J. Maine Med. Assoc., 66:224–232, 1975.

Jacobson, D. H.; and Gorman, C. A.: Endocrine ophthalmopathy: Current ideas concerning etiology, pathogenesis and treatment. Endocr. Rev., 5:200–220, 1984.

Jansson, R.; Dahlberg, P. A.; Johansson, H.; and Linstrom, B.: Intrathyroidal concentrations of methimazole in patients with Graves' disease. J. Clin. Endocrinol. Metab., 28:1432, 1983.

Jortso E.; Lennquist, S.; Lundstrom, B.; Norrbyk, K.; and

Smeds, S.: The influence of remnant size, antithyroid anti-bodies, thyroid morphology, and lymphocytic infiltration on thyroid function after subtotal resection for hyperthyroidism. World J. Surg., 11:365–370, 1987.

Kampmann, J. P.; Johansen, K.; Hansen, J. M.; and Helweg, J.: Propylthiouracil in human milk: Revision of a dogma. Lancet, 1:736–738, 1980.

Kaplan, M. M.: Clinical and laboratory assessment of thyroid abnormalities. Med. Clin. North Am., 69:863–880, 1985.

Kriss, J. P.; Pleshakov, V.; Rosenblum, A.; and Sharp, G.: Therapy with occlusive dressings of pretibial myxedema with fluocinolone acetonide. J. Clin. Endocrinol. Metab., 27:595–604, 1967.

Ladenson, P. W.; Goldenhein, P. D.; and Ridgway, E. C.: Rapid pituitary and peripheral tissue responses to intravenous L-triiodothyronine in hypothyroidism. J. Clin. Endocrinol. Metab., 56:1252–1259, 1983.

Larsen, P. R.: Feedback regulation of thyrotropin secretion by thyroid hormones. N. Engl. J. Med., 306:23–32, 1982.

MacKenzie, C. G.; and MacKenzie, J. B.: Effect of sulfon-amides and thioureas on the thyroid gland and basal metabo-lism. Endocrinology, 32:185–209, 1943.

MacKenzie, J. B.; MacKenzie, C. G.; and McCollum, E. V.: The effect of sulfanilylguanidine on the thyroid of the rat. Science, 94:518–519, 1941.

Marchant, B.; Brownlie, B. E. W.; Hart, D. M.; Horton, P. W.; and Alexander, W. D.: The placental transfer of pro-pylthiouracil, methimazole, and carbimazole. J. Clin. Endo-crinol. Metab., 45:1187–1193, 1977.

Martino, E.; Aghini-Lombardi, F.; Marioti, S.; Lenziardi, M.; Baschieri, L.; Braverman, L. E.; and Pinchera, A.: Treat-ment of amiodarone associated thyrotoxicosis by simultane-ous administration of potassium perchlorate and methima-zole. J. Endocrinol. Invest., 9:201–207, 1986.

Mashio, Y.; Beniko, M.; Mizumoto, H.; and Konita, H.: Treat-ment of hyperthyroidism with a small single daily dose of methimazole. Acta Endocrinol., 119:139–144, 1988.

McConahey, W. M.; Hay, I. D.; Woolner, L. B.; van Heerden, J. A.; and Taylor, W. F.: Papillary thyroid cancer treated at the Mayo Clinic, 1946 through 1970: Initial manifestations, pathologic findings, therapy, and outcome. Mayo Clin. Proc., 61:978–996, 1986.

Milham, S. Jr.; and Elledge, W.: Maternal methimazole and congenital defects in children. Teratology, 5:125, 1972.

Mulaisho, C.; and Utiger, R. D.: Serum thyroxine binding glob-ulin: Determination by competitive ligand-binding assay in thyroid disease and pregnancy. Acta Endocrinol., 85:314–324, 1977.

Nikolai, T. F.; Coombs, G. J.; McKenzie, A. K.; Miller, R. W.; and Weir, J. Jr.: Treatment of lymphocytic thyroiditis with spontaneously resolving hyperthyroidism (silent thyroi-ditis). Arch. Intern. Med., 142:2281–2283, 1982.

Northcutt, R. C.; Stiel, J. N.; Hollifield, J. W.; and Stant, E. G. Jr.: The influence of cholestyramine on thyroxine ab-sorption. J.A.M.A., 208:1857–1861, 1969.

Oppenheimer, J. L.: Role of plasma proteins in the binding, distribution, and metabolism of the thyroid hormones. N. Engl. J. Med., 278:111253–111262, 1968.

Pekonen, F.; Teramo, K.; Ikonen, E.; Osterlund, K.; Makinen, T.; and Lamberg, B.-A.: Women on thyroid hormone ther-apy: Pregnancy course, fetal outcome, and amniotic fluid thyroid hormone level. Obstet. Gynecol., 63:635–638, 1984.

Potter, J. D.: Hypothyroidism and reproduction failure. Surg. Gynecol. Obstet., 150(2):251–255, 1980.

Ratanachaiyavong, S.; and McGregor, A. M.: Immunosuppres-sion effects of antithyroid drugs. Clin. Endocrinol. Metab., 14:449–466, 1985.

Richter, C. P.; and Clisby, K. H.: Toxic effects of the bitter-tasting phenylthiocarbamide. Arch. Pathol., 33:46–57, 1942.

Robbins, J.: Thyroid Storm. In, Current Therapy in Endocri-nology and Metabolism-3 (Bardin, C. W., ed.). B. C. Decker, Toronto, pp. 66–69, 1988.

Ross, D. S.: Subclinical hyperthyroidism: Possible danger of overzealous thyroxine replacement therapy. Mayo Clin. Proc., 63:1223–1229, 1988.

Ross, D. S.; Daniels, G. H.; de Stefano, P.; Maloof, F.; and Ridgway, E. C.: Use of adjunctive potassium iodide follow-ing radioactive iodine (131I) treatment of Graves' hyperthy-roidism. J. Clin. Endocrinol. Metab., 57:250–253, 1983.

Saenger, E. L.; Thoma, G. E.; and Tompkins, E. A.: Incidence of leukemia following treatment of hyperthyroidism: Prelimi-nary report of the Cooperative Thyrotoxicosis Therapy Follow-Up Study. J.A.M.A., 205:147–154, 1968.

de los Santos, E. T.; Starich, G. H.; and Mazzaferri, M. D.: Sensitivity, specificity, and cost-effectiveness of the sensitive thyrotropin assay in the diagnosis of thyroid disease in ambu-latory patients. Arch. Intern. Med., 149:526–532, 1989.

Sawin, C. T.: Hypothyroidism. Med. Clin. North Am., 69:989–1004, 1985.

Schimmel, M.; and Utiger, R. D.: Thyroidal and peripheral production of thyroid hormones. Review of recent findings and their clinical implications. Ann. Intern. Med., 87:760–768, 1977.

Shen, D.-C.; Wu, S.-Y.; Chopra, I. J.; Huang, H.-W.; Shian, L.-R.; Bian, T.-Y.; Jeng, C.-Y.; and Solomon, D. H.: Long term treatment of Graves' hyperthyroidism with sodium ipo-date. J. Clin. Endocrinol. Metab., 61:723, 1985.

Shulkin, B. C.; Peele, M. E.; and Utiger, R. D.: Beta-adrenergic antagonist inhibition of hepatic 3,5,3'-triiodo-thyronine production. Endocrinology, 115:858–861, 1984.

Silva, J. E.: Effects of iodine and iodine containing compounds on thyroid function. Med. Clin. North Am., 69:881–898, 1985.

Smith, D. A.; Fraser, S. A.; and Wilson, G. M.: Hyperthyroid-ism and calcium metabolism. Clin. Endocrinol. Metab., 2: 333–354, 1973.

Spencer, C. A.; LoPresti, J. S.; Patel, A.; Guttler, R. B.; Eigen, A.; Shen, D.; Gray, D.; and Nicoloff, J. T.: Applications of a new chemiluminometric thyrotropin assay to subnormal measurement. J. Clin. Endocrinol. Metab., 70:453–460, 1990.

Sridama, V.; McCormick, M.; Kaplan, E. L.; Fauchet, R.; and DeGroot, L. J.: Long-term follow-up study of compensated low-dose 131I therapy for Graves' disease. N. Engl. J. Med., 311:426–432, 1984.

Stoffer, S. S.; and Szpunar, W. E.: Potency of brand name and generic levothyroxine products. J.A.M.A., 244:1704–1705, 1980.

Surks, M. I.; Shadlow, A. R.; and Oppenheimer, J. H.: A new radioimmunoassay for plasma-L-triiodothyronine: Measure-ments in thyroid disease and in patients maintained on hor-monal replacement. J. Clin. Invest., 51:3104–3113, 1972.

Takaichi, Y.; Tamai, H.; Honda, K.; Nagai, K.; Kuma, K.; and Nakagawa, T.: The significance of antithyroglobulin and antithyroidal microsomal antibodies in patients with hyper-thyroidism due to Graves' disease treated with antithyroid drugs. J. Clin. Endocrinol. Metab., 68:1097–1100, 1989.

Tubiana, M.; Haddard, E.; Schlumberger, M.; Hill, C.; Rou-gier, P.; and Sarrazin, D.: External radiotherapy in thyroid cancers. Cancer, 55:2062–2071, 1985.

Vickery, A. L. Jr.; Wang, C.; and Walker, A. M.: Treat-ment of intrathyroidal papillary carcinoma of the thyroid. Cancer, 60:2587–2595, 1987.

Volpe, R.: Subacute (de Quervain's) thyroiditis. Clin. Endocri-nol. Metab., 8:81–95, 1979.

Weitzman, S. A.; Stossel, T. P.; Harmon, D. C.; Daniels, G.; Maloof, F.; and Ridgway, E. C.: Antineutrophilic antibodies in Graves' disease. Implications of thyrotropin binding to neutrophils. J. Clin. Invest., 75:119–123, 1985.

Wiersinga, W. M.; and Touber, J. L.: The influence of beta-adrenergic blocking agents on plasma thyroxine and tri-iodothyronine. J. Clin. Endocrinol. Metab., 45:293–298, 1977.

Wolff, J.; and Chaikoff, K.: Plasma inorganic iodide as a ho-meostatic regulator of thyroid function. J. Biol. Chem., 174: 555–564, 1948.

Zakarija, M.; and McKenzie, J. M.: Pregnancy-associated changes in the thyroid-stimulating antibody of Graves' dis-ease and the relationship to neonatal hyperthyroidism. J. Clin. Endocrinol. Metab., 57:1036–1040, 1983.

15

Treatment of Endocrine Disorders: Lipids

Fredric B. Kraemer

Chapter Outline

The Lipoproteins
  Normal Lipoprotein Metabolism
  Lipoprotein Abnormalities as Risk Factors
  Specific Lipoprotein Abnormalities
Therapy of Lipoprotein Abnormalities
  Bile Acid Sequestrants

Fibric Acids
HMG-CoA Reductase Inhibitors
Nicotinic Acid (Niacin)
Probucol
Other Drugs

Lipoprotein and lipid abnormalities are disorders that commonly occur in the general population. There has been a long-standing interest in lipid and lipoprotein metabolism since lipoproteins were first detected as constituents of normal plasma in the early 20th century. This interest was further fueled by evidence suggesting a relationship between cholesterol and atherosclerosis. The tremendous advances over the last 35 years in the understanding of the pathophysiologic bases of lipoprotein abnormalities have allowed the results from epidemiologic and interventional studies in humans linking hyperlipidemia to disease processes, particularly atherosclerosis, to move the treatment of lipid and lipoprotein disorders to the forefront in strategies of preventive medicine. This chapter reviews normal lipoprotein metabolism and the pathophysiology of lipoprotein disorders. Then each of the classes of drugs that are available for the treatment of lipoprotein disorders is discussed in terms of its pharmacology and indications, with particular emphasis on efficacy demonstrated in clinical trials involving primary or secondary prevention of disease.

THE LIPOPROTEINS

Normal Lipoprotein Metabolism

Lipoproteins are macromolecules that are responsible for transporting lipids (cholesteryl esters and triglycerides) from their sites of synthesis to their sites of utilization (Jackson et al., 1976; Schaefer et al., 1978; Scanu and Landsberger, 1980; Mahley et al., 1984). All classes of lipoproteins share the same general structure, consisting of a core of nonpolar lipids (cholesteryl esters and triglycerides) surrounded by a monolayer of phospholipids, unesterified cholesterol, and various apolipoproteins. The apolipoproteins are essential for maintaining the structure of the lipoproteins and for directing the metabolism of the particle. The amphipathic properties (hydrophobic and hydrophilic orientation) of the phospholipid and apolipoprotein surface components allow the otherwise water-insoluble lipids to be transported in plasma. While the overall structure of lipoproteins is similar, differences in the chemical and apolipoprotein compositions of the particles result in various classes of lipoproteins. The classification of lipoproteins is generally based on their physical properties and can be viewed as a continuous spectrum of particles with a changing pattern of lipid and protein composition. Lipoproteins are conventionally separated by their densities during ultracentrifugation but also can be separated by electrophoresis on paper or agarose or by size on column chromatography.

Chylomicrons. The first class of lipoproteins is chylomicrons, which are derived from dietary lipids and are usually found only in postprandial plasma and not in the plasma of fasting normal subjects. Chylomicrons float in the cold without centrifugation, having a density <0.94 and remain at the origin during electrophoresis (Table 15–1). They are the largest lipoproteins, ranging from 70 to 120 nm and larger. Chylomicrons are formed in the intestinal epithelial cells. Following the hydrolysis of dietary lipids in the intestinal lumen, the absorbed fatty acids and cholesterol are reesterified in these cells to triglycerides and cholesterol esters and then packaged with polar lipids and structural apolipoproteins (B-48, AI, AII). The low-molecular-weight apolipoprotein B-48 that the intestine produces is found only in chylomicrons in humans and can be used as a

Table 15-1. LIPOPROTEIN CLASSIFICATION

CLASS	ULTRACENTRIFUGAL DEFINITION (DENSITY)	ELECTROPHORETIC DEFINITION	DIAMETER (NM)
Major			
Chylomicrons	<0.94	Remain at origin	70–120
Very-low-density lipoproteins (VLDLs)	<1.006	Pre-β mobility	30–70
Intermediate-density lipoproteins (IDLs)	1.006–1.019	β mobility	23–30
Low-density lipoproteins (LDLs)	1.019–1.063	β mobility	18–23
High-density lipoproteins (HDLs)	1.063–1.215	α mobility	5–12
Minor			
Lipoprotein(a)	1.050–1.080	Pre-β mobility	23–26
β-Very-low-density lipoproteins (β-VLDLs)	<1.006	β mobility	30–70

marker of lipoproteins of intestinal origin. Chylomicrons are very triglyceride-rich lipoproteins, consisting of 90% to 95% triglycerides and small amounts of cholesterol esters, unesterified cholesterol, phospholipids, and apolipoproteins (Table 15-2). Chylomicrons are initially secreted into lymph and then enter the peripheral circulation where they acquire apolipoproteins E and C (CI, CII, CIII) from circulating high-density lipoproteins (HDLs). In the circulation, chylomicrons are acted on by the enzyme lipoprotein lipase, which is located on the surface of capillary endothelium. Lipoprotein lipase is activated by apolipoprotein CII and hydrolyzes the triglycerides of the chylomicrons. The fatty acids released are used by cells for energy or reesterified and stored in adipocytes as triglyceride. During hydrolysis of the triglycerides, phospholipids and apolipoprotein Cs are lost from chylomicrons. The resulting particles (chylomicron remnants) are smaller, triglyceride- and apolipoprotein C–poor, and cholesteryl ester– and apolipoprotein E–rich since other apolipoproteins and cholesteryl esters are not lost during hydrolysis by lipoprotein lipase. Chylomicron remnants are rapidly cleared from the circulation by parenchymal cells of the liver via recognition of apolipoprotein E by a specific remnant or apolipoprotein E receptor (Herz et al., 1988). The bound chylomicron remnant particles are internalized by the hepatic cells and degraded in lysosomes with release of free fatty acids and unesterified cholesterol.

Very-Low-Density Lipoproteins. While chylomicron production occurs in the intestine and is dependent on dietary fat intake, the second major class of lipoproteins, very-low-density lipoproteins (VLDLs), are triglyceride-rich lipoproteins that are produced by the liver. VLDLs are smaller than chylomicrons (range 30–70 nm), have a density <1.006 (the density of plasma), and exhibit pre-β mobility on electrophoresis (Table 15–1). Although they are triglyceride-rich lipoproteins (50% to 60% triglyceride), VLDLs contain significant amounts of cholesteryl esters (15% to 20%), with the remainder consisting of phospholipid and apolipoproteins (Table 15-2). VLDL production is dependent on the availability of substrate for triglyceride synthesis by the liver, that is, circulating free fatty acids or chylomicron triglyceride uptake. The newly synthesized triglycerides are packaged with cholesterol, phospholipids, and apolipoprotein B-100 (a high-molecular-weight apolipoprotein B that is synthesized exclusively by the liver in humans), apolipoprotein Cs, and apolipoprotein E. Following secretion, VLDLs can be directly removed by the liver via low-density lipoprotein (LDL) receptors (see below) or can acquire more C apolipoproteins from HDLs and then be hydrolyzed in the peripheral circulation by lipoprotein lipase in a similar fashion to chylomicrons.

As the triglycerides of VLDLs become depleted, VLDL remnants or intermediate-density lipoproteins (IDLs; density = 1.006–1.019, β mo-

Table 15-2. COMPOSITION OF LIPOPROTEINS

	CHYLOMICRONS (%)	VLDLs (%)	LDLs (%)	HDLs (%)
Triglyceride	80–95	45–65	4–8	2–7
Cholesterol esters	2–4	16–22	45–50	15–20
Free cholesterol	1–3	4–8	6–8	3–5
Phospholipid	3–6	15–20	18–24	26–32
Protein	1–2	6–10	18–22	45–55
Apolipoprotein species	B-48, AI, AIV, CI, CII, CIII, E	B-100, CI, CII CIII, E	B-100	AI, AII, CI, CII, CIII, D, E

bility) are formed that are triglyceride- and apolipoprotein C-poor and cholesterol- and apolipoprotein E-rich. The IDLs are metabolized by one of two different pathways: either (1) they are removed from the circulation by the liver via recognition of apolipoprotein E by the LDL receptor or (2) they are converted to LDLs by a poorly defined processing mechanism involving hepatic lipase. Under normal conditions, approximately half the IDL is removed by the liver and half is converted to LDL. A decreased expression of hepatic LDL receptors results in less clearance of IDL by the liver and greater conversion to LDL. Conversely, with increased expression of hepatic LDL receptors, more IDL is removed by the liver and less is converted to LDL. Therefore, an inverse relationship exists between the amount of IDL converted to LDL (i.e., LDL production) and the number of LDL receptors expressed by the liver.

Low-Density Lipoproteins. Thus, LDLs, which are the major cholesterol-carrying lipoproteins in humans (responsible for ~70% of total cholesterol in plasma), are the catabolic product of VLDLs. The LDLs have a density of 1.019 to 1.063 and exhibit β mobility on electrophoresis. Approximately 50% of the mass of LDLs consists of cholesteryl esters, while the remainder comprises equal amounts of phospholipids and apolipoproteins, with apolipoprotein B-100 being the predominant (>95%) species. LDLs provide cholesterol to extrahepatic cells for membrane synthesis in dividing cells and for steroid hormone production in the adrenals and gonads. Although all nucleated cells are capable of de novo synthesis of cholesterol, cholesterol derived from LDL is preferentially utilized when available. Approximately 60% to 80% of LDL catabolism occurs through uptake by the liver and the remainder by extrahepatic tissues. The LDLs are catabolized primarily via specific cell surface receptors (LDL receptors) that recognize apolipoprotein B-100 and apolipoprotein E. Following binding, LDLs are internalized by adsorptive endocytosis. The resultant endosome is delivered to and fuses with lysosomes. Within the lysosome, the protein moiety of LDL is degraded by proteases to amino acids and the lipid moieties are hydrolyzed by acid lipases to unesterified cholesterol and free fatty acids. The unesterified cholesterol liberated by hydrolysis from cholesterol esters enters the cytoplasmic compartment, where it serves three key functions: (1) it inhibits the activity of 3-hydroxy-3-methylglutaryl coenzyme A (HMG-CoA) reductase, the rate-limiting enzyme in cholesterol biosynthesis, (2) it stimulates the activity of fatty acyl coenzyme A:cholesterol acyltransferase, the enzyme that reesterifies cholesterol for

storage as nonpolar cholesteryl esters, and (3) it decreases the number of LDL receptors expressed by the cells and consequently suppresses the further uptake of LDL.

High-Density Lipoproteins. The fourth class of lipoproteins is HDLs, which are a heterogeneous group of small lipoprotein particles (range 5-12 nm) with densities of 1.063 to 1.215 and α mobility on electrophoresis (Table 15-1). While considered cholesterol-rich lipoproteins, HDLs are composed predominantly of phospholipids and apolipoproteins with 20% of the mass consisting of cholesteryl esters (Table 15-2). Apolipoprotein AI (70%) and apolipoprotein AII (20%) account for most of the protein of HDLs, with small amounts of apolipoprotein Cs, apolipoprotein D, and, in the lighter-density HDL particles, apolipoprotein E comprising the remainder. Along with the physical and compositional heterogeneity of HDLs, HDLs are metabolically heterogeneous. HDLs are derived from two major pathways: (1) by direct secretion from the liver and intestine and (2) by formation from excess surface components produced during the hydrolysis of chylomicrons and VLDLs by lipoprotein lipase. Intact HDLs are probably not secreted or formed directly, but HDLs are first found as discoidal phospholipid-apolipoprotein bilayers that acquire unesterified cholesterol on efflux from peripheral cells. The unesterified cholesterol is then converted to cholesteryl esters in the HDL core by the plasma enzyme lecithin:cholesterol acyltransferase, which is activated by apolipoprotein AI. The cholesteryl esters in HDLs can then be transferred to "acceptor" lipoproteins, for example, chylomicron remnants, VLDL, and LDL, by a poorly defined process requiring lipid-transfer protein. Thus, HDL plays an important role in transporting cholesterol from peripheral tissues to the liver, the process of *reverse cholesterol transport*. Both HDL and apolipoprotein AI are catabolized primarily by the liver and the kidneys by unknown mechanisms.

Minor Lipoproteins. In addition to the major classes of lipoproteins, several other minor lipoproteins exist that are important in normal or disease states. Of these, lipoprotein(a) has received attention recently because of the positive relationship of concentrations of lipoprotein(a) with coronary heart disease (Morissett et al., 1987). Lipoprotein(a) has a density of 1.050 to 1.080, a composition relatively similar to that of LDL but with slightly more protein and less cholesterol, and pre-β mobility on electrophoresis. The apolipoproteins in lipoprotein(a) are apolipoprotein B-100 and a unique apolipoprotein, apolipoprotein(a), which displays structural homology to plasminogen (Utermann, 1989). Lipoprotein(a) is produced by the liver and catabolized via poorly understood mechanisms. There is no apparent metabolic interconversion of lipoprotein(a) with any other lipoproteins. Another lipoprotein class of importance is β-VLDLs, which are lipoproteins occurring in patients with familial dysbetalipoproteinemia, occasionally in patients with diabetes mellitus or uremia, and in a variety of animal species during cholesterol feeding (Mahley, 1982). The β-VLDLs have a density < 1.006, similar to that of normal VLDLs, but migrate on electrophoresis with β mobility. The β-VLDLs resemble "remnant" particles, being both cholesterol- and apolipoprotein E–rich and triglyceride- and apolipoprotein C–poor.

Lipoprotein Abnormalities as Risk Factors

The diagnosis of a lipoprotein abnormality is based, for the most part, on the results of laboratory testing. However, unlike other conditions in which a diagnosis is dependent solely on the results of laboratory tests, the range of normal values for serum lipids and lipoproteins is not defined by the 90% to 95% confidence limits of a normal reference population. *Principle: When an identifiable parameter of health places an entire population or a significant percentage of that population at increased risk for a disease, the definition of* **abnormal** *should be adjusted to include all individuals at risk.* Normal or, more appropriately, desirable lipid and lipoprotein levels have been established on the basis of experimental and epidemiologic studies that have demonstrated relationships between particular lipid concentrations and the development of specific diseases such as atherosclerosis.

Serum LDL Cholesterol. This is best illustrated by a large number of epidemiologic studies that have documented a strong, positive relationship between serum cholesterol (LDL) values and the incidence of atherosclerotic, coronary heart disease (Kannel et al., 1971; Rose and Shipley, 1986; Martin et al., 1986). The Multiple Risk Factor Intervention Trial (MRFIT) has the greatest discriminatory power of these studies since it is the largest, having evaluated more than 350,000 middle-aged men over a period of 6 years (Martin et al., 1986; Stamler et al., 1986). The results from MRFIT display a nonlinear, continuously graded rise of mortality from coronary heart disease with increasing concentrations of serum cholesterol, without evidence of a threshold phenomenon. Thus, an ever-increasing relative risk is observed, beginning with cholesterol levels of 150 mg/dl (Fig. 15–1).

Even though fewer studies have examined co-horts that do not consist of middle-aged men, it appears that the relationship between serum cholesterol concentrations and coronary heart disease still holds in women (Harris et al., 1988) and older individuals (Barrett-Conner et al., 1984; Denke and Grundy, 1990). Based on these analyses, current recommendations propose a screening measurement of serum cholesterol in all adults over the age of 20 (The Expert Panel, 1988). If the cholesterol value obtained on screening is elevated, the serum cholesterol concentration should be reassessed, along with measurement of plasma triglyceride and HDL cholesterol concentrations in order to define the lipoprotein abnormality present and to determine the concentration of LDL cholesterol (see below).

The established goal is to reduce total and LDL cholesterol in all individuals to ≤ 200 mg/dl and ≤ 130 mg/dl, respectively. Individuals with total and LDL cholesterol values ≥ 240 mg/dl and ≥ 160 mg/dl, respectively, who do not respond to diet therapy are advised to undergo treatment with lipid-lowering drugs. Likewise, individuals with total cholesterol values between 200 and 240 mg/dl and LDL cholesterol concentrations between 130 and 160 mg/dl who have known coronary artery disease or who have two or more additional cardiovascular risk factors (male sex, family history of premature coronary artery disease, cigarette smoking, hypertension, low HDL cholesterol, diabetes mellitus, history of cerebrovascular or peripheral vascular disease, or extreme obesity) are advised to be treated with hypocholesterolemic agents if an adequate response is not observed with diet. Some authors have suggested that therapeutic goals should be set even lower in those patients with known vascular disease or with significant additional cardiovascular risk factors, with total cholesterol concentrations ≤ 180 mg/dl and LDL cholesterol concentrations ≤ 100 mg/dl being recommended (Witztum, 1989; Garg and Grundy, 1990). *Principle: Therapy should be more aggressive in individuals who manifest a disease than in individuals in whom treatment is instituted as a potential preventive measure.*

Serum Triglyceride Concentrations. While there is reasonable unanimity of opinion regarding the relationship between serum cholesterol concentrations and coronary heart disease, the relationship between triglyceride values and coronary heart disease is much more controversial (Austin, 1989). Some large epidemiologic studies have found a strong correlation between triglyceride concentrations and coronary heart disease (Bottiger and Carlson, 1980; Aberg et al., 1985), while others have been unable to detect such a relationship (Hulley, 1980). Part of this con-

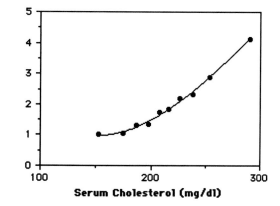

Fig. 15-1. Relationship between serum cholesterol concentration and relative risk of death from coronary heart disease over 6 years. Adapted from data from the Multiple Risk Factor Intervention Trial (Stamler, 1986).

troversy stems from the fact that the statistical significance of the correlation between serum triglyceride concentrations and coronary heart disease is often lost when examined by multivariant analysis. This is particularly true when HDL cholesterol values are considered since HDL cholesterol values are, in general, inversely related to serum triglyceride concentrations (Phillips et al., 1981). *Principle: When parameters are physiologically interrelated, whether one factor (triglycerides) is mechanistically involved with the disease process (atherogenesis) is less important than its clinical value as a marker or predictor of that disease.*

Nonetheless, whether elevations of triglyceride concentrations directly contribute to the development of atherosclerosis or simply reflect other, possibly unmeasured, contributory factors, it appears that triglyceride concentrations do correlate with the incidence of coronary heart disease in some well-defined settings. Specifically, the incidence of coronary heart disease in patients with diabetes mellitus appears to be related strongly to elevations in serum triglyceride concentrations (West et al., 1983; Fontbonne et al., 1989). Since the relationship of hypertriglyceridemia to coronary heart disease has not been definitively established, it has been difficult for agreement to be reached on a definition of hypertriglyceridemia (Consensus Conference, 1984). Nonetheless, triglyceride measurements are required for the calculation of LDL cholesterol in most laboratories according to the formula: LDL cholesterol = total cholesterol − HDL cholesterol − triglycerides/5 (Friedewald et al., 1972). This calculation is reasonably accurate provided triglyceride concentrations do not exceed 300 mg/dl and the patient does not have type III (dysbetalipoproteinemia) hyperlipoproteinemia (see below). Moreover, all available evidence substantiates a strong relationship between triglyceride values greater than 1000 mg/dl and the development of

one disease, namely, acute pancreatitis. Based on the variability of triglyceride measurements, a triglyceride concentration of 500 mg/dl or more is considered abnormal and warrants therapy for the prevention of pancreatitis. Patients with triglyceride values between 250 and 500 mg/dl should be considered for therapy in light of the presence or absence of other cardiovascular risk factors (see above). If significant cardiovascular risk factors are present in addition to hypertriglyceridemia, hypolipidemic therapy is probably indicated. Although this approach is a compromise, it emphasizes the need for therapeutic decisions to be determined on an individual basis and with respect to the patient as a whole. *Principle: Not one, but all relevant factors should be considered when deciding to initiate preventive therapy for a disease.*

Specific Lipoprotein Abnormalities

Hypertriglyceridemia.   Hypertriglyceridemia occurs when there are elevations in plasma values of triglyceride-rich lipoproteins, that is, chylomicrons, VLDLs, or both chylomicrons and VLDLs. The excessive accumulation of these lipoprotein particles can result from increased production, decreased removal, or both.

Chylomicronemia.   Chylomicrons are not usually present in normal fasting plasma. Fasting hyperchylomicronemia or type I hyperlipoproteinemia in the Fredrickson classification (Fredrickson et al., 1967) is due to deficiency in lipoprotein lipase or, rarely, to deficiency of apolipoprotein CII, the cofactor that activates lipoprotein lipase (Brunzell, 1989). In either case there is a severe defect in the catabolism of chylomicrons. Chylomicronemia is a rare disorder, with the homozygous affected individuals occurring with a frequency of about 1 in 1 million in the population. Type I hyperlipoproteinemia usually presents in childhood with pancreatitis,

hepatosplenomegaly, eruptive xanthoma, and li-
pemia retinalis. Since chylomicrons are derived
entirely from dietary fat, treatment consists of a
marked reduction of dietary fat to 5% to 15% of
total calories, which generally leads to a highly
efficacious therapeutic response. No hypolipidemic agents are indicated in the therapy of this
disorder, and there is no evidence for an increase
in risk for atherosclerosis.

*Increased VLDL or Increased VLDL and Chy-
lomicron Concentrations.* Hypertriglyceridemia
due to elevated concentrations of VLDLs of normal composition (type IV hyperlipoproteinemia)
is the most common lipid abnormality observed
in the general population. When VLDL values
increase to triglyceride values greater than 500
mg/dl, chylomicrons also begin to accumulate in
plasma since VLDLs and chylomicrons share similar removal mechanisms. The differentiation between type IV hyperlipoproteinemia and the accumulation of increased amounts of VLDLs and
chylomicrons (type V hyperlipoproteinemia) is
determined by the absence or presence of chylomicrons, which is a reflection of the severity of
the hypertriglyceridemia or of the patient's diet
more than differences in the underlying pathophysiology. Types IV and V hyperlipoproteinemia are heterogeneous disorders that may occur
secondarily to a number of diseases or polygenetic
causes. This heterogeneity has contributed to the
controversy surrounding the relationship of hypertriglyceridemia and atherosclerosis.

Secondary causes of hypertriglyceridemia include diabetes mellitus, uremia, nephrotic syndrome, alcohol abuse, estrogen use, glucocorticoid excess (endogenous or exogenous), metabolic
stress (including trauma, burns, infections, and
sepsis), glycogen storage disease, dysglobulinemia, pregnancy, and lipodystrophies. Individuals without evidence of secondary causes
have familial or sporadic hypertriglyeridemia.
The hypertriglyeridemia in familial and most secondary causes (excluding type I insulin-dependent
diabetes mellitus and uremia) is due to increased
production of VLDLs (Olefsky et al., 1974). The
factors leading to the increased production of
VLDLs are probably multiple; however, familial
and secondary causes of hypertriglyceridemia
share several metabolic features. In particular, all
the conditions, including familial hypertriglyceridemia, in which patients are almost invariably
overweight, are characterized by insulin resistance
(Reaven, 1988). This has allowed a unifying hypothesis to be formulated: the basic defect in
these patients is insulin resistance, leading to hyperinsulinemia and increased free fatty acid flux.
In response to the increased free fatty acid concentrations (precursor) and stimulation by hyperinsulinemia, the liver increases triglyceride and
VLDL production, resulting in elevations in
plasma VLDL concentrations. Thus, it is vital for
initial therapy in these patients to be directed toward decreasing free fatty acid flux and insulin
resistance by weight loss and/or correction of the
underlying disease before pharmacologic intervention is considered.

Hypercholesterolemia. Hypercholesterolemia,
in the absence of elevated triglyceride concentrations, is due to elevations in LDL concentrations
(type IIa hyperlipoproteinemia). The one important exception to this generalization is the person
with hyperalphalipoproteinemia who has normal
values of LDL cholesterol, but increased values
of HDL (Glueck et al., 1975). In contrast to the
typical hypercholesterolemic patients, these patients are not at increased risk for coronary heart
disease and, consistent with the definition of hypercholesterolemia as an elevated LDL cholesterol concentration (see above), do not require
therapy to lower their total cholesterol concentrations.

Patients with type IIa hyperlipoproteinemia
comprise a heterogeneous group consisting of
several different monogenetic and polygenetic abnormalities. The best studied of these abnormalities is familial hypercholesterolemia, in which defects in the LDL receptor lead to elevations of
LDL cholesterol concentrations (Goldstein and
Brown, 1983). Familial hypercholesterolemia is
an autosomal recessive disorder with heterozygotes constituting approximately 1 out of 500 in
the population and homozygotes about 1 in 1 million people. Affected patients are characterized
by hypercholesterolemia, tendon xanthomas, and
an increased risk of coronary heart disease. There
are a number of different molecular defects that
have been described that cause an abnormal expression of LDL receptors (Russell et al., 1989).
The decreased expression of LDL receptors results in a defective catabolism of LDL from
plasma. In addition, because LDL receptors also
mediate the removal of VLDL and VLDL remnants from plasma, there is a concomitant increase in the production of LDL secondary to an
increased conversion from uncleared VLDL and
VLDL remnants. Thus, elevated LDL concentrations occur because of a combination of increased
production and decreased removal.

Recently, another genetic abnormality causing hypercholesterolemia has been described in
which LDL receptors are normal. In these patients there is a mutation in apolipoprotein B-100,
termed familial defective apolipoprotein B-100
(Innerarity et al., 1987). This alteration in apolipoprotein B-100 diminishes the affinity of LDL for
its receptor, leading to decreased catabolism
of LDL but a normal production rate since apo-

lipoprotein E–mediated removal of VLDLs and VLDL remnants remains normal. While these genetic defects have been studied extensively, the majority of patients with hypercholesterolemia do not have these highly specific genetic defects.

Some patients have hypercholesterolemia that occurs secondarily to an underlying disease, such as hypothyroidism, nephrotic syndrome, dysglobulinemia, glucocorticoid excess, anorexia nervosa, or acute intermittent porphyria; evaluation of these possibilities should be pursued in the appropriate clinical setting. However, most patients have an array of metabolic (polygenetic) causes that are characterized by an increased rate of LDL production in some, perhaps influenced by obesity (Kesaniemi and Grundy, 1983), and by a decreased rate of LDL removal without apparent defects in LDL receptors or apolipoprotein B-100 in others (Vega and Grundy, 1986).

Combined Hypercholesterolemia and Hypertriglyceridemia. Not infrequently, hypercholesterolemia and hypertriglyceridemia coexist in the same individual or within the same family. When this occurs, it can be secondary to an underlying disease, that is, diabetes mellitus, nephrotic syndrome, use of corticosteroids, and so forth, or due to a genetic abnormality. Patients with combined hypercholesterolemia and hypertriglyceridemia fall into two classifications: type IIb hyperlipoproteinemia and type III hyperlipoproteinemia.

Type IIb Hyperlipoproteinemia. Patients with type IIb hyperlipoproteinemia, also known as familial combined hyperlipidemia (or dyslipidemia) or hyperapobetalipoproteinemia, represent a heterogeneous group of subjects (Grundy et al., 1987). This disorder is an extremely common abnormality (Williams et al., 1988) in which patients display multiple lipoprotein phenotypes, with individuals or family members having hypertriglyceridemia, hypercholesterolemia, or both hypertriglyceridemia and hypercholesterolemia at any given time. Thus, patients with type IIb hyperlipoproteinemia are often erroneously classified as having type IV or type IIa hyperlipoproteinemia. As opposed to patients with type IV hyperlipoproteinemia, in which the relationship to atherosclerosis is controversial, persons with familial combined hyperlipidemia, whether hypertriglyceridemic, hypercholesterolemic, or both, are at increased risk for coronary heart disease (Goldstein et al., 1973). Independent of the prevailing lipoprotein phenotype, patients with type IIb hyperlipoproteinemia are characterized by elevated concentrations of apolipoprotein B. An increased rate of VLDL apolipoprotein B and VLDL triglyceride production are observed in hypertriglyceridemic individuals (Kissebah et al., 1981), while an increased production rate of LDL apolipoprotein B is seen in all these patients (Teng et al., 1986). Rates of removal of LDLs are normal. The increase in LDL production is probably due to multiple underlying metabolic and genetic abnormalities causing decreased direct hepatic uptake of VLDLs and VLDL remnants (IDL) that leads to increased conversion to LDLs. Genetic traits that can predispose persons to develop familial combined hyperlipidemia include heterozygous expression of lipoprotein lipase deficiency (Babirak et al., 1989), as well as nephrotic syndrome and non-insulin-dependent diabetes mellitus.

Type III Hyperlipoproteinemia or Dysbetalipoproteinemia. Type III hyperlipoproteinemia or familial dysbetalipoproteinemia is a rare disorder caused by the accumulation of cholesterol-rich VLDLs in plasma that results in elevations of triglyceride and cholesterol concentrations. This disorder cannot be detected using routinely performed lipid analyses but requires direct analysis of VLDL composition using ultracentrifugation or apolipoprotein E phenotype using isoelectric focusing electrophoresis. The diagnosis of familial dysbetalipoproteinemia should be considered in any patient with elevations of both cholesterol and triglyceride values. However, particular attention should be directed at those patients with both hypercholesterolemia and hypertriglyceridemia who have evidence of accelerated atherosclerosis or a strong family history of atherosclerosis and hyperlipidemia.

The cholesterol-rich VLDLs, or β-VLDLs, that accumulate in these patients are remnant particles that are not cleared normally by the liver (Brewer et al., 1983). Polymorphism of apolipoprotein E is the reason for this defect in catabolism of β-VLDLs. There are three common alleles in humans encoding three isoforms of apolipoprotein E — E-2, E-3, and E-4, which differ from each other by a single amino acid (Davignon et al., 1988). Apolipoprotein E-3 is the most common isoform, followed by E-4 and then E-2, with only 1% of the population homozygous for apolipoprotein E-2. When compared with apolipoprotein E-3 or E-4, apolipoprotein E-2 has a markedly decreased affinity for binding to the LDL receptor or the chylomicron remnant receptor (Weisgraber et al., 1982). Therefore, apolipoprotein E-2–containing lipoprotein particles, whose removal is dependent on receptor recognition of apolipoprotein E, display a decreased clearance. However, this defect in catabolism is not sufficient to cause type III hyperlipoproteinemia, since less than 5% of individuals who are homozygous for apolipoprotein E-2 are hyperlipidemic even though all homozygotes have β-VLDLs that display decreased binding affinity (Rall et al., 1983). Thus, an additional abnormality is required in order to develop type III hyperlipoproteinemia. The additional abnormality can vary from metabolic disorders, such as non-insulin-dependent diabetes mellitus, hypothyroidism, nephrotic syndrome, steroids (glucocorticoids and estrogens), or obesity, to inherited disorders, such as familial hypertriglyceridemia or familial combined hyperlipidemia; the common feature of these disorders is an increase in VLDL production.

THERAPY OF LIPOPROTEIN ABNORMALITIES

The therapeutic approach to a patient with hyperlipidemia is predicated on establishing the type of lipid abnormality the patient has and then tailoring therapy toward altering the underlying pathophysiology. Establishing a patient's lipoprotein abnormality entails not only determining which lipoprotein classes are elevated, but also determining whether the lipid abnormality is primary (genetic, environmental) or secondary to another underlying disorder. *Principle: Therapy toward an underlying disease should be maximized prior to initiating treatment of a symptom or sign of the disease.*

If an underlying disease that can contribute to the hyperlipidemia is uncovered, therapy should be directed at correcting the causative disorder before instituting specific therapy for the lipid abnormality. This is particularly important if hypothyroidism or diabetes mellitus is discovered since these are relatively common disorders that dramatically affect lipoprotein metabolism and can be directly treated effectively. Indeed, achievement of euthyroidism and normalization or improvement in glucose control frequently results in correction of the hyperlipidemia in these instances.

Once secondary causes of hyperlipidemia are eliminated or properly treated, the initial therapy for all patients with hyperlipidemias should be dietary modification. Dietary modifications generally entail a reduction in total fat intake, particularly a reduction in saturated fat, a decrease in dietary cholesterol, and frequently caloric restriction in overweight patients. Specific dietary recommendations, and the scientific bases on which they are founded, are beyond the scope of this chapter. The reader is referred to recent reviews on this topic (Ad Hoc Committee to Design a Dietary Treatment of Hyperlipoproteinemia, 1984; Grundy, 1987; Conner and Conner, 1989; and chapter 10) for further information. A period of 3 to 6 months of dietary intervention should be undertaken before pharmacologic therapy is considered. Since the rationale for treatment is to lower the risk of development and progression or to increase the regression of atherosclerosis by decreasing concentrations of atherogenic lipoproteins, therapy is planned to proceed for many years. Therefore, it is essential to consider risks and benefits carefully when prescribing hypolipidemic agents. *Principle: When therapy is planned to extend over the lifetime of a patient for the purpose of potentially preventing a disease, the cumulative risk (morbidity, mortality, and quality of life) of the treatment must be carefully weighed against the effectiveness of the intervention.*

If hypercholesterolemia persists after dietary restrictions, present recommendations are to treat with bile acid sequestrants, followed, in order, by trials of niacin, HMG-CoA reductase inhibitors, gemfibrozil and probucol (The Expert Panel, 1988). However, given their efficacy and the rapidly increasing clinical experience with their use, HMG-CoA reductase inhibitors seem to be becoming the agents to add after bile acid sequestrants. If hypertriglyceridemia persists after dietary restriction, gemfibrozil and niacin are the drugs of choice, with HMG-CoA reductase inhibitors having possible utility in some clinical settings. The use of each of these agents, singly or in combination, is discussed in the following sections.

Bile Acid Sequestrants

History. The bile acid sequestrants were the first agents successfully developed for the treatment of hyperlipidemia. Because of findings in the early 1950s that feeding ferric chloride can attenuate the hypercholesterolemia induced by dietary cholesterol in chickens through its ability to precipitate bile acids in the GI tract (Siperstein et al., 1953), nontoxic agents that bind bile acids were sought. Cholestyramine, a nonabsorbable anion-exchange resin that avidly binds bile acids, was developed in 1960 (Tennent et al., 1960). Later, a second bile acid–binding resin with a different structure (colestipol) was developed (Parkinson et al., 1970).

Mechanism of Action. In order to understand the mechanism of action of bile acid sequestrants, it is necessary first to review bile metabolism briefly (Packard and Shepherd, 1982). Bile secreted by the liver consists of bile acids, phospholipids, and unesterified cholesterol (biliary cholesterol) solubilized by the detergent effects of bile acids and phospholipids. Bile acids are the principal oxidative product of hepatic cholesterol metabolism. The two major bile acids, cholic and chenodeoxycholic acid, are produced from 7α-hydroxycholesterol, which is formed from cholesterol by the action of 7α-hydroxylase, the rate-limiting enzyme in bile acid synthesis. Bile acid synthesis is under feedback regulation, with cholic and chenodeoxycholic acids inhibiting the activity of 7α-hydroxylase. In humans, approximately 30% of the bile acids and 20% of the biliary cholesterol are derived from newly synthesized cholesterol, the vast majority being derived from lipoprotein cholesterol. After bile is secreted into the intestine, the bile acids undergo further metabolism by the bacterial flora. Normally, 95% of the bile acids secreted into the intestine are reabsorbed by the terminal ileum and returned via the portal system to the liver, where they are reutilized. Nonetheless, the bile acids and biliary cholesterol that are not reabsorbed represent the major route of removal of cholesterol from the body.

Through their ability to bind bile acids and form an insoluble complex, cholestyramine and colestipol interrupt the enterohepatic circulation of bile acids and promote sterol excretion in the feces (Fig. 15–2B). As bile acids are sequestered by bile acid resins, the feedback inhibition of 7α-hydroxylase activity is released, leading to a 3- to 10-fold increase in bile acid synthesis (Fig. 15–2B). This increase in bile acid synthesis allows a new steady state to be reached so that the total bile acid pool is not significantly depleted by bile acid sequestrant therapy. The increased diversion of cholesterol into bile acid synthesis causes an apparent decrease in the pool of intracellular cholesterol. The depletion of intracellular, unesterified cholesterol removes the feedback inhibition on HMG-CoA reductase activity and LDL-receptor expression, resulting in increased cholesterol synthesis and increased LDL uptake mediated via LDL receptors (Brown and Gold-

stein, 1983). In parallel, there is an increase in triglyceride synthesis in some, but not all, subjects, suggesting some integration of bile acid metabolism with triglyceride, as well as cholesterol synthesis. Thus, a fall in plasma LDL concentration occurs because of a greater catabolism of LDL by the liver; however, this effect is attenuated in part by the compensatory increases in cholesterol and triglyceride syntheses that give rise to increases in VLDL production.

Pharmacokinetics. Cholestyramine (Questran) is the chloride salt of a quartenary ammonium anion-exchange resin in which the basic groups are attached by carbon bonds to a styrene-divinyl benzene copolymer skeleton. Colestipol (Colestid) is an anion-exchange resin that is a copolymer of diethylenetriamine and 1-chloro-2,3-epoxypropane. Neither cholestyramine nor colestipol is soluble in water, nor is either absorbed from the intestine to any appreciable degree (<0.02%). In addition to a powder, cholestyramine is also available as a "granola" bar (Cholybar) that some patients find more palatable. No matter what formulation, both agents must be taken with water or a suitable liquid. The dose of cholestyramine ranges from 8 to 24 g/day, and the dose of colestipol from 15 to 30 g/day; however, some patients display adequate responses to lower doses. The bile acid sequestrants should be taken with meals in order to coincide with the times of maximum bile acid secretion. Although cholestyramine has a slightly higher capacity on a weight per weight basis (4 g of cholestyramine being roughly equivalent to 5 g of colestipol), both agents bind bile acids similarly to form insoluble complexes. The bile acid sequestrants have a greater affinity for chenodeoxycholate than

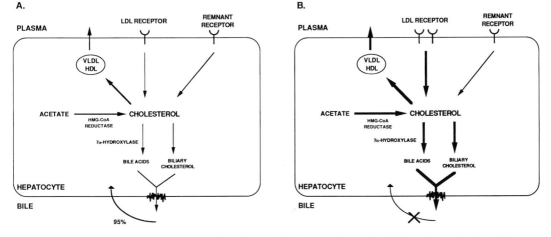

Fig. 15–2. (A) Schematic representation of normal hepatic cholesterol and bile acid metabolism. (B) Mechanisms of action of bile acid sequestrants. See text for full explanation.

cholate. This increased affinity for chenodeoxy-cholate, combined with the greater induction of cholic acid synthesis than chenodeoxycholic acid synthesis, causes a marked alteration in bile composition. While these changes in the species of bile acids occur, there are no alterations in the ratio of total bile acids to biliary cholesterol or phospholipid; thus, the lithogenicity of bile remains unchanged (chapter 9).

Indications and Efficacy. The bile acid sequestrants are indicated in the treatment of hypercholesterolemia due to elevations in LDL concentrations (type II hyperlipoproteinemia). A large number of controlled trials have established the safety and efficacy of bile acid sequestrants (Heel et al., 1980; Illingworth and Bacon, 1989; Witztum, 1989). These studies have shown that treatment with bile acid sequestrants results in a 15% to 35% reduction in serum cholesterol concentrations that is due entirely to a reduction in LDL cholesterol concentrations. In parallel to the reduction in LDL cholesterol concentrations, there is a fall in apolipoprotein B values; however, the reduction in cholesterol concentrations is greater than the fall in apolipoprotein B concentrations, as a consequence of a change in the composition of the lipoproteins (Witztum et al., 1985). Plasma triglyceride values are generally unchanged or increased, and no consistent alterations in HDL cholesterol values are observed with bile acid sequestrants. Similarly, no changes in lipoprotein(a) concentrations occur (Vessby et al., 1982). The Lipid Research Clinics Primary Prevention Trial (Lipid Research Clinics Program, 1984a, 1984b) showed that when cholestyramine monotherapy was compared with placebo in 3800 middle-aged men with serum cholesterol concentrations ≥ 265 mg/dl and serum triglyceride concentrations ≤ 300 mg/dl, there was a 12% reduction in LDL cholesterol concentrations and a 19% reduction in coronary artery disease over 7 years. However, total mortality was unchanged because of an increased number of accidental and violent deaths. Similarly, the Type II Coronary Intervention Study organized by the NHLBI (National Heart, Lung and Blood Institute) found a lower incidence of progression of coronary artery lesions by angiography in patients treated with cholestyramine (Brensike et al., 1984; Levy et al., 1984). Based on the efficacy demonstrated in these studies and on the absence of long-term adverse effects, bile acid sequestrants are the drugs of first choice for initiation of therapy of hypercholesterolemia after failure of dietary restriction (The Expert Panel, 1988). *Principle: The ideal agent for lifelong preventive intervention should be effective and have no systemic adverse effects. Unfortunately, few such preventive agents have been found.*

The cholesterol-lowering effects of the bile acid sequestrants are synergistic with those of other hypolipidemic agents. A variety of drug combinations involving bile acid sequestrants are efficacious and discussed in later sections. Patients with homozygous familial hypercholesterolemia who are LDL-receptor-negative do not respond to bile acid sequestrants. Since the bile acid sequestrants are not absorbed, they are likely to be safe for pregnant and nursing women, as well as children. However, these groups of patients have not been extensively studied, and attention to the nutritional availability of fat-soluble vitamins is warranted in these subjects. The bile acid sequestrants are contraindicated in patients with marked elevations in plasma triglyceride concentrations since these drugs may accentuate the hypertriglyceridemia. However, bile acid sequestrants can be used in these patients if, after an initial response to a triglyceride-lowering agent, they manifest elevations in LDL cholesterol concentrations.

In addition to their effects as hypocholesterolemic agents, bile acid sequestrants are effective in reducing pruritis in patients with partial, but not complete, biliary obstruction by depleting the bile acid pool. *Principle: There are few gross derangements in biochemical physiology that are manifest clinically by a single sign or symptom. If the clinical derangement can be reversed, do not be surprised to find several of its signs reversed.*

Adverse Effects and Drug Interactions. Since the bile acid sequestrants are not absorbed from the GI tract, there are no appreciable systemic side effects. There was, however, a small, but statistically significant, increase in the concentrations of aspartate aminotransferase (AST; previously SGOT) and alkaline phosphatase and a small decrease in the concentration of serum carotene noted in the Lipid Research Clinics Primary Prevention Trial (Lipid Research Clinics Program, 1984a). With these minor exceptions that have no apparent clinical sequelae, the major side effects of bile acid sequestrants are confined to the GI system. Constipation is the primary adverse effect, with an incidence reported between 10% and 50%, and that increases at higher doses and in patients over 60 years. In addition, minor-to-severe complaints of flatulence, abdominal discomfort, nausea, vomiting, and poor palatability are encountered. There is no evidence for any increased risk for GI or other malignancies. Because the total bile acid pool is not significantly depleted during therapy, fat malabsorption is unusual but may be seen at the highest doses. Similarly, concentrations of fat-soluble vitamins are not usually disturbed and do not require supplementation; however, vitamin K–responsive hypoprothrombinemia has been reported. Because the bile acid sequestrants are anion-exchange resins, it is possible for increases in chloride absorption to predispose to hyperchloremic metabolic acidosis, particularly in children. Furthermore, the resins are capable of binding acidic and basic substances in addition to bile acids and thus impairing the absorption of many drugs. Although the interaction of the bile acid sequestrants with a few drugs has been assessed, the number of drugs studied is limited. Therefore, it is prudent to assume that the bile acid sequestrants will interfere with another drug's absorption and to give other drugs at least 1 hour before or 4 hours after the dose of the bile acid sequestrant. *Principle: Once a fundamental mechanism of drug interaction has been demonstrated with a few pairs of drugs, the burden of proof as to whether it more broadly applies lies with the physician, not with the "system" or the industry.*

Fibric Acids

History. In screening chemicals for hypolipidemic activity, a series of α-aryloxyisobutyric acid compounds were found to lower cholesterol concentrations in rats; the most potent of these was ethyl 2-(*p*-chlorophenoxy)-2-methylisobutyrate (CPIB) (Thorp, 1962). Originally, CPIB, or clofibrate as it was later named, was thought to

exert its action through a synergistic effect with the adrenal steroid androsterone. Therefore, the first formulation included clofibrate in combination with androsterone (Atromid); however, when it became apparent that the hypolipidemic effects of Atromid were due solely to the actions of clofibrate, androsterone was deleted from the preparation and it was renamed Atromid-S. After the successful introduction of clofibrate as a hypolipidemic agent, several other analogs were produced. Of these fibric acids, gemfibrozil, a substituted xylyloxyvaleric acid, is the only other one available in the United States, while bezafibrate, fenofibrate, and others are in use in Europe or are in clinical development (Fig. 15–3).

Mechanism of Action. Although the fibric acids have been in use for over 25 years, their mechanism of action is not fully understood. Indeed, there is evidence suggesting that almost each step in every pathway of lipid and lipoprotein metabolism is affected by fibric acids (Grundy and Vega, 1987). Nevertheless, it seems likely that many of these changes observed with fibric acids are not primary effects of the agents but occur secondarily to their principal actions. The major action of the fibric acids is to decrease

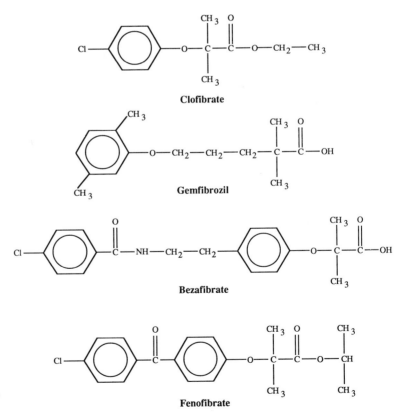

Fig. 15–3. Chemical structures of fibric acids.

Clofibrate

Gemfibrozil

Bezafibrate

Fenofibrate

VLDL concentrations, which kinetic studies have shown is due to an increase in catabolism of VLDLs (Kesaniemi and Grundy, 1984). The fibric acids appear to promote the catabolism of VLDLs by stimulating lipoprotein lipase activity (Nikkila et al., 1977); however, the mechanism responsible for this effect on lipoprotein lipase is unknown. While an increase in catabolism of VLDLs explains most of the reduction in concentrations of VLDLs, gemfibrozil and, in some patients, clofibrate also decrease VLDL triglyceride and apolipoprotein B production. The reason for the decline in production of VLDLs is not fully understood but has been attributed to several mechanisms of the fibric acids: inhibition of hepatic acetyl-CoA carboxylase, an important enzyme in triglyceride synthesis (Rodney et al., 1976); and suppression of lipolysis and free fatty acid flux (Kissebah et al., 1974).

The effects of the fibric acids on LDL metabolism are quite variable. In patients with hypertriglyceridemia, fibric acids frequently increase LDL values by decreasing LDL catabolism with no change or small decreases in production of LDLs (Vega and Grundy, 1985). This alteration probably is not a direct effect of fibric acids but occurs secondarily to the enhanced catabolism of VLDLs and the resultant down-regulation of LDL receptors in the liver induced by the increased clearance of VLDLs and VLDL remnants (IDLs). In patients with hypercholesterolemia and normal triglyceride concentrations, fibric acids have been reported to increase receptor-mediated catabolism of LDL slightly, without affecting production of LDLs (Stewart et al., 1982). The mechanism of this effect is unknown, but inhibition of cholesterol synthesis has been observed with fibric acids and might up-regulate hepatic LDL receptors (Grundy et al., 1972); however, no direct effects of fibric acids on cholesterol synthesis have been observed. The fibric acids, particularly gemfibrozil, raise HDL cholesterol and apolipoprotein AI values by increasing the production rate of apolipoprotein AI by unknown mechanisms (Saku et al., 1985). All the fibric acids increase biliary cholesterol concentrations and decrease bile acid secretion, leading to a saturated or lithogenic state that predisposes to formation of gallstones (Palmer, 1987; chapter 9).

Pharmacokinetics. The fibric acids presently available in the United States are clofibrate and gemfibrozil. They are prescribed in doses of 0.5 to 1.0 g and 300 to 600 mg twice daily, respectively. Because it is generally more efficacious and usually associated with fewer adverse effects (see below), gemfibrozil is more frequently recommended. Both clofibrate and gemfibrozil are readily absorbed from the GI tract. Clofibrate is very highly (90%–95%) protein-bound and has a plasma half-life of 7 to 8 hours, while gemfibrozil has a half-life of only 1.5 hours (Okerholm et al., 1976). The only metabolism of clofibrate that occurs is conjugation of clofibric acid with subsequent renal excretion. In contrast, gemfibrozil undergoes hydroxylation and conjugation before renal excretion.

Indications and Efficacy. Although fibric acids have been used as hypocholesterolemic agents for over 25 years, they are primarily indicated in the treatment of patients with various forms of hypertriglyceridemia since their major effect is to lower VLDL values. In general, the fibric acids cause a 25% to 60% reduction in triglyceride concentrations, while lowering cholesterol values 5% to 25% (Hunninghake and Peters, 1987). The HDL cholesterol concentrations usually increase 10% to 20% with fibric acids; however, the LDL cholesterol response is quite variable, with decreases of 10% to 20% occurring in some patients, and increases of 5% to 20% occurring in others. The response of LDL cholesterol appears to be dependent on the underlying hyperlipidemia's being treated. Increases in LDL concentrations generally occur in patients with primary hypertriglyceridemia (type IV hyperlipoproteinemia), while modest decreases in LDL concentrations occur in patients with hypercholesterolemia (type II hyperlipoproteinemia) or in patients with combined hypertriglyceridemia and hypercholesterolemia (type IIb hyperlipoproteinemia). Apolipoprotein values usually parallel the lipid changes observed, apolipoprotein B values either fall or remain unchanged, and apolipoprotein AI values usually increase.

Fibric acids also reverse the abnormalities in lipoprotein composition seen in hypertriglyceridemia (Eisenberg et al., 1984). Because fibric acids reduce both triglyceride and cholesterol concentrations in patients with type IIb hyperlipoproteinemia, they are useful in other patients with elevations of VLDL and LDL concentrations, such as diabetic dyslipidemia and nephrotic syndrome (Garg and Grundy, 1989; Groggel et al., 1989). Indeed, fibric acids might improve glucose tolerance (Kobayashi et al., 1988); however, their use in nephrotic syndrome should be undertaken with caution since renal insufficiency predisposes to some of their adverse effects (see below). Additionally, fibric acids are very effective in patients with type III hyperlipoproteinemia (dysbetalipoproteinemia) because of their ability to lower VLDL concentrations (Brewer et al., 1983).

Clofibrate and gemfibrozil have been used in combination with other hypolipidemic agents, including bile acid sequestrants, HMG-CoA reductase inhibitors (see below), and niacin (see below)

(East et al., 1988; Groggel et al., 1989). These combinations are generally considered when patients with type IV or type IIb hyperlipoproteinemia have a good hypotriglyceridemic response to a fibric acid, but a rise in LDL cholesterol concentrations is observed. While these combinations can be effective, an increase in adverse effects may be seen with HMG-CoA reductase inhibitors (see below) and probucol (see below), but not with bile acid sequestrants. Fibric acids have not been studied in women during pregnancy or lactation. Studies in animals have shown no teratogenicity of fibric acids, but embryotoxicity and carcinogenesis have been observed at high doses. Thus, fibric acids are not routinely recommended during pregnancy but can be used cautiously in women with severe hypertriglyceridemia that is exacerbated by pregnancy. Since fibric acids are excreted in breast milk, they should also be used cautiously during lactation.

Clofibrate and gemfibrozil have been employed in several long-term primary and secondary prevention trials. In the largest primary prevention trial, sponsored by the World Health Organization (WHO), 10,000 men with moderate hypercholesterolemia (mean cholesterol concentrations ~270 mg/dl) were randomized to clofibrate or placebo (Committee of Principal Investigators, 1978). After 5 years of follow-up, clofibrate reduced cholesterol concentrations by 9% and decreased nonfatal myocardial infarction (MI) by 25%; however, no differences in fatal MI were noted. Most disturbing, clofibrate was associated with a 25% increase in overall mortality, due primarily to diseases of the GI tract (see below). Following discontinuation of therapy, the excess mortality in the clofibrate treated group did not continue (Committee of Principal Investigators, 1984).

In a secondary prevention trial of men with previous MIs, 1100 men were randomized to clofibrate (The Coronary Drug Project Research Group, 1975). These men had multiple risk factors including hypertension, cigarette smoking, glucose intolerance, and hyperlipidemia; hypertriglyceridemia was the most prevalent abnormality, with serum cholesterol concentrations averaging ~250 mg/dl and serum triglyceride concentrations averaging ~550 mg/dl. After 5 years of follow-up, serum cholesterol concentrations fell 6.5% and serum triglyceride concentrations 22% with clofibrate. However, no differences in MI (fatal or nonfatal) or in overall mortality were noted. On the contrary, clofibrate was associated with an increased incidence of thromboembolic disease, arrhythmias, claudication, and the development of angina. Based on the results of the WHO and the Coronary Drug Project studies, the use of clofibrate has declined and its use cannot be generally recommended.

In contrast to the results with clofibrate, the findings of a primary prevention trial with gemfibrozil have been more encouraging (Frick et al., 1987). Over 4000 men with a variety of lipoprotein abnormalities (mean cholesterol concentration 289 mg/dl and mean triglyceride concentration 178 mg/dl), but all with non-HDL cholesterol values ≥200 mg/dl, were randomized to gemfibrozil or placebo for 5 years. At the completion of the study there were 10% and 35% declines in cholesterol and triglyceride concentrations, with an 11% increase in HDL concentrations (Manninen et al., 1988). These changes were associated with a 34% reduction in the incidence of coronary heart disease but no differences in overall mortality due to an increase in accidental and violent deaths. The improvement in the incidence of coronary heart disease was greatest for patients with type IIb hyperlipoproteinemia and correlated best with the extent of increase of HDL concentrations. Thus, with the results of the various intervention trials to date, gemfibrozil can be recommended as a first-line agent for the treatment of hypertriglyceridemia and as a secondary agent for the treatment of several other hyperlipidemias. *Principle: Before using a surrogate end point as the sole measure of efficacy, the clinician must be assured that the surrogate correlates very well with the ultimate efficacy being sought.*

Adverse Effects and Drug Interactions. The number and incidence of reported adverse effects is more extensive with clofibrate than gemfibrozil; however, the clinical experience with clofibrate also is greater. Thus, any of the adverse effects observed with clofibrate should be considered as potential adverse effects of gemfibrozil. *Principle: An overlapping spectrum of adverse effects should be expected to be observed with new agents that are chemically related to widely used compounds with known adverse effects.*

The most common adverse effects with fibric acids involve the GI tract. Abdominal pain, diarrhea, nausea, and vomiting are seen in some patients, with reversible elevations in hepatic transaminases also observed. Therefore, liver function should be routinely evaluated in patients taking fibric acids, and their use is contraindicated in patients with preexisting liver disease. The most serious adverse effect is an approximately twofold increase in gallstones with clofibrate (The Coronary Drug Project Research Group, 1977; Committee of Principal Investigators, 1978). This incidence of gallstones has not been observed with gemfibrozil (Frick, 1987); however, gemfibrozil does alter the lithogenicity of bile, as does clofibrate, and a trend toward a greater prevalence of gallstones has been observed. Fibric acids should be avoided in patients with cholelithiasis. Other complications observed during long-term therapy include an increased incidence of thromboembolic events and a trend toward an increased mortality from GI disease, particularly with clofibrate (as described above).

The syndrome of inappropriate antidiuretic hormone with hyponatremia has been reported with clofibrate. Furthermore, clofibrate and gemfibrozil are associated with myositis and rhabdomyolysis, which are more likely to develop in patients with renal insufficiency, possibly since the fibric acids are cleared primarily by the kidneys. In addition, the combination of fibric acids with HMG-CoA reductase inhibitors appears to predispose to a greater incidence of myositis (see below). Finally, major interactions of the fibric acids with other drugs occur, specifically with oral anticoagulants. Clofibrate and gemfibrozil potentiate the action of oral anticoagulants, necessitating close monitoring of the prothrombin time and adjustment of doses to achieve appropriate anticoagulation. *Principle: The most important interactions on which to focus are between drugs with narrow therapeutic indices. Such interactions are especially problematic when indications for the interacting drugs are the same.*

HMG-CoA Reductase Inhibitors

History. From the time that elevations in serum cholesterol concentrations were first noted to be associated with the development of atherosclerosis in experimental animals and later in epidemiologic studies in humans, many efforts have been directed toward developing inhibitors of cholesterol synthesis as a strategy for lowering serum cholesterol concentrations and preventing or reversing atherosclerosis. Initial efforts in this direction were undertaken at a time prior to the sophistication of understanding of cholesterol and lipoprotein metabolism that exists today. The early compounds that were successfully developed as inhibitors of cholesterol synthesis proved to cause serious metabolic side effects (many of which could have been predicted based on the present understanding of cholesterol metabolism). In the early 1950s, Δ^4-cholestenone was noted to act through an unknown mechanism as a potent inhibitor of cholesterol biosynthesis (Tomkins et al., 1953). However, it was clear that cholestenone was not clinically useful, since it causes the accumulation of dihydrocholesterol, a compound that was as atherogenic as cholesterol (Steinberg et al., 1958). In 1959, the first compound (triparanol, or MER-29) was developed that had a known site of action (Blohm and MacKenzie, 1959). Triparanol blocks the final step in cholesterol synthesis, the conversion of desmosterol to cholesterol (Avigan et al., 1960). While triparanol caused significant reductions in concentrations of serum cholesterol in humans, there were reciprocal elevations of desmosterol concentrations (Steinberg et al., 1961) that proved to be associated with the development of *accelerated* atherosclerosis in rabbits and cataracts in humans (Avigan and Steinberg, 1962; Laughlin and Carey, 1962; Kirby, 1967). These experiences led investigators to be wary of inhibitors of cholesterol synthesis that lead to overproduction of toxic intermediates. The search began for compounds that would inhibit an early step of cholesterol biosynthesis before the formation of sterol intermediates. *Principle: By inhibiting an early step in a biosynthetic pathway, the accumulation of toxic intermediates can be avoided.*

While searching for potential inhibitors of cholesterol synthesis among products of microorganisms, Endo and colleagues (Endo et al., 1976a, 1976b) reported the isolation of several metabolites from *Penicillium citrinum* that inhibit HMG-CoA reductase, the rate-limiting step in cholesterol biosynthesis (Fig. 15-4). One of the metabolites, ML-236B, was termed *compactin* since it was also isolated from the fungus *Penicillium brevicompactin* (Brown et al., 1976). Compactin lowered serum cholesterol values effectively in several animals and humans (Yamamoto et al., 1980). Shortly after the discovery of compactin, a closely related compound was isolated from *Aspergillus terreus* (mevinolin) and from *Monascus ruber* (monacolin K) (Endo and Monakolin, 1979; Alberts et al., 1980). Mevinolin (lovastatin) differs from compactin by the substitution of a methyl group for a hydrogen at carbon 6 (Fig. 15-5) that is associated with a twofold increase in affinity for HMG-CoA reductase. After early clinical trials, compactin was never developed for the marketplace (the reasons for this decision were not revealed); however, lovastatin was released in 1987 in the United States. Several newer agents (simvastatin and pravastatin) have been synthesized by chemical modifications of lovastatin and compactin (Fig. 15-5). These and other HMG-CoA reductase inhibitors are presently under investigation.

Mechanism of Action. These agents (of which lovastatin is presently the only one available) act as competitive inhibitors of HMG-CoA reductase, the rate-limiting enzyme in cholesterol biosynthesis. This enzyme catalyzes the conversion of HMG-CoA to mevalonate (Fig. 15-4). HMG-CoA, the natural substrate of the enzyme, has a K_m of $\sim 10 \ \mu M$, while lovastatin has a K_i of ~ 1 nM, or approximately a 10,000-fold greater affinity. This very high affinity of the inhibitors for HMG-CoA reductase results from their binding to two separate sites on the enzyme (Nakamura

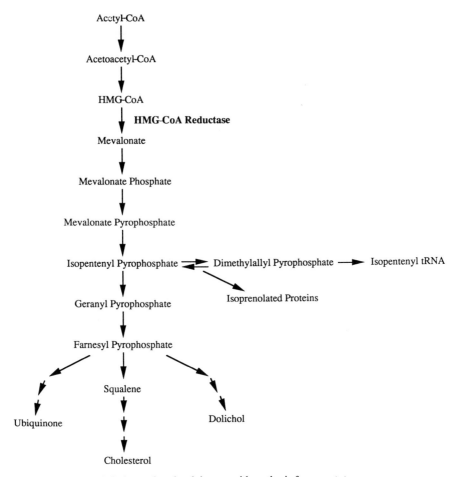

Fig. 15-4. Pathway of cholesterol and polyisoprenoid synthesis from acetate.

and Abeles, 1985). By inhibiting HMG-CoA reductase, these compounds inhibit the synthesis of cholesterol and other polyisoprenoid products (compounds containing multiple copies of the five-carbon isopentenyl pyrophosphate) of mevalonate metabolism (Fig. 15-4) in vitro. However, at the doses used clinically, no significant suppression of synthesis of noncholesterol polyisoprenoids is expected or found since much higher doses and more complete inhibition of HMG-CoA reductase are required to achieve such an effect (Brown and Goldstein, 1980). *Principle: If an agent is developed to inhibit an early step in a biosynthetic pathway, depletion of other, nontargeted, products of the pathway can potentially cause adverse effects.*

In vivo studies using sterol balance or urinary excretion of mevalonate to assess total body cholesterol synthesis have shown that maximal reduction of lipoprotein values is associated with only modest suppression of total body cholesterol synthesis, suggesting that mechanisms other than inhibition of cholesterol synthesis are involved in lipoprotein-lowering effects (Grundy and Bilheimer, 1984; Parker et al., 1984; Pappu et al., 1989). The modest reduction in cholesterol synthesis produced by HMG-CoA reductase inhibitors can be explained, in part, by the fact that these competitive inhibitors induce the expression of HMG-CoA reductase in vitro and in vivo, which tends to attenuate their effects (Brown et al., 1978; Stone et al., 1989).

The mechanism whereby a modest suppression of cholesterol synthesis causes a large reduction of lipoprotein values appears to be due to normal homeostatic responses (Fig. 15-6); suppression of cholesterol synthesis results in a fall in intracellular cholesterol concentration, which then triggers an increase in the expression of LDL receptors (Ma et al., 1986). This enhanced expression of LDL receptors by the liver causes an increased catabolic clearance of LDLs and a fall in plasma

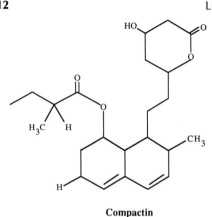

Compactin

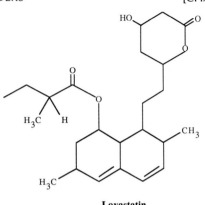

**Lovastatin
(mevinolin)**

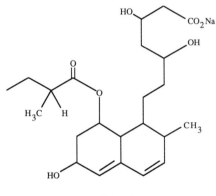

Pravastatin

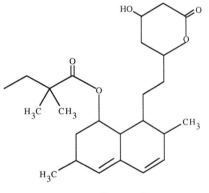

Simvastatin

Fig. 15–5. Chemical structures of HMG-CoA reductase inhibitors.

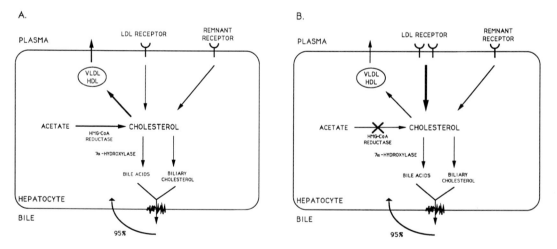

Fig. 15–6. (A) Schematic representation of normal hepatic cholesterol and bile acid metabolism. (B) Mechanisms of action of HMG-CoA reductase inhibitors. See text for full explanation.

LDL values (Bilheimer et al., 1983). Some studies have failed to observe an increase in catabolism of LDLs but instead have found a decrease in LDL production (Grundy and Vega, 1985). This finding is compatible with an enhanced expression of LDL receptors increasing the receptor-mediated clearance of VLDLs and IDL (VLDL remnants), resulting in a reduction of both triglyceride values and the rate of production of LDLs. In addition, it has been proposed that HMG-CoA reductase inhibitors might directly inhibit the hepatic formation of lipoproteins (Ginsberg et al., 1987). The HMG-CoA reductase inhibitors do not consistently alter bile metabolism and, therefore, are not associated with any consistent changes in net excretion of sterol from the body.

Pharmacokinetics. All the HMG-CoA reductase inhibitors are given orally. Approximately 30% of an oral dose of lovastatin is absorbed from the GI tract in animal species. Lovastatin and simvastatin are prodrugs. They are in a lactone form that is inactive and are metabolized by the liver to their corresponding β-hydroxyacids, which are the active drugs. In contrast, pravastatin is delivered as an open acid. The lactone nature of lovastatin and simvastatin allows the active forms of the drugs to be targeted to the liver, where the majority of drug is metabolized during its first pass. In animal studies, 16% or less of active drug is found in extrahepatic tissues (Alberts, 1988). Although pravastatin does not require hepatic metabolism to activate the drug, in vitro studies suggest that it is preferentially taken up by the liver.

After oral administration approximately 10% of lovastatin is excreted in the urine and the remainder is found in feces, representing unabsorbed drug and hepatically metabolized drug that is excreted in bile. Because lovastatin is metabolized in the liver by cytochrome P450 enzymes, it is possible for its metabolism to be modified by other drugs. In vitro studies suggest that cimetidine inhibits and phenobarbital increases its metabolism (Vyas, 1990). Therefore, even though no in vivo interactions have yet been reported, cimetidine might be expected to blunt the response to lovastatin by preventing its conversion to active drug. Lovastatin has no effect on antipyrine kinetics. Lovastatin and its metabolites are highly protein-bound (>95%) and cross both the blood–brain barrier and the placenta. Plasma concentrations of drug and metabolites peak between 2 to 4 hours after an oral dose and return toward baseline by 24 hours. Steady-state levels are achieved by 2 to 3 days; however, since lipoprotein values do not stabilize for 2 to 4 weeks, adjustments of dose should not be made more

frequently than every 4 weeks. Concentrations in plasma are one third higher when the drug is given with meals. Thus, the drug can generally be given once per day (usually at night), but twice-a-day dosing is required at higher doses. The dosage range for lovastatin is 20 to 80 mg/day.

Indications and Efficacy. HMG-CoA reductase inhibitors are indicated in the treatment of all types of hypercholesterolemia since they are the single most effective agents for lowering cholesterol concentrations. However, they are generally not recommended as initial therapy because of the relatively limited experience with their long-term use. *Principle: The more efficacious an agent, the more likely one is to accept adverse side effects of that agent. However, when lifelong therapy is considered, a drug with slightly less overall efficacy may be preferred if it also produces fewer serious side effects.*

HMG-CoA reductase inhibitors are indicated in patients with elevations of LDL concentrations due to heterozygote familial hypercholesterolemia (type II hyperlipoproteinemia), as well as polygenic forms of hypercholesterolemia. Given as a single agent, HMG-CoA reductase inhibitors decrease LDL cholesterol values between 30% and 40% (Illingworth and Bacon, 1989). In addition, consistent decreases in VLDL cholesterol concentrations and reductions in triglyceride concentrations range between 10% and 30%, and generally increases in HDL cholesterol of 2% to 15% are seen. The decline in LDL and VLDL concentrations is paralleled by reduction of LDL and VLDL apolipoprotein B values. No changes in lipoprotein(a) concentrations occur (Kostner et al., 1989).

When HMG-CoA reductase inhibitors are combined with bile acid sequestrants, reductions in LDL cholesterol values of 40% to 55% are observed. Similar falls in LDL cholesterol values are seen when HMG-CoA reductase inhibitors are combined with niacin; however, this combination should be used cautiously because of potential adverse effects (see below). When HMG-CoA reductase inhibitors are combined with bile acid sequestrants and niacin, a 67% reduction of LDL cholesterol values has been observed (Malloy et al., 1987). Thus, HMG-CoA reductase inhibitors are an important part of therapeutic regimens designed to normalize severely and moderately elevated values of LDL cholesterol.

Patients with homozygous familial hypercholesterolemia who are LDL-receptor-negative do not respond to HMG-CoA reductase inhibitors, but a response may be seen in some individuals with decreased expression of LDL receptors (Stein, 1989). Since the HMG-CoA reductase inhibitors have been teratogenic in animals, they should not be used in premenopausal women unless the probability of pregnancy is very low. Likewise, nursing mothers should not be treated with HMG-CoA reductase inhibitors since they are excreted in milk. To date there have been no substantive studies in children, but it may be appropriate to use HMG-CoA reductase inhibitors in severely hypercholesterolemic children and adolescents. *Principle: When drugs tested in adults are used in children, the need for extraordinary surveillance of these children is obvious. Most important, the clinician must be willing to consider the development of any unexpected event as due to the drug until proved otherwise.*

In addition to their primary indications for patients with elevations of LDL cholesterol, HMG-CoA reductase inhibitors are very effective in other lipoprotein abnormalities. Lovastatin reduces triglyceride and cholesterol values markedly in patients with type III hyperlipoproteinemia (dysbetalipoproteinemia) by increasing the catabolism and decreasing the production of β-VLDLs (Vega et al., 1988). Furthermore, conditions in which both VLDL and LDL concentrations are raised, for example, familial combined hyperlipidemia, diabetic dyslipidemia, and nephrotic syndrome, appear to respond well to HMG-CoA reductase inhibitors. Treatment of a small number of patients with familial combined hyperlipidemia with compactin caused a 25% and 20% reduction in cholesterol and triglyceride concentrations, respectively (Yamamoto et al., 1980). Hyperlipidemic patients with non-insulin-dependent diabetes mellitus responded to lovastatin with a 25% and 30% reduction of cholesterol and triglyceride concentrations, respectively (Garg and Grundy, 1988), while patients with nephrotic syndrome have shown a 30% to 35% reduction of cholesterol and triglyceride concentrations (Vega and Grundy, 1988b). Because hypertriglyceridemia frequently predominates in these conditions characterized by both elevated VLDL and elevated LDL concentrations, gemfibrozil or niacin is commonly used initially. Addition of an HMG-CoA reductase inhibitor may yield further benefit, but these combinations should be used cautiously (see below). No long-term intervention studies have yet been completed with HMG-CoA reductase inhibitors.

Adverse Effects and Drug Interactions. At the time of its release in 1987, lovastatin had been given to only 1500 patients in clinical trials (chapters 34, 35, 39, 40). Since that time it has been prescribed to over 1 million patients and has undergone extensive postmarketing clinical trials and postmarketing surveillance. Lovastatin and the other HMG-CoA reductase inhibitors are very well tolerated medications with few known adverse side effects. The major adverse effect necessitating discontinuation of the drug has been abnormalities in liver function tests. Elevations in transaminase concentrations to values greater than three times the upper limits of normal occur in less than 2% of patients. There appears to be a dose dependency to this effect since the incidence is 0.1% at 20 mg/day and increases progressively to 1.5% at 80 mg/day (Tobert et al., 1990). The majority of increases in transaminase concentrations have occurred within 48 weeks of initiation of therapy. All have returned to normal upon discontinuation of lovastatin. In addition to increases in transaminase concentrations, reversible, symptomatic hepatitis, manifested by cholestatic or hepatocellular changes, has been reported in some patients. Thus, it is important to follow liver function tests on a regular basis.

The most worrisome adverse effect is myopathy, which is defined as diffuse muscle pain or weakness with elevations of creatine kinase concentrations greater than 10 times the upper limits of normal. This occurs in <0.2% of patients and usually within the first 48 weeks of therapy. Several patients have demonstrated frank rhabdomyolysis with renal failure. Most, but not all, of the patients manifesting severe myopathy received concomitant therapy with cyclosporine, gemfibrozil, or niacin. Cyclosporine particularly appears to increase the incidence, since 28% of those patients on both cyclosporine and lovastatin manifest myopathy. Cyclosporine seems to interfere with the metabolism of lovastatin, raising plasma concentrations three- to fourfold. Thus, in individuals receiving cyclosporine for immunosuppressive therapy, lovastatin should be prescribed cautiously and not in doses exceeding 20 mg/day. The association of myopathy with the combination of gemfibrozil and lovastatin appears to be due to the myopathic effects of each agent and not to any effects of gemfibrozil on lovastatin kinetics. Since approximately 5% of patients taking this combination develop myopathy, it should be used with caution. Approximately 2% or less of patients receiving niacin and lovastatin are reported to develop myopathy. The underlying mechanism for this interaction is unclear since niacin does not affect lovastatin metabolism and is not associated with myopathy when given as a single agent. Nonetheless, levels of creatine kinase should be regularly evaluated in patients taking lovastatin and particularly when those patients are on additional medications that might predispose to myopathy. However, normal concentrations of creatine kinase do not mean that the patient is protected from developing myopathy, only that no evidence of myopathy is present at that point in time. Myopathy can develop rapidly without any increases in creatine kinase concentrations presaging its onset.

Other, less serious, adverse effects include skin

rash in <0.3%, with hypersensitivity reactions presenting as anaphylaxis, lupuslike syndromes, or urticaria reported in a few patients, GI complaints in <0.3%, with constipation the major manifestation; and insomnia in 0.1%. There are possible interactions of lovastatin with warfarin since elevated prothrombin times have been reported in some patients.

Postmarketing studies have focused on investigating the possible relationship of lovastatin with the development of cataracts. This concern is based on the history of cataract development with the cholesterol-synthesis inhibitor triparanol (see above), and on the finding of cataracts in dogs treated with high doses of lovastatin (MacDonald et al., 1988). However, no increase in lens opacification beyond that expected with normal aging has been noted to date. Since the HMG-CoA reductase inhibitors can block the end products of mevalonate metabolism, deficiencies of cholesterol, ubiquinone, and dolichol, as well as isoprenylated proteins, are possible. Evidence suggests that this is not the case at the doses of inhibitors used in humans. Both adrenal and gonadal steroid hormone production from their precursor, cholesterol, are normal, as is bile acid production (Grundy, 1988). Ubiquinone participates in mitochondrial functions, and its concentrations are not altered by compactin. Likewise, no deficiencies in glycoproteins have been observed that could be referable to changes in dolichol concentrations, since dolichol is required for glycoprotein synthesis. Thus, HMG-CoA reductase inhibitors have been reasonably well tolerated with few short-term adverse side effects; nonetheless, longer periods of observation are required to determine whether adverse effects secondary to alterations in mevalonate metabolism might occur. *Principle: Most targets of drug therapy have complex physiologic roles that often are incompletely understood. When drugs cause unexpected and severe adverse effects, use those signals to expand your knowledge of the drug's mechanism of action. In the case of cholesterol, do not be surprised if effects related to alterations in concentrations of cellular cholesterol or other isoprenoid products of mevalonate metabolism appear overt while using HMG-CoA reductase inhibitors.*

Nicotinic Acid (Niacin)

History. Nicotinic acid was first produced in 1867 from the oxidation of nicotine, derived from the leaves of the plant nicotiana that had been introduced into France from America by Count Nicot (Altschul, 1964). In the early 20th century nicotinic acid (Fig. 15–7) was directly isolated from foodstuffs and suggested to be a nutrient; however, it was not until the mid-1930s that nicotinic acid was shown to be a vitamin and to cure pellagra. It was at that time that nicotinic acid and its amidated form, nicotinamide, were identified as components of nicotinamide adenine dinucleotide (NAD) and nicotinamide adenine dinucleotide phosphate (NADP) and, thus, important cofactors in a variety of metabolic pathways utilizing oxidative processes. In 1942, nicotinic acid was renamed niacin (**ni**cotinic **ac**id vitam**in**) in order to avoid confusion with nicotine, especially in food labeling. Based on nicotinic acid's involvement in oxidative processes and on an earlier observation that an increased oxygen tension could lower serum cholesterol concentrations, Altschul et al. (1955) gave large doses of nicotinic acid in an attempt to lower serum cholesterol concentrations by increasing its oxidation. In subjects with cholesterol concentrations >250 mg/dl, a decline in total cholesterol

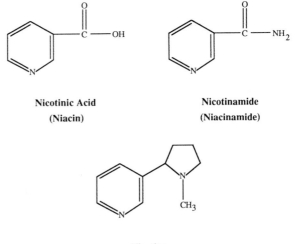

Nicotinic Acid
(Niacin)

Nicotinamide
(Niacinamide)

Nicotine

Fig. 15–7. Chemical structures of nicotinic acid, nicotinamide, and nicotine.

concentrations of up to 21% was observed with nicotinic acid, but no effects were seen with nicotinamide. This led to niacin's becoming the first agent to be used widely for reducing concentrations of cholesterol in serum. Later, its ability to lower triglyceride concentrations was observed (Carlson and Oro, 1962), leading to one of its major therapeutic indications.

Mechanism of Action. Even though niacin has been used as a hypolipidemic agent for over 35 years, its mechanisms of action in reducing lipoprotein values are not fully understood. The major action of niacin is to decrease the hepatic production of VLDLs without affecting their catabolism (Grundy et al., 1981). This decrease in VLDL production is due principally to a fall in production of triglycerides with a decrease in the triglyceride content of VLDLs; however, a decrease in apolipoprotein B production also appears to occur with a decline in the number of VLDL particles. Furthermore, the rate of production of LDLs, but not their catabolism, is also reduced (Levy et al., 1972). The working model to explain these effects is depicted in Fig. 15–8. Nicotinic acid exerts its primary effect in adipose tissue, where it causes a rapid suppression of lipolysis with a fall in circulating free fatty acids (Carlson and Oro, 1962). Interestingly, nicotinamide, which is ineffective as a hypolipidemic agent, does not suppress lipolysis. The actions of nicotinic acid on the fat cell are mediated by nicotinic acid "receptors" on the cell surface that are coupled to inhibitory G proteins. Activation of these receptors leads to the inhibition of adenylate cyclase activity, decreasing the accumulation of cyclic AMP and thus inhibiting lipolysis. The decrease in free fatty acid flux lowers the amount of precursor (fatty acids) available to the liver for triglyceride synthesis (reesterification) and VLDL production. Since VLDLs are the precursors of LDLs, a fall in VLDL production then leads to a subsequent decline in LDL production. While this model might explain the actions of nicotinic acid

on lipoprotein metabolism, it is not the sole explanation, since there is escape from the suppression of free fatty acids by nicotinic acid. In fact, daylong values of free fatty acids are not significantly lower in patients treated with niacin. Thus, a direct effect of nicotinic acid to inhibit VLDL (triglyceride) synthesis by the liver has been proposed. Indeed, nicotinic acid has been reported to decrease cholesterol (hepatic) synthesis, but the mechanism for this action is unclear (Miettinen, 1968). Nicotinic acid increases the concentration of HDL cholesterol and apolipoprotein AI by decreasing apolipoprotein AI catabolism (Shepherd et al., 1979); however, the underlying mechanism for this effect also is not known. Nicotinic acid does not appear to have any consistent effects on fecal sterol excretion or on the composition of bile.

Pharmacokinetics. Niacin is part of the water-soluble vitamin B complex. It is rapidly and completely absorbed from the intestine following oral administration of even high doses. However, time-released preparations have a delayed absorption and lower peak concentrations. While 15 mg is the daily requirement of niacin as a vitamin, hypolipidemic effects are not seen until doses over 1 g are reached, and up to 6.5 g may be needed for full therapeutic effects. No additional benefit is seen at even higher doses. After absorption, niacin is cleared by first-pass hepatic metabolism; however, since hepatic clearance saturates, a greater percentage of unaltered nicotinic acid enters the systemic circulation with increasing doses (Weiner and van Eys, 1983). The half-life of nicotinic acid in plasma is approximately 45 minutes. It distributes to all tissues in the body, where it acts as a vitamin cofactor. Nicotinic acid is first amidated to nicotinamide, which is active as a vitamin, but not as a hypolipidemic agent. Nicotinamide is further metabolized by N-methylation and 2-pyridone derivatization (Bicknell and Prescott, 1953). The major metabolic derivative of nicotinic acid is nicotinuric acid, its glycine conjugate. The amounts of unaltered nicotinic acid and

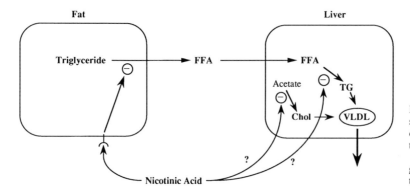

Fig. 15–8. Schematic representation of the mechanisms of action of nicotinic acid. See text for full explanation. FFA = free fatty acids; TG = triglycerides; Chol = cholesterol.

of nicotinuric acid appearing in the urine increase progressively at higher doses. When niacin therapy is initiated, dosing should begin at 100 mg given three times daily and increase progressively every 5 to 7 days until a therapeutic effect is achieved.

Indications and Efficacy. Niacin is indicated as a first-line agent in the treatment of all forms of hypertriglyceridemia and hypercholesterolemia. When therapeutic doses are achieved (3–6.5 g/day), niacin generally decreases plasma triglyceride (VLDL) values by 20% to 80%, with the greatest falls seen in subjects with the highest initial elevations. In parallel, cholesterol concentrations fall 10% to 40% because of reductions in VLDL cholesterol and LDL cholesterol; HDL cholesterol concentrations increase 10% to 30%. The decline in VLDL cholesterol concentrations is greater in patients with hypertriglyceridemia and is primarily responsible for the reduction of serum cholesterol concentrations in these patients. In normotriglyceridemic subjects, the decline in VLDL concentrations is relatively small, and most of the fall in serum cholesterol concentrations occurs in the LDL fraction. In concert with these changes in lipid values, niacin causes a decrease in apolipoprotein B values, reflecting fewer circulating VLDL and LDL particles, and an increase in apolipoprotein AI, reflecting an increase in HDLs. Interestingly, niacin is the only agent reported to lower lipoprotein(a) values (Gurakar et al., 1985). Since its major action is to decrease VLDL production, niacin is particularly effective in patients with type IV and type V hyperlipoproteinemia, as well as patients with type III hyperlipoproteinemia (Levy and Langer, 1972). Furthermore, since niacin effectively lowers VLDL and LDL levels, it is useful as a single agent in patients in whom both VLDL and LDL concentrations are raised, for example, in those with familial combined hyperlipidemia (Grundy et al., 1981), diabetic dyslipidemia, and nephrotic syndrome. However, its use in diabetes has been associated with worsened glucose control in some patients, and its use in the nephrotic syndrome has not been thoroughly evaluated.

Although no studies have been conducted to evaluate the long-term efficacy of niacin in patients with hypertriglyceridemia, the Coronary Drug Project (The Coronary Drug Project Group, 1975) compared niacin with placebo in men who had previously had a documented MI. These men had multiple risk factors including hypertension, cigarette smoking, glucose intolerance, and hyperlipidemia; in the group, hypertriglyceridemia was the most prevalent abnormality with serum cholesterol concentrations averaging ~250 mg/dl and serum triglyceride concentra-

tions averaging ~550 mg/dl. After 5 years of follow-up, serum cholesterol concentrations fell 10% and serum triglyceride concentrations 26% with niacin. This was associated with a 27% reduction in nonfatal MI but no differences in overall mortality compared with placebo. However, 15-year follow-up revealed an 11% reduction in overall mortality with niacin (Canner et al., 1986). *Principle: Absence of a positive "long-term" effect when the drug has been given for a reasonably brief period does not exclude the "long-term" effect when studies are sufficiently lengthened.*

While niacin causes only modest reductions in cholesterol and LDL concentrations when given as a single agent, it is very effective when used in combination with other hypolipidemic agents. Since bile acid sequestrants increase LDL catabolism but their actions are attenuated by an increase in VLDL production, the ability of niacin to suppress VLDL production results in a synergistic effect. Indeed, a combination of bile acid sequestrant and niacin can normalize LDL cholesterol values in patients with heterozygous familial hypercholesterolemia (Kane et al., 1981). A combination of colestipol and niacin was compared with placebo in the Cholesterol-Lowering Atherosclerosis Study to examine the effects of cholesterol lowering on the progression of atherosclerosis in men who have had coronary artery bypass surgery (Blankenhorn et al., 1987). At entry these men were principally hypercholesterolemic with mean cholesterol values of 246 mg/dl and triglyceride values of 151 mg/dl. After 2 years there was a 26% decrease in cholesterol concentrations with a 43% decrease in LDL cholesterol concentrations, a 22% decrease in triglyceride concentrations, and a 47% increase in HDL cholesterol concentrations that was associated with significantly less progression and greater regression of atherosclerotic lesions on coronary angiography. In another randomized secondary prevention trial, niacin was used in combination with clofibrate in men with previous MIs (Carlson and Rosenhamer, 1988). After 5 years of follow-up, serum cholesterol and triglyceride concentrations decreased 13% and 19%, respectively, from initial values of approximately 230 and 210 mg/dl, respectively. This was associated with a decrease in mortality from ischemic heart disease of 36% and in overall mortality of 26%. Thus, niacin has been shown to be a very effective agent, singly and in combination, for reducing triglyceride and cholesterol concentrations in a variety of hyperlipoproteinemias. Moreover, it is the only hypolipidemic agent to date that has been associated with a decrease in overall mortality. Unfortunately, its usefulness as a hypolipidemic agent is frequently limited by its adverse effects.

Adverse Effects and Drug Interactions. At the large doses used for hypolipidemic effects, niacin has a considerable number of adverse effects that are not observed at the low doses taken as a vitamin (Hotz, 1983). The most obvious and dramatic adverse effect is an intense cutaneous flush, with or without pruritis, that occurs within a few minutes to hours after an oral dose. This cutaneous flush is part of a generalized vasodilatory effect of niacin that appears to be mediated via prostaglandins. Aspirin is effective in preventing the flush and can be given 30 minutes preceding a dose to prevent symptoms; however, aspirin is often not required since tachyphalaxis develops to the vasodilatory effects of the drug with diminution of the symptoms over time while the same doses are continued. Other skin changes such as dryness, hyperpigmentation, and acanthosis nigracans occur occasionally. Additionally, the incidence of atrial fibrillation and ventricular ectopy increases with niacin.

The most serious adverse effect of niacin is hepatic dysfunction, with elevations of alkaline phosphatase and transaminase concentrations commonly occurring at doses above 3 g. Occasionally, symptomatic hepatitis with jaundice is seen. The hepatic abnormalities are reversible upon discontinuation of the drug; however, hepatic fibrosis has been reported (Kohn and Montes, 1969). An inhibitory effect of the high doses of niacin on normal NAD synthesis is the presumed mechanism of the hepatotoxicity. Niacin increases gastric acid secretion and is contraindicated in patients with peptic ulcer disease. It also is associated with other GI effects, such as abdominal discomfort, nausea, and diarrhea. Time-released preparations are associated with less cutaneous flushing but appear to have a greater incidence of elevation of liver function tests (Knopp et al., 1985).

Another adverse effect is a deterioration of glucose tolerance that generally occurs in patients with preexisting impaired glucose tolerance. The impairment of glucose tolerance is probably due to changes in the glucose–fatty acid cycle induced by the suppression of lipolysis, with a resultant increase in insulin resistance. Hyperuricemia secondary to increases in purine metabolism and decreases in renal clearance may occur, occasionally with precipitation of gouty arthritis. No interactions of niacin with other medications have been described; however, decreased levels of total thyroxine due to low thyroxine-binding globulin have been observed in patients on the combination of colestipol and niacin even though thyroid function tests are normal on either agent alone (Cashin-Hemphill et al., 1987).

Probucol

History and Pharmacokinetics. Probucol is a bis-phenol — (4,4′-[(1-methylethylidene)bis(thio)] bis[2,6-bis(1,1-dimethylethyl)phenol] — whose structure is unlike that of any other hypolipidemic agent (Fig. 15–9). Probucol was discovered to have hypolipidemic action during screening of various chemicals for nontoxic hypocholesterolemic effects (Barnhart et al., 1970). Probucol is given in a fixed dose of 500 mg twice daily even though no clearcut dose effect is observed at doses greater than 375 mg/day (Heel et al., 1978). It is poorly and variably absorbed from the GI tract with peak concentrations occurring at 8 to 24 hours that represent only 0.7% to 14% of the administered dose. Steady-state plasma concentrations are not reached for 3 to 4 months. Probucol is lipophilic and distributes into lipoproteins and adipose tissue. Its elimination occurs primarily via biliary excretion without evidence of metabolism. The half-life of the elimination of probucol after a single dose is 23 days, but this is further prolonged with chronic administration so that patients who receive drug for 1 year have plasma concentrations of probucol that are still 20% of steady-state concentrations 6 months after discontinuation of the drug. With its long half-life, maximum lipid-lowering effects of probucol are not observed for several months.

Mechanism of Action. The cholesterol-lowering mechanisms of probucol are not well understood, although it is clear that probucol can decrease the plasma concentrations of LDLs and HDLs. Kinetic studies examining probucol's effects have been inconsistent but suggest that the

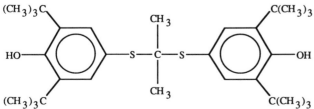

Fig. 15–9. Chemical structure of probucol.

probucol-induced fall in LDL cholesterol is due to increased catabolism of LDLs via non-receptor-mediated pathways without any effects on production of LDLs (Bilheimer, 1986). How probucol affects non-receptor-mediated clearance is unknown. The decline in HDL cholesterol observed with probucol is due to a decrease in the synthesis of apolipoproteins AI and AII; the mechanism for this action is unknown. Probucol does not appear to have any consistent effects on cholesterol synthesis or bile acid and fecal sterol excretion. Recently, probucol was shown to be a potent antioxidant (Parthasarathy et al., 1986), an action that might have very important implications in the therapy of atherosclerosis. There is accumulating evidence that the oxidation of lipoproteins might be one of the essential mechanisms in the process of atherogenesis (Steinberg et al., 1989). Since probucol is a lipophilic antioxidant that is incorporated into lipoproteins, it prevents the oxidation of lipoproteins. Its potential use in this regard is illustrated by the ability of probucol to prevent the development of atherosclerosis in spontaneously hypercholesterolemic rabbits without significantly affecting serum cholesterol concentrations (Kita et al., 1987; Carew et al., 1987). Whether this action has clinical implications in humans remains to be established. *Principle: An agent often is developed on the basis of one specific action (e.g., lowering cholesterol concentrations), but often has an effect on a specific disease process (atherogenesis) that is due to an action that was not initially known and that is independent of the action for which it was initially developed.*

Indications and Efficacy. Probucol is presently considered a secondary agent in the treatment of hypercholesterolemia due to elevations in LDL concentrations. As a single agent it usually results in a 10% to 20% reduction in total serum cholesterol concentrations that is secondary to a 5% to 15% fall in LDL cholesterol concentrations and a 10% to 30% decline in HDL cholesterol concentrations without any consistent changes in triglyceride concentrations (Heel et al., 1978; Durrington and Miller, 1985; Fellin et al., 1986). Apolipoprotein B and apolipoprotein AI values are reduced in parallel to the changes in LDL and HDL concentrations. Thus, probucol has a more pronounced effect in reducing HDL than LDL concentrations. It is indicated only in some patients with elevations of LDL cholesterol concentrations and has no place in the therapy of hypertriglyceridemic patients. Interestingly, probucol promotes regression of xanthomas and small reductions in LDL cholesterol concentrations in patients with homozygous familial hypercholesterolemia (Yamamota et al., 1986) and, thus, might be useful in this clinical setting.

Probucol has been used in combination with other hypolipidemic agents, particularly bile acid sequestrants; it has been suggested that the soft stools associated with probucol counteract the constipating effects of bile acid sequestrants, leading to improvement in patient compliance and the tolerability of both agents (Dujovne et al., 1984). The combination of probucol with clofibrate is contraindicated since this combination appears to result in a markedly decreased concentration of HDL cholesterol, often below 15 mg/dl (Davignon, 1986). The use of probucol during pregnancy and lactation has not been explored. Because probucol might have a greater effect of preventing atherosclerosis (see above) than its relatively modest effects on lowering cholesterol values, a fall in the concentration of cholesterol might not be the most appropriate end point to follow in order to evaluate its efficacy.

Adverse Effects and Drug Interactions. Probucol is very well tolerated with few adverse effects. Thus, less than 3% of subjects discontinue the drug due to adverse effects. The most common side effects are GI effects, primarily diarrhea or loose stools, but flatulence, abdominal pain, nausea and vomiting are also reported (Heel et al., 1978). Eosinophilia has been reported in approximately 10% of patients. The most serious adverse effect is a prolongation of the QT interval with the occurrence of serious ventricular arrhythmias or bradyarrhythmias. For this reason, probucol is contraindicated in patients taking medications that can prolong the QT interval or delay AV conduction, such as antiarrhythmics, tricyclic antidepressants, phenothiazines, β blockers, or digoxin. Excluding these combinations, no specific drug interactions have been reported with probucol. Any systemic adverse effects that develop with probucol can be expected to persist for long periods of time due to the prolonged half-life of elimination of the drug.

Other Drugs

There are several other drugs that are used as hypolipidemic agents, but they should be considered as alternative therapy; others have been used as hypolipidemic agents in the past and cannot be recommended for use at the present time.

Neomycin, Activated Charcoal, and Psyllium Hydrophilic Mucilloid. These drugs have been used as hypocholesterolemic agents with modest benefit. Neomycin, a poorly absorbed aminoglycoside antibiotic, was serendipitously discovered in 1959 to lower serum cholesterol concentrations

(Samuel and Steiner, 1959). Further studies have shown that neomycin, 2 g/day in divided oral doses, causes a 10% to 30% reduction in total and LDL cholesterol concentrations with no change or an increase in triglyceride concentrations (Samuel, 1979). Neomycin forms an insoluble complex with bile acids in the GI tract, inhibiting their reabsorption, consequently having actions similar to the bile acid sequestrants. Neomycin has been employed singly and in combination with other hypolipidemic agents in the treatment of hypercholesterolemia, that is, the same clinical indications as bile acid sequestrants. Neomycin is associated with abdominal discomfort, diarrhea, and interference with drug absorption, specifically digoxin. However, it has not been widely used because of its potential ototoxicity and nephrotoxicity, particularly in patients with preexisting renal insufficiency. Nevertheless, neomycin therapy can be considered in select individuals who do not tolerate bile acid sequestrants.

Activated charcoal has been used in a small number of hypercholesterolemic subjects in doses of 8 g three times daily; it decreases total and LDL cholesterol concentrations by 25% and 40%, respectively (Kuusisto et al., 1986). It appears to act by mimicking the actions of bile acid sequestrants (Neuvonen et al., 1989); however, with the limited clinical experience using it and its potential for interference with drug absorption, the drug cannot presently be recommended as a hypolipidemic agent.

Finally, psyllium hydrophilic mucilloid (e.g., Metamucil) exerts an effect similar to that of bile acid sequestrants (Bell et al., 1989). Psyllium hydrophilic mucilloid at doses of 3.4 g three times daily reduces total and LDL cholesterol concentrations by 5% to 15%. Given the beneficial effects of fiber, psyllium hydrophilic mucilloid or other sources high in fiber appear to provide a reasonable adjunct therapy but cannot be recommended as primary therapy for hypercholesterolemia.

β-Sitosterol. In the past, this phytosterol (plant sterol) was used as a hypocholesterolemic agent. It structurally resembles cholesterol but is not normally absorbed significantly from the gut (Salen et al., 1970). β-Sitosterol appears to interfere with the absorption of cholesterol and is used in doses of 3 g with meals to cause a small, variable decrease in cholesterol values. Some patients readily absorb β-sitosterol and develop β-sitosterolemia and xanthomas containing β-sitosterol (Bhattacharyya, 1974). Given its relative lack of efficacy and potential side effects, β-sitosterol should not be presently recommended.

D-Thyroxine. This optical isomer of thyroid hormone was previously used as a hypocholester-

olemic agent. Its mechanism of action is thought to be mediated by its effects as a thyromimetic agent that has a greater ability to lower serum lipids than to increase the overall metabolic rate. Thyroid hormone increases the number of LDL receptors (Chait et al., 1979) and, thus, the catabolism of LDLs (Thompson et al., 1981). D-Thyroxine causes a 10% decrement in the plasma concentration of LDL cholesterol with a 10% to 20% decrease in triglyceride (VLDL) concentrations. The Coronary Drug Project (The Coronary Drug Project Research Group, 1972) in comparing D-thyroxine with placebo in men who had previously had a documented MI found that D-thyroxine was associated with an increased incidence of MIs, angina, and fatal arrhythmias, and a greater overall mortality, necessitating discontinuation of the study. Therefore, its use is not recommended in adults; however, it can possibly be considered as secondary therapy in children or individuals without evidence of coronary artery disease. Interestingly, it has been suggested that newer analogs of thyroid hormone can be synthesized that are preferentially taken up by the liver to yield a greater differential effect on hepatic cholesterol metabolism than on myocardial metabolism and oxygen demand (Underwood, 1986; Leeson et al., 1989). These newer agents might be very beneficial if they are proved to be safe. *Principle: An agent that is effective, but limited by adverse effects, can potentially be altered to eliminate tissue-specific side effects while maintaining efficacy.*

REFERENCES

Aberg, H.; Lithell, H.; Selinus, I.; and Hedstrand, H.: Serum triglycerides are a risk factor for myocardial infarction but not for angina pectoris: Results from a 10-year follow-up of Uppsala primary preventive study. Atherosclerosis, 54:89–97, 1985.

Ad Hoc Committee to Design a Dietary Treatment of Hyperlipoproteinemia: Recommendations for treatment of hyperlipidemia in adults. A joint statement of the Nutrition Committee and the Council on Arteriosclerosis. Circulation, 69:1067A–1090A, 1984.

Alberts, A.: Discovery, biochemistry and biology of lovastatin. Am. J. Cardiol., 62:10J–15J, 1988.

Alberts, A. W.; Chen, J.; Kuron, G.; Hunt, V.; Huff, J.; Hoffman, C.; Rothrock, J.; Lopez, M.; Joshua, H.; Harris, E.; Patchett, A.; Monaghan, R.; Currie, S.; Stapley, E.; Albers-Schonberg, G.; Hensons, O.; Hirschfield, J.; Hoogsteen, K.; Liesch, J.; and Springer, J.: Mevinolin: A highly-potent competitive inhibitor of hydroxymethylglutaryl-coenzyme A reductase and a cholesterol-lowering agent. Proc. Natl. Acad. Sci. U.S.A., 77:3957–3961, 1980.

Altschul, R.: Influence of nicotinic acid (niacin) on hypercholesterolemia and hyperlipemia and on the course of atherosclerosis. In, Niacin in Vascular Disorders and Hyperlipemia (Altschul, R., ed.). Charles C Thomas, Springfield, Ill., pp. 3–135, 1964.

Altschul, R.; Hoffer, A.; and Stephen, J. D.: Influence of nicotinic acid on serum cholesterol in man. Arch. Biochem. Biophys., 54:558–559, 1955.

Austin, M. A.: Plasma triglyceride as a risk factor for coronary heart disease: The epidemiologic evidence and beyond. Am. J. Epidemiol., 129:249–259, 1989.

Avigan, J.; and Steinberg, D.: Deposition of desmosterol in the lesions of experimental atherosclerosis. Lancet, 1:572, 1962.

Avigan, J.; Steinberg, D.; Vroman, H. E.; Thompson, M. J.; and Mosettig, E.: Studies of cholesterol biosynthesis: I. The identification of demosterol in serum and tissues of animals and man treated with MER-29. J. Biol. Chem., 235:3123–3126, 1960.

Babirak, S. P.; Iverius, P.-H.; Fujimoto, W. Y.; and Brunzell, J. D.: The detection and characterization of the heterozygote state for lipoprotein lipase deficiency. Arteriosclerosis, 9: 326–334, 1989.

Barnhart, J. W.; Sefranka, J. A.; and McIntosh, D. D.: Hypocholesterolemic effect of 4,4′-(isopropylidenedithio)-bis (2,6-di-t-butylphenol) (probucol). Am. J. Clin. Nutr., 23:1229–1233, 1970.

Barrett-Conner, E.; Suzrez, L.; Khaw, K.; Criqui, M. H.; and Wingard, D. L.: Ischemic heart disease risk factors after age 50. J. Chronic Dis., 37:903–908, 1984.

Bell, L. P.; Hectorne, K.; Reynolds, H.; Balm, T. K.; and Hunninghake, D. B.: Cholesterol-lowering effects of psyllium hydrophilic mucilloid. Adjunct to a prudent diet for patients with mild to moderate hypercholesterolemia. J.A.M.A., 261:3419–3423, 1989.

Bhattacharyya, A. K.; and Conner, W. E.: β-Sitosterolemia and xanthomatosis. A newly described lipid storage disease in two sisters. J. Clin. Invest., 53:1033–1043, 1974.

Bicknell, F.; and Prescott, F.: Nicotinic acid. In, The Vitamins in Medicine. Grune & Stratton, New York, pp. 333–389, 1953.

Bilheimer, D. W.: Lipoprotein fractions and receptors: A role for probucol? Am. J. Cardiol., 57:7H–15H, 1986.

Bilheimer, D. W.; Grundy, S. M.; Brown, M. S.; and Goldstein, J. L.: Mevinolin and colestipol stimulate receptor-mediated clearance of low density lipoprotein from plasma in familial hypercholesterolemia heterozygotes. Proc. Natl. Acad. Sci. U.S.A., 80:124–128, 1983.

Blankenhorn, D. H.; Nessim, S. A.; Johnson, R. L.; Sanmarco, M. D.; Azen, S. P.; and Cashin-Hemphill, L.: Beneficial effects of combined colestipol-niacin therapy on coronary atherosclerosis and coronary venous bypass grafts. J.A.M.A., 257:3233–3240, 1987.

Blohm, T. R.; and MacKenzie, R. D.: Specific inhibition of cholesterol biosynthesis by a synthetic compound (MER-29). Arch. Biochem. Biophys., 85:245–249, 1959.

Bottiger, L.-E.; and Carlson, L. A.: Risk factors for ischaemic vascular death for men in the Stockholm prospective study. Atherosclerosis, 36:389–408, 1980.

Brensike, J. F.; Levy, R. I.; Kelsey, S. F.; Passamani, E. R.; Richardson, J. M.; Loh, I. K.; Stone, N. J.; Aldrich, R. F.; Battaglini, J. W.; Moriarty, D. J.; Fisher, M. R.; Friedman, L.; Friedewald, W.; Detre, K. M.; and Epstein, S. E.: Effects of therapy with cholestyramine on progression of coronary arteriosclerosis: Results of the NHLBI type II coronary intervention study. Circulation, 69:313–324, 1984.

Brewer, B. H. Jr.; Zech, L. A.; Gregg, R. E.; Schwartz, D.; and Schaeffer, E. J.: Type III hyperlipoproteinemia: Diagnosis, molecular defects, pathology, and treatment. Ann. Intern. Med., 98:623–640, 1983.

Brown, M. S.; and Goldstein, J. L.: Lipoprotein receptors in the liver: Control signals for plasma cholesterol traffic. J. Clin. Invest., 72:743–747, 1983.

Brown, M. S.; and Goldstein, J. L.: Multivalent feedback regulation of HMG CoA reductase, a control mechanism coordinating isoprenoid synthesis and cell growth. J. Lipid Res., 21:505–517, 1980.

Brown, M. S.; Faust, J. R.; Goldstein, J. L.; Kaneko, I.; and Endo, A.: Induction of 3-hydroxy-3-methylglutaryl coenzyme A reductase activity in human fibroblasts incubated with compactin (ML-236B), a competitive inhibitor of the reductase. J. Biol. Chem., 253:1121–1128, 1978.

Brown, A. G.; Smale, T. C.; King, T. J.; Hasenkamp, R.; and Thompson, R. H.: Crystal and molecular structure of compactin, a new antifungal metabolite from Penicillium brevicompactum. J. Chem. Soc. Perkin., 1:1165–1170, 1976.

Brunzell, J. D.: Familial lipoprotein lipase deficiency and other causes of the chylomicronemic syndrome. In, The Metabolic Basis of Inherited Disease, 6th ed. (Scriver, C. R.; Beaudet, A. L.; Sly, W. S.; Valle, D.; eds.). McGraw-Hill, New York, pp. 1165–1180, 1989.

Canner, P. L.; Berge, K. G.; Wenger, N. K.; Stamler, J.; Freidman, L.; Prineas, R. J.; Friedewald, W.; for the Coronary Drug Project Research Group: Fifteen year mortality in Coronary Drug Project patients: Long-term benefit with niacin. J. Am. Coll. Cardiol., 8:1245–1255, 1986.

Carew, T. E.; Schwenke, D. C.; and Steinberg, D.: Antiatherogenic effect of probucol unrelated to its hypocholesterolemic effect: Evidence that antioxidants in vivo can selectively inhibit low density lipoprotein degradation in macrophage-rich fatty streaks and slow the progression of atherosclerosis in the Watanabe heritable hyperlipidemic rabbit. Proc. Natl. Acad. Sci. U.S.A., 84:7725–7729, 1987.

Carlson, L. A.; and Oro, L.: The effect of nicotinic acid on plasma free fatty acids. Demonstration of a metabolic type of synapthicolysis. Acta Med. Scand., 172:641–645, 1962.

Carlson, L. A.; and Rosenhamer, G.: Reduction of mortality in the Stockholm Ischaemic Heart Disease Secondary Prevention Study by combined treatment with clofibrate and nicotinic acid. Acta Med. Scand., 223:405–418, 1988.

Cashin-Hemphill, L.; Spencer, C. A.; Nicoloff, J. T.; Blankenhorn, D. H.; Nessim, S. A.; Chin, H. P.; and Lee, N. A.: Alterations in serum thyroid hormonal indices with colestipol-niacin therapy. Ann. Intern. Med., 107:324–329, 1987.

Chait, A.; Bierman, E. L.; and Albers, J. J.: Regulatory role of triiodothyronine in the degradation of low density lipoprotein by cultured human skin fibroblasts. J. Clin. Endocrinol. Metab., 48:887–889, 1979.

Committee of Principal Investigators: WHO cooperative trial on primary prevention of ischaemic heart disease with clofibrate to lower serum cholesterol: Final mortality follow-up. Lancet, 2:600–604, 1984.

Committee of Principal Investigators: A co-operative trial in the primary prevention of ischaemic heart disease using clofibrate. Br. Heart J., 40:1069–1118, 1978.

Connor, W. E.; and Connor, S. L.: Dietary treatment of familial hypercholesterolemia. Arteriosclerosis, 9(suppl. 1):I.91–I.105, 1989.

Consensus Conference: The treatment of hypertriglyceridemia. J.A.M.A., 251:1196–1200, 1984.

The Coronary Drug Project Research Group: Gallbladder disease as a side effect of drugs influencing lipid metabolism. Experience in the Coronary Drug Project. N. Engl. J. Med., 296:1185–1190, 1977.

The Coronary Drug Project Research Group: Clofibrate and niacin in coronary heart disease. J.A.M.A., 231:360–381, 1975.

The Coronary Drug Project Research Group: The Coronary Drug Project. Findings leading to further modifications of its protocol with respect to dextrothyroxine. J.A.M.A., 220: 996–1008, 1972.

Davignon, J.: Medical management of hyperlipidemia and the role of probucol. Am. J. Cardiol., 57:22H–28H, 1986.

Davignon, J.; Gregg, R. E.; and Sing, C. F.: Apolipoprotein E polymorphism and atherosclerosis. Arteriosclerosis, 8:1–21, 1988.

Denke, M. A.; and Grundy, S. M.: Hypercholesterolemia in elderly persons: Resolving the treatment dilemma. Ann. Intern. Med., 112:779–791, 1990.

Dujovne, C. A.; Krehbiel, P.; Decoursey, S.; Jackson, B.; Chernoff, S. B.; Pitterman, A.; and Garty, M.: Probucol with colestipol in the treatment of hypercholesterolemia. Ann. Intern. Med., 10:477–482, 1984.

Durrington, P. N.; and Miller, J. P.: Double-blind, placebo-controlled, cross-over trial of probucol in heterozygous familial hypercholesterolaemia. Atherosclerosis, 55:187–194, 1985.

East, C.; Bilheimer, D. W.; and Grundy, S. M.: Combination

therapy for familial combined hyperlipidemia. Ann. Intern. Med., 109:25–32, 1988.

Eisenberg, S.; Gavish, D.; Oschry, Y.; Fairaw, M.; and Deckelbaum, R. G.: Abnormalities in very low, low, and high density lipoproteins in hypertriglyceridemia. Reversal toward normal with bezafibrate treatment. J. Clin. Invest., 74:470–482, 1984.

Endo, A.: Monakolin K, a new hypocholesterolemic agent produced by a monascus species. J. Antibiot., 32:852–854, 1979.

Endo, A.; Kurdo, M.; and Tanzawa K.: Competitive inhibition of 3-hydroxy-3-methylglutaryl coenzyme A reductase by ML-236A and ML-236B, fungal metabolites having hypocholesterolemic activity. FEBS Lett., 72:323–326, 1976a.

Endo, A.; Kuroda, M.; and Tsujita, Y.: ML-236A, ML-236B, and ML-236C, new inhibitors of cholesterogenesis produced by *Penicillium citrinum*. J. Antibiot., 29:1346–1348, 1976b.

The Expert Panel: Report of the National Cholesterol Education Program expert panel on detection, evaluation, and treatment of high blood cholesterol in adults. Arch. Intern. Med., 148:36–69, 1988.

Fellin, R.; Gasparotto, A.; Valerio, G.; Baiocchi, M. R.; Padrini, R.; Lamon, S.; Vitale, E.; Baggio, G.; and Crepaldi, G.: Effect of probucol treatment on lipoprotein cholesterol and drug levels in blood and lipoproteins in familial hypercholesterolemia. Atherosclerosis, 59:47–56, 1986.

Fontbonne, A.; Eschwege, E.; Cambien, F.; Richard, J.-L.; Ducimetiere, P.; Thibult, N.; Warnet, J.-M.; Claude, J.-R.; and Rosselin, G. E.: Hypertriglyceridaemia as a risk factor of coronary heart disease mortality in subjects with impaired glucose tolerance or diabetes. Diabetologia, 32:300–304, 1989.

Fredrickson, D. S.; Levy, R. I.; and Lees, R. S.: Fat transport in lipoproteins: An integrated approach to mechanism and disorders. N. Engl. J. Med., 27:34–43, 94–103, 148–156, 215–224, 273–281, 1967.

Frick, M. H.; Elo, O.; Haapa, K.; Heinonen, O. P.; Heinsalmi, P.; Helo, P.; Huttunen, J. K.; Kaitaniemi, P.; Manninen, V.; Maenpaa, H.; Malkonen, M.; Manttari, M.; Norola, S.; Pasternack, A.; Pikkarainen, J.; Romo, M.; Sjoblom, T.; and Nikkila, E. A.: Helsinki Heart Study: Primary prevention trial with gemfibrozil in middle-aged men with dyslipidemia. Safety of treatment, changes in risk factors, and incidence of coronary heart disease. N. Engl. J. Med., 317:1237–1245, 1987.

Friedewald, W. T.; Levy, R. I.; and Fredrickson, D. S.: Estimation of the concentration of low density lipoprotein cholesterol in plasma, without use of the preparative ultracentrifuge. Clin. Chem., 18:499–502, 1972.

Garg, A.; and Grundy, S. M.: Management of dyslipidemia in NIDDM. Diabetes Care, 13:153–169, 1990.

Garg, A.; and Grundy, S. M.: Gemfibrozil alone and in combination with lovastatin for treatment of hypertriglyceridemia in NIDDM. Diabetes, 38:364–372, 1989.

Garg, A.; and Grundy, S. M.: Lovastatin for lowering cholesterol levels in non-insulin-dependent diabetes mellitus. N. Engl. J. Med., 318:81–86, 1988.

Ginsberg, H. N.; Le, N.-A.; Short, M. P.; Ramakrishnan, R.; and Desnick, R. J.: Suppression of apolipoprotein B production during treatment of cholesteryl storage disease with lovastatin: Implications for regulation of apolipoprotein B synthesis. J. Clin. Invest., 80:1692–6297, 1987.

Glueck, C. J.; Fallat, R. W.; Millett, F.; Gartside, P.; Elston, R. C.; and Go, R. C. P.: Familial hyper-alpha-lipoproteinemia: Studies in eighteen kindreds. Metabolism, 24:1243–1265, 1975.

Goldstein, J. L.; and Brown, M. S.: Familial hypercholesterolemia. In, The Metabolic Basis of Inherited Disease, 5th ed. (Stanbury, J. B.; Wyngaarden, J. B.; Fredrickson, D. S.; Goldstein, J. L.; and Brown, M. S., eds.). New York, McGraw-Hill, pp. 672–712, 1983.

Goldstein, J. L.; Schrott, H. G.; Hazzard, W. R.; Bierman, E. L.; and Motulsky, A. G.: Hyperlipidemia in coronary heart disease: II. Genetic analysis of lipid levels in 176 families and delineation of a new inherited disorder, combined hyperlipidemia. J. Clin. Invest., 52:1544–1568, 1973.

Groggel, G. C.; Cheung, A. K.; Ellis-Benigni, K.; and Wilson, D. E.: Treatment of nephrotic hyperlipoproteinemia with gemfibrozil. Kidney Int., 36:266–271, 1989.

Grundy, S. M.: HMG-CoA reductase inhibitors for treatment of hypercholesterolemia. N. Engl. J. Med., 319:24–33, 1988.

Grundy, S. M.: Dietary treatment of hyperlipidemia. In, Hypercholesterolemia and Atherosclerosis (Steinberg, D.; and Olefsky, J. M., eds.). Churchill Livingstone, New York, pp. 169–193, 1987.

Grundy, S. M.; and Bilheimer, D. W.: Inhibition of 3-hydroxy-3-methylglutaryl-CoA reductase by mevinolin in familial hypercholesterolemia heterozygotes: Effects on cholesterol balance. Proc. Natl. Acad. Sci. U.S.A., 81:2538–2542, 1984.

Grundy, S. M.; and Vega, G. L.: Fibric acids: Effects on lipids and lipoproteins. Am. J. Med., 83(suppl. 5B):9–20, 1987.

Grundy, S. M.; and Vega, G. L.: Influence of mevinolin on metabolism of low density lipoproteins in primary moderate hypercholesterolemia. J. Lipid Res., 26:1464–1475, 1985.

Grundy, S. M.; Chait, A.; and Brunzell, J. D.: Familial Combined Hyperlipidemia Workshop. Arteriosclerosis, 7:203–207, 1987.

Grundy, S. M.; Mok, H. Y. I.; Zech, L.; and Berman, M.: Influence of nicotinic acid on metabolism of cholesterol and triglycerides in man. J. Lipid Res., 22:24–36, 1981.

Grundy, S. M.; Ahrens, E. H. Jr.; Salen, G.; Schriebman, P. H.; and Nestel, P. J.: Mechanisms of action of clofibrate on cholesterol metabolism in patients with hyperlipemia. J. Lipid Res., 13:531–551, 1972.

Gurakar, A.; Hoeg, J. M.; Kostner, G.; Papadopoulos, N. M.; and Brewer, H. B. Jr.: Levels of lipoprotein Lp(a) decline with neomycin and niacin treatment. Atherosclerosis, 57:293–301, 1985.

Harris, T.; Cook, E. F.; Kannel, W. B.; and Goldman, L.: Proportional hazards analysis of risk factors for coronary heart disease in individuals aged 65 or older. The Framingham Heart Study. J. Am. Geriatr. Soc., 36:1023–1028, 1988.

Heel, R. C.; Brogden, R. N.; Pakes, G. E.; Speight, T. M.; and Avery, G. S.: Colestipol: A review of its pharmacological properties and therapeutic efficacy in patients with hypercholesterolaemia. Drugs, 19:161–180, 1980.

Heel, R. C.; Brogden, R. N.; Speight, T. M.; and Avery, G. S.: Probucol: A review of its pharmacological properties and therapeutic use in patients with hypercholesterolaemia. Drugs, 15:409–428, 1978.

Herz, J.; Hamann, U.; Rogne, S.; Myklebost, O.; Gausepohl, H.; and Stanley, K. K.: Surface location and high affinity for calcium of a 500-kd liver membrane protein closely related to the LDL-receptor suggest a physiological role as lipoprotein receptor. Eur. Mol. Biol. Lab., 7:4119–4127, 1988.

Hotz, W.: Nicotinic acid and its derivatives: A short survey. Adv. Lipid Res., 20:195–217, 1983.

Hulley, S. B.; Rosenman, R. H.; Bawol, R. D.; and Brand, R. J.: Epidemiology as a guide to clinical decisions. The association between triglyceride and coronary heart disease. N. Engl. J. Med., 302:1383–1389, 1980.

Hunninghake, D. B.; and Peters, J. R.: Effect of fibric acid derivatives on blood lipid and lipoprotein levels. Am. J. Med., 83(suppl. 5B):44–49, 1987.

Illingworth, D. R.; and Bacon, S.: Treatment of heterozygous familial hypercholesterolemia with lipid-lowering drugs. Arteriosclerosis, 9(suppl. I):I.121–I.134, 1989.

Innerarity, T. L.; Weisgraber, K. H.; Arnold, K. S.; Mahley, R. W.; Krauss, R. M.; Vega, G. L.; and Grundy, S. M.: Familial defective apolipoprotein B-100: Low density lipoproteins with abnormal receptor binding. Proc. Natl. Acad. Sci. U.S.A., 84:6919–6923, 1987.

Jackson, R. L.; Morrisett, J. D.; and Gotto, A. M. Jr.: Lipoprotein structure and metabolism. Physiol. Rev., 56:259–316, 1976.

Kane, J. P.; Malloy, M. J.; Tun, P.; Phillips, N. R.; Freedman, D. D.; Williams, M. L.; Rowe, J. S.; and Havel, R. J.: Normalization of low-density-lipoprotein levels in heterozygous familial hypercholesterolemia with a combined drug regimen. N. Engl. J. Med., 304:251–258, 1981.

Kannel, W. B.; Castelli, W.; Gordon, T.; and McNamara, P. M.: Serum cholesterol, lipoproteins, and risk of coronary heart disease: The Framingham Study. Ann. Intern. Med., 74:1–12, 1971.

Kesaniemi, Y. A.; and Grundy, S. M.: Influence of gemfibrozil on metabolism of cholesterol and plasma triglycerides in man. J.A.M.A., 251:2241–2246, 1984.

Kesaniemi, Y. A.; and Grundy, S. M.: Increased low density lipoprotein production associated with obesity. Arteriosclerosis, 3:170–177, 1983.

Kirby, T. J.: Cataracts produced by triparanol (MER/29). Trans. Am. Ophthalmol. Soc., 65:493–543, 1967.

Kissebah, A. H.; Alfarsi, A.; and Adams, P. W.: Integrated regulations of very low density lipoprotein triglyceride and apolipoprotein B kinetics in man: Normolipemic subjects, familial hypertriglyceridemia and familial combined hyperlipidemia. Metabolism, 30:856–868, 1981.

Kissebah, A. H.; Adams, P. W.; Harrigan, P.; and Wynn, V.: The mechanism of clofibrate and tetranicotinyl fructose (Bradilan) on the kinetics of plasma free fatty acids and triglyceride transport in type IV and type V hypertriglyceridemia. Eur. J. Clin. Invest., 4:163–174, 1974.

Kita, T.; Nagano, Y.; Ishii, K.; Kume, N.; Ooshima, A.; Yoshida, H.; and Kawai, C.: Probucol prevents the progression of atherosclerosis in Watanabe heritable hyperlipidemic rabbit, an animal model for familial hypercholesterolemia. Proc. Natl. Acad. Sci. U.S.A., 84:5928–5931, 1987.

Knopp, R. H.; Ginsberg, J.; Albers, J. J.; Hoff, C.; Ogilvie, J. T.; Warnick, R.; Burrows, E.; Retzlaff, B.; and Poole, M.: Contrasting effects of unmodified and time-release forms of niacin on lipoproteins in hyperlipidemic subjects: Clues to mechanism of action of niacin. Metabolism, 34:642–650, 1985.

Kobayashi, M.; Shigeta, Y.; Hirata, Y.; Omori, Y.; Sakaota, N.; Namby, S.; and Baba, S.: Improvement of glucose tolerance in NIDDM by clofibrate: Randomized double-blind study. Diabetes Care, 11:495–499, 1988.

Kohn, R. M.; and Montes, M.: Hepatic fibrosis following long acting nicotinic acid therapy: A case report. Am. J. Med. Sci., 258:94–99, 1969.

Kostner, G. M.; Gavish, D.; Leopold, B.; Bolzano, K.; Weintraub, M. S.; and Breslow, J. L.: HMG CoA reductase inhibitors lower LDL cholesterol without reducing Lp(a) levels. Circulation, 80:1313–1319, 1989.

Kuusisto, P.; Heikki, V.; Manninen, V.; Huttunen, J. K.; and Huttunen, P. J.: Effect of activated charcoal on hypercholesterolaemia. Lancet, 2:366–367, 1986.

Laughlin, R. C.; and Carey, T. F.: Cataracts in patients treated with triparanol. J.A.M.A., 181:339–340, 1962.

Leeson, P. D.; Emmett, J. C.; Shah, V. P.; Showell, G. A.; Novelli, R.; Prain, H. D.; Benson, M. G.; Ellis, D.; Pearce, N. J.; and Underwood, A. H.: Selective thyromimetics. Cardiac-sparing thyroid hormone analogues containing 3′-arylmethyl substituents. J. Med. Chem., 32:320–336, 1989.

Levy, R. I.; and Langer, T.: Hypolipidemic drugs and lipoprotein metabolism. Adv. Exp. Med. Biol., 27:155–163, 1972.

Levy, R. I.; Brensike, J. F.; Epstein, S. E.; Kelsey, S. F.; Passamani, E. R.; Richardson, J. M.; Loh, I. K.; Stone, N. J.; Aldrich, R. F.; Battaglini, J. W.; Moriarty, D. J.; Fisher, M. L.; Freidman, L.; Friedewald, W.; and Detre, K. M.: The influence of changes in lipid values induced by cholestyramine and diet on progression of coronary artery disease: Results of the NHLBI type II coronary intervention study. Circulation, 69:325–337, 1984.

Levy, R. I.; Fredrickson, D. S.; Shulman, R.; Bilheimer, D. W.; Breslow, J. L.; Stone, N. J.; Lux, S. E.; Sloan, H. R.; Krauss, R. M.; and Herbert, P. N.: Dietary and drug treatment of primary hyperlipoproteinemia. Ann. Intern. Med., 77:267–294, 1972.

Lipid Research Clinics Program: The Lipid Research Clinics Coronary Primary Prevention Trial results: I. Reduction in incidence of coronary heart disease. J.A.M.A., 251:351–364, 1984a.

Lipid Research Clinics Program: The Lipid Research Clinics Coronary Primary Prevention Trial results: II. The relationship of reduction in incidence of coronary heart disease to cholesterol lowering. J.A.M.A., 251:365–374, 1984b.

Ma, P. T. S.; Gil, G.; Sudhof, T. C.; Bilheimer, D. W.; Goldstein, J. L.; and Brown, M. S.: Mevinolin, an inhibitor of cholesterol synthesis, induces mRNA for low density lipoprotein receptor in livers of hamsters and rabbits. Proc. Natl. Acad. Sci. U.S.A., 83:8370–8374, 1986.

MacDonald, J. S.; Gerson, R. J.; Kornbrust, D. J.; Kloss, M. W.; Prahalada, S.; Berry, P. H.; Alberts, A. W.; and Bokelman, D. L.: Preclinical evaluation of lovastatin. Am. J. Cardiol., 62:16J–27J, 1988.

Mahley, R. W.: Atherogenic hyperlipoproteinemia. The cellular and molecular biology of plasma lipoproteins altered by dietary fat and cholesterol. Med. Clin. North Am., 66:375–402, 1982.

Mahley, R. W.; Innerarity, T. L.; Rall, S. C. Jr.; and Weisgraber, K. H.: Plasma lipoproteins: Apolipoprotein structure and function. J. Lipid Res., 25:1277–1294, 1984.

Malloy, M. J.; Kane, J. P.; Kunitake, S. T.; and Tun, P.: Complimentarity of colestipol, niacin, and lovastatin in treatment of severe familial hypercholesterolemia. Ann. Intern. Med., 107:616–623, 1987.

Manninen, V.; Elo, O.; Frick, H.; Haapa, K.; Heinonen, O. P.; Heinsalmi, P.; Helo, P.; Huttenen, J. K.; Kaitaniemi, P.; Koskinen, P.; Maenpaa, H.; Malkonen, M.; Manttari, M.; Norola, S.; Pasternack, A.; Pikkarainen, J.; Romo, M.; Sjoblom, T.; and Nikkila, E. A.: Lipid alterations and decline in the incidence of coronary heart disease in the Helsinki Heart Study. J.A.M.A., 260:641–651, 1988.

Martin, M. J.; Hulley, S. B.; Browner, W. S.; Kuller, L. H.; and Wentworth, D.: Serum cholesterol, blood pressure, and mortality: Implications from a cohort of 361,662 men. Lancet, 2:933–936, 1986.

Miettinen, T. A.: Effect of nicotinic acid on catabolism and synthesis of cholesterol in man. Clin. Chim. Acta, 20:43–51, 1968.

Morrisett, J. D.; Guyton, J. R.; Gaubatz, J. W.; and Gotto, A. M. Jr.: Lipoprotein (a): Structure, metabolism and epidemiology. In, Plasma Lipoproteins (Gotto, A. M. Jr., ed.). Elsevier Science, Amsterdam, pp. 129–152, 1987.

Nakamura, C. E.; and Abeles, R. H.: Mode of interaction of β-hydroxy-β-methylglutaryl coenzyme A reductase with strong binding inhibitors: Compactin and related compounds. Biochemistry, 24:1364–1376, 1985.

Neuvonen, P. J.; Kuusisto, P.; Manninen, V.; Vapaatalo, H.; and Miettinen, T. A.: The mechanism of the hypocholesterolaemic effect of activated charcoal. Eur. J. Clin. Invest., 19:251–254, 1989.

Nikkila, E. A.; Huttunen, J. K.; and Ehnholm, C.: Effect of clofibrate on postheparin plasma triglyceride lipase activities in patients with hypertriglyceridemia. Metabolism, 26:179–186, 1977.

Okerholm, R. A.; Keeley, F. J.; Peterson, F. E.; and Glazko, A. J.: The metabolism of gemfibrozil. Proc. R. Soc. Med., 69(suppl. 2):11–14, 1976.

Olefsky, J. O.; Farquhar, J. W.; and Reaven, G. M.: Reappraisal of the role of insulin in hypertriglyceridemia. Am. J. Med., 57:551–560, 1974.

Packard, C. J.; and Shepherd, J.: The hepatobiliary axis and lipoprotein metabolism: Effects of bile acid sequestrants and ileal bypass surgery. J. Lipid Res., 23:1081–1098, 1982.

Palmer, R. H.: Effects of fibric acid derivatives on biliary lipid composition. Am. J. Med., 83(suppl. 5B):37–43, 1987.

Pappu, S. D.; Illingworth D. R.; and Bacon, S.: Reduction in plasma low-density lipoprotein cholesterol and urinary mevalonic acid by lovastatin in patients with heterozygous familial hypercholesterolemia. Metabolism, 38:542–549, 1989.

Parker, T. S.; McNamara, D. J.; Brown, C. D.; Kolb, R.;

Ahrens, E. H.; Alberts, A. W.; Tobert, J.; Chen, J.; and DeSchepper, P. J.: Plasma mevalonate as a measure of cholesterol synthesis in man. J. Clin. Invest., 74:795–804, 1984.

Parkinson, T. M.; Gundersen, K.; and Nelson, N. A.: Effects of colestipol (U-26,597A), a new bile acid sequestrant, on serum lipids in experimental animals and man. Atherosclerosis, 11:531–537, 1970.

Parthasarathy, S.; Young, S. G.; Witztum, J. L.; Pittman, R. C.; and Steinberg, D.: Probucol inhibits oxidative modification of low density lipoprotein. J. Clin. Invest., 77:641–644, 1986.

Phillips, N. R.; Havel, R. J.; and Kane, J. P.: Levels and interrelationships of serum and lipoprotein cholesterol and triglycerides. Association with adiposity and the consumption of ethanol, tobacco, and beverages containing caffeine. Arteriosclerosis, 1:13–24, 1981.

Rall, S. C.; Welsgraber, K. H.; Innerarity, T. L.; and Mahley, R. W.: Identical structural and receptor binding defects in apolipoprotein E2 in hypo-, normo- and hypercholesterolemic dysbetalipoproteinemia. J. Clin. Invest., 71:1023–1031, 1983.

Reaven, G. M.: Role of insulin resistance in human disease. Diabetes, 37:1595–1607, 1988.

Rodney, G.; Uhlendorf, P.; and Maxwell, R. E.: The hypolipidaemic effect of gemfibrozil (CI-719) in laboratory animals. Proc. R. Soc. Med., 69(suppl. 2):6–10, 1976.

Rose, G.; and Shipley, M.: Plasma cholesterol concentration and death from coronary heart disease: 10 year results of the Whitehall study. Br. Med. J., 293:306–307, 1986.

Russell, D. W.; Esser, V.; and Hobbs, H. H.: Molecular basis of familial hypercholesterolemia. Arteriosclerosis, 9:8–12, 1989.

Saku, K.; Gartside, P. S.; Hynd, B. A.; and Kashyap, M. D.: Mechanism of action of gemfibrozil on lipoprotein metabolism. J. Clin. Invest., 75:1702–1712, 1985.

Salen, G.; Ahrens, E. H. Jr.; and Grundy, S. M.: Metabolism of β-sitosterol in man. J. Clin. Invest., 49:952–967, 1970.

Samuel, P.: Treatment of hypercholesterolemia with neomycin—A time for reappraisal. N. Engl. J. Med., 301:595–597, 1979.

Samuel, P.; and Steiner, A.: Effect of neomycin on serum cholesterol level in man. Proc. Soc. Exp. Biol. Med., 100:193–195, 1959.

Scanu, A. M.; and Landsberger, F. R. (eds.): Lipoprotein structure. Ann. N.Y. Acad. Sci., 348:1–434, 1980.

Schaefer, E. J.; Eisenberg, S.; and Levy, R. L.: Lipoprotein apoprotein metabolism. J. Lipid Res., 19:667–687, 1978.

Shepherd, J.; Packard, C. J.; Patsch, J.; Gotto, A. M. Jr.; and Taunton, O. D.: Effects of nicotinic acid therapy on plasma high density lipoprotein distribution and composition and on apolipoprotein A metabolism. J. Clin. Invest., 63:858–867, 1979.

Siperstein, M. D.; Nichols, C. W. Jr.; and Chaikoff, I. L.: Effects of ferric chloride and bile on plasma cholesterol and atherosclerosis in the cholesterol-fed bird. Science, 117:386–389, 1953.

Stamler, J.; Wentworth, D.; and Neaton, J.: Is the relationship between serum cholesterol and risk of death from CHD continuous or graded? J.A.M.A., 256:2823–2828, 1986.

Stein, E. A.: Treatment of familial hypercholesterolemia with drugs in children. Arteriosclerosis, 9(suppl. 1):I.145–I.151, 1989.

Steinberg, D.; Parthasarathy, S.; Carew, T. E.; Khoo, J. C.; and Witztum, J. L.: Beyond cholesterol: Modifications of low density lipoprotein that increase its atherogenicity. N. Engl. J. Med., 320:915–924, 1989.

Steinberg, D.; Avigan, J.; and Feigelson, E. B.: Effects of triparanol (MER-29) on cholesterol biosynthesis and on blood sterol levels in man. J. Clin. Invest., 40:884–893, 1961.

Steinberg, D.; Fredrickson, D. S.; and Avigan, J.: Effects of Δ⁴-cholestenone in animals and in man. Proc. Soc. Exp. Biol. Med., 97:784–790, 1958.

Stewart, J. M.; Packard, C. J.; Lorimer, A. R.; Boag, D. E.; and Shepherd, J.: Effects of bezafibrate on receptor-mediated and receptor-independent low density lipoprotein catabolism in type II hyperlipoproteinemic subjects. Atherosclerosis, 44:355–365, 1982.

Stone, B. G.; Evans, C. D.; Prigge, W. F.; Duane, W. C.; and Gebhard, R. L.: Lovastatin treatment inhibits sterol synthesis and induces HMG-CoA reductase activity in mononuclear leukocytes of normal subjects. J. Lipid Res., 30:1943–1952, 1989.

Teng, B.; Sniderman, A. D.; and Soutar, A. K.: Metabolic basis of hyperapobetalipoproteinemia: Turnover of apolipoprotein B in low density lipoprotein and its precursors and subfractions compared with normal and familial hypercholesterolemia. J. Clin. Invest., 77:663–672, 1986.

Tennent, D. M.; Siegel, H.; Zanetti, M. E.; Kuron, G. W.; Ott, W. H.; and Wolf, F. J.: Plasma lowering action of bile acid binding polymers in experimental animals. J. Lipid Res., 1:469–473, 1960.

Thompson, G. R.; Soutar, A. K.; Spengel, F. A.; Jadhav, A.; Gavingan, S. J.; and Myant, N. B.: Defects of receptor-mediated low density lipoprotein catabolism in homozygous familial hypercholesterolemia and hypothyroidism in vivo. Proc. Natl. Acad. Sci. U.S.A., 78:2592–2595, 1981.

Thorp, J. M.; and Waring, W. S.: Modification of metabolism and distribution of lipids by ethyl chlorophenoxyisobutyrate. Nature, 194:948–949, 1962.

Tobert, J. A.; Shear, C. L.; Chremos, A. N.; and Mantell, G. E.: Clinical experience with lovastatin. Am. J. Cardiol., 65:23F–26F, 1990.

Tomkins, G. M.; Sheppard, H.; and Chaikoff, I. L.: Cholesterol synthesis by liver: IV. Suppression by steroid administration. J. Biol. Chem., 203:781–786, 1953.

Underwood, A. H.; Emmett, J. C.; Ellis, D.; Flynn, S. B.; Leeson, P. D.; Benson, G. M.; Novelli, R.; Pearce, N. J.; and Shah, V. P.: A thyromimetic that decreases plasma cholesterol levels without increasing cardiac activity. Nature, 324:425–429, 1986.

Utermann, G.: The mysteries of lipoprotein (a). Science, 246:904–910, 1989.

Vega, G. L.; and Grundy, S. M.: Lovastatin therapy in nephrotic hyperlipidemia: Effects on lipoprotein metabolism. Kidney Int., 33:1160–1168, 1988.

Vega, G. L.; and Grundy, S. M.: In vivo evidence for reduced binding of low density lipoproteins to receptors as a cause of primary moderate hypercholesterolemia. J. Clin. Invest., 78:1410–1414, 1986.

Vega, G. L.; and Grundy, S. M.: Gemfibrozil therapy in primary hypertriglyceridemia associated with coronary heart disease. Effects on metabolism of low-density lipoproteins. J.A.M.A., 253:2398–2403, 1985.

Vega, G. L.; East, C.; and Grundy, S. M.: Lovastatin therapy in familial dysbetalipoproteinemia: Effects on kinetics of apolipoprotein B. Atherosclerosis, 70:131–143, 1988.

Vessby, B.; Kostner, G.; Lithell, H.; and Thomis, J.: Diverging effects of cholestyramine on apolipoprotein B and lipoprotein Lp(a): A dose-response study of the effects of cholestyramine in hypercholesterolaemia. Atherosclerosis, 44:61–71, 1982.

Vyas, K. P.; Kari, P. H.; Wang, R. W.; and Lu, A. Y. H.: Biotransformation of lovastatin: III. Effects of cimetidine and famotidine on in vitro metabolism of lovastatin by rat and human liver microsomes. Biochem. Pharmacol., 39:67–73, 1990.

Weiner, M.; and van Eys, J.: Nicotinic Acid. Nutrient-Cofactor-Drug. Marcel Dekker, New York, 1983.

Weisgraber, K. H.; Innerarity, T. L.; and Mahley, R. W.: Abnormal lipoprotein receptor–binding activity of the human apoE apoprotein due to cysteine–arginine interchange at a single site. J. Biol. Chem., 257:2518–2521, 1982.

West, K. M.; Ahuja, M. S.; Bennett, P. H.; Czyzyk, A.; de Acosta, O. M.; Fuller, J. H.; Grab, B.; Grabauskas, V.; Jarrett, J.; Kosaka, K.; Keen, H.; Krolewski, A. S.; Miki, E.; Schliack, V.; Teuscher, A.; Watkins, P. J.; and Stober, J. A.: The role of circulating glucose and triglyceride concentrations and their interactions with other "risk factors" as determinants of arterial disease in nine diabetic populations samples from the WHO multinational study. Diabetes Care, 6:361–369, 1983.

Williams, R. R.; Hunt, S. C.; Hopkins, P. N.; Stults, B. M.; Wu, L. L.; Hasstedt, S. J.; Barlow, G. K.; Stephenson, S. H.; Lalouel, J.-M.; and Kuida, H.: Familial dyslipidemic hypertension. Evidence from 58 Utah families for a syndrome present in approximately 12% of patients with essential hypertension. J.A.M.A., 256:3579–3586, 1988.

Witztum, J. L.: Current approaches to drug therapy for the hypercholesterolemic patient. Circulation, 80:1101–1114, 1989.

Witztum, J. L.; Young, S. G.; Elam, R. L.; Carew, T. E.; and Fisher, M.: Cholestyramine-induced changes in low density lipoprotein composition and metabolism: I. Studies in the guinea pig. J. Lipid Res., 26:92–103, 1985.

Yamamoto, A.; Matsuuzawa, Y.; Yokoyama, S.; Funahashi, T.; Yamamura, T.; and Bun-Ichiro, K.: Effects of probucol on xanthomata regression in familial hypercholesterolemia. Am. J. Cardiol., 27:29H–35H, 1986.

Yamamoto, A.; Sudo, H.; and Endo, A.: Therapeutic effects of ML-236B in primary hypercholesterolemia. Atherosclerosis, 35:259–266, 1980.

16

Treatment of Endocrine Disorders: Diabetes Mellitus

Fredrick L. Dunn and Diana B. McNeill

Chapter Outline

Pathophysiology and Classification of
  Diabetes
  Type I Diabetes Mellitus
  Type II Diabetes Mellitus
  Other Types of Glucose Intolerance
Treatment
  Insulin
  Glucagon
  Sulfonylureas

Biguanides
Aldose Reductase Inhibitors
Immunosuppression
Summary
Examples of Choices in Therapeutics
  Diabetic Ketoacidosis
  Nonketotic Hyperosmolar Coma
  Brittle Diabetes
  Hypoglycemia

PATHOPHYSIOLOGY AND CLASSIFICATION OF DIABETES

Diabetes mellitus is a common disease of insulin and glucose metabolism characterized by either destruction of the pancreatic islets due to an autoimmune process (Type I) or decreased insulin action combined with inadequate release of insulin from the pancreas (Type II) (Palmer and Lernmark, 1990; Khan and Porte, 1990). Patients with Type I diabetes must take exogenous insulin in order to prevent diabetic ketoacidosis and control their hyperglycemia. On the other hand, most patients with Type II diabetes can be adequately treated without exogenous insulin. Type II diabetes is characterized by insulin resistance and often occurs in obese persons. In these patients, sensitivity to endogenous insulin may be increased toward normal as they lose weight. Still some patients with Type II diabetes require either an oral hypoglycemic agent or insulin to control their hyperglycemia.

Diabetes mellitus is a major health problem in the United States and Europe. In the United States, it is estimated that diabetes affects approximately 10 to 15 million people, or >5% of the American population. Diabetes remains the leading cause of blindness and accounts for over 80% of major limb amputations performed in this country. In addition, diabetic patients are 3 to 4 times more likely to develop coronary artery disease or suffer a cerebrovascular accident as nondiabetic persons, and 17 times more likely to

develop chronic renal failure. *Principle: The therapist must distinguish between features of the disease that are modifiable by existing therapy and those that seem to be resistant to therapy in order to establish realistic goals for therapy.*

The goals of treatment in patients with diabetes are to relieve symptoms, to improve the quality of life, and to prevent ketoacidosis and hyperosmolar coma. These are easily attainable with today's therapeutics. The chronic sequelae of diabetes, including retinopathy, neuropathy, nephropathy, and premature atherosclerosis, may be much more resistant to traditional therapeutic modalities. Evidence accumulated from biochemical and animal experiments, epidemiologic surveys, and short-term prospective clinical trials suggests that chronic hyperglycemia is an important factor in the development of most of the long-term diabetic complications (Pirart, 1978; Feldt-Rasmussen et al., 1986; Raskin and Rosenstock, 1986; Rosenstock et al., 1986; Greene et al., 1987; Krolewski et al., 1987; Brownlee et al., 1988; Chase et al., 1989). Whether these long-term complications can be prevented by rigorously normalizing blood glucose metabolism is currently being investigated by a national multicenter study, the Diabetes Control and Complications Trial (The DCCT Research Group, 1986, 1987).

In 1979, the National Diabetes Data Group recommended new guidelines for the diagnosis and classification of diabetes based on the underlying pathophysiology of the disorders (National

426

Diabetes Data Group, 1979). They carefully defined the criteria for "normal" and "diabetic" glucose tolerance tests and included a third category of glucose intolerance falling between these two. This new category is called *impaired glucose tolerance*. The National Diabetes Data Group also clarified the difference between the two major types of diabetes. Previously, the two largest categories were called *juvenile-onset* and *maturity-onset* diabetes. The nomenclature was changed because the age of onset does not always identify the type of diabetes. The new categories were called *Type I*, or insulin-dependent, diabetes mellitus (IDDM) and *Type II*, or non-insulin-dependent, diabetes mellitus (NIDDM).

Type I Diabetes Mellitus

Type I diabetes, or IDDM, tends to occur in younger individuals (less than 30 years of age, but it can occur at any age) who are usually thin. These patients are deficient in their production and reserves of insulin. Insulin therapy is essential to treat their diabetes, and they will ultimately develop diabetic ketoacidosis if they are not treated.

The cause of Type I diabetes is thought to be genetically linked autoimmune destruction of the pancreas (Eisenbarth, 1986; Krolewski et al., 1987). Greater than 80% of patients who develop Type I diabetes have one or both of the HLA antigen types DR3 and DR4, whereas the prevalence of these antigens in the general population is only 40%. Although most individuals with these HLA types do not develop diabetes, inheritance of DR3 or DR4 appears to place an individual at higher risk of developing Type I diabetes.

Development of Type I diabetes is heralded and initiated by the production of antibodies against the insulin-producing β cells within the pancreatic islets. These islet cell antibodies produce an inflammation of the pancreas in the region of the β cells. The "insulitis" gradually destroys the β cells, resulting in a progressive decrease in insulin production and reserve. Antibodies against the body's own insulin (autoinsulin antibodies) also are formed during the very early stages of Type I diabetes. Finally, usually long after the destructive process starts and when less than 10% of the β cells remain, hyperglycemia and clinically noticeable symptoms of diabetes develop. Eventually, there is complete destruction of the β cells, and the patient is truly and completely insulin-deficient. These islet cell and autoinsulin antibodies are early markers of the actual presence of Type I diabetes and identify patients destined to develop Type I diabetes before they develop hyperglycemia (Ziegler et al., 1990). *Principle: When markers of a disease identify those who* *are predisposed and later those in the group who actually have early signs of the disease, they can be used to put the therapist in a position to prevent complications of the disease that previously were only the target of ameliorative therapy. In the case of Type I diabetic patients, the therapist's focus may well shift from replacing insulin to preventing the loss of insulin-producing capacity.*

Type II Diabetes Mellitus

Type II diabetes, or NIDDM, tends to occur in obese persons, although thin persons may also develop NIDDM. NIDDM is much more common than IDDM and accounts for about 85% of patients with diabetes. Unlike patients with Type I diabetes, most patients with Type II diabetes are not deficient in insulin production or reserve. They initially retain significant insulin secretory capacity in their pancreas. In general, most of these patients do not develop ketoacidosis, even through they have no access to exogenous insulin. However, during the stress of serious illness, even patients with Type II diabetes can develop ketoacidosis. Type II diabetes usually is treated with diet and/or an oral hypoglycemic agent, but some patients may require insulin to control hyperglycemia.

Because many Type II diabetic patients have "normal" or "high" concentration of insulin in their plasma, the pathogenetic concept evolved that Type II diabetes is due to resistance to insulin's effects (DeFronzo et al., 1983). This resistance to insulin has been postulated to occur at two levels: defects of the insulin receptor itself and defects distal to the insulin–receptor interaction (*post-insulin receptor*) (Olefsky et al., 1985). The insulin receptor is a heterotetrameric transmembrane glycoprotein that is present on a wide variety of cells. A number of factors can modulate insulin receptors, including insulin concentrations in the cell's environment. High concentrations of insulin in plasma down-regulate the number of insulin receptors. Diet, exercise, certain drugs (sulfonylurea, glucocorticoids, oral contraceptives), the menstrual cycle, and pregnancy all have independent effects on insulin-receptor availability (Kahn, 1980; Reddy and Kahn, 1988). The insulin resistance of obesity is associated with a decreased number of insulin receptors on peripheral cells. This is thought to be one reason why there is a high association between obesity and Type II diabetes (Bogardus et al., 1985). In general, however, NIDDM is associated with a post-receptor rather than receptor defect (Eriksson et al., 1989).

A second metabolic abnormality in Type II diabetes is relative insulin deficiency, reflecting a progressive loss of β-cell responsiveness to increased blood glucose concentrations, and eventually a progressive decrease in the functioning of the β cell (O'Rahilly et al., 1986; Temple et al., 1989). Although plasma concentrations of insulin often are normal or high in patients with early Type II diabetes, once fasting hyperglycemia develops, insulin secretion is reduced compared with that of nondiabetic persons of similar weight and with similar degrees of hyperglycemia (DeFronzo, 1988). Eventually, the peripheral resistance to insulin and chronic hyperglycemia lead to β-cell "exhaustion" and diminished insulin secretion (Leahy et al., 1986; Rossetti et al., 1987).

Other Types of Glucose Intolerance

There are three other categories of glucose intolerance. There are a number of patients with impaired glucose tolerance who are neither normal nor diabetic. This group of patients had previously been labeled chemical diabetics or prediabetics. Many of these patients have a greatly exaggerated insulin response to a glucose challenge. Despite this reactive hyperinsulinemia, postprandial glucose concentrations are higher than normal, indicating that these patients are insulin-resistant (Reaven, 1988). Yet only about 1% to 3% per year of patients with impaired glucose tolerance develop frank diabetes mellitus. In fact, one third eventually revert to a normal glucose tolerance test. If they were to have been treated, then insulin and not regression to the mean could be credited with the reversal to normality. *Principle: During treatment, the clinician is understandably tempted to attribute observed improvement to treatment and to continue that treatment, needed or not. Frequent review of the data and reconsideration of the need to treat are sensible strategies to ascertain the need to treat.* These patients rarely develop the classic microvascular complications characteristic of diabetes, but they have an increased risk of developing atherosclerosis, perhaps as a result of their chronic hyperinsulinemia. Thus, impaired glucose tolerance has been identified as an independent risk factor for coronary artery disease (Fuller et al., 1983).

An additional group of patients have hyperglycemia due to diseases other than diabetes or due to drug therapy. Diseases affecting the pancreas that can cause diabetes include pancreatectomy, chronic pancreatitis, carcinoma, cystic fibrosis, and hemochromatosis. Hyperglycemia secondary to hypersecretion of hormones that antagonize the action of insulin occurs in Cushing disease, acromegaly, pheochromocytoma, primary aldosteronism, and glucagonoma. A number of drugs also can impair glucose tolerance. The most common are glucocorticoids, thiazide diuretics, oral contraceptives, phenytoin, phenothiazines, tricyclic antidepressants and β blockers. Diabetes mellitus is also associated with several unusual genetic syndromes, such as myotonic dystrophy, leprechaunism, and lipoatrophic diabetes.

Finally, gestational diabetes is a type of diabetes that develops during pregnancy and disappears after the pregnancy. It is usually detected during the second or third trimester when insulin resistance develops secondary to high concentrations of hormones that are antagonistic to the action of insulin. Human chorionic somatomammotropin, cortisol, estrogen, and progesterone are included in that group. Many such pregnant women are genetically predisposed to develop diabetes later in life (usually Type II diabetes), and about 50% of these women will develop diabetes within 10 years of the episode experienced during pregnancy. Although gestational diabetes is usually mild, it may have significant effects on the fetus, including macrosomia, increased mortality, respiratory distress syndrome, congenital anomalies, and neonatal hypoglycemia (Landon and Gabbe, 1988). Prompt detection and treatment of gestational diabetes is important to prevent these effects on the fetus.

TREATMENT

One of the first steps in treating any patient with diabetes is to design an appropriate diet (American Diabetes Association, 1987). That recommended by the American Diabetes Association reduces the amount of saturated fat and cholesterol in the diet to reduce the risk of atherosclerosis due to hypercholesterolemia (Dunn, 1988). The diet allows an increase in the amount of complex carbohydrates and fiber. However, simple carbohydrates, such as concentrated sweets, are limited, because they increase postprandial hyperglycemia (see chapter 10).

Current dietary recommendations emphasize the different needs of patients with Type II versus Type I diabetes (Bantle, 1988). In obese patients with Type II diabetes, the primary goal is to reduce caloric intake to produce weight loss that can, in some instances, restore normoglycemia (Savage et al., 1979; Stanik and Marcus, 1980). In contrast, patients with Type I diabetes or those with insulin-requiring Type II diabetes require a more complex diet, since insulin and food intake must be balanced throughout the day. For this diet, the size, timing, composition, and spacing of meals are important. An exchange system that allows a greater number of choices of food and planned snacks that prevent hypoglycemia when long-acting insulin is peaking has been developed for these patients (Wood and Bierman, 1986).

Exercise is a useful adjunct in the treatment

program for diabetic patients (Horton, 1988). In patients with Type II diabetes, exercise can improve the body's sensitivity to insulin. In patients with insulin-requiring diabetes, exercise can have variable effects on absorption of subcutaneous insulin and requirements for glucose. The exercise should be timed in relation to meals and/or supplemental snacks to prevent hypoglycemia. In IDDM, hypoglycemia can occur several hours after finishing exercise because glucose in blood is gradually used to replenish depleted hepatic glycogen stores. Hypoglycemia may also occur unexpectedly if the insulin has been injected into a limb that is involved in vigorous exercise, since the increased blood flow to the limb may result in more rapid absorption of the insulin.

When the pancreas of patients with Type II diabetes is unable to secrete insulin in sufficient quantity to overcome the insulin resistance, an oral hypoglycemic agent may be added to a patient's regime to achieve acceptable control of blood glucose concentrations. Insulin is required for all patients with Type I (ketosis-prone) diabetes and patients with Type II diabetes whose hyperglycemia is refractory to control with diet, exercise, and oral hypoglycemic agents. Insulin is also used in patients with gestational diabetes, since sulfonylureas may produce hypoglycemia in the fetus or newborn (see chapter 29).

Insulin

Prior to the introduction of insulin therapy by Banting and Best in 1922, it was difficult even to ameliorate the symptoms of diabetes (Burrow et al., 1982). Most patients with insulin-dependent diabetes died from ketoacidosis within 6 months. Early preparations of insulin were relatively impure and short-acting. Several injections were needed each day. Advances in the purification and pharmaceutical preparations of insulin have resulted in products with improved purity, varying durations of action, and even structure similar to human insulin (Tables 16–1 and 16–2) (Skyler, 1988; Zinman, 1989). The major characteristics distinguishing insulin preparations today are the degree of purity, the concentration of the insulin,

the time course of action, and the species from which the insulin derives.

Degree of Purity. Insulin preparations have been purified from extracts of beef and pork pancreas and crystallized with zinc. Progressive improvements in the extraction procedure to remove pancreatic enzymes and other animal proteins combined with two recrystallization steps have improved the purity of commercially available preparations of insulin. The result is a "standard" insulin preparation that in the early 1970s was 92% pure and contained 8% noninsulin substances or 20,000 ppm of proinsulin (a marker of noninsulin proteins). Repeated recrystallization and the use of gel chromatography in the purification process, introduced in 1972, resulted in "single-peak" insulin that was 99% pure and contained 2000 ppm of proinsulin. In the late 1970s, the addition of molecular sieving and ion-exchange chromatography into the manufacturing process resulted in "purified" insulins that contained less than 10 ppm of proinsulin. Today, "standard" insulin contains less than 20 ppm of proinsulin and "purified" insulin preparations contain less than 1 ppm of proinsulin (Skyler, 1988). These improvements in the purity of today's insulin preparations have resulted in a reduction of many adverse effects including allergy, lipoatrophy, and immunologic-induced insulin resistance associated with the use of insulin (Kahn and Rosenthal, 1979).

Concentration. The potency of insulin is measured in units, defined by a rabbit bioassay. Since the late 1920s, insulin has been prepared in concentrations of 40 and 80 units/ml, known as U-40 and U-80 insulin. In the 1970s, U-100 insulin (100 units/ml) was introduced. Although U-100 insulin has become the standard strength used in the United States and Canada, it is still not available worldwide. Highly concentrated U-500 regular insulin (500 units/ml) is also available for special circumstances, such as antibody-mediated insulin resistance in which exceptionally high doses of insulin may be required (Nathan et al., 1981). *Principle: Bioassays of drug preparations may be variably (1) related to the pharmacologic effect sought in humans and (2) affected by impurities in the preparations. When using bioassayed preparations, be especially willing to retitrate the effect of new preparations in given patients.*

Types of Insulin. Commonly used types of insulin are classified according to their onset and length of action (Table 16–2). Rapid (regular, Semilente), intermediate (neutral protamine Hagedorn [NPH], Lente), and long-acting (Ultralente, protamine zinc insulin [PZI]) preparations are widely available. The rationale for the

Table 16–1. DIFFERENCES BETWEEN AMINO ACID SEQUENCES OF BEEF, PORK, AND HUMAN INSULINS

SPECIES	α CHAIN		β CHAIN
	α8	α10	β30
Beef	Alanine*	Valine*	Alanine*
Pork	Threonine	Isoleucine	Alanine*
Human	Threonine	Isoleucine	Threonine

* Indicates difference from human.

Table 16–2.   INSULIN PREPARATIONS

| TYPES | PREPARATIONS | ACTION (HOURS)* | | | PROTAMINE CONTENT† (MG/100 U) | ZINC CONTENT† (MG/100 U) |
		ONSET	PEAK	DURATION		
Short-Acting	Regular	0.25–1	2–4	5–8	None	0.01–0.04
	Semilente	0.5–1	4–6	8–12	None	0.12–0.25
Intermediate	NPH	2–4	6–10	12–24	0.3–0.5	0.01–0.04
	Lente	2–4	6–10	12–24	None	0.12–0.25
Long-Acting	PZI	3–4	14–20	24–36	1–1.5	0.15–0.25
	Ultralente	3–4	14–20	24–36	None	0.12–0.25

* Data from Schade et al., 1983.
† Data from Galloway and deShazo, 1990.

development of different types of insulin preparations was to create insulin with prolonged biologic activity so that once-a-day injections could be feasible. The difference in pharmacokinetics between the types is created by complexing insulin with different substances or altering the physical form of the insulin to delay its absorption and prolong its excretion, thereby prolonging the action of a single dose.

Regular or crystalline zinc insulin (CZI) is unmodified insulin. After a subcutaneous injection, the onset of hypoglycemic activity occurs within 15 to 60 minutes, peaks at 2 to 4 hours, and lasts only 5 to 8 hours. Because of regular insulin's relatively short duration of action, it must be given three to four times per day subcutaneously in order to maintain adequate insulin effects throughout the day. Regular insulin is the only type of insulin available that is in solution. It can also be given as an IV or IM injection. When given as an IV bolus, the peak insulin concentrations are seen within 2 to 4 minutes and the plasma half-life is 3 to 6 minutes. As a consequence, IV infusions must be continuous when used in the treatment of diabetic ketoacidosis, management of the acutely ill patient in an intensive care unit, or during surgery or labor and delivery.

Protamine zinc insulin (PZI) was introduced in 1936 and was the first stable preparation of insulin with prolonged action. Its duration of action is 48 to 72 hours. Because of an excess of protamine in the preparation, it cannot be mixed with regular insulin, as mixing converts regular insulin into PZI. Although still available, it is no longer widely used.

Neutral protamine Hagedorn (NPH) insulin became available in the late 1940s. This preparation mixes insulin and protamine in an equal ratio at neutral pH with a small amount of zinc and phenol. The NPH insulin's action peaks in 8 to 12 hours and persists for 18 to 24 hours. In the United States, NPH is the most widely used insulin.

Insulin zinc suspensions (*Lente* insulins) were

introduced in the early 1950s. These preparations do not use modifying proteins but complex the insulin with zinc in acetate buffer at physiologic pH. There are two physical forms of this series, crystalline (UltraLente) and amorphous (Semi-Lente), which are mixed together to form Lente insulin. The time course of action of Lente insulin is similar to that of NPH. Ultralente is similar to PZI. Semilente is intermediate in effect between regular and NPH.

Species of Origin. Until recently, commercially available insulin preparations were obtained exclusively from either beef or pork pancreas. Most commercially available "standard" preparations are either mixtures of beef and pork insulins or beef monospecies. So-called purified preparations are pork or sometimes beef monospecies. With the development of recombinant DNA technology, human insulin became widely available, and it is gradually replacing the use of animal insulins (Brogden and Heel, 1987).

Insulin is synthesized in the β cells of the pancreas from a single precursor polypeptide, called proinsulin. The connecting (C-) peptide is enzymatically cleaved from proinsulin within the β cells, resulting in the production of mature insulin. Insulin consists of two amino acid chains, a 21–amino acid α chain and 30–amino acid β chain. These chains are connected by two disulfide bridges; there is a third disulfide bridge within the α chain. The amino acid composition of the two chains is relatively similar across mammalian species. The sequence of pork insulin differs by only one amino acid (amino acid 30 on the β chain) from human insulin, and beef insulin differs by three amino acids from human insulin (Table 16–1). The greater similarity between human and pork insulin probably explains why pork insulin may be less antigenic than beef insulin.

Human insulin is manufactured by two different methods: by enzymatic conversion of pork insulin (semisynthetic); or by recombinant DNA technology (biosynthetic). Novolin (Novo-Nordisk) is pork insulin that has the β30-position alanine enzymatically cleaved and replaced with threonine (Karam and Etzwiler, 1983). Humulin (Eli Lilly) is manufactured by recombinant DNA technology: a human proinsulin gene is inserted into bacteria, proinsulin is produced and isolated, and human insulin is formed from the cleavage products (Skyler, 1982). Since recombinant DNA production requires no animal source of insulin, it provides a potentially unlimited supply of insulin.

The main advantage of human insulin is that it is substantially less antigenic than beef or pork insulin, and slightly less antigenic than "purified" pork preparations. The use of human insulin results in lower titers of insulin antibodies than when animal insulins are used. Insulin-binding antibodies can alter the pharmacokinetics of insulin. The peak activity of the insulin may be delayed, and its clearance from the circulation may be prolonged (Van Heaften et al., 1987). These factors can contribute to an increased risk of hypoglycemia and impairment in recovery from the hypoglycemia (Bolli et al., 1984). Insulin antibodies also cross the placenta (Leiper et al., 1986). Use of human insulin during pregnancy decreases the likelihood of transfer of antibody-bound insulin from the mother to the fetus, thereby decreasing the risk of fetal macrosomia (Menon et al., 1990). There is no evidence, however, that insulin antibodies are related to long-term microvascular complications of diabetes. *Principle: When factors other than the direct response to a drug alter requirements for the drug, the clinician must determine the mechanism of altered response in order to readjust dosage adequately and at appropriate intervals.*

Another advantage of human insulin is that it is absorbed more quickly after subcutaneous injection than pork insulin. Therefore, it may have enhanced value in improving glycemic control after meals (Gulan et al., 1987). The more rapid absorption probably also accounts for human NPH insulin's shorter duration of action, compared with NPH insulins made from other animal sources. The mechanism of more rapid absorption of human insulin is thought to be related to increased solubility, which is caused by loss of a hydroxyl group when the alanine is replaced with threonine at position B30. The enhanced absorption from the subcutaneous site may have some disadvantages. Switching patients from animal to human insulin may result in faster-than-expected development of hypoglycemia. If the drop in glucose concentration is fast enough, early warning symptoms of low blood glucose concentrations may be masked (Berger et al., 1989).

There are several other reasons for preferring the use of human insulin over other animal insulins. Human insulin should be less allergenic, and

fewer skin allergies and instances of immunologic resistance to insulin should result. To take advantage of this property, human insulin should be started in patients who need insulin for the first time. For patients requiring temporary insulin therapy, such as during gestational diabetes or in patients with Type II diabetes undergoing surgery, human insulin is the preparation of choice because starting and stopping insulin increases its antigenic potential. Another preferred indication for the use of human insulin is during intensive insulin therapy, because human insulin is more rapidly absorbed after subcutaneous injection than insulins from other animals, and this factor improves control of postprandial hyperglycemia. The lower titer of insulin–antibody complexes also reduces the risk of insulin-induced hypoglycemia. *Principle: There are almost always good reasons to choose between preparations of the same drug for the same indications in given patients. Often the choice relates to properties of the drug preparation that are not focused on its primary pharmacologic actions.*

Stability. Insulin is best stored in the refrigerator, but it is stable for several weeks at room temperature. It should not be exposed to extremes of temperature. With the exception of regular insulin, vials of insulin contain suspensions, not solutions. They must be mixed gently to ensure uniform distribution of the insulin. Two different types of insulin can be mixed together in the same syringe, but the stability of the mixture varies with the types of insulins used. For example, regular and NPH insulins can be mixed together in various proportions and still retain their separate action profiles. On the other hand, when regular is mixed with Lente insulin, the regular interacts with the excess zinc in the Lente, delaying the onset of the short-acting insulin.

Indications for Insulin Therapy. Insulin is required for the treatment of IDDM to prevent ketosis, maintain the patient free of symptoms, help maintain ideal body weight, and assist in the prevention of certain complications, particularly infections of the skin, vagina, and urinary tract. For example, the incidence of urinary tract infections in diabetic patients is directly related to the amount of glucose excreted in the urine per 24 hours. Similar relationships for skin and vaginal infections have been claimed. Insulin is also necessary in the control of symptoms in patients with diabetes secondary to pancreatectomy and chronic pancreatitis, and in some Type II diabetic patients who fail to respond to oral hypoglycemic therapy.

The prevention of other complications of diabetes by insulin therapy has been argued since the advent of this method of treatment. Although a number of studies have suggested that rigid control of the blood glucose concentration forestalls the onset of vascular complications, many were inadequately controlled and designed. Tight control of the diabetic pregnant woman can prevent malformations in the offspring. At the present time, there is as yet no scientifically acceptable and convincing evidence that any particular form of treatment is better than any other for the prevention of these complications. Additional controlled studies are needed to determine that the advantages of careful control outweigh its disadvantages, although evidence is slowly mounting in support of this hypothesis.

In the absence of unequivocal demonstration of superiority of a single preparation or dosage schedule for the insulins, the physician may select the drug form, degree of control, and dosage schedule felt to be optimal for the individual patient. This selection may take into consideration the patient's ability to cooperate, his or her age, and other factors outlined below.

Because insulin therapy *alone* cannot prevent the progression of atherosclerosis or other vascular complications of diabetes, realistic objectives should be set for its use. Most important, the therapist should make sure the patient avoids detrimental hypoglycemic episodes. Positive overall objectives for the use of insulin are to protect the patient from ketoacidosis and to allow him or her to live as normal a life as possible. The therapist who concentrates on narrow and precise management of the glucose concentrations in blood often is only treating himself or herself and making the patient's life miserable. Above all, the therapist must not inadvertently complicate the course of the disease by unnecessarily introducing drugs that make management impossible, or mistake sudden unmanageable swings in concentrations of glucose in blood as disease-induced when additional drugs are responsible for the problem.

Conventional Insulin Therapy. There are several different insulin regimens that are commonly used to control concentrations of glucose in blood throughout the day. The simplest is a single injection of NPH or Lente insulin given in the morning. This is most often used in patients with Type II diabetes or in patients with Type I diabetes who are relatively early in the course of their disease, since both these types of patients have some endogenous insulin secretion. Sometimes regular insulin is added to the morning injection to help cover postbreakfast hyperglycemia. After several years of Type I diabetes, most patients become severely insulin-deficient, and the single morning injection of insulin will no longer last throughout the day. In this situation, a second injection in

the evening or at bedtime is needed. A second injection may also be needed in patients with Type II diabetes who require large amounts of insulin. If both regular and intermediate insulins are used for both injections, it is called a *split-mix* regime.

Intensive Insulin Therapy. In the attempt to achieve more physiologic control in patients with diabetes, there has been increasing interest in using complicated and sophisticated insulin regimens that more closely mimic normal secretion of insulin in the nondiabetic individual (Schade et al., 1983; Nathan, 1988). One type of intensive insulin therapy involves the use of a portable external insulin-infusion pump. These devices deliver continuous amounts of insulin subcutaneously, mimicking the nondiabetic person's basal insulin secretion. Boluses of insulin are added before meals to control postprandial hyperglycemia. The additional insulin is administered by the patient 20 to 30 minutes before each meal directly with the insulin-infusion pump. Since only regular insulin is used in these devices, the absorption of insulin from the subcutaneous tissues is more predictable than when intermediate or long-acting insulins are used in the same site. Similar insulin profiles can also be obtained without using insulin-infusion pumps, if the patient is willing to take three to four injections of insulin each day. These therapies using insulin are called *multiple daily injections* (MDIs). The regimen consists of UltraLente insulin to provide basal insulin needs; injections of regular insulin are then given before each meal. When such a protocol is used, excursions in concentrations of serum glucose can be greatly minimized.

Unfortunately, the use of insulin-infusion pumps or MDIs does not automatically normalize the blood glucose profiles. The regimens must be combined with self-monitoring of glucose concentrations in blood (an essential component of intensive insulin therapy programs). Intensive insulin therapy requires patients to alter their insulin dose several times a day in response to their measured blood glucose concentrations or in anticipation of changes in diet or exercise. Adjustment of each insulin dose is made according to an individualized algorithm used in conjunction with the self-monitoring blood glucose result. The goals of intensive insulin therapy are to maintain the fasting and preprandial blood glucose concentrations between 70 and 120 mg/dl, postprandial concentrations < 180 mg/dl, and 3 A.M. concentrations > 65 mg/dl. Long-term control can be judged by measuring glycosylated hemoglobin (Hb A_{1c}), which provides an estimate of average glycemia during the previous 2 to 3 months. These therapies can be effective in improving control of blood glucose concentrations in properly selected and motivated patients (The DCCT Research Group, 1987). The major adverse effect of using these therapies is a substantially increased risk of hypoglycemic reactions, which can carry substantial morbidity (Cryer and Gerich, 1985). *Principle: There must be very good reason to require pharmacologic precision of a patient such as described with intensive insulin therapy. So far, the size of the pumps, the distraction of a patient's attention to comply to instructions, and the lack of definitive data of the efficacy of this approach in reducing complications of diabetes should limit the use of this device to appropriately motivated patients.* A significant minority of patients benefit from use of a pump in terms of their lifestyle, prevention of unpredictable hypoglycemia, and wide swings of their blood glucose concentrations.

Implantable Insulin Pumps. Because of the limitations of the external insulin pump (Pietri and Raskin, 1981; Mecklenburg et al., 1985), there has been considerable interest in the development of implantable insulin-infusion pumps that are capable of delivering intraperitoneal or IV insulin. These implantable pumps offer the advantage of more predictable absorption of insulin than is possible by the subcutaneous route, as well as the potential advantage of restoring the normal portal/systemic insulin gradient when insulin is delivered by the intraperitoneal route. Although these devices are effective in improving metabolic control in select IDDM patients, long-term technical problems of the pumps have not been completely solved (Point Study Group, 1988; Saudek et al., 1989; Cafferty et al., 1990). A major problem is obstruction of intraperitoneal catheters due to peritoneal or omental reaction. In addition, insulin's tendency to form high-molecular-weight aggregates when subjected to motion or body temperature for prolonged periods has impaired the development of implantable insulin pump delivery systems. The use of additives, such as glycerol or polymers, to the insulin preparation or different formulations of insulin is currently being explored (Grau and Saudek, 1987). These same problems with insulin aggregation occur less frequently with external insulin pumps, and a special buffered regular insulin for use in external pumps is available.

Nasal Insulin. Intranasal delivery of insulin offers the potential of providing postprandial insulin requirements without injections (Salzman et al., 1985). Intranasal aerosolized insulin results in a rapid increase in insulin concentrations in plasma within 15 minutes. Its maximal action on lowering plasma glucose in fasting IDDM patients is at 120 minutes, and its effects last 3 to 4 hours.

This form of insulin delivery can closely mimic the endogenous insulin response in a normal person after a meal. Although this approach is useful for controlling postprandial hyperglycemia, basal insulin requirements must still be administered by subcutaneous injection of a long-acting preparation. Because the insulin molecule is relatively large, adjuvants such as bile salts and nonionic detergents are required to facilitate transnasal absorption. A major complication has been mucosal irritation due to the adjuvant. *Principle: Unconventional routes of drug administration must be evaluated not only in usual conditions, but under most conditions the patient is likely to encounter and over protracted periods. This is particularly true if the administered drug has a narrow therapeutic index.*

Glucagon

Glucagon is a hormone secreted by the α cells of the pancreas in response to hypoglycemia. The primary action of glucagon under normal circumstances is to maintain plasma concentrations of glucose in the postabsorptive state by stimulating hepatic glycogenolysis and gluconeogenesis (Unger and Orci, 1990). During diabetic ketoacidosis, high concentrations of glucagon in plasma (associated with low concentrations of insulin) invoke hepatic metabolism toward oxidation of fatty acids into ketone bodies (Foster and McGarry, 1983). The main pharmacologic use of glucagon is by patients' families to treat hypoglycemia unresponsive to oral intake of glucose and before medical attention is available to insulin-requiring diabetic patients. When glucagon is injected subcutaneously in a patient with hypoglycemia, it is effective within 15 minutes, raising the plasma concentration of glucose by stimulating hepatic glycogenolysis. When a physician is available to the severely hypoglycemic patient, IV glucose is the drug of choice.

Hypoglycemic Reactions in the Diabetic Patient. Once other causes of hypoglycemia are ruled out (Table 16-3) and a diabetic patient is placed on insulin or other drugs, he or she must be warned of the symptoms of hypoglycemia. The symptoms vary with the preparation used. When intermediate-acting insulin preparations are used, hypoglycemia develops relatively slowly; mild CNS symptoms predominate and may not be recognized as hypoglycemia. Rapid-acting insulin preparations produce symptoms referable to sympathetic discharge. Hypoglycemia occurring at night may go unnoticed by the patient and may be accompanied only by abnormalities in the sleep pattern: frequent nightmares, night sweats, morning headache, and enuresis in children.

**Table 16-3.   CLASSIFICATION
OF HYPOGLYCEMIA***

I. Spontaneous hypoglycemia
  A. Fasting hypoglycemia
    1. Deficient glucose production
      a. Lack of available glucose or its precursors
        (1) Inadequate caloric intake
        (2) Impaired absorption or excessive loss
        (3) Inborn errors of amino acid metabolism†
        (4) Ketotic hypoglycemia†
      b. Congenital liver disease†
        (1) Glycogen storage disease (types I, III, VI)
        (2) Glycogen synthetase deficiency
        (3) Fructose 1,6-diphosphatase deficiency
      c. Acquired liver disease
    2. Increased glucose utilization
      a. Hyperinsulinism
        (1) Insulinoma and islet cell hyperplasia
        (2) Infants of diabetic mothers
      b. Extrapancreatic tumors (mesenchymal tumors, hepatomas, adrenocortical carcinoma, etc.)
        (1) Excessive synthesis of insulinlike growth factor (IGF)-II
        (2) Excessive glucose catabolism
    3. Deficiencies in hormonal regulation
      a. Adrenocortical insufficiency
      b. Growth hormone deficiency
      c. Glucagon deficiency
  B. Reactive hypoglycemia
    1. Induced by glucose
      a. Functional or idiopathic
      b. Postgastric surgery
      c. Chemical diabetes mellitus
    2. Induced by other sugars or amino acids
      a. Galactosemia
      b. Hereditary fructose intolerance
II. Pharmacologic or toxic causes of hypoglycemia
  A. Exogenous insulin administration (factitious or iatrogenic)
  B. Sulfonylureas (factitious or iatrogenic)
  C. Ethanol
  D. Other drugs or chemical compounds

---

* Modified from Ensinck, J. W.; and Williams, R. H.: Disorders causing hypoglycemia. In, Textbook of Endocrinology, 5th ed. (Williams, R. H., ed.). W.B. Saunders, Philadelphia, pp. 627–659, 1974. Used in 2nd edition of this text.
†Causes of hypoglycemia seen frequently or exclusively in children.

The most effective and appropriate therapy for hypoglycemic reactions is the IV administration of glucose. Since the glucose is often utilized very rapidly, treatment should be followed by additional dietary carbohydrates and protein over the next few hours. Administration of glucose orally during an acute hypoglycemic episode is less reliable, because gastric emptying and absorption may be inadequate as a result of autonomic dysfunction in the hypoglycemic period. Intramuscular glucagon may be helpful, particularly when

IV therapy is difficult, but glucagon therapy has two disadvantages. (1) The immediate effect of glucagon on raising the concentration of glucose in blood depends on adequate stores of liver glycogen. In some diabetic subjects with hypoglycemic episodes, hepatic glycogen is insufficient. (2) Glucagon stimulates release of insulin from the pancreatic islets. In patients with Type II diabetes with some remaining islet cell function, this effect of glucagon may be disadvantageous. *Principle: Glucose therapy is the treatment of choice for hypoglycemic reactions in the diabetic patient and may necessarily be prolonged depending upon the severity of the reaction, the time of onset in relation to the dose of insulin, and the type of insulin used.*

Sulfonylureas

In most patients with mild Type II diabetes, a diet that results in weight loss and an exercise program are all that is required to control their disease. However, some patients are not able to achieve satisfactory control of their diabetes with diet and exercise alone. This group may benefit from the use of a sulfonylurea drug. Sulfonylureas improve diabetic control by two mechanisms: they increase insulin secretion and they improve insulin action on target cells (Gerich, 1989).

History. In 1946, Loubatiere noticed that a sulfonamide-containing drug caused hypoglycemia in normal dogs but had no effect in the pancreatectomized animal (Loubatiere, 1957). If blood from the treated dogs was perfused into the pancreatectomized animals, hypoglycemia occurred. Loubatiere hypothesized that the sulfonamide-containing drug augmented insulin secretion from the pancreas, and that sulfa drugs might have potential use in the treatment of Type II diabetic patients.

By the mid-1960s, four compounds were in use: tolbutamide, acetohexamide, tolazamide and chlorpropamide (Table 16-4). The drugs were widely used until the University Group Diabetes Program (UGDP) reported an increase in cardiovascular mortality associated with tolbutamide (University Group Diabetes Program, 1970, 1976). Sulfonylurea use subsequently declined. Thereafter, a number of reevaluations of the UGDP results criticized the conclusions of the study on the basis of patient selection (including inclusion of nondiabetic subjects), the choice of treatments used (fixed-dose medication), failure to control blood glucose concentrations, a high rate of noncompliance, and ascertainment bias (Feinstein, 1971; Seltzer, 1972). In addition, possible failure of the randomization process may have occurred that resulted in a spuriously low

Table 16-4. SULFONYLUREAS*

CHARACTERISTIC	TOLBUTAMIDE	ACETOHEXAMIDE	TOLAZAMIDE	CHLORPROPAMIDE	GLIPIZIDE	GLYBURIDE
Relative potency	1	2.5	5	6	100	150
Duration of action (h)	6–10	12–18	16–24	24–72	16–24	18–24
Protein binding	Ionic and nonionic	Ionic and nonionic	Ionic and nonionic	Ionic and nonionic	Nonionic	Nonionic
Activity of metabolites	Weak	More active	Moderate	Weak	Inactive	Moderate
Urinary excretion of active drug (%)	2	<2	7	20	3	3
Bile excretion of active drug (%)	<1	<1	<1	<1	12	50
Dose range (mg/d)	500–3000	250–1500	100–1000	100–500	2.5–40	1.25–20
Doses/day	2–3	2	1–2	1	1–2	1–2
Initial dose (mg)	500	250	100	100	5	2.5

* Modified from Gerich, 1989.

cardiovascular death rate in the placebo group (Kilo et al., 1980). These criticisms may explain why the conclusions of the UGDP have not been supported by other studies (Lebovitz, 1990). On the basis of the presently available data, the American Diabetes Association has recommended that restrictions on the use of sulfonylureas are unwarranted (American Diabetes Association, 1979). Nevertheless, the Food and Drug Administration continues to require a warning on the use of sulfonylureas concerning the possible increased risk of cardiovascular mortality (see chapter 34). *Principle: All too often, willingly or unwillingly, "authorities" influence practice without a well-founded basis.*

In the late 1970s, sulfonylureas again became widely used. In 1984, a new generation of sulfonylureas, glyburide and glipizide, which had been available in Europe for several years, was approved for use in the United States. Today, sales of glyburide, glipizide, and chlorpropamide constitute 75% of the oral hypoglycemic market, with nearly 40% of all patients with Type II diabetes being managed with a sulfonylurea plus nonpharmacologic adjunctive approaches (Kennedy et al., 1988).

Mechanism of Action. To work, sulfonylureas require endogenous synthesis of insulin by the β cells. Sulfonylureas exert their effect by enhancing the secretion of preformed insulin. Binding of a sulfonylurea to receptors on the β-cell membrane stimulates the release of insulin in the absence of other secretagogues (Grodsky et al., 1977). In addition to stimulating release of insulin in the absence of glucose, sulfonylureas also potentiate glucose-mediated release of insulin. These effects occur without increasing insulin synthesis. All sulfonylureas have the same mechanism of action but differ in potency based on their affinity to the sulfonylurea receptor (Gaines et al., 1988). The second-generation sulfonylureas, glipizide and glyburide, bind more tightly to the receptors than do the first-generation agents, and therefore are equally effective at lower dosages (Feldman, 1985).

High-affinity plasma membrane receptors on the β-cell membranes are closely linked to ATP-sensitive potassium-ion channels (Boyd, 1988). Binding of a sulfonylurea to these receptors inhibits K^+ from leaving the cell, leading to depolarization of the membrane and opening of voltage-dependent calcium-ion channels. Thus, extracellular calcium enters the cell (Schmid-Antomarchi et al., 1987). It is this increase in intracellular calcium that stimulates cytoplasmic granules to secrete insulin through the plasma membrane. Sulfonylureas also inhibit the release of glucagon (Pfeifer et al., 1983), but decreased glucagon secretion may be due to improved β-cell

function rather than to a direct effect of the drug.

Sulfonylureas also reduce hyperglycemia in NIDDM by mechanisms other than enhanced insulin secretion (Beck-Nielsen et al., 1988). However, these possible extrapancreatic effects require the presence of intact islet cells; the drugs do not work in patients with nonfunctioning β cells (Simonson et al., 1987). Long-term treatment with sulfonylurea improves tissue sensitivity to insulin and possibly increases insulin-receptor binding (Olefsky and Reaven, 1976; Koltermann et al., 1984). Sulfonylurea therapy enhances the ability of insulin to inhibit production of glucose by the liver and to stimulate utilization of glucose. This improvement in hepatic and muscle cell sensitivity to insulin in patients taking sulfonylureas also may be partly explained by the effects of the drug to reduce the hyperglycemic threshold for insulin secretion (Rossetti et al., 1987; Yki-Jarvinen et al., 1987). *Principle: Drugs that have multiple mechanisms of action may be easier to use to achieve a given clinical result than drugs that do not have as many separate pharmacologic mechanisms. Second-generation drugs of a given type (e.g., β-adrenergic antagonists, sulfonylureas, etc.) often have focused mechanisms of action. They cannot be assumed to have the same efficacy or toxicity as their progenitors until such is proved.*

Pharmacokinetics. The sulfonylureas differ in dosage, duration of action, adverse effects, and presence of active metabolites. A recent review of oral hypoglycemic agents has summarized these differences (Gerich, 1989). All sulfonylureas should be taken 15 to 30 minutes before meals. Studies using glipizide show 30% less activity when the medication is taken after a meal (Sartor et al., 1978). Plasma concentrations of the sulfonylurea peak 2 to 4 hours after administration, but there is considerable variability of concentrations between patients. Serum concentrations of sulfonylurea are not routinely measured because it is easier and clinically more meaningful to measure blood glucose concentrations to assess drug efficacy and the adequacy of a given dosage regimen.

All sulfonylureas are extensively protein-bound. The first-generation agents bind by ionic and nonionic interactions. The second-generation agents are 98% nonionically bound, which decreases their interaction with other drugs that bind ionically to plasma proteins (Jackson and Bressler, 1981). All the sulfonylureas undergo hepatic metabolism to inactive or less active metabolites except acetohexamide, which is converted by the liver to a metabolite that is more pharmacologically active than the parent drug. Liver disease reduces inactivation, prolongs the half-life, and thereby enhances the risk of hypoglycemia for all sulfonylureas except acetohexamide. Hypoalbuminemia reduces protein binding, making more free drug available, for any given dose. These mechanisms increase the hypoglycemic action of given doses of these agents in patients with liver disease. Most of the active drug and its metabolites is excreted in the urine, with the remainder eliminated in the feces.

Therapeutic Indications. The use of sulfonylurea in the treatment of Type II diabetes should be considered when normal glycemic control cannot be achieved with weight loss, exercise, and modification of the diet. Since sulfonylureas require β-cell function of some degree, Type I diabetics (IDDM) should not be treated with these oral hypoglycemic agents. The medications should not be used during pregnancy or lactation because they cross the placenta and are secreted in milk, and may cause severe hypoglycemia in the fetus and/or newborn (see chapter 29). Allergy to sulfa drugs and/or hepatic dysfunction also are contraindications to use of sulfonylureas. Finally, the medications may not be effective in particularly stressful situations such as surgery, acute myocardial infarction, or trauma. The patient who will most likely respond satisfactorily to sulfonylurea therapy is the Type II diabetic who is obese, has a short duration of diabetes (less than 5–10 years), has the onset of diabetes after age 40, and has never required insulin for control of hyperglycemia.

When a patient with NIDDM is hospitalized for surgery or for an acute illness, it is usually necessary to institute insulin therapy. An adequate source of calories must also be supplied. If the patient is unable to take oral nourishment, an IV solution of dextrose must be administered in addition to the insulin. When the patient is ready for discharge, insulin often can be discontinued and the oral hypoglycemic agent may be restarted. The physician must be certain to ascertain the ability of the reinstated oral hypoglycemic agent to work. If it is not effective, it may be necessary to continue insulin for several weeks until the patient is eating and exercising regularly. Then the oral hypoglycemic agent should once again be tested for its efficacy.

First-Generation Agents. Selecting a particular sulfonylurea depends on the patient's other medical problems and medications. *Tolbutamide* is the least potent agent, has the shortest duration of action, and is metabolized by the liver to products that are mostly inactive. It is given two to three times a day (500–3000 mg/day) since its effective duration of action is 6 to 10 hours. The drug may be particularly useful in patients with renal insufficiency because of its weaker hypogly-

cemic effects and shorter duration of action (compared with other sulfonylureas), and it may result in fewer serious adverse effects. In addition, it is converted into relatively inactive compounds by the liver before renal excretion.

Acetohexamide is slightly more potent than tolbutamide and intermediate in duration of action (12–18 hours). It is given once or twice daily in a dose range of 250 to 1500 mg/day. It is metabolized by the liver to a compound more active than the parent drug. This hypoglycemic metabolite is excreted in the urine. Therefore, this drug should not be used in patients with impaired renal function. It also has diuretic activity and is a powerful uricosuric agent. *Principle: When multiple drugs can produce the same efficacy, sometimes the choice between them depends on their effects in patients with coexisting diseases.*

Tolazamide is intermediate in hypoglycemic activity and duration of action (16–24 hours). Its dosage range is 100 to 1000 mg/day, and it can be given once or twice a day. It is metabolized by the liver to weakly active metabolites that are excreted in the urine. Therefore, the drug should be used cautiously in patients with renal insufficiency.

Chlorpropamide is the longest-acting sulfonylurea. It has effective duration of action of up to 72 hours. Usual dosages range from 100 to 500 mg/day. Dosages should not be adjusted more than once a week, since it takes 7 to 10 days to reach steady-state concentrations of drug in plasma. It is much more potent than tolbutamide, and due its very long plasma half-life, it can be given as a single daily dose. It is partially metabolized by the liver to moderately active metabolites that are excreted in the urine along with the parent drug. The risk of hypoglycemia from chlorpropamide is relatively high because it has a substantial long duration of action and it requires renal excretion. It should be used cautiously, if at all, in the elderly and should not be used in patients with impaired renal function. Chlorpropamide causes water retention and hyponatremia due to its potentiation of the effect of antidiuretic hormone. It is also the sulfonylurea most frequently associated with alcohol-induced flushing. Doses greater than 500 mg/day increase the risk of jaundice.

Second-Generation Agents. The second-generation sulfonylureas available in the United States are glyburide (Micronase and Diabeta) and glipizide (Glucotrol). These agents are 100 to 150 times more potent than tolbutamide, and because of nonionic protein binding have minimal interactions with drugs (such as warfarin, salicylates, and phenylbutazone) that bind ionically to plasma proteins.

Glyburide is the most potent sulfonylurea currently available. It is metabolized in the liver to several metabolites, one of which (4-hydroxyglyburide) retains significant hypoglycemic activity. Fifty percent of glyburide is excreted in the bile, with the remainder excreted in the urine. When patients with decreased renal function are treated with glyburide, caution should be used since 4-hydroxyglyburide accumulates in such settings. The dosage range is 2.5 to 20 mg/day, and the effective duration of action is 24 hours or longer. It can be given once a day, but often the dose is divided when it exceeds 10 mg/day. Glyburide is more effective than glipizide in decreasing basal hepatic glucose production and therefore may be more effective in controlling fasting hyperglycemia (Groop et al., 1987).

Glipizide is slightly less potent on a weight basis than glyburide but is equally effective in controlling hyperglycemia. It has a dosage range of 5 to 40 mg/day. Its duration of action is 16 to 24 hours, and the dose is usually divided when more than 15 mg/day is required. The effect of the medication is increased when it is given at least 30 minutes before a meal (Sartor et al., 1978). Glipizide results in a greater increase in acute-phase insulin release compared with glyburide and may be more effective in controlling postprandial hyperglycemia than fasting hyperglycemia (Groop et al., 1987). Glipizide is metabolized by the liver into inactive metabolites. Because of this, its wide dosage range, and its shorter duration of action, glipizide may produce less hypoglycemia than glyburide in older patients and in those with renal insufficiency.

Combination Therapy with Insulin. Whether patients who are unable to achieve satisfactory glycemic control with sulfonylureas can achieve better control with combination therapy (insulin plus a sulfonylurea) than with insulin alone has been the subject of numerous clinical trials (Bailey and Mezitis, 1990). Many of these studies were not adequately controlled, did not use objective end points, and/or used suboptimal insulin regimes. In some studies, the glycosylated hemoglobin concentration was modestly decreased ($< 10\%$) with combination therapy compared with insulin therapy alone, and in other studies, comparable glycemic control was maintained with about 20% less insulin with combined therapy (Gerich, 1989). Lebovitz has suggested that a subset of NIDDM patients who are mildly to moderately obese, have adequate endogenous insulin secretory reserve, and are in poor glycemic control despite twice-daily insulin injections (> 70 units/day), may benefit from combined insulin-sulfonylurea therapy (Lebovitz and Pasmantier, 1990). However, combining a sulfonylurea with an ineffective insulin regime may still not achieve as good glycemic control as optimal insulin therapy (Garvey et al., 1985). Most patients with NIDDM can be adequately controlled with either insulin or sulfonylurea (Nathan et al., 1988), and combination therapy is generally not needed.

Biguanides

The two drugs in this class of oral hypoglycemic agents, phenformin and metformin, are currently not available in the United States. Phenformin was withdrawn in 1975 because it was associated with a high frequency of lactic acidosis (Williams and Palmer, 1975). Metformin is currently available in Canada and Europe, and it is undergoing clinical trials in the United States. Metformin differs from the sulfonylureas in several important aspects (Vigneri and Goldfine, 1987): it is not bound to plasma proteins, it is excreted without metabolism solely by the kidney, it rarely causes hypoglycemia, and its use does not appear to be associated with weight gain. Its mechanism of action is not well understood, but it does not stimulate insulin secretion. In patients with NIDDM, its most important action may be to reduce hepatic glucose overproduction, probably by inhibiting gluconeogenesis (Nosadini et al., 1987; Jackson et al., 1987). Other proposed mechanisms of action include direct stimulation of glycolysis in peripheral tissues, slowing of glucose absorption from the GI tract, and increased insulin binding to insulin receptors. Metformin appears to be as effective as glyburide in control of hyperglycemia and may be useful even in patients in whom sulfonylurea therapy has failed.

Aldose Reductase Inhibitors

A new series of compounds, aldose reductase inhibitors, are being investigated for their effect on the prevention and management of complications in the diabetic patient (Raskin and Rosenstock, 1987). These drugs inhibit the enzyme aldose reductase, which is the rate-limiting enzyme in tissues that controls the conversion of glucose to sorbitol. Hyperglycemia leads to increased intracellular concentrations of glucose. In tissues with aldose reductase (e.g., eye, nerves, and kidney), glucose is converted to sorbitol by the polyol pathway (Gabbay, 1973). Accumulation of intracellular sorbitol is thought to be one mechanism by which hyperglycemia leads to the microvascular complications of diabetes (Greene et al., 1988). Aldose reductase inhibitors block the conversion of intracellular glucose into sorbitol and offer the potential of preventing certain diabetic complications independent from attempts at improving concentrations of glucose in blood.

Three different aldose reductase inhibitors (sorbinil, tolrestat, and statil) are undergoing clinical trials to determine their efficacy and safety. Studies to date suggest that these agents improve nerve conduction velocity in asymptomatic diabetic patients (Judzewitch et al., 1983) and are helpful in the symptomatic control of painful diabetic neuropathy (Jaspan et al., 1983; Young et al., 1983). Unfortunately, many of these early studies were performed with sorbinil, a drug that causes a high rate of severe dermatologic adverse effects that are attributed to the hydantoin structure of the drug.

Immunosuppression

Our improved understanding of the autoimmune etiology of Type I diabetes has stimulated interest in the use of immunosuppression to alter the natural history of IDDM. Since the etiology of IDDM is immune-mediated, it may be possible to prevent or delay the onset of diabetes by altering immune function in persons who are at high risk for developing diabetes. Several different immunotherapies have been tried in patients who have recently developed diabetes, including plasmapheresis, monoclonal antibodies, antithymocyte γ-globulins, prednisone, azathioprine, and niacinamide, but no modality has generally been effective when used alone (Pozzilli, 1988). The combination of azathioprine and prednisone was partially effective, but the efficacy was temporary and may not be worth the adverse effects associated with the treatment (Silverstein et al., 1988).

Recently, a large multicenter randomized controlled trial reported that cyclosporin treatment increased the rate of remission and enhanced β-cell function during the first year of IDDM (The Canadian-European Randomized Control Trial Group, 1988). However, cyclosporin was most effective in patients who had the best preservation of β-cell function and when it was begun as early as possible after diagnosis (<3 months) (Bougneres et al., 1988). The improvement lasted only as long as the patient took the medication. However, cyclosporin has been associated with nephrotoxicity when taken at the currently recommended doses for long periods of time. With our improved ability to detect predisposition to and actual autoimmune β-cell destruction at an early stage of the disease (no clinical signs or symptoms of abnormal glucose metabolism), it may be possible to start immunotherapy before there is complete β-cell destruction (Ziegler et al., 1990). The use of lower doses of agents such as cyclosporin started prior to the development of overt diabetes may allow a higher likelihood of preventing diabetes with lower risk of toxicity from the drugs. *Principle: There is little in therapeutics as exciting as redirecting attention from treatment of a dis-* *ease to prevention itself. Early studies of prevention could not have been expected to produce dramatic results if the criteria for inclusion in the study were advanced clinical signs of disease. We already know that the clinical signs require the destructive process to have proceeded to almost complete destruction of the β cells. Look for progress in this area, and perhaps management of other autoimmune diseases as well.*

Summary

Clearly, homeostasis of glucose, in both the normal and the hyperglycemic state, invokes a large number of complex interrelated control mechanisms, which feed back on one another in primary, secondary, and tertiary modes. The complexity of these compensatory mechanisms makes it difficult to determine which of the many observed derangements is primary to the genesis of a given hyperglycemic state. The situation is least ambiguous in the minority of diabetic patients in whom massive destruction of β cells results in lack of insulin and a series of predictable metabolic consequences. In the majority of diabetic patients, in whom major destruction of the β cell does not occur, many abnormalities have been described in all aspects of the system, but designation of any one of these as the primary defect appears to be premature. The relationship of the late complications of diabetes that occur in these patients to their abnormalities of glucose and insulin regulation as well as to abnormalities of basement membranes is a subject of ongoing and intense research. In the meantime, it is more than prudent to believe that control of hyperglycemia is important. To do this, the therapeutic dicta seem to say that when the benefits of therapy to the health and comfort of the patient clearly outweigh the side effects of hypoglycemia, and so forth, they should be pursued. In addition, there can be no excuse for a diabetic patient to be left uncontrolled or unnecessarily be left to face ketoacidosis. Even in the Diabetic Control and Complication Trial, the patients randomized to conventional therapy had an average hemoglobin A1c in the 9% range. No one recommends uncontrolled diabetes!

EXAMPLES OF CHOICES IN THERAPEUTICS

Diabetic Ketoacidosis

Patients with diabetic ketoacidosis (DKA) have an absolute deficiency of the action of insulin (Foster and McGarry, 1983). While most of those who develop DKA are Type I diabetic patients, Type II diabetic patients can rarely develop DKA when stressed. The most common presentation of ketoacidosis is polyuria, polydipsia, vomiting, and weakness with or without an altered sensorium. Abdominal pain and other symptoms are less common. Although ketoacidosis can occur in adolescents who have omitted an injection of insulin, the clinician should look for other precipitating causes in all patients with DKA. The most common underlying causes include infections (especially of the urinary tract and upper respiratory systems), both viral and bacterial. The DKA itself does not cause fever but can cause leukocytosis. Therefore, unlike leukocytosis, the presence of fever implies infection. Moreover, infection often is present in diabetic patients who do not demonstrate a fever. Symptoms of sinusitis should be pursued to rule out the presence of mucormycosis, a devastating and potentially lethal infection. In adult patients, myocardial infarction must be considered, since diabetic patients are at special risk for developing silent ischemia. Patients with DKA are prone to develop vascular thromboses and cerebral edema that typically occur during the recovery phase.

Physical examination of such patients may demonstrate signs of dehydration and Kussmaul-type hyperventilation, and stupor or coma may evolve with severe hyperosmolality. Laboratory studies reveal hyperglycemia and an anion gap acidosis. The serum sodium concentration is depressed by 1.6 mEq/l for each 100 mg/dl of glucose > 100 mg/dl. Hypertriglyceridemia may also be present and further lower the measured serum sodium concentration.

Diabetic ketoacidosis is a medical emergency. Therapy consists of IV fluids and IV regular insulin. Most adults have a 3- to 5-liter volume deficit. Initially, 1 liter of normal saline per hour for the first 2 to 3 hours is given, followed by one half normal saline as needed. Insulin should be administered as an IV bolus of 0.1 to 0.2 units/kg per hour (10–20 units) of regular human insulin, followed by 0.1 unit/kg per hour (5–10 units/hr) of regular human insulin by continuous IV infusion. If the acidosis does not begin to improve within 3 to 4 hours, the infusion rate of the insulin should be increased. Modified insulins should not be given during DKA, and subcutaneous insulin should be avoided because absorption from this site is uncertain in a severely dehydrated patient. If necessary, hourly injections of IM regular insulin can be given, but even this site is not one from which insulin will be predictably absorbed.

The key laboratory tests that can be used to monitor progress are the serum ketone concentrations and pH; the serum glucose concentrations may fall rapidly when fluids and insulin are given. When the glucose concentration falls below 250 mg/dl, 5% to 10% dextrose should be added to the infusion. Intravenous insulin should be continued until serum ketone tests are negative; ketonuria and a mild hyperchloremic acidosis may persist for many hours after the resolution of DKA (Oh et al., 1978). When the DKA has resolved and the patient is able to consume a normal diet, subcutaneous insulin may be resumed. However, it is important to give the subcutaneous insulin injection 1 to 2 hours before discontinuing its IV infusion. Because of the extremely short half-life of IV insulin, concentrations of insulin in serum will quickly fall to extremely low levels until the subcutaneous insulin is absorbed. As a result, the patient can slip back into ketoacidosis.

When a diabetic patient presents with DLA, the concentration of serum potassium may be low, normal, or high (Adrogue et al., 1986). However, total body potassium stores are depleted in all patients with DKA. The average deficit is 3 to 5 mmol/kg of body weight. Patients with low serum potassium concentrations should receive IV replacement of potassium at a rate of 20 to 40 mmol/h. In patients with normal or high initial serum potassium concentrations, potassium replacement should begin 2 to 4 hours later, as the potassium concentrations will fall when insulin therapy increases its flux into cells. Serum potassium concentrations should be monitored regularly. Serum phosphate values usually are depressed in patients with DKA. The average deficit is 0.5 to 1.5 mmol/kg body weight. However, it is not necessary to replace phosphate acutely in well-nourished patients (Fisher and Kitabchi, 1983).

The use of bicarbonate therapy in DKA is controversial, with most recent studies suggesting that it is not indicated when the initial pH is > 7.10 (Morris et al., 1986). Most endocrinologists administer sodium bicarbonate when the acidosis is more severe, but there is no evidence that such therapy is beneficial. Alkali therapy may rapidly lower the serum concentrations of potassium and theoretically cause paradoxical increases in CSF acidosis.

Nonketotic Hyperosmolar Coma

Nonketotic hyperosmolar coma usually occurs in elderly patients who may or may not have a prior history of diabetes (Khardori and Soler, 1984). Patients have a level of consciousness ranging from fully alert to completely comatose. Every conceivable neurologic sign can be manifest, and patients are often mistakenly diagnosed as having had a stroke. The clinical presentation is similar to that of DKA, with patients or family members noting polyuria, polydipsia, and increasing lethargy. Precipitating events are almost always found and include infections (especially pneumonia and urosepsis), renal insufficiency, GI bleed, and stroke (Wachtel et al., 1987). Because of the seriousness of the underlying condition and the age of the typical patient, mortality is very high.

These patients are severely dehydrated and often hypotensive. The volume deficit averages approximately one quarter of normal total body water, or one eighth of total body weight. By definition, patients are not ketotic, so serum ketone tests are negative or only weakly positive. The pH is usually > 7.25, but lactic acidosis or uremic acidosis may occur concurrently and lower the pH. The plasma concentration of glucose usually is > 900 mg/dl. Serum osmolality can be estimated by using the following formula:

$$\text{Serum osmolality} = 2[\text{serum Na}^+] + \frac{[\text{glucose}]}{18} + \frac{[\text{BUN}]}{3}$$

where [serum Na$^+$] is concentration of serum Na$^+$ in mEq/l, [glucose] is concentration of glucose in milligrams per deciliter, and [BUN] is concentration of BUN in milligrams per deciliter.

Resuscitative therapy consists of using insulin and fluids in a manner similar to that used when managing DKA. However, one half normal saline should be given initially to patients in nonketotic hyperosmolar coma. Approximately one half of the volume deficit should be replaced in the first 12 hours and the remainder in the ensuing 24 hours. Plasma glucose concentrations may fall very rapidly when fluids are given, so frequent determinations of the plasma glucose concentrations must be obtained and followed.

Brittle Diabetes

Brittle diabetes refers to wide variations in blood glucose concentrations seen in some Type I diabetic patients treated with insulin. These patients are often precariously balanced between severe hypoglycemic reactions and episodes of ketoacidosis. The cause of this variation is generally unknown, but changes in diet and exercise, inaccuracies in insulin administration (sometimes because the patient is blind), mild infections, and emotional factors have been incriminated. Changes in the concentrations of circulating insulin antibodies have also been suspected. Of these factors, occult infection is the most common, and careful examination for occult infections, such as sinusitis, osteomyelitis, and prostatitis, is necessary in all patients with apparent resistance to insulin.

The treatment of the brittle diabetic patient is difficult and frustrating because of the uncertainties of causal factors. A number of treatment programs have met with some success in individual patients. Attempts should be made to control

physical activity and diet. The use of frequent small feedings throughout the day and evening is particularly useful in this circumstance. Intensive insulin therapy is usually difficult to manage in these patients, and the general principle that frequent hypoglycemic attacks are more dangerous than hyperglycemia might favor loose control in some patients. Nevertheless, intensive insulin therapy often is the only form of therapy that can prevent severe and disabling hypoglycemia. The patients must be taught to take regular insulin before each meal using self-adjustment of their insulin dose based on their premeal glucose concentration, meal size, and anticipated activity. This type of adjustment is not "tight" control of hyperglycemia. Usually the emphasis should be on raising the target premeal blood glucose concentrations to prevent hypoglycemia.

The patient whose requirement for insulin appears to be steadily increasing without obtaining successful control may be exhibiting the *Somogyi effect*. In some Type I diabetic patients, when morning blood tests are used to guide the dosage of insulin, increasing the dose of insulin often is used to "cover" morning hyperglycemia. In some of these patients, unnoticed hypoglycemic reactions may occur during the early morning or late evening, leading to excessive release of catecholamines in response to the hypoglycemia. This may then in turn lead to a subsequent hyperglycemia, lipolysis, and positive urine ketone tests, particularly in the early morning. In these patients, less insulin rather than more insulin is required (to avoid the hypoglycemic reactions and the subsequent hyperglycemia). Careful questioning of patients for subtle symptoms of hypoglycemia (morning headache, night sweats, paresthesias, frequent nightmares) and frequent determinations of glucose concentrations in blood (sometimes during the evening hours) are important in determining whether the Somogyi effect is present.

Hypoglycemia

The diagnosis of hypoglycemia is usually readily apparent, as it is uncommon for normal persons to have fasting plasma glucose values less than 60 to 70 mg/dl. However, the range of "normal" plasma glucose concentrations after a prolonged (< 48 hour) fast is very broad, with men being able to maintain their plasma glucose levels far better than women (Merimee and Tyson, 1974). The most common cause of "hypoglycemia" (i.e., low plasma glucose concentrations in the absence of symptoms) in hospital is iatrogenic, that is, starvation. One liter of 5% dextrose contains 200 kcal, and hospitalized patients who receive no enteral nutrition are often given only 2 to 3 liters of this solution IV each day. The clinical diagnosis of true hypoglycemia should fulfill Whipple's triad: *clinical symptoms* of hypoglycemia should occur simultaneously with *low concentrations of glucose* in plasma, and the *symptoms should then resolve* when glucose is administered. Diabetic patients with severe autonomic neuropathy may be unaware of the adrenergic symptoms of hypoglycemia (Kleinbaum and Shamoon, 1983; Havel and Taborsky, 1989). For the same reason, one should administer β-adrenergic blocking agents with extreme caution to diabetic patients. In general, it is not safe to aim for tight control of plasma glucose concentrations in patients who are insensitive to the symptoms of hypoglycemia.

Hypoglycemia represents one of the most dangerous long-term problems for insulin-treated diabetic patients, for the neurologic consequences of repeated bouts of severe hypoglycemia can be devastating. Diabetic patients often present to the emergency room with hypoglycemia due to insulin overdose or inadequate feeding in the face of the patient's usual oral hypoglycemic or insulin therapy (Arem and Zoghbi, 1985). In general, patients with hypoglycemia due to excessive short-acting insulin can be treated with dextrose infusions and released, but the following evaluation is mandatory before discharging the patient:

1. An eye examination for visual acuity to determine if the patient has cataracts or has had a recent retinal hemorrhage and as a result inadvertently took too much insulin.
2. A consideration for the development of deteriorating renal function. Patients with uremia may be anorexic, and the half-life of insulin is decreased in renal insufficiency. Patients with renal failure often require much less insulin.
3. A dietary history to rule out the presence of gastroparesis that can delay absorption of nutrients. It is very difficult to maintain tight glucose control in these patients without causing frequent bouts of hypoglycemia.

Patients whose hypoglycemia is caused by oral hypoglycemic agents or large doses of modified insulin (or by ethanol, salicylates and other drugs) may have profound and long-lasting depression of the plasma glucose concentrations. Such patients may become hypoglycemic again after receiving dextrose infusions. Therefore, they should be observed in hospital.

REFERENCES

Adrogue, H. J.; Lederer, E. D.; Suki, W. N.; and Eknoyan, G.: Determinants of plasma potassium levels in diabetic ketoacidosis. Medicine, 65:163–172, 1986.

American Diabetes Association: Policy Statement: The UGDP Controversy. Diabetes Care, 2:1–3, 1979.

American Diabetes Association: Nutritional recommendations and principles for individuals with diabetes mellitus: 1986. Diabetes Care, 10:126–132, 1987.

Arem, R.; and Zoghbi, W.: Insulin overdose in eight patients: Insulin pharmacokinetics and review of the literature. Medicine, 64:232–332, 1985.

Bailey, T. S.; and Mezitis, N. H. E.: Combination therapy with insulin and sulfonylureas for type II diabetes. Diabetes Care, 13:687–695, 1990.

Bantle, J. P.: The dietary treatment of diabetes mellitus. Med. Clin. North Am., 72:1285–1299, 1988.

Beck-Nielsen, H.; Hother-Nielsen, O.; and Pederson, O.: Mechanism of action of sulfonylureas with special references to the extrapancreatic effect: An overview. Diabetic Med., 5: 613–620, 1988.

Berger, W.; Honegger, B.; Keller, U.; and Jaeggi, E.: Warning symptoms of hypoglyceamia during treatment with human and porcine insulin in diabetes mellitus. Lancet 1:1041–1044, 1989.

Bogardus, C.; Lillioja, S.; Mott, D.; Hollenbeck, C.; and Reaven, G.: Relationship between degree of obesity and in vivo insulin action in man. Am. J. Physiol., 248:E286–E291, 1985.

Bolli, G. B.; Dimitriadis, G. D.; and Pehling, G. B.: Abnormal glucose counterregulation after subcutaneous insulin in insulin-dependent diabetes mellitus. N. Engl. J. Med., 310: 1706–1711, 1984.

Bougneres, P. F.; Carel, J. C.; Castano, L.; Boitard, C.; Gardin, J. P.; Landais, P.; Hors, J.; Mihatsch, M. J.; Paillard, M.; Chaussain, J. L.; and Bach, J. F.: Factors associated with early remission of type I diabetes in children treated with cyclosporin. N. Engl. J. Med., 318:663–670, 1988.

Boyd, A. E. III: Sulfonylurea receptors, ion channels, and fruit flies. Diabetes, 37:847–850, 1988.

Brogden, R. N.; and Heel, R. C.: Human insulin: A review of its biological activity, pharmacokinetics, and therapeutic use. Drugs, 34:350–371, 1987.

Brownlee, M.; Cerami, A.; and Vlassara, H.: Advanced glycosylation end products in tissue and the biochemical basis of diabetic complications. N. Engl. J. Med., 318:1315–1321, 1988.

Burrow, G. N.; Hazlett, B. E.; and Phillips, M. J.: A case of diabetes mellitus. N. Engl. J. Med., 306:340–343, 1982.

Cafferty, M.; Dunn, F. L.; Eaton, R. P.; Fogel, H.; Micossi, P.; Pinget, P.; Reeves, M.; and Salem, J. L.: Treatment of IDDM with a totally implantable programmable insulin infusion device. Diabetes, 39(suppl. 1):112A, 1990.

The Canadian-European Randomized Control Trial Group: Cyclosporin-induced remission of IDDM after early intervention. Association of 1 yr of cyclosporin treatment with enhanced insulin secretion. Diabetes, 37:1574–1582, 1988.

Chase, H. P.; Jackson, W. E.; Hoops, S. L.; Cockerham, R. S.; Archer, P. G.; and O'Brien, D.: Glucose control and the renal and retinal complications of insulin-dependent diabetes. J.A.M.A., 261:1155–1160, 1989.

Cryer, P. E.; and Gerich, J. E.: Glucose counterregulation, hypoglycemia and intensive insulin therapy in diabetes mellitus. N. Engl. J. Med., 313:232–241, 1985.

The DCCT Research Group: Diabetes Control and Complications Trial (DCCT): Results of feasibility study. Diabetes Care, 10:1–19, 1987.

The DCCT Research Group: The Diabetes Control and Complications Trial (DCCT): Design and methodologic considerations for the feasibility phase. Diabetes, 35:530–545, 1986.

DeFronzo, R. A.; Ferrannini, E.; and Koivisto, V.: New concepts in the pathogenesis and treatment of noninsulin-dependent diabetes mellitus. Am. J. Med., 74(suppl. 1A):52–81, 1983.

DeFronzo, R. A.: The triumverate: Beta-cell, muscle, liver: A collusion responsible for NIDDM. Diabetes, 37:667–687, 1988.

Dunn, F. L.: Treatment of lipid disorders in diabetes mellitus. Med. Clin. North Am., 72:1379–1398, 1988.

Eisenbarth, G. S.: Type I diabetes mellitus: A chronic autoimmune disease. N. Engl. J. Med., 314:1360–1368, 1986.

Eriksson, J.; Franssila-Kallunki, A.; Ekstrand, A.; Saloranta, C.; Widen, E.; Schalin, C.; and Groop, L.: Early metabolic defects in persons at increased risk for non-insulin-dependent diabetes mellitus. N. Engl. J. Med., 321:337–343, 1989.

Feinstein, A. R.: Clinical biostatistics: VIII. An analytic appraisal of the University Group Diabetes Program (UGDP) study. Clin. Pharmacol. Ther., 12:167–191, 1971.

Feldman, J. M.: Glyburide: A second-generation sulfonylurea hypoglycemic agent. History, chemistry, metabolism, pharmacokinetics, clinical use and adverse effects. Pharmacotherapy, 5:43–62, 1985.

Feldt-Rasmussen, B.; Mathiesen, E.; and Deckert, T.: Effect of two years of strict metabolic control on progression of incipient nephropathy in insulin-dependent diabetes. Lancet, 2:1300–1304, 1986.

Fisher, J. N.; and Kitabchi, A. E.: A randomized study of phosphate therapy in the treatment of diabetic ketoacidosis. J. Clin. Endocrinol. Metab., 57:177–180, 1983.

Foster, D. W.; and McGarry, J. D.: The metabolic derangements and treatment of diabetic ketoacidosis. N. Engl. J. Med., 309:159–169, 1983.

Fuller, J. H.; Shipley, M. J.; Rose, G.; Jarrett, R. J.; and Keen, H.: Mortality from coronary heart disease and stroke in relation to degree of glycaemia: The Whitehall Study. Br. Med. J., 287:861–870, 1983.

Gabbay, K. H.: The sorbital pathway and the complications of diabetes. N. Engl. J. Med., 288:831–836, 1973.

Gaines, K. L.; Hamilton, S.; and Boyd, A. E.: Characterization of the sulfonylurea receptor on beta cell membranes. J. Biol. Chem., 263:2589–2592, 1988.

Galloway, J. A.; and deShazo, R. D.: Insulin chemistry, pharmacology, dosage, algorithms, and the complications of insulin treatment. In, Ellenberg and Rifkin's Diabetes Mellitus. Theory and Practice (Rifkin, H.; and Porte, D. Jr., eds.). Elsevier Science Publishing, New York, pp. 497–513, 1990.

Garvey, W. T.; Olefsky, J. M.; Griffin, J.; Hamman, R. F.; and Kolterman, O. G.: The effect of insulin treatment on insulin secretion and insulin action in type II diabetes mellitus. Diabetes, 34:222–234, 1985.

Gerich, J. E.: Oral hypoglycemic agents. N. Engl. J. Med., 321:1231–1243, 1989.

Grau, U.; and Saudek, C. D.: Stable insulin preparation for implanted insulin pumps. Laboratory and animal trials. Diabetes, 36:1453–1459, 1987.

Greene, D. A.; Lattimer, S. A.; and Sima, A. A.: Are disturbances of sorbitol, phosphoinositide, and Na^+-K^+-ATPase regulation involved in pathogenesis of diabetic neuropathy? Diabetes, 37:688–693, 1988.

Greene, D. A.; Lattimer, S. A.; and Sima, A. A. F.: Sorbitol, phosphoinositides, and sodium-potassium-ATPase in the pathogenesis of diabetic complications. N. Engl. J. Med., 316:599–606, 1987.

Grodsky, G. M.; Epstein, G. H.; Fanska, R.; and Karam, J. H.: Pancreatic action of the sulfonylureas. Fed. Proc., 36:2714–2719, 1977.

Groop, L.; Luzi, L.; Melander, A.; Groop, P.-H.; Ratheiser, K.; Simonson, D. C.; and DeFronzo, R. A.: Different effects of glyburide and glipizide on insulin secretion and hepatic glucose production in normal and NIDDM subjects. Diabetes, 36:1320–1328, 1987.

Gulan, M.; Gottesman, I. S.; and Zinman, B.: Biosynthetic human insulin improves post prandial glucose excursions in type 1 diabetes mellitus. Ann. Intern. Med., 107:506–509, 1987.

Havel, P. J.; and Taborsky, G. J. Jr.: The contribution of the autonomic nervous system to changes of glucagon and insulin secretion during hypoglycemic stress. Endocrine Rev., 10:332–350, 1989.

Horton, E. S.: Exercise and diabetes mellitus. Med. Clin. North Am., 72:1301–1321, 1988.

Jackson, J. E.; and Bressler, R.: Clinical pharmacology of sulfonylurea hypoglycemic agents. Drugs, 22:211–245, 295–320, 1981.

Jackson, R. A.; Hawa, M. I.; Jaspan, J. B.; Sim, B. M.; DiSilvio, L.; Featherbe, D.; and Kurtz, A. B.: Mechanism of metformin action in non-insulin-dependent diabetes. Diabetes, 36:632–640, 1987.

Jaspan, J.; Masselli, R.; Herold, K.; and Bartkus, C.: Treatment of severely painful diabetic neuropathy with an aldose reductase inhibitor: Relief of pain and improved somatic and autonomic nerve function. Lancet, 2:758–762, 1983.

Judzewitsch, R. G.; Jaspan, J. B.; Polonsky, K. S.; Weinberg, C. R.; Halter, J. B.; Halar, E.; Pfeifer, M. A.; VuKadinovic, C.; Bernstein, L.; Schneider, M.; Liang, K. Y.; Gabbay, K. H.; Rubenstein, A. H.; and Porte, D. Jr.: Aldose reductase inhibition improves nerve conduction velocity in diabetic patients. N. Engl. J. Med., 308:119–125, 1983.

Kahn, C. R.: Role of insulin receptors in insulin-resistant states. Metabolism, 29:455–466, 1980.

Kahn, C. R.; and Rosenthal, A. S.: Immunologic reactions to insulin: Insulin allergy, insulin resistance, and the autoimmune insulin syndrome. Diabetes Care, 2:283–295, 1979.

Kahn, S. E.; and Porte, D. Jr.: Pathophysiology of type II (non-insulin-dependent) diabetes mellitus: Implications for treatment. In, Ellenberg and Rifkin's Diabetes Mellitus. Theory and Practice (Rifkin, H.; and Porte, D. Jr., eds.). Elsevier Science Publishing, New York, pp. 436–456, 1990.

Karam, J. H.; and Etzwiler, D.: International symposium on human insulin. Diabetes Care, 6(suppl. 1): 1983.

Kennedy, D. L.; Piper, J. M.; and Baum, C.: Trends in use of oral hypoglycemic agents, 1964–1986. Diabetes Care, 11:558–562, 1988.

Khardori, R.; and Soler, N. G.: Hyperosmolar hyperglycemic nonketotic syndrome. Report of 22 cases and brief review. Am. J. Med., 77:899–904, 1984.

Kilo, C.; Miller, J. P.; and Williamson, J. R.: The crux of the UGDP: Spurious results and biologically inappropriate data analysis. Diabetologia, 18:179–185, 1980.

Kleinbaum, J.; and Shamoon, H.: Impaired counterregulation of hypoglycemia in insulin-dependent diabetes mellitus. Diabetes, 32:493–498, 1983.

Koltermann, O. G.; Gray, R. S.; Shapiro, G.; Scarlett, J. A.; Griffin, J.; and Olefsky, J. M.: The acute and chronic effects of sulfonylurea therapy in type II diabetic subjects. Diabetes, 33:346–354, 1984.

Krolewski, A. S.; Warram, J. H.; Rand, L. I.; and Kahn, C. R.: Epidemiologic approach to the etiology of type I diabetes mellitus and its complications. N. Engl. J. Med., 317:1390–1398, 1987.

Landon, M. B.; and Gabbe, S. G.: Diabetes and pregnancy. Med. Clin. North Am., 88:1493–1511, 1988.

Leahy, J. L.; Cooper, H.; Deal, D. A.; and Weir, G. C.: Chronic hyperglycemia is associated with impaired glucose influence on insulin secretion: A study of normal rats using chronic in vivo glucose infusions. J. Clin. Invest., 77:908–915, 1986.

Lebovitz, H. E.: Oral hypoglycemic agents. In, Ellenberg and Rifkin's Diabetes Mellitus. Theory and Practice (Rifkin, H.; and Porte, D. Jr., eds.). Elsevier Science Publishing, New York, pp. 554–574, 1990.

Lebovitz, H. E.; and Pasmantier, R.: Combination insulin-sulfonylurea therapy. Diabetes Care, 13:667–675, 1990.

Leiper, J. M.; Paterson, K. R.; Lunan, C. B.; and MacCuish, A. C.: A comparison of biosynthetic human insulin with porcine insulin in the blood glucose control of diabetic pregnancy. Diabetic Med., 3:49–51, 1986.

Loubatiere, A.: The hypoglycemic sulfonamides: History and development of the problem from 1942 to 1955. Ann. N.Y. Acad. Sci., 71:4–11, 1957.

Mecklenburg, R. S.; Benson, E. A.; Benson, J. W. Jr.; Blumenstein, B. A.; Fredlund, P. N.; Guinn, T. S.; Metz, R. J.; and Nielsen, T. L.: Long-term metabolic control with insulin pump therapy. Report of experience with 127 patients. N. Engl. J. Med., 313:465–468, 1985.

Menon, R. K.; Cohen, R. M.; Sperling, M. A.; Cutfield, W. S.; Mimouni, F.; and Khoury, J. C.: Transplacental passage of insulin in pregnant women with insulin-dependent diabetes mellitus. It role in fetal macrosomia. N. Engl. J. Med., 323:309–315, 1990.

Merimee, T. J.; and Tyson, J. E.: Stabilization of plasma glucose during fasting. N. Engl. J. Med., 291:1275–1278, 1974.

Morris, L. R.; Murphy, M. B.; and Kitabchi, A. E.: Bicarbonate therapy in severe diabetic ketoacidosis. Ann. Intern. Med., 105:836–840, 1986.

Nathan, D. N.: Modern management of insulin-dependent diabetes mellitus. Med. Clin. North Am., 72:1365–1378, 1988.

Nathan, D. M.; Roussel, A.; and Godine, J. E.: Glyburide or insulin for metabolic control in non-insulin-dependent diabetes mellitus. A randomized, double-blind study. Ann. Intern. Med., 108:334–340, 1988.

Nathan, D. M.; Axelrod, L.; Flier, J. S.; and Carr, D. B.: U-500 insulin in the treatment of antibody-mediated insulin resistance. Ann. Intern. Med., 94:653–656, 1981.

National Diabetes Data Group: Classification and diagnosis of diabetes mellitus and other categories of glucose intolerance. Diabetes, 28:1039–1057, 1979.

Nosadini, R.; Avogaro, A.; Trevisan, R.; Valerio, A.; Tessari, P.; Duner, E.; Tiengo, A.; Velussi, M.; DelPrato, S.; DeKreutzenberg, S.; Muggeo, M.; and Crepaldi, G.: Effect of metformin on insulin-stimulated glucose turnover and insulin binding to receptors in type II diabetes. Diabetes Care, 10:62–67, 1987.

O'Rahilly, S. P.; Nugent, Z.; Rudenski, A. S.; Hosker, J. P.; Burnett, M. A.; Darling, P.; and Turner, R. C.: Beta-cell dysfunction, rather than insulin insensitivity, is the primary defect in familial type 2 diabetes. Lancet, 2:360–364, 1986.

Oh, M. S.; Carroll, H. J.; Goldstein, D. A.; and Fein, I. A.: Hyperchloremic acidosis during the recovery phase of diabetic ketosis. Ann. Intern. Med., 89:925–927, 1978.

Olefsky, J. M.; and Reaven, G. M.: Effects of sulfonylurea therapy on insulin binding to mononuclear leukocytes of diabetic subjects. Am. J. Med., 60:89–95, 1976.

Olefsky, J. M.; Ciaraldi, T. P.; and Kolterman, O. G.: Mechanisms of insulin resistance in non-insulin-dependent (type II) diabetes. Am. J. Med., 79(suppl. 3B):12–22, 1985.

Palmer, J. P.; and Lernmark, A.: Pathophysiology of type I (insulin-dependent) diabetes. In, Ellenberg and Rifkin's Diabetes Mellitus. Theory and Practice (Rifkin, H.; and Porte, D. Jr., eds.). Elsevier Science Publishing, New York, pp. 414–435, 1990.

Pfeifer, M. A.; Beard, J. C.; Halter, J. B.; Judzewitsch, R.; Best, J. D.; and Porte, D. Jr.: Suppression of glucagon secretion during a tolbutamide infusion in normal and noninsulin-dependent diabetic subjects. J. Clin. Endocrinol. Metab., 56: 586–591, 1983.

Pietri, A.; and Raskin, P.: Cutaneous complications of chronic continuous subcutaneous insulin infusion therapy. Diabetes Care, 4:624–626, 1981.

Pirart, J.: Diabetes mellitus and its degenerative complications: A prospective study of 4,400 patients observed between 1947 and 1973, Diabetes Care, 1:252–263, 1978.

Point Study Group: One-year trial of a remote-controlled implantable insulin infusion system in type I diabetic patients. Lancet, 2:866–869, 1988.

Pozzilli, P.: Immunotherapy in type I diabetes. Diabetic Med., 5:734–738, 1988.

Raskin, P.; and Rosenstock, J.: Aldose reductase inhibitors and diabetic complications. Am. J. Med., 83:298–306, 1987.

Raskin, P.; and Rosenstock, J.: Blood glucose control and diabetic complications. Ann. Intern. Med., 105:254–263, 1986.

Reaven, G. M.: Role of insulin resistance in human disease. Diabetes 37:1595–1607, 1988.

Reddy, S. S.-K.; and Kahn, C. R.: Insulin resistance: A look at the role of insulin receptor kinase. Diabetic Med., 5:621–629, 1988.

Rosenstock, J.; Friberg, T.; and Raskin, P.: Effect of glycemic control on microvascular complications in type I diabetes mellitus. Am. J. Med., 81:1012–1018, 1986.

Rossetti, L.; Smith, D.; Shulman, G.; Papachristou, D.; and DeFronzo, R.: Correction of hyperglycemia with phlorizin normalizes tissue sensitivity to insulin in diabetic rats. J. Clin. Invest., 79:1510–1515, 1987.

Salzman, R.; Manson, J. E.; Griffing, G. T.; Kimmerle, R.; Ruderman, N.; McCall, A.; Stoltz, E. I.; Mullin, C.; Small, D.; Armstrong, J.; and Melby, J. C.: Intranasal aerosolized insulin: Mixed-meal studies and long-term use in type I diabetes. N. Engl. J. Med., 312:1078–1084, 1985.

Sartor, G.; Schersten, B.; and Melander, A.: Effects of glipizide and food intake on the blood levels of glucose and insulin in diabetic patients. Acta Med. Scand., 203:211–214, 1978.

Saudek, C. D.; Salem, J.-L.; Pitt, H. A.; Waxman, K.; Rubio, M.; Jeandidier, N.; Turner, D.; Fischell, R. E.; and Charles, M. A.: A preliminary trial of the programmable implantable medication system for insulin delivery. N. Engl. J. Med., 321: 574–579, 1989.

Savage, P. J.; Bennion, L. J.; and Bennett, P. H.: Normalization of insulin and glucagon secretion in ketosis resistant diabetes mellitus with prolonged diet therapy. J. Clin. Endocrinol. Metab., 3:830–833, 1979.

Schade, D. S.; Santiago, J. V.; Skylar, J. S.; and Rizza, R. A.: Intensive Insulin Therapy. Medical Examination Publishing, Princeton, 1983.

Schmid-Antomarchi, H.; deWeille, J.; Fosset, M.; and Lazdunski, M.: The receptor for antidiabetic sulfonylurea controls the activity of the ATP-modulated K^+ channel in insulin secreting cells. J. Biol. Chem., 292:15840–15844, 1987.

Seltzer, H. S.: A summary of criticisms of the findings and conclusions of the University Group Diabetes Program (UGDP) study. Clin. Pharmacol. Ther. 12:167–191, 1972.

Silverstein, J.; Maclaren, N.; Riley, W.; Spillar, R.; Radjenovic, D.; and Johnson, S.: Immunosuppression with azathioprine and prednisone in recent-onset insulin-dependent diabetes mellitus. N. Engl. J. Med., 319:599–604, 1988.

Simonson, D. C.; Delprato, S.; Castellino, P.; Groop, L.; and DeFronzo, R. A.: Effect of glyburide on glycemic control, insulin requirement, and glucose metabolism in insulin-treated diabetic patients. Diabetes, 36:136–146, 1987.

Skyler, J. S.: Insulin pharmacology. Med. Clin. North Am., 72:1337–1354, 1988.

Skyler, J. S.: Symposium on human insulin of recombinant DNA origin. Diabetes Care, 5(suppl. 2):1982.

Stanik, S.; and Marcus, R.: Insulin secretion improves following dietary control of plasma glucose in severely hyperglycemic obese patients. Metabolism, 29:346–350, 1980.

Temple, R. C.; Carrington, C. A.; and Luzio, S. D.: Insulin deficiency in noninsulin-dependent diabetes. Lancet, 1:293–295, 1989.

Unger, R. H.; and Orci, L.: Glucagon. In, Ellenberg and Rifkin's Diabetes Mellitus. Theory and Practice (Rifkin, H.; and Porte, D. Jr., eds.). Elsevier Science Publishing, New York, pp. 104–120, 1990.

University Group Diabetes Program: A study of the effects of hypoglycemic agents on vascular complications in patients with adult-onset diabetes: VI. Supplementary report on nonfatal events in patients treated with tolbutamide. Diabetes, 25:29–53, 1976.

University Group Diabetes Program: A study of the effects of hypoglycemic agents on vascular complications in patients with adult onset diabetes: II. Mortality results. Diabetes, 19: 789–830, 1970.

Van Heaften, T. W.; Heiling, V. J.; and Gerich, J. E.: Adverse effects of insulin antibodies on postprandial plasma glucose and insulin profiles in diabetic patients with immune insulin resistance: Implications for intensive insulin regimes. Diabetes, 36:305–309, 1987.

Vigneri, R.; and Goldfine, I. D.: Role of metformin in treatment of diabetes mellitus. Diabetes Care, 10:118–122, 1987.

Wachtel, T. J.; Silliman, R. A.; and Lamberton, P.: Predisposing factors for the diabetic hyperosmolar state. Arch. Intern. Med., 147:409–501, 1987.

Williams, R. H.; and Palmer, J. P.: Farewell to phenformin for treating diabetes mellitus. Ann. Intern. Med., 83:567–568, 1975.

Wood, F. C. Jr.; and Bierman, E. L.: Is diet the cornerstone in management of diabetes? N. Engl. J. Med., 315:1224–1227, 1986.

Yki-Jarvinen, H.; Helve, E.; and Koivisto, V. A.: Hyperglyce-mia decreases glucose uptake in type I diabetes. Diabetes, 38:892–896, 1987.

Young, R. J.; Ewing, D. J.; and Clarke, B. F.: A controlled trial of sorbinil, an aldose reductase inhibitor, in chronic painful diabetic neuropathy. Diabetes, 32:938–942, 1983.

Ziegler, A. G.; Herkowitz, R. D.; Jackson, R. A.; Soeldner, J. S.; and Eisenbarth, G. S.: Predicting type I diabetes. Diabetes Care, 13:762–765, 1990.

Zinman, B.: The physiologic replacement of insulin. An elusive goal. N. Engl. J. Med., 321:363–370, 1989.

17

Treatment of Endocrine Disorders: Estrogens and Progestins

Andrew R. Hoffman and Robert Marcus

PHYSIOLOGY OF THE MENSTRUAL CYCLE

Hypothalamic–Pituitary–Ovarian Axis

The normal menstrual cycle is characterized by a carefully orchestrated, complex neuroendocrine secretory output that is modulated by a variety of ovarian steroids and peptides. Cells in the anterior hypothalamus secrete gonadotropin-releasing hormone (GnRH, also known as luteinizing hormone–releasing hormone, LHRH) in a pulsatile manner. GnRH interacts with receptors on the gonadotrope cells of the anterior pituitary to stimulate the release of both LH and follicle-stimulating hormone (FSH). These pituitary hormones induce maturation of the oocyte and stimulate the ovarian follicles, which are composed of theca and granulosa cells, to synthesize estrogens and progestins as well as the peptide hormone inhibin. Estrogens and progestins directly inhibit GnRH and pituitary gonadotropin secretion and thus inhibit further stimulation of the ovary. Inhibin is a recently cloned and characterized peptide, synthesized primarily in ovary and testis. It is a heterodimer, with α and β chains. Inhibin-$\alpha\beta$ selectively inhibits FSH secretion from the pituitary gland. Preliminary studies indicate that inhibin $\beta\beta$ (called *activin*) may act as a FSH-releasing factor (Ying, 1988).

Physiology of the Ovarian Follicle

Ovarian folliculogenesis begins at the very end of the luteal phase of the preceding menstrual cycle and terminates at the beginning of the midcycle surge of LH (DiZerga and Hodgen, 1981). The initiation of follicular growth is independent of gonadotropins. Even in the hypophysectomized woman, limited follicular development into the early preantral stages occurs. During pregnancy, when the pituitary gonadotrope cells are suppressed by placental and fetal hormone production, follicular development continues to the preantral stage. In the preantral follicle, the oocyte enlarges and is surrounded by the zona pellucida. Granulosa cells mature into a multilayered compartment, and the theca layer appears in the periphery. The two-cell, two-gonadotropin theory of steroidogenesis suggests that a complex paracrine system cooperates in the synthesis of estrogens: LH stimulates the theca cells to synthesize androgens, which are obligate precursors for the synthesis of natural estrogens. The androgens are secreted from the theca and interact with the nearby granulosa cells, which are the major target cells for FSH. Rising FSH concentrations stimulate aromatase, the enzyme that converts androgenic steroids to estrogens by aromatizing the A ring of the steroid nucleus.

In the early part of the menstrual cycle, FSH secretion causes an increase in the number of FSH receptors on the granulosa cell membranes. In fact, FSH concentrations may begin to rise 1 day prior to the onset of menstruation of the preceding cycle. Together with the estrogen being produced by the granulosa cells, FSH exerts a mitogenic action and stimulates proliferation of granulosa cells. An estrogenic environment is needed for further development of the follicle; a relatively androgenic environment may cause arrest of folliculogenesis at an immature stage, as in so-called polycystic ovarian disease syndrome (PCOD).

The fluid in the follicular antrum is produced under the influence of FSH and estrogen, and it provides a hormone-rich milieu that is unique for each follicle. The greater the rate of proliferation of granulosa cells, the higher the estrogen concentration. The exact constituents of the antral fluid, which has steroid and peptide concentrations manyfold higher than the circulating values, may have important implications for further development of the particular ovum. While estrogen may enhance FSH activity within the follicle, it, along with inhibin, also suppresses pituitary FSH secretion, thereby withdrawing support to developing follicles.

The larger follicles have undergone greater granulosa cell proliferation and therefore have higher antral estrogen levels. As FSH secretion declines, the larger follicles may thus be at a relative survival advantage, resulting in selection of the fittest follicle(s). However, the dominant follicle is still dependent upon serum FSH, the concentration of which is declining under the influence of its own increasing estrogen production. Thus, the dominant follicle acts as an ovarian dictator, enriching itself as it suppresses its sister follicles.

The Midcycle Surge and Luteal Phase

Estrogen exerts biphasic feedback upon pituitary secretion of gonadotropin. Early in the cycle when the concentration of estrogen is relatively low, estrogen *inhibits* LH secretion. However, as the gonadotropes are primed by estradiol and as the concentration of estradiol increases in midcycle, *positive* feedback occurs, and LH pulse frequency and amplitude increase dramatically. This positive feedback occurs in women when estradiol concentrations approach approximately 200 pg/ml and are maintained for 2 days or more. Estradiol concentrations peak at 24 to 36 hours before ovulation occurs. This final increase in estradiol results in the LH surge that leads to ovulation of the dominant follicle, but atresia of the other follicles. Ovulation typically occurs on day 14 of the typical 28-day cycle. Progesterone concentrations begin to increase significantly 12 to 24 hours before ovulation. The LH surge causes reinitiation of meiosis, luteinization of the granulosa cells, and local synthesis of prostaglandins; it also coincides with a transient decrement in estradiol levels.

The period after ovulation is known as the luteal phase. It is characterized by a decreasing LH pulse frequency and a lower serum LH concentration. The corpus luteum is formed from lipid-laden granulosa cells along with some theca cells derived from the dominant follicle. The function of the corpus luteum is to make progesterone. The survival of the corpus luteum is dependent upon continued LH (or in pregnancy, human chorionic gonadotropin [hCG]) stimulation, and upon low-density lipoproteins (LDLs) as a source of cholesterol, the precursor of progesterone and estrogens. Progesterone inhibits further follicular development by inhibiting gonadotropin secretion, and, possibly, by intraovarian mechanisms as well. The rise in serum progesterone concentrations is associated with an increase in the basal body temperature of 0.3 to 0.5°C. Progesterone concentrations peak approximately 7 to 8 days after ovulation and then decline unless pregnancy has ensued. Progesterone is necessary for nidation of the fertilized ovum and for maintenance of the developing embryo. The progesterone antagonist mifepristone (RU 486) is an effective contraceptive and abortifacient medication (Nieman et al., 1987).

Unlike the situation with most other endocrine organs, the normal functioning of the ovary is frequently deliberately interrupted in order to effect contraception or to treat an estrogen- or progesterone-dependent disease. Ovarian function is usually interrupted by suppression of ovulation, thereby inhibiting the normal cyclic expression of estrogens and progesterone. The hypothalamic–gonadotrope axis can be inhibited by the exogenous administration of sex steroids (estrogens, androgens, or progestational agents) or by the use of superpotent GnRH analogs that desensitize the pituitary to endogenous GnRH stimulation (see chapter 18). For general references on the physiology of the menstrual cycle, see Filicori et al., 1986, and Knobil, 1980.

OVARIAN STEROID PHARMACOLOGY

Estrogens

Active steroids (estrogens and progestins) and nonsteroidal estrogens (e.g., diethylstilbestrol) are used to suppress ovulation, to replace inadequate production of ovarian steroids in hypogonadal individuals, and to counter the effects of excessive androgen secretion in women. The most active estrogenic hormone secreted by women during their reproductive years is 17β-estradiol, which is synthesized predominantly in the ovary. After the menopause, ovarian production of estradiol falls to less than 20 μg/ day. In postmenopausal women, estrone is the most abundant estrogen; it is derived from peripheral conversion of androstenedione, which is synthesized by the zona reticularis of the adrenal cortex. These natural estrogens are extremely potent suppressors of gonadotropin secretion, but difficulties may be encountered when they are used as drugs.

Intramuscular injections of estradiol valerate or cypionate can provide high concentrations in serum. Following absorption from the GI tract, orally administered estradiol is rapidly metabolized by the liver to inactive metabolites. As a result, higher doses of estrogen than the ovaries normally secrete must be given orally to produce the needed pharmacologic effect. For example, micronized estradiol (Estrace) is usually given in a dose of 1 to 2 mg/day, while endogenous production of estradiol ranges between approximately 60 and 600 μg/day. Most of the estradiol given by mouth is converted to estrone in the intestine, and a large fraction of the absorbed estrone is rapidly conjugated or degraded by the liver. A substantial fraction of the conjugated estrogens is then excreted into the bile, but estrogenic activity may be recovered through enterohepatic recirculation (Stumpf, 1990).

Estradiol can also be absorbed through the skin and thereby escape the first-pass hepatic metabolism. Estradiol-containing patches are designed to deliver the equivalent of 50 to 100 μg/day of estradiol. Transdermal estradiol increases circulating concentrations of both estradiol and estrone. Like conjugated oral estrogens, transdermal estrogen lowers urinary calcium excretion. However, transdermal estradiol may not exert the pharmacologic action on hepatic metabolism that is characteristic of oral conjugated estrogens. Thus, transdermal estradiol is less potent at lowering serum lipoprotein concentrations; it does not increase concentrations of angiotensinogen or steroid-binding globulins (Chetkowski et al., 1986).

Conjugated equine estrogens (Premarin; Estra tab) are natural estrogens recovered from the urine of pregnant mares. The active estrogens include estrone sulfate, equilin sulfate, and 17α-dihydroequilin sulfate. The equilins have aromatic A and B rings, and they have prolonged active half-lives because they are very lipophilic

and therefore accumulate in adipose tissue (Bhavnani, 1988).

Another approach to providing nonparenteral estrogen therapy has been to utilize synthetic derivatives of estradiol that are less actively metabolized by the liver: 17α-ethinyl estradiol and its 3-methyl ether, mestranol. Approximately one half of the mestranol is demethylated in the liver to form the active steroid, ethinyl estradiol, and these two synthetic estrogens have essentially identical pharmacokinetics. The addition of the ethinyl group decreases hepatic hydroxylation and conjugation, thereby enhancing oral activity. Ethinyl estradiol is far more active than natural estrogens in inducing hepatic globulin synthesis. The nonsteroidal estrogens diethylstilbestrol and chlorotrianisene are also active orally. In addition to suppressing gonadotropin secretion, these estrogenic compounds duplicate the effects of native estrogens on both reproductive and nonreproductive tissues.

Progestins

Progesterone is the major progestin secreted by the corpus luteum. Like estradiol, it is rapidly metabolized in the liver when taken orally. Therefore, oral micronized progesterone must be administered in high doses. Medroxyprogesterone acetate is a synthetic progestin that is effective when taken orally. Moreover, a variety of derivatives of 19-nortestosterone have progestational activity in vivo when they are administered orally. Five of these derivatives are currently used, primarily as components of oral contraceptives. However, some of these derivatives retain variable amounts of androgenic activity, making some combination birth control pills less useful in the treatment of hyperandrogenic disorders (Table 17-1). Other progestational compounds, like cyproterone acetate, are effective antiandrogens (Whitehead et al., 1990).

Each class of steroid hormone interacts most avidly with a specific type of steroid hormone receptor. Thus, estrogens bind to estrogen re-

Table 17-1.   RELATIVE POTENCY OF ORAL PROGESTINS

PROGESTIN	RELATIVE PROGESTATIONAL POTENCY	ANDROGENICITY
Micronized progesterone	0.003	Low
Medroxyprogesterone acetate	0.1	Low
Norethindron	1	Low
Norethindrone acetate	1	High
Ethynodiol diacetate	1	Low
Norgestrel	5–10	High
Levonorgestrel	10–20	High

ceptors with greater affinity than they do to androgen receptors. Depending on concentrations available, a steroid of one class may "overlap" into the receptors of other types of steroid hormones and act as an agonist or an antagonist for that system. This phenomenon is most pronounced for progestins, which interact not only with the progesterone receptor, but also with the androgen, estrogen, and glucocorticoid receptors.

ORAL CONTRACEPTIVES

Types of Oral Contraceptives

A wide variety of oral contraceptives are available worldwide (Table 17-2). Most are formulations consisting of 21 pills per month containing fixed doses of a synthetic estrogen and a synthetic progestin. Formulations containing less than 50 μg of estrogen are considered "low-dose" pills, those with 50 μg of estrogen are called "regular" birth control pills, and those containing more than 50 μg are considered "high-dose" pills. In order to avoid some of the complications seen in women who have used oral contraceptives, the amount of estrogen in birth control pills has been steadily declining since the 1970s, and the vast majority of patients are now treated with low doses of estrogen. More recently, variable-dose combination pills have been devised. In these oral contraceptives, the steroid doses are adjusted to mimic the amounts of estrogen and progestin made in the normal menstrual cycle; for some combinations, the variable dosing results in less total progestin ingested during the month. There are also three formulations of progestin-only oral contraceptives ("minipills") available (Mishell, 1989). In addition, capsules of levonorgestrel (Norplant) may be implanted subdermally to provide prolonged contraception (Sivin, 1988). *Principle: It is advantageous to use the lowest possible dose of synthetic sex steroids to achieve the desired therapeutic goal. Higher doses of the steroids may result in a higher incidence of adverse effects without adding to the therapeutic efficacy.*
In addition to inhibiting ovulation by suppressing the hypothalamic–gonadotrope axis, combination oral contraceptives directly alter the cervical mucus and thereby inhibit sperm penetration. Moreover, the oral contraceptives inhibit the normal development of the endometrium, preventing implantation. While the precise contraceptive mechanism of the progestogen-only pill has not been fully determined, the minipills have a similar spectrum of action on the neuroendocrine network and on the endometrium as do the combination oral contraceptives. *Principle: Fixed-dose combination products seldom offer a better op-* *portunity for optimal therapy than do drugs administered alone. The birth control pill is an example of an exception to this rule.*

Postcoital contraception (a "morning-after pill") may be achieved by administering relatively high doses of estrogen-progestin combination contraceptive pills on the day following intercourse. The steroids in these formulations may inhibit normal hypothalamic-gonadotrope secretion and thereby interrupt the functioning of the corpus luteum, but there may be a significant failure rate using this regimen. The progesterone antagonist mifepristone (RU 486) is a very effective and safe method for terminating early pregnancy (Couzinet et al., 1986).

Effects on Other Organ Systems

The steroids in the oral contraceptive medications also have a wide range of metabolic actions on a variety of nonreproductive organ systems. In the liver, estrogen induces the synthesis of a number of different proteins, including coagulation factors (leading to an increased incidence of thromboembolic complications), thyroxine–binding and sex steroid–binding globulins, and angiotensinogen. The increase in angiotensinogen production has been causally implicated in the mild hypertension seen in some patients taking oral contraceptives, even those taking lose-dose estrogen formulations (Meade, 1982). Rare patients develop idiosyncratic hypertension of greater severity. The two components of the combination pills have different effects on serum lipid values: estrogens exert a salutary action, raising high-density lipoprotein (HDL) and lowering LDL concentrations, while progestins, especially the more androgenic compounds, have an opposite effect (Knopp et al., 1982). All estrogen-containing oral contraceptives raise the concentrations of serum triglycerides by increasing the concentrations of VLDLs. The progestin component of the oral contraceptive is responsible for the decrease in glucose tolerance and occasionally development of insulin resistance seen in treated patients. The hyperinsulinemia that develops in these women could contribute to the risk of developing hypertension (Reaven and Hoffman, 1987). In patients with diabetes mellitus or with a predisposition to develop diabetes, it would be prudent to choose a combination pill with low progestational activity.

Much of the epidemiologic literature concerning cardiovascular sequelae in women taking birth control pills is based on the first-generation oral contraceptives that contained higher doses of steroids than are now generally used. There is an increased risk of myocardial infarction in users

Table 17-2. AVAILABLE ORAL CONTRACEPTIVES

BRAND	PROGESTIN	ESTROGEN	COMPANY
Norethindrone			
Nor-QD	Norethindrone 0.35 mg	None	Syntex
Micronor	Norethindrone 0.35 mg	None	Ortho
Ovcon 35	Norethindrone 0.4 mg	Ethinyl estradiol 35 μg	Mead Johnson
Brevicon	Norethindrone 0.5 mg	Ethinyl estradiol 35 μg	Syntex
Genora 0.5/35	Norethindrone 0.5 mg	Ethinyl estradiol 35 μg	Rugby
Modicon	Norethindrone 0.5 mg	Ethinyl estradiol 35 μg	Ortho
Norinyl 1 + 35	Norethindrone 1.0 mg	Ethinyl estradiol 35 μg	Syntex
Norethin 1/35	Norethindrone 1.0 mg	Ethinyl estradiol 35 μg	Schiapparelli Searle
Norcept-E 1/35	Norethindrone 1.0 mg	Ethinyl estradiol 35 μg	GynoPharma
Ortho-Novum 1/35	Norethindrone 1.0 mg	Ethinyl estradiol 35 μg	Ortho
Genora 1/35	Norethindrone 1.0 mg	Ethinyl estradiol 35 μg	Rugby
Ovcon 50	Norethindrone 1.0 mg	Ethinyl estradiol 50 μg	Mead Johnson
Genora 1/50	Norethindrone 1.0 mg	Mestranol 50 μg	Rugby
Ortho-Novum 1/50	Norethindrone 1.0 mg	Mestranol 50 μg	Ortho
Norethin 1/50	Norethindrone 1.0 mg	Mestranol 50 μg	Schiapparelli Searle
Norinyl 1 + 50	Norethindrone 1.0 mg	Mestranol 50 μg	Syntex
Ortho-Novum 1/80	Norethindrone 1.0 mg	Mestranol 80 μg	Ortho
Ortho-Novum 2 mg	Norethindrone 2.0 mg	Mestranol 100 μg	Ortho
Tri-Norinyl	Norethindrone 0.5 mg	Ethinyl estradiol 35 μg (X7d)	Syntex
	Norethindrone 1.0 mg	Ethinyl estradiol 35 μg (X9d)	
	Norethindrone 0.5 mg	Ethinyl estradiol 35 μg (X5d)	
Ortho-Novum 7/7/7	Norethindrone 0.5 mg	Ethinyl estradiol 35 μg (X7d)	Ortho
	Norethindrone 0.75 mg	Ethinyl estradiol 35 μg (X7d)	
	Norethindrone 1.0 mg	Ethinyl estradiol 35 μg (X7d)	
Ortho-Novum 10/11	Norethindrone 0.5 mg	Ethinyl estradiol 35 μg (X10d)	Ortho
	Norethindrone 1.0 mg	Ethinyl estradiol 35 μg (X11d)	
Norethindrone Acetate			
Loestrin 1/20	Norethindrone acetate 1.0 mg	Ethinyl estradiol 20 μg	Parke-Davis
Loestrin 1.5/30	Norethindrone acetate 1.5 mg	Ethinyl estradiol 30 μg	Parke-Davis
Ethynodiol Diacetate			
Demulin 1/35	Ethynodiol diacetate 1.0 mg	Ethinyl estradiol 35 μg	Searle
Demulin 1/50	Ethynodiol diacetate 1.0 mg	Ethinyl estradiol 50 μg	Searle
Norgestrel			
Lo/Ovral	Norgestrel 0.3 mg	Ethinyl estradiol 30 μg	Wyeth-Ayerst
Ovral	Norgestrel 0.5 mg	Ethinyl estradiol 50 μg	Wyeth-Ayerst
Ovrette	Norgestrel 0.075 mg	None	Wyeth-Ayerst
Levonorgestrel			
Nordette	Levonorgestrel 0.15 mg	Ethinyl estradiol 30 μg	Wyeth-Ayerst
Levelen	Levonorgestrel 0.15 mg	Ethinyl estradiol 30 μg	Berlex
Tri-Levelen	Levonorgestrel 0.05 mg	Ethinyl estradiol 30 μg (X6d)	Berlex
	Levonorgestrel 0.075 mg	Ethinyl estradiol 40 μg (X5d)	
	Levonorgestrel 0.125 mg	Ethinyl estradiol 30 μg (X10d)	
Tri-Phasil	Levonorgestrel 0.05 mg	Ethinyl estradiol 30 μg (X6d)	Wyeth-Ayerst
	Levonorgestrel 0.075 mg	Ethinyl estradiol 40 μg (X5d)	
	Levonorgestrel 0.125 mg	Ethinyl estradiol 30 μg (X10d)	

of birth control pills. Although this risk is very low in normal young women, it is enhanced in smokers and in those who use pills containing high progestational activity and/or ≥ 50 μg of estrogen (Mann et al., 1976). The incidence of stroke is also increased in women who use oral contraceptives; this enhanced risk is multiplied severalfold in women who smoke and who have hypertension (Stadel, 1981). Birth control pills, therefore, should not be prescribed to smokers over the age of 35.

Although estrogens may accelerate the progression of gallbladder disease, pills containing low doses of estrogen are not associated with an increased risk for cholelithiasis. Nausea and breakthrough bleeding (bleeding between menstrual periods) are not uncommon in the early cycles of use of oral contraceptives. Women may note breast enlargement and tenderness, particularly if they are taking pills with ≥ 50 μg of estrogen. A sense of bloating, edema, abdominal cramps, and emotional lability and irritability are thought to be progestin-related side effects.

Numerous beneficial effects of oral contraceptives have also been documented. In addition to regulating the periodicity of menstrual bleeding, the use of oral contraceptives results in decreased blood loss with each cycle, thereby decreasing the incidence of iron deficiency states. Women taking oral contraceptives have fewer ectopic pregnancies, functional ovarian cysts, benign disease of the breast, and pelvic inflammatory disease. The incidence of endometrial and ovarian cancers is diminished. Long-term users of oral contraceptives have increased lumbar spine bone density.

The existence of oral contraceptive–induced "postpill amenorrhea" remains somewhat controversial. The vast majority of women *who had normal menstrual periods before starting birth control pills* resume normal menses within 3 months of discontinuing the oral contraceptive. While prolactin concentrations in serum may be slightly elevated in some women taking oral contraceptives, there is no association between the use of oral contraceptives and the development of pituitary adenomas (Pituitary Adenoma Study Group, 1983). Many women with oligomenorrhea or amenorrhea are given oral contraceptives in order to regularize menstrual bleeding. In general, the oral contraceptive does not treat the fundamental cause of this menstrual disturbance, which may become manifest again when the oral contraceptive is discontinued. *Principle: The development of abnormal menstrual cycles may reflect pathophysiologic functioning of the hypothalamic–pituitary axis, ovarian dysfunction or other endocrine disease, a gynecologic pathologic lesion, or a systemic illness. Prolonged amenorrhea or severe oligomenorrhea mandates careful* *clinical evaluation and treatment. The use of oral contraceptives frequently masks the menstrual disturbance without treating the underlying disease.*

Interactions and Contraindications

Oral contraceptives are an exceptionally effective method of preventing pregnancy. However, a number of drugs induce hepatic cytochrome P450 enzymes. If given concomitantly with oral contraceptives, these medications can increase the metabolism of estrogens and effectively inactivate the contraceptive action of the birth control pill. The antibiotic rifampin and anticonvulsant medications have commonly been implicated (see chapters 1, 40). The use of oral contraceptives is contraindicated in women with coronary or cerebrovascular disease, thrombophlebitis or a history of thromboembolic disease, estrogen-dependent neoplasms (e.g., breast or endometrium), hepatic adenomas, jaundice, or undiagnosed unusual genital bleeding. Oral contraceptives are contraindicated during pregnancy. Pregnancy itself is more hazardous than any currently accepted method of birth control, and the oral contraceptives are clearly better than any other method of contraception with regard to preventing pregnancy. The patient must be informed of the hazards as well as the benefits of their use and, in that way, participate in the decision to use this medication. An extensive discussion of the complications associated with the use of oral contraceptives must be a part of the decision to use or disregard the drug. The process of the discussion should help both the doctor and the patient with this decision. *Principle: The relative rates of efficacy and toxicity between varying therapeutic regimens or modalities are not necessarily static. They may vary with the patient's age, habits, or coincidental illnesses. Compliance is influenced by information promulgated by newspapers and popular magazines as well as by the physician's attitude concerning the relative cost/benefit ratio of the modality. The therapist must keep abreast of the lay literature, to understand the political ramifications of contraceptive therapy used only by women, and to appreciate how patients interpret scientific data. Certainly, as women learn more about the incidence of toxicity caused by oral contraceptives, use patterns will continue to change.*

TREATMENT OF SPECIFIC SYNDROMES

Turner Syndrome

Ovarian hypofunction occurs when sex steroids or oocytes are not produced, either because of a deficiency of GnRH or gonadotropins or because of intrinsic ovarian disease. Primary ovarian failure may be caused by gonadal dysgenesis (Turner syndrome), by autoimmune mechanisms, by surgical, radiation, or chemotherapy-induced castration, and by menopause. The serum concentrations of gonadotropins are elevated because of a lack of feedback inhibition of ovarian hormones, both steroids and peptides, on the hypothalamic-gonadotrope axis. Since FSH and LH remain high even in those patients who are treated with estrogen and progestin replacement therapy, it has been proposed that ovarian peptides would be needed in addition to sex steroids to inhibit gonadotropin secretion completely.

In Turner syndrome, there is a deletion of all or a portion of one of the X chromosomes, resulting in a 45/XO karyotype (Hall et al., 1982). As many as 1/2500 live female infants has gonadal dysgenesis, but the vast majority of fetuses with this genotype are aborted. In fact, 45/XO is the most common abnormal karyotype in spontaneous abortuses. While these individuals have a near normal complement of primitive oocytes in early fetal life, oocyte number declines rapidly. In effect, these girls undergo menopause before entering menarche. The girls are often born with lymphedema and may have a webbed neck, shield chest, and other abnormalities. Short stature is universal in this condition. Coarctation of the aorta, dissecting aortic aneurysm, diabetes mellitus, and hypothyroidism are associated with Turner syndrome. It is rare for a patient with gonadal dysgenesis to have menstrual periods, and therefore these individuals remain sexually immature and require replacement therapy with sex hormones. In order to induce secondary sex characteristics and to increase linear growth (Copeland, 1988), girls should be treated with sex steroids to induce puberty. It is advantageous to start therapy with estrogen alone for 6 to 12 months, since progesterone has an antiestrogen effect. Since initial menstrual periods are usually anovulatory, this form of therapy mimics normal physiologic development. Progestens should be added after this initial period to provide normal menstrual cycling; it is often useful to use combination oral contraceptives.

Menopausal Syndrome

Menopause is defined as the permanent cessation of menstrual periods. The number of oocytes is sharply reduced, and follicles no longer undergo maturation. In the United States, menopause normally occurs at age 51. Early menopause is defined as the permanent cessation of menses before the age of 35. Patients with the autoimmune polyglandular endocrine deficiency syndrome may develop autoimmune ovarian disease and stop menstruating in their early twenties. The age of menopause is not determined by prior use of oral contraceptive medications nor by the number of pregnancies.

A persistently elevated serum FSH concentration is the best biochemical marker for the menopause. Concentrations of total estrogens in serum are decreased, and the serum estradiol/estrone ratio, which is >1 in premenopausal women, is reversed. Serum concentrations of adrenal androgens do not fall substantially until the zona reticularis involutes (so-called adrenopause), an event that generally occurs several years after natural menopause.

Symptoms. Estrogen deficiency manifests as hot flashes, genital atrophy, diminished libido, and osteoporosis. Hot flashes occur in sexually mature individuals who have been castrated or have undergone menopause; they can also occur in patients who have been treated with exogenous estrogen or androgen therapy when that therapy is discontinued. The hot flash is a vasomotor flush that ascends over the upper trunk and is accompanied by sweating and an unpleasant sensation of warmth. Typical flushes last from 30 seconds to 5 minutes and may recur many times each day. While many women tolerate the flush with minimal discomfort, others may report that their daily habits, and even their sleep, are frequently and severely interrupted. The majority of women report that the discomfort associated with hot flashes lasts for more than 1 year following the menopause; it is not uncommon for hot flashes to continue to occur for as long as five years after cessation of menses. It has been postulated that withdrawal from sex steroid initiates the vasomotor flush through hypothalamic mechanisms. Although hot flashes are associated with a subsequent pulse in serum LH concentration, the gonadotropin is not responsible for the vasomotor flush because people without pituitary glands also suffer from hot flashes when hormone replacement is discontinued; similarly, GnRH cannot be implicated as the etiologic agent because hot flashes are experienced by patients with Kallmann syndrome, a GnRH deficiency syndrome. In most cases, hot flashes can be ameliorated by estrogen or estrogen plus progestin replacement therapy in women (or testosterone replacement in men) (Sherwin and Gelfand, 1984). Medroxyprogesterone alone may suffice in women who cannot take estrogens. Clonidine may also be effective (Clayden et al., 1974).

Genital atrophy may result in substantial morbidity. In the absence of estrogen, the vagina becomes foreshortened and its walls become thin and pale. Secretions are diminished, and there is an increased risk of vaginal infection and ulceration. As the urethra becomes atrophic, patients may complain of dysuria, urgency, and frequency. With the decreased vaginal lubrication, patients suffer from dyspareunia and often choose to reduce their sexual activity. Estrogen therapy restores normal vaginal secretion. The role of sex steroid replacement in enhancing libido, however, has long been debated, but current data suggest that estrogen and progestin therapy do not significantly influence sexual arousal in healthy postmenopausal women (Myers et al., 1990).

Osteoporosis. Loss of bone is an inevitable consequence of aging. The clinical entity, *osteoporosis*, is considered to be the end result of this loss. Osteoporotic fractures occur in thousands of individuals every year, and they constitute a major and growing public health problem for older women and men. Currently it is fashionable to define osteoporosis as a critical reduction in bone mass to the point that fracture vulnerability increases. In this sense, osteoporosis is analogous to anemia defined as a low red blood cell mass. However, this definition is not strictly accurate. Osteoporosis consists not only of a reduction in bone mass but also of important changes in trabecular microarchitecture, such as trabecular perforation and loss of connectivity. This section will consider the effect of estrogen deprivation and replacement on bone. Other aspects of prevention of osteoporosis and treatment are discussed in chapter 20.

Formidable evidence supports an important role for gonadal function in the acquisition and maintenance of bone mass. Hypogonadal boys and girls have substantial deficits in both cortical and trabecular bone mineral. The loss of endogenous androgen or estrogen during adult life regularly leads to accelerated loss of bone mineral, an effect that is particularly striking when it occurs at an early age, such as after oophorectomy in a young woman.

In women, the loss of estrogen has dual effects. Decreased efficiency of intestinal and renal calcium homeostasis increases the level of calcium intake necessary to maintain calcium balance. In addition, recent evidence shows that estrogen directly affects bone cell function (Gray et al., 1985; Eriksen et al., 1988; Komm et al., 1988), and it is this interaction that is thought to underlie an early acceleration in the rate of bone loss in estrogen deficiency. In terms of the specific dynamics of bone remodeling, estrogen deficiency permits osteoclasts to resorb bone with greater efficiency. This may lead to perforation of trabeculae, with no scaffold left for initiation of bone formation. Thus, entire trabecular elements may be eliminated. It is important to note that the interruption

or cessation of menses with consequent estrogen deficiency may have an overwhelming influence on bone mass even when adequate attention is given to other important influences on bone health. For example, women athletes who experience interruption of menstrual function lose bone, despite regular exercise at high intensity (Marcus et al., 1985).

Replacement of estrogen at menopause protects bone mass and affords significant protection against risk for osteoporotic fractures (Recker et al., 1977; Weiss et al., 1980; Lindsay, 1988). The largest published experience has been with conjugated equine estrogens, for which it appears that 0.625 mg/day is a minimally effective dose. There has been less experience with the 17β-estradiol transdermal patch, and there is no published information regarding the use of transcutaneous estradiol and the incidence of osteoporotic fracture. However, patients who use the 50-mg estradiol patch have decreased urinary excretion of calcium and hydroxyproline and decreased circulating concentrations of the bone turnover marker, osteocalcin, so it appears likely that transdermal estrogen provides adequate skeletal protection.

The use of estrogen for skeletal protection requires long-term therapy. Some evidence suggests that fracture risk is reduced only after 5 years of treatment. In addition, cessation of estrogen replacement at any time leads to acceleration in bone loss. *Principle: Since the rate of bone loss increases during the first few years after menopause, the optimal time to initiate replacement therapy is as close to the cessation of ovarian function as possible.*

However, this principle does not imply that older women do not benefit from estrogen replacement. The early randomized estrogen intervention trials that demonstrated the efficacy of estrogen replacement therapy included women who were well into their seventh decades, far beyond the initial 5 years after menopause. In addition, there are extraskeletal effects of estrogen that may indirectly influence bone health. For example, in a group of women whose average age was 64 years, estrogen increased circulating concentrations of 1,25-dihydroxyvitamin D_3, the active vitamin D metabolite (Cheema et al., 1989).

For women who have not undergone hysterectomy, it is normal practice to use cyclic or continuous progestin therapy in addition to estrogen replacement in order to prevent endometrial hyperplasia and carcinoma. The progestational agent most commonly used in the United States is medroxyprogesterone acetate. When prescribed in conventional doses of 10 mg/day for 12 days, this agent does not interfere with the actions of estrogen on mineral metabolism. The androgenic progestins, such as norethisterone, actually reduce urinary calcium excretion and provide skeletal protection on their own. Thus, the use of cyclic or continuous progestins should theoretically not mitigate the skeletal protective effects of estrogen.

Finally, it should be acknowledged that many women choose not to take estrogen. The factors that go into such a decision are complex and transcend skeletal protection. However, it must be emphasized that the effects of estrogen deficiency cannot be avoided by overzealous attention to the other factors that regulate bone mass. For example, osteoporosis in women who are in early menopause does not respond nearly as well to calcium supplementation as to estrogen replacement (Riis et al., 1987), and the experience with amenorrheic athletes supports the conclusion that abundant exercise will not prevent estrogen-dependent bone loss (Marcus et al., 1985).

Cardiovascular Effects of Estrogen. One of the least appreciated aspects of women's health is the fact that ischemic heart disease is the leading cause of hospitalization and mortality for elderly women in the United States. Age-specific mortality rates due to coronary heart disease exceed by severalfold those for breast cancer, hip fracture, and uterine cancer. Furthermore, powerful epidemiologic evidence supports the conclusion that estrogen replacement is associated with an important reduction in risk for coronary heart disease, the magnitude of which may be as great as 50% (Nachtigall et al., 1979; Stampfer et al., 1985; Bush et al., 1987; Henderson et al., 1988; Sullivan et al., 1988). The magnitude of protection appears to be similar regardless of obesity, blood pressure, and tobacco use (Bush et al., 1987). In addition, this protective effect appears to extend to cerebrovascular disease (Paganini-Hill et al., 1988). Most importantly, estrogen replacement is associated with major reductions in all-cause mortality (Bush et al., 1987; Criqui et al., 1988).

The mechanisms by which cardiovascular risk protection is conferred are not clear. However, a model based on lipoprotein metabolism has substantial scientific support. Circulating concentrations of HDL cholesterol are inversely related to risk of coronary disease in women, and estrogen administration is associated with simultaneous increases in concentrations of HDL cholesterol and reductions in concentrations of LDL cholesterol. It must be emphasized that a causal relationship between these effects on lipoprotein metabolism and cardiovascular risk protection has not been established. Nonetheless, the possibility that such a relationship exists raises important practical issues. For example, although the lower-dose (50

mg) estradiol patch adequately controls vasomotor instability and decreases urinary calcium excretion, it does not mimic the effects of oral estrogen on HDL or LDL cholesterol concentrations. Thus, to whatever extent lipoprotein concentrations underlie a reduced cardiovascular risk, transcutaneous estrogen may not be as effective as oral estrogen.

A second, and related, issue concerns the use of progestin cycling. The androgenic progestins have the capacity to modulate lipoprotein metabolism in the opposite direction as estrogens, that is, they may elevate the concentrations of LDL cholesterol and decrease the concentrations of HDL cholesterol. The widely used progestin medroxyprogesterone, on the other hand, does not directly alter circulating lipoprotein concentrations but may blunt the beneficial effects of estrogen on these constituents. The possibility arises, therefore, that progestin cycling, particularly if carried out on a monthly basis, might jeopardize the cardioprotective benefits of estrogen. Since the incidence and morbidity associated with uterine cancer are far less than those of ischemic heart disease, the overall public health impact of progestin cycling may be deleterious. It is stressed that this issue remains strictly theoretical, and that longitudinal randomized intervention trials currently in progress should help to resolve it in the near future. For the moment, however, one should note that the only randomized clinical intervention trial to date (Nachtigall et al., 1979) demonstrated *protection* against myocardial infarction with the combined use of estrogens and progestin.

A more troublesome issue is the potential effect of estrogen replacement on the risk of breast cancer. A large body of epidemiologic work has addressed this question over the past several decades. In most studies, it appears as though little if any overall effect of estrogen on breast cancer risk can be demonstrated (Brinton et al., 1986). However, several other reports indicate a modest, but significant, rise in breast cancer risk among women who received estrogen replacement (Ross et al., 1980) so this issue cannot be considered closed. A recent Swedish study (Bergkvist et al., 1989) has been widely cited to argue that there is a progressive increase in breast cancer risk with duration of estrogen use. However, it should be noted that the primary mode of hormone replacement for Swedish women is a combination of estrogen and androgenic progestin rather than estrogen alone or with cyclic progestin. These results may therefore not be applicable to North American treatment patterns. Nevertheless, concerns about breast cancer risk must be addressed before it will be possible to endorse a global policy of hormone replacement for menopausal women.

Hirsutism

Physiology and Pathophysiology. The relationship between hair growth and sex steroids is complex. Steroid hormones are unimportant in the development and growth of hair on the scalp, the forearms, the lower legs, and the eyebrows and eyelashes. Serum concentrations of the weak androgens, dehydroepiandrosterone (DHEA), DHEA-S, and androstenedione, increase in boys and girls when the zona reticularis of the adrenal cortex matures just before puberty. These relatively low concentrations of androgens are responsible for development of axillary hair and the hair in the lower pubic triangle. Hair appears in the upper pubic triangle, beard, mustache, nasal tips, ears, chest, and back only with the higher concentrations of androgens normally seen in sexually mature men. Adult male concentrations of testosterone may also cause male-pattern balding, with temporal recession and hair loss on the vertex. While androgens increase the number of cells in the papilla of the hair and may increase the diameter of the hair shaft, no new follicles can be induced to develop. Hair follicles are not destroyed during postnatal development, but their density decreases as body surface area increases during normal growth. Hair tends to grow faster in summer than in winter. Scalp hair grows faster in women, while body hair usually grow faster in men.

Hirsutism is defined as the development of dark terminal hairs in androgen-dependent areas in women or prepubertal children. The presence of hirsutism may indicate excessive production of androgens from the ovaries (as in the polycystic ovarian disease syndrome) or from the adrenals (in childhood or adult-onset congenital adrenal hyperplasia). In many hirsute patients, however, androgen concentrations in serum are normal. These women may have hair follicles with increased sensitivity to androgenic stimulation. In some ethnic groups (e.g., Italians), women commonly develop some hair on the upper lip, chin, and sideburns, while in some groups (e.g., Chinese), any hair in these areas is distinctly unusual, and such hair growth commonly indicates an underlying endocrinopathy.

Exposure to very high levels of androgens results in *virilization*: hirsutism, baldness, atrophy of the breasts, deepening of the voice, clitoromegaly, and increased muscle mass. *Hypertrichosis* is defined as excessive growth of lanugo or vellus hairs (soft, unmedullated, usually unpigmented hair) in a pattern different from male hair distribution. It is seen in anorexia nervosa, porphyria cutanea tarda, and hypothyroidism, and as an effect of some drugs, like phenytoin, corticosteroids, and diazoxide. Hypertrichosis is not caused by increased androgen concentrations and does not respond to hormonal therapy.

Treatment. Hirsutism should be treated by addressing the underlying cause when possible. Ovarian tumors or large steroid-producing cysts may be surgically excised. In the polycystic ovarian disease syndrome (Barnes and Rosenfeld, 1989), ovarian androgen production (primarily testosterone) can be halted by inhibiting the hypothalamic–gonadotrope axis with estrogens alone, with oral contraceptives containing a weakly androgenic progestin such as ethynodiol diacetate or norethindrone, or with a long-acting GnRH agonist (see chapter 18). The estrogen in the birth control pills increases the concentration of the sex hormone–binding globulin and may thereby decrease the concentration of freely circulating, biologically active testosterone. Adrenal androgen concentrations may be elevated in Cushing syndrome, in adrenal neoplasms, or in congenital adrenal hyperplasia (CAH), which is most commonly caused by 21-hydroxylase or 11-hydroxylase deficiency. Pituitary and adrenal tumors that result in Cushing syndrome and hyperandrogenism should be surgically removed if possible.

If the tumors are not resectable, steroid production can be decreased by the antifungal agent ketoconazole, an imidizole that inhibits a range of steroidogenic cytochrome P450 enzymes (Feldman, 1986). High doses of ketoconazole also inhibit cortisol synthesis, so exogenous glucocorticoids may have to be given simultaneously to avoid the development of addisonian crisis. In patients with CAH, adrenal steroid production can be inhibited by administering glucocorticoids, which inhibit production of ACTH. The goal is to give just enough glucocorticoid to inhibit adrenal androgen secretion but not enough to cause iatrogenic Cushing syndrome. *Principle: Glucocorticoid inhibition of the hypothalamic–pituitary–adrenal (HPA) axis is dependent upon the timing of glucocorticoid administration. A given dose of glucocorticoid inhibits the HPA axis more effectively when it is given at midnight than when it is given at 8 A.M. (Nichols et al., 1965). In treating CAH, therefore, part or all of the glucocorticoid should be given at night. When glucocorticoids are used for their anti-inflammatory or immunosuppressive effects, however, it is best to administer the drug in the morning to minimize suppression of the HPA axis.*

Another pharmacologic approach to ameliorate hirsutism is to block androgen action at the level of its receptor. The potassium-sparing diuretic spironolactone was developed as a mineralocorticoid antagonist. In practice, it was soon learned that men taking spironolactone frequently developed gynecomastia and, less often, diminished libido and potency. Spironolactone competitively inhibits the binding of dihydrotestosterone to the androgen receptor and thereby acts as an antiandrogen. As a result, it has been a safe, effective agent in the treatment of mild hirsutism. Nonpharmacologic methods for treating hirsutism include bleaching, epilation by plucking or waxing, shaving, depilatories, and electrolysis. Androgen production is increased in obesity, and patients often find that hair growth decreases with weight loss.

REFERENCES

Barnes, R.; and Rosenfeld, R. L.: The polycystic ovary syndrome: Pathogenesis and treatment. Ann. Intern. Med., 110: 386–399, 1989.

Bergkvist, L.; Adami, H.-O.; Persson, I.; Hoover, R.; and Schairer, C.: The risk of breast cancer after estrogen and estrogen-progestin replacement. N. Engl. J. Med., 321:293–297, 1989.

Bhavnani, B. R.: The saga of the ring B unsaturated equine estrogens. Endocr. Rev., 9:396–416, 1988.

Brinton, L. A.; Hoover, R.; and Fraumeni, J. F. Jr.: Menopausal oestrogens and breast cancer risk: An expanded-case control study. Br. J. Cancer, 54:825–832, 1986.

Bush, T. L.; Barrett-Connor, E.; Cowan, L. D.; Criqui, M. H.; Wallace, R. B.; Suchindran, C. M.; Tyroler, H. A.; and Rifkind, B. A.: Cardiovascular mortality and noncontraceptive use of estrogen in women: Results from the Lipid Research Clinics Program Follow-up Study. Circulation, 75: 1102–1109, 1987.

Cheema, C.; Grant, B. F.; and Marcus, R.: Effects of estrogen on circulating "free" and total 1,25-dihydroxy vitamin D and on the parathyroid-vitamin D axis in post menopausal women. J. Clin. Invest., 83:537–542, 1989.

Chetkowski, R. J.; Meldrum, D. R.; Steingold, K. A.; Randle, D.; Lu, J. K.; Eggena, P.; Hershman, J. M.; Alkjaersig, N. K.; Fletcher, A. P.; and Judd, H. L.: Biologic effects of transdermal estradiol. N. Engl. J. Med., 314:1615–1620, 1986.

Clayden, J. R.; Bell, J. W.; and Pollard, P.: Menopausal flushing: Double-blind trial of a non-hormonal medication. Br. Med. J., 1:409–412, 1974.

Copeland, K. C.: Effects of acute high dose and chronic low dose estrogen on plasma somatomedin-C and growth in patients with Turner's syndrome. J. Clin. Endocrinol. Metab., 66:1278–1282, 1988.

Couzinet, B.; Le Strat, N.; Ulmann, A.; Baulieu, E. E.; and Schaison, G.: Termination of early pregnancy by the progesterone antagonist RU 486 (mifepristone). N. Engl. J. Med., 315:1565–1570, 1986.

Criqui, M. H.; Suarez, L.; Barrett-Connor, E.; McPhillips, J.; Wingard, D. L.; and Garland, C.: Postmenopausal estrogen use and mortality. Results from a prospective study in a defined, homogeneous community. Am. J. Epidemiol., 128: 606–614, 1988.

DiZerga, G. S.; and Hodgen, G. D.: Folliculogenesis in the primate ovarian cycle. Endocr. Rev., 2:27–49, 1981.

Eriksen, E. F.; Colvard, D. S.; Berg, N. J.; Graham, M. L.; Mann, K. G.; Spelsberg, T. C.; and Riggs, B. L.: Evidence of estrogen receptors in normal human osteoblast-like cells. Science, 241:84–86, 1988.

Feldman, D.: Ketoconazole and other imidazole derivatives

as inhibitors of steroidogenesis. Endocr. Rev., 7:409–420, 1986.

Filicori, M.; Santoro, N.; Merriam, G. R.; and Crowley, W. F. Jr.: Characterization of the physiological pattern of episodic gonadotropin secretion throughout the human menstrual cycle. J. Clin. Endocrinol. Metab., 62:1136–1144, 1986.

Gray, T. K.; Flynn, T. C.; Gray, K. M.; and Nabell, L. M.: 17β-Estradiol acts directly on the clonal osteoblast cell line UMR 106. Proc. Natl. Acad. Sci. U.S.A., 84:62–67, 1985.

Hall, J. G.; Sybert, V. P.; Williamson, R. A.; Fisher, N. L.; and Reed, S. D.: Turner's syndrome. West. J. Med., 137:32–44, 1982.

Henderson, B. E.; Paganini-Hill, A. N.; and Ross, R. K.: Estrogen replacement therapy and protection from acute myocardial infarction. Am. J. Obstet. Gynecol., 159:312–317, 1988.

Knobil, E.: The neuroendocrine control of the menstrual cycle. Rec. Prog. Horm. Res., 36:53–88, 1980.

Knopp, R. H.; Walden, C. E.; Wahl, P. W.; and Hoover, J. J.: Effects of oral contraceptives on lipoprotein triglyceride and cholesterol: Relationships to estrogen and progestin potency. Am. J. Obstet. Gynecol., 142:725–731, 1982.

Komm, B. S.; Terpenening, C. M.; Benz, D. J.; Graeme, K. A.; Gallegos, A.; Korc, M.; Green, S. L.; O'Malley, B. W.; and Haussler, M. R.: Estrogen binding, receptor mRNA, and biologic response in osteoblast-like osteosarcoma cells. Science, 241:81–84, 1988.

Lindsay, R.: Sex steroids in the pathogenesis and prevention of osteoporosis. In, Osteoporosis, Etiology, Diagnosis, and Management (Riggs, B. L.; and Melton, L. J.; eds.). Raven Press, New York, pp. 333–359, 1988.

Mann, J. I.; Doll, R.; Thorogood, M.; Vessey, M. P.; and Waters, W. E.: Risk factors for myocardial infarction in young women. Br. J. Prev. Soc. Med., 30:94–100, 1976.

Marcus, R.; Cann, C.; Madvig, P.; Minkoff, J.; Goddard, M.; Bayer, M.; Martin, M.; Gaudiani, L.; Haskell, W.; and Genant, H.: Menstrual function and bone mass in elite women distance runners: Endocrine metabolic features. Ann. Intern. Med., 102:158–163, 1985.

Meade, T. W.: Oral contraceptives, clotting factors, and thrombosis. Am. J. Obstet. Gynecol., 142:758–761, 1982.

Mishell, D. R. Jr.: Contraception. N. Engl. J. Med., 320:777–787, 1989.

Myers, L. S.; Dixen, J.; Morrissette, D.; Carmichael, M.; and Davidson, J. M.: Effects of estrogen, androgen, and progestin on sexual psychophysiology and behavior in postmenopausal women. J. Clin. Endocrinol. Metab., 70:1124–1131, 1990.

Nachtigall, L.; Nachtigall, R. H.; Nachtigall, R. D.; and Beckman, E. M.: Estrogen replacement therapy: II. A prospective study in the relationship to carcinoma and cardiovascular and metabolic problems. Obstet. Gynecol., 54:74–80, 1979.

Nichols, T.; Nugent, C. A.; and Tyler, F. H.: Diurnal variation in suppresssion of adrenal function by glucocorticoids. J. Clin. Endocrinol., 25:343–349, 1965.

Nieman, L. K.; Choate, T. M.; Chrousos, G. P.; Healy, D. L.; Morin, M.; Renquist, D.; Merriam, G. R.; Spitz, I. M.; Bardin, C. W.; Baulieu, E.-E.; and Loriaux, D. L.: The progesterone antagonist RU 486. A potential new contraceptive agent. N. Engl. J. Med., 316:187–191, 1987.

Paganini-Hill, A.; Ross, R. K.; and Henderson, B. E.: Postmenopausal oestrogen treatment and stroke: A prospective study. Br. Med. J., 297:519–522, 1988.

Pituitary Adenoma Study Group: Pituitary adenomas and oral contraceptives: A multicenter case-control study. Fertil. Steril., 39:753–760, 1983.

Reaven, G. M.; and Hoffman, B. B.: A role for insulin in the aetiology and course of hypertension? Lancet, 2:435–437, 1987.

Recker, R. R.; Saville, P. D.; and Heaney, R. P.: Effect of estrogens and calcium carbonate on bone loss in postmenopausal women. Ann. Intern. Med., 87:649–655, 1977.

Riis, B.; Thomsen, K.; and Christiansen, C.: Does calcium supplementation prevent postmenopausal bone loss? A double-blind controlled clinical study. N. Engl. J. Med., 316:173–177, 1987.

Ross, R. K.; Paganini-Hill, A.; Gerkins, V. R.; Mack, T. M.; Pfeffer, R.; Arthur, M.; and Henderson, B. E.: A case-control study of menopausal estrogen therapy and breast cancer. J.A.M.A., 243:1635–1639, 1980.

Sherwin, B. B.; and Gelfand, M. M.: Effects of parenteral administration of estrogen and androgen on plasma hormone levels and hot flushes in the surgical menopause. Am. J. Obstet. Gynecol., 148:552–557, 1984.

Sivin, I.: International experience with Norplant and Norplant-2 contraceptives. Stud. Fam. Plan., 19:81–94, 1988.

Stadel, B. V.: Oral contraceptives and cardiovascular disease. N. Engl. J. Med., 305:612–618; 672–677, 1981.

Stampfer, M. J.; Willett, W. C.; Colditz, G. A.; Rosner, B.; Speizer, F. E.; and Hennekens, C. H.: A prospective study of postmenopausal estrogen therapy and coronary heart disease. N. Engl. J. Med., 313:1044–1049, 1985.

Stumpf, P. G.: Pharmacokinetics of estrogen. Obstet. Gynecol., 75:9S–14S, 1990.

Sullivan, J. M.; Vander Zwaag, R.; Lemp, G. F.; Hughes, J. P.; Maddock, V.; Kroetz, F. W.; Ramanathan, K. B.; and Mirvis, D. M.: Postmenopausal estrogen use and coronary atherosclerosis. Ann. Intern. Med., 108:358–363, 1988.

Weiss, N. S.; Ure, C. L.; Ballard, J. H.; Williams, A. R.; and Daling, J. R.: Decreased risk of fractures of the hip and lower forearm with postmenopausal use of estrogen. N. Engl. J. Med., 303:1195–1198, 1980.

Whitehead, M. I.; Hillard, T. C.; and Crook, D.: The role and use of progestogens. Obstet. Gynecol., 75:59S–76S, 1990.

Ying, S.-Y.: Inhibins, activins, and follistatins: Gonadal proteins modulating the secretion of follicle-stimulating hormone. Endocr. Rev., 9:267–293, 1988.

18

Treatment of Endocrine Disorders: Hypothalamic Hormones

Steven A. Lieberman and Andrew R. Hoffman

The discovery of the hypothalamic peptides that are released into the hypothalamic-hypophyseal portal circulation has greatly expanded our understanding of endocrine control mechanisms and the means by which the CNS can communicate with the anterior pituitary and the rest of the peripheral endocrine system. In addition, analogs of these hormones have been synthesized and are now used as pharmaceutic agents for a wide variety of illnesses. This section will discuss the pharmacology of gonadotropin-releasing hormone, growth hormone–releasing hormone, and somatostatin. No significant therapeutic use has yet been found for thyrotropin-releasing hormone or corticotropin-releasing hormone. Vasopressin and its analogs have been used for the treatment of diabetes insipidus, GI bleeding, and defects of hemostasis, and their use in these conditions is discussed elsewhere (see chapters 9, 11, and 22).

GONADOTROPIN-RELEASING HORMONE (GnRH) AND GnRH ANALOGS

Physiology of GnRH

The pituitary hormones responsible for regulation of gonadal function are the glycoprotein heterodimers luteinizing hormone (LH) and follicle-stimulating hormone (FSH). In the male, LH stimulates the Leydig cell of the testes to synthesize testosterone, while FSH (1) stimulates the Sertoli cells to synthesize inhibin and androgen-binding protein and (2) in conjunction with high intratesticular concentrations of testosterone, initiates and maintains spermatogenesis. In females,

LH interacts primarily with the theca cells to stimulate androgen synthesis, and FSH increases aromatase (estrogen synthase) activity and inhibin synthesis in the granulosa cells. Both LH and FSH are released from the gonadotrope cells of the anterior pituitary in response to the hypothalamic hormone GnRH (also known as LH-releasing hormone, LHRH). Human GnRH is a decapeptide with the following primary structure:

$$\underset{1}{\text{Pyro Glu}}\text{-}\underset{2}{\text{His}}\text{-}\underset{3}{\text{Trp}}\text{-}\underset{4}{\text{Ser}}\text{-}\underset{5}{\text{Tyr}}\text{-}\underset{6}{\text{Gly}}\text{-}\underset{7}{\text{Leu}}\text{-}\underset{8}{\text{Arg}}\text{-}\underset{9}{\text{Pro}}\text{-}\underset{10}{\text{Gly}}\text{-NH}_2$$

The peptide is synthesized in the medial preoptic area and the tuberal region of the hypothalamus in neurons whose projections go to the median eminence, where they abut capillaries of the hypothalamic-hypophyseal portal circulation. While high concentrations of GnRH are present in the portal circulation, very little hormone escapes into the peripheral circulation. In the systemic circulation, GnRH has a half-life of < 10 minutes, as it is rapidly degraded, with initial proteolysis catalyzed by an endopeptidase between amino acids 6 and 7, and subsequently catalyzed by a carboxyamide peptidase between amino acids 9 and 10 (Handelsman and Swerdloff, 1986).

The hormone GnRH is necessary for normal pubertal development and for the initiation and maintenance of fertility. In mice with a deletional mutation of the gene encoding GnRH, gonadotropin secretion is low and gonadal maturation does not progress (Mason et al., 1986). Physiologic GnRH deficiency also occurs in humans, manifesting as congenital or acquired hypogonadotropic hypogonadism. When GnRH was initially isolated, characterized, and chemically synthesized, several groups decided to treat men with idiopathic hypogonadotropic hypogonadism (IHH) and other hypothalamic lesions by GnRH replacement therapy. Since most peptides are degraded when ingested orally, GnRH was administered by subcutaneous injection. Although large boluses of hormone were injected several times daily for months, gonadotropin and testosterone concentrations in plasma rarely increased into the normal range. In general, infrequent injections of native synthetic GnRH could not induce or maintain pubertal development in these patients. The reasons for this therapeutic failure were not readily apparent, but it was suggested that native GnRH had too short a half-life to be an effective therapeutic agent (Hoffman, 1985).

Within several years of the discovery of GnRH, numerous very potent, long-acting GnRH analogs were synthesized. In designing analogs, a strategy of substituting a bulky, hydrophobic D-amino acid at position 6 was employed to inhibit proteolysis; in many cases, the terminal amino acid was truncated with the addition of ethylamide to the proline at position 9. These synthetic peptides have a longer duration of action and a greater affinity for pituitary GnRH receptors than the native peptide (Karten and Rivier, 1986). Several investigators used these analogs in an attempt to induce puberty in men with IHH. While serum gonadotropin concentrations rose initially, the increase in hormone secretion could not be maintained for more than several months, even when the dose of analog or the frequency of its administration was increased.

This failure of GnRH and its analogs to induce and maintain pubertal changes led to a reexamination of the normal physiology of the control of gonadotropin secretion. It had long been recognized that LH is secreted into the circulation in discrete pulses and not in a continuous manner. Knobil and his colleagues (Belchetz et al., 1978) reasoned that the pulsatile secretion of LH reflects episodic release of GnRH from the hypothalamus, and they demonstrated that only pulsatile administration of GnRH results in normal gonadotrope responsiveness. These workers studied castrated rhesus monkeys whose GnRH neurons had been stereotactically ablated. When these monkeys received IV boluses of GnRH, gonadotropin concentrations increased and remained elevated. A continuous infusion of GnRH, however, could not sustain this increase in gonadotropin secretion. When the timing of GnRH administration was altered from the known physiologic pulsatile frequency, the increased gonadotropin concentrations were not maintained. Subsequent studies demonstrated

that continuous infusions of native GnRH ultimately inhibit LH secretion in normal persons by desensitizing the pituitary gonadotrophs. *Principle: Cells may respond in a physiologic manner to intermittent exposure to an agonist, but fail to respond to more frequent or continuous exposure to the same agent. Desensitization is most likely to occur during constant exposure to an agonist. One takes therapeutic advantage of such observations either by mimicking the natural release patterns to mimic the effect of native substances or by deliberately desensitizing the receptors if inhibition of the effect of the native substance becomes desirable.*

These studies provided an explanation for the previous failure to induce puberty using GnRH and its analogs and suggested a rational basis for designing drug schedules for GnRH replacement therapy. On a chronic basis, the gonadotrope responds only to pulsatile exposure to GnRH, and not to a continuous infusion of the peptide. Moreover, the GnRH pulses must be delivered in a near-physiologic frequency in order for the pituitary to recognize the stimulatory signal. Thus, infrequent boluses of native GnRH cannot induce normal pubertal development because they do not lead to sufficient LH secretion to maintain testicular secretion. The pituitary is programmed to respond best to approximately 60- to 120-minute interpulse intervals of this hypothalamic hormone. Because of their long serum half-lives and greater duration of binding to the GnRH receptor, the GnRH analogs provide, in effect, a continuous, nonfluctuating level of GnRH bioactivity: a bolus injection of a long-acting agonist is pharmacodynamically similar to a constant infusion of the short-acting native hormone. In normal persons, the potent GnRH analogs initially stimulate gonadotropin secretion; however, by 4 weeks, gonadotrope function is suppressed, serum LH and FSH concentrations fall, and gonadal function declines markedly. This pharmacologic induction of hypogonadotropic hypogonadism has been termed a "medical castration," and, as described below, the GnRH analogs have become extremely useful agents for lowering sex steroid concentrations in clinical settings (Vickery, 1986). *Principle: All hormones are secreted in a pulsatile manner. However, in order for the receptor to experience pulsatile, intermittent exposure to an agonist, the interval between two pulses of hormone secretion (or drug administration) must be substantially longer than the half-life of the agonist.*

GnRH Replacement Therapy

Induction of Puberty in Males with IHH. After appreciating the implications of pulsatile hormone delivery in the hypothalamic–pituitary–gonadal network, it became possible to design treatment schedules for replacement of GnRH. Frequent, round-the-clock administration of hormone is achieved with the use of a portable infusion pump that can be programmed to deliver subcutaneous boluses of GnRH. Men with IHH are treated with 25 to 300 ng of GnRH per kilogram of body weight every 2 hours. On this treatment regimen, distinct pulses of GnRH are evident in the patient's serum. Pulsatile LH and FSH secretion is induced, testosterone concentrations reach the normal range for adult males, testicular size increases, and spermatogenesis ensues in most individuals. Rarely, antibodies against GnRH may be induced that block hormone action, leading to decreased gonadotropin secretion (Hoffman and Crowley, 1982). The success in restoring normal gonadal function in these men by administering GnRH at a physiologic frequency provides further evidence that IHH is in fact a disease of aberrant GnRH synthesis or secretion.

Induction of Ovulation in Women with Hypothalamic Amenorrhea. Abnormalities or deficits in GnRH synthesis or secretion have been implicated in the menstrual disturbances and infertility associated with hypothalamic tumors, IHH, hyperprolactinemia, anorexia nervosa, "stress-" and weight-loss-associated amenorrhea, athletes' amenorrhea, and some forms of the polycystic ovarian disease syndrome. In a series of elegant experiments, Knobil (1980) and his associates demonstrated that pulsatile GnRH administration can induce ovulation in immature rhesus monkeys. Crowley and McArthur (1980) replicated this finding in women with IHH, inducing normal ovulatory cycles by administering a fixed dose of GnRH subcutaneously at a frequency of every 2 hours. In normal women, the frequency of gonadotropin secretion varies throughout the menstrual cycle. By altering the interval between doses of GnRH administration to women with hypo-

thalamic amenorrhea, it is possible to induce a menstrual cycle with daily sex steroid concentrations similar to those seen in a natural cycle. When the doses are given by IV or subcutaneous route via a portable infusion pump, ovulation and fertility can be achieved. This form of therapy provides important advantages over the traditional method of ovulation induction with human gonadotropins. The GnRH therapy induces the secretion of the individual's own gonadotropin; this secretion is further modified by feedback from ovarian steroids and, potentially, inhibin and other ovarian peptides. By taking advantage of this physiologic feedback inhibition and regulation, one can largely avoid the hyperstimulation syndrome and multiple births seen with other methods of ovulation induction.

Clinical Applications of GnRH Analogs

After an initial stimulatory phase, GnRH analogs suppress the pituitary–gonadal axis by desensitizing the gonadotrope, down-regulating GnRH receptors, and inhibiting postreceptor events. In addition, the ratio of bioactive to immunoreactive LH declines with chronic administration of agonist. A variety of GnRH analogs with agonist properties have been used in clinical studies, and preparations are, or will soon be, available that can be administered by subcutaneous injection, nasal spray, and long-acting polymer implant, or microsphere depots (Table 18–1). Efficacious dosing schedules are dependent upon the particular analog and the rate of administration.

Central Precocious Puberty. In normal children, puberty is heralded by the appearance of nocturnal gonadotropin secretion. Although it is not known what CNS events initiate the pubertal process, activation of GnRH-secreting neurons is believed to be the final neural pathway leading to sexual maturation. The diagnosis of idiopathic precocious puberty is made when puberty begins before the age of 8 in children who lack other

Table 18–1.   GnRH ANALOGS WITH AGONIST ACTIVITY

STRUCTURE	GENERIC NAME	PHARMACEUTICAL COMPANY
9–Amino Acid Analogs		
[D-Trp^6, Pro^9 Net] GnRH	Deslorelin	Salk Institute
[D-Trp^6, NMeLeu^7, Pro^9 Net] GnRH	Lutrelin	Wyeth
[D-Leu^6, Pro^9 Net] GnRH	Leuprolide	Abbott
[D-His(Bzl)^6, Pro^9 Net] GnRH	Histerelin	Ortho
[D-Ser(t-But)^6, Pro^9 Net] GnRH	Buserelin	Hoechst
10–Amino Acid Analogs		
Native GnRH	Gonadorelin	Ayerst
	Lutrepulse	
[D-Naphthyl-Ala (2)^6] GnRH	Nafarelin	Syntex
[D-Ser(t-But)^6, AzaGly^{10}] GnRH	Goserelin	ICI
[D-Trp^6] GnRH	Tryptorelin	Debiopharm

obvious causes (e.g., hypothalamic lesions or gonadotropin-independent adrenal or gonadal hypersecretion). The early onset of pubertal levels of sex steroids may lead to premature closure of the epiphyses and ultimate short stature, and the adolescent behavior triggered by the hormonal changes can cause profound social difficulties for the child and his or her family and school. Attempts to suppress the pubertal process, including inhibiting gonadotropin release with medroxyprogesterone, met with limited success. Long-acting GnRH analogs, however, have been extremely effective in desensitizing the gonadotropes in patients with idiopathic precocious puberty. Within several weeks of therapy, gonadotropin concentrations fall and sex steroid concentrations decline back into the prepubertal range. Menses may cease in girls, and boys may experience a decrease in testicular size. The abnormally accelerated rate of skeletal growth may also return to that appropriate for the child's chronologic age. Striking amelioration of behavioral difficulties has also been reported. Children can be treated with a GnRH analog for several years, and, when its use is discontinued, normal puberty begins. No long-term adverse sequelae have been encountered so far (Pescovitz et al., 1986).

Prostate Cancer and Benign Prostatic Hypertrophy. Since prostatic carcinoma is an androgen-dependent tumor, attempts to ablate testicular function have long been used for palliative therapy. Both castration and high-dose diethylstilbestrol (a potent estrogen that suppresses the hypothalamic–pituitary–testicular axis) are effective in the majority of patients with metastatic disease. However, castration is not acceptable to many men, and pharmacologic amounts of estrogens are associated with gynecomastia, thromboembolism, and an increased risk for coronary ischemic events. The use of a GnRH analog to inhibit gonadotrope function has proved to be as effective a therapy as estrogen (The Leuprolide Study Group, 1984). While GnRH analogs do not cause feminizing side effects, patients treated with these agents complain of hot flashes, diminished libido, and, in some cases, impotence. During the first week of therapy, GnRH analogs stimulate the pituitary, and as a result, testosterone concentrations transiently increase, before falling to castrate values (approximately 5%–10% of normal adult concentrations) by 1 month. This initial, transient rise is associated with a flare in bone pain and other symptoms in approximately 10% of patients treated with the GnRH analogs alone. Furthermore, adrenal androgen secretion, which is not inhibited by GnRH analogs, continues, providing significant stimulation to the prostatic cancer. Therefore, in order to inhibit androgen ac-

tion during the initial stimulatory phase of GnRH analog action and to ablate the effects of adrenal androgens, the antiandrogen flutamide, a nonsteroidal compound that competes with testosterone for binding to the androgen receptor, is often added to the regimen (Crawford et al., 1989). *Principle: Desensitization caused by an agonist is preceded by agonist activity. Often, independent pharmacologic measures not dependent upon desensitization must be instituted to treat the disease until receptor desensitization is completed.*

Benign prostatic hypertrophy (BPH) is a universal finding in the aging male population. It leads to urinary retention, bladder outlet obstruction, and if untreated, renal failure. More than 300,000 prostatectomies are performed each year in the United States. The GnRH analogs decrease the size of the prostate and relieve symptoms of outlet obstruction after 4 months of treatment in the majority of patients. While GnRH therapy is effective in decreasing prostate size and in controlling symptoms in patients with BPH, these effects are reversed after the drug is discontinued; thus chronic administration is required if the disease is to be managed using these analogs (Peters and Walsh, 1987). Since the accompanying hypogonadism has significant adverse effects (e.g., decreased bone mineral content, impotence), the general usefulness of GnRH therapy for treating BPH has been limited.

Gynecologic Disease. The GnRH analogs can also be used to inhibit menstrual function and produce a severely hypoestrogenic state. Endometriosis is an ectopic proliferation of endometrial tissue that results in pain and infertility. Since endometrial tissue is estrogen-dependent, the medical castration effected by the GnRH analogs has proved to be an effective treatment that allows avoidance of both surgery and the use of androgenic steroids that can cause virilization (Meldrum et al., 1982). Uterine fibroids are also dependent upon estrogen and may shrink with GnRH analog therapy (Healy et al., 1986). The GnRH analogs are also used to inhibit secretion of endogenous gonadotropins prior to the start of exogenous gonadotropin therapy in some women with infertility. As with men, chronic use of the analogs causes hot flashes. In addition, the prolonged hypoestrogenemia may result in osteoporosis, vaginal dryness, and dyspareunia.

Since all GnRH agonist analogs briefly stimulate pituitary gonadotropin secretion before causing desensitization, sex hormone–dependent diseases may flare during the initial treatment period. Several GnRH analogs that act as direct and immediate *antagonists* are currently under development and may ultimately replace these high-potency agonist GnRH analogs (Pavlou et al., 1989).

GROWTH HORMONE–RELEASING HORMONE (GHRH)

Chemistry and Physiology

Growth hormone (GH) is secreted by the somatotrophs of the anterior pituitary in discrete pulses with an increase in pulse amplitude and frequency occurring during sleep. These pulses result from the interaction of a number of influences on both the hypothalamus and the pituitary. Two hypothalamic peptides, GH-releasing hormone (GHRH) and somatostatin (somatotropin release–inhibiting hormone), are the principle stimulatory and inhibitory factors, respectively. Secretion of these regulatory peptides is modified by a number of influences, including the CNS (mediated by several neurotransmitters) and feedback inhibition by GH and the GH-dependent insulinlike growth factors (Ceda et al., 1987).

Hypothalamic GHRH occurs in two forms: 40- and 44-amino acid peptides, both of which have their biologic activity residing in amino-terminal residues 1 to 29. Synthetic GHRH (1–44) and (GHRH 1–40) as well as a truncated form (GHRH 1–29) have been studied in humans. Except for a higher incidence of formation of nonblocking antibodies found with the 1-to-29 form (Gelato et al., 1985), no differences in the three peptides have been reported following administration to humans.

In contrast to chronic GnRH administration, in which desensitization follows initial release of gonadotropins, long-term use of GHRH results in continued augmentation of the GH response. In adults, two consecutive boluses of GHRH result in a lower GH peak following the second dose (Ghigo et al., 1989). However, continued GHRH administration in either children or adults enhances the GH response. The amplitude and frequency of GH peak and total GH secretion increases, regardless of the timing or route of administration of GHRH (Vance et al., 1985; Hulse et al., 1986; Rochiccioli et al., 1986; Sassolas et al., 1986; Martha et al., 1988). While several studies have shown a diminished GH peak when a GHRH bolus is given after various periods of GHRH administration (Gelato et al., 1985; Vance et al., 1985; Hulse et al., 1986), it is unclear whether this is due to partial desensitization to GHRH, depletion of pituitary stores of GH, or some other mechanism (Ceda and Hoffman, 1985).

The pulsatile nature of secretion of growth hormone is retained during continuous infusion of GHRH (Gelato et al., 1985; ; Vance et al., 1985; Hulse et al., 1986; Rochiccioli et al., 1986; Sassolas et al., 1986) but is lost following administration of anti-GHRH antibodies (Wehrenberg et al., 1982). Thus, GHRH is necessary but not wholly responsible for these pulsations. Furthermore, chronic administration of equal doses of GHRH every 3 hours does not abolish the sleep-entrained increase in GH secretion (Martha et al., 1988). The nocturnal increase in GH secretion occurs 1 to 2 hours after the onset of deep (stage III or IV) sleep. *Principle: When multiple factors (e.g., other than GHRH) are involved in the production of a pulsatile event (e.g., GH secretion), the relative contributions of other factors (e.g., somatostatin, the CNS, and negative feedback by GH and/or IGFs) must be taken into account in any attempt at clinical intervention.*

GHRH Therapy

Many children with short stature due to GH deficiency secrete GH in response to GHRH, implicating a hypothalamic rather than pituitary defect in these patients. Several studies have demonstrated acceleration of growth in patients treated with GHRH, with a sustained effect throughout study periods of up to 18 months (Ross et al., 1987; Low et al., 1988; Thorner et al., 1988). Various schedules of subcutaneous administration have been examined, including once, twice, and three times a day, pulses every 3 hours (administered by pump), pulses only at night, and continuous subcutaneous infusion. The degree of growth acceleration appears to depend more on the total daily dose than on the dosing schedule (Gelato et al., 1985) with one exception: the nocturnal pulse regimen has produced slower growth acceleration and higher failure rates (Thorner et al., 1988). Only one study has compared the efficacy of GHRH therapy directly with GH therapy in GH-deficient children (Butenandt and Staudt, 1989). The seven patients all responded to GHRH with an increase in GH concentrations. Only two of the patients had a significant increase in growth rate, and in only one did the growth rate reach the normal range. The number of patients studied was small, so a potential role for GHRH therapy has not been ruled out at this point.

Evans et al. (1985) found the bioavailability of subcutaneously and intranasally administered GHRH (1–40) to be one sixtieth and one five-hundredth, respectively, that of IV-administered hormone. The distribution half-life of GHRH (1–40) is 7.6 minutes, and the elimination half-life is 41 to 52 minutes. The precise role of GHRH in the therapy of growth hormone deficiency, including optimum dosing and administration, remains to be determined.

SOMATOSTATIN

History and Chemistry

Somatostatin is a phylogenetically ancient peptide that is found in all vertebrate classes, many invertebrates, and even protozoa (Berelowitz et al., 1982). Its name derives from the fact that it was initially discovered as an inhibitor of GH secretion by the anterior pituitary. Further study has revealed a wide range of biologic functions. The first evidence of its existence came in studies aimed at finding a GH-releasing factor (Krulich et al., 1968). Isolation and purification of hypothalamic fractions yielded a cyclic tetradecapeptide (14 amino acids) whose ring structure is the result of a disulfide bond between the 3rd and 14th residues from the amino terminus (Fig. 18–1). Biologic activity resides in the carboxy terminus and is partially lost when the disulfide bond is reduced. Receptor binding occurs at amino acids 7 through 10 (Veber et al., 1981). While somatostatin-14 appears to be the major form in humans and other animals, other biologically active, naturally occurring forms of somatostatin have been discovered. The most common of these, somatostatin-28, contains a 14–amino acid extension at the amino terminus. In neurons and perhaps in other tissues, alternate forms derive from a common preprohormone, with variation in structure resulting from posttranslational processing in the Golgi apparatus and in secretory granules (Reichlin, 1983). The relative amounts of the hormones secreted vary from tissue to tissue.

Distribution

Somatostatin is widely distributed in the body, in concordance with its multiple physiologic roles. Hypothalamic nuclei involved in regulation of secretion of GH release somatostatin into the hypothalamic-hypophyseal portal circulation, providing high concentrations of somatostatin in the anterior pituitary. Other somatostatin-containing neurons project from the hypothalamus to areas of the limbic system, brainstem, and spinal cord. Somatostatin is also found in the cerebral cortex and a variety of peripheral neurons, particularly those involved in sensory systems (Reichlin, 1983). Its role in these systems is unclear.

The GI tract is the other principal location of somatostatin. It is secreted by D cells in the intestinal epithelium and pancreatic islets as well as by

elements of the visceral autonomic nervous system. The concentration of D cells in gut epithelium is highest in the stomach and duodenum and gradually decreases to the distal colon. In the pancreas, D cells are found in close association with A and B cells that secrete glucagon and insulin, respectively. Other tissues found to contain somatostatin in humans include the salivary glands, thyroid C cells, adrenal medulla, and placenta (Wass, 1989). *Principle: Somatostatin operates in several modes, functioning as an autocrine, paracrine, or endocrine factor; a neurotransmitter; or a neuromodulator in different tissues.*

Receptors for somatostatin also are found in many organs, with some differences among species. In humans, the receptors have so far been demonstrated in the anterior pituitary, cerebral cortex, limbic system, basal ganglia, cerebellum, and A, B, and D cells of the pancreatic islets. Receptor affinity for the various naturally occurring and synthetic forms of somatostatin is tissue-specific. There is evidence for several mechanisms of signal transduction in somatostatin-responsive cells: (1) inhibition of cAMP generation, (2) diminishing of the intracellular calcium concentration, and (3) inhibition of phosphoinositide metabolism (Gespach et al., 1980; Toro et al., 1988). These multiple potential mechanisms inhibit the release of secretory granules in various endocrine cells. *Principle: Through variations in hormone structure, receptor affinity, and postreceptor signaling events, somatostatin can modify a wide range of physiologic functions to varying degrees in different organs. Other "ubiquitous" hormones likely can behave similarly.*

Physiology

Administration of somatostatin inhibits the secretion of a wide variety of peptide hormones, as seen in Table 18–2. In the anterior pituitary, somatostatin suppresses the physiologic nocturnal GH surge, spontaneous daytime peaks of GH secretion, and secretion of GH in response to virtually all known stimuli including GHRH, insulin-induced hypoglycemia, arginine infusion, and exercise (Hall et al., 1973; Prange-Hansen et al., 1973). Somatostatin also inhibits the TSH response to infusion of TRH, though its effect on

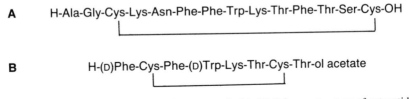

A   H-Ala-Gly-Cys-Lys-Asn-Phe-Phe-Trp-Lys-Thr-Phe-Thr-Ser-Cys-OH

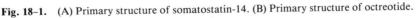

B   H-(D)Phe-Cys-Phe-(D)Trp-Lys-Thr-Cys-Thr-ol acetate

Fig. 18–1. (A) Primary structure of somatostatin-14. (B) Primary structure of octreotide.

Table 18-2. INHIBITION OF HORMONE SECRETION BY SOMATOSTATIN

Hypothalamic hormones
  GHRH

Anterior pituitary hormones
  GH
  TSH

Pancreatic hormones
  Insulin
  Glucagon
  Gastrin
  Cholecystokinin (CCK)
  Secretin
  Pepsin
  Motilin
  Pancreatic polypeptide (PP)
  Gastrointestinal peptide (GIP)
  Vasoactive intestinal polypeptide (VIP)

Kidney hormones
  Renin

basal TSH levels is variable (Weeke et al., 1974, 1975). In the pancreas, somatostatin suppresses glucagon secretion more potently than insulin secretion, although the effect on insulin is of greater duration. Thus, administration of somatostatin-14 in humans produces mild but transient hyperglycemia (Rizza et al., 1979).

In addition to its effects on endocrine organs, somatostatin inhibits many other physiologic activities, including gastric acid secretion, gastric motility, gallbladder emptying, pancreatic enzyme and bicarbonate secretion, visceral blood flow, and intestinal absorption of glucose, amino acids, triglycerides, and water. This multitude of effects suggests both therapeutic potential and real potential for toxicity for somatostatin. A number of characteristics of the native hormone make it unsuitable for clinical use. Its elimination half-life of 1 to 3 minutes necessitates continuous infusion to sustain its effects, and rebound hypersecretion follows the initial suppression of the release of many hormones following a bolus dose. Because of these limitations, a search for analogs with longer duration of action, lack of rebound effects, and narrowed spectra of action has been undertaken.

Octreotide—A Long-Acting Somatostatin Analog

One somatostatin analog, octreotide, has been studied in detail and is currently approved for clinical use in the United States. Octreotide is a cyclic octapeptide with the sequences shown in Fig. 18-1. When administered IV, it has a volume of distribution of 18 to 30 liters, a distribution half-life of 9 to 14 minutes, and an elimination half-life of 70 to 100 minutes (Kutz et al., 1986). Octreotide is rapidly and completely absorbed following subcutaneous administration, with peak concentrations occurring in 30 to 60 minutes. Its half-life following subcutaneous administration is 90 to 115 minutes, and the drug is detectable for up to 12 hours following a 1 mg/kg dose. From 30% to 40% of the drug is metabolized by the liver, 11% is excreted unchanged in the urine, and less than 2% is excreted in the feces (Kutz et al., 1986; Longnecker, 1988). The remainder of the peptide appears to undergo proteolytic degradation in the bloodstream and other tissues.

Octreotide produces almost all the effects of the native hormone, although to varying degrees. In rhesus monkeys, comparisons with somatostatin-14 showed the inhibitory effect of octreotide to be 45 times greater on GH secretion and 11 times greater on glucagon secretion, but only 1.3 times greater on insulin secretion (Bauer et al., 1982). As with the native hormone, both spontaneous and induced GH pulses are inhibited; however, there is no rebound phenomenon. Glucagon secretion is rapidly suppressed, as are basal and postprandial concentrations of insulin. Placebo-controlled studies in normal volunteers demonstrated a delayed and heightened postprandial peak in blood glucose concentrations that persisted for 4 hours after the meal. The delay in elevation of blood glucose concentrations is attributed to slowing of nutrient absorption from the gut, while insulin suppression accounts for the exaggerated peak (Fuessl et al., 1987). Postprandial pancreatic polypeptide, GI peptide, and motilin concentrations are inhibited to a greater degree than the gastrin concentration. The latter shows a rebound hypersecretion 3 to 4 hours postprandially (Fuessl et al., 1987).

Therapeutic Uses of Octreotide. Its suppressive effects on pituitary somatotrophs and various cells of the gastroenteropancreatic system make octreotide a promising agent for treatment of tumors derived from these cells. At present, however, the United States Food and Drug Administration has approved the use of octreotide in only two conditions: metastatic carcinoid tumors and tumors secreting vasoactive intestinal polypeptide (VIP).

Carcinoid tumors may secrete a variety of hormones, either singly or in combinations, and can cause a variety of endocrine syndromes. The carcinoid syndrome itself consists of cutaneous flushing, diarrhea, and hypotension sometimes associated with bronchospasm. Most of the tumors producing this syndrome arise in portions of the GI tract drained by the portal vein. Because serotonin and other tumor-derived factors are inactivated by the liver, such tumors rarely produce symptoms until extensive hepatic metastases are present. Thus, therapy in most cases is necessarily medical and palliative.

Uncontrolled studies of octreotide in the carcinoid syndrome report significant symptomatic relief, with improvement in flushing and/or diarrhea in approximately 80% of patients on doses of 100 to 600 mg/day (Battershill and Clissold, 1989). However, patients may experience recurrence of symptoms despite continued therapy. Blood concentrations of serotonin and to a lesser extent urinary excretion of 5-hydroxyindole acetic acid (5-HIAA, the major metabolite of serotonin and a marker of disease activity) decrease in the majority of patients, although not to the normal range. Studies examining octreotide's effect on tumor size have found shrinkage to be uncommon (Kvols et al., 1986; Souquet et al., 1987). The therapeutic effects of octreotide may be transient in some patients, with tumors becoming insensitive to its hormone-suppressing effects after several months of therapy.

As treatment of carcinoid tumors is palliative, control of symptoms is paramount. Given the generally slow growth of these tumors (even after metastases are present) and the incomplete evidence regarding risks of chronic octreotide administration, initial symptomatic therapy with other time-tested medications (e.g., antiadrenergic, antiserotonergic, antihistamine, and antidiarrheal) seems most appropriate. Octreotide can be used as an effective second-line agent should these fail. Patients with aggressive tumors should be considered for more aggressive therapy: hepatic artery ligation, hepatic artery embolization, and/or systemic chemotherapy (Vinik et al., 1989; Kvols, 1989).

As with carcinoid tumors, tumors secreting VIP usually are metastatic at the time of initial diagnosis. Patients present with profuse watery diarrhea, hypokalemia, hypochlorhydria, and acidosis. Octreotide in doses of 100 to 600 mg/day produces a striking and rapid reduction in stool volume, much greater than the more modest reduction in blood VIP concentrations (Wood et al., 1985; Maton et al., 1986). With prolonged therapy, some patients experience slowly increasing concentrations of VIP, and diarrhea may subsequently recur. Again, few patients have reduction in tumor size (Battershill and Clissold, 1989).

Studies of the effects of octreotide in other gastroenteropancreatic tumors, including gastrinomas, glucagonomas, and insulinomas, have similarly reported alleviation of symptoms, partial reduction in circulating hormone concentrations, diminishing effect with long-term treatment in some patients, and, infrequently, reduction in tumor size. *Principle: The degree of clinical improvement is frequently greater than the degree of suppression of target hormone concentrations, suggesting greater complexity in octreotide's mechanism(s) of action than simple inhibition of hormone release.*

Chronic hypersecretion of GH produces the clinical syndrome of acromegaly: enlargement of the hands, feet, and jaw; sweating; hypertension; glucose intolerance; arthropathy; and paraesthesias. The vast majority of cases are caused by benign pituitary adenomas. If the condition is diagnosed early, resection of the tumor can be curative. However, the insidious onset of this disease often prevents early detection, requiring additional nonsurgical therapy in many cases.

Octreotide has been studied in a large number of acromegalic patients, with generally favorable results. Many symptoms, including fatigue, sweating, headaches, and paraesthesias, respond within days. The characteristic soft tissue changes respond more slowly. Octreotide effectively suppresses concentrations of GH and insulin-like growth factor I (IGF-I, or somatomedin C, a hormone that modulates many of the effects of GH) in most patients. The peak effect on GH concentration occurs 2 to 5 hours after administration and lasts up to 10 hours. One report showed an average 64% reduction in circulating GH concentrations over 10 hours (Lamberts et al., 1985). Increasing the dose of octreotide has produced a longer duration of effect in some studies and a greater magnitude of effect in others (Lamberts and Del Pozo, 1986; George et al., 1987).

In doses of 75 to 1500 mg/day, octreotide has brought about normalization of IGF-I concentrations in approximately 50% of patients studied (Battershill and Clissold, 1989). Patients with lower pretreatment concentrations of GH generally have a better response rate (Ho et al., 1990). Modest degrees of tumor shrinkage (20%–30%) have been reported in up to one third of patients (Battershill and Clissold, 1989). While one long-term study has shown greater suppression of GH after 18 to 24 months of treatment than at 6 to 12 months (Lamberts et al., 1987), others report diminishing effectiveness with continued therapy, similar to that found in the carcinoid syndrome and VIP-secreting tumors. Rebound hypersecretion of GH may occur between doses. Continuous subcutaneous infusion of octreotide can prevent this rebound. No desensitization of its GH-inhibiting effect has been noted with continuous administration (Wilson and Hoffman, 1986). At present, octreotide cannot be considered first-line therapy for acromegaly but is a useful adjunct in patients whose acromegaly has not reponded to other modes of treatment. The patients who respond best to octreotide (low GH levels, small tumors) also have the highest rate of surgical cure and should receive surgery as the primary treatment. In surgical failures or nonsurgical patients, the use of octreotide, bromocriptine, or radiation therapy must be considered on an individual basis. *Principle: Unlike the gonadotrope, the somatotrope is not routinely desensitized in vivo by chronic exposure to its tropic or inhibiting hormones.*

The nonendocrine effects of native somatostatin have prompted investigation of the use of octreotide in a number of other conditions. Octreotide significantly reduces output from small bowel and pancreatic fistulas and promotes early closure of such fistulas (Nubiola-Calonge et al., 1987; DeBois et al., 1988). Preliminary reports suggest that octreotide may be beneficial in the treatment of upper GI bleeding from gastric or duodenal ulcers or esophageal varices. Secretory diarrhea and cryptosporidium infection (a frequent cause of diarrhea in patients with AIDS) have also responded favorably to octreotide (Katz et al., 1988). Two studies have examined octreotide in the treatment of orthostatic hypotension of various etiologies (Hoeldtke et al., 1986; Hoeldtke and Israel, 1989). Though the number of patients studied is small ($n = 8$, $n = 28$ in the two studies), about three fourths of patients had an increase in sitting postprandial or semirecumbent blood pressure following a low dose of octreotide (0.2–0.4 μg/kg). Higher doses (up to 1.6 μg/kg) yielded a dramatic effect in exercise tolerance in about half of the patients, allowing them to walk for up to 100 minutes. Adverse events in these studies included recumbent hypertension and abdominal cramping, particularly in patients with diabetic autonomic neuropathy. A few patients who did not respond to octreotide alone did improve with the combination of octreotide and dihydroergotamine.

While such reports are promising, the precise role of octreotide in the treatment of these conditions is still undefined. Recently, an increased incidence of gallstones in acromegalic patients treated with octreotide has been reported (Ho et al., 1990). This significant side effect presumably results from inhibition of cholecystokinin secretion and gallbladder contraction by octreotide, actions shared by native somatostatin. Other adverse effects of octreotide therapy include abdominal cramping, bloating, nausea, diarrhea, steatorrhea, and flatulence. Again, these effects are not surprising, given the known actions of native somatostatin in GI physiology. *Principle: Analogs of somatostatin with narrowed spectra of action to produce specific targeted actions while minimizing effects on other physiologic functions are targets of ongoing investigation.*

REFERENCES

Battershill, P. E.; and Clissold, S. P.: Octreotide. Drugs, 38: 658–702, 1989.

Bauer, W.; Briner, U.; Doepfner, W.; Haller, R.; and Huguenin, R.: SMS 201-995: A very potent and selective octapeptide analog of somatostatin with prolonged action. Life Sci., 31:1133–1140, 1982.

Belchetz, P. E. T.; Plant, T. M.; Nakai, Y.; Keough, E. J.; and Knobil, E.: Hypophyseal responses to continuous and intermittent delivery of hypothalamic gonadotropin-releasing hormone. Science, 202: 631–633, 1978.

Berelowitz, M.; LeRoith, D.; and Von Schenk, H.: Somatostatin-like immunoreactivity and biological activity is present in *Tetrahymena pyriformis*, a ciliated protozoan. Endocrinology, 110:1939–1944, 1982.

Butenandt, O.; and Staudt, B.: Comparison of growth hormone releasing therapy and growth hormone therapy in growth hormone deficiency. Eur. J. Pediatr., 148(5):393–395, 1989.

Ceda, G. P.; and Hoffman, A. R.: Growth hormone–releasing factor desensitization in rat anterior pituitary cells in vitro. Endocrinology, 116:1334–1340, 1985.

Ceda, G. P.; Davis, R. G.; Rosenfeld, R. G.; and Hoffman, A. R.: The growth hormone (GH) releasing hormone (GHRH)-GH-somatomedin axis: Evidence for rapid inhibition of GHRH-elicited GH release by insulin-like growth factors I and II. Endocrinology, 120:1658–1662, 1987.

Crawford, E. D.; Eisenberger, M. A.; McLeod, D. G.; Spaulding, J. T.; Benson, R.; Dorr, F. A.; Blumenstein, B. A.; Davis, M. A.; and Goodman, P. J.: A controlled trial of leuprolide with and without flutamide in prostatic carcinoma. N. Engl. J. Med., 321:419–424, 1989.

Crowley, W. F. Jr.; and McArthur, J. W.: Stimulation of the normal menstrual cycle in Kallmann's syndrome by pulsatile administration of luteinizing hormone–releasing hormone (LHRH). J. Clin. Endocrinol. Metab., 51:173–175, 1980.

DeBois, M. H. W.; Bosman, C. H. R.; DeGraaf, P.; and Van Hoogenhuijze, J.: Closure of a high-output pancreatic fistula by SMS 201-995, a long-acting analog of somatostatin. Neth. J. Med., 32:293–297, 1988.

Evans, W. S.; Vance, M. L.; Kaiser, D. L.; Sellers, R. P.; Borges, J. L. C.; Downs, T. R.; Frohman, L. A.; Rivier, J.; Vale, W.; and Thorner, M. O.: Effects of intravenous, subcutaneous, and intranasal administration of growth hormone–releasing hormone-40 on serum GH concentrations in normal men. J. Clin. Endocrinol. Metab., 61:846–850, 1985.

Fuessl, H. S.; Burrin, J. M.; Williams, G.; Adrian, T. E.; and Bloom, S. R.: The effect of a long-acting somatostatin analog (SMS 201-995) on intermediary metabolism and gut hormones after a test meal in normal subjects. Aliment. Pharmacol. Ther., 1:321–330, 1987.

Gelato, M. C.; Malozowski, S.; Pescovitz, O. H.; Cassorla, F.; Loriaux, D. L.; and Merriam, G. R.: Growth hormone–releasing hormone: Therapeutic perspectives. Pediatrician, 14:162–167, 1987.

Gelato, M. C.; Rittmaster, R. S.; Pescovitz, O. H.; Nicoletti, M. C.; Nixon, W. E.; D'Agata, R.; Loriaux, D. L.; and Merriam, G. R.: GH responses to continuous infusions of growth hormone–releasing hormone. J. Clin. Endocrinol. Metab., 61:223–228, 1985.

George, S. R.; Hegele, R. A.; and Burrow, G. N.: The somatostatin analog SMS 201-995 in acromegaly: Prolonged, preferential suppression of growth hormone but not pancreatic hormones. Clin. Invest. Med., 10:309–315, 1987.

Gespach, C.; Dupont, C.; Bataille, D.; and Rosseling, G.: Selective inhibition by somatostatin of cyclic AMP production in rat gastric glands. FEBS Lett., 114:247–252, 1980.

Ghigo, E.; Goffi, S.; Mazza, E.; Arvat, E.; Procopio, M.; Bellone, J.; Muller, E.; and Camanni, F.: Repeated GH-releasing hormone administration unravels different GH secretory patterns in normal adults and children. Acta Endocrinol., 120:598–601, 1989.

Hall, R.; Schally, A. V.; and Evered, D.: Action of growth

hormone release inhibitory hormone in healthy men and acromegaly. Lancet, 2:581–584, 1973.

Handelsman, D. J.; and Swerdloff, R. S.: Pharmacokinetics of gonadotropin-releasing hormone and its analogs. Endocr. Rev., 7:95–105, 1986.

Healy, D. L.; Lawson, S. R.; Abbott, M.; Baird, D. T.; and Fraser, H. M.: Toward removing uterine fibroids without surgery: Subcutaneous infusion of a luteinizing hormone-releasing hormone agonist commencing in the luteal phase. J. Clin. Endocrinol. Metab., 63:619–625, 1986.

Ho, K. Y.; Weissberger, A. J.; Marbach, P.; and Lazarus, L.: Therapeutic efficacy of the somatostatin analog SMS 201-995 in acromegaly. Ann. Intern. Med., 112:173–181, 1990.

Hoeldtke, R. D.; and Israel, B. C.: Treatment of orthostatic hypotension with octreotide. J. Clin. Endocrinol. Metab. (United States), 68(6):1051–1059, 1989.

Hoeldtke, R. D.; O'Dorisio, T. M.; and Boden, G.: Treatment of autonomic neuropathy with a somatostatin analogue SMS-201-995. Lancet, 2(8507):602–605, 1986.

Hoffman, A. R.: Fertility induction in hypothalamic hypogonadism. Ann. Intern. Med., 102:643–657, 1985.

Hoffman, A. R.; and Crowley, W. F. Jr.: Induction of puberty in men by long-term pulsatile administration of low dose gonadotropin-releasing hormone. N. Engl. J. Med., 307:1237–1241, 1982.

Hulse, J. A.; Rosenthal, S. M.; Cuttler, L.; Kaplan, S. L.; and Grumbach, M. M.: The effect of pulsatile administration, continuous infusion, and diurnal variation on the GH response to growth hormone–releasing hormone in normal men. J. Clin. Endocrinol. Metab., 63:872–878, 1986.

Karten, M. J.; and Rivier, J. E.: Gonadotropin-releasing hormone analog design. Structure-function studies toward the development of agonists and antagonists: Rationale and perspective. Endocr. Rev., 7:44–66, 1986.

Katz, M. D.; Erstad, B. L.; and Rose, C.: Treatment of severe cryptosporidium-related diarrhea with octreotide in a patient with AIDS. Drug Intell. Clin. Pharm., 22:134–136, 1988.

Knobil, E.: The neuroendocrine control of the menstrual cycle. Recent Prog. Horm. Res., 36:53–88, 1980.

Krulich, L.; Dhariwal, A. P. S.; and McCann, S. M.: Stimulatory and inhibitory effects of purified hypothalamic extracts on growth hormone release from rat pituitary in vitro. Endocrinology, 83:783–790, 1968.

Kutz, K.; Nuesch, E.; and Rosenthaler, J.: Pharmacokinetics of SMS 201-995 in healthy subjects. Scand. J. Gastroenterol., 21(suppl. 119):65–72, 1986.

Kvols, L. K.: Therapy of the malignant carcinoid syndrome. Endocrinol. Metab. Clin. North Am. (United States) 18(2):557–568. 1989.

Kvols, L. K.; Moertel, C. G.; O'Connell, M. J.; Schutt, A. J.; and Rubin, J.: Treatment of the malignant carcinoid syndrome: Evaluation of a long-acting somatostatin analog. N. Engl. J. Med., 315:663–666, 1986.

Lamberts, S. W. J.; and Del Pozo, E.: Acute and long-term effects of SMS 201-995 in acromegaly. Scand. J. Gastroenterol., 21(suppl. 119):141–148, 1986.

Lamberts, S. W. J.; Uitterlinden, P.; and Del Pozo, E.: SMS 201-995 induces a continuous decline in circulating growth hormone and somatomedin-C levels during therapy of acromegalic patients for over two years. J. Clin. Endocrinol. Metab., 65:703–710, 1987.

Lamberts, S. W. J.; Oosterom, R.; Neufeld, M.; and Del Pozo, E.: The somatostatin analog SMS 201-995 induces long-acting inhibition of growth hormone secretion without rebound hypersecretion in acromegalic patients. J. Clin. Endocrinol. Metab., 60:1161–1165, 1985.

The Leuprolide Study Group: Leuprolide versus diethylstilbestrol for metastatic prostate cancer. N. Engl. J. Med., 311:1281–1286, 1984.

Longnecker, S. M.: Somatostatin and octreotide: Literature review and description of therapeutic activity in pancreatic neoplasia. Drug Intell. Clin. Pharm., 22:99–106, 1988.

Low, L. C.; Wang, C.; Cheung, P. T.; Ho, P.; Lam, K. S.;

Young, R. T.; Yeung, C. Y.; and Ling, N.: Long term pulsatile growth hormone (GH)-releasing hormone therapy in children with GH deficiency. J. Clin. Endocrinol. Metab., 66:611–617,1988.

Martha, P. M.; Blizzard, R. M.; Mc Donald, J. A.; Thorner, M. O.; and Rogol, A. D.: A persistent pattern of varying pituitary responsivity to exogenous growth hormone–releasing hormone in GH-deficient children: Evidence supporting periodic somatostatin secretion. J. Clin. Endocrinol. Metab., 67:449–454, 1988.

Mason, A. J.; Hayflick, J. S.; Zoeller, R. T.; Young, W. S.; Phillips, H. S.; Nikolics, K.; and Seeburg, P. H.: A deletion truncating the gonadotropin-releasing hormone gene is responsible for hypogonadism in the hpg mouse. Science, 234:1366–1371, 1986.

Maton, P. N.; O'Dorisio, T. M.; O'Dorisio, M. S.; Malarkey, W. B.; and Gower, W. R.: Successful therapy of pancreatic cholera with the long-acting somatostatin analog SMS 201-995: Relation between plasma concentrations of drug and clinical and biochemical responses. Scand. J. Gastroenterol., 21(suppl. 119):181–186, 1986.

Meldrum, D. R.; Chang, R. J.; Lu, J.; Vale, W.; Rivier, J.; and Judd, H. L.: "Medical oophorectomy" using a long-acting GnRH agonist – a possible new approach to the treatment of endometriosis. J. Clin. Endocrinol. Metab., 54:1081–1083, 1982.

Nubiola-Calonge, P.; Sancho, J.; Segura, M.; Badia, J. M.; and Cril, M. J.: Blind evaluation of the effect of octreotide on small bowel fistula output. Lancet, 2:672–674, 1987.

Pavlou, S. N.; Wakefield, G.; Schlechter, N. L.; Lindner, J.; Souza, K. H.; Kamilaris, T. C.; Konidaris, S.; Rivier, J. E.; Vale, W. W.; and Toglia, M.: Mode of suppression of pituitary and gonadal function after acute or prolonged administration of a luteinizing hormone–releasing hormone antagonist in normal men. J. Clin. Endocrinol. Metab., 68:446–454, 1989.

Pescovitz, O. H.; Comite, F.; Hench, K.; Barnes, K.; McNemar, A.; Foster, C.; Kenigsberg, D.; Loriaux, D. L.; and Cutler, G. B.: The NIH experience with precocious puberty: Diagnostic subgroups and response to short-term luteinizing hormone–releasing hormone analogue therapy. J. Pediatr., 108:47–54, 1986.

Peters, C. A.; and Walsh, P. C.: The effect of nafarelin acetate, a luteinizing-hormone-releasing hormone agonist, on benign prostatic hyperplasia. N. Engl. J. Med., 317:599–604, 1987.

Prange-Hansen, A.; Orskov, H.; Seyer-Hansen, K.; and Lundbaek, K.: Some actions of growth hormone release inhibiting factor. Br. Med. J., 3:523–524, 1973.

Reichlin, S.: Somatostatin. N. Engl. J. Med., 309:1495–1501, 1556–1563, 1983.

Rizza, R.; Verdonk, C.; and Miles, J.: Somatostatin does not cause sustained fasting hyperglycemia in man. Horm. Metab. Res., 11:643–644, 1979.

Rochiccioli, P. E.; Tauber, M. T.; Uboldi, F.; Coude, F. X.; Morre, M.: Effect of overnight constant infusion of human growth hormone releasing hormone (1-44) on 24 hour GH secretion in children with partial GH deficiency. J. Clin. Endocrinol. Metab., 63:1100–1105, 1986.

Ross, R. J.; Rodda, C.; Tsagarakis, S.; Davies, P. S.; Grossman, A.; Rees, L. H.; Preece, M. A.; Savage, M. O.; and Besser, G. M.: Treatment of growth-hormone deficiency with growth-hormone-releasing hormone. Lancet, 1(8523):5–8, 1987.

Sassolas, G.; Garry, J.; Cohen, R.; Bastuji, H.; Vermeulen, E.; Cabrera, P.; Roussel, B.; and Jouvet, M.: Nocturnal continuous infusion of growth hormone–releasing hormone results in a dose-dependent accentuation of episodic GH secretion in normal men. J. Clin. Endocrinol. Metab., 63:1016–1022, 1986.

Souquet, J.; Sassolas, G.; Forichon, J.; Champetier, P.; and Partensky, C.: Clinical and hormonal effects of a long-acting somatostatin analog in pancreatic endocrine tumors and in carcinoid syndrome. Cancer, 59:1654–1660, 1987.

Thorner, M. O.; Rogol, A. D.; Blizzard, R. M.; Klingensmith, G. J.; Najjar, J.; Misra, R.; Burr, I.; Chao, G.; Martha, P.; McDonald, J.; Pezzoli, S.; Chitwood, J.; Furlanetto, R.; River, J.; Vale, W.; Smith, P.; and Brook, C.: Acceleration of growth rate in growth hormone–deficient children treated with growth hormone–releasing hormone. Pediatr. Res., 24: 1245–1251, 1988.

Toro, M. J.; Birnbaumer, L.; Redonm, M. C.; and Montoya, C.: Mechanism of action of somatostatin. Horm. Res., 29: 59–64, 1988.

Vance, M. L.; Kaiser, D. L.; Evans, W. S.; Furlanetto, R.; Vale, W.; Rivier, J.; and Thorner, M. O.: Pulsatile GH secretion in normal man during a continuous 24-hour infusion of human growth hormone releasing factor (1-40). J. Clin. Invest., 75:1584–1590, 1985.

Veber, D. F.; Freidinger, R. M.; and Schwenk-Perlow, D.: A potent cyclic hexapeptide analog of somatostatin. Nature, 292:55–58, 1981.

Vickery, B.: Comparison of the potential for therapeutic utilities with gonadotropin-releasing hormone agonists and antagonist. Endocr. Rev., 7:115–124, 1986.

Vinik, A. I.; McLeod, M. K.; Fig, L. M.; Shapiro, B.; Lloyd, R. V.; and Cho, K.: Clinical features, diagnosis, and localization of carcinoid tumors and their management. Gastroenterol. Clin. North Am. (United States), 18(4):865–896, 1989.

Wass, J. A. H.: Somatostatin. In, Endocrinology, 2nd ed. (DeGroot, L. J., ed.). W. B. Saunders, Philadelphia, pp. 152–166, 1989.

Weeke, J.; Hansen, A. P.; and Lundbaek, K.: Inhibition by somatostatin of basal levels of serum thyrotropin (TSH) in normal men. J. Clin. Endocrinol. Metab., 41:168–171, 1975.

Weeke, J.; Hansen, A. P.; and Lundbaek, K.: The inhibition by somatostatin of the thyrotropin response to thyrotropin-releasing hormone in normal subjects. Scand. J. Clin. Lab Invest., 33:101–103, 1974.

Wehrenberg, W. B.; Brazeau, P.; Luben, R.; Bohlen, P.; and Guillemin, R.: Inhibition of the pulsatile secretion of GH by monoclonal antibodies to the hypothalamic growth hormone releasing factor (GRF). Endocrinology, 111:2147–2148, 1982.

Wilson, D. M.; and Hoffman, A. R.: Reduction of pituitary size by the somatostatin analog SMS 201-995 in a patient with an islet cell tumor secreting growth hormone releasing factor. Acta Endocrinol., 113:23–28, 1986.

Wood, S. M.; Kraenzlin, S. E.; Adrian, T. E.; and Bloom, S. R.: Treatment of patients with pancreatic endocrine tumors using a new long-acting somatostatin analog: Symptomatic and peptide responses. Gut, 26:438–444, 1985.

19

Rheumatic Disorders

Elliot Ehrich, R. Elaine Lambert, and James L. McGuire

PATHOGENESIS OF IMMUNE-MEDIATED RHEUMATIC DISEASES

The pathogenic mechanisms that result in autoimmune disease are incompletely defined. Investigation into specific components of the immune response at different phases of the disease has elucidated pathological steps that contribute to cell injury and organ dysfunction.

The interaction of antigen with either an antibody or a human leukocyte antigen (HLA) recognition molecule of an antigen-presenting cell is the primary triggering event in the immune response. These interactions are understood to initiate mechanisms of immunologically mediated diseases (McDermott and McDevitt, 1988). In the case of allergy, the foreign antigen often is known and the IgE antibody response to it well characterized. In autoimmune disorders, including rheumatoid arthritis and systemic lupus erythematosus (SLE), the initiating antigens, whether self or foreign, are essentially unknown. In addition to antigenic stimulus, genetic susceptibility alleles (e.g., HLA type), environmental factors, and hormonal milieu are important determinants of disease expression. The diversity of susceptibility factors limits prognostic and therapeutic generalizations because of variability among individual patients. It is of note that successful therapies for many rheumatic diseases were discovered empirically with little knowledge of basic disease mechanisms. Indeed, it is challenging to explain efficacy of existing therapies in light of a growing understanding of the immune response. *Principle: As the pharmacologic effects of empirically efficacious drugs are revealed, elements of the pathophysiology of the diseases they ameliorate may be revealed.*

Rheumatoid Arthritis

Rheumatoid arthritis is a destructive joint disease that is often accompanied by a variety of extraarticular features. The etiology of rheumatoid arthrits is not known, but activation of T and B cells, presumably in response to an antigen, occurs early in the disease (Harris, 1990). Genetically determined factors, including HLA subtypes DR1 and DR4, may play critical roles in this response and ultimately may enable clinicians to predict the severity or susceptibility to disease.

Within the joint lining (synovium) of rheumatoid arthritis patients, an intensely proliferative lymphocytic inflammatory infiltrate develops. Synovial macrophages and fibroblasts proliferate and secrete proteolytic enzymes such as collagenase and stromelysin. Macrophages and lymphocytes secrete cytokines, including interleukin-1 and tumor necrosis factor, both of which stimulate an array of cellular responses that perpetuate the disease. The synovial fluid is highly cellular with a predominance of neutrophils. In the later stages of disease, irreversible destruction of cartilage and bony erosions are prominent.

Systemic Lupus Erythematosus

Systemic lupus erythematosus (SLE) is a variable multisystem disorder that is characterized by rash, arthritis, mucositis, nephritis, serositis, cytopenias, and cerebritis. Though the initiating events or inciting antigens in susceptible individuals are unknown, complement deficiencies (C2, C4) and the presence of HLA-DR2 and HLA-DR3 as well as exposure to ultraviolet light, infectious agents, and certain drugs have been identified with risk of development of disease. Early pathogenic events are associated with B-cell hyperactivity and autoantibody production, particularly antinuclear antibodies. Immune complexes are deposited or formed in blood vessels and other tissues, which presumably accounts for many of the clinical manifestations of SLE.

Vasculitis

Vasculitis is a broad term signifying inflammation within and surrounding blood vessels. Vasculitis can occur as part of a multisystem rheumatic disorder such as SLE or rheumatoid arthritis, or exist as a primary disorder. Classified by size of involved vessels (small, medium, or large), several clinical syndromes have been characterized (Conn, 1990). Immune complexes have been implicated in the pathogenesis of fibrinoid necrosis, granulomas, and giant cell reactions that are observed within the vessel wall in various forms of vasculitis. The antigen bound within the immune complex is known for only a few types of vasculitis. These include hepatitis B and certain drug-induced vasculitides.

Drug-Induced Immune Disease

Drug-induced immune disease is caused by one or another of two principal pathologic mechanisms. Drugs can act as a foreign antigen that incites a direct immune response. Clinical expression of this type of process may include anaphylaxis and vasculitis. Alternatively, drugs can induce alterations of endogenous macromolecules so that they become antigenic to the host immune system. Drug-induced lupus erythematosus (DILE) is thought to be induced by this mechanism (McGuire and Lambert, in press). Most commonly, DILE presents with pleuropericarditis, rash, and/or arthritis. Involvement of the kidneys and CNS is distinctly uncommon. Many patients taking DILE-inducing drugs develop a positive antinuclear antibody (ANA) in the absence of clinical symptoms. Hydralazine and procainamide are the drugs most frequently associated with DILE. Other drugs implicated in DILE are listed in Table 19-1. Complete reversal of the disease usually occurs following discontinuation of the offending drug, although exceptions have been reported.

Table 19-1. MEDICATIONS ASSOCIATED WITH DRUG-INDUCED LUPUS ERYTHEMATOSUS

DEFINITE ASSOCIATION	POSSIBLE ASSOCIATION	
Procainamide	Acebutolol	Metoprolol
Hydralazine	Atenolol	Nitrofurantoin
Chlorpromazine	Captopril	Penicillamine
Isoniazid	Carbamazepine	Phenylbutazone
Methyldopa	Ethosuximide	Phenytoin
	Labetolol	Primadone
	L-Dopa	Propylthiouracil
	Lithium	Quinidine
	Mephenytoin	Trimethadione

Reproduced with permission from McGuire and Lambert, in press.

DRUGS USED TO TREAT IMMUNE-MEDIATED RHEUMATIC DISEASES

The drugs that are most commonly used in the management of rheumatoid arthritis, SLE, vasculitis, and DILE are reviewed in this section. Though antirheumatic drugs demonstrate a variety of immunomodulatory properties, the precise mechanism of their clinical benefit in immune-mediated rheumatic diseases remains largely unknown. Moreover, study of the immunologic effects of these agents in rheumatic diseases is complicated by underlying immune abnormalities that are inherent in these diseases. Nonsteroidal anti-inflammatory drugs (NSAIDs) are frequently used in the treatment of rheumatic diseases. The clinical pharmacology of NSAIDs is discussed in detail in chapter 20.

Gold

Elemental gold was used in ancient times as a topical agent for skin disorders. Koch (1890) observed that gold cyanide inhibits the growth of *Mycobacterium tuberculosis*. Since rheumatoid arthritis was believed at that time to be a manifestation of tuberculosis or a related infectious process, chrysotherapy was attempted. Forestier (1935) reported a favorable response in 70% to 80% of 550 patients with polyarthritis and is generally recognized as the pioneer of gold therapy for rheumatoid arthritis.

Parenteral gold compounds are water-soluble and contain the monovalent aurous ion (Au^+) stabilized by attachment to a sulfur-containing ligand. Gold sodium thiomalate (GST) and aurothioglucose (ATG) are the two most commonly used parenteral compounds in North America. Both are approximately 50% gold by weight and are administered IM. Despite differences in their chemical composition, GST and ATG are generally indistinguishable in terms of their distribution, biologic activity, and clinical efficacy. The ATG is prepared as a sesame oil suspension whereas GST is available as an aqueous solution.

Despite the widespread use of gold as a disease-modifying agent in rheumatoid arthritis, its mechanisms of action are poorly understood. Gold is present in high concentration in monocytes and macrophages, including synovial macrophages, where it is sequestered within lysosomal-like bodies termed *aurosomes* (Ghadially et al., 1978). Several pharmacologic effects of gold compounds are known, though the explicit role of each in modifying disease activity in rheumatoid arthritis is unclear. These include (1) inhibition of lysosomal enzymes (Ennis et al., 1968; Persellin and Ziff, 1966), (2) inhibition of macrophage and polymorphonuclear leukocyte phagocytic function (Jessop et al., 1973), (3) deactivation of superoxide free radicals (Corey et al., 1987), (4) reduction of immune globulins, including rheumatoid factor (Gottlieb et al., 1975), (5) inactivation of C1 in the classic complement pathway (Schultz et al., 1974), (6) inhibition of the amplification loop of the alternative complement pathway (Burge et al., 1978), and (7) inhibition of antigen- and mitogen-induced lymphocyte proliferation (Lipsky and Ziff, 1977).

After a single IM injection of GST (50 mg), a peak serum concentration of about 700 mg/dl is reached within 2 hours (Gottlieb et al., 1974). The ATG has a slower absorption rate and lower peak serum concentration because of its oil-based vehicle. The concentration then declines to half the peak value over 7 days. With continued weekly administration, serum gold concentrations plateau after 6 to 8 weeks. Gold is slowly eliminated in the urine and feces (Gottlieb and Gray, 1981). After termination of treatment, traces of gold in the serum can be detected for at least a year.

Gold therapy is typically initiated with successive weekly doses of 10 and 25 mg, followed by 50 mg for 20 weeks or until major clinical improvement has occurred. Dosing intervals may then be lengthened if the clinical response is maintained. Maintenance gold therapy may be continued indefinitely.

The incidence of toxicity from parenteral gold compounds is high. During a standard 20-injection course of gold, approximately 35% of patients experience adverse effects. About 15% of patients require discontinuation of the gold because of the severity of adverse effects (Richter et al., 1980). The most common complications are minor and consist primarily of localized dermatitis or stomatitis (accounting for 60%–80% of all adverse reactions), and transient hematuria or mild proteinuria. The most serious adverse effect is bone marrow aplasia, which can be fatal but fortunately is quite rare (see Table 19–2). Membranous glomerulonephritis with nephrotic syndrome occurs in 0.2% to 2.6% of patients but has a good prognosis for full recovery (Silverberg et al., 1970). Vasomotor reactions are observed within 5 to 10 minutes following injection, whereas a postinjection inflammatory flare with transient arthralgias, myalgias, and malaise may appear within 6 to 24 hours. Vasomotor reactions and inflammatory flare occur less commonly with ATG, probably because of its slower rate of absorption.

Most toxicities induced by parenteral gold, if detected early, can be managed by discontinuing the drug. Evidence for toxicity should be evaluated before every injection. This should include regular monitoring of complete blood count and urinalysis (see Table 19–3). A flow-sheet record of these values should be maintained for each patient. Mild or local rashes may be managed with topical corticosteroids, but a generalized rash requires discontinuation of therapy. Proteinuria of greater than 800 mg per 24 hours or hematologic abnormalities also necessitate immediate

Table 19–2. TOXICITIES ASSOCIATED WITH PARENTERAL GOLD COMPOUNDS

Mucocutaneous:	Stomatitis, pruritus, dermatitis (typically discrete pruritic lesions located in cutaneous folds), urticaria, exfoliative dermatitis, toxic epidermal neurolysis, trophic nail changes with yellow discoloration, gray or blue skin discoloration, alopecia, photosensitivity
Postinjection reactions:	Vasomotor or nitritoid reaction (weakness, dizziness, nausea, vomiting, sweating, flushing, palpitations, malaise, hypotension), anaphylaxis, syncope, myalgias, arthralgias
Renal:	Proteinuria, hematuria, nephrotic syndrome, membranous glomerulonephritis, renal insufficiency
Hematologic:	Eosinophilia, thrombocytopenia, granulocytopenia, lymphocytopenia, hypogammaglobulinemia, pancytopenia, aplastic anemia
Pulmonary:	Diffuse pulmonary infiltrates, interstitial fibrosis, acute respiratory distress syndrome
Gastrointestinal:	Metallic taste, enterocolitis (diarrhea, abdominal pain, nausea, vomiting, fever), cholestatic jaundice, elevated transaminase and alkaline phosphatase concentrations
Neurologic:	Headache, myokymia, peripheral and cranial neuropathies, encephalopathy
Ocular:	Corneal or lens chrysiasis (benign)

Table 19–3.   DRUG-MONITORING SCHEDULES*

A. *NSAIDs*
   Initial: CBC, Cr, U/A, K^+, ASAT every 1–3 months
   Stable: CBC, Cr, U/A, K^+, ASAT every 3–12 months†

B. *Gold Salts (injectable)*
   Initial: CBC, platelet count or estimate; U/A every 1–2 weeks
   Stable: CBC; platelet count or estimate; U/A every other injection, no less than once per month

C. *Gold Salts (oral)*
   Initial: CBC, platelet count or estimate, U/A every 2 weeks
   Stable: CBC, platelet count or estimate, U/A every 4 weeks

D. *Penicillamine*
   Initial: CBC, platelet count, U/A every 1–2 weeks
   Stable: CBC, platelet count, U/A every 4–6 weeks; CK every 4–6 months

E. *Antimalarials*
   Initial: Baseline eye exam before or during first month
   Stable: CBC, eye exam every 6 months

F. *Azathioprine*
   Initial: CBC, platelet count or estimate every 1–2 weeks, LFTs every 6–12 weeks
   Stable: CBC, platelet count or estimate every 1–3 months, LFTs every 3–6 months

G. *Methotrexate*
   Initial: CBC, platelet count or estimate every 1–2 weeks, LFTs every 2–4 weeks, Cr every 3–12 months
   Stable: CBC, platelet count or estimate every month, LFTs every 1–3 months, Cr every 3–12 months, CXR every 6–12 months

H. *Cyclophosphamide*
   Initial: CBC, platelet count or estimate, U/A every 1–2 weeks
   Stable: CBC, platelet count or estimate, U/A every month

I. *Corticosteroids*
   Low–dose (10 mg/day prednisone): As needed for signs and symptoms
   High–dose (30 mg/day prednisone): CBC, K^+, glucose every 1–3 months

---

* CBC = complete blood count, CXR = chest x-ray, ASAT = serum aspartamine aminotransferase, LFTs = liver function tests (serum bilirubin, alanine and aspartamine aminotransferase, alkaline phosphatase), Cr = serum creatinine, U/A = urinalysis, CK = serum creatine kinase, K^+ = serum potassium.
† During continuous treatment with unchanging dosage.
Reproduced with permission from Campbell and Wilske, 1986, p. 24.

cessation of gold therapy (Lorber, 1985). Systemic corticosteroids may ameliorate gold-induced rashes, nephrosis, and pulmonary toxicity. Because of the prolonged excretion of gold compounds after chronic administration, many toxic effects may continue weeks to months after therapy is stopped. Gold therapy should be avoided in patients with a history of bone marrow depression or renal insufficiency. However, patients with rheumatoid arthritis and Felty syndrome with disease-induced neutropenia generally tolerate chrysotherapy without increased rates of toxicity.

A major inconvenience of gold therapy had been the need for parenteral administration. Consequently, an orally active gold compound was sought and developed. Auranofin is approximately 29% gold by weight and is lipid-soluble compared with its water-soluble parenteral counterparts.

Auranofin has anti-inflammatory and immunomodulatory properties that differ from those of other gold compounds. These include reduction in extracellular release of lysosomal enzymes (DiMartino et al., 1974) and interference with the release of mediators in hypersensitivity reactions (Walz et al., 1976). The reasons for distinct pharmacologic properties in auranofin are not well understood (Blocka and Paulus, 1987).

Approximately 25% of auranofin is absorbed from the GI tract. The mean terminal half-life of auranofin is about 26 days. Elimination of absorbed auranofin is similar to that of parenteral gold compounds.

Auranofin has a lower incidence of adverse effects compared with parenteral gold compounds (Todd, 1987). Despite the lower toxicity, patients who have had serious toxicities from parenteral gold should not receive auranofin. The most common adverse reaction is diarrhea or loose stools that may occur in up to 40% of patients but necessitates discontinuation in only 3%. Other GI toxicities include nausea, vomiting, anorexia, and abdominal cramps. These adverse effects are related to the poor GI absorption of auranofin. Rash, stomatitis, and conjunctivitis are common but rarely require cessation of therapy. Rare toxicities include alopecia, proteinuria, microscopic hematuria, thrombocytopenia, leukopenia, metallic taste, aplastic anemia, cholestatic jaundice, and interstitial pneumonitis. In a retrospective review of 3082 patients, only 11% discontinued auranofin due to adverse effects (Blodgett et al., 1984). *Principle: The strategy for discontinuation of a drug with a long half-life is to do so as quickly as seems reasonable. The longer the drug is given up to the time of steady state, the longer it will take for the adverse effect to reverse. The strategy for discontinuation should be clear and objective before therapy is initiated.*

Antimalarials

In 1820, Pelletier and Caventau isolated the active ingredients of quinine and cinchonine from the bark of the Peruvian cinchona tree. Extracts of the bark had been used to treat fevers and, in particular, malaria (Webster, 1985). The antirheumatic properties of antimalarial drugs were first reported by Payne (1894), who found quinine to be effective in treating skin lesions of lupus, and later by Page (1951) in the treatment of rheumatoid arthritis. Chloroquine and hydroxychloroquine are the two derivatives of quinine that are still used clinically.

Although the mechanisms responsible for the antirheumatic effects of antimalarial drugs are unknown, these agents have a multitude of actions, such as to (1) decrease production of prostaglandin because of inhibition of phospholipase A_2, (2) interfere with lysosomal enzyme function, (3) inhibit nucleic acid biosynthesis, (4) inhibit polymorphonuclear cell chemotaxis and phagocytosis, (5) inhibit platelet aggregation, (6) interfere with macrophage and lymphocyte function, (7) interfere with immune complex formation, and (8) absorb ultraviolet light (Wickens and Paulus, 1987; Rynes, 1989). Theoretically, all these effects could contribute to the clinical benefits of the drug.

After oral administration, antimalarials are rapidly and completely absorbed (Page, 1951). Concentrations increase until steady state is reached in 3 to 4 weeks. Plateau concentrations in plasma may be reached more quickly by giving twice the anticipated maintenance dose within the first week. Antimalarials are concentrated in the intracellular compartment of all tissues. Chloroquine is detectable in urine up to 119 days following a single 300-mg dose (Gustafsson et al., 1983).

In humans, hydroxychloroquine has been found to be about half as toxic as chloroquine on a weight basis (Scherbel et al., 1958). This finding, as well as reports that chloroquine-induced retinopathy can begin or progress after discontinuation of the drug (Bruns, 1966), has led to the preference for use of hydroxychloroquine in countries such as Canada, Australia, and the United States. The incidence of untoward adverse effects varies widely depending on daily dose. Gastrointestinal upset and rash are uncommon adverse effects (see Table 19-4). Retinal pigment deposition, the most feared toxicity of the antimalarials, is related to total daily dose. The daily dose of hydroxychloroquine and chloroquine is therefore limited to 400 and 250 mg, respectively. Ophthalmologic monitoring should be performed every 6 months. If changes in retinal pigmentation or visual field are detected, the drug should be discontinued or dosage reduced with frequent repeated ophthalmologic testing to determine the progress of the lesion (Easterbrook, 1988).

Sulfasalazine

Sulfasalazine is a conjugate of 5-aminosalicylic acid linked by an azo bond to sulfapyridine.

Table 19-4. TOXICITIES OF ANTIMALARIAL DRUGS

GI:	Anorexia, bloating, cramps, nausea, vomiting, diarrhea, weight loss
Skin and Hair:	Alopecia, bleaching of hair, dryness of skin, skin pigmentation (especially sun-exposed areas), pruritus, rash, exacerbation of psoriasis
Ocular:	Corneal deposits, diplopia, defects in accommodation, loss of corneal reflex, retinopathy (decrease in visual acuity, color vision, or visual field testing)
Neuromuscular:	Neuromyopathy (muscle weakness and diminished deep tendon reflexes), nervousness, insomnia, headache, confusion, ototoxicity, myasthenic reaction, tardive dyskinesia
Others:	Blood dyscrasias, hemolytic anemia with glucose-6-phosphate dehydrogenase deficiency, birth defects, exacerbation of porphyria

Svartz and colleagues synthesized the drug in the 1930s as a treatment for rheumatoid arthritis, which at the time was thought to be a granulomatous disease with a probable infectious cause (Hirschburg and Paulus, 1987). With its antibacterial and anti-inflammatory constituents, sulfasalazine has many pharmacologic properties and possible mechanisms of action (see Table 19-5). In inflammatory bowel disease, the 5-aminosalicylate is likely the active moiety. It also is therapeutically as effective as sulfasalazine and more effective than sulfapyridine (Klotz et al., 1980). In rheumatoid arthritis, however, sulfapyridine appears to be the active component (Neumann et al., 1986).

To minimize gastric irritation, enteric coated tablets of sulfasalazine are the preferred formulation. The azo bond in sulfasalazine is reduced by intestinal bacteria. Peak concentrations of

Table 19-5. POSTULATED MECHANISMS OF ACTION OF SUFASALAZINE

Alteration of action of enteric microbial agents
Inhibition of folate absorption and metabolism[a]
Inhibition of prostaglandin synthesis and degradation[b]
Reduction of leukotriene production[c]
Inhibition of leukocyte mobility[d]
Inhibition of mast cell degranulation[e]
Decrease in circulating activated lymphocytes[f]
Scavenging of oxidants[g]
Reduction in B-cell galactotransferase activity[h]

[a] Selhub et al., 1978.
[b] Stenson and Lobos, 1983.
[c] Hoult and Moore, 1980.
[d] Rhodes et al., 1981.
[e] Barrett et al., 1985.
[f] Symmons et al., 1988.
[g] Aruoma et al., 1987.
[h] Axford et al., 1987.

Table 19-6. ADVERSE REACTIONS ATTRIBUTED TO SULFASALAZINE

GI:	Nausea, vomiting, indigestion, abdominal discomfort or cramps, diarrhea, flatulence, anorexia, stomatitis
CNS:	Irritability, headache, dizziness, depression, confusion, vertigo, insomnia, ataxia, hearing loss, tinnitus, seizures, peripheral neuropathy
Pulmonary:	Allergic interstitial pneumonitis, fibrosing alveolitis, bronchospasm
Mucocutaneous:	Nonspecific drug rash, urticaria, bluish discoloration of the skin
Hematologic:	Neutropenia, agranulocytosis, aplastic anemia, macrocytosis, megaloblastic anemia in folate deficiency, thrombocytopenia, hemolytic anemia with glucose-6-phosphate dehydrogenase deficiency, methemoglobinemia
Hypersensitivity or autoimmune reactions:	Stevens–Johnson syndrome, toxic epidermal necrolysis, hepatitis with immune complex formation, photosensitization, arthralgia, polyarteritis nodosa, lupuslike disease, pancreatitis, lymphadenopathy
Other:	Male infertility (reversible)

sulfapyridine occur in 3 to 5 hours. The half-life is about 6 hours (Kimberly and Plotz, 1989). Sulfapyradine undergoes acetylation in the liver (Das and Dubin, 1976). Slow acetylators have a higher incidence of adverse effects (Das et al., 1973) (see chapter 32).

Adverse reactions attributed to sulfasalazine are listed in Table 19-6. Most will occur in the first 3 months of drug use. Gastrointestinal distress is the most common, occurring in up to one third of patients. Treatment is initiated at 500 mg/day with a gradual increase to 2 to 3 g/day over several weeks. This gradual increase in dose enhances patient tolerance with regard to GI adverse effects.

Penicillamine

Penicillamine is a five carbon sulfhydryl amino acid structural analog of cysteine that initially was derived from penicillin by acid hydrolysis. More recently, penicillamine is synthetically prepared in the preferable D-isomer form. It was initally demonstrated to be clinically useful as a copper-chelating agent in Wilson disease (Walshe, 1956). Subsequently, Jaffe (1965) discovered that penicillamine lowers the titer of rheumatoid factor and also has beneficial effects on clinical and laboratory markers of disease activity in patients with rheumatoid arthritis.

The aminothiol group of penicillamine is largely responsible for its biochemical activities that include (1) chelation of copper and other divalent cations (Walshe, 1956), (2) thiazolidine binding that results in antagonism of vitamin B_6 (Kuchinskas and du Vigaud, 1957) and inhibition of collagen cross-linking and collagen biosynthesis (Nimni and Bavetta, 1965), and (3) sulfhydryl disulfide exchange (Tabachnik et al., 1954). Whether any of these properties are responsible for penicillamine's efficacy in rheumatoid arthritis is unknown. Inhibition of collagen cross-linking has led to its use in the treatment of scleroderma. Penicillamine is neither cytotoxic nor

anti-inflammatory (Jaffe, 1989a, 1989b). Although its effects on the cellular immune response are not well understood, the drug suppresses antibody synthesis and enhances clearance of immune complexes (Jaffe, 1975; Lipsky, 1981). Penicillamine also has antiviral properties (Loddo and Marcialis, 1974).

Gastrointestinal absorption of penicillamine is rapid but may be reduced by as much as 50% if it is taken postprandially. Oral iron and antacids also decrease absorption (Osman et al., 1983). Penicillamine is highly protein-bound in plasma and cleared by the kidney. Penicillamine-cysteine mixed disulfide may be detected for up to 3 months after the drug is stopped, suggesting a tissue-bound compartment, possibly the skin (Wei and Sass-Kortsak, 1970).

The numerous and varied adverse effects of penicillamine have limited its clinical usefulness (see Table 19-7). Some of the effects are dose-

Table 19-7. TOXICITIES OF PENICILLAMINE

Mucocutaneous:	Pruritus, maculopapular rash, urticaria, eczematous rash, bullous rash similar to pemphigus, stomatitis
GI:	Dysgeusia, hypogeusia, anorexia, nausea, vomiting, diarrhea, cholestasis, hepatotoxicity
Renal:	Proteinuria, nephrotic syndrome, hematuria, immune complex glomerulonephritis (Goodpasture syndrome)
Pulmonary:	Hemorrhagic pneumonitis (Goodpasture syndrome), bronchiolitis obliterans, fibrosing alveolitis
Hematologic:	Thrombocytopenia, agranulocytosis, aplastic anemia, hemolytic anemia, thrombotic thrombocytopenic purpura
Neuromuscular:	Myasthenia gravis, polymyositis, dermatomyositis, peripheral neuropathy, neuromyotonia
Others:	Fever, breast enlargement, galactorrhea, DILE

related whereas others are idiosyncratic. The most common adverse effects are pruritus and rash that typically occur early in the course of treatment. Bullous dermatosis can occur as late as the second year of treatment and necessitates immediate and permanent discontinuation of penicillamine. The incidence of change or loss of taste is as high as 25% at 6 weeks of therapy, but this problem usually disappears within 6 to 8 more weeks despite continued drug administration. Bone marrow depression may be abrupt and occur at any time during therapy, necessitating close hematologic monitoring (see Table 19–3). The use of penicillamine may lead to the development of other autoimmune diseases such as pemphigus, Goodpasture syndrome, polymyositis, myasthenia gravis, or lupus. This induction of immune phenomena may be due to hapten formation or "immune dysregulation" (Noguchi and Nishitani, 1976; Troy et al., 1981). Penicillamine is also associated with the appearance of a number of autoantibodies including antinuclear, anti-double-stranded DNA, anti-acetylcholine receptor, anti-striated muscle, and anti-cardiac muscle (Crouzet et al., 1974; Zilko et al., 1977). Rheumatoid arthritis patients with HLA-DR3 and B8 are at a greater risk for developing penicillamine-induced nephropathy. Conversely, HLA-DR2 is associated with a substantially reduced incidence of this toxicity (Stockman et al., 1986).

Corticosteroids

The development of corticosteroids heralded a new era in the treatment of inflammatory diseases. Mason et al. (1936) isolated cortisone (compound E) from adrenal glands. As early as 1929, P. S. Hench noted that patients with rheumatoid arthritis experienced substantial relief from their joint symptoms when they became pregnant or were jaundiced, starved, subjected to surgery, or treated with estrogens or androgens. He postulated that an adrenocortical hormone might be the antirheumatic substance responsible for such clinical improvement and thus began trials with compound E. The therapeutic success of cortisone was dramatic in patients with rheumatoid arthritis, and the impact on the medical community was like a "scientific bombshell" (Freyberg, 1953). Hench and E. C. Kendall received the Nobel Prize for their work in 1950, only 1 year after their preliminary report on the use of cortisone in rheumatic diseases (Hench et al., 1949).

Cortisol, the naturally secreted glucocorticoid of the adrenal cortex, is a 17-hydroxycorticoid compound. Normal production of cortisol ranges from 8 to 25 mg/day in humans (Baxter and Tyrrell, 1987).

As catabolic hormones, glucocorticoids have multiple metabolic effects that regulate homeostasis. When overproduction or administration of exogenous corticosteroids leads to high steroid concentrations in the plasma, accentuation of these metabolic effects results in toxicity. Corticosteroids are the most powerful anti-inflammatory agent available. Effects of corticosteroid on inflammatory and immune responses are numerous and varied (Parillo and Fauci, 1979). They include (1) increased circulating neutrophils, (2) decreased circulating lymphocytes and monocytes, (3) inhibition of accumulation of neutrophils and macrophages at inflammatory sites, (4) suppression of the delayed hypersensitivity reaction, (5) suppression of T-cell-mediated and spontaneous cytotoxicity, (6) inhibition of interleukin-1 production, (7) decreased lysosomal enzyme release, (8) mild decrease in immunoglobulin levels, but without decrease in specific antibody production, (9) decreased reticuloendothelial clearance of antibody-coated cells, and (10) decreased synthesis of prostaglandins, leukotrienes, and bradykinins.

Corticosteroids are absorbed in the upper jejunum, and peak concentrations in plasma occur in 30 minutes to 2 hours. Eighty percent of circulating cortisol is bound to transcortin, a corticosteroid-binding globulin. Hepatic metabolism of corticosteroids by reduction and conjugation with glucuronic acid enhances renal excretion. Small structural differences in the synthetic analogs of cortisol result in striking differences in potency and duration of action (see Table 19–8).

Prolonged administration of corticosteroid may adversely affect virtually every organ system within the body (see Table 19–9). Patients treated with corticosteroids exhibit a wide range of susceptibility to adverse effects likely relating to individual differences in plasma protein binding and variations in metabolism and clearance of synthetic corticosteroids (Behrens and Goodwin, 1989). The major differences between iatrogenic and spontaneous Cushing syndrome relate primarily to increased mineralocorticoid and androgen concentrations in the spontaneous syndrome (Axelrod, 1976).

Osteoporosis is a potentially devastating adverse effect of corticosteroids. The incidence appears to correlate with cumulative dose and length of administration rather than daily dose. Supplemental vitamin D, calcium, and estrogens have been employed to attempt to reduce the risk of osteoporosis due to corticosteroids (see chapters 17 and 20). Corticosteroid use leads to an insidious myopathy that initially affects the proximal musculature. It is not associated with elevation in concentrations of muscle enzymes in the plasma.

The true ulcerogenic potential of corticoste-

Table 19-8. CORTICOSTEROID PREPARATIONS

DRUG	BIOLOGIC HALF-LIFE (H)	APPROXIMATE PLASMA HALF-LIFE (MIN)	ANTI-INFLAMMATORY POTENCY	EQUIVALENT DOSE (MG)	SODIUM-RETAINING POTENCY
Hydrocortisone	8–12	90	1	20	2+
Cortisone	8–12	30	0.8	25	2+
Prednisone	12–36	60	4	5	1+
Prednisolone	12–36	200	4	5	0
Methylprednisolone	12–36	180	5	4	0
Triamcinolone	12–36	300	5	4	0
Betamethasone	36–54	100–300	20–30	0.6	0
Dexamethasone	36–54	100–300	20–30	0.75	0

Adapted with permission from Garber, E.K.; Targoff, C.; Paulus, H.E.: Corticosteroids in the rheumatic diseases. In, Drugs for Rheumatic Disease (Paulus, H.E.; Furst, D.E.; Droomgoole, S.H., eds.). Churchill Livingstone, New York, 1987.

roids remains controversial. In an analysis of pooled data from 71 controlled clinical trials, it was determined that 1.8% of corticosteroid-treated patients developed peptic ulcers compared with 0.8% of controls, a significant difference (Messer et al., 1983). Psychiatric symptoms from corticosteroids include euphoria, depression, insomnia, nervousness, and frank psychosis. They are reversible with reduction in dose or discontinuation of therapy. Estimation of the true incidence of corticosteroid-induced infections is difficult. This is because corticosteroids often are prescribed for diseases that independently predispose patients to infections. Moreover, corticosteroids are frequently used concomitantly with immunosuppressive agents (Ginzler et al., 1978). The incidence of posterior subcapsular cataracts correlates with dosage and the duration of therapy. Corticosteroids increase intraocular pressure in up to 40% of patients (Dujovne and Azarnoff, 1975). Many of the known atherosclerosis risk factors, including hypertension, hyperlipidemia, glucose intolerance, and obesity, are induced or exacerbated by corticosteroids, leading to the increased incidence of atherosclerotic complications. Despite the potential for more serious complications, the most distressing effects of corticosteroids to the patient often are cushingoid appearance with buffalo hump formation, moon facies, acne, striae, weight gain, and easy bruising.

Patients with underlying diabetes mellitus, osteoporosis, glaucoma, peptic ulcer disease, tuberculosis or other chronic infections, hypertension, or cardiovascular disease are all at increased risk of developing corticosteroid toxicity.

Corticosteroids use is considered relatively safe during pregnancy (see chapter 29). Impaired intrauterine growth or adrenal insufficiency in the neonate are rare complications even with chronic high-dose maternal corticosteroid use (Lee, 1985). A placental enzyme (11-β-OH-dehydrogenase) inactivates corticosteroids and leads to low concentrations of active drug in the fetus. Prednisone and prednisolone are more susceptible to this enzymatic inactivation compared with betamethasone and dexamethasone. The former agents are therefore preferred in pregnant women

Table 19-9. ADVERSE EFFECTS OF GLUCOCORTICOIDS

Very Common and Should Be Anticipated in All Patients
 Negative calcium balance leading to osteoporosis
 Increased appetite
 Centripetal obesity
 Impaired wound healing
 Increased risk of infection
 Suppression of hypothalamic–pituitary–adrenal axis
 Growth arrest in children
Frequently Seen
 Myopathy
 Avascular necrosis
 Hypertension
 Plethora
 Thin, fragile skin or striae or purpura
 Edema secondary to sodium and water retention
 Hyperlipidemia
 Psychiatric symptoms, particularly euphoria
 Diabetes mellitus
 Posterior subcapsular cataracts
Uncommon, but Important to Recognize Early
 Glaucoma
 Benign intracranial hypertension
 "Silent" intestinal perforation
 Peptic ulcer disease (often gastric)
 Hypokalemic alkalosis
 Hyperosmolar nonketotic coma
 Gastric hemorrhage
Rare
 Pancreatitis
 Hirsutism
 Panniculitis
 Secondary amenorrhea
 Impotence
 Epidural lipomatosis
 Allergy to synthetic steroids

Reproduced with permission from Behrens and Goodwin, 1989, p. 163.

(Gabbe, 1983). With the substantial toxicities noted above, one wonders whether the Nobel Prize was awarded prematurely. It is always dangerous to predict the toxicity of a drug at the earliest time its efficacy is apparent.

If, after careful consideration, corticosteroids are indeed felt to be necessary for therapy, the minimal effective dose should be given for the shortest possible time to reduce toxicity. Alternate-day dosing of corticosteroids is preferred when clinically feasible as this minimizes growth retardation, infectious complications, myopathy, obesity, cushingoid appearance, and glucose intolerance (Axelrod, 1976).

As exogenous corticosteroids suppress the hypothalamic–pituitary–adrenal (HPA) axis, abrupt withdrawal can lead to adrenal insufficiency (addisonian crisis). Excessively rapid taper of drug may also lead to relapse of disease activity. Nonetheless, it is generally desirable to attempt to decrease or discontinue use of glucocorticosteroids when clinically feasible due to their adverse effects. The rate at which a dose can be decreased is influenced by the dose of drug, duration of therapy, and severity of underlying disease. Patients in whom steroids are lowered too rapidly may complain of malaise, arthralgias, myalgias, or fatigue or develop manifestations of adrenal insufficiency such as nausea, vomiting, and hypotension.

Azathioprine

Azathioprine, a purine analog, has been used for many years in the treatment of rheumatic disease. Taken orally, it is readily absorbed from the GI tract and metabolized sequentially to 6-mercaptopurine and 6-thioinosinic acid. These two metabolites function as purine antagonists. Though the mechanism responsible for the therapeutic effects of azathioprine is unknown, it is believed that its primary mode of action is to inhibit DNA synthesis. Rapidly cycling cells undergoing active DNA synthesis presumably are most sensitive to this effect of azathioprine (chapter 23). Metabolites of azathioprine are excreted by the kidney. Alternative metabolic pathways of azathioprine exist, although their therapeutic relevance is uncertain.

Experimentally, azathioprine possesses a variety of immunomodulatory activities. Patients with rheumatic disease taking therapeutic doses of azathioprine develop moderate lymphopenia with a decrease in absolute numbers of both T and B lymphocytes (Yu et al., 1974). Independent of its antiproliferative activity, azathioprine causes striking inhibition of the mixed lymphocyte reaction (Al-Safi and Maddocks, 1985). Azathioprine also decreases B lymphocyte immune

globulin production (Levy et al., 1972) but does not consistently depress delayed-type hypersensitivity responses.

The major toxicity of azathioprine is myelosuppression, particularly lymphopenia and granulocytopenia. Complete blood counts including the platelet count must be monitored frequently during therapy, especially during the first months of treatment (Table 19–3). Gradual, progressive macrocytic anemia is commonly seen, though this may not have clinical importance. As with any immunomodulatory agent, there is an increased risk of infection. Viral, fungal, mycobacterial, and protozoal infections in association with azathioprine have been reported. Gastrointestinal upset is common. Hepatitis with or without biliary stasis; stomatitis; dermatitis; and a flulike syndrome are infrequent complications. Azathioprine is associated with an increased risk of lymphoreticular malignancies in renal transplant patients, although an increased risk in patients with rheumatic diseases has been more difficult to document (Singh et al., 1989).

Allopurinol inhibits metabolism of 6-mercaptopurine to 6-thioxanthine. Severe myelosuppression may result when azathioprine and allopurinol are used together. When it is necessary to use both drugs simultaneously, reduction of the azathioprine dose by 75% is usually required and vigilant hematologic monitoring is particularly important. *Principle: The interaction of allopurinol and azathioprine illustrates the high threshold that physicians have for using data that warn against lethal and common drug interactions. Initially allopurinol was developed as a xanthine oxidase inhibitor. It was hoped that the drug might prolong the half-life of antineoplastic purine analogs. Not only was there a potential for allopurinol's prolonging the half-life of any purine analog that required xanthine oxidase for metabolism (detoxification), but the scientists who discovered the series of drugs warned of the need to carefully think out the drug combinations before and during their administration (Elion, 1989). Nonetheless, repeated reports of "unsuspected" severe azathioprine-plus-allolpurinol-induced bone marrow depression occurred and continue to occur. The reports are not about our ignorance of unanticipated drug effects but of our inability to translate even the strongest scientific observations on drug effects into clinical actions (Venning, 1983; Melmon, 1984).*

Methotrexate

In 1948, folic acid antagonists were first reported to induce temporary remission in acute lymphoblastic leukemia (Farber et al., 1948) (see chapter 23). In the years that followed, the folate antagonists, including methotrexate, were studied in the treatment of nonmalignant inflammatory disorders. Early experience with psoriasis revealed that methotrexate not only improves skin lesions but also reduces joint symptoms in patients with psoriatic arthritis (see chapter 21). Since the early 1980s, methotrexate has been used on an increasingly widespread basis for the treatment of rheumatoid arthritis and other rheumatic disorders.

Dihydrofolate reductase (DHFR) is an enzyme that catalyzes the hydrogenation of dihydrofolate (folic acid) to tetrahydrofolate, which then can accept a variety of one-carbon units. Such bioactive folates are required for purine metabolism and biosynthesis of pyrimidine and glycine. Methotrexate, a folate analog, functions intracellularly as a competitive inhibitor of DHFR, preventing the reduction of folic acid to tetrahydrofolate. This folate antagonist activity confers cytotoxicity on methotrexate. Cytotoxicity is readily demonstrable as tumor shrinkage and marrow suppression following high doses employed in the chemotherapy of malignancy. In the therapy of rheumatic disease, however, methotrexate is generally administered in relatively low doses (5–20 mg), orally or IM, on a weekly basis. In this dose range, reduction in absolute numbers of lymphocytes is not usually observed. The therapeutic effects of methotrexate in rheumatic disease may be unrelated to cytotoxicity.

Potentially more relevant to its use in autoimmune disease, methotrexate functions in vivo as an immunomodulator. In patients with rheumatoid arthritis treated with methotrexate, IgG production and IgM rheumatoid factor synthesis are decreased (Olsen et al., 1987). Primary delayed hypersensitivity responses are inhibited by methotrexate, although preexisting delayed hypersensitivity responses are unaffected (O'Callaghan et al., 1986). Methotrexate often improves arthritic symptoms within 1 to 2 months subsequent to initiation of therapy. This rapid effect may represent a direct anti-inflammatory activity, although this has yet to be demonstrated.

Methotrexate is eliminated almost entirely by the kidney. Renal function should therefore be assessed prior to initial use. Significant potentiation of toxicity has been observed even with mild renal impairment. The NSAIDs, commonly used in conjunction with methotrexate in the setting of inflammatory arthritis, may similarly potentiate toxicity through their adverse effects on renal function.

Insidious hepatic fibrosis leading to cirrhosis during low-dose, weekly methotrexate therapy given over years has been demonstrated in patients treated for psoriasis (see chapter 21). Risk factors for accelerated fibrosis in this population include obesity, advanced age, use of alcohol, and presence of diabetes mellitus (Weinstein et al., 1973). As a result, serial liver biopsies have been advocated to detect early fibrosis. The direct applicability of this experience and role of liver biopsies in patients receiving methotrexate for rheumatoid arthritis is uncertain (Kremer, 1989). However, it is prudent to avoid using methotrexate in patients with coexistent hepatitis or exposure to hepatotoxins such as alcohol. Although frequent monitoring of liver function tests is recommended (Table 19–3), it has been repeatedly demonstrated that fibrosis can progress despite normal serum laboratory values (Robinson et al., 1980). *Principle: Using a laboratory test of a drug's effects that does not truly reflect toxicity-induced organ dysfunction creates a false sense of security and likely increases the damage that does occur once toxicity begins, because the drug will not be discontinued early.*

Acute pneumonitis, manifested by malaise, dyspnea, and fever, may be caused by methotrexate and may require treatment with corticosteroids. Other toxicities include nausea, GI upset, oral ulceration, headache, and a sensation of lightheadedness. Leukopenia and thrombocytopenia may occur. Regular monitoring of complete blood count is warranted (Table 19–3). Concurrent administration of folic acid or folinic acid does not convincingly alter the therapeutic index of methotrexate.

Methotrexate is highly teratogenic. Patients receiving methotrexate must use reliable birth control during reproductive years. Methotrexate should be discontinued at least 4 months before attempting to conceive.

Cyclophosphamide

Cyclophosphamide, a derivative of nitrogen mustard, was first used clinically as a cancer chemotherapeutic agent (chapter 23). During the past 2 decades, cyclophosphamide has been employed with increasing frequency for severe or refractory rheumatic illness. As therapy for rheumatic disease, cyclophosphamide is generally administered either in a daily oral dose or monthly in a "pulse" IV infusion. It is metabolized in the liver by the mixed function oxidase system to 4-hydroxycyclophosphamide. Metabolites of 4-hydroxycyclophosphamide are active alkylating agents that cross-link DNA and other cellular macromolecules. As a result, they exhibit greatest toxicity to rapidly dividing cells. The serum half-life of cyclophosphamide following IV administration is reported to be in the range of 4 to $6\frac{1}{2}$ hours although active metabolites may persist in the circulation for a considerably longer time. Renal excretion is the principal route of elimination of cyclophosphamide's metabolites. A reduction in dose is therefore generally required in the presence of renal failure.

As a potent cytotoxic agent, cyclophosphamide induces absolute reductions in both B- and T-lymphocyte populations. In addition to lymphopenia, numerous immunomodulatory effects are observed with cyclophosphamide. These include decreased immunoglobulin concentrations (Hurd and Ziff, 1974) and diminished B-cell responsiveness to mitogenic stimuli (Cupps et al., 1982). Patients with SLE receiving monthly infusions of cyclophosphamide develop subtle alterations of a T-lymphocyte activation pathway (McCune et al., 1988).

Cyclophosphamide has a low therapeutic index. Toxicity generally is expected with therapy even with low doses used for the treatment of rheumatic disease. Bone marrow suppression manifested by anemia, leukopenia, and thrombocytopenia is commonly encountered and may be dose-dependent. Frequent monitoring of complete blood count is mandatory (Table 19–3). When the drug is given as monthly pulses, the nadir of the leukopenia occurs at 8 to 15 days following infusion, and recovery takes up to 28 days. Prednisone, which is often used in combination with cyclophosphamide, may exert a "protective" effect on the leukocyte depression by increasing leukocyte demargination and possibly by altering the hepatic metabolism of cyclophosphamide (Hayakawa et al., 1969). Reversible alopecia is common with prolonged therapy, especially when the drug is administered daily. Nausea during or following infusion of IV cyclophosphamide may require treatment with antiemetics. An increased incidence of infection must be anticipated, particularly if leukopenia develops, although there is evidence to suggest that risk of infection may be more directly related to concurrent use of corticosteroids (Balow et al., 1987). *Principle: When multiple drugs can lead to the same toxicity, there is a tendency to focus on the drug that produces a surrogate effect (e.g., leukopenia) as the culprit rather than on those that produce the problem without laboratory warning.*

Hemorrhagic cystitis has been reported to occur in up to 17% of patients with rheumatic disease who are treated with oral cyclophosphamide (Plotz et al., 1979). Adequate hydration should be maintained during both oral and IV therapy to ensure dilution of metabolites in the urinary system. Less common adverse effects include hepatitis, stomatitis, and fluid retention.

Cyclophosphamide may induce malignancies. Prolonged oral administration to patients with rheumatic disease results in an approximately twofold increased risk of skin, bladder, and hematopoietic malignancies (Baker et al., 1987).

The relative risk of developing bladder cancer is particularly high and may correlate with prior episodes of hemorrhagic cystitis. Experience with IV pulse cyclophosphamide in rheumatic patients is not yet sufficient to determine whether the risk of malignancy with this form of therapy is increased.

Cyclophosphamide is highly mutagenic and teratogenic and must be discontinued several months before patients attempt to conceive. Even following discontinuation of therapy, azoospermia and ovarian failure are common and may be irreversible. *Principle: Distinguishing reversible from irreversible important toxicities of a drug before commencing therapy is a key responsibility of the clinician in building a contract with the patient.*

Experimental and Future Immunomodulatory Therapeutics

Cyclosporin A, a fungal-derived cyclic polypeptide, is a potent immunomodulatory agent. Unlike the cytotoxic agents, it induces neither myelosuppression nor mutagenesis. Increase in serum creatine concentrations is seen in virtually every patient treated with cyclosporin. Numerous clinical trials have demonstrated the effectiveness of cyclosporin in the treatment of rheumatoid arthritis (Shand and Richardson, 1988). Because of the incidence of renal toxicity, cyclosporin remains an experimental therapy solely for refractory disease.

Other experimental therapies for autoimmune diseases have employed monoclonal antibodies directed against lymphocyte cell surface molecules such as CD4 and major histocompatibility antigens (Herzog et al., 1987; Sany, 1988). These monoclonal antibody therapies are intended to interfere with the autoimmune process by eliminating the responsible effector cells. However, entire subsets of lymphocytes are affected, and the antibodies lack specificity for the particular cells responsible for triggering autoimmunity. Consequently, they cause a degree of nonspecific immunosuppression. As the precise immunologic events that precipitate autoimmune diseases are better understood, therapies with antibodies or peptides that interfere with the initial presentation of specific inciting antigens to T lymphocytes may be possible (Wraith et al., 1989).

Interleukin-1 is a peptide produced mainly by macrophages that is important in activation of the immune system. Recently, an endogenous inhibitor of interleukin-1 has been isolated and cloned (Eisenberg et al., 1990). This inhibitor or other interleukin inhibitors might conceivably be used to block immune activation in autoimmune disease. *Principle: When efficacy based on a clear mechanism of action begins to emerge, look for apparently phenotypically unrelated diseases with similar pathogenesis to be the next targets of equivalent therapy.*

CLINICAL THERAPEUTICS OF RHEUMATIC DISEASE

Rheumatoid Arthritis

General Approach. Current treatment of rheumatoid arthritis is primarily directed toward reduction of pain and disability and secondarily at improving survival. For the past several decades, NSAIDs have been considered the standard initial pharmacologic therapy of rheumatoid arthritis. Because rheumatoid arthritis is a chronic, persistent inflammatory disorder, NSAIDS with longer serum half-lives such as naproxen, piroxicam, and sulindac are favored. The long half-lives enhance compliance and simplify dosing regimens. Long-half-life drugs permit sustained concentrations through the night, which may decrease morning stiffness that is characteristic upon awakening in the untreated patient.

Aspirin, used extensively in the past, is no less effective than other NSAIDs. Aspirin therapy, however, requires frequent dosing. A complete discussion of NSAIDs is included in chapter 20. Adequate rest, nutrition, physical and occupational therapy, and regular exercise programs remain the nonpharmacologic mainstays of therapy.

When patients are unresponsive or have persistent symptoms despite maximally tolerated NSAID therapy and use of other measures, so-called disease-modifying antirheumatic drugs (DMARDs) are added to the therapeutic regimen. The term *DMARDs* derives from a perception that they alter the course of disease (e.g., retard the progression of joint destruction). Though effective when monitored over months to a few years, there is no clear evidence that DMARDs improve the ultimate long-term outcome of rheumatoid arthritis either in terms of functional disability or mortality. Examples of DMARDs include gold compounds, methotrexate, sulfasalazine, hydroxychloroquine, azathioprine, and penicillamine.

In the past, DMARDs had been started only after several months of therapy with NSAIDs had failed to produce an adequate response. They were used sequentially according to their relative potential toxicity. NSAID therapy followed by sequential use of DMARDs with increasing toxicity has been termed *pyramid* therapy. Recent long-term analysis of patients with rheumatoid arthritis suggests that this pyramid approach has not reduced mortality associated with rheumatoid arthritis nor has it prevented irreversible damage to cartilage (Pincus and Callahan, 1986). These findings have prompted proposals to invert the traditional pyramid by initiating more toxic but potentially more efficacious DMARD therapy earlier in the course of disease (Healy and Wilske, 1989). Clinicians have speculated that the disease process might be slowed before irreversible joint damage has taken place. Thus DMARDs would truly be disease-modifying by decreasing mortality and long-term disability.

In current practice, the presence of bony erosions on radiographs and strong family history of deforming arthritis prompts early therapy with DMARDs. Other features including the immunogenetic profile of the patient (e.g., HLA type) may be used in the future to predict which patients are most likely to progress to severe disease. These would then be prime candidates for early aggressive therapy with DMARDs. *Principle: Beware of acronyms of theraputics (e.g., those used for combinations of antineoplastic and antitumor agents, or those applying to anti-inflammatory drugs like DMARDs). They are almost never what they appear to be. Given the need to oversimplify, they usually promise more than has been demonstrated, incorrectly connote homogeneity of pharmacologic effects, and downplay the values in individualization of therapy.*

The selection of a specific DMARD for a patient requires a variety of considerations. These include the severity and pace of the arthritis, cost of the drug and laboratory tests needed to follow it, the route of administration, particular susceptibility to adverse effects, and history of adverse reactions. Some of these considerations are outlined in Table 19–10. Individual DMARDs are discussed below.

Methotrexate. Methotrexate has been used with increasing frequency by clinicians as a DMARD. Short-term placebo-controlled studies have clearly demonstrated that weekly oral therapy with doses of 7 to 15 mg improves arthritic symptoms and objective measurements of severity within 12 to 18 weeks (Weinblatt et al., 1985; Williams et al., 1985). In a long-term study, the clinical improvement conferred by methotrexate was observed to plateau by 6 months and was sustained through 53 months of clinical follow-up (Kremer and Lee, 1988). Although radiographic improvement of skeletal erosions was initially seen in a number of patients in this study, longer follow-up revealed reversal of this trend and progression of erosions.

Gold. Parenteral gold compounds are used primarily in patients with progressive polyarticular rheumatoid arthritis. The benefit of gold therapy has been well established over the past 50 years. A 30-month double-blind study with GST

Table 19-10. **PRINCIPLES OF DMARD THERAPY**

Intramuscular Gold Salts	
Advantages:	Reported to be effective in erosive disease.
	Many decades of clinical experience.
Disadvantages:	Weekly IM injection and laboratory monitoring.
	Clinical improvement may require several months of therapy.
Methotrexate	
Advantages:	Oral administration.
	Onset of clinical effects within weeks.
	Effective in severe and erosive disease.
Disadvantages:	Hepatotoxicity cannot be fully assessed without liver biopsy.
Azathioprine, Penicillamine	
Advantages:	Effective alternatives to gold and methotrexate.
Disadvantages:	Frequent, numerous, and varied adverse effects (penicillamine).
	Potential for induction of malignancy (azathioprine).
	Clinical improvement may require 6 months of therapy.
Auranofin, Hydroxychloroquine, Sulfasalazine	
Advantages:	Lower incidence of toxicity relative to other DMARDs.
	Require less frequent clinical and laboratory monitoring for adverse effects.
Disadvantages:	Probably less effective in severe and erosive arthritis.

showed a significant reduction in the radiographic progression of rheumatoid arthritis when compared with placebo treatment (Sigler et al., 1974). In this study, improvement required at least 3 months of treatment and sometimes took 9 months. In some patients, improvement has been evident only after 18 months of therapy (Srinivasan et al., 1979). *Principle: The longer it takes to show efficacy, the bigger the problem with compliance, and the more important that legitimate expectations of the therapy be understood by both the physician and the patient.*

Auranofin, an oral gold preparation, is generally used in rheumatoid arthritis with early or modestly aggressive disease. Standard therapy is 6 mg/day in divided doses. Increased efficacy may be achieved with 9 mg/day although with increased toxicity. In one study, radiographs of the hands and wrists of auranofin-treated patients showed a definite reduction in the advancement of erosive disease after 1 year of therapy (Gofton et al., 1984).

Antimalarials. Both open and controlled studies have confirmed the therapeutic effectiveness of antimalarials in rheumatoid arthritis. Adams et al. (1983) observed that 65% of patients treated with 400 mg of hydroxychloroquine daily showed a significant improvement in morning stiffness and articular index at 6 months. Freedman and Steinberg (1960) demonstrated general improvement in 80% of patients with rheumatoid arthritis receiving chloroquine 400 mg/day for 1 year. The patients with earlier onset of rheumatoid arthritis or those in whom disease is not rapidly progressive show the most marked improvement. Beneficial effects are generally not observed until treatment is given for at least 6 to 12 weeks.

Sulfasalazine. The primary clinical uses of sulfasalazine are in rheumatoid arthritis and inflammatory bowel disease; however, its use is increasing in spondyloarthropathies such as ankylosing spondylitis, Reiter syndrome, and psoriatic arthritis. Use in rheumatoid arthritis has waxed and waned coordinate with favorable and unfavorable reports of its clinical efficacy. In 1989, a double-blind comparative study of hydroxychloroquine and sulfasalazine in patients with rheumatoid arthritis demonstrated similar efficacy of the two drugs at 48 weeks but an earlier response (approximately 8 weeks) in the sulfasalazine group (Nuver-Zwart et al., 1989).

Penicillamine. The efficacy of penicillamine in rheumatoid arthritis was first definitively established by a placebo-controlled, multicenter trial in the United Kingdom (Multi-Centre Trial Group, 1973). The pattern of improvement of synovitis with penicillamine is slow, and clinical efficacy may not be observed until 6 months of therapy. Extraarticular manifestations of rheumatoid arthritis, particularly vasculitis, rheumatoid lung disease, Felty syndrome, amyloidosis, and nodulosis, may be responsive to penicillamine. Penicillamine is begun at 125 or 250 mg/day and increased by 125- or 250-mg increments at intervals of 8 to 12 weeks. Evidence for toxicity must be monitored before increasing the dose. Most responders are controlled on 500 mg/day or less, although some patients require 1000 mg/day (Lyle, 1979). The numerous and varied adverse reactions and the long periods of drug buildup in the body associated with penicillamine have limited its clinical usefulness.

Azathioprine. Azathioprine has been used for many years as a DMARD in the treatment of rheumatoid arthritis. A randomized double-blind controlled study using azathioprine in doses of 2 to 2.5 mg/kg per day demonstrated modest improvement in symptoms compared with placebo. The improvement persisted over a 2-year follow-up period (Hunter et al., 1975). Azathioprine has been directly compared with several other DMARDs including gold, penicillamine, hydroxychloroquine, and methotrexate. In none of these studies has azathioprine been judged to be superior. For this reason, and because of concerns regarding immunosuppression and possible induction of malignancy, azathioprine is generally used after other DMARDs have failed to have sufficient efficacy.

Cyclophospamide. Cyclophosphamide in oral doses averaging 1.25 mg/kg per day is an effective treatment of rheumatoid arthritis (Townes et al., 1976). Toxicity including myelosuppression, infertility, and induction of malignancy prohibit routine use of cyclophosphamide in rheumatoid arthritis. Certain complications of rheumatoid disease such as vasculitis or pericarditis may warrant cyclophosphamide therapy.

Prednisone. Prednisone in low doses can be a useful addition to the therapeutic regimen in aggressive rheumatoid arthritis (Docken, 1989). A single morning dose over about 7.5 mg of prednisone may provide reasonable anti-inflammatory and analgesic effects with significantly less toxicity and fewer adverse effects than occur with higher doses of prednisone. Higher-dose regimens may, however, be required for the treatment of extraarticular manifestations of rheumatoid disease such as vasculitis, pericarditis, or pneumonitis.

SLE

Treatment of SLE is influenced by the principal organs that are involved in any given patient. When disease is limited to skin and joints, NSAIDs and/or hydroxychloroquine 200 to 400 mg/day usually provide adequate therapy. If these symptoms are not fully controlled or additional systemic problems develop such as fever, fatigue, and lymphadenopathy, steroids equivalent to 0.5 mg/kg per day of prednisone in divided doses are usually effective. As soon as control of the symptoms is achieved, a steady taper of steroids is begun with the goal at 1 month being

a single 10-mg dose of prednisone given in the morning.

With life-threatening organ involvement, notably in the kidney, CNS, and/or heart (pericardium), more aggressive therapy may be required. High doses of prednisone (1 mg/kg per day) alone may suffice. When disease activity progresses despite high-dose steroid therapy or relapses as steroids are tapered, addition of a cytotoxic agent such as azathioprine or cyclophosphamide generally becomes necessary. Controlled studies concerning the use of cytotoxic agents in SLE involving the CNS do not exist. *Principle: When a rare disease is lethal, one cannot expect controlled double-blind randomized studies to help choose between useful agents or even define a useful agent. Such situations require the clinician to plan the experiment (see chapters 35 and 36).*

In patients with SLE and nephritis, a trend toward decreased mortality and preservation of renal function with azathioprine and cyclophosphamide compared with prednisone was noted in a long-term study (Austin et al., 1986). In that study, therapy with IV monthly "pulse" cyclophosphamide ($0.5–1.0$ g^2), and combined therapy with oral cyclophosphamide and azathioprine revealed that preservation of renal function was superior compared with therapy with prednisone or azathioprine alone. These observations have been generalized so that cyclophosphamide is now frequently used for other life-threatening, steroid-resistant complications of SLE including CNS involvement. In the treatment of steroid-responsive complications of lupus, addition of azathioprine (2–2.5 mg/kg per day) may permit a more rapid taper of corticosteroids and thus exert a steroid-sparing effect (Ginzler et al., 1975). In this way the multiple complications of prolonged high-dose steroid therapy can be minimized.

Vasculitis

The rational treatment of vasculitis is similar to that of SLE because organ involvement and risk to life dictates the aggressiveness of the therapy. For instance, small-vessel vasculitis confined to the skin may be treated with a NSAID. A potentially lethal vasculitis involving the kidney or lung, such as Wegener granulomatosis or polyarteritis nodosa, may require an alkylating agent such as cyclophosphamide in addition to high-dose daily corticosteroids. These forms of aggressive vasculitis may relapse unless an alkylating agent is given for a period of months.

Giant cell arteritis, a granulomatous large vessel vasculitis of the elderly, is generally very responsive to high daily doses of glucocorticoid alone. Permanent visual loss, a potential consequence of giant cell arteritis, is prevented with this therapy (Huston and Hunder, 1980). Following a month of high-dose steroids (prednisone 1 mg/kg per day), the dose is tapered. Lower maintenance doses of steroids are usually required for at least 2 years to prevent relapse of disease. Alternate-day steroids or a "steroid-sparing agent" such as methotrexate in the maintenance phase has recently been advocated to minimize the almost inevitable complications of long-term steroid use in the elderly. *Principle: Caution must be exercised when an agent that enables less use of another drug may be as dangerous as the drug whose dose you are trying to minimize.*

Drug-Induced Lupus Erythematosus

The fundamental treatment of DILE is to discontinue the offending medication. If the symptoms are initially severe or persist after discontinuation of the drug, administration of oral glucocorticoids may be indicated (Harmon and Portanova, 1982). The dose of glucocorticoids depends on the particular organ systems involved. A prolonged course of DILE is generally effectively controlled by the use of NSAID, hydroxychloroquine, or glucocorticoids, either alone or in combination.

REFERENCES

Adams, E. M.; Yocum, D. E.; and Bell, C. L.: Hydroxychloroquine in the treatment of rheumatoid arthritis. Am. J. Med., 75:321–326, 1983.

Al-Safi, S. A.; and Maddocks, J. L.: Strength of the human mixed lymphocyte reaction (MLR) and its suppression by azathioprine or 6-mercaptopurine. Br. J. Clin. Pharmacol., 19:105–107, 1985.

Aruoma, O. I.; Wasil, M.; Halliwell, B.; Hoey, B. M.; and Butler, J.: The scavenging of oxidants by sulfasalazine and its metabolites. Biochem. Pharmacol., 36:3739–3742, 1987.

Austin, H. A.; Klippel, J. H.; Balow, J. E.; LeRiche, N. G. H.; Steinberg, A. D.; Plotz, P. H.; and Decker, J. L.: Therapy of lupus nephritis. Controlled trial of prednisone and cytotoxic drugs. N. Engl. J. Med., 314:614–619, 1986.

Axelrod, L.: Glucocorticoid therapy. Medicine, 55:39–65,1976.

Axford, J. S.; MacKenzie, L.; Lydyard, P. M.; Hay, F. C.; Isenberg, D. A.; and Roitt, I. M.: Reduced B-cell galactotransferase activity in rheumatoid arthritis. Lancet, 2:1486–1488, 1987.

Baker, G. L.; Kahl, L. E.; Zee, B. C.; Stolzer, B. L.; Agarwal, A. K.; and Medsger, T. A. Jr.: Malignancy following treatment of rheumatoid arthritis with cyclophosphamide. Am. J. Med., 83:1–9, 1987.

Balow, J. E.; Austin, H. A.; Tsokos, C. G.; Antonovych, T. T.; Steinberg, A. D.; and Klippel, J. H.: NIH conference: Lupus nephritis. Ann. Intern. Med., 106:79–94, 1987.

Barrett, K. E.; Tashof, T. L.; and Metcalf, D. D.: Inhibition of IgE mediated mast cell degranulation by sulphasalazine. Eur. J. Pharmacol., 107:279–281, 1985.

Baxter, J. D.; and Tyrell, J. B.: The adrenal cortex. In, Endocrinology and Metabolism, 2nd ed. (Felig, P.; Baxter J. D.; Broadus, A. E.; and Frohman, L. A., eds.). McGraw-Hill, New York, pp. 511–650, 1987.

Behrens, T. W.; and Goodwin, J. S.: Glucocorticoids. In, Arthritis and Allied Conditions: A Textbook of Rheumatology (McCarty, D. J., ed.). Lea & Febiger, Philadelphia, pp. 604–621, 1989.

Blocka, K.; and Paulus, H. E.: The clinical pharmacology of the gold compounds. In, Drugs for Rheumatic Disease (Paulus, H. E.; Furst, D. E.; and Dromgoole, S. H., eds.). Churchill Livingstone, New York, pp. 49–83, 1987.

Blodgett, R. C. Jr.; Hauer, M. A.; and Pietrusko, R. G.: Auranofin: A unique oral chrysotherapeutic agent. Semin. Arthritis Rheum., 13:255–275, 1984.

Bruns, R. P.: Delayed onset of chloroquine retinopathy. N. Engl. J. Med., 275:695–696, 1966.

Burge, J. J.; Fearon, D. T.; and Austin, K. F.: Inhibition of the alternative pathways of complement by gold sodium thiomalate in vitro. J. Immunol., 120:1626–1630, 1978.

Campbell, X. X.; and Wilske, X. X.: Guidelines for Reviewers of Rheumatic Disease Care. Council on Rheumatic Care of the American Rheumatism Association Inc., 1986.

Conn, D. L.: Vasculitic syndromes. Rheum. Dis. Clin. North Am., 16:251–490, 1990.

Corey, E. J.; Mehrotra, M. M.; and Kahn, A. U.: Antiarthritic gold compounds effectively quench electronically excited singlet oxygen. Science, 236:68–69, 1987.

Crouzet, J.; Camus, J. P.; Leca, A. P.; Guillien, P.; and Lievre, J. A.: Lupus induit par la D-penicillamine au cours du traitement de la polyarthrite rhumatoile: Deux observations et étude immunologique systematique au cours de ce traitement. Ann. Med. Interne, 125:71–79, 1974.

Cupps, T. R.; Edgar, L. C.; and Fauci, A. S.: Suppression of human B lymphocyte function by cyclophosphamide. J. Immunol., 128:2453–2457, 1982.

Das, K. M.; and Dubin, R.: Clinical pharmacokinetics of sulphasalazine. Clin. Pharmacokinet., 1:406–425, 1976.

Das, K. M.; Eastwood, M. A.; McManus, J. P. A.; and Sircus, W.: Adverse reactions during salicylazosulfapyridine therapy and the relation with drug metabolism and acetylator phenotype. N. Engl. J. Med., 289:491–495, 1973.

DiMartino, M. J.; Walz, D. T.; Wolff, C. E.; and Mahn, W. A.: Inhibition of lysosomal enzyme release from rat leukocytes by a new gold compound SK&FD-39162 (abstract). Fed. Proc., 33:558, 1974.

Docken, W. P.: Low dose prednisone therapy. Rheum. Dis. Clin. North Am., 15:569–575, 1989.

Dujovne, C. A.; and Azarnoff, D. L.: Clinical complications of corticosteroid therapy: A selected review. In, Steroid Therapy (Azarnoff, D. L., ed.). W. B. Saunders Co., Philadelphia, 1975.

Easterbrook, M.: Ocular effects and safety of antimalarial agents. Am. J. Med., 85 (suppl. 4A):23–29, 1988.

Eisenberg, S. P.; Evans, R. J.; Arend, W. P.; Verderber, E.; Brewer, M. T.; Hannum, C. H.; and Thompson, R. C.: Primary structure and functional expression from complementary DNA of a human interleukin-1 receptor antagonist. Nature, 343:341–346, 1990.

Elion, G. B.: The purine pathway to chemotherapy. Science, 244:41–47, 1989.

Ennis, R. S.; Granda, J. L.; and Posner, A. S.: Effect of gold salts and other drugs in the release and activity of lysosomal hydrolases. Arthritis Rheum., 11:756–765, 1968.

Farber, S.; Diamond, L. K.; Mercer, R. D.; Sylvester, R. F. Jr.; and Wolff, J. A.: Temporary remission in acute leukemia in children produced by folic acid antagonist 4-aminopteroyl-glutamic acid (aminopterin). N. Engl. J. Med., 238:787–793, 1948.

Forestier, J.: Rheumatoid arthritis and its treatment with gold salts. J. Lab. Clin. Med., 20:827–840, 1935.

Freedman, A.; and Steinberg, V. L.: Chloroquine in rheumatoid arthritis, a double blindfold trial of treatment for one year. Ann. Rheum. Dis., 19:243–250, 1960.

Freyberg, R. H.: Corticotropin, cortisone and hydrocortisone. In, Arthritis and Allied Conditions (Hollander, J. L., ed.). Lea & Febiger, Philadelphia, 1953.

Gabbe, S. G.: Drug therapy in autoimmune disease. Clin. Obstet. Gynecol., 26:635–641, 1983.

Ghadially, F. N.; DeCouteau, W. E.; Huang, S.; and Thomas, I.: Ultrastructure of the skin of patients treated with sodium aurothiomalate. J. Pathol., 124:77–83, 1978.

Ginzler, E.; Diamond, H.; Kaplan, D.; Weiner, M.; Schlesinger, M.; and Seleznick, M.: Computer analysis of factors influencing frequency of infection in systemic lupus erythematosus. Arthritis Rheum., 21:37–44, 1978.

Ginzler, E.; Sharon, E.; Diamond, H.; and Kaplan, D.: Long term maintenance therapy with azathioprine in systemic lupus erythematosus. Arthritis Rheum., 18:27–34, 1975.

Gofton, J. P.; O'Brien, W. M.; Hurley, J. N.; and Scheffler, B. J.: Radiographic evaluation of erosion in rheumatoid arthritis: Double blind study of auranofin vs. placebo. J. Rheumatol., 11:768–771, 1984.

Gottlieb, N. L.; and Gray, R. G.: Pharmacokinetics of gold in rheumatoid arthritis. Agents Actions, 8 (suppl.):529–538, 1981.

Gottlieb, N. L.; Kiem, I. M.; Penneys, N. S.; and Schultz, D. R.: The influence of chrysotherapy on serum protein and immunoglobulin levels, rheumatoid factor and antiepithelial antibody titers. J. Lab. Clin. Med., 86: 962–972. 1975.

Gottlieb, N. L.; Smith, P. M.; and Smith, E. M.: Pharmocodynamics of 197Au and of 195Au labeled authiomalate in blood: Correlation with course of rheumatoid arthritis, gold toxicity and gold excretion. Arthritis Rheum., 17:171–183, 1974.

Gustafsson, L. L.; Walker, O.; Alvan, G.; Beerman, B.; Estevez, F.; Gleisner, L.; Lindstrom, B.; and Sjoqvist, F.: Disposition of chloroquine in man after single intravenous and oral doses. Br. J. Clin. Pharmacol., 15:471–479, 1983.

Harmon, C. E.; and Portanova, J. P.: Drug induced lupus: Clinical and serologic studies. Clin. Rheum., 8:121–135, 1982.

Harris, E. D. Jr.: Rheumatoid arthritis—pathophysiology and implications for therapy. N. Engl. J. Med., 322:1277–1289, 1990.

Hayakawa, T.; Kanai, N.; Yamada, R.; Kuroda, R.; Higashi, H.; Mogami, H.; and Jinnai, D.: Effect of steroid hormone on activation of endoxan (cyclophosphamide). Biochem. Pharmacol., 18:129–135, 1969.

Healy, L. A.; and Wilske, K. R.: Reforming the pyramid: A plan for treating rheumatoid arthritis. Rheum. Dis. Clin. North Am., 15:615–620, 1989.

Hench, P. S.; Kendall, E. C.; Slocomb, C. H.; and Polley, H. E.: The effect of a hormone of the adrenal cortex (17-hydroxy-11-dehydrocorticosterone: compound E) and of pituitary adrenocorticotropic hormone on rheumatoid arthritis: Preliminary report. Proc. Staff Meetings. Mayo Clin., 24: 181–197, 1949.

Herzog, C.; Walker, C.; Pichler, W.; Aeschlimann, A.; Wassner, P.; Stockinger, H.; Knupp, W.; Rieber, P.; and Muller, W.: Monoclonal anti-CD4 in arthritis. Lancet, 2:1461–1463, 1987.

Hirschburg, J.; and Paulus, H. E.: Immunomodulators and other disease modifying antirheumatic drugs. In, Drugs for Rheumatic Disease (Paulus, H. E.; Furst, D. E.; and Dromgoole, S. H., eds.). Churchill Livingstone, New York, pp. 187–201, 1987.

Hoult, J. R. S.; and Moore, P. K.: Effects of sulphasalazine and its metabolites on prostaglandin synthesis inactivation and acting on smooth muscle. Br. J. Pharmacol., 68:719–730, 1980.

Hunter, T.; Urowitz, M. B.; Gordon, D. A.; Symthe, H. A.; and Ogyslo, M. O.: Azathioprine in rheumatoid arthritis: A long term follow-up study. Arthritis Rheum., 18:15–20, 1975.

Hurd, E. R.; and Ziff, M.: Parameters of improvement in patients with rheumatoid arthritis treated with cyclophosphamide. Arthritis Rheum., 17:72–78, 1974.

Huston, K. A.; and Hunder, G. G.: Giant cell (cranial) arteritis: A clinical review. Am. Heart J., 100:99–105, 1980.

Jaffe, I. A.: Penicillamine. In, Textbook in Rheumatology (Kelley, W. N.; Harris, E. D. Jr.; Ruddy, S.; and Sledge, C. B., eds.). W. B. Saunders, Philadelphia, pp. 824–832, 1989a.

Jaffe, I. A.: Penicillamine. In, Arthritis and Allied Conditions: A Textbook of Rheumatology, 11th ed. (McCarty, D. J., ed.). Lea & Febiger, Philadelphia, pp. 593–603, 1989b.

Jaffe, I. A.: The technique of penicillamine administration in rheumatoid arthritis. Arthritis Rheum., 18:513–514, 1975.

Jaffe, I. A.: The effect of penicillamine on the laboratory parameters in rheumatoid arthritis. Arthritis Rheum., 8:1064–1079, 1965.

Jessop, J. D.; Vernon-Roberts, B.; and Harris, J.: Effects of gold salts and prednisolone on inflammatory cells. Ann. Rheum. Dis., 32:294–300, 1973.

Kimberly, R. P.; and Plotz, P. H.: Salicylates including aspirin and sulfasalazine. In, Textbook of Rheumatology (Kelley, W. N.; Harris, E. D. Jr.; Ruddy, S.; and Sledge, C., eds.). W. B. Saunders, Philadelphia, pp. 739–764, 1989.

Klotz, U.; Maier, K.; Fischer, G.; and Heinkel, K.: Therapeutic efficacy of sulfasalazine and its metabolites in patients with ulcerative colitis and Crohn's disease. N. Engl. J. Med., 303: 1499–1502, 1980.

Koch, R.: Ueber bacteriologische forschung. Dtsch. Med. Wochenschr., 16:756, 1890.

Kremer, J. M.: Methotrexate therapy in the treatment of rheumatoid arthritis. Rheum. Dis. Clin. North Am., 15:533–556, 1989.

Kremer, J. M.; and Lee, J. K.: A long term prospective study of the use of methotrexate in rheumatoid arthritis. Arthritis Rheum., 31:577–589, 1988.

Kuchinskas, E. J.; and du Vigneaud, V.: An increased vitamin B_6 requirement in the rat on a diet containing L-penicillamine. Arch. Biochem., 66:1–9, 1957.

Lee, P.: Anti-inflammatory therapy during pregnancy and lactation. Clin. Invest. Med., 8:328–332, 1985.

Levy, J.; Barnett, E. V.; MacDonald, N. S.; Klinenberg, J. R.; and Pearson, C. M.: The effect of azathioprine on gammaglobulin synthesis in man. J. Clin. Invest., 51:2233–2238, 1972.

Lipsky, P. E.: Modulation of human antibody production in vitro by D-penicillamine and $CuSO_4$: Inhibition of T cell function. J. Rheumatol., 7 (suppl.):69–73, 1981.

Lipsky, P. E.; and Ziff, M.: Inhibition of antigen- and mitogen-induced human lymphocyte proliferation by gold compounds. J. Clin. Invest., 59:455–466, 1977.

Loddo, B.; and Marcialis, M. A.: Characteristics of the inhibitory action of D-penicillamine on the growth of poliovirus. Postgrad. Med. J., 50 (suppl. 2):45–50, 1974.

Lorber, A.: Gold salt therapy. In, Rheumatic Therapeutics (Roth, S. H.; Calabro, J. J.; Paulus, H. E.; Willkens, R. F., eds.). McGraw-Hill, New York, pp. 437–439, 1985.

Lyle, W. H.: Penicillamine. Clin. Rheum. Dis., 5:569–601, 1979.

Mason, H. L.; Myers, C. S.; and Kendall, E. C.: Chemical studies of the suprarenal cortex. The identification of a substance which possesses the qualitative action of cortin. J. Biol. Chem., 116:267–276, 1936.

McCune, W. J.; Golbus, J.; and Zeldes, W.: Clinical and immunologic effects of monthly administration of intravenous cyclophosphamide in severe systemic lupus erythematosus. N. Engl. J. Med., 318:1423–1431, 1988.

McDermott, M.; and McDevitt, H. O.: The immunogenetics of rheumatic diseases. Bull. Rheum. Dis., 38:1–10, 1988.

McGuire, J. L.; and Lambert, R. E.: Lupus erythematosus. In, Textbook of Internal Medicine, 2nd ed. (Kelly, W., ed.). J. B. Lippincott, Philadelphia, in press.

Melmon, K. L.: Will the sighted physician see? Pharos, 47:2–6, 1984.

Messer, J.; Rutman, D.; Sacks, H. S.; Smith, H. Jr.; and Chalmers, T. C.: Association of adrenocorticosteroid therapy and peptic ulcer disease. N. Engl. J. Med., 309:21–24, 1983.

Multi-Centre Trial Group: Controlled trial of D-penicillamine in severe rheumatoid arthritis. Lancet, 1:275–280, 1973.

Neumann, V. C.; Taggart, A. J.; LeGallez, P.; Astbury, C.; Hill, J.; and Bird, H. A.: A study to determine the active moiety of sulfasalazine in rheumatoid arthritis. J. Rheumatol., 13:285–287, 1986.

Nimni, M. E.; and Bavetta, L. A.: Collagen defect induced by penicillamine. Science, 150:905–907, 1965.

Noguchi, S.; and Nishitani, H.: Immunologic studies of a case of myasthenia gravis associated with pemphigus vulgaris after thymectomy. Neurology, 26:1075–1080, 1976.

Nuver-Zwart, I. H.; Van Riel, P. L. C. M.; Van de Putt, L. B. A.; and Gribnaw, F. W. J.: A double-blind comparative study of sulfasalazine and hydroxychloroquine in rheumatoid arthritis: Evidence of an earlier effect of sulfasalazine. Ann. Rheum. Dis., 48:389–395, 1989.

O'Callaghan, J. W.; Bretscher, P.; and Russel, A. S.: The effect of low-dose chronic intermittent parenteral methotrexate on delayed type hypersensitivity and acute inflammation in a mouse model. J. Rheumatol., 13:710–714, 1986.

Olsen, N. J.; Callahan, L. F.; and Pincus, T.: Immunologic studies of rheumatoid arthritis patients treated with methotrexate. Arthritis Rheum., 30:481–488, 1987.

Osman, M. A.; Patel, R. B.; Schuna, A.; Sundstrom, W. R.; and Welling, P. G.: Reduction in oral penicillamine absorption by food, antacid and ferrous sulfate. Clin. Pharmacol. Ther., 33:465–470, 1983.

Page, F.: Treatment of lupus erythematosus with mepacrine. Lancet, 2:755–758, 1951.

Parillo, J. E.; and Fauci, A. S.: Mechanism of glucocorticoid action on immune processes. Ann. Rev. Pharmacol. Toxicol., 19:179–208, 1979.

Payne, J. P.: A post-graduate lecture on lupus erythematosus. Clin. J., 4:223–229, 1894.

Persellin, R. H.; and Ziff, M.: The effect of gold salts on lysosomal enzymes of the peritoneal macrophage. Arthritis Rheum., 9:57–65, 1966.

Pincus, T.; and Callahan, L. F.: Taking mortality in rheumatoid arthritis seriously—predictive markers, socioeconomic status and comorbidity. J. Rheumatol., 13:841–845, 1986.

Plotz, P. H.; Lippel J. H.; and Decker, J. L.: Bladder complications in patients receiving cyclophosphamide for systemic lupus erythematosus or rheumatoid arthritis. Ann. Intern. Med., 91:221–223, 1979.

Rhodes, J. M.; Bartholomew, T. C.; and Jewell, D. P.: Inhibition of leukocyte motility by drugs used in ulcerative colitis. Gut, 22:642–647, 1981.

Richter, J. A.; Runge, J. A.; Runge L. A.; Pinals, R. S.; and Oates, R. P.: Analysis of treatment terminations with gold and antimalarial compounds in rheumatoid arthritis. J. Rheumatol., 7:153–159, 1980.

Robinson, J. K.; Baughman, R. D.; Auerback, R.; and Cimis, R. J.: Methotrexate hepatotoxicity in psoriasis—Consideration of liver biopsies at regular intervals. Arch. Dermatol., 116:413–415, 1980.

Rynes, R. I.: Antimalarial drugs. In, Textbook of Rheumatology (Kelley, W. N.; Harris, E. D. Jr.; Ruddy, S.; and Sledge, C. B., eds.). W. B. Saunders, Philadelphia, pp. 792–803, 1989.

Sany, J.: Treatment of rheumatoid arthritis by antibodies directed against class II MHC antigens. Scand. J. Rheumatol. Suppl. 76:289–295, 1988.

Scherbel, A. L.; Harrison, J. W.; and Atdjian, M.: Further observations in the use of 4-aminoquinoline compounds in patients with rheumatoid arthritis or related diseases. Cleve. Clin. Q., 25:95–111, 1958.

Schultz, D. R.; Volanakis, J. E.; Arnold, P. I.; Gottlieb, N. L.; Sakai, K.; and Stroud, R. M.: Inactivation of C1 in rheumatoid synovial fluid, purified C1 and C1 esterase by gold compounds. Clin. Exp. Immunol., 17:395–406, 1974.

Selhub, J.; Dhar, G. J.: and Rosenberg, I. H.: Inhibition of folate enzymes by sulfasalazine. J. Clin. Invest., 61:221–224, 1978.

Shand, N.; and Richardson, B.: Sandimmun^R (cyclosporin A): Mode of action and clinical results in rheumatoid arthritis. Scand. J. Rheumatol. Suppl., 76:265–278, 1988.

Sigler, J. W.; Bluhm, G. B.; Duncan, H.; Sharp, J. T.; Ensign, D. S.; and McCrum, W. R.: Gold salts in the treatment of rheumatoid arthritis: A double-blind study. Ann. Intern. Med., 80:21–26, 1974.

Silverberg, D. S.; Kidd, E. G.; and Shnitka, T. K.: Gold nephropathy: A clinical and pathologic study. Arthritis Rheum., 13:812–825, 1970.

Singh, G.; Fries, J. F.; Spitz, P.; and Williams, C. A.: Toxic effects of azathioprine in rheumatoid arthritis: A national post-marketing perspective. Arthritis Rheum., 32:837–843, 1989.

Srinivasan, R.; Miller, B. L.; and Paulus, H. E.: Long-term chrysotherapy in rheumatoid arthritis. Arthritis Rheum., 22:105–110, 1979.

Stenson, W. F.; and Lobos, E.: Inhibition of platelet thromboxane synthetase by sulfasalazine. Biochem. Pharmacol., 32:2205–2209, 1983.

Stockman, A.; Zilko, P. J.; Major, G. A.; Tait, B. D.; Property, D. N.; Mathews, J. D.; Hannach, M. C.; McClusky, J.; and Muirden, K. A.: Genetic markers in rheumatoid arthritis: Relationship to toxicity from D-penicillamine. J. Rheumatol., 13:269–273, 1986.

Symmons, D.; Salmon, M.; Farr, M.; and Bacon, P. A.: Sulfasalazine treatment and lymphocyte function in patients with rheumatoid arthritis. J. Rheumatol., 15:575–579, 1988.

Tabachnik, M.; Eisen, H. N.; and Levine, B.: New mixed disulphide penicillamine-cysteine. Nature, 174:701–702, 1954.

Todd, P. A.: Auranofin in rheumatoid arthritis. In, Auranofin in Rheumatoid Arthritis (Gottlieb, N. L., ed.). ADIS Press, Langhorne, Pa., pp. 78–106, 1987.

Townes, A. S.; Sowa J. M.; and Shulman, L. E.: Controlled trial of cyclophosphamide in rheumatoid arthritis. Arthritis Rheum., 19:563–573, 1976.

Troy, J. L.; Silvers, D. N.; Grossman, M. E.; and Jaffe, I. A.: Penicillamine associated pemphigus: Is it really pemphigus? J. Am. Acad. Dermatol., 4:547–555, 1981.

Venning, G. R.: Identification of adverse reactions to new drugs. B. Med. J., 286:199–202, 289–292, 365–368, 458–460, 544–547, 1983.

Walz, D. T.; DiMartino, M. J.; Chakrin, L. W.; Sutton, B. M.; and Misher, A.: Antiarthritic properties and unique pharmacologic profile of a potential chrysotherapeutic agent: SK&FD-39162. J. Pharmacol. Exp. Ther., 197:142–152, 1976.

Walshe, J. M.: Wilson's disease: New oral therapy. Lancet, 1:25, 1956.

Webster, L. T.: Drugs used in the chemotherapy of protozoal infections, malaria. In, The Pharmacological Basis of Therapeutics, 7th ed. (Gilman, A. J.; Goodman, L. S.; Rall, T. W.; and Murad, F., eds.). Macmillan Publishing, New York, pp. 1029–1048, 1985.

Wei, P.; and Sass-Kortsak, A.: Urinary excretion and renal clearance of D-penicillamine in humans and the dog (abstract). Gastroenterology, 58:288, 1970.

Weinblatt, M. E.; Colbyn, J. S.; Fox, D. A.; Fraser, P. A.; Holdsworth, D. E.; Glass, D. N.; and Trentham, D. E.: Efficacy of low-dose methotrexate in rheumatoid arthritis. N. Engl. J. Med., 312:818–822, 1985.

Weinstein, G.; Rocnigk, H. H.; Mailback, K.; Cosmides, J.; and Halprin, K.: Psoriasis-liver methotrexate interactions. Arch. Dermatol., 108:36–42, 1973.

Wickens, and Paulus, H. E.: Autimalarial drugs. In, Drugs for Rheumatic Disease (Paulus, H. E.; Furst, D. E.; and Dromgoole, S. H., eds.). Churchill Livingstone, New York, pp. 113–133, 1987.

Williams, H. F.; Wilkens, R. F.; Samuelson, C. O.; Dahl, S. R.; Egger, M. J.; Reading, J. C.; Ward, J. R.; Alarcon, G. S.; Guttadauria, M.; Yarboro, C.; Polisson, R. P.; Weiner, S. R.; Luggen, M. E.; and Billingsly, L. M.: Comparison of low-dose oral pulse methotrexate and placebo in the treatment of rheumatoid arthritis: A controlled clinical trial. Arthritis Rheum., 28:721–730, 1985.

Wraith, D. C.; McDevitt, H. O.; Steinman, L; and Acha-Orbea, H.: T cell recognition as the target for immune intervention in autoimmune disease. Cell, 57:709–715, 1989.

Yu, D. T.; Clemens, P. J.; Peter, J. B.; Levy, J.; Paulus, H. E.; and Barnett, E. V.: Lymphocyte characteristics in rheumatic patients and the effect of azathioprine therapy. Arthritis Rheum., 17:37–45, 1974.

Zilko, P. J.; Dawkins, R. L.; and Cohen, M. L.: Penicillamine treatment of rheumatoid arthritis: Relationship of proteinuria and autoantibodies to immune status. Proc. R. Soc. Med., 70 (suppl. 3):118–122, 1977.

20

Metabolic and Degenerative Disorders of Connective Tissue and Bone

Tammi L. Shlotzhauer, R. Elaine Lambert, and James L. McGuire

PATHOGENESIS OF SPECIFIC DISEASES

Musculoskeletal disorders in which the immune system does not have a primary role include osteoarthritis, osteoporosis, and gout. Osteoarthritis (OA) is caused by the progressive loss of articular cartilage and reactive changes at joint margins and subchondral bone. These changes result in dysfunction of the joint primarily affecting weight-bearing joints of the spine and lower extremities. Osteoporosis is the most common metabolic bone disease and presents as either symptomatic fracture or asymptomatic loss of bone density found on incidental radiographs. Gout is a disorder of uric acid metabolism that involves abnormal production and/or reduced renal excretion of uric acid.

Osteoarthritis

Osteoarthritis (OA) is the most common form of degenerative joint disease (DJD). The etiology of the cartilage abnormalities is not known. Cartilage is a complex matrix composed of collagen, mostly type II, and proteoglycans that together surround isolated islands of active chondrocytes (Mankin and Brandt, 1989). The chondrocytes control both the synthesis and the extracellular turnover of the matrix. During the course of the disease, proteoglycans including hyaluronic acid decrease both in absolute amount and in their ability to aggregate. In addition to abnormalities in the cartilage, the subchondral bone stiffens and may cause bony outgrowths called osteophytes.

Within the joint space, the cartilage debris usually evokes an inflammatory response.

Osteoporosis

Osteoporosis can be a devastating illness presenting clinically as multiple fractures, chronic back pain, or loss of height. Predominantly seen in women, osteoporosis has been linked to lack of estrogen because of its temporal association with ovarian failure occurring either naturally or surgically. The cause of excessive bone loss in postmenopausal women is complex and involves decreases in both mineral content and structural strength. Bone density is lost rapidly after the menopause, driven by bone resorption in excess of bone formation. Estrogens probably have a protective role against excessive resorption (Riggs and Melton, 1986). Additionally, many patients with osteoporosis have decreased intestinal absorption of calcium that may be partially estrogen-dependent.

The mechanical rigidity that confers resistance to compressive loads in trabecular bone depends on the longitudinal trabeculae with stabilization by horizontal struts. Loss of the cross struts results in weaker bone at any given density.

The potential development of osteoporosis relates, in part, to the initial bone density at the onset of menopause. A low value at that time suggests a failure to attain maximal bone mass before age 30.

Medications can cause osteoporosis. Administration of corticosteroids results in excess resorption of bone and excretion of calcium in the urine. Additionally, decreases in bone formation and intestinal calcium absorption have been observed in patients receiving corticosteroids (Lukert and Raisz, 1990). Other drugs that adversely affect bone metabolism include phenytoin, barbiturates, thyroxine, and heparin. Moreover, certain loop diuretics can further aggravate a negative calcium balance by causing continuous hypercalciuria (Marcus, 1990).

Gout

Gout is associated with the extracellular precipitation of monosodium urate (MSU) crystals, the predominant salt of uric acid found at physiologic pH. The acute gouty attack characteristically affects the first metatarsophalangeal joint, but other joints are frequently involved. Some patients have additional subcutaneous deposits of urate called tophi. Clinical gout usually occurs after years of hyperuricemia and most commonly presents in men in their 40s and in women in their 60s. Normal serum uric acid concentrations are 4 to 7 mg/dl in males and slightly lower in females.

Uric acid can be synthesized from ingested or endogenously produced purines (see Fig. 20–1). There is a prominent recapture mechanism to provide purines for nucleic acid synthesis. Two main mechanisms of persistent hyperuricemia exist (Kelly et al., 1989). First, uric acid can be overproduced. In most patients, de novo synthesis accounts for the majority of the uric acid produced with a lesser component derived from dietary purines. Certain genetic enzyme defects, notably deficient hypoxanthine-guanine phosphoribosyltransferase (HGPRT) or overactive 5-phosphoribosyl-1-pyrophosphate (PRPP) synthetase, account for some cases of overproduction of uric acid. Large urate loads can be produced from rapid cell death during chemotherapy for neoplasia (see chapter 23). Second, the majority of patients with gout have abnormal renal tubular handling of urate, resulting in decreased clearance of uric acid, which leads to accumulation of uric

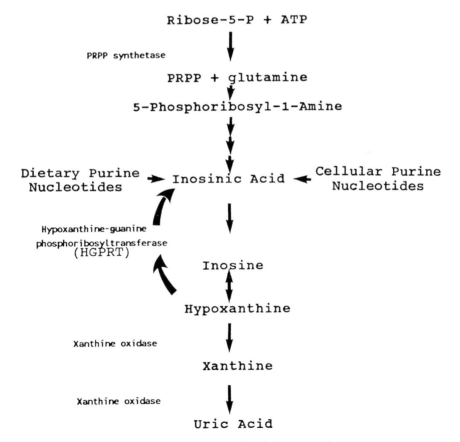

Fig. 20–1. Purine metabolism. PRPP = phosphoribosyl-1-pyrophosphate.

acid in the body. Certain drugs, including thiazides, furosemide, ethanol, and low doses of salicylate, have been associated with hyperuricemia and decreased urinary clearance of uric acid.

The mechanism of an acute attack of gout is unknown. Tissue precipitation, crystal dispersion within a joint, and acute inflammation are important components. The coating of MSU crystals with IgG and complement may facilitate phagocytosis by neutrophils (Terkeltaub and Ginsberg, 1988). A variety of chemotactic factors and cytokines, particularly interleukin-1, perpetuate the inflammation and lysosomal enzyme release from neutrophils, both of which contribute to the intensity of the attack.

PHARMACOLOGY OF IMPORTANT DRUGS

Drugs Used to Treat Osteoarthritis

Nonsteroidal Anti-Inflammatory Drugs. The NSAIDs, including salicylate derivatives, have been the cornerstone of treatment for rheumatic disease for decades by virtue of their anti-inflammatory and analgesic properties (see Table 20–1). They have been used widely in osteoarthritis, rheumatoid arthritis, crystal-induced arthritis, spondyloarthropathies, soft tissue rheumatism, and other systemic connective tissue diseases. The utility of these agents as analgesics in nonrheumatic acute and chronic pain disorders is well known.

Mechanism of Action. The NSAIDs inhibit the production of prostaglandins (PGs) that play a major role in inflammation. Inhibition of the cyclooxygenase pathway of arachidonic acid metabolism has been the accepted explanation for the NSAIDs' anti-inflammatory, analgesic, and antipyretic properties. The result of this inhibition is to decrease the generation of two unstable cyclic endoperoxidases, PGG_2 and PGH_2, that ordinarily are further metabolized to the stable prostaglandins (PGE_2, PGF_2, or PGD_2), thromboxanes, prostacyclin (PGI_2), and toxic oxygen radicals (see Fig. 20–2). Inhibition of synthesis occurs via irreversible acetylation of cyclooxygenase by aspirin, or by reversible inhibition by other NSAIDs. Nonacetylated salicylates have some ability to inhibit prostaglandin synthesis, but markedly less than other NSAIDs.

The ability of PGs to potentiate inflammation led early investigators to believe that cyclooxygenase inhibition is the sole mechanism of action of NSAIDs. However, the lipoxygenase pathway of arachidonic acid metabolism that leads to the production of leukotrienes and lipoxins also has been under evaluation in relation to the effects of NSAIDs. Leukotrienes are potent mediators of inflammation. Their production can be decreased by certain NSAIDs in vitro (Forrest and Brooks,

1988). Inhibition of 5-lipoxygenase in vivo, however, has not been clearly demonstrated. The clinical significance of this finding is unclear.

Additionally, NSAID effects on neutrophil function have been suggested to explain part of their anti-inflammatory activity (Abramson and Weissman, 1989). Inhibition of neutrophil activation, aggregation, and adhesion by NSAIDs has been observed. Inhibition of the release of lysosomal enzymes and superoxide radicals from neutrophils as well as from monocytes and macrophages has also been shown. Decreased lipopolysaccharide-induced leakage and neutrophil-dependent edema can be demonstrated (Forrest and Brooks, 1988; Hochberg, 1989).

Although NSAIDs have not yet demonstrated clinical effects on the normal immune system, secondary immunomodulatory effects via PGE_2s ability to alter cell- and humoral-mediated immune responses may exist. Goodwin (1984) reviews PGE_2 effects that include induction of suppressor T cells; suppression of mitogen responsiveness, clonal proliferation, and lymphocyte cytotoxicity; and inhibition of secretory responses of neutrophils. He suggests that PGE_2 may represent a protective, feedback inhibitor of cellular immune response that may be adversely affected by NSAIDs. Alternatively, pathologic immunoglobulin production, which is dependent on cellular immune function, may be favorably decreased in the setting of inhibited PG synthesis. Analogous immunomodulatory roles of other mediators of inflammation also have been attributed to histamine and to some extent to the β-adrenergic effects of catecholamines (Rocklin, 1990). They are not controlled by catecholamines. *Principle: As evidence accumulates about an effect of an endogenous mediator or drugs that affect it, comments often are made about there being "no evidence" of corresponding clinical effects. The clinician should not be reassured by such statements that these effects have been sought and ruled out or that they will not ultimately be sought and found. In the meantime, the physician may be in the best position to detect such effects when drugs given for a different indication modulate a phenomenon that they were not "approved for."*

Pharmacokinetics. The NSAIDs may be classified according to their chemical structure (see Table 20–1). Differentiating these drugs on the basis of their pharmacokinetic differences, such as half-life and clearance, may have more clinical importance (see Table 20–2).

The NSAIDs are weak acids with a pK_a that is typically less than 5 (Verbeeck, 1988). They are well absorbed orally with some variability in the rate of absorption and time to peak concentrations in plasma (see Table 20–2). Enteric-coated NSAIDs such as diclofenac are absorbed more slowly. Indomethacin may be used as a supposi-

Table 20-1. DOSES OF AVAILABLE NSAID

CLASS AGENT	DOSE FREQUENCY	TOTAL ANALGESIC DOSE‡ (MG/DAY)	TOTAL ANTI- INFLAMMATORY DOSE‡ (MG/DAY)
Salicylates (Acetylated)			
Aspirin*	Variable	1200–3600	4000–6000
Salicylates (Nonacetylated)			
Salsalate*	b.i.d.–q.i.d	NI	1500–5000
Trilisate	b.i.d.–q.i.d.	NI	1500–4000
Salicylate Derivatives			
Diflunisal	b.i.d.–t.i.d.	500–1000	1000
Anthranilic Acids (Fenamates)			
Meclofenamate*	t.i.d.–q.i.d.	200–300	200–400
Mefenamic acid	q.i.d.	1000	NI
Proprionic Acids			
Ibuprofen*	3–6 X	800–2400	1200–3200
Fenoprofen	3–6 X	800–1200	900–3200
Naproxen	b.i.d.–t.i.d.	750–1000	750–1250
Naproxen Na	b.i.d.–t.i.d.	550–1375	550–1375
Flurbiprofen	b.i.d.–t.i.d.	150–300	200–300
Ketoprofen	b.i.d.–q.i.d.	75–200	150–300
Carprofen	b.i.d.–t.i.d.	NI	300–600
Arylacetic Acids			
Diclofenac	b.i.d.–t.i.d.	50–150	100–200
Heteroarylacetic Acids			
Tolmetin Na	t.i.d.–q.i.d.	NI	600–1800
Indole and Indene Acetic Acids			
Indomethacin*	b.i.d.–t.i.d.	NI	75–200
Sulindac†	b.i.d.	NI	300–400
Oxicams			
Piroxicam	qd	NI	20
Pyrazoles			
Phenylbutazone*	qd–q.i.d.	NI	100–600

* Generic available.
† Expected generic 1991.
‡ NI = not indicated.

tory. The NSAIDs are lipid-soluble, are strongly bound to plasma albumin, and have a volume of distribution (V_d) that is mostly confined to the actual V_d of albumin (Verbeeck, 1988). The most clinically relevant pharmacokinetic differences among NSAIDs lie in their different half-lives of elimination. These drugs can be roughly divided into those with half-lives greater than 5 hours and those with half-lives less than 5 hours (Table 20-2).

The NSAIDs with long half-lives can be administered once or twice daily; examples include piroxicam, sulindac, naproxen, and diflunisal. Using these drugs allows construction of a simplified regimen and results in increased compliance. Drugs with long half-lives have less peak-to-trough fluctuation of concentration in plasma when compared with those with short half-lives given at the same interval between doses. The longer period of relatively steady high concentration of drug may favor less breakthrough pain

during the later part of the day and in the early morning. In addition, drugs with long half-lives may more readily produce higher, sustained concentrations of drug in synovial fluid; diffusion of NSAIDs into joint fluid is generally slow, and the longer serum concentrations are high, the more time the drug has to enter the fluid.

The NSAIDs with short half-lives usually are administered every 6 to 8 hours but should be given less frequently if they are used as analgesics rather than as anti-inflammatory drugs. Commonly used agents in this group includes ibuprofen, fenoprofen, indomethacin, diclofenac, ketoprofen, meclofenamate, flurbiprofen, and tolmetin sodium. These agents have the advantage of rapidly producing peak concentrations in plasma. Most of these agents are excellent analgesics and have equivalent anti-inflammatory efficacy compared with those with longer half-lives (see Table 20-1). *Principle: Drugs with truly identical pharmacologic properties except for their*

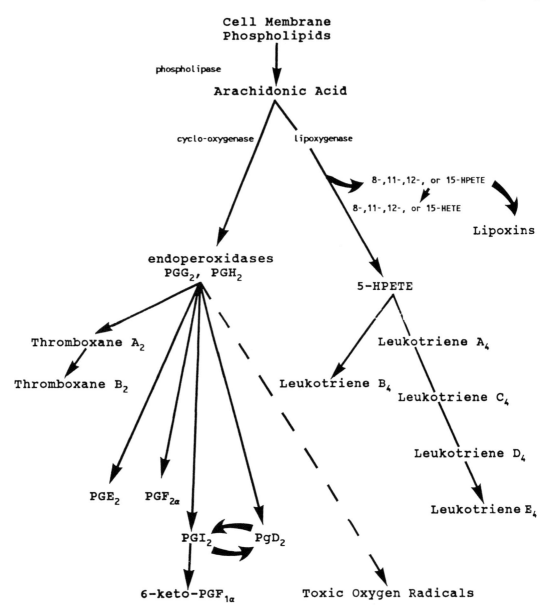

Fig. 20-2. Arachidonic acid metabolism. HPETE = Hydroperoxyeicosatetraenoic Acid.

pharmacokinetics can be chosen for the latter properties to aid compliance. However, if there is some difference between both the pharmacodynamic and pharmacokinetic properties and the former is advantageous, adjusting the dose and dose intervals and explaining to your patient why adhering to a more difficult regimen is important may be quite sufficient to equalize pharmacokinetic differences.

It has been suggested that there may be less relative toxicity with short-half-life agents. How-

ever, differences in toxicity (if there are any) may be more related to compliance and the relative degrees of cyclooxygenase inhibition brought about by standard dosage regimens than to reduced innate toxicity of the shorter-acting agents. Clinically significant differences between agents can be ascribed to their rates of clearance by the kidney and liver. Most NSAIDs are eliminated predominantly by hepatic biotransformation. This process may include glucuronide formation as it does with naproxen, ketoprofen, carprofen,

Table 20-2. PHARMACOKINETIC DATA FOR COMMON NSAIDs

	T_{max} (H)	$T_{1/2}$ (H)	CLEARANCE (ML/MIN)	CHANGE IN CLEARANCE WITH†		
				RI	HI	E
$T_{1/2}$ < 5 hours						
Diclofenac	2–3	2	260 (IV)	↔◆	↔◆	↔↓
Fenoprofen	1–2	2–3	40–90	↓	?	↔◆
Flurbiprofen	1.5	5.7	20	?	?	↔◆
Ibuprofen	1–2	1.8–2.5	50	↔	↔	↔↓
Indomethacin	1–2	4.5	70–140	↓	↓	↓
Indocin SR	2–4	4.5–6.0	70–140	↓	↓	?
Ketoprofen	0.5–2	2–4	80–90	↓	?	↓
Meclofenamate Na	0.5–1	2–3	?	?	?	?
Mefenamic acid	2–4	2–4	?	?	?	?
Tolmetin Na	0.5–1.0	1–1.5	125	?	?	↔
$T_{1/2}$ > 5 hours						
Carprofen	1–3	2–13	20–40	↓	↔	↔
Diflunisal	2–3	11–15	5–15	↓	?	↓
Naproxen	2–4	12–15	5	↓	↓	↓
Naproxen Na	1–2	12–13	5	↓	↓	↓
Piroxicam	3–5	30–86	2–3	↔	?	↔
Phenylbutazone	2–5	45–93	1–2	?	?	↔
Sulindac	1–2	7.8 (16.4*)	?	↔	↓	↓

* Active sulfide.

† RI = renal insufficiency; ◆ = single-dose pharmacokinetic studies; HI = hepatic insufficiency; ↔ = no change in clearance; E = elderly; ↓ = decreased clearance.

Adapted from Verbeeck et al., 1983; Woodhouse and Wynne, 1987; Day et al., 1988; and Olin, 1990, p. 251.

fenoprofen, indomethacin, and diflunisal. Patients with renal failure retain these labile acyl glucuronide metabolites that may be easily transformed back to the parent NSAID with potential for toxic accumulation (Day et al., 1988). Since decreased binding to plasma albumin with increased free-drug concentration (Verbeeck, 1988) may also exist in this group of drugs, it is prudent to avoid using these agents in patients with renal insufficiency. Although the products of biotransformation of all NSAIDs are excreted via the kidney, renal insufficiency does not appear to result in retention of the metabolites equally with all agents (see Table 20-2). As will be discussed below, this does not ensure the safety of any NSAID in renal failure, since most renal toxicity is largely secondary to inhibition of the synthesis of renal PGs with a lesser contribution of toxicity due to accumulation of metabolites.

Substantial amounts of sulindac, diclofenac, carprofen, meclofenamate, and indomethacin are secreted in the bile and feces. In most situations, the hepatic clearance is much greater than the renal clearance. Despite the central role of the liver in metabolism of NSAIDs, little is known about the effect of liver disease on the pharmacokinetics of NSAIDs. The clearance of ibuprofen, diclofenac, and salicylates is not generally modified by liver disease. However, accumulation of metabolites of sulindac is increased in patients with liver disease (Day et al., 1988). Clearance of indometh-

acin and naproxen is also decreased with liver disease (Verbeeck et al., 1983; Table 20-2).

Renal clearance of NSAIDs in the elderly is a clinically important issue that has been extensively reviewed (Woodhouse and Wynne, 1987). No change in clearance has been found in elderly women taking ibuprofen, or after single doses of flurbiprofen and fenoprofen. Healthy elderly patients generally can take piroxicam, salicylates, phenylbutazone, and indomethacin without unusual dose adjustments. Decreased clearance has been demonstrated with naproxen, ketoprofen, sulindac, and diflunisal in both elderly men and elderly women, and in elderly men taking ibuprofen. Studies that measure clearance after single doses of a NSAID may not be clinically relevant.

Aspirin and Other Salicylates. This class of agents is notable for its wide array of formulations. Aspirin (acetyl salicylic acid) is the classic inexpensive analgesic, anti-inflammatory agent that has been in use for over 100 years. Plain aspirin, a weak acid, rapidly crosses the gastric mucosa often resulting in GI distress (see chapter 8). Many formulations attempt to expedite its transit into the small intestine to decrease direct gastric irritation. These formulations, including enteric coating and timed-release preparations, also slow the onset of action.

After absorption, aspirin is rapidly hydrolyzed to salicylic acid. Salicylic acid is eliminated by renal excretion. When aspirin is used in small doses, salicylate has a half-life of approximately 4 hours. However, when aspirin is used in doses needed for anti-inflammatory effects (4–6 g/day) with salicylate concentrations in serum reaching 200 to 300 mg/l, salicylate half-life increases to 12–25 hours. This indicates that the kinetics of salicylate clearance are nonlinear (see chapter 37). Changes in urinary pH importantly affect the excretion of salicylates, with an alkaline urine favoring excretion. Thus, absorption and excretion kinetics can be highly variable depending on the preparation, dose, or individual to whom it is given. Monitoring concentrations of salicylate in plasma is important when using large anti-inflammatory doses (see chapters 1, 37, 38).

Although the nonacetylated salicylates are less effective analgesics than aspirin (because of their relative inability to easily inhibit synthesis of PG), they can be potent anti-inflammatory agents when concentrations are kept at therapeutic salicylate concentrations. Several nonacetylated salicylates are available including salicylsalicylic acid (salsalate), magnesium salicylate, sodium salicylate, choline salicylate, and choline magnesium salicylate. Regardless of the parent salicylate compound, once absorbed, they are all rapidly hydrolyzed to salicylic acid. Again, because salicylic acid metabolism is capacity-limited, the apparent half-life can be prolonged as saturation of the more efficient excretory pathway occurs. Large intermittent doses can be used to decrease the frequency of administration and increase compliance when salicylates are used for their anti-inflammatory properties.

Diflunisal is a difluorophenyl derivative of salicylic acid whose metabolism is similar to that of salicylic acid. No salicylic acid is formed. It also exhibits dose-dependent pharmacokinetics, with concentrations in plasma increasing more than proportionally as the dosage is increased. Diflunisal is a potent inhibitor of cyclooxygenase, unlike the other nonacetylated salicylates.

Accumulation of salicylate may result in nausea, emesis, diarrhea, hyperventilation, flushing, or headache. Severe salicylism can present as confusion, seizure, pulmonary edema, coma, respiratory alkalosis, metabolic acidosis, respiratory failure, or cardiovascular collapse. Suspicion should be increased in the elderly, in whom symptoms may mimic other conditions and the history of excessive self-medication may not be known to the physician.

Adverse Effects of NSAIDs and Salicylates. The most common adverse effects of NSAIDs focus on the GI tract, kidney, and platelets. All are largely secondary to inhibition of PG synthesis. Several, less common adverse effects are listed in Table 20–3.

Table 20–3. **COMMON ADVERSE EFFECTS OF NSAIDs***

GI:	Gastritis, ulcer, hemorrhage, diarrhea (meclofenamate), pancreatitis (sulindac)
Neurologic:	Headache (indomethacin), confusion, dizziness, ataxia, aseptic meningitis (ibuprofen), ocular problems, tinnitus (salicylates)
Renal:	Interstitial nephritis (fenoprofen), nephrotic syndrome, acute renal failure, fluid and electrolyte changes, papillary necrosis, hematuria
Hepatic:	Increased transaminase concentrations, hepatitis, cholestasis, hepatic necrosis
Skin:	Rash, photosensitivity (piroxicam), erythema multiforme, vasculitis, bullous disease, Stevens-Johnson syndrome, exfoliative dermatitis, toxic epidermal necrolysis
Hematologic:	Platelet effects, neutropenia, thrombocytopenia, aplastic anemia (phenylbutazone), hemolytic anemia (fenamates), pancytopenia
Allergic:	Fever, rash, urticaria, angioedema, pulmonary infiltrates, asthma, anaphylaxis

* Major offending agent for particular toxicity in parentheses.

GI Toxicity. Gastric mucosal ulceration or irritation is the most frequent adverse effect and can be severe (Semble and Wu, 1987). The mucosal damage appears to be related to the loss of cytoprotective effects of PGs on the gastric mucosa. The gastric ulceration, unlike the acid-mediated duodenal peptic ulcer, usually is not accompanied by pain. The elderly are particularly susceptible to the silent ulceration that can be life-threatening (Griffin et al., 1988). Bleeding associated with NSAIDs can be large in the absence of pain. The onset of bleeding can occur as early as after very few doses, or after a chronic regimen that has been well tolerated. The incidence of serious bleeding caused by NSAIDs was anticipated to be rather high based on their premarketing testing (about 6%), but subsequent to marketing the frequency has settled into the 1% range (Inman and Rawson, 1983). This rate of bleeding still is quite high, when one considers the potential consequences. Corticosteroids, aspirin, and other NSAIDs find themselves on a restricted list, while there are few data to help the clinician decide whether bleeding caused by one such agent predisposes to bleeding caused by others. Patients with rheumatoid arthritis who cannot use NSAIDs or corticosteroids are left only with remittive agents that have less analgesic activity and potential for equally serious adverse effects (see chapter 19).

One strategy to circumvent this dilemma is to use nonacetylated salicylates (with the exception of diflunisal) that have less ability to inhibit cyclooxygenase and presumably cause less gastropathy and bleeding (Inman and Rawson, 1983). Another and more promising approach is to consider using misoprostol, a synthetic methyl analog of PGE_1, in conjunction with NSAIDs. Misoprostol may decrease the risk of bleeding from NSAID ulceration (see chapter 8). Early data show that this combination is effective in protecting the gastric mucosa and preventing gastric bleeding caused by NSAIDs. The cytoprotective role of PG is presumed to be secondary to stimulation of secretion of mucus and bicarbonate by gastric mucosa, increasing mucosal blood flow, and inhibiting secretion of gastric acid (Graham et al., 1988). There are more potent PGs being developed for the same purpose. Likely, the choice between them largely will depend on their relative efficacy as cytoprotective agents, but also on their potential to cause other undesired local or systemic effects. ***Principle: Basic literature on new chemical entities often contains the findings that lead to additive uses of the entity or to strategies that counter some of their serious effects.*** In the case of the GI bleeding caused by NSAIDs, cytoprotective effects of locally acting PGs were known to prevent bleeding in rats many years before they were even tried in humans.

All NSAIDs have serious gastropathic potential. Aspirin appears to have additional local toxic effects, which when coupled with irreversible platelet acetylation, promote bleeding. Drugs with increased enterohepatic circulation such as indomethacin, sulindac, and meclofenamate may increase the risk of small bowel ulceration because more of the drug is exposed to the GI tract per dose than others with no enterohepatic component of clearance. Sulindac is associated with the largest degree of enterohepatic circulation and has been associated with pancreatitis (Goldstein et al., 1980).

Nephrotoxicity. The renal syndromes associated with NSAID use have been well described (Clive and Stoff, 1984; see chapter 11). A common abnormality is sodium retention leading to edema that can occasionally be severe. Hyponatremia occurs if decreased free-water clearance exceeds sodium retention. Significant hyponatremia has been described in patients on NSAIDs and thiazides. In general, however, effects of thiazide diuretics are inhibited by NSAIDs in proportion to their ability to inhibit cyclooxygenase (see chapter 11).

Rarely, marked increases in serum potassium concentrations can be caused by NSAIDs. Patients at risk for this effect include the elderly, those with preexisting kidney disease, and those who are taking potassium-sparing diuretics. The use of NSAIDs in patients with hyporeninemic hypoaldosteronism induced by β-adrenergic receptor antagonists or angiotensin-converting enzyme (ACE) inhibitors also can result in significant but reversible hyperkalemia (see chapters 2, 5, 11). Thus, patients at high risk should have serum potassium concentrations checked within 1 to 2 weeks of initiation of a NSAID.

A form of hemodynamic renal failure is occasionally produced if NSAIDs are given to patients with elevated concentrations of angiotensin II. At risk are those with hypovolemia, functional hypovolemia (congestive heart failure, cirrhosis, nephrotic syndrome), chronic renal failure, and high renin-angiotensin states (i.e., renal artery stenosis). Renal failure in this setting is rapid in onset and largely reversible after the drug is discontinued. Nonacetylated salicylates rarely cause this type of renal failure (Clive and Stoff, 1984). Sulindac may be somewhat less likely to alter renal blood flow and glomerular filtration rate, but the "renal sparing" effect is relative and most likely dose-related, as shown in more recent studies on high-risk patients with preexisting renal insufficiency (Klassen et al., 1989). Thus, patients at high risk starting NSAIDs should have their creatinine concentrations checked after approximately 2 weeks of therapy.

In the elderly, there is an increased risk that renal function may be compromised. Before treatment with a NSAID is started, and shortly after a chronic regimen has been established, renal function should be checked and the dose adjusted appropriately. In addition, to minimize the potential for accumulation of drug in the elderly, it may be more prudent to initiate therapy with a short-acting agent before considering using longer acting preparations. There are factors other than potential drug accumulation that make the elderly more prone to the toxicity of NSAIDs. These include physiologic changes in their GI tract, decreased concentrations of albumin in the serum, increased numbers of coexisting diseases and greater potential for drug interactions.

The NSAIDs also can damage the renal parenchyma. Chronic renal injury secondary to papillary necrosis is one form of drug induced injury. This form of "analgesic nephropathy" has been associated most commonly with combination aspirin-phenacetin preparations. It also occurs with NSAID combinations and rarely when only a single NSAID is used. This damage is the least reversible of the renal effects of NSAIDs.

An idiosyncratic interstitial nephritis with or without nephrotic syndrome can occur. Often presenting with flank pain, an "active" urinary sediment, high eosinophil counts in the urine, proteinuria, increased creatinine concentration, or systemic evidence of hypersensitivity, the condition is almost always reversible. This adverse effect is reported most commonly with fenoprofen but can occur with all NSAIDs (Scharschmidt and Feinfeld, 1989).

Hepatotoxicity. Although less commonly recognized, elevation of liver transaminase concentrations in plasma can be induced by NSAIDs. Clinically significant hepatitis or cholestasis, or irreversible liver injury may occur, or even rare cases of fatal hepatic necrosis. These consequences may be due to accumulation of toxic metabolites, or to idiosyncratic or hypersensitivity reactions. In anti-inflammatory doses, salicylates appear to be direct hepatotoxins, particularly in women with connective tissue disease and children with juvenile rheumatoid arthritis (Zimmerman, 1981). All NSAIDs have been associated with hepatotoxicity, but some appear to carry increased risk. Higher-risk agents reported by Prescott (1986) include diclofenac, sulindac, phenylbutazone, and salicylates. Although patient demography does not predict hypersensitivity-related liver disease, advanced age, use of many drugs, prolonged or high-dose therapy, decreased renal function, systemic lupus erythematosus (SLE), and juvenile rheumatoid arthritis are factors that are associated with increased risk of liver damage by NSAIDs (Paulus, 1982). After initial close observation, some physicians recommend checking liver as well as renal function every 3 months in patients chronically taking NSAIDs. Those with significant concurrent disease, including renal or hepatic insufficiency, may need closer observation. The NSAIDs should be discontinued if transaminase concentrations increase more than three times normal or if evidence of systemic hypersensitivity develops.

Hematologic Toxicity. Although several potential hematologic adverse effects can be caused by NSAIDs (see Table 20–3), the most predictable are related to effects on platelets. With the exception of nonacetylated salicylates, impairment of thromboxane-mediated platelet aggregation routinely leads to prolonged bleeding time. Aspirin irreversibly acetylates platelets; other NSAIDs produce only transient inactivation of the cyclooxygenase. Therefore, aspirin should be discontinued at least 2 weeks before and after surgery. Other NSAIDs should be stopped the equivalent of 5 to 6 half-lives for that particular agent before surgery (see Table 20–2). Patients with a high risk of bleeding or those taking anticoagulants should be given nonacetylated salicylates if they need anti-inflammatory agents. Phenylbutazone can cause agranulocytosis and aplastic anemia. This agent should be reserved for severe disease unabated by all other NSAIDs.

CNS Toxicity. All NSAIDs can cause CNS effects. Indomethacin is the most notorious for these adverse reactions. A wide range of nonspecific symptoms can be evoked (see Table 20–3). A rare form of aseptic meningitis has been described in patients with lupuslike diseases and in some normal patients using NSAIDs, particularly ibuprofen.

Idiosyncratic Reactions. Idiosyncratic or hypersensitivity reactions fortunately are rare. Patients with other nondrug allergic diseases appear to have a higher incidence of these reactions while taking NSAIDs than those who do not have such propensity. Patients with bronchial asthma, nasal polyps, and urticaria are at relatively high risk to develop sensitivity to aspirin, which may manifest itself with a life-threatening asthmatic attack (Stevenson and Simon, 1988). This adverse response may be linked to inhibition of PG synthesis leading to shunting down the lipoxygenase pathway of the arachidonic acid cascade (see Fig. 20–2). This pathogenetic hypothesis is strengthened by the patients' cross-sensitivity to all NSAIDs that significantly inhibit cyclooxygenase. Nonacetylated salicylates with the exception of diflunisal do not produce as extensive cross-sensitivity, but they must still be used with great care if at all in patients who are sensitive to aspirin.

Editors' Note: This latter observation throws some doubt on the hypothesis since nonacetylated salicylates are still reasonable inhibitors of cyclooxygenase. But old and comfortable theories die slowly.

Drug Interactions. The NSAIDs can interact with other drugs via two major mechanisms. A NSAID can change the clearance of another drug or it can displace it from plasma protein. Some pharmacodynamic interferences with the efficacy of an interacting drug have already been described (Table 20–4). For a complete review, see Tonkin and Wing (1988).

So far we have grouped NSAIDs as if they all had common fundamental mechanisms of efficacy and toxicity and little besides their half-lives that could be used to choose between them for the treatment of specific disorders. In some situations, this generalization may be valid. For example, different proprionic acid derivatives appear to have equal efficacy and toxicity profiles in the treatment of rheumatoid arthritis. The differences between their routes of metabolism and clearance from the body have been discussed as a basis for drug choice in a given patient. However, serious therapeutic discretion is lost if one thinks that the validity of the generalization about equal efficacy of proprionic acid derivatives necessarily holds for use of these drugs for other indications. For instance, proprionic acid derivatives with rapid onset of action may be more efficacious in the treatment of dysmenorrhea. In addition, there appears to be great interpatient variability be-

Table 20-4.   COMMON DRUG INTERACTIONS INVOLVING NSAIDs

AFFECTED DRUG	INTERFERING NSAID	CLINICAL EFFECT
Oral anticoagulants	Phenylbutazone All NSAIDs	Increased anticoagulant effect Increased risk of bleeding
Lithium	All NSAIDs except sulindac, salicylates	Decreased clearance; increased concentration in plasma
Oral hypoglycemic agents	Phenylbutazone Salicylates	Decreased clearance $t_{1/2}$ of oral hypoglycemic agents leading to hypoglycemia Direct potentiation of hypoglycemia
Phenytoin	Phenylbutazone Other NSAIDs	Increased concentrations of phenytoin in plasma Decreased total concentrations in plasma with no change in unbound concentration (see chapter 12)
Digoxin	All NSAIDs	Potential decreased clearance of digoxin, increased plasma concentration (see chapter 4)
Aminoglycosides	All NSAIDs	Potential decreased clearance, increased plasma concentrations (see chapter 24)
Antihypertensives	All NSAIDs ?except sulindac	Decreased hypotensive effect (see chapter 2)
Diuretic agents	All NSAIDs ?except sulindac	Decreased natriuretic and diuretic effects (see chapter 11)
Potassium-sparing diuretics; ACE inhibitors; β blockers	All NSAIDs	Potential hyperkalemia (see chapters 2, 11)
Uricosurics	Salicylates, diflunisal	Decreased uricosuric effect

Adapted with permission from Tonkin and Wing (1988).

tween individuals being treated for the same condition with the same agent. *Principle: Chemically related drugs may share some pharmacologic effects but very likely will not have identical pharmacologic profiles. Do not assume that because a class of chemically related entities has almost equivalent efficacy for one indication, they will have equivalent effects for all indications for all patients.*

Such an assumption was made when zomepirac (simply considered one among many NSAIDs because it was related to tolmetin) was taken off the market because it was suspected of causing anaphylactoid reactions and severe hepatitis. The drug was discontinued without much debate partially because other NSAIDs were not suspected of causing similar adverse effects. When the committee on drug safety in the United Kingdom was asked to retrospectively review the validity of the decision to ban the drug, they found no epidemiologic data to support the suspicion that the drug caused the adverse effects it had been accused of (Inman and Rawson, 1983). More important epidemiologic data were developed to hypothesize that the drug had unexpected efficacy in the prevention of stroke, pulmonary emboli, and myocardial infarction (Inman and Rawson, 1983). The possible tragedy crystalized when it was later found that no other NSAIDs shared these valuable properties. But it was too late, for zomepirac had already been taken off the market and for

many nonmedical reasons is not likely to return to medical use (Inman and Rawson, 1983). *Principle: The most important signals of alternative efficacy or unexpected toxicity of marketed drugs often may only appear while they are being used in the field* (see chapters 35 and 41).

Drugs Used to Treat or Prevent Osteoporosis

Calcium Supplements. Calcium supplements have traditionally been included in regimens to prevent and treat postmenopausal osteoporosis. In the 1970s a few studies suggested that calcium supplements reduce postmenopausal bone loss (Horsman et al., 1977). More recent studies have not confirmed a benefit on trabecular bone loss with calcium use. A *small* positive effect on cortical bone was suggested (Riis et al., 1987). However, a possible benefit is suggested when calcium supplements are used in combination with estrogen or fluorides (Riggs et al., 1982). The mechanism of action of calcium supplements on bone is not known. Clearly, the supplements ensure adequate substrate availability for bone mineralization in patients with low intestinal absorption of calcium. Calcium absorption appears to decline with age, especially with achlorhydric patients (Bullamore et al., 1970). The role of deficiency of 1,25-dihydroxyvitamin D in this malabsorption is uncertain (Slovick et al., 1981; Francis et al., 1984) (see chapter 17).

Table 20–5.   **ORAL CALCIUM PREPARATIONS**

DRUG	PERCENT CALCIUM	TABLET SIZE (MG)	EQUIVALENT OF 1 G CALCIUM PER DAY (TABLETS)
Calcium carbonate	40	600	4
	40	500	5
	40	1250	2
Calcium gluconate	9	600	18.5
	9	1000	11
Calcium lactate	13	600	12
	13	300	24
Dibasic calcium phosphate	31	500	7
Chelated calcium	20	750	7
Calcium citrate	20	950	5

Adapted with permission from Medical Letter 24:106,1982.

There are several different calcium preparations available for oral administration (see Table 20–5) including salts of gluconate, lactate, citrate, and phosphate. Calcium carbonate preparations provide the highest amount of elemental calcium per tablet. Absorption of this preparation is improved when taken with food, particularly in the elderly, who may have decreased gastric acid secretion (Peck et al., 1987). The recommended daily requirement of calcium for adults over 24 years of age is 800 mg (see chapter 10). After menopause, the amount of calcium intake required to maintain neutral calcium balance rises from about 1000 to nearly 1500 mg/day (Heaney, 1982). This intake can be accomplished with a combination of supplements and diet (see Tables 20–5 and 20–6).

Some adverse effects of calcium supplementation are linked to absorption of calcium. Hypercalcemia is rare in the absence of concurrent use of vitamin D or presence of renal failure (milk alkali syndrome) (see chapter 11). Hypercalciuria occurs more frequently and may cause nephrolithiasis in some patients. Citrate is a natural inhibitor of stone formation, so the use of this calcium salt is reasonable in patients requiring calcium supplementation who have a history of nephrolithiasis. An increased constipating effect of the calcium carbonate preparations may be seen in the elderly. This can usually be ameliorated by divided doses, increased water intake, or change to a different preparation.

Vitamin D. The role of vitamin D in the treatment of osteoporosis is even less clear than that of calcium supplements. The primary mechanism of action of the vitamin is to improve intestinal absorption of calcium, again ensuring adequate availability of calcium and phosphate for bone mineralization. Vitamin D, or more likely one of its active metabolites, 25-hydroxyvitamin D or 1,25-dihydroxyvitamin D, may have a direct role in the bone cell (Rasmussen and Bordier, 1978). Although most adults have adequate vitamin D generation from exposure to sun and eating a balanced diet, the elderly are often more susceptible to deficiency because of their limited outside recreation and poorer diets (Peck et al., 1987). Some

Table 20–6.   **CALCIUM CONTENT OF FOODS**

FOOD	SERVING SIZE	CALCIUM CONTENT (MG)
Vanilla shake (Burger King)	1 average	479
Parmesan, grated	1 oz	390
Sardines (canned in oil)	8 medium-sized	354
Yogurt (low-fat)	1 cup	345
Milk, skim	1 cup	303
Milk, whole (3.5% fat)	1 cup	288
Cheddar cheese (American)	1 oz	211
Creamed cottage cheese	1 cup	211
Muenster cheese	1 oz	203
American cheese, processed	1 oz	195
Taco (Taco Bell)	1 average	120
Chocolate fudge pudding	$3\frac{1}{2}$ oz	100

Adapted with permission from Medical Letter 29:76, 1987.

elderly osteoporotic patients presenting with fe- mur fractures have had bone biopsy consistent with osteomalacia (Aaron et al., 1974). These pa- tients would likely be helped by supplementation with vitamin D.

The recommended dose of vitamin D (actually D_2) for treatment of osteoporosis has decreased dramatically. In the 1970s daily recommended dosages were in the 10,000-unit range, usually taken orally as 50,000 units once or twice a week. Currently, 400 units daily seems prudent and is consistent with nutritional recommendations (see chapter 10). An intake of significantly more than this involves the risk of stimulating bone resorp- tion (Nordin et al., 1980). The administration of 50,000 units once per month is probably effective, since vitamin D compounds, D_2 and D_3, are stored for prolonged periods in fat cells (Mawer et al., 1972). There is little evidence that 25- hydroxyvitamin D and 1,25-dihydroxyvitamin D should be used in preference to the less expensive D_2 despite their approved indication for treatment of renal osteodystrophy. *Principle: Similar dis- eases with different pathogenesis should not be treated with similar regimens unless there is proof that such treatment is optimal. Think about this in terms of treatment of different forms of hyperten- sion, asthma, bacterial pneumonia, and so forth.*

The adverse effects of vitamin D therapy are reflected in hypercalcemia and hypercalciuria that may result in the formation of kidney stones or rarely renal failure (Schwartzman et al., 1987). Concentrations of calcium and creatinine in plas- ma and calcium in urine should be monitored ev- ery 3 to 6 months in patients receiving high doses of vitamin D. Glucocorticoid therapy has been advocated for severe cases of hypervitaminosis D, but usually discontinuation of the drug and ade- quate hydration are sufficient.

Estrogens. Estrogen therapy started at the time of menopause can prevent bone loss and de- crease the rate of fractures of major weight- bearing bones (Ettinger et al., 1985). The pharma- cology of estrogens is discussed in chapter 17.

Fluoride. The use of fluorides has been associ- ated with increased radiographic density of bone, called fluorosis. Fluoride can stimulate osteo- blastic-directed bone formation (Farley et al., 1983). Additionally, fluoride can be incorporated into the central crystal structure of bone, hy- droxyapatite.

The degree of GI absorption of fluoride prepa- rations correlates with the solubility of the vari- ous fluoride compounds. The major route of ex- cretion of fluoride is by the kidneys; additional losses occur in sweat, breast milk, and GI secre- tions.

The therapeutic oral dose of sodium fluoride (NaF) for the formation of bone ranges between 20 and 80 mg daily. This dosage is much higher than the 1 part per million concentration found in most fluorinated public water systems to prevent dental caries. The currently available tablet of NaF is 2.2 mg. Clinical trials using a 20-mg timed-release tablet are in progress (Pak et al., 1989).

Several studies have demonstrated increased vertebral bone density induced by fluoride. How- ever, a recent blinded study suggested that verte- bral fractures are not decreased with NaF mono- therapy (Riggs and Melton, 1990). In fact, there was an increased number of fractures in the pe- ripheral skeleton. Fluoride given in combination with calcium and estrogen appeared to protect against vertebral fractures (Riggs et al., 1982). Additional long-term studies are necessary to evaluate the optimal use of those drug combina- tions.

The adverse effects of NaF include GI distress, tendinitis, and lower extremity synovitis, particu- larly of the knees and ankles. The cause of the synovitis may be related to new bone formation around the joint or to microfractures that might be enhanced by the drug. Large doses of fluorides cause skeletal fluorosis and osteomalacia. Fluo- rides should not be used or should be used with frequent adjustment of dosage in patients with renal insufficiency because fluoride may accumu- late and cause toxicity. Other contraindications include active peptic ulcer disease and pregnancy. *Principle: When only small gains are produced by drugs used to treat common diseases, the decision to treat often rests on the likelihood of toxicity. If the gains are attended by toxicities that may be as bad as the disease, the decision to use the drug becomes very difficult to defend.*

Calcitonin. Calcitonin (CT) is a 32–amino acid peptide that inhibits osteoclast-mediated re- sorption of bone. Calcitonin is secreted by the C cells of thyroid and seems to have relatively little physiologic effect on mineral homeostasis in hu- mans. Salmon CT is a more potent inhibitor of bone resorption than is the human peptide. The salmon preparation has been used effectively to treat Paget disease of bone and hypercalcemia of malignancy. Human CT is approved for use in Paget disease but not for osteoporosis.

Therapy with CT can result in increased density of vertebral bone and an increase in total calcium body burden (Gruber et al., 1984). These positive effects need to be confirmed by long-term studies to determine if fracture rates are reduced. The CT is given by injection, either subcutaneously or IM, at dosages of 50 to 100 units daily. The disadvantages to using CT are its high cost and many patients' reluctance to take repeated injections for non-life-threatening illnesses.

The adverse effects of CT relate to the need for repeated injections of the peptides. Local and systemic allergic reactions can occur. Some patients may experience flushing, nausea, or a marked increase in sodium and water excretion in the early postinjection period. These effects diminish with continual treatment. Human CT is less immunogenic and should be used as an alternative to salmon CT if efficacy is lost because of the formation of neutralizing antibodies.

Drugs Used to Treat or Prevent Gout

Colchicine. Extracts from the seeds of *Colchicum autumnale* have been used in the treatment of inflammatory conditions since the sixth century A.D. Colchicine was first isolated in 1820 and has remained an important drug in the treatment of gout (Chang et al., 1987). In general, colchicine is a weak anti-inflammatory agent and has no analgesic or antipyretic properties, nor does it affect the serum or urine concentration of uric acid. The effectiveness of colchicine lies in its ability to modify polymorphonuclear neutrophil (PMN) functions leading to a decrease in the inflammatory response induced by urate crystals. Colchicine binds to tubulin and prevents its polymerization into functional microtubules that are involved in maintaining cell structure and movement. Microtubular disaggregation results in decreased PMN motility and chemotaxis, impaired release of chemotactic factors, interference with formation of digestive vacuoles, and impaired lysosomal degranulation (Chang et al., 1987).

Colchicine is readily absorbed from the GI tract, reaching peak concentrations in plasma within 0.5 to 2 hours (Wallace and Ertel, 1973). The drug rapidly enters cells and accumulates in peripheral blood leukocytes, where measurable concentrations may be present as long as 10 days after administration (Ertel and Wallace, 1973). There is no evidence that colchicine undergoes metabolism. It is excreted in urine, bile, and feces (Chang et al., 1987).

The primary clinical uses of colchicine are to decrease the inflammatory response in acute gouty arthritis and decrease the frequency and intensity of recurrent attacks. Colchicine has also been beneficial in the management of acute episodes and the prophylactic treatment of pseudogout (calcium pyrophosphate dihydrate deposition disease) as well as hypersensitivity (leukocytoclastic) vasculitis, palindromic rheumatism, Behçet syndrome, sarcoidosis, Sweet syndrome, calcific tendonitis, and prevention of amyloidosis and acute attacks of familial Mediterranean fever (Chang et al., 1987).

The effectiveness of colchicine in treating acute gouty arthritis is maximal when it is given within a few hours of the beginning of the symptoms of gout. The dramatic and rapid improvement that typically occurs has allowed its use as a diagnostic aid when gout is suspected in cases when synovial fluid is not easily obtainable. The oral and IV routes of administration are available for colchicine. Gastrointestinal toxicity including nausea, vomiting, diarrhea, and abdominal cramping is a predictable side effect in patients who take a full oral therapeutic dosage for acute gout. The IV route avoids these GI side effects and allows a more rapid action, usually 4 to 12 hours, compared with 12 to 36 hours with oral administration (Chang et al., 1987).

Adverse reactions to colchicine are a function of dosage since cumulative toxicity occurs. These reactions include urticaria, dermatitis, alopecia, purpura, hyponatremia, hypocalcemia, aplastic anemia, agranulocytosis, disseminated intravascular coagulation, muscle weakness, peripheral neuropathy, amenorrhea, dysmenorrhea, oligospermia, or azoospermia. Local extravasation may result in tissue necrosis when it is given IV. Roberts et al. (1987) formulated the following recommendations for the prevention of toxic reactions and death while using IV colchicine: (1) closely monitor the drug, because it is infrequently used and has potential for mortal effects if dosing is excessive, (2) separate IV from oral therapy in time whenever possible, (3) give elderly patients smaller than usual doses even when renal and hepatic function appear normal, (4) treat patients with liver and kidney disease very conservatively, and (5) do not substitute IV colchicine milligram for milligram for oral colchicine, that is, the maximal IV dosage should never exceed 4 mg (Roberts et al., 1987).

Probenecid. Probenecid was developed to help prolong and sustain concentrations of penicillin in plasma by competing for its renal excretion. Later, the drug became the first widely used uricosuric agent. The uricosuric effect of probenecid is attributed to its inhibition of the renal tubular reabsorption of filtered urate. However, even large dosages of probenecid do not increase the clearance of uric acid beyond 50% of the filtered load (Dayton et al., 1963).

Probenecid is rapidly and completely absorbed, and uricosuria begins as early as 40 minutes after a single oral dose (Sirota et al., 1952). The half-life in plasma is dose-dependent and ranges from 6 to 12 hours. Probenecid is extensively protein-bound (89%–94%) and remains primarily extracellular (Dayton et al., 1963). The majority of probenecid is metabolized in the liver, with only 5% of the administered dose appearing in the urine within 24 hours. In acidic urine, excretion of probenecid is negligible (Weiner et al., 1960).

The primary clinical uses of probenecid are to lower serum uric acid values in patients with gout, and to promote sustained plasma concentrations of penicillin. Probenecid has been demonstrated to decrease the size of tophi, inhibit formation of tophi, and diminish frequency of attacks of acute gouty arthritis. Gutman and Yu (1951) demonstrated that probenecid dosages of 500 to 2000 mg/day would control patient gout in 85% of cases. Probenecid becomes progressively less effective with advancing renal insufficiency, requiring increased dosage at creatinine clearances less than 20 ml/min (Gutman, 1951).

Probenecid is remarkably well tolerated, with only rare serious adverse effects. Gastrointestinal intolerance with nausea, vomiting, and anorexia is the most common toxicity with an approximately 3% incidence, whereas skin rashes, fever, and acute allergic reactions (with urticaria or anaphylaxis) are much less common (Boger and Strickland, 1955). Other reported toxicities include headache, dizziness, gingival tenderness, hepatic necrosis, nephrotic syndrome, alopecia, flushing, aplastic anemia, leukopenia, and hemolytic anemia. Urate nephrolithiasis can be minimized by excluding patients with excessive urate production, starting therapy at low doses, encouraging fluid intake, and if necessary, alkalinizing the urine to a pH greater than 6.0 (Sirota et al., 1952).

Probenecid inhibits the renal tubular secretion of a number of drugs, and alters hepatic clearance of still others. See Table 20-7 for a summary of these effects.

Allopurinol. Allopurinol is a purine analog of hypoxanthine and a potent inhibitor of xanthine oxidase, the enzyme responsible for oxidation of xanthine and hypoxanthine to uric acid (see Fig. 20-1). Both allopurinol and its major metabolite, oxipurinol, effectively inhibit the formation of uric acid regardless of the mechanism that may have led to its accumulation. Allopurinol is completely absorbed by the GI tract. Most of the allopurinol is metabolized to oxipurinol. The biologic half-life of allopurinol is 2 to 3 hours, whereas oxipurinol's half-life is as long as 18 to 33 hours (Elion et al., 1966). The renal clearance of allopurinol and oxipurinol ranges from 14 to 20 ml/minute and 23 to 31 ml/minute, respectively (Hande et al., 1978). Uricosuric drugs increase renal excretion of oxipurinol, whereas renal insufficiency reduces its excretion. See Table 20-8 for dosing of allopurinol in patients with various levels of renal function (Hande et al., 1984).

In most patients 50% reductions in both serum and urinary uric acid concentrations can be antici-

Table 20-7. EFFECTS OF PROBENECID ON OTHER DRUGS

Decreased Renal Tubular Excretion
  Penicillin
  Indomethacin
  Other β-lactam antibiotics
  Salicylic acid
  Dapsone
  Naproxen
  Paraminosalicylic acid
  Sulfinpyrazone
  Acyclovir
  Acetozolamide
  Furosemide
  Thiazides
Reduced Volume of Distribution
  Ampicillin
  Nafcillin
  Cephaloridine
Decreased Renal Excretion
  Heparin
Decreased Plasma Protein Binding and Inhibition of Biliary Excretion
  Methotrexate
Inhibition of Hepatic Uptake
  Rifampin
Inhibition of Biliary Excretion
  Indomethacin
Inhibition of Hepatic Metabolism
  Azathioprine
  Naproxen
  Ketoprofen

Adapted from Weinberger and Paulus, 1987.

pated when taking doses of allopurinol ranging between 200 and 500 mg/day. These reductions reach their maximum in 4 to 14 days and then remain stable (Yu and Gutman, 1964). The average dose required to maintain serum uric acid concentrations of 6.0 to 6.9 mg/dl in patients with normal renal function is 300 mg/day (Hande et al., 1984). Rapid and major changes in concentrations of urate in serum may precipitate an acute attack of gout. Thus, one should begin allopurinol with low dosage and gradually increase it

Table 20-8. RECOMMENDED MAINTENANCE DOSE OF ALLOPURINOL BASED ON CREATININE CLEARANCE

CREATININE CLEARANCE (ML/MIN)	DOSE OF ALLOPURINOL (MG)
100	300
80	250
60	200
40	150
20	100
10	100 every 2 days
0*	100 every 3 days

* If on hemodialysis, dosing should follow dialysis since both allopurinol and oxipurinol are dialyzable.
Reproduced with permission from Hande et al., 1984.

to reduce this risk. Dosages of allopurinol may be adjusted to approach the patient's target urate concentration. The drug is effective when given as a single daily dose because of the prolonged half-life of oxipurinol.

The effectiveness of allopurinol in treating and preventing gout, mobilizing tophi, and decreasing the incidence of urate nephropathy and nephrolithiasis has been known for greater than 20 years (Rundles, 1985). Allopurinal is generally well tolerated, though serious and even fatal adverse effects have been reported. Toxic effects tend to occur more frequently in patients with renal insufficiency and in those concurrently taking thiazide diuretics (Boston Collaborative Drug Surveillance Program, 1970). Table 20–9 summarizes allopurinol's known direct toxicities. A constellation of findings, including fever, skin rash, eosinophilia, hepatitis, and progressive renal insufficiency has been referred to as an allopurinol hypersensitivity syndrome. This syndrome is quite rare but has a significant risk of death due to systemic vasculitis (Hande et al., 1984). The potential severity of this allergic reaction emphasizes the need to restrict allopurinol therapy to those patients with a specific indication for its use (see the section on clinical therapeutics below). Skin rashes are more frequent and serious in patients receiving concomitant ampicillin or amoxicillin (Young et al., 1974). In patients with preexisting liver disease, periodic liver function tests are recommended during the early stages of therapy. If renal insufficiency is present, monitoring parameters of renal function is essential in order to adjust allopurinol dosages appropriately (see Table 20–8).

Table 20–9. POTENTIAL ADVERSE EFFECTS OF ALLOPURINOL

Systemic:	Fever
Skin:	Urticaria, maculopapular rash, exfoliative dermatitis, purpura, Stevens-Johnson syndrome, hypersensitivity vasculitis, toxic epidermal necrolysis, icthyosis, alopecia
GI:	Nausea, diarrhea, abdominal pain, loss of taste, abnormal liver function tests, cholestatic jaundice, acute cholangitis, granulomatous hepatitis, hepatic necrosis
Respiratory:	Epistaxis
Renal/ Urologic:	Interstitial nephritis, renal insufficiency, xanthine stones
Musculoskeletal:	Precipitation of acute gouty arthritis, arthralgias, myopathy
Neurologic:	Headache, drowsiness, peripheral neuropathy, retinal lesions
Hematologic:	Eosinophilia, leukocytosis, bone marrow suppression

The biologic activities of purine analog such as azathioprine and 6-mercaptopurine are potentiated by allopurinol-induced inhibition of xanthine oxidase (Elion et al., 1963). The dose of azathioprine and 6-mercaptopurine should be reduced to 25% of its usual dose if allopurinol is used concurrently with the purine analog (see chapter 23). The toxicity of other cytotoxic agents such as cyclophosphamide also appears to be increased when they are used with allopurinol, though the mechanism is unclear and no specific guidelines exist for adjusting doses of these agents. Allopurinol prolongs the half-life of coumarin and probenecid. Thus patients receiving concomitant coumarin and allopurinol therapy should have their prothrombin times monitored closely and either of the drugs adjusted appropriately.

CLINICAL THERAPEUTICS

Osteoarthritis

The treatment of osteoarthritis is multifaceted. Weight reduction, instruction in joint protection, physical therapy, surgery, and drug therapy play important roles in the management of this disease. The NSAIDs provide anti-inflammatory effects if used in appropriate doses (see Table 20–1). Agents with the best analgesic profile include aspirin, the propionic acid class derivatives, and diflunisal (Brogden, 1986). Additional benefit may be derived from acetaminophen or other analgesics. Depending on the age and renal function of the patient, a NSAID that is convenient to take (once or twice a day) and has a low adverse-effect profile usually constitutes initial therapy. The availability of over-the-counter NSAIDs (ibuprofen, salicylates) and the goal of adequate analgesia should alert the clinician to the potential problems that might be created by self-medication. General guidelines for laboratory monitoring of patients on NSAIDs suggested by the American College of Rheumatology include a complete blood cell count (CBC), urinalysis, and measurement of concentrations of creatinine, potassium, and aspartate aminotransferase (AST) every 1 to 3 months initially, then a CBC, urinalysis, and measurement of concentrations of creatinine, potassium, and AST every 3 to 12 months while a stable dose is being taken (see specific recommendations for high-risk patients in the NSAID toxicity section). *Principle: For diseases that are common and symptomatic, there are over-the-counter and over-the-fence therapies available for patients to consider, but not necessarily to discuss with their physician. Consider the possibility that unusual and unexpected changes in the course of such disease are the result of unprescribed therapy.*

The NSAIDs are usually continued indefinitely in osteoarthritis. In vitro studies suggest that some NSAIDs may have adverse effects on proteoglycan synthesis (Bjelle, 1989). This finding is worrisome, but the clinical experience so far in those treated with NSAIDs is not consistent with acceleration of the progression of the disease. *Principle: Following the progress of a disease when symptoms are relieved may be difficult from the vantage of the psychology of both the patient and physician. Nevertheless, surrogate end points should never be used in lieu of more definitive end points if the drug has a chance of worsening the pathologic condition while ameliorating symptoms.*

Osteoporosis

Therapy for osteoporosis is divided into prevention of bone loss and reversal of bone loss in patients with established osteoporosis. Prevention has two phases. First, women must attain maximal bone mass throughout their teens and early twenties. This may be best accomplished by a combination of adequate daily intake of calcium (1200 mg) by a combination of diet and calcium supplements if necessary (see Tables 20–5 and 20–6), and regular physical activity. Second, women can be protected against impending loss of bone associated with the start of menopause. Conjugated estrogen in the daily dose range of 0.625 to 1.25 mg is effective in preventing much of the obligatory bone loss phase early after menopause (Ettinger et al., 1985). Most bone specialists and gynecologists favor cycling estrogen with a progestin for women with a uterus. Some postmenopausal patients may derive favorable effects on bone from supplementation with calcium (Riggs and Melton, 1990). Thiazides are known to cause calcium retention and have been suggested to increase the mineral content of bone (Wasnich et al., 1983). Whether this has a preventive role for osteoporosis will require controlled, prospective trials. Any preventive program should include an exercise program to help maintain bone mass.

Patients who already have osteoporosis diagnosed, either by low bone mass (measured by densitometry or quantitative computer tomography) or by a history of bone fracture, require therapy. However, the current regimens have not been dramatically successful in reversing severe osteopenia in many of these patients. Calcium supplements at doses of 1000 mg/day can be justified in light of decreased absorption of calcium with aging (Bullamore et al., 1970). Whether this is beneficial is uncertain. The efficacy of estrogen therapy in treating established osteoporosis is unclear. Sodium fluoride may increase the formation of bone in doses of 20 to 80 mg daily but should not be used alone (Riggs et al., 1990). Earlier studies suggest that combinations of all three, namely estrogen, fluoride, and calcium, may reduce the fracture rate in osteoporotic women (Riggs et al., 1982). Sodium fluoride will be used in clinical investigation for osteoporosis, but widespread use is not advised at this time. Modest exercise in the elderly can result in increased bone-mineral content and should be advised in the asymptomatic patient with osteoporosis (Smith et al., 1981).

In summary, prevention is still the best avenue for both idiopathic and steroid-induced osteoporosis. For confirmed osteoporosis, agents that stimulate new bone mass including growth hormones, androgen, and insulin-like growth factors are currently being investigated. *Principle: Physicians frequently must make therapeutic decisions with inadequate or only partial information at hand. If you decide to treat, use drugs that are least toxic, treat for limited periods; follow signs of definitive changes as noninvasively as possible; perhaps most important, follow the literature very carefully so that aggressive or conservative approaches can be justified in a timely manner.*

Gout

Therapy for gout has two distinct phases. First, the inflammation and severe pain associated with an acute attack must be controlled. Second, elevated serum urate concentrations should be lowered to prevent further episodes of acute gout. The acute joint disease has historically been treated with colchicine. Oral colchicine (0.6 mg) given hourly until a maximum dose of 4 mg is reached is very effective in aborting an attack. Intravenous colchicine at doses of 1 to 2 mg also is effective with less GI upset than the oral preparation.

The NSAIDs in high doses also are effective in the treatment of an acute gouty episode. If an attack has been present for more than 24 hours, NSAIDs may be the agents of choice. Indomethacin currently is the most popular NSAID because of its short time to peak concentration and rapid clearance. Fortunately, the GI and CNS adverse effects are generally tolerable during a course of indomethacin of 150 to 200 mg daily in divided doses for 1 to 2 days. All other NSAIDs in high doses, with the exception of salicylate and its derivatives such as diflunisal, can be effective in controlling the acute attack (see Table 20–2). Salicylates actually may worsen the attack because they can induce fluxes in serum and tissue urate stores. Furthermore, allopurinol and probenecid have no place in the therapy of an acute attack because of the flux in concentrations of urate in plasma they can create.

After the acute phase of gout has subsided, the patient should be evaluated by determining the 24-hour urinary uric acid excretion in order to distinguish overproduction from renal under-excretion of urate as the dominant cause of the hyperuricemia. During the evaluation period, colchicine (0.6 mg once or twice per day) may be used to prevent further acute episodes. The finding of 24-hour urinary urate excretion greater than 800 mg suggests overproduction, whereas values less than 500 mg are consistent with decreased clearance, providing that such patients are not receiving drugs that can affect excretion of uric acid.

Overproduction of uric acid in a gouty patient usually warrants treatment with allopurinol. Allopurinol is also the drug of choice in patients with tophi, nephrolithiasis, or renal insufficiency. In the patient with normal renal function who has a dimished clearance of urate, probenecid is the drug of choice in view of its safety; its effects must be monitored so that appropriate doses are used. Probenecid should not be used in patients who overexcrete uric acid in view of the risk of inducing uric acid stones in urine.

Several special situations exist that warrant allopurinol therapy in a patient who does not have clinical gout. They include patients undergoing cancer chemotherapy in whom a large purine load is anticipated from cell death due to therapy. Here, prophylaxis with allopurinol is given to prevent acute urate nephropathy. In addition, patients who have calcium nephrolithiasis associated with hyperuricosuria can benefit from allopurinol. Finally, a person with a serum uric acid values above 13 mg/dl probably should be treated because of their substantially increased potential of experiencing nephrolithiasis or gout. However, asymptomatic hyperuricemia of lesser levels does not warrant treatment.

The initiation of treatment with urate-lowering drugs can cause rapid fluxes of urate in tissue, blood, and synovial compartments. These shifts can precipitate further acute attacks. Therefore, allopurinol is started at 100 mg daily and increased by 100 mg at the end of each month until a dose of 300 mg (or the maximum adjusted dose for renal insufficiency) is reached. At this time a serum uric acid concentration is determined. Values of 2 mg/dl below the upper limit of normal for the laboratory are the goal. Allopurinol is then continued as a single daily dose indefinitely. If hyperuricemia persists, further increases in dose in 100-mg increments are given monthly until a satisfactory response is achieved. Probenecid is started at 250 mg twice daily and increased by 500-mg increments at 4-week intervals to a maximum of 1000 mg twice daily or until the desired serum urate concentration is obtained. When therapy with either allopurinol or probenecid is initiated and until a stable dose is attained, prophylactic colchicine or an NSAID should be co-administered.

REFERENCES

Aaron, J. E.; Gallagher, J. C.; Anderson, J.; Stasiak, L.; Longton, E. B.; Nordin, B. E. C.; and Nicholson, M.: Frequency of osteomalacia and osteoporosis in fractures of the proximal femur. Lancet, 1:229–233, 1974.

Abramson, S. B.; and Weissman, G.: The mechanism of action of non-steroidal anti-inflammatory drugs. Arthritis Rheum., 32:1–9, 1989.

Bjelle, A.: NSAIDS and cartilage metabolism. Scand. J. Rheumatol. Suppl. 77:43–52, 1989.

Boger, W. P.; and Strickland, S. C.: Probenecid (Benemid): Its uses and side effects in 2502 patients. Arch. Intern. Med., 95:83–92, 1955.

Boston Collaborative Drug Surveillance Program: Excess of ampicillin rashes associated with allopurinol or hyperuricemia. N. Engl. J. Med., 286:505–507, 1972.

Brogden, R. N.: Non-steroidal anti-inflammatory analgesics other than salicylates. Drugs, 32(suppl. 4):27–45, 1986.

Bullamore, J. R.; Gallagher, J. C.; and Wilkinson, R.: Effect of age in calcium absorption. Lancet, 2:535–537, 1970.

Chang, Y. H.; Silverman, S. L.; and Paulus, H. E.: Colchicine. In, Drugs in Rheumatic Diseases (Paulus, H. E.; Furst, D. E.; and Dromgoole, S. H., eds.). Churchill Livingstone, New York, pp. 431–442, 1987.

Clive, D. M.; and Stoff, J. S.: Renal syndromes associated with nonsteroidal antiinflammatory drugs. N. Engl. J. Med., 310: 563–572, 1984.

Day, R. O.; Graham, G. G.; and Williams, K. M.: Pharmacokinetics of non-steroidal anti-inflammatory drugs. Bailliere's Clin. Rheumatol., 2:363–393, 1988.

Dayton, P. G.; Yu, T. F.; and Chen, W.: The physiological disposition of probenecid including renal clearance in man, studied by an improved method for its estimation in biological material. J. Pharmacol. Exp. Ther., 140:278–286, 1963.

Elion, G. B.; Kovensky, A.; and Hitchings, G. H.: Metabolic studies of allopurinol, an inhibitor of xanthine oxidase. Biochem. Pharmacol., 15:863–880, 1966.

Elion, G. B.; Callahan, S.; Nathan, H.; Bieber, S.; Rundles, R. W.; and Hitchings, G. H.: Potentiation by inhibition of drug degradation: 6-Substituted purine and xanthine oxidase. Biochem. Pharmacol., 12:85–93, 1963.

Ertel, N. H.; and Wallace, S. L.: Measurement of colchicine in urine and peripheral leukocytes (abstract). Clin. Res., 19:348, 1973.

Ettinger, B.; Genant, H. K.; and Cann, C. E.: Long-term estrogen replacement therapy prevents bone loss and fractures. Ann. Intern. Med., 102:319–324, 1985.

Farley, J. R.; Wergedal, J. E.; and Baylink, D. J.: Fluoride directly stimulates proliferation and alkaline phosphatase activity of bone-forming cells. Science, 222:330–332, 1983.

Forrest, E.; and Brooks, P. M.: Mechanisms of action of non-steroidal anti-rheumatic drugs. Bailliere's Clin. Rheumatol., 2:275–291, 1988.

Francis, R. M.; Peacock, M.; Taylor, G. A.; Storer, J. H.; and Nordin, B. E.: Calcium malabsorption in elderly women with vertebral fractures: Evidence for resistance to the action of vitamin D metabolites on the bowel. Clin. Sci., 66(1):103–107, 1984.

Goldstein, J.; Laskan, B. A.; and Ginsberg, G. H.: Sulindac associated with pancreatitis. Ann. Intern. Med., 93:151, 1980.

Goodwin, J.: Immunologic effects of nonsteroidal anti-inflammatory drugs. Am. J. Med., 77:7–14, 1984.

Graham, D. Y.; Agrawal, N. M.; and Roth, S. H.: Prevention of NSAID induced gastric ulcer with misoprostol: Multicentre, double-blind placebo-controlled trial. Lancet, 1(8597): 1277–1280, 1988.

Griffin, M. R.; Ray, W. A.; and Schaffner, W.: Nonsteroidal anti-inflammatory drug use and death from peptic ulcer in elderly patients. Ann. Intern. Med., 108:359–363, 1988.

Gruber, H. E.; Ivey, J. L.; Baylink, D. J.; Matthews, M.; Nelp, W. B.; Sisan, K.; and Chestnut, C. H. III: Long-term calcitonin therapy in postmenopausal osteoporosis. Metabolism, 33: 295–303, 1984.

Gutman, A. B.: Uricosuric drugs, with special reference of probenecid and sulfinpyrazone. Adv. Pharmacol., 4:91–142, 1951.

Gutman, A. B.; and Yu, T. F.: Benemid (*p*-{di-*n*-propylsulfamyl}-benzoic acid) as uricosuric agent in chronic gouty arthritis. Trans. Assoc. Am. Physicians, 64:279, 1951.

Hande, K. R.; Noone, R. M.; and Stone, W. J.: Severe allopurinol toxicity. Description and guidelines for prevention in patients with renal insufficiency. Am. J. Med., 76:47–56, 1984.

Hande, K.; Reed, E.; and Chabner, B.: Allopurinol kinetics. Clin. Pharmacol. Ther., 23:598–605, 1978.

Hochberg, M. C.: NSAIDs: Mechanisms and pathways of action. Hosp. Pract., 24:185–198, 1989.

Heaney, R. P.: Calcium intake requirement and bone mass in the elderly. J. Lab. Clin. Med., 100:309–312, 1982.

Horsman, A.; Gallagher, J. C.; Simpson, M.; and Nordin, B. E. C.: Prospective trial of oestrogen and calcium in postmenopausal women. Br. Med. J., 2:789–792, 1977.

Inman, W. K.; and Rawson, N. S.: Zomepirac and cardiovascular deaths. Lancet, 2:908, 1983.

Klassen, D. K.; Stout, R. L.; Spilman, P. S.; and Whelton, A.: Sulindac kinetics and effects on renal function and prostaglandin excretion in renal insufficiency. J. Clin. Pharmacol., 29:1037–1042, 1989.

Kelly, W. N.; Fox, I. H.; and Palella, T. D.: Gout and related disorders of purine metabolism. In, Textbook of Rheumatology, 3rd ed. (Kelly, W. N.; Harris, E. D. Jr.; Ruddy, S.; and Sledge, C., eds.). W. B. Saunders, Philadelphia, pp. 1395–1435, 1989.

Lukert, B. P.; and Raisz, L. G.: Glucocorticoid-induced osteoporosis: Pathogenesis and management. Ann. Intern. Med., 112:352–364, 1990.

Mankin, H. J.; and Brandt, K. D.: Pathogenesis of osteoarthritis. In, Textbook of Rheumatology, 3rd ed. (Kelly, W. N.; Harris, E. D. Jr.; Ruddy, S.; and Sledge, C., eds.). W. B. Saunders, Philadelphia, pp. 1469–1471, 1989.

Marcus, R.: Secondary forms of osteoporosis. In, Disorders of Bone and Mineral Metabolism, 1st ed. (Coe, F. L. and Favus, M. J., eds.). Raven Press, New York, 1990 (In press).

Mawer, E. B.; Backhouse, J.; Holman, C. A.; Lumb, G. A.; and Stansbury, S. W.: The distribution and storage of vitamin D and its metabolites in human tissue. Clin. Sci., 43: 413–431, 1972.

Nordin, B. E. C.; Horsman, A.; Crilly, R. G.; Marshall, D. H.; and Simpson, M.: Treatment of spinal osteoporosis in postmenopausal women. Br. Med. J., 280:451–454, 1980.

Olin, B. R. (ed.-in-chief): Facts and Comparisons. J. B. Lippincott, Philadelphia, p. 251. 1990.

Pak, C. Y. C.; Sakhaeek, K.; Zerwekh, J. E.; Parcel, C.; Peterson, R.; and Johnson, K.: Safe and effective treatment of osteoporosis with intermittent slow-release fluoride: Augmentation of vertebral bone mass and inhibition of fractures. J. Clin. Endocrinol. Metab., 68:150–159, 1989.

Peck, W. A.; Riggs, B. L.; and Bell, N. H.: In, Physician's Resource on Osteoporosis: A Decision-Making Guide. National Osteoporosis Foundation, Medica, 1987.

Paulus, H. E.: FDA arthritis advisory committee meeting. Arthritis Rheum., 25(9):1124–1125, 1982.

Prescott, L. F.: Effects of non-narcotic analgesics on the liver. Drugs, 32(suppl. 4):129–147, 1986.

Rasmussen, H.; and Bordier, P.: Vitamin D and bone. Metab. Bone Dis. Relat. Res., 1:7–13, 1978.

Riggs, B. L.; and Melton, L. J. III: Clinical heterogeneity of involutional osteoporosis: Implications for preventive therapy. J. Clin. Endocrinol. Metab., 70:1229–1232, 1990.

Riggs, B. L.; and Melton, L. J. III: Involutional osteoporosis. N. Engl. J. Med., 314:1676–1686, 1986.

Riggs, B. L.; Hodgson, S. F.; O'Fallen, W. M.; Chao, E. Y. S.; and Melton, L. J.: Effect of fluoride treatment on fracture rate in postmenopausal women with osteoporosis. N. Engl. J. Med., 322:810–815, 1990.

Riggs, B. L.; Seeman, E.; Hodgson, S. F.; Taves, D. R.; and O'Fallen, W. M.: Effect of the fluoride/calcium regimen on vertebral fracture occurrence in postmenopausal osteoporosis. N. Engl. J. Med., 306:446–450, 1982.

Riis, B.; Thomsen, K.; and Christiansen, C.: Does calcium supplementation prevent postmenopausal bone loss? N. Engl. J. Med., 316:173–177, 1987.

Roberts, W. N.; Liang, M. H.; and Stern S. H.: Colchicine in acute gout: Reassessment of risks and benefits. J.A.M.A., 257:1920–1922, 1987.

Rocklin, R. E. (ed): Histamine and H_2 Antagonists in Inflammation and Immunodeficiency. Vol. I. Marcel Dekker, New York, Basel, 1990.

Rundles, R. W.: The development of allopurinol. Arch. Intern. Med., 145:1492–1503, 1985.

Scharschmidt, L. A.; and Feinfeld, D. A.: Renal effects of nonsteroidal anti-inflammatory drugs. Hosp. Physician, 25: 29–33, 1989.

Schwartzman, M. S.; and Franck, W. A.: Vitamin D toxicity complicating the treatment of senile, postmenopausal and glucocorticoid-induced osteoporosis. Am. J. Med., 82:224–230, 1987.

Semble, E. L.; and Wu, W. C.: Antiinflammatory drugs and gastric mucosal damage. Semin. Arthritis Rheum., 16:271–286, 1987.

Sirota, J. H.; Yu, T. F.; and Gutman, A. B.: Effect of benemid on urate clearance and other discrete renal functions in gouty subjects. J. Clin. Invest., 31:692–701, 1952.

Slovick, D. M.; Adams, J. S.; Neer, R. M.; Holick, M. F.; and Potts, J. T. Jr.: Deficient production of 1,25-dihydroxyvitamin D in elderly osteoporotic patients. N. Engl. J. Med., 305: 372–374, 1981.

Smith, E. L. Jr.; Redden, W.; and Smith, P. E.: Physical activity and calcium modalities for bone mineral increase in aged women. Med. Sci. Sports Exerc., 13:60–64, 1981.

Stevenson, D. D.; and Simon, R. A.: Aspirin sensitivity: Respiratory and cutaneous manifestations. In, Allergy: Principles and Practice, 3rd ed. (Klein, E. A., ed.). C. V. Mosby, St. Louis, pp. 1537–1554, 1988.

Terkeltaub, R. A.; and Ginsberg, M. H.: The inflammatory reaction to crystals. Rheum. Dis. Clin., 14:353–364, 1988.

Tonkin, A.; and Wing, L. M. H.: Interactions of non-steroidal antiinflammatory drugs. Bailliere's Clin. Rheumatol., 2:455–483, 1988.

Verbeeck, R. K.: Pathophysiologic factors affecting the pharmacokinetics of nonsteroidal antiinflammatory drugs. J. Rheumatol. Suppl. 17 16:44–57, 1988.

Verbeeck, R. K.; Blackburn, J. L.; and Loewen, G. R.: Clinical pharmacokinetics of non-steroidal anti-inflammatory drugs. Clin. Pharmacol., 8:297–331, 1983.

Wallace, S. L.; and Ertel, N. H.: Plasma levels of colchicine after oral administration of a single dose. Metabolism, 22: 749–753, 1973.

Wasnich, R. D.; Benfante, R. J.; Yano, K.; Heilbrun, L; and Vogel, J. M.: Thiazide effect on the mineral content of bone. N. Engl. J. Med., 309:344–347, 1983.

Watts, N. B.; Harris, S. T.; Genant, H. K.; Wasnich, R. D.; Miller, P. D.; Jackson, R. D.; Licata, A. A.; Ross, P.; Woodson, G. C. III; Yanover, M. J.; Mysiw, W. J.; Kohse, L.; Rao, M. B.; Steiger, P.; Richmond, B.; Chestnut, Ch. H. III: Intermittent cyclical etidronate treatment of post menopausal osteoporosis. N. Engl. J. Med., 323(2):73–79, 1990.

Weiner, J. M.; Washington, J. A.; and Mudge, G. H.: On the mechanism of action of probenecid on renal tubular secretion. Bull. Johns Hopkins Hosp., 106:333–361, 1960.

Weinberger, A.; and Paulus, H. E.: Uric acid lowering drugs. In, Drugs for Rheumatic Disease (Paulus, H. E.; Furst,

D. E.; Dromgoole, S. H., eds.). Churchill Livingstone, New York, pp. 17–47, 1987.

Woodhouse, K. W.; and Wynne, H.: The pharmacokinetics of non-steroidal anti-inflammatory drugs in the elderly. Clin. Pharmacol., 12:111–122, 1987.

Young, J. L. Jr.; Boswell, R. B.; and Nies, A. S.: Severe allopurinol hypersensitivity. Association with thiazides and prior renal compromise. Arch. Intern. Med., 134(3):553–558, 1974.

Yu, T. F.; and Gutman, A. B.: Effect of allopurinol on serum and urinary uric acid in primary and secondary gout. Am. J. Med., 37:885–898, 1964.

Zimmerman, H. J.: Effects of aspirin and acetominophen on the liver. Arch. Intern. Med., 141:333–342, 1981.

21

Dermatologic Disorders

Marc E. Goldyne

Discussions about the therapy of cutaneous diseases are often introduced by citing the skin's role as a supportive interface between humans' external and internal milieu and as a barrier to potentially harmful agents in the environment. Because our knowledge regarding therapeutically relevant details of the skin's complex organization and functions are relatively limited, we must often satisfy ourselves with such introductory statements. Unfortunately, on a pharmacologic level, such statements are meaningless unless the barrier properties of the skin or the pathophysiologic events that lead to skin disease can be described in a way that assists therapeutic decisions. If the physician challenges the worn out clichés regarding dermatologic therapy and attempts to understand how the skin may be interacting not only with the external milieu but with the internal milieu as well, he or she may begin to appreciate the need for actively thinking about the therapy of dermatologic diseases.

The fact that most dermatologic disorders are not life-threatening (but often significantly debilitating) should not lessen a physician's responsibility for having to make as correct a therapeutic decision as is currently possible. A lapse in this responsibility is exemplified by a fungal infection that is clinically misdiagnosed as eczema and inappropriately (and also ineffectually) treated with cóstly topical steroids and systemic antibiotics because of failure to perform a simple skin scraping and microscopic inspection for fungal hyphae. Less than thorough evaluation in relation to simple dermatologic problems will not automatically change when problems become more complex. Furthermore, when knowledge of the science of dermatology stops, the need to practice the art of

medicine is as essential as ever. If the therapy causes more problems than the disease, the physician is not practicing good medicine. The message sounds self-evident, but ensuring its implementation can be challenging.

The drugs and the therapeutic principles reviewed in this chapter will focus on four common dermatologic diagnoses for which a large number of drug prescriptions are written. To attempt more would be presumptuous since entire books are currently devoted to each of the diseases to be discussed as well as to the specific subject of dermatologic therapy. The diagnoses addressed in this chapter include acne, eczema, psoriasis, and drug-induced skin reactions. It will be in the context of discussing each diagnosis that relevant principles of dermatologic therapy will be discussed. To associate these principles with specific diseases hopefully puts them in a more applicable context for the clinician.

ACNE

Pathogenesis

The specific genotype that permits the development of the disease called acne is unknown. The fact that acne provides a spectrum of clinical presentations suggests a combination of endogenous as well as exogenous determinants. Nevertheless, knowledge of some of the factors that appear to contribute to each clinical presentation helps justify choosing a specific therapeutic protocol.

Acne is a disease of the pilosebaceous follicle. The interaction of three conditions appears essential to the evolution of acne: (1) altered keratinization of the infundibulum of the pilosebaceous duct (Knutson, 1974; Plewig, 1974), (2) overproduction of sebum by the sebaceous glands (Pochi and Strauss, 1964), and (3) proliferation of the anaerobic diphtheroid *Propionibacterium acnes* within retained sebum (Leyden et al., 1975).

Altered keratinization and desquamation of the ductal epithelium lead to impaction of the pilosebaceous duct with a mixture of sebum and keratin. The combination of ductal plugging and increased sebum generation leads to distension of the follicular duct, which can be appreciated microscopically as a microcomedo. As the microcomedo expands it forms either (1) an open comedo (blackhead) if the follicular orifice dilates or (2) a closed comedo if the orifice remains microscopic. The factors favoring the formation of closed versus open comedones are not known. The closed comedo has particular clinical significance because the escape channel for sebum is totally blocked. This condition sets the stage for inflammation.

Within the closed comedo, the lipid-rich sebum provides an ideal growth medium for the proliferation of *P. acnes*, an anaerobic diphtheroid normally found within the pilosebaceous duct. Data show that the lipase activity of *P. acnes* converts triglycerides in sebum to free fatty acids as well as free glycerol, which may function as a growth substrate for the bacteria (Rebello and Hawk, 1978). The fatty acids themselves are comedogenic in animal models and may contribute to the chemotactic activity of sebum; they may also possess cytotoxic activity (Shalita, 1974; Puhvel and Sakamoto, 1978; Tucker et al., 1980).

The inflammation in acne is associated with the rupture of the closed comedo due to (1) the continued secretion of sebum with resultant thinning of the follicular epithelium and (2) release by *P. acnes* of low-molecular-weight chemotactic factors that diffuse through the thinned follicular wall and attract neutrophils that migrate through the follicular epithelium, ingest the *P. acnes*, and simultaneously release hydrolytic enzymes that attack the follicular epithelium, causing it to rupture (Webster et al., 1979a; Webster and Leyden, 1980).

When the contents of the ruptured comedo enter the dermis, various inflammatory signals are triggered. Activation of the classic and alternate complement pathways by *P. acnes* leads to complement-derived (e.g., C5a) chemotactic factor generation (Webster et al., 1979b), and a foreign body response is generated by comedonal contents (Dalziel et al., 1984). The fact that acne runs an inflammatory gamut from mild pustular comedones to large, multilocular, disfiguring cysts supports differences in individual host response to the factors so far described. *Principle: The genotypic reasons for such host differences are as yet unknown. However, the factors already impli-* *cated in the pathogenesis of acne provide a rational basis for current therapy.*

Therapy

The therapy of acne is guided by knowledge of the factors contributing to the clinical presentation. The therapy can be divided into noninflammatory and inflammatory categories.

Noninflammatory Acne. If noninflamed comedones, open or closed, constitute the majority of lesions, the abnormal keratinization and desquamation of the pilosebaceous orifice is the causative factor on which to focus. Therapy should accordingly be aimed at normalizing the altered keratinization and desquamation process. The drug that appears to accomplish this best is topical tretinoin (Kligman et al., 1969).

Topical tretinoin (retinoic acid) is the acid form of vitamin A (retinol). It is applied as a cream (0.025%, 0.05%, and 0.1%), a gel (0.01% and 0.025%), or a 0.05% solution to affected skin once per day. It is recommended that application be done at bedtime since some animal data suggest that retinoic acid may enhance the tumorigenic potential of sunlight (Olsen, 1982). There is less than 10% absorption of topically applied tretinoin into the circulation, where it is metabolized in the liver and excreted in bile and in urine. The therapeutic efficacy of tretinoin as a comedolytic agent stems from its ability to decrease the cohesiveness of the follicular epithelium and accelerate epithelial cell turnover (Wolff et al., 1975). These actions allow eventual expulsion of comedonal contents and prevention of new microcomedo formation.

Optimal treatment with tretinoin requires that the patient be informed about the potential side effects of therapy as well as the time frame in which the patient can expect to see improvement. A frequent cause of treatment failure is an uninformed patient who, experiencing some cutaneous irritation, stops therapy because of the fear that an allergic reaction to the medication has occurred or stops because 48 hours of therapy has not produced any improvement. Both these frequent compliance problems can be prevented by a physician's stressing the following points: (1) skin irritation may occur following initiation of tretinoin therapy; if this occurs, application should be stopped for 48 hours and then initiated again (alternatives are to lower the concentration of tretinoin, change the vehicle—cream has the least potential for irritation—or try initial alternate-day therapy); (2) exacerbation of lesions may occur during the first 2 to 3 weeks of therapy; this should not serve as an indication to stop application of tretinoin; (3) 6 to 12 weeks of therapy are required before maximal benefit, and therefore clinical efficacy, can be determined (Olsen, 1982); and (4) use of a sunscreen is strongly encouraged if prolonged exposure to ultraviolet light is contemplated since tretinoin, at least in animal studies, appears to enhance the tumorigenic potential of ultraviolet light.

A patient must be told, repeatedly if necessary, that the aim of acne therapy is to control the disease; a cure, even with oral isotretinoin (to be described) cannot be guaranteed, but excellent control can be achieved with proper therapy and compliance. *Principle: Inappropriate patient expectations can sabotage compliance with therapy and preclude the possibility of a beneficial clinical response. The physician's obligations to the patient in this regard become obvious.*

Inflammatory Acne. The presence of inflammatory papules, pustules, and cysts should suggest not only that follicular plugging is present but that the bacterial contribution to acne must be treated. This may be accomplished with a variety of topical or systemic antibiotics that are capable of controlling the proliferation of *P. acnes* and therefore the *P. acnes*-induced inflammatory stimuli reviewed above. The most frequently used agents include topical benzoyl peroxide, topical erythromycin or clindamycin, and systemic tetracycline or erythromycin.

Topical benzoyl peroxide is bactericidal for *P. acnes* as well as being mildly comedolytic (Burke et al., 1983). Its mechanism of action has not been established, whereas its clinical efficacy has been confirmed. When applied to the skin as a $2\frac{1}{2}\%$, 5%, or 10% lotion, cream, or gel, less than 5% of the dose is absorbed through the skin over 8 hours (Nacht et al., 1981). Within the skin, it is completely metabolized to benzoic acid that enters the circulation as benzoate and is excreted by the kidneys unchanged (Yeong et al., 1983). Available data suggest that the drug is safe to use in pregnancy (Rothman and Pochi, 1988). Because benzoyl peroxide can be potentially irritating, therapy should begin with the lowest concentration applied once per day to the affected areas of skin and progression to higher concentrations made if some therapeutic benefit is perceived.

Combining the use of topical tretinoin at night with the morning application of benzoyl peroxide can provide the benefits of both the more potent comedolytic properties of the first agent and the antibacterial effects of the second agent. It is important to inform patients that if using both topical agents, they should not be applied at the same time since the benzoyl peroxide will oxidatively inactivate the tretinoin (Hurwitz, 1979). Benzoyl peroxide may induce allergic contact dermatitis after several weeks of use in up to 2.5% of patients (Haustein et al., 1985). *Principle: The efficacy of combination drug regimens may depend crucially on timing and sequencing. While acne may not be life-threatening, cancers are, and the proper sequencing of drug therapy can make the difference between life and death* (see chapter 23).

Topical clindamycin phosphate and *erythromycin base* are the two most frequently employed antibiotics for topical use in the therapy of mild acne when inflammatory papules and pustules, but not cysts, are the predominant lesions. Whereas topical benzoyl peroxide is bactericidal, clindamycin and erythromycin are bacteriostatic, functioning as competitive inhibitors of ribosomal protein synthesis. Use of these antibiotics is indicated when a patient cannot tolerate benzoyl peroxide because of irritation or contact allergy; they appear to be equally effective and are applied twice a day to all areas where acne lesions exist or where they have the potential to erupt (Shalita et al., 1984). The topical antibiotics are generally well tolerated with the major side effects being vehicle-related dryness and irritation. Because topical erythromycin and clindamycin are bacteriostatic, their use may result in development of resistant strains (Eady et al., 1989). Clinically this is suggested by the patient's complaint that an initial beneficial response to topical erythromycin or clindamycin is not continuing. In response to topical clindamycin there have been several cases of pseudomembranous colitis reported, but it is a rare complication (Milstone et al., 1981; Parry and Rha, 1986). Nevertheless, any patient developing diarrhea while using topical clindamycin should be advised to stop treatment. *Principle: While we are accustomed to considering the skin as a barrier to the environment, we should not lose sight of the fact that many substances applied at high concentrations for prolonged periods will reach the systemic circulation. Expect systemic effects of topically applied drugs.*

If an 8-week trial of a topical antibiotic, applied twice per day, fails to provide clinical improvement, systemic antibiotics should be considered if inflammatory lesions are the major clinical finding.

Tetracycline hydrochloride and *erythromycin base* are the most frequently employed systemic antibiotics for acne. Studies show that both drugs significantly decrease bacterial counts of *P. acnes* and the levels of skin surface free fatty acids (Strauss and Pochi, 1966; Akers et al., 1975). In a controlled trial with 200 patients, both antibiotics have proved equally effective in treating papulopustular acne (Gammon et al., 1986). However, closed comedo counts did decrease more rapidly in patients treated with tetracycline. The initial quantity of antibiotic should be at least 1 g/day divided into either two or four doses. In more severe inflammatory acne, the benefit of doses of tetracycline greater than 1 g/day (e.g., 2 g/day) has been documented (Baer et al., 1976). Other oral antibiotics such as minocycline (50 mg twice per day) have also shown efficacy in treating inflammatory acne, but because of higher cost, minocycline is often reserved for cases refractory to therapy with tetracycline or erythromycin. ***Principle: It is avoiding to reality to believe that the cost of a prescription is not a factor in compliance and the eventual outcome of a therapeutic regimen.***

As with topical antibiotics, judgment of the clinical efficacy of systemic antibiotics should not be made until an 8-week treatment program has been completed. A major cause of apparent treatment failure is the physician's failure to inform the patient with acne that maximum improvement will not be seen for approximately 6 to 8 weeks. The anxious patient, expecting a 24-hour cure, stops the drug after a few days because improvement is not evident and then at a follow-up visit or, more likely, to a new physician, the frustrated patient reports that systemic antibiotics failed to help. This problem can be avoided by proper instruction to the patient. ***Principle: When a physician is told that a particular therapy has failed, it is crucial to make sure that it was indeed the drug and not some other factor that caused the failure.***

If an adequate period of therapy does result in improvement, consideration can be given to decreasing the dose of systemic antibiotic to no less than 500 mg/day as long as improvement is maintained. It is essential to understand that it is not solely the antibiotic properties of these drugs that appear to provide therapeutic efficacy; for example, the oral antibiotics mentioned also appear to inhibit leukocyte chemotaxis and inhibit bacterial lipase activity without significantly affecting bacterial colony counts (Shalita and Wheatly, 1970; Cunliffe et al., 1973; Esterly et al., 1978).

The inevitable question asked by the patient with acne is how long oral antibiotic therapy needs to be continued. Once therapeutic benefit is documented, the goal of subsequent therapy is to switch from a systemic to a topical antibiotic. The topical preparation should be introduced while the patient is still taking the minimum dose of the systemic antibiotic required for control of the acne. Then the systemic antibiotic can be withdrawn after a week's overlap to see if topical therapy will suffice to maintain control. Other schedules can be tried with the ultimate criterion for change being the clinical response of the patient.

A concern often raised by physicians is how long one can safely maintain systemic antibiotic therapy. Studies have shown that treatment with tetracycline for 3 to 4 years in otherwise healthy patients with acne has not led to major morbidity from resistant organisms or opportunistic infections (Bjornberg and Roupe, 1972; Akers et al., 1975; Gould and Cunliffe, 1978; Adams et al., 1985).

The major side effect of systemic antibiotic therapy is modification of the GI flora; in roughly 5% of patients, this may lead to colic and/or diarrhea (Gould and Cunliffe, 1978; Adams et al., 1985). In women, candida vaginitis may infrequently occur (Bjornberg and Roupe, 1972; Gammon et al., 1986). Several cases of gram-negative folliculitis that resemble pustular acne but are unresponsive to continuing tetracycline therapy have also been documented (Fulton et al., 1968). There have also been several cases of benign intracranial hypertension reported in patients using oral tetracycline (Walters and Gubbay, 1981).

In regard to treating acne in pregnant women, tetracycline therapy is definitely contraindicated because of its association with maternal hepatic toxicity as well as with staining of deciduous teeth and with cataract formation in the developing fetus (Rothman and Pochi, 1988).

In patients with severe nodulocystic acne involving the face and back, in patients with less severe inflammatory acne who have not responded to adequate therapeutic trials of the drugs heretofore discussed, or in patients suffering from significant dysmorphophobia in regard to their acne, systemic *isotretinoin* (13-*cis*-retinoic acid) therapy is the treatment of choice (Jones, 1989). This derivative of vitamin A acid is well absorbed, is virtually totally protein-bound, and is excreted by both the kidneys and GI tract. Its elimination half-life is 10 to 20 hours. The majority of responding patients receive between 1 and 2 mg/kg per day in a b.i.d. schedule over a period of 15 to 20 weeks. The remarkable effectiveness of isotretinoin (sold under the name Accutane) appears to stem from its influence on all the major etiologic factors associated with acne: (1) sebum secretion is reduced by 90% at 4 weeks (Jones et al., 1983), (2) pilosebaceous ductal cornification is normalized (Cunliffe et al., 1985), (3) microbial colonization of the skin is significantly reduced (King et al., 1982), and (4) inflammation is decreased (Camisa et al., 1982).

The major concern with isotretinoin therapy is its teratogenic potential in pregnant women (Lammer et al., 1985). Of 154 women inadvertently exposed to isotretinoin during the first trimester of pregnancy, 95 pregnancies ended in elective abortion while 12 ended in spontaneous abortion. Whereas 26 infants were born without major malformations noted at birth, 21 infants were born with major anomalies involving craniofacial structures, the heart, and the thymus. Therefore, isotretinoin must not be given to women of childbearing age unless the physician establishes by serum pregnancy testing that the female patient is not pregnant prior to initiating therapy, is on an effective form of birth control during, and for 1 month following cessation of, therapy, and understands the risks to a fetus should she become pregnant during therapy. *Principle: We should be learning a lot about human nature when, in spite of the known toxicity of a highly efficacious drug, laxity in ensuring patient protection almost forced the FDA to remove this drug from the market.*

Other relatively common effects of isotretinoin therapy include dryness of the skin and mucous membranes (the latter sometimes leading to epistaxis) and elevation of serum triglyceride and high-density lipoprotein (HDL) concentrations. Hepatic transaminase concentrations in plasma are temporarily elevated in approximately 20% of patients taking isotretinoin. They return to normal despite continued therapy (DiGiovanna and Peck, 1987). Less commonly seen are thinning of hair, muscle and joint pains, headache, corneal opacities, pseudotumor cerebri, inflammatory bowel disease, and anorexia. These problems are all reversible on discontinuation of therapy. Note that in the rare patient whose serum triglyceride concentrations increase to around 800 mg/dl, isotretinoin therapy should be stopped because in such cases, acute hemorrhagic pancreatitis as well as eruptive xanthomas have been reported (Shalita et al., 1983). Consequently, pretreatment evaluation of liver function and of plasma lipid concentrations should be obtained, periodically reevaluated during the 15 to 20 weeks of therapy, and then 2 weeks following cessation of therapy to document normalization. In selected patients, a second course of therapy may be considered if several weeks following an initial course, acne lesions begin to appear. The same precautions are indicated during retreatment. Need for retreatment appears to correlate with the use of less than a 1 g/kg dosage for initial therapy. Nevertheless, lower dosages are sometimes justified because an individual may find the adverse effects of the optimum dose too uncomfortable.

ECZEMA

Eczema (derived from the Greek word *ekzein* = "to boil out") is not a disease, but a manifestation of a variety of skin diseases. Therefore, if the physician makes a diagnosis of eczema, he or she must still determine its underlying cause. The identification of the cause is the key to rational therapy.

Acute eczema presents either as a localized or as a more generalized condition, the severity of which may depend on the cause. The skin develops patches of erythema, papulation, and vesiculation with oozing of serous fluid, and crusting. Chronic eczema exhibits features of erythema, scaling, thickening of the skin with prominence of skin lines (lichenification), and hyper- or hypopigmentation. Vesiculation, weeping, and oozing are not features of chronic eczema.

Pathogenesis

Eczema is found most often in association with atopy, allergic contact dermatitis, or chemical and physical irritation of the skin. The common thread that appears to explain the clinically similar cutaneous manifestations of these different diseases is the disruption of the barrier function of the stratum corneum of the epidermis. Normally the lipid composition of this region serves to control transepidermal water loss (Elias and Finegold, 1988). By excoriating the skin in response to the pruritus and/or inflammation induced by underlying disease, the patient disrupts the lipid barrier, leading to an increase in transepidermal water loss (to be differentiated from eccrine sweating). Through a yet-to-be-delineated mechanism, the abnormal transepidermal water loss lowers the threshold for pruritus, with the resultant initiation of an itch–scratch cycle. In the particular case of atopy, altered barrier function appears to be an integral part of the disease (Strauss and Pochi, 1961).

Atopy. Atopy is the name applied to a symptom complex that may include asthma, hay fever, and eczema associated with the findings of elevated serum concentrations of IgE (80% of patients), suppressed in vitro mitogenic response of peripheral blood T cells, altered leukocyte cyclic AMP responses, significantly increased incidence of skin colonization with *Staphylococcus aureus*, and susceptibility to cutaneous spread of infections with herpes and vaccinia viruses (Leyden et al., 1974; Aly et al., 1977; Parker et al., 1977).

The eczema associated with atopy appears to result from the physical excoriation of the skin in response to the characteristically severe pruritus that is associated with the disease (Rajka, 1968). The eczema appears in characteristic localizations from infancy (face, scalp, and extensor surfaces) through childhood (flexural folds of arms, legs, feet, and wrists, plus the skin of the eyelids and of the back and sides of the neck) to adulthood (more generalized to face, scalp, chest, neck, extremities, hands, and feet).

Allergic Contact Eczema. This form of eczema results from a delayed hypersensitivity reaction (cell-mediated or type IV hypersensitivity) to a low-molecular-weight (<1000) sensitizing agent that comes into contact with the skin (Roitt et al., 1985). The inciting molecules (haptens), which must be fat-soluble in order to traverse the stratum corneum of a susceptible patient, must become covalently or noncovalently bound to normal epidermal proteins in order to serve as antigenic determinants (epitopes) capable of eliciting T-cell recognition specific for the hapten–protein conjugate. Of central importance to this response is the epidermal Langerhans cell that serves as the Ia-bearing, antigen-presenting cell (Wolff and Stingl, 1983). In contrast to tuberculin-type hypersensitivity that is primarily dermal in location, contact hypersensitivity is primarily epidermal.

The papulovesicles initially developing at sites of antigen contact most probably result from the T-cell-mediated cytotoxicity and consequent edema occurring within the epidermis. The pruritus associated with this reactivity invites excoriation of the involved skin, leading to the clinical picture of acute eczema. Table 21–1 lists the most frequently implicated allergens encountered and their sources. Occasionally, a hapten will only become sensitizing following alteration by ultraviolet light; this type of reaction is suggested by a "photodistribution" of the eczema.

Chemical and Physical Irritant Eczema. Occupational or recreational exposure to various solvents or detergents, or repeated hand washing, can alter the lipid barrier of the epidermis leading to both enhanced transepidermal water loss and enhanced penetration of potentially irritating substances. When this involves the hands, the induced pruritus and scratching in addition to continued contact with the offending agents can result in the generation of acute and chronic eczema commonly referred to as hand or housewife's eczema. When other areas of skin are involved, both acute and chronic round (coin-shaped) patches of eczema can occur; this clinical presentation has been labeled nummular eczema from the Latin *numisma* meaning "coin." Some people develop a habit tic that involves the repeated excoriation of one skin site because of a perceived local pruritus that can be precipitated and propagated by stress. The resultant eczema, which is clinically distinct only because of its singular location, is referred to as localized neurodermatitis; this chronic lesion that often shows lichenification as a prominent feature is referred to as lichen simplex chronicus.

A unique form of hand and foot eczema that appears to be induced by stress in susceptible persons begins as an eruption of grouped tiny pruritic vesicles that have the appearance of tapioca kernels and erupt along the lateral margins of the fingers, and the thenar eminences. In more severe cases it can also involve the soles of the feet and the toes. Scratching of these pruritic vesicles leads to a clinical picture of acute eczema that with time may take on the features of chronic eczema. This condition has been given the name dyshidrotic eczema or pompholyx because of the misconception that the vesicles are the result of trapped eccrine sweat. The actual cause of the vesicles is unclear.

Xerotic eczema is the term used for eczema arising from pruritus-induced excoriation of dry skin. This disease is most frequently seen in elderly persons who, because of a presumed decline in surface lipids, demonstrate clinically dry skin due to increased transepidermal water loss. The episodes of eczema increase during the winter months (hence the term *winter eczema* is sometimes used) because of the increased drying of the skin that results from the drop in indoor humidity because of increased use of heating. The episodes of itching usually occur more frequently at night after clothing that has maintained higher local humidity of the covered skin is removed exposing

Table 21–1.   ALLERGIC CONTACT ECZEMA FREQUENT OFFENDERS

HAPTEN	SOURCES
Urushiol (pentadecylcatechol)	Poison oak, ivy, sumac oleoresin
Paraphenylenediamine	Hair dyes
Nickel	Earrings, necklaces, watchbands, zippers, metal buttons, coins
Ethylenediamine	Stabilizer in Mycolog cream (not in ointment); may get drug eruption from aminophylline and ethylenediamine-related antihistamines
Dichromates	Leather dyes, preservatives, cement
Tetramethylthiuram, mercaptobenzothiazole	Rubber materials
Neomycin sulfate	Topical antibiotic
Benzocaine	Topical anesthetic
Formalin	Textile finishes
Balsam Peru	Perfumes
Parabens	Preservatives in topical medicament creams

the skin to a much lower humidity level. Combining this condition with hot soapy showers or baths that further delipidize the skin leads to increased dryness, concomitant pruritus, and excoriation. The result is a patient presenting with acute and chronic eczema who provides a history of increasingly itchy skin primarily involving the extremities that is more symptomatic at night.

Therapy

Therapy of eczema has to be approached from three aspects: (1) suppression of inflammation, (2) eradication of superinfection if present, and (3) suppression and prevention of pruritus. The third aspect is conceptually the most important and most challenging to accomplish because if the physician does not achieve control of the pruritus, the patient will continue to scratch, the scratching will generate the eczema as the skin's response to repeated excoriation, and in the case of atopic eczema, superinfection of the eczematized skin will more than likely occur.

Suppression of Inflammation. Localized eczema that shows the acute signs of weeping, oozing, and crusting initially requires drying and debridement, since the serous fluid and epidermal debris can foster bacterial proliferation and, especially in atopic patients, infection with *S. aureus*. The first steps must be accomplished along with more specific anti-inflammatory therapy.

Drying of acute eczema is actually achieved through the application of water to the affected skin. By removing occlusive crusts and proteinaceous debris, as well as by delipidizing keratin, endogenous transepidermal water loss can be further enhanced at sites of eczema. The effect is drying. For localized eczema this is best achieved with cool or tepid tap water compresses with clean, closely woven cotton cloth (old bed sheets or T-shirts) for 20 to 30 minutes twice to three times a day. The use of dilute *aluminum acetate solution* (e.g., Domeboro powder or tablets dissolved in water) for use in compresses is a more effective astringent, and it also provides bacteriostasis. For more generalized eczema, drying of weeping lesions can be accomplished by tepid water baths to which can be added an *oilated colloid* [e.g., oilated oatmeal (Aveeno)]. Once the weeping and oozing of acute eczema has been controlled, the physician needs to consider more specific suppression of inflammation.

The efficacy of *topical corticosteroids* in suppressing cutaneous inflammation is undisputed. The mechanism(s) involved have yet to be definitively established. Data show that corticosteroids (1) stabilize and prevent lysosomal enzyme release (Weissman and Fell, 1962; Frichot and Zelickson,

1972), (2) inhibit the synthesis of inflammatory mediators like prostaglandins and leukotrienes (eicosanoids) by inducing a phospholipase A_2 inhibitory protein (lipocortin) that blocks release of the arachidonic acid required for eicosanoid synthesis (Hammerstrom et al., 1977; Blackwell et al., 1980; DiRosa et al., 1984), (3) deplete skin mast cells (Lavker and Schecter, 1985), and (4) prevent intravascular margination of neutrophils and therefore their diapedesis into inflammatory sites (Allison et al., 1955).

The decisions that must be made by the physician in regard to topical corticosteroid therapy in eczema as well as in other topical steroid–responsive skin diseases are the potency of corticosteroid to use, the appropriate vehicle to use, the frequency of use, and the duration of treatment. By convention, the potency of various topical corticosteroid preparations (over 100 available) has been expressed in terms of relative capacity to constrict the dermal vessels of normal skin under given test conditions (McKenzie and Stoughton, 1962; Gibson et al., 1984; Tan et al., 1986; Stoughton and Cornell, 1987). While there are inherent weaknesses in this system, it has provided acceptable correlation with clinical potency (Barry and Woodford, 1978; Cornell and Stoughton, 1985; Shah et al., 1989). *Principle: Standardization of drugs by bioassay may not necessarily provide direct correlation with clinical potency.*

Table 21–2 lists some representative corticosteroids in the different potency categories along with average wholesale prices based on listing in the *Drug Topics Red Book 1988*. The most recently introduced superpotent steroids (*clobetasol propionate, betamethasone dipropionate,* and *difluorasone diacetate*) are over 1000 times more potent than hydrocortisone (Stoughton and Cornell, 1987).

In treating eczema, the question of which potency of corticosteroid to use should be related to the extent and relative responsiveness to steroid of the particular form of eczema. For example a localized plaque of neurodermatitis (lichen simplex chronicus), localized hand eczema, or localized allergic contact eczema could be most efficaciously treated with a superpotent topical corticosteroid because the area of skin that is involved requires far less than the recommended maximum of 50 g/week for therapy. Furthermore, the more potent the steroid in this setting, the more rapid should be the resolution. On the other hand, a patient with atopic dermatitis or xerotic eczema scattered over the arms and legs (roughly 54% of the adult body surface) requires roughly 30 g/day (see Fig. 21-1) of a steroid preparation. The wholesale cost to the pharmacist (not the patient) would amount to approximately $20 per day for a superpotent steroid versus approximately $4 per

Table 21-2. TOPICAL CORTICOSTEROIDS: RELATIVE POTENCIES AND COST[a]

CORTICOSTEROID	GENERIC	VS. BRAND[b]	VEHICLE[c]
Lowest Potency[d]			
Hydrocortisone 1%	1.77		C/O/L
Hydrocortisone 2.5%	2.71		C
Low Potency[d]			
Desonide 0.05%			
Desowen (Owen)		6.72	C
Tridesilon (Miles)		7.61	C/O
Triamcinolone 0.025%	1.09		C/O/L
Aristocort (Lederle)		4.48	C
Kenalog (Squibb)		4.68	C/O
Intermediate Potency[e]			
Betamethasone valerate 0.1%	3.07		C
	3.19		O
	2.27		L
Valisone (Schering)		8.70	C/O
		8.06	L
Desoximetasone 0.05%	6.65		C
Topicort (Hoechst-Roussel)		7.50	G
Fluocinolone acetonide 0.025%	2.17		C/O
Fluonid (Herbert)		8.94	C/O
Halcinonide 0.025%			
Halog (Princeton)		7.36	C
Triamcinolone acetonide 0.1%	1.49		C/O
	2.34		L
Aristicort (Lederle)		5.66	C/O
Kenalog (Squibb)		5.57	C/O/L
High Potency[f]			
Amcionide 0.1%			
Cyclocort (Lederle)		9.26	C/O
Betamethasone dipropionate 0.05%	4.95		C/O
	2.67		L
Diprosone (Schering)		11.04	C/O
(20 ml)		13.56	L
Alphatrex (Savage)		6.62	C/O
(60 ml)		15.50	L
Fluocinonide 0.05%			
Lidex (Syntex)		14.36	C/O/G
Triamcinolone acetonide 0.5%	3.41		
Aristocort A (Lederle) (15 gm)		22.90	C
Kenalog (Squibb) (20 gm)		22.29	C/O
Superpotency[f]			
Betamethasone dipropionate 0.05%			
Diprolene (Schering)		12.91	C/O
Clobetasol propionate 0.05%			
Temovate (Glaxo)		17.86	C/O
Diflorasone diacetate 0.05%			
Psorcon (Dermik)		14.26	O

[a] Based on manufacturers' listing in *Drug Topics Red Book 1988.*
[b] Average cost in dollars to pharmacist; cost to patient will be higher.
[c] Vehicle abbreviations: C = cream; O = ointment; L = lotion; G = gel.
[d] Cost of 15 g.
[e] Cost of 15 g (cream or ointment) or 15 ml (lotion).
[f] Cost of 30 g (cream or ointment).

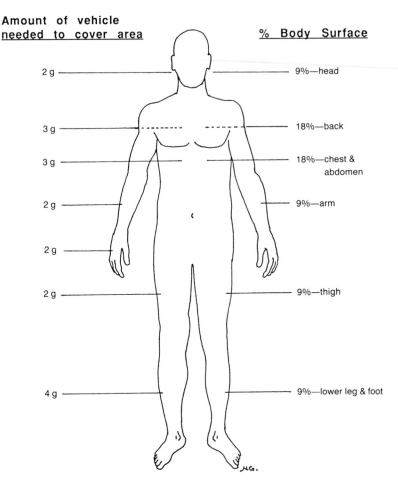

Amount of vehicle needed to cover area

% Body Surface

2 g — 9%—head

3 g — 18%—back

3 g — 18%—chest & abdomen

2 g — 9%—arm

2 g

2 g — 9%—thigh

4 g — 9%—lower leg & foot

Fig. 21-1. Application of topical corticosteroids. Whole-body coverage requires approximately 30 to 60 g of cream or ointment or 120 ml of lotion per application.

day for a generic intermediate-strength steroid such as *triamcinolone acetonide. Principle: Consider total surface area of treated skin as an area of potential absorption of drug into the systemic circulation.*

Because of the more generalized nature of atopic dermatitis or xerotic eczema, use of the more potent steroid preparations would rapidly produce systemic concentrations that would significantly suppress pituitary-adrenal axis function. For example, studies using a superpotent topical corticosteroid showed that covering at least 30% of the body surface of adults with psoriasis or atopic dermatitis with 0.5% clobetasol dipropionate cream or ointment for 1 week resulted in depressed A.M. cortisol concentrations (<5 μg/dl) in 75% of patients receiving 7 g per day, 22% of patients receiving 3.5 g per day, and 11% of patients receiving 2 g per day (Olsen and Cornell, 1986). Thus, some patients receiving the recommended maximum weekly dosage of 50 g

per week demonstrated pituitary-adrenal axis suppression. However, it should also be noted that in all studies so far conducted, return of A.M. plasma cortisol concentrations to within normal limits occurred within 2 to 7 days. Nevertheless, it is important to remember that for a given period of application, the greater the surface area to be treated, the greater the probability for pituitary-adrenal axis suppression to occur with any topical corticosteroid.

It is helpful to remember, in a practical context, that the recommended use of superpotent topical steroids is for a maximum of 50 g per week of a 0.05% preparation (cream or ointment) for not longer than 2 weeks. Also, because of inherent regional variations in absorption of topically applied corticosteroids through the skin, certain sites (scrotal skin, facial skin, intertriginous skin) are more susceptible to beneficial therapy with lower-strength preparations than sites such as the palm or sole (McKenzie and Stoughton, 1962).

Furthermore, eczematized skin or psoriatic skin even though clinically and histologically thicker shows enhanced penetration of topically applied corticosteroids. *Principle: The fact that skin shows regional changes in anatomy and therefore in drug absorptive properties has been considered in the development of transdermal drug delivery systems. Be aware of this when such systems are used.*

In the specific case of allergic contact dermatitis, the discomfort produced by the acute eczematous response to widespread contact with an allergen (e.g., poison oak's oleoresin) may require systemic therapy with oral *prednisone*, especially if facial edema is present and pronounced. Systemic therapy in this case must be initiated by a high enough dose of prednisone (at least 60–80 mg per day single A.M. dose) and tapered over 21 days to avoid flare-up of the skin lesions when a shorter course of systemic therapy is followed. For more localized cases of allergic contact dermatitis, the superpotent topicals appear to be the most beneficial.

Several principles can guide the physician who is deciding on an appropriate vehicle for treating eczema: (1) use a cream or lotion on acute eczema, because the water base of the cream or lotion will not prevent the desired dehydration of weeping, oozing lesions, (2) use a cream on intertriginous skin because the apposition of skin surfaces in intertriginous areas already provides sufficient occlusion, and (3) use an ointment on very dry and thick eczema since, by maximally hydrating the skin, it not only enhances penetration of the corticosteroid, but it helps alleviate the xerosis and accompanying pruritus.

The frequency of application of any topical steroid should not exceed three times per day. Most importantly, if the patient with eczema complains after a week of steroid therapy that his or her skin is still itchy and dry, the physician should not interpret this situation as an indication for more frequent use of a topical steroid or for a more potent steroid. Instead, the physician should increase the frequency of application of an appropriate emollient to increase hydration of the skin. This approach is supported by studies showing that applying a corticosteroid six times per day was not clinically more efficacious than a three-times-per-day schedule (Eaglestein et al., 1974). Furthermore, a study in monkeys by Wester et al. (1977) showed that a single application of [^{14}C]hydrocortisone (13.3 μg/cm^2) in acetone to a fixed area on the ventral surface of the forearm produced the same total percent absorption (based on radioactivity applied and recovered in the urine) as did three applications of this same dose to the same site at 6-hour intervals. However

when 40 μg/cm^2 was applied, a substantial increase in percent absorption was seen compared to either the single or triple application of 13.3 μg/cm^2. These data suggest that there may be local effects induced by the initial application of a corticosteroid that significantly affect the absorption kinetics of a subsequent application to the same area if done within a specific time. In fact, acute tachyphylaxis to the vasoconstrictive and antimitotic effects of topically applied corticosteroids has been documented, which abates after 96 drug-free hours (de Vivier, 1976). Consequently, in the patient with eczema, a single application of a topical steroid with adequately repeated application of an appropriate emollient may, in some instances, be as efficacious as use of the corticosteroid two or three times per day. *Principle: Careful observation often reveals that more drug may not be needed or advantageous. Consider the case of continuous administration of nitroglycerin, or β-adrenergic agonists, and increasing doses and duration of administration of antibiotics, antiarrhythmics, phenothiazines, and tricyclic antidepressants. The example with corticosteroids illustrates how important it is to have a strategy to quantitate the effects of therapy rather than simply "sitting back" and expecting a cure.*

Once the potency of, and vehicle for, the corticosteroid to be used has been determined, the physician is faced with the question of how long a given potency can be safely used before unwanted side effects occur [e.g., pituitary–adrenal axis suppression, skin atrophy, striae, steroid acne, allergic contact dermatitis to the corticosteroid itself (Reitamo et al., 1986)]. This question cannot be answered easily because absorption and bioavailability of different preparations vary depending on the vehicle used, the absorption characteristics of different skin sites, and disease-related alterations in skin barrier function, all of which can significantly affect absorption of the drug (McKenzie and Stoughton, 1962; Jackson et al., 1989). Some studies indicate that outpatients treated for chronic skin disease over several years with daily application of potent fluorinated steroids showed little or no evidence of suppression of the pituitary–adrenal axis when occlusion therapy was avoided (occlusion of skin with impermeable plastic wrap can increase cutaneous absorption 10-fold) (Munro and Clift, 1973; Wilson et al., 1973). However more recent studies on topical *halcinonide, desoximetasone,* and *betamethasone valerate* have documented depression of endogenous cortisol secretion (Gomez et al., 1977; Cornell and Stoughton, 1981). Furthermore, skin atrophy, the result of epidermal thinning, is evident histologically *after 1 week* of occlusive therapy with a potent fluorinated steroid ointment (Kirby and Monroe, 1976). Since occlusion may enhance steroid penetration 10-fold, one might expect several weeks of nonocclusive topical therapy with a potent fluorinated steroid to be permissible. Consequently, one principle to be followed by the physician using potent or super-potent steroids in a patient for longer than 2 weeks is appropriate follow-up to document by inspection and appropriate laboratory work the absence of noticeable skin atrophy, steroid acne, or striae, as well as suppression of the pituitary–adrenal axis. Signs of skin atrophy, if found, often disappear within 6 months following discontinuation of the topical corticosteroid.

Eradication of Superinfection. In eczema associated with atopy, there is both a higher than normal carriage rate and high lesional counts of *S. aureus* (Leyden et al., 1974; Aly et al., 1977). More recent studies have also documented increased colonization of nonatopic hand eczema with *S. aureus*. The reasons for altered bacterial flora in the forms of eczema studied are not well understood. Normal skin has efficient defense mechanisms that seem to discourage foreign organisms from colonizing. These include desiccation, the antibacterial effect of certain skin-surface fatty acids, surface pH, and the presence of a resident microflora (Noble, 1981). However, these mechanisms may be disturbed in eczema. For example, IgG and fibronectin may be present in the exudate associated with acute eczema, and the protein A in the cell wall of *S. aureus* has a high affinity for IgG and fibronectin (Forsgren et al., 1966; Ryden et al., 1983). Thus staphyloccal colonization could be propagated by these interactions.

For the physician confronting acute eczema, especially in the atopic patient, an important question is whether the lesions are not only pruritic but painful or tender. These latter two symptoms may signify superinfection of eczema even in the absence of frank pustulation. Under these circumstances empiric systemic antibiotic therapy should be considered part of the required therapy of the eczema. Many dermatologists initially treat all cases of acute atopic eczema with a 10-day course of *erythromycin* or a semisynthetic penicillinase-resistant penicillin (e.g., *dicloxicillin*). Culturing the lesions is encouraged only if an appropriate course of empirical therapy is ineffective, since initial culture of the lesions almost always grows out *S. aureus*. It should also be remembered that the presence of punched-out erosions at sites of eczema in atopic patients should raise the possibility of herpes simplex infection, and

appropriate therapy (acyclovir) should be instituted based on viral culture.

The anti-inflammatory and immunosuppressive effects of corticosteroids sometimes become a theoretical cause for concern in treating eczema colonized with *S. aureus*. However, studies have shown that the application of superpotent clobetasol propionate to hand eczema in both atopic and nonatopic patients caused a significant reduction or complete elimination of *S. aureus* in association with eliminating the eczematous skin changes (Nilsson et al., 1986). The reason(s) for these findings have yet to be found. Thus, in acute nonatopic eczema, the use of bacteriostatic compresses (e.g., aluminum acetate) plus a potent topical steroid cream may be sufficient without the need for antibiotic therapy. *Principle: Infection in the skin or elsewhere is not an automatic indication for antibiotic therapy.*

Suppression and Prevention of Pruritus. Since pruritus plays a pivotal role in the evolution and propagation of eczema, controlling or possibly eliminating it is the key to ultimate success in treating eczema. Unfortunately, despite a variety of approaches, this remains the most difficult aspect of eczema to treat.

Based on the premise that altered cutaneous-barrier function (with increased transepidermal loss of water) and endogenous release of histamine are contributing factors to pruritus, the use of various emollients and oral antihistamines constitutes the major therapeutic approach to managing pruritus.

The proper use of emollients in the therapy of atopic eczema, xerotic eczema, nummular eczema, and localized neurodermatitis cannot be overemphasized. As previously mentioned, the acute stage of eczema should be handled with topical medications in creams or lotion vehicles, the dry eczema and associated dry skin should be handled with more frequent application of creams (e.g., Eucerin) or if tolerated, very thinly applied ointments (e.g., white petrolatum). The physician must be specific in telling patients that frequency of application, not the brand of emollient, is the most crucial aspect of therapy.

Because so many cosmetics and OTC topical medications are used by society without any specific directions or cosmetic consequences, a less-than-attentive attitude on the part of the patient in regard to applying a topical emollient will only increase the chances of therapeutic failure. The patient needs to be told that when pruritus occurs, applying the appropriate emollient, not scratching, is the proper response. Furthermore, since bathing or showering, especially with soap, leads to increased dryness of the skin, especially in atopic but also nonatopic xerotic skin, washing should be minimized and when required should be accompanied by immediate application of an appropriate emollient to the still-wet skin followed by gentle pat drying. *Principle: The clinician who focuses on the drug alone, ignoring so-called adjunctive measures, often creates impossible obstacles for the drug to overcome. While therapeutic failure may easily be attributed to the drug, it is the doctor who really has failed and the patient who really pays.*

The use of oral antihistamines for pruritus may be effective only in so far as the associated sedation discourages the physical effort to scratch. While there is definite evidence that concentrations of free histamine are elevated in atopic skin and that histamine release may be more labile among atopic mast cells or basophils, the use of newer potent H_1 antagonists (e.g., *astemizole, terfenadine*) that have little or no sedative effect have not been shown to be efficacious in managing pruritus (Julin, 1967; Ring et al., 1980; Krause and Shuster, 1983). Furthermore, H_2-receptor antagonists such as *cimetidine* do not provide any significant therapeutic benefit for pruritus associated with atopic dermatitis (Foulds and MacKie, 1981). Since the sedative effect of the most widely used H_1 antagonists [e.g., *diphenhydramine* (Benadryl), *hydoxyzine hydrochloride* (Atarax)] appears to be the important property for combating pruritus associated with eczema, the patients must be warned about this drug effect if driving or working with dangerous machinery is part of their daily routine. Sometimes, suggesting that the patient take a leave of absence from work is most appropriate, since work-related stress may work against the best therapies for relieving severe pruritus related to eczema.

The chronic use of topical antihistamines (e.g., *diphenhydramine, promethazine hydrochloride*) available in OTC anti-itch preparations or the *benzocaine*-containing topical anesthetic ointments should be discouraged because of their potential to induce allergic contact dermatitis.

In summary, successful treatment of eczema fully depends on identifying its cause and then instituting appropriate topical and systemic therapies as outlined. Failure to respond should lead the physician to first document patient compliance with the prescribed therapy and then reevaluate the suspected cause. The most frequently missed diagnosis that may sometimes present as eczema is tinea corporis, which requires appropriate antifungal therapy. Diagnosis of tinea depends on the finding of typical hyphae on microscopic examination of scales (so-called potassium hydroxide or KOH preparation) as well as on culture for the fungus.

PSORIASIS

Psoriasis is a skin disease characterized by a chronic relapsing eruption of scaling papules that so rapidly coalesce that the physician usually only finds erythematous, scaly plaques by the time the patient seeks consultation. It is estimated to affect roughly 7 million Americans with approximately 200,000 new cases occurring each year.

The classic predilection for plaques of psoriasis to appear symmetrically on the elbows and knees assists in the diagnosis. However, patients can present a broad clinical spectrum from only scalp involvement to scattered plaques on the trunk and extremities to, in the most serious cases, a generalized erythroderma accompanied by a rheumatoid factor–negative symmetric arthritis. In all these cases, the finding of very small pits in the nail plates of the hands and feet, the presence of gluteal "pinking" (erythema and slight scaling of the intergluteal cleft), and the occurrence of lesions conforming to specific sites of skin trauma (isomorphic response, or Koebner phenomenon) help secure a clinical diagnosis. A skin biopsy can help to confirm the diagnosis in cases in which lichen simplex chronicus, chronic nummular eczema, or severe seborrhea of the scalp may not be readily excluded on examination alone.

Acute guttate (Latin *gutta* = a "drop") psoriasis is a unique presentation of the disease that follows a minor streptococcal infection; it presents as an eruption of small 1- to 3-mm erythematous, scaly papules in a generalized distribution that slowly enlarge to more closely resemble generalized plaque psoriasis (Whyte and Baughman, 1964). The multiple clinical presentations coupled with familial inheritance suggest that psoriasis is dominantly inherited with variable penetrance of the phenotype.

Pathogenesis

The factors regulating the phenotypic expression of psoriasis are unclear. While studies have explored alterations in cyclic nucleotide function, eicosanoid metabolism, polyamine synthesis, and a variety of other metabolic parameters, none of the alterations so far identified have been shown to be unique to involved psoriatic skin. Studies have documented markedly accelerated in vivo turnover of epidermal cells in the involved skin of patients with psoriasis (approximately 4 days) versus normal epidermal cells (approximately 28 days) (Van Scott and Ekel, 1963; Weinstein and Frost, 1968) and consequently postulated an inherent epidermal defect. However, there is a distinct possibility that the altered epidermal kinetics in psoriasis may, in fact, stem from pathologic stimulation of a normal epidermis by dermal fibroblasts (Saiag et al., 1985). Furthermore, the recent identification of a novel fibroblast-derived keratinocyte growth factor (KGF) that stimulates keratinocyte proliferation suggests that alterations in the production of such cytokines within the dermis could contribute to skin diseases characterized by a hyperproliferative epidermis (Rubin et al., 1989).

Interestingly, β-adrenergic receptor blocking agents can exacerbate psoriasis (Gold et al., 1988). Whether this adverse effect is providing insight into the pathogenesis of psoriasis remains to be determined. Currently, however, the therapies that have evolved for psoriasis focus on the hyperproliferative epidermis. *Principle: When a drug unexpectedly modulates a disease, think carefully about what follow-up you want in order to establish new understanding in regard to pathogenesis or to document drug efficacy.* In this case, we would want to know whether the β-adrenergic antagonists are working by their blocking properties. If so, we might then expect to see studies on the effects of absorbable β-adrenergic agonists on the disease.

Therapy

The therapy of psoriasis must be tailored to the type of clinical presentation that the physician encounters. Localized disease can be handled by a variety of topical therapies. More generalized disease may require different topical therapies with the additional consideration of systemic therapies in recalcitrant cases that cause serious morbidity for the patient.

Topical Therapy. For isolated hyperkeratotic plaques, the use of potent or superpotent topical corticosteroids probably is the most widely used initial treatment. The use of the superpotent *clobetasol propionate* 0.05% ointment has been shown to be superior to one of the high-potency steroid ointments both in terms of faster improvement and longer remission (Jacobson et al., 1986). If no more than the recommended 50 g/week of the superpotent topical corticosteroids is required, a 2-week course should be tried with these preparations (see previous section on use of topical corticosteroids). If less than 50 g/week is required over the initial 2 weeks, the physician can consider, especially for very thick plaques, alternate-day therapy first, with the superpotent corticosteroid alternating with a less potent corticosteroid (0.05% *fluocinonide* or 0.1% *triamcinolone* ointment on the off days). Another alternative is to apply a 1%, 2%, or 5% *crude coal tar* ointment to the lesions on the days when steroids are not administered. Some experienced clinicians

feel that coal tar alone may have a steroid-sparing effect (Lowe, 1988).

Once the lesions are flat and the erythema has significantly diminished, daily application of some of the commercially available coal tars can be used until the lesions are totally clear. Some of the available preparations include Estar Gel, Psorigel, Bakers PS and plus Gel, and T Derm Tar Oil. The reason for the therapeutic benefit of coal tar in psoriasis is unclear even though it was introduced 65 years ago to treat psoriasis in combination with hot quartz (ultraviolet B, UVB) light therapy (Goeckerman, 1925). Coal tar is a by-product of coking ovens, and its specific composition depends on the type of coal burned, the temperature, and efficiency of the coking ovens (Gruber et al., 1970). One of the lingering concerns with using coal tar is its demonstrated carcinogenicity in laboratory animals (Rasmussen, 1978). However, an international survey conducted in 1976 was able to identify only 3 out of 135,000 psoriatic patients that appeared to have skin cancer related to use of coal tar (Farber, 1977). A more recent study of long-term use of topical coal tar in psoriasis was likewise unable to uncover an increased incidence of skin cancer (Pittlekow et al., 1981).

Another effective topical agent for use on isolated, noninflamed, thick plaques of psoriasis is *anthralin* (or dithranol). It is commercially available in different concentrations in both cream (Drithocreme 0.1%, 0.25%, 0.5%, and 1.0%) and ointment (Anthra-Derm 0.1%, 0.25%, 0.5%, and 1.0%) vehicles and is a coal tar derivative that appears to exert an antimitotic effect on the hyperproliferative epidermis (Swanbeck and Liden, 1966). Because of its irritant effect on normal skin, most protocols employ a thick paste vehicle with the application of petrolatum around the involved skin to protect the normal skin. The drug is then left on the skin for the entire day. While effective (daily application often produces clearing of plaques within an average period of 3 weeks), irritation of the normal skin as well as staining of clothing and bed sheets by anthralin can create problems with compliance of outpatients. More recent studies have demonstrated a more rapid absorption of anthralin through psoriatic epidermis and have therefore explored short exposure (10–30 minutes) of plaques to anthralin (Shaefer et al., 1980; Runne and Kunze, 1982; Lowe et al., 1984). While taking an average of 4 to 6 weeks of therapy, the short exposure is efficacious in resolving localized plaques while minimizing the chance for skin irritation, especially if the physician begins with the lowest concentration of anthralin and increases the concentration as tolerated.

For more generalized disease, the topical therapies just reviewed may become too cumbersome and lead to lack of patient compliance. While these therapies may still be applied to localized sites where plaques may by especially hypertrophic, the most widely used therapy for generalized psoriasis is the combination of topical coal tar applications with UVB light (290- to 320-nm wavelength). This treatment, initiated by Goeckerman in the 1920s (still referred to as *Goeckerman therapy*), consists of combining topical coal tar treatment (in the form of ointments or tar solutions mixed into bathwater) three times per day with interspersed use of increasing exposures to UVB light to induce a mild erythema. In the 1950s the so-called Ingram method was introduced, replacing coal tar with anthralin (Ingram, 1953). Both these therapies, while initially delivered in an inpatient setting, have, because of the increasing costs of inpatient care, been successfully transferred to the setting of so-called ambulatory psoriasis treatment centers, or psoriasis day care centers (Bohm and Voorhees, 1985).

Systemic Therapy. For the population of psoriasis patients who suffer from generalized disease that is recalcitrant to the above therapies or for whom recurrence rates seriously interfere with occupational or other living demands, systemic therapies have been developed, again primarily based on suppressing the markedly increased epidermal cell proliferation. However, the increased risk of potentially adverse effects associated with these therapies can only be justified by the degree of morbidity that more extensive cases of psoriasis can occasionally produce. These systemic approaches include (1) oral *8-methoxypsoralin* combined with subsequent exposure to *ultraviolet A* (UVA) light, so-called *PUVA* therapy (Melski et al., 1977), (2) oral or IM *methotrexate*, a folic acid antagonist that interferes with DNA, RNA, and protein synthesis (Roenigk et al., 1988) (see chapter 23), (3) oral *hydroxyurea*, a DNA-synthesis inhibitor (Leavell and Yarbro, 1970) (see chapter 23), (4) oral *etretinate*, a vitamin A derivative that inhibits epidermal ornithine decarboxylase and thereby interferes with polyamine metabolism required for cell growth (Lowe et al., 1982; Kaplan et al., 1983), (5) a combination of the retinoid etretinate and PUVA (so-called *REPUVA*) therapy that may shorten the required course of PUVA therapy, thereby decreasing its potential long-term hazards (Honigsmann and Wolff, 1989), and (6) *cyclosporin A*, which, in addition to its immunosuppressive effects, appears to suppress keratinocyte DNA synthesis (Ellis et al., 1986; Furure et al., 1988; Meinardi and Bos, 1988).

A detailed discussion of the systemic therapies is beyond the scope of this chapter. Needless to say, treatment of the more severe cases of psoriasis should be handled by clinicians experienced with the systemic therapies for psoriasis and their potential hazards [e.g., hepatotoxicity and hematologic side effects of methotrexate (O'Connor et al., 1989); macrocytic anemia, leukopenia, and thrombocytopenia associated with hydroxyurea therapy; teratogenicity, hyperlipidemia, skeletal hyperostoses, and hepatotoxicity associated with etretinate therapy (Matt et al., 1989); cataracts and skin cancers associated with PUVA (Gupta and Anderson, 1987); and nephrotoxicity with cyclosporin A (Picascia et al., 1988)]. *Principle: From a therapeutic perspective, the best justification for subspecialization is to be found in the use of drugs that, because of the substantial toxicity that may accompany therapeutic efficacy, mandate expertise in their delivery.*

SKIN REACTIONS INDUCED BY SYSTEMIC MEDICATIONS

Drug-induced skin reactions may occur in approximately 2% to 3% of medical inpatients (60,000-90,000 reactions per year nationwide) (Shapiro et al., 1969). Roughly 1 in 44 inpatients may be expected to develop a morbilliform, urticarial, or other exanthem. The highest rates of reaction were noted for the combination of trimethoprim and sulfamethoxazole (59 per 1000 recipients) followed closely by ampicillin (52 per 1000 recipients) (Arndt and Jick, 1976). With the exception of ampicillin and other semisynthetic penicillins (50% occur after 1 week of administration) cutaneous reactions usually occur within 1 week of beginning therapy with the offending drug.

Pathogenesis

Untoward reactions of the skin to drugs administered systemically can be classified on the basis of etiology if known, but clinical morphology still remains the basis for categorizing most cutaneous reactions to systemic medications (Wintroub, 1985). If an immunologic mechanism can be found that explains a skin reaction, the term *allergic drug reaction* is appropriate. However, nonimmunologic drug reactions can also be identified wherein a given drug can activate specific effector pathways without invoking participation of the immune system. An example of such nonimmunologic activation of effector pathways is the direct release of histamine and activation of complement in the absence of antibody by radiocontrast media (Lasser, 1968; Arroyave et al., 1976). However, radiocontrast media themselves can produce a bullous skin reaction (Grunwald et al., 1985) as well as a necrotizing vasculitis (Kerdel et al., 1984). It thus becomes clear that any given systemically administered drug may be responsible for both immunologically and nonimmunologically mediated skin reactions depending on host factors yet to be accurately identified. Consequently the following discussion will focus on morphologic patterns of skin response to drugs, those drugs most frequently associated with a given morphology, and approaches to therapy of drug reactions in the presence or absence of a defined etiology.

Urticarial Reactions. Urticaria, sometimes accompanied by angioedema, probably is one of the most common cutaneous manifestations of an allergic drug reaction. In the vast majority of clinical cases of urticaria or angioedema, the cause cannot be identified (Champion et al., 1969). Urticaria or angioedema occurring within minutes of drug ingestion is termed an *immediate reaction*; a response manifesting itself 12 to 36 hours following drug exposure is termed an *accelerated reaction*. The term *chronic urticaria* is used to describe urticaria that lasts more than 6 weeks.

Urticaria can represent an IgE-mediated response in which drug or drug–metabolite protein conjugates bind to hapten-specific IgE attached to Fc^E receptors on the surface of mast cells or basophils. Bridging of Fc^E receptors through binding of antigen by the resident IgE molecules leads to mast cell or basophil degranulation. The released mediators can induce vasodilation (e.g. histamine, prostaglandin D_2, platelet-activating factor (PAF) and vascular permeability (e.g., leukotriene C_4) that are the pathophysiologic markers of urticaria.

Urticaria also can be a frequent manifestation of serum sickness and in this context occurs within 7 to 12 days following initial exposure to the offending drug. Accompanying fever, arthralgias, myalgias, and lymphadenopathy can help solidify the diagnosis. Data support IgG immune complex deposition in the cutaneous postcapillary venules with resultant complement activation and mast cell degranulation (Yancy and Lawley, 1984) as an etiologic mechanism for the urticaria.

The drugs most frequently associated with urticaria or angioedema include penicillin and related derivatives that retain the 6-aminopenicillinic acid nucleus, sulfa drugs, barbiturates (especially phenobarbital), anticonvulsants, salicylates, allergy extracts, opiate analgesics, and, as mentioned, radiocontrast materials.

Morbilliform Reactions. This is probably the most frequent type of skin reaction to systemically administered drugs and presents as a generalized fine maculopapular eruption resembling measles (hence *morbilliform*). It can be difficult to distinguish from viral exanthems. The mechanism underlying this type of reaction is unknown. It may be induced by a wide variety of drugs, penicillin and its derivatives being the most common inducers, with blood products (e.g., whole human blood, packed red blood cells, blood platelets) next highest in frequency (Arndt and Jick, 1976).

Erythema Multiforme (EM). This skin eruption is characterized by the acute appearance of annular erythematous lesions, most having a central erythematous papule or bulla that gives the appearance of a marksman's target to the lesions (hence the term *target lesion*). Lesions are often generalized and can involve the palms and soles. *EM minor* is the term used for eruptions that involve the skin and/or one mucosal surface without systemic symptoms. *EM major* (*Stevens-Johnson syndrome*) is a more severe form of the eruption and is characterized by erosive mucous membrane lesions most prominent in the conjunctiva and mouth as well as systemic symptoms of fever and malaise.

Drug reactions have been cited as responsible for up to 60% of EM cases, though this may be an overestimate since some of the drugs are used to treat the viral infections that may in themselves induce EM (Bianchine et al., 1968). Long-acting sulfonamides are the drugs most frequently implicated in EM (Carroll et al., 1966), with barbiturates, sulindac, and fenoprofen also frequently implicated (Hardie and Savin, 1979). Whereas the pathogenesis of EM is not firmly established, an immune complex–mediated vasculitis may be implied from studies on herpes simplex– and *Mycoplasma pneumonia*–associated EM (Kazmierowski and Wuepper, 1978; Wuepper et al., 1980; Tonnesen et al., 1983).

Toxic Epidermal Necrolysis (TEN). This severe cutaneous reaction is clinically characterized by diffuse erythema with tenderness, fever, and malaise followed by widespread sloughing of the epidermis resembling a scalding injury. Mucous membranes show erythema, erosions, and bullae. While associated with a variety of etiologic factors (Lyell, 1967), drugs that are definitely implicated include sulfonamides, butazones, hydantoins, barbiturates, and penicillin (Hardie and Savin, 1979).

Toxic epidermal necrolysis must be differentiated for both prognostic and therapeutic reasons from *staphyloccal scalded skin syndrome* (SSSS), which is caused by infection with specific strains of *S. aureus* and requires a different therapeutic approach (Elias et al., 1977). Clinically, SSSS may defy differentiation from TEN. An exfoliative cytology preparation obtained at the bedside and stained with Giemsa shows primarily nucleated squamous cells in SSSS but cell debris, leukocytes, and only occasional squamous cells in TEN. These differences are due to the fact that in SSSS the epidermal cleavage is due to a circulating bacterial epidermolytic exotoxin that attacks the epidermis at or below the stratum granulosum with little to be found as far as an inflammatory cell infiltrate; the bacteria are not present in the skin lesions but can be readily cultured from the nares. In drug-induced TEN, however, the full thickness of epidermis is destroyed in a reaction associated with numerous leukocytes (Amon and Diamond, 1975).

Other Morphologic Forms of Cutaneous Reactions to Systemic Drugs. While the cutaneous eruptions heretofore described represent the most common as well as clinically most consequential, there are a variety of other adverse cutaneous responses to systemic drugs that would require far more space for complete discussion. These are covered in a reference devoted solely to such reactions (Wintroub et al., 1987).

Therapy

The treatment of drug-induced skin reactions ultimately depends on identification and immediate cessation of therapy with the offending drug. If possible an alternate, structurally unrelated substitute should be found. In the case of a relatively asymptomatic morbilliform skin rash, the offending drug may be continued if it is absolutely essential. Resolution of morbilliform eruptions in the presence of continuing therapy has occurred. However, if evolution to a more symptomatic erythroderma appears possible by careful and repeated inspection by the physician, the offending drug should be immediately discontinued and every effort made to find adequate alternative therapy.

The therapy of urticarial drug reactions depends on the accompanying symptoms. In the extreme case of urticaria or angioedema as manifestations of an anaphylactic response, appropriate emergency procedures should be instituted including IM epinephrine, maintenance of airway, and other appropriate measures. When pruritus is the only symptom, treatment with H_1-antagonist antihistamines (e.g., hydroxyzine or diphenhydramine) may provide benefit if histamine is the major causative mediator. If pruritus is the major source of discomfort, these antihistamines may be beneficial through their sedative properties, even if the urticaria itself does not immediately respond.

In cases of chronic urticaria (>6 weeks) when there is a history of aspirin or NSAID sensitivity or penicillin sensitivity in the form of urticaria, chronic exposure to trace salicylates or penicillin derivatives present in various fruits, vegetables, and dairy products may be occurring. Attempts to remove potential dietary sources of these offending agents should be attempted. Recent studies have also suggested that some of the long-acting non-sedating H_1 antihistamines provide benefit in chronic urticaria. *Astemazole* (Hismanal) and *terfenadine* (Seldane) may offer greater relief in chronic urticaria than the shorter-acting sedating antihistamines (Cainelli et al., 1986; Bernstein and Bernstein, 1986).

The cutaneous reactions that carry a significant associated morbidity and mortality are EM major and TEN. The differentiation of TEN from SSSS is important since the former reaction has a mortality rate of 25% to 50% and is unaffected or possibly made worse if treated with an antibiotic that cross-reacts with the offending drug. Conversely, SSSS is associated with about a 4% mortality and responds to appropriate antistaphylococcal drugs; systemic corticosteroids are contraindicated (Elias et al., 1977). Because of the loss of significant areas of epidermis in EM major and TEN, treatment must focus on immediate cessation of therapy with the suspected drug, prevention of superinfection, and maintenance of fluid balance following the same procedures that one would for a burn patient. Patients with EM major or TEN should be managed in a hospital setting. The use of steroids in these patients is controversial.

REFERENCES

Adams, S. J.; Cunliffe, W. J.; and Cooke, M. J.: Long-term antibiotic therapy for acne vulgaris: Effects on the bowel flora of patients and their relatives. J. Invest. Dermatol., 85: 35–37, 1985.

Akers, W. A.; Allen, A. M.; Burnett, J. W.; Freinkel, R. K.; Horvath, P. N.; Lazar, P.; Leyden, J. J.; Maibach, H. I.; Marples, R. R.; O'Quinn, S. E.; Pochi, P. E.; Smith, E. B.; and Taplin, D.: Systemic antibiotics for treatment of acne vulgaris: Efficacy and safety. Arch. Dermatol., 111:1630–1636, 1975.

Allison, F.; Smith, M. R.; and Wood, W. B.: Studies on the pathogenesis of acute inflammation: II. The action of cortisone on the inflammatory response to thermal injury. J. Exp. Med., 102:669–675, 1955.

Aly, R.; Maibach, H. I.; and Shinefeld, H. R.: Microbial flora of atopic dermatitis. Arch. Dermatol., 113:780–782, 1977.

Amon, R. B.; and Diamond, R. L.: Toxic epidermal necrolysis: Rapid differentiation between staphylococcal- and drug-induced disease. Arch. Dermatol., 111:1433–1437, 1975.

Arndt, K. A.; and Jick, H.: Rates of cutaneous reactions to drugs. J.A.M.A., 235:918–923, 1976.

Arroyave, C. M.; Bhatt, K. N.; and Crown, N. R.: Activation of the alternative pathway of the complement system by radiocontrast media. J. Immunol., 117:1866–1869, 1976.

Baer, R. L.; Leshan, S. M.; and Shalita, A. R.: High dose tetracycline therapy in severe acne. Arch. Dermatol., 112: 479–481, 1976.

Barry, B.; and Woodford, R.: Activity and bioavailability of topical steroids. In vivo/in vitro correlations for the vasoconstrictor test. J. Clin. Pharmacol., 3:43–65, 1978.

Bernstein, I. L.; and Bernstein, D. I.: Efficacy and safety of Astemizole, a long acting and nonsedating H1 antagonist for the treatment of chronic idiopathic urticaria. J. Allerg. Clin. Immunol., 77:37–42, 1986.

Bianchine, J. R.; Macaraeg, P. V. J.; Lasagna, L.; Azarnoff, D. L.; Brunk, S. F.; Hvidberg, E. F.; and Owen, J. A. Jr.: Drugs as etiologic factors in Stevens-Johnson syndrome. Am. J. Med., 44:390–405, 1968.

Bjornberg, A.; and Roupe, G.: Susceptibility to infections during long term treatment with tetracyclines in acne vulgaris. Dermatologica, 145:334–337, 1972.

Blackwell, G. J.; Carnuccio, R.; DiRosa, M.; Flower, R. J.; Parente, L.; and Persico, P.: Macrocortin: A polypeptide causing the anti-phospholipase effect of glucocorticoids. Nature, 287:147–149, 1980.

Bohm, M. L.; and Voorhees, J. J.: Role of ambulatory psoriasis treatment center. J. Am. Acad. Dermatol., 12:740–747, 1985.

Burke, B.; Eady, E. A.; and Cunliffe, W. J.: Benzoyl peroxide versus topical erythromycin in the treatment of acne vulgaris. Br. J. Dermatol., 108:199–204, 1983.

Cainelli, T.; Seidenari, S.; Valsecchi, R.; and Mosca, M.: Double blind comparison of astemizole and terfenadine in the treatment of chronic urticaria. Pharmatherapeutica, 4:679–686, 1986.

Camisa, C.; Eisenstadt, B.; Ragoz, A.; and Weissmann, G.: The effects of retinoids on neutrophil functions in vitro. J. Am. Acad. Dermatol., 6:620–629, 1982.

Carroll, O. M.; Bryan, P. A.; and Robinson, R. J.: Stevens-Johnson syndrome associated with long acting sulfonamides. J.A.M.A., 195:691–693, 1966.

Champion, R. H.; Roberts, S. O. B.; Carpenter, R. G.; and Roger, J. H.: Urticaria and angio-edema: A review of 554 patients. Br. J. Dermatol., 81:88–97, 1969.

Cornell, R. C.; and Stoughton, R. B.: Correlation of the vasoconstriction assay and clinical activity in psoriasis. Arch. Dermatol., 121:63–67, 1985.

Cornell, R. C.; and Stoughton, R. B.: Six month controlled study of effects of desoximetasone and betamethasone 17-valerate on the pituitary-adrenal axis. Br. J. Dermatol., 105:91–95, 1981.

Cunliffe, W. J.; Jones, D. H.; Pritlove, J.; and Parkin, D.: Long-term benefit of isotretinoin in acne. In, Retinoids: New Trends in Research and Therapy (Saurat, J. H., ed.). S. Karger, Basel, pp. 242–251, 1985.

Cunliffe, W. J.; Forster, R. A.; Greenwood, N. D.; Heatherington, C.; Holland, K. T.; Holmes, R. L.; Khan, S.; Roberts, C. D.; Williams, M.; and Williamson, B.: Tetracycline and acne vulgaris: A clinical and laboratory investigation. Br. Med. J., 2:332–335, 1973.

Dalziel, K.; Dykes, P. J.; and Marks, R.: Inflammation due to intracutaneous implantation of stratum corneum. Br. J. Exp. Pathol., 65:107–115, 1984.

de Vivier, A.: Acute tolerance to effect of topical glucocorticoids. Br. J. Dermatol., 94 (suppl. 12):25–32, 1976.

DiGiovanna, J. J.; and Peck, G. L.: Retinoid toxicity. Prog. Dermatol., 21(3):1–8, 1987.

DiRosa, M.; Flower, R. J.; Hirata, F.; Parente, L.; and Russo-Marie, F.: Nomenclature announcement. Anti-phospholipase protein. Prostaglandins, 28:441–442, 1984.

Eady, E. A.; Cove, J. H.; Holland, K. T.; and Cunliffe, W. J.: Erythromycin resistant propionibacteria in antibiotic treated acne patients: Association with therapeutic failure. Br. J. Dermatol., 121:51–57, 1989.

Eaglestein, W. H.; Farzad, A.; and Capland, L.: Topical corticosteroid therapy: Efficacy of frequent application. Arch. Dermatol., 110:955–956, 1974.

Elias, P. M.; and Finegold, K.: Lipid-related barriers and gradients in the epidermis. Ann. N.Y. Acad. Sci., 548:4–13, 1988.

Elias, P. M.; Fritsch, P.; and Epstein, E. H. Jr.: Staphyloccal scalded skin syndrome: Clinical features, pathogenesis, and recent microbiological and biochemical developments. Arch. Dermatol., 113:207–219, 1977.

Ellis, C. N.; Gorsulowsky, D. C.; Hamilton, T. A.; Billings, J. K.; Brown, M. D.; Headington, J. T.; Cooper, K. D.;

Baadsgaard, O.; Duell, E. A.; Annesley, T. M.; and Voorhees, J. J.: Cyclosporine improves psoriasis in a double blind study. J.A.M.A., 256:3110–3116, 1986.

Esterly, N. B.; Furey, N. L.; and Flanagan, L. E.: The effect of antimicrobial agents on leukocyte chemotaxis. J. Invest. Dermatol., 70:51–55, 1978.

Farber, E. (ed.): International Psoriasis Bulletin, 4(4):1–6, 1977.

Forsgren, A.; and Sjoquist, J.: "Protein A" from S. aureus: I. Pseudo immune reaction with human gamma-globulin. J. Immunol., 97:822–827, 1966.

Foulds, I. S.; and MacKie, R. M.: A double-blind trial of the H2 receptor antagonist cimetidine and the H1 receptor antagonist promethazine hydrochloride in the treatment of atopic dermatitis. Clin. Allergy, 11:319–323, 1981.

Frichot, B. C. 3rd; and Zelickson, A. S.: Steroids, lysosomes and dermatitis. Acta. Derm. Venereol. (Stockh.), 52:311–319, 1972.

Fulton, J. E.; Marples, R.; McGinley, K.; and Leyden, J. J.: Gram negative folliculitis in acne vulgaris. Arch. Dermatol., 98:349–353, 1968.

Furure, M.; Gaspari, A.; and Katz, S. T.: The effect of cyclosporin A on epidermal cells: II. Cyclosporin A inhibits proliferation of normal and transformed keratinocytes. J. Invest. Dermatol., 90:796–800, 1988.

Gammon, W. R.; Meyer, C.; Lantis, S.; Shenefelt, P.; Reizner, G.; and Cripps, D. J.: Comparative efficacy of oral erythromycin versus oral tetracycline in the treatment of acne vulgaris. J. Am. Acad. Dermatol., 14:183–186, 1986.

Gibson, J. R.; Kirsch, J. M.; Darley, C. R.; Harvey, S. G.; Burke, C. A.; and Hanson, M. E.: An assessment of the relationship between vasoconstrictor assay findings, clinical efficacy and skin thinning effects of a variety of undiluted and diluted corticosteroid preparations. Br. J. Dermatol. 111 (suppl. 27):204–212, 1984.

Goeckerman, W. H.: The treatment of psoriasis. Northwest Med., 24:2–9, 1925.

Gold, M. H.; Holy, A. K.; and Roenigk, H. H.: Beta-blocking drugs and psoriasis: A review of cutaneous side effects and retrospective analysis of their effects on psoriasis. J. Am. Acad. Dermatol., 19:837–841, 1988.

Gomez, E. C.; Kaminester, L.; and Frost, P.: Topical halcinonide and betamethasone valerate effects on plasma cortisol: Acute and subacute usage studies. Arch. Dermatol., 113:1196–1202, 1977.

Gould, D. J.; and Cunliffe, W. J.: The long term treatment of acne vulgaris. Clin. Exp. Dermatol., 3:253–257, 1978.

Gruber, M.; Klein, R.; and Foxx, M.: Chemical standardization and quality assurance of whole crude coal tar USP utilizing GLC procedures. J. Pharm. Sci., 59(6):830–834, 1970.

Grunwald, M. H.; David, M.; and Feuerman, E. J.: Coexistence of psoriasis vulgaris and bullous diseases. J. Am. Acad. Dermatol., 13:224–228, 1985.

Gupta, A. K.; and Anderson, T. F.: Psoralen photochemotherapy. J. Am. Acad. Dermatol., 17:703–734, 1987.

Hammarstrom, S.; Hamberg, M.; Duell, E.; Stawiski, M.; Anderson, T. F.; and Voorhees, J. J.: Glucocorticocoids in inflammatory proliferative skin disease reduces arachidonic acid hydroxyeicosatetraenoic acids. Science, 197:994–995, 1977.

Hardie, R. A.; and Savin, J. A.: Drug-induced skin diseases. Br. Med. J., 1:935–937, 1979.

Haustein, U. F.; Tegetmeyer, L.; and Ziegler, V.: Allergic and irritant potential of benzoyl peroxide. Contact Dermatitis, 13:252–257, 1985.

Honigsmann, H.; and Wolff, K.: Results of therapy for psoriasis using retinoid and photochemotherapy (REPUVA). Pharmacol. Ther., 40:67–73, 1989.

Hurwitz, S.: Acne vulgaris. Current concepts of pathogenesis and treatment. Am. J. Dis. Child., 133:536–544, 1979.

Ingram, J. T.: The approach to psoriasis. Br. Med. J., 2:591–594, 1953.

Jackson, D. B.; Thompson, C.; McCormack, J. R.; and Guin, J. D.: Bioequivalence (bioavailability) of generic topical corticosteroids. J. Am. Acad. Dermatol., 20:791–796, 1989.

Jacobson, C.; Cornell, R. C.; and Savin, R. C.: A comparison of clobetasol propionate 0.05 percent ointment and an optimized betamethasone dipropionate 0.05 percent ointment in the treatment of psoriasis, Cutis, 37:213–220, 1986.

Jones, D. H.: The role and mechanism of action of 13-*cis*-retinoic acid in the treatment of severe (nodulocystic) acne. Pharmacol. Ther., 40:91–106, 1989.

Jones, D.; King, K.; Miller, A.; and Cunliffe, W. J.: A dose-response study of 13-*cis*-retinoic acid in acne vulgaris. Br. J. Dermatol., 103:333–343, 1983.

Julin, L.: Localization and content of histamine in normal and diseased skin. Acta Derm. Venereol. (Stockh.), 42:218–229, 1967.

Kaplan, R. P.; Russell, D. H.; and Lowe, N. J.: Etretinate therapy for psoriasis: Clinical responses, remission times, epidermal DNA and polyamine responses. J. Am. Acad. Dermatol., 8:95–102, 1983.

Kazmierowski, J. A.; and Wuepper, K. D.: Erythema multiforme: Immune complex vasculitis of the superficial cutaneous microvasculature. J. Invest. Dermatol., 71:366–369, 1978.

Kerdel, F. A.; Fraker, D. L.; and Haynes, H. A.: Necrotizing vasculitis from radiographic contrast media. J. Am. Acad. Dermatol., 10:25–29, 1984.

King, K.; Jones, D. H.; Daltry, D. C.; and Cunliffe, W. J.: A double-blind study of the effects of 13-*cis*-retinoic acid on acne sebum excretion rate and microbial population. Br. J. Dermatol., 107:583–590, 1982.

Kirby, J. D.; and Monroe, D. D.: Steroid induced atrophy in an animal and human model. Br. J. Dermatol., 94 (suppl. 12):11–19, 1976.

Kligman, A. M.; Fulton, J. E.; and Plewig, G.: Topical vitamin A acid in acne vulgaris. Arch. Dermatol., 99:469–476, 1969.

Knutson, D. D.: Ultrastructural observations in acne vulgaris: The normal sebaceous follicle and acne lesions. J. Invest. Dermatol., 62:288–307, 1974.

Krause, L.; and Shuster, S.: Mechanism of action of antipruritic drugs. Br. Med. J., 287:1199–1200, 1983.

Lammer, E. J.; Chen, D. T.; Hoar, R. M.; Acnish, N. O.; Benke, P. J.; Braun, J.; Curry, C. J.; Fernhoff, P. M.; Grix, A. W. Jr.; Lott, I. T.; Richard, J. M.; and Sun, S. C.: Retinoic acid embryopathy. N. Engl. J. Med., 313:837–841, 1985.

Lasser, E. G.: Basic mechanisms of contrast media reactions. Radiology, 91:63–65, 1968.

Lavker, R. M.; and Schecter, N.: Cutaneous mast cell depletion results from topical corticosteroid usage. J. Immunol., 135:2368–2373, 1985.

Leavell, U. W. Jr.; and Yarbro, J. W.: Hydroxyurea: A new treatment for psoriasis. Arch. Dermatol., 102:144–150, 1970.

Leyden, J. J.; Marples, R. R.; and Kligman, A. M.: *Staphylococcus aureus* in the lesions of atopic dermatitis. Br. J. Dermatol., 90:525–530, 1975.

Leyden, J. J.; McGinley, K. J.; Mills, O.; and Kligman, A. M.: Propionibacterium levels in patients with and without acne vulgaris. J. Invest. Dermatol., 65:382–384, 1974.

Lowe, N. J.: Psoriasis. Semin. Dermatol., 7(1):43–47, 1988.

Lowe, N. J.; Ashton, R. E.; Koudsi, H.; Verschoore, M.; and Schaefer, H.: Anthralin for psoriasis: Short-contact anthralin therapy compared with topical steroid and conventional anthralin. J. Am. Acad. Dermatol., 10:69–72, 1984.

Lowe, N. J.; Kaplan, R.; and Breeding, J.: Etretinate treatment for psoriasis inhibits epidermal ornithine decarboxylase. J. Am. Acad. Dermatol., 6:697–698, 1982.

Lyell, A.: A review of toxic epidermal necrolysis in Britain. Br. J. Dermatol., 79:662–671, 1967.

Matt, L.; Lazarus, V. N.; and Lowe, N. J.: Newer retinoids for psoriasis — Early clinical studies. Pharmacol. Ther., 40:157–169, 1989.

McKenzie, A. W.; and Stoughton, R. T.: Method for comparing absorption of steroids. Arch. Dermatol., 86:608–610, 1962.

Melski, J. W.; Tanenbaum, L.; Parrish, J. A.; Fitzpatrick, T. B.; and Bleich, H. L.: Oral methoxsalen photochemotherapy for the treatment of psoriasis: A cooperative clinical trial. J. Invest. Dermatol., 68:328–335, 1977.

Meinardi, M. M.; and Bos, J. D.: Cyclosporine maintenance therapy in psoriasis. Transplant Proc., 20(3) (suppl. 4):42–49, 1988.

Milstone, E. B.; McDonald, A. J.; and Scholhamer, C. F.: Pseudomembranous colitis after topical application of clindamycin. Arch. Dermatol., 117:154–155, 1981.

Munroe, D. D.; and Clift, D. C.: Pituitary-adrenal function after prolonged use of topical corticosteroids. Br. J. Dermatol., 88:381–385, 1973.

Nacht, S.; Young, D.; Beasley, J. N.; Anjo, M. D.; and Maibach, H. I.: Benzoyl peroxide percutaneous penetration and metabolic disposition. J. Am. Acad. Dermatol., 4:31–37, 1981.

Nilsson, E.; Henning, C.; and Hjorleifsson, M-L.: Density of microflora in hand eczema before and after topical treatment with a potent corticosteroid. J. Am. Acad. Dermatol., 15:192–197, 1986.

Noble, W. C.: Microbiology of Human Skin, 2nd ed., Lloyd-Luke, London, pp. 3–106, 1981.

O'Connor, G. T.; Olmstead, E. M.; Zug, K.; Baughman, R. D.; Beck, J. R.; Dunn, J. L.; Seal, P.; and Lewandowski, J. F.: Detection of hepatotoxicity associated with methotrexate therapy for psoriasis. Arch. Dermatol., 125:1209–1217, 1989.

Olsen, E. A.; and Cornell, R. C.: Topical clobetasol-17-propionate: Review of its clinical efficacy and safety. J. Am. Acad. Dermatol., 15:246–255, 1986.

Olsen, T. G.: Therapy of acne. Med. Clin. North. Am., 66:851–871, 1982.

Parker, C. W.; Kennedy, S.; and Eisen, A. Z.: Leukocyte and lymphocyte cyclic AMP responses in atopic eczema. J. Invest. Dermatol., 68:302–306, 1977.

Parry, M. F.; and Rha, C. K.: Pseudomembranous colitis caused by topical clindamycin phosphate. Arch. Dermatol., 122:583–584, 1986.

Picascia, D. D.; Garden, J. M.; Freinkel, R. K.; and Roenigk, H. H. Jr.: Resistant severe psoriasis controlled with systemic cyclosporine therapy. Transplant Proc., 20(3) (suppl. 4):58–62, 1988.

Pittelkow, M. R.; Perry, H. O.; Muller, S. A.; and Nanghan, W. Z.: Skin cancer in patients with psoriasis treated with coal tar. A 25-year follow-up study. Arch. Dermatol., 117:465–468, 1981.

Plewig, G.: Follicular keratinization. J. Invest. Dermatol., 62:308–315, 1974.

Pochi, P. E.; and Strauss, J. S.: Sebum production, casual sebum levels, titratable acidity of sebum, and urinary fractional 17-ketosteroid excretion in males with acne. J. Invest. Dermatol., 43:383–388, 1964.

Puhvel, S. M.; and Sakamoto, M.: The chemoattractant properties of comedonal components. J. Invest. Dermatol., 71:324–329, 1978.

Rajka, G.: Itch duration of uninvolved skin of atopic dermatitis (prurigo Besnier). Acta Derm. Venereol. (Stockh.), 48:320–321, 1968.

Rasmussen, J. E.: The crudeness of coal tar. Prog. Dermatol., 12(5):23–29, 1978.

Rebello, T.; and Hawk, J. L. M.: Skin surface glycerol levels in acne vulgaris. J. Invest. Dermatol., 70:352–354, 1978.

Red Book 1988, Annual Pharmacist's Reference. Medical Economics, Oradell, NJ, 1988.

Reitamo, S.; Lauerma, A. I.; Stubb, S.; Kayhko, K.; Visa, K.; and Forstrom, L.: Delayed hypersensitivity to topical corticosteroids. J. Am. Acad. Dermatol., 14:582–589, 1986.

Ring, J.; Allen, D. H.; Mathison, D. A.; and Spiegelberg, H. L.: In vitro releasibility of histamine and serotonin: Studies in atopic patients. J. Clin. Immunol., 3:85–91, 1980.

Roenick, H. N. Jr.; Auerbach, R.; Maibach, H. I.; and Weinstein, G. D.: Methotrexate in psoriasis: Revised guidelines. J. Am. Acad. Dermatol., 19:145–156, 1988.

Roitt, I. M.; Brostoff, J.; and Male, D. K.: Immunology, Gower Medical Publishing, London, pp. 22.1–22.3, 1985.

Rothman, K. F.; and Pochi, P. E.: Use of oral and topical agents for acne in pregnancy. J. Am. Acad. Dermatol., 16: 431–442, 1988.

Rubin, J. S.; Osada, H.; Finch, P. W.; Taylor, W. G.; Rudikoff, S.; and Aaronson, S. A.: Purification and characterization of a newly identified growth factor specific for epithelial cells. Proc. Natl. Acad. Sci. U.S.A., 86:802–806, 1989.

Runne, U.; and Kunze, J.: Short duration ("minutes") therapy with dithranol for psoriasis: A new outpatient regimen. Br. J. Dermatol., 106:135–139, 1982.

Ryden, C.; Rubin, K.; Speziale, P.; Hook, M.; Lindberg, M.; and Wadstrom, T.: Fibronectin in receptors from *Staphylococcus aureus*. J. Biol. Chem., 258:3396–3401, 1983.

Saiag, P. B.; Coulomb, B.; Lebreton, C.; Bell, E.; and Dubertret, L.: Psoriatic fibroblasts induce hyperproliferation of normal keratinocytes in a skin equivalent model in vitro. Science (Washington), 230:669–672, 1985.

Schaefer, H.; Farber, E. M.; Goldberg, L.; and Schalla, W.: Limited application period for dithranol in psoriasis. Br. J. Dermatol., 102:571–573, 1980.

Shah, V. P.; Peck, C. C.; and Skelly, J. P.: "Vasoconstriction"—Skin blanching—Assay for glucocorticoids—A critique. Arch. Dermatol., 125:1558–1563, 1989.

Shalita, A. R.: Genesis of free fatty acids. J. Invest. Dermatol., 62:332–335, 1974.

Shalita, A. R.; and Wheatly, V.: Inhibition of pancreatic lipase by tetracycline. J. Invest. Dermatol., 54:413–416, 1970.

Shalita, A. R.; Smith, E. B.; and Bauer, E.: Topical erythromycin v clindamycin therapy for acne. A multicenter double-blind comparison. Arch. Dermatol., 120:351–355, 1984.

Shalita, A. R.; Cunningham, W. J.; Leyden, J. J.; Pochi, P. E.; and Strauss, J. S.: Isotretinoin treatment of acne and related disorders: An update. J. Am. Acad. Dermatol., 9: 629–638, 1983.

Shapiro, S.; Slone, D.; Siskind, V.; Lewis, G. P.; and Jick, H.: Drug rash with ampicillin and other penicillins. Lancet, 2: 969–972, 1969.

Stoughton, R. B.; and Cornell, R. C.: Review of super-potent topical corticosteroids. Semin. Dermatol., 6(2):72–76, 1987.

Strauss, J. S.; and Pochi, P. E.: Effect of orally administered antibacterial agents on titratable acidity of human sebum. J. Invest. Dermatol., 47:577–581, 1966.

Strauss, J. S.; and Pochi, P. E.: The quantitative gravimetric determination of sebum production. J. Invest. Dermatol., 36: 293–298, 1961.

Swanbeck, G.; and Liden, S.: The inhibitory effect of dithranol (anthralin) on DNA synthesis. Acta Derm. Venereol. (Stockh.), 66:228–230, 1966.

Tan, P. L.; Barnett, G. L.; Flowers, F. P.; and Araujo, O. E.: Current topical corticosteroid preparations. J. Am. Acad. Dermatol., 14:79–93, 1986.

Tonnesen, M. G.; Harrist, T. J.; Wintroub, B. U.; Mihm, M. C.; and Soter, N. A.: Erythema multiforme: Microvascular damage and infiltration of lymphocytes and basophils. J. Invest. Dermatol., 80:282–286, 1983.

Tucker, S. B.; Rogers, R. S.; Winkelmann, R. K.; Privett,

O. S.; and Jordon, R. E.: Inflammation in acne vulgaris. Leukocyte attraction and cytotoxicity by comedonal material. J. Invest. Dermatol., 74:21–25, 1980.

Van Scott, E. J.; and Ekel, T. M.: Kinetics of hyperplasia in psoriasis. Arch. Dermatol., 88:373–380, 1963.

Walters, B. N. J.; and Gubbay, S. S.: Tetracycline and benign intracranial hypertension: Report of five cases. Br. Med. J., 282:19–20, 1981.

Webster, G. F.; and Leyden, J. J.: Characterization of serum independent polymorphonuclear leukocyte chemotactic factors produced by *Propionibacterium acnes*. Inflammation, 4: 261–269, 1980.

Webster, G. F.; Tsai, C. C.; and Leyden, J. J.: Neutrophil lysosomal release in response to *Propionibacterium acnes*. J. Invest. Dermatol., 72:209, 1979a. Abstract.

Webster, G. F.; Leyden, J. J.; and Nilsson, U. R.: Complement activation in acne vulgaris: Consumption of complement by comedones. Infect. Immun., 26:183–186, 1979b.

Weinstein, G. D.; and Frost, P.: Abnormal cell proliferation in psoriasis. J. Invest. Dermatol., 50:254–259, 1968.

Weissman, G.; and Fell, H. B.: The effect of hydrocortisone on the response of fetal rat skin to ultraviolet irradiation. J. Exp. Med., 116:365–380, 1962.

Wester, R. C.; Noonan, P. K.; and Maibach, H. I.: Frequency of application on percutaneous absorption of hydrocortisone. Arch. Dermatol., 113:620–622, 1977.

Whyte, H. J.; and Baughman, R. D.: Acute guttate psoriasis and streptococcal infection. Arch. Dermatol., 89:350–356, 1964.

Wilson, L.; Williams, D. I.; and Marsh, S. D.: Plasma corticosteroid levels in out patients treated with topical steroids. Br. J. Dermatol., 88:373–380, 1973.

Wintroub, B. U.: Cutaneous drug reactions. J. Am. Acad. Dermatol., 13:167–179, 1985.

Wintroub, B. U.; Stern, R. S.; and Arndt, K. A.: Cutaneous reactions to drugs. In, Dermatology in General Medicine, 3rd ed. (Fitzpatrick, T. B.; Eisen, A. Z.; Wolff, K.; Freedberg, I. M.; and Austen, K. F., eds.). McGraw-Hill Book Co., New York, pp. 1353–1366, 1987.

Wolff, H. H.; Plewig, G.; and Braun-Falco, O.: Ultrastructure of human sebaceous follicles and comedones following treatment with vitamin A acid. Acta. Derm. Venereol. Suppl. (Stockh.), 55:90–110, 1975.

Wolff, K.; and Stingl, G.: The Langerhans cell. J. Invest. Dermatol., 80 (suppl.):17s–21s, 1983.

Wuepper, K. D.; Watson, P. A.; and Kazmierowski, J. A.: Immune complexes in erythema multiforme and the Stevens-Johnson syndrome. J. Invest. Dermatol., 74:368–371, 1980.

Yancy, K. B.; and Lawley, T. J.: Circulating immune complexes: Their immunochemistry, biology, and detection in selected dermatologic and systemic diseases. J. Am. Acad. Dermatol., 10:711–731, 1984.

Yeong, D.; Nacht, S.; Bucks, D.; and Maibach, H. I.: Benzoyl peroxide: Percutaneous penetration and metabolic disposition: II. Effect of concentration. J. Am. Acad. Dermatol., 9: 920–924, 1983.

22

Hematologic Disorders

Peter L. Greenberg, Robert Negrin, and George M. Rodgers

OVERVIEW OF HEMOPOIESIS: BIOLOGIC FEATURES

Therapy of hemopoietic disorders has evolved impressively over the 2 decades since the discovery of a family of hemopoietic growth factors (HGFs) that are involved in the regulation of bone marrow function. Clonogenic in vitro marrow cell cultures enabled definition of hemopoietic progenitor and stem cells and their responsiveness to HGFs, including their induced proliferation and directed differentiation to cells of various lineages. Because these HGFs are derived from cells, they are called cytokines. Cytokines having either stimulatory or inhibitory functions have been discovered. The HGFs have subsequently been biochemically defined, functionally characterized, and ultimately produced in pure form by recombinant gene-cloning tech-

niques. When they became available in larger quantities, in vivo studies demonstrating their biologic effects could be performed. The HGFs are clinically effective for patients with a variety of hemopoietic disorders. They also improve bone marrow recovery after chemotherapy. This section will focus on characterizing the biologic nature of growth factors and their therapeutic applications.

Hemopoietic Stem Cells and Progenitor Cells

Cultures of bone marrow cells have demonstrated the existence of committed myeloid progenitor cells, defined as colony forming units (CFUs)—granulocyte, macrophage (CFU-GM), granulocyte (CFU-G), or macrophage (CFU-M). These progenitor cells can be induced to differentiate to granulocyte-monocyte, granulocytic, or monocytic cells, respectively, under the influence of specific myeloid HGFs termed colony-stimulating factors (CSFs) (Sachs, 1978; Metcalf, 1986). Studies evaluating molecular control of granulocyte–monocyte and macrophage production in vitro have identified a family of glycoproteins capable of stimulating formation of maturing colonies consisting of these types of cells, hence the generic term CSFs for this group of regulators. The main cell type in the bone marrow stimulated by the CSFs is indicated by a prefix. For example, G-CSF is primarily stimulatory for granulocyte formation, M-CSF for monocyte and macrophage formation, GM-CSF for both cell types, and multi-CSF (or interleukin-3, IL-3) for these cells as well as megakaryocytes. In combination with erythropoietin, IL-3 stimulates erythroid cells (Fig. 22–1). Erythroid burst-forming units (BFU-E) and colony-forming units (CFU-E) are clonogenic precursors of erythroid cells, with the CFU-E more mature progeny of the BFU-E. Megakaryocyte precursors (BFU-Meg and CFU-Meg) engender morphologically identifiable megakaryocytes and platelets.

Multipotential hemopoietic stem cells (CFU-GEMM [granulocyte, erythroid, monocyte, megakaryocyte]) generate lineage-restricted progenitor cells and form colonies consisting of cells of the myeloid, erythroid, and megakaryocytic line (Fauser and Messner, 1979). As described below, these in vitro findings have been recapitulated in vivo upon stimulation of marrow with specific HGFs. Although stem and progenitor cells are present mainly in bone marrow, they also circulate (except for CFU-E) in low number in peripheral blood of normal persons. Hemopoietic precursor cells have been enriched by a variety of

physical and immunologic techniques and have been demonstrated to be low-density nonadherent cells lacking markers for T or B lymphocytes with morphologic characteristics similar to those of transitional lymphoid cells or blasts (Moore et al., 1973).

In basal conditions, 30% to 50% of progenitor cells and <5% of CFU-GEMM are in active cell cycle, a fraction that is augmented by a variety of proliferative stimuli. More primitive stem cells, less mature than previously described colony-forming cells, have been defined as cells that repopulate marrow in vivo (Bertoncello et al., 1985). In mice, these cells include in vivo spleen-colony-forming cells (CFU-S) and early stem cells (Bertoncello et al., 1985; Spangrude et al., 1988; Ploemacher and Brons, 1989). In human and murine assays, the CFU-blast and high-proliferative-potential colony-forming cells (HPP-CFC) also possess marrow-repopulating activity (Brandt J. et al., 1988; McNiece et al., 1990). These cells regenerate new stem cells, including CFU-GEMM and committed progenitor cells. Primitive stem cells are dependent upon multiple rather than single growth factors for their proliferation; in contrast to more mature progenitor cells, they may lack HLA-DR (Brandt J. et al., 1988).

Hemopoietic Stimulatory and Inhibitory Growth Factors

Hemopoietic stem cells and progenitor cells undergo extensive proliferation and differentiation in vitro under the influence of a variety of hemopoietic growth factors. These glycoprotein HGFs and their unique cell-surface receptors have been biochemically defined (Table 22–1) and their

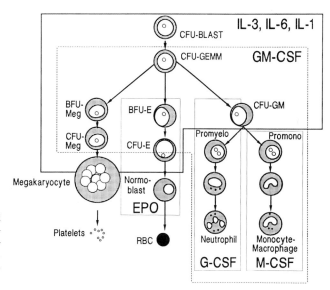

Fig. 22–1. Hemopoietic growth factors and regeneration of hemopoietic cell development. Overlapping interactions between regulatory molecules and target cells are depicted. Adapted with permission from Griffin, 1988. S. Karger AG, Basel, publisher.

Table 22–1.   HUMAN HEMOPOIETIC GROWTH FACTORS AND RECEPTORS

	GROWTH FACTOR			RECEPTOR	
FACTOR	ALTERNATE NAME*	MOLECULAR MASS (KD)	GENE LOCATION	MOLECULAR MASS (KD)	GENE LOCATION‡
Interleukin-3	Multi-CSF	15–30	5q23-31	140	
GM-CSF	Pluripoietin α, CSF-α, MGI-1	18–30	5q23-31	45, 84	X, Y PAR‡
G-CSF	Pluripoietin β, CSF-β	20	17q11-21	150	
M-CSF	CSF-1	70–90, 45–50	5q23-33	160†	5q23-34
Interleukin-1	Hemopoietin-1, MRA	17	2q13-21	68, 80	
Interleukin-6	β_2-Interferon, MGI-2, BCSF-2	21	5	80	
Erythropoietin	EPO	39	7q11-22	55–60	19p
Interferon α		17–25	9	110–130	21
Interferon β		17–25	9	110, 130	21
Interferon γ		17–25	12	54	6

* MRA = monocyte-derived recruiting activity; MGI = macrophage-granulocyte inducer; BCSF-2 = B-cell-stimulating factor 2.
† Receptor–ligand interaction induces tyrosine kinase–mediated autophosphorylation.
‡ PAR = pseudoautosomal region of X, Y chromosomes.

functional characteristics described (Kawasaki et al., 1985; Lee et al., 1985; Wong et al., 1985; Souza et al., 1986; Yang et al., 1986; Sieff, 1987; Wong et al., 1987). Such peptide regulatory factors have some degree of lineage specificity. However, as defined initially in vitro and recently confirmed by in vivo studies, they generally overlap in their ability to stimulate cells of various lineages and differentiation stages (Fig. 22–1). In concert with IL-6 and IL-1, IL-3 induces proliferation of the early hemopoietic precursor cells; in combination with the more differentiating factors such as GM-CSF, G-CSF, M-CSF, and erythropoietin, IL-3 induces myeloid and erythroid growth in vitro (Suda et al., 1985).

GM-CSF has mainly proliferative activity with modest differentiative potential for myeloid precursor cells, inducing granulocytic and monocytic maturation. G-CSF is more potent for induction of granulocytic differentiation of myeloid precursors as well as having myeloid proliferative effects. Both GM-CSF and G-CSF may act synergistically with erythropoietin to enhance erythropoiesis (Sieff, 1987). M-CSF (also known as CSF-1) enhances the differentiation of myeloid precursor cells to undergo monocytic differentiation. Both GM-CSF and M-CSF also augment production of HGFs by monocytes and other accessory cells (Sisson and Dinarello, 1988; Metcalf, 1989). Erythroid burst-promoting activity (BPA), together with erythropoietin, stimulates BFU-E-related erythropoiesis in vitro, whereas erythropoietin alone stimulates the more mature CFU-E and the morphologically definable erythroid precursor cells. Megakaryocyte CSF (Meg-CSF) enhances megakaryocyte colony formation (Shimizu et al., 1987) and thrombopoiesis, although these stimuli and the megakaryocyte precursors

(CFU-Meg) have been less well characterized than those of the other hemopoietic lineages. Combinations of IL-6 and IL-3, possibly potentiated by GM-CSF and IL-1, stimulate thrombopoiesis in vitro and in vivo (Long et al., 1988; Bruno et al., 1988; Ishibashi et al., 1989; Warren et al., 1989; Hill et al., 1990).

Factors that act synergistically to enhance hemopoiesis in vitro and in vivo with these well-defined HGFs have been demonstrated. Interleukin-6 increases the ability of IL-3 to cause proliferation and survival of the CFU-GEMMs and blast-CFUs (Ikebuchi et al., 1987; Leary et al., 1988; Koike et al., 1988; Kishimoto, 1989) as well as augmenting megakaryocytic proliferation (Asano et al., 1990). One of the functions of IL-3 is to enhance survival of these cells by altering glucose transport and ATP generation (Whetton et al., 1984). In vivo, IL-1 can alter hemopoiesis and is radiation-protective (Neta et al., 1986 and 1988). Studies suggest that IL-1 acts either directly by altering responsiveness of early precursor cells to regulatory factors or indirectly by enhancing production of HGFs from accessory marrow cells (or by both mechanisms) (Segal et al., 1987; Fibbe et al., 1988; Herrmann et al., 1988; Kauschansky et al., 1988; Zhou et al., 1988; Johnson et al., 1989). After 5-fluorouracil treatment in mice, IL-1 synergizes with G-CSF to stimulate stem cell recovery and hemopoietic regeneration (Moore and Warren, 1987). Tumor necrosis factors α and β (cachectin and lymphocytoxin, respectively) are referred to as TNF and have a close functional relation. The TNF induces differentiation of human myeloid cell lines (Beutler and Cerami, 1987) and also provokes HGF production by stromal cells (Broudy et al., 1986). Both IL-1 and TNF are active mediators of the inflammatory response (Dinarello, 1986; Beutler and Cerami, 1987).

Both IL-1 and TNF-α are produced mainly by macrophages, whereas TNF-β is a product of lymphoid cells. Stromal cells such as fibroblasts and endothelial cells, as well as T lymphocytes and natural killer (NK) cells, are triggered by IL-1 and TNF to produce CSFs as their state of activation is altered (Bagby et al., 1981; Munker et al., 1986; Zucali et al., 1986; Tosato and Jones, 1990) (Fig. 22–2). Cellular contact, bacterial challenge or antigens cause T cells and NK cells to produce stimulatory HGFs, interferon γ and other inhibitory substances. In contrast, IL-2 causes resting T and NK cells to produce erythroid BPA but not GM-CSFs (Skettino et al., 1988), whereas such activated cells can be induced to produce both these factors as well as the inhibitory substance interferon γ (Degliantoni et al., 1985). Both IL-3 and IL-6 are produced by stimulated T cells,

whereas GM-CSF, G-CSF, M-CSF, and IL-6 are normally produced by activated monocytes, fibroblasts, and endothelial cells (Nathan et al., 1978; Greenberg et al., 1980; Mangan et al., 1982; Ascensao et al., 1984; Sieff, 1987; Tosato and Jones, 1990). Analysis of results of in vivo infusions of purified recombinant HGFs into rodents and nonhuman primates has demonstrated the physiologic roles for many of these substances (Metcalf, 1986 and 1989) and the ability of bacterial and antigenic stimuli to produce the HGFs.

In addition to the stimulatory substances named above, a number of factors that inhibit hemopoiesis have been defined (Fig. 22–3). These factors modulate the actions of the stimulatory factors, thus providing an inhibitory arc to regulatory control of hemopoiesis. Prostaglandin E (PGE), produced by macrophages, inhibits the proliferation of CFU-GM while enhancing the growth of BFU-E in vitro. Interferons α and γ

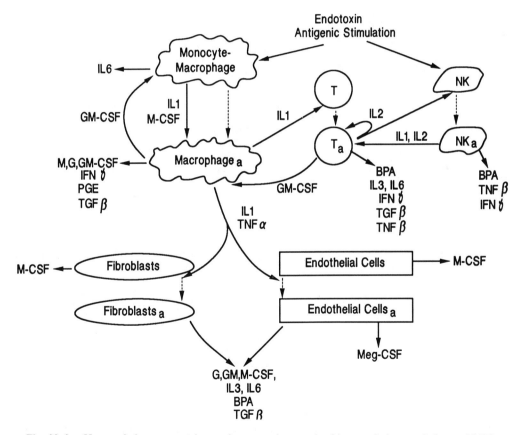

Fig. 22–2. Hemopoietic marrow microenvironmental network of hemopoietic growth factor (HGF) production. Constitutive low-level production of IL-1 and M-CSF occurs and is augmented upon activation of accessory cells (e.g., macrophage$_a$, T lymphocyte$_a$, etc.) by antigenic or bacterial challenge. The accessory cells, activated by this means or by cell contact or their cytokines (e.g., IL-1, TNF), generate HGFs (including M-CSF, G-CSF, GM-CSF, IFNγ, PGE, TGFβ, IL3, and TNF) from adjacent microenvironmental cells. IFN = interferon, TGF = transforming growth factor.

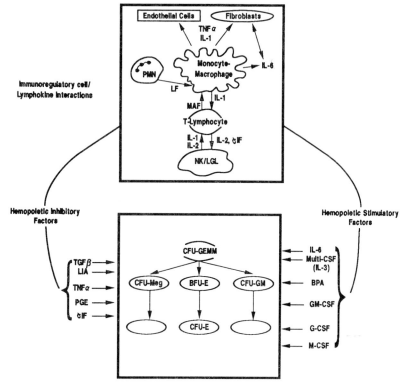

Hemopoietic Cell/Growth Factor Interactions

Fig. 22–3. Interacting marrow cells and humoral factors regulating hemopoiesis. One marrow "compartment" includes accessory cells [lymphocytes, large granular lymphocytes (LGL), NK cells, monocyte-macrophages, endothelial cells] and their production of cytokines activating and amplifying these cells. Once activated, these accessory cells (many of which are immunoregulatory) produce HGFs possessing stimulatory or inhibitory influences on cells within the hemopoietic stem-progenitor cell compartment. The stimulatory factors (CSFs, BPA, IL-6) have proliferative and/or differentiative influences on the progenitor cells, causing their lineage-specific expansion and maturation. Inhibitory influences include lactoferrin, secreted by polymorphonuclear neutrophils (which inhibit IL-1 production by macrophages), prostaglandin E (which inhibits CFU-GM proliferative responses and enhances BFU-E growth), and leukemia-associated inhibitory activity (LIA), TGF-β and γ-interferon (γIF) (which diminish normal stem-progenitor cell proliferation). These cell compartments are comingled within the bone marrow microenvironment; thus these regulatory influences are generally of a local (paracrine) nature. The HGFs act via their binding to specific cell-surface receptors on the hemopoietic cells, permitting selective functions of these humoral factors. See text for details. Adapted with permission from Greenberg, 1986.

inhibit proliferation of myeloid, erythroid, and megakaryocytic cells and cause monocytic differentiation (Greenberg and Mosny, 1977; Broxmeyer et al., 1983). Tumor necrosis factor α inhibits myeloid colony formation in addition to its ability to enhance myeloid differentiation and increase production of CSFs by stromal cells (Peetre et al., 1986; Murase et al., 1987). Transforming growth factor β (TGF-β), produced ubiquitously by monocytic, neutrophilic, stromal, and lymphoid cells and by platelets (Sporn et al., 1987; Grotendorst et al., 1989) inhibits early multipotent hemopoietic stem cell proliferation in vitro (Massague, 1987; Sing et al., 1988; Axelrad, 1990). An acidic isoferritin, termed leukemia-associated inhibitory activity (LIA) (Broxmeyer et al., 1981), prominently found within leukemic bone marrow, peripheral blood, and spleen, inhibits normal more than leukemic hemopoiesis in vitro (Olofsson and Olsson 1980; Axelrad, 1990). Lactoferrin, a substance present within the specific granules of mature neutrophils, inhibits GM-CSF production by accessory cells by suppressing monocyte release of IL-1 (Zucali et al., 1989). Integration of the role of these inhibitors into the model of hemopoietic regulation requires much further study. However, these inhibitors are now being evaluated for their ability to modify hemopoiesis in vivo.

Stem cell commitment into the various lineages may occur by stochastic (random) processes or by induction of differentiation determined by the balance of HGFs present in the marrow microenvironment. Receptors for multiple HGFs are present on early stem cells. Some receptors are lost as lineage-specific markers appear concomitant with differentiation (Nicola, 1987). The HGFs are produced by accessory cells within the marrow and tend to act locally (have paracrine-type actions) on adjacent cells. Each cell line appears to require at least two factors for optimal growth, one predominantly proliferative and the other mainly differentiative. For example, GM-CSF and G-CSF are stimulatory for granulocytic cells, GM-CSF and M-CSF for monocytic cells, BPA and erythropoietin for erythroid cells, and Meg-CSF and synergistic thrombopoietic substances (including IL-6 and IL-1 in combination) for megakaryocytes, thus making them attractive potential therapeutic agents. In addition, the biologic effects of HGFs include their ability to augment survival and function of hemopoietic precursors and their end cells. Enhanced differentiation may alter commitment and self-renewal of stem cells. Early-acting stimuli, such as IL-3 and IL-6, enhance self-renewal of early stem cells, whereas the later-acting G-CSF and M-CSF are more lineage-restricted and provide differentiation and commitment of these cells, thereby decreasing self-renewal.

In addition to these cytokines, a number of other hormones modulate the effects of the specific CSFs for hemopoietic cell proliferation and differentiation. Insulin and insulin-like growth factors (IGFs), produced by stromal cells and present in serum, have recently been shown to cause proliferation of myeloid and erythroid cells in vitro and in vivo and to enhance responsiveness of these cells to GM-CSF and erythropoietin (Kurtz et al., 1983 and 1985; Daniak and Kreczko, 1985; Oksenberg et al., 1990). Specific and distinct cell-surface receptors for insulin and the IGFs as well as for the CSFs are present on human leukemic cells (Pepe et al., 1987; Oksenberg et al., 1990).

In adults, hemopoiesis normally occurs exclusively in the bone marrow where specific localization of hemopoietic cells of various lineages occurs (Coulombel et al., 1983; Gordon et al., 1980). In long-term marrow cultures, growth of hemopoietic cells occurs in association with an adherent layer of stromal cells (Dexter et al., 1977). The hemopoietic microenvironment, composed of stromal cells, HGFs, and extracellular matrix (ECM), is crucial for the growth and differentiation of hemopoietic cells. Determinants expressed on the stem cell surface may be important in targeting these cells to hemopoietic sites, as well as in mediating specific interactions with stromal cells of ECM in the marrow. Studies have suggested that murine marrow stem cells utilize specific membrane lectins that act as "homing" receptors for supportive marrow stroma. Leukemic cells from patients with chronic myeloid leukemia (CML) often establish extramedullary sites of hemopoiesis; they also have a lowered affinity for and adhesivity to stromal cells in vitro in comparison with normal hemopoietic precursors (Gordon et al., 1987). Specific membrane lectins on murine CFU-GM have been found that are capable of binding to supportive stroma. They may be involved in the homing of hemopoietic stem cells to specific niches within hemopoietic tissues (Tavassoli and Hardy, 1990).

The human cell-adhesion molecule [H-CAM (CD44)] plays a role in multiple cell–cell and cell–substrate adhesion events throughout the body, including lymphocyte homing (Jalkanen et al., 1987; Picker et al., 1989a, 1989b). This antigen is expressed at high concentrations on human bone marrow CFUs-GM and BFUs-E (Lewinsohn et al., 1990). These findings define H-CAM expression as an additional phenotypic marker of human hemopoietic progenitor cells and raise the possibility that this CAM may play an important compartmentalizing role in the interaction of hemopoietic progenitor cells with elements of the bone marrow microenvironment. Expression of these receptors can be modified by CSFs.

Mechanisms of Hemopoietic Growth Factor Action

As hemopoietic cells are exposed to a multiplicity of HGFs within the marrow microenvironment, competing demands exist on the hemopoietic progenitor target cells for proliferative, differentiative, and inhibitory influences that contribute to determining the intensity and direction of hemopoiesis (Wolf, 1979). Distinctive receptors have been defined for each of the CSFs (Table 22–1), and expression of these receptors changes with cell differentiation (Sherr et al., 1985; Nicola, 1987; Gearing et al., 1989; Itoh et al., 1990; Fukunaga et al., 1990). The HGF activation of these receptors initiates message transduction for genetic programs intrinsic to the specific cell lineage. Although each factor has distinct plasma membrane receptors on responding cells, different CSF receptors can interact after activation by specific hormones. A unidirectional hierarchical organization of CSF binding to receptors for murine stem cells exists in which IL-3 transmodulates receptors for GM-CSF, G-CSF, and M-CSF. The GM-CSF down-regulates receptors for G-CSF and M-CSF, and G-CSF down-modulates receptors for M-CSF (Walker et al., 1985). These findings suggest a coupling between the early-acting (proliferative) and later-acting (differentiative) CSF-receptor systems. It is not yet clear whether similar interactions occur for human hemopoietic cells.

Both low- and high-affinity GM-CSF receptors have been defined that have significant sequence homologies with other HGF receptors including those for IL-3, IL-6, and erythropoietin (Gasson et al., 1986; Park et al., 1986; DiPersio et al., 1988; Gearing et al., 1989; Itoh et al., 1990). The M-CSF receptor possesses intrinsic tyrosine kinase activity and phosphorylates protein substrates upon hormone–receptor binding, whereas the IL-3, GM-CSF, and G-CSF receptors lack intrinsic tyrosine kinase and belong to a cytokine receptor family. Cellular activation of CSFs also alters expression of a number of nuclear oncogenes, including *myc, myb, fos,* and *fms* (Gonda and Metcalf, 1984; Kastan et al., 1989). Induction of differentiation causes decreased levels of *myc* and *myb* mRNA expression (Kastan et al., 1989). The role of these oncogenes for proliferation or differentiation programs and their possible alterations in normal versus leukemic cells remain to be defined.

MYELOPOIESIS

Disordered Marrow Regulation in Hemopoietic Diseases

Altered production and responsiveness to HGFs contribute to pathogenetic mechanisms underlying many hemopoietic disorders. These diseases include the myeloid clonal hemopathies (acute myeloid leukemia, myeloproliferative disorders, and myelodysplastic syndromes) as well as many congenital and acquired nonmalignant neutropenias.

Acute Myeloid Leukemia. Acute myeloid leukemia (AML) is the prototypical disorder of abnormal hemopoietic regulation, illustrating the most striking combination of defective differentiation and excessive proliferation by hemopoietic cells. Patients with AML have blastic proliferation in the marrow, often with blasts evident in the peripheral blood. This is generally associated with severe decreases in neutrophils, platelets, and red blood cells. Pancytopenia leads to clinical problems of infections, bleeding, and anemia. Clinical management requires intensive chemotherapy to eradicate the leukemic clone in order to permit emergence of residual normal clones. Clonogenic cultures have provided methods for analyzing the underlying biologic lesions in this and related disorders and have generated insights into the role of CSFs in these potential treatments. Abnormalities in growth patterns of myeloid clonogenic cells, including defective myeloid differentiation, are observed in vitro (Metcalf, 1973; Moore et al., 1973). Colonies grown in culture have the same abnormal karyotypic abnormalities as native leukemic cells, suggesting their clonal leukemic nature.

Regulatory abnormalities have been documented in AML. Compared with normal cells, leukemic blood and marrow cells produce more LIA, and leukemic hemopoietic precursor cells are less responsive to inhibition by this factor and to PGE (Pelus et al., 1980; Broxmeyer et al., 1981). Leukemic cells are not autonomous in vitro, requiring exogenous CSFs for their proliferation, and may have increased proliferative responsiveness to GM-CSF (Metcalf et al., 1974). Decreased production or altered responsiveness to differentiation-inducing factors [G-CSF, macrophase-granulocyte inducer 2 (MGI-2)] have been demonstrated in certain murine models of AML (Metcalf, 1982). The blasts from some patients with AML also express mRNAs for a variety of CSFs, IL-1, IL-6, and TNF (Griffin et al., 1987; Young et al., 1987; Oster et al., 1989). Whether this degree of CSF production or synergistic activity generated (i.e., IL-1, IL-6) is adequate for stimulating cell growth in vivo remains to be determined. Autocrine production of CSFs may define a subset of patients with more aggressive disease. In addition, receptor modulation by GM-CSF is less effective for leukemic blasts than for normal precursor cells.

Consequently, in AML an uncoupling between proliferative and differentiative programs occurs, and this may relate to pathogenesis of the disease (Lotem and Sachs, 1982). These findings of differential responses by leukemic compared with normal precursors to proliferative, inhibitory, and differentiative factors provide a growth advantage for leukemic cells. In murine model systems, leukemic cell clonogenicity and tumorigenesis in vivo are diminished upon exposure of leukemic cells to differentiation factors such as G-CSF (Lotem and Sachs 1981, 1984; Metcalf, 1982; Begley et al., 1987). Such findings provide a rationale for considering use of HGFs that stimulate differentiation for treating myeloid leukemia and related disorders.

Myeloproliferative Disorders. The myeloproliferative disorders (MPDs) and myelodysplastic syndromes (MDS) are clonal hemopathies characterized by relatively indolent clinical courses, but having the potential for aggressive evolution to an acute blastic transformation stage (Fialkow et al., 1977). These diseases demonstrate differing proliferative versus differentiative abilities of their hemopoietic precursors. In MPD, excessive proliferation of selected cell lineages is the major clinical feature with attendant elevated peripheral blood counts, whereas in MDS, defective differentiation predominates associated with low blood counts. The lesion underlying these defects resides predominantly at the level of the hemopoietic stem cell, and phenotypic expression of such aberrant cells is clonal. In vitro analysis of hemopoietic stem-progenitor cell compartments and the humoral factors involved with regulating their proliferation and differentiation have provided insights into pathogenetic mechanisms underlying these disorders.

A dominant abnormal stem cell clone arises in the MPDs, which may subsequently demonstrate definable genetic abnormalities such as the Philadelphia (Ph) chromosome in CML. The dominant stem cell clone may have a proliferative advantage over normal polyclonal cells (Fialkow et al., 1981). Patients with MPDs, such as CML, polycythemia vera, or essential thrombocythemia, generally have increased numbers of marrow and circulating blood CFUs associated with elevated blood counts, predominantly of the dominant hematologic lineage describing the disease (leukocytes, red blood cells, or platelets, respectively) (Goldman et al., 1974; Ash et al., 1982; Vainchenker et al., 1982; Partanen et al., 1983). Cells from marrow or peripheral blood from patients with MPDs also exhibit "endogenous" colony formation activity (CFU-GM and BFU-E) in the absence of added CSFs or erythropoietin (EPO) (Zanjani et al., 1977; Eaves and Eaves, 1978; Lutton and Levere, 1979; Lipton et al., 1981; Cashman et al., 1983; Eridani et al., 1983). Although one possible implication of this finding is that the precursor cells in these disorders are autonomous, they appear to be more sensitive to CSFs and EPO, and accessory cells within the marrow of these patients release excesses of CSFs or IL-1 (Bagby et al., 1986). "Endogenous" colony formation, increased responsiveness of MPD hemopoietic progenitor cells to positive (CSF) humoral signals, and diminished responsiveness of CML hemopoietic precursors to negative humoral signals (e.g., PGE and LIA) are biologic features that help explain the growth advantage of the abnormal cells in MPDs (Metcalf, 1973; Pelus et al., 1980; Oloffson and Olsson, 1980; Broxmeyer et al., 1981; Oloffson et al., 1984).

As the precursor cells in MPDs maintain their ability to differentiate, there is less accumulation of blasts and interference with effective blood counts. However, progressive changes in these parameters develop as the disease evolves toward blastic transformation. The major clinical manifestations of these diseases (hypermetabolic symptoms, hyperviscosity, or thromboembolic phenomena) relate to the degree of elevation of these blood cells.

Management of these disorders has generally entailed lowering the blood counts by using cytotoxic therapy. Understanding regulatory abnormalities underlying these disorders has recently permitted use of inhibitory cytokines such as interferon α to treat some patients. Interferons are inhibitory in vitro to hemopoietic cells from CML and normal subjects (Greenberg and Mosny, 1977; Broxmeyer et al., 1983) and diminish the excessive endogenous marrow cell production of and precursor responsiveness to proliferative stimuli in CML and other MPDs (see below). Determining the cell(s) responsible for producing these factors and modifying their function will be a critical step in attempting to diminish the proliferative aspects of these disorders. ***Principle: When a field suddenly expands its knowledge base, potential therapies show themselves. The prepared clinician understands the leads and gaps in knowledge that appear as endogenous regulatory substances make the transition to potential therapeutics.***

Myelodysplastic Syndrome. Abnormal myeloid hemopoietic growth patterns similar to those existing in AML occur in the MDSs. MDSs represent a spectrum of relatively indolent clonal hemopathies. The clonal nature of these disorders has been defined by biologic abnormalities demonstrated with cytogenetics and in vitro studies of marrow culture. Such clones are similar to those occurring in AML and demonstrate critical neoplastic features initially, indicating that a neoplastic clone is likely to be established from onset of the disease.

The MDS patients are characterized clinically by having refractory cytopenias with associated cellular dysfunction and marrow morphology demonstrating specific defective myeloid maturation and dysplasia of at least two and generally three hemopoietic cell lines. Approximately 10% to 40% of these patients evolve into AML.

Morphologic categorizing of MDS patients has been useful for evaluating prognosis and potential evolution to AML (Foucar et al., 1985). Biologic parameters, such as marrow culture and marrow cytogenetics, have provided prognostic information (Strueli et al., 1980; Greenberg, 1983 and 1986). Abnormal clonogenic findings include decreased CFUs-GM and abortive myeloid cluster formation (Greenberg and Mara, 1979; Greenberg, 1983). As these patients enter a more acute phase, such growth abnormalities become more pronounced. The MDS marrow cells (as well as those from patients with AML and CML) have decreased responsiveness to the inhibitory effects of PGE and LIA. Recent studies in MDS with G-CSF and GM-CSF demonstrated that both factors had potential for enhancing in vitro differentiation without increasing clonal self-generation, although G-CSF had greater differentiation effects and smaller proliferative effects than GM-CSF in MDS cells (Nagler et al., 1990a and 1990b). This contrasts with the finding of minimal differentiative potential of G-CSF or GM-CSF in AML. Because of the differentiation-inducing effects of the CSFs, these studies suggested the possible therapeutic utility of growth factors for MDS patients with severe cytopenias. *Principle: Examination of the origin of a therapeutic hypothesis often helps to establish the seriousness with which one will follow subsequent experiments.*

Molecular Basis of Abnormal Regulatory Responses. Certain alterations occur within marrow that appear to be related to the defined nonrandom marrow cytogenetic abnormalities in the myeloid clonal hemopathies. Both MDS and AML are often associated with characteristic marrow cell chromosomal abnormalities in a high proportion of patients, the predominant finding being deletion of part or loss of chromosomes 5 or 7 (Le Beau et al., 1986a). Such cytogenetic abnormalities have negative prognostic implications (Jacobs et al., 1986).

The abnormalities of chromosome 5 are situated in a specific banding region in the long arm of the chromosome. The connection between this finding and information being generated about human chromosome constitution, detecting the oncogenes coding for growth factors or growth factor receptors, is striking. The demonstration that the M-CSF receptor is an oncogene (c-*fms*) product that possesses tyrosine kinase activity (Sacca et al., 1986) suggests potential for altered control of cell growth in the MDSs. The genes coding for the M-CSF receptor, and for GM-CSF and IL-3 are present in the 5q chromosomal banding region (Sherr et al., 1985; Le Beau et al., 1986a and 1986b; Yang et al., 1988). This region is deranged following chemotherapy and is deleted in the MDS disorder 5q− syndrome (Nienhuis et al., 1985) (Table 22–1). The gene coding for G-CSF is located on chromosome 17 proximal to the breakpoint of the t(15;17) translocation characteristic of acute promyelocytic leukemia (Simmers et al., 1987). These data provide a molecular framework defining possible mechanisms for abnormal growth factor responsiveness or production contributing to the dysplastic marrow cell growth and differentiation occurring in MDS, MPD, and leukemic patients.

Nonmalignant Neutropenias. In nonmalignant neutropenias, myeloid precursor cells have suboptimal proliferative response (in vitro) due to qualitative or quantitative abnormalities of their stem cells or suboptimal production of CSFs. In patients with congenital and acquired chronic neutropenias, such as idiopathic neutropenias or Kostmann syndrome, hemopoietic progenitor cells are present and responsive to CSFs in vitro, suggesting that decreased provision of differentiation or proliferative signals contribute to the disease (Barak et al., 1971; Mintz and Sachs, 1973; Greenberg et al., 1980). In cyclic neutropenia, oscillation in the number of stem cells responsive to CSF has been demonstrated (Greenberg et al., 1976b). In contrast, most patients with aplastic anemia have low numbers of CFU-GM (Greenberg and Schrier, 1973; Singer and Brown, 1978). However, a subgroup of these patients demonstrated enhanced colony formation upon T-cell depletion, suggesting the presence of adequate stem cells inhibited by T cells (Abdou et al., 1978). Therapeutic responses with antithymocyte globulin (ATG) and other immunosuppressive agents have been demonstrated. In addition to the immune suppressive mechanism of ATG, this agent may enhance production of HGFs. These data suggest yet another therapeutic hypothesis: the possible efficacy of CSFs for treating patients with these illnesses.

Clinical Applications of CSFs

Preliminary Studies. The isolation and cloning of the genes encoding the hemopoietic growth factors GM-CSF, G-CSF, IL-3, and M-CSF have resulted in the production of sufficient quantities of these recombinant proteins to administer them to patients. The CSFs have been administered either by IV continuous infusion, IV bolus, or subcutaneous injection. All three methods of administration have resulted in clinical effects.

Clinical pharmacokinetic studies have been performed using G-CSF and GM-CSF administered to patients with advanced cancer who were also treated with chemotherapy. In one study G-CSF was given by IV infusion over 20 to 30 minutes in doses of 1 to 60 μg/kg (Mortsyn et al., 1988). Immediately after the infusion of CSF a fall in absolute neutrophil count (ANC) was observed, followed by a rise to above-normal values after approximately 4 hours. A similar initial fall in circulating neutrophils was observed following the subcutaneous administration of GM-CSF (Lieschke, 1989b). This drop was then followed by a 10-fold rise in neutrophil counts over a 10-day dosing period. The immediate effects of CSFs are probably related to a demargination of neutrophils out of the blood compartment.

Biphasic elimination of G-CSF after IV administration was noted with a $t_{1/2\alpha}$ of 8 minutes and a $t_{1/2\beta}$ of 110 minutes. When GM-CSF was given subcutaneously, peak serum concentrations were found 3.8 to 6.3 hours after dosing; measurable concentrations persisted for 14 to 24 hours (Thompson et al., 1989). Although both IV and subcutaneous dosing have shown clinical effects, the prolonged effect and ease of the latter mode of drug delivery, as well as the chronic nature of many of the diseases that are treated with these agents, has made subcutaneous administration the preferred route. *Principle: Early studies of a new chemical entity in humans are not likely to optimize a dosage regimen. This may be particularly true when the entity is an endogenous substance whose ordinary kinetics are not defined.*

The CSFs have been used in a variety of clinical settings for the purpose of stimulating hemopoiesis and improving blood counts (Table 22–2). The broadest clinical experience is with GM-CSF and G-CSF. Both these agents raise the neutrophil count and in some instances also enhance erythropoiesis without enhancing the platelet count. The GM-CSF increases the numbers of eosinophils, monocytes, and lymphocytes as well as neutrophils, whereas G-CSF has a more specific effect in enhancing neutrophil counts. In addition to increasing the actual neutrophil count, both agents enhance a variety of neutrophil functions such as phagocytosis, bactericidal activity and superoxide generation. However, their effect on neutrophil chemotaxis differ, as GM-CSF but not G-CSF decreases this function in vivo (Peters et al., 1988). Whether this effect is clinically important remains to be determined.

Adjunct to Chemotherapy. The use of CSFs to reduce the myelotoxicity of chemotherapy has been studied extensively. The premise is that the CSFs can decrease the period of neutropenia, thereby decreasing the risk of infection and limiting or avoiding the need for antibiotics and hospitalization. If these effects were observed, it might be possible to deliver more vigorous chemotherapy with possibly improved clinical efficacy. One significant concern is that the use of CSFs could stimulate tumor growth because many different tumor cell lines express receptors for these factors (Tomonaga et al., 1986; Vellenga et al., 1987; Berdel et al., 1989). However, this potential problem has not been clinically apparent. *Principle: Early observations of the absence of a potentially menacing effect of a new drug are heartening but should not justify the sense of safety that results from testing in adequate numbers in people who live for long periods.*

Several studies have demonstrated the clinical efficacy of administration of G-CSF and GM-CSF following high-dose chemotherapy for a variety of cancers (Bronchud et al., 1987; Mortsyn et al., 1988; Antman et al., 1988; Gabrilove et al., 1988; Hermann et al., 1989; Gianni et al., 1990). In these studies, improved leukocyte counts, decreased length of neutrophil nadirs, and decreased febrile episodes compared with historical subjects were noted (Fig. 22–4).

In one instance decreased mucositis was also observed. In one recent study in which patients were treated with 7 g/m^2 of cyclophosphamide, a

Table 22–2. CLINICAL STUDIES DEMONSTRATING NEUTROPHIL-ENHANCING EFFECTS OF CSFs

	G-CSF*	GM-CSF*	M-CSF*	IL-3*	REFERENCES
Acquired Neutropenias					
Chemotherapy-induced	+	+		+	Bronchud et al., 1987; Mortsyn et al., 1988; Antman et al., 1988; Gabrilove et al., 1988; Hermann et al., 1989; Ganser et al., 1989; Gianni et al., 1990
Bone marrow transplantation	+	+	+		Brandt et al., 1988; Sheridan et al., 1989; Taylor et al., 1989; Masaoka et al., 1988
AIDS	+	+			Groopman et al., 1987; Mitsuyasu et al., 1988; Miles et al., 1989
Myelodysplastic syndromes	+	+		+	Vadhan-Raj et al., 1987; Ganser et al., 1989; Hermann et al., 1989; Thompson et al., 1989; Negrin et al., 1990; Ganser et al., 1990
Aplastic anemia	+	+ / −		+	Vadhan-Raj et al., 1988a & b; Champlin et al., 1989; Nissen et al., 1988; Kojima et al., 1991
Congenital Neutropenias					
Cyclic neutropenia	+	−			Hammond et al., 1989
Congenital agranulocytosis (Kostmann syndrome)	+	−			Bonilla et al., 1989

* + = positive neutrophil response; − = no neutrophil response.

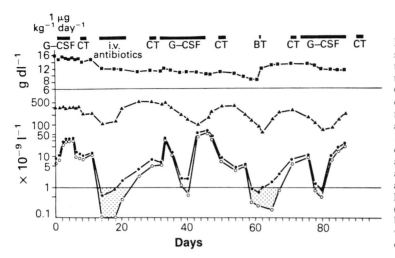

Fig. 22-4. Hematologic response in days following G-CSF therapy before and after chemotherapy (CT). Treatment with G-CSF was at 1 μg/kg per day; chemotherapy included ifosfamide 5 g/m^2, mesna 8 g/m^2, adriamycin 50 mg/m^2, all on day 1, and etoposide 120 mg/m^2 on days 1, 2, and 3. The shaded areas represent the total time of absolute neutropenia. Symbols are (■) hemoglobin, (▲) platelets, (●) white blood cells, and (±) neutrophils. BT indicates blood transfusion. Reprinted with permission from Bronchud et al., 1987.

dose that causes reversible but sustained myelosuppression, decreased neutrophil nadirs were noted following 14 days of continuous IV infusion of GM-CSF at the well-tolerated dose of 5.5 μg/kg per day (Gianni et al., 1990). In general, these beneficial effects were noted in a dose-dependent manner and lasted only as long as the factor was administered. Phase III studies, currently in progress, will determine the ultimate role of these agents as adjuncts to chemotherapy.

In studies using GM-CSF and G-CSF, the responses that have been noted are largely limited to the myeloid series. There has been no consistent improvement in the duration of thrombocytopenia, and erythroid responses have been rare. In patients treated with GM-CSF, a rise in eosinophil and monocyte counts is commonly associated with improved neutrophil counts. Interleukin-3, which stimulates an earlier progenitor cell, appears to have the broadest effects. Preliminary data suggest that this CSF may increase platelet counts and leukocytes in patients without damaged marrows (Ganser et al., 1989). Data in primates suggest that the use of multiple CSFs, such as IL-3 and GM or G-CSF, may result in synergistic responses (Pacquette et al., 1988; Donahue et al., 1988). Fortunately, the in vitro activities of the CSFs closely predict their clinical effects in different cell lines. *Principle: Relevant in vitro models of clinical diseases greatly facilitate moving new pharmaceutical products from bench to bedside.*

Bone Marrow Transplantation. Bone marrow transplantation has emerged as the treatment of choice for several hematolymphoid malignancies. In this form of treatment, lethal doses of chemotherapy and/or radiation therapy are administered, followed by IV administration of bone marrow cells. These donor cells may be previously harvested from an HLA-compatible donor (allogeneic), or from the patient himself or herself (autologous). Following the infusion of bone marrow cells, 20 to 30 days are generally required before there is sufficient engraftment and hematologic reconstitution to protect the individual from infection. During this period of pancytopenia there is great risk for infection and bleeding, as well as the need for prolonged hospitalization. Both GM-CSF and G-CSF have been administered in an effort to shorten this recovery period and thereby decrease the morbidity and perhaps mortality of the procedure.

The GM-CSF has been administered by continuous IV infusion at doses between 2 and 32 μg/kg per day for 14 days following autologous bone marrow transplantation. The total white blood cell (WBC) count after 14 days was significantly elevated in a dose-dependent manner compared with historical controls (Brandt S. J., et al., 1988) (Fig. 22-5). Toxicity was acceptable at doses below 16 μg/kg per day; however, at 32 μg/kg per day, edema, weight gain, pleural effusions and hypotension was observed. In this study, when the infusion of GM-CSF was discontinued, there was an immediate drop in the WBC count to control values followed by a gradual rise. *Principle: During testing of a new therapeutic entity, do not be distracted by a transient surrogate effect from focus on the ultimate desired effect.*

Similar improvements in the rate of WBC reconstitution were seen using G-CSF at doses up to 60 μg/kg per day after autologous bone marrow transplantation (Sheridan et al., 1989; Taylor et al., 1989). Compared with historical controls, there was reduced period of neutropenia and fewer days of antibiotic treatment. Generally, the rate of return of platelets and red cells was not changed by the administration of CSF.

Following bone marrow transplantation M-CSF has also been used (Masaoka et al., 1988). In a study of 51 patients, there was an accelerated rate of WBC return compared with historical controls. No change in relapse rates of their underlying malignancies or in the incidence or severity of graft-versus-host disease in the allotransplants was noted. Randomized controlled trials, currently in progress, will be needed to confirm and extend these findings.

Unexpectedly, administration of GM-CSF or G-CSF in patients with malignancies produces dramatic rises (up to 100-fold) in hematologic progenitor cells in the peripheral blood (Soconski et al., 1988; Duhrsen et al., 1988). This raised the possibility that patients could be pretreated with CSFs prior to peripheral stem cell collections, which could then be reinfused after the preparative regimen. In one study, patients were pretreated with GM-CSF followed by peripheral stem cell collections 8 days later. Following high-dose chemotherapy, the stored autologous bone marrow and peripheral stem cells were reinfused along with GM-CSF. In these patients the number of days of severe neutropenia (ANC < 100) appeared to be decreased. *Principle: Even when a drug's mechanism of action is known, its optimal timing and dosing becomes clear only after extensive clinical experience.*

AIDS. The acquired immunodeficiency syndrome (AIDS) results in severe leukopenia and

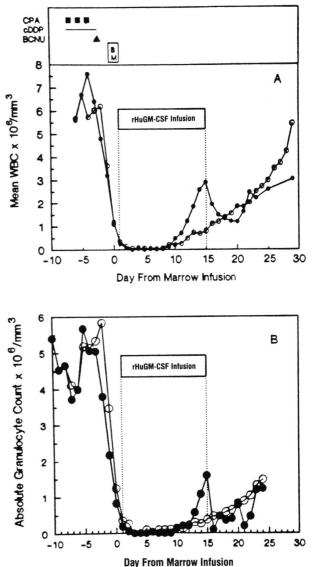

Fig. 22–5. Effects of GM-CSF therapy following chemotherapy and autologous bone marrow transplantation for breast cancer. Mean leukocyte (WBC) and absolute granulocyte counts in four patients who received 16 μg/kg per day of GM-CSF (●) IV, compared with 24 historical control patients. Reprinted with permission of the New England Journal of Medicine, from Brandt SJ, et al. 318:869–876, 1988.

opportunistic infections. These patients are often anemic as a result of treatment with agents such as azidothymidine (AZT). The CSFs have been used in an attempt to reverse the hematologic deficiencies. In one study of 16 patients with AIDS and leukopenia, GM-CSF was administered by continuous IV infusion over 14 days. A dose-dependent rise in the number of neutrophils, eosinophils, and monocytes was observed (Groopman et al., 1987). There were no changes in reticulocyte or platelet counts. In a companion study, neutrophil function was assessed before, during, and after the administration of GM-CSF. Most patients had normal in vitro neutrophil function. In all patients, including the two who were initially deficient in phagocytosis and intracellular killing, the neutrophils appeared functional (Baldwin et al., 1988).

When 15 of these patients were treated with maintenance subcutaneous administration of GM-CSF at doses ranging from 0.25–8 μg/kg per day, all had at least a threefold rise in total WBCs, neutrophils, and eosinophils, with most patients also having a rise in total lymphocyte counts (Mitsuyasu et al., 1988). One potential concern is that the activation of monocytes may allow increased replication of the human immunodeficiency virus (HIV). This problem has not been evident thus far in clinical trials; no increase in p24 levels has been noted. These studies indicate that patients with AIDS may respond to GM-CSF and the positive effects can be maintained for up to 6 months.

Patients who are treated with AZT often develop neutropenia and a transfusion-dependent anemia. Initial studies have indicated that GM-CSF or G-CSF and EPO can improve these low counts (Miles et al., 1989). Longer-term trials are required to determine the clinical value of this approach.

Myelodysplasia. Patients with MDSs have refractory cytopenias associated with cellular dysfunction and morphologic evidence of defective maturation. These patients often require transfusions and are at increased risk for infection, bleeding, and conversion to acute leukemia (Greenberg, 1983). Treatment options for this disease are limited because many of these patients are elderly and not ideal candidates for bone marrow transplantation. Also, patients who progress to a leukemic phase are less responsive to standard chemotherapeutic agents (Mertelsmann et al., 1980). Allogeneic bone marrow transplantation has been successful in approximately 30% to 40% of younger patients (Appelbaum et al., 1990). Various agents such as pyridoxine, androgens, danazol, and corticosteroids have had limited benefit (Najean and Pecking, 1977). Attempts at inducing maturation of these abnormal cells with agents such as cytosine arabinoside or retinoids have not resulted in improved survival in controlled series (Koeffler et al., 1988; Miller, 1988).

The use of CSFs in this disorder has been studied in limited numbers of patients. Their use is complicated by the chronic nature of the cytopenias as well as the inherent potential for conversion to acute leukemia. Several groups of investigators have reported results using GM-CSF in the treatment of patients with MDSs. These studies have generally reported short-term treatment (several repeated 7- to 14-day courses) administered either by IV infusion or subcutaneous injection (Vadhan-Raj et al., 1987; Ganser et al., 1989; Hermann et al., 1989; Thompson et al., 1989). In one study of eight patients, an increase in total WBC count (5- to 70-fold) and ANC (5- to 373-fold) was noted (Vadhan-Raj et al., 1987). The GM-CSF was administered over 14 days by continuous IV infusion over a dose range of 30 to 500 μg/m^2. The absolute number of monocytes, eosinophils, and lymphocytes also rose in these patients. Three of eight patients had a rise in platelet count (2- to 10-fold), and two of three patients dependent on red cell transfusion had a decrease in this requirement over the study period. An increase in bone marrow cellularity and a decrease in the percentage of myeloblasts was also noted in five responding patients. Adverse effects were generally mild except for bone pain in some patients associated with elevated WBC counts. In a similar study, a dose-dependent rise in total WBC count and ANC was noted in 10 of 11 patients (Ganser et al., 1989). In five patients, all with >15% marrow myeloblasts at entry to the study, progression to AML was found either during or within 1 month of treatment. *Principle: In a disease caused by defective marrow cell maturation and complicated by acute leukemia, only careful clinical trials can identify the subset of patients for whom benefits of treatment will ultimately outweigh risks.*

Subcutaneous administration of GM-CSF has also been used to treat 16 patients with MDS at doses ranging from 0.3 to 10 μg/kg per day, with 11 patients having a response (Thompson et al., 1989). Five of these patients were then begun on a daily maintenance schedule of GM-CSF. However, despite therapy, these patients had a fall in ANC after several weeks. One patient progressed to AML, and one patient developed an antibody to GM-CSF.

In combining data from these five studies, 38 of 45 patients treated with GM-CSF responded with a rise in total leukocyte count and ANC. Several patients have had a decrease in transfusion requirement of red blood cells, and a rare patient also had a rise in platelet count. Conversion to leukemia occurred in seven patients after short-term treatment with GM-CSF.

The use of GM-CSF with other agents such as low doses of cytosine arabinoside has been explored in preliminary studies. A minority of patients have experienced a persistent beneficial response; however, thrombocytopenia has been an appreciable problem.

Treatment of patients with MDS with G-CSF has also been explored. Eighteen patients were treated with daily subcutaneous injections of G-CSF; 16 patients responded with improved (5- to 40-fold) neutrophil counts (Negrin et al., 1989, 1990). Dosages required to obtain a response varied between 0.3 and 5 µg/kg per day. When treatment was stopped, blood counts returned to baseline values over 2 to 4 weeks. To maintain responses, 11 patients were treated with daily subcutaneous injections of G-CSF for periods up to 16 months (Negrin et al., 1990) (Fig. 22–6). Persistent responses were noted in 10 patients. Four patients had a decrease in red cell transfusion requirements or an improvement in anemia. In addition, a decrease in serious bacterial infections was found in responding patients. Three patients in this study have developed leukemia.

An interesting question in the treatment of MDS patients with CSFs is whether the enhanced neutrophil counts are due to maturation of the normal or abnormal clone of cells. Cytogenetic analysis of dividing cells suggests that the improvement in neutrophil counts is due to maturation of the abnormal clone because cytogenetic abnormalities, when present before treatment, persist (Vadhan-Raj et al., 1987; Negrin et al., 1989, 1990). Another approach to this question involves the analysis of restriction-fragment-length polymorphisms in female patients who are heterozygous for an allele on the X chromosome (Vogelstein et al., 1987). Clonal hematopoiesis can be demonstrated in approximately 35% of evaluable patients with MDSs (Janssen et al., 1989). In one patient who demonstrated clonal hematopoiesis prior to treatment, the same clonal pattern was found in the mature neutrophils following treatment with G-CSF (Negrin et al., 1990). In contrast, polyclonal hemopoiesis following treatment with GM-CSF was found in another patient who initially had a clonal pattern (Vadhan-Raj et al., 1989). *Principle: A randomized controlled study is needed to establish the value of an entity that appears to have efficacy, but also theoretically could contribute to the disease's worst complications and end points.*

Aplastic Anemia. Patients who develop aplastic anemia have peripheral pancytopenia with bone marrow hypocellularity and are at risk for infection and bleeding. Treatment for this disorder has included antithymocyte globulin (ATG), corticosteroids, and more recently cyclosporin A. Allogeneic bone marrow transplantation is the treatment of choice for patients with severe disease who have an HLA-matched sibling donor.

The CSFs have been used in this disorder with mixed results. In one study of 10 moderately severe aplastic patients treated with a 14-day continuous infusion of GM-CSF between the doses of 60 and 500 µg/m^2 per day, all patients responded with an increase in numbers of neutrophils (1.5- to 20-fold), eosinophils (12- to >70-fold), and monocytes (2- to 32-fold) (Vadhan-Raj et al., 1988a and 1988b). No change in reticulocyte or platelet counts was noted in these patients. In addition, bone marrow cellularity improved. However, several patients developed bacterial infections despite improvements in peripheral WBC counts.

In a similar study, 10 of 11 patients responded. However, the incremental rises in neutrophil counts were much larger for those patients who began treatment with neutrophil counts >300/mm^3 (Champlin et al., 1989). One patient in this study had a rise in hemoglobin values and platelet count. The GM-CSF was well tolerated at doses below 16 µg/kg per day.

In a small study of four patients with severe aplastic anemia that was refractory to ATG, only one patient responded to treatment with GM-CSF using doses up to 32 µg/kg per day (Nissen et al., 1988). Once the drug was stopped, the blood counts reverted to the pretreatment baseline values, indicating the need for continuous exposure to the drug. Similar short-term myeloid responses to G-CSF have been reported in children with aplastic anemia (Kojima et al., 1991).

These data demonstrate the limits of growth factor treatment in this disease. Possibly agents such as IL-3, which stimulate a more immature precursor cell, or combinations of growth factors may be more effective in producing a multilineage response. *Principle: Testing the effects of only one among many factors that can interact to produce a desirable effect often underplays the real value of the single factor.*

Idiopathic Neutropenias. The CSFs have been used to treat a variety of other conditions characterized by chronic neutropenias. Perhaps the best example is the rare disorder of congenital agranulocytosis (Kostmann syndrome). In this disorder, maturational arrest at the promyelocyte stage in the development of neutrophils is evident in the bone marrow (Kostmann, 1975). These patients have numerous bacterial infections at a young age leading to frequent morbidity and mortality. In one study of five patients with Kostmann

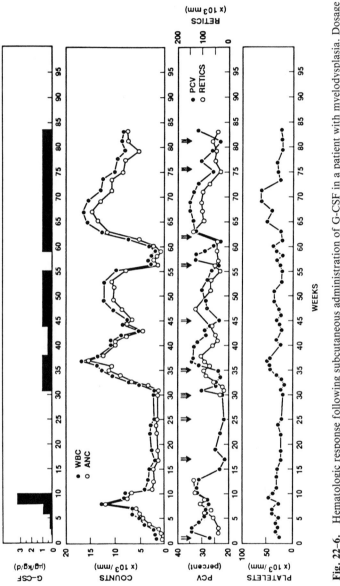

Fig. 22-6. Hematologic response following subcutaneous administration of G-CSF in a patient with myelodysplasia. Dosage of G-CSF varied between 0.1 and 3.0 μg/kg per day as denoted by the solid bars. Total WBC count, ANC, and packed cell volume (PCV) were measured. Arrows denote red blood cell transfusions.

syndrome, improvements in neutrophil counts were noted 8 to 9 days after administration of G-CSF but not of GM-CSF (Bonilla et al., 1989). Relatively high doses of G-CSF (10 to 60 μg/kg) were required initially, followed by maintenance therapy (3–18 μg/kg per day). Marrow aspirations obtained 14 days after beginning treatment showed that maturation had progressed to the mature neutrophil stage. These improvements in neutrophil counts were associated with a decrease in chronic infections and antibiotic usage. The G-CSF was well tolerated, although splenomegaly occasionally developed.

The CSFs have also been used to treat the neutropenia of other disorders such as cyclic neutropenia. In this disease patients have characteristic 21-day fluctuations in the numbers of circulating neutrophils (Page and Good, 1973; Guerry et al., 1973) and frequently develop infectious complications during periods of neutrophil nadirs. In six patients, G-CSF, but not GM-CSF, has been successfully used to treat this disorder (Hammond et al., 1989). The G-CSF was administered by IV or subcutaneous injection at a dose of 3 to 10 μg/kg per day. Interestingly, the cyclic nature of the neutrophil counts persisted; however, the number of days of severe neutropenia was significantly reduced. These improvements in WBC counts were associated with a decrease in the frequency of mouth ulcerations frequently seen in these patients.

Toxicity of CSFs. Therapy with CSFs has generally been well tolerated. The major dose-limiting toxicity with both G-CSF and GM-CSF appears to be bone pain that usually occurs at higher doses when the WBC count is elevated. A transient leukopenia has been noted within the first few minutes of an IV infusion of either G-CSF or GM-CSF (Devereux et al., 1987; Bronchud et al., 1987). A curious syndrome consisting of flushing, tachycardia, hypotension, musculoskeletal pain, and dyspnea has been noted after the first dose of IV GM-CSF in 13 of 42 patients (Lieschke et al., 1989a). When GM-CSF is given in doses above 16 μg/kg per day, fever, malaise, myalgias, arthralgias, fluid retention, and pleural and pericardial effusions have been noted (Vadhan-Raj et al., 1987; Groopman et al., 1987; Mitsuyasu et al., 1988; Brandt SJ, et al., 1988; Antman et al., 1988).

Treatment with G-CSF has generally been associated with few problems. One patient treated with G-CSF developed a neutrophilic infiltration of the skin (Sweet syndrome), and another patient with a history of psoriasis developed a flare of that disease (Glaspy et al., 1988; Negrin et al., 1989).

To date only a few patients have developed nonneutralizing antibodies to these recombinant proteins. Despite initial concern that treatment with CSFs might result in exhaustion of the bone marrow, there is no evidence at present that this has yet occurred. *Principle: When new drugs are evaluated in low numbers of patients (usually a few hundred) in phase I and II clinical trials, it is unlikely that infrequent adverse reactions will be observed.*

Clinical Applications of Interferons

Background. The interferons are classified into three distinct types termed α, β, and γ, all of which have been used clinically. Interferons β and γ are encoded by single genes located on chromosomes 9 and 12, respectively. There are at least 23 distinct interferon α genes, all located on chromosome 9, which encode for 15 different proteins (Balkwill, 1989) (Table 22–1). The various α subtypes appear to have similar activity because mixtures of all α types and recombinant interferon α have similar in vitro and in vivo activities.

Receptors for the interferons are found in a variety of tissues. Interferons α and β appear to share a common receptor of 110 to 130 kd molecular mass, the gene for which is located on chromosome 21. The interferon γ receptor, the gene for which is located on chromosome 6, has a molecular mass of 54 kd (Auget et al., 1988). When interferon binds to its receptors, a variety of poorly understood events take place that eventually influence the expression of several genes including the oncogene c-*myc* (Kimchi, 1987). In addition, the interferons have a variety of immunoregulatory activities that are partially regulated by increased expression of cell-surface proteins of the major histocompatibility complex (MHC). All three types of interferons increase the expression of class I molecules, whereas interferon γ also increases expression of class II MHC molecules. Interferons also induce the expression of cell-surface receptors for the Fc domain of immunoglobulins and enhance secretion of other cytokines.

The biologic effects of the interferons have been studied extensively in animals and humans. Interferon α appears to have the greatest antitumor effects, whereas interferon γ is the most potent immunomodulator. The inhibitory effects of the interferons for normal and leukemic hemopoiesis have been discussed.

Hairy Cell Leukemia. The interferons have been used to treat a variety of different tumors. Interferon α has shown significant activity in the treatment of a variety of hematolymphoid malignancies. The disease most responsive to interferon is the rare form of B-cell malignancy termed hairy cell leukemia (HCL). In this disease, response rates as high as 90% have been reported in patients treated with interferon α (Quesada et al., 1984; Golomb, 1987). From 5% to 15% of these responses have been complete. These results led to FDA approval in the United States in 1986 of interferon α (Roferon A, Intron A) for the treatment of HCL. The initial dose of interferon α is 3×10^6 units/m^2 per day administered by IM or subcutaneous injection. Studies using 2×10^6 units/m^2 three times weekly have been used with similar responses. Responses can be slow and may not be apparent for several weeks or months after initiating treatment. Continued treatment is required in most patients to maintain the responses. However, up to 24% of patients have developed antibodies to the drug, some of which are neutralizing and limit the effectiveness of interferon treatment (Steis et al., 1988). Recently, the drug deoxycoformycin (Pentostat IV) has also shown major activity in the treatment of HCL. Randomized clinical trials comparing these two drugs are being conducted.

CML. Interferon α also has demonstrated activity in the treatment of CML. In one study of chronic-phase patients with cells positive for Philadelphia chromosome, 13 of 17 patients experienced complete hematologic remissions (Talpaz et al., 1986). The dose used in this study was 5×10^6 units/m^2 per day administered by 1M injection. In a longer follow-up of this study, a 71% complete response rate was seen in 51 patients at doses between 3 and 9×10^6 units/m^2 per day with 18 patients treated for longer than 6 months (Talpaz et al., 1986). In another study of 82 patients, a 68% response rate and 46% complete response rate was observed using 2 to 5×10^6 units/m^2 three times weekly (Alimena et al., 1990). Longer-term follow-up of these and other studies will be needed to determine whether treatment of CML with interferon α alters the natural history of this disease by delaying or preventing progression to blast crisis.

Multiple Myeloma. Interferon α has also been used to treat patients with multiple myeloma. Responses in 10% to 25% of patients have been observed when the drug was used as a single agent. In a recent study, 101 chemotherapy-responsive patients were randomized either to observation or interferon α (3×10^6 units/m^2 subcutaneously three times weekly) at the completion of initial chemotherapy. Those patients who received interferon α had longer durations of response (26 vs. 14 months, $p < 0.0002$) and longer survival (52 vs. 39 months $p = 0.05$) (Mandelli et al., 1990).

Other Malignancies. Patients with non-Hodgkin lymphoma, renal cell carcinoma, and Kaposi sarcoma have also responded to interferon α therapy. In patients with non-Hodgkin lymphoma, response rates of 35% to 54% for low-grade and 15% for high-grade tumors have been observed (Foon et al., 1984; Quesada and Gutterman, 1986). In patients with renal cell carcinoma, response rates of approximately 20% have been noted. However, doses of as high as 20×10^6 units/m^2 per day were required (Quesada et al., 1985). Patients with Kaposi sarcoma also respond to interferon α. However, the responses are usually partial and the high doses required have been associated with considerable toxicity (Real et al., 1982; Krown et al., 1983). Patients with breast, colon, and lung cancer do not appear to respond to interferon α.

These studies demonstrate that treatment with interferon α can result in clinical responses, usually partial rather than complete. Clinical trials with combination chemotherapeutic regimens that include interferon α are in process and may demonstrate a significant role for this drug in the treatment of cancer.

Infectious Diseases. Interferon γ has also been used to treat patients with several different infectious diseases. Children with the rare hereditary disorder termed chronic granulomatous disease, which is characterized by dysfunctional phagocytic cells leading to frequent infections, have been treated successfully with interferon γ (Ezekowitz et al., 1988). In addition to clinical improvement, enhanced phagocytic activity was demonstrated in vitro. Interferon γ has also been used to treat patients with condylomata acuminata and lepromatous leprosy (Eron et al., 1986; Nathan et al., 1986) (see chapter 24).

Toxicity. Treatment with interferon α has been associated with significant toxicity. At lower doses (1–9×10^6 units/m^2 per day) the drug is relatively well tolerated. However, fever, fatigue, myalgias, malaise, and headaches are common symptoms, and in elderly patients mental confusion can be debilitating. At higher doses (20–120×10^6 units/m^2 per day) high fever, rigors, peripheral cyanosis, vasoconstriction, nausea, vomiting, severe headaches, and fatigue are serious problems. Doses above 50×10^6 units/m^2 per day are not usually tolerable.

ERYTHROPOIESIS

Physiology of Red Cell Production

The major function of red blood cells is to transport and deliver oxygen from the lungs to peripheral tissues. The function is accomplished through the complex interaction of molecular oxygen, hemoglobin, and 2,3-diphosphoglycerate (DPG). The loading and unloading of oxygen is influenced by factors such as the partial pressure of CO_2, temperature, pH, concentration of DPG, and the oxidation state of the iron atom in hemoglobin. Effective oxygen delivery requires optimization of all these factors, as well as a sufficient number of red blood cells and adequate cardiac output. A variety of feedback loops allow control and optimization of this system.

The marrow can increase its red cell production six- or sevenfold above the normal level. Clinically, one assesses the rate of red cell production by the reticulocyte count and by the cellularity and morphology of the bone marrow, and occasionally by changes in the saturation of the serum iron-binding capacity.

The best understood regulator of erythropoiesis is the peptide hormone EPO. This molecule was initially discovered in the 1950s and purified in 1977 (Miyake et al., 1977; Erslev, 1983). Subsequently, the gene for human EPO was cloned and sufficient quantities of this agent became available for clinical trials (Lee-Huang, 1984; Jacobs et al., 1985; Lin et al., 1985; Powell et al., 1986). Recently, EPO has received FDA approval in the United States for the treatment of anemia associated with chronic renal failure (see below).

Role of EPO. Human EPO is a glycoprotein with a molecular mass of 39,000 d containing 166 amino acid residues. There are two forms of EPO, designated α and β, which differ only in their glycosylation patterns (Miyake et al., 1977). The degree of glycosylation plays a central role in the biologic half-life of the molecule, as the desialylation of EPO results in significant loss in biologic activity and rapid clearance by the liver (Goldwasser et al., 1974; Sasaki et al., 1987). The importance of glycosylation of EPO has become apparent as the recombinant EPO produced in *Escherichia coli* was found to be inactive in vivo. Therefore, expression in mammalian cells is critical for the production of clinically useful material (Sasaki et al., 1987).

The pharmacokinetics of EPO have been studied extensively in animals. Biphasic clearance has been found with an initial distribution $t_{1/2}$ of 0.2 hours and an elimination $t_{1/2}$ of 3 to 8 hours (Sasaki et al., 1987; Lim et al., 1989). Interestingly, in one study the mean elimination half-life decreased from 8 to 5 hours after 8 weeks of treatment (24 doses). The volume of distribution was found to be 4.1 liters, which closely approximates plasma volume (Lim et al., 1989). Erythropoietin is produced by the kidney in response to renal hypoxia (Jacobson et al., 1957).

There is increased production and release of EPO in times of relative hypoxia, and release is suppressed during hyperoxia (Fig. 22–7). Erythropoietin is normally detectable in blood, and injections with antibodies to EPO result in suppression of erythropoiesis; it is likely that EPO plays a role in the control of normal red blood cell production (Schooly and Mahlmann, 1972; Zanjani et al., 1974).

Erythropoietin modulates several steps in the production and differentiation of erythroid precursors. In addition, EPO induces hemoglobin synthesis and increases the release of reticulocytes into the peripheral blood (Spivak and Graber, 1980; Finch, 1982). A prompt and sustained increase in synthesis and release of red blood cells occurs upon treatment with EPO.

The development of recombinant human erythropoietin (r-HuEPO) has permitted clinical trials to study the effects of this hormone in patients with anemia caused by low endogenous serum EPO values, as may occur in chronic renal failure, inflammation, or tumor. The pharmacokinetics of EPO administered subcutaneously are substantially different from EPO administered IV, presumably due to the hydrophobic nature of the protein. The slow absorption, or "depot" effect, of subcutaneously injected EPO is therapeutically useful because self-administration by patients is possible. Erythropoietin acts via specific high-affinity receptors on the surface of its target cells. It promotes quiescent but committed erythroid progenitor cells to enter active cell cycle, maintains the survival of these cells, enhances their differentiation, and causes the expansion of the erythroid progenitor cell pool.

Normal Destruction of Erythrocytes. A normal erythrocyte survives in the blood for approximately 120 days before the cell is removed by the reticuloendothelial system (RES) and destroyed. The iron atom is salvaged, and the heme moiety of cellular hemoglobin is degraded into biliverdin and unconjugated (indirect) bilirubin. Indirect bilirubin is bound to albumin and transferred to the liver, where it is conjugated and directed into bile. The hemoglobin that escapes this route of elimination is complexed with haptoglobin and then is cleared by the RES. Therefore, at times of increased red cell destruction (hemolysis) there are increased concentrations of bilirubin (indirect) and lactic dehydrogenase (present in red blood cells), and a low haptoglobin concentration in the serum. Measurements of red blood cell survival such as radiolabeling cells with ^{51}Cr can be performed but rarely are necessary.

Nutritional Requirements. A variety of minerals and vitamins are required for effective eryth-

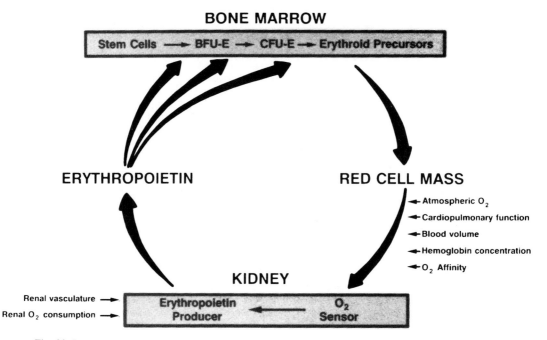

Fig. 22-7. Erythropoiesis: feedback control mechanism of red cell production mediated by hemoglobin oxygen in one limb and EPO in the other. (Adapted from Erslev and Gabuzda, 1985.)

ropoiesis. Iron is needed for hemoglobin synthesis, vitamin B_6 (pyridoxine) for heme synthesis, amino acids for globin synthesis, and vitamin B_{12} and folic acid for nucleic acid synthesis. Nutritional deficiencies caused either by inadequate intake or impaired absorption can lead to profound anemia.

Correct diagnosis of hematologic disorders is essential to rational therapy. Thorough evaluation of such disorders is extremely important because abnormalities of the blood frequently reflect underlying disease. For example, iron deficiency anemia may be the clue to blood loss from a carcinoma of the GI tract; a normocytic anemia may indicate serious renal disease. Simply treating the anemia without a thorough investigation of its cause may prove disastrous for the patient. *Principle: The use of "shotgun" hematinics has no place in clinical medicine.* Specific replacement therapy is cheaper, confirms the diagnosis when successful, and if not successful, suggests a mistaken diagnosis.

Treatment of Iron Deficiency

Iron Metabolism. A single atom of iron is required for each hemoglobin chain. Iron metabolism is tightly controlled, and the ability to increase the absorption of iron is limited, leading to the frequent occurrence of a deficiency state.

There is between 3.5 and 5 g of elemental iron in the body, of which 70% is found in red cells, 30% in storage, and a small amount in myoglobin and iron-containing enzymes.

Iron is absorbed from the GI tract in the duodenum and requires an acidic environment for optimal absorption. Partial gastrectomy, achlorhydria, or agents that suppress gastric acidity (i.e., H_2 antagonists, antacids) can interfere with the efficient uptake of iron in the small intestine. Under usual conditions 5% to 10% of orally ingested iron is absorbed. Oral bioavailability can increase to approximately 20% during periods of iron deficiency, enhanced erythropoiesis, or pregnancy.

In the average adult male approximately 1 mg of elemental iron is absorbed from a nonsupplemented diet per day. This approximately equals the amount lost through the daily turnover of tissues. In menstruating women, blood loss results in dietary requirements that are approximately twice those of men. During pregnancy, needs for iron are even greater because of the expanded blood volume and red cell mass as well as the iron requirements of the fetus and placenta. In addition, blood loss during delivery and iron loss during lactation add to the iron deficit of approximately 1 g per completed pregnancy. Because of the limited dietary content of iron and its low bioavailability, iron supplementation is advisable during pregnancy.

Iron absorption is a multistep process. Dietary iron is initially taken up into the mucosal cells of the small intestine and prepared for transfer into plasma. The amount of iron that is absorbed is greater than that eventually transferred, and this may be under regulatory control. The remainder of the mucosal iron is sloughed into the bowel with turnover of enterocytes. The major plasma protein that is responsible for iron transport is transferrin; it has a molecular mass of 79,500 d and can bind up to two molecules of iron with high affinity. Iron is then taken up from plasma by cells via the transferrin receptor, which internalizes the bound complex by receptor-mediated endocytosis (Huebers and Finch, 1984). Iron is then disassociated from the transferrin in vacuoles. Iron stored in tissue is associated with a cellular protein called ferritin, with the liver serving as the principal storage site. Ferritin has a molecular mass of approximately 480,000 d and can bind several thousand iron atoms. Ferritin can also be measured in the serum by a radioimmunoassay and is a sensitive indicator of total body stores (Lipschitz et al., 1974). Storage iron is also normally present in the form of hemosiderin in the bone marrow. Therefore, absence of iron staining on a bone marrow aspirate specimen indicates significant iron deficiency.

Iron Deficiency. Iron deficiency is a common cause of anemia and is usually due to blood loss from the GI tract or by menstruation and during and at the end of pregnancy. If inadequate dietary intake of iron occurs, iron stores are depleted followed by impaired synthesis of hemoglobin. Under these conditions iron absorption can increase up to approximately 2 to 4 mg/day (Finch and Huebers, 1982).

The diagnosis of iron deficiency can be made by morphologic examination of the peripheral blood smear; the red blood cells may appear small (microcytic) and contain decreased amounts of hemoglobin (hypochromic). However, it should be recognized that normochromic, normocytic cells may be present unless the iron deficiency is prolonged. Typically a low mean red cell volume (MCV) is found along with decreased values of serum iron and ferritin, an increased iron-binding capacity (mainly transferrin), and a low reticulocyte count. In classic iron deficiency anemia, the red blood cell count is below normal, which helps distinguish this disorder from the thalassemic traits (red blood cell count usually is elevated in these disorders). When treatment with iron produces an appropriate increase in numbers of reticulocytes and hemoglobin values, the diagnosis of iron deficiency anemia is confirmed.

The determination of the cause of iron deficiency is central to the appropriate management of these patients. In men, if no obvious bleeding source can be determined, investigation to search for occult blood loss, especially from the GI tract, must be done to rule out the possibility of a malignancy. In women, normal menstruation and pregnancy may account for the anemia. However, a detailed history and physical exam as well as additional evaluation should be performed if the cause for blood loss is unclear.

Iron Supplementation. Supplementation with iron is often a clinical challenge because of the unpleasant effects of oral iron in some patients. Iron should be administered in a fasting state or given with juice containing ascorbic acid that maximizes absorption. A useful technique is to use a liquid iron preparation starting at a low dose and escalating the frequency of administration as tolerated by the patient. Alternatively, ferrous sulfate tablets can be administered orally. The optimal dose is 180 mg of elemental iron per day (i.e., three tablets of 360-mg ferrous sulfate). At this daily dose, 10 to 20 mg of elemental iron may be absorbed per day.

Rarely it may be necessary to administer iron parenterally. This can be accomplished by either IM or IV injection of a parenteral iron formulation containing dextran. The IM route is often painful and produces a discoloration of the skin at the injection sites. The IV administration allows the rapid replacement of iron stores. However, hypotension and anaphylactoid reactions may occur; this problem mandates careful monitoring of all patients who receive iron IV. A test dose should be given prior to the administration of a therapeutic dose (usually 100 mg/day) to make sure that an anaphylactoid reaction does not occur. With careful counseling, oral iron replacement can be successfully accomplished.

Iron replacement causes a prompt rise in reticulocyte counts and hemoglobin values. If these do not occur, several issues must be entertained. The physician should consider the possibility that the diagnosis of iron deficiency is incorrect, the patient may not be taking the iron as directed, the patient is taking the medication with food or antacids, bleeding is continuing, or other vitamin deficiencies (i.e., folic acid or B_{12}) may be present concurrently (chapter 10).

Treatment of Vitamin B_{12} Deficiency

Vitamin B_{12} Metabolism. Vitamin B_{12} is required for efficient nucleic acid biosynthesis, acting as a coenzyme for several reactions involving the metabolism of single-carbon groups and folate. It is also necessary for nervous system function. The adult daily requirement of this vitamin is 0.6 to 1.2 μg (Chung, 1961; Heysel, 1966). An average diet contains sufficient vitamin B_{12}, and a deficiency state from inadequate supply of this vitamin is extremely rare, being found in only the strictest of vegetarians. Dietary vitamin B_{12} is complexed to several other proteins during the absorptive process. After oral administration in food, oral B_{12} is complexed to several salivary proteins termed *R proteins*. These are degraded by trypsin and chymotrypsin, releasing the vitamin in the intestines (Allen et al., 1978). A glycoprotein termed *intrinsic factor* secreted by the parietal cells of the stomach then binds the B_{12} (Corcino, 1972). This complex is absorbed in the terminal ilium. Once absorbed, vitamin B_{12} is transported in the plasma by transcobalamin II. The complexed vitamin B_{12} is then taken up by many tissues.

Vitamin B_{12} Deficiency. The main storage site for vitamin B_{12} is the liver. Adequate stores are available to sustain an individual for approximately 1 year even if dietary intake ceases. Deficiencies in vitamin B_{12} can occur due to the lack of intrinsic factor (pernicious anemia), malabsorption of B_{12}, deficiencies in the diet (rare), or metabolism of B_{12} by intestinal parasites.

The clinical presentation of vitamin B_{12} deficiency is typically a megaloblastic anemia (elevated MCV) with hypersegmented polymorphonuclear leukocytes (PMNs). Atrophy of the tongue and glossitis can occur. Neuropathy may also be present in some patients, with parasthesias being the most common and earliest neurologic symptom. If left untreated, loss of vibratory sense, ataxia, weakness, and spasticity may develop. Mental impairment may also be prominent (Shorvon et al., 1980).

The diagnosis of vitamin B_{12} deficiency is confirmed by a low plasma concentration of the vitamin. This test, though usually accurate, can be falsely low in severe folate deficiency, during the third trimester of pregnancy, or in patients who have recently received radioisotopes such as technetium.

Once a deficiency of vitamin B_{12} has been found, its cause should be determined. A standard approach involves the use of the Schilling test, in which absorption of ^{57}Co-labeled vitamin B_{12} is measured. In this test a 1-μg dose of the radiolabeled material is administered orally after a 1-mg dose of unlabeled vitamin B_{12} is given IM. This parenteral dose of the vitamin saturates serum binding sites, permitting full excretion of the orally absorbed B_{12} in the urine. Urine is collected over a 24-hour period and the amount of radiolabeled B_{12} excreted is determined. If less than 10% of the oral dose is recovered, an abnormality of absorption exists. The Schilling test can then be repeated with an oral dose of intrinsic factor given with the radiolabeled B_{12}. If the coadministration of intrinsic factor normalizes vitamin B_{12} absorption, a diagnosis of pernicious anemia is made. If abnormal B_{12} absorption is uncorrected by intrinsic factor, then either destruction of B_{12} in gut or a more generalized malabsorption disorder should be considered (Chanarin, 1976). Poor renal function may cause decreased excretion of B_{12}.

Vitamin B_{12} Supplementation. Prompt replacement of vitamin B_{12} is indicated in patients who are found to be deficient. A rise in numbers of reticulocytes generally occurs within 4 to 6 days. Vitamin B_{12} is given as a 1-mg dose each week for approximately 6 weeks, and then monthly for life. The relative risk of gastric cancer is increased in patients with pernicious anemia, although the absolute risk is still quite low. A GI series may be indicated depending upon the clinical circumstances. In cases of malabsorption or pancreatic insufficiency, the etiology of these disorders must be determined and treated appropriately.

Treatment of Folic Acid Deficiency

Folic Acid Metabolism. Folic acid, or, more correctly, the coenzyme forms of folic acid, are required for purine and thymidylate synthesis and cell replication. Folic acid, a stable, therapeutically useful folate, does not occur naturally and is probably an artifact of isolation. Reduced folates, particularly N^{10}-formyltetrahydrofolate, N^5-methyltetrahydrofolate, and their polyglutamates, are probably the major folates found in the diet. Fresh fruits and vegetables, liver, and kidney are major sources of the vitamin. The fate of ingested folates and their polyglutamates is not yet clear; however, studies with the polyglutamate forms of folic acid have demonstrated that conjugase enzymes in the intestinal mucosa convert the polyglutamates to the monoglutamate form before or during absorption. Intestinal conjugase activity may be inhibited in patients receiving either oral contraceptives or phenytoin (Hoffbrand and Necheles, 1968; Streiff, 1969).

Absorption of folates probably occurs throughout the small intestine. The average daily folate requirement in adults is estimated to be 25 to 50 μg/day. Requirements are increased during infancy and pregnancy and when blood cell production is increased; in these circumstances folate supplementation may be necessary. Folates are stored in liver as polyglutamates. These stores are sufficient for only 1 to 2 months if folate intake ceases, thus explaining the rapidity with which folate deficiency can occur, as contrasted with vitamin B_{12} deficiency (see chapter 10).

Folate coenzymes play an important role in cell metabolism in the transfer of one-carbon units to acceptor molecules for the synthesis of purines, thymidylate, and methionine. Methionine biosynthesis is of particular importance in that a vitamin B_{12} coenzyme (methylcobalamin) is also required. The involvement of coenzymes of both B_{12} and folate in this reaction may explain the hematologic response of B_{12}-deficient patients to large doses of folate and vice versa. Folic acid deficiency results when dietary sources or intestinal absorption is inadequate to meet demands.

Folic Acid Deficiency. Deficiency can occur in persons who adhere to "fad" diets devoid of foods containing folic acid, malnourished individuals, and alcoholics. Ingestion of ethanol appears to interfere with folate metabolism (Lane et al., 1976). Other causes of folate deficiency include poor absorption due to inflammatory bowel disease, intestinal resection, diabetic enteropathy, or diphenylhydantoin ingestion. A variety of drugs such as methotrexate, trimethoprim, and pyrimethamine share the ability to inhibit the enzyme dihydrofolate reductase, thereby interfering with folate metabolism.

Folate concentrations can be readily measured in the serum; these values reflect recent folate intake. A more useful measure may be that of red blood cell folate values, as these more closely reflect tissue stores. In severe vitamin B_{12} deficiency, folate values can also be low due to poor absorption and anorexia.

Folic Acid Supplementation. Therapy for folate deficiency simply involves oral replacement with folic acid. A dose of 1 mg/day usually results in a rise in reticulocytes in 4 to 6 days. The hypersegmented neutrophils typically disappear after 10 to 14 days (Nath and Lindenbaum, 1979). Parenteral folic acid may be necessary if small-bowel disease or malabsorption was the cause for the deficiency state.

Treatment of Anemia of Chronic Renal Failure

Hypoproliferative anemia with generally normocytic red blood cells develops in most patients with chronic renal failure, impairing the success of maintenance dialysis therapy, particularly hemodialysis (see chapter 11). Anemia can be a complication of the hemodialysis procedure itself, because of associated blood loss. Increased hemolysis, a comparatively mild factor in the anemia of chronic dialysis patients, may be related to retention of products of protein metabolism, hypersplenism, hypophosphatemia, or drugs. However, the primary cause of anemia in the chronic dialysis patient is decreased erythropoie-

sis. The most important mechanism leading to decreased erythropoiesis involves the production of subnormal amounts of EPO by the damaged kidney.

Because more than 90% of EPO is produced by endothelial cells lining the peritubular capillaries in the cortex and outer medulla of the kidneys (the liver synthesizes approximately 10% in adults) (Lacombe et al., 1988), chronic renal failure results in decreased production of the hormone. Renal disease interferes with the normal erythropoietic response to renal hypoxia and thus results in low EPO release, despite the stimulus of anemia (Caro et al., 1979). Radioimmunoassay methods have provided more precise determinations of serum EPO concentrations and have shown that anemic patients with chronic renal failure have much lower values than anemic patients with normal kidney function (Cotes, 1982). Other factors such as iron deficiency (from reduced dietary intake or bleeding), folate deficiency (removed during dialysis), hyperparathyroidism, systemic infections, and aluminum toxicity may also contribute to the hypoproductive anemia in some patients.

Treatment Options. There are several traditional treatment options for anemia in these patients: transfusions; supplemental iron or folic acid when indicated; a change to peritoneal dialysis; and administration of androgens. None of these treatments has proved to be satisfactory, and some, such as transfusions and androgen therapy, may have serious adverse effects. Administration of EPO (r-HuEPO) is very effective in treating the anemia associated with chronic renal failure.

Iron Therapy. In patients with anemia related to end-stage renal disease, the state of iron balance should be established. Administering oral iron supplements may be helpful in treating iron deficiency or maintaining iron stores. On the rare occasions that iron is administered parenterally, IV delivery (Imferon) is preferred to IM delivery because amounts of iron can be more readily delivered although rare anaphyilactoid reactions may occur, for which patients require careful monitoring. Avoid IM injections in uremic patients with underlying platelet dysfunction or those receiving anticoagulants in conjunction with dialysis therapy. Both oral and parenteral iron administration have been used for patients who required iron supplementation in conjunction with r-HuEPO therapy.

Dialysis. Patients undergoing hemodialysis have lower hematocrits and higher transfusion requirements than patients undergoing chronic ambulatory peritoneal dialysis (CAPD). However, patients receiving CAPD generally are anemic. With the use of r-HuEPO, this problem may be lessened by raising the hematocrits in both types of dialysis patients to near-normal values.

Androgens. The use of androgens has been another pharmacologic approach to the treatment of the anemia of patients with renal insufficiency. Nandrolone decanoate administered parenterally (200–300 mg administered IM once a week) enhances erythropoiesis in some dialysis patients. Patients who may be helped with androgens can be identified by evaluating changes in either hematocrit or transfusion requirement after drug administration for 3 to 6 months. If the anemia is not improved after 6 months, androgen therapy should be discontinued. The drug is thought to act by stimulating both renal and extrarenal EPO production and may have direct effects on enhancing hemopoietic stem cell proliferation. Androgens have been associated with several adverse effects, most notably masculinizing effects (hirsutism, acne, changes in muscle distribution) in female patients and priapism in male patients. Hepatic dysfunction, including cholestasis and liver function test abnormalities, also occurs. Because r-HuEPO is more effective and less toxic, androgens are rarely used for this indication. *Principle: Drugs of choice for any indication are not static. Newer drugs are especially useful when older drugs exhibit marginal efficacy and marked toxicity.*

Transfusions. Until recently, the treatment of choice for the anemia of many patients on dialysis has been routine use of transfusions to maintain an adequate hematocrit. Washed leukocyte-poor red cells have usually been administered rather than whole blood, although the type of transfusion used has varied depending on availability and transplant protocol. However, there are major clinical consequences associated with such frequent transfusions. With each transfusion, the patient receives about 250 mg of iron; after many transfusions this iron load may lead to the development of hemochromatosis with iron deposition in and damage to the liver, heart, and other tissues. Chelating agents have been proposed for treating iron overload; in most protocols, deferoxamine has been given in dosages of 40 to 90 mg/kg per week and has been removed either via the usual dialysis sessions or with the use of hemofiltration. These trials have met with mixed clinical results.

Another disadvantage of the liberal use of transfusions has been the risk of transmission of viral diseases. Blood-screening programs have resulted in great strides toward minimizing the risk of transmission of the hepatitis B virus and HIV, but the incidence of non-A non-B hepatitis has remained high among patients who receive multiple transfusions.

EPO Therapy. Sustained dose-dependent increases in hematocrit are achieved in at least 95% of anemic patients with chronic renal failure treated with r-HuEPO, with improvement in quality of life, exercise tolerance, cardiac function, decrease in total body iron stores, and virtual elimination (40-fold reduction) of transfusion requirements (Winearls et al., 1986; Eschbach et al., 1987). To date, anti-EPO antibodies have not been detected in patients treated with this hormone. In adequate doses, EPO generally increases hematocrit values to normal within 2 months, with iron replacement therapy needed in most patients. The response in anemic predialysis patients is similar to that in those who require dialysis.

The usual initial IV dose is 150 to 300 units/kg administered thrice weekly. Subcutaneous dose requirements appear to be approximately one third less than the IV dose. Eschbach et al. (1989a,b) administered EPO to 25 anemic patients receiving chronic hemodialysis over a dose range of 1.5 to 500 units/kg body weight three times a week for up to 12 weeks. A dose of 150 units/kg and higher increased the hematocrit in all but one patient to normal values within 12 weeks. The rate and intensity of hematocrit responses were dose-related (Fig. 22–8).

Recently, in a larger study, more than 300 anemic patients receiving hemodialysis were treated with a dose of 150 to 300 units/kg of r-HuEPO three times a week for up to 4 months (Eschbach et al., 1989a). The dosage was reduced to 75 units/kg three times a week to maintain a hematocrit of 35%. In 95% of patients, the hematocrit rose to target values within 2 weeks. All patients became transfusion-free within two months. Only six patients, five of whom had indications of iron-deficiency anemia, failed to respond. Transfusions were virtually no longer required. Increased blood pressure was the only significant toxicity noted. Lim et al. (1989) treated 14 uremic patients and demonstrated a dose-dependent 41% rise of hematocrit levels (from 27% to 38%) after 8 weeks of treatment.

Erythropoietin has no intrinsic pressor or coagulant activity of its own, but exacerbation of preexisting hypertension, new-onset hypertension, seizures, and clotting of vascular access sites have been observed in end-stage renal failure patients with and without the hormone. These complications have not been an issue in other types of patients, but the number of patients studied to date is small. Whether a significant relation exists

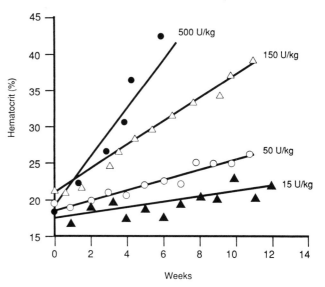

Fig. 22–8. Improvement in hematocrit in anemic patients with renal failure on dialysis following various dosages of r-HuEPO (units/kg). Mean weekly values for all evaluable patients (adapted from Eschbach et al., 1987).

between these adverse experiences and r-HuEPO therapy is unknown.

Although the mechanisms for the blood pressure abnormalities associated with EPO are unknown, hypertension appears to occur early during the hormone's administration and may be associated with changes in the red cell mass relative to the plasma volume and the rate of change of the hematocrit. Consequently, these events may be secondary to the underlying disease state in patients with chronic renal disease, exacerbated by increased microvascular viscosity associated with the higher hematocrits (Raine, 1988). Gradual and careful introduction of r-HuEPO and blood pressure monitoring are necessary and should prevent hypertension from becoming problematic.

Changes in renal function associated with EPO therapy have been minimal. Although studies of rats with preexisting renal disease demonstrated further renal dysfunction with increasing hematocrit after EPO treatment (Garcia et al., 1988), there is no evidence at present that renal failure is accelerated in predialysis patients who receive the hormone.

Treatment of Other Anemias

Recombinant human EPO is effective in increasing red cell mass not only in patients with end-stage renal disease, but also in patients with chronic inflammatory disorders such as AIDS, rheumatoid arthritis, or cancer.

AIDS Patients Receiving AZT. Peripheral blood cytopenias are frequent in AIDS patients (Spivak et al., 1984). Azidothymidine (zidovudine) is associated with several adverse effects, the most important of which is bone marrow suppression. Pancytopenia may result, but anemia and leukopenia are most common. Of AIDS patients treated with AZT, 31% had hemoglobin values less than 7.5 g/100 ml; about one half of these patients required transfusions (Richman et al., 1987). A recent clinical trial has demonstrated that r-HuEPO is beneficial in treating this type of anemia. Sixty-three patients with AIDS undergoing treatment with AZT were randomized to receive either 100 units/kg of r-HuEPO or placebo IV three times a week for up to 12 weeks (Fischl et al., 1990). In patients with a low baseline endogenous serum values of EPO (i.e., < 500 units/l) significantly fewer r-HuEPO-treated patients required red blood cell transfusions, and fewer units were transfused. Patients with high baseline endogenous EPO values did not benefit from r-HuEPO therapy.

Patients with Cancer or Arthritis. Erythropoietin therapy may be of special benefit to cancer patients receiving platinum-based chemotherapy, nearly all of whom develop a transfusion requirement after 3 to 4 doses of platinum (Wood et al., 1988). Trials in these patients, as well as those receiving other forms of chemotherapy, and in patients with anemia due to malignancy, have been initiated. In a recent study of 20 patients with cancer, nearly half had improved hemoglobin values after EPO treatment (Ludwig et al., 1989). Anemic patients with rheumatoid arthritis have also responded to r-HuEPO (Means et al., 1989).

Thus, r-HuEPO is capable of alleviating the anemias of the majority of patients with low endogenous values of EPO and intrinsically normal marrow erythropoietic cells. This has been trans-lated into major improvement in the clinical sta-tus of these patients, with less use and complica-tions of red blood cell transfusions (Casati et al., 1987). Current studies will help to determine the role of EPO for treating patients with anemias of other causes as well. *Principle: Any new chemical entity will pass through a period of expanding indications and toxicities. When the drug repre-sents a highly unusual entity (e.g., proteins have not been used much as pharmacologic agents), there may be more of a tendency to exaggerate claims and underestimate problems because of the enthusiasm for the new class of drugs. Here the clinician is well served to review the primary liter-ature as thoroughly as possible and to be guided by data, rather than the excitement of peers.*

Editors Note: Hematology is the major dis-cipline through which development of recombi-nant DNA products are appearing in medicine. Proteins as drugs represent new pharmacologic challenges. Recombinant products represent very sharp therapeutic tools with unprecedented po-tential. History is allowing the student of thera-peutics to witness an age and stage of drug devel-opment that also is unprecedented. Therefore, we considered the length and detail of this chapter carefully and feel it is utterly justified.

OVERVIEW OF HEMOSTASIS

The hemostatic mechanism consists of seven major components: coagulation proteases and their inhibitors, platelets and their adhesive pro-teins, fibrinolytic proteases and their inhibitors, and the blood vessel wall. All these components normally function in concert to maintain the blood in a fluid state and to preserve vascular integrity. However, the hemostatic mechanism is rapidly activated in response to vascular perturba-tion or injury. Following thrombus formation and cessation of bleeding, the fibrinolytic mecha-nism dissolves the intravascular thrombus.

The hemostatic and fibrinolytic mechanisms are continually active. For example, in response to minimal vascular injury that causes local gener-ation of thrombin and platelet activation, com-pensatory regulating mechanisms limit thrombin formation and platelet aggregation. Thrombi that are formed are lysed by the fibrinolytic system. Abnormalities in components of the hemostatic mechanism may result in either a bleeding or a thrombotic disorder, necessitating specific ther-apy to correct the hemostatic defect. This section will briefly review the hemostatic mechanism, common bleeding and thrombotic disorders, and the therapeutic agents available to treat disorders of hemostasis.

The Blood Coagulation Mechanism

The major event in blood coagulation is genera-tion of the enzyme thrombin. As illustrated in Fig. 22–9, thrombin is formed from prothrombin when serine protease zymogens are transformed into active enzymes in a cascade mechanism. Co-agulation reactions occur on cell surfaces ("phos-pholipid"), where assembly of a serine protease, substrate zymogen, and nonenzymatic cofactor protein occurs, with or without calcium ions (Fig. 22–9).

The cofactor proteins in the blood coagulation mechanism are high-molecular-weight kininogen (HMW kininogen), factors V and VIII, and tissue factor. Although two mechanisms for initiation of coagulation are depicted (contact pathway in-volving factor XII; tissue factor pathway involv-ing tissue factor and factor VII), most data sug-gest that tissue factor is the primary initiator of coagulation (Nemerson, 1988). Initiation of coag-ulation occurs when blood is exposed to cells that have been induced to express tissue factor activity (vascular endothelium and monocytes) or to non-vascular cells that constitutively express tissue factor activity (fibroblasts). Once thrombin is generated, coagulation is enhanced due to throm-bin feedback-activation of factors V and VIII (not shown). This thrombin amplification mecha-nism may be the target for the anticoagulant ef-fect of heparin.

The major activity of thrombin is to cleave fi-brinogen, initiating formation of the fibrin clot. Thrombin also activates platelets to induce their aggregation, and activates factor XIII to initiate fibrin cross-linking and generation of the insolu-ble fibrin clot (Fig. 22–9). The hemostatic plug formed as a result of thrombin's action on fi-brinogen, factor XIII, and platelets consists of a meshwork of fibrin, erythrocytes, and platelet aggregates. Additional hemostatic events, includ-ing platelet secretion of the vasoconstrictor sero-tonin and platelet-mediated clot retraction, result in consolidation of the hemostatic plug and cessa-tion of hemorrhage. Laboratory studies useful in evaluating the coagulation mechanism have re-cently been reviewed (Rodgers, 1990).

Fibrinolysis

Localized fibrinolysis is essential for mainte-nance of vascular patency. Defects in fibrinolysis may lead to bleeding or thrombosis; these defects may be inherited or acquired. As with the coagu-lation mechanism, the fibrinolytic pathway con-sists of serine proteases that activate substrate zy-mogens, and fibrinolytic inhibitors that regulate the extent of fibrinolysis. A detailed discussion of mechanisms of fibrinolysis has recently been

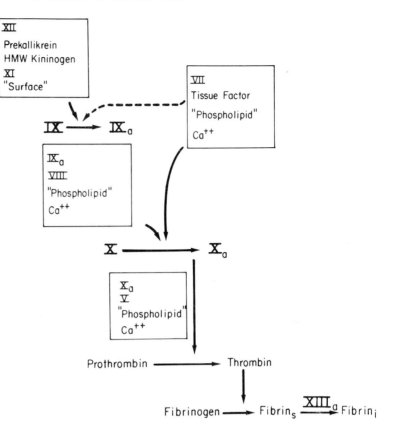

Fig. 22-9. The blood coagulation mechanism. Initiation of coagulation occurs either by the factor XII (contact) pathway or by the tissue factor pathway. Surface complexes (within boxes) are assembled to promote activation of substrate zymogens by serine proteases. The tissue factor–factor VII complex can activate both factor IX and factor X. Thrombin converts fibrinogen into soluble fibrin (fibrin$_s$); factor XIII$_a$ converts soluble fibrin into insoluble fibrin (fibrin$_i$). HMW = high molecular weight. Modified from Rodgers (1988), with permission.

presented (Francis and Marder, 1990). In the setting of thrombosis, physiologic fibrinolysis begins with thrombin-mediated secretion of plasminogen activators from vascular endothelium (tissue plasminogen activator, TPA) or from renal cells (urokinase, UK). Fibrin binding of endogenous plasminogen activator plays a major role in regulating fibrinolysis; both plasminogen and its endogenous activator bind to fibrin to limit plasmin production and fibrinolytic activity to the clot. The major inhibitor of fibrinolysis, α_2-antiplasmin, rapidly inactivates circulating plasmin to prevent disseminated fibrinolysis.

Normal Platelet Function

The major actions of platelets in hemostasis are to promote thrombin generation and to participate in formation of the hemostatic plug (George et al., 1984). Hemostatic plug formation consists of three events; *therapeutic agents are available to interrupt each phase of platelet function listed*:

1. *Adhesion* of platelets to subendothelial structures (e.g., collagen) exposed by vascular injury. Glycoprotein Ib on the platelet surface and

plasma von Willebrand factor are required for normal platelet adhesion.

2. *Secretion* of platelet granular contents resulting in release of ADP, serotonin, and vasoactive prostaglandins, including thromboxane A$_2$. Thromboxane A$_2$ is an eicosanoid released by platelets. It is generated from arachidonic acid metabolism by cyclooxygenase. It is a potent stimulus to platelet aggregation; ADP is also an important platelet agonist.

3. *Aggregation* of platelets with resultant formation of the primary hemostatic plug. This event is mediated by the glycoprotein IIb-IIIa complex on the platelet surface, which when expressed binds fibrinogen to initiate platelet aggregation.

In addition to secretion and aggregation, platelets also participate in the coagulation mechanism by expression of receptors for clotting factors on their surface membrane. The thrombin generated results in fibrin formation, which reinforces the primary platelet aggregate. As platelets retract these fibrin strands into a clot, hemostatic plug formation is complete. Platelet membrane components and metabolic pathways relevant to antiplatelet therapy are discussed in detail below.

Platelets and their function are evaluated clinically with a peripheral blood smear (for estimated number and morphology), by automated cell counting, and by measuring a standardized bleeding time to assess the overall integrity of the platelet-vascular phase of hemostasis. Platelet aggregation studies, in which platelet agonists (collagen, ADP, epinephrine) are added to platelet-rich plasma and their aggregation responses measured, may be useful in selected patients.

Regulation of Hemostasis

Figure 22–10 summarizes the mechanisms that regulate hemostasis, including inhibitors of coagulation and platelet activation, and the fibrinolytic mechanism and its inhibitors. These hemostatic mechanisms are presented in the context of the blood vessel wall that plays a major role in regulation of hemostasis (Rodgers, 1988). Vascular endothelial cells actively maintain resistance to thrombosis by expressing several antithrombotic substances that are summarized in Fig. 22–10A.

Fig. 22–10. Hemostatic properties of the vessel wall. (A) Antithrombotic properties. Major vascular antithrombotic properties are depicted within boxes. Heparin-like glycosaminoglycans (GAG) present on the vascular surface catalyze the inactivation of several coagulation proteases, including thrombin by antithrombin III (AT III), and by heparin cofactor II (not shown). Formation of the thrombin-thrombomodulin complex generates activated protein C (APC). Binding of APC to endothelial cell-bound protein S promotes inactivation of factors V_a and VIII_a, which inhibits coagulation. Prostacyclin (PGI$_2$) secretion limits platelet thrombus formation at sites of vascular injury, as does secretion of endothelium-derived relaxing factor (not shown). Tissue plasminogen activator (TPA) is released in response to thrombin formation to initiate fibrinolysis. (B) Prothrombotic properties. Major vascular prothrombotic properties are depicted within boxes. Injured endothelial cells may initiate coagulation by expression of a factor XII activator, or more importantly, tissue factor. Binding sites for coagulation proteases promote factor X activation. Arterial endothelial cells synthesize and express factor V on the vascular surface, resulting in increased factor X_a-catalyzed prothrombin activation. An endothelial cell activator of factor V (EC protease) also increases thrombin formation. Vascular injury also promotes platelet adhesion and thrombus formation by exposure of subendothelial von Willebrand factor (vWf) and endothelial cell secretion of platelet-activating factor (PAF). Thrombin generated by the vessel wall activates platelets and cleaves fibrinogen, resulting in the fibin clot. Tissue plasminogen activator (TPA) inhibitor secretion stabilizes the fibrin clot by inhibiting fibrinolysis. From Rodgers (1988), with permission.

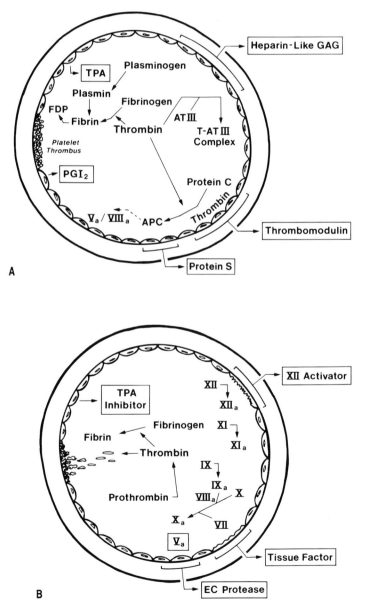

A

B

Endothelial cell synthesis of prostacyclin (PGI_2) inhibits platelet activation, limiting platelet thrombus formation. Another antiplatelet substance not shown in the figure is endothelium-derived relaxing factor (nitric oxide).

Anticoagulant substances are also expressed by endothelium, including synthesis of glycosaminoglycans such as heparan sulfate that catalyze the inactivation of coagulation proteases by antithrombin III. In addition to antithrombin III, a second heparin-dependent inhibitor of thrombin has been described, heparin cofactor II. Another important vascular anticoagulant mechanism is the protein C pathway that consists of two plasma proteins, proteins C and S, and an endothelial cell receptor for protein C termed thrombomodulin (Esmon, 1987). When thrombin is generated in response to vascular injury, thrombin binds to thrombomodulin, forming a complex that activates protein C. Activated protein C serves as a potent anticoagulant by inactivation of factors V_a and VIII_a; proteolysis of these coagulation cofactors by activated protein C requires protein S (Fig. 22–10A).

An additional vascular antithrombotic substance is TPA, secreted in response to thrombin or other inflammatory mediators. When TPA is secreted in response to thrombin-mediated fibrin clot formation, TPA cleaves plasminogen to generate plasmin and initiate fibrinolysis.

Prothrombotic properties of the vessel wall are depicted in Fig. 22–10B. The most important of these prothrombotic substances is tissue factor. Platelet adhesion to damaged vessel wall (subendothelium) requires an adhesive glycoprotein, von Willebrand factor. Fibrin clot stability is enhanced by secretion of an inhibitor to TPA that prevents fibrinolysis.

THERAPY OF COAGULATION DISORDERS

Bleeding disorders may result from deficiencies in or inhibitors of certain coagulation proteins, vascular disorders, or quantitative or qualitative abnormalities of platelets. Table 22–3 summarizes etiologies of common inherited and acquired bleeding disorders. This discussion will briefly review the three most common inherited bleeding disorders (von Willebrand disease, factors VIII and IX deficiencies) and the three most common coagulation-type acquired bleeding disorders [vitamin K deficiency, liver disease, and disseminated intravascular coagulation (DIC)]. Platelet-type bleeding disorders (thrombocytopenia, thrombocytosis, disorders of platelet function) are discussed in the platelet section of this chapter. A detailed discussion of these and other bleeding disorders has recently been presented (Rodgers, 1990).

Inherited Disorders

Von Willebrand disease (vWD), deficiency of factor VIII, and deficiency of factor IX are the most common causes of inherited bleeding disorders. A minimum of 2 to 3 patients per 10,000 population will be found to have one of these disorders (Rodgers, 1990). An Italian epidemiologic study found that about 0.8% of that population had vWD (Rodeghiero et al., 1987). The laboratory evaluation of these disorders has recently been reviewed (Rodgers, 1990); the primary screening test for patients with significant clinical bleeding due to vWD or factors VIII or IX deficiency is an isolated, prolonged partial thromboplastin time (PTT). Because certain patients may develop inhibitors (antibodies) to these clotting factor proteins, and because the presence of an inhibitor may alter patient management, inhibitors should be routinely sought in evaluation of bleeding patients with prolonged PTT values.

vWD. Von Willebrand disease is a bleeding disorder inherited in autosomal dominant fashion in which plasma von Willebrand factor (vWf) is decreased or qualitatively abnormal. The vWf is required for platelet adhesion to vascular subendothelium following vascular injury; diminished vWf activity results in a bleeding disorder of the platelet-vascular type (mucosal hemorrhage). The vWf serves as the carrier molecule for factor VIII in plasma, so that severe vWf protein deficiency is also associated with factor VIII deficiency and a clinical picture similar to that of hemophilia. The laboratory evaluation of vWD involves assays of factor VIII properties in patients suspected of having the disease, including factor VIII coagulant activity, vWf antigen concentration, ristocetin cofactor activity, and qualitative analysis of the structure of vWf (Rodgers, 1990).

Two therapies are available to correct the hemostatic defect of vWD: blood products (primarily cryoprecipitate, also plasma and certain commercial factor VIII concentrates) or a nontransfusional therapy, 1- desamino-8-D-arginine vasopressin (DDAVP, desmopressin acetate). Cryoprecipitate is obtained by slowly thawing frozen human plasma; the insoluble material remaining (cryoprecipitate) is enriched in certain coagulation proteins—vWf, factor VIII, fibrinogen, and factor XIII. Cryoprecipitate is standard therapy for patients who are severely deficient in these proteins.

In calculating the optimal dose of cryoprecipitate for patients with inherited bleeding disorders, it is usually necessary to calculate the patient's plasma volume and to determine the

Table 22–3. A CLASSIFICATION OF COMMON BLEEDING DISORDERS*

DISORDERS OF COAGULATION	DISORDERS OF PLATELETS	DISORDERS OF THE BLOOD VESSEL
Inherited	*Quantitative Disorders*	*Inherited* (rare)
von Willebrand disease	Thrombocytopenia	Connective tissue disorders
Factor VIII deficiency	Platelet destruction (immune, infec-	Hereditary hemorrhagic telangiectasia
Factor IX deficiency	tion, DIC)	
	Splenic sequestration	*Acquired*
Acquired	Hemodilution	Scurvy
Vitamin K deficiency	Diminished marrow production	Senile purpura
Liver disease	(aplastic anemia, marrow infiltra-	
DIC	tion)	
	Thrombocytosis	
	Myeloproliferative disorders	
	Qualitative Disorders	
	Inherited (rare — Glanzmann thrombasthenia)	
	Acquired	
	Uremia	
	Platelet activation (immune disorders, artificial surfaces)	

* Emphasis on the most common. When a category of disease is listed (e.g., platelet destruction), specific examples of diseases within that category are listed in parentheses. A comprehensive listing of disorders of hemostasis is presented in Williams (1990). Reproduced with permission of McGraw-Hill, Inc., from Williams (1990).

baseline plasma concentration of the deficient factor. The approximate dosage can then be determined based on the therapeutic objective (desired plasma concentration) and the estimated V_d (plasma volume in this case). For example, major bleeding usually requires 50% to 100% of normal activity of a given coagulation protein (e.g., factor VIII); this is equivalent to 0.5 to 1 unit of factor VIII per milliliter of plasma. If the patient has severe factor VIII deficiency ($< 1\%$ factor VIII value), has a plasma volume of 2500 ml, and is scheduled for major surgery, a loading dose of 2500 units of factor VIII is required to achieve a 100% value [LD $= V_d \times C_p = (2500$ ml) (1 unit/ml) $\doteq 2500$ units, where LD is loading dose, V_d is volume of distribution, and C_p is concentration of factor VIII in plasma]. Laboratory measurement of the pertinent factor concentration provides confirmatory data to guide dosage adjustment. *Principle: Clinical pharmacokinetic calculations of loading dose, and a target concentration strategy, apply equally well to blood products used as drugs.*

The activity of vWf is not routinely quantitated in cryoprecipitate; consequently, the dosage regimen of cryoprecipitate in treating vWD is arbitrary, 10 bags of cryoprecipitate every 12 to 24 hours for the average adult, with the frequency of infusion dependent on the severity of disease and type of bleeding or surgery expected. Correction of all of the abnormal hemostasis tests associated with vWD may not occur following appropriate therapy; therefore, posttreatment laboratory monitoring is not routinely done for vWD patients (Rodgers, 1990).

An alternative therapy for vWD is DDAVP, usually reserved for patients with mild disease who are having minor surgical procedures. The advantage of DDAVP therapy is that it corrects the hemostatic defect in these patients without exposing them to the risks of therapy with blood products. Prior to treating a vWD patient with DDAVP, the vWD type of vWD needs to be classified (discussed in Rodgers, 1990); DDAVP therapy is most appropriate for type I vWD. The compound DDAVP is an analog of 8-arginine vasopressin; its primary use is for antidiuretic hormone replacement therapy in patients with central diabetes insipidus. *Principle: Proteins and polypeptides, like more traditional drugs, may have indications far different from their primary or initial indications.*

Infusions of DDAVP induce short-term increases in plasma vWf and factor VIII concentrations in healthy volunteers and in patients with mild vWD and factor VIII deficiency (Mannucci, 1988). And DDAVP may also be useful in reducing blood loss after cardiac surgery (Salzman et al., 1986) and in reducing bleeding due to uremia or other qualitative platelet disorders (Mannucci, 1988). Extrarenal vasopressin V_2 receptors have been implicated in mediation of the hemostatic effect of DDAVP (Bichet et al., 1988).

The recommended dosage of DDAVP is 0.3 $\mu g/kg$ infused IV over 30 minutes (Mannucci, 1988). Recent data indicate that the subcutaneous route of administration of DDAVP is therapeutically equivalent to the IV route (Mannucci et al., 1987). The percentage increase of factor VIII and vWf values in patients with mild vWD and hemophilia A was not significantly different from that seen in normal persons following an infusion of DDAVP; factor VIII values generally rise at least threefold over baseline values and have a half-life of 8 to 12 hours. Consequently, DDAVP infusions may be repeated at 12 to 24 hour intervals, although tachyphylaxis may occur with repeated daily dosage. Once patients are diagnosed with mild to moderate hemophilia A or vWD (type I), DDAVP should be administered to document the extent and duration of the patient's hemostatic response. When DDAVP is used to prevent excessive bleeding following oral surgery, the addition of an antifibrinolytic agent is suggested. Therapy with DDAVP is not appropriate for patients with severe vWD or hemophilia A, or for patients with mild disease who have a major hemorrhage.

Infusion of DDAVP is usually associated with minimal toxicity; headaches and flushing are the most commonly noted adverse effects. Hypertension and hyponatremia are seen infrequently. Recent anecdotal reports indicate that older patients, especially those with vascular disease, may experience thrombosis associated with DDAVP therapy (Bond and Bevan, 1988). Consequently, DDAVP should be used with caution in patients with advanced vascular disease (atherosclerosis, diabetes); cryoprecipitate may be more appropriate therapy for these patients.

Most commercial factor VIII concentrates have little vWf activity; however, a recent study identified two factor VIII products (Koate-HS, Humate-P) that have a composition adequate for achieving hemostasis in patients with vWD (Bona et al., 1989). The advantages of using these commercial products over cryoprecipitate in treating vWD patients include sterility and more rapid availability in emergent situations. The use of cryoprecipitate (and other blood products) is associated with a risk of transmitting non-A non-B hepatitis and HIV infection and requires several hours for blood bank personnel to prepare.

Factor VIII Deficiency (Hemophilia A). Factor VIII deficiency is a sex-linked recessive disorder in which plasma factor VIII coagulant concentrations are decreased. Factor VIII is required for the factor IX_a-catalyzed activation of factor X (Fig. 22–9); absence of this coagulant activity results in a bleeding disorder of the coagulation type (soft tissue hemorrhage, hemarthroses, visceral hemorrhage). The laboratory evaluation of hemophilia A is straightforward, with low factor VIII coagulant activity ($< 30\%$ of normal) and normal vWf antigen values being diagnostic of the disorder. Since about 10% of patients with hemophilia A have antibodies to factor VIII, laboratory studies to exclude a factor VIII inhibitor should be performed. Details of laboratory testing and diagnosis of factor VIII deficiency are reviewed elsewhere (Rodgers, 1990).

Both recombinant and plasma-derived coagulation products are available to treat patients with hemophilia A. Table 22–4 summarizes therapeutic options available to treat hemorrhage in patients with hemophilia A. Most patients are currently treated with plasma-derived products, especially commercial concentrates. Viral trans-

Table 22–4.   **THERAPEUTIC AGENTS USED TO TREAT FACTOR VIII DEFICIENCY***

THERAPY	COMMENTS
Plasma-Derived Products	
Commercial factor VIII concentrates	Factor VIII prepared by virus inactivation and monoclonal antibody purification is favored by most practitioners.
Cryoprecipitate, fresh-frozen plasma	Not useful for the majority of patients with factor VIII deficiency; risk of viral transmission exists.
Prothrombin-complex concentrates	Useful for patients with high-titer antibodies to factor VIII.
Activated prothrombin-complex concentrates	Probably no advantage over standard prothrombin-complex concentrates; DIC has been reported with their use.
Porcine factor VIII	Useful for patients with high-titer antibodies to factor VIII; no risk of virus transmission; antibodies to porcine factor VIII may develop.
Recombinant Coagulation Proteins	
Factor VIII	Undergoing clinical trials; cost will be a consideration in determining how widely this product is used.
Factor VII_a	A new agent that may be particularly useful in patients with inhibitors.
Pharmacologic Agents	
DDAVP	Recommended only for patients with mild to moderate disease who require only short-term improvement in hemostasis.
Antifibrinolytic agents (EACA, tranexamic acid)	Useful as adjunctive therapy for oral surgery.

* Modified from Rodgers (1990).
EACA = ε–aminocaproic acid.

Table 22–5. THERAPEUTIC OBJECTIVES IN HEMOPHILIAS A AND B*

BLEEDING EVENT	PEAK FACTOR LEVEL DESIRED (%)	FREQUENCY OF TREATMENT	DURATION (DAYS)	OTHER THERAPY
HEMOPHILIA A (Factor VIII)				
Oral surgery	30	Daily	1–2	Antifibrinolytic therapy useful; patients with mild disease may respond to DDAVP therapy.
Hemarthrosis	30–50	Daily	1–2	—
Major surgery	50–100	Twice daily	10–14	—
HEMOPHILIA B† (Factor IX)				
Oral surgery	30 (15–20)	Daily	1–2	Antifibrinolytic agents (not used with PCC).
Hemarthrosis	30 (15–30)	Daily	1–2	—
Major surgery	(50) (30–40)	Daily	10–14	—

* Information contained in this table was derived from Kasper and Dietrich (1985). For patients being treated for major bleeding, specific factor assays for factors VIII or IX should be obtained to document adequacy of response. For hemophilia B therapy,† percentages for peak factor IX levels using prothrombin complex concentrate (PCC) are given in parentheses. The percentage not in parentheses represents the desired level using fresh-frozen plasma. From Rodgers (1990), with permission.

mission with these agents is low due to use of viral-inactivation techniques and affinity-purification methods (Brettler and Levine, 1989).

The role of proteins isolated using recombinant DNA techniques has not yet been defined. If these newer agents have a prohibitive cost and standard commercial concentrate therapy is demonstrated to be free from virus in long-term studies, recombinant proteins may have limited routine clinical use. Patients with antibodies (Inhibitors) to factor VIII should benefit from a variety of therapies, including standard or activated prothrombin-complex concentrates, porcine factor VIII, and recombinant factor VII$_a$. Details of the use of these agents in patients with and without inhibitors is discussed elsewhere (Kasper, 1989; Rodgers, 1990). Table 22–5 summarizes the therapeutic objectives and dosage recommendations for patients with factor VIII deficiency. Infused factor VIII remains within the vascular space; therefore calculated plasma values usually agree quite well with factor VIII laboratory measurements. The half-life of infused factor VIII is 8 to 12 hours. *Principle: For a few drugs such as factor VIII, the apparent volume of distribution corresponds well with a readily apparent physiologic space—the total plasma volume.*

Factor IX Deficiency. Hemophilia B is the third most common inherited bleeding disorder. In terms of inheritance and clinical symptoms, factor IX deficiency is indistinguishable from factor VIII deficiency. Decreased values of plasma factor IX coagulant activity establish the diagnosis.

Compared with factor VIII deficiency, there

are fewer therapeutic options available for treating factor IX–deficient patients. Dosage calculation for these therapies is done as described above, using the patient's plasma volume, baseline factor IX value, and the target factor IX value. Therapeutic guidelines for factor IX deficiency are summarized in the lower portion of Table 22–5. Fresh-frozen plasma is used to treat patients with mild factor IX deficiency who have minor bleeding. Prothrombin-complex concentrates are the primary therapy because most patients have severe disease, and therapy with fresh-frozen plasma alone cannot provide adequate hemostatic values of factor IX for these patients. Because factor IX is a lower-molecular-weight protein than factor VIII, it distributes to both intra- and extravascular compartments (i.e., larger V_d). The initial loading dose of factor IX required to achieve 100% of normal plasma factor IX values should, therefore, be calculated using an assumed V_d that is 1.5- to 2-fold greater than the patient's plasma volume. The thrombogenicity of prothrombin-complex concentrates (compared with factor VIII concentrates) results in lower doses of prothrombin-complex concentrates being required to achieve hemostasis (Table 22–5). These aspects of factor IX therapy make dosage estimates of the optimal loading dose uncertain, and monitoring of the patient's postinfusion factor IX values is important to ensure appropriate dosing.

Complications of therapy with prothrombin-complex concentrate include thrombogenicity and virus transmission. The risk of DIC with these agents means that patients receiving prothrombin-complex concentrates should not receive concomitant antifibrinolytic therapy. In fact, some practitioners routinely add small amounts of heparin (about 5 units) to each milliliter of reconstituted prothrombin-complex concentrate to minimize thrombogenicity (Kasper and Dietrich, 1985).

Prothrombin-complex concentrates are not as likely to be sterile as factor VIII concentrates because not all manufacturers use solvent-detergent methods in preparing these products. This policy should change soon in the United States, so that all commercial concentrates (factor VIII and prothrombin complex) can be expected to be sterile. Additionally, factor IX concentrates obtained by monoclonal purification techniques are now available; these highly purified concentrates do not exhibit the thrombogenicity of standard prothrombin-complex concentrates and are safer products for hemophilia B patients.

Acquired Disorders

Acquired coagulation disorders are more common than the inherited disorders. A detailed discussion of their laboratory diagnosis and management has been presented (Rodgers, 1990). This section will focus on the therapy of the three most common acquired coagulation disorders, vitamin K deficiency, liver disease, and DIC.

Vitamin K Deficiency and Liver Disease. These two acquired disorders are discussed together because of the link between hepatocellular function and vitamin K metabolism. Vitamin K is a fat-soluble vitamin required for the posttranslational modification of a variety of proteins, including coagulation proteins (prothrombin; factors VII, IX, and X; protein C; protein S; a noncoagulation bone matrix protein (osteocalcin); and a variety of other plasma and tissue proteins. Protein synthesis in parenchymal liver cells initially produces vitamin K–dependent coagulation proteins. A posttranslational modification of these proteins, γ-carboxylation of specific glutamic acid residues, then occurs (Olson, 1987). This modification allows these proteins to bind both calcium and phospholipid, permitting assembly of coagulation proteins on cell surfaces where activation of coagulation normally occurs. Failure of γ-carboxylation, whether caused by hepatocellular disease or vitamin K deficiency, results in incomplete synthesis of the vitamin K–dependent coagulation proteins, inability of these proteins to participate in coagulation, and a bleeding tendency. The structure of vitamin K and the vitamin K cycle are depicted in Fig. 22–11.

Vitamin K deficiency occurs when body stores are depleted as a result of dietary restriction, malabsorption, hepatobiliary disease, or use of broad-spectrum antibiotics. Hospitalized patients may develop vitamin K deficiency because of a combination of poor nutrition (usually in the postoperative state) and antibiotic therapy, especially with use of the newer β-lactam antibiotics (Brown et al., 1986; Cohen et al., 1988). An additional mechanism by which these antibiotics induce hypoprothrombinemia is by their *N*-methyl-

Fig. 22–11. (A) Structures of vitamin K and warfarin sodium. (B) The vitamin K cycle. The active species of vitamin K is the reduced form (hydroquinine). Reduced vitamin K mediates γ-carboxylation of certain glutamic acid residues of the vitamin K–dependent proteins, resulting in production of vitamin K epoxide. Regeneration of vitamin K from vitamin K epoxide occurs via an epoxide reductase and is critical to maintain availability of vitamin K necessary for the γ-carboxylation mechanism. Warfarin antagonizes γ-carboxylation primarily by inhibiting the epoxide reductase, and also by inhibiting the vitamin K reductase. (Data from Fasco et al., 1983.)

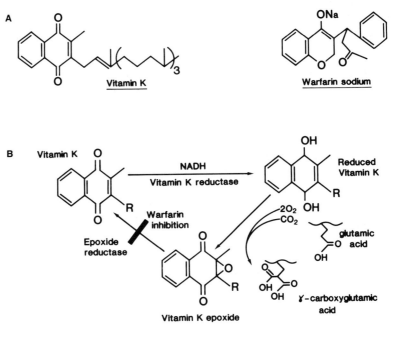

thiotetrazole side chain; in vitro studies suggest that this side chain directly inhibits γ-carboxylation of glutamic acid (Lipsky, 1983). Patients with mild vitamin K deficiency exhibit an isolated prolonged prothrombin time (PT); severe vitamin K deficiency results in prolongation of both the PT and the PTT. Exclusion of DIC by assaying fibrinogen and D dimer confirm the diagnosis of vitamin K deficiency in appropriate clinical settings. Treatment of vitamin K deficiency with vitamin K (10 mg subcutaneously daily, for 3 days) corrects the coagulopathy within 12 to 24 hours in patients with normal hepatic function. Intravenous administration of vitamin K has been associated with anaphylactoid reactions (de la Rubia et al., 1989) and is not recommended. Patients with malnutrition who are receiving broad-spectrum antibiotics should receive prophylactic vitamin K, 5 mg twice weekly, orally or subcutaneously.

The coagulopathy associated with liver disease may result from several abnormalities: deficient hepatic synthesis of coagulation proteins, decreased liver clearance function, a qualitative platelet defect, and thrombocytopenia due to portal hypertension and hypersplenism. Distinguishing the coagulopathy of liver disease from DIC may be difficult. Both disorders usually are associated with prolonged PT and PTT values and thrombocytopenia. However, the D-dimer test is strongly positive and fibrinogen values are low in DIC, while D-dimer values are minimally elevated and fibrinogen levels are normal to elevated in liver disease. Patients with liver disease who have positive tests for DIC have a coexisting illness (cancer, sepsis) frequently associated with DIC (van de Water et al., 1986). A practical consideration in evaluating bleeding patients who have liver disease is that structural bleeding may be important (varices, ulcers), and that primary importance should be placed on addressing potential structural lesions.

Although patients with mild liver disease may have their coagulopathy reversed by the administration of parenteral vitamin K, patients with severe liver disease will not respond. For the latter group of patients, therapy with fresh-frozen plasma may be useful. Fresh-frozen plasma may partially correct the coagulopathy for treatment of minor bleeding episodes; however, since most patients with severe liver disease do not have reversible disease, long-term therapy with plasma is not effective. Such patients may be candidates for prothrombin-complex concentrate therapy; however, the risk of DIC and thrombosis associated with giving these patients prothrombin-complex concentrates is particularly high. The addition of small amounts of heparin and plasma (as a source of antithrombin III) to the reconstituted product may help to avoid thrombosis induced by pro-

thrombin-complex concentrates (Kasper and Dietrich, 1985). Short-term improvement in hemostasis may be achieved in severe liver disease with the use of DDAVP. This agent appears to improve platelet function in these patients. The dosage is as described earlier for patients with vWD or hemophilia A.

DIC. Persistent intravascular generation of thrombin is the hallmark of DIC, which may be divided into two clinical syndromes—acute and chronic. Patients with acute DIC have a clinical picture in which bleeding predominates. Acute DIC is associated with diseases such as gram-negative sepsis and acute promyelocytic leukemia. The clinical picture of chronic DIC is dominated by thrombosis, as is seen in patients with adenocarcinomas. Extensive reviews of the clinical and laboratory aspects of acute and chronic DIC are available (Sack et al., 1977; Colman et al., 1979). The key laboratory tests in confirming the diagnosis of DIC are elevated fibrin degradation products and D-dimer assays.

The major therapeutic objective in DIC is to treat the underlying disease that initiated intravascular coagulation. This may involve appropriate antibiotics for sepsis-associated DIC, or chemotherapy for tumor-associated DIC. Heparin therapy is most useful in preventing thrombotic complications of chronic DIC (Sack et al., 1977). In these patients, full therapeutic dosages of IV heparin are necessary to inhibit intravascular coagulation. Patients with chronic DIC who experience venous thromboembolism should receive a standard therapeutic heparin regimen; long-term prophylaxis for these patients should be with subcutaneous heparin rather than warfarin (Sack et al., 1977). Sack et al. reported that about one third of patients with chronic DIC associated with malignancy experienced recurrent thromboembolism when warfarin was used for long-term anticoagulation; such recurrences were not seen when heparin anticoagulation was used. One hypothesis to explain these observations is that DIC seen with malignancy is initiated by unique cancer procoagulants not affected by inhibition of vitamin K. For example, cancer cells may contain thrombin-like enzymes that directly clot fibrinogen; such enzymes would not be inhibited by warfarin.

Therapy with heparin for patients with acute DIC is controversial (Colman et al., 1979). Because these patients primarily experience bleeding, there is reluctance to use heparin to treat acute DIC. Most patients are given therapy to address their underlying illness; if bleeding persists, the coagulopathy is then treated with blood products. Hypofibrinogemia can be treated with cryoprecipitate. One bag of cryoprecipitate contains about 250 mg of fibrinogen; the replacement dosage of cryoprecipitate is calculated as described above using the patient's plasma volume and baseline plasma fibrinogen value. Adequate hemostasis can be achieved with fibrinogen concentrations >100 mg/dl. One group of patients with acute DIC who apparently benefit from heparin therapy is those with acute promyelocytic leukemia (Collins et al., 1978). Patients with acute DIC due to prostate cancer may benefit from ketoconazole therapy (Litt et al., 1987) or antiandrogenic therapy (Martinez et al., 1988); the antitumor effects of these agents may be helpful in treating clinical DIC associated with prostate cancer.

Antithrombin III (AT III) concentrates are now available for clinical use, and their utility in treating DIC has been investigated. The rationale for the use of AT III concentrates is that this inhibitor of thrombin may be consumed in DIC; replacement therapy with AT III should resolve the hypercoagulable state. However, no clear benefit of AT III concentrates has yet been demonstrated in DIC (Buller and ten Cate, 1989; Schwartz et al., 1989). The AT III concentrates should be most useful in prophylaxis of patients with inherited deficiency of AT III (Menache et al., 1990) and may also be useful in patients with acquired AT III deficiency and thrombosis who require AT III replacement for heparin anticoagulation to be successful. Pharmacokinetic studies indicate that the half-life of AT III is 3 days in patients with inherited deficiency receiving AT III concentrate therapy. Concurrent heparin treatment shortens the half-life of AT III. The therapeutic objective is to maintain plasma AT III values at about 80% of normal; dosage calculations can be done using the patient's plasma volume and baseline AT III value. The manufacturer recommends a loading dose to achieve values about 120% of normal. Plasma AT III values should be measured before and after AT III is given to ensure appropriate therapy. Patients being treated for inherited AT III deficiency should have normal AT III values maintained for several days to prevent thromboembolic disease.

The use of antifibrinolytic agents in DIC is also controversial. These agents are discussed below in detail in the section on fibrinolytic and antifibrinolytic therapy. Administration of inhibitors of fibrinolysis to patients with ongoing thrombin generation and fibrin formation induces disseminated thrombosis (Naeye, 1962). The patients with DIC most likely to benefit from antifibrinolytic therapy are those with genitourinary tumors, DIC, and hyperfibrinolysis (Taylor et al., 1985) and those with acute promyelocytic leukemia. When antifibrinolytic therapy is used in the presence of DIC, concomitant heparin administration is mandatory to prevent thrombosis.

Novel therapies for sepsis-associated DIC have been developed. Recombinant mutants of human α_1-antitrypsin have been produced; these enzymes inhibit key coagulation proteases associated with sepsis-induced DIC. These agents are discussed below in the section on novel antithrombotic therapy.

THERAPY OF THROMBOTIC DISORDERS

Overview

Thrombotic disorders, including myocardial infarction (MI), thrombotic stroke, and pulmonary embolism, account for more patients' deaths and morbidity in the United States than any other group of diseases. Vital statistics indicate that over 900,000 people died in 1986 from these disorders, which account for about 40% of all deaths annually in this country. Nonfatal thrombotic disorders, such as transient ischemic attacks, venous thrombosis, and other vascular disorders take an additional toll in patient morbidity and health care costs. One study estimated that 300,000 patients are treated annually for venous thromboembolism alone. Consequently, successful prophylaxis and treatment of these disorders would be expected to have a major impact on morbidity and mortality figures. This section will focus on the common thrombotic disorders and the therapeutic modalities available for their prophylaxis and treatment.

Three major factors contribute to arterial and venous thrombosis: stasis of blood, alterations in the coagulability of blood (hypercoagulability), and vascular abnormalities. Arterial thrombosis is most frequently associated with underlying vascular disease, especially atherosclerosis, while venous thrombosis is most commonly associated with stasis or hypercoagulable states. Hypercoagulability may be either inherited or acquired, with acquired thrombotic disorders being the more common (Rodgers and Shuman, 1986).

Arterial thrombotic disorders include MI, thrombotic stroke, peripheral vascular disease, and transient ischemic attacks. In general, the pathologic basis of these arterial thrombotic disorders involves atherosclerotic vascular disease associated with platelet thrombi. Although platelets can interact with one another and with the vessel wall independent of coagulation proteases, recent evidence strongly suggests that thrombin is a major mediator of platelet-dependent arterial thrombosis (discussed below). Consequently, pharmacologic modalities for prevention of arterial thrombi include agents with antiplatelet or antithrombin activity. In contrast to arterial thrombosis, venous thrombosis usually occurs in the setting of a normal vessel wall, with stasis of blood and/or hypercoagulable states. A fibrin-rich thrombus is the typical pathologic finding; platelets are of lesser importance in venous thrombosis. Therefore, drugs that prevent thrombin formation or that lyse fibrin clots are of major importance in preventing or treating venous thrombi.

Better characterization of the physiology of platelets, hemostasis, and fibrinolysis has led to the identification of mechanisms of thrombosis in many patients. Table 22-6 summarizes the etiologies of thrombosis to be considered in patients with thrombotic disorders. It is important to establish whether or not an inherited or acquired disorder is present because the type and duration of anticoagulant therapy may depend on this distinction (discussed below).

Heparin

Pharmacology. Heparin is a naturally occurring, highly sulfated glycosaminoglycan widely distributed in a variety of normal human tissues. While studying the procoagulant activity of tissue lipids, McLean (1916) isolated heparin from ox liver and identified its anticoagulant properties. His original term for the anticoagulant fraction was "heparphosphatid."

Unfractionated heparin is commercially obtained from either bovine lung or porcine intestinal mucosa and consists of a heterogenous mixture of polysaccharides with molecular weights ranging from 4000 to 40,000. Polysaccharides with anticoagulant activity constitute about 30% by weight of commercial heparin preparations (Lam et al., 1976; Wessler and Gitel, 1979). Both sodium and calcium salts of heparin are available.

Heparin consists of alternating residues of uronic acid and glucosamine that may be variably sulfated (Rosenberg, 1987). Figure 22-12 illustrates the structure of common saccharides found in commercially used heparin. The negative charge imparted by sulfation appears to be an important determinant of the anticoagulant effect of a given heparin preparation. Vascular endothelium synthesizes and expresses a related heparin species, termed heparan sulfate; this glycosaminoglycan is probably important in regulating natural anticoagulant mechanisms (Rosenberg and Rosenberg, 1984).

Heparin is not by itself an anticoagulant; rather, it requires the plasma protein cofactor AT III to express anticoagulant activity. Antithrombin III is a member of the serine protease inhibitor (SERPIN) family and regulates coagulation by inactivating activated coagulation proteases, such as factor X_a and thrombin, by irreversible complex formation (Rosenberg, 1987). Heparin exerts its anticoagulant effect by binding to AT III so as to allosterically enhance AT III inactivation of coagulation proteases. Heparin-mediated activation of AT III (and inactivation of coagulation) occurs instantaneously in vitro. In this mechanism, heparin acts as a catalyst and is not consumed. Recent in vitro data suggest that heparin exerts its major anticoagulant effect by enhancing the ability of AT III to suppress thrombin-dependent amplification reactions. The importance of AT III in vivo is emphasized by the thrombotic tendency seen in patients with inherited and acquired deficiency of this protease inhibitor (Marciniak et al., 1974). Many patients with AT III deficiency and thrombosis may be

Table 22-6.   ETIOLOGIES OF INHERITED AND ACQUIRED THROMBOTIC DISORDERS*

Inherited†	Acquired
1. Deficiency or qualitative abnormality of inhibitors of activated coagulation factors	1. Hematologic disorders
Low antithrombin III activity	Myeloproliferative disorders
Low heparin cofactor II activity	Paroxysmal nocturnal hemoglobinuria
Low protein C activity	Lupus anticoagulant
Low protein S activity	Thrombotic thrombocytopenic purpura
2. Abnormal fibrinogen	Heparin-associated thrombocytopenia
3. Certain fibrinolytic defects	2. Malignancy
Low plasminogen activity	3. Pregnancy, estrogen use
Decreased secretion of TPA	4. Vascular disorders
Increased fibrinolytic inhibitors	Artificial surfaces
4. Homocystinuria	Vasculitis
	Diabetes
	Atherosclerosis
	5. Postoperative state, immobilization
	6. Other disorders
	Nephrotic syndrome
	Inflammatory bowel disease

* Information in this table is summarized from Rodgers and Shuman (1986).

† Inherited defects of coagulation proteins may result either from a quantitative deficiency of the protein or from qualitative abnormality of the protein causing defective function.

TPA = tissue plasminogen activator

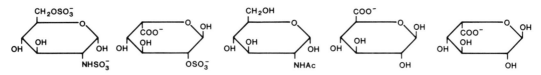

Fig. 22-12. Structure of common saccharides found in commercial heparin. Heparin consists of heterogeneous, straight-chain polymeric structures termed glycosaminoglycans; constituent subunits are termed saccharides. This figure illustrates the structures of the major saccharide units present in commercial heparin, in order of decreasing frequency (left to right). From left to right, the saccharide structures are 2-deoxy-2-sulfamino-α-D-glucose 6-sulfate; α-L-iduronic acid 2-sulfate; 2-acetamido-2-deoxy-α-D-glucose; β-D-glucuronic acid; and α-L-iduronic acid.

difficult to anticoagulate with heparin until they are first given AT III replacement therapy (Rodgers and Shuman, 1986). With adequate plasma AT III values and sufficient concentrations of heparin, anticoagulation is readily achieved in these patients.

In addition to its anticoagulant activity, heparin exhibits additional and unrelated biologic effects (Jaques, 1982). For example, heparin releases vascular endothelial cell–bound lipoprotein lipase into the blood resulting in hydrolysis of triglycerides from chylomicrons and very-low-density lipoproteins (Bengtsson-Olivecrona and Olivecrona, 1985). Other actions of heparin include effects on aldosterone and thyroxine metabolism, suppression of cell-mediated immunity, and activation of platelets. Platelet activation may be important in heparin-associated thrombocytopenia (discussed below). *Principle: As the pharmacology of a molecule becomes fully defined, the clinician must decide whether the combined actions add to or subtract from the effects that contribute to its intended efficacy.*

Pharmacokinetics. Because heparin is a highly charged molecule and is transported poorly across biologic membranes, parenteral administration is recommended, either IV or subcutaneously. The likelihood of hematoma formation precludes the IM route of administration.

The average half-life of an IV heparin dose is 1 to 1.5 hours (Wessler and Gitel, 1979; deSwart et al., 1982). The half-life appears to be dose-dependent, apparent half-life increasing with increasing dosage (Nyman et al., 1974). Extensive thrombosis appears to increase the clearance of heparin, thereby decreasing its half-life (Hirsh et al., 1976). Heparin is cleared from the circulation by the reticuloendothelial system and metabolized in the liver. Metabolic products are excreted in the urine. However, given the variability of response to heparin administration, dosage adjustment is not usually required in patients with underlying renal or liver disease (Wessler and Gitel, 1979) but rather is based on the anticoagulant

response as measured by coagulation testing (see below). Measurement of plasma concentrations of heparin is not done routinely, because measurement of clotting times is more useful. However, therapeutic plasma concentrations of heparin range from 0.3 to 0.6 units/ml. Evidence suggests that calcium heparin may have greater bioavailability than sodium heparin (Doyle et al., 1987).

Therapeutic Indications. There are two indications for heparin administration: therapy of thromboembolic disease using high-dose anticoagulation, and prophylaxis of disease using low-dose anticoagulation. The basis for therapeutic high-dose heparin anticoagulation is that patients with established thrombotic disease require large doses to neutralize large amounts of thrombin generated during intravascular coagulation and thrombosis. In contrast, patients at risk but who have not yet developed thrombosis can avoid the occurrence of thrombosis with smaller doses of heparin. The cascade nature of the coagulation mechanism suggests that inactivation of coagulation proteases generated prior to thrombin (e.g., factors IX_a and X_a) can be accomplished with lower heparin concentrations than that required for patients with established thrombosis.

Specific indications for the use of high-dose heparin therapy include prophylaxis and therapy of deep venous thrombosis and pulmonary embolism, prevention of mural thrombosis in patients with acute transmural anterior MI, arterial thrombosis (Second American College of Chest Physicians Conference on Antithrombotic Therapy, 1989; Turpie et al., 1989), and certain cases of DIC (Sack et al., 1977; Collins et al., 1978). In all these disorders, activation of coagulation has occurred and thrombin has been generated in the blood.

Heparin is also indicated for use in maintenance of catheter patency, dialysis procedures, and as an anticoagulant for extracorporeal circulation (cardiopulmonary bypass). The use of heparin to prevent stroke progression in acute partial stroke is of unestablished efficacy.

Studies done before the introduction of routine anticoagulant therapy indicated that 20% of patients with untreated venous thrombosis died of pulmonary embolism (Zilliacus, 1946). A controlled trial using heparin followed by an oral anticoagulant demonstrated a dramatic reduction in deaths from pulmonary embolism and in nonfatal recurrences in high-risk patients (Barritt and Jordan, 1960). These and other studies (summarized in Hirsh et al., 1987) provide convincing evidence that anticoagulants are very effective in preventing extension of venous thrombosis and pulmonary embolism in patients with documented venous thrombotic disease.

Administration. The dosage of heparin used to treat established thromboembolic disease is designed to achieve a therapeutic anticoagulant response, determined using a functional coagulation assay as an intermediate end point. Most investigators recommend the activated PTT assay to monitor heparin anticoagulation (Hirsh et al., 1987). An initial dose of heparin is chosen, and subsequent dosage adjustments are guided by PTT assays. For example, it is recommended that patients with proximal deep venous thrombosis be given a bolus loading dose of heparin of 5000 units IV followed by a continuous infusion of heparin on the order of 20 to 25 units/kg per hour. The goal is to rapidly achieve prolongation of the PTT between 1.5 and 2.5 times the laboratory control PTT. A prospective study of the relation between the degree of prolongation of the PTT and recurrence of venous thromboembolism found that recurrence was rare if the PTT was prolonged to 1.5 or more times the control values at all times, and if this prolongation was achieved within 24 hours.

Adjusting the PTT into the therapeutic range may require altering the hourly infusion rate and repeating the heparin bolus injection. It is important to rapidly achieve adequate anticoagulation since until the PTT is therapeutically prolonged, the patient is at risk for thrombus extension and/ or embolization. Consequently, rigorous use of heparin therapy coupled with frequent monitoring of PTT values (every 4–6 hours until the PTT is within the therapeutic range, then daily) is mandatory. Patients with pulmonary emboli or massive venous thrombosis should be initially treated with a heparin bolus of 10,000 units IV, followed by a continuous infusion of heparin of 25 to 30 units/kg per hour. After successful anticoagulation is achieved, daily PTT values should be obtained since heparin requirements may diminish with cessation of the hypercoagulable state.

Although some physicians believe that intermittent IV heparin injections every 4 to 6 hours represent an acceptable alternative therapy, continuous IV infusion offers the advantages of consistent therapeutic anticoagulation and may decrease the rate of bleeding complications (Salzman et al., 1975; Glazier and Crowell, 1976). Coagulation tests other than the PTT (whole-blood clotting time, activated clotting time) may be used to monitor anticoagulation; however, regardless of the test chosen for monitoring heparin dosage, unless the coagulation test is prolonged by heparin therapy, the patient is not adequately anticoagulated. Current recommendations are to administer heparin for a period of 7 to 10 days (Hirsh et al., 1987). It is believed that with therapeutic heparin 7 days is the minimum time necessary for a venous thrombus to become immobilized to the vessel wall; consequently, prevention of thrombus extension and embolization during this period of time is crucial. A recent study indicated that a 5-day course of heparin was as effective as a 10-day course in treating deep venous thrombosis (Hull et al., 1990). Both the 5-day and 10-day patient groups experienced a 7% rate of recurrence of venous thromboembolism. If warfarin were begun earlier and the duration of heparin therapy were reduced to 5 days for the routine treatment of deep venous thrombosis, the length of hospital stays for these patients would be markedly shortened, and substantial amounts of money would be saved in health care costs.

Another therapeutic use of heparin is in patients who require long-term anticoagulation, but who have contraindications to warfarin (pregnancy, inability to be monitored with coagulation tests, etc.). A safe and effective outpatient heparin regimen is available for these patients. Hull et al. (1982a) reported that administration of heparin subcutaneously was as efficacious and safe as low-intensity warfarin therapy. After the patient has received 5 to 7 days of therapeutic heparin IV, a subcutaneous regimen is begun (10,000–20,000 every 12 hours), with the goal being to achieve a PTT value (6 hours after subcutaneous injection) of 1.5 times the laboratory control PTT. After 2 to 3 injections, the optimal subcutaneous regimen is arrived at and additional coagulation monitoring is generally not necessary.

Heparin is also used to prevent deep vein thrombosis and pulmonary embolism in high-risk patients, such as those scheduled for general or gynecologic surgical procedures. The American Heart Association recommends using heparin in this setting, giving 5000 units subcutaneously 2 hours before surgery, then 5000 units subcutaneously every 12 hours until the patient is ambulatory (American Heart Association, 1977). Such a regimen reduces venous thrombosis by 67% and fatal pulmonary emboli by about 90% (Kakkar et al., 1975). A recent analysis of more than 70 randomized trials that studied 16,000 patients reported that prophylactic use of heparin reduced the risk of pulmonary embolism by 47%, and deep vein thrombosis by 67% (Collins et al., 1988). Prophylactic heparin is not recommended for patients undergoing urologic, neurosurgical, or orthopedic procedures. Patients undergoing a urologic or neurosurgical procedure should receive external pneumatic leg compression, while patients undergoing orthopedic procedures should receive more intense anticoagulant prophylaxis, such as warfarin therapy or adjusted-dose subcutaneous heparin (Second American College of Chest Physicians Conference on Antithrombotic Therapy, 1989). Patients bedridden with significant medical illnesses (congestive heart failure, MI, pneumonia) also benefit from prophylactic heparin.

Contraindications. Heparin use is contraindicated in patients with underlying thrombocytopenia or coagulopathy, trauma, CNS disease, or active bleeding. Heparin is thought to be safe for use in pregnancy (discussed below).

Complications. Heparin is a commonly used medication, and numerous adverse effects have been described. The most frequent toxicity is bleeding, usually presenting as epistaxis, hematuria, melena, or ecchymosis. One large survey of drug-related deaths among medical inpatients found that heparin was the major drug responsible for drug-related deaths in patients considered to be reasonably healthy (Porter and Jick, 1977). Actual hemorrhage caused by heparin is usually associated with overdosage or misuse of the drug and can be decreased by paying attention to the following details:

1. Patients on heparin should be carefully monitored with a coagulation test to ensure adequate, but not excessive, heparin dosage.

2. Patients who have absolute contraindications to therapeutic anticoagulation should not receive heparin; these conditions include an underlying coagulopathy, thrombocytopenia, surgery within the preceding 2 weeks, intracranial disease, and severe hypertension. If such patients require anticoagulation for deep vein thrombosis, they should undergo a procedure to interrupt the inferior vena cava. Patients needing prophylactic heparin therapy, but who have a contraindication, should receive external pneumatic compression therapy of the lower extremities. Heparin is considered to be safe for use in pregnant women because it does not cross the placental barrier; heparin is preferred to warfarin for therapy of venous thrombotic disease during the first trimester of pregnancy because warfarin crosses the placenta and has teratogenic effects (Ginsberg et al., 1989).

3. Medications that impair platelet function (aspirin, NSAIDs) should not be used with therapeutic dosages of heparin. Intramuscular injections should not be given during heparin therapy.

4. Older patients, especially older women, may be more sensitive to heparin anticoagulation. Smaller loading doses and maintenance infusions should be considered.

5. Patients receiving therapeutic doses of heparin should have hematocrits and platelet counts checked regularly to detect occult bleeding and thrombocytopenia. Routine urinalyses and stool guaiac examinations are also useful in this regard.

Hemorrhage associated with heparin therapy has made many practitioners overly cautious with respect to its proper use. A recent study reviewed heparin usage in patients with thromboembolic disease in a major medical center (Wheeler et al., 1988). Two major problems in the use of heparin were identified: delays in initiating therapeutic anticoagulation, and inadequate heparin dosage during initial anticoagulation. The authors concluded that many physicians were excessively concerned about hemorrhagic complications of heparin therapy and were reluctant to use heparin promptly and in effective doses. Attention to the above details should prevent significant bleeding complications from occurring in patients treated with therapeutic heparin and should prevent thrombotic complications resulting from delayed or inadequate heparin administration (Barritt and Jordan, 1960; Wheeler et al., 1988). *Principle: The fear of toxicity may be hard to overcome when the administration of an efficacious drug is complicated. But the fear of toxicity is not an excuse for inadequate administration of the drug.*

Another adverse effect that has received increased attention during the past few years is heparin-associated thrombocytopenia, with or without arterial thrombosis. Although early studies suggested that as many as 30% of patients receiving heparin would develop simple thrombocytopenia, an analysis of 12 prospective studies including more than 1500 patients indicated that about 6% of patients receiving heparin developed thrombocytopenia and that no patient in this group developed heparin-associated thrombocytopenia and thrombosis (incidence of the latter syndrome calculated to be <0.2%) (Levine et al., 1987). Heparin-associated thrombocytopenia appears to be immunologic in nature, occurs more commonly with bovine heparin than porcine heparin, requires 6 to 12 days to develop, occurs with heparin given therapeutically or prophylactically, and is usually reversible when heparin is discontinued. Heparin-associated thrombocytopenia is usually moderate with platelet counts rarely falling below 50,000 per cubic millimeter. Diagnosis of heparin-associated thrombocytopenia is based on clinical grounds because therapeutic decisions must be made immediately, and confirmation by laboratory testing may take 24 hours or longer.

The rare and dramatic complication of heparin-associated thrombocytopenia with thrombosis can be prevented by using porcine heparin, monitoring platelet counts, and starting warfarin therapy within 1 to 2 days after therapeutic heparin anticoagulation has begun. Consequently, if heparin-associated thrombocytopenia and thrombosis occur in a patient requiring anticoagulation, warfarin will provide adequate prophylaxis when heparin is discontinued. The future use of low-molecular-weight heparin (LMWH) species and heparinoids as substitutes for current commercial heparin preparations may also prevent this complication (discussed below).

Other complications caused by heparin are much less frequent and include allergy and osteoporosis. Patients who exhibit hypersensitivity to one preparation of commercial heparin (e.g., bovine heparin) should receive another preparation (porcine heparin). The advent of LMWH preparations should further diminish this adverse effect of heparin. Osteoporosis is seen only in the infrequent patients who receive large doses of heparin (>10,000 units per day) for periods greater than 3 to 4 months. This adverse effect results from increased bone resorption induced by heparin. Patients who receive adjusted-dose subcutaneous heparin prophylaxis for prolonged periods may be at risk for this complication.

Heparin can also decrease plasma AT III activity (Marciniak and Gockerman, 1977). Abrupt withdrawal of heparin in such patients could lead to a hypercoagulable state; however, since most patients are given warfarin anticoagulation before discontinuing heparin, this complication of heparin therapy may not be clinically important. •

Treatment of Heparin Overdosage.

Patients who receive therapeutic doses of heparin, have PTT values above the therapeutic range ($>2.5 \times$ baseline), and have little or no bleeding should have heparin infusion rates diminished or briefly curtailed. The short half-life of heparin (1-1.5 hour) ensures rapid correction of the prolonged PTT. Care should be taken to avoid loss of therapeutic anticoagulation if heparin is temporarily discontinued.

Patients who sustain a major hemorrhage associated with heparin use are candidates for immediate reversal of heparin anticoagulation with protamine sulfate. The anticoagulant effect of heparin (strongly negatively charged) is promptly neutralized by protamine sulfate (strongly positively charged). Protamine is given by IV infusion; a loading dose is calculated using the assumption that 1 mg of protamine will neutralize about 100 units of heparin. Given the short half-life of heparin, an estimate of the quantity of heparin in the body at the time of the protamine infusion should be made so that excess protamine is not administered. A protamine sulfate infusion is not without adverse effects; administration should be by slow IV infusion; otherwise anaphylactoid reactions may occur. Protamine is infused over a 10-minute period. Several studies suggest that patients allergic to fish, or patients who receive insulin containing protamine are at increased risk of developing a true anaphylactic reaction to protamine infusion. In addition, positively charged proteins when infused rapidly may lead to mast cell degranulation; histamine may cause severe hypotension. Excess protamine administration should be avoided since it can result in a "paradoxical" bleeding diathesis. The mechanism of paradoxical bleeding following excess protamine administration is drug-induced platelet aggregation and thrombocytopenia, and interference with fibrin formation by protamine. *Principle: Seek surrogate end points when administering an antidote that can cause the problem it is being used to correct.*

Low-Molecular-Weight Heparins and Heparinoids.

In contrast to commercial preparations of heparin, which have components that are heterogeneous in molecular weight (range 4000–40,000) and anticoagulant activity, LMWHs are more homogeneous (molecular weight range 1000–15,000) and possess higher specific activity. The LMWH species are isolated from traditional commercial heparin preparations by fractionation methods, chemical hydrolysis or depolymerization techniques, or oligosaccharide synthesis. Heparinoids are low-molecular-weight glycosaminoglycans not derived from heparin. These agents have been extensively investigated in Europe since 1985. Emphasis is placed on discussion of this new group of anticoagulants because they have the potential to replace heparin in the therapy of thromboembolic disease. Table 22–7 summarizes information on LMWHs and a heparinoid, and results of controlled clinical trials with them.

Interest in these compounds arose from the observation that a highly-active heparin species could be obtained with only a pentasaccharide sequence (Choay et al., 1983). The pharmacokinetics of LMWHs are markedly different from those of treatment preparations of heparin; for example, the half-life of these molecules is twice as long as that of commercial heparin (Thomas, 1986), and the half-life of LMWHs is not dose-dependent. Additionally, bioavailability is in-

Table 22–7. RESULTS OF MAJOR CLINICAL TRIALS WITH LOW-MOLECULAR-WEIGHT HEPARIN AND HEPARINOID COMPOUNDS*

COMPOUND†	MANUFACTURER	MEAN MW	TYPE OF SURGERY	PERCENT OF PATIENTS WITH DVT		REFERENCE
				LMWH	CONTROL	
CY216	Choay	4500	Abdominal	2.5‡	(CH)7.5	Kakkar and Murray, 1985
K2165	KabiVitrum	5000	Abdominal	6.4‡	(CH)4.3	Bergqvist et al., 1986
			Abdominal	5.0‡	(CH)9.2	Bergqvist et al., 1988
			Abdominal	3.1‡	(CH)3.7	Caen, 1988
			Abdominal	4.2‡	(Placebo)15.9	Ockelford et al., 1989
PK10169	Pharmuka	4500	Hip replacement	10.8‡	(Placebo)51.3	Turpie et al., 1986
			Hip replacement	12.5‡	(CH)25.0	Planes et al., 1988
Org 10172	Organon	6400	Nonhemorrhagic Stroke	4.0‡	(Placebo)28.0	Turpie et al., 1987

* Eight representative, controlled randomized clinical studies comparing LMWH or heparinoid compounds with commercial heparin (CH) or placebo are presented. Modified with permission from ten Cate et al. (1988) Clinical studies with low-molecular-weight heparin(oid)s: An interim analysis. Am J Hematol. 27:146–153, © 1988, Wiley-Liss.
† Org10172 is a heparinoid compound; the others are LMWHs.
‡ Statistically different from control ($p < 0.05$)
DVT = deep venous thrombosis
MW = molecular weight

creased three- to fourfold after subcutaneous injections compared with commercial heparin. Early studies indicated that LMWHs acted primarily to inhibit thrombosis by inhibition of factor X_a and not thrombin, suggesting that these compounds would be more active, more specific, and potentially less toxic (with regard to hemorrhage) than commercial heparin. These expectations have not been completely realized; however, clinical trials continue to indicate that LMWHs are useful anticoagulants (Levine and Hirsh, 1988). It is important to recognize the distinctions between LMWHs and commercial heparin in terms of understanding results of published clinical trials:

1. Assay methods and definitions of anticoagulant activity are major variables in comparing one LMWH preparation with another. This problem does not exist in studies of commercial heparin preparations. Most studies report LMWH dosages in terms of anti-factor X_a activity units; routine coagulation tests (PTT) are not affected by these compounds. Standardization of assay techniques has only recently been recognized to be a problem in these clinical trials (Barrowcliffe et al., 1988; Thomas, 1989).

2. The LMWHs are not pharmacokinetically equivalent. This observation may explain why similar dosages of different preparations yield dramatically different clinical effects (ten Cate et al., 1988).

3. Optimal dosage and treatment intervals have not been firmly established (Salzman, 1986).

Most studies have reported on LMWH prophylactic regimens in surgical patients (ten Cate et al., 1988), but recent studies have also investigated the efficacy of these preparations in treating established venous thrombosis (Albada et al., 1989). Clinical studies have compared these agents with placebo (Turpie et al., 1986; Ockelford et al., 1989), as well as with standard heparin regimens (Koller et al., 1986; Caen, 1988). Additionally, LMWHs have been useful for anticoagulating patients in whom standard anticoagulant therapy was contraindicated because of heparin-associated thrombocytopenia (Harenberg et al., 1983) or bleeding with standard therapy (Harenberg and Heene, 1988). Although additional clinical studies are necessary to establish optimum dosage and treatment schedules for various LMWH preparations, it is clear that these agents hold great promise for both prophylaxis and therapy of thrombotic disease. *Principle: New drugs "closely related" to older products may differ considerably with respect to pharmacokinetics, pharmacodynamics, and pharmacologic properties. When they are compared, the comparison must be between reproducible and medically meaningful identical end points if their relative effects are to be known.*

Warfarin

The discovery of warfarin dates back to the 1920s, when cattle fed spoiled sweet clover were found to develop a hemorrhagic disorder. Identification of the agent in clover by Campbell and

Link (1941) as bishydroxycoumarin (dicoumarol) led to the development of synthetic derivatives such as warfarin. Independent studies by others led to the discovery of vitamin K and its role in coagulation. Initial enthusiasm for warfarin as therapy for a large variety of thrombotic disorders waned in the 1970s because of hemorrhage associated with the drug (Hirsh and Levine, 1987); however, recent awareness of the variability in laboratory assays used to monitor warfarin therapy, and a variety of controlled clinical studies, have led to a resurgence in use of oral anticoagulants (Second American College of Chest Physicians Conference on Antithrombotic Therapy, 1989).

Chemistry and Pharmacology of Warfarin. The chemistry and pharmacokinetics of the oral anticoagulants have been summarized in previous review articles (O'Reilly, 1974; Breckenridge, 1978). Oral anticoagulants are derivatives of either coumarin or indanedione. This discussion will focus on warfarin because it is the primary oral anticoagulant used in the United States.

The structures of warfarin and vitamin K are shown in Fig. 22–11. Also shown is a summary of the vitamin K cycle that is essential to understanding the mechanism of warfarin activity. Structure-function studies indicate that the 4-hydroxycoumarin structure with an alkyl substituent in the carbon 3 position results in an active anticoagulant molecule. The carbon 3 position in warfarin is asymmetric with the levorotatory (S) form being more active than the dextrorotatory (R) form. Commercially available warfarin is a racemic mixture of both forms.

Warfarin is well absorbed; individual differences in absorption are not important as a cause of altered drug response. Warfarin binds extensively to plasma proteins, chiefly albumin. Hepatic metabolism converts warfarin to inactive products that are subsequently conjugated to glucuronic acid. These inactive metabolites undergo enterohepatic recirculation and are ulti-

mately excreted in urine and stool. The half-life of warfarin in blood is about 36 hours (O'Reilly, 1974). Plasma concentrations of warfarin in patients with adequately prolonged PTs are about 2 μg/ml. Although liver disease is well recognized to enhance warfarin's anticoagulant effect, renal disease does not increase the response to warfarin. As discussed below, monitoring of warfarin therapy is done using functional coagulation tests; obtaining plasma warfarin concentrations is reserved for the unusual patient who does not respond to standard warfarin therapy and in whom malabsorption, noncompliance, or inherited drug resistance is an issue.

Warfarin acts as an inhibitor to epoxide reductase and vitamin K reductase (Fig. 22–11), two enzymes in the vitamin K cycle responsible for recycling oxidized vitamin K to the reduced form. Warfarin thereby prevents generation of the reduced form of vitamin K, blocking γ-carboxylation of key coagulation (and other) proteins.

Warfarin does not directly inhibit vitamin K–dependent coagulation proteins, but rather prevents their synthesis. The anticoagulant effect of warfarin results from disappearance of the normal γ-carboxylated forms of these proteins from the blood. The rates of disappearance of these proteins are inversely related to their elimination half-lives. The decrease in concentrations of prothrombin, and factors VII, IX, and X following institution of warfarin therapy is illustrated in Fig. 22–13. An important conclusion can be drawn from these data: factor X and prothrombin have half-lives >2 days, so reduction of *all* vitamin K–dependent coagulation protein values into the therapeutic range (about 20% of normal) requires 4 to 5 days. This fact is the basis for the recommendation that patients given warfarin should be anticoagulated with therapeutic heparin for at least 5 days to provide complete anticoagulant prophylaxis until the therapeutic effect of warfarin is achieved (O'Reilly, 1974). Cessation of heparin therapy before completing 5 days of

Fig. 22-13. Effects of standard warfarin therapy on the plasma vitamin K–dependent procoagulant coagulation proteins. Administration of warfarin, 5 to 10 mg daily, results in inhibition of synthesis of functional vitamin K–dependent proteins. Coagulant activity of these proteins in plasma declines as a function of their half-life. The half-lives of the procoagulant vitamin K–dependent coagulation proteins—factors VII, IX, X, and prothrombin—are 6, 24, 40, and 60 hours, respectively. Although 1 to 2 days of warfarin therapy prolongs the PT assay (because of the rapid fall in factor VII concentrations), therapeutic anticoagulation takes 4 to 5 days. (Data from O'Reilly, 1974.)

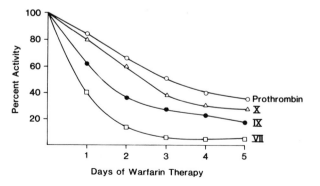

warfarin treatment may subject the patient to recurrent thromboembolism.

As a practical matter, it is advantageous to initiate warfarin therapy as soon as therapeutic heparinization is achieved. Should heparin-associated thrombocytopenia (with or without thrombosis) occur in such patients necessitating discontinuation of heparin, early warfarin therapy would permit safe cessation of heparin in such patients. Additionally, because dosage adjustments of warfarin are usually necessary, early institution of warfarin therapy may prevent delays in converting the patient to oral anticoagulation. For example, if a patient is not begun on warfarin therapy until the third to fourth day of heparin therapy, and 5 days of heparin overlap is mandatory while warfarin anticoagulation is achieved, the patient will receive a total of 8 to 9 days of therapeutic heparin, which may unnecessarily prolong hospitalization.

The dose of warfarin required for anticoagulation has important intra- and interpatient variability; dose is influenced by the patient's vitamin K intake and stores, liver function, coexisting medical disorders, and concurrent medications. Most patients are initially given 5 to 10 mg orally daily for 2 to 3 days; larger loading doses are unnecessary and inappropriate (O'Reilly, 1974). The warfarin maintenance dose is adjusted according to the patient's PT (Loeliger et al., 1985). The PT assay is the most useful coagulation test available to monitor warfarin therapy because three of the five coagulation proteins (prothrombin, and factors VII and X) measured by the PT are vitamin K–dependent. The PT is particularly sensitive to deficiency of factor VII, the vitamin K–dependent protein with a half-life of 4 to 6 hours. Within 1 day of receiving warfarin, the PT is prolonged, primarily as a result of decreased factor VII values (Fig. 22–13). However, as related above, therapeutic anticoagulation is not achieved until after 4 to 5 days of warfarin therapy. There is no clinical advantage to giving patients larger initial doses of warfarin (O'Reilly, 1974). This practice does not accelerate therapeutic anticoagulation and may, in fact, predispose to an unusual warfarin toxicity–warfarin skin necrosis (see below). *Principle: When drug therapy is maintained by following a laboratory test, the test itself must be thoroughly understood by the physician if he or she is to apply test results in a rational manner.*

Some patients have been described who require very large doses of warfarin (≥ 50 mg daily) to achieve adequate anticoagulation. The term *warfarin resistance* has been applied to these patients (O'Reilly et al., 1964). Patients refractory to warfarin-induced anticoagulation may be candidates for adjusted-dose subcutaneous heparin therapy (Hull et al., 1982a).

Monitoring Warfarin Therapy. Crucial to the understanding of monitoring warfarin therapy is the concept of the international normalized ratio (INR), a method that standardizes coagulation assays used to monitor patients taking warfarin. Use of the INR permits safe, effective oral anticoagulation. Variations in reagents used in the PT assay led to excessive warfarin anticoagulation and hemorrhagic complications in patients treated in the United States during the 1970s. Recognition of this important variable in warfarin therapy led to clinical trials using less-intense warfarin therapy (Hull et al., 1982b). The basic finding of this and other trials using less-intense warfarin therapy is that such regimens are as effective as previous warfarin regimens in preventing recurrence of thromboembolic disease but are associated with substantially fewer bleeding complications. A recent National Institutes of Health consensus panel has recommended less intense warfarin therapy for a variety of indications (Second American College of Chest Physicians Conference on Antithrombotic Therapy, 1989). Table 22–8 summarizes the most common indications for warfarin therapy and recommended intensity of treatment. For a review of these recommendations, the reader is referred to Stults et al. (1989) and the Second American College of Chest Physicians Conference on Antithrombotic Therapy (1989).

In order for practitioners to translate the recommended INR intensity into appropriate dosage regimens for their patients, the hospital coagulation laboratory can be helpful by conveying to the physician the PT ratio (PT of patient on warfarin divided by the control PT) necessary to achieve the appropriate INR value (Fig. 22–14). Another consideration in using the PT assay to monitor warfarin therapy is that heparin therapy exerts an unpredictable effect on the PT. Consequently, before discharging a patient taking oral anticoagulant therapy, the physician should measure the PT after heparin has been discontinued to ensure appropriate oral anticoagulant intensity.

A new assay that has the potential to decrease complications associated with standard PT-monitored warfarin therapy has been described (Furie et al., 1990). A radioimmunoassay that specifically measures native prothrombin antigen (normal γ-carboxylated prothrombin) was used in a randomized trial in which patients were monitored either by this radioimmunoassay or by standard PT assays. Patients monitored by the radioimmunoassay had an 85% reduction in complications (bleeding and thrombosis) compared with the group of patients monitored by conventional PT assays. Whether this assay can be adopted for routine use in the typical hospital

Table 22–8. RECOMMENDATIONS FOR LONG-TERM ANTICOAGULATION WITH WARFARIN*

THROMBOEMBOLIC DISORDER	RECOMMENDED INR INTENSITY	DURATION	COMMENTS
Proximal deep venous thrombosis or pulmonary embolus	2.0–3.0	3 months	Longer duration of therapy required for recurrence, or until risk factors resolve.
Calf vein thrombosis	2.0–3.0	3 months	Noninvasive monitoring for proximal extension is an acceptable substitute for anticoagulation.
Chronic atrial fibrillation (AF)	2.0–3.0	Until sinus rhythm restored	
With embolism	3.0–4.5	1 year	Reduce INR intensity to 2.0–3.0 after 1 year.
Cardioversion	2.0–3.0	3 weeks before, then 2 weeks afterward	
Myocardial infarction			
Transmural anterior MI MI with AF or congestive failure	2.0–3.0	3 months	
Valvular heart disease			
Bioprosthetic valve	2.0–3.0	3 months	
Mechanical valve	3.0–4.5	Lifetime	
Mitral valve prolapse (MVP)			No therapy needed for asymptomatic MVP.
With embolism	3.0–4.5	1 year	Reduce INR intensity to 2.0–3.0 for life.
Mitral stenosis or regurgitation			Reduce INR intensity to 2.0–3.0 for life.
With embolism	3.0–4.5	1 year	

* Modified from Stults et al. (1989). For most laboratories, an INR intensity of 2.0–3.0 corresponds to a PT ratio of 1.3–1.5; however, practitioners should check with their hospital coagulation laboratory for the appropriate PT ratio at that institution.

laboratory remains to be determined. ***Principle: Improved methods for monitoring drug therapy can lead to improved safety, and also to new indications as risk/benefit ratios.***

Duration of warfarin therapy depends on whether the risk factor(s) for thrombosis continue (i.e., inherited disorders, prolonged immobilization). If no continuing risk factors are identified, a routine 3-month course of warfarin therapy is recommended (Coon and Willis, 1973; Second American College of Chest Physicians Conference on Antithrombotic Therapy, 1989). Shorter treatment intervals may be as useful, but large-scale studies are necessary to demonstrate their effectiveness. Patients with thrombosis due to an inherited disorder should receive therapeutic warfarin for life (Rodgers and Shuman, 1986).

Indications for Warfarin Use. The primary use of warfarin is in the long-term prophylaxis

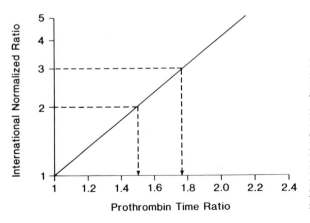

Fig. 22–14. Relationship between a patient's PT ratio on warfarin therapy and the corresponding INR value (data from Hirsh and Levine, 1987). The slope of the line reflects the particular preparation of thromboplastin used in that laboratory's PT assay. The laboratory performs PT assays to obtain the PT ratio. In this example, for standard low-intensity warfarin therapy (INR = 2.0–3.0), a PT ratio between 1.5 and 1.75 would be required. If the laboratory PT control is 12.0 sec, then warfarin sufficient to prolong the patient's PT to 18–21 seconds would be required using this laboratory's assay.

against new or recurrent venous thrombotic disease and pulmonary embolism. Numerous studies have documented warfarin's efficacy in these settings (Hull et al., 1979; Second American College of Chest Physicians Conference on Antithrombotic Therapy, 1989). The appreciation of diminished toxicity of low-intensity warfarin regimens has led to clinical trials studying additional uses for warfarin. For example, recent studies indicate that low-dose warfarin is effective in preventing embolic events in patients with atrial fibrillation (Peterson et al., 1989; Preliminary report of the Stroke Prevention in Atrial Fibrillation Study, 1990). A low-dose warfarin regimen has been successfully used to prevent postoperative thromboembolic complications in orthopedic patients (Francis et al., 1983). Another low-dose regimen has been reported to increase catheter patency in patients requiring chronic venous access (Bern et al., 1990). The effectiveness of warfarin in anticoagulating patients with bioprosthetic heart valves has also been demonstrated (Turpie et al., 1988). Although heparin is effective in treating DIC patients in whom thrombosis predominates, there is unsatisfactory experience with warfarin for this indication. Chronic DIC and thrombosis associated with malignancy have been reported to respond better to heparin than warfarin (Sack et al., 1977).

Contraindications. Patients with underlying coagulopathy, thrombocytopenia, recent surgery or trauma, CNS disease, active bleeding, or uncontrolled hypertension have contraindications to the use of anticoagulants, including warfarin. Pregnant patients should not receive warfarin because it is teratogenic and crosses the placental barrier (discussed below and chapter 29). Patients who are unable or unwilling to comply with dosage recommendations or laboratory monitoring should not receive warfarin. Poor compliance by outpatients is the major cause of unstable anticoagulation with warfarin (Kumar et al., 1989).

Complications of Warfarin Therapy. As with all anticoagulant therapy, the major complication when using warfarin is hemorrhage. Use of recommended low-intensity dosage regimens dramatically lowers the risk of bleeding. When bleeding occurs in patients with therapeutic PT assays, this often results from warfarin-induced structural bleeding (Zweifler, 1962). In these cases, warfarin-associated bleeding is not diffuse hemorrhage, but rather related to preexisting polyps, ulcers, carcinomas, and so forth. Consequently, patients receiving warfarin who develop genitourinary or GI bleeding while their PT assays are optimal should be evaluated for occult disease.

A recent study identified five independent risk factors for bleeding in outpatients beginning warfarin therapy: age > 65 years; atrial fibrillation; comorbid disorders (MI, renal insufficiency); and history of stroke or GI bleeding (Landefeld and Goldman, 1989).

Reversal of warfarin-induced bleeding depends on the severity of the bleeding and whether or not resumption of anticoagulation will be necessary following the bleeding episode. Patients receiving warfarin who develop bruising or other minor bleeding associated with PT values outside the therapeutic range should have their dosage tapered or withheld for a short time (1–2 days) until the PT value falls into the appropriate range. Patients with more emergent bleeding because of excessive warfarin anticoagulation and who are nearing completion of their period of anticoagulation can be easily treated by stopping their warfarin and administering vitamin K. Parenteral vitamin K can totally correct prolonged PT values due to warfarin within 12 to 24 hours. For such patients, 5 to 10 mg of vitamin K_1 is given, preferably by the subcutaneous route. Administration by the IV route has been associated with rare but severe episodes of anaphylactoid reactions (de la Rubia et al., 1989) and has no advantage over the subcutaneous route of administration. The IM route may be associated with formation of hematoma, especially in patients who have a profound coagulopathy due to warfarin excess. Vitamin K therapy is reserved for patients who will not require continued anticoagulation, because administration of vitamin K makes resumption of warfarin therapy very difficult to achieve.

For patients with life-threatening bleeding in whom a 12- to 24-hour delay for PT correction is inappropriate, or in patients in whom resumption of warfarin anticoagulation is indicated, the use of fresh-frozen plasma (3–4 units for a 70-kg patient) provides rapid correction of the PT without inducing refractoriness to subsequent warfarin therapy.

Vitamin K–dependent proteins mediate events other than coagulation. This fact is borne out by a tragic complication of warfarin therapy—embryopathy. This toxicity occurs when pregnant mothers receive warfarin during the first trimester. An important bone matrix protein, osteocalcin, is vitamin K–dependent; during embryogenesis, vitamin K deficiency results in fetal bone malformations. Other fetal abnormalities have also been associated with warfarin use during pregnancy (Hall et al., 1980; Iturbe-Alessio et al., 1986). For this reason, warfarin therapy is contraindicated during the first trimester of pregnancy. In fact, most practitioners recommend adjusted-dose subcutaneous heparin for patients requiring anticoagulation during pregnancy. Heparin appears to be a safe anticoagulant during pregnancy

(Ginsberg et al., 1989). Women receiving warfarin should be informed of its teratogenic effect and should avoid becoming pregnant while taking the drug. Warfarin is not found in breast milk of nursing mothers taking the drug (Breckenridge, 1978).

Warfarin-induced skin necrosis is an unusual but devastating complication of warfarin therapy, usually occurring within a week of initiating the drug. The basis for this complication is thought to be rapid reduction in plasma concentrations of proteins C or S in patients with deficiency of one of these vitamin K–dependent anticoagulant proteins. Patients deficient in proteins C or S would experience a hypercoagulable state following warfarin therapy when concentrations of the vitamin K–dependent anticoagulant proteins C or S fall faster than concentrations of vitamin K–dependent procoagulant proteins. This complication can be prevented by ensuring that patients are therapeutically anticoagulated with heparin prior to initiation of warfarin therapy and that large loading doses of warfarin are not used.

In contrast to the indanedione oral anticoagulants (primarily used in Europe), warfarin causes immune-mediated reactions (e.g., rash, cytopenias) very uncommonly. Patients exhibiting this complication can be given another coumarin drug such as dicoumarol or changed to adjusted-dose subcutaneous heparin.

One beneficial effect of warfarin therapy is the increase in plasma AT III activity that occurs in some patients receiving the drug. This is a particularly useful effect in patients with inherited AT III deficiency, many of whom have exhibited increased AT III values while receiving warfarin (Marciniak et al., 1974). The mechanism for this effect is not known.

Interactions of Warfarin with Other Drugs and Medical Conditions.

Breckenridge (1978) identified three mechanisms by which individuals may show variable responses to oral anticoagulant therapy. These include altered receptor affinity, as typified by patients with an inherited resistance to warfarin (O'Reilly et al., 1964); variability in vitamin K availability (diet, production by intestinal bacteria, liver disease), and variable warfarin pharmacokinetics (absorption, distribution, metabolism). These last two mechanisms for variable responses to warfarin form the basis for the widely recognized difficulty in managing patients on warfarin therapy, namely the large number of potential adverse interactions with other drugs and diseases. Patients receiving warfarin frequently have underlying diseases (other than thrombosis) and take additional medications. Physician awareness of these interactions between warfarin and other medications or medical disorders will help the patient avoid excessive or inadequate anticoagulation. Extensive reviews of this subject have been published (O'Reilly, 1974; Breckenridge, 1978; Stults et al., 1989). Table 22–9 summarizes medical conditions and drugs that interact with warfarin to either enhance or reduce the anticoagulant effect, as well as the mechanisms involved in these interactions. Appendix II also summarizes many of these drug interactions.

Because of the numerous potential interactions, patients taking warfarin should be told to notify the physician when *any* other medication is begun or discontinued, or when a new illness occurs. If a potentially interacting drug must be added to or deleted from the patient's regimen, the dose of warfarin should be changed appropriately and the physician should closely monitor the PT to determine whether further adjustment of warfarin dosage is indicated. Patients taking warfarin should wear Med-Alert bracelets or other forms of identification stating that they are anticoagulated, so that emergency personnel can take appropriate precautions should the patient become acutely ill.

FIBRINOLYTIC AND ANTIFIBRINOLYTIC THERAPY

Therapeutic agents are available both to initiate fibrinolysis in patients with certain thrombotic disorders (plasminogen activator therapy), and to inhibit excessive fibrinolysis in patients with certain bleeding disorders (antifibrinolytic therapy). The recent availability of new plasminogen activators including recombinant TPA and modified streptokinase has resulted in large-scale clinical studies to define the role of these agents in therapy of thrombotic disorders and to determine whether they are superior to the older fibrinolytic agents, streptokinase and urokinase.

One important consideration in using these agents to treat thrombosis or hemorrhagic disorders is that their use may be associated with substantial morbidity and mortality, especially when practitioners not familiar with their use administer them indiscriminantly. For example, when antifibrinolytic agents are used inappropriately to treat hemorrhage in patients with unrecognized intravascular coagulation (DIC), disseminated thrombosis may result (Naeye, 1962). Similarly, use of plasminogen activator therapy in patients with intracranial disease or bleeding disorders may be associated with catastrophic hemorrhagic complications, including stroke. Consequently, careful thought should be given to the correct indications and contraindications for using these agents as discussed below.

Therapy with Plasminogen Activators

Streptokinase (SK) is obtained from cultures of β-hemolytic streptococci. This protein has no in-

Table 22-9. SOME DRUGS AND MEDICAL CONDITIONS AFFECTING THE POTENCY OF WARFARIN*

ANTICOAGULANT EFFECT	MECHANISM
	INCREASED
Drugs	
Antibiotics	Induce vitamin K deficiency when combined with reduced vitamin K in diet.
	Newer β-lactam antibiotics may also directly interfere with the vitamin K cycle, inducing a warfarin-like defect.
Aspirin	Displaces warfarin bound to albumin
	Also:
	Low doses: impair platelet function.
	High doses: induce hypoprothrombinemia directly.
Cimetidine	Inhibits warfarin metabolism.
Clofibrate	Impairs platelet function, increases turnover of vitamin K–dependent coagulation factors.
Disulfiram	Inhibits warfarin metabolism.
Metronidazole	Prolongs half-life of levowarfarin.
Phenylbutazone	Displaces warfarin bound to albumin. Inhibits levowarfarin metabolism.
Sulfinpyrazone	Prolongs half-life of levowarfarin.
Conditions	
Age	Increases metabolism of vitamin K–dependent coagulation proteins.
Biliary disease or malabsorption	Decreases absorption of vitamin K.
Congestive heart failure	Impairs liver function.
Fever	Increases metabolism of vitamin K–dependent coagulation proteins.
Hyperthyroidism	
Malnutrition	Decreases dietary intake of vitamin K.
	DECREASED
Drugs	
Barbiturates	Increase warfarin metabolism.
Cholestyramine	Decreases warfarin absorption.
Diuretics	Improve liver synthetic function following diuresis in patients with congestive heart failure.
Glutethimide	Increases warfarin metabolism.
Rifampin	Increases warfarin metabolism.
Conditions	
Excess dietary vitamin K	Antagonizes warfarin's effect to reduce vitamin K levels.
Hereditary resistance to warfarin	Altered hepatic receptor affinity for warfarin.
Hypothyroidism	Decreased metabolism of vitamin K–dependent coagulation factors.
Nephrotic syndrome	Hypoalbuminemia.

* Information in this table was obtained from O'Reilly (1974) and Breckenridge (1978).

trinsic enzymatic activity; however, following IV infusion, it combines with plasminogen to form a complex capable of activating additional plasminogen molecules to plasmin. Although SK can lyse fibrin thrombi, it does not selectively degrade fibrin, and its therapeutic use results in systemic fibrinolysis and a "lytic state," due to degradation of fibrinogen and other coagulation proteins (factors V and VIII), as well as perturbation of platelet function (Marder and Bell, 1987). Although the lytic state may predispose patients to bleeding complications, the potential benefit of decreased blood viscosity that results from the lytic state may be therapeutically important.

More than 20 years of clinical experience has been obtained with SK and UK. The half-life of SK is about 20 minutes; metabolites of SK have not been identified (Marder and Francis, 1990). Since SK is a bacterial product, patients with previous streptococcal infections may have sufficient antistreptococcal antibody in blood to neutralize the fibrinolytic activity of SK. Consequently, it is important to monitor the patient after the initial infusion to ensure attainment of the lytic state (discussed below). Another potential complication of SK therapy is allergic reactions to the bacterial protein, which occurs in about 6% of patients. The risk of anaphylactic shock during use of SK is about 0.1% (Sharma et al., 1982).

Urokinase is obtained from human renal cell cultures, and consequently, UK therapy is not associated with hypersensitivity or neutralization complications. Like SK, UK does not selectively degrade fibrin and also produces a lytic state. The half-life of IV UK is about 20 minutes; clearance is predominantly by the liver.

A modified SK has been recently introduced. Anisoylated plasminogen SK activator complex (APSAC) is without enzymatic activity until deacylation of the active site occurs in vivo following infusion (Smith et al., 1981). Production of the lytic state is required for therapeutic fibrinolysis induced by APSAC. This modified SK has a fourfold longer plasma half-life than SK or UK, indicating that IV-bolus APSAC therapy may be effective. Hypersensitivity and neutralization reactions occur with APSAC since bacterial SK is used in production of this agent (Marder and Francis, 1990). APSAC is one of the most recently available fibrinolytic agents. However, it is likely that APSAC will have similar utility as SK in treating thrombotic disease, with the potential benefit of not requiring continuous infusion (Marder et al., 1986).

Two additional fibrinolytic agents are TPA and prourokinase (Pro-UK; single-chain UK). They are obtained either from cultured human cells or by recombinant techniques. In vitro studies, animal thrombosis models, and initial human studies suggested that these agents had specificity for fibrin (Weimar et al., 1981) and had superior potential efficacy when compared with SK, raising the possibility that fibrinolysis could be achieved without induction of the lytic state and a bleeding tendency. Prourokinase and TPA activate plasminogen by distinct mechanisms (Collen, 1987; Gurewich, 1988). Unfortunately, clinical trials with these agents (especially TPA) indicate that dosages sufficient to lyse pathologic thrombi routinely induce both a lytic state and a bleeding tendency. The half-lives of infused TPA and pro-UK are 5 to 10 minutes. Liver metabolism is important for the clearance of TPA (Loscalzo and Braunwald, 1988). Table 22–10 summarizes the recommended dosages of available fibrinolytic agents for treatment of venous thromboembolism and MI, and costs for such treatment in the United States. *Principle: The long process of drug development produces many surprises. New and exciting indications may be found, but potential advantages hoped for in new drugs may fail to materialize.*

Monitoring of Fibrinolytic Therapy. Because all fibrinolytic agents available require induction of the lytic state in order to lyse pathologic thrombi, laboratory evaluation to measure attainment of the lytic state ensures adequate dosage of the agent. This is especially important in SK and UK therapy of venous thromboembolism in which infusions of 12 to 72 hours are used. The potential presence of neutralizing anti-SK antibodies is another reason laboratory evaluation is important during therapy with SK and APSAC. The lytic state is most simply monitored with the thrombin time assay; prolongation of the thrombin time to values between two- and fivefold over baseline indicates the presence of the lytic state

(Bell and Meek, 1979). Because there is no correlation between efficacy of therapy and changes in coagulation or fibrinolytic assays, if an appropriate increase in the thrombin time occurs, no further testing is necessary and therapy is continued (Marder and Sherry, 1988). Following cessation of SK or UK infusion, the thrombin time decreases to less than twice the baseline value within 4 to 6 hours and returns to normal by 24 hours. For patients with MI who receive short-term infusions of fixed-dose thrombolytic therapy, monitoring may be less important, with the exception of those receiving SK or APSAC.

Indications. Recent clinical studies that demonstrate the benefit of early fibrinolytic therapy in patients with acute MI, combined with the introduction of newer fibrinolytic agents, have led to increased use of these agents in a variety of thrombotic disorders. Fibrinolytic agents have been shown to be useful as therapy for early acute MI (within 6 hours of onset of symptoms), pulmonary embolism with hemodynamic compromise, massive deep venous thrombosis, and peripheral arterial thrombosis or embolism, and for restoring patency of obstructed venous catheters. Less common thrombotic diseases for which these agents may be useful are described elsewhere (Marder and Sherry, 1988). The use of these agents for treatment of routine deep venous thrombosis or submassive pulmonary embolism is controversial. Those who favor routine use of fibrinolytic therapy for the latter conditions point to the benefits of rapid resolution of thrombi (improved pulmonary diffusion capacity, prevention of the postphlebitic syndrome) (Arnesen et al., 1978; Sharma et al., 1980; Sasahara et al., 1982) as well as the potential benefit of lysing venous thrombi that produced the embolus. Other investigators have argued that the potential risk of serious bleeding complications may outweigh potential benefits in patients in whom venous thromboembolism does not represent a life-threatening situation (Hirsh et al., 1987).

Venous Thrombosis. A summary of trials comparing SK to heparin in patients with acute venous thrombosis was published recently (Sidorov, 1989). The conclusion of the individual reports was that SK was more effective than heparin in the resolution of venous thrombosis as measured by venography. Such early resolution of venous thrombi by fibrinolytic agents may help prevent long-term sequelae of thrombosis such as pulmonary embolism and the postphlebitic syndrome. However, the data supporting the use of routine fibrinolytic therapy in venous thrombosis are inconclusive (Siderov, 1989). Lack of definitive information may explain why fibrinolytic

Table 22–10. DOSAGE AND COST (U.S. DOLLARS) OF FIBRINOLYTIC AGENTS USED TO TREAT VENOUS THROMBOEMBOLISM AND MI*

FIBRINOLYTIC AGENT	DEEP VENOUS THROMBOSIS OR PULMONARY EMBOLISM			ACUTE MI		
	DOSAGE	COST	REFERENCE	DOSAGE	COST	REFERENCE
SK	250,000-unit bolus 100,000 units/h for 24–72 h	$160/24 h	USET (1974)	1.5×10^6 units over 1 h	$72	Gruppo Italiano (1986)
UK	4400 units/kg bolus, 4400 u/kg/h for 12 h	$2340/70 kg	USET (1974)	3.0×10^6 units over 1 h	$1625	Neuhaus et al. (1988)
TPA	40–100 mg IV over 2–7 h	$1100/50 mg	Goldhaber et al. (1988)	100 mg over 1 h	$2200	Wilcox et al. (1988)
Anisoylated Plasminogen SK Activator complex	10- to 30-mg bolus	$1650/30 mg	Vander Sande et al. (1988)	30-mg bolus	$1650	Marder et al. (1986)
Prourokinase	?	?		80 mg over 1 h	?	PRIMI Trial Study Group (1989)

* Current recommended dosages. Approximate pharmacy cost at University of Utah Medical Center Hospital Pharmacy May, 1990. Less information is available for the use of prourokinase.

571

therapy has not been more widely used for this indication (Hirsh et al., 1987).

Recent trials have studied recombinant TPA in treating venous thrombosis. A randomized trial comparing TPA, TPA plus heparin, and heparin alone was reported (Goldhaber et al., 1990). The TPA was much more effective in lysis of venous thrombi than heparin alone, and addition of heparin to TPA did not enhance clot lysis. However, the only major complication in this study was one intracranial hemorrhage occurring in a patient receiving TPA. The fundamental question of whether enhanced clot lysis is an important goal remains unanswered.

Pulmonary Embolism. The advantage of routine fibrinolytic therapy (SK or UK) over heparin therapy in management of pulmonary embolism was demonstrated in the 1970s in two multicenter trials (Sasahara et al., 1973; Urokinase-Streptokinase Embolism Trial, 1974). The end points of these trials were accelerated resolution of pulmonary embolism documented by angiography, hemodynamic measurements, and lung scanning. The benefits of fibrinolytic therapy were most evident after 1 to 2 days, but not at later intervals; in particular, there was no difference in mortality between patients receiving heparin and those receiving fibrinolytic agents.

The earliest reported use of TPA in treating a patient with massive pulmonary embolism resulted in dramatic angiographic resolution of the thrombus without evidence of development of the lytic state (Bounameaux et al., 1985). A subsequent clinical trial compared TPA with UK in treatment of pulmonary embolism (Goldhaber et al., 1988). This latter study indicated that TPA lysed emboli more rapidly and with less bleeding than UK. A smaller study compared TPA plus heparin with heparin therapy alone for treatment of acute pulmonary embolism and found less benefit for TPA (PIOPED Investigators, 1990), although a lower dosage of TPA was used.

There still are no data supporting a long-term advantage for routine use of fibrinolytic therapy in patients with pulmonary embolism. Lack of substantive data indicating a survival advantage for routine fibrinolytic therapy has led most practitioners to reserve these agents for use in patients with hemodynamically significant, massive pulmonary embolism, and to treat patients with less severe embolism with anticoagulants alone (Hirsh et al., 1987).

Peripheral Arterial Occlusion. Convincing data support the use of fibrinolytic therapy, especially UK, in restoring patency of peripheral arteries or grafts occluded by thrombi or emboli. Urokinase has been demonstrated to be effective for this indication (McNamara, 1987). When UK is infused at 4000 units/min for an average of 18 hours, >80% patients experienced complete clot lysis; a 4% rate of major bleeding complications was noted. Heparin was used concomitantly in this regimen (McNamara, 1987). The reason for the superiority of UK over SK in treating peripheral arterial occlusion is unknown. Less information is available on the use of other fibrinolytic agents for this indication.

MI. The extensive literature concerning this indication for fibrinolytic therapy has been reviewed recently (Marder and Sherry, 1988; Collen and Gold, 1990). Despite the documented efficacy of these agents in MI, only a minority of patients (about 20%) will be found eligible for treatment (Lee et al., 1989). Streptokinase has had the widest clinical use of all the fibrinolytic agents to treat MI. Trials using SK have highlighted important factors:

1. Therapy is much more effective if given within a few hours of initial symptoms of acute MI (Gruppo Italiano, 1986).
2. Intravenous SK is as effective as intracoronary SK therapy (Schroder, 1983). The benefits of SK therapy on mortality prevention continue for at least 1 year after treatment (Rovelli et al., 1987).
3. Addition of aspirin to SK further improves the fibrinolytic benefit of SK, presumably by preventing platelet-mediated reocclusion (ISIS-2, 1988).
4. Major bleeding complications occur in less than 1% of patients receiving SK (Collen and Gold, 1990). The incidence of bleeding appears to be related both to the dose and duration of therapy and appears to be similar for both SK and TPA (TIMI Study Group, 1985).

Recent trials have compared TPA to SK for treatment of acute MI (reviewed in Collen and Gold, 1990); however, definitive information on which agent is superior is not yet available. Results of a comparative study involving over 12,000 patients with acute MI demonstrated very similar mortality data for patients receiving TPA and SK (8.7% and 9.2%, respectively) (Gruppo Italiano, 1990). The final analysis of data from this and other large multicenter studies should provide definitive information to guide practitioners in selecting an appropriate fibrinolytic agent. There is less information available on the use of APSAC or pro-UK in treating MI (Marder et al., 1986; van de Werf et al., 1986), but APSAC therapy may be advantageous given the ease of bolus administration and its prolonged half-life, while pro-UK may be most useful in low-dose combination fibrinolytic therapy (discussed below).

Contraindications to Fibrinolytic Therapy. Absolute contraindications include intracranial disease, coagulopathy or thrombocytopenia, recent surgery or trauma, and active internal bleeding. Relative contraindications include uncontrolled hypertension, pregnancy, and mural thrombus. As with any other potentially hazardous therapy, the risks and benefits of fibrinolytic agents should be carefully weighed before initiating use in a specific patient.

Practical Aspects of Fibrinolytic Therapy. After the decision has been made to use fibrinolytic therapy, baseline coagulation tests (PT, PTT, thrombin time), hematocrit, and platelet count should be performed. If SK or APSAC is to be used, hydrocortisone (100 mg, IV) should be given first to help prevent minor allergic complications occasionally seen with these agents. Following administration of the fibrinolytic agent, the thrombin time assay should be repeated to confirm adequate dosage (thrombin time value 2-5 times baseline). Precautions should be taken to avoid invasive procedures during the period of the lytic state (arterial punctures, IM injections). If heparin therapy is to begin following fibrinolytic therapy, it should be started when the thrombin time value is less than two times over baseline values (usually 4-6 hours following cessation of fibrinolytic therapy). For these patients, loading doses of heparin may not be necessary. In order for the PTT assay to be a valid test to monitor heparin anticoagulation, the patient's fibrinogen concentration should be at least 100 mg/dl. Certain protocols (specifically for acute MI) may require the simultaneous administration of heparin. Drugs that impair platelet function should not be given to patients receiving fibrinolytic therapy for venous thromboembolism. Hematocrit values should be followed to monitor occult blood loss.

Complications of Fibrinolytic Therapy. As with anticoagulant therapy, the major complication of fibrinolytic therapy is bleeding. Both SK and APSAC therapy may also be associated with allergic reactions and hypotension that may occur in up to 10% of patients.

Despite initial enthusiasm for the new "fibrin-selective" agents, clinical trials clearly demonstrate a bleeding risk with all fibrinolytic therapy. More recently, it has been appreciated that fibrinolytic agents cannot distinguish between fibrin in pathologic thrombi and fibrin in useful hemostatic plugs present, for example, in the gastric or cerebral vasculature. This nonselective fibrinolytic action, combined with the lack of predictive laboratory tests for bleeding in treated patients, makes it mandatory to carefully evaluate patients before initiating fibrinolytic therapy.

If major bleeding occurs in patients receiving fibrinolytic therapy, the agent should be discontinued and cryoprecipitate administered (to reverse drug-induced hypofibrinogenemia). If heparin has been administered, reversal with protamine sulfate should be considered. For emergent bleeding, the use of antifibrinolytic agents (discussed below) should also be considered.

Perspective. The profusion of recent clinical trials with these agents, combined with claims of superiority of one fibrinolytic agent over another, makes it difficult for practitioners to objectively evaluate which agent to use in patients with thrombotic disorders. Some factors that should be considered in this decision include the following:

1. **Age of the Clot.** For venous thromboembolism, clots older than 7 days are less likely to lyse in response to SK or UK (and probably APSAC) therapy. Older clots may, however, respond to TPA. Consequently, patients with venous thromboembolism who are deemed candidates for fibrinolytic therapy should benefit from any fibrinolytic agent if they come to medical attention shortly after symptoms occur. Patients presenting much later should probably receive TPA. For patients with acute MI who present more than 6 to 8 hours after symptoms begin, the benefits of fibrinolytic therapy are reduced (Gruppo Italiano, 1986).

2. **Bleeding Risks Induced by Fibrinolytic Agents.** As discussed, all fibrinolytic agents that lyse pathologic thrombi induce the lytic state and a bleeding tendency. There appears to be a relationship between increased bleeding risks associated with increased dosage of a fibrinolytic agent. There does not seem to be a major difference in bleeding risks between these drugs when they are used as single agents (Collen, 1990). Consequently, other factors (efficacy, cost, ease of administration) should be considered when deciding which agent to use. Recent clinical trials using low-dose combination fibrinolytic therapy suggest that bleeding risks may be reduced without loss of efficacy (discussed below).

3. **Differences in Efficacy.** Some (Marder and Sherry, 1988), but not all (Collen, 1990), investigators believe no fibrinolytic agent has conclusively been demonstrated to be superior to other agents. Large-scale multicenter randomized trials directly comparing the effect of these agents on mortality from acute MI should provide a definitive answer to this controversial question.

4. **Price.** As indicated in Table 22-10, the cost of fibrinolytic therapy can vary dramatically with the agent chosen. Given the fact that the largest randomized study that compared SK to TPA us-

ing mortality as an end point failed to show a clear advantage of either agent (Gruppo Italiano, 1990), drug cost may be a relevant issue in selection of a fibrinolytic agent.

Major problems remaining in fibrinolytic therapy for acute MI include (1) optimizing the fibrinolytic effect, (2) obtaining more relative clot lysis of thrombi without affecting hemostatic plugs, and (3) preventing reocclusion of coronary arteries following fibrinolytic therapy. Novel pharmacologic approaches are being developed to address these issues.

A promising development in optimizing fibrinolytic therapy is the use of two fibrinolytic agents that activate plasminogen by different mechanisms (TPA, pro-UK) (Collen, 1987; Gurewich, 1988). The resulting effect is synergistic fibrinolysis, an effect achieved using lower doses of the individual agents than would be required if they were used alone. Preliminary clinical trials of TPA and pro-UK combination therapy indicate that fibrinolytic synergy does occur in humans, raising the possibility of more effective fibrinolysis with a decrease in the lytic state (Bode et al., 1990). Even if synergistic therapy is not ultimately shown to be superior to standard therapy, it may be more cost-effective. The current approval of TPA and pro-UK as individual fibrinolytic agents and the promise of safe, effective combination therapy with these agents suggest that this new regimen may be rapidly incorporated into routine fibrinolytic treatment. The observation that SK can be made less allergenic by treatment with polyethylene glycol (Rajagopalan et al., 1985) suggests that safer forms of currently useful fibrinolytic agents can also be developed.

Substantial interest exists in producing mutant plasminogen activators in order to achieve better fibrinolytic agents (Haber et al., 1989). The most useful property of a novel plasminogen activator would be the ability to distinguish between fibrin associated with a recent thrombus (e.g., in a coronary artery), and fibrin associated with an aged thrombus (e.g., in a cerebral artery).

As discussed in the section on novel antithrombotic therapies, the ability of a variety of agents to prevent arterial reocclusion following fibrinolytic therapy is being investigated. Antiplatelet and antithrombin peptides, monoclonal antibodies, and other antithrombotics are currently being evaluated in clinical trials to determine their effectiveness in preventing platelet-dependent arterial thrombosis. *Principle: Prospects of new indications and more sharply focused pharmacologic agents arise when a drug representing new chemistry and efficacy becomes available. The clinician's major responsibility in a rapidly changing situation is to understand the basis of claims of differ-* *ences in indications or effects of similar chemical entities.*

Guidelines for Treating Patients with Massive Pulmonary Embolism or Patients with Contra-indications to Standard Therapy. Patients with venous thromboembolism frequently have contraindications to antithrombotic therapy. For example, conditions such as coagulopathy, marked thrombocytopenia, recent bleeding, or surgery are absolute contraindications to anticoagulant therapy and complicate treatment decisions for these patients. Suggested guidelines for treating patients with contraindications to standard therapy are summarized as follows (Miller et al., 1977; Hirsh et al., 1987):

1. Patients with venous thrombosis and/or submassive pulmonary embolism and an *absolute* contraindication to anticoagulation should undergo a procedure to interrupt the inferior vena cava (e.g., placement of a Greenfield filter). While this will not prevent extension of thrombus, it should protect the patient against subsequent pulmonary embolism. Patients who do not respond clinically to anticoagulation (embolism during "adequate therapy") should also be considered for caval interruption.

2. Fibrinolytic therapy should be considered for patients with massive pulmonary embolism and hemodynamic compromise. Those patients with massive embolism who have contraindications to fibrinolytic therapy, or in whom maintenance of blood pressure is difficult, should be considered for embolectomy if appropriate personnel to perform this procedure are available. *Principle: Although drugs should have similar effects no matter where given geographically, procedures in different places almost always have different outcomes associated with them.*

3. Patients with venous thrombosis and/or submassive embolism and a *relative* contraindication to anticoagulation (e.g., mild thrombocytopenia) may be managed using less intensive heparin therapy (prolongation of PTT $1.5 \times$ control).

Figure 22-15 depicts an algorithm suggesting one strategy for determining when fibrinolytic therapy or surgical embolectomy may be helpful.

Antifibrinolytic Therapy

Excessive fibrinolysis is seen in a variety of inherited disorders, including deficiency of α_2-plasmin inhibitor or plasminogen activator inhibitor, or excessive secretion of TPA. Several acquired disorders may also be associated with excessive fibrinolysis, including primary fibrinolysis (usually seen in patients with genitourinary malignancy), DIC with secondary hyperfibrinolysis,

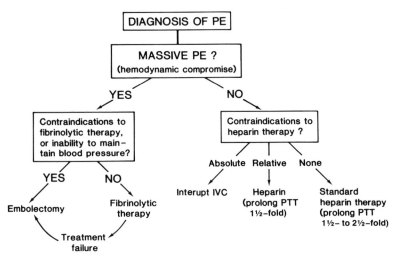

Fig. 22-15. One approach to evaluating therapeutic options for patients with massive pulmonary embolism (PE) or patients with contraindications to standard therapy. Following the diagnosis of venous thromboembolism by objective testing, consider whether massive PE is present; if not, contraindications to heparin therapy are considered. If none exist, the standard heparin regimen is used; if a relative contraindication (mild thrombocytopenia) exists, heparin is given to achieve anticoagulation at the low therapeutic range ($1\frac{1}{2}$-fold $= 1\frac{1}{2}$-times control PTT). The presence of an absolute contraindication to anticoagulation means that a procedure to interrupt the inferior vena cava (IVC) should be performed. If massive PE is present (defined as the presence of hemodynamic compromise), the existence of contraindications to fibrinolytic therapy is evaluated; if present, surgical embolectomy is recommended. Patients who are deemed too hemodynamically unstable to tolerate fibrinolytic therapy or patients who have failed fibrinolytic therapy should also be considered for embolectomy. If the patient has no contraindications and is relatively stable, fibrinolytic therapy should be administered.

and local excessive secretion of plasminogen activator (postprostatectomy) (Marder and Francis, 1990). Suppression of excessive fibrinolysis by antifibrinolytic agents may be clinically indicated in many of these disorders. In addition, patients with certain nonfibrinolytic bleeding disorders (hemophilia, von Willebrand disease, thrombocytopenia) may benefit from antifibrinolytic agents, especially to prevent bleeding associated with oral surgery. Prior to using these agents, the physician should understand the mechanism of the underlying hyperfibrinolytic disorder in order to prevent potentially catastrophic thrombotic complications caused by misuse of antifibrinolytic drugs. The utility of these agents is in their potential to reduce bleeding and to limit or avoid transfusion of blood products that might otherwise be required to treat hemorrhage.

Two antifibrinolytic agents are currently available for clinical use, ϵ-aminocaproic acid (EACA) and tranexamic acid. The structures of these synthetic agents are shown in Fig. 22-16. Both agents suppress fibrinolysis by inhibiting activation of plasminogen. Plasminogen contains lysine-binding sites important for plasminogen-fibrin interactions. Tranexamic acid and EACA have a structure similar to that of lysine; both drugs bind to lysine-binding sites on plasminogen, blocking plasminogen from associating with fibrin. Because fibrinolysis requires plasminogen (and plasmin) binding to fibrin, fibrinolysis is inhibited. Tranexamic acid is 6 to 10 times more potent than EACA in inhibition of fibrinolysis.

Pharmacokinetics. The half-lives of elimination of EACA and tranexamic acid following oral administration are 77 and 120 minutes, respectively. Both drugs are eliminated by the kidney, with minimal metabolism occurring before excretion (Nilsson, 1980).

The short half-life of EACA means that frequent administration is necessary to suppress fibrinolysis. In patients with inherited disorders of coagulation, EACA is given to prevent bleeding following oral surgery. The usual dose is 4 to 6 g every 4 to 6 hr with a maximal dosage of 24 g/day. The EACA can be given in tablet or liquid form. Therapy of active bleeding requires loading doses of EACA (5 g). Tranexamic acid is administered either orally (25 mg/kg every 6-8 hours or IV (10 mg/kg every 6-8 hours). Dosage reduction is necessary in patients with renal insufficiency.

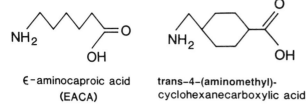

ε-aminocaproic acid
(EACA)

trans-4-(aminomethyl)-
cyclohexanecarboxylic acid
(tranexamic acid)

Fig. 22-16. Structures of the two antifibrinolytic agents ε-aminocaproic acid and tranexamic acid. The similarity of these structures to lysine permits the antifibrinolytic agents to bind to lysine-binding sites on plasminogen, inhibiting fibrinolysis.

Indications. Therapy with EACA may be useful in preventing or suppressing hemorrhage due to enhanced fibrinolysis in the following conditions: deficiency of α_2-plasmin inhibitor or of plasminogen activator inhibitor, excessive secretion of TPA, primary fibrinolytic syndromes, DIC with hyperfibrinolysis, and postsurgical conditions associated with excessive bleeding (prostatectomy, nephrectomy). Additionally, patients with inherited or acquired hemostatic defects (von Willebrand disease, hemophilia) who are scheduled for oral surgery benefit from suppression of fibrinolytic activity in oral secretions (Griffin and Ellman, 1978). Patients who have thrombocytopenia on the basis of bone marrow failure or immune destruction have been shown to benefit from EACA (Gardner and Helmer, 1980; Bartholomew et al., 1989). The use of EACA has also been advocated for patients with a variety of other conditions, including acute promyelocytic leukemia (APL) and liver disease; these patients may have severe α_2-plasmin inhibitor deficiency associated with these disorders. However, DIC associated with APL needs to be monitored carefully and treated with heparin in addition to EACA if the latter agent is used. It has been reported that EACA is useful in treating traumatic hyphema (Kutner et al., 1987), and the coagulopathy associated with vascular malformations (Ortel et al., 1988). Lastly, these agents have been suggested as possibly beneficial in reversing the activity of excessive therapeutic fibrinolytic agents (SK, TPA). The use of antifibrinolytic therapy in treating subarachnoid hemorrhage is not established; in fact, tranexamic acid appears to be contraindicated in these patients because of anecdotal reports of drug-related cerebral infarction (Fodstad, 1980). Tranexamic acid should be useful for the same indications as listed for EACA. These agents must not be used in DIC without concomitant heparin as indicated above. Renal obstruction due to thrombosis is a complication when these drugs are used to treat upper urinary tract bleeding. Hypotension is seen with both drugs if they are infused rapidly. Tranexamic acid has been associated with retinal degeneration when used for prolonged periods of time. A detailed ophthalmologic examination should be performed on patients receiving tranexamic acid for more than 4 to 5 days.

PLATELET DISORDERS

Platelet disorders can be divided into two broad categories: those associated with abnormal platelet counts and those associated with qualitative abnormalities in platelet function. Functional disorders may be inherited or acquired.

Disorders of Platelet Function

Inherited Disorders. Congenital qualitative platelet disorders are rare and can be divided into disorders of adhesion (Bernard-Soulier syndrome) in which there is deficiency or abnormality in platelet glycoprotein Ib, disorders of aggregation (Glanzmann thrombasthenia) in which there is deficiency or abnormality in platelet glycoprotein IIb-IIIa, and disorders of platelet secretion (storage pool disease, cyclooxygenase deficiency). Clinical manifestations vary from mild mucocutaneous bleeding to severe hemorrhage. Laboratory diagnosis is based on studies of platelet aggregation. Platelet transfusion is effective in patients not previously immunized against transfused platelets. In certain inherited qualitative platelet disorders DDAVP therapy is effective in improving hemostasis (Mannucci, 1988).

Acquired Disorders. The most common acquired qualitative platelet disorder is due to uremia; approximately 20% of patients with advanced renal failure exhibit abnormal bleeding. The nature and treatment of the hemostatic defect of uremia has been reviewed (Rodgers, 1990) (chapter 11). The uremic platelet defect is manifested by a prolonged bleeding time with a normal platelet count, thought to result from an abnormality in platelet arachidonic acid metabolism leading to decreased production of thromboxane A_2 (Smith and Dunn, 1981). The uremic metabolite responsible for platelet dysfunction is unknown. Other possible contributory factors to uremic bleeding include defective vascular prostaglandin metabolism, anemia, and changes in vWF (Rodgers, 1990). A role for endothelium-derived relaxing factor (nitric oxide) in the hemostatic defect of uremia has also been identified (Remuzzi et al., 1990).

In evaluating uremic patients with bleeding, the clinician must remember that in addition to aspirin and the NSAIDs, other widely used drugs possess antiplatelet activity that may contribute to bleeding in these patients (Steiner et al., 1979). All such medications should be discontinued. Other reversible disorders (such as vitamin K deficiency) should be treated. Optimal dialysis improves the hemostatic defect in most uremic patients. Maintenance of the patient's hematocrit at a level of 30% using red cell transfusions or treatment with EPO also improves hemostasis. If bleeding persists despite these measures, a modality that enhances vWF is indicated. For example, DDAVP will provide short-term correction of the hemostatic defect. Emergent bleeding should respond to cryoprecipitate (Rodgers, 1990). A newly described therapy useful in preparing uremic patients for surgery is administration of conjugated estrogens. This modality takes about 1 week for maximal hemostatic improvement to occur and is useful in elective surgery. Conjugated estrogens are infused at a dosage of 0.6 mg/kg daily for 5 days (Livio et al., 1986). Oral estrogens have also been reported to be effective in improving hemostasis in renal failure (Shemin et al., 1990).

Less common causes of bleeding due to acquired platelet dysfunction are platelet activation due to artificial surfaces, severe liver disease, and certain myeloproliferative disorders. Exposure of platelets to artificial surfaces (e.g., during bypass surgery) may activate them, inducing degranulation and resulting in an acquired storage pool defect. Platelet transfusion may be helpful if given after exposure to the artificial surface. Therapy of the acquired platelet defect associated with myeloproliferative disorders is discussed below.

Diminished liver function may result in failure to clear fibrin and fibrinogen degradation products. These molecules act as inhibitors to platelet function and may contribute to defective hemostasis in patients with liver disease, especially those with hypersplenism-induced thrombocytopenia. It has been shown that DDAVP is transiently useful in correcting this hemostatic defect.

Thrombocytopenia

The normal platelet count ranges from 150,000 to 400,000/mm³; thrombocytopenia is defined as a platelet count less than 150,000/mm³. Four major etiologies of thrombocytopenia include defective or reduced bone marrow platelet production (because of infiltrative marrow disorders or myelosuppressive chemotherapy), increased platelet destruction (because of immune or nonimmune mechanisms), splenic sequestration, or hemodi-

lution. Drug therapy is most useful when thrombocytopenia is due to immune-mediated platelet destruction, typified by idiopathic thrombocytopenic purpura (ITP; discussed below). Not all thrombocytopenic patients require treatment; major hemorrhage is unusual with platelet counts >20,000/mm³ unless platelet dysfunction is also present. The underlying mechanism for the thrombocytopenia determines the therapeutic approach. For example, discontinuing a marrow-suppressant drug suffices in some patients, whereas treating an underlying disease causing DIC and thrombocytopenia is necessary in others.

ITP. Idiopathic thrombocytopenic purpura may cause thrombocytopenia in children and adults. While immune thrombocytopenia may be associated with certain drugs, connective tissue disorders, malignancy, or infection, the term *ITP* is, by definition, reserved for immune thrombocytopenia occurring in the absence of known predisposing factors. Childhood ITP frequently occurs after a viral infection, is an acute, self-limited illness, and may not require treatment. In contrast, ITP in adults is generally a chronic illness that may last for years and virtually always requires treatment. The mechanism of development of thrombocytopenia in ITP is production of autoantibodies to target platelet antigens; binding of antibody to platelets leads to their removal from the circulation by macrophages of the spleen and liver (McMillan et al., 1987). In addition to causing thrombocytopenia, the interaction of antibody with platelets may induce platelet activation and degranulation. Thus, ITP may result in a bleeding disorder both from quantitative and qualitative platelet defects. There also is recent evidence that platelet production may be impaired in some patients with ITP (Ballem et al., 1987). The diagnosis of ITP is made by excluding other causes of immune and nonimmune thrombocytopenia (hypersplenism, DIC, drug-induced, infection, connective tissue disorder), and by a compatible bone marrow examination (increased megakaryocytes, absence of a primary hematologic disorder). Some authorities recommend determining antiplatelet antibody values; however, results of this test are not immediately available in time to make clinical decisions about treating emergent thrombocytopenia, and antiplatelet antibody values may be elevated in nonimmune disorders.

Initial therapeutic efforts are usually directed toward attaining a complete response, that is, a normal platelet count. If these efforts are not successful, or if the patient is not a candidate for aggressive therapy, treatment should be directed at maintaining a platelet count that would normally be considered safe or adequate (≥30,000/mm³). In certain circumstances, severe, life-threatening ITP requires emergent therapy, independent of sustained treatment that is later directed toward obtaining a complete response. This discussion will first review therapeutic agents or modalities available to treat ITP and then summarize how therapy may be used in treating emergent ITP, inducing a complete response, or achieving adequate platelet counts in refractory patients.

Table 22–11 lists available therapies used in treating patients with ITP. Emergent treatment involves administration of IV IgG (1 g/kg over 4- to 5-hour IV infusion) followed by a platelet transfusion (Baumann et al., 1986). Infusion of platelets in patients with immune thrombocytopenia results in rapid platelet removal secondary to antibody coating of the platelets and clearance

by the RES. Administration of high-dose IgG prior to infusion of platelets results in blockade of the RES and longer survival of transfused platelets. Patients with ITP who do not have life-threatening bleeding should be treated with prednisone (1 mg/kg per day p.o.) and maintained on that dosage, if tolerated, until normalization of the platelet count occurs, or for a total of 4 to 6 weeks. If a normal platelet count is achieved, the dose of prednisone is gradually decreased. One recent report found that a lower dose of prednisone (0.25 mg/kg per day) was as effective as the higher dose (Bellucci et al., 1988). Additional studies are needed to confirm this report. Patients who do not respond to prednisone, or those who relapse when the dose of prednisone is decreased, should undergo splenectomy. Accessory splenic

Table 22–11. STANDARD THERAPEUTIC AGENTS AND MODALITIES USED IN TREATMENT OF ITP

AGENTS OR MODALITY	DOSAGE	COMMENT
Splenectomy		Results in a higher complete response rate (about 60%) than any other therapy; a small number of unresponsive patients have accessory splenic tissue.
Platelet transfusions		Indicated only for emergent bleeding; most useful after IV IgG is given; risk of transmitting infectious disease.
Immunosuppressive Drugs		
Prednisone	1 mg/kg/day p.o. for 4–6 weeks; if a normal platelet count is achieved, a flow taper is done (6–8 weeks) to maintain the response. A lower dose (0.25 mg/kg/day) may be as effective.	Standard initial therapy; only about 10% of patients obtain a normal platelet count with steroids alone; improves hemostasis in absence of an increase in platelet count (vascular effect); inexpensive; toxicity: weight gain, hypertension, diabetes.
Cyclophosphamide	100–200 mg p.o. daily; response may take several weeks.	Toxicity: myelosuppression, hemorrhagic cystitis, sterility, possible induction of neoplasia; complete response rate about 20%; most effective in postsplenectomy patients.
Azathioprine	200–400 mg p.o. daily.	Toxicity: myelosuppression, GI distress; about 10% complete response rate.
Vincristine	0.02 mg/kg slow IV infusion every week for 4–6 weeks.	Toxicity: neuropathy. Both vinca alkaloids result in a rapid, but transient improvement of the platelet count in about 50% of patients. Complete response rate about 10%–20%.
Vinblastine	0.1 mg/kg slow IV infusion every week for 4–6 weeks.	Toxicity: myelosuppression.
Other Useful Agents		
Danazol	200 mg p.o. t.i.d. or q.i.d.; lower-dose regimens (50 mg/day) may be effective, but take longer to achieve a response.	Toxicity: weight gain, acne, liver dysfunction; complete response rate about 30%; expensive.
IV IgG	Emergent use: 1 g/kg IV slow infusion prior to platelet transfusion. Routine use: 0.4 g/kg IV slow infusion.	A nontoxic, but expensive therapy most useful in emergent ITP or in pregnancy-associated ITP when other therapies are less desirable.
ε-Aminocaproic acid	5-g loading dose IV or p.o., then 4–6 g every 6 h.	Used to control mucosal bleeding in refractory patients when a complete response is not obtained; inhibits fibrinolysis; toxicity: thrombosis, DIC must be excluded before using.

* From Ahn et al., 1983; Baumann et al., 1986; Bellucci et al., 1988; Bussel et al., 1988; Berchtold and McMillan, 1989.

Table 22-12. EXPERIMENTAL THERAPIES FOR ITP*

AGENT	DOSE	COMMENT
Colchicine	0.6 mg t.i.d. or q.i.d.	Toxicity: diarrhea; an unproven therapy, but lack of toxicity makes this agent potentially useful.
Ascorbic acid	2 g p.o. daily	Inexpensive and nontoxic, but only one report exists supporting its use (Brox et al., 1988).
Interferon α	3×10^6 units s.c. 3 times weekly for 4 weeks	Toxicity: myelosuppression; few studies exist and responses are transient; expensive.
Cyclosporin	2–6 mg/kg/day p.o. b.i.d.	Limited clinical use; expensive; toxicity: renal insufficiency, induction of neoplasia.

* Therapies listed in this table should be reserved for patients with refractory ITP in whom standard agents have failed. These therapies may also be useful in younger patients with nonsevere thrombocytopenia in whom cytotoxic agents pose the threat of acute and late toxicity.

tissue should be sought and removed at laparotomy. Approximately 60% to 70% of patients are cured with prednisone or by splenectomy. The remaining one third of patients are considered refractory and are candidates for other agents, including vinca alkaloids (Ahn et al., 1984), danazol (Ahn et al., 1983, 1987), cyclophosphamide, and azathioprine (Berchtold and McMillan, 1989). These agents are frequently tried in this order, the least toxic utilized first. For a detailed discussion of the pharmacology of these agents, the reader is referred to chapter 23.

Three unproven or experimental therapies that appear to be nontoxic also can be considered, especially in young patients in whom platelet counts are not dangerously low (Table 22-12). These therapies are colchicine (Strother et al., 1984), ascorbate (Brox et al., 1988), and interferon α (Proctor et al., 1989). Additional studies are required before these agents can be recommended as standard therapies. Chronic IV administration of IgG can also be used, but this therapy is expensive (Bussel et al., 1988). Detailed discussions of therapeutic approaches to ITP are presented elsewhere (Pizzuto and Ambriz, 1984; Berchtold and McMillan, 1989).

Thrombocytosis

Thrombocytosis is defined as a platelet count greater than 400,000/mm^3. Elevated platelet counts may be reactive (secondary) to a variety of underlying conditions (solid tumors, infections or inflammatory disorders, postsplenectomy), or due to autonomous (primary) bone marrow production of platelets (myeloproliferative disorders). Elevated platelet counts in patients with reactive thrombocytosis are not associated with abnormal hemostasis and resolve with treatment of the underlying disorder. In contrast, primary thrombocytosis (also termed thrombocythemia) may be associated with either bleeding or thrombosis and frequently requires specific therapy. The reason for this clinical distinction is that platelet function is normal in reactive thrombo-

cytosis, while platelets from patients with myeloproliferative disorders are qualitatively abnormal.

Symptomatic thrombocythemia seen with the myeloproliferative disorders (CML, polycythemia vera, myelofibrosis, essential thrombocythemia) is generally associated with platelet counts of 1,000,000/mm^3 or greater. Thrombocythemia may be associated with thrombosis (30%), bleeding (50%), or no hemostatic abnormalities (20%) (Silverstein, 1983). Management of patients with thrombocythemia must include a risk–benefit analysis, given the number of asymptomatic patients and the potential adverse effects of available therapeutic agents. For cases of emergent hemorrhage or thrombosis associated with thrombocythemia, the treatment of choice to rapidly lower the platelet count and reduce symptoms is plateletpheresis (Shafer, 1984). More permanent lowering of the platelet count can be accomplished by a variety of therapeutic modalities.

Cytoreductive Therapy. Radioactive phosphorus (^{32}P), 2.3 to 2.9 mCi/m^2 (possibly repeated after 3 months), and several alkylating agents (melphalan 10 mg/day for 5 days, then 2 mg/day; busulfan 4–6 mg/day; uracil mustard 1–2 mg/day for 14 days; phenylalanine mustard 1–4 mg/day all result in predictable and effective (70%–90%) reduction in platelet counts, although lowering the platelet count with these agents may require several weeks. Consequently, these agents are most useful in treatment of chronic symptomatic thrombocythemia (Bellucci et al., 1986). All these agents are associated with a risk of secondary malignancy, especially acute leukemia; the estimated 10-year risk following low-dose melphalan therapy is approximately 2%. This complication makes use of these agents less desirable in younger patients (<50 years of age) (Berk et al., 1981).

Hydroxyurea (15–30 mg/kg per day) is effective in 90% of patients in controlling thrombocythemia, with responses that may persist even after discontinuation of long-term treatment (Lofvenberg and Wahlin, 1988). This drug does not appear to cause secondary malignancies and is therefore an acceptable form of treatment in younger patients.

Experimental Therapy. Recombinant interferon α_{2a} (induction dose 3–18 $\times$ 10^6 units/day; maintenance dose 1.5 $\times$ 10^6 to 9 $\times$ 10^6 units/day) causes an effective (70%–100%) response in thrombocythemia (Tichelli et al., 1989). The adverse effects of interferon, the high cost of this drug, and the need for continual treatment are disadvantages that preclude use of this drug as a first-line agent. However, certain theoretical considerations (the potential of interferon to induce hematologic and cytogenetic remissions in CML) justify its further use and investigation in thrombocythemia (Talpaz et al., 1986).

Anagrelide is a member of the imidazo (2,1-β) quinazolin-2-one series of compounds, available as experimental therapy from the National Institutes of Health in the United States. Based on limited clinical experience, anagrelide is effective in 90% of patients in controlling thrombocythemia (Silverstein et al., 1988). Its mechanism of action is unknown but may involve inhibition of formation of megakaryocyte colonies. Effective doses are 1.0 to 1.5 mg orally every 6 hours initially, followed by maintenance therapy of 0.5 mg twice daily to 1.0 mg four times daily, based on achievement of the desired platelet count. Erythrocyte and granulocyte number are not affected by anagrelide therapy, and mutagenesis has not been documented. Toxicity is usually minor; common side effects are headache and nausea. Larger clinical studies with long-term follow-up are necessary before anagrelide therapy can be considered standard therapy for thrombocythemia.

Use of Antiplatelet Drugs in Thrombocythemia. The use of aspirin and other antiplatelet agents in thrombocythemia is controversial. Patients with increased platelet counts associated with bleeding should not receive these drugs because they may further increase the risk of bleeding. In contrast, patients with thrombocythemia associated with thrombotic phenomena (gangrene, transient ischemic attacks) may benefit acutely from drugs that inhibit platelet formation, while other modalities are used to lower the platelet count. One report described the use of aspirin (325–650 mg) daily to treat pregangrenous symptoms (digital ischemia) or transient ischemic attacks associated with thrombocythemia; 15 of 16 patients responded to antiplatelet therapy, most within hours of starting aspirin therapy (Preston, 1983).

ANTIPLATELET DRUGS

Platelets have been implicated in the pathogenesis of many vascular disorders, including unstable angina and MI, transient ischemic attacks (TIAs), and strokes, as well as limb and mesenteric ischemia. The significant morbidity and mortality associated with these syndromes has prompted the evaluation of antiplatelet agents in multiple primary and secondary prevention trials. A recent summary (metaanalysis) of 25 of these trials noted the efficacy of antiplatelet treatment; overall mortality due to vascular disease was decreased by 15%, and nonfatal vascular events were reduced by 30% in treated patients (Antiplatelet Trialists' Collaboration, 1988). Figure 22–17 illustrates the pathways modified by antiplatelet agents.

Aspirin

Aspirin (acetylsalicylic acid) is the prototypical antiplatelet drug; it exerts its antithrombotic activity by irreversibly acetylating platelet cyclooxygenase (Roth and Majerus, 1975), preventing the synthesis of thromboxane A_2, with resultant impaired platelet secretion and aggregation. Aspirin is the least expensive antiplatelet agent and has been the most widely studied of this group of drugs. The structure of aspirin is shown in Fig. 22–18.

Pharmacology. Aspirin is rapidly absorbed from the upper GI tract, resulting in peak plasma salicylate concentrations within 1 hour. The effects of aspirin on platelet function occur within 1 hour and last for the duration of the affected platelets' life span (about 1 week). The toxic effects of aspirin appear to be dose-related; this is a major reason why clinical studies have attempted to find the lowest effective antithrombotic dose. Major complications of aspirin use are GI distress, occult GI blood loss, and risk of hemorrhage. Adverse drug interactions with aspirin in patients receiving anticoagulants have been discussed earlier. Although most clinical trials have used 325 mg/day of aspirin, recent data suggest that 80 mg/day is effective, both in providing an antithrombotic effect and in maintaining prostacyclin production by vascular tissue.

Unstable Angina. Three large double-blind trials clearly documented a benefit from aspirin in patients with unstable angina; a 50% risk reduction in MI and sudden death was observed (chapters 2–6). Aspirin doses of 325 to 1300 mg/day were used in these studies. Therapy was initiated within the first hours to 8 days of symptoms and was continued for 12 weeks to 8 months

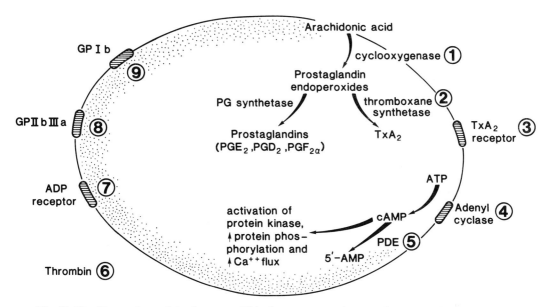

Fig. 22–17. Targets for antiplatelet agents. This diagram summarizes certain aspects of platelet function relevant to antiplatelet therapy. Platelet metabolic pathways, membrane receptors, and enzymes are depicted with specific therapeutic targets enumerated. Four target categories for antiplatelet drugs are the arachidonic acid pathway that regulates production of prostaglandins and thromboxanes, the cyclic-AMP mechanism that modulates important metabolic events, platelet membrane glycoproteins that act as receptors for platelet agonists, and thrombin, a key stimulus to platelet activation. Specific targets for anti-platelet therapies are

1. Cyclooxygenase is the target of acetylation and irreversible inactivation by aspirin, as well as reversible inactivation by the NSAIDs, including sulfinpyrazone.
2. Inhibitors to thromboxane (Tx) synthetase such as dazoxiben and imidazole analogs prevent generation of Tx-A$_2$.
3. An example of a Tx-A$_2$ receptor antagonist is BM 13177.
4. Infusion of PGE$_1$ or stable analogs of prostacyclin [iloprost, (5 Z)-carbacyclin] increases platelet concentrations of cyclic AMP (cAMP) via stimulation of adenylate cyclase.
5. Dipyridamole increases platelet cAMP concentrations by inhibition of cyclic nucleotide phosphodiesterase (PDE).
6. Since thrombin is the most potent stimulus to platelet activation, inhibitors of thrombin (heparin, hirudin, antithrombin peptides) may be important agents in preventing platelet-dependent thrombosis.
7. Ticlopidine inhibits platelet activation, probably by inhibition of ADP-induced aggregation.
8. Monoclonal antibodies or peptides directed against the glycoprotein (GP) IIb-IIIa complex inhibit fibrinogen binding to platelets and subsequent platelet aggregation.
9. Inhibitors to the vWf receptor (GPIb) are being developed to prevent platelet adhesion.

(Lewis et al., 1983; Cairns et al., 1985; Theroux et al., 1988). Over 2000 patients were studied in these trials. In one study, the addition of sulfinpyrazone to ASA provided no additional benefit (Cairns et al., 1985).

Secondary Prevention of MI. Eight studies have investigated the efficacy of aspirin in preventing recurrence of MI following the initial thrombotic event (reviewed in Antiplatelet Trialists' Collaboration, 1988). The aggregate data obtained from these studies involving over 10,000 patients demonstrated a reduction in both recur-

rent MI and cardiovascular death in patients given aspirin.

TIAs and Stroke. Aspirin is the primary treatment for prophylaxis of stroke in patients with TIAs, although trials comparing ticlopidine to aspirin for this disorder suggest that ticlopidine may be more efficacious (discussed below). The efficacy of aspirin is based on two large clinical studies that found that patients who received aspirin after experiencing a TIA had about a 50% reduction in stroke and stroke-related deaths (The Canadian Cooperative Study Group, 1978; Bousser

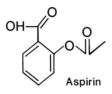

Fig. 22–18. Structure of aspirin (acetylsalicylic acid).

et al., 1983; also reviewed in Antiplatelet Trialists' Collaboration, 1988). The former study demonstrated beneficial effects of aspirin for male patients only, while Bousser et al. (1983) found benefit for both male and female patients. The daily dosage of aspirin approved by the FDA in the United States for this indication is based on the dosage used in these two trials, 1300 mg/day. However, a British trial comparing 300 mg with 1200 mg daily found similar beneficial effects for both aspirin dosages in stroke prevention; the lower dose was associated with less gastric toxicity (UK-TIA Study Group, 1988). *Principle: Large studies that demonstrate efficacy of a drug for a new indication often cannot assure the clinician of optimal dose. That ultimately will be determined by examining multiple studies with reasonably homogeneous patient bases.*

The TIAs due to carotid vascular disease are thought to be more responsive to aspirin therapy than TIAs due to vertebrobasilar disease. Additionally, aspirin therapy is often given following carotid endarterectomy (Fields et al., 1988). Aspirin has not been shown to benefit patients with completed stroke.

Primary Prevention of MI. Two large clinical trials have recently studied whether aspirin therapy could prevent first MIs in healthy patients but reached opposite conclusions. An American trial recently reported that aspirin 325 mg every other day reduced the risk of MI by 44%; this benefit was apparent for subjects 50 years of age and older (Physicians' Health Study Research Group, 1989). Aspirin use was associated with a nonstatistically significant increased risk of hemorrhagic stroke. In contrast, a similar British trial found that administration of aspirin 500 mg/day showed no benefit in preventing MI in healthy subjects (Peto et al., 1988). However, the British study had fewer subjects and used a higher aspirin dosage; both these variables may explain the observed lack of benefit. Many physicians are using the results of the American trial to justify treating patients who are healthy, but who have risk factors for coronary artery disease (Fields et al., 1988). Whether this approach is efficacious is currently unknown.

Evolving MI. The ISIS-2 trial (1988) that was discussed above in the section on fibrinolytic therapy also evaluated the effects of aspirin alone versus placebo in patients with acute MI (chapters 2–6). The group receiving aspirin (162 mg/day for 1 month) experienced a 23% reduction in vascular mortality (ISIS-2, 1988) without an associated increased hemorrhagic risk. The same study also identified the benefit of adding ASA to SK therapy in these patients.

Peripheral Vascular Disease. One randomized clinical trial evaluated antiplatelet therapy in preventing progression of peripheral vascular disease in patients with preexisting disease (Hess et al., 1985). Aspirin (330 mg/day) and aspirin (330 mg/day) plus dipyridamole (75 mg/day) were compared with placebo therapy. The combination of antiplatelet agents was effective in delaying progression of arterial occlusive disease.

Dipyridamole and Sulfinpyrazone

These antiplatelet agents have been studied alone or in combination with aspirin for prophylaxis and therapy of a variety of arterial vascular disorders. The structure of dipyridamole is shown in Fig. 22–19. Dipyridamole exerts antiplatelet activity, at least in part, by inhibiting the phosphodiesterase that metabolizes cAMP. Increased accumulation of cAMP potentiates the antiplatelet activity of prostacyclin. Dipyridamole also inhibits platelet uptake of adenosine; adenosine activates specific adenosine receptors on the platelet's surface that increase cAMP accumulation in the platelets (FitzGerald, 1987). Peak plasma concentrations of dipyridamole are achieved within 1 to 2 hours of oral administration; the half-life is about 10 hours. The only indication for dipyridamole currently approved by the FDA is as adjunctive therapy with warfarin anticoagulation for the prevention of thromboembolic complica-

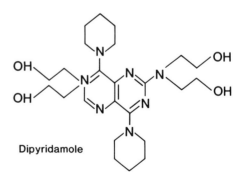

Fig. 22–19. Structure of dipyridamole.

tions of cardiac valve replacement. The recommended dose is 75 to 100 mg four times daily (Sullivan et al., 1971).

Additional studies have suggested benefit from dipyridamole in patients with peripheral vascular disease (Hess et al., 1985), coronary bypass grafts (Chesebro et al., 1982), or those undergoing angioplasty (Barnathan et al., 1987). Dipyridamole appears to have no role as a prophylactic agent in prevention of stroke or MI (Fields et al., 1988). Dipyridamole's toxicity is generally mild, with common adverse effects including GI distress, dizziness, and headache.

The pharmacology of sulfinpyrazone is discussed in chapter 19; this agent has mild anti-inflammatory properties and is a reversible inhibitor of cyclooxygenase. Clinical trials have indicated that sulfinpyrazone is not beneficial as monotherapy or as an adjunct with aspirin in the prophylaxis of coronary artery disease or TIA (Fields et al., 1988). Its role as an antithrombotic agent in other vascular disorders is unproved.

Ticlopidine

Ticlopidine is a promising experimental platelet inhibitor currently being evaluated in clinical trials for efficacy in patients with a variety of vascular or thrombotic disorders. Ticlopidine has a distinct mechanism of action in inhibition and is structurally distinct from other antiplatelet agents (Fig. 22–20).

Mechanism of Action. The primary effect of ticlopidine on platelet function is inhibition of ADP-induced aggregation and prevention of fibrinogen receptor expression (Feliste et al., 1987). Ticlopidine additionally modifies platelet responses to other agonists, including arachidonic acid, collagen, epinephrine, and calcium ionophore, suggesting that a "thrombasthenic defect" is induced by the drug (Di Minno et al., 1985). This effect is most pronounced in platelets obtained from animals or human subjects given the drug rather than when the drug is added to platelets in vitro, which raises the possibility that active metabolites, rather than the parent drug, mediate its effects (Di Minno et al, 1985). Ticlopidine has

no effect on platelet cyclooxygenase activity or thromboxane generation.

Pharmacokinetics. Ticlopidine is well absorbed orally ($\sim 90\%$) with peak plasma concentrations achieved after 1 to 3 hours. Following an oral dose, 60% of ticlopidine is recovered in urine and 25% in stool. Elimination half-lives of 20 to 30 hours have been reported. The drug is extensively metabolized; the true half-life is not known (Saltiel and Ward, 1987). Pharmacokinetic studies in patients with hepatic and renal disease have not been reported.

Effects on Hemostasis. Ticlopidine is a potent inhibitor of platelet function, exerting diverse effects on platelets obtained from human subjects given the drug (reviewed in Saltiel and Ward, 1987). Volunteers given ticlopidine exhibit a two- to fivefold prolongation of their bleeding time, an effect much greater than that exerted by any other antiplatelet agent. Platelet activation (measured by serotonin release, malondialdehyde and thromboxane production, and fibrinogen binding to platelets) is markedly reduced when platelets are studied ex vivo from patients given ticlopidine. The most consistent effect of ticlopidine on platelet function is a dose-related inhibition of ADP-induced platelet aggregation; inhibition of both the primary and secondary waves of aggregation occurs. These effects begin within 1 to 2 days and peak by about 5 days following administration of the drug. Another antithrombotic effect of ticlopidine is reduction in plasma fibrinogen values and decreased blood viscosity seen in patients taking the drug (Palareti et al., 1988). Blood concentrations of ticlopidine do not correlate with its antiplatelet effect.

Therapeutic Indications. Exact indications for ticlopidine are being established. It has been investigated in a variety of cardiovascular disorders, including peripheral vascular disease (diabetic and atherosclerotic), angina, MI, cerebrovascular disease, and prosthetic vascular grafts, as well as sickle cell disease. In addition to determining whether ticlopidine has efficacy in these disorders, it will be important to determine whether it is superior to currently available antiplatelet agents. An exhaustive review of clinical studies of ticlopidine has been published (Saltiel and Ward, 1987). A brief summary of available data includes the following:

1. **Peripheral Vascular Disease.** Ticlopidine appears to be more beneficial in nondiabetic peripheral vascular disease (claudication syndromes,

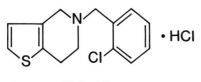

Ticlopidine

Fig. 22–20. Structure of ticlopidine.

Reynaud phenomenon, leg ulcers) than in diabetic peripheral vascular disease (Saltiel and Ward, 1987; Balsano et al., 1989).

2. **Cardiac Disease.** Ticlopidine does not benefit patients with chronic stable angina. Patients with acute MI who received ticlopidine normalized platelet survival and experienced reduced infarct size (Knudsen et al., 1985). However, no data are available concerning whether ticlopidine reduces mortality from MI or whether it is superior to other antiplatelet agents.

3. **Cerebrovascular Disease.** Most large studies investigating the effectiveness of ticlopidine have focused on the effects of this agent on the prevention of stroke in high-risk patients. Three studies reported in 1984 investigated ticlopidine in treatment of subarachnoid hemorrhage, TIA, and stroke (reviewed in Saltiel and Ward, 1987). Positive results favoring ticlopidine therapy in these disorders led to two large clinical trials, one comparing ticlopidine with aspirin in patients with TIA (Hass et al., 1989), the other comparing ticlopidine to placebo in patients with recent stroke (Gent et al., 1989). In the former study, ticlopidine and aspirin were associated with a rate of stroke (fatal and nonfatal) of 10% and 13%, respectively. In the latter study, efficacy analysis (event rate for stroke, MI, vascular death) indicated that ticlopidine was associated with a 10.8% event rate compared with a 15.3% event rate in the placebo group. In both large studies, the antithrombotic benefit of ticlopidine was evident in both men and women; this contrasts with earlier studies with aspirin that failed to show benefit for women (The Canadian Cooperative Study Group, 1978). The positive results of these two studies of ticlopidine involving >4000 patients suggest that cerebrovascular disease may be the first indication for which ticlopidine is approved. The only caveat to the widespread use of ticlopidine is the toxicity associated with the drug (discussed below).

4. **Prosthetic Vascular Grafts.** A number of clinical situations involving graft-induced thrombosis have been investigated using ticlopidine to maintain vascular patency. Efficacy has been demonstrated in patients undergoing arteriovenous shunt or fistula placement when the drug is started prior to surgery. Patients undergoing open heart surgery who received preoperative ticlopidine had higher platelet counts and required fewer platelet transfusions than patients who received placebo. Studies in which ticlopidine was given to prevent vascular occlusion in aortocoronary bypass grafts or prosthetic vascular grafts have yielded mixed results, with benefit depending upon the type of graft material used (Saltiel and Ward, 1987).

5. **Sickle Cell Disease.** Two controlled studies compared ticlopidine to placebo in patients with sickle cell disease using frequency of pain crises or improvement in cardiopulmonary status as clinical end points. Ticlopidine appeared to have efficacy in both these studies; decreased blood viscosity induced by ticlopidine may play a major role in the efficacy of the drug in patients with sickle cell disease (reviewed in Saltiel and Ward, 1987).

Dosage Regimens. Most studies, including the two most recent large clinical trials investigating ticlopidine use for cerebrovascular disease, have used doses of 250 mg twice daily. It should be remembered that ticlopidine must be given for several days before maximal inhibition of platelet function occurs. This fact is most important when the drug is used to provide prophylaxis for patients undergoing vascular graft procedures.

Toxicity. Unlike other antithrombotic agents that are associated with bleeding as a major complication of therapy, bleeding appears to be less of a problem with ticlopidine. Approximately 10% to 20% of patients experience other forms of toxicity with ticlopidine therapy. Common adverse effects include GI discomfort (diarrhea, nausea) and skin rash (Hass et al., 1989). Less commonly but potentially more significant are hematologic toxicities, especially neutropenia; cases of ticlopidine-induced agranulocytosis have been described. The large clinical studies suggest an incidence of neutropenia of about 1% (Gent et al., 1989). The GI and dermatologic toxicities are mild and reversible. Other described toxicities include abnormal liver function tests and increased serum cholesterol concentrations (Saltiel and Ward, 1987).

Concomitant administration of aspirin results in an additive antiplatelet effect without inducing a marked bleeding tendency. Corticosteroids reverse the prolonged bleeding time associated with ticlopidine use without affecting ex vivo platelet dysfunction (Saltiel and Ward, 1987). *Principle: When the indication for use of a new drug is a disease that is often treated with other drugs, or associated with other common diseases, or both, the clinician should seek postmarketing surveillance data that verifies possible alternative indications and unanticipated drug interactions of the new chemical entity.*

Other Antiplatelet Drugs

Newer antiplatelet agents targeted to the arachidonic acid pathway have been developed and studied in clinical trials (Oates et al., 1988; Nicosia and Patrono, 1989). Two groups of agents under active investigation are thromboxane synthetase inhibitors, and thromboxane A_2

(Tx-A$_2$) receptor antagonists (Fiddler and Lumley, 1990). Compared with aspirin that inhibits production of both Tx-A$_2$ and other prostaglandins, Tx synthetase inhibitors (typified by dazoxiben and other imidazole compounds) selectively prevent synthesis of Tx-A$_2$ and therefore might be considered superior to aspirin as antiplatelet therapy. However, as summarized in a review of clinical studies with these agents, there are no data thus far indicating that Tx synthetase inhibitors have greater efficacy than aspirin (Fiddler and Lumley, 1990).

The other group of drugs that are targeted to arachidonic acid metabolites is Tx-A$_2$-receptor antagonists. These agents appear to have more promise as antithrombotic agents. One of the more widely studied Tx-A$_2$ receptor antagonists is BM 13,177, which appears to have greater antithrombotic activity than aspirin (Fiddler and Lumley, 1990). A longer-acting Tx-A$_2$ receptor antagonist, GR 32191, is under investigation (Thomas and Lumley, 1990).

Picotamide, a recently developed drug, acts both as a Tx synthetase inhibitor and Tx-A$_2$-receptor antagonist in human platelets (Gresele et al., 1989). While there are theoretical reasons suggesting that the antithrombotic activity of picotamide might be superior to that of other antiplatelet agents, clinical studies are needed to test this hypothesis.

NOVEL ANTITHROMBOTIC THERAPY

Detailed characterization of components of the hemostatic mechanism combined with advances in recombinant DNA technology have led to substantial progress in the development of novel antithrombotic agents. Hemostatically active agents in venoms and other animal secretory products have been identified. In addition, the design of synthetic peptides and the production of monoclonal antibodies offers the promise of more potent and selective antithrombotic agents. The rapid pace of these investigations suggests that many of these newer agents may be available for use in clinical trials, if not routine clinical use, in the next few years. The potential clinical importance of these agents cannot be overemphasized since they are targeted for use in treating diseases that cause substantial mortality and morbidity including MI, thrombotic stroke, and venous thromboembolic disease. A brief description of these novel antithrombotic strategies is presented below with a summary of their potential clinical uses.

Inhibitors to Thrombin and Factor X$_a$

A variety of selective thrombin inhibitors have been studied including natural and recombinant hirudin (Markwardt et al., 1989), and synthetic peptides such as D-phenylalanyl-L-prolyl-L-arginyl chloromethyl ketone (FPRCH$_2$Cl) (Hanson and Harker, 1988), argatroban (Jang et al., 1990), and MCI-9038 (Eidt et al., 1989). Many studies have investigated the utility of hirudin, an anticoagulant peptide produced in the salivary glands of the medicinal leech, *Hirudo medicinalis* (Markwardt, 1985). Recombinant hirudin is now available, permitting investigation of the therapeutic utility of this extremely potent thrombin inhibitor. Most studies have compared the abilities of hirudin with heparin to prevent thrombotic reocclusion in experimental animal models of arterial thrombosis. In a variety of arterial thrombosis models, hirudin is more effective than heparin in preventing arterial reocclusion (Kaiser et al., 1990). This agent is effective after either IV or subcutaneous administration (Markwardt et al., 1989; Kaiser et al., 1990).

The peptide FPRCH$_2$Cl has been reported to prevent platelet thrombosis in a vascular graft experimental model in which heparin was ineffective in preventing thrombotic occlusion (Hanson and Harker, 1988). Other recently discovered synthetic thrombin inhibitors have also been reported to be superior to heparin as well (Eidt et al., 1989; Jang et al., 1990). One of these reagents, argatroban (MCI-9038), has been studied in clinical trials in Japan as an anticoagulant (Kumon et al., 1984). The ability of these specific thrombin inhibitors to suppress platelet–arterial interactions suggests that thrombin is a major mediator of platelet-dependent thrombosis. The apparent superiority of these agents over heparin may relate to the requirement of heparin to associate with antithrombin III before anticoagulant activity is expressed; these smaller inhibitors interact directly with thrombin. It is possible that an early use of these antithrombin agents will be to prevent arterial thrombosis following angioplasty or thrombolytic therapy in patients with coronary artery disease.

Antistasin is another interesting peptide, secreted by the Mexican leech (*Haementeria officinalis*), that selectively inhibits factor X$_a$ (Nutt et al., 1988). Another specific factor X$_a$ inhibitor, tick anticoagulant peptide, has also been described (Waxman et al., 1990). The efficacy of these inhibitors and their role as potential antithrombotic agents are not yet defined.

Other Novel Anticoagulants

Two key components of the protein C anticoagulant pathway are thrombomodulin, the thrombin-binding protein that activates protein C, and activated protein C, an anticoagulant protease. Recombinant DNA technology has produced both these proteins; a soluble thrombomodulin fragment has been developed that acts as a potent inhibitor of thrombin when tested in an animal model of DIC (Gomi et al., 1990). Activated protein C was demonstrated to prevent DIC and death associated with gram-negative sepsis in a primate model (Taylor et al., 1987) and to prevent platelet-dependent thrombosis in a primate graft model (Gruber et al., 1990).

An additional novel therapy for sepsis-associated DIC has been presented. A mutant variant of human α_1-antitrypsin (Met^{358} → Arg) has been produced by recombinant techniques and found to inhibit key proteases involved in contact pathway–mediated activation of coagulation, which may be an important mechanism in sepsis-induced DIC (Schapira et al., 1985; Scott et al., 1986). This agent is useful in ameliorating lethal affects of septic shock in an animal model of gram-negative sepsis (Colman et al., 1988). These data suggest that these agents may be of clinical use in DIC, especially sepsis-induced DIC. Routine use of heparin anticoagulation in acute DIC is controversial and not generally recommended because of the risk of hemorrhagic complications (Colman et al., 1979). The natural anticoagulant proteins (thrombomodulin, activated protein C) appear to inhibit thrombin activity without inducing a bleeding tendency. Similarly, the recombinant mutant α_1-antitrypsin molecules appear to be selective inhibitors of coagulation and have not been associated with bleeding. Clinical trials of these promising agents will define their possible role as antithrombotic agents.

Novel Antiplatelet Agents

The role of platelet–platelet and platelet–vessel wall interactions in arterial thrombotic disease is well established. A wide variety of antiplatelet drugs has been developed, including inhibitors of the Tx-A$_2$ receptor, synthetic peptide inhibitors, a monoclonal antibody to the fibrinogen receptor, and synthetic peptide inhibitors to the vWf receptor. Preliminary clinical information has been obtained on the pharmacokinetics of the monoclonal antibody to the fibrinogen receptor. Infusion of this agent in humans markedly prolongs the bleeding time and inhibits platelet aggregation in vitro (Coller et al., 1988). Use of this antibody in an animal model of coronary thrombosis prevented reocclusion following thrombolytic therapy (Yasuda et al., 1988). Clinical trials of this agent are underway. Potential adverse effects relate to the fact that this agent is a murine antibody, and immunogenicity may be a problem.

Another group of novel antiplatelet agents is the family of synthetic peptides derived from snake venoms that inhibit fibrinogen-receptor

function (Gan et al., 1988; Dennis et al., 1990). These peptides exhibit potent antiplatelet activity both in vitro and in animals in vivo. These agents have potential advantages over antibody blockade of the fibrinogen receptor, particularly since their actions are readily reversible, although there is little clinical experience with them. Initial investigation of inhibitors of the receptor for platelet vWf is also in progress.

Perspective on Novel Antithrombotic Agents

The rapid developments in this area of investigation, with numerous drugs being studied for antithrombotic efficacy, should be put in perspective. It is likely that many of these novel agents will be demonstrated to have potent antithrombotic activity. However, the key question will be whether or not these agents will exhibit advantages over drugs currently available. For example, will the novel anticoagulants be preferable to standard or LMWH, and will the novel antiplatelet agents have advantages over aspirin? Additionally, will combinations of standard therapy (e.g., thrombolytic therapy plus aspirin) be preferable?

Results of recent studies suggest that the novel anticoagulants may indeed be superior to standard heparin therapy, or be useful for clinical situations in which heparin is not effective (Hanson and Harker, 1988; Colman et al., 1988). However, definitive recommendations must await additional clinical studies. Our current knowledge of the efficacy and toxicity of these newer agents is incomplete. Studies comparing newer agents to more traditional drugs for use in a variety of thrombotic conditions are only just beginning to appear.

REFERENCES

Abdou, M.; Abdou, N.; and Robinson, M.: Aplastic anemia associated with bone marrow suppressor T-cell hyperactivity: Successful treatment with antithymocyte globulin. Am. J. Haematol., 5:25–32, 1978.

Ahn, Y. S.; Mylvaganam, R.; Garcia, R. O.; Kim, C. I.; Palow, D.; and Harrington, W. J.: Low-dose danazol therapy in idiopathic thrombocytopenic purpura. Ann. Intern. Med., 107:177–181, 1987.

Ahn, Y. S.; Harrington, W. J.; Mylvaganam, R.; Allen, L. M.; and Pall, L. M.: Slow infusion of vinca alkaloids in the treatment of idiopathic thrombocytopenic purpura. Ann. Intern. Med., 100:192–196, 1984.

Ahn, Y. S.; Harrington, W. J.; Simon, S. R.; Mylvaganam, R.; Pall, L. M.; and So, A. G.: Danazol for the treatment of idiopathic thrombocytopenic purpura. N. Engl. J. Med., 308:1396–1399, 1983.

Albada, J.; Nieuwenhuis, H. K.; and Sixma, J. J.: Treatment of acute venous thromboembolism with low molecular weight heparin (Fragmin): Results of a double-blind randomized study. Circulation, 80:935–940, 1989.

Alimena, G.; Morra, E.; Lazzarino, M.; Liberati, A. M.; Montefusco, E.; Inverardi, D.; Bernasconi, P.; Mancini, M.; Donti, E.; Grignani, F.; Bernasconi, C.; Dianzani, F.; and

Mandelli, F.: Maintenance treatment with recombinant interferon alpha-2b in patients with multiple myeloma responding to conventional induction chemotherapy. N. Engl. J. Med., 322:1430–1434, 1990.

Allen, R. H.; Seetharam, B.; Podell, E.; and Alpers, D. H.: Effect of proteolytic enzymes on the binding of cobalamin to R protein and intrinsic factor. J. Clin. Invest., 61:47–54, 1978.

American Heart Association: Special report: Prevention of venous thromboembolism in surgical patients by low-dose heparin. Circulation, 55:423A–426A, 1977.

Antiplatelet Trialists' Collaboration: Secondary prevention of vascular disease by prolonged antiplatelet treatment. Br. Med. J., 296:320–331, 1988.

Antman, K. S.; Griffin, J. D.; Elias, A.; Socinski, M. A.; Ryan, L.; Cannistra, S. A.; Oette, D.; Whitley, M.; Frei, E.; III; and Schnipper, L. E.: Effects of recombinant human granulocyte-macrophage colony-stimulating factor on chemotherapy induced myelosuppression. N. Engl. J. Med., 319: 593–598, 1988.

Appelbaum, F. R.; Barrall, J.; Storb, R.; Fisher, L. D.; Schoch, G.; Ramberg, R. E.; Shulman, H.; Anasetti, C.; Bearman, S. I.; Beatty, P.; Bensinger, W. I.; Buckner, C. D.; Clift, R. A.; Hansen, J. A.; Martin, P.; Petersen, F. B.; Sanders, J. E.; Singer, J.; Stewart, P.; Sullivan, K. M.; Witherspoon, R. P.; and Thomas, E. D.: Bone marrow transplantation for patients with myelodysplasia. Pretreatment variables and outcome. Ann. Intern. Med., 112: 590–597, 1990.

Arnesen, H.; Heilo, A.; Jakobsen, E.; Ly, B.; and Skaga, E.: A prospective study of streptokinase and heparin in the treatment of venous thrombosis. Acta Med. Scand., 203:457–463, 1978.

Asano, S.; Okano, A.; Ozawa, K.; Nakahatra, T.; Ishibashi, T.; Koike, K.; Kimura, H.; Tanioka, Y.; Shibuya, A.; Hirano, T.; Kishimoto, T.; Takaku, F.; and Akiyama, Y.: In vitro effects of recombinant human interleukin-6 in primates: Stimulated production of platelets. Blood, 75:1602–1605, 1990.

Ascensao, J. L.; Vercellotti, G. M.; Jacob, H. S.; and Zanjani, E. D.: Role of endothelial cells in human hematopoiesis: Modulation of mixed colony growth in vitro. Blood, 63:553–558, 1984.

Ash, R. C.; Detrick, R. A.; and Zanjani, E. D.: In vitro studies of human pluripotential hematopoietic progenitors in polycythemia vera: Direct evidence of stem cell involvement. J. Clin. Invest., 69:1112–1118, 1982.

Auget, M.; Dembric, Z.; and Merlin, G.: Molecular cloning and expression of the human interferon-gamma receptor. Cell, 55:273–280, 1988.

Axelrad, A.: Some hemopoietic negative regulators. Exp. Hematol., 18:143–150, 1990.

Bagby, G. C. Jr.; Dinarello, C. A.; Wallace, P.; Wagner, C.; Hefeneider, S.; and McCall, E.: Interleukin-1 stimulates granulocyte macrophage colony-stimulating activity release by vascular endothelial cells. J. Clin. Invest., 78:1316–1323, 1986.

Bagby, G. C. Jr.; Rigas, V. B.; Bennett, R.; Vandenbark, A. A.; and Garewal, H. S.: Interaction of lactoferrin, monocytes, and T-lymphocyte subsets in the regulation of steady state granulopoiesis in vitro. J. Clin. Invest., 68:56–63, 1981.

Baldwin, G. C.; Gasson, J. C.; Quan, S. G.; Fleischmann, J.; Weisbart, R.; Oette, D.; Mitsuyasu, R. T.; and Golde, D. W.: Granulocyte-macrophage colony-stimulating factor enhances neutrophil function in acquired immunodeficiency syndrome patients. Proc. Natl. Acad. Sci. U.S.A., 85:2763–2766, 1988.

Balkwill, F. R.: Interferons. Lancet, 1:1060–1063, 1989.

Ballem, P. J.; Segal, G. M.; Stratton, J. R.; Gernsheimer, T.; Adamson, J. W.; and Slichter, S. J.: Mechanisms of thrombocytopenia in chronic autoimmune thrombocytopenic purpura: Evidence of both impaired platelet production and increased platelet clearance. J. Clin. Invest., 80:33–40, 1987.

Balsano, F.; Coccheri, S.; Libretti, A.; Nenci, G. G.; Catalano, M.; Fortunato, G.; Grasselli, S.; Violi, F.; Hellemans, H.; and Vanhove, P. H.: Ticlopidine in the treatment of intermittent claudication: A 21-month double-blind trial. J. Lab. Clin. Med., 114:84–91, 1989.

Barak, Y.; Paran, M.; Levin, S.; and Sachs, L.: In vitro induction of myeloid proliferation and maturation in infantile genetic agranulocytosis. Blood, 38:74–80, 1971.

Barnathan, E. S.; Schwartz, J. S.; Taylor, L.; Laskey, W. K.; Kleaveland, J. P.; Kussmaul, W. G.; and Hirschfield, J. W.: Aspirin and dipyridamole in the prevention of acute coronary thrombosis complicating coronary angioplasty. Circulation, 76:125–134, 1987.

Barritt, D. W.; and Jordan, S. C.: Anticoagulant drugs in the treatment of pulmonary embolism. A controlled trial. Lancet, 1:1309–1312, 1960.

Barrowcliffe, T. W.; Curtis, A. D.; Johnson, E. A.; and Thomas, D. P.: An international standard for low molecular weight heparin. Thromb. Haemost., 60:1–7, 1988.

Bartholomew, J. R.; Salgia, R.; and Bell, W. R.: Control of bleeding in patients with immune and nonimmune thrombocytopenia with aminocaproic acid. Arch. Intern. Med., 149: 1959–1961, 1989.

Baumann, M. A.; Menitove, J. E.; Aster, R. H.; and Anderson, T.: Urgent treatment of idiopathic thrombocytopenic purpura with single-dose gammaglobulin infusion followed by platelet transfusion. Ann. Intern. Med., 104:808–809, 1986.

Begley, C. G.; Metcalf, D.; and Nicola, N. A.: Purified colony stimulating factors (G-CSF and GM-CSF) induce differentiation in human HL60 leukemic cells with suppression of clonogenicity. Int. J. Cancer, 39:99–105, 1987.

Bell, W. R.; and Meek, A. G.: Guidelines for the use of thrombolytic agents. N. Engl. J. Med., 301:1266–1270, 1979.

Bellucci, S.; Charpak, Y.; Chastang, C.; Tobelem, G.; and the Cooperative Group on Immune Thrombocytopenic Purpura: Low doses v conventional doses of corticoids in immune thrombocytopenic purpura (ITP): Results of a randomized clinical trial in 160 children, 223 adults. Blood, 71:1165–1169, 1988.

Bellucci, S.; Janvier, M.; Tobelem, G.; Flandrin, G.; Charpak, Y.; Berger, R.; and Boiron, M.: Essential thrombocythemias: Clinical evolutionary and biological data. Cancer, 58:2440–2447, 1986.

Bengtsson-Olivecrona, G.; and Olivecrona, T.: Binding of active and inactive forms of lipoprotein lipase to heparin: Effects of pH. Biochem. J., 226:409–413, 1985.

Berchtold, P.; and McMillan, R.: Therapy of chronic idiopathic thrombocytopenic purpura in adults. Blood, 74:2309–2317, 1989.

Berdel, W. E.; Dahauser-Riedl, S.; Steinhauser, G.; and Winton, E. F.: Various human hematopoietic growth factors (interleukin-3, GM-CSF, G-CSF) stimulate clonal growth of nonhematopoietic tumor cells. Blood, 73:80–83, 1989.

Berk, P. D.; Goldberg, J. D.; Silverstein, M. N.; Weinfeld, A.; Donovan, P. B.; Ellis, J. T.; Wandau, S. A.; Saszlo, J.; Najean, Y.; Pisciotta, A. V.; and Wasserman, L. M.: Increased incidence of acute leukemia in polycythemia vera associated with chlorambucil therapy. N. Engl. J. Med., 304: 441–447, 1981.

Bergqvist, D.; Matzsch, T.; Burmark, U. S.; Frisell, J.; Guilbaud, O.; Hallbook, T.; Horn, A.; Lindhagen, A.; Ljungner, H.; Ljungstrom, K.-G.; Onarheim, H.; Risberg, B.; Torngren, S.; and Ortenwall, P.: Low molecular weight heparin given the evening before surgery compared with conventional low-dose heparin in prevention of thrombosis. Br. J. Surg., 75:888–891, 1988.

Bergqvist, D.; Burmark, U. S.; Frisell, J.; Hallbook, T.; Lindblad, B.; Risberg, B; Torngren, S.; and Wallin, G.: Low molecular weight heparin once daily compared with conventional low-dose heparin twice daily: A prospective double-blind multicentre trial on prevention of postoperative thrombosis. Br. J. Surg., 73:204–208, 1986.

Bern, M. M.; Lokich, J. J.; Wallach, S. R.; Bothe, A.; Benotti, P. N.; Arkin, C. F.; Greco, F. A.; Huberman, M.; and

Moore, C.: Very low doses of warfarin can prevent thrombosis in central venous catheters. A randomized prospective trial. Ann. Intern. Med., 112:423–428, 1990.

Bertoncello, I.; Hodgson, G. S.; and Bradley, T. R.: Multiparameter analysis of transplantable hemopoietic stem cells: I. The separation and enrichment of stem cells homing to marrow and spleen on the basis of rhodamine-123 fluorescence. Exp. Hematol., 13:999–1006, 1985.

Beutler, B.; and Cerami, A.: Cachectin: More than a tumor necrosis factor. N. Engl. J. Med., 316:379–385, 1987.

Bichet, D. G.; Razi, M.; Lonergan, M.; Arthus, M.-F.; Papukna, V.; Kortas, C.; and Barjon, J.-N.: Hemodynamic and coagulation responses to 1-desamino [8-D-arginine] vasopressin in patients with congenital nephrogenic diabetes insipidus. N. Engl. J. Med., 318:881–887, 1988.

Bode, C.; Schuler, G.; Nordt, T.; Schonermark, S.; Baumann, H.; Richardt, G.; Dietz, R.; Gurewich, V.; and Kubler, W.: Intravenous thrombolytic therapy with a combination of single-chain urokinase-type plasminogen activator and recombinant tissue-type plasminogen activator in acute myocardial infarction. Circulation, 81:907–913, 1990.

Bona, R. D.; Rickles, F. R.; Hanna, W. T.; Weinstein, R. E.; Carta, C. A.; Zimmerman, C. E.; and Rousell, R.: Characterization of von Willebrand factor in factor VIII products. Blood, 74(suppl. 1):38a, 1989.

Bond, L.; and Bevan, D.: Myocardial infarction in a patient with hemophilia treated with DDAVP. N. Engl. J. Med., 318:121, 1988.

Bonilla, M. A.; Gillo, A. P.; Ruggeiro, M.; Kernan, N. A.; Brochstein, J. A.; Abboud, M.; Fumagalli, L.; Vincent, M.; Gabrilove, J. L.; Welte, K.; Souza, L. M.; and O'Reilly, R. J.: Effects of recombinant human granulocyte colony-stimulating factor on neutropenia in patients with congenital agranulocytosis. N. Engl. J. Med., 320:1574–1580, 1989.

Bounameaux, H.; Vermylen, J.; and Collen, D.: Thrombolytic treatment with recombinant tissue-type plasminogen activator in a patient with massive pulmonary embolism. Ann. Intern. Med., 103:64–65, 1985.

Bousser, M. G.; Eschwege, E.; Haguenau, M.; Lefaucconnier, J. M.; Thibult, N.; Touboul, D.; and Touboul, P. J.: AICLA controlled trial of aspirin and dipyridamole in the secondary prevention of athero-thrombotic cerebral ischemia. Stroke, 14:5–14, 1983.

Brandt, J.; Baird, N.; Lu, L.; Srour, E.; and Hoffman, R.: Characterization of a human hematopoietic progenitor cell capable of forming blast cell containing colonies in vitro. J. Clin. Invest., 82:1017–1027, 1988.

Brandt, S. J.; Peters, W. P.; Atwater, S. K.; Kurtzberg, J.; Borowitz, M. J.; Jones, R. B.; Shpall, E. J.; Bast, R. C.; Gilbert, C. J.; and Oette, D. H.: Effect of recombinant human granulocyte-macrophage colony-stimulating factor on hematopoietic reconstitution after high-dose chemotherapy and autologous bone marrow transplantation. N. Engl. J. Med., 318:869–876, 1988.

Breckenridge, A.: Oral anticoagulant drugs: Pharmacokinetic aspects. Semin. Hematol., 15, 19–26, 1978.

Brettler, D. B.; and Levine, P. H.: Factor concentrates for treatment of hemophilia: Which one to choose? Blood, 73: 2067–2073, 1989.

Bronchud, M. H.; Scarffe, J. H.; Thatcher, N.; Crowther, D.; Souza, L. M.; Alton, N. K.; Testa, N. G.; and Dexter, T. M.: Phase I/II study of recombinant human granulocyte colony-stimulating factor in patients receiving intensive chemotherapy for small cell lung cancer. Br. J. Cancer, 56:809–813, 1987.

Broudy, V. C.; Kaushansky, K.; Segal, G. M.; Harlan, J. M.; and Adamson, J. W.: Tumor necrosis factor type alpha stimulates human endothelial cells to produce granulocyte/macrophage colony-stimulating factor. Proc. Natl. Acad. Sci. U.S.A., 83:7467–7471, 1986.

Brown, R. B.; Klar, J.; Lemeshow, S.; Teres, D.; Pastides, H.; and Sands, M.: Enhanced bleeding with cefoxitin or moxalactam: Statistical analysis within a defined population of 1493 patients. Arch. Intern. Med., 146:2159–2164, 1986.

Brox, A. G.; Howson-Jan, K.; and Fauser, A. A.: Treatment of idiopathic thrombocytopenic purpura with ascorbate. Br. J. Haematol., 70:341–344, 1988.

Broxmeyer, H. E.; Lu, L.; Platzer, E.; Feit, C.; Juliano, L.; and Rubin, B. Y.: Comparative analysis of the influence of human gamma, alpha, and beta interferons on human multipotential, erythroid and granulocyte-macrophage progenitor cells. J. Immunol., 131:1300–1305, 1983.

Broxmeyer, H. E.; Bognacki, J.; and Dormer, M. H.: Identification of leukemia-associated inhibitory activity as acidic isoferritins. A regulatory role for acidic isoferritins in the production of granulocytes and macrophages. J. Exp. Med., 152:1426–1444, 1981.

Bruno, E.; Briddell, R.; and Hoffman, R.: Effect of recombinant and purified hematopoietic growth factors on human megakaryocyte colony formation. Exp. Hematol., 16:371–377, 1988.

Buller, H. R.; and ten Cate, J. W.: Acquired antithrombin III deficiency: Laboratory diagnosis, incidence, clinical implications, and treatment with antithrombin III concentrate. Am. J. Med., 87 (suppl. 3B):44S–48S, 1989.

Bussel, J. B.; Pham, L. C.; Aledort, L.; and Nachman, R.: Maintenance treatment of adults with chronic refractory immune thrombocytopenic purpura using repeated intravenous infusions of gammaglobulin. Blood, 72:121–127, 1988.

Caen, J. P.: A randomized double-blind study between a low molecular weight heparin Kabi 2165 and standard heparin in the prevention of deep vein thrombosis in general surgery: A French multicenter trial. Thromb. Haemost., 59:216–220, 1988.

Cairns, J. A.; Gent, M.; Singer, J.; Finnie, K. J.; Froggatt, G. M.; Holder, D. A.; Jablonsky, G.; Kostuk, W. J.; Melendez, L. J.; Myers, M. G.; Sackett, D. L.; Sealey, B. J.; and Tanser, P. H.: Aspirin, sulfinpyrazone, or both in unstable angina: Results of a Canadian multicenter trial. N. Engl. J. Med., 313:1369–1375, 1985.

Campbell, H. A.; and Link, K. P.: Studies on the hemorrhagic sweet clover disease: IV. The isolation and crystallization of the hemorrhagic agent. J. Biol. Chem., 138:21–33, 1941.

The Canadian Cooperative Study Group: A randomized trial of aspirin and sulfinpyrazone in threatened stroke. N. Engl. J. Med., 299:53–59, 1978.

Caro, J.; Brown, S; Miller, O.; Murray, T.; and Erslev, A. J.: Erythropoietin levels in uremic nephric and anephric patients. J. Lab. Clin. Med., 93:449–458, 1979.

Casati, S.; Passerini, P.; Campise, M. R.; Grazani, G.; Cesana, B.; Perisic, M.; and Ponticelli, C.: Benefits and risks of protracted treatment with human recombinant erythropoietin in patients having hemodialysis. Br. Med. J., 295:1017–1020, 1987.

Cashman, J.; Henkelman, D.; Humphries, K.; Eaves, C.; and Eaves, A.: Individual BFU-E in polycythemia vera produce both erythropoietin dependent and independent progeny. Blood, 61:876–884, 1983.

Champlin, R. E.; Nimer, S. D.; Ireland, P.; Oette, D. H.; and Golde, D. W.: Treatment of refractory aplastic anemia with recombinant human granulocyte-macrophage colony-stimulating factor. Blood, 73:694–699, 1989.

Chanarin, I.: Investigation and management of megaloblastic anemia. Clin. Haematol., 5:747–763, 1976.

Chesbro, J. H.; Clements, I. P.; Fuster, V.; Elveback, L. R.; Smith, H. C.; Bardsley, W. T.; Frye, R. L.; Holmes, D. R.; Vlietstra, R. E.; Pluth, J. R.; Wallace, R. B.; Puga, F. J.; Orszulak, T. A.; Piehler, J. M.; Schaff, H. V.; and Danielson, G. K.: A platelet-inhibitor-drug trial in coronary-artery bypass operations: Benefit of perioperative dipyridamole and aspirin therapy on early postoperative vein-graft patency. N. Engl. J. Med., 307, 73–78, 1982.

Choay, J.; Petitou, M.; Lormeau, J. C.; Sinay, P.; and Casu, B.; Gatti, G.: Structure-activity relationship in heparin: A synthetic pentasaccharide with high affinity for antithrombin III and eliciting high anti-factor X_a activity. Biochem. Biophys. Res. Commun., 116:492–499, 1983.

Chung, A. S. M.; Pearson, W.; Darby, W.; Miller, O.; and

Goldsmith, G.: Folic acid, vitamin B_6, pantothenic acid and vitamin B_{12} in human dietaries. Am. J. Clin. Nutr., 9:573–582, 1961.

Cohen, H.; Scott, S. D.; Mackie, I. J.; Shearer, M.; Bax, R.; Karran, S. J.; and Machin, S.: The development of hypoprothrombinemia following antibiotic therapy in malnourished patients with low serum vitamin K_1 levels. Br. J. Haematol., 68:63–66, 1988.

Collen, D.: Coronary thrombolysis: Streptokinase or recombinant tissue-type plasminogen activator? Ann. Intern. Med., 112:529–538, 1990.

Collen, D.: Molecular mechanisms of fibrinolysis and their application to fibrin-specific thrombolytic therapy. J. Cell. Biochem., 33:77–86, 1987.

Collen, D. C.; and Gold, H. K.: New developments in thrombolytic therapy. Thromb. Res., 10(suppl.):105–131, 1990.

Coller, B. S.; Scudder, L. E.; Berger, H. J.; and Iuliucci, J. D.: Inhibition of human platelet function in vivo with a monoclonal antibody: With observations on the newly dead as experimental subjects. Ann. Intern. Med., 109:635–638, 1988.

Collins, A. J.; Bloomfield, C. D.; Peterson, B. A.; McKenna, R. W.; and Edson, J. R.: Acute promyelocytic leukemia: Management of the coagulopathy during daunorubicin-prednisone remission induction. Arch. Intern. Med., 138:1677–1680, 1978.

Collins, R.; Scrimgeour, A.; Yusuf, S.; and Peto, R.: Reduction in fatal pulmonary embolism and venous thrombosis by perioperative administration of subcutaneous heparin: Overview of results of randomized trials in general, orthopedic, and urologic surgery. N. Engl. J. Med., 318:1162–1173, 1988.

Colman, R. W.; Flores, D. N.; de la Cadena, R.; Scott, C. F.; Cousens, L.; Barr, P. J.; Hoffman, I. B.; Kueppers, F.; Fisher, D.; Idell, S.; and Pisarello, J.: Recombinant α_1-antitrypsin Pittsburgh attenuates experimental gram-negative septicemia. Am. J. Pathol., 130:418–426, 1988.

Colman, R. W.; Robboy, S. J.; and Minna, J. D.: Disseminated intravascular coagulation: A reappraisal. Ann. Rev. Med., 30:359–374, 1979.

Coon, W. W.; and Willis, P. W.: Recurrence of venous thromboembolism. Surgery, 73:823–827, 1973.

Corcino, J. J.: Absorption and malabsorption of vitamin B_{12}. Am. J. Med., 52:679–689, 1972.

Cotes, P. M.: Immunoreactive erythropoietin in serum: I. Evidence for the validity of the assay method and the physiological relevance of estimates. Br. J. Haematol., 50:427–438, 1982.

Coulombel, L.; Eaves, A. C.; and Eaves, C. J.: Enzymatic treatment of long-term human marrow cultures reveals the preferential location of primitive hemopoietic progenitors in the adherent layer. Blood, 62:291–297, 1983.

Daniak, N.; and Kreczko, S.: Interactions of insulin, insulin-like growth factor II and platelet-derived growth factor in erythropoietic culture. J. Clin. Invest., 76:1237–1242, 1985.

de la Rubia, J.; Grau, E.; Montserrat, I.; Zuazu, I.; and Paya, A.: Anaphylactic shock and vitamin K_1. Ann. Intern. Med., 110:943, 1989.

Degliantoni, G.; Perussia, B.; Mangoni, L.; and Trinchieri, G.: Inhibition of bone marrow colony formation by human natural killer cells by natural killer cell–derived colony-inhibiting activity. J. Exp. Med., 161:1152–1168, 1985.

Dennis, M. S.; Henzel, W. J.; Pitti, R. M.; Lipari, M. T.; Napier, M. A.; Deisher, T. A.; Bunting, S.; and Lazarus, R. A.: Platelet glycoprotein IIb-III$_a$ protein antagonists from snake venoms: Evidence for a family of platelet-aggregation inhibitors. Proc. Natl. Acad. Sci. U.S.A., 87:2471–2475, 1990.

deSwart, C. A. M.; Nijmeyer, B.; Roelofs, J. M. M.; and Sixma, J. J.: Kinetics of intravenously administered heparin in normal humans. Blood, 60:1251–1258, 1982.

Devereux, S.; Linch, Campos-Costa, D.; Spittle, M. F.; and Jellife, A. M.: Transient leukopenia induced by granulocyte-macrophage colony-stimulating factor. Lancet, 2:1523–1524, 1987.

Dexter, T. M.; Allen, T. D.; and Lajtha, L. G.: Conditions controlling the proliferation of hemopoietic stem cells in vitro. J. Cell. Physiol., 91:335–344, 1977.

Di Minno, G.; Cerbone, A. M.; Mattioli, P. L.; Turco, S.; Iovine, C.; and Mancini, M.: Functionally thrombasthenic state in normal platelets following the administration of ticlopidine. J. Clin. Invest., 75:328–338, 1985.

Dinarello, C. A.: Multiple biological properties of recombinant human interleukin 1 (beta). Immunobiology, 172:301–315, 1986.

DiPersio, J.; Billing, P.; Kaufman, S.; Eghtesady, P.; Williams, R. E.; and Gasson, J. C.: Characterization of the human granulocyte-macrophage colony-stimulating factor (GM-CSF) receptor. J. Biol. Chem., 263:1834–1841, 1988.

Donahue, R. E.; Seehra, J.; Metzger, M.; Lefebvre, D.: Human IL-3 and GM-CSF act synergistically in stimulating hematopoiesis in primates. Science, 241:1820–1823, 1988.

Doyle, D. J.; Turpie, A. G. G.; Hirsh, J.; Best, C.; Kinch, D.; Levine, M. N.; and Gent, M.: Adjusted subcutaneous heparin or continuous intravenous heparin in patients with acute deep vein thrombosis: A randomized trial. Ann. Intern. Med., 107:441–445, 1987.

Duhrsen, U.; Villeval, J. L.; Boyd, J.; Kannourakis, G.; Mortsyn, G.; and Metcalf, D.: Effects of recombinant human granulocyte colony-stimulating factor on hematopoietic progenitor cells in cancer patients. Blood, 72:2074–2081, 1988.

Eaves, C. J.; and Eaves, C.: Erythropoietin dose–response curves for three classes of erythroid progenitors in normal human marrow and in patients with polycythemia vera. Blood, 52:1196–1210, 1978.

Eidt, J. F.; Allison, P.; Noble, S.; Ashton, J.; Golino, P.; McNatt, J.; Buja, L. M.; and Willerson, J. T.: Thrombin is an important mediator of platelet aggregation in stenosed canine coronary arteries with endothelial injury. J. Clin. Invest., 84:18–27, 1989.

Eridani, S.; Batten, S.; and Sawyer, B.: Erythroid colony formation in primary thrombocythaemia: Evidence of hypersensitivity to erythropoietin. Br. J. Haematol., 55:157–161, 1983.

Eron, L. J.; Judson, F.; Tucker, S.; Prawer, S.; Mills, J.; Murphy, K.; Hickey, M.; Rogers, M.; Flannigan, S.; Hien, N.; Katz, H. I.; Goldman, S.; Gottlieb, A.; Adams, K.; Burton, P.; Tanner, D.; Taylor, E.; and Peets, E.: Interferon therapy for condylomata acuminata. N. Engl. J. Med., 3:1059–1064, 1986.

Erslev, A. J.: Humoral regulation of red cell production. Blood, 8:349–357, 1983.

Erslev, A. J.; and Gabuzda, T. G.: Pathophysiology of Blood, 3rd ed. W. B. Saunders, Philadelphia, 1985.

Eschbach, J. W.; Abdulhadi, M. H.; Brown, J. K.; Delano, B. G.; Downing, M. R.; Egrie, J. C.; Evans, R. N.; Friedman, E. A.; Graber, S. E.; Haley, N. R.; Korbet, S.; Krantz, S. B.; Lundin, A. P.; Nisson A. R.; Ogden, D. A.; Paganini, E. P.; Rader, B.; Rutsky, E. A.; Stivelman, J.; Stone, W. J.; Techan, P.; Van Stone, J. C.; Van Wyck, D. P.; Zuckerman, K.; and Adamson, J. W.: Recombinant human erythropoietin in anemic patients with end-stage renal disease: Results of a phase III, multicenter clinical trial. Ann. Intern. Med., 111(12):992–1000, 1989a.

Eschbach, J. W.; Kelly, M. R.; Haley, N. R.; Abels, R. I.; and Adamson, J. W.: Treatment of the anemia of progressive renal failure with recombinant human erythropoietin. N. Engl. J. Med., 321:158–163, 1989b.

Eschbach, J. W.; Egrie, J. C.; Downing, M. R.; Browne, J. K.; and Adamson, J. W.: Correction of the anemia of end-stage renal disease with recombinant human erythropoietin: Results of a combined phase I and II clinical trial. N. Engl. J. Med., 316:73–78, 1987.

Esmue, C. T.: The regulation of natural anticoagulant pathways. Science, 235, 1348–1352, 1987.

Ezckowitz, R. A. B.; Dinauer, M. C.; Jaffe, H. S.; Orkin, S. H.; and Newburger, P. E.: Partial correction of the phagocytic defect in patients with chronic granulomatous disease by subcutaneous interferon gamma. N. Engl. J. Med., 319: 146–151, 1988.

Fasco, M. J.; Principe, L. M.; Walsh, W. A.; and Friedman, P. A.: Warfarin inhibition of vitamin K 2,3-epoxide reductase in rat liver microsomes. Biochemistry, 22: 5655–5660, 1983.

Fauser, A. A.; and Messner, H. A.: Identification of megakaryocytes, macrophages and eosinophils in colonies of human bone marrow containing neutrophilic granulocytes and erythroblasts. Blood, 53:1023–1027, 1979.

Feliste, R.; Delebassee, D.; Simon, M. F.; Chap, H.; Defreyn, G.; Vallee, E.; Douste-Blazy, L.; and Maffrand, J. P.: Broad spectrum anti-platelet activity of ticlopidine and PCR 4099 involves the suppression of the effects of released ADP. Thromb. Res., 48:403–415, 1987.

Fialkow, P. J.; Martin, P. J.; Najfeld, V.; Penfold, G.; Jacobson, R.; and Hansen, J.: Evidence for a multistep pathogenesis of chronic myelogenous leukemia. Blood, 58:158–163, 1981.

Fialkow, P. J.; Jacobson, R. J.; and Papayannopoulou, T.: Chronic myelocytic leukemia: Clonal origin in a stem cell common to the granulocyte, erythrocyte, platelet and monocyte/macrophage. Amer. J. Med., 63:125–130, 1977.

Fibbe, W. E.; Van Damme, J.; Billiau, A.; Goselink, H. M.; Voogt, P. J.; vanEeden, G.; Ralph, P.; Altrock, B. W.; and Falkenberg, J. H.: Interleukin 1 induces human marrow stromal cells in long-term culture to produce granulocyte colony-stimulating factor and macrophage colony-stimulating factor. Blood, 71:430–435, 1988.

Fiddler, G. I.; and Lumley, P.: Preliminary clinical studies with thromboxane synthase inhibitors and thromboxane receptor blockers: A review. Circulation, 81 (suppl. I):I-69–I-78, 1990.

Fields, W. S.; Goldhaber, S. Z.; and Lewis, H. D.: Who should have prophylactic aspirin? Patient Care, 22:28–39, 1988.

Finch, C. A.: Erythropoiesis, erythropoietin and iron. Blood, 60:1241–1246, 1982.

Finch, C. A.; and Huebers, H.: Perspectives in iron metabolism. N. Engl. J. Med., 306:1520–1528, 1982.

Fischl, M.; Galpin, J. E.; Levine, J. D.; Groopman, J. E.; Henry, D. H.; Kennedy, P.; Miles, S.; Robbins, W.; Starrett, B.; Zalusky, R.; Abels, R. I.; Tsai, H. C.; and Rudnick, S. A.: Recombinant human erythropoietin for patients with AIDS treated with zidovudine. N. Engl. J. Med., 322:1488–1493, 1990.

FitzGerald, G. A.: Dipyridamole. N. Engl. J. Med., 316:1247–1255, 1987.

Fodstad, H.: Tranexamic acid (AMCA) in aneurysmal subarachnoid hemorrhage. J. Clin. Pathol., 33 (suppl. 14):68–73, 1980.

Foon, K. A.; Sherwin, S. A.; Abrams, P. G.; Longo, D. L.; Fer, M. F.; Stevenson, H. C.; Ochs, J. J.; Bottino, G. C.; Schoenberger, C. S.; Zeffren, J.; Jaffe, E. S.; and Oldham, R. K.: Treatment of advanced non-Hodgkin's lymphoma with recombinant leukocyte A interferon. N. Engl. J. Med., 311:1148–1152, 1984.

Foucar, K.; Langdon, R. M.; and Armitage, J. O.: Myelodysplastic syndromes: A clinical and pathologic analysis of 109 cases. Cancer, 56:553–561, 1985.

Francis, C. W.; and Marder, V. J.: Mechanisms of fibrinolysis. In, Hematology, 4th ed. (Williams, W. J.; Beutler, E.; Erslev, A. J.; Lichtman, M. A., eds.). McGraw-Hill Book Co., New York, pp. 1313–1321, 1990.

Francis, C. W.; Marder, V. J.; Evarts, M.; and Yaukoolbodi, S.: Two-step warfarin therapy: Prevention of post-operative venous thrombosis without excessive bleeding. J.A.M.A., 249:374–378, 1983.

Fukunaga, R.; Ishizaka-Ikeda, E.; Seto, Y.; and Nagata, S.: Expression cloning of a receptor for murine granulocyte colony-stimulating factor. Cell, 61:341–350, 1990.

Furie, B.; Diuguid, C. F.; Jacobs, M.; Diuguid, D. L.; and Furie, B. C.: Randomized prospective trial comparing the native prothrombin antigen with the prothrombin time for monitoring oral anticoagulant therapy. Blood, 75:344–349, 1990.

Gabrilove, J. L.; Jakubowski, A.; Scher, H.; Sternberg, C.; Wong, G.; Grous, J.; Yagoda, A.; Fain, K.; Moore, M. A. S.; Clarkson, B.; Oettgen, H. F.; Alton, K.; Welte, K.; and Souza, L.: Effect of granulocyte colony-stimulating factor on neutropenia and associated morbidity due to chemotherapy for transitional-cell carcinoma of the urothelium. N. Engl. J. Med., 318:1414–1422, 1988.

Gan, Z.-R.; Gould, R. J.; Jacobs, J. W.; Friedman, P. A.; and Polokoff, M. A.: Echistatin: A potent platelet aggregation inhibitor from the venom of the viper, Echis carinatus. J. Biol. Chem., 263:19827–19832, 1988.

Ganser, A.; Volkers, B.; Greher, J.; Ottmann, O. G.; Walther, F.; Becher, R.; Bergmann, L.; Schulz, G.; and Hoelzer, D.: Recombinant human granulocyte-macrophage colony-stimulating factor in patients with myelodysplastic syndromes — A phase I/II trial. Blood, 73:31–37, 1989.

Ganser, A.; Seipelt, G.; and Lindemann, A.: Effects of recombinant interleukin 3 in patients with myelodysplastic syndromes. Blood, 76:455–460, 1990.

Garcia, D. L.; Anderson, S.; Rennke, H. G.; and Brenner, B. M.: Anemia lessens and its prevention with recombinant human erythropoietin worsens glomerular injury and hypertension in rats with reduced renal mass. Proc. Natl. Acad. Sci. U.S.A., 85:6142–6146, 1988.

Gardner, F. H.; and Helmer, R. E.: Aminocaproic acid. Use in control of hemorrhage in patients with amegakaryocytic thrombocytopenia. J.A.M.A., 243:35–37, 1980.

Gasson, J. C.; Kaufman, S. E.; Weisbart, R. H.; Kaufman, S. E.; Clark, D. W.; Hewick, R. M.; Wong, G. G.; and Golde, D. W.: High-affinity binding of granulocyte-macrophage colony-stimulating factor to normal and leukemic human myeloid cells. Proc. Natl. Acad., Sci. U.S.A., 83: 669–673, 1986.

Gearing, D. P.; King, J. A.; Gough, N. M.; and Nicola, N. A.: Expression cloning of a receptor for human granulocyte-macrophage colony-stimulating factor. EMBO J., 8:3667–3676, 1989.

Gent, M.; Blakely, J. A.; Easton, J. D.; Ellis, D. J.; Hachinski, V. C.; Harbison, J. W.; Panak, E.; Roberts, R. S.; Sicurella, J.; Turpie, A. G. G.; and the CATS Group: The Canadian American Ticlopidine Study (CATS) in thromboembolic stroke. Lancet, 1:1215–1220, 1989.

George, J. N.; Nurden, A. T.; and Phillips, D. R.: Molecular defects in interactions of platelets with the vessel wall. N. Engl. J. Med., 311:1084–1098, 1984.

Gianni, A. M.; Bregni, M.; Siena, S.; Orazi, A.; Stern, A. C.; Gandola, L.; and Bonadonna, G.: Recombinant human granulocyte-macrophage colony-stimulating factor reduces hematologic toxicity and widens clinical applicability of high-dose cyclophosphamide treatment in breast cancer and non-Hodgkin's lymphoma. J. Clin. Oncol., 8:768–777, 1990.

Ginsberg, J. S.; Hirsh, J.; Turner, D. C.; Levine, M. N.; and Burrows, R.: Risks to the fetus of anticoagulant therapy during pregnancy. Thromb. Haemost., 61:197–203, 1989.

Glaspy, J. A.; Baldwin, G. C.; Robertson, P. A.; Souza, L.; Vincent, M.; Ambersley, J.; and Golde, D. W.: Therapy for neutropenia in hairy cell leukemia with recombinant human granulocyte colony-stimulating factor. Ann. Intern. Med., 109:789–795, 1988.

Glazier, R. L.; and Crowell, E. B.: Randomized prospective trial of continuous vs intermittent heparin therapy. J.A.M.A., 236: 1365–1367, 1976.

Goldhaber, S. Z.; Meyerovitz, M. F.; Green, D.; Vogelzang, R. L.; Citrin, P.; Heit, J.; Sobel, M.; Wheeler, H. B.; Plante, D.; Kim, H.; Hopkins, A.; Tufte, M.; Stump, D.; and Braunwald, E.: Randomized controlled trial of tissue plasminogen activator in proximal deep venous thrombosis. Am. J. Med., 88:235–240, 1990.

Goldhaber, S. Z.; Kessler, C. M.; Heit, J.; Markis, J.; Sharma, G. V. R. K.; Dawley, D.; Nagel, J. S.; Meyerovitz, M.; Kim, D.; Vaughan, D. E.; Parker, J. A.; Tumeh, S. S.; Drum, D.; Loscalzo, J.; Reagan, K.; Selwyn, A. P.; Anderson, J.; and Braunwald, E.: Randomised controlled trial of recombinant tissue plasminogen activator versus urokinase in the treatment of acute pulmonary embolism. Lancet, 2:293-298, 1988.

Goldman, J. M.; Th'ng, K. H.; and Lowenthal, R. M.: In vitro colony forming cells and colony stimulating factor in chronic granulocytic leukemia. Br. J. Cancer, 30:1-12, 1974.

Goldwasser, E.; Kung, C. K.; and Eliason, J.: On the mechanism of erythropoietin-induced differentiation: XIII. The role of sialic acid in erythropoietin action. J. Biol. Chem., 249:4202-4206, 1974.

Golomb, H.: The treatment of hairy cell leukemia. Blood, 69: 979-983, 1987.

Gomi, K.; Zushi, M.; Honda, G.; Kawahara, S.; Matsuzaki, O.; Kanabayashi, T.; Yamamoto, S.; Maruyama, I.; and Suzuki, K.: Antithrombotic effect of recombinant human thrombomodulin on thrombin-induced thromboembolism in mice. Blood, 75:1396-1399, 1990.

Gonda, T. J.; and Metcalf, D.: Expression of *myb*, *myc* and *fos* proto-oncogenes during the differentiation of a murine myeloid leukaemia. Nature, 310:249-251, 1984.

Gordon, L. I.; Miller, W. J.; Branda, R.; Zanjani, E.; and Jacob, H.: Regulation of erythroid colony formation by bone marrow macrophages. Blood, 55:1047-1050, 1980.

Gordon, M. Y.; Riley, G. P.; Watt, S. M.; and Greaves, M. F.: Compartmentalization of a haematopoietic growth factor (GM-CSF) by glycosaminoglycans in the bone marrow microenvironment. Nature, 326:403-405, 1987.

Greenberg, P. L.: In vitro culture techniques defining biologic abnormalities in the myelodysplastic syndromes and myeloproliferative disorders. Clin. Haematol., 15:973-993, 1986.

Greenberg, P. L.: The smoldering myeloid leukemic states: Clinical and biologic features. Blood, 61:1035-1044, 1983.

Greenberg, P. L.; and Mara, B.: The preleukemic syndrome: Correlation of in vitro parameters of granulopoiesis with clinical features. Am. J. Med., 66:951-958, 1979.

Greenberg, P. L.; and Mosny, S.: Cytotoxic effects of interferon in vitro on granulocytic progenitor cells. Cancer Res., 37:1794-1799, 1977.

Greenberg, P. L.; and Schrier, S. L.: Granulopoiesis in neutropenic disorders. Blood, 41:753-769, 1973.

Greenberg, P. L.; Mara, B.; Steed, S. M.; and Boxer, L.: The chronic idiopathic neutropenia syndromes: Correlation of clinical features with in vitro parameters of granulocytopoiesis. Blood, 55:915-921, 1980.

Greenberg, P. L.; Mara, B.; Bax, I.; Brossel, R.; and Schrier, S.: The myeloproliferative disorders: Correlation between clinical evolution and alterations of granulopoiesis. Am. J. Med., 61:878-891, 1976a.

Greenberg, P. L.; Bax, I.; Levin, J.; and Andrews, T. M.: Alteration of colony stimulating factor output endotoxemia and granulopoiesis in cyclic neutropenia. Am. J. Hematol., 1:275-385, 1976b.

Gresele, P.; Deckmyn, H.; Arnout, J.; Nenci, G. G.; and Vermylen, J.: Characterization of N,N-bis(3-picolyl)-4-methoxy-isophtalamide (picotamide) as a dual thromboxane synthase inhibitor/thromboxane A_2 receptor antagonist in human platelets. Thromb. Haemost., 61:479-484, 1989.

Griffen, J. D.: Clinical applications of colony stimulating factors. Oncology, 2:15-21, 1988.

Griffin, J. D.; and Ellman, L.: Epsilon-aminocaproic acid (EACA). Semin. Thromb. Hemost., 5:27-40, 1978.

Griffin, J. D.; Rambaldi, A.; Vellenga, E.; Young, D. C.; Ostapovicz, D.; and Cannistra, S. A.: Secretion of interleukin-1 by acute myeloblastic leukemia cells in vitro induces endothelial cells to secrete colony stimulating factors. Blood, 70: 1218-1221, 1987.

Groopman, J. E.; Mitsuyasu, R. T.; Deleo, M. J.; Oette, D. H.; and Golde, D. W.: Effect of recombinant human granulocyte-macrophage colony-stimulating factor on myelopoiesis in the acquired immunodeficiency syndrome. N. Engl. J. Med., 317:593-598, 1987.

Grotendorst, G. R.; Smale, G.; and Pencev, D.: Production of transforming growth factor beta by human peripheral blood monocytes and neutrophils. J. Cell. Physiol., 140:396-402, 1989.

Gruber, A.; Hanson, S. R.; Kelly, A. B.; Yan, B. S.; Bang, N.; Griffin, J. H.; and Harker, L. A.: Inhibition of thrombus formation by activated recombinant protein C in a primate model of arterial thrombosis. Circulation, 82:578-585, 1990.

Gruppo Italiano per lo studio della sopravvenza nell'infarto miocardico GISSI-2: A factorial randomised trial of alteplase versus streptokinase and heparin versus no heparin among 12,490 patients with acute myocardial infarction. Lancet, 2: 65-71, 1990.

Gruppo Italiano per lo studio della streptochinasi nell'infarto miocardico (GISSI): Effectiveness of intravenous thrombolytic treatment in acute myocardial infarction. Lancet, 1:397-402, 1986.

Guerry, D. W.; Dale, D. C.; Omine, M.; Perry, S.; and Wolff, S. M.: Periodic hematopoiesis in human cyclic neutropenia. J. Clin. Invest., 53:3220-3230, 1973.

Gurewich, V.: Pro-urokinase: Physiochemical properties and promotion of its fibrinolytic activity by urokinase and by tissue plasminogen activator with which it has a complementary mechanism of action. Semin. Thromb. Hemost., 14:110-115, 1988.

Haber, E.; Quertermous, T.; Matsueda, G. R.; and Runge, M. S.: Innovative approaches to plasminogen activator therapy. Science, 243:51-56, 1989.

Hall, J. A. G.; Pauli, R. M.; and Wilson, K. M.: Maternal and fetal sequelae of anticoagulation during pregnancy. Am. J. Med., 68:122-140, 1980.

Hammond, W. P. IV; Price, T. H.; Souza, L. M.; and Dale, D. C.: Treatment of cyclic neutropenia with granulocyte colony-stimulating factor. N. Engl. J. Med., 320:1306-1311, 1989.

Hanson, S. R.; and Harker, L. A.: Interruption of acute platelet-dependent thrombosis by the synthetic antithrombin D-phenylalanyl-L-prolyl-L-arginyl chloromethyl ketone. Proc. Natl. Acad. Sci. U.S.A., 85:3184-3188, 1988.

Harenberg, J.; and Heene, D. L.: Pharmacology and special clinical applications of low-molecular-weight heparins. Am. J. Hematol., 29:233-240, 1988.

Harenberg, J.; Zimmerman, R.; Schwarz, F.; and Kubler, W.: Treatment of heparin-induced thrombocytopenia with thrombosis by new heparinoid. Lancet, 1:986-987, 1983.

Hass, W. K.; Easton, J. D.; Adams, H. P. Jr.; Pryse-Phillips, W.; Molony, B. A.; Anderson, S.; and Kamm, B.: A randomized trial comparing ticlopidine hydrochloride with aspirin for the prevention of stroke in high-risk patients. N. Engl. J. Med., 321:501-507, 1989.

Herrmann, F.; Lindemann, A.; Klein, H.; Lubbert, M.; Schulz, G.; and Mertelsmann, R.: Effect of recombinant granulocyte-macrophage colony-stimulating factor in patients with myelodysplastic syndrome with excess blasts. Leukemia, 3: 335-338, 1989.

Herrmann, F.; Oster, W.; Meuer, S. C.; Lindemann, A.; and Mertelsmann, R. H.: Interleukin-1 stimulates T lymphocytes to produce granulocyte-monocyte colony-stimulating factor. J. Clin. Invest., 81:1415-1418, 1988.

Hess, H.; Mietaschk, A.; and Deichsel, G.: Drug-induced inhibition of platelet function delays progression of peripheral occlusive arterial disease: A prospective double-blind arteriographically controlled trial. Lancet, 1:415-419, 1985.

Heysel, R. M.: Vitamin B_{12} turnover in man — the assimilation of vitamin B_{12} from natural foodstuff by man and estimates of minimal daily dietary requirements. Am. J. Clin. Nutr., 18:176-184, 1966.

Hill, R. J.; Warren, M. K.; and Levin, J.: Stimulation of thrombopoiesis in mice by human recombinant interleukin 6. J. Clin. Invest., 85:1242-1247, 1990.

Hirsh, J.; and Levine, M. N.: The optimal intensity of oral anticoagulant therapy. J.A.M.A., 258:2723-2726, 1987.

Hirsh, J.; Marder, V. J.; Salzman, E. W.; and Hull, R. D.: Treatment of venous thromboembolism. In, Hemostasis and Thrombosis: Basic Principles and Clinical Practice, 2nd ed. (Colman, R. W.; Hirsh, J.; Marder, V. J.; Salzman, E. W., eds.). J. B. Lippincott Co., Philadelphia, pp. 1266-1272, 1987.

Hirsh, J.; van Aken, W. G.; Gallus, A. S.; Dollery, C. T.; Cade, J. F.; and Yung, W. L.: Heparin kinetics in venous thrombosis and pulmonary embolism. Circulation, 53:691–695, 1976.

Hoffbrand, A. V.; and Necheles, T. F.: Mechanisms of folate deficiency in patients receiving phenytoin. Lancet, 2:528–530, 1968.

Huebers, H. A.; and Finch, C. A.: Transferrin: Physiologic behavior and clinical applications. Blood, 64:763–767, 1984.

Hull, R. D.; Raskob, G. E.; Rosenbloom, D.; Panju, A. A.; Brill-Edwards, P.; Ginsberg, J. S.; Hirsh, J.; Martin, G. J.; and Green, D.: Heparin for 5 days as compared with 10 days in the initial treatment of proximal venous thrombosis. N. Engl. J. Med., 322:1260–1264, 1990.

Hull, R.; Delmore, T.; Carter, C.; Hirsh, J.; Genton, E.; Gent, M.; Turpie, G.; and McLaughlin, D.: Adjusted subcutaneous heparin versus warfarin sodium in the long-term treatment of venous thrombosis. N. Engl. J. Med., 306:189–194, 1982a.

Hull, R.; Hirsh, J.; Jay, R.; Carter, C.; England, C.; Gent, M.; Turpie, A. G. G.; McLoughlin, D.; Dodd, P.; Thomas, M.; Raskob, G.; and Ockelford, P.: Different intensities of oral anticoagulant therapy in the treatment of proximal-vein thrombosis. N. Engl. J. Med., 307:1676–1681, 1982b.

Hull, R.; Delmore, T.; Genton, E.; Hirsh, J.; Gent, M.; Sackett, D.; McLoughlin, D.; and Armstrong, P.: Warfarin sodium versus low-dose heparin in the long-term treatment of venous thrombosis. N. Engl. J. Med., 301:855–858, 1979.

Ikebuchi, K.; Wong, G. G.; Clark, S. C.; Ihle, J. N.; Hirai, Y.; and Ogawa, M.: Interleukin 6 enhancement of interleukin 3-dependent proliferation of multipotential hemopoietic progenitors. Proc. Natl. Acad. Sci. U.S.A., 84:9035–9039, 1987.

Ishibashi, T.; Kimura, H.; Shikama, Y. H.; Uchida, T.; Kariyone, S.; Hirano, T.; Kishimoto, T.; Takatsuki, F.; and Akiyama, Y.: Interleukin-6 is a potent thrombopoietic factor in vivo in mice. Blood, 74:1241–1244, 1989.

ISIS-2 (Second International Study of Infarct Survival) Collaborative Group: Randomised trial of intravenous streptokinase, oral aspirin, both or neither among 17,187 cases of suspected myocardial infarction. Lancet, 2:349–360, 1988.

Itoh, N.; Yonehara, S.; Schreurs, J.; Gorman, D. M.; Maruyama, K.; Ishii, A.; Yahara, I.; Arai, K.-I.; and Miyajima, A.: Cloning of an interleukin-3 receptor gene: A member of a distinct receptor gene family. Science, 247:324–327, 1990.

Iturbe-Alessio, I.; del Carmen Fonseca, M.; Mutchinik, O.; Santos, M. A.; Zajarias, A.; and Salazar, E.: Risks of anticoagulant therapy in pregnant women with artificial heart valves. N. Engl. J. Med., 315:1390–1393, 1986.

Jacobs, R. H.; Cornbleet, M. A.; Vardiman, J. W.; Larson, R. A.; LeBeau, M. M.; and Rowley, J. F.: Prognostic implications of morphology and karyotype in primary myelodysplastic syndromes. Blood, 67:1765–1772, 1986.

Jacobs, K.; Shoemaker, C.; Rudersdorf, R.; Neill, S. D.; Kaufman, R. J.; Mufson, A.; Seehra, J.; Jones, S. S.; Hewick, R.; Fritsch, E. F.; Kawakita, M.; Shimizu, T.; and Miyake, T.: Isolation and characterization of genomic and cDNA clones of human erythropoietin. Nature, 313:806–810, 1985.

Jalkanen, S.; Bargatze, R. F.; de los Toyos, J.; and Butcher, E. C.: Lymphocyte recognition of high endothelium: Antibodies to distinct epitopes of an85-95-kD glycoprotein antigen differentially inhibit lymphocyte binding to lymph node, mucosal, or synovial endothelial cells. J. Cell. Biol., 105:983–990, 1987.

Jang, I.-K.; Gold, H. K.; Ziskind, A. A.; Leinbach, R. C.; Fallon, J. T.; and Collen, D.: Prevention of platelet-rich arterial thrombosis by selective thrombin inhibition. Circulation, 81:219–225, 1990.

Janssen, J. W. G.; Buschle, M.; Layton, M.; Drexler, H. G.; Lyons, J.; van den Berghe, H.; Heimpel, H.; Kubanek, B.; Kleihauer, E.; Mufti, G. J.; and Bartram, C. R.: Clonal analysis of myelodysplastic syndrome: Evidence of multipotent stem cell origin. Blood, 73:248–254, 1989.

Jaques, L. B.: Heparin: A unique misunderstood drug. Trends Pharmacol. Sci., 3:289–291, 1982.

Johnson, C. S.; Keckleer, D. J.; Topper, M. C.; Braunschwei-

ger, P. G.; and Furmanski, P.: In vivo hematopoietic effects of recombinant interleukin-1 alpha in mice: Stimulation of granulocytic, monocytic, megakaryocytic, and early erythroid progenitors, suppression of late-stage erythropoiesis, and reversal of erythroid suppression with erythropoietin. Blood, 73:678–683, 1989.

Kaiser, B.; Simon, A.; and Markwardt, F.: Antithrombotic effects of recombinant hirudin in experimental angioplasty and intravascular thrombolysis. Thromb. Haemost., 63:44–47, 1990.

Kakkar, V. V.; and Murray, W. J. G.: Efficacy and safety of low-molecular weight heparin (CY 216) in preventing postoperative venous thromboembolism: A cooperative study. Br. J. Surg., 72:786–791, 1985.

Kakkar, V. V.; Corrigan, T. P.; and Fossard, D. P.: Prevention of fatal post-operative pulmonary embolism by low doses of heparin: An international multicentre trial. Lancet, 2:45–51, 1975.

Kasper, C. K.: Treatment of factor VIII inhibitors. Prog. Hemost. Thromb., 9:57–86, 1989.

Kasper, C. K.; and Dietrich, S. L.: Comprehensive management of haemophilia. Clin. Haematol., 14:489–512, 1985.

Kastan, M. B.; Stone, K. D.; and Civin, C. I.: Nuclear oncoprotein expression as a function of lineage, differentiation stage, and proliferative status of normal human hematopoietic cells. Blood, 74:1517–1524, 1989.

Kaushansky, K.; Lin, N.; and Adamson, J. W.: Interleukin 1 stimulates fibroblasts to synthesize granulocyte-macrophage and granulocyte colony-stimulating factors. J. Clin. Invest., 81:92–97, 1988.

Kawasaki, E. S.; Ladner, M. B.; Wang, A. W.; Van Arsdell, J.; Warren, M. K.; Coyne, M. Y.; Schweickart, V. L.; Lee, M. T.; Wilson, K. J.; Boosman, A.; Stanley, E. R.; Ralph, P.; and Mark, D. F.: Molecular cloning of a complementary DNA encoding human macrophage-specific colony-stimulating factor (CSF-1). Science, 230:291–296, 1985.

Kimchi, A.: Autocrine interferon and the suppression of the c-*myc* nuclear oncogene. Interferon, 8:86–110, 1987.

Kishimoto, T.: The biology of interleukin 6. Blood, 74:1–10, 1989.

Kojima, S.; Fukuda, M.; Miyajima, Y.; Mutsayama, T.; and Horibe, K.: Treatment of aplastic anemia in children with recombinant G-CSF. Blood, 77:937–941, 1991.

Knudsen, J. B.; Kjoller, E.; Skagen, K.; and Gormsen, J.: The effect of ticlopidine on platelet functions in acute myocardial infarction: A double-blind controlled trial. Thromb. Haemost., 53:332–336, 1985.

Koeffler, H. P.; Hetjan, D.; Mertelsmann, R.; Kolitz, J. E.; Schulman, P.; Itri, L.; Gunter, P.; and Besa, E.: Randomized study of 13-*cis* retinoic acid vs. placebo in the myelodysplastic disorders. Blood, 71:703–708 1988.

Koike, K.; Nakahata, T.; Takagi, M.; Kobayashi, T.; Ishiguro, A.; Tsuji, K.; Naganuma, K.; Okano, A.; Akiyama, Y.; and Akabane, T.: Synergism of BSF-2/interleukin 6 and interleukin 3 on development of multipotential hemopoietic progenitors in serum-free culture. J. Exp. Med., 168:879–890, 1988.

Koller, M.; Schoch, U.; Buchmann, P.; Largiader, F.; von Felten, A.; and Frick, P. G.: Low molecular weight heparin (KABI 2165) as thromboprophylaxis in elective visceral surgery: A randomized, double blind study versus unfractionated heparin. Thromb. Haemost., 56:243–246, 1986.

Kostmann, R.: Infantile genetic agranulocytosis: A review with presentation of ten new cases. Acta Paediatr. Scand., 64:362–368, 1975.

Krown, S. E.; Real, F. X.; Cunningham-Rundles, S.; Myskowski, P. L.; Koziner, B.; Fein, S.; Mittelman, A.; Oettgen, H. F.; and Safai, B.: Prelimianry observations on the effect of recombinant leukocyte A interferon in homosexual men with Kaposi's sarcoma. N. Engl. J. Med., 308:1071–1076, 1983.

Kumar, S.; Haigh, J. R. M.; Rhodes, L. E.; Peaker, S.; Davies, J. A.; Roberts, B. E.; and Feely, M. P.: Poor compliance is a major factor in unstable outpatient control of anticoagulant therapy. Thromb. Haemost., 62:729–732, 1989.

Kumon, K.; Tanaka, K.; Nakajima, N.; Naito, Y.; and Fujita,

T.: Anticoagulation with a synthetic thrombin inhibitor after cardiovascular surgery and for treatment of disseminated intravascular coagulation. Crit. Care Med., 12:1039–1043, 1984.

Kurtz, A.; Hartl, W.; Helkmann, W.; Zaft, J.; and Bauer, C.: Activity in fetal bovine serum that stimulates erythroid colony formation in fetal mouse livers in insulin-like growth factor. J. Clin. Invest., 76:1643–1648, 1985.

Kurtz, A.; Jelkmann, W.; and Bauer, C.: Insulin stimulates erythroid colony formation independently of erythropoiesis. Br. J. Haematol., 53:311–316, 1983.

Kutner, B.; Fourman, S.; Brein, K.; Hobson, S.; Mrvos, D.; Sheppard, J.; and Weisman, S.: Aminocaproic acid reduces the risk of secondary hemorrhage in patients with traumatic hyphema. Arch. Ophthalmol., 105:206–208, 1987.

Lacombe, C.; Da Silva, J.-L.; Bruneval, P.; Fournier, J.-G.; Wendling, F.; Casadevall, N.; Camilleri, J.-P.; Bariety, J.; Varet, B.; and Tambourin, P.: Peritubular cells are the site of erythropoietin synthesis in the murine hypoxic kidney. J. Clin. Invest., 81:620–623, 1988.

Lam, L. H.; Silbert, J. E.; and Rosenberg, R. D.: The separation of active and inactive forms of heparin. Biochem. Biophys. Res. Commun., 69:570–577, 1976.

Landefeld, C. S.; and Goldman, L.: Major bleeding in outpatients treated with warfarin: Incidence and prediction by factors known at the start of outpatient therapy. Am. J. Med., 87:144–152, 1989.

Lane, F.; Goff, P.; McGuffin, R.; Eichner, E. R.; and Hillman, R. S.: Folic acid metabolism in normal, folate deficient and alcoholic man. Br. J. Haematol., 34:489–500, 1976.

Leary, A. G.; Ikebuchi, K.; Hirai, Y.; Wong, G. G.; Yang, Y. C.; Clark, S. C.; Ogawa, M.; and VA Medical Center, Charleston, S.C.: Synergism between interleukin 6 and interleukin 3 in supporting proliferation of human hemopoietic stem cells: Comparison with interleukin 1α. Blood, 71:1759–1763, 1988.

Le Beau, M. M.; Albain, K. S.; Larson, R. A.; Vardiman, J. W.; Davis, E. M.; Blough, R. R.; Golomb, H. M.; and Rowley, J. D.: Clinical and cytogenetic correlations in 63 patients with therapy-related myelodysplastic syndromes and acute non-lymphocytic leukemia: Further evidence for characteristic abnormalities of chromosomes no. 5 and 7. J. Clin. Oncol., 4:325–345, 1986a.

Le Beau, M. M.; Westbrook, C. A.; Diaz, M. O.; Larson, R. A.; Rowley, J. D.; Gasson, J. C.; Golde, D. W.; and Sherr, C. J.: Evidence for the involvement of GM-CSF and fms in the deletion (5q) in myeloid disorders. Science, 231:984–987, 1986b.

Lee, T. H.; Weisberg, M. C.; Brand, D. A.; Rouan, G. W.; and Goldman, L.: Candidates for thrombolysis among emergency room patients with acute chest pain: Potential true- and false-positive rates. Ann. Intern. Med., 110:957–962, 1989.

Lee, F.; Yokota, T.; Otsuka, T.; Gemmell, L.; Larson, N.; Lun, J.; Arai, K.; Rennick, D.; and DNAX Research Institute of Molecular & Cellular Biology, Palo Alto, CA: Isolation of a cDNA for a human granulocyte-macrophage colony-stimulating factor by functional expression in mammalian cells. Proc. Natl. Acad. Sci. U.S.A., 82:4360–4364, 1985.

Lee-Huang, S.: Cloning and expression of human erythropoietin cDNA in *Escherichia coli*. Proc. Natl. Acad. Sci. U.S.A., 81:2708–2712, 1984.

Levine, M. N.; and Hirsh, J.: Clinical use of low molecular weight heparins and heparinoids. Semin. Thromb. Hemost., 14:116–125, 1988.

Levine, M. N.; Hirsh, J.; and Kelton, J. G.: Hemorrhagic complications of antithrombotic therapy. In, Hemostasis and Thrombosis: Basic Principles and Clinical Practice, 2nd ed. (Colman, R. W.; Hirsh, J.; Marder, V. J.; Salzman, E. W., eds.). J. B. Lippincott Co., Philadelphia, pp. 873–885, 1987.

Lewinsohn, D.; Nagler, A.; Greenberg, P.; and Butcher, E.: Hemopoietic progenitor cell expression of the H-CAM (CD44) homing associated adhesion molecule. Blood, 75:589–595, 1990.

Lewis, H. D. Jr.; Davis, J. W.; Archibald, D. G.; Steinke, W. E.; Smitherman, T. C.; Doherty, J. E.; Schnaper, H. W.;

LeWinter, M. M.; Linares, E.; Pouget, J. M.; Sabharwal, S. C.; Chesler, E.; and DeMots, H.: Protective effects of aspirin against acute myocardial infarction and death in men with unstable angina. Results of a Veterans Administration cooperative study. N. Engl. J. Med., 309:396–403, 1983.

Lieschke, G. J.; Cebon, J.; and Mortsyn, G.: Characterization of the clinical effects after the first dose of bacterially synthesized recombinant human granulocyte-macrophage colony-stimulating factor. Blood, 74:2634–2643, 1989a.

Lieschke, G. J.; Maher, D.; Cebon, J.; O'Connor, M.; Green, M.; Sheridan, W.; Boyd, A.; Rallings, M.; Bonnem, E.; Metcalf, D.; Burgess, A. W.; McGrath, K.; Fox, R. M.; and Morstyn, G.: Effects of bacterially synthesized recombinant human granulocyte-macrophage colony-stimulating factor in patients with advanced malignancy. Ann. Intern. Med., 110:357–364, 1989b.

Lim, V. S.; DeGowin, R. L.; Zavala, D.; Kirchner, P.; Abels, R.; Perry, P.; and Fangman, J.: Recombinant human erythropoeitin treatment in pre-dialysis patients. A double-blind placebo controlled trial. Ann. Intern. Med., 110:108–114, 1989.

Lin, F.-K.; Suggs, S.; Lin, C.-H.; Browne, J. K.; Smalling, R.; Egrie, J. C.; Chen, K. K.; Fox, G. M.; Martin, F.; Stablinsky, Z.; Badrawi, S. M.; Lai, P. H.; and Goldwasser, E.: Cloning and expression of the human erythropoietin gene. Proc. Natl. Acad. Sci. U.S.A., 82:7580–7584, 1985.

Lipschitz, D. A.; Cook, J. D.; and Finch, C. A.: A clinical evaluation of serum ferritin as an index of iron stores. N. Engl. J. Med., 290:1213–1216, 1974.

Lipsky, J. J.: N-methyl-thio-tetrazole inhibition of the gamma carboxylation of glutamic acid: Possible mechanism for antibiotic-associated hypoprothrombinaemia. Lancet, 2:192–193, 1983.

Lipton, J. M.; Kudish, M.; and Nathan, D. G.: Response of three classes of human erythroid progenitors to the absence of erythropoietin in vitro as a measure of progenitor maturity. Exp. Hematol., 9:1035–1041, 1981.

Litt, M. R.; Bell, W. R.; and Lepor, H. A.: Disseminated intravascular coagulation in prostatic carcinoma reversed by ketoconazole. J.A.M.A., 258:1361–1362, 1987.

Livio, M.; Mannucci, P. M.; Vigano, G.; Mingardi, G.; Lombardi, R.; Mecca, G.; and Remuzzi, G.: Conjugated estrogens for the management of bleeding associated with renal failure. N. Engl. J. Med., 315:731–735, 1986.

Loeliger, E. A.; van den Besselaar, A. M. H. P.; and Lewis, S. M.: Reliability and clinical impact of the normalization of the prothrombin times in oral anticoagulant control. Thromb. Haemost., 53:148–154, 1985.

Lofvenberg, E.; and Wahlin, A.: Management of polycythaemia vera, essential thrombocythemia and myelofibrosis with hydroxyurea. Eur. J. Haematol., 41:375–381, 1988.

Long, M. W.; Hutchinson, R. J.; Gragowski, L. L.; Heffner, C. H.; and Emerson, S. G.: Synergistic regulation of human megakaryocyte development. J. Clin. Invest., 82:1779–1786, 1988.

Loscalzo, J.; and Braunwald, E.: Tissue plasminogen activator. N. Engl. J. Med., 319:925–931, 1988.

Lotem, J.; and Sachs, L.: Control of in vivo differentiation of myeloid leukemia cells: IV. Inhibition of leukemia development by myeloid differentiation-inducing protein. Int. J. Cancer, 33:147–154, 1984.

Lotem, J.; and Sachs, L.: Mechanisms that uncouple growth and differentiation in myeloid leukemia cells: Restoration of requirement for normal growth-inducing protein without restoring induction of differentiation-inducing protein. Proc. Natl. Acad. Sci. U.S.A., 79:4347–4351, 1982.

Lotem, J.; and Sachs, L.: In vivo inhibition of the development of myeloid leukemia by injection of macrophage and granulocyte-inducing protein. Int. J. Cancer, 28:375–386, 1981.

Ludwig, H.; Fritz, E.; Kotzmann, H.; Hocker, P.; Gisslinger, H.; and Barnas, U.: Erythropoietin treatment for chronic anemia of malignancy. Blood, 74(suppl. 1):16a, 1989.

Lutton, J. D.; and Levere, R. D.: Endogenous erythroid colony formation by peripheral blood mononuclear cells from patients with myelofibrosis and polycythaemia vera. Acta Hematol., 62:94–99, 1979.

Mandelli, F.; Avrisati, G.; Amadori, S.; Boccadoro, M.; Gernone, A.; Lauta, V. M.; Marmont, F.; Petrucci, M. T.; Tribalto, M.; Vegna, M. L.; Dammacco, F.; and Pileri, A.: Maintenance treatment with recombinant interferon alpha-2b in patients with multiple myeloma responding to conventional induction chemotherapy. N. Engl. J. Med., 322:1430–1434, 1990.

Mangan, K. F.; Chikkappa, K. F.; Bieler, L. Z.; Scharfman, W. B.; and Parkinson, D. R.: Regulation of human blood erythroid burst-forming unit proliferation by T-lymphocyte subpopulations. Blood, 59:990–996, 1982.

Mannucci, P. M.: Desmopressin: A non-transfusional form of treatment of congenital and acquired bleeding disorders. Blood, 72:1449–1455, 1988.

Mannucci, P. M.; Vicente, V.; Alberca, I.; Sacchi, E; Longo, G.; Harris, A. S.; and Lindquist, A.: Intravenous and subcutaneous administration of desmopressin (DDAVP) to hemophiliacs: Pharmacokinetics and factor VIII responses. Thromb. Haemost., 58:1037–1039, 1987.

Marciniak, E.; and Gockerman, J. P.: Heparin-induced decrease in circulating antithrombin III. Lancet, 2:581–584, 1977.

Marciniak, E.; Farley, C. H.; and DeSimone, P. A.: Familial thrombosis due to antithrombin III deficiency. Blood, 43: 219–231, 1974.

Marder, V. J.; and Bell, W. R.: Fibrinolytic therapy. In, Hemostasis and Thrombosis: Basic Principles and Clinical Practice, 2nd ed. (Colman, R. W.; Hirsh, J.; Marder, V. J.; Salzman, E. W., eds.). J. B. Lippincott Co., New York, pp. 1393–1437, 1987.

Marder, V. J.; and Francis, C. W.: Clinical aspects of fibrinolysis. In, Hematology, 4th ed. (Williams, W. J.; Beutler, E.; Erslev, A. J.; Lichtman, M. A., eds.). McGraw-Hill Book Co., New York, pp. 1543–1558, 1990.

Marder, V. J.; and Sherry, S.: Thrombolytic therapy: Current status (parts 1 and 2). N. Engl. J. Med., 318:1512–1520, 1585–1595, 1988.

Marder, V. J.; Rothbard, R. L.; Fitzpatrick, P. G.; and Francis, C. W.: Rapid lysis of coronary artery thrombi with anisoylated plasminogen: Streptokinase activator complex: Treatment by bolus intravenous injection. Ann. Intern. Med., 104:304–310, 1986.

Markwardt, F.: Pharmacology of hirudin: One hundred years after the first report of the anticoagulant agent in medicinal leeches. Biomed. Biochim. Acta, 44:1007–1013, 1985.

Markwardt, F.; Kaiser, B.; and Nowak, G.: Studies on antithrombotic effects of recombinant hirudin. Thromb. Res., 54:377–388, 1989.

Martinez, J. F. T.; Redondo, M. D. T.; Silva, I. A.; and Lopez-Borrasca, A.: Disseminated intravascular coagulation in prostatic carcinoma reversed by anti-androgenic therapy. J.A.M.A., 260:2507, 1988.

Masaoka, T.; Motoyoshi, K.; Takaku, F.; Kato, S.; Harada, M.; Kodera, Y.; Kanamaru, A.; Moriyama, Y.; Ohno, R.; Ohria, M.; Shibata, H.; and Inoue, T.: Administration of human urinary colony stimulating factor after bone marrow transplantation: Overall findings. Bone Marrow Transplant., 3:121–7 1988.

Massague, J.: The TGF-beta family of growth and differentiation factors. Cell, 49:437–438, 1987.

McLean, J.: The thromboplastic action of cephalin. Am. J. Physiol., 41:250–257, 1916.

McMillan, R.; Tani, P.; Millard, F.; Berchtold, P.; Renshaw, L.; and Woods, V. L.: Platelet-associated and plasma antiglycoprotein autoantibodies in chronic ITP. Blood, 70:1040–1045, 1987.

McNamara, T. O.: Role of thrombolysis in peripheral arterial occlusion. Am. J. Med., 83 (suppl. 2A):6–10, 1987.

McNiece, I. K.; Bertoncello, I.; Kriegler, A. B.; and Quesenberry, P. J.: Colony-forming cells with high proliferative potential (HPP-CFC). Int. J. Cell Clon., 8:146–160, 1990.

Means, R. T. Jr.; Olsen, N. J.; Krantz, S. B.; Dessypris, E. N.; Graber, S. E.; Stone, W. J.; O'Neil, V. L.; and Pincus, T.: Treatment of the anemia of rheumatoid arthritis with recombinant human erythropoietin: Clinical and in vitro trials. Arthritis Rheum., 32:638–642, 1989.

Menache, D.; O'Malley, J. P.; Schorr, J. B.; Wagner, B.; Williams, C.; and the Cooperative Study Group (Alving, B. M.; Ballard, J. O.; Goodnight, S. H.; Hathaway, W. E.; Hultin, M. B.; Kitchens, C. S.; Lessner, H. E.; Makary, A. Z.; Manco-Johnson, M.; McGehee, W. G.; Penner, J. A.; and Sanders, J. E.): Evaluation of the safety, recovery, half-life, and clinical efficacy of antithrombin III (human) in patients with hereditary antithrombin III deficiency. Blood, 75:33–39, 1990.

Mertelsmann, R.; Tzvi Thaler, T.; To, L.; Gee, T. S.; McKenzie, S.; Schauer, P.; Friedman, A.; Arline, Z.; Cirrincione, C.; and Clarkson, B.: Morphological classification, response to therapy and survival in 263 adult patients with acute non-lymphoblastic leukemia. Blood, 56:773–781, 1980.

Metcalf, D.: Haemopoietic growth factors. Lancet, 1:825–827, 1989.

Metcalf, D.: Regulator-induced suppression of myelomonocytic leukemic cells: Clonal analysis of early cellular events. Int. J. Cancer, 30:203–210, 1982.

Metcalf, D.: The molecular biology and functions of the granulocyte-macrophage colony-stimulating factors. Blood, 67:257–267, 1986.

Metcalf, D.: Human leukemia: Recent tissue culture studies on the nature of myeloid leukemia. Br. J. Cancer, 27:191–202, 1973.

Metcalf, D.; Moore, M.; and Sheridan, J.: Responsiveness of human granulocytic leukemic cells to colony-stimulating factor. Blood, 43:847–859, 1974.

Miles, S.; Glaspy, J.; and Chung, Y.: Recombinant granulocyte colony stimulating factor (r-met HuG-CSF) increase neutrophil number and function but does not alter HIV expression in patients with AIDS (abstract). In, V International Conference on AIDS: The Scientific and Social Challenge. Montreal, p. 558, 1989.

Miller, G. A. H.; Hall, R. J. C.; and Paneth, M.: Pulmonary embolectomy, heparin, and streptokinase: Their place in the treatment of acute massive pulmonary embolism. Am. Heart J., 93:568–574, 1977.

Miller, K.; Kim, K.; and Morrison, F.: Evaluation of low dose ara C vs. supportive care in the treatment of myelodysplastic syndrome. Blood, 72 (suppl. 1): 215a, 1988.

Mintz, U.; and Sachs, L.: Normal granulocyte colony-forming cells in the bone marrow of Yemenite Jews with genetic neutropenia. Blood, 41:745–751, 1973.

Mitsuyasu, R.; Levine, J.; Miles, S. A.; DeLeo, M.; Oette, D.; Golde, D.; and Groopman, J.: Effects of long term subcutaneous (sc) administration of recombinant granulocyte-macrophage colony-stimulating factor (GM-CSF) in patients with HIV-related leukopenia. Blood, 72(suppl. 1):356a, 1988.

Miyake, T.; Kung, C. K.; and Goldwasser, E.: Purification of human erythropoietin. J. Biol. Chem., 252:5558–5564, 1977.

Moore, M.; and Warren, D. J.: Synergy of interleukin 1 and granulocyte colony stimulating factor: In vivo stimulation of stem-cell recovery and hemopoietic regeneration following 5-fluorouracil treatment of mice. Proc. Natl. Acad. Sci. U.S.A., 84:7134–7138, 1987.

Moore, M.; Williams, N.; and Metcalf, D.: In vitro colony formation by normal and leukemic human hemopoietic cells. Characterization of the colony forming cells. J. Natl. Cancer Inst., 50:603–623, 1973.

Mortsyn, G.; Campbell, L.; Souza, L. M.; Alton, N. K.; Keech, J.; Green, M.; Sheridan, W.; Metcalf, D.; and Fox, R.: Effect of granulocyte colony stimulating factor on neutropenia induced by cytotoxic chemotherapy. Lancet, 1:667–672, 1988.

Munker, R.; Gasson, J.; Ogawa, M.; and Koeffler, H. P.: Recombinant human TNF induces production of granulocyte-monocyte colony-stimulating factor. Nature, 323:79–82, 1986.

Murase, T.; Hotta, T.; Saito, H.; and Ohno, R.: Effect of recombinant human tumor necrosis factor on the colony growth of human leukemia progenitor cells and normal hematopoietic progenitor cells. Blood, 69:467–472, 1987.

Naeye, R. L.: Thrombotic state after a hemorrhagic diathesis, a possible complication of therapy with epsilon-aminocaproic acid. Blood, 19:694–701, 1962.

Nagler, A.; Ginzton, N.; Bangs, C.; Donlon, T.; and Greenberg, P. L.: In vitro differentiative and proliferative effects of human recombinant colony stimulating factors on marrow hemopoiesis in myelodysplastic syndromes. Leukemia, 4: 193–202, 1990a.

Nagler, A.; Mackichan, M. L.; Negrin, R.; Bangs, C.; Donlon, T.; and Greenberg, P.: Impact of marrow cytogenetics and morphology on in vitro hemopoiesis in the myelodysplastic syndromes: Comparison between recombinant human granulocyte colony stimulating factor and granulocyte-monocyte colony stimulating factor. Blood, 76:1299–1307, 1990b.

Najean, Y.; and Pecking, A.: Refractory anemia with excess of myeloblasts in the bone marrow: A clinical trial of androgens in 90 patients. Br. J. Haematol., 37:25–33, 1977.

Nath, B. J.; and Lindenbaum, J.: Persistence of neutrophil hypersegmentation during recovery from megaloblastic granulopoiesis. Ann. Intern. Med., 90:757–760, 1979.

Nathan, C. F.; Kaplan, G.; Levis, W. R.; Nusrat, A.; Witner, M. D.; Sherwin, S. A.; Job, C. K.; Path, F. R. C.; Horowitz, C. R.; Steinman, R. M.; and Cohn, Z. A.: Local and systemic effects of intradermal recombinant interferon-gamma in patients with lepromatous-leprosy. N. Engl. J. Med., 315:6–15, 1986.

Nathan, D. G.; Chess, L.; Hillman, D. G.; Clarke, B.; Breard, J.; Merler, E.; and Housman, D. E.: Human erythroid burst-forming units: T cell requirement for proliferation in vitro. J. Exper. Med., 147:324–339, 1978.

Negrin, R. S.; Haeuber, D. H.; Nagler, A.; Olds, L. C.; Donlon, T.; Souza, L. M.; and Greenberg, P. L.: Treatment of myelodysplastic syndromes with recombinant human granulocyte colony-stimulating factor. A phase I/II trial. Ann. Intern. Med., 110:976–984, 1989.

Negrin, R. S.; Haeuber, D. H.; Nagler, A.; Kobayashi, Y.; Sklar, J.; Doulou, T.; Vincent, M.; and Greenberg, P. L.: Maintenance treatment of patients with myelodysplastic syndromes using recombinant human granulocyte colony-stimulating factor. Blood, 76:36–43, 1990.

Nemerson, Y.: Tissue factor and hemostasis. Blood, 71:1–8, 1988.

Neta, R.; Oppenheim, J. J.; and Douches, S. D.: Interdependence of the radioprotective effects of human recombinant interleukin 1 alpha, tumornecrosis factor alpha, granulocyte colony-stimulating factor, and murine recombinant granulocyte-macrophage colony-stimulating factor. J. Immunol., 140:108–111, 1988.

Neta, R.; Douches, S.; and Oppenheim, J. J.: Interleukin 1 is a radioprotector. J. Immunol., 136:2483–2485, 1986.

Neuhaus, K.-L.; Tebbe, U.; Gottwik, M.; Weber, M. A. J.; Feuerer, W.; Niederer, W.; Haerer, W.; Praetorius, F.; Grosser, K.-D.; Huhmann, W.; Hoepp, H.-W.; Alber, G.; Sheikhzadeh, A.; and Schneider, B.: Intravenous recombinant tissue plasminogen activator (rt-PA) and urokinase in acute myocardial infarction: Results of the German Activator Urokinase Study (GAUS). J. Am. Coll. Cardiol., 12:581–587, 1988.

Nicola, N. A.: Why do hemopoietic growth factor receptors interact with each other? Immunol. Today, 8:134–140, 1987.

Nicosia, S.; and Patrono, C.: Eicosanoid biosynthesis and action: Novel opportunities for pharmacological intervention. FASEB J., 3:1941–1948, 1989.

Nienhuis, A. W.; Bunn, H. F.; Turner, P.; Gopal, T. V.; Nash, W. G.; O'Brien, S. J.; and Sherr, C. J.: Expression of the human c-fms proto-oncogene in hematopoietic cells and its deletion in the 5q– syndrome. Cell, 42:421–428, 1985.

Nilsson, I. M.: Clinical pharmacology of aminocaproic and tranexamic acids. J. Clin. Pathol., 33(suppl. 14):41–47, 1980.

Nissen, C.; Tichelli, A.; Gratwohl, A.; Speck, B.; Milne, A.; Gordon-Smith, E. C.; and Schaedelin, J.: Failure of recombinant human granulocyte-macrophage colony-stimulating factor therapy in aplastic anemia patients with very severe neutropenia. Blood, 72:2045–2047, 1988.

Nutt, E.; Gasic, T.; Rodkey, J.; Gasic, G. J.; Jacobs, J. W.; Friedman, P. A.; and Simpson, E.: The amino acid sequence of antistasin: A potent inhibitor of factor X_a reveals a repeated internal structure. J. Biol. Chem., 263:10162–10167, 1988.

Nyman, D.; Thurnherr, N.; and Duckert, F.: Heparin dosage in extracorporeal circulation and its neutralization. Thromb. Diath. Haemorrh., 33:102–104, 1974.

O'Reilly, R. A.: The pharmacodynamics of the oral anticoagulant drugs. Prog. Hemost. Thromb., 2:175–213, 1974.

O'Reilly, R. A.; Aggeler, P. M.; Hoag, M. S.; Leong, L. S.; and Kropatkin, M. L.: Hereditary transmission of exceptional resistance to coumarin anticoagulant drugs: The first reported kindred. N. Engl. J. Med., 271:809–815, 1964.

Oates, J. A.; FitzGerald, G. A.; Branch, R. A.; Jackson, E. K.; Knapp, H. R.; and Roberts, L. J.: Clinical implications of prostaglandin and thromboxane A_2 formation. N. Engl. J. Med., 319:689–698, 1988.

Ockelford, P. A.; Patterson, J.; and Johns, A. S.: A double-blind randomized placebo controlled trial of thromboprophylaxis in major elective general surgery using once daily injections of a low molecular weight heparin fragment (Fragmin). Thromb. Haemost., 62:1046–1049, 1989.

Oksenberg, D.; Dieckmann, B.; and Greenberg, P. L.: Functional interactions between granulocyte-monocyte colony stimulating factor and the insulin hormone family in human myeloid leukemic cells. Cancer Res., 50:6471–6477, 1990.

Olofsson, T.; and Olsson, I.: Suppression of normal granulopoiesis in vitro by a leukemia-associated inhibitor (LAI) of acute and chronic leukemia. Blood, 55:975–982, 1980.

Olofsson, T.; Nilsson, E.; and Olsson, I.: Characterization of the cells in myeloid leukemia that produce leukemia-associated inhibitor (LAI) and demonstration of LAI-producing cells in normal bone marrow. Leukemia Res., 48:387–396, 1984.

Olson, R. E.: Vitamin K. In, Hemostasis and Thrombosis: Basic Principles and Clinical Practice, 2nd ed. (Colman, R. W.; Hirsh, J.; Marder, V. J.; Salzman, E. W., eds.). J. B. Lippincott Co., Philadelphia, pp. 846–860, 1987.

Ortel, T. L.; Onorato, J. J.; Bedrosian, C. L.; and Kaufman, R. E.: Antifibrinolytic therapy in the management of the Kasabach-Merritt syndrome. Am. J. Hematol., 29:44–48, 1988.

Oster, W.; Cicco, N. A.; Klein, H.; Hirano, T.; Kishimoto, T.; Lindemann, A.; Merteslmann, R. H.; and Herrmann, F.: Participation of the cytokines interleukin 6, tumor necrosis factor-alpha, and interleukin 1-beta secreted by acute myelogenous leukemia blasts in autocrine and paracrine leukemia growth control. J. Clin. Invest., 84:451–457, 1989.

Pacquette, R. L.; Zhou, J. Y.; Yang, Y. C.; Clark, S. C.; and Koeffler, H. P.: Recombinant gibbon interleukin-3 acts synergistically with recombinant human G-CSF and GM-CSF in vitro. Blood, 71:1596–1600, 1988.

Page, A. R.; and Good, R. A.: Studies on cyclic neutropenia: A clinical and experimental investigation. Am. J. Dis. Child., 94:623–626, 1973.

Palareti, G.; Poggi, M.; Torricelli, P.; Balestra, V.; and Coccheri, S.: Long-term effects of ticlopidine on fibrinogen and haemorheology in patients with peripheral arterial disease. Thromb. Res., 52:621–629, 1988.

Park, L. S.; Friend, P.; Gillis, S.; and Urdal, D. L.: Characterization of the cell receptor for human granulocyte/macrophage colony-stimulating factor. J. Exp. Med., 164:251–262, 1986.

Partanen, S.; Ruutu, T.; and Vuopio, P.: Haemopoietic progenitors in essential thrombocythaemia. Scand. J. Haematol., 30:130–134, 1983.

Peetre, C.; Gullberg, U.; Nilsson, E.; and Olsson, I.: Effects of recombinant tumor necrosis factor on proliferation and differentiation of leukemic and normal hemopoietic cells in vitro: Relationship to cell surface receptor. J. Clin. Invest., 78:1694–1700, 1986.

Pelus, L. M.; Broxmeyer, H. E.; Clarkson, B. D.; and Moore, M. A.: Abnormal responsiveness of granulocyte-macrophage committed colony-forming cells from patients with chronic myeloid leukemia to inhibition by prostaglandin E. Cancer Res., 40:2512–2515, 1980.

Pepe, M.; Ginzton, N.; Lee, P.; Hintz, R.; and Greenberg, P.: Receptor binding and mitogenic effects of insulin and insulin-like growth factors for human myeloid leukemic cells. J. Cell Physiol., 133:219–227, 1987.

Peters, W. P.; Stuart, A.; Affronti, M. L.; Kim, C. S.; and Coleman, R. E.: Neutrophil migration is defective during recombinant human granulocyte-macrophage colony-stimulating factor infusion after autologous bone marrow transplantation in humans. Blood 72:1310–1315, 1988.

Petersen, P.; Boysen G.; Godtfredsen, J.; Andersen, E. D.; and Andersen, B.: Placebo-controlled, randomised trial of warfarin and aspirin for prevention of thromboembolic complications in chronic atrial fibrillation. The Copenhagen AFASAK study. Lancet, 1:175–179, 1989.

Peto, R.; Gray, R.; Collins, R.; Wheatley, K.; Hennekens, C.; Jamrozik, K.; Warlow, C.; Hafner, B.; Thompson, E.; Norton, S.; Gilliland, J.; and Doll, R.: Randomised trial of prophylactic daily aspirin in British male doctors. Br. Med. J., 296:313–316, 1988.

Physicians' Health Study Research Group: Final report on the aspirin component of the ongoing Physicians' Health Study. N. Engl. J. Med., 321:129–135, 1989.

Picker, L. J.; de los Toyos, J.; Telen, M. J.; Haynes, B. F.; and Butcher, E. C.: Monoclonal antibodies against the CD4[In(Lu)-related p80] and Pgp-1 antigens in man recognize the Hermes class of lymphocyte homing receptors. J. Immunol., 142:2046–2051, 1989a.

Picker, L. J.; Nakache, M.; and Butcher, E. C.: Monoclonal antibodies to human lymphocyte homing receptors define a novel class of adhesion molecules on diverse cell types. J. Cell Biol., 109:927–937, 1989b.

PIOPED Investigators: Tissue plasminogen activator for the treatment of acute pulmonary embolism. Chest, 97:528–533, 1990.

Pizzuto, J.; and Ambriz, R.: Therapeutic experience on 934 adults with idiopathic thrombocytopenic purpura: Multicentric trial of the Cooperative Latin American Group on Hemostasis and Thrombosis. Blood, 64:1179–1183, 1984.

Planes, A.; Vochelle, N.; Mazas, F.; Mansat, C.; Zucman, J.; Landais, A.; Pascariello, J. C.; Weill, D.; and Butel, J.: Prevention of postoperative venous thrombosis: A randomized trial comparing unfractionated heparin with low molecular weight heparin in patients undergoing total hip replacement. Thromb. Haemost., 60:407–410, 1988.

Ploemacher, R. E.; and Brons, R. H. C.: Separation of CFU-S from primitive cells responsible for reconstitution of the bone marrow hemopoietic stem cell compartment following irradiation: Evidence for a pre-CFU-S cell. Exp. Hematol., 17: 263–266, 1989.

Porter, J.; and Jick, H.: Drug-related deaths among medical inpatients. J.A.M.A., 237:879–881, 1977.

Powell, J. S.; Berkner, K. L.; Lebo, R. V.; and Adamson, J. W.: Human erythropoietin gene: High level expression in stably transfected mammalian cells and chromosome localization. Proc. Natl. Acad. Sci. U.S.A., 83:6465–6469, 1986.

Preliminary report of the Stroke Prevention in Atrial Fibrillation Study. N. Engl. J. Med., 322:863–868, 1990.

Preston, F. E.: Aspirin, prostaglandins, and peripheral gangrene. Am. J. Med., 74:55–60, 1983.

PRIMI Trial Study Group: Randomised double-blind trial of recombinant pro-urokinase against streptokinase in acute myocardial infarction. Lancet, 1: 863–868, 1989.

Proctor, S. J.; Jackson, G.; Carey, P.; Stark, A.; Finney, R.;

Saunders, P.; Summerfield, D. G.; Maharaj, D.; and Youart, A.: Improvement of platelet counts in steroid-unresponsive idiopathic immune thrombocytopenic purpura after short-course therapy with recombinant α-2b interferon. Blood, 74: 1894–1897, 1989.

Quesada, J. R.; and Gutterman, J. U.: Alpha interferons in B-cell neoplasma. Br. J. Haematol., 64:639–646, 1986.

Quesada, J. R.; Swanson, D. A.; and Gutterman, J. U.: Phase II study of alpha interferon in metastatic renal cell carcinoma. A progress report. J. Clin. Oncol., 3:1086–1092, 1985.

Quesada, J. R.; Reuben, J.; Manning, J. T.; Hersh, E. M.; and Gutterman, J. U.: Alpha interferon for induction of remission of hairy cell leukemia. N. Engl. J. Med., 310:15–18, 1984.

Raine, A. E. G.: Hypertension, blood viscosity, and cardiovascular morbidity in renal failure: Implications of erythropoietin therapy. Lancet, 1:97–100, 1988.

Rajagopalan, S.; Gonias, S. L.; and Pizzo, S. V.: A nonantigenic covalent streptokinase-polyethlene glycol complex with plasminogen activator function. J. Clin. Invest., 75:413–419, 1985.

Real, F. X.; Oettgen, H. F.; and Krown, S. E.: Kaposi's sarcoma and the acquired immunodeficiency syndrome: treatment with high and low doses of recombinant leukocyte A interferon. J. Clin. Oncol., 4:544–557, 1982.

Remuzzi, G.; Perico, N.; Zoja, C.; Corna, D.; Macconi, D.; and Vigano, G.: Role of endothelium-derived nitric oxide in the bleeding tendency of uremia. J. Clin. Invest., 86:1768–1771, 1990.

Richman, D. D.; Fischl, M. A.; Grieco, M. H.; Gottlieb, M. S.; Volberding, P. A.; Laskin, O. L.; Leedom, J. M.; Groopman, J. E.; Mildvan, D.; Hirsch, M. S.; Jackson, G. G.; Durack, D. T.; Phil, D.; Nusinoff-Lehrman, S.; and the AZT Collaborative Working Group: The toxicity of azidothymidine (AZT) in the treatment of patients with AIDS and AIDS-related complex: A double-blind, placebo-controlled trial. N. Engl. J. Med., 317:192–197, 1987.

Rodeghiero, F.; Castaman, G.; and Dini, E.: Epidemiological investigation of the prevalence of von Willebrand's disease. Blood, 69:454–459, 1987.

Rodgers, G. M.: Common clinical bleeding disorders. In, Contemporary Management in Internal Medicine – Update on Hemostasis (Stein, J. H., ed.). Vol. 1, No. 2. Churchill Livingstone, New York, pp. 75–120, 1990.

Rodgers, G. M.: Hemostatic properties of normal and perturbed vascular cells. FASEB J., 2:116–123, 1988.

Rodgers, G. M.; and Shuman, M. A.: Congenital thrombotic disorders. Am. J. Hematol., 21:419–430, 1986.

Rosenberg, R. D.: The heparin-antithrombin system: A natural anticoagulant mechanism. In, Hemostasis and Thrombosis: Basic Principles and Clinical Practice, 2nd ed. (Colman, R. W.; Hirsh, J.; Marder, V. J.; Salzman, E. W., eds.). J. B. Lippincott Co., Philadelphia, pp. 1373–1392, 1987.

Rosenberg, R. D.; and Rosenberg, J. S.: Natural anticoagulant mechanisms. J. Clin. Invest., 74:1–6, 1984.

Roth, G. J.; and Majerus, P. W.: The mechanism of the effect of aspirin on human platelets: I. Acetylation of a particulate fraction protein. J. Clin. Invest., 56:624–632, 1975.

Rovelli, F.; DeVita, C.; Feruglio, G. A.; Lotto, A.; Selvini, A.; and Tognoni, G.: GISSI trial: Early results and late follow up. J. Am. Coll. Cardiol., 10:33B–39B, 1987.

Sachs, L.: Annotation: The differentiation of myeloid leukemia cells: new possibilities for therapy. Br. J. Haematol., 40:509–517, 1978.

Sack, G. H.; Levin, J.; and Bell, W. R.: Trousseau's syndrome and other manifestations of chronic disseminated coagulopathy in patients with neoplasms: Clinical, pathophysiologic, and therapeutic features. Medicine, 56:1–37, 1977.

Saltiel, E.; and Ward, A.: Ticlopidine: A review of its pharmacodynamic and pharmacokinetic properties, and therapeutic efficacy in platelet-dependent disease states. Drugs, 34:222–262, 1987.

Salzman, E. W.: Low-molecular-weight heparin: Is small beautiful? N. Engl. J. Med., 315:957–959, 1986.

Salzman, E. W.; Weinstein, M. J.; Weintraub, R. M.; Ware, J. A.; Thurer, R. L.; Robertson, L.; Donovan, A.; Gaffney, T.; Bertele, V.; Troll, J.; Smith, M.; and Chute, L. E.: Treatment with desmopressin acetate to reduce blood loss after cardiac surgery: A double-blind randomized trial. N. Engl. J. Med., 314:1402–1406, 1986.

Salzman, E. W.; Deykin, D.; Shapiro, R. M.; and Rosenberg, R. D.: Management of heparin therapy: Controlled prospective trial. N. Engl. J. Med., 292:1046–1050, 1975.

Sasahara, A. A.; Sharma, G. V. R. K.; Tow, D. E.; McIntyre, K. M.; Parisi, A. F.; and Cella, G.: Clinical use of thrombolytic agents in venous thromboembolism. Arch. Intern. Med., 142:684–688, 1982.

Sasahara, A. A.; Hyers, T. M.; Cole, C. M.; Ederer, F.; Murray, J. A.; Wenger, N. K.; Sherry, S.; and Stengle, J. M.: The urokinase pulmonary embolism trial: A national cooperative study. Circulation, 47(suppl. II):1–108, 1973.

Sasaki, H.; Bothner, B.; Dell, A.; and Fukada, M.: Carbohydrate structure of erythropoietin expressed in Chinese hamster ovary cells by a human erythropoietin cDNA. J. Biol. Chem., 262:12059–12076, 1987.

Schapira, M.; Ramus, M.-A.; Jallat, S.; Carvallo, D.; and Courtney, M.: Recombinant α_1-antitrypsin Pittsburgh (Met $^{358}\rightarrow$Arg) is a potent inhibitor of plasma kallikrein and activated factor XII fragment. J. Clin. Invest., 76:635–637, 1985.

Schooly, J. C.; and Mahlmann, L. J.: Studies with antierythropoietin. In, Regulation of Erythropoiesis (Gordon, A. S.; Condorelli, M.; Peschle, C., eds.). Ponte, Milan, Italy, pp. 167–176, 1972.

Schroder, R.: Systemic versus intracoronary streptokinase infusion in the treatment of acute myocardial infarction. J. Am. Coll. Cardiol., 1:1254–1261, 1983.

Schwartz, R. S.; Bauer, K. A.; Rosenberg, R. D.; Kavanaugh, E. J.; Davies, D. C.; and Bogdanoff, D. A.: Clinical experience with antithrombin III concentrate in treatment of congenital and acquired deficiency of antithrombin. Am. J. Med., 87 (suppl. 3B):53S–60S, 1989.

Scott, C. F.; Carrell, R. W.; Glaser, C. B.; Kueppers, F.; Lewis, J. H.; and Colman, R. W.: Alpha-1-antitrypsin-Pittsburgh: A potent inhibitor of human plasma factor XI_a, kallikrein, and factor XII_f. J. Clin. Invest., 77:631–634, 1986.

Second American College of Chest Physicians Conference on Antithrombotic Therapy. Chest, 95 (suppl.):1S–162S, 1989.

Segal, G. M.; McCall, E.; Stueve, T.; and Bagby, G. C.: Interleukin 1 stimulates endothelial cells to release multilineage human colony-stimulating factors. J. Clin. Invest., 138:1772–1778, 1987.

Shafer, A. I.: Bleeding and thrombosis in the myeloproliferative disorders. Blood, 64:1–12, 1984.

Sharma, G. V. R. K.; Cella, G.; Parisi, A. F.; and Sasahara, A. A.: Thrombolytic therapy. N. Engl. J. Med., 306:1268–1276, 1982.

Sharma, G. V. R. K.; Burleson, V. A.; and Sasahara, A. A.: Effect of thrombolytic therapy on pulmonary-capillary blood volume in patients with pulmonary embolism. N. Engl. J. Med., 303:842–845, 1980.

Shemin, D.; Elnour, M.; Amarantes, B.; Abuelo, J. G.; and Chazan, J. A.; Oral estrogens decrease bleeding time and improve clinical bleeding in patients with renal failure. Am. J. Med., 89:436–440, 1990.

Sheridan, W. P.; Mortsyn, G.; Wolf, M.; Dodds, A.; Lusk, J.; Maher, D.; Layton, J. E.; Green, M. D.; Souza, L.; and Fox, R. M.: Granulocyte colony-stimulating factor and neutrophil recovery after high-dose chemotherapy and autologous bone marrow transplantation. Lancet, 2:891–895, 1989.

Sherr, C. J.; Rettenmier, C. W.; Sacca, R.; Roussel, M. F.; Look, A. T.; Stanley, E. R.; and the Department of Tumor Cell Biology, St. Jude Children's Hospital, Memphis, TN: The c-*fms* proto-oncogene product is related to the receptor for the mononuclear phagocyte growth factor, CSF-1. Cell, 41:665–676, 1985.

Shimizu, T.; Whitacre, C.; Katao, T.; Mizoguchi, H.; and Miyake, T.: Purification of human sialylated megakaryocyte colony stimulating factor (abstract). Exp. Hematol., 15:140, 1987.

Shorvon, S. D.; Carney, M. W. P.; Chanarian, I.; and Reynolds, E. A.: The neuropsychiatry of megaloblastic anemia. Br. J. Med., 81:1036–1040, 1980.

Sidorov, J.: Streptokinase vs heparin for deep venous thrombosis. Can lytic therapy be justified? Arch. Intern. Med., 149:1841–1845, 1989.

Sieff, C. A.: Hematopoietic growth factors. J. Clin. Invest., 79:1549–1557, 1987.

Silverstein, M. N.: Primary thrombocythemia. In, Hematology, 3rd ed. (Williams, W. J.; Beutler, E.; Erslev, A. J.; Lichtman, M. A., eds.). McGraw-Hill Book Co., New York, pp. 218–221, 1983.

Silverstein, M. N.; Petitt, R. M.; Solberg, L. A.; Fleming, J. S.; Knight, R. C.; and Schacter, L. P.: Anagrelide: A new drug for treating thrombocytosis. N. Engl. J. Med., 318:1292–1294, 1988.

Simmers, R. N.; Webber, L. M.; Shannon, M. F.; Garson, O. M.; Wong, G.; Vadas, M. A.; and Sutherland, G. R.: Localization of the G-CSF gene on chromosome 17 proximal to the breakpoint in the t(15:17) in acute promyelocytic leukemia. Blood, 70:330–332, 1987.

Sing, G. K.; Keller, J. R.; Ellingsworth, J. R.; and Ruscetti, F. W.: Transforming growth factor beta selectively inhibits normal and leukemic human bone marrow cell growth in vitro. Blood, 72:1504–1511, 1988.

Singer, J. W.; and Brown, J. E.: In vitro marrow culture techniques in aplastic anemia and other disorders. Clin. Haematol., 7:487–499, 1978.

Sisson, S. D.; and Dinarello, C. A.: Production of interleukin-1α, interleukin-1β and tumor necrosis factor by human mononuclear cells stimulated with granulocyte-macrophage colony-stimulating factor. Blood, 72:1368–1374, 1988.

Skettino, S.; Phillips, J.; Lanier, L.; and Greenberg, P.: Selective generation of erythroid burst promoting activity by recombinant interleukin 2-stimulated T-lymphocytes and natural killer cells. Blood, 71:907–914, 1988.

Smith, M. C.; and Dunn, M. J.: Impaired platelet thromboxane production in renal failure. Nephron, 29:133–137, 1981.

Smith, R. A. G.; Dupe, R. J.; English, P. D.; and Green, J.: Fibrinolysis with acyl-enzymes: A new approach to thrombolytic therapy. Nature, 290:505–508, 1981.

Soconski, M. Y.; Elias, A.; Schnipper, L.; Cannistra, S. A.; Antman, K. H.; and Griffin, J. D.: Granulocyte-macrophage colony-stimulating factor expands the circulating hematopoietic progenitor cell compartment in man. Lancet, 1:1194–1198, 1988.

Souza, L. M.; Boone, T. C.; Gabrilove, J.; Lai, P. H.; Zsebo, K. M.; Murdock, D. C.; Chazin, V. R.; Bruszewski, J.; Lu, H.; Chen, K. K.; Barendt, J.; Platzer, E.; Moore, M. A. S.; Mertelsmann, R.; and Welke, K.: Recombinant human granulocyte colony-stimulating factor: Effects on normal and leukemic myeloid cells. Science, 232:61–65, 1986.

Spangrude, G.; Heimfeld, S.; and Weissman, I.: Purification and characterization of mouse hematopoietic stem cells. Science, 241:58–62, 1988.

Spivak, J. L.; and Graber, S. E.: Erythropoietin and the regulation of erythropoeisis. Johns Hopkins Med. J., 146:311–320, 1980.

Spivak, J. L.; Bender, B. S.; and Quinn, T. C.: Hematologic abnormalities in the acquired immune deficiency syndrome. Am. J. Med., 77:224–228, 1984.

Sporn, M. B.; Roberts, A. B.; Wakefield, L. M.; and Cromburgghe, B.: Some recent advances in the chemistry and biology of transforming growth factor-beta. J. Cell Biol., 195:1039–1045, 1987.

Steiner, R. W.; Coggins, C.; and Carvalho, A. C. A.: Bleeding time in uremia: A useful test to assess clinical bleeding. Am. J. Hematol., 7:107–117, 1979.

Steis, R. G.; Smith, J. W.; Urba, W. J.; Clark, J. W.; Itri, L. M.; Evans, L. M.; Schoenberger, C.; and Longo, D. L.: Resistance to recombinant interferon alfa-2a in hairy cell leukemia associated with neutralizing anti-interferon antibodies. N. Engl. J. Med., 318:1409–1413, 1988.

Streiff, R. R.: Malabsorption of polyglutamic folic acid secondary to oral contraceptives. Clin. Res., 17:345, 1969.

Streuli, R. A.; Testa, J. R.; Vardiman, J. W.; Mintz, U.; Golomb, H. M.; and Rowley, J. D.: Dysmelopoietic syndrome: Sequential clinical and cytogenetic studies. Blood, 55:636–644, 1980.

Strother, S. V.; Zuckerman, K. S.; and LoBuglio, A. F.: Colchicine therapy for refractory idiopathic thrombocytopenic purpura. Arch. Intern. Med., 144:2198–2200, 1984.

Stults, B. M.; Dere, W. H.; and Caine, T. H.: Long-term anticoagulation: Indications and management. West. J. Med., 151:414–429, 1989.

Suda, T.; Suda, J.; Ogawa, M.; and Ihle, J. N.: Permissive role of IL3 in proliferation and differentiation of multipotential hemopoietic progenitors in culture. J. Cell Physiol., 124:182–190, 1985.

Sullivan, J. M.; Harken, D. E.; and Gorlin, R.: Pharmacologic control of thromboembolic complications of cardiac-valve replacement. N. Engl. J. Med., 284:1391–1394, 1971.

Talpaz, M.; Kantarjian, H. M.; McCredie, K.; Trujillo, J. M.; Keating, M. J.; and Gutterman, J. U.: Hematologic remission and cytogenetic improvement induced by recombinant human interferon alpha$_A$ in chronic myelogenous leukemia. N. Engl. J. Med., 314:1065–1069, 1986.

Tavassoli, M.; and Hardy, C.: Molecular basis of homing of intravenously transplanted stem cells to the marrow. Blood, 76:1059–1070, 1990.

Taylor, F. B.; Chang, A.; Esmon, C. T.; D'Angelo, A.; Vigano-D'Angelo, S.; and Blick, K. E.: Protein C prevents the coagulopathic and lethal effects of *Escherichia coli* infusion in the baboon. J. Clin. Invest., 79:918–925, 1987.

Taylor, K. M.; Jagannath, S.; Spitzer, G.; Spinolo, J. A.; Tucker, S. L.; Fogel, B.; Cabanillas, F. F.; Hagemeister, F. B.; and Souza, L. M.: Recombinant human granulocyte colony-stimulating factor hastens granulocyte recovery after high-dose chemotherapy and autologous bone marrow transplantation in Hodgkin's disease. J. Clin. Oncol., 7:1791–1799, 1989.

Taylor, R. N.; Lacey, C. G.; and Shuman, M. A.: Adenocarcinoma of Skene's duct associated with a systemic coagulopathy. Gynecol. Oncol., 22:250–256, 1985.

ten Cate, H.; Henny, C. P.; ten Cate, J. W.; and Buller, H. R.: Clinical studies with low-molecular-weight heparin(oid)s: An interim analysis. Am. J. Hematol., 27:146–153, 1988.

Theroux, P.; Ouimet, H.; McCans, J.; Latour, J.-G.; Joly, P.; Levy, G.; Pelletier, E.; Juneau, M.; Stasiak, J.; DeGuise, P.; Pelletier, G. B.; Rinzler, D.; and Waters, D. D.: Aspirin, heparin, or both to treat unstable angina. N. Engl. J. Med., 319:1105–1111, 1988.

Thomas, D. P.: Biologicals, standards and heparin. Thromb. Haemost., 62:648–650, 1989.

Thomas, D. P.: Current status of low molecular weight heparin. Thromb. Haemost., 56:241–242, 1986.

Thomas, M.; and Lumley, P.: Preliminary assessment of a novel thromboxane A$_2$ receptor-blocking drug, GR 32191 in healthy subjects. Circulation, 81(suppl. I):153–158, 1990.

Thompson, J. A.; Lee, D. J.; Kidd, P.; Rubin, E.; Kaufmann, J.; Bonner, E. M.; and Fefer, A.: Subcutaneous granulocyte-macrophage colony-stimulating factors in patients with myelodysplastic syndrome: Toxicity, pharmacokinetics and hematologic effects. J. Clin. Oncol., 7:629–637, 1989.

Tichelli, A.; Gratwohl, A.; Berger, C.; Lori, A.; Würsch, A.; Dieterle, A.; Thomssen, C.; Nissen, C.; Holdener, E.; and Speck, B.: Treatment of thrombocytosis in myeloproliferative disorders with interferon alpha-2a. Blut, 58:15–19, 1989.

TIMI Study Group: The Thrombolysis in Myocardial Infarction (TIMI) Trial: Phase I findings. N. Engl. J. Med., 312:932–936, 1985.

Tomonaga, M.; Golde, D. W.; and Gasson, J. C.: Biosythetic (recombinant) human granulocyte-macrophage colony-stimulating factor: Effect on normal bone marrow and leukemia cell lines. Blood, 67:31–36, 1986.

Tosato, G.; and Jones, K.: Interleukin 1 induces IL6 production in peripheral blood monocytes. Blood, 75:1305–1310, 1990.

Turpie, A. G. G.; Robinson, J. G.; Doyle, D. J.; Mulji, A. S.; Mishkel, G. J.; Sealey, B. J.; Cairns, J. A.; Skingley, L.; Hirsh, J.; and Gent, M.: Comparison of high-dose with low-dose subcutaneous heparin to prevent left ventricular mural thrombosis in patients with acute transmural anterior myocardial infarction. N. Engl. J. Med., 320:352–357, 1989.

Turpie, A. G. G.; Gunstensen, J.; Hirsh, J.; Nelson, H.; and Gent, M.: Randomised comparison of two intensities of oral anticoagulant therapy after tissue heart valve replacement. Lancet, 1:1242–1245, 1988.

Turpie, A. G. G.; Levine, M. N.; Hirsh, J.; Carter, C. J.; Jay, R. M.; Powers, P. J.; Andrew, M.; Magnani, H. N.; Hull, R. D.; and Gent, M.: Double-blind randomised trial of ORG 10172 low-molecular-weight heparinoid in the prevention of deep-vein thrombosis in thrombotic stroke. Lancet, 1:523–526, 1987.

Turpie, A. G. G.; Levine, M. N.; Hirsh, J.; Carter, C. J.; Jay, R. M.; Powers, P. J.; Andrew, M.; Hull, R. D.; and Gent, M.: A randomized controlled trial of a low-molecular-weight heparin (enoxaparin) to prevent deep-vein thrombosis in patients undergoing elective hip surgery. N. Engl. J. Med., 315:925–929, 1986.

UK-TIA Study Group.: United Kingdom Transient Ischaemic Attack (UK-TIA) aspirin trial: Interim results. Br. Med. J., 296:316–320, 1988.

Urokinase-streptokinase embolism trial (USET). Phase 2 results: A cooperative study. J.A.M.A., 229:1606–1613, 1974.

Vadhan-Raj, S.; Broxmeyer, H. E.; Spitzer, G.; LeMaistre, A.; Hultman, G.; Ventura, G.; Tigaud, J.-D.; Cork, M. A.; Trujillo, J. M.; Gutterman, J. U.; and Hittelman, W. N.: Stimulation of nonclonal hematopoiesis and suppression of the neoplastic clone after treatment with recombinant human granulocyte-macrophage colony-stimulating factor in a patient with therapy-related myelodysplastic syndrome. Blood, 74:1491–1498, 1989.

Vadhan-Raj, S.; Buescher, S.; Broxmeyer, H. E.; LeMaistre, A.; Lepe-Zuniga, J. L.; Ventura, G.; Juha, S.; Horwitz, L. J.; Trujillo, J. M.; Gillis, S.; Hittelman, W. N.; and Gutterman, J. U.: Stimulation of myelopoiesis in patients with aplastic anemia by recombinant human granulocyte-macrophage colony-stimulating factor. N. Engl. J. Med., 319:1628–1634, 1988a.

Vadhan-Raj, S.; Buescher, S.; LeMaistre, A.; Keating, M.; Walters, R.; Ventura, C.; Hittelman, W.; Broxmeyer, H. E.; and Gutterman, J. U.: Stimulation of hematopoiesis in patients with bone marrow failure and in patients with malignancy by recombinant human granulocyte-macrophage colony-stimulating factor. Blood, 72:134–141, 1988b.

Vadhan-Raj, S.; Keating, M.; LeMaistre, A.; Hittelman, W. N.; McCredie, K.; Trujillo, J. M.; Broxmeyer, H. E.; Henney, C.; and Gutterman, J. U.: Effects of recombinant human granulocyte-macrophage colony-stimulating factor in patients with myelodysplastic syndromes. N. Engl. J. Med., 317:1545–1552, 1987.

Vainchenker, W.; Gulchard, J.; Deschamps, J.; Bouguet, J.; Titleux, B. M.; Chapman, J.; McMichael, A. J.; and Breton-Gorius, J.: Megakaryocyte cultures in the chronic phase and in the blast crisis of chronic myeloid leukaemia: Studies on the differentiation of the megakaryocyte progenitors and on the maturation of megakaryocytes in vitro. Br. J. Haematol., 51:131–146, 1982.

van de Water, L.; Carr, J. M.; Aronson, D.; and McDonagh, J.: Analysis of elevated fibrin(ogen) degradation product levels in patients with liver disease. Blood, 67:1468–1473, 1986.

van de Werf, F.; Nobuhara, M.; and Collen, D.: Coronary thrombolysis with human single-chain, urokinase-type plasminogen activator (pro-urokinase) in patients with acute myocardial infarction. Ann. Intern. Med., 104:345–348, 1986.

Vander Sande, J.; Bossaert, L.; Brochier, M.; Charbonnier, B.; Serradigmini, A.; Elias, A.; Pintens, H.; and Lauwers, M. C.: Thrombolytic treatment of pulmonary embolism with APSAC. Eur. Respir. J., 1:721–725, 1988.

Vellenga, E.; Young, D. C.; Wagner, K.; Wiper, D.; Ostapoicz, D.; and Griffin, J. D.: The effects of GM-CSF and G-CSF in promoting growth of clonagenic cells in acute myelogenous leukemia. Blood, 69:1771–1776, 1987.

Vogelstein, B.; Fearon, E. R.; Hamilton, S. R.; Preisinger, A. C.; Willard, H. F.; Michelson, A. M.; Riggs, A. D.; and Orkin, S. H.: Clonal analysis using recombinant DNA probes from the X chromosomes. Cancer Res., 47:4806–4813, 1987.

Walker, F.; Nicola, N. A.; Metcalf, D.; and Burgess, A. W.: Hierarchical down-modulation of hemopoietic growth factor receptors. Cell, 43:269–276, 1985.

Warren, M. K.; Conroy, L. B.; and Rose, J. S.: The role of interleukin 6 and interleukin 1 in megakaryocyte development. Exp. Hematol., 17:1095–1099, 1989.

Waxman, L.; Smith, D. E.; Arcuri, K. E.; and Vlasuk, G. P.: Tick anticoagulant peptide (TAP) is a novel inhibitor of blood coagulation factor X_a. Science, 248:593–596, 1990.

Weimar, W.; Stibbe, J.; van Seyen, A. J.; Billiau, A.; De Somer, P.; and Collen, D.: Specific lysis of an iliofemoral thrombus by administration of extrinsic (tissue-type) plasminogen activator. Lancet, 2:1018–1020, 1981.

Wessler, S.; and Gitel, S. N.: Heparin: New concepts relevant to clinical use. Blood, 53:525–544, 1979.

Wheeler, A. P.; Jaquiss, R. D. B.; and Newman, J. H.: Physician practices in the treatment of pulmonary embolism and deep venous thrombosis. Arch. Intern. Med., 148:1321–1325, 1988.

Whetton, A.; Brazil, G.; and Dexter, T. M.: Haemopoietic cell growth factor mediates cell survival via its action on glucose transport. EMBO J., 3:409–413, 1984.

Wilcox, R. G.; von der Lippe, G.; Olsson, C. G.; Jensen, G.; Skene, A. M.; and Hampton, J. R.: Trial of tissue plasminogen activator for mortality reduction in acute myocardial infarction. Anglo-Scandinavian Study of Early Thrombolysis (ASSET). Lancet, 2:525–530, 1988.

Williams. W. J.: Classification and clinical manifestations of disorders of hemostasis. In, Hematology, 4th ed. (Williams. W. J.; Beutler, E.; Erslev, A. J.; and Lichtman, M. A., eds.). McGraw-Hill Book Co., New York, pp. 1338–1342, 1990.

Winearls, C. G.; Oliver, D. O.; Pippard, M. J.; Reid, C.; Downing, M. R.; and Cotes, P. M.: Effect of human erythropoietin derived from recombinant DNA on the anaemia of patients maintained by chronic haemodialysis. Lancet, 2: 1175–1177, 1986.

Wolf, N.: The haemopoietic microenvironment. Clin. Haematol., 8:469–500, 1979.

Wong, G. G.; Temple, P. A.; Leary, A. C.; Witek-Giannotti, J. S.; Yang, Y. C.; Ciarletta, A. B.; Chung, M.; Murtha, P.; Kriz, R.; Kaufman, R. S.; Ferenz, C. R.; Sibley, B. S.; Turner, K. J.; Hewick, R. M.; Clark, S. C.; Yanai, N.; Yakota, H.; Yamada, M.; Saito, M.; Motoyoshi, K.; and Takaku, F.: Human CSF-1: Molecular cloning and expression 4-kb cDNA encoding the human urinary protein. Science, 235:1504–1509, 1987.

Wong, G. G.; Witek, J.; Temple, P. A.; Wilkens K. M.; Leary,

A. C.; Luxemberg, D. P.; Jones, S. S.; Brown, E. L.; Kay, R. M.; Orr, E. C.; Shoemaker, C.; Golde, D. W.; Kaufman, R. J.; Hewick, R. M.; Wang, E. A.; and Clark, S. C.: Human GM-CSF: Molecular cloning of cDNA and purification of natural and recombinant proteins. Science, 228:810–815, 1985.

Wood, P.; Nygaard, S.; and Hrushesky, W.: Cisplatin-induced anemia is correctable with erythropoietin (abstract). Blood, 72(suppl.1): 52a, 1988.

Yang, Y.-C.; Kovacic, S.; Kriz, R.; Wolf, S.; Clark, S. C.; Wellems, T. E.; Nienhuis, A.; and Epstein, N.: The human genes for GM-CSF and IL3 are closely linked in tandem on chromosome 5. Blood, 71:958–961, 1988.

Yang, Y.-C.; Ciarletta, A. B.; Temple, P. A.; Chung, M. P.; Kovacic, S.; Witcek-Giannotti, J. S.; Leary, A. C.; Kriz, R.; Donaheu, R. E.; Wong, G. G.; and Clark, S. C.: Human IL-3 (multi-CSF): Identification by expression cloning of a novel hemapoietic growth factor related to murine IL-3. Cell, 47:3–10, 1986.

Yasuda, T.; Gold, H. K.; Fallon, J. T.; Leinbach, R. C.; Guerrero, J. L.; Scudder, L. E.; Kanke, M.; Shealy, D.; Ross, M. J.; Collen, D.; and Coller, B. S.: Monoclonal antibody against the platelet glycoprotein (GP) II_b/III_a receptor prevents coronary artery reocclusion after reperfusion with recombinant tissue-type plasminogen activator in dogs. J. Clin. Invest., 81:1284–1291, 1988.

Young, D. C.; Wagner, K.; and Griffin, J. D.: Constitutive expression of the granulocyte-macrophage colony-stimulating factor gene in acute myeloblastic leukemia. J. Clin. Invest., 79:100–106, 1987.

Zanjani, E. D.; Lutton, J. D.; and Hoffman, R.: Erythroid colony formation by polycythemia vera bone marrow in vitro. J. Clin. Invest., 59:841–848, 1977.

Zanjani, E. D.; Mann, L. I.; Burlington, H.; Gordon, A. S.; and Wasserman, L. R.: Evidence for a physiologic role of erythropoietin in fetal erythropoeisis. Blood, 44:285–290, 1974.

Zhou, Y. Q.; Stanley, E. R.; Clark, S. C.; Hatzfeld, J. A.; Levesque, J. P.; Federici, C.; Watt, S. M.; Hatzfeld, A.; and the Laboratory of Cellular and Molecular Biology of Growth Factors, Hospital Paul, Brousse, Villejuif, France: Interleukin-3 and interleukin-1 alpha allow earlier bone marrow progenitors to respond to human colony-stimulating factor I. Blood, 72:1870–1874, 1988.

Zilliacus, H.: On the specific treatment of thrombosis and pulmonary embolism with anticoagulants, with particular reference to the post-thrombotic sequelae. Acta Med. Scand. Suppl., 171:1–221, 1946.

Zucali, J. R.; Broxmeyer, H. E.; Levy, D.; and Morse, C.: Lactoferrin decreases monocyte-induced fibroblast production of myeloid colony-stimulating activity by suppressing monocyte release of interleukin-1. Blood, 74:1531–1536, 1989.

Zucali, J. R.; Dinarello, C. A.; Oblon, D. J.; Gross, M. A.; Anderson, L.; and Weiner, R. S.: Interleukin-1 stimulates fibroblasts to produce granulocyte-macrophage colony-stimulating activity and prostaglandin E_2. J. Clin. Invest., 77: 1857–1863, 1986.

Zweifler, A. J.: Relation of prothrombin concentration to bleeding during oral anticoagulant therapy: Its importance in detection of latent organic lesions. N. Engl. J. Med., 267: 283–285, 1962.

23

Antineoplastic Drugs

J. R. Bertino

The modern era of cancer chemotherapy began in 1941, when C. Huggins and C. U. Hodges demonstrated that administration of diethylstilbestrol ameliorated carcinoma of the prostate. A host of drugs was subsequently introduced for chemotherapy. Because the history of this field is short, a rational basis for drug therapy of malignancies has developed only recently and is in a state of rapid evolution. Since qualitative, exploitable differences in the biochemistry of malignant cells versus normal cells are rare, most of the drugs available to the cancer chemotherapist affect normal cells, especially those that are replicating.

Drug treatment of rapidly growing malignancies has been one of the major accomplishments of cancer chemotherapy. Long-term disease-free remissions and probable cures are now possible for patients with acute lymphocytic leukemia, Hodgkin disease, diffuse intermediate-grade or high-grade lymphomas, testicular cancer, and certain childhood tumors. Although the cure rate of these malignancies with chemotherapy is high, failure due to drug resistance still occurs in some patients, especially those with a large tumor volume at presentation. In addition, short-term and

long-term toxicities due to treatment (chemotherapeutic agents and/or irradiation) remain important problems.

Complete remissions are also commonly obtained after drug treatment in patients with other neoplasms, such as ovarian cancer and acute myeloid leukemia (AML). With these tumors, however, the number of useful drugs and therefore effective combinations are limited, and drug resistance limits the curability of these diseases. Other malignancies, such as breast cancer, and head and neck cancer, and the chronic hematologic malignancies [chronic lymphocytic leukemia (CLL), myeloma, chronic myelogenous leukemia (CML), low-grade lymphomas], respond, but usually not completely to anticancer drug treatment. Chemotherapy is rarely curative in these instances, although it may improve survival.

This chapter emphasizes the principles of chemotherapy of malignant diseases. Because this field is rapidly changing, detailed information on drug usage is not provided. Instead, generalizations regarding classes of drugs and principles of their use are stressed. The reader may obtain more detailed information on the pharmacology of anticancer drugs from other sources (Calabresi and Parks, 1985; Black and Livingston, 1990; Chabner and Collins, 1990). Specific examples of how therapeutic programs might be formulated for certain diseases are given in these sources.

THEORETICAL CONSIDERATIONS

Tumor and Normal Stem Cell Kinetics

The growth rate of a tumor is a function of the number of stem or *clonogenic* cells (the so-called growth fraction), the generation time of these cells, and the rate of cell loss. In tissues that normally renew themselves frequently (i.e., the bone marrow), the rate of production of cells is exquisitely balanced by the rate of loss of cells. The balance results in a steady state with no net growth of the organ. Tumors grow (at variable rates) if the birth rate of tumor cells exceeds the death rate. It also follows that the rate of growth of a tumor, usually expressed as the doubling time, does not provide insight into the dynamics of tumor growth; for example, a "slow"-growing tumor may have a high growth fraction and a short generation time, but these processes may be balanced by a high rate of loss of cells (Schackney and Ritch, 1982).

Cell-Kill Hypothesis

In experimental tumor systems, especially transplanted mouse tumors (e.g., the L1210 leukemia), most available chemotherapeutic agents increase the survival of tumor-bearing mice by killing a proportion of stem cells (Skipper, 1967). In the L1210 system, a single stem cell can eventually cause death at a predictable time when a critical tumor size is reached (about 10^9 cells); the increase in survival that occurs when animals bearing a known tumor burden are treated is therefore related to the number of tumor cells left after treatment. The use of this model system has made it possible to show that a given treatment will produce a relatively constant certain *cell kill*, regardless of the number of tumor cells initially present. For example, if 10^5 cells could be killed by a given treatment, cure is possible if 10^4 cells are present, but will not occur if 10^6 or a greater number of cells are present.

Because most chemotherapy tends to kill a fraction of normal cell populations (e.g., bone marrow, gut epithelium) as well as abnormal cells, the problems in chemotherapy become twofold; first, one tries to attain as large a difference as possible in cell kill between malignant and normal cell populations, and, second, one needs to manage any complications that arise from destruction of normal cells.

How do we obtain "selective" cell kill? For the cure of the L1210 tumor in mice, up to 10^9 cells must be killed (Skipper et al., 1964). It has been estimated that a 20-kg child, dying of acute lymphoblastic leukemia (ALL), has 10^{12} malignant cells (Frei, 1984). Assuming that a tumor weighing 1 g is the smallest detectable size and that it contains 10^9 cells, chemotherapy must eradicate the entire malignant population of 10^9 cells. This must be accomplished without producing an intolerable deficit of normal cells, such as in the bone marrow and gut epithelium. An estimate of the *logs of kill* that these normal cell compartments can withstand has been obtained (Bruce and Bergsagel, 1967). In humans, 450 rad of whole-body irradiation is probably lethal; 600 rad is lethal for mice. As 600 rad produces 2 logs of reduction of hemopoietic stem cells in mice, the lethality of 450 rad in humans may be related to the same factor of reduction (Alexander, 1965). With intensive support therapy, perhaps another log of normal stem cells can be killed and may be tolerated and reversed. Therefore, a successful treatment program must eradicate 9 to 12 logs of cells (whether by surgery, x-ray, and/or drugs, and/or immunotherapy) while decreasing normal stem cells by only 2 to 3 logs.

Cycle-Specific and Non-Cycle-Specific Drugs

To approach the problem of selectivity, a model system in an experimental animal was devised to quantitate the effects of chemotherapeutic agents on both normal and malignant cells (Bruce et al., 1966). The study revealed a linear relationship between the number of hemopoietic stem cells injected into irradiated mice and the macroscopic colonies produced (Till and McCulloch, 1961). Similarly, transplantable AKR lymphoma cells produced macroscopic colonies in the spleens of syngeneic mice in direct relationship to the number of cells inoculated (Bruce et al., 1966). This assay has allowed measurements of the effects of dose and duration of treatment on both tumor cell and hemopoietic stem cell proliferation. On the basis of effects on these two compartments of stem cells, drugs were classified into three groups (Bruce et al., 1966). The first group of drugs [which included nitrogen mustard, 1,3-bis-2-chloroethyl-1-nitrosourea (BCNU) and x-ray; Fig. 23–1] decimated both the normal hemopoietic stem cells and the tumor cells to the same degree. However, the second and third classes of drugs, also given over a 24-hour period, decimated the tumor population to a much greater extent than the normal stem cells. When some of the drugs in the third class were given at high doses, they produced as much as a 10,000-fold greater kill of lymphoma cells than of normal stem cells. This class included drugs such as

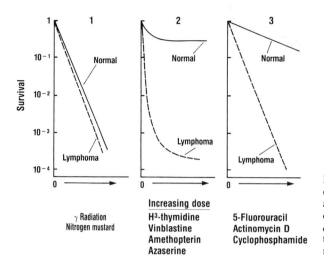

Fig. 23-1. Dose–survival curves for nine different anticancer agents tested (24-hour exposure) against normal hemopoietic and lymphoma colony-forming cells. Class 1 are *non-cycle-active* drugs; class 2 and 3 agents are considered to be *cycle-active* agents. (Reproduced with permission from Bruce, 1967).

cyclophosphamide (Fig. 23-1), actinomycin D, and 5-fluorouracil. The remaining drugs tested (methotrexate, vinblastine, azaserine, 6-mercaptopurine, and high-specific-activity tritiated thymidine [^{3}H]TdR) still achieved a marked differential cell kill (500-fold), but the differences diminished as the dose of drugs increased.

The selectivity of the agents in the last two classes was attributed to a differential effect of the agents on proliferating versus nonproliferating cells. Hemopoietic stem cells were in a state of low proliferative activity compared with the lymphoma cells. However, the susceptibility of the normal stem cells to agents of the second and third class increased when their proliferative activity increased (e.g., after sublethal irradiation or drug treatment) and reverted to usual only when this increased rate of proliferation returned to near normal (Valeriote and Bruce, 1967; Bruce et al., 1969). Bruce suggested that class II and III agents were capable of killing cells only if the drug was present when these cells were engaged in active proliferation (DNA synthesis and mitosis). The cells that were not killed by therapy were considered quiescent during the time of exposure to drug. On implantation into animals, however, these cells actively proliferated and produced splenic colonies. The proliferating cells killed by the class II and III agents were said to be in *cycle*. Agents that killed both the normal and tumor cells irrespective of their proliferative state (class I) have been referred to as *non-cycle-specific* agents, and agents of the second and third class have been called *cycle-specific* agents. Cycle-specific agents may be further characterized in some instances on the basis of studies of cell killing that used synchronous populations. Some agents (e.g., methotrexate, cytosine arabinoside, hydroxyurea) kill cells in the S phase of the cell cycle, during which DNA synthesis occurs. Other agents, for example, bleomycin and the vinca alkaloids, affect cells during the G_2-M phase of the cell cycle as cells undergo mitosis.

The classification of chemotherapeutic agents into cycle-specific or non-cycle-specific subgroups has been useful in terms of certain generalizations that may be made concerning the properties of these drugs (Table 23-1). *Principle: Cycle-active agents are* **schedule dependent**, *that is, antitumor and toxic results are dependent more on the duration of exposure than the dose.*

Very large doses of cycle-active drugs may be given if the duration of exposure is short and the interval between retreatment is sufficiently long. For example, in high-dose methotrexate (MTX) regimens, 20 g/m^2 of MTX is safe and effective versus acute lymphocytic leukemia (ALL) if the duration of exposure is kept to 36 hours or less

Table 23-1. EXAMPLES OF CYCLE-SPECIFIC AND NON-CYCLE-SPECIFIC CHEMOTHERAPEUTIC AGENTS

I. Cycle-specific drugs
    S-phase specific
        Methotrexate (MTX)
        Ara-C
        Hydroxyurea
    G_2-M-phase specific
        Bleomycin
        Vinca alkaloids
    Non-phase specific
        Anthracyclines
        Cyclophosphamide
        Fluorouracil

II. Non-cycle-specific drugs
    Alkylating agents
    Nitrosoureas
    Platinum compounds

by using leucovorin rescue, and the treatment is not repeated more than weekly or biweekly (Ackland and Schilsky, 1987; Allegra, 1990). In contrast, 20 *mg*/m^2 per day of MTX is highly toxic to normal bone marrow and GI mucosa if given as a 5-day continuous infusion. The explanation for this difference in the relative toxicity of these two regimens is that short-term exposure to antimetabolites spares bone marrow stem cells, which subsequently proliferate and replenish the decimated proliferating and differentiating compartment, while longer exposures (48 hours or longer) begin to kill stem cells that have been recruited into cycle. *Principle: It follows that agents that damage or stress the marrow (previous x-ray, chemotherapy, infection) that result in recruitment of stem cells into cycle may predispose patients to toxicity with antimetabolites.* Consequently, treatment of patients with ALL using high-dose intermittent pulse dose of antimetabolite regimens may be safe as well as effective if instituted while the patient is in bone marrow remission, while similar treatment of patients with infection or who are in bone marrow relapse may cause serious marrow toxicity.

In contrast to the relative selectivity that may be obtained with antimetabolites in the treatment of rapidly proliferating malignancies, non-cycle-active agents have a steeper dose response, and less of a selective action in relation to marrow toxicity. *Principle: Total dose, rather than dose schedule, is important for non-cycle-active agents.* The choice of schedule used with non-cycle-active agents may depend on other toxic effects, rather than marrow toxicities; for example, doxorubicin delivered as a continuous infusion (over 48–96 hours) or as a pulse (every 3 weeks) has similar marrow toxicity at the same total dose, but continuous infusions of doxorubicin may be less cardiotoxic (Legha et al., 1982).

Effect of Size on Growth Rate of a Tumor

The concepts developed thus far have assumed that the rate of tumor growth is constant. However, in most circumstances, when the size of the tumor increases, its rate of growth slows. This may be due to an increase in the generation time of the tumor, a decrease in the growth fraction of the tumor, and/or an increase in the death rate of the tumor cells (Steel, 1967). These changes may result from overcrowding and decreased nutrition of the tumor, but the process is poorly understood. In this phase of growth the tumor population is not in so active a proliferative state; both tumor and normal cells may be in a resting state, and the differential cell kill of cycle-specific agents is lost. Indeed, if marrow involvement with tumor or infection is present, the normal cells of the marrow may be in a more active proliferative phase than are the tumor cells; in this setting, even greater toxicity than usual may be produced with drug therapy.

The DNA synthesis in cells in a plateau phase of growth is less sensitive to the action of cycle-specific drugs than are cells in the logarithmic phase of growth (Hryniuk et al., 1969). Therefore, when tumors are large and growth has plateaued, attempts to decrease tumor size by the use of non-cycle-active agents, surgery, or x-ray therapy should be considered. The use of a non-cycle-active agent is of value if recovery of normal tissue is more rapid than is recovery of the tumor tissue. Since this dose–response curve of these agents is steep, a maximum dose should be administered to kill as may cells as possible, keeping in mind the narrow therapeutic index of these compounds. If sufficient tumor kill of cells is obtained, the logarithmic phase of tumor growth may be reestablished and the cycle-specific agents may regain their value.

Compartmentalization of Cells

Not all tumor-bearing compartments are affected to the same degree by a course of therapy (Skipper, 1965). In animal model systems, as well as in humans, cells in the CNS are least affected by chemotherapy, owing to failure of certain drugs to pass readily through the blood–brain barrier.

The failure to achieve cell kill in the CNS may account for relapses in leukemia. Intrathecal administration of chemotherapeutic agents is necessary in patients with manifest CNS involvement. In contrast, similar cells in the blood are most sensitive to effects of antimetabolites (at least when methotrexate is used) (Hryniuk and Bertino, 1969b). Furthermore, sensitivity of tumor cells in different organs (e.g., leukemia cells in the spleen, kidney, or liver) may vary depending on the drug employed. Organ-specific differences in sensitivity of cells may be related to binding or metabolism of the drug in the different tissues or to biochemical influences of the organ on growth or metabolism of cells.

Drug Resistance

During the past decade, the genetic basis for the phenotypic expression of drug resistance has been elucidated in tumor cell lines for many drugs. Table 23-2 lists the observed mechanisms of drug resistance to anticancer drugs and the genetic basis for this resistance. Less is known about the cause of drug resistance in human cancers, although progress is being made in this regard, especially in patients with leukemia (Sobrero and Bertino, 1986).

**Table 23–2.   MECHANISMS OF
DRUG RESISTANCE TO ANTICANCER DRUGS**

GENETIC MECHANISM	PHENOTYPIC EXPRESSION
1. Gene amplification	Increase in target enzyme activity
	Increase in a catabolic enzyme activity
	Decreased uptake of drug
2. Mutation or deletion	Decrease in target enzyme activity
	Decreased binding of drug to enzyme or receptor
	Decreased uptake of drug

Of great current interest is a type of resistance called multidrug resistance (Riordan and Ling, 1985; Tsuruo, 1988). When tumor cell lines were made resistant to certain drugs, they were found to be cross-resistant to other classes of drugs they had not been exposed to. Although drugs sharing this resistance phenotype have entirely different structures and mechanisms of cytotoxicity, they share a common transport mechanism. They are mainly toxic alkaloids that are actively pumped out of the cell as a consequence of expression of a protein of molecular weight of 170,000. Some drugs that have been shown to be involved in this multidrug resistance phenotype are the anthracyclines, the vinca alkaloids, etoposide (VP-16), and actinomycin D. Since these medicines are extensively used in the treatment of malignancies, it

will be important to determine if multidrug resistance is a mechanism of natural or acquired resistance to these agents in the clinic.

CLINICAL PHARMACOLOGY OF DRUGS USED IN CANCER TREATMENT

Antimetabolites

Folate Antagonists (Aminopterin, MTX)

History.   The folate antagonist aminopterin was the first drug shown to induce complete remissions in children with ALL (Farber, 1966). It was soon appreciated that these remissions were short-lived, as a result of the development of resistance of the leukemia to subsequent courses of this drug. In the 1950s MTX supplanted aminopterin in the clinic, based on experimental studies showing it had an improved therapeutic index compared with aminopterin. The structures of folic acid (the vitamin), aminopterin, and MTX are shown in Fig. 23–2.

Mechanism of Action.   The major mechanism of action of MTX is to powerfully inhibit the enzyme dihydrofolate reductase (DHFR), the enzyme that catalyses the reduction of dihydrofolate to tetrahydrofolate, the coenzyme form of folic acid (Bertino, 1989; Allegra, 1990). As a consequence of this inhibition, the levels of intracellular folate coenzymes are rapidly depleted. Since folate coenzymes are required for thymidylate biosynthesis as well as purine biosynthesis, DNA synthesis is blocked and cell replication stops. In

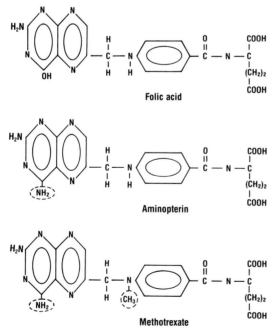

Fig. 23–2.   Structures of folic acid, aminopterin, and methotrexate.

addition, MTX blocks uptake of reduced folates, and thus restoration of folate stores is also impaired. Recent work has shown that MTX is retained in certain cells for long periods, as a consequence of an enzymatic process that adds additional glutamates (up to five) to the antifolate (for review, see Allegra, 1990). This may be an important determinant of MTX selectively, since cells capable of this conversion (e.g., lymphoblasts) may be expected to be more susceptible to cell kill by this drug (Whitehead et al., 1987).

Acquired resistance to MTX in tumor cells has been shown to be due to one or more of several mechanisms: increased concentrations of DHFR as a consequence of gene amplification, defective polyglutamylation, impaired uptake, or an alteration in the target enzyme, DHFR (for review, see Sobrero and Bertino, 1986).

Clinical Pharmacology. When administered orally in low doses (5–10 mg) MTX is well absorbed, but when doses exceed 30 mg, oral bioavailability decreases, with significant interpatient variation (Henderson et al., 1965). Therefore, doses of MTX of 30 mg or greater should be administered IV, IM, or subcutaneously. After IV injection, the disappearance of MTX from plasma is triphasic. The distribution phase (α) $t_{1/2}$ is 30 to 45 minutes, the renal clearance phase (β) $t_{1/2}$ is 3 to 4 hours, and the $t_{1/2}$ of the third phase, probably representing reabsorption from the gut and excretion, is 6 to 20 hours.

Methotrexate is excreted primarily unchanged by the kidneys by both glomerular filtration and active tubular secretion. With larger doses, a significant amount of the drug (7%–30%) is excreted in the urine as the major metabolite 7-hydroxymethotrexate, formed principally in the liver by the action of the enzyme aldehyde oxidase. A small amount of 2,4-diamino-N^{10}-methylpteroic acid has also been noted in plasma and urine, presumably due to cleavage of the peptide bond by enzymes present in bacteria in the large intestine. Patients with renal impairment ordinarily should not be treated with MTX, since the prolonged plasma concentrations that may result may lead to increased hematologic and GI toxicity. In some patients renal toxicity may occur following MTX treatment, especially high-dose regimens, and thus the excretion of the drug may be delayed. In this circumstance leucovorin (folinic acid, N^5-formyl tetrahydrofolate) should be administered until concentrations of MTX decrease to nontoxic values (Tattersall et al., 1975a; Ackland and Schilsky, 1987; Allegra, 1990). In the presence of effusions, MTX may accumulate in this "third space," acting as a storage depot, potentially increasing toxicity by maintaining plasma concentrations over longer periods of time.

Adverse Effects. The dose-limiting toxicities of MTX are myelosupression and GI toxicity. These adverse effects usually occur 7 to 10 days after treatment. An early sign of MTX toxicity to the GI tract is mucositis, involving the oral mucosa. Severe toxicity may be manifest by diarrhea, due to small-bowel damage, that can progress to ulceration and bleeding.

Less common toxic effects caused by MTX are skin rash, pleuritis, and hepatitis. Hepatitis is reversible in most patients, but low-dose chronic administration may lead to fibrosis and cirrhosis of the liver in a small percentage of patients. Renal toxicity is uncommon with conventional doses of MTX but has been a problem with high-dose regimens (>0.5 g/m^2) in adults. Alkalinization and hydration, as well as monitoring MTX serum concentrations are important prophylactic measures to avoid and detect this potential problem (Allegra, 1990). Leucovorin, the antidote used to treat potential toxic effects of MTX overdose, is also used as part of high-dose MTX regimens as planned "rescue." Table 23–3 describes some high-dose MTX regimens used in the clinic and guidelines for monitoring these patients. *Principle: Monitoring of MTX serum concentrations in patients receiving high-dose therapy is essential for safe use of this agent.*

Therapeutic Uses. Methotrexate continues to be a key drug in combination regimens used to treat ALL, and it is used widely in combination therapy of intermediate-grade and high-grade lymphomas, breast cancer, cancer of the head and neck, osteogenic sarcoma, and bladder cancer (Table 23–4). It is also used intrathecally to treat meningeal involvement of leukemia or of carcinomas. Methotrexate is also used to treat certain nonmalignant diseases, including psoriasis and rheumatoid arthritis.

Fluoropyrimidines (5-Fluorouracil and 5-Fluorodeoxyuridine)

History. The development of 5-fluorouracil (5-FU) as an antitumor drug is a marvelous example of the rational design of drugs. Heidelberger et al. (1957) observed that uracil was salvaged more efficiently by certain malignant cells than by normal tissues and designed 5-FU and its deoxy and ribose nucleosides (Fig. 23–3).

Mechanism of Action. 5-Fluorouracil may exert its cytotoxic effects by inhibition of DNA synthesis or by incorporation into RNA, thus inhibiting RNA processing and function (for review, see Grem, 1990). The active metabolite of 5-FU that inhibits DNA synthesis via potent inhibition of thymidylate synthetase is 5-fluorodeoxyuridylate (5-FdUMP).

In rapidly growing tumors, inhibition of thy-

Table 23–3. HIGH-DOSE MTX TREATMENT (> 0.5 g/m²)

Prehydration and Alkalinization of Urine

8–12 h before treatment, give patients 1.5 l/m² of saline or 5% glucose with 100 mEq of HCO_3^- and 20 mEq of KCL per liter. Continue until pH of urine is 7.0 or greater at time of MTX administration.

MTX Administration

1. 0.5–3.0 g/m² as 20- to 30-min bolus. At 24 h begin leucovorin, 15 mg/m², q6h × 6 doses.
2. Jaffe regimen: 1.2–6 g/m² over 6 h IV, with continued IV hydration for an additional 18 h. Begin leucovorin 2 h after MTX infusion, 15 mg/m², q6h × 7 doses.
3. 36-h infusion: Give MTX, 50 mg/m², as bolus, followed by infusion of MTX over 36 h at dose of 1.5 g/m². Start leucovorin rescue at end of infusion: 200 mg/m² over 12 h as infusion, then 25 mg/m² IM q6h × 6.

Drug Monitoring

Monitor MTX concentrations at 24 h for regimen 1, or 48 h for regimens 2 and 3. Determine serum creatinine concentrations before treatment, and at 24 h and 48 h.

For regimen 1, 24-h concentrations of MTX of greater than $1 \times 10^{-6} M$ require additional leucovorin rescue; for regimens 2 and 3, 48-h MTX concentrations above $5 \times 10^{-7} M$ should receive additional leucovorin rescue. The dose of leucovorin should be increased to 100 mg/m² q6h for blood concentrations of 1×10^{-6} to $5 \times 10^{-6} M$, and concentrations above $5 \times 10^{-6} M$ should receive doses of 200 mg/m² or higher. MTX concentrations should be monitored daily and leucovorin continued (in decreasing doses as the blood concentration of MTX falls) until the plasma concentration of MTX is below $1 \times 10^{-8} M$.

---

midylate synthase appears to be the key mechanism of cell death caused by 5-FU; however, in other tumors, cell death is better correlated with incorporation of 5-FU into RNA.

"Modulation" of 5-FU Action. The ternary complex formed by FdUMP, the bioactive folate N^5, N^{10}-methylenetetrahydrofolate, and thymidylate synthase has been noted to dissociate slowly, with a half-life of several hours. The presence of excess bioactive folate ensures maximal ternary-complex formation and in addition retards the dissociation of FdUMP from the complex. Based on this understanding, recent clinical trials have employed high doses of folinic acid (leucovorin, N^5-formyltetrahydrofolate), a stable reduced folate precursor of N^5, N^{10}-methylenetrahydrofolate, followed by 5-FU treatment, in the hope of maximizing ternary-complex formation in malignant cells, and subsequent cell death. This approach, as well as sequential MTX–5-FU treatment, has led to an increase in response rate in certain solid tumors, notably colon cancer (Mini et al., 1990).

Methotrexate pretreatment may increase 5-FU cytotoxicity by increasing 5-phosphoribosyl-1-pyrophosphate (PRPP) concentrations in cells, thus increasing 5-FU nucleotide formation. Increased PRPP concentrations are a consequence of the ability of MTX to inhibit purine biosynthesis. In addition, inhibition of dihydrofolate reductase by MTX leads to an increase in dihydrofolate polyglutamates in cells, thereby enhancing FdUMP binding to thymidylate synthase (Fernandez and Bertino, 1980).

Other strategies to modulate 5-FU cytotoxicity are also being tested in the clinic; these include pretreatment with the de novo pyrimidine synthesis inhibitor phosphonacetyl-L-aspartate (PALA);

the use of dipyrimadole, an inhibitor of nucleoside salvage; and uridine "rescue" (Table 23–5).

Clinical Pharmacology. The clinical pharmacology of 5-FU has been reviewed recently (Grem, 1990). 5-Fluorouracil is absorbed erratically after oral administration and therefore is administered IV. The drug has a short plasma half-life (10–15 minutes), and after a pulse dose with conventional doses (600 mg/m²), cytotoxic concentrations (> 1 μM) are maintained in blood for only 6 hours or less. Cytotoxicity depends on the efficiency of conversion of 5-FU to its active metabolites, FdUMP and FUTP; the concentrations of the competing substrate, dUMP; the concentrations of the folate coenzyme, N^5, N^{10}-methylenetetrahydrofolate; the concentration of the target enzyme, thymidylate synthase, in the malignant cell; and possibly the extent of incorporation of 5-FU into RNA. Various dosage schedules of 5-FU have been investigated, including bolus treatment daily for 5 days once a month, weekly bolus treatment, and infusions of 5-FU lasting 24, 48, 120 hours or longer.

When infusions of 5-FU are administered, the major toxicity is GI, while bolus treatment usually produces leukopenia and thrombocytopenia as limiting toxicity. The drug distributes freely into third spaces (e.g., CSF, ascites). Metabolism occurs mainly in the liver to dihydrofluorouracil, and further breakdown products, fluoroureidoproprionic acid and CO_2. Because of its metabolism by liver, 5-FU has also been infused into the hepatic artery or administered intraperitoneally; this method achieves high local concentrations, with decreased systemic toxicity. 5-Fluorodeoxyuridine (5-FUdR) is even more rapidly metabolized by the liver than is 5-FU. Thus, administration of this drug into the intrahepatic artery is

Table 23-4. ANTIMETABOLITES

DRUG	CYCLE-ACTIVE	TOXICITY			ANTITUMOR RESULTS		
		BONE MARROW	GI	OTHER	EXCELLENT	GOOD	FAIR
Methotrexate (amethopterin)	Yes	++	++	Renal toxicity (high doses) Liver toxicity (chronic use) Skin rash	Choriocarcinoma Burkitt lymphoma ALL	Head and neck cancer Osteogenic sarcoma Large-cell lymphoma Breast Bladder	Lung Cervix
Fluorouracil (5-FU)	Yes	++	++			GI tract Breast	Bladder Prostate Head and neck
Cytosine arabinoside (Ara-C)	Yes	++	+	CNS toxicity (high doses)	Acute leukemias		Non-Hodgkin lymphoma
Mercaptopurine (6-MP)	Yes	++	+	Hepatic fibrosis	ALL	AML CML	
6-Thioguanine (6-TG)	Yes	++	±	Hepatic fibrosis	ALL	AML CML	

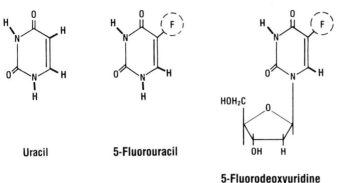

| Uracil | 5-Fluorouracil | 5-Fluorodeoxyuridine |

Fig. 23–3. Structures of uracil, its antimetabolite 5-fluorouracil, and the nucleoside 5-fluorodeoxyuridine (5-FUdR).

used to treat isolated hepatic metastases from colon cancer.

Adverse Effects. The major dose-limiting toxicities of 5-FU and 5-FUdR are marrow toxicity and GI toxicity (Table 23–4). Stomatitis and diarrhea usually occur 4 to 7 days after treatment. Further treatment should be withheld until recovery occurs. The nadir of leukopenia and thrombocytopenia usually occurs 7 to 10 days after a single dose or a 5-day course of the drug, and recovery usually takes place in 14 days. The dose-limiting toxicity of infusions of 5-FUdR via the hepatic artery is transient liver toxicity, occasionally resulting in biliary sclerosis.

Less common toxicities noted with 5-FU after systemic administration are skin rash, cerebellar symptoms (with single-pulse doses greater than 800 mg/m^2), and conjunctivitis and tearing. Myocardial infarction has also been reported in association with 5-FU administration, but a clear causal relationship has not been established.

Therapeutic Uses. Both 5-FU and 5-FUdR have antitumor activity against several solid tumors, most notably colon cancer, breast cancer,

and head and neck cancer. A preparation containing 5-FU is also used topically to treat skin hyperkeratosis and superficial basal cell carcinomas.

Cytosine Arabinoside

History and Chemistry. Cytosine arabinoside (ara-C, 1-β-D-arabinofuranosylcytosine) is an antimetabolite analog of deoxycytidine (Fig. 23–4). The difference between deoxycytidine and the analog ara-C is that in the analog the OH group at the 2′ position in the sugar ring is in the arabinose configuration. This compound was first isolated from the sponge *Cryptothethya crypta*.

Mechanism of Action. Cytosine arabinoside is converted to the nucleotide triphosphate (ara-CTP) intracellularly; this latter compound both is an inhibitor of DNA polymerase and is incorporated into DNA (Kufe et al., 1984). The latter event is considered to cause the lethal action of ara-C, as incorporation has been known to result in a defect in ligation of newly synthesized fragments of DNA.

Both ara-C and its mononucleotide may be inactivated by two intracellular enzymes, cytidine deaminase and deoxycytidylate deaminase, respectively (for review, see Pallavincini, 1984). The

Table 23–5. "MODULATION" OF 5-FU ACTION IN CELLS

MODULATING AGENT	MECHANISM
Folinic acid (leucovorin) pretreatment	Increases folate cofactor in cells, increasing ternary complex formation.
PALA pretreatment	Blocks de novo pyrimidine synthesis; increases 5-FU nucleotide formation.
Thymidine	Enhances 5-FU incorporation into RNA; delays 5-FU breakdown.
MTX pretreatment	Increases PRPP, thus increasing FU nucleotide levels; increases dihydrofolate polyglutamates in cells.
Uridine posttreatment	Protects normal cells from 5-FU toxicity; mechanism not clear.

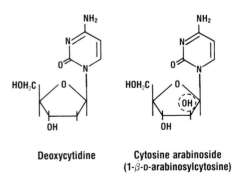

| Deoxycytidine | Cytosine arabinoside (1-β-D-arabinosylcytosine) |

Fig. 23–4. Structures of deoxycytidine and the antimetabolite cytosine arabinoside (ara-C).

ara-U (uracil arabinoside) formed from ara-C is more slowly cleared from plasma than ara-C and may slow subsequent metabolism of ara-C in high-dose regimens (Capizzi et al., 1985).

Resistance. Although several mechanisms for acquired resistance to ara-C have been elucidated in experimental tumor systems, an explanation for acquired resistance in leukemia cells of patients is still not clear. A decrease of deoxycytidine kinase activity, an increased pool size of CTP, and increased activity of cytidine deaminase have been described to occur in ara-C-resistant cell lines. Evidence for the decrease of deoxycytidine kinase activity, or an increase of cytidine deaminase activity, has been reported in human leukemia (Steward and Burke, 1971; Tattersall et al., 1974), but other studies have not confirmed these results (Chang et al., 1979). The level of ara-CTP formation after dosing has been reported to be useful in monitoring drug efficacy (Liliemark et al., 1985).

Clinical Pharmacology. Since it is poorly absorbed orally, ara-C is administered IV as a pulse dose or a continuous infusion. The drug distributes rapidly into body water, and a high concentration (50% of the plasma value) occurs in the CSF 2 hours after IV administration. The ara-C disappears rapidly from plasma with a $t_{1/2}$ of 7 to 20 minutes. With higher doses, a longer half-life is found, presumably due to inhibition of metabolism of ara-C by ara-U. The formation of ara-U occurs in plasma, liver, granulocytes, and other tissues of the body (Pallavincini, 1984; Capizzi et al., 1985). Most of the drug is excreted in the urine in the form of the inactive metabolite ara-U. As in the case of MTX, single-bolus infusions of doses as high as 5 g/m^2 (given over 1–3 h) produce little marrow toxicity because of its rapid clearance, while doses of 1 g/m^2 given IV over 48 hours may produce severe marrow toxicity (Spriggs et al., 1988).

Adverse Reactions. In conventional doses (100–200 mg/m^2 per day for 5–10 days), the dose-limiting toxicity of ara-C is myelosuppression (see Table 23–4). Some nausea and vomiting is seen with these doses, which increases markedly when high doses are employed, although repeated administration of the drug results in some tolerance to this adverse affect. Leukopenia and thrombocytopenia nadirs occur at about day 10, and marrow injury is rapidly reversible. In addition to increased nausea and vomiting noted with high-dose ara-C, neurologic, GI, and liver toxicity have been observed when high-dose regimens are used (Rudnick et al., 1979; Spriggs et al., 1988). The severity of these effects increases with increasing duration of therapy. High doses (2–3 g/m^2) given every 12 hours for a total of 6 doses may be as effective as 12 doses, and lower doses

of ara-C (0.5–1 g/m^2) given over 2 hours every 12 hours may be as effective as higher doses.

Intrathecal ara-C is usually well tolerated, but adverse neurologic effects, such as seizures and alterations in mental status, have been reported.

Therapeutic Uses. Cytosine arabinoside remains the drug of choice for the treatment of AML. When used together with an anthracycline drug (daunomycin, mitoxantrone), remissions may be achieved in 60% to 80% of patients with this disease. This drug is also used in combination to treat other hematologic malignancies, but its exact role in the treatment of these neoplasms is less well defined. Cytosine arabinoside is also used intrathecally to treat meningeal leukemia.

Purine Analogs (6-Mercaptopurine and 6-Thioguanine)

History. The purine analogs 6-mercaptopurine (6-MP) and 6-thioguanine (6-TG) were synthesized by Elion et al. (1952) and introduced into the clinic soon after MTX by Burchenal et al. (1953). Other purine analogs are also used clinically, including azathioprine, a 6-MP *prodrug* that is a potent immunosuppressive agent; allopurinol, an inhibitor of xanthine oxidase, useful in the prevention of uric acid nephropathy; and antiviral compounds such as ara-A (adenine arabinoside) (McCormack and Johns, 1990). Deoxycoformycin (Fig. 23–5), a potent inhibitor of adenosine deaminase, has also been found to be a useful agent in the treatment of T-cell malignancies as well as hairy cell leukemia. Another purine analog, 2-chlorodeoxyadenosine, has also been reported to be extremely effective in the treatment of hairy cell leukemia, and its use in low-grade lymphomas is being tested (Piro et al., 1990).

Mechanism of Action of 6-Thiopurines. Both 6-MP and 6-TG have a thiol group substitution for the 6-hydroxy group found in hypoxanthine or guanine, respectively (Fig. 23–5). Both compounds are converted to nucleotides by the enzyme hypoxanthine-guanine phosphoribosyl transferase (HPRT). Despite considerable investigation, the exact mechanism whereby these analogs exert their cytotoxic effects is not known (Elion, 1967; Tidd and Paterson, 1974; McCormack and Johns, 1990). De novo purine synthesis is blocked by the 6-thiopurine nucleotides, which are also incorporated into DNA after conversion to the triphosphates. This incorporation may also contribute to the cytotoxic effects of the thiopurines.

In experimental tumor cells, resistance is most commonly found to be a consequence of markedly decreased activity of the activating enzyme HPRT (Brockman, 1963). In human ALL, resistance was found to be associated with an increase

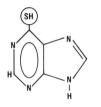

6-Mercaptopurine

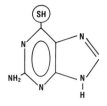

6-Thioguanine

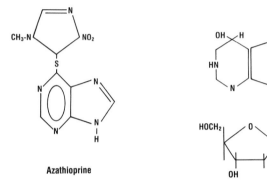

Azathioprine

2'Deoxycoformycin

Fig. 23–5. Chemical structures of purines and purine analogs 6-MP, 6-TG, azathioprine, and 2'-deoxycoformycin.

in activity of alkaline phosphatase, found in membranes, and capable of degrading the nucleotides of the 6-thiopurines (Rosman et al., 1974; Scholar and Calabresi, 1979). Absence of HPRT activity was a rare cause of resistance in patients with AML; an alteration of this enzyme leading to decreased thiopurine binding to this enzyme was found in the blast cells of some patients (Rosman and Williams, 1973).

Clinical Pharmacology. Both 6-MP and 6-TG are given orally, although absorption is erratic and variable (LePage and Whitecar, 1971). A recent study indicates that clinical benefit may reflect the concentrations of drug in blood that were achieved; therefore, dosages may require adjusting in individual patients (Koren et al., 1990). **Principle: Monitoring blood concentrations of potent anticancer agents may be required to be sure that adequate dose intensity is achieved.**

6-Mercaptopurine is metabolized primarily by xanthine oxidase to 6-thiouric acid, a reaction that is inhibited by allopurinol, while 6-TG is principally methylated, followed eventually by oxidation and elimination of the sulfur moiety. Therefore, a 6-MP dosage reduction of 75% is recommended when allopurinol is used with this drug; no dose reduction is necessary when 6-TG and allopurinol are administered together. An-

other difference between these two drugs is GI toxicity; 6-TG causes less nausea and vomiting than does 6-MP, presumably because of metabolism of this latter drug by the GI mucosa.

Adverse Reactions. Except for less GI toxicity from 6-TG compared with 6-MP, both drugs have equivalent toxicity to the bone marrow, the limiting toxicity (see Table 23–4). Mild hepatotoxicity may be noted after treatment with either of these compounds but usually is rapidly reversible. Treatment with 6-MP has been implicated as a cause for cirrhosis in patients on long-term therapy with this drug.

Therapeutic Use. Both 6-MP and 6-TG are used for the treatment of ALL and AML as part of combination regimens.

Vinca Alkaloids

History. Vinblastine and vincristine are alkaloids isolated from the leaves of the Madagascar periwinkle plant (*Catharanthus roseus*). Vinca alkaloids are asymmetric diametric compounds (Fig. 23–6). The small difference in the structure of vincristine compared with vinblastine results in important differences in the spectrum of antitumor activity as well as toxicity.

Mechanism of Action. The vinca alkaloids

exert their cytotoxic action via binding to tubulin, a dimeric protein found in the cytoplasm of cells. Microtubules are essential for forming the spindle along which the chromosomes migrate during mitosis, and for maintaining cell structure. Binding of the vinca alkaloids to tubulin leads to inhibition of the process of assembly and dissolution of the mitotic spindle (Ludena et al., 1977). As a consequence, cells are arrested in metaphase; cell kill may also occur in late S phase.

Resistance to vinca alkaloids has been reported to be due to an alteration in the structure of tubulin, resulting in decreased binding of the drugs. Another important mechanism of resistance to the vinca alkaloids is the multidrug resistance phenotype (Riordan and Ling, 1985; Tsuruo, 1988), resulting in increased drug efflux.

Clinical Pharmacology. The clinical pharmacology of both drugs has been reviewed recently (Bender et al., 1990). Both vincristine and vinblastine are administered IV. After a rapid distribution phase ($t_{1/2} = 7$ minutes), vincristine disappears from the plasma with a half-life of 164 minutes (Bender et al., 1977). Vinblastine's distribution phase is 4 minutes, and subsequent breaks in the curve have half-lives of 53 minutes and 20 hours. For clinical purposes and for calculation of doseage and doseage intervals, the half-lives of vincristine and vinblastine are 2 hours and 1 hour, respectively. Almost 70% of a dose of vincristine is metabolized by the liver and excreted in the feces. Metabolism of vinblastine is also the major route of inactivation of this drug, but details of the site of metabolism and metabolic products are lacking. Most investigators decrease the dose of vincristine or vinblastine in patients with hepatic impairment, although information on this subject is not complete. A 50% decrease in dose is recommended for patients with a bilirubin concentration greater than 3 mg/dl, while no decrease in dose is advocated for patients with impaired renal function.

Adverse Reactions. The dose-limiting toxicity to vincristine is neurotoxicity (see Table 23–6). The initial signs of neurotoxicity are paresthesias of the fingers and lower extremities, and loss of deep tendon reflexes. Continued use may lead to more advanced neurotoxicity, which includes profound weakness of motor strength, in particular dorsiflexion of the foot. Occasionally cranial nerve palsies and severe jaw pain are noted with vincristine administration. At high doses of vincristine (>3 mg total single dose), autonomic neuropathy may be noted, leading to obstipation and paralytic ileus. Sensory changes and reflex abnormalities slowly improve when treatment is stopped; however, motor impairment improves less rapidly and may be irreversible. In addition to these commonly observed toxicities, inappropriate antidiuretic hormone (ADH) release may occur, which can lead to marked hyponatremia. While marrow suppression is not commonly noted with vincristine, some additive marrow toxicity may be noted in patients with impaired or recovering marrow function.

The primary toxicity of vinblastine is leukopenia, which reaches a nadir at day 6 to 7 after treatment and is rapidly reversible. Mucositis is occasionally observed when vinblastine is taken at higher doses (>8 mg/m²), or when it is used in combination with drugs that also have the potential for this toxic effect. Neurotoxicity is rarely observed at conventional doses with vinblastine. Both drugs cause severe pain and local toxicity if extravasated. ***Principle: Neither drug should be given intrathecally, since deaths have been reported from vincristine administered inadvertently into the CSF.***

Therapeutic Uses. Of the three alkaloids tested extensively in the past 2 decades (vinblastine, vincristine, and vindesine), only the former two are now available for use in the United States. These drugs are used widely in the treatment of malignant neoplasms (see Table 23–6); vinblastine

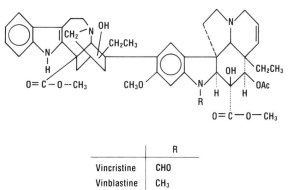

Fig. 23–6. Structures of vinblastine and vincristine.

Table 23-6. VINCA ALKALOIDS

DRUG	CYCLE-ACTIVE	TOXICITY			ANTITUMOR RESULTS		
		BONE MARROW	GI	OTHER	EXCELLENT	GOOD	FAIR
Vinblastine (Velban)	Yes	++	±	Vesicant if extravasates	Hodgkin disease	Choriocarcinoma Testicular cancer	Kidney Bladder
Vincristine (Oncovin)	Yes	±	±	Neuropathy Severe constipation Inappropriate ADH release Vesicant	ALL Wilms tumor Lymphoma	Ewing sarcoma Neuroblastoma	Breast

Table 23-7. PODOPHYLLOTOXINS

DRUG	CYCLE-ACTIVE	TOXICITY			ANTITUMOR RESULTS		
		BONE MARROW	GI	OTHER	EXCELLENT	GOOD	FAIR
Etoposide (VP-16)	Yes	++	+	Hypotensive episodes if administered rapidly	Hodgkin disease Large-cell lymphoma Testicular cancer	ALL Lung cancer	
Tenoposide (VM-26)	Yes	++	–		ALL		

because of its activity in the treatment of testicular cancer, bladder cancer, and Hodgkin disease, and vincristine for its activity in lymphoma, lymphatic leukemia, and in Wilms tumor (Bender et al., 1990).

Podophyllotoxins

History and Chemistry. Although the cytotoxic properties of podophyllin have been known since 1946, this compound is too toxic for systemic use. A large synthetic program led to the synthesis and testing of two derivatives, etoposide (VP-16) and tenoposide (VM-26) (Fig. 23–7). Etoposide has received a much more extensive clinical evaluation than tenoposide, and the latter drug is not yet approved by the FDA for use as an anticancer agent in the United States.

Mechanism of Action. The mechanism of action of these compounds is not clear; induction of single-stranded breaks in DNA has been demonstrated in cells, possibly due to its interaction with topoisomerase II (Ross et al., 1984). Resistance to etoposide may also occur via the multidrug-resistant phenotype (Riordan and Ling, 1985; Tsuruo, 1988). Recent studies also show that resistance may be a consequence of an alteration in topoisomerase II, leading to decreased binding of etoposide (Pommier et al., 1986).

Clinical Pharmacology. Etoposide may be administered either orally or IV. When it is administered orally, 50% of the dose is absorbed. After a single IV dose of etoposide, the plasma half-lives are 2.8 and 15.1 hours. Approximately one half of the dosage is excreted in the urine, with one third as a metabolite. The remainder of the drug is excreted in the feces and further metabolized by the liver. The drug's pharmacokinetics have been reviewed recently (Creaven, 1984; Bender et al., 1990).

Adverse Effects. When administered IV, etoposide should be administered over a 30-minute period to avoid hypotensive episodes. The major toxicity is leukopenia, which is rapidly reversible (see Table 23–7). Thrombocytopenia may also occur but is much less common. Nausea and vomiting are common with IV drug administration. Alopecia is also common, while other toxicities such as fever, mild elevation of liver tests, or peripheral neuropathy are relatively uncommon. Because the major toxicity of etoposide is limited to the marrow, this drug is under extensive investigation as part of treatment with high-dose regimens followed by marrow transplantation.

Therapeutic Uses. Etoposide has significant clinical activity in several malignancies, including Hodgkin disease, diffuse lymphomas, leukemias, lung cancer, and testicular cancer.

Alkylating Agents

General Comments. Alkylating agents are important in the treatment of various malignancies either as single agents or as components of effective combination regimens. This important role may be a result of their non-cycle-active action, and there appears to be little or no cross-resistance of alkylating agents with other classes of drugs. The alkylating agents may be classified as bifunctional or monofunctional agents (Fig. 23–8). Examples of the first class are cyclophosphamide, nitrogen mustard, thiotepa, melphalan, busulfan, chlorambucil, and the nitrosoureas (Farmer, 1987). Bifunctional agents have two reactive sites on the molecule and thus are capable of cross-linking important biologic molecules, in particular DNA. The most susceptible region for alkylation of DNA is the N-7 position of guanine. Other DNA-reacting drugs, such as procarbazine and dacarbazine (DTIC, ditriazenoimidazolecarboxamide), may be thought of as monofunctional agents and therefore do not cross-link DNA but may produce breaks in single strands of DNA.

Resistance may be specific for certain alkylat-

Podophyllotoxin

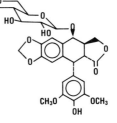

R = CH$_3$ **Etoposide (VP-16)**

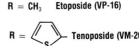

R = ⟨S⟩– **Tenoposide (VM-26)**

Fig. 23–7. Structures of podophyllotoxin, VP-16 (etoposide) and VM-26 (tenoposide).

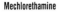

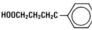

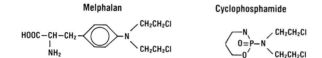

Fig. 23-8. Structures of alkylating agents in clinical use: mechlorethamine, melphalan, chlorambucil, cyclophosphamide, and ifosfamide are nitrogen mustards; thiotepa is an ethylenimine; and busulfan is an alkylsulfonate.

ing agents, for example, impaired uptake of nitrogen mustard as a consequence of an alteration in the carrier for the natural substrate choline (Goldenberg et al., 1970). Resistance may also be common to alkylating agents, for example, increased degradation associated with an increase in intracellular sulfhydryl compounds, and increased repair of DNA damage.

For purposes of discussion, these agents may be further classified according to chemical structures, and a brief discussion of each agent is given below.

Nitrogen Mustards. The prototype of this class of alkylating agent is mechlorethamine (mustine, nitrogen mustard, HN_2), first studied by Gilman and colleagues in 1946, developed as a result of chemical warfare research in World War II (for review, see Gilman, 1963).

Mechlorethamine

CLINICAL PHARMACOLOGY. Mechlorethamine is a highly reactive compound that immediately after mixing may be administered IV. It is a potent vesicant, and care must be taken in mixing and administering the drug. Intramolecular cyclization produces ethylenimonium products, and these reactive intermediates rapidly bind to various nucleophiles, especially sulfydryl compounds and DNA.

ADVERSE REACTIONS. Adverse effects include severe nausea and vomiting, occurring within minutes to hours after administration; marrow suppression with a nadir of 10 to 14 days; and alopecia (see Table 23-8). Mechlorethamine causes severe tissue damage if extravasation occurs, and immediate treatment with sodium thiosulfate into the same IV site may help to decrease

potential tissue damage by reacting with the active intermediates of mechlorethamine.

CLINICAL USES. Mechlorethamine is almost exclusively used in the treatment of Hodgkin disease, especially as part of combination regimens such as MOPP (mechlorethamine, vincristine, procarbazine, and prednisone) (DeVita et al., 1972). This drug is also used to control pleural and pericardial effusions by intracavitary administration, and is also applied topically in dilute solution to treat mycosis fungoides (Vonderheid, 1984).

Cyclophosphamide

INTRODUCTION. This alkylating agent was first described in 1958 and represents an effort to selectively activate a drug at the tumor site. This drug has a wide spectrum of antitumor activity and is also used as an immunosuppressant.

MECHANISM OF ACTION AND CLINICAL PHARMACOLOGY. Most of the parent compound, which is inactive, is metabolized by the P450 system in vivo, generating active metabolites, in particular phosphoramide mustard, from its precursor 4-hydroxycyclophosphamide (Colvin and Hilton, 1981). This latter compound is also used to selectively kill leukemia and lymphoma cells in bone marrow in autologous transplant programs ("purging").

The plasma half-life is 16 hours (Sladek et al., 1984), and 80% or more of the administered dose is eliminated by metabolism. Some dose adjustment may be required in patients with renal impairment, inasmuch as the parent drug and the metabolites are excreted in the urine (Juma et al., 1979).

Cyclophosphamide may be administered orally or IV. In low doses, 75% or more of the dose is

Table 23-8. ALKYLATING AGENTS

DRUG	TOXICITY				ANTITUMOR RESULTS		
	CYCLE-ACTIVE	BONE MARROW	GI	OTHER	EXCELLENT	GOOD	FAIR
Mechlorethamine (nitrogen mustard, Mustargen, HN$_2$)	No	++	++	Vesicant	Hodgkin disease	Lymphoma	Cervix Head and neck Lung
Cyclophosphamide (Endoxan, Cytoxan)	Yes	++	+	Alopecia Chemical cystitis	Burkitt lymphoma Hodgkin disease Non-Hodgkin lymphoma Breast	ALL Myeloma Neuroblastoma Retinoblastoma Breast	Lung Melanoma Head and neck Cervix
Ifosfamide	Yes(?)	+	+	Chemical cystitis	Ovary	Lymphoma Testis	Lung Breast
Melphalan (Alkeran, PAM)	No	++	±	–	–	Breast Myeloma	Melanoma
Chlorambucil (Leukeran)	No	++	±	–	Lymphoma CLL	Breast	
Thiotepa	No	++	±	–	Bladder (intravesical)	Breast Lymphoma	
Busulfan (Myleran)	No	++	±	Pulmonary fibrosis Skin pigmentation	CML		

absorbed, and the drug is tolerated well (Grochow and Colvin, 1979). Higher doses (500 mg or greater) may produce nausea and vomiting. When the drug is administered IV, extravasation does not produce tissue injury as in the case of mechlorethamine.

ADVERSE EFFECTS. As with all alkylating agents, bone marrow suppression is the limiting adverse effect of this drug (nadir 10–14 days after a single dose) (see Table 23–8). This drug is relatively platelet-sparing, and leukopenia is the major limiting toxicity. Hemorrhagic cystitis is occasionally seen with this drug, caused by the metabolite acrolein that accumulates in the bladder. Vigorous hydration, especially when high doses of the drug are used, helps to decrease the incidence of this problem. With larger doses (500 mg/m^2 or greater), severe nausea and vomiting are seen, typically 8 to 12 hours after drug is administered and presumably due to conversion of cyclophosphamide to active metabolites. Pulmonary toxicity (fibrosis) and cardiac toxicity (acute hemorrhagic carditis) may occur, especially with larger doses of this drug as used in these regimens. The total dose of cyclophosphamide in a single course is usually limited to 200 mg/kg (Muggia et al., 1983).

Other uncommon toxicities are the inappropriate ADH syndrome (Buckner et al., 1972) and hiccups. Long-term toxicities include infertility and carcinogenesis. Cyclophosphamide appears to be less carcinogenic than other alkylating agents, in particular when compared with melphalan.

CLINICAL USE. Cyclophosphamide is used in combination regimens to treat lymphoma, lymphoid leukemia, breast cancer, small-cell lung cancer, and ovarian cancer. It has an important use as part of high-dose regimens in bone marrow transplantation programs. Cyclophosphamide is also used widely as an immunosupressant (Growchow and Colvin, 1979).

Ifosfamide

INTRODUCTION. This compound has recently been approved for use in the United States. It differs from cyclophosphamide only in the location of a chloroethyl moiety (Fig. 23–8). As with cyclophosphamide, activation occurs in the liver predominantly by the P450 mixed-function oxidase system, generating ifosphamide mustard.

MECHANISM OF ACTION AND CLINICAL PHARMACOLOGY. Activation of ifosfamide also occurs predominantly in liver, by the P450 mixed-function oxidase system. Ifosfamide mustard, the active compound, is generated. Acrolein and chloroacetic acid are the principal toxic metabolites (Colvin, 1982). The plasma disappearance of

ifosfamide is slightly longer than that of cyclophosphamide, and some of the compound is excreted unchanged in the urine (Allen et al., 1976).

ADVERSE REACTIONS. The dose-limiting toxicity of this drug is bladder toxicity, presumably due to accumulation of acrolein and chloroacetic acid in the bladder (Creaven et al., 1976) (see Table 23–8). Dose fractionation and vigorous hydration with diuretics decreases this toxic effect. Mesna, a thiol that is excreted in the urine, is now used routinely in ifosfamide-containing regimens, because of its ability to inactivate the toxic metabolites of ifosfamide in the bladder (see section on miscellaneous drugs). Mesna is generally well tolerated but may cause some nausea and vomiting. The nausea and vomiting produced by ifosfamide is less than that observed with large doses of cyclophosphamide, as is the degree of myelosuppression (Table 23–8). Central nervous system toxicity is occasionally seen in patients treated with high doses of ifosfamide and mesna and is manifested by changes in mental status, cerebellar dysfunction, and even seizures (Pratt et al., 1986).

CLINICAL USE. Ifosfamide, like cyclophosphamide, has a broad spectrum of activity. Antitumor effects are seen in patients with lymphomas, ovarian cancer, and testicular cancer, and in various solid tumors. Its role in combination therapy is still under investigation (Brade et al., 1987).

Melphalan

INTRODUCTION. Melphalan (Fig. 23–8) is a bifunctional alkylating agent, and similar to others in this class causes interstrand, intrastrand, and DNA–protein cross-links (Sarosy et al., 1988). Melphalan, like cyclophosphamide is active orally, although an IV preparation is available as an investigational drug.

MECHANISM OF ACTION AND CLINICAL PHARMACOLOGY. Studies indicate that this drug is absorbed erratically (Alberts et al., 1979c). *Principle: Patients receiving this drug should receive a dose resulting in a fixed end point (e.g., leukopenia) or have concentrations measured in the blood to be certain that an effective dose is obtained.*

ADVERSE EFFECTS. In the usual therapeutic doses administered orally, melphalan is well tolerated, and its major limiting toxicity is myelosuppression (see Table 23–8). Alopecia is sometimes seen, and pulmonary fibrosis has been reported to occur in patients on this drug for long periods of time. High-dose IV regimens used with autologous bone marrow transplantation rescue cause more serious GI toxicity (nausea, vomiting, diarrhea, mucositis), as well as the expected more profound marrow toxicity (Hersh et al., 1983; Lazarus et al., 1987).

CLINICAL USE. Melphalan is the drug of choice with prednisone to treat myeloma. It is also used in the treatment of ovarian and breast cancer, but it has been mainly supplanted in the treatment of these latter tumors by cyclophosphamide.

Chlorambucil

INTRODUCTION. Chlorambucil, like melphalan, is an orally administered alkylating agent (Fig. 23–8). Its mechanism of action is believed to be similar to that of the other nitrogen mustards.

CLINICAL PHARMACOLOGY AND ADVERSE EFFECTS. The absorption of this slow-acting nitrogen mustard is usually consistent (Alberts et al., 1979b). It is well tolerated, usually without nausea and vomiting, even when used as pulse treatment (5 days once a month) or in continuous daily administration. The dose-limiting toxicity is myelosuppression; occasional liver abnormalities and pulmonary fibrosis have been reported with long-term use (Cole et al., 1978). Like all the alkylating agents, this drug can cause secondary leukemias and sterility.

CLINICAL USE. The major use of chlorambucil is to treat patients with CLL or low-grade non-Hodgkin lymphoma (Portlock et al., 1987) (Table 23–8).

Ethylenimine Derivatives

Thiotepa. Thiotepa (triethylenethiophosphoramide) is an ethylenimine type of alkylating agent (Fig. 23–8). It has the attribute of being lipophilic and thus is able to penetrate the CNS to achieve high concentrations (Edwards et al., 1979).

MECHANISM OF ACTION AND CLINICAL PHARMACOLOGY. This drug also is believed to act by alkylation of DNA, similar to the nitrogen mustards. It may be administered both orally and parenterally, and has been given intravesically, intraarterially, and IM, since it is not a vesicant. When it is used by local instillation to treat superficial bladder cancer and malignant effusions, absorption and toxicity is possible.

CLINICAL USE. There is a resurgence of interest in this drug since it may be used in high doses with other agents followed by autologous bone marrow rescue. In addition to dose-limiting myelosuppression, other adverse effects may be seen with these high doses, including mucositis, skin rash, and CNS toxicity (Lazarus et al., 1987) (see Table 23–8).

CLINICAL USE. Although early studies showed antitumor effects in breast, lung, ovarian, and hematologic malignancies, its use, except for marrow transplantation, is generally restricted to in-travesicular administration for superficial bladder cancer.

Alkyl Sulphonates

Busulfan. Busulfan is an alkyl sulfonate type of alkylating agent (Fig. 23–8).

CLINICAL PHARMACOLOGY. Busulfan is available for oral use; it is well absorbed with an elimination half-life of about 2 to 5 hours and is excreted mainly as metabolites in the urine (Ehrsson et al., 1983).

ADVERSE EFFECTS. Dose-limiting toxicity is myelosuppression, primarily of the myeloid elements. Other less common adverse effects are mild nausea, gynecomastia, hyperpigmentation, and transient elevation of liver enzyme concentrations. Long-term treatment may cause pulmonary fibrosis.

CLINICAL USE. The only indication for use of busulfan is to treat CML (Table 23–8). It can reduce the leukocytosis and splenomegaly associated with this disease but does not delay the onset of transformation to blast crisis.

Nitrosoureas

Carmustine and Lomustine

History. Carmustine (BCNU, bischloroethyl-nitrosourea) was the first of the nitrosourea compounds in clinical trial to receive extensive clinical evaluation (Fig. 23–9). An unusual feature of these highly reactive compounds is their lipid solubility and thus their ability to cross the blood-brain barrier (Walker, 1973).

Lomustine [CCNU, 1-(2-chloroethyl)-3-cyclohexyl-1-nitrosourea] (Fig. 23–9) is similar to carmustine in its mechanism of action and clinical activity. It is administered orally and is rapidly absorbed and biotransformed (Woolley, 1983).

Mechanism of Action. The nitrosoureas, in particular carmustine and lomustine, have been extensively studied in animal tumor models and in the clinic (Schein et al., 1984). The nitrosoureas show some degree of cross-resistance with other alkylating agents, and recent studies indicate that these compounds are primarily alkylating agents. A base-catalyzed decomposition of these compounds generates the alkylating chloroethyldiazonium hydroxide entity (Colvin et al., 1976).

Clinical Pharmacology. After IV administration, carmustine disappears from plasma with an initial half-life of 6 minutes and an elimination $t_{1/2}$ of 68 minutes.

Toxicity. The nitrosoureas, like other alkylating agents, are potent bone marrow toxins (Table 23–9). However, the hemopoietic depression produced by the nitrosoureas occurs later than that seen with other alkylating agents. Leukocyte and

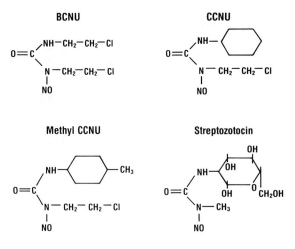

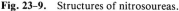

Fig. 23-9. Structures of nitrosoureas.

platelet nadirs occur 4 to 5 weeks after administration of the drugs. Thus the nitrosoureas appear to damage a primitive stem cell. The late marrow depression and cumulative toxicity make these drugs difficult to use clinically. Nausea and vomiting occur frequently with the nitrosoureas. Nephrotoxicity may also result from treatment with a nitrosurea. Both drugs may produce hepatotoxicity; this adverse effect is less common with lomustine. A large adjuvant study of lomustine plus 5-FU by the Gastrointestinal Tumor Study Group has shown that treatment with this combination was associated with an increased incidence of acute leukemia, presumably attributable to the nitrosourea (Boice et al., 1983).

Therapeutic Uses. Nitrosoureas have a reasonably broad spectrum of activity, and currently they are used in the treatment of lymphoma as well as certain solid tumors, in particular brain tumors. Their use in the treatment of GI cancer has been diminishing.

Streptozotocin

Introduction. Streptozotocin is a nitrosourea that has been in clinical trials since 1967 (for review, see Weiss, 1982).

Mechanism of Action and Clinical Pharmacology. Like the other nitrosoureas, this drug functions as an alkylating agent. Its plasma half-life is short (35 minutes), and it is excreted in the urine as metabolites (Adolphe et al., 1975). This drug selectively destroys β-islet cells of the pancreas and causes diabetes in animals.

Adverse Effects. The dose-limiting adverse effect of streptozotocin is nephrotoxicity (see Table 23-9). Drug-induced diabetes is not seen in humans as a result of this drug, but mild glucose intolerance may occur as a result of its use. As

with the other nitrosoureas, nausea and vomiting may be severe. Unlike the result of therapy with carmustine and lomustine, little or no bone marrow depression is seen after giving this drug, thus allowing it to be used in combinations.

Clinical Use. The major use for streptozotocin is to treat carcinoid and islet cell tumors (Table 23-9). It has also been used in combinations to treat Hodgkin disease and colon cancer, but its contribution to the antitumor effects seen is not well defined.

Platinum Compounds

Cisplatin

History. Cisplatin (diamminodichloroplatinum, DDP) is a platinum coordination complex that has broad-spectrum antitumor activity in humans (Fig. 23-10). The story of its discovery is one of serendipity and the prepared scientific mind.

Dr. B. Rosenberg noted that in experiments with bacteria, a toxic substance was being produced by platinum electrodes. He found this material to be the platinum coordination complex, *cis*-diamminodichloroplatinum (Rosenberg et al., 1965). He subsequently investigated its cytotoxic effects on bacteria as well as mammalian tumor cells. These results prompted a clinical trial in humans, and despite some antitumor activity in early phase I trials, further trials were stopped because of renal toxicity. The drug was then found to be relatively safe when administered with forced hydration.

Mechanism of Action. Cisplatin is a reactive molecule and is able to form inter- and intrastrand links with DNA to cross-link proteins with DNA.

Table 23–9. NITROSOUREAS

		TOXICITY			ANTITUMOR RESULTS		
DRUG	CYCLE-ACTIVE	BONE MARROW	GI	OTHER	EXCELLENT	GOOD	FAIR
Carmustine (BCNU)	No	++	±	Renal toxicity	Lymphoma	Glioblastoma	Colon cancer
Lomustine (CCNU)	No	++	±	Renal toxicity	Lymphoma	Glioblastoma	Colon cancer
Semustine (Methyl CCNU)	No	++	±	Renal toxicity	Lymphoma	Glioblastoma GI tract	
Streptozotocin	No	+	+	Renal toxicity Diabetes mellitus		Islet-cell tumors of pancreas Carcinoid tumor	

Table 23–10. PLATINUM COMPOUNDS

		TOXICITY			ANTITUMOR RESULTS		
DRUG	CYCLE-ACTIVE	BONE MARROW	GI	OTHER	EXCELLENT	GOOD	FAIR
Cisplatin	No	±	++	Renal Neurologic	Testicular cancer Ovarian cancer	Head and neck cancer Bladder cancer Lung cancer	Lymphoma Breast cancer
Carboplatin	No	++	±			Same as above	

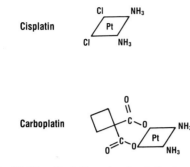

Fig. 23–10. Cisplatin and carboplatin structures.

Drug-resistant cell lines have been produced, and resistance has been attributed to various mechanisms including decreased uptake, an increase in repair of DNA lesions, and an increase of the metal-binding protein metallothionine.

Clinical Pharmacology. Cisplatin is administered IV with forced hydration. Following administration, the drug is rapidly bound to protein and persists in serum for long periods of time, with only 20% to 40% excreted in the urine within the first few days following drug administration. High concentrations of platinum, as measured by atomic absorption, persist in the liver, intestines, and kidney (Reed and Kohn, 1990).

Adverse Effects. The dose-limiting toxicity of cisplatin is nephrotoxicity due to tubular injury (see Table 23–10). This complication may be largely but not completely avoided by vigorous hydration, before and after administration of cisplatin. The use of 3% sodium chloride may allow even higher doses to be safely administered, since chloride ion may decrease activation of this compound and renal injury (Ozols et al., 1984). Hypomagnesemia may also result from tubular damage (Schilsky et al., 1982).

Severe nausea and vomiting caused by this drug recently has been shown to be controlled by antiemetic therapy (Hubbard and Jenkins, 1990).

Myelosuppression is not a major problem caused by this drug, although anemia has been noted frequently in patients receiving multiple courses of the drug. Neurotoxicity including peripheral neuropathy and ototoxicity, especially high-frequency hearing loss, is a problem in patients receiving multiple courses of the drug (Mead et al., 1982). Rarely Ig-mediated hypersensitivity reactions have occurred (Hood, 1986).

Therapeutic Uses. Cisplatin has significant antitumor effects in ovarian, testicular, lung, bladder, and head and neck carcinomas (Table 23–10). Of great importance is its ability, when used in combination, to give additive or syner-

gistic activity. The use of cisplatin with vinblastine and bleomycin, or more recently with etoposide, has led to a high cure rate (77%) in patients with advanced testicular cancer. In combination with cyclophosphamide, it is the treatment of choice in the treatment of ovarian cancer, leading to a high response rate (70%), and some cures (~10%). Cisplatin and 5-FU infusions also are highly effective in causing tumor regressions in patients with squamous cell carcinoma of the head and neck, although the remissions produced are only temporary.

Carboplatin. This platinum complex has recently been approved by the FDA in the United States for the treatment of ovarian cancer. It has the same mechanism of action as cisplatin, and exhibits some cross-resistance with that drug. A major advantage of carboplatin over cisplatin is its lack of nephrotoxicity; it may be administered without the need for hydration. The limiting toxicity is bone marrow depression (Table 23–10).

Triazenes

Dacarbazine. Although dacarbazine (DTIC, ditriazenoimidazolecarboxamide) is structurally similar to the purine precursor 5-aminoimidazole-4-carboxamide, DTIC acts primarily as an alkylating agent (Bono, 1976). Its structure is shown in Fig. 23–11.

Mechanism of Action and Clinical Pharmacology. Dacarbazine is activated by the hepatic cytochrome P450 system as an alkylating moiety is generated. The elimination $t_{1/2}$ is about 5 hours; about half the drug is excreted in the urine unchanged and the rest as metabolites.

Adverse Reactions. Severe nausea and vomiting occur when therapeutic doses of DTIC are used. Myelosuppression is uncommon after the usual doses are used but occasionally can be severe. Other toxic effects are a flulike syndrome and facial flushing (Spiegel, 1981). Hepatotoxicity has occasionally been noted (Frosch et al., 1979). Dacarbazine may cause severe pain and tissue necrosis if infiltration occurs.

Clinical Use. Dacarbazine is used in combination with doxorubicin (Adriamycin), bleomycin, and vinblastine (ABVD regimen) to treat Hodg-

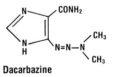

Dacarbazine

Fig. 23–11. Chemical structure of dacarbazine.

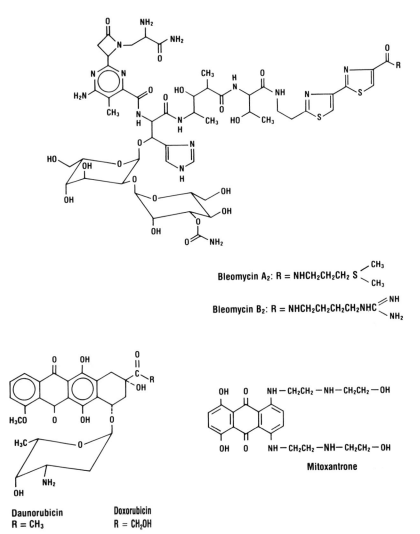

Fig. 23–12.   Chemical structures of antitumor antibiotics bleomycins and anthracyclines.

kin disease, and is also used to treat soft tissue sarcoma and malignant melanoma.

Antitumor Antibiotics

Bleomycin.   Bleomycin is a mixture of peptides (Fig. 23–12). It is produced by the fungus *Streptomyces verticillus*, first isolated by Umezawa et al. (1966).

Mechanism of Action.   Bleomycin causes both single- and double-strand breaks in DNA, as a consequence of production of an Fe(II) complex that generates free radicals (Burger et al., 1986). The reason for the tumor specificities and toxicities of this drug may be the presence or absence

of a bleomycin-inactivating enzyme (bleomycin hydrolase) (Umezawa et al., 1974; Lazo and Humphreys, 1983). Of interest is the lack of activity of this enzyme in the lung and skin, two normal organs that are damaged by this drug. Cell killing is maximal in cells in the G_2 phase of the cell cycle. The drug may be considered a cycle-active agent (Table 23–11).

Clinical Pharmacology.   Bleomycin may be administered either IV or IM for treatment of tumors, and intrapleurally or intraperitoneally for control of malignant effusions (Alberts et al., 1978, 1979a; Howell et al., 1987). Some preclinical data support the use of this drug in a continuous infusion, but definitive data on this point are

Table 23-11. ANTITUMOR ANTIBIOTICS

| DRUG | CYCLE-ACTIVE | TOXICITY | | | ANTITUMOR RESULTS | | |
		BONE MARROW	GI	OTHER	EXCELLENT	GOOD	FAIR
Bleomycin	Yes	−	±	Skin changes Pulmonary fibrosis	Lymphoma Embryonal testicular tumors	Head and neck Skin	Cervix Esophagus
Doxorubicin (Adriamycin)	Yes	+ +	+	Cardiac toxicity Alopecia Vesicant	Acute leukemia Breast Sarcoma Lymphoma	Thyroid Bladder Ewing Wilms Rhabdomyosarcoma	Head and neck Cervix Ovary Lung
Daunorubicin	Yes	+ +	+	Cardiac toxicity Alopecia Vesicant	Acute leukemia	—	—
Mitoxantrone	?	+ +	±	?Less cardiotoxic	Acute leukemia	Breast	—
Actinomycin D (dactinomycin, Cosmegen)	Yes	+ +	+ +	Radiation recall Vesicant Alopecia	Choriocarcinoma Wilms tumor	Rhabdomyosarcoma Osteosarcoma Testicular tumors	Soft tissue sarcomas
Mitomycin C	?	+ +	+	Hemolytic uremic syndrome (rare)	—	Lung Colon cancer Gastric cancer	—
Mithramycin	?	+ +	+ +	Liver toxicity Hypocalcemia Bleeding	—	Embryonal testicular tumors	Glioblastoma

lacking in humans (Carlson and Sikic, 1983; Vogelzang, 1984). After a single IV injection, the drug disappears rapidly with over half the dose excreted in the urine in 24 hours. The elimination half-life has been estimated to be about 2 to 3 hours. Although there are no exact guidelines for the use of this drug in patients with renal impairment, reduction of the dose should be considered.

Adverse Effects. As mentioned, bleomycin has little or no effect on normal marrow; however, in patients given other myelosuppressive drugs or recovering from marrow toxicity from these agents, additional mild myelosuppression may be observed (Table 23–11).

The two major toxicities that may result from bleomycin are pulmonary fibrosis and skin changes. The risk of pulmonary toxicity is related to the cumulative dose and increases to 10% of patients administered more than 450 mg (Blum et al., 1973). Risk is also greater in patients over the age of 70; in those with underlying lung disease, particularly when they are receiving oxygen; and when they take large single doses of the drug (25 mg/m^2 or more). However, a small percentage of patients (2%–3%) without these risk factors may develop pulmonary toxicity, even at relatively low doses of this drug. Some improvement of the lung lesion may be seen on discontinuation of the drug, but there always is substantial irreversible pulmonary fibrosis. Steroids have been used to counter this toxicity with probable benefit (Yagoda et al., 1972).

The toxic effects of bleomycin on skin also are dose-related. When the drug is given in conventional daily doses for longer than 2 to 3 weeks, erythema, hyperkeratosis, and even frank ulceration may occur. Areas of skin pressure, especially on the hands, fingers, and joints, are initially affected. Nail changes and alopecia also may occur with continued use of the drug. In combination regimens where bleomycin is used intermittently in lower doses (e.g., ABVD regimen) these skin toxicities usually are not seen.

Fever and malaise are common symptoms caused by the drug and may be alleviated with acetaminophen. Hypersensitivity reactions have also been observed with bleomycin therapy. A peculiar type of idiosyncratic cardiovascular collapse has been noted particularly in lymphoma patients but it is rare. A 1-mg test dose in these patients may be useful in detecting patients who may be at risk to this problem (Bennett and Reich, 1979).

Therapeutic Uses. Bleomycin is a "selective" drug, that is, it can exert antitumor effects with little or no marrow toxicity. The drug is used as part of a combination regimen (ABVD) to treat Hodgkin disease, non-Hodgkin lymphomas, and testicular cancer.

Anthracyclines. The three anthracyclines approved for clinical use are doxorubicin, daunorubicin, and mitoxantrone. The former two compounds are alkaloids produces by various *Streptomyces* species, while mitoxantrone is a synthetic compound, not containing a sugar moiety (Fig. 23–12).

Mechanism of Action. These drugs appear to exert their effects via binding to DNA and intercalation (Ghione, 1975). In addition, doxorubicin and daunorubicin affect preribosomal RNA synthesis and bind to membranes (Powis, 1987).

The anthracylines enter cells via a passive transport process and are pumped out of cells by the P-glycoprotein system that is increased in activity in multidrug-resistant cells (Tsuruo, 1988). Other mechanisms for anthracycline resistance have also been reported, including increased DNA repair (Capranico et al., 1987) and an alteration in topoisomerase II (Glisson et al., 1986).

Because of their clinical utility, a large number of analogs have been synthesized, and many are in clinical trial.

Clinical Pharmacology. After an IV bolus dose of doxorubicin, the drug disappears in three phases (Myers and Chabner, 1990). An initial rapid distribution phase lasts approximately 15 minutes; a second phase due to metabolism and elimination lasts several hours; and a prolonged third phase of 24 to 48 hours may represent release of drug from binding sites. Both daunorubicin and doxorubicin are metabolized primarily in liver to daunomycinol and doxorubicinol, respectively, compounds that are less toxic than the parent drugs. Modification of the dose has been recommended for patients with hepatic impairment, using bilirubin concentrations as a guideline. There is no firm basis for this recommendation.

The usual dose of doxorubicin used as a single agent is 60 to 75 mg/m^2 given as a single dose every 3 to 4 weeks. Some evidence supports the use of dose schedules that employ more frequent, lower doses, given either weekly or by constant infusion over 48 to 96 hours. These modifications can result in less cardiac toxicity by avoiding high peak concentrations in plasma. When given in combination with other myelotoxic agents such as cyclophosphamide, the dose of doxorubicin usually is decreased by one third. While daunorubicin has been used as the anthracycline of choice in the treatment of AML (usually in combination with cytosine arabinoside), recent evidence indicates that doxorubicin and mitoxantrone may be equally effective (Walters et al., 1988).

Toxicity. Myelosuppression usually occurs with a nadir 10 days after administration of a single dose (see Table 23–11). Recovery usually occurs within 3 weeks. The drugs cause tissue necrosis if they extravasate, and alopecia. Mitoxantrone usually does not cause these toxic effects and produces less nausea and vomiting than is seen with daunomycin or doxorubicin. Doxorubicin may cause mucositis, especially when it is used in maximally tolerated divided doses given over 2 to 3 days, or when used in combination with other drugs that cause mucositis. These drugs also may cause a recall reaction in previously irradiated tissues, especially when they are administered just prior to (up to 3 weeks), or following, irradiation.

In addition to myelosuppression, the other significant toxic effect of doxorubicin and daunorubicin is cardiac toxicity (Von Hoff et al., 1982). Both acute effects, manifested by arrhythmias and conduction abnormalities, and a "pericarditis-myocarditis syndrome," as well as chronic effects may occur. Cardiac biopsy demonstrates a dose-dependent effect of doxorubicin on the viability of myocardial cells (Billingham et al., 1978). Measurements of ejection fraction have been extremely helpful as a noninvasive technique that can demonstrate a drug-induced decline in myocardial function. When the problem appears, the anthracycline therapy must be discontinued.

Most patients will tolerate total doses of 450 to 550 mg/m^2 of doxorubicin or daunorubicin before the risk of cardiac damage is significant (>5%). Once clinically overt cardiac toxicity occurs, usually manifested by congestive heart failure, the mortality rate may be as high as 50%. Congestive heart failure usually occurs during, or within 1 month following, therapy; rarely, heart failure may occur months to years later. Other anthracycline analogs such as mitoxantrone may produce less cardiac toxicity, but the data with this drug are less complete than with doxorubicin.

Therapeutic Uses. Doxorubicin has a broad spectrum of activity in neoplastic disease. It is an important drug for the treatment of hematologic malignancies, especially ALL, Hodgkin disease, and the non-Hodgkin lymphomas. It is also used in combination to treat solid tumors, especially breast cancer, lung cancer, bladder cancer, and certain childhood tumors. Daunomycin is used almost exclusively in the treatment of AML. Recently, mitoxantrone has been approved for the treatment of AML.

Actinomycin D (Dactinomycin). Dactinomycin is an antibiotic with antineoplastic activity that is produced by *Streptomyces parvullus*. It is composed of a phenoxazone ring structure, to which two identical cyclic peptide chains are bound (Fig. 23–13).

Mechanism of Action. Dactinomycin binds to DNA, with the polypeptide chains binding in the minor grove of the DNA helix (Sobell et al., 1971). Intercalation is a result of a specific interaction between these chains and deoxyguanosine.

Few data are available on mechanisms of resistance to actinomycin D in patients, or the basis for natural or inherent resistance or sensitivity to this drug. In experimental systems, actinomycin D participates in the multidrug-resistance phenotype (Diddens et al., 1987).

Clinical Pharmacology. The drug is rapidly cleared from the blood after an IV dose. Most is excreted unchanged in bile and urine. After an initial rapid disappearance phase from plasma (minutes), a slower phase (36-hour half-life) occurs (Tattersall et al., 1975b).

Adverse Effects. The major dose-limiting toxicities to this drug are leukopenia and thrombocytopenia (Frei, 1974). These effects reach a nadir 2 to 3 weeks after a course of therapy. Nausea and vomiting also are common acute toxicities that begin within a few hours of treatment and may last as long as 24 hours. Other side effects noted with full doses of actinomycin D are stomatitis, cheilitis, glossitis, and proctitis (see Table 23–11). Actinomycin may cause radiation recall, that is, cutaneous erythema, desquamation, and hyperpigmentation in previously irradiated areas (D'Angio et al., 1959). Cellulitis and pain also can result if the drug extravasates. Alopecia and severe skin toxicity may occasionally be seen.

Clinical Use. Actinomycin D is still used to treat Wilms tumor, gestational choriocarcinoma, and embryonal rhabdomyosarcoma. Some regimens for osteosarcoma also include actinomycin D. While this drug has significant activity in the treatment of testicular cancer, it has been supplanted by other more effective drugs.

Mitomycin C. Mitomycin C is a quinone antibiotic, isolated from cultures of *Streptomyces caespitosus* (Fig. 23–13). The drug requires reduction to produce an activated molecule that can cross-link DNA strands, similar to an alkylating agent (Reddy and Randerath, 1987; Tomasz et al., 1987).

Clinical Pharmacology. After IV administration there is a rapid half-life of distribution (2–10 minutes) followed by an elimination half-life of 25 to 90 minutes (Dorr, 1988).

Adverse Effects. In addition to nausea and vomiting that is commonly seen with administration of the drug, the major toxicity of mitomycin C is bone marrow suppression that usually is cumulative (see Table 23–11). The nadir of blood element decrease is 3 to 5 weeks. Extravasation results in severe tissue damage. Less common side effects are the hemolytic uremic syndrome, which may be fatal; interstitial pneumonitis; and cardiomyopathy.

Clinical Use. Mitomycin C is used in combi-

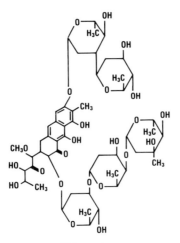

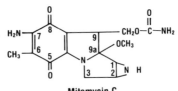

Mitomycin C

Mithramycin

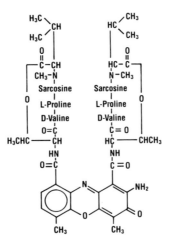

Actinomycin D

Fig. 23–13. Chemical structures of antitumor antibiotics mithramycin, mitomycin C, and actinomycin D.

nation regimens in the treatment of lung and GI cancers.

Mithramycin. Mithramycin (Plicamycin) was isolated from *Streptomyces plicatus* (Fig. 23–13). Its major use is to treat hypercalcemia caused by malignancy. Although this drug was used to treat patients with embryonal carcinoma of the testis, other more effective and less toxic drugs have replaced it in the clinic.

Mechanism of Action. The precise mechanism of action of mithramycin is not fully known, but it forms complexes with DNA and subsequently inhibits DNA-dependent synthesis of RNA (Miller et al., 1987).

Clinical Pharmacology. In a single patient studied with tritium-labeled drug, plasma radioactivity declined slowly over 14 hours.

Toxicity. Severe adverse effects were seen fol-

lowing the daily dosing with mithramycin that was used to treat patients with malignancy. Less toxicity was seen with an alternate-day regimen (Kennedy, 1970). A severe hemorrhagic syndrome associated with thrombocytopenia, prolonged clotting and prothrombin times, and hepatotoxicity was rather common using the daily high-dose regimen. Common adverse effects include nausea and vomiting (see Table 23–11). The severe side effects noted with the doses and schedules used to treat embryonal carcinoma are not seen with the doses used (15–25 μg/kg) at weekly intervals to treat hypercalcemia (Stewart, 1983).

Enzymes

L-Asparaginase

History. Kidd (1953) noted that the growth of certain transplantable lymphomas in the mouse were inhibited by guinea pig serum but not by other mammalian sera. After intensive investigation Broome and co-workers in 1963 isolated the factor responsible for this antilymphoma activity and found it to be L-asparaginase (Broome, 1963).

Mechanism of Action. This enzyme catalyzes the hydrolysis of asparagine to aspartic acid and ammonia. It rapidly depletes the serum of asparagine, which is necessary for growth of certain lymphoid cells (Capizzi et al., 1970).

Clinical Pharmacology. L-asparaginase is administered either IV or IM. After a single IV or IM dose, concentrations of drug in serum are detectable for several days. The concentrations of the enzyme fall quickly (within minutes of injection) below detectable levels and begin to be measurable again 7 to 10 days after a single dose. The half-life of the enzyme in plasma is 14 to 24 hours.

Toxicity. A major problem with administration of L-asparaginase is hypersensitivity (Weiss and Bruno, 1981). Reactions to the first dose are uncommon, but after the second or subsequent doses, allergic reactions may occur. These reactions vary from urticaria to anaphylaxis and may include hypotension, laryngospasm, and cardiac arrest. Skin testing to predict allergic reactions is only partially helpful. Hypersensitive patients may have serum antibodies to L-asparaginase. However, more than half the patients with such antibodies will not display an allergic reaction to the drug.

Patients who are treated with L-asparaginase should be observed carefully for several hours after dosing. Epinephrine should be available in case an anaphylactic reaction occurs. If an anaphylactic reaction occurs with the enzyme purified from *Escherichia coli*, the patient may still be treated with the enzyme from *E. carotovora* since there is no cross-sensitivity between these preparations.

Additional major toxic effects caused by L-asparaginase are due to its ability to transiently inhibit protein synthesis in normal tissues. Inhibition of protein synthesis in the liver results in hypoalbuminemia, decreases in clotting factors, and decreases in serum lipoproteins. The clotting function abnormalities that are regularly observed as a consequence of treatment with L-asparaginase include prolongation of the prothrombin, partial thromboplastin, and thrombin times. A marked fall in plasma fibrinogen concentrations and a decrease in clotting factors IX and XI may also be observed. Despite continued treatment with this enzyme, these effects are transient. Other complications of L-asparaginase treatment when used in high-dose schedules are confusion, stupor, coma, and acute pancreatitis,

which in some patients may progress to severe hemorrhagic pancreatitis. Inhibition of the production of insulin may lead to hyperglycemia.

Therapeutic Uses. The enzyme L-asparaginase is used to treat lymphoid malignancies, in particular ALL (null cell), T-cell leukemia, and T-cell lymphomas (Table 23–12) (Chabner, 1990). This is one of the few circumstances in the chemotherapy of malignant disease in which a biochemical basis for selectivity is clear. These lymphoid malignancies are all asparagine auxotrophs, that is, they require exogenous L-asparagine for growth, and they obtain this amino acid primarily from the liver.

Use in Combination Chemotherapy. Since L-asparaginase has no or little toxicity to bone marrow or GI mucosa, the drug has been used in combination with other drugs. L-asparaginase ameliorates the toxic effects of drugs that inhibit DNA synthesis (e.g., MTX and ara-C). The reduction of toxicity probably results from the inability of cells to enter the S phase because of the block of protein synthesis caused by the enzyme, making them less susceptible to the killing effects of S-phase-specific agents. Based upon the observation that null cells and T cells are not rescued from MTX treatment by L-asparaginase, while normal stem cells are, Capizzi (1975) devised a regimen in which MTX is followed 24 hours later by L-asparaginase. This combination is effective even in acute leukemia refractory to conventional doses of MTX (Lobel et al., 1979). The interval of treatment of MTX followed by L-asparaginase is ideally 10 days, since as mentioned it takes 7 to 10 days for the L-asparagine concentrations in the blood to recover after a single dose of L-asparaginase. At that time, the leukemia cells begin to proliferate and may be more sensitive to a repeat course of this treatment.

Miscellaneous Agents

Several useful chemotherapeutic drugs have been introduced into clinical practice that do not fall into the categories mentioned above are listed in Table 23–12. The structures of some of these compounds are shown in Fig. 23–14.

Mitotane. Mitotane, *o,p'*-DDD [1,1-dichloro-2-(*o*-chlorophenyl)-2-(*p*-chlorophenyl)ethane] (Fig. 23–14), a derivative of the insecticides DDT and DDD, is useful in only one neoplastic disease, adrenocortical carcinoma. However, as a prototype agent that has selective action, it is of great interest, since its dose-limiting toxicities are not on the bone marrow, but relate to GI disturbances (nausea and vomiting) and effects on the CNS. This drug was introduced into the clinic based on toxicity studies in dogs with the insecticide DDD.

Table 23-12. MISCELLANEOUS AGENTS

| | CYCLE-ACTIVE | TOXICITY | | | ANTITUMOR RESULTS | | |
		BONE MARROW	GI	OTHER	EXCELLENT	GOOD	FAIR
L-Asparaginase	?	–	+	Liver toxicity Pancreatitis Allergic reactions	ALL	Lymphocytic lymphoma	–
Mitotane (Lysodren, o,p'-DDD)	?	±	+ +	CNS toxicity Skin rash	–	Adrenocortical carcinoma	–
Procarbazine (Natulan)	No	+ +	+	CNS toxicity	Hodgkin disease	–	Lung
Hydroxyurea (Hydrea)	Yes	+ +	±		CML	Acute leukemia	Head and neck cancer Melanoma

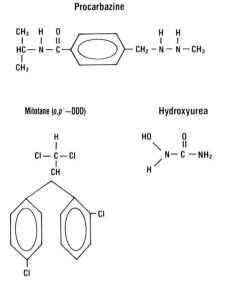

Fig. 23-14. Chemical structures of three miscellaneous agents.

It was noted that adrenal cortical necrosis occurred, because of the presence of the *o,p'* isomer of DDD. Transient regression of tumor is obtained in about one third of patients with adrenocortical carcinoma (Hutter and Kayhoe, 1966) (Table 23-12).

Procarbazine. This drug (Fig. 23-14) requires activation by the P450 cytochrome system in liver to produce several active metabolites that produce effects on DNA similar to those of classic alkylating agents (Weikam and Shiba, 1982).

Clinical Pharmacology and Adverse Effects. Procarbazine is administered orally and is well absorbed. The drug equilibrates rapidly between plasma and the CSF. The half-life of the parent compound is 10 minutes. The drug is excreted mainly in the urine in the form of metabolites (Breithaupt et al., 1982). Nausea and vomiting commonly occur with the use of this drug, but tolerance rapidly develops to these adverse effects. The major toxic effect, myelosuppression, is dose-related. Foods with a high tyramine content may precipitate a reaction that includes severe headache since this drug is a weak monoamine oxidase inhibitor (DeVita et al., 1967). Interactions with sympathomimetic amines, tricyclic antidepressants, and alcohol have also been reported (Weiss et al., 1974; Warren and Bender, 1977). Neurotoxicities that include dizziness, ataxia, paresthesia, headache, insomnia, and nightmares occur, especially in patients who are receiving CNS-acting drugs (Weiss et al., 1974).

Clinical Use. The major indication for procarbazine is as part of the MOPP regimen for the treatment of Hodgkin disease (see Table 23-12) (DeVita et al., 1970). Procarbazine also has been used to treat other neoplasms including non-Hodgkin lymphoma, lung cancer, and brain tumors.

Hydroxyurea. Hydroxyurea is a substituted urea that was first synthesized in 1969 by Dresler and Stein (Fig. 23-14).

Mechanism of Action. Hydroxyurea inhibits ribonucleotide reductase, the enzyme that converts ribonucleotides at the diphosphate level to deoxyribonucleotides (Yarbro et al., 1965). Resistance to the drug has been associated with an increase in enzyme activity and/or an alteration of binding of hydroxyurea to the iron-containing subunit of this enzyme (for review, see Wright, 1989).

Clinical Pharmacology. Hydroxyurea is well absorbed even in large oral doses. Plasma concentrations reach a maximum after 1 hour; these fall rapidly. The drug is excreted mainly unchanged by the kidney (Donehower, 1990).

Adverse Reactions. The major toxicity of hydroxyurea is bone marrow suppression, primarily leukopenia (see Table 23-12). Little other toxicity has been observed with this drug, even when large doses are administered. Hydroxyurea is an S-phase-specific drug. Single large doses have little toxicity. The nadir in the leukocyte count occurs 6 to 7 days after a single dose of drug and then recovers rapidly.

Therapeutic Uses. Hydroxyurea is used for the treatment of myeloproliferative diseases, in particular CML. It appears to be equally as effective as busulfan, with potentially less toxicity. In addition, it is used to treat patients with head and neck cancer. Hydroxyurea can be used to rapidly lower the blast count in patients with acute blast crisis of CML.

PRACTICE OF CHEMOTHERAPY: GENERAL CONSIDERATIONS

Combination Chemotherapy

Pharmacotherapy of human cancer has rapidly evolved since the introduction of nitrogen mustard and aminopterin into the clinic in the late 1940s. As new agents were evaluated in humans, it became clear that resistance would occur in a matter of months when single-agent therapy was used. The introduction of effective combination chemotherapy for ALL and Hodgkin disease in the 1960s was the outgrowth of experimental studies that showed that combinations of effective drugs gave additive cell kill and delayed or prevented the onset of drug resistance. In these regimens, "selective agents" (Table 23–13) were able to be used in full dosage because of nonoverlapping toxicities. A second important concept in the use of combination chemotherapy is the initial use of alkylating agents or non-cycle-specific drugs, followed by or used together with cycle-active agents. The concept involves the non-cycle-active drug's converting a plateau-phase tumor population to a logarithmically growing one, thus increasing the cells' susceptibility to antimetabolites. An example of this strategy is the COMLA [cyclophosphamide, Oncovin®(vincristine), metrotexate, leucovorin, ara-C] regimen used to treat diffuse lymphoma (Berd et al., 1975). Current strategies emphasize the use of drug combinations used in sequence given in high doses (with autologous marrow reinfusion) or with protection by hemopoietic cytokines (IL-1, IL-3, G-CSF, GM-CSF; see Chapter 22).

Attempts to recruit tumor cells into S phase, thus making them more vulnerable to cycle-specific agents have in a large measure failed because of the difficulty in synchronizing human tumor cells, but the concept of combination does have value.

Other lessons from experimental tumor models should be considered when drug combinations are used. *Principle: When two drugs are combined that both have marrow suppression as the limiting toxicity, it is usually possible to use 66% of the optimum dose of each drug without increasing the net toxicity.* If both drugs are equally effective, then the effective total dose delivered is 1.5 times the dose of the single drug. However, if both drugs are not effective, then subadditive results may occur. Some experimental evidence that drugs used in combination have additive or synergistic effects rather than antagonistic effects must be obtained before the combination is used. The sequence of drug administration may be important in this regard. For example, when MTX and L-asparaginase are used together, L-asparaginase will block the cytotoxicity of MTX; when MTX administration precedes L-asparaginase adminis-

tration by 24 hours, then drug synergy is observed in the treatment of ALL if the interval of treatment is 10 to 14 days (Capizzi, 1975).

The disadvantages of combination therapy are that it may be difficult to ascertain which of the drugs is of value if a positive antitumor effect is produced. If resistance occurs, it may not be to all the drugs used in the combination. If toxicity occurs, it may be difficult to adjust subsequent doses of individuals drugs, since the major offending agent may not be obvious.

Recently, the idea of using alternating cycles of two or more drug combinations has evolved. The theoretical considerations behind the concepts is based on probabilities that drug-resistant cells are less likely to survive alternating drug combinations compared with repeated dosing with a fixed combination (Goldie et al., 1982). An example of this concept is the use of alternating cycles of MOPP, [mechlorethamine, Oncovin®(vincristine), prednisone, procarbazine], and ABVD [Adriamycin®(doxorubicin), bleomycin, vinblastine and DTIC (dacarbazine)] (see Table 23–14) in the treatment of Hodgkin disease (Bonnadonna et al., 1986). However attractive, this concept remains unproved in the clinic. Current efforts are being directed toward short-term, intense chemotherapy with drug combinations used sequentially.

Dose Intensity

An important consideration in the treatment of curable malignancies is optimal intensity of the dose (Hryniuk, 1987). *Principle: If cure is possible, then full doses of drugs should be used.* For responsive malignancies that have features of poor risk (e.g., a large tumor burden), intensification of the dose may be achieved by the use of doses of chemotherapy that ablate the bone marrow followed by bone marrow rescue either with autologous marrow or marrow from a histocompatible donor. This approach has led to encouraging results in the treatment of refractory leukemia and lymphoma.

Adjuvant Chemotherapy

The use of adjuvant chemotherapy in treating tumors in humans when the surgeon or radiotherapist has eradicated all clinically evident tumor has a firm experimental basis. Both in certain experimental models and in humans, the likelihood of tumor recurrence can be predicted with accuracy (Schabel, 1975). When this possibility is high, then adjuvant chemotherapy may be used, and the risks may be justifiable. Several advanced transplantable or spontaneous neoplasms in laboratory animals can be cured by chemotherapy if all palpable disease is removed by surgery;

Table 23–13.   DRUGS USED TO TREAT ALL

Selective Drugs (lack significant marrow toxicity):
  Prednisone
  Vincristine
  L-Asparaginase

Effective Drugs (with significant marrow toxicity):
  MTX
  6-MP
  Doxorubicin
  Etoposide, tenoposide
  Ara-C

surgery alone or chemotherapy alone is not curative (Fugman et al., 1970; Schabel, 1975). Reducing the tumor cell burden by surgery or irradiation decreases the residual tumor cell number that must be dealt with by adjuvant chemotherapy (and/or immunotherapy). In addition, the growth fraction of the surviving cells increases, thus making the relatively small tumor cell populations that remain in the primary site or in the distant metastasis more vulnerable to destruction by cycle-active agents, especially the antimetabolite drugs (Schabel, 1975). Intermittent, high-dose treatment with these agents (alone or in combination with alkylating agents) is then more effective against neoplastic cells than against normal stem cells. In addition, intermittent therapy may allow the opportunity for normal immune mechanisms to recover between doses.

The role of immunotherapy for treating patients with cancer has not been adequately defined. However, data from several experimental systems indicate that the use of this modality will be useful only when the residual tumor cell mass is small (Bast et al., 1974). *Principle: Large, bulky tumors defeat the chemotherapist because of large numbers of tumor cells and the consequent development of drug resistance. Chemotherapy is most effective when the number of remaining cells is small and growth of tumor is logarithmic.*

Special Methods to Deliver High Concentrations of Drugs to Isolated Areas

Regional Perfusion and Infusion. The rationale for administering drugs to a tumor via its arterial blood supply is that high concentrations of drug may be delivered to the neoplasm. Since there may be a dose effect in tumor cell kill, the same amount of drug administered intraarterially rather than IV may produce better results by producing a higher concentration of drug in the tumor. Intraarterial therapy has been used either to treat tumors in areas of the body that are difficult to treat by surgical procedures or by x-ray therapy, or to definitively manage tumors that perhaps may be cured by chemotherapy without requiring amputation or disfigurement. Such lesions have been located in the head and neck, the brain, the extremities, the liver, and the organs of the lower abdomen (the rectum, cervix, and bladder).

Infusion refers to the administration of drug via the artery supplying a tumor without attempting to isolate the venous return. Thus, circulation of the drug beyond the tumor is allowed. This technique is more commonly used than perfusion and is associated with fewer exacting technical problems.

Perfusion therapy, that is, administering a drug into the arterial blood supply of a tumor via a closed circuit in which the tumor's venous return is recirculated via a pump, has a great potential advantage: the therapeutic index should be very wide and systemic toxicity should be minimal. Even in settings of perfusion of the extremities, this ideal is difficult to achieve practically since some leakage of drug into the systemic circulation usually occurs.

These dramatic procedures have received a great deal of attention in the past decade. Most of the technical problems of intraarterial administration have been solved. However, much more research needs to be done on selection and scheduling drugs, how to use these procedures as an adjuvant to surgical x-ray therapy, and what the effect of this type of treatment on the subsequent biologic behavior of the tumor is.

Antimetabolites have an advantage over alkylating agents for intraarterial use in that local toxicity may be more selective, that is, limited to replicating tissue. For example, the continuous intraarterial administration of low doses of fluorouracil into the external carotid artery produces regional mucositis as its major toxicity. Long-term administration of antimetabolites, by encompassing the generation time of most of the tumor cells, may produce the greatest therapeutic benefit. Several approaches have been used to minimize systemic toxicity of antimetabolites: (1) using low concentrations of drug (i.e., enough to produce an appreciable concentration of the agent in the blood supply of the tumor, but not enough to reach the systemic circulation) and (2) using a drug that is rapidly metabolized by blood or liver, such as 5-FU or 5-FUdR (Kemeny et al., 1989).

The role of intraarterial chemothrapy as an adjunct to radiation therapy and/or surgery is being evaluated in several centers. Although the response of the tumor to intraarterial therapy often is impressive, the ultimate value of this combined approach has not been demonstrated. *Principle: Even the most logically sound therapeutic intervention must be confirmed by testing in appropriate patients. A critical study allows rejection of logical and rational but ineffective interventions and establishes the efficacy of others.*

Intrathecal and Intraventricular Administration of Drugs. The delivery of drugs into the CSF via the intrathecal or intraventricular route has limited usefulness. The principal indication for administration of an antineoplastic drug directly into the CSF is to treat tumors that grow in suspension in the CSF and/or involve the meninges and are nourished by the CSF (Moore et al., 1960). The advantage of intrathecal or intraventricular administration of drug in these circumstances is considerable, since high concentrations of drug are achieved, producing less systemic toxicity than would be seen if comparable concentrations were produced by giving the drug systemically. That is, when given systemically, many drugs do not cross the blood–brain barrier to get into the brain. Systemic use of the folate antagonist MTX in conventional doses is ineffective for treatment of neoplasms in the meninges. In contrast, intrathecal MTX is effective in treating meningeal leukemia (Rieselbach et al., 1963). High doses of MTX (i.e., > 500 mg/m^2, IV) followed by leucovorin rescue achieve concentrations of MTX in the CNS that are cytocidal (Tattersall et al., 1975a). However, the blood–brain barrier is unidirectional for MTX as well as for most other drugs. The MTX directly administered intrathecally diffuses into the systemic circulation, and systemic toxicity can be produced if a high dose is administered intrathecally.

Inasmuch as most solid tumors of the brain derive their nourishment from the arterial circulation rather than from the CSF, intraventricular administration of drugs is usually not effective for the treatment of brain tumors. Delivery of drugs via the arterial circulation to brain tumors has been attempted but has met with only limited success.

Intracavitary Administration of Drug. Chemotherapeutic agents often are administered into the pleural space, peritoneum, or pericardial sac to control malignant effusions. Several irritating agents including radioisotopes, mechlorethamine, quinacrine, tetracycline, and even talc cause pleural adhesions that obliterate the pleural space. This inflammatory effect does not depend on any specific antitumor property of the drug. Nonetheless, absorption of the drug can occur, and systemic toxicity has been produced after nitrogen mustard was instilled intrapleurally. Pleural drainage using large tubes that are left in place for 2 to 3 days also can obliterate the pleural space without using sclerosing agents (Lambert et al., 1967). For a young patient with poor bone marrow reserve, drainage might be preferred. In a "fragile" patient or a patient with defects of blood clotting, intracavitary therapy with drugs might be safer. *Principle: When apparently equivalent alternative means to the same therapeutic goal are available, they should carefully be weighed for relative toxicities and advantages in the individual patient.*

Evaluation of Drug Therapy in Humans

Measurement of Normal Stem Cells. Techniques for accurate measurement of tumor and hemopoietic stem cell kill in the mouse have provided valuable information about differential cell kill, dose response, and rates of recovery of these tissues. The recent development of methods for growing human bone marrow cells in vitro may allow the eventual development of an assay to measure normal hemopoietic stem cells before and during therapy. Thus far there is no satisfactory assay for marrow stem cells. However, progenitor cells (for example, colony forming units, or CFU) may be assayed for cell lines such as granulocytes or macrophages (CFU$_{GM}$).

Some predictive estimate of the eventual effect of chemotherapy on the stem cell of the marrow and the epithelium of the gut can be made by assessing the early consequences of cell kill in either of these tissues. The reduction in granulocyte, reticulocyte, and platelet counts directly relates to the killing of the stem cells of the bone marrow. If the counts of blood cells are carefully performed, they can be used to accurately determine concentrations of granulocytes as low as 100/mm^3. When serial counts of granulocytes are plotted on a logarithmic scale, changes in cell counts over several orders of magnitude can be quantitated. Thus, evaluation of the intensity of therapy on the bone marrow can be made from its effects on peripheral blood (Hryniuk and Bertino, 1969a, 1969b).

Mucositis produced by therapy should be graded on a scale of 1 to 4+. Although this manifestation of drug effect can only be semiquantitative, it crudely relates to the logarithm of the mucosal cell kill. *Principle: Although there may not be precise means of following a drug's effects, reliable albeit semiquantitative measures can be used in the development of a dosage strategy. Using the available information in a semiquantitative manner permits usable estimates of response and provides a solid basis for comparison of one patient with others or one treatment schedule with others.*

Evaluation of Tumor Cell Kill

Reliable techniques to measure the reduction of tumor cells in humans have not been developed. Whenever possible, semiquantitative estimates of the mass of tumor should be performed. This estimate of the volume of tumor is usually the best available guide by which to follow the response to therapy. By using measurements of volume of tumor, the therapist can estimate the change in cell number, assuming that 1 ml of cells represents approximately 10^9 cells. However, a change in the size of a tumor mass may not accurately or solely reflect the amount of kill of tumor cells. For example, in an experimental mouse tumor, 3 logs (99.9%) of cell kill was obtained by cyclophosphamide therapy, yet no measurable change in tumor size occurred because the removal of dead tumor cells was slow and once removed they were rapidly replaced with new cells (Wilcox et al., 1965).

By analogy with the quantitation of normal granulocytes as an indirect correlate with hemopoietic stem cell kill, accurate measurement of the peripheral count of blast cells plotted on a logarithmic scale may be helpful in assessing the results of treatment in patients with leukemia. A decrease of as much as 3 logs (orders of magnitude) may be measured (e.g., reduction from 100,000 to 100). However, quantitation of changes in cell content of the bone marrow by "marrow counts" (the more important compartment) is less satisfactory.

When tumors produce characteristic enzymes or hormones, sometimes measurements of these products in blood may be valuable in guiding therapy. If the amount of substance produced is a direct function of the number of tumor cells, and if therapy produces a decrease in the concentrations of these substances only by killing cells, then the concentration of the product may be directly reflective of cell kill. The measurement of urinary chorionic gonadotropin titers in patients with choriocarcinoma or embryonal testicular tumors has been extemely useful in this regard, and accurate quantitation of very low concentrations is possible by using a radioimmunoassay. Quantitation of urinary paraproteins in patients with myeloma (Alexanian et al., 1969; Salmon and Smith, 1970) and concentrations of lysozymes in serum and urine from patients with monocytic leukemia (Osserman and Lawlor, 1966; Perillie et al., 1968) may be useful to assess cell kill, or changes in cell mass. Quantitation by sensitive assays of hormones produced by other endocrine and nonendocrine tumors may provide similarly useful information to guide treatment (Rees and Landon, 1976).

However, a hormone marker may not be a perfect reflection of tumor mass. Tumors such as the carcinoid tumor or tumors of neural crest origin make different hormones at varying rates and different times, and different metabolites of the hormones at different times seemingly independent of gross tumor size. Furthermore, some hormones may be carried in the blood by factors that are sensitive to the chemotherapeutic agent. Thus when 5-FU is given to patients with carcinoid syndrome, the concentration of serotonin in blood decreases whether or not the tumor size changes. The diminution of the concentration of serotonin in blood is more reflective of drug effect on platelets where the serotonin is stored than of effect on the size of the tumor where the serotonin is made (Melmon, 1974).

PRACTICE OF CHEMOTHERAPY: SPECIFIC EXAMPLES

After the patient's general condition has been evaluated, the histology of the tumor should be identified (pathologic staging) and some estimate should be made of the progression and amount of tumor present (clinical staging). Then the chemotherapist is ready to consider a specific individualized drug regimen and the ancillary measures necessary to optimize its effects.

In vitro tests have not been developed to the point where response of a patient's tumor cells to drugs is predictive of what will occur in vivo; therefore, the initial judgment of the sensitivity of the tumor to antitumor agents must be made on the basis of previous trials with various drugs in other patients. Aside from the kinetic considerations previously discussed, and a few exceptions, the reasons for the differences in tumor sensitivity to certain drugs are poorly understood (Bertino et al., 1989).

Once a drug or drug combination has been selected as likely to be active, the dose, duration, and route of administration of each compound must then be considered. The therapist must understand the metabolism of the drug, as well as any possible alterations in its metabolism caused by the patient's condition (involvement of liver or kidney by the disease or concurrent disease unrelated to neoplasm) or by concurrent use of other drugs. The feasible goals of therapy before starting treatment must be decided on. The type of tumor and its histologic and clinical staging are important considerations in establishing goals. *Principle: The patient and physician should be aware of the toxic potential of the drug(s), and the acceptable limits of the intensity of therapy should be set before therapy commences. When cure is possible, as in choriocarcinoma, only near-lethal toxicity (i.e., greater than the LD_{10}) may be prohibitive. However, if the expected gain is minimal, as in the routine treatment of carcinoma of the colon with 5-FU, even moderate morbidity may not be acceptable.*

Rapidly Growing Tumors: Single-Agent Cure

Human tumors, even those caused by a single clone of cells, have variable growth rates. Nonetheless a few tumors are characterized by rapid doubling times and relatively homogeneous behavior. These are choriocarcinoma, Burkitt lymphoma, ALL, and diffuse histiocytic lymphoma. In their early stages, two of these neoplams (Burkitt and choriocarcinoma) can be cured by a single therapeutic agent. The other two require combination chemotherapy for long-term, disease-free survival.

Choriocarcinoma. Several important lessons may be derived from consideration of this disseminated neoplastic disease in humans that was first made curable by chemotherapy. Although MTX (or aminopterin, its predecessor) was available since 1949 for clinical use, the initial evidence demonstrating that this rapidly growing tumor could be cured by the drug was not obtained until 1956. In order to obtain cures, maximally tolerated doses of methotrexate or actinomycin D were necessary (Goldstein, 1972; Hertz, 1972). Thus, effective drugs may be available for long periods before their optimal employment is discovered. *Principle: When potential long-term remission or cure is possible, the risks necessary to obtain these benefits may be justified.*

The value of a marker reflecting the presence of a tumor-cell (i.e., human chorionic gonadotropin, hCG) in assessing cell kill was clearly demonstrated in the treatment of these patients. The marker can be used as a guide to the choice of therapy, the quantity necessary, the efficacy or failure of therapy, and the point at which treatment should be stopped. Thus the patient is spared unnecessary risks of treatment (Fig. 23–15).

When the hCG titer in urine was used as a measure of the cell mass in tumors, it was found that the larger the tumor cell burden was demonstrated to be, the more difficult it became to obtain regression of total tumor cell mass. The hCG titer, the duration of the disease, and the clinical staging of these patients (e.g., whether brain or liver was involved) have allowed predictive separation of groups of patients who will not respond to drugs from those who should be treated aggressively (Hammond et al., 1973).

The experience with treating this disease also established the value of intensive, intermittent therapy that allowed time for the immune response to recover. The latter observation is especially important for the patient whose tumor is strongly likely to alter immune responses. This same concept has subsequently been used to plan several other programs of chemotherapy (Mitchell et al., 1969).

Fig. 23–15. Chemotherapy of a patient with metastatic choriocarcinoma. The vertical arrows indicate 5-day courses of MTX and actinomycin D (ACT). This patient presented with a urinary chorionic gonadotropin (UCG) titer of 20,000,000; with the sensitive assays available, this titer was followed down through 7 logs, allowing therapy to be closely monitored.

Methotrexate produced 2 logs of decrease in the UCG titer, but despite continued therapy with this drug, the titer began to rise, indicating that resistance was developing. Guided by this rise in UCG titer rather than by the chest x-ray film (which did not change), therapy was rapidly changed to actinomycin D. This drug decreased the UCG titer markedly, each course resulting in 1 to 2 logs of decrease of UCG titer and presumably of tumor cells. The patient was then treated until the titer was within the normal range.

The patient has remained free of disease since 1962. Although the effects on normal tissue are not shown here, the therapy was intensive, and each course of MTX or ACT was given to the limit of tolerable toxicity (usually 2 logs of granulocyte or platelet decrease, or mucositis), and therapy was resumed immediately on recovery from toxicity (granulocyte count greater than 1500/mm³, platelet count greater than 100,000/mm³, no liver function abnormalities).

Supportive care for this type of regimen must be optimal to avoid drug-related deaths; in a series of 50 patients, including this patient, 37 presumable "cures" were obtained with the use of sequential MTX and actinomycin D therapy (or vice versa), with only 1 death due to MTX toxicity. (From Ross, G.T.; Goldstein, D.P.; Hertz, R.; Lipsett, M.B.; and Odell, W.D.: Sequential use of methotrexate and actinomycin D in the treatment of metastatic choriocarcinoma and related trophoblastic diseases in women. *Am. J. Obstet. Gynecol,* 93:223–29, 1965, with permission.)

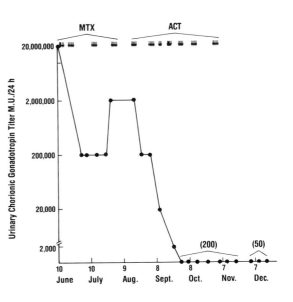

Patients who have survived long periods and are therefore potentially cured after treatment with either MTX or actinomycin D or both in sequence have not developed any long-term adverse effects from this therapy. Many have had normal pregnancies (Hertz, 1972).

Burkitt Lymphoma. Burkitt lymphoma is the other example of a human neoplasm that may be cured in a significant percentage of patients who are given single-agent chemotherapy. This tumor, which can grow extremely rapidly (doubling time 12–14 hours), may have the highest growth fraction of any human tumor (Ziegler, 1973). Its etiology, epidemiology, and therapy have been extensively studied (Burkitt and Burchenal, 1969; Ziegler, 1973). The tumor is unusually sensitive to cyclophosphamide, and large doses (40 mg/kg of body weight given intermittently) can produce cure. As noted for choriocarcinoma, curability decreases as the clinical stage advances.

Rapidly Growing Tumors: Use of Combination Chemotherapy

Therapy of Patients with ALL. The cure of children with ALL has been one of the major triumphs of chemotherapy (Steinherz, 1987). The evolution of curative treatment has been a painfully slow process and has depended upon understanding the biology of this disease, including tumor cell kinetics and subsets of ALL; development of effective agents; and an understanding of the pharmacology of combined drugs (Frei, 1984). At the present time most centers are reporting 5-year disease-free survivals of over 60%; adults with ALL have a lower cure rate (30%).

Drugs Used to Treat ALL. The first drug used to treat ALL was aminopterin. Complete remissions were reported by Farber (1966). It was soon realized that drug resistance developed rapidly, and despite continued treatment with maximally tolerated doses, patients relapsed in several months. Corticosteroids and then 6-MP were also introduced into the clinic; single-agent treatment produced remissions in patients, but again resistance rapidly developed.

Combinations of prednisone and 6-MP or prednisone and MTX were found to be more effective than aminopterin in animal studies and were then tested in humans. A higher percentage of complete remissions was produced, and the duration of those remissions was longer. *Principle: Agents with different mechanisms of action and different toxicities may be combined in full dose.*

A benchmark study was then reported by the acute leukemia B study group: a combination of MTX with 6-MP was found to be more effective than either drug alone. The introduction of vin-

cristine into the clinic then provided the clinician with another "selective" drug in addition to prednisone. The combination of prednisone and vincristine allowed the successful induction of 80% to 90% of patients into complete remission without serious marrow toxicity and risk of bleeding and infection during treatment. After remission induction with these drugs, antimetabolites 6-MP and MTX may be used in high doses with less chance of serious toxicity to normal marrow. Longer remissions were regularly produced with this regimen, and some cures, but most patients continued to relapse, particularly in the CNS.

An important breakthrough came when irradiation therapy to the craniospinal axis, or irradiation to the brain plus intrathecally administered MTX, was added to this treatment regimen. For the first time, a substantial (50%) number of children were now rendered disease-free. Current treatment programs now utilize additional effective agents in the total therapy of childhood ALL; these include L-asparaginase especially in combination with MTX (see section on L-asparaginase) and tenoposide (VM-26) with ara-C, a synergistic combination in animal models of leukemia (see Table 23–13). High-dose regimens of MTX with leucovorin rescue have also been shown to be an alternative to radiation of the brain, since at high doses of MTX (>0.5 g/m^2), concentrations of MTX are achieved in the CNS that are cytocidal to ALL blasts ($>10^{-7}$ M). Some newer regimens also include doxorubicin, which may be added to vincristine and prednisone in the induction phase without compromising dosage. *Principle: Drug distribution may play a key role in the therapeutic outcome.*

The Importance of Dose Intensity. Several studies have demonstrated that outcome depends upon adequate dose intensity. The suggestion has been made that patients receiving MTX and 6-MP should have concentrations of drug in blood monitored to be sure that adequate doses are given. *Principle: Ideally, patients should be treated to achieve a desired plasma concentration in order to achieve maximum therapeutic benefit.*

Several questions still remain to be fully answered in the treatment of ALL: (1) What is the optimum treatment regimen for standard-risk versus "high-risk" patients, (2) how long should the patient be treated, and (3) what are the long-term toxic effects of the various treatment programs? For example, some recent data indicate that doxorubicin, even in cumulative doses not thought to be cardiotoxic, can cause effects on the myocardium in children. The adverse effects are not detectable until these children are examined several years after cure. *Principle: Expect adverse-effect profiles of very potent antitumor drugs to extend after they are used to produce cures.*

Therapy of Patients with Hodgkin Disease.
This disease is used as a paradigm for a human cancer that is curable, even when it is first seen in an advanced stage. Clinical and pathologic staging have played a major role in determining the extent of disease and developing effective treatment. In order to treat this disease optimally, the cooperation and expertise of medical oncologists, radiotherapists, and pathologists skilled in the evaluation and treatment of lymphoma are required.

Drugs Used to Treat Advanced Hodgkin Disease. Early-stage Hodgkin disease (stage I or II, disease in one lymph node area, or two or more lymph node areas, respectively, above or below the diaphragm) is treated with irradiation therapy alone, usually after exploratory laparatomy to confirm that the patient does not have more advanced disease. The 5-year cure rates with extended field irradiation [x-ray therapy to the involved lymph node region(s) plus to the contiguous nodes] are in the range of 80% to 90%. Patients who relapse may be "salvaged" with combination chemotherapy. Thus approximately 95% of patients with early-stage Hodgkin disease may be expected to be cured. There are, however, concerns about the long-term effects of irradiation, in particular an increased incidence of secondary malignancies. Therefore, in several centers, chemotherapy regimens (not containing alkylating agents) alone or in combination with limited irradiation (covering only the involved field) are being explored as alternatives.

More advanced stages of Hodgkin disease (stage III, lymph node involvement above and below the diaphragm; stage IV, extranodal organ involvement) are less likely to be cured by x-ray therapy. In these settings, combination chemotherapy is required.

The first combination demonstrated to be curative in advanced-stage Hodgkin disease was MOPP (Table 23–14). This four-drug combination was formulated on principles outlined in the first part of the chapter: "selective" drugs (vincristine, prednisone) were used in full dosage, with scheduled doses of two additional effective drugs

Table 23–14. DRUG COMBINATIONS USED TO TREAT HODGKIN DISEASE

1.	MOPP
	Mechlorethamine
	Vincristine (Oncovin)
	Prednisone
	Procarbazine
2.	ABVD
	Doxorubicin (Adriamycin)
	Bleomycin
	Vinblastine
	Dacarbazine

that both produced marrow toxicity. The treatment was given in divided doses on days 1 and 8 and was repeated again on day 28, when toxicity especially to the bone marrow subsided (DeVita et al., 1967). None of these drugs used singly in full doses was curative. However the combination of these four agents prevented the emergence of drug-resistant clones, and in 50% to 60% of patients, long-term remissions (>15 years) have been produced. The major long-term toxicities associated with this combination have been sterility and secondary cancer, in particular leukemia and lymphoma in 1% to 5% of patients.

When additional effective drugs against Hodgkin disease were introduced into the clinic in the 1970s, a second four-drug combination (ABVD) was devised, with results equal to or perhaps better than the MOPP regimen in untreated patients (Table 23–14). Long-term adverse effects, in particular secondary malignancies and sterility, with this ABVD program were much reduced, thus increasing the therapeutic index (Bonnadonna et al., 1986).

Inasmuch as a substantial percentage (30%–40%) of patients with advanced Hodgkin disease are not cured, attempts have been directed toward further improving the cure rate, especially by defining a "poor-risk" group that may require even more aggressive treatment. Alternating or hybrid combinations of MOPP and ABVD are being tested, as well as combinations of chemotherapy and x-ray treatment. More recently, the use of autologous marrow rescue following high-dose treatment, and the use of cytokines to stimulate marrow recovery, are being explored. ***Principle: The optimum treatment of a malignancy is cure with as few adverse effects as possible. However, the possibility of cure should not be compromised to decrease the adverse effects.***

Treatment of Solid Tumors with Moderate Growth Rates

Therapy of Patients with Breast Cancer. The chemotherapeutic treatment of patients with cancer of the breast requires that the physician be knowledgeable about the biology of the disease, the physical and mental condition of the patient, and the properties of, as well as the concepts involved in, the use of drugs used to treat these patients. This is a disease with a wide variation in its clinical behavior.

Drugs and Hormones Used to Treat Advanced or Metastatic Breast Cancer. A large number of hormones as well as chemotherapeutic agents are available to treat patients with breast cancer. However, even with protocols for combination chemotherapy, cure of patients with advanced breast cancer has not been achieved. The estrogen antagonist tamoxifen has replaced ablative surgery (ovariectomy, adrenalectomy, hypophysectomy) as a means of decreasing estrogen activity in patients with breast cancer. Treatment with this drug is relatively nontoxic and is effective in 60% to 70% of patients with elevated amounts of estrogen receptor (ER) and progestin receptor (PR) proteins in their tumors. Responses usually last 10 to 12 months; relapse may occur because ER-negative tumor cells emerge. Other effective hormonal agents include high doses of progestins, estrogens, or androgens. The inhibitor of corticosteroid synthesis, aminogluthethimide, may also be effective in patients who have previously responded to other hormonal manipulations. In elderly patients with ER- or PR-positive metastatic breast cancer, it may be possible to obtain several years of relatively "good" life with sequential use of these agents.

Several drugs also have been shown to be effective when used as single agents in the treatment of patients with breast cancer (Table 23-15). Combinations of these drugs are more effective than single agents, but the number of complete responders is small, and cure is rare (Henderson, 1984). For certain patients (minimal or no disease following treatment with these regimens) the value of additional intense chemotherapy (e.g., high-dose melphalan) with reinfusion of autologous bone marrow is under investigation. The major problem that limits the usefulness of chemotherapy in this disease is development of drug resistance. Optimization of drug combinations and scheduling may partially overcome this problem, but development of additional active new agents or therapies may be required before cure of advanced breast cancer is achieved.

Operable Breast Cancer and the Use of Adjuvant Chemotherapy. In patients who have breast cancer that is "operable" (that is, the surgeon is able to remove all gross tumor and axillary lymph nodes), the ultimate prognosis is deter-

mined by (1) the size of the tumor, (2) the number of axillary nodes involved, and (3) the ER and PR status (Bonadonna and Valagussa, 1988). The goals of treatment with hormonal agents or chemotherapy are to reduce the risk of recurrence presumably by eradicating metastatic foci not detectable at the time of surgery. For example, in node-negative (N_0), ER- or PR-positive patients, treatment may not be indicated because this group of patients may do very well without further therapy [90% disease-free survival (DFS) at 5 years]. Treatment for N_0, ER- or PR-*negative* patients may be warranted, since the 5-year DFS is approximately 70%. Obviously, if the treatment itself is associated with mortality in some patients or has significant long-term morbidity (cardiac or lung problems, secondary leukemia or cancer associated with cyclophosphamide, MTX, and 5-FU), then even in this group adjuvant therapy may not be justified. However, if adjuvant therapy has minimal risks (as with the combination of MTX sequenced with 5-FU), then the risk/benefit ratio favors treatment in this subset of patients. The deletion of an alkylating agent from the treatment program may decrease long-term risks (Fisher et al., 1989). *Principle: Treatment intensity (and therefore risk) should reflect the potential benefit expected.*

In patients with 10 or more positive nodes at mastectomy, current chemotherapy programs, even those containing doxorubicin, are only moderately effective in improving the DFS (from 20% to 40% at 5 years). Therefore, even more aggressive therapy that includes high-dose chemotherapy regimens with autologous bone marrow transfusion, despite the increase in morbidity, is currently under study, especially in young (premenopausal) women.

Postmenopausal patients (over 50 years of age) have not obtained the same benefit as premenopausal patients from the use of adjuvant chemotherapy. One possible explanation is that these patients are not able to be treated with the same dosage intensity as the younger patient. Standard practice is to treat these patients with the estrogen antagonist tamoxifen if they are ER-positive, rather than with chemotherapy. However, there are many clinical trials in progress utilizing different chemotherapy regimens with or without tamoxifen that may further improve the modest change in DFS in postmenopausal patients treated with tamoxifen alone.

Slower-Growing Tumors

Certain tumors, by virtue of their extremely long doubling time, may be classified as "slow-growing," or chronic, neoplasms. Examples of these diseases are multiple myeloma, CLL, nodu-

Table 23-15. DRUGS USED TO TREAT BREAST CANCER

1. Hormones
   Prednisone
   Estrogens
   Progestins
   Androgens

2. Hormone antagonists
   Tamoxifen
   Aminoglutethimide

3. Chemotherapeutic Agents
   Alkylating agents (cyclophosphamide, melphalan)
   MTX
   5-FU
   Anthracyclines (doxorubicin)

lar lymphocytic lymphoma, and certain other well-differentiated solid tumors. One of these tumors is discussed in some detail, to illustrate the principles of drug thrapy for this type of condition.

Multiple Myeloma. Multiple myeloma is a neoplastic disease caused by proliferation of malignant plasma cells. They usually produce γ-globulin and may be detected by an increase in the concentration of a γ-globulin in the serum called myeloma globulin. A spectrum of clinical syndromes ranging from an asymptomatic increase in the concentration of myeloma proteins to rapidly progressive disease characterized by destruction of bone, hematologic abnormalities, and renal impairment is associated with this disease. *Principle: The clinician should be prepared to treat not only the neoplasia but also the secondary manifestations that may result as a consequence of the tumor (i.e., hyperviscosity, hypercalcemia, and renal failure).*

Proliferation of plasma cells is slow when compared with the rate of proliferation of other malignancies in humans. The mass of tumor cells may be estimated by measuring the turnover of the total body pool of myeloma globulins in vivo (Salmon and Smith, 1970). Thus, effect of therapy on the mass of malignant cells can be accurately quantitated. Patients with myeloma in relapse have as many as 10^{12} tumor cells. "Remission" occurs when this mass of tumor cells is reduced by as little as 1 to 2 logs. These measurements make it clear that before a cure can be obtained additional effective therapies must be developed, for there is no logical way to lull one into thinking one has cured a patient who still has 10^{10} malignant cells. These studies also demonstrate that when the mass of tumor cells is reduced by chemotherapy, the growth fraction significantly increases. Thus cycle-active agents might be of value after the alkylating agents have had a chance to reduce the total mass of malignant cells.

Because of the large burden of tumor cells usually present in patients when they seek medical aid, and the slow doubling time of this tumor, it is not surprising that cycle-active agents are generally ineffective when they are used alone or before alkylating agents. In particular phenylalanine mustard (melphalan, PAM) and cyclophosphamide have been used most widely as initial or sole therapy. Approximately 50% of patients benefit from therapy with alkylating agents. When adrenocortical steroids are added to the regimen, the remission rates are higher, but survival may not be improved (Bergsagel and Rider, 1985). Because of the serious effects of chronic administration of steroids, they are generally used in short pulses of 4 or 5 days every 4 to 6 weeks in combination with the alkylating agent, which is used either in pulses or daily. There is no superiority of either dose schedule of the alkylating agents. The median survival of patients has improved since using therapy with alkylating agents.

Additional agents are being tested for their efficacy. A nitrosourea (lomustine) and procarbazine may be useful in managing myeloma. In addition, proper sequencing of cycle-active agents with the therapeutic regimen (e.g., vincristine and ara-C) is being tested (Gore et al., 1989).

In summary, slow-growing tumors may be sensitive to alkylating agents. Since recovery of normal cells in the bone marrow is more rapid than recovery of tumor cells, the drugs may have some selectivity. Further understanding of cell kinetics in this disease may lead to improved therapy by appropriate introduction of cycle-specific antitumor drugs.

REFERENCES

Ackland, S. P.; and Schilsky, R. L.: High dose methotrexate: A critical reappraisal. J. Clin. Oncol., 5(12):2017–2031, 1987.

Adolphe, A. B.; Glasofer, E. D.; Troetel, W. M.; Zeigenfuss, J.; Stambaugh, J. E.; Weiss, A. J.; and Manthei, R. W.: Fate of streptozotocin (NSC-85998) in patients with advanced cancer. Cancer Chemother. Rep., 59:547–556, 1975.

Alberts, D. S.; Chen, H.-S. G.; Mayersohn, M.; Perrier, D.; Moon, T. E.; and Gross, J. F.: Bleomycin pharmokinetics in man: II. Intracavitary administration. Cancer Chemother. Pharmacol., 2:127–132, 1979a.

Alberts, D. S.; Chang, S. Y.; Chen, H.-S. G.; Larcom, B. J.; and Jones, S. E.: Pharmacokinetics and metabolism of chlorambucil in man: A preliminary report. Cancer Treat. Rev., 6(suppl.):9–17, 1979b.

Alberts, D. S.; Chang, S. Y.; Chen, H.-S. G.; and Moon, T. E.: Oral melphalan kinetics. Clin. Pharmacol. Ther., 26: 737–745, 1979c.

Alberts, D. S.; Chen, H.-S. G.; Liu, R.; Himmelstein, K. J.; Mayersohn, M.; Perrier, D.; Gross, J.; Moon, T.; Broughton, A.; and Salmon, S. E.: Bleomycin pharmacokinetics in man: I. Intravenous administration. Cancer Chemother. Pharmacol., 1:177–181, 1978.

Allegra, C. J.: Antifolates. In, Cancer Chemotherapy: Principles and Practice (Chabner, B. A.; and Collins, J. M., eds.). J. B. Lippincott, Philadelphia, pp. 110–153, 1990.

Alexander, P.: Atomic Radiation and Life, 2nd ed. Penguin Books, Middlesex, England, 1965.

Alexanian, R.; Haut, A.; Khan, A. U.; Lane, M.; McKelvey, E. M.; Migliore, P. J.; Stuckey, W. J. Jr.; and Wilson, H. E.: Treatment for multiple myeloma. Combination chemotherapy with different melphalan dose regimens. J.A.M.A., 208:1680–1685, 1969.

Allen, L. M.; Creaven, P. J.; and Nelson, R. L.: Studies on the human pharmacokinetics of isophosphamide (NSC-109724). Cancer Treat. Rep., 60:451–458, 1976.

Bast, R. C.; Zbar, G.; Borsos, T.; and Rapp, H. J.: BCG and cancer. N. Engl. J. Med., 290:1413–1420;1458–1469, 1974.

Bender, R. A.; Hamel, E.; and Hande, K. P.: Plant alkaloids. In, Cancer Chemotherapy: Principles and Practice (Chabner, B. A.; and Collins, J. M., eds.). J. B. Lippincott, Philadelphia, pp. 253–275, 1990.

Bender, R. A.; Castle, M. C.; Margileth, D. A.; and Oliverio, V.: The pharmacokinetics of [³H] vincristine in man. Clin. Pharmacol. Ther., 22:430–435, 1977.

Bennett, J. M.; and Reich, S. D.: Bleomycin. Ann. Intern. Med., 90:945–948, 1979.

Berd, D.; Cornog, J.; DeConti, R. C.; Levitt, M.; and Bertino, J. R.: Long term remission in diffuse histiocytic lymphoma treated with combination sequential chemotherapy. Cancer, 35:1050–1054, 1975.

Bergsagel, D. E.; and Rider, W. D.: Plasma cell neoplasms. In, Cancer: Principles and Practice of Oncology, 2nd ed. (DeVita, V. T.; Hellman, S.; and Rosenberg, S. A., eds.). J. B. Lippincott, Philadelphia, pp. 1753–1795, 1985.

Bertino, J. R.: The general pharmacology of methotrexate. In, Methotrexate Therapy in Rheumatic Diseases (Wilke, W. S., ed.). Marcel Dekker, New York, pp. 11–23, 1989.

Bertino, J. R.; Lin, J. T.; Pizzorno, G.; Li, W. W.; and Chang, Y. M.: The basis for intrinsic drug resistance or sensitivity to methotrexate. Adv. Enzyme Reg., 29:277–285, 1989.

Billingham, M. E.; Mason, J. W.; Bristow, M. R.; and Daniels, J. R.: Anthracycline cardiomyopathy monitored by morphologic changes. Cancer Treat. Rep., 62:865, 1978.

Black, D. J.; and Livingston, R. B.: Antineoplastic drugs in 1990. Drugs, 39:489–501; 652–673, 1990.

Blum, R. H.; Carter, S. K.; and Agnes, K.: A clinical review of bleomycin—A new antineoplastic agent. Cancer, 31:903–914, 1973.

Boice, J. D. Jr.; Greene, M. H.; Killen, J. Y. Jr.; Ellenberg, S. S.; Klein, R. J.; McFadden, E.; Chen, T. T.; and Fraumeni, J. F. Jr.: Leukemia and preleukemia after adjuvant treatment of gastrointestinal cancer with semustine (BCNU). N. Engl. J. Med., 309:1079–1084, 1983.

Bonadonna, G.; and Valagussa, P.: Current status of adjuvant chemotherapy for breast cancer. Semin. Oncol., 14:8–22, 1988.

Bonadonna, G.; Valagussa, P.; and Santoro, A.: Alternating non-cross resistant combination chemotherapy or MOPP in stage IV Hodgkin's disease. Ann. Intern. Med., 104:739–746, 1986.

Bono, V. H. Jr.: Studies on the mechanism of action of DTIC (NSC-45388). Cancer Treat. Rep., 60:141–148, 1976.

Brade, W.; Nagel, G. A.; and Seeber, S. (eds): Ifosamide in Tumor Therapy. Vol. 26. Karger, Basel, 1987.

Breithaupt, H.; Dammann, A.; and Aigner, K.: Pharmacokinetics of dacarbazine (DTIC) and its metabolite 5-aminoimidazole-4-carboxamide (AIC) following different dose schedules. Cancer Chemother. Pharmacol., 9:103–109, 1982.

Brockman, R. W.: Mechanism of resistance to anticancer agents. Adv. Cancer Res., 7:129, 1963.

Broome, J. R.: Evidence that L-asparaginase of guinea pig serum is responsible for its antilymphoma effects. J. Exp. Med., 118:99–120, 1963.

Bruce, W. R.: The action of chemotherapeutic agents at the cellular level and the effects of these agents on hematopoietic and lymphomatous tissue. In, Canadian Cancer Conference: Proceedings of the Seventh Canadian Cancer Research Conference. Pergamon Press, Elmsford, N. Y., pp. 53–64, 1967.

Bruce, W. R.; and Bergsagel, D. E.: On the application of results from a model system to the treatment of leukemia in man. Cancer Res., 27:2646–2649, 1967.

Bruce, W. R.; Meeker, B. E.; Powers, W. E.; and Valeriote, F. A.: Comparison of the dose and time-survival curves for normal hematopoietic and lymphoma colony-forming cells exposed to vinblastine, vincristine, arabinosylcytosine, and amethopterin. J. Natl. Cancer Inst., 42:1015–1023, 1969.

Bruce, W. R.; Meeker, B. E.; and Valeriote, F. A.: Comparison of the sensitivity of normal hematopoietic and transplanted lymphoma colony-forming cells to chemotherapeutic agents and administered in vivo. J. Natl. Cancer Inst., 37:233–245, 1966.

Buckner, C. D.; Rudolph, R. H.; Fefer, A.; Clift, R. A.; and Epstein, R. B.: High dose cyclophosphamide for malignant disease. Cancer, 50:357–365, 1972.

Burchenal, J. H.; Murphy, M. L.; Ellison, R. R.; Sykes, M. P.; Tan, T. C.; Leone, L. A.; Karnofsky, D. A.; Craver, D. H. W.; and Rhoads, C. P.: Clinical evaluation of a new antimetabolite, 6-mercaptopurine, in the treatment of acute leukemia and allied diseases. Blood, 8:965–999, 1953.

Burger, R. M.; Projan, S. J.; Horwitz, S. B.; and Peisach, J.: The DNA cleavage mechanism of iron-bleomycin. J. Biol. Chem., 261:15955–15959, 1986.

Burkitt, D. P.; and Burchenal, J. H. (eds.): Treatment of Burkitt's Tumor. Springer-Verlag, New York, 1969.

Calabresi, P.; and Parks, R. E. Jr.: Chemotherapy of Neoplastic Diseases. In, The Pharmacological Basis of Therapeutics (Gilman, A. G.; Goodman, L. S.; Raul, T. W.; and Murad, F., eds.). MacMillan, New York, pp. 1240–1307, 1985.

Capizzi, R.: Improvement in the therapeutic index of L-asparaginase by methotrexate. Cancer Chem. Rep., (3)6:37–41, 1975.

Capizzi, R. L.; Yang, J. L.; Rathmell, J. P.; White, J. C.; Cheng, E.; Cheng, Y. C.; and Kute, T.: Dose related pharmacologic effects of high dose ara-C and its self potentiation. Semin. Oncol., 12:65–74, 1985.

Capizzi, R. L.; Bertino, J. R.; and Handschumacher, R. E.: L-asparaginase. Ann. Rev. Med., 21:433–444, 1970.

Capranico, G.; Riva, A.; Tinnelli, S.; Dasdia, T.; and Zunino, F.: Markedly reduced levels of anthracycline-induced DNA strand breaks in resistant P388 leukemia cells and isolated nuclei. Cancer Res., 47:3752–3756, 1987.

Carlson, R. W.; and Sikic, B. I.: Continuous infusion or bolus injection in cancer chemotherapy. Ann. Intern. Med., 99:823–833, 1983.

Chang, P.; Wiernik, P. H.; Reich, S. D.; Coleman, C. N.; Stoller, R. G.; Hande, K. R.; Chabner, B. A.; and Bachur, N. R.: Prediction of response to cytosine arabinoside and daunorubicin. In, Acute Non-Lymphocytic Leukemia, Therapy of Acute Leukemias (Manduli, F., ed.). Proceedings of 2nd International Symposium. Lonbardo Editore, Rome, pp. 148–156, 1979.

Chabner, B. A.: Enzyme therapy: L-Asparaginase. In, Cancer Chemotherapy: Principles and Practice (Chabner, B. A.; and Collins, J. M., eds.). J. B. Lippincott, Philadelphia, pp. 397–407, 1990.

Chabner, B. A.; and Collins, J. M.: Cancer Chemotherapy: Principles and Practice. J. B. Lippincott, Philadelphia, 1990.

Cole, S. R.; Myers, J. J.; and Klatsky, A. U.: Pulmonary disease with chlorambucil therapy. Cancer, 41:455–459, 1978.

Colvin, M.: The comparative pharmacology of cyclophosphamide and ifosfamide. Semin. Oncol., 9(suppl. 1):2–7, 1982.

Colvin, M.; and Hilton, J.: Pharmacology of cyclophosphamide and metabolites. Cancer Treat. Rep., 65(suppl. 3):89–95, 1981.

Colvin, M.; Brundett, R. B.; Cowens, J. L.; Jardine, I.; and Ludlum, D. B.: A chemical basis for the antitumor activity of chloroethylnitrosoureas. Biochem. Pharmacol., 25:695–699, 1976.

Creaven, P. J.: The clinical pharmacology of etoposide (VP-16) in adults. In, Etoposide (VP-16) (Issell, B. F.; Maggia, R. M.; and Carter, S. K., eds.). Academic Press, pp. 103–115, 1984.

Creaven, P. J.; Allen, L. M.; Cohen, M. H.; and Nelson, R. L.: Studies on the clinical pharmacology and toxicology of isophosphamide (NSC-109724). Cancer Treat. Rep., 60:445–449, 1976.

D'Angio, G. J.; Farber, S.; and Maddock, C. L.: Potentation of x-ray effects by actinomycin D. Radiology, 73:175–177, 1959.

Diddens, H.; Gekeler, V.; Neumann, M.; and Niethammer, D.: Characterization of actinomycin-D resistant CHO cell lines exhibiting a multidrug-resistance phenotype and amplified DNA sequences. Int. J. Cancer, 40:635–642, 1987.

DeVita, V. T.; Canellos, G. P.; and Moxley, J. H. III: A decade of combination chemotherapy of advanced Hodgkin's disease. Cancer, 30:1495–1504, 1972.

DeVita, V. T.; Serpick, A. A.; and Carbone, P. P.: Combination chemotherapy in the treatment of advanced Hodgkin's disease. Ann. Intern. Med., 73:881–895, 1970.

DeVita, V. T.; Denham, C.; Davidson, J.; and Oliverio, V. T.: The physiological disposition of carcinostatic 1,3-bis(2-

chloroethyl)-1-nitrosourea (BCNU) in man and animals. Clin. Pharmacol. Ther., 8:566–577, 1967.

Donehower, R. C.: Hyroxyurea. In, Cancer Chemotherapy: Principles and Practice (Chabner, B. A.; and Collins, J. M., eds.). J. B. Lippincott, Philadelphia, pp. 225–233, 1990.

Dorr, R. T.: New findings in pharmacokinetics, metabolic and drug-resistance aspects of mitomycin-C. Semin. Oncol., 15(suppl. 4):32–41, 1988.

Dresler, W. F. C.; and Stein, R.: Über den hydroxyl Harnstoff. Liebigs Ann. Chem., 150:242–252, 1969.

Edwards, M. S.; Levin, V. A.; Seager, M. L.; Pischer, T. L.; and Wilson, C. B.: Phase II evaluation of thiotepa for treatment of central nervous system tumors. Cancer Treat. Rep., 63:1419–1421, 1979.

Ehrsson, H.; Hassan, M.; Ehrnbo, M.; and Beran, M.: Busulfan kinetics. Clin. Pharmacol. Ther., 34:86–89, 1983.

Elion, G. B.: Biochemistry and pharmacology of purine analogs. Fed. Proc., 26:898–964, 1967.

Elion, G. B.; Bargi, E.; and Hitchings, G. H.: Studies on condensed pyrimidine systems: IX. The synthesis of some 6-substituted purines. J. Am. Chem. Soc., 74:411–414, 1952.

Farber, S.: Chemotherapy in the treatment of leukemia and Wilm's tumor. J.A.M.A., 198:826–836, 1966.

Farmer, P. B.: Metabolism and reactions of alkylating agents. Pharmacol. Ther., 35:301–358, 1987.

Fernandes, D. J.; and Bertino, J. R.: 5-Fluorouracil-methotrexate synergy. Enhancement of 5-fluorodeoxyuridylate binding to thymidylate synthetase by dihydropteroyl polyglutamates. Proc. Natl. Acad. Sci. U.S.A., 77:5663–5667, 1980.

Fisher, B.; Redmond, C.; Dimitrov, N. V.; Bowman, D.; Legault-Poisson, S.; Wickerham, D. L.; Wolmark, N.; Fisher, E. R.; Margolese, R.; Sutherland, C.; Glass, A.; Foster, R.; and Caplan, R.: A randomized clinical trial evaluating sequential methotrexate and fluorouracil in the treatment of patients with node negative breast cancer who have estrogen receptor tumors. N. Engl. J. Med., 320:473–478, 1989.

Frei, E. III: Acute leukemia in children: Model for the development of scientific methodology for clinical therapeutic research in cancer. Cancer, 53:2013–2025, 1984.

Frei, E. III: The clinical use of actinomycin. Cancer Chemother. Rep., 58:49–54, 1974.

Frosch, P. J.; Czarnetzki, B. M.; Macher, E.; Grundman, E.; and Gottschalk, I.: Hepatic failure in patients treated with dacarbazine (DTIC) for malignant melanoma. J. Cancer Res. Clin. Oncol., 95:281–286, 1979.

Fugman, R. A.; Martin, D. S.; Hayworth, P. E.; and Stolfi, R. L.: Enhanced cures of spontaneous mammary carcinoma with surgery and five compound combination chemotherapy and their immunotherapeutic interrelationship. Cancer Res., 30:1931–1936, 1970.

Ghione, M.: Development of adriamycin (NSC-123127). Cancer Chem. Rep., 6:83–89, 1975.

Glisson, B.; Gupta, R.; Hodges, P.; and Ross, W.: Cross resistance to intercalating agents in an epipodophyllotoxin-resistant chinese hamster ovary cell line: Evidence for a common intracellular target. Cancer Res., 46:1939–1942, 1986.

Gilman, A.: The initial clinical trial of nitrogen mustard. Am. J. Surg., 105:574–578, 1963.

Goldie, J. H.; Coldman, A. J.; and Gudauskas, G. A.: Rationale for the use of alternating non-cross resistant chemotherapy. Cancer Treat. Rep., 66:439–449, 1982.

Goldenberg, G. J.; Vanstone, C. L.; Israels, L. G.; Ilse, D.; and Bihler, I.: Evidence for a transport carrier of nitrogen mustard in nitrogen mustard–sensitive and resistant L5178Y cells. Cancer Res., 30:2285–2291, 1970.

Goldstein, D. P.: The chemothrapy of trophoblastic disease. J.A.M.A., 220:209–213, 1972.

Gore, M. E.; Selby, P. J.; Viner, C.; Clark, P. I.; Meldrum, M.; Millar, B.; Bell, J.; Maitland, J. A.; Milan, S.; Judson, I. R.; Zuiable, A.; Tillyer, C.; Selvin, M.; Malpasss, J. S.; and McElwain, T. J.: Intensive treatment of multiple myeloma and criteria for complete remission. Lancet, 2:879–882, 1989.

Grem, J. L.: Fluorinated pyrimidines. In, Cancer Chemotherapy: Principles and Practice (Chabner, B. A.; and Collins, J. M., eds.). J. B. Lippincott, Philadelphia, pp. 180–224, 1990.

Grochow, L. B.; and Colvin, M.: Clinical pharmacokinetics of cyclophosphamide. Clin. Pharmacokinet., 4:380–394, 1979.

Hammond, C. B.; Borchet, L. G.; Tyrey, L.; Creesman, N. T.; and Parker, R. T.: Treatment of metastatic trophoblastic disease: Good and poor prognosis. Am. J. Obstet. Gynecol., 115:451–457, 1973.

Heidelberger, C.; Chaudhuari, N. K.; Danenberg, P.; Mooren, D.; Griesbach, L.; Duschiwsky, R.; Schnitzer, R. J.; Pleven, E; and Scheiner, J.: Fluorinated pyrimidines: A new class of inhibitory compounds. Nature, 179:663–666, 1957.

Henderson, E. S.; Adamson, R. H.; and Oliverio, V. T.: The metabolic fate of tritiated methotrexate: II. Absorption and excretion in man. Cancer Res., 25:1018–1024, 1965.

Henderson, I. C.: Chemotherapy for advanced disease. In, Breast Cancer: Diagnosis and Management (Bonadonna, G., ed.). John Wiley & Sons, New York, pp. 247–280, 1984.

Hersh, M. R.; Ludden, T. M.; Kuhn, J. G.; and Knight, W. A. III: Pharmacokinetics of high dose melphalan. Invest. New Drugs, 1:331–334, 1983.

Hertz, R.: Gestational trophoblastic neoplasia, Hosp. Pract., 1:157–164, 1972.

Hood, A. F.: Cutaneous side effects of cancer chemotherapy. Med. Clin. North Am., 70:187–209, 1986.

Howell, S. B.; Schiefer, M.; Andrews, P. A.; Markham, M.; and Abramson, I.: The pharmacology of intraperitoneally administered bleomycin. J. Clin. Oncol., 5:2009–2016, 1987.

Hryniuk, W. M.: Average relative dose intensity and the impact on design of clinical trials. Semin. Oncol., 14:65–74, 1987.

Hryniuk, W. M.; and Bertino, J. R.: Rationale for the selection of chemotherapeutic agents. Adv. Intern. Med., 15:267–298, 1969a.

Hryniuk, W. M.; and Bertino, J. R.: The treatment of leukemia with large doses of methotrexate and folinic acid: Clinical-biochemical correlates. J. Clin. Invest., 48:2140–2155, 1969b.

Hryniuk, W. M.; Fisher, G. A.; and Bertino, J. R.: S Phase cells of rapidly growing and resting populations. Differences in response to methotrexate. Mol. Pharmacol., 5:557–564, 1969.

Hubbard, S. M.; and Jenkins, J. F.: Chemotherapy administration. In, Cancer Chemotherapy: Principles and Practice (Chabner, B. A.; and Collins, J. M., eds.). J. B. Lippincott, Philadelphia, pp. 449–464, 1990.

Hutter, A. M. Jr.; and Kayhoe, D. E.: Adrenal colon carcinoma. Results of treatment with o,p-DDD in 138 patients. Am. J. Med., 41:581–592, 1966.

Juma, F. D.; Rogers, H. J.; and Trounce, J. R.: Pharmacokinetics of cyclophosphamide and alkylating activity in man after intravenous and oral administration. Br. J. Clin. Pharmacol., 8:209–217, 1979.

Kemeny, N.; Cohen, A.; Bertino, J. R.; Sigurdson, E. R.; Botet, J.; and Oderman, P.: Continuous intrahepatic infusion of floxuridine and leucovorin through an implantable pump for the treatment of hepatic metatases from colorectal carcinoma. Cancer, 65:2446–2450, 1989.

Kennedy, B. J.: Mithramycin therapy in advanced testicular neoplasms. Cancer, 26:755–766, 1970.

Kidd, J. G.: Regression of transplanted lymphomas induced in vivo by means of normal guinea pig serum. J. Exp. Med., 98:565–582, 1953.

Koren, G.; Ferrazini, O.; Sulh, A. M.; Langevin, A. M.; Kapelushnik, J.; Klein, J.; Giesbrecht, E.; Soldin, S.; and Greenberg, M.: Systemic exposure to mercaptopurine as a prognostic factor in acute lymphocytic leukemia in children. N. Engl. J. Med., 323:17–21, 1990.

Kufe, D. W.; Monroe, D.; Herrick, D.; Egan, E.; and Spriggs, D.: Effects of 1-D-arabinofuranosylcytosine incorporation on eukaryotic DNA template function. Mol. Pharmacol., 26:128–134, 1984.

Lambert, C. J.; Shad, H. H.; Urschel, H. C. Jr.; and Paulson,

D. L.: The treatment of malignant pleural effusions by closed trocar tube drainage. Ann. Thorac. Surg., 3:1–5, 1967.

Lazarus, H. M.; Reed, M. D.; Spitzer, T. R.; Rab M. S.; and Blumer, J. L.: High-dose IV thiotepa and cryopreserved autologous bone marrow transplantation for therapy of refractory cancer. Cancer Treat. Rep., 71:689–695, 1987.

Lazo, J. S.; and Humphreys, C. J.: Lack of metabolism as the biochemical basis of bleomycin-induced pulmonary toxicity. Proc. Natl. Acad. Sci. U.S.A., 80:3064–3068, 1983.

Legha, S. S.; Benjamin, R. S.; Mackay, B.; Ewer, M.; Wallace, S.; Valdivieso, M.; Rasmussen, S. L.; Blumenschein, G. R; and Freireich, E. J.: Reduction of doxorubicin cardiotoxicity by prolonged continuous intravenous infusion. Ann. Intern. Med., 96:133–139, 1982.

LePage, G. A.; and Whitecar, J. P.: The pharmacology of 6-thioguanine in man. Cancer Res., 31:1627–1631, 1971.

Liliemark, J. O.; Plunkett, W.; and Dixon, D. O.: Relationship of 1-D-arabinofuranosylcytosine-5-triphosphate levels in leukemia cells during treatment with high dose 1-D-arabinofuranosylcytosine. Cancer Res., 45:5952–5957, 1985.

Lobel, J. S.; O'Brien, R. T.; McIntosh, S.; Aspnes, G. T.; and Capizzi, R. L.: Methotrexate and asparaginase combination chemotherapy in refractory acute lymphoblastic leukemia of childhood. Cancer, 43:1089–1094, 1979.

Luduena, R. F.; Shooter, E. M.; and Wilson, L.: Structure of the tubulin dimer. J. Biol. Chem., 252:7006–7014, 1977.

McCormack, J. J.; and Johns, D. G.: Purine and purine nucleoside antimetabolites. In, Cancer Chemotherapy: Principles and Practice (Chabner, B. A.; and Collins, J. M., eds.). J. B. Lippincott, Philadelphia, pp. 234–252, 1990.

Mead, G. M.; Arnold, A. M.; and Green, J. A.: Epileptic seizures associated with cisplatin administration. Cancer Treat. Rep., 66:1719–1722, 1982.

Melmon, K. L.: The endocrinologic manifestations of the carcinoid tumor. In, Textbook of Endocrinology (Williams, R. H., ed.). W. B. Saunders, Philadelphia, pp. 1084–1104, 1974.

Miller, D. M.; Polansky, D. A.; Thomas, S. D.; Ray, R.; Campbell, V. W.; Sanchez, J.; and Koller, C. A.: Rapid communication: Mithramycin selectively inhibits transcription of GC containing DNA. Am. J. Med. Sci., 294:388–394, 1987.

Mini, E.; Trave, F.; Rustum, Y. M.; and Bertino, J. R.: Enhancement of the anti-tumor effects of 5-fluorouracil by folinic acid. Pharmacol. Ther., 47:1–19, 1990.

Mitchell, M. S.; Wade, M. E.; DeConti, R. C.; Bertino, J. R.; and Calabresi, P.: Immunosuppressive effects of cytosine arabinoside and methotrexate in man. Ann. Intern. Med., 70:535–547, 1969.

Moore, E. W.; Thomas, L. B.; Shaw, R. K.; and Freireich, E. J.: The central nervous system in acute leukemia: A postmortem study of 117 consecutive cases, with particular reference to hemorrhage, leukemic infiltrations and the syndrome of meningeal leukemia. Arch. Intern. Med., 105:451–468, 1960.

Muggia, F. M.; Louie, A. C.; and Sikic, B. I.: Pulmonary toxicity of antitumor agents. Cancer Treat. Rev., 10:221–243, 1983.

Myers, C. E.; and Chabner, B. A.: Anthracyclines. In, Cancer Chemotherapy: Principles and Practice (Chabner, B. A.; and Collins, J. M., eds.). J. B. Lippincott, pp. 356–381, 1990.

Osserman, E. F.; and Lawlor, D. P.: Serum and urinary lysozyme (muramidase) in monocytic and monomyelocytic leukemia. J. Exp. Med., 124:921–952, 1966.

Ozols, R. F.; Corden, B. J.; and Jacob J.: High-dose cisplatin in hypertonic saline. Ann. Intern. Med., 100:19–24, 1984.

Pallavincini, M. G.: Cytosine arabinoside, molecular, pharmacokinetic and cytokinetic considerations. Pharmacol. Ther., 25:207–238, 1984.

Perillie, P. E.; Kaplan, S. S.; Lefkowitz, E.; Rogaway, W.; and Finch, S. C.: Studies of muramidase (lysozyme) in leukemia. J.A.M.A., 203:317–322, 1968.

Piro, L. D.; Carrera, C. J.; Carson, D. A.; and Beutler, E.: Lasting remissions in hairy-cell leukemia induced by a single infusion of 2-chlorodeoxyadenosine. N. Engl. J. Med., 322:1117–1121, 1990.

Pommier, Y.; Kerrigan, D.; Schwartz, R. E.; Swack, J. A.; and McCurdy, A.: Altered DNA topoisomerase II activity in chinese hamster cells resistant to topoisomerase II inhibitors. Cancer Res., 46:3075–3081, 1986.

Portlock, C. S.; Fischer, D. S.; Cadman, E.; Lundberg, W. B.; Levy, A.; Bobrow, S.; Bertino, J. R.; and Farber, L.: High-dose pulse chlorambucil in advanced low grade non-Hodgkins lymphoma. Cancer Treat. Rep., 71:1029–1031, 1987.

Powis, G.: Metabolism and reactions of quinoid anti-cancer agents. Pharmacol. Ther., 35:57–162, 1987.

Pratt, C. B.; Green, A. A.; and Horowitz, M. E.: Central nervous system toxicity, following the treatment of pediatric patients with ifosfamide/mesna. J. Clin. Oncol., 4:1253–1261, 1986.

Reddy, M. V.; and Randerath, K.: Analysis of DNA products in somatic and reproductive tissues of rats tested with the anticancer antibiotic mitomycin C. Mutat. Res., 179:75–88, 1987.

Reed, E.; and Kohn, K. W.: Platinum analogs. In, Cancer Chemotherapy: Principles and Practice (Chabner, B. A.; and Collins, J. M., eds.). J. B. Lippincott, Philadelphia, pp. 465–490, 1990.

Rees, L. H.; and Landon, J.: Biochemical abnormalities in some human neoplasms: Inappropriate biosynthesis of hormones by tumors. In, Scientific Foundations of Oncology (Symington, T.; and Carter, R. L., eds.). William Heineman, London, pp. 107–116, 1976.

Rieselbach, R. E.; Morse, E. E.; Rall, D. P.; Frei, E. III; and Freireich, E. J.: Intrathecal aminopterin therapy of meningeal leukemia. Arch. Intern. Med., 111:620–630, 1963.

Riordan, J. R.; and Ling, V.: Genetic and biochemical characterization of multidrug resistance. Pharmacol. Ther., 28:51–75, 1985.

Rosenberg, B.; Van Camp, L.; and Krigas, T.: Inhibition of division in E. coli by electrolysis products from a platinum electrode. Science, 698–699, 1965.

Rosman, M.; and Williams, H. E.: Leukocyte purine phosphoribosyltransferases in human leukemias sensitive and resistant to 6-thiopurines. Cancer Res., 33:1202–1209, 1973.

Rosman, M.; Lee, M. H.; Creasey, W. A.; and Sartorelli, A. C.: Mechanisms of resistance to 6-thiopurines in human leukemia. Cancer Res., 34:1952–1956, 1974.

Ross, W.; Rowe, T.; Glisson, B.; Yalowich, J.; and Liu, L.: Role of toperisomerase II in mediating epidophyllotoxin-induced DNA cleavage. Cancer Res., 44:5857–5860, 1984.

Ross, G. T.; Goldstein, D. P.; Hertz, R.; Lipsett, M. B.; and Odell, W. D.: Sequential use of methotrexate and actinomycin D in the treatment of metastatic choricarcinoma and related trophoblastic diseases in women. Am. J. Obstet. Gynecol., 93:223–229, 1965.

Rudnick, S. A.; Cadman, E. C.; Capizzi, R. L.; Skeel, R. T.; Bertino, J. R.; and McIntosh, S.: High-dose cytosine (HDARAC) arabinoside in refractory acute leukemia. Cancer, 44:1189–1193, 1979.

Salmon, S. E.; and Smith, B. A.: Immunoglobulin synthesis and total body tumor cell number in IgG multiple myeloma. J. Clin. Invest., 49:1114–1121, 1970.

Sarosy, G.; Leyland-Jones, B.; Soochan, P.; and Chesson, B. D.: The systemic administration of intravenous melphalan. J. Clin. Oncol., 6:1768–1782, 1988.

Schabel, F. M. Jr.: Concepts for systemic treatment of micrometastases. Cancer, 35:15–24, 1975.

Schackney, S. E.; and Ritch, P. S.: Cell kinetics. In, Pharmacologic Principles of Cancer Treatment (Chabner, B. A., ed.). W. B. Saunders, Philadelphia, pp. 45–76, 1982.

Schein, P. S.; Tew, K. D.; and Mathe, G.: Pharmacology of nitrosourea anti-cancer agents. In, Clinical Chemotherapy: Antineoplastic Chemotherapy (Bukarda, B.; Karrer, K.; and Mathe, G., eds.). Vol. 3. Thieme-Stratton, pp. 264–282, 1984.

Schilsky, R. L.; Barlock, A.; and Ozols, R. F.: Persistent hypomagnesemia following cisplatin chemotherapy for testicular cancer. Cancer Treat. Rep., 66:1767–1769, 1982.

Scholar, E. M.; and Calabresi, P.: Increased activity of alkaline phosphatases in leukemia cells from patients resistant to thiopurine. Biochem. Pharmacol., 28:445–446, 1979.

Skipper, H. E.: Experimental evaluation of potential anticancer agents: XXI. Scheduling of arabinosylcytosine to take advantage of its S-phase specificity against leukemia cells. Cancer Chemother. Rep., 51:125–165, 1967.

Skipper, H. E.: Experimental evaluation of potent anticancer agents: XIV. Further study of certain basic concepts underlying chemotherapy of leukemia. Cancer Chemother. Rep., 45: 5–28, 1965.

Skipper, H. E.; Schabel, F. M. Jr.; and Wilcox, W.: Experimental evaluation of potential anticancer agents: XIII. On the criteria kinetics associated with "curability" of experimental leukemia. Cancer Chemother. Rep., 35:3–111, 1964.

Sladek, N. E.; Doeden, D.; Powers, J. F.; and Krivit, W.: Plasma concentrations of 4-hydroxycyclophosphamide and phosphoramide mustard in patients given repeatedly high dose of cyclophosphamide in preparation for bone marrow transplantation. Cancer Treat. Rep., 68:1247–1254, 1984.

Sobell, H. M.; Jain, S. C.; Sakore, T. D.; and Nordman, C. E.: Stereo chemistry of actinomycin-DNA binding. Nature, New Biol., 231:200–205, 1971.

Sobrero, A.; and Bertino, J. R.: Clinical aspects of drug resistance. Cancer Surveys, 5:93–107, 1986.

Spiegel, R. J.: The acute toxicities of chemotherapy. Cancer Treat. Rev., 8:197–207, 1981.

Spriggs, D. R.; Robbins, G.; Arthur, K.; Mayer, R. J.; and Kufe, D.: Prolonged high dose ara-C infusions in acute leukemia. Leukemia, 2:304–306, 1988.

Steel, G. G.: Cell loss as a factor in the growth of human tumors. Eur. J. Cancer, 3:381–387, 1967.

Steinherz, P. G.: Acute lymphoblastic leukemia of childhood. Hematol./Oncol. Clin. North Am., 1:549–566, 1987.

Steuart, C. D.; and Burke, P. J.: Cytidine deaminase and the development of resistance to arabinocytosine. Nature, New Biol., 233:109–110, 1971.

Stewart, A. F.: Therapy of malignancy-associated hypercalcemia. Am. J. Med., 74:475–480, 1983.

Tattersall, M. H. N.; Parker, L. M.; and Pittman, S.: Clinical pharmacology of high dose methotrexate (NSC-740). Cancer Chemother. Rep., 6:25–29, 1975a.

Tattersall, M. H. N.; Sodegren, J. E.; Sengupta, S. K.; Trites, D. H.; Modest, E. J.; and Frei, E. III: Pharmacokinetics of actinomycin D in patients with malignant melanoma. Clin. Pharmacol. Ther., 17:701–708, 1975b.

Tattersall, M. H. N.; Ganeshaguru, K.; and Hoffbrand, A. V.: Mechanisms of resistance of human acute leukemia cells to cytosine arabinoside. Br. J. Haematol., 27:39–46, 1974.

Tidd, D. M.; and Paterson, A. R. P.: A biochemical mechanism for the delayed cytotoxic reaction of 6-mercaptopurine. Cancer Res., 34:738–746, 1974.

Till, J. E.; and McCulloch, E. A.: A direct measurement of the radiation sensitivity of normal mouse marrow cells. Radiat. Res., 14:213–222, 1961.

Tomasz, M.; Lipman, R.; Lee, M. S.; Verdine, G. L.; and Nakanishi, K.: Reaction of acid-activated mitomycin C with calf thymus DNA and model guanines: Elucidation of the base-catalyzed degradation of N^7 alkylguanine nucleosides. Biochemistry, 26:2010–2027, 1987.

Tsuruo, T.: Mechanisms of multidrug resistance and implications for therapy. Jpn. J. Cancer Res., 79:285–296, 1988.

Umezawa, H.; Hori, S.; Sawa, T.; Yoshioka, T.; and Takeuchi, T.: A bleomycin-inactivating enzyme in mouse liver. J. Antibiot. (Tokyo), 27:419–424, 1974.

Umezawa, H.; Maeda, K.; Takeuchi, T.; and Okaris, Y.: New Antibiotics: Bleomycin A and B. J. Antibiot. (Tokyo), 19: 200–209, 1966.

Valeriote, F. A.; and Bruce, W. R.: Comparison of the sensitivity of hematopoietic colony-forming cells in different proliferative states to vinblastine. J. Natl. Cancer Inst., 38:393–399, 1967.

Vogelzang, N. J.: Continuous infusion chemotherapy: A critical review. J. Clin. Oncol., 2:289–304, 1984.

Vonderheid, E. C.: Topical mechlorethamine chemotherapy. Int. J. Dermatol., 23:180–186, 1984.

Von Hoff, D. D.; Rosenczweig, M.; and Piccart, M.: The cardiotoxicity of anticancer agents. Semin. Oncol., 9:23–33, 1982.

Walker, M. D.: Nitrosoureas in central nervous system tumors. Cancer Chemother. Rep. 4(part 3):21–26, 1973.

Walters, R. S.; Kantarjian, H. M.; Keating, M. J.; Plunkett, W. K.; Estey, E. H.; Andersson, B.; Beran, M.; McCredie, K. B.; and Freireich, E. J.: Mitoxantrone and high-dose cytosine arabinoside in refractory acute myelogenous leukemia. Cancer, 62:677–682, 1988.

Warren, R. D.; and Bender, R. A.: Drug interactions with antineoplastic agents. Cancer Treat. Rep., 61:1231–1241, 1977.

Weikam, R. J.; and Shiba, D. A.: Non-classical alkylating agents: Procarbazine. In, Pharmacologic Principles of Cancer Treatment (Chabner, B. A., ed.). W. B. Saunders, Philadelphia, pp. 340–349, 1982.

Weiss, H. D.; Walker, M. D.; and Wiernik, P. H.: Neurotoxicity of commonly used antineoplastic agents. N. Engl. J. Med., 291:75–81; 127–133, 1974.

Weiss, R. B.: Streptozocin: A review of its pharmacology, efficacy, and toxicity. Cancer Treat. Rep., 66:427–438, 1982.

Weiss, R. B.; and Bruno, S.: Hypersensitivity reactions to cancer chemotherapy. Ann. Intern. Med., 94:66–72, 1981.

Whitehead, V. M.; Kalman, T. I.; Rosenblatt, D. S.; Vuchich, M. J.; and Beaulieu, D.: Methotrexate polyglutamate synthesis in lymphoblasts from children with acute lymphoblastic leukemia. Dev. Pharmacol. Ther., 10:443–448, 1987.

Wilcox, W. S.; Griswold, D. P.; Laster, W. R. Jr.; Schabel, F. M. Jr.; and Skipper, H. E.: Experimental evaluation of potential anticancer agents: XVII. Kinetics of growth and regression after treatment of certain solid tumors. Cancer Chemother. Rep., 47:27–39, 1965.

Woolley, P. V.: Hepatic and pancreatic damage produced by cytotoxic drugs. Cancer Treat. Rev., 10:117–137, 1983.

Wright, J. A.: Altered mammalian ribonucleoside diphosphate reductase from mutant cell lines. In, Inhibitors of Ribonucleoside Diphosphate Reductase Activity (Cory, J. G.; and Cory, A. H., eds.). Pergamon Press, Elmsford, N.Y., pp. 89–111, 1989.

Yagoda, A.; Mukherji, B.; Young, C.; Etcubanas, E.; Lamonte, C.; Smith, J. R.; Tan, C. T.; and Krakoff, J. H.: Bleomycin an antitumor antibiotic. Clinical experience in 274 patients. Ann. Intern. Med., 77:861–870, 1972.

Yarbro, J. W.; Kennedy, B. J.; and Barnum, C. P.: Hydroxyurea inhibition of DNA synthesis in ascites tumor. Proc. Natl. Acad. Sci. U.S.A., 53:1033–1035, 1965.

Ziegler, J. L.: Burkitt's tumor. In, Cancer Medicine (Holland, J. F.; and Frei, E. III, eds.). Lea & Febiger, Philadelphia, pp. 1321–1330, 1973.

24

Infectious Disorders

Peter D. O'Hanley, Janice Y. Tam, and Mark Holodniy

Chapter Outline

Infectious diseases comprise those illnesses that are caused by microorganisms or their products. Clinical manifestations of infection occur only when sufficient tissue injury has been inflicted directly by microbial products (e.g., endotoxins and exotoxins), or indirectly by host responses involving its cellular products (e.g., cytokines and hydrolytic enzymes released by polymorphonuclear leukocytes). Too often in the practice of medicine, insufficient attention is paid to the rationale of therapeutics in the management of patients with infectious diseases. Physicians frequently neglect to consider preventive measures (e.g., education or immunoprophylaxis) even though it is obvious from patient-care and economic perspectives that preventing diseases is preferable to treating it. Despite the extraordinary recent advances that have occurred in therapeutics for infectious diseases, there are a number of basic principles that should be followed in order to appropriately prescribe antimicrobials and vaccines. This chapter deals with the broader issues of treating infectious diseases, while providing a number of practical clinical examples to demonstrate rational therapeutics.

The therapeutic strategy in the management of proven or suspected infectious diseases must focus on the following:

1. Performing a detailed history and physical examination, and obtaining appropriate laboratory specimens to determine whether a specific infectious disease process exists

2. Choosing cost-effective and safe therapy to interrupt the infectious process

The authors recognize the major contribution of the previous authors of this chapter, Richard Root and Walter J. Hierholzer, Jr.

3. Assessing the role of host factors in modifying the course of infection during therapy

4. Recognizing the failure of a therapeutic plan and its causes

5. Applying available methods to prevent an infectious disease before it occurs

The primary problems that clinicians encounter usually stem from the first four points. The general importance of such decision making is highlighted by the fact that antimicrobials are among the most prescribed of all drugs on a worldwide basis. Antibiotics may account for one of five new and refill prescriptions each year (Stolley et al., 1972). Furthermore, hospital purchases of antibiotics usually represent 25% to 30% of the annual drug budget for the institution (Barriere, 1985; Col and O'Connor, 1987; Lebow, 1987). Tertiary care hospitals in the United States typically spend more than $1 million per annum on antibiotic purchases alone. Given this tremendous utilization of antimicrobials, it is disturbing that numerous carefully performed surveys at private and university-affiliated facilities indicate that the majority of hospitalized patients had no evidence of infection to justify antimicrobial usage or were treated with inappropriate dosage or inappropriate antimicrobials with respect to the infectious disease process (Kunin et al., 1973; Maki and Schunna, 1978; Craig et al., 1978; Coleman et al., 1990).

Precise data are not available on usage of antibiotics in the outpatient setting; however, the number of clinicians who prescribe antibiotics for the "common cold" and who select inappropriate antibiotics for treatment of various infectious disease syndromes is considerable. These examples of excessive utilization and misuse of antibiotics justify ongoing educational programs related to improving usage of antimicrobials (Kunin, 1985; Jeffrey and Mahone, 1987; Woodward et al., 1987; Avorn et al., 1987, 1988). Furthermore, the financial considerations for hospitals, health insurance companies, and patients related to the costs of antibiotics represent a potentially serious misuse of health care resources to the extent that compromises are made in delivery of other patient care services. If the physician does not recognize and respond to this problem, bureaucratic policies regarding utilization may be instituted (Wenneberg et al., 1984). *Principle: The physician's strategies do not go completely unnoticed. Those that are inappropriate and costly may well be changed by those who do not understand medicine or assume responsibility for the consequence of their policy.*

The decision to initiate antimicrobial therapy for a patient must be made in the context of treating a known or highly likely specific infectious disease. Therapies should not be undertaken without serious and often aggressive attempts to document the etiologic agent by appropriate examination of the patient and possibly smears, cultures, skin testing, and/or histologic procedures. The choice of the antimicrobial should be based on the likelihood of efficacy to cure rather than a demonstration of in vitro testing that documents microbial inhibition of growth or killing. Clinical "cure" is a function of the pharmacology of the drug and its ability to reach the tissue site in concentrations adequate to kill the microorganism. Furthermore, the physician must be familiar with host factors that may significantly modify the pharmacologic properties of drugs or alter their ability to effect a cure at a given site. The potential for a given drug to produce toxicity or to promote superinfection by selecting out resistant flora must always be assessed when other drugs could be administered or when the infectious process is not serious enough to justify therapy. Finally, when efficacy and toxicity of different compounds are equivalent, cost should dictate drug selection.

Once treatment has begun, consideration must be given to correct abnormal anatomy or aberrant host defense mechanisms that might promote infection or hinder cure. The interplay between the natural history of an infectious process and the ability of host defenses to eradicate the microorganism versus the ability of host defenses to produce cellular injury at a given tissue site and the propensity for relapse or superinfection is crucial for deciding what measures for monitoring efficacy are necessary and what the duration of treatment should be.

EPIDEMIOLOGIC AND VIRULENCE FACTORS IN INFECTIOUS DISEASES

Epidemiologic Considerations

Before appropriate therapy can be given for an infectious disease, consideration of epidemiologic factors is essential. This section does not fully discuss the epidemiology of infectious diseases (a subject that deals with the determinants, occurrence, distribution, and control of health and disease). However, there are a number of basic principles and historical points that are worth emphasizing. *Principle: Evaluation of epidemiologic considerations, including the patient's contact with or the physician's isolation of an organism, is pivotal in deciding which types of infection merit therapeutic intervention.*

Basic Principles of Transmission. Infectious disease results from the interaction between an infectious agent and a susceptible host. The agent may be transported from an external source to the host (exogenous infection); or because of changes in the agent–host relationship, a normally occurring, usually innocuous, microbial agent on mucosal surfaces can produce disease (endogenous infection). The relationships between the agent, transmission, and host represent the chain of infection. In general, the greatest risk for developing infections in the immunocompetent individual is related to acquisition of pathogenic exogenous flora (e.g., *Shigella*); among immunocompromised patients (e.g., leukemic patients undergoing chemotherapy), indigenous flora (e.g., staphylococci) are more likely the cause of disease. *Principle: In infectious diseases, understanding how the disease was initiated greatly influences the scope of therapeutic considerations for patients and their friends, family, and co-workers.*

Acquisition. Humans usually acquire their first exposure to microorganisms at birth during passage through the vagina. Thereafter, acquisition, carriage, and clearance of microorganisms are basic facts of life. There are four main routes of acquisition of microorganisms: (1) contact, (2) inhalation, (3) common-vehicle, and (4) vector-borne. Table 24–1 outlines the source, route of acquisition, and portal of entry of microorganisms causing certain specific diseases. The route for contact involves direct transfer of the agent to the susceptible host from person to person or via fomite or droplet. For transmission by inhalation, the agent is truly airborne in small particles (≤ 5 μm diameter). In contrast, contact droplet spread occurs when large droplets (≥ 5 μm diameter) are physically transmitted directly onto surfaces of the respiratory tract. Streptococcal and measles infections are examples of droplet-spread disease. They usually occur when multiple persons are exposed to a single index patient who comes in close contact with susceptible hosts. In contrast, transmission by inhalation occurs when susceptible hosts are exposed to aerosols containing microbes. Direct-proximity contact is not necessary. Tuberculosis is an example of spread by

inhalation from human to human; psittacosis and Q fever represent transmission from animal to human by inhalation transmission. A common inanimate vehicle usually serves to transmit an agent to multiple hosts. The most frequently involved common vehicles are food and water that can transmit a number of different pathogens (e.g., enteric bacillary pathogens and hepatitis A). Contaminated needles are an important common vehicle for transmitting HIV agent and hepatitis B virus among IV drug users. These three common vehicles provide effective and complete "mechanical transmission" of viable agents directly to a susceptible host.

For some agents, maturation and multiplication through intermediate host(s) (e.g., arthropod vectors) are necessary preliminaries for transmission to humans. Vector-borne diseases (e.g., malaria) are termed *biologically transmitted* diseases. Their routes of acquisition, sources of contact, and sites of entry constitute important factors around which rational therapy of infectious diseases has developed.

Patient Information. Information relative to epidemiologic considerations must be collected from patients suspected of having infection. In *community-acquired* infections, critical points of information include age, gender, place of residence, family and other personal contacts (including the history of these contacts with disease), occupation, hobbies, contacts with animals, travel history, exposure to parenteral drugs or blood products, sexual habits, dietary habits, other active medical problems, and medications. Obviously, the thoroughness with which this information should be collected needs to be tailored to the particular situation. However, routine careful scrutiny to seemingly insignificant issues might suggest appropriate diagnostic considerations that would otherwise have been missed.

In *hospital-acquired* infections, important points of epidemiologic information that should

Table 24–1. TRANSMISSION OF SPECIFIC DISEASES

INFECTIOUS VECTOR	ROUTE OF ACQUISITION	PORTAL OF ENTRY	SPECIFIC DISEASE
Lesion exudate	Contact (sexual intercourse)	Genital mucosa	Gonorrhea, syphilis
Contaminated water	Contact (fomite – razor blade)	Broken skin	Carbuncles, *Pseudomonas* cellulitis
Respiratory secretions	Contact (droplets)	Respiratory tract	Streptococci, measles, "common cold"
Respiratory aerosols	Inhalation	Respiratory tract	Tuberculosis, psittacosis, Q fever
Contaminated food	Common vehicle (ingestion)	GI	*Shigella, Salmonella,* hepatitis A
Blood	Common vehicle (IV "street-drug" needle)	Bloodstream	AIDS, hepatitis B
Blood	Vector-borne (arthropod)	Broken skin	Malaria, yellow fever, epidemic typhus

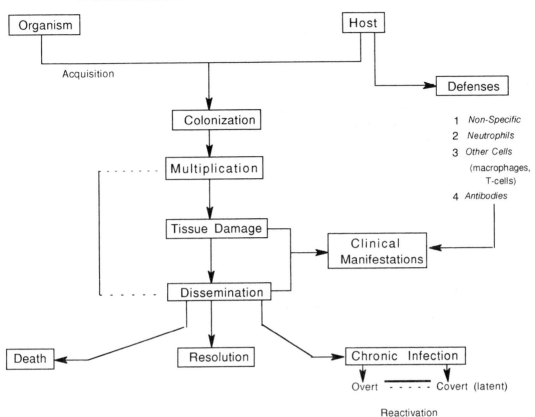

Fig. 24-1. The interplay between the microorganism and host factors. These processes may be interrupted at any stage in the prevention or therapy of infectious disease.

be sought include the types of infectious complications that are associated with different procedures or conditions in general, and that occur specifically in the particular institution; possible previous exposure of patients to antimicrobials; the concomitant use of other medications that might alter host defense or the manifestations of disease (e.g., corticosteroids); the history of transfusion or parenteral use of medication; the incidence and type of infections in other patients or personnel who have been in contact with the patient; and the nature of the hospital's flora and their susceptibility to antimicrobials. The decisions involved in empirical selection of antimicrobials to treat hospital-acquired infections are much more complex. They must be based on a credible data base that is continually being reviewed for new trends in infectious diseases in a particular hospital. In general, this task is assigned to an infection surveillance and control committee in the hospital (Joint Commission on Accreditation of Hospitals, 1987). Despite the importance of such local groups in establishing standards for prevention and in providing rational

guidelines for treatment of nosocomial infections (Haley, 1978), most practitioners are unaware of their recommendations.

Infectivity

The sequence of acquisition followed by colonization and multiplication (Fig. 24–1) is termed the *infectivity* of the organism. Individuals harbor a varied population of microorganisms that have different potentials to produce disease. The endogenous flora of people periodically includes a number of organisms that are commonly described as *virulent* and called *pathogens*. The names are apt because the organisms have been clearly identified as major causative agents of disease. For example, strains of *Neisseria meningitidis* are a leading cause of bacterial meningitis in infants, children, and adults but are often found in the nasopharynx of healthy individuals of all ages (e.g., 25%–40% of normal young adults). Carriers can be properly thought of as being "infected" with a potentially virulent organism; yet, because of host and other immunologic factors, a harmless carrier state exists (Griffiss and Brandt, 1986). In fact, this carrier state is probably crucial for eliciting protective immunity in individuals and the population. Other "pathogens" that can be carried for long periods of time without their hosts developing disease include pneumococci, group A streptococci, *Staphylococcus aureus*, salmonellae, and many viruses including herpes group agents. When host defenses are altered, infections may develop not only with these recognized pathogens but with other organisms usually considered harmless. In the absence of selected host defense factors, some pathogens are so virulent that when acquired they virtually always produce disease. For example, in a classic epidemiologic study of persons who lacked protective antibody and were colonized with rubeola virus in the upper respiratory tract, the attack rate of measles exceeded 90% (Christiansen, 1952–1953). *Principle: Knowledge of the infectivity and virulence of microorganisms is important in determining the likelihood of infection. Mere documentation of the presence of a potential pathogen is not alone sufficient reason to institute treatment unless disease is present or the threat of disease is great. The concept is no different from that of simple abnormalities (e.g., elevated uric acid concentrations) not being sufficient reason to treat the disease that may or may not accompany them.*

Virulence Factors

Microbial factors that regulate pathogenicity or virulence include the size of the infective dose, the duration of exposure of the host to the microbe, competition from surrounding flora, and the ability to elaborate compounds that cause tissue injury. For example, the pathogenesis of ascending, nonobstructive *Escherichia coli* pyelonephritis in women with anatomically normal urinary tracts exemplifies a number of important characteristics and will be discussed in some detail as an example. This infection may be viewed as a culmination of a sequence of events mediated by specific determinants of microbial virulence (Table 24–2). In brief, pyelonephritogenic *E. coli* strains usually originate in the colon (Turck and Petersdorf, 1962). From the stool, they are translocated to the vaginal introitus and/or the periurethral region.

Bacterial colonization of these areas may ensue, eventually leading to uroepithelial colonization of the periurethral and bladder mucosa (Fowler and Stamey, 1977). Due to normal vesicoureteric reflux, bacteria ascend the urinary tract and colonize the renal pelvic epithelia. Once they are able to colonize and proliferate in sufficient numbers, other determinants of bacterial virulence produce or cause tissue injury, cellular inflammation, and dissemination.

Pyelonephritogenic *E. coli* appear to constitute a pathogenic phenotype. They usually belong to a restricted number of O and K antigen serogroups (Vosti et al., 1964; Evans et al., 1981; Svanborg-Eden and deMan, 1987; Plos et al., 1990); they are resistant to the bactericidal action of normal human serum (Olling, 1972; Olling et al., 1973); they secrete hemolysin (Minshew et al., 1978; Cavalieri et al., 1984; O'Hanley et al., 1985a) and produce colicin V (O'Hanley et al., 1985a; Harber et al., 1986); and they attach to uroepithelial cells by specific adhesins (Vaisanen-Rhen et al., 1984; Svanborg-Eden and deMan, 1987; Archambaud et al., 1988). These virulence factors occur together in pyelonephritogenic *E. coli* more frequently than in normal enteric strains. These data suggest that strains of pyelonephritogenic *E. coli* are derived from a limited number of clones or that virulent transposon elements were transferred to susceptible strains (Orskov and Orskov, 1983; Arthur et al., 1989).

Uropathogenic *E. coli* colonize epithelial surfaces by elaborating proteinaceous appendages termed *pili* that bind host receptor carbohydrates (Beachey, 1981; Schoolnik et al., 1985). The binding appears to be the crucial first step in the pathogenesis of ascending *E. coli* urinary tract infection. Therapeutic strategies that block this binding step protect the host from disease. Subinhibitory concentrations of antibiotics, particularly those that act on the bacterial ribosome, appear to interfere with normal synthesis or expression of the adhesin proteins (Eisenstein, 1979; Kristiansen, 1983). This phenomenon could be therapeutically relevant since antibiotics on mucosal surfaces at sublethal concentrations might reduce the colonizing capacity of pathogenic bacteria. Also, antimicrobial usage might enable pathogenic strains to readily colonize mucosal

Table 24–2.   UROPATHOGENESIS OF *Escherichia coli* PYELONEPHRITIS

PATHOGENIC STEP	MICROBIAL DETERMINANT	HOST DEFENSES
Colonization	Pap pili	Bile, urine flow, antibody
Proliferation	Colicin V	Acute-phase reactants
Invasion or cellular injury	?Invasion proteins, hemolysin, lipopolysaccharide	Phagocytes, antibody–complement lysis, antibody neutralization
Dissemination	K antigens, serum resistance	Phagocytes, antibody, complement lysis

surfaces by interfering with the colonization ability of normal flora (Freter, 1981). These possible effects of antibiotic usage illustrate their potential beneficial and deleterious effects. Also, pili vaccines have been developed and tested for efficacy (Roberts et al., 1984; Pecha et al., 1989). Specific anti-pili IgG antibody in the urine is correlated with protection against infection by preventing subsequent *E. coli* colonization of the kidney. The antibody-coated bacteria may be more readily cleared from the urinary tract as aggregates.

Once uropathogenic *E. coli* strains are able to colonize the renal epithelium, a number of determinants of virulence are required to eventually produce disease. The colicin V product is important for the organism to sequestrate iron effectively; iron is crucial for cellular growth of this bacterial species and that of most other pathogenic bacteria. After sufficient bacterial proliferation on the mucosa, a number of other functions are required to injure host cells or allow bacteria to invade the parenchyma. Hemolysin released from the *E. coli* injures renal epithelial cells by producing pores in their plasma membranes (Bhakdi et al., 1986; Bhakdi and Tranum-Jensen, 1988; Benz et al., 1989). Adhesin and hemolysin are responsible for stimulating leukocytes to release inflammatory mediators (e.g., leukotriene and histamine) (Konig et al., 1989; Ventur et al., 1990). The inflammatory process appears important as an endogenous mechanism to eradicate intrarenal bacteria; however, the cellular products from the leukocytes associated with the inflammatory response are also responsible for a significant amount of the parenchymal injury. Possibly, the microorganism can directly penetrate cells by means of invasin, which is a protein on the outer membrane of some enteric bacteria (Isberg et al., 1987).

Once the bacterial organism dies, its lipopolysaccharides are released and produce a dramatically intense polymorphonuclear leukocyte response. This inflammatory response might be contributory to the tissue injury observed in renal infection and is attributed to release of lysosomal enzymes from leukocytes. Finally, once the organism has invaded the renal parenchyma, uropathogenic *E. coli* strains are likely to disseminate. Factors that facilitate this process include K antigens that constitute the acid polysaccharide component of the capsule and serum resistance. The K antigen interferes with polymorphonuclear leukocyte phagocytosis of the bacteria, whereas serum resistance is associated with the bacteria's ability to evade the normal killing effects of serum.

In summary, the pathogenic process of microbial disease is orderly and requires sequential steps for disease. Virulence factors enable the microbial pathogen to establish, proliferate, damage, and disseminate in niches of the host. These determinants of bacterial virulence probably are under the control of a regulatory system that enables the microorganism to adapt to local host environments (Miller et al., 1989; Relman and Falkow, 1990). Relatively little is known about either the specific environmental signals (e.g., temperature, pH, calcium, iron, amino acids) to which these systems respond or the rationale for these responses. The regulatory system usually involves a pair of proteins: one protein acts as a sensor of environmental stimuli and transmits a signal to the other protein, usually by means of phosphorylation; the second protein, once stimulated, acts to regulate gene expression.

There might be many regulatory systems in the genetic element(s) of the microorganism that are operable and that respond independently to a variety of environmental stimuli. However, coordinated control of a group of operons is under the domain of a regulon. A regulon provides a means by which many genes can respond in a coordinated fashion to a particular environmental stimulus. The regulon exerts its regulatory functions by *trans*-acting regulatory loci that exert positive or negative expression on a number of virulence factors (e.g., *vir* in *Bordetella pertussis* (Weiss and Falkow, 1984) and *virR* in *Shigella* (Maurelli and Sansonetti, 1988). These determinants mediate their regulatory function at the level of transcription. Another mechanism by which bacteria can regulate expression of virulence and thereby invade host defenses is DNA rearrangements. A well-studied example of this is the expression of flagellin genes in *Salmonella typhimurium* (Simon et al., 1980). By this mechanism, *S. typhimurium* expresses either H1 or H2 flagellins, thereby evading possible host antibody responses. *Principle: Understanding of the molecular pathogenesis of bacterial virulence offers the possibility of new therapeutic strategies that could not have been deliberately considered without such information.*

HOST FACTORS

The ability of a microorganism to produce disease in the host is a function of the interplay between the virulence of the microorganism and host factors. Host factors that interfere with a microorganism's ability to colonize, proliferate, invade, or injure include nonspecific and specific defense mechanisms (Table 24–3). Nonspecific responses represent primitive protective mechanisms that are not specifically directed to the microorganism and do not involve immunologic memory. In contrast, specific host defense mechanisms involve lymphocytes that kill micro-

Table 24–3.   HOST FACTORS ASSOCIATED WITH DEFENSE AGAINST MICROORGANISMS*

Nonspecific	Normal flora
	Tissue tropism
	Epithelial barriers (substances and cells)
	Excretory secretions and flows
	Natural antibodies
	Cytokines and other acute-phase reactants
	Phagocytosis by leukocytes
	Alternative complement system
	Hormones
Specific	Antibodies
	Classic complement system
	T cells

* From Tramont, 1990.

organisms specifically or that elicit antibody production. Specific antibodies bind to selected microbial antigens and, in coordination with the classic complement system, eventually kill microorganisms. These specific host defense mechanisms involve immunologic memory and have extensively been described as important for host immunity to subsequent exposure or infection by microorganisms. Defects in any of the host's armamentarium for defense provide a risk of the host's susceptibility to infection. It must also be stressed that although a majority of infections are associated with microbial evasion of host factors, the elicited host responses (e.g., cytokines) to microorganisms can account for considerable host injury. *Principle: In considering the pathogenesis of infection, it is crucial to assess the defects in host defenses that contributed to disease. The goal of treatment is to correct these abnormalities so that a successful clinical outcome will occur and disease will not worsen or reoccur after therapeutic intervention. Conversely, when host defense mechanisms contribute to injury during infection, modulation of host factors may be required for successful outcomes.*

Some important host factors that are not generally considered in discussions of immunity include normal flora, tropism, and cytokines. Microorganisms that usually produce disease must come in contact with or penetrate the skin or mucosal surfaces. The integrity of skin and mucous membrane barriers constitutes a major line of defense against microorganisms. The majority of infections among leukemic patients undergoing chemotherapy occur only when these surfaces are broken, thereby allowing indigenous flora to invade deeper structures and cause disease. Under normal conditions, the flora that usually colonize epithelial surfaces (e.g., skin and GI tract) also protect the host from microbial invasion by exogenous pathogens. The nonspecific mechanisms of

this protection include competition for the same nutrients, competition for host receptors for colonization, and production of bacteriocins that are toxic to other microbes. The result of these mechanisms is to limit the ability of a "foreign microbe" to colonize and proliferate on these surfaces.

Normal flora are influenced by a number of factors including diet, hormones, sanitary conditions, hygienic habits, and exposure to toxins and antibiotics. Indiscriminate use of antimicrobials is a common problem; the resulting changes in indigenous flora may produce deleterious effects in the host. Antibiotic concentrations at these epithelial surfaces can be sufficient to kill microorganisms directly or to affect their physiology. The overall effects of antibiotics on normal flora are to decrease their number or their ability to persist on these surfaces. These changes enable potential pathogens to colonize the epithelial surfaces.

Normal flora also are crucial for continuous "priming" of the immune system. The continuous influx of products from normal flora across epithelial surfaces represents a constant priming signal for macrophages to process these substances. In germ-free animals and newborns, there is an overall lack of antigen processing by the host, as exemplified by the low levels of class II histocompatibility (DR) molecule expression on macrophages (Steinman et al., 1980; Stiehm et al., 1984; Tramont, 1990). However, once indigenous flora are established on epithelial mucosal surfaces, there are marked increases in expression of DR in macrophages. Therefore, the constant exposure of host macrophages and T cells to antigens from indigenous flora enables the host to be primed for immune responses. The maintenance of the normal flora is crucial for health. *Principle: The indiscriminate use of antibiotics can have deleterious effects on the host by eliminating or adversely affecting the physiology of the normal flora.*

The ability of microorganisms to colonize specific epithelial surfaces is linked to the presence of microbial adhesins and host receptors that permit attachment. Most microorganisms whether indigenous or pathogens preferentially colonize certain tissues; this phenomenon is referred to as *tissue tropism*. Host receptors for attachment of microorganisms vary depending on the tissue (e.g., esophagus vs. colon), cellular mixture (e.g., epithelial cells vs. stromal constituents), and conditions of health (e.g., during menstruation) or disease (e.g., following viral and bacterial infections).

Table 24–4 lists selected *E. coli* adhesins and host receptor moieties. These receptor compounds usually are located on epithelial surfaces and enable the microorganism to colonize organ tissue sites. For example, type 1 pili of uropatho-

Table 24-4. SELECTED *E. coli* ADHESINS AND HOST RECEPTORS

E. COLI ADHESIN	HOST COMPOUND OR RECEPTOR
Type 1 pili	D-mannose (Tamm-Horsfall uromucoid)
Pap pili	α-D-Gal$p$-(1→4)-β-D-Gal$p$
K88 pili	GM_1 ganglioside
K99 pili	β-D-Gal$p$-(1→4)-β-D-Glc$p$-(1-1)-ceramide
CFA pili	GM_2 ganglioside
S pili	Sialic acid (glycophorin)
MN pili	*N*-acetylneuraminic acid

genic *E. coli* strains can bind to uroepithelia because D-mannose is bound to these cells (O'Hanley et al., 1985a). However, the host possesses a natural defense factor to prevent epithelial mucosal binding by this adhesin under normal conditions. Renal tubular cells secrete the Tamm-Horsfall uromucoid, a highly mannosylated glycoprotein (Orskov et al., 1980). This uromucoid interferes with attachment of bacteria with this mannose adherence specificity to the uroepithelium because the uromucoid binds bacterial adhesins when the microorganism is in the urinary stream. The binding of the bacterial adhesin by D-mannose moieties in the uromucoid represents an important normal host factor that prevents bacteriuria. There are a number of other host excretory and secretory substances (e.g., saliva, tears, fibronectin, mucus) that hinder colonization of mucosal surfaces by microbes. Also, in conjunction with normal processes (e.g., GI peristalsis, the ciliary movement of the respiratory epithelia, cough, and micturition), microorganisms are readily cleared from the host.

The use of soluble receptor analogs to prevent microorganism attachment to target host cells is a new therapeutic strategy. For example, administration of soluble CD4 molecule prevents HIV attachment to T-helper cells in vitro, thus abrogating viral invasion of these cells. The usefulness of this strategy in clinical conditions requires complete inhibition of virus attachment to host cells and effective clearance of the microorganism from the host. This exciting new direction in disease prevention has been possible only by elucidating the basis of the attachment of microorganisms to the host at a molecular level (viz., tropism). *Principle: The ability of microorganisms to attach to cells is crucial to the pathogenesis of microbial disease. Interference at this step has therapeutic potential.*

Considerable progress within the last decade has elucidated the chemical basis of regulation of host immunity. It appears that cytokines are responsible for many of the host's responses to microorganisms, accounting for acute inflamma-

tion and long-term immunity. Table 24-5 summarizes the major biologic effects of cytokines.

These proteins are produced locally by a variety of stromal cells. They are secreted in small quantities and have short (viz., seconds to minutes) systemic half-lives. They act in a complicated network producing a cascade of events (Tracey et al., 1987; O'Garra et al., 1990). Several inflammatory cytokines (e.g., IL-1, IL-6, and TNF-α) appear to contribute to physiologic events that can result in death. Numerous studies have demonstrated the correlation between elevated concentrations of inflammatory cytokines with death due to bacterial septicemia (Girardin et al., 1988; Waage et al., 1989a, 1989b). Perhaps modulation of acute inflammatory cytokines by use of anticytokine antibodies and analogs that inhibit their synthesis or secretion will become part of the management of life-threatening infections that produce shock. Investigations in relevant animal models of human sepsis have demonstrated the efficacy of anti-TNF-α antibody and anti-TNF synthesis analog (viz., pentoxyfylline) against fatal gram-negative bacterial sepsis (Tracey et al., 1987; Harada et al., 1989). Further work is required to elucidate the kinetics of inflammatory cytokine responses and approaches to modulate their physiologic response. Clearly, different types of immune deficiency states are associated by common infectious syndromes (Table 24-6).

DOCUMENTATION OF INFECTION

Review of the patient's history and symptoms provides essential clues concerning the possibilities for acquisition of infectious agents and the development of an infectious disease. Documentation of the cause of infection is usually derived from objective tests and examinations. The information provided may be of a specific or nonspecific nature.

Nonspecific Methods

Few reliable nonspecific methods exist for documentation of infection. Symptoms and physical signs are frequently supportive of a diagnosis but rarely are pathognomonic. For example, the activation of the acute inflammatory response is the most common way in which the clinical manifestations of infection become apparent. However, noninfectious conditions may also activate the same inflammatory mechanisms; therefore, the symptoms and signs of inflammation are by no means specific for infection.

Granulocytosis and the appearance of immature neutrophilic forms in the circulation with toxic granulation are typical of moderate to severe acute bacterial infections. This type of inflammatory response is related to the organism

Table 24–5. SOURCE AND BIOLOGIC PROPERTIES OF CYTOKINES*

CYTOKINE	NATURAL SOURCE	MAJOR BIOLOGICAL EFFECTS (IN VITRO AND IN VIVO)
Interleukin-1 (IL-1)	Macrophages Fibroblasts Keratinocytes Other endothelial, epithelial, and hemopoietic cells	Induces fever, shock, synthesis of acute-phase proteins, bone resorption, prostaglandin E (PGE) release, nonspecific bacterial resistance in animal models, and endothelial cell activation Stimulates cytokine production from macrophages and T cells, proliferation of thymocytes, hemopoietic cell growth and differentiation, and granulocyte and natural killer (NK) cell activity. Costimulates proliferation of B and T cells, antibody secretion
Interleukin-2 (IL-2)	T cells	Activates NK cells, cytotoxic T cells, macrophages, and endothelial cells Stimulates proliferation of T cells and thymocytes, cytokine production from T cells, cytotoxicity, proliferation of NK cells, and differentiation of T cells to lymphokine-activated killer (LAK) cells Costimulates proliferation of B cells, antibody secretion, and antitumor activity Has antitumor activity
Interleukin-3 (IL-3)	T cells	Supports survival, growth, and differentiation of stem cells and hemopoietic progenitor cells Supports proliferation of mast cell lines and growth of pre-B cells lines
Interleukin-4 (IL-4)	T cells Mast cells	Induces IgG1 and IgE secretion in LPS-activated B cells Activates resting B cells and macrophages Stimulates proliferation of mast cells and activated T cells, cytotoxic T-cell activity Costimulates proliferation of thymocytes and activated B cells Suppresses TNF-α, IL-1, IL-6, and PGE$_2$ in monocytes Inhibits or enhances other cytokine activities in hemopoietic progenitors Has antitumor activity
Interleukin-5 (IL-5)	T cells	Induces IgA production from LPS-activated B cells, IgM secretion from activated B cells, proliferation and differentiation of eosinophils from bone marrow precursors, and differentiation of cytotoxic T cells (with IL-2)
Interleukin-6 (IL-6)	Monocytes T cells Fibroblasts Myelomas Epithelial-type cells	Induces synthesis of acute-phase proteins, antibody secretion, and differentiation of cytotoxic T cells Stimulates proliferation and differentiation of hemopoietic precursors, proliferation of megakaryocytes, and plasmacytoma growth Costimulates T-cell and thymocyte proliferation
Interleukin-7 (IL-7)	Stromal cells Thymus	Stimulates proliferation and differentiation of pre-B cells, and proliferation of thymocytes
? Neutrophil-activating protein (IL-8)	Blood monocyte (mouse)	Is chemotactic for neutrophils and T cells
? P40 (IL-9)	T cells (mouse)	Induces antigen-independent growth of helper T cells
? Cytokine synthesis inhibitory factor (IL-10)	T cells (mouse)	Inhibits production of IL-2, IL-3, TNF, IFN, and GM-CSF

(continued)

Table 24–5. *(CONTINUED)*

CYTOKINE	NATURAL SOURCE	MAJOR BIOLOGICAL EFFECTS (IN VITRO AND IN VIVO)
Interferon (IFN-α)	T cells NK cells	Activates macrophages, NK cells, cytotoxic T cells, and endothelial cells Stimulates LAK activity, secretion of IgG2 from activated B cells Costimulates human B-cell proliferation Inhibits T-cell proliferation, IL-4-induced IgE secretion, and FC receptor (CD23) in LPS-stimulated B cells, and viral replication and cell growth Has antitumor activity
Tumor necrosis factor (TNF-α)	T cells Macrophages	Induces fever, shock, and synthesis of acute-phase proteins Activates macrophages and endothelial cells Stimulates granulocyte-eosinophil activity, chemotaxis, B- and T-cell proliferation, angiogenesis, and bone resorption Inhibits viral replication Has antitumor activity; is cytotoxic to many cells
Lymphotoxin (TNF-β)	T cells	Activates endothelial cells Stimulates granulocyte activity, B-cell proliferation, and bone resorption Inhibits angiogenesis and viral replication Has antitumor activity; is cytotoxic to many cells
Granulocyte-colony-stimulating factor (G-CSF)	T cells	Stimulates hemopoiesis and granulocyte differentiation and activity
Macrophage CSF (M-SCF)	T cells Macrophages	Stimulates macrophage growth and activity
Granulocyte-Macrophage CSF (GM-CSF)	T cells Endothelial cells	Stimulates hemopoiesis, macrophage, and granulocyte-eosinophil growth and activity, T-cell proliferation, and chemotaxis

Reproduced by permission of Hope Rugo.

that is causing infection, the marrow reserves of the host, and other features of the host. In contrast, neutropenia may be a feature of any patient with overwhelming gram-negative bacterial sepsis or of patients, particularly alcoholics, with severe bacterial pneumonia caused by gram-positive organisms. Neutrophilic leukocytosis or leukopenia may be seen during the active phases of vasculitis, systemic lupus erythematosus, or acute drug reac-

tions, all of which can mimic the host response to infections.

Measures that attempt to enhance the specificity of an examination of granulocyte responses for bacterial infection by incubating blood with nitroblue tetrazolium dye (NBT test) and counting the percentage of cells with reduced dye are not reliable (Steigbeigel et al., 1974). At present, the major value of the NBT test is in the screening

Table 24–6. COMMON INFECTIOUS SYNDROMES ASSOCIATED WITH IMMUNE DEFICIENCY

DEFECT	SYNDROME
Local: Loss of mucosal membrane integrity	Bacterial septicemia in leukemic patients with GI ulceration, staphylococcal catheter infections
Phagocytic cells: Decreased number or function (e.g., chronic granulomatous disease)	Infections due to bacteria and opportunistic fungi, especially catalase-positive bacteria and *Nocardia, Candida, Aspergillus*
Complement	Neisserial septicemia, infection due to encapsulated bacteria
B lymphocytes	Infections due to encapsulated bacteria, *Pneumocystis carinii,* recurrent viral infections
T lymphocytes	Disseminated infection to intracellular microorganisms, protracted diarrheal syndromes, mucocutaneous candidiasis

of selected subjects for chronic granulomatous disease of childhood or one of its variants (Ochs and Igo, 1973). Similar comments can be applied to the appearance of immature lymphocytes in the circulation during fever. Initially thought to be specific for infectious mononucleosis, this finding is now known to appear with regularity in patients with other disorders including cytomegalovirus infection, adenovirus infection, and occasionally toxoplasmosis (Ho, 1982; Horwitz, 1987; McCabe et al., 1987). Such lymphocytes also may be difficult to differentiate from the immature forms of cells seen in patients with acute lymphocytic leukemia. Certainly, a single nonspecific laboratory test (e.g., examination of peripheral blood cells) that is simply a marker of the activation of the acute inflammatory response is a poor way to demonstrate the presence or absence of infection.

Certain laboratory tests add information by helping to define abnormalities in the organ systems of the infected host. Since many microorganisms have tissue tropism, these nonspecific methods of organ function may narrow the search for the site of infection. An abnormality in biochemical tests usually related to liver function (e.g., elevated concentrations of transaminases) and a tender liver on physical examination strongly suggest hepatitis but obviously do not differentiate among the many causes of inflammation of the liver. The limitations of nonspecific diagnostic methods as they apply to infectious diseases are outlined in Table 24-7 (Evans, 1976). When the spectrum of noninfectious disorders that can mimic infections is included in these considerations, the possibilities for misdiagnosis and misapplied therapy become legion. Therefore, more specific methods are required to document infection so that rational therapy can ensue. *Principle: Antimicrobial therapy for infectious diseases should not be chosen on the basis of nonspecific methods of diagnosis and "probabilities" alone. Such treatment may cause more harm than good. A reasonable attempt at specific diagnostic methods is mandatory before instituting therapy. A "diagnostic trial" of treatment is the least reliable way of revealing the specific nature of infections*

Table 24-7.   EVANS'S FIVE REALITIES

1. The same syndrome is caused by a variety of agents.
2. The same agent produces a variety of syndromes.
3. The predominant agent for a syndrome may vary with year, population, geography, and age.
4. The identification of the agent is frequently impossible by clinical findings alone.
5. The cause of a large portion of infectious disease syndromes is still unknown.

and is often synonymous with therapeutic misadventure.

Specific Methods

The sampling of host tissues and body fluids for biochemical, histologic, and microbiologic testing remains the cornerstone of accurate documentation and diagnosis of a specific infection. Performance of such studies provides a data base to direct rational therapy and is mandatory in the seriously ill patient. The lack of adequate sampling of appropriate sites and the failure to adequately transport specimens to the laboratory are the most frequent and unrecognized reasons for failure to document the etiologic agents of an infectious disease. For example, an improperly collected urine sample (not placed in a sterile container and delayed in delivery to the laboratory) often will be contaminated by large numbers of bacteria bearing little relationship to the presence or number of the true urinary tract pathogen (Kunin, 1974).

The host site to be sampled for the microbiologic identification of infecting agents is critical (Table 24-8). Since many epithelial surfaces have their own commensal flora, enumeration of organisms per sample volume and weight may be important in differentiating the commensals from pathogens. For example, the presence of 10^5 and 10^3 colony-forming units (CFU) per milliliter of clean catch midstream-voided urine is widely recognized as representing significant bacteriuria in women and men, respectively. However, fewer bacteria can be in urine that still is infected. Studies have conclusively demonstrated that acute dysuria in women with cystitis can be caused by as few as 10^2 CFU of enteric gram-negative rods per milliliter of urine (Stamm et al., 1982). Therefore, it is always important for the clinician to correlate the microbiologic data with the patient's symptoms and physical signs. If dissemination has taken place, samples taken from distant sites may be helpful. Thus, pneumococcal pneumonia may be documented by sampling respiratory secretions, but the strength of the diagnosis is increased by the finding of pneumococci in blood cultures (Barrett-Connor, 1971).

The usual sites recommended for sampling for bacteriologic, mycologic, and virologic organisms in given clinical situations are presented in Tables 24-8 and 24-9. Blood cultures are frequently submitted when any evidence of dissemination is suggested by systemic signs and symptoms. Any collections of fluid associated with the signs of infection should be sampled for similar microbiologic determinations. Tissue biopsy may be indicated for certain types of infections. This is

Table 24–8. SUGGESTED SPECIMENS TO BE SUBMITTED FOR BACTERIOLOGIC AND MYCOLOGIC DIAGNOSIS

SITE OF INFECTION OR SUBJECT	SPECIMEN SOURCE FOR CULTURE						SPECIAL OR TISSUE BIOPSY
	BLOOD	URINE	STOOL	THROAT	SPUTUM	CSF	
Upper respiratory	+			+			
Lower respiratory	+	+			+		Pleural fluid or biopsy, lung biopsy
Enteric illness	+	+	+				GI or rectal biopsy, liver biopsy
CNS disease	+					+	Brain biopsy
Genitourinary	+	+					
Sexually transmitted	+	+	+	+			
Exanthem	+					+	Vesicular fluid
Arthritis	+						Synovial fluid or biopsy
Immunocompromised	+	+	+	+	+	+	
Newborn or FUO	+	+	+	+	+	+	
Hepatitis	+						Liver biopsy

FUO = Fever of unknown origin.

653

Table 24-9. SUGGESTED SPECIMENS TO BE SUBMITTED FOR VIRAL DIAGNOSIS

DIAGNOSTIC CONSIDERATION	SOURCE FOR CULTURE*						SEROLOGIC STUDY
	NASAL OR THROAT	STOOL OR RECTAL	URINE	CSF	SKIN	SPECIAL	
Respiratory	+++		+†			Lung, bronchial, pleural	+
Enteric							
Gastroenteritis		+++‡					+
Hepatitis			+				+
Central Nervous System							
Aseptic meningitis	++	++	+§		++	Blood+¶,	+
Encephalitis	++	++		++		Brain+++	+
Exanthemas							
Maculopapular	++	+	+				++
Vesciluar					++		++
Myocarditis or pericarditis	++	++				Pericardial fluid, tissue	+
Orchitis or parotitis or pancreatitis	++	+	++				+
Newborn with probable intrauterine infection	++	++	++	++			
Genitourinary							
Genital	+	+	++		++	Cervicovaginal tissue	+
Acute hematuria							+

* +++ = indicated, valuable; ++ = usually valuable; + = sometimes valuable; no indication implies not a valuable test.
† If cytomegalovirus is suspected.
‡ If electron microscopy or indirect (e.g., ELISA) techniques are available.
§ If mumps virus is suspected.
¶ If toga or bunya viral meningitis is suspected.

particularly important in identifying the pathogens in infected immunocompromised patients (e.g., patients with AIDS or neoplastic disease) since the number of possible pathogens in these patients is much greater than in other, noncompromised patients. The necessity for these biopsies is also influenced by weighing the seriousness of the disease against the risk of the biopsy procedure per se. With a biopsy, histologic examination with special staining techniques augments the classic microbiologic laboratory testing.

Proper transport of specimens to the laboratory requires prompt delivery under appropriate conditions to protect and allow survival of the organisms for laboratory growth or identification. Although many organisms require only the minimum moisture and nutrients of "routine" carrying media, fastidious organisms may require complicated special media for transfer. Anaerobic microorganisms may be sufficiently fragile to require oxygen-free transport systems to ensure their survival. Viral agents may require special solutions containing antibiotics to suppress bacterial growth, and ultralow temperatures for transfer and storage before inoculation into susceptible cell systems for identification. The clinician must be aware of the requirements for collecting and transporting clinical specimens correctly so that the best chances of a definitive diagnosis of infection can be developed. Discussion with laboratory personnel provides the most efficient method for ensuring that the most appropriate steps are taken.

Histologic examinations of stained smears remain the most rapid, inexpensive, and useful method of preliminary recognition of classes of infectious agents. The classic Gram stain allows differentiation of microorganisms into certain groups by size, form, and staining characteristics. This rough classification combined with other nonspecific data may provide sufficient information to allow appropriate therapy before a definitive diagnosis (culture) is confirmed. Other commonly used, inexpensive, and simple rapid-staining techniques include acid-fast staining for mycobacteria, methylene blue stains and KOH preparations for fungi, and India ink preparations for the recognition of cryptococci. Dark-field microscopic examination for spirochetes, wet preparations for motile organisms, and phase contrast examination are other convenient methods that take advantage of distinctive biologic characteristics of living microorganisms for their identification. Cytologic examination utilizing standard stains of infected cells scraped from body surfaces may identify intracellular pathogens (e.g., *Chlamydia trachomatis*) and inclusion bodies that indicate infection by selected intracellular microorganisms. Cytomegalovirus, herpes-

virus, and measles virus are among those agents that commonly cause formation of inclusion bodies. In addition, the use of fluorescent-labeled antibodies that bind to determinants of pathogenic microorganisms provides a rapid, definitive histologic test to confirm infection by a specific etiologic agent including herpesviruses, *Legionella* species, and *C. trachomatis*. There has been increasing interest in developing new laboratory tests for the diagnosis of infectious diseases (Tam, 1984; Kingsburg and Falkow, 1985; Brooks and York, 1986). This rapidly evolving field is based on the availability of new reagents derived from molecular biology and on the ability to automate testing. Ultimately, cost effectiveness will dictate whether these new diagnostic tests will be commonly employed. However, molecular biologic techniques have enabled investigators to produce monoclonal antibodies and genetic probes for a number of fastidious or difficult-to-detect microorganisms. Diagnostic kits that employ these new reagents may be superior to the current conventional tests, especially when these tests incorporate improved antibody-antigen detection and genetic amplification (e.g., the polymerase chain reaction) techniques. Their ultimate value remains to be evaluated in terms of sensitivity, specificity, and predictive value compared with conventional culture tests to detect pathogenic microorganisms. *Principle: The rational choice of an efficacious treatment for infectious diseases is dependent upon diagnostic accuracy. The physician must be certain that the appropriate specimens have been obtained and that they have been properly transported and processed to ensure accuracy and reliability.*

Serologic Approaches to Documentation of Infection. Cultures of selected microorganisms may be unavailable because the methodology is not available or adequate (e.g., viral hepatitis), is unsafe for laboratory personnel (e.g., rickettsiae), or is impractical (e.g., *Chlamydia* species or certain viruses). A common reason for negative cultures is the use of antimicrobial agents before the culture was taken. Under these circumstances, a serologic approach to documentation of infection might be diagnostically or epidemiologically important. As outlined in Fig. 24–1, the host mounts nonspecific and specific defenses against various infective agents (e.g., humoral antibodies). There are many nonspecific (e.g., VDRL for syphilis) and specific antibody (e.g., streptolysin O for group A streptococci) tests that are important diagnostic tools. It is not within the scope of this section to list the many available specific serologic tests. In general, the presence of specific IgM antibodies in high titer indicates a very recent or current infection and has been particularly useful in diagnosing some viral infections and toxoplasmosis (Ruskin and Remington, 1976). Acute and convalescent sera demonstrating a fourfold rise in specific IgG antibody are also useful indicators of recent infection. Sera should be obtained at an interval of 2 to 3 weeks to permit adequate time to lapse for the formation of detectable amounts of IgG antibodies. The presence of IgG antibody in a single serum specimen, while indicating exposure to the agent, is usually of little assistance in diagnosing a current illness. In general, serologic testing is indicated in those patients who will require therapeutic intervention. Such tests are not necessary for the majority of viral infections when the natural history of disease is self-limiting and short (e.g., rotavirus). Serologic tests are particularly important in patients suspected of having syphilis, HIV infection, rickettsial diseases, invasive parasitic diseases, and fungal diseases (e.g., coccidioidomycosis).

Measurements of Cell-Mediated Immunity. The appearance of specific cell-mediated immunity is a commonly measured specific change in a host's response to infection. Although there are several sophisticated measurements of T-lymphocyte function to document prior exposure to an antigen, the intradermal skin test remains the simplest, cheapest, and most-used measurement of this aspect of immune function. It evaluates specific T cells that mediate delayed-type hypersensitivity reactions (Snider, 1982; Collins, 1982; deShazo et al., 1987). Properly performed, this test provides an indication of prior exposure to (or current infection with) the antigen injected. However, intradermal skin tests of delayed-type hypersensitivity provide no indication of current activity of infection by an agent. A change from a negative to a positive test usually indicates new exposure during the interval between tests and may be correlated with active infection.

The tuberculin test with purified protein derivative (PPD) is the prototype of this type of test. It has proven utility in detecting exposure to *Mycobacterium tuberculosis* (Snider, 1982). There are other commonly employed skin tests for screening for histoplasmosis, blastomycosis, coccidioidomycosis, and candidiasis. However, results from these tests have not been clinically useful. The primary reasons for this failure are the high percentage of positive responders who do not have clinical disease, and the ubiquitous nature of exposure to these antigens by persons living in zones where hyperendemic rates of these diseases occur.

The dose of antigen and the skin reaction's size are critical in avoiding misinterpretation of cross-reactivity with other related agents (e.g., atypical mycobacteria). False-negative tests (i.e., negative reactions to skin tests in the presence of true in-

fection) may occur because of defects in any of the afferent or efferent arms of the cell-mediated immune system or faulty preparation or application of the antigen. False-negative tests have been seen in overwhelming tuberculous infection, intercurrent viral infections including those with live-virus vaccines, immunosuppressant therapy, malnutrition, sarcoidosis, or various cancers and leukemias that suppress immune function (Twomey et al., 1975; Fauci et al., 1976; Nussenzweig, 1982; Chandra, 1983; Rouse and Horohov, 1986). *Principle: Positive serologic and delayed-type hypersensitivity reactions indicate prior exposure to selected antigens. These tests have limited confirmatory value to document acute infection and provide only circumstantial evidence for active infection that demands treatment. There is no substitute for culture or detection of the organism in clinical specimens to document the presence of infection.*

ANTIMICROBIAL THERAPY: GENERAL PRINCIPLES

A wide variety of antimicrobial agents is available to treat established infections caused by bacteria, fungi, or parasites. In contrast, there are relatively few effective therapies to eradicate viruses once infection has occurred. Because of the considerable recent efforts to control HIV, it is plausible to anticipate that many more effective antiviral agents will become available soon. Primary efforts to control viral infections must currently be directed at augmenting host defenses by means of active or passive immunization. This section will cover the general principles of antimicrobial therapy and will also include illustrative clinical problems to emphasize proper decision making in using antimicrobials.

Determinants of Antimicrobial Efficacy

Measurement of Antimicrobial Activity In Vitro. Susceptibility testing is indicated for any pathogen warranting chemotherapy if its susceptibility cannot be predicted from knowledge of the pathogen's identity. Drugs that irreversibly destroy the ability of an organism to replicate, and perhaps in the process destroy the structural integrity of the organism, are *microbicidal*. Drugs that reversibly impair replicating ability, with this function being restored when drug concentrations fall below critical inhibitory levels, are *microbistatic*. In quantitative assays of in vitro antimicrobial activity, an organism is stated to be "sensitive" to an antimicrobial when in vitro microbicidal or microbistatic concentrations of drug are equivalent to those that may be easily achieved in vivo.

Most quantitative assays express this property

in terms of the concentrations in the blood that can be reached with standard forms of administration of drug. Assays that do not correlate in vitro activity with their potential in vivo therapeutic values have been abandoned. Detailed discussions of antimicrobial sensitivity testing can be found elsewhere (Marr et al., 1988; Sahm et al., 1988; Washington, 1988; National Committee for Clinical Laboratory Standards, 1990). Discussion of susceptibility tests will be confined to the two most commonly employed assays for aerobic bacteria: disk and broth dilution sensitivity testing.

Susceptibility testing for anaerobic bacteria, mycobacteria, fungi, and viruses usually should be performed by reference laboratories since technologic difficulties are formidable and interpretation of the data is not always straightforward. The susceptibility testing of these microorganisms is highly specialized. Since there are a number of effective antibiotics for anaerobic bacteria, it is not necessary to regularly assess the susceptibility of anaerobic bacteria to a variety of agents. It is important that susceptibility testing be performed in serious or persistent infections including bacteremia, brain abscess, and infections of the eyes, joints, and bones.

Disk Sensitivity Testing. Disk diffusion tests (e.g., Kirby-Bauer) are the most widely used type of susceptibility test. This method has been standardized for rapidly growing pathogens including Enterobacteriaceae, *Staphylococcus*, *Pseudomonas*, *Acinetobacter*, some streptococci such as *Streptococcus pneumoniae*, *Hemophilus*, and *Neisseria* species. This method is not appropriate for anaerobic bacteria, slow-growing organisms, or organisms that show marked strain-to-strain variation.

Assays that measure the ability of drug to inhibit a microorganism's growth by this method are done by placing drug-impregnated paper disks on a "lawn" of organisms inoculated on the surface of agar plates. While disk sensitivity testing is simple and inexpensive, it has been standardized only for the testing of bacteria that can easily be grown on agar surfaces. Broth dilution techniques must be used to measure antimicrobial activity against more fastidious bacteria and fungi.

The quantitative technique most commonly employed was developed in 1966 (Bauer et al., 1966). With diffusion of the antibiotic through the agar, a decreasing gradient of antibiotic concentrations develop around the disk. If the antibiotic is active against the organism tested, a growth-free zone surrounds the disk. Provided that a standard amount of active antibiotic and standard bacterial inocula are used, the size of the zone of growth inhibition can be correlated directly with broth dilution assays that measure minimal inhibitory concentrations. Thus, when the diameter of the inhibitory zone is greater than a certain size, there is a correlation with antibiotic concentrations in the blood that will be inhibitory to the organism; as in these cases, the organism is said to be *sensitive* to the antimicrobial. When the zone diameter is below a defined size, then in vivo concentrations of antibiotic are not likely to inhibit the organism and it is said to be *resistant*. Results are labeled *intermediate sensitivity* when the size of the zone indicates that antibiotic concentrations that are inhibitory to the organisms might be reached in vivo, provided that high dosages are used or that the infection is localized to an area where concentrations of antibiotic may exceed those in the blood (e.g., in the urine). The reliability of the Kirby-Bauer technique depends upon adequate growth of bacteria on Mueller-Hinton agar, a standardized inoculum size, specific concentrations of active antibiotic in the antimicrobial disk, and standardized growth conditions. Any alteration of these specifications can invalidate the results. The Kirby-Bauer technique does not provide information on whether the drug is bactericidal.

Broth Dilution Sensitivity Testing. The broth dilution technique is a well-known method to measure quantitatively the in vitro activity of an antimicrobial agent against a particular bacterial isolate. It is more expensive to perform and technically more sophisticated than disk diffusion tests. There are very few indications for mandatory use of broth dilution testing since information derived from disk diffusion tests is adequate in the majority of common bacterial infections. Broth dilution studies should be performed when it is critical for the practitioner to prescribe antibiotics that will effectively kill the pathogen. Bactericidal antibiotics are required to treat endocarditis, meningitis, septic arthritis, osteomyelitis, and infections in immunocompromised patients.

Tubes of broth containing specified serial dilutions of antibiotic are inoculated with a known number of organisms; the tubes are incubated for a sufficient time to permit visual growth of the organism (usually 16 to 24 hours). The lowest concentration of antibiotic that inhibits bacterial replication (as defined by no visual growth in the tube) is stated to be the *minimal inhibitory concentration* (MIC). A *minimal microbicidal concentration* (MBC) can be determined by subculturing tubes that show no visual growth on antibiotic-free agar or in broth. The lowest concentration of antimicrobial that prevents growth on subculture indicates the MBC.

In the case of bacteriostatic drugs, no MBC will be found, since the growth of the organism is only temporarily impaired by the presence of the antibiotic. With most bactericidal drugs, the MBC usually is within 1 or 2 dilutions (twofold) of the MIC. The data derived from these tests can be coupled with the knowledge of expected or measured antibiotic concentrations in vivo to predict efficacy of the antibiotic. These tests are considerably more time-consuming and expensive than are disk sensitivity testing techniques and are not suitable for mass testing techniques unless an automated apparatus is used. Test reproducibility depends on standardized inoculum sizes and incubation conditions. The tests provide the clinician with a direct measure of antimicrobial concentrations that should inhibit microbial replication in vivo. Unless automation is employed, measurements of antimicrobial MICs and MBCs against a specific organism usually are reserved for patients with serious systemic infections such as endocarditis, in which antibiotic efficacy is a more critical factor than host defenses in eradicating the infection. Both dilution tests are also useful in evaluating causes of treatment failure.

Other Sensitivity-Testing Techniques. Another technique for measuring antimicrobial activity in vitro that lends itself to mass testing combines aspects of both the above assays. Mueller-Hinton, or some other agar, is prepared with known concentrations of antibiotic; fixed amounts of the different organisms for testing are inoculated on the surface using a replicator (Steers et al., 1959). The MICs can then be determined from the concentration of antibiotic that inhibits visible growth of the organisms on the surface of the agar. Results of these assays usually correlate well with tube dilution MICs and can be reported to the clinician along with the information as to which sites in the body are likely to have antimicrobial concentrations in excess of such MICs (using standard doses of a given antimicrobial). This technique provides a better in vitro correlation with in vivo efficacy of antimicrobials than does the Kirby-Bauer method. For example, many "intermediate" and some "resistant" organisms defined by the Kirby-Bauer methodology may be eradicated from the urinary tract if the renal route is the major pathway of excretion and higher concentrations of drug are present in the urine than in the blood.

The serum bactericidal test is another sensitivity test employed that is a simple variation of the broth dilution test. It is performed in the same manner except serial dilutions of a sample of serum from the patient are used instead of the various concentrations of antimicrobial agents. The serum is obtained from the patient during antimicrobial therapy and diluted. The tubes or wells are then inoculated with a standardized suspension of the pathogen isolated from the patient.

After appropriate growth, the tubes are examined and the serum's inhibiting titer is determined. All samples are subsequently subcultured. The serum bactericidal titer is that dilution of serum that shows >99.9% killing of the initial inoculum. The use of the serum bactericidal test is controversial, the controversy focusing on the technology and the clinical significance of the results. To date there is no conclusive recommendation as to its utility in predicting antimicrobial efficacy in vivo. The serum bactericidal test may be useful in several conditions including bacterial endocarditis, bacteremia in cancer patients, osteomyelitis, septic arthritis, monitoring combinations of antibiotics, and a guide when changing from parenteral to oral therapy in infected patients (Wilson et al., 1975; Klastersky et al., 1977; Prober and Yeager, 1979; Parker and Fossieck, 1980; Jordan and Kawochi, 1981; Tuomanen et al., 1981; Stratton, 1984; Robinson et al., 1985).

Selection of Antimicrobial Agents

Agents selected for inclusion in susceptibility testing panels should be chosen carefully, since information obtained from these tests encourages the practitioner to use the agent(s) likely to have in vivo efficacy. Suggested guidelines for selecting agents to be tested against common bacterial pathogens are listed in Table 24–10. Changes in this list can be anticipated as improved and cost-effective agents are developed.

Deliberately selective reporting of the results of antibiotic susceptibility tests by the laboratory also provides a useful method to promote efficacious and cost-effective use of antimicrobials. For example, if an *E. coli* blood isolate is sensitive to gentamicin, there is no reason to report susceptibility to the other aminoglycosides unless the patient has a hypersensitivity reaction to gentamicin. Reporting of the susceptibility results for the other aminoglycosides in this case might encourage physicians to prescribe a more costly aminoglycoside agent when it is not necessary. Such reasoning is particularly important for the large group of β-lactam antibiotics. Close coordination between the microbiology laboratory and hospital drug formulary committee provides a rational basis for antibiotic selection. *Principle: Reports of in vitro sensitivity tests do not guarantee that the antibiotic selected will work in vivo. The drug must reach the site of infection in concentrations adequate to reproduce the in vitro effects when coupled with the host's own defense mechanisms.*

Pharmacologic Factors Regulating Antibiotic Activity

A major goal in antimicrobial therapy is to choose an agent that is selectively active for the

Table 24–10. SUGGESTED GROUPINGS OF ANTIMICROBIAL AGENTS THAT SHOULD BE CONSIDERED FOR ROUTINE TESTING AND REPORTING BY CLINICAL MICROBIOLOGY LABORATORIES AND A GUIDE FOR APPROPRIATE ANTIBIOTIC USAGE*

	ENTEROBACTERIACEAE	Pseudomonas	STAPHYLOCOCCI	ENTEROCOCCI	STREPTOCOCCI NOT INCLUDING ENTEROCOCCI	Hemophilus
Group 1 Routine tests (all clinical specimens)	Ampicillin Cephalothin Cefazolin Gentamicin	Mezlocillin or ticarcillin Gentamicin	Penicillin G Oxacillin or methicillin Cephalothin Cefazolin Erythromycin Clindamycin	Penicillin G or ampicillin	Penicillin G	Ampicillin Trimethoprim-sulfamethoxazole
Group 2 Selected reporting (if resistance in group 1; from CSF, blood, or special procedure, i.e., bone biopsy)	Ticarcillin or mezlocillin or piperacillin Ampicillin-sulbactam Amoxicillin-clavulanic acid Ticarcillin-clavulanic acid Cefotetan Cefoxitin Cefoperazone Cefuroxime or cefamandole or cefonicid Cefotaxime or ceftazidime or ceftizoxime or ceftriaxone Aztreonam Tobramycin or amikacin or kanamycin or netilmicin Trimethoprim-sulfamethoxazole	Azlocillin or piperacillin Cefoperazone or ceftazidime Aztreonam Ticarcillin-clavulanic acid Imipenem Ciprofloxacin Tobramycin or amikacin or kanamycin or netilmicin	Vancomycin	Vancomycin	Cephalothin Erythromycin Clindamycin Tetracycline Chloramphenicol Vancomycin	Amoxicillin-clavulanic acid Ampicillin-sulbactam Cefuroxime sodium (parenteral) Cefaclor Cefixime Cefuroxime axetil (oral) Cefotaxime or ceftazidime or ceftizoxime or ceftriaxone Chloramphenicol
Group 3 Supplemental selected reporting (if resistance in groups 1 and 2)	Imipenem Tetracycline Chloramphenicol Ciprofloxacin	Cefotaxime or ceftriaxone Chloramphenicol Trimethoprim-sulfamethoxazole	Imipenem Chloramphenicol Ciprofloxacin Rifampin			Cefamandole Cefonicid Rifampin
Group 4 Selected reporting for urinary isolates (if resistance in group 3)	Cinoxacin Norfloxacin Nitrofurantoin Trimethoprim Sulfisoxazole	Ceftizoxime Norfloxacin Tetracycline Sulfisoxazole	Nitrofurantoin Norfloxacin Trimethoprim Sulfisoxazole	Ciprofloxacin Norfloxacin Tetracycline Nitrofurantoin	Norfloxacin Nitrofurantoin	

* Adapted from National Committee for Clinical Laboratory Standards, 1990.

most likely infecting microorganism(s) at the site of infection. Pharmacologic factors that affect antimicrobial drug efficacy include absorption of the drug(s) from the site of administration, delivery by the circulation to the infected region, diffusion from the plasma through tissues, penetration to the site of infection, and maintenance of adequate amounts of active drug at that site. If antibiotics only inhibit the growth of organisms rather than kill them, the host's defense mechanisms must be sufficiently effective to eradicate the pathogenic microorganism to attain a therapeutic success (Yourtee and Root, 1984). If this is not the case, microbicidal agents should be employed. In selected clinical syndromes (e.g., bacteremia in a neutropenic leukemic patient undergoing chemotherapy), sufficient bactericidal drug must be administered so that a cure will be produced, while in the vast majority of infections antimicrobial agents are required only to augment host defenses to effect cure. Table 24–11 lists commonly used agents according to microbicidal or microbistatic status. *Principle: Consideration of the patient's physiologic resilience as a determinant of efficacy is a key factor in choice of drug in a panoply of disease settings.*

Absorption of Antimicrobials. Determining the most effective route of administration to achieve adequate concentrations in the blood and tissue is important in choosing an antimicrobial (Table 24–12). Although oral administration of many antibiotics is preferred because of ease, safety, and cost, parenteral administration is mandatory when treating any infection that poses a serious threat to life.

Parenteral administration helps ensure that adequate concentrations of drug are achieved in the blood. Two important considerations in choosing the route of administration of a drug are the plasma concentration of drug that can be achieved by oral versus parenteral administration, and the location and severity of the infection. For example, penicillin G has an oral bioavailability of only 20% to 30%. Resulting plasma concentrations may be inadequate to treat serious infections, particularly when the infections are located in tissues resistant to penetration by the antibiotics (e.g., brain or endocardium). The use of a variety of tests to measure drug concentration in plasma is appropriate when there are questions as to the adequacy of those concentrations in seriously ill patients. *Principle: In treating any infection that poses a serious threat to life, it is unwise to de-*

Table 24–11. SYSTEMIC ANTIMICROBIAL DRUGS BY CLASS AND ACTION

	MICROCIDAL	MICROSTATIC
Antibacterial agents	Penicillins Cephalosporins Aminoglycosides Vancomycin Teicoplanin Quinolones Nitrofurantoin Methenamine Metronidazole Carbapenems (Imipenem) Monobactams (Aztreonam)	Chloramphenicol Clindamycin Erythromycin Tetracyclines Trimethoprim Sulfonamides
Antituberculous agents	Isoniazid Rifampin Streptomycin Pyrazinamide	p-Aminosalicylic acid Ethambutol Ethionamide Cycloserine
Antifungal agents	Amphotericin B Flucytosine Clotrimazole Nystatin Griseofulvin	Ketoconazole Fluconazole Itraconazole
Antiviral agents	Idoxuridine Cytarabine Amantadine Rimantadine Acyclovir AZT Vidarabine	

Table 24-12. CLASSIFICATION OF ANTIMICROBIAL AGENTS

CLASS	ROUTE*	COMMON TRADE NAME	SPECTRUM OF ACTIVITY
			ANTIBACTERIAL
β-Lactam Antibiotics			
Penicillins			
Natural Penicillins			
Penicillin G	IV, IM, p.o.	Various	Active against most strains of streptococci, pneumococci, meningococci, anaerobes except *Bacterioides fragilis*, spirochetes, *Listeria monocytogenes*, *Corynebacterium* spp., and *Bacillus* spp.
Penicillin V	p.o.	Various	
Aminopenicillins			
Ampicillin	IV, IM, p.o.	Omipen	Less active than penicillin G against streptococci; increased activity against enterococci and gram-negative organisms: *Escherichia coli*, *Hemophilus influenzae*, and *Proteus mirabilis*.
Amoxicillin	p.o.	Amoxil	
Bacampicillin	p.o.	Spectrobid	
Hetacillin	p.o.	Verspen	
Penicillinase-Resistant Penicillins			
Methicillin	IV, IM	Staphcillin, Celbenin	Active against penicillinase-producing and nonproducing strains of *Staphylococcus aureus*; less active than penicillin G against other organisms.
Nafcillin	IV, IM	Unipen	
Oxacillin	IV, IM	Bactocil, Prostaphlin	
Dicloxacillin	IM, p.o.	Dycill	
Cloxacillin	p.o.	Tegopen	
Carboxypenicillins			
Carbenicillin	IV, IM, p.o.	Geopen, Geocillin	Good activity against *Proteus vulgaris*, *Serratia* spp., and *Pseudomonas aeruginosa*; less activity than penicillin G against gram-positive organisms.
Ticarcillin	IV, IM	Ticar	
Ureidopenicillins			
Azlocillin	IV	Azlin	Greater activity than carboxypenicillins against enterococci, *Bacteroides* spp., and certain aerobic gram-negative organisms: *P. aeroginosa* (azlocillin, piperacillin), *Klebsiella* spp., *Serratia marcescens*, and *E. coli*.
Mezlocillin	IV, IM	Mezlin	
Piperacillin	IV, IM	Piperacil	
Combinations with β-Lactamase Inhibitors			
Amoxacillin + clavulanic acid	p.o.	Augmentin	Addition of β-lactamase inhibitor generally increases activity against β-lactamase-producing strains of *S. aureus*, *H. influenzae*, *B. fragilis*, and *Branhamella catarahalis*. No enhanced activity against *P. aeruginosa*, *Enterobacter* spp., *Serratia* spp., *Acinetobacter* spp., and methicillin-resistant *S. aureus*.
Ticarcillin + clavulanic acid	IV	Timentin	
Ampicillin + sulbactam	IV, IM	Unasyn	

(continued)

Table 24–12. CLASSIFICATION OF ANTIMICROBIAL AGENTS (continued)

CLASS	COMMON TRADE NAME	ROUTE*	SPECTRUM OF ACTIVITY
			ANTIBACTERIAL
β-Lactam Antibiotics (continued)			
Cephalosporins			
First-generation			
Cephradine	Velosef	IV, IM, p.o.	Excellent activity against streptococcus (except *Streptococcus faecalis*) and *S. aureus*; good activity against many strains of *P. mirabilis*, *E. coli*, and *Klebsiella* spp., minimal activity against *Bacteroides* spp.
Cephalexin	Keflex, Keflet	p.o.	
Cefadroxil	Duricef, Ultracef	p.o.	
Cephalothin	Seffin	IV, IM	
Cephapirin	Cefadyl	IV, IM	
Cefazolin	Ancef, Kefzol	IV, IM	
Second-generation			
Cefamandole	Mandol	IV, IM	Excellent activity against *Streptococcus* (except *S. faecalis*); cefmandole, cefuroxime, and cefmetazole have good activity against *S. aureus*; good activity against most members of Enterobacteriaceae family including *Proteus* spp., *E. coli*, and *Klebsiella* spp.; cefotetan, cefonicid, cefamandole, and cefuroxime have good activity against *H. influenzae*; cefotetan has extended activity against some strains of *Serratia* spp. and indole-positive *Proteus* spp.; cefoxitin, cefotetan, and cefmetazole are active against *B. fragilis*; cefuroxime has good CSF penetration.
Cefoxitin	Mefoxin	IV, IM	
Cefuroxime	Zinacef, Ceftin	IV, IM, p.o.	
Cefonicid	Monocid	IV, IM	
Ceforanide	Precef	IV, IM	
Cefotetan	Cefotan	IV, IM	
Cefaclor	Ceclor	p.o.	
Cefmetazole	Zefazone	IV	
Third-generation			
Cefotaxime	Claforan	IV, IM	Excellent activity against *Streptococcus* and good activity against *Staphylococcus* with the exception of moxalactam and ceftazidime; excellent activity against Enterobacteriaceae family including *Proteus* spp., *E. coli*, *Klebsiella* spp., *Salmonella* spp., and *Shigella* spp. Good activity against *Serratia*, *Enterobacter*, *Citrobacter*. Both ceftazidime and cefoperazone are active against *Pseudomonas aeruginosa*; moxalactam has good activity against *B. fragilis*; most agents have good CSF penetration.
Ceftizoxime	Ceftizox	IV, IM	
Ceftriaxone	Rocephin	IV, IM	
Ceftazidime	Fortaz, Tazicef	IV, IM	
Cefoperazone	Cefobid	IV	
Moxalactam	Moxam	IV, IM	
Cefixime	Suprax	p.o.	
Carbapenems			
Imipenem	Primaxin	IV, IM	Excellent activity against both gram-positive and gram-negative aerobes and anaerobes; should be reserved for multidrug-resistant *P. aeruginosa*, *Enterobacter*, or *Citrobacter* infections; unpredictable activity against methicillin-resistant staphylococci, some enterococci, *Xanthomonas maltophilia*, and *Pseudomonas cepacia*.

β-Lactam Antibiotics (continued)

Monobactams

Aztreonam — Azactam — IV, IM — Excellent activity against most members of the Enterobacteriaceae family including *E. coli, Klebsiella* spp., *Serratia* spp., *Citrobacter* spp., and *Enterobacter* spp.; no activity against aerobic gram-positive and anaerobic organisms.

Aminoglycosides

Amikacin — Amikin — IV, IM
Gentamicin — Various — IV, IM
Netilmicin — Netromycin — IV, IM
Tobramycin — Nebcin — IV, IM

Excellent activity against aerobic gram-negative organisms; gentamicin and tobramycin are very similar in activity with the exception that tobramycin is more active against *P. aeruginosa* and gentamicin is more active against *S. marcescens*; aminoglycosides have been used in combination with β-lactams for synergy in treatment of staphylococcal and enterococcal infections (gentamicin is preferred).

Protein Synthesis Inhibitors

Erythromycin — Ilotycin, E.E.S., Erygel — IV, p.o., T — Good activity against streptococcus (except enterococcus), *Legionella, Mycoplasma,* and *Chlamydia trachomatis.*

Clindamycin — Cleocin — IM, IV, p.o. — Good activity against aerobic gram-positive organisms including staphylococci and nonenterococcal streptococci; moderate activity against *B. fragilis* and other anaerobes.

Chloramphenicol — Chloromycetin — IV, p.o., T — Good activity against aerobic gram-positive organisms including staphylococci and nonenterococcal streptococci; good activity against most members of the Enterobacteriaceae family including *E. coli, Klebsiella* spp., *Proteus* spp., *H. influenzae, Serratia* spp., *Salmonella, Shigella,* meningococcus and *Neisseria gonorrhoeae;* excellent activity against *B. fragilis* and other anaerobes.

Tetracyclines

Doxycycline — Vibramycin — IV, p.o.
Minocycline — Minocin — IV, p.o.
Tetracycline — Achromycin, Sumycin — IV, p.o.

Excellent activity against *Mycoplasma pneumoniae* and *C. trachomatis;* good activity against most of aerobic gram-positive organisms including staphylococci and nonenterococcal streptococci; good activity against *E. coli* and *Klebsiella* spp.; most strains of *Proteus* and *Serratia* spp. are resistant; minimal activity against anaerobes including *B. fragilis.*

Folate Inhibitors

Trimethoprim — Trimpex — p.o. — Good activity against aerobic gram-positive including staphylococci and streptococci; also active against many members of the Enterobacteriaceae family including *E. coli, H. influenzae, Proteus* spp., and *Serratia* spp.; minimal activity against anaerobes.

(continued)

663

Table 24-12. CLASSIFICATION OF ANTIMICROBIAL AGENTS (continued)

ANTIBACTERIAL

CLASS	ROUTE*	COMMON TRADE NAME	SPECTRUM OF ACTIVITY
Sulfonamides			
Sulfamethoxazole	p.o.	Gantanol	Good activity against aerobic gram-positive, including staphylococci and streptococci; excellent activity against many members of the Enterobacteriaceae family including *E. coli, Klebsiella* spp., *H. influenzae, P. mirabilis, Enterobacter* spp., *Salmonella,* and *Shigella;* also active against *Nocardia asteroides* and *Toxoplasma gondi;* minimal activity against anaerobes.
Sulfisoxazole	p.o.	Gantrisin	
Sulfadiazine	p.o.	Microsulfon	
Quinolones			
Naldixic acid	p.o.	Negram	Excellent activity against aerobic gram-negative bacilli including *E. coli, Klebsiella* spp., *Enterobacter* spp., *Citrobacter* spp., *P. mirabilis,* and *P. aeruginosa;* good activity against staphylococci including methicillin-resistant *S. aureus;* poor activity against anaerobes; clinically unreliable against streptococci.
Ciprofloxacin	IV, p.o.	Cipro	
Norfloxacin	p.o.	Noroxin	
Ofloxacin*	IV, p.o.	Oflox	
Pefloxacin*			
Miscellaneous			
Metronidazole	IV, p.o.	Flagyl	Excellent activity against both anaerobic gram-positive and gram-negative organisms including *B. fragilis, Clostridia* spp., *Peptococcus, Peptostreptococcus,* and *Propionibacterium;* good activity against *Trichomonas vaginalis, Giardia lamblia,* and *Entamoeba histolytica;* little to no activity against aerobic organisms.
Glycopeptides			
Vancomycin	IV, p.o.	Vancocin	Excellent activity against aerobic gram-positive organisms including pneumococci, enterococci, and methicillin-resistant staphylococci.
Teicoplanin†	IV		

ANTIVIRAL

CLASS	ROUTE*	COMMON TRADE NAME	MAJOR INDICATION
Acyclovir	IV, p.o., T	Zovirax	Herpes simplex virus, varicella-zoster virus
Ganciclovir	IV	Cytovene	Cytomegalovirus
Amantadine	p.o.	Symmetrel	Influenza A virus
Azidothymidine	p.o.	Retrovir	HIV-1
Vidarabine	IV	Vira-A	Second-line agent for life-threatening herpesvirus or varicella-zoster infection
Ribavirin	Inh	Virazole	Respiratory syncytial virus

CLASS	ROUTE*	COMMON TRADE NAME	MAJOR INDICATION
Isoniazid	p.o.	Nydrazid	Primary
Rifampin	IV, p.o.	Rifadin, Rimactane	Primary
Streptomycin	IM	Streptomycin	Primary
Ethambutol	p.o.	Myambutol	Primary
Pyrazinamide	p.o.	Pyrazinamide	Primary CNS or secondary
Capreomycin	IM	Capastat	Secondary or atypical
Kanamycin	IM	Kantrex	Secondary
Cycloserine	p.o.	Seromycin	Secondary
Ethionamide	p.o.	Trecator-SC	Secondary or atypical
Aminosalicylic acid	p.o.	P.A.S.	Secondary
Clofazimine	p.o.	Lamprene	Atypical in HIV patient
Rifabutin	p.o.	Ansamycin	Atypical in HIV patient

ANTIFUNGAL

CLASS	ROUTE*	COMMON TRADE NAME	MAJOR INDICATION
Polyenes			
Amphotericin B	IV	Fungizone	Agent of choice for deep-seated candidiasis, aspergillosis, mucormycosis, coccidioidomycosis, cryptococcosis, and extracutaneous sporotrichosis.
Nystatin	p.o., T	Nilstat, Mycostatin	Mucosal and vaginal candidiasis.
Imidazoles			
Ketoconazole	p.o., T	Nizoral	Esophageal candidiasis; alternate agent for chronic mucocutaneous candidiasis, paracoccidiomycosis, blastomycosis, histoplasmosis, and coccidioidomycosis; also effective when used orally in the treatment of dermatophytoses including *Trichophyton* and *Microsporum* spp.
Miconazole	IV, p.o., T	Monistat	Topical and oral miconazole is used for the treatment of dermatophytoses, and vaginal candidiasis; IV miconazole can be used for the treatment of disseminated candidiasis, coccidioidomycosis, and paracoccidioidomycosis.
Clotrimazole	T	Mycelex, Lotrimin	Mucosal and vaginal candidiasis.
Triazoles			
Fluconazole	IV, p.o.	Diflucan	Esophageal and vaginal candidiasis; alternate agent for treatment and suppressive therapy of cryptococcosis.
Miscellaneous			
Flucytosine	p.o.	Ancobon	Usually in combination with amphotericin B for cryptococcosis and candidiasis, seldom used alone due to rapid development of resistance.
Griseofulvin	p.o.	Fulvicin, Gris-PEG	Dermatophytes including *microsporum* and *trichophyton* spp.

* IV = intravenous; p.o. = oral; T = topical; IM = intramuscular; Inh = inhaled.
† Investigational agent as of October 1, 1990.

Table 24–13. FACTORS AFFECTING TISSUE PENETRATION OF ANTIMICROBIALS

1. Concentration of antimicrobial in blood
2. Molecular size of antimicrobial
3. Protein binding of antimicrobial in plasma
4. Lipid solubility of antimicrobial
5. Ionic charge of antimicrobial
6. Antimicrobial binding to exudate or tissue
7. Presence or absence of inflammation
8. Active transport mechanisms
9. Pathways of excretion of antimicrobial

pend on oral absorption, especially in the presence of vomiting or GI dysfunction. A parenteral formulation is usually indicated.

Tissue Distribution of Antimicrobials. Once an antimicrobial is in the blood, its ability to reach an infected site depends on the interplay of the factors outlined in Table 24–13. The most important are those of protein and tissue binding. Biologic activity of an antimicrobial is best correlated with the concentration of free (rather than total) drug in a protein-rich medium (Kunin, 1965; Merrikin et al., 1983). Extensive protein binding of an antimicrobial may not only reduce its biologic activity but also restrict its distribution into tissues, its penetration into interstitial and inflammatory spaces, and its excretion by glomerular filtration (Craig and Kunin, 1976; Wise et al., 1980; Wise, 1983). Likewise, extensive tissue binding of drugs (e.g., the polymyxins) also may restrict distribution and penetration to sites of infection (Kunin and Bugg, 1971; Kucers and Bennett, 1989). The development of an inflammatory response at the site of bacterial infection,

with an increase in blood flow and capillary permeability, presumably counteracts some of the restrictive effects of protein binding. Furthermore, most drugs in clinical use can be given in dosages that are adequate to overcome their potentially "negative" binding characteristics.

Antimicrobial concentrations in soft tissues, joint spaces, and body fluids are usually adequate to inhibit microbial growth. However, there are some special situations in which the tissue-penetrating characteristics of drugs may be particularly important in determining clinical responses to treatment. Such situations include suppurative meningitis, bacterial endocarditis, and septic arthritis. Critical concentrations of antibiotics in plasma for the treatment of other infections have not been established, but it is usually recommended that plasma concentrations exceed the MIC by 10-fold or greater. This practice ensures a margin of safety such that less-than-optimal distribution of drug to site of action can be overcome.

Pathways of Excretion. Taking into account the pharmacokinetics of excretion of an antibiotic is a determinant of therapeutic success (Tables 24–14 and 24–15). This point is amply illustrated by the ability of nalidixic acid to sterilize the urinary tract in spite of the fact that concentrations of drug in plasma are ineffective against common urinary pathogens (Kunin, 1974). Tetracyclines that do not accumulate well in the urine (e.g., minocycline or doxycycline) may be less effective in the treatment of urinary tract infection than is tetracycline itself, which is predominantly excreted in the urine (Steigbeigel et al., 1968). When

Table 24–14. PENETRATION OF ANTIMICROBIAL AGENTS INTO CEREBROSPINAL FLUID*

THERAPEUTIC ANTIBIOTIC CONCENTRATIONS				
OBTAINED WITHOUT INFLAMED MENINGES	LIKELY WITH INFLAMED MENINGES		NOT LIKELY REGARDLESS OF STATE OF MENINGES	
Trimethoprim	Penicillin G	Ceftizoxime	Amikacin	First-generation
Sulfonamides	Ampicillin	Ceftazidime†,‡	Streptomycin	cephalosporins
Chloramphenicol	Nafcillin	Ceftriaxone	Gentamicin	Cefamandole
Isoniazid	Ticarcillin	Imipenem†,‡	Tobramycin	Cefoxitin
Rifampin	(± clavulinic	Aztreonam†,‡	Lincomycin	Cefotetan
Flucytosine	acid)	Ciprofloxacin and	Clindamycin	Cefmetazole
	Carbenicillin	other quino-		Vancomycin
	Mezlocillin	lones†,‡		Amphotericin B
	Piperacillin	Fluconazole and		
	Cefuroxime	other bis-triazoles		
	Cefotaxime	*p*-Aminosalicylic		
		acid		
		Ethambutol		

* Reproduced by permission from Applied Therapeutics: The Clinical Use of Drugs, fourth edition, edited by Lloyd Yee Young and Mary Anne Koda-Kimble, published by Applied Therapeutics, Inc., Vancouver, Washington ©, 1988.
† Does not have FDA approval for treatment of CNS infection.
‡ Limited data available.

ANTIMICROBIAL THERAPY: GENERAL PRINCIPLES**667**

Table 24–15. PENETRATION OF ANTIMICROBIAL AGENTS INTO URINE

Therapeutic antibiotic concentrations obtained in urine:

- Amoxacillin (± clavulanic acid)
- Ampicillin
- Carboxypenicillins (carbenicillin, ticarcillin)
- Ureidopenicillins (azlocillin, mezlocillin, piperacillin)
- First-generation cephalosporins (cefazolin, cephalothin, cefadroxil, cephalexin, cephradine)
- Second-generation cephalosporins (cefonicid, ceforanide, cefamandole, cefoxitin, cefotetan, cefuroxime)
- Third-generation cephalosporins (cefotaxime, ceftriaxone, ceftazidime, ceftizoxime, cefoperazone, moxalactam)
- Carbapenem (imipenem)
- Monobactam (aztreonam)
- Aminoglycosides (amikacin, tobramycin, gentamicin, streptomycin, kanamycin)
- Quinolones (nalidixic acid, ciprofloxacin, norfloxacin, ofloxacin, and enoxacin)
- Methenamine*
- Nitrofurantoin*
- Doxycycline
- Tetracycline†
- Sulfonamides
- Trimethoprim
- Vancomycin
- Flucytosine
- Fluconazole
- Ethambutol
- Cycloserine

* Ineffective in patients with renal failure.
† Avoid in renal failure because of increased azotemia.

the normal pathway of excretion of tetracycline is impaired, therapeutic success is reduced. This is particularly true in patients with renal failure, when delivery of drugs to urine is decreased. For instance, in such patients not only is tetracycline rendered ineffective in treating urinary tract infections, but standard doses become more toxic (Kucers and Bennett, 1989). Similarly, in patients with biliary tract obstruction, the concentrations of antimicrobials in bile are decreased; this may be a factor in the failure of treatment (Schoenfield, 1971; Sande and Mandell, 1985; Kucers and Bennett, 1989).

Toxicity of Antimicrobial Therapy

Mechanisms of Toxicity. The mechanisms associated with common adverse reactions to antimicrobials include dose-related toxicity that occurs in a certain fraction of patients when a critical plasma concentration or total dose is exceeded, and toxicity that is unpredictable and mediated through allergic or idiosyncratic mechanisms. For example, certain classes of drugs, such as the aminoglycosides, are associated with dose-related toxicity. In contrast, the major toxicity of the penicillins and cephalosporins is due to allergic reactions (see chapter 39). These differences are explained in part by the relative ability of a specific drugs to inhibit enzymatic pathways in the host versus their stimulation of specific immune response. Table 24–16 summarizes some of the major toxicities of various antimicrobials.

Not included in these lists is mention of the subtle adverse effects of a number of antibiotics on the host immune response. Antibiotics can reduce the efficacy of the host response to microbial pathogens. They can diminish chemotaxis, phagocytosis, neutrophil- and macrophage-mediated microbial killing, lymphocyte transformation, delayed hypersensitivity reactions, and production of antibody (Hauser and Remington, 1982; Mandell, 1982). For example, doxycycline decreases chemotaxis, phagocytosis, lymphocyte transformation, delayed hypersensitivity reactions, and production of antibody. The antimicrobial effects on immune responses observed in vitro may or may not be clinically relevant; however, these data reinforce the concept that antimicrobials have potential to produce deleterious effects that are related to their pharmacologic effects independent of their actions on bacteria or viruses.

A consideration of the relative toxicities of different antimicrobials in relationship to their efficacy is critical to the appropriate choice of antimicrobials. If two antibiotics have equivalent efficacy, the less toxic antibiotic should be chosen. The therapeutic index of an antimicrobial compares the plasma concentration of drug at which host toxicity appears with that which is effective in the treatment of the infectious disease. This ratio varies with the properties of the different drugs and the amount of antibiotic necessary to inhibit the organism in vivo at the site of infection. It may also vary with host factors that alter susceptibility to drug toxicity.

For example, gentamicin and nafcillin both exhibit in vitro activity against staphylococci. However, the therapeutic index of gentamicin in most patients is quite narrow, whereas that of nafcillin is relatively wide. Accordingly, nafcillin or other penicillinase-resistant penicillins are the treatment of choice for staphylococcal infections (in subjects not allergic to penicillin). Similarly, because of their wide therapeutic indices, the penicillins and the cephalosporins are the preferred agents in the treatment of any serious infection caused by susceptible organisms in which bactericidal therapy is preferred.

The picture changes dramatically in the case of

Table 24-16. ADVERSE EFFECTS AND TOXICITIES

ANTIBIOTICS*

AGENT	ADVERSE EFFECTS	COMMENTS
β-Lactams (penicillins, cephalosporins, monobactams, penems)	Allergic: anaphylaxis, urticaria, serum sickness, rash, fever	Patients with "ampicillin rash" have no cross-reactivity with other penicillins; ampicillin rash most common in patients with mononucleosis or patients receiving allopurinol.
		The likelihood of cross-reactivity between penicillins and cephalosporins approximately 3%–7%; extensive cross-reactivity between penicillins and imipenem; no cross-reactivity between aztreonam and penicillins.
	Diarrhea	Particularly common with ampicillin, ceftriaxone, cefoperazone. Pseudomembranous colitis can occur with most β-lactams.
	Hematologic (anemia, thrombocytopenia, antiplatelet activity, hypoprothrombinemia)	Hemolytic anemia more common with higher doses and is associated with idiosyncratic reactions.
		Antiplatelet activity most common with the antipseudomonal penicillins and high serum levels of other β-lactams, especially moxalactam.
		Hypoprothrombinemia is more associated with those cephalosporins with the methylthiotetrazole side chain (cefamandole, cefotetan, cefoperazone, cefmetazole, moxalactam); the reaction is preventable and reversible with vitamin K.
	Hepatitis	Most common with oxacillin.
	Seizure activity	Associated with high levels of β-lactams (e.g., in renal failure patients) particularly penicillins and imipenem in patients with prior history of seizure.
	Sodium load	Carbenicillin, ticarcillin.
	Interstitial nephritis	Most common with methicillin; however, reported for most other β-lactams.
	Disulfiram reaction	Associated with cephalosporins with methylthiotetrazole side chain (cefamandole, cefotetan, cefoperazone, cefmetazole, moxalactam).
	Hypotension, nausea	Associated with fast infusion of imipenem.
Aminoglycosides (gentamicin, tobramycin, amikacin, netilmicin)	Nephrotoxicity	Averages 10%–15% incidence, increased in patients that are acidotic, dehydrated, or receiving furosemide; generally reversible < 5 days treatment.
	Ototoxicity	1%–5% incidence, generally irreversible; cochlear and/or vestibular toxicity occur involving high-frequency loss.
		Netilmicin may be less ototoxic than other aminoglycosides.
	Neuromuscular paralysis	Rare; most common in patients with myasthenia gravis, parkinsonism, receiving blood, or receiving neuromuscular blocking drugs or large volumes of citrated blood.
Clindamycin	Diarrhea	Most common adverse effect; high association with pseudomembranous colitis, which is effectively treated with oral metronidazole.
Erythromycin	Nausea, vomiting	Oral administration.
	Cholestatic jaundice	Reported for all erythromycin salts, but most common with estolate.
	Ototoxicity	Most common with high doses in patients with renal and/or hepatic failure; usually transient.

Drug	Toxicity	Comments
Vancomycin	Ototoxicity	Primarily with high serum levels ($>50\mu g$/ml).
	Nephrotoxicity	Little to no nephrotoxicity observed with the current preparations of vancomycin; may increase the nephrotoxicity of aminoglycosides.
	Hypotension, flushing (Red man syndrome)	Associated with rapid infusion of vancomycin.
	Phlebitis	Needs large volume dilution.
Tetracyclines (TC)	Allergic	Rash, anaphylaxis, urticaria, fever.
	Photosensitivity	Common.
	Teeth or bone deposition and discoloration	Avoid in pediatrics.
	GI	Nausea, diarrhea, most common with oxytetracycline usage.
	Hepatitis	Primarily with high IV doses in pregnancy.
	Renal (azotemia)	Tetracyclines have an antianabolic effect and should be avoided usually in those patients with decreased renal function; doxycycline can be used in patients with renal failure.
	Vestibular	Associated with minocycline.
Chloramphenicol	Anemia	Idiosyncratic irreversible aplastic anemia (rare); reversible dose-related anemia (common).
	Gray baby syndrome	Due to inability of neonates to conjugate chloramphenicol.
Sulfonamides	GI	Nausea, diarrhea.
	Hepatic	Cholestatic hepatitis; increased incidence in AIDS.
	Rash	Photosensitization, exfoliative dermatitis, drug fever (common); Stevens-Johnson syndrome (rare in AIDS patients).
	Bone marrow	Neutropenia and thrombocytopenia occur (more common in AIDS patients).
	Kernicterus	Due to increased unbound drug in the neonate because the premature liver is unable to conjugate bilirubin; sulfonamide displaces bilirubin from protein, resulting in excess free bilirubin and kernicterus.
Trimethoprim	Skin	Rash in $>20\%$ of patients receiving 400 mg/day.
	Hematologic	Thrombocytopenia and leukopenia occur; neutropenia rare.
	GI	Nausea, vomiting, diarrhea.
	CNS	Altered mental status, confusion, seizures.
Quinolones (norfloxacin, ciprofloxacin, enoxacin)	Cartilage toxicity	Avoid in children.
Metronidazole	Hepatic insufficiency	Associated with rapidly deteriorating liver functions in patients with decompensated liver disease.
	Neurologic	Headaches and paresthesias common; ataxia and seizure rare.
	Disulfiram reaction	Common.

(continued)

* Modified with permission from Applied Therapeutics: The Clinical Use of Drugs, fourth edition, edited by Lloyd Yee Young and Mary Anne Koda-Kimble, published by Applied Therapeutics, Inc., Vancouver, Washington © , 1988.

Table 24-16. ADVERSE EFFECTS AND TOXICITIES *(continued)*

AGENT	ADVERSE EFFECTS	COMMENTS
ANTIFUNGAL AGENTS		
Amphotericin B	Headache, fever, nausea, vomiting, chills, malaise, and hypotension	Associated with IV infusion; antipyretic, antiemetic, and antihistamine drugs may be used to provide some symptomatic relief.
	Nephrotoxicity	Decreased glomerular filtration rate and renal tubular acidosis; usually reversible; permanent renal impairment occurs when the total dose exceeds 4 to 5 g.
	Electrolyte disturbances	Hypokalemia and hypomagnesemia.
	Hematologic (anemia, thrombocytopenia)	Generally reversible.
Ketoconazole	GI	Nausea, vomiting.
	Hepatic	Transient (generally reversible) elevations of serum transaminase or alkaline phosphatase concentrations.
	Endocrine	Gynecomastia, decreased testosterone synthesis.
Miconazole	GI	Nausea, vomiting.
	Neurotoxicity	Tremors, confusion, hallucination, and grand mal seizures.
	Hematologic (anemia)	Appears to be dose-related. Generally reversible.
Fluconazole	GI	Nausea, vomiting, diarrhea.
	Hepatic	Elevation of serum transaminase level. Generally reversible.
Flucytosine	GI	Vomiting, abdominal pain, diarrhea.
	Hematologic (anemia, neutropenia, thrombocytopenia)	Generally occurs with prolonged high serum levels >100–150 µg/ml.
Griseofulvin	GI	Nausea, vomiting, diarrhea.
	Neurotoxicity	Headache, fatigue, confusion, and peripheral neuritis.
ANTIVIRAL AGENTS		
Acyclovir	GI	Nausea, vomiting, and abdominal pain.
	Nephrotoxicity	Increased serum BUN and creatinine concentrations; occurs in about 10% of patients receiving parenteral acyclovir therapy.
	Crystal nephropathy	Generally reversible.
	Neurotoxicity	Lethargy, agitation, tremor, and disorientation (uncommon and generally reversible).
Ganciclovir	Hematologic (neutropenia, thrombocytopenia)	Neutropenia is more common in AIDS patients but still a problem in 40% of patients.
	CNS	Confusion, convulsions, and headache occur in <5%.

Drug	System	Comments
Amantadine	CNS	Nervousness, insomnia, dizziness occur in 33%; increased incidence with daily dose of 300 mg, with renal failure, or in elderly.
Vidarabine	Hematologic (anemia, thrombocytopenia, and neutropenia)	Usually reversible.
	GI	Nausea and vomiting.
	Neurotoxicity	Tremor, dizziness, confusion, and hallucination can occur.
Zidovudine	GI	Nausea, vomiting, and diarrhea can occur.
	Hematologic	Neutropenia and megaloblastic anemia are generally reversible.
	Headache	Meningoencephalitis is common (20%), especially in those with prior history of encephalopathy; generally disappears with prolonged therapy.

ANTITUBERCULAR AGENTS

Drug	System	Comments
Isoniazid (INH)	CNS	Peripheral neuropathy occurs with increased incidence in slow acetylators, pregnancy, chronic alcoholics, malnourished patients, elderly diabetes patients, and chronic liver diseases; prevented by daily pyridoxine 10 mg.
	Hepatitis	Elevated transaminase level occurs with increased risk >35 years of age; usually occur within first 6 months of therapy.
Rifampin	Hepatitis	Elevated transaminase level is uncommon, occurring in 1% of patients; generally mild and reversible.
	Reddish discoloration of urine and other body fluids	
	Flulike syndrome	Usually occurs with intermittent high-dosage therapy (1200 mg twice weekly).
Pyrazinamide (PZA)	Hepatotoxicity	Elevated transaminase level generally occurs with doses >40–50 mg/kg day.
	Hyperuricemia	Increased serum uric acid level, occasionally precipitating clinical gout.
Ethambutol (ETH)	Retrobulbar neuritis	Blurred vision and red-green color blindness; usually reversible upon discontinuation and associated with doses >25 mg/kg/day.
Rifabutin	Hematologic	Leukopenia and thrombocytopenia common.
Clofazimine	GI	Abdominal pain in >50%.
	Skin	Increased pigmentation changes (pink–black range); dermatitis and pruritus can occur; conjunctival irritation.

penicillin allergy, when microgram amounts of these drugs may lead to fatal anaphylaxis. The one notable exception to this principle is the finding that anaphylactic reactions to penicillin do not occur on exposure to the monobactams (e.g., aztreonam) (Saxton et al., 1984; Adkinson et al., 1984). Otherwise, an anaphylactic reaction to one penicillin usually precludes administration of any other β-lactam antibiotic. Appropriate substitution therapy in the event of penicillin allergy is discussed in the section on specific antimicrobial drugs.

In any untoward event during antimicrobial therapy, the potential deleterious role of the drug must always be considered. For example, patients who are receiving parenteral amphotericin B should have a baseline potassium, magnesium, blood urea nitrogen (BUN), and creatinine concentration, urinalysis, and peripheral blood count determined before therapy is initiated. These values should be checked frequently (such as every 3 days) so that appropriate adjustments of dosage can be made or the drug stopped in the event of serious toxicity. Such close monitoring is not necessary when less toxic antimicrobials are used, although in any patient receiving prolonged therapy it is wise to follow blood counts and renal function, examine the skin for rashes as a check for allergic manifestations that may not be readily apparent on casual questioning, and measure body temperature to check for drug-induced fever. *Principle: There are few clinical settings as confusing as in infectious disease, when the drug used to treat infection causes fever.*

Toxicity Due to Altered Host Factors. Elimination of antibiotics may be modified by genetic factors, concomitant treatment with other drugs, or disorders that alter normal elimination pathways (see chapters 32 and 40). Furthermore, the change in indigenous flora that occurs as a result of antimicrobial treatment can lead to unfavorable reactions. For example, any antimicrobial that affects aerobic bacteria can alter the normal gut flora, thereby promoting selection for anaerobic *Clostridium difficile* superinfection of the GI lumen (Gorbach and Bartlett, 1977). This organism produces a potent cytotoxin that can result in a pseudomembranous colitis. The potential contribution of these factors to both therapeutic efficacy and drug toxicity must be taken into consideration when selecting antimicrobials and monitoring patients for the effects of treatment.

Host Conditions Associated with Altered Drug Metabolism. The exposure of pregnant women and neonates to certain drugs poses several problems that may have serious consequences to the fetus or infant (see chapters 29 and 30). Some drugs readily cross the placental barrier and can produce toxicity in the fetus. Examples of fetal toxicity include dental staining or tooth malformation (e.g., tetracyclines), ototoxicity (e.g., aminoglycosides), arthropathy (e.g., quinolones), and displacement of bilirubin from serum albumin with the production of kernicterus at birth (e.g., sulfonamides). Accordingly, these drugs should not be used during pregnancy nor should they be given to neonates.

Newborns, particularly if premature, have a relative deficiency of the hepatic enzyme glucuronyl transferase and cannot inactivate chloramphenicol (Nyphan, 1961; Kucers and Bennett, 1989). Their reduced clearance of chloramphenicol leaves neonates susceptible to a potentially lethal syndrome characterized by flaccidity, ashen color, and cardiovascular collapse (the "gray baby" syndrome). The use of chloramphenicol in neonates should be avoided, or if clearly and exclusively needed, given in dosages limited to no more than 25 mg/kg per day for premature babies, and 50 mg/kg per day for full-term infants while frequently monitoring the concentrations in blood. Subjects with glucose-6-phosphate dehydrogenase deficiency may develop hemolysis when given drugs with oxidant activities; drugs to be avoided include nitrofurantoin, chloramphenicol, the sulfonamides, furazolidone, naladixic acid, aminosalicylic acid, and primaquine. The physician must also recognize that there is a considerable lack of knowledge on the safety of a variety of newer antimicrobials in the pregnant woman. Therefore, it is always prudent to use these drugs with restraint and only when clearly necessary.

Reactions Secondary to Drug Interactions. Certain combinations of drugs may lead to inactivation or to an exaggeration of the effects of antimicrobials (see chapter 40). For example, concomitant administration of antacids containing calcium or magnesium, or the administration of ferrous sulfate, can prevent absorption of tetracycline from the gut. Chloramphenicol inhibits the activity of certain liver enzymes, and it interferes with biotransformation of barbiturates, phenytoin, warfarin, and tolbutamide (Rose et al., 1977). Simultaneous administration of these drugs can exaggerate the effects of both groups of compounds. Isoniazid with phenytoin and sulfonamides with sulfonylureas similarly compete for the same enzymatic inactivating systems (Christensen et al., 1963; Kabins, 1972). The practitioner must be aware of all drugs and dietary substances ingested by his or her patient and be able to anticipate the presence of clinically important drug interactions. *Principle: Whenever more than one drug is given to a patient, the po-*

tential for toxicity is increased through known or unknown interactions. Polypharmacy should be avoided unless the indications for it are compelling.

Reactions Due to Impaired Excretion. Almost all antimicrobials are excreted to some extent by the kidney; some are cleared predominantly by the liver. Whenever renal or hepatic failure is present, the physician should be aware of necessary alterations of dosage in order to avoid dose-related toxicity. The degree of change in the regimen is determined by the potential of a compound to cause dose-related toxicity, the drug's route of clearance, and the magnitude of the renal or hepatic impairment. Table 24–17 provides a guide to modifications of dose necessary for different classes of drugs in the presence of renal failure. The major principles upon which these recommendations are made include the following:

1. The concentration of drug in plasma (C_p) after an initial dose is a function of the dose and the rate of absorption of the drug versus the rates of distribution to tissues and excretion. If the rate of absorption is much faster than the distribution and excretion of the drug, then slow excretion in renal failure will not appreciably alter initial concentrations of drug in blood. This is the situation that prevails with most antibiotics with significant dose-related toxicity (e.g., aminoglycosides). Therefore, the initial doses of these drugs require no modification in patients with renal failure.

2. After the initial dose of drug is given, the clearance becomes the important determinant of the rate of decline of concentrations in plasma. Subsequent dosing must be reduced to correspond to slowed elimination. These reductions of dose can be achieved by lengthening the interval between doses or by reducing the dose administered at a fixed interval.

These points can be illustrated by using gentamicin as an example. The drug is excreted by glomerular filtration and is handled in the kidney similar to the handling of creatinine. Consequently, creatinine clearance can be used as a guide to adjustment of the maintenance dose. In some patients, especially elderly ones, serum creatinine concentrations may be within normal values even when there is significant renal insufficiency or failure (see chapters 1 and 11). The administration of drugs at dose intervals that are two to three times their half-life in the plasma usually is adequate to maintain concentrations in plasma within a four- or eightfold therapeutic range. Gentamicin has a half-life that varies from 2 to 4 hours in subjects with normal renal function. Us-

ing these points, one suggested dosage regimen for gentamicin makes use of the serum creatinine as follows (McHenry et al., 1971):

1. **Initial (Loading) Dose:** Administer 1.7 mg/kg IM or IV to produce a peak plasma concentration of 7 to 8 μg/ml in most patients.
2. **Subsequent Maintenance Doses:** Administer a dose of 1.0 to 1.7 mg/kg every 8 hours (about three half-lives) if the creatinine concentration is 1 mg/dl or less (i.e., normal renal function). To extend the dose interval in patients with renal compromise, multiply the usual dose interval (8 hours) by the patient's serum creatinine concentration. Higher doses would be reserved for patients with serious infections outside the urinary tract, in which cases one cannot take advantage of the concentrating ability of the kidney to provide high concentrations at the site of infection.

The above dosing guidelines are not precise. Patients vary in the plasma concentrations that are achieved with a given loading dose of gentamicin (intrapatient variation in volume of distribution V_d). In some, the excretion of compounds may be more rapid than the creatinine clearance would suggest; in others, it is slower. When the serum creatinine concentration is above 3 mg/dl and the interval between doses is more than 24 hours, some patients may have lower-than-therapeutic concentrations for a substantial period of time (McHenry et al., 1971).

The second approach is to administer the second and subsequent doses of gentamicin at the usual fixed interval of every 8 hours, reducing the amount of drug according to a formula based on the serum creatinine value:

$$\text{Maintenance dose} = \left(\frac{1.0 \text{ to } 1.7 \text{ mg/kg}}{[\text{serum creatinine}]} \right)$$

$$\text{IM or IV q8h}$$

The total amount of gentamicin administered over a given period would be as indicated in the above formula, but the smaller doses given more frequently would ensure against subtherapeutic concentrations of the drug near the end of a dose interval. Other formulas for dosage of gentamicin have been suggested; however, there is no documentation that they offer a more reliable method for safe and effective treatment than is provided by the above formula. *Principle: Formulas are only approximations; individual patients vary in their distribution and clearance of antibiotics despite apparently comparable degrees of renal or hepatic impairment. Thus, in any patient with significant impairment in excretion or metabolism of an antimicrobial, direct measurements of drug in plasma should be performed, particularly if the*

Table 24-17. PHARMACOKINETICS AND DOSAGE OF ANTIMICROBIAL AGENTS IN RENAL FAILURE*

DRUG	MAJOR ROUTE OF ELIMINATION	HALF-LIFE†		NORMAL DOSING INTERVAL (H)	ADJUSTMENT FOR RENAL FAILURE‡ CRCL (ML/MIN)			METHOD§	DIALYSIS¶
		NL	ESRD		>50	10-50	<10		
β-Lactam									
Penicillin G	Renal / Hepatic	0.5	6-20	6-8	6-8	8-12	12-16	I	Yes (H) / No (P)
Ampicillin	Renal / Hepatic	0.8-1.5	7-20	4-6	6	6-12	12-16	I	Yes (H) / No (P)
Amoxacillin	Renal / Hepatic	0.9-2.3	5-20	4-6	6	6-12	12-16	I	Yes (H) / No (P)
Methicillin	Renal / Hepatic	0.5-1.0	4	4-6	4-6	6-8	8-12	I	No (H, P)
Nafcillin	Hepatic / Renal	0.5-1.0	1.2	6	Unch	Unch	Unch	D	No (H)
Dicloxacillin	Renal / Hepatic	0.8	1-2	6	Unch	Unch	Unch	I	No (H)
Cloxacillin	Renal / Hepatic	0.5	1	6	Unch	Unch	Unch	D	No (H)
Carbenicillin	Renal / Hepatic	1.2-1.5	10-20	4-6	8-12	12-24	24-48	I	Yes (H)
Ticarcillin	Renal / Hepatic	1.2	16	4-6	8-12	12-24	24-48	I	Yes (H) / No (P)
Azlocillin	Renal / Hepatic	0.8-1.5	5-6	4-6	4-6	6-8	8	I	Yes (H)
Mezlocillin	Renal / Hepatic	0.6-1.2	2.6-5.4	4-6	4-6	6-8	8	I	Yes (H)
Piperacillin	Renal / Hepatic	0.8-1.5	3.3-5.1	6	4-6	6-8	8	I	Yes (H)
Cephalosporins									
Cephradine	Renal	1.3	6-15	6	100	50	25	D	Yes (H, P)
Cephalexin	Renal	1	20-40	6	6	6	8-12	I	Yes (H, P)
Cefadroxil	Renal	1.5	20-25	8	8	12-24	24-48	I	Yes (H)
Cephalothin	Renal	0.5-1	3-18	6	6	6-8	12	I	Yes (H)
Cephapirin	Renal / Hepatic	0.6-0.8	2.4-2.7	6	6	6-8	12	I	Yes (H)

Drug	Elimination	t½ Normal (h)	t½ ESRD (h)					Method	Dialysis
Cefazolin	Renal	1.8–2	40–70	8	8	12	24–48	I	Yes (H)
Cefamandole	Renal	1	11	4–6	6	6–8	8	I	No (P)
Cefoxitin	Renal	1	13–20	6–8	6–8	8–12	24–48	I	Yes (H)
Cefuroxime	Renal	1.1–1.4	17	6–8	45–100	10–45	5–10	D	Yes (H)
Cefonicid	Renal	3.5–4.5	17–56	24	50	20–50	10–20	D	No (P)
Ceforanide	Renal	2.2–3	25	12	12	24–48	48–72	I	Yes (H)
Cefaclor	Renal	0.6–1	3	8	100	50–100	33	D	Yes (H)
Cefmetazole	Renal	1.2–1.5		6–12	6–12	16–24	48	I	Yes (H, P)
Cefotaxime	Renal / Hepatic	1.0	2.6	6–8	6–8	8–12	12–24	I	Yes (H)
Ceftizoxime	Renal	1.4–1.7	30	8–12	50–100	15–50	10–15	D	Yes (H)
Ceftriaxone	Hepatic	7–9	12–24	12–24	Unch	Unch	Unch	D	No (H)
Ceftazidime	Renal	1.2–2	13	8–12	8–12	24–48	48–72	I	Yes (H)
Cefoperazone	Hepatic	1.6–2.4	2.1	12	Unch	Unch	Unch	I	No (P)
Moxalactam	Renal / Hepatic	2–2.3	18–23	8	8	12	12–24	I	Yes (H)
Imipenem	Renal	1.0	3.7	6–8	Unch	50	NTE: 500 mg every 12 h	D	Yes (H, P)
Aztreonam	Renal / Hepatic	1.5–2.9	6–8	8–12	Unch	50–75	25	D	Yes (H, P)
Erythromycin	Hepatic / Renal	1.4	5–6	6	Unch	Unch	50–75	D	No (H, P)
Clindamycin	Hepatic	2–4	3–5	6	Unch	Unch	Unch	D	No (H, P)
Metronidazole	Hepatic	6–14	8–15	8	8	8–12	12–24	I	Yes (H), No (P)
Chloramphenicol	Hepatic / Renal	1.6–4	3–7	6	Unch	Unch	Unch	D	No (H, P)
Tetracycline	Hepatic / Renal	6–10	57–108	6	8–12	12–24	24	I	No (H, P)
Doxycycline	Hepatic	15–24	18–25	24	Unch	Unch	Unch	I	No (H, P)
Minocycline	GI / Renal	12–16	12–18	12	Unch	Unch	Unch	D	No (H, P)

(continued)

Table 24-17. PHARMACOKINETICS AND DOSAGE OF ANTIMICROBIAL AGENTS IN RENAL FAILURE *(continued)*

DRUG	MAJOR ROUTE OF ELIMINATION	HALF-LIFE†		NORMAL DOSING INTERVAL (H)	ADJUSTMENT FOR RENAL FAILURE‡ CRCL (ML/MIN)			METHOD§	DIALYSIS¶
		NL	ESRD		>50	10–50	<10		
Trimethoprim	Renal	9–13	20–49	12	12	18	24	I	Yes (H)
Sulfamethoxazole	Hepatic Renal	9–11	20–50	12	12	18	24	I	Yes (H) No (P)
Sulfisoxazole	Hepatic Renal Hepatic	3–8	6–12	6	6	8–12	12–24	I	Yes (H, P)
Quinolones									
Naldixic acid	Hepatic	6–7	21	6	Unch	Avoid	Avoid	D	?
Ciprofloxacin	Hepatic	0.65–0.8	0.9–1	12	Unch	50	50	D	?
Enoxacin	Hepatic	6–9	<30	24	Unch	Unch	25	D	?
Vancomycin	Renal	6–10	200–250	6–12	24–72	72–240	240	I	No (H, P)
Antifungal Agents									
Amphotericin B	Hepatic Nonrenal	24	24	24	24	24	24–36	I	No (H, P)
Ketoconazole	Hepatic	1.5–8	1.8	24	Unch	Unch	Unch	D	No (H)
Miconazole	Hepatic	20–24	20–24	8	Unch	Unch	Unch	D	No (H, P)
Fluconazole	Renal	22–30	?	24	100	50	25	D	Yes (H)
Itraconazole	Hepatic	17	?	12	Unch(?)	Unch(?)	Unch(?)	I	?
Flucytosine	Renal	3–6	75–200	6	6	12–24	24–48	I	Yes (H, P)
Antitubercular Agents									
Isoniazid	Hepatic	0.7–4	17	8	8	8	8	I	Yes (H, P)
Rifampin	Hepatic	1.5–5	1.8–3.1	24	Unch	Unch	Unch	I	No (H)
Ethambutol	Renal	4	7–15	24	24	24–36	48	I	Yes (H, P)
Cycloserine	Renal	12–20	?	12	24	Avoid	Avoid	I	Yes (H)
Aminosalicyclic acid	Hepatic	1.5	23	8	8	12	Avoid	I	Yes (H)

* Modified from Bennett, 1988.
† ESRD = end-stage renal disease; NL = normal.
‡ Unch = unchanged.
§ I = interval extension method; D = dose reduction method.
¶ H = hemodialysis; P = peritoneal dialysis.

*agents have a low therapeutic index. Such proce-
dure ensures that the concentrations achieved are
in the therapeutic, nontoxic range.*

When patients with severe renal failure are
given antimicrobials, consider whether they are
undergoing dialysis, and if so, by what technique.
Some drugs such as gentamicin are appreciably
removed by hemodialysis, whereas their removal
by peritoneal dialysis usually is quantitatively less
and unpredictable (Kucers and Bennett, 1989).
Conversely, most penicillins and cephalosporins
are not removed well by either method of dialysis,
since no dialysis apparatus comes close to the
penicillin-secreting function of the renal tubule
(Bennett et al., 1974). Table 24–17 lists the removal and need for replacement of the various
antibiotics during different types of dialysis. The
physician should refer to standard texts or consult
with infectious disease physicians to determine
whether replacement dosing is indicated after dialysis.

In the neonate, particularly a premature one,
pathways of metabolism or excretion may not be
fully developed and modifications of dosages may
be required (see chapters 29 and 30). Furthermore, some classes of drugs may cause toxicity in
neonates but not in older persons [e.g., chloramphenicol and the tetracyclines (Moffett, 1975)].
*Principle: Impaired excretion or metabolic path-
ways may lead to extraordinarily high plasma
concentrations of antibiotics, which may cause
significant toxicity. It is critical to know both the
manifestations of dose-related toxicity and the
normal elimination pathways of drugs, so that
required dosage modifications can be made when
antimicrobial clearance is impaired.*

**Reactions Due to Changes in Indigenous
Flora.** Whenever the natural flora is suppressed
by the administration of an antimicrobial, other
organisms proliferate (e.g., *C. difficile*). The
emergence or overgrowth of flora resistant to a
given antibiotic may cause superinfections that
are more severe than the original infection itself
(e.g., enterococci that develop high aminoglycoside resistance, or methicillin-resistant staphylococci).

Some of the more striking effects of this phenomenon were observed during the 1950s and
early 1960s when tetracyclines commonly were
given prior to abdominal surgery. As a consequence, normal flora were suppressed and some
patients developed a fulminant form of enterocolitis caused by tetracycline-resistant staphylococci
(Thaysen and Eriksen, 1955–1956; Lundsgaard-
Hansen et al., 1960). Failure to promptly recognize this complication contributed to death.

More recently, we have recognized that several
commonly used antibiotics (e.g., clindamycin and

many β-lactams) produce a pseudomembranous
colitis that may also be fatal if the meaning of
the characteristically profuse diarrhea is unrecognized (Bartlett, 1984; Lyerly et al., 1988). Strains
of *C. difficile* that produce a cytotoxin are most
commonly associated with antibiotic-associated
colitis. Staphylococci and *C. perfringens* type C
also may produce a similar syndrome.

Changes in bowel flora may lead to decreased
absorption of vitamin K with resultant bleeding
in patients already receiving oral anticoagulants
(Bentley and Meganathan, 1982). However, controversy remains as to whether antibiotic-induced
killing of intestinal bacteria results in hypoprothrombinemia (Smith and Lipsky, 1983). Apparently, the vitamin K produced by these bacteria
is not responsible for synthesis of clotting factors. Perhaps multiple factors are involved in the
vitamin K–responsive hypoprothrombinemia observed in patients receiving antimicrobials.

Prolonged administration of oral neomycin
may cause malabsorption; whether this is due to
an alteration in normal bowel flora or to direct
mucosal toxicity is not known (Jacobson and
Faloon, 1961; Lindenbaum et al., 1976). Another consequence of altered flora is the rising
incidence of severe superinfections caused by
fungi, especially in patients with cancer who
receive treatment with broad-spectrum antimicrobials. Excellent discussions of the factors involved in superinfections occurring in patients
receiving antimicrobial therapy are available in
most standard textbooks of medicine and infectious diseases.

Use of Combinations of Antimicrobials

Combinations of antimicrobials are frequently
used to treat infection; rational combinations are
chosen after carefully considering several important principles. For a specific organism or organisms causing infection, combinations of antibiotic
may be synergistic, antagonistic, or indifferent
(see Fig. 24–2). All too frequently, antibiotic
combinations are used to provide "broad-spectrum" coverage in response to the physician's insecurity rather than the medical need. In some situations, broad-spectrum coverage is appropriate
because either mixed infection or a rapidly lethal
infection is likely from pathogens whose precise
identification is in progress. Combination therapy
beyond these situations is unwarranted. *Principle:
Appropriate uses of antimicrobial combinations
include necessary synergy against an infecting organism, initial empiric treatment of life-threatening infections, or treatment of mixed infections.
Use of combinations for other conditions except
use of combination therapy for treatment of tuberculosis and leprosy to prevent development of*

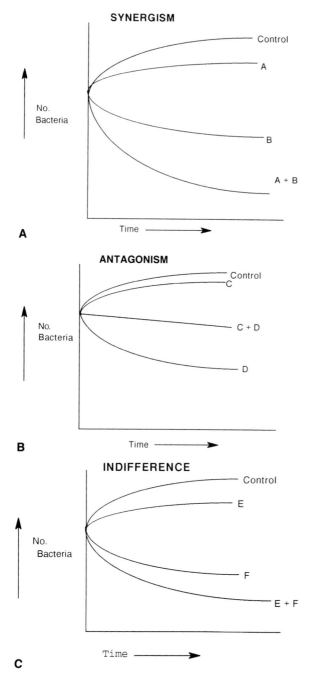

Fig. 24–2. Possible effects on bacterial killing by combination therapy. (A) Synergism; (B) antagonism; (C) indifference (additive). Reproduced with permission from Moellering, 1972.

drug resistance is not justified and unnecessarily increases the risk of toxicity to the patient.

Synergy. Antimicrobials may exert synergistic effects (see Fig. 24–2A) if they work at two different sites, involving either the same or different metabolic pathways in an organism (Jawetz,

1968; Moellering, 1972). Examples of synergistic combinations of antibiotics are the combined use of penicillins (or cephalosporins) with aminoglycosides for killing aerobic bacteria. The mechanism of this synergy has been best elucidated in enterococci. The resistance of enterococci to aminoglycosides may be mediated by either of two mechanisms. One is the failure of the compounds to enter the microbial cell in amounts sufficient to bind to ribosomes and thereby alter translation of the genetic code by ribosomal RNA. The other mechanism occurs when entry is adequate but ribosomal binding and altered translation do not occur. In the former situation, the potential for synergy between penicillins, cephalosporins, or vancomycin and the aminoglycosides exists since the "cell-wall-active" compounds act to facilitate entry of the aminoglycoside into the bacterial cell (Moellering and Weinberg, 1971; Moellering et al., 1971; Gale et al., 1972; Watanakunakorn and Bakie, 1973). The same principles probably apply to the mechanism of synergy between other cell-wall-active agents and the aminoglycosides in their action against staphylococci or gram-negative rods (Andriole, 1974; Steigbeigel et al., 1975). The major determining factors in these situations are some activity of the cell-wall-active antibiotic against the organism and ribosomal activity of the aminoglycoside.

Another example of synergism of antibiotics is seen when amphotericin B is combined with flucytosine against fungi (Kobayashi et al., 1974). Much of the synergistic effect is related to facilitated entry of the companion drug by amphotericin B.

Synergy potentially exists when two drugs are active against an organism at different points along the same vital biologic pathway. An example of this mechanism is the use of a dihydrofolate reductase inhibitor (trimethoprim and pyrimethamine) together with a sulfonamide. Both classes of drugs inhibit bacterial dihydrofolate reductase which ultimately prevents the transfer of methyl groups used in purine synthesis. When these drug combinations are used, a microbicidal action frequently results (Darrell et al., 1968; Gordon et al., 1975).

Despite suggestive in vitro data, convincing clinical evidence that synergistic drug combinations are superior to single drugs exists only for treatment of enterococcal endocarditis, and when the combination trimethoprim-sulfamethoxasole is used. There is considerable in vitro data that suggest that most antimicrobial combinations are associated with antagonism (e.g., rifampin plus penicillins for staphylococci) or indifference (e.g., chloramphenicol plus rifampin for selected *Hemophilus influenzae* strains) (Van der Auwera et al., 1983; Jadavji et al., 1984). Therefore, unless there is clear need or documentation of synergism, combination therapy should not be used. *Principle: The use of synergistic combinations may be essential to manage some severe infections (e.g., endocarditis) caused by partially resistant bacteria, or those that occur in severely impaired hosts.*

Extended Antimicrobial Spectrum. Another indication (often abused) for the use of combinations of antimicrobials is to provide broad-spectrum "coverage" in the early empiric treatment of presumed life-threatening infections such as bacterial septicemia. The use of a combination such as a penicillinase-resistant penicillin or a cephalosporin with an aminoglycoside is based on the presumption that almost all organisms potentially causing the septicemic picture will be treated and that failure to treat could result in rapid death. The potential for abuse of this type of reasoning is that all too often it is applied in clinical situations either as a substitute for adequate collection of data, or to treat the physician's insecurity. Furthermore, a second type of abuse may be observed in patients who respond to treatment and who eventually are found to have clinical isolates that are affected by only one member of the combination. Despite this evidence, antibiotic combinations are frequently continued to the ultimate disadvantage of the patient, using the faulty reasoning that one does not like to tamper with "success." Besides the potential harm to the patient offered by continued application of toxic or inappropriate drugs, this type of approach may be particularly deleterious in the hospital setting, where selecting out flora resistant to multiple drugs can be lethal. *Principle: Broad-spectrum coverage with antibiotics should not be a substitute for adequate collection of data. In most cases, single drugs with a selective spectrum of activity will provide adequate coverage for a successful outcome and will avoid the potential for toxic interactions or the selection of a highly resistant flora. In life-threatening situations, broad-spectrum coverage is justified initially; once the pathogen is identified, selective single-drug treatment is highly preferable.*

Prevention of Resistance. Another indication for the use of a combination of antibiotics is to prevent the emergence of strains of bacteria that are resistant to one or more of the drugs employed. The reasoning behind such an approach is simply an application of probability statistics. If the probability of an event (i.e., spontaneous mutation to a resistant strain) is known for two different antibiotics given separately (e.g., P_1 and P_2), then the probability that resistance to two drugs will occur simultaneously is the product of those two probabilities ($P_{\text{simultaneous resistance}} = P_1 \times P_2$). This rationale has been applied most successfully to the treatment of tuberculosis, since the rates of development of resistance to single drugs are high.

Treatment of Mixed Infections. Combination therapy is appropriate for the treatment of mixed infections. Such combinations may be useful even when the doses chosen exhibit antagonism. For example, one such combination involves ampicillin and chloramphenicol used together for the treatment of mixed infections in the abdominal cavity (Gorbach and Bartlett, 1974). If an organism happens to be sensitive to both drugs, the use of chloramphenicol (which slows bacterial growth) inhibits the effect of the penicillin, which requires active cell wall synthesis to be effective (Jawetz et al., 1951). Since chloramphenicol alone is an effective drug for many infections, the combination is often of little therapeutic benefit. Chloramphenicol and ampicillin similarly have been used together in pediatric patients as initial therapy for meningitis of unproven bacterial cause. Here the possibility of an ampicillin-resistant *H. influenzae* type B infection exists (Nelson, 1974). Despite the potential for antagonistic activity of this combination of chloramphenicol with ampicillin against all three bacterial species that commonly cause meningitis in children (*H. influenzae*, pneumococci, and meningococci), these patients generally respond to treatment. The explanation is that chloramphenicol is a highly effective drug by itself in the treatment of meningitis caused by these susceptible organisms. This contrasts with an earlier trial in which treatment with tetracycline plus penicillin was compared with treatment with penicillin alone for pneumococcal meningitis. The group receiving the combination fared much worse than that given penicillin alone, because penicillin's effects were antagonized by tetracycline and tetracycline was not an effective agent to treat meningitis, except that caused by *H. influenzae* (Lepper and Dowling, 1951; Nelson et al., 1972). Chloramphenicol also may antagonize the activity of aminoglycosides; this is usually of no clinical consequence, unless host factors that are involved in eradication of the organism during bacteriostatic therapy have been substantially inhibited (Sande and Overton, 1973). Table 24–18 provides some examples of appropriate antimicrobial combinations. *Principle: As with any combination of drugs, theory must be backed by clinical hypothesis testing. Beware of potential antagonistic combinations of antimicrobials when selecting therapy for mixed infections. The least "active" drug in a combination must be adequate to treat potential pathogens by itself in case of overlapping sensitivities, particularly if compromised host factors are of overriding importance in the determination of a successful outcome.*

Treatment Schedules

Treatment schedules must be designed to ensure adequate delivery of active antimicrobials to the site of infection for a sufficient time to promote a cure. In treating infections that pose a serious threat to life, or that are in sites where high plasma concentrations of antimicrobials are necessary to ensure penetration of tissue (e.g., in the endocardium and brain), parenteral antibiotics are required initially. In minor infections with highly sensitive organisms and excellent delivery of antimicrobials into tissues, oral administration of drugs can be employed (e.g., most urinary tract infections and streptococcal pharyngitis).

The duration of therapy with antibiotics is determined by the amount of antibiotic that must be administered over a given time to effect a cure of an active infection and prevent a relapse of the infection. The precise duration of therapy required for different infectious diseases to meet these criteria is poorly documented.

A few generalizations based on clinical observations and pathogenetic principles can be made and applied to specific clinical situations. The critical points in these considerations of duration of treatment revolve around (1) the ability of the

Table 24–18.　SOME EXAMPLES OF APPROPRIATE COMBINATIONS OF ANTIMICROBIALS

RATIONALE	EXAMPLE
1. Synergy	
a) Empiric treatment for gram-negative shock	Aminoglycoside and semi-synthetic or anti-pseudomonal penicillin (e.g., mezlocillin) (change to specific drugs once organism identified and clinical condition improves)
b) Life-threatening infection of undetermined cause	Aminoglycoside and imipenem (change to specific drugs once organisms identified)
c) Serious enterococcal infection (e.g., endocarditis)	Gentamicin and penicillin or ampicillin
d) Serious *Pseudomonas aeruginosa* infections (e.g., septicemia associated with pneumonia)	Aminoglycoside and semi-synthetic or anti-pseudomonal penicillin versus third-generation cephalosporin or imipenem if necessary
2. Serious mixed aerobic–anaerobic infection (e.g., intraabdominal sepsis)	Aminoglycoside and metronidazole
3. Decrease rate of antimicrobial resistance	Isoniazid and rifampin for tuberculosis

Table 24–19.   SUGGESTED TREATMENT REGIMENS FOR DEFINED INFECTIONS

SITE OF INFECTION	THERAPEUTIC OPTION	DURATION OF THERAPY
Urinary Tract		
Cystitis	Oral or parenteral drugs that are renally excreted	One dose or 3 days
Pyelonephritis		10 to 14 days
Respiratory Tract		
Pneumonia		
Pneumococcal	Parenteral penicillin G	Minimum of 5 days
Aerobic gram-negative	Parenteral drugs	21 days or longer
Legionnaire's disease	Erythromycin parenterally	21 days
Staphylococcal	Nafcillin or vancomycin parenterally	21 days
Bronchitis in COPD	Trimethoprim-sulfamethoxazole	5 to 7 days
Abscess	Penicillin or clindamycin parenterally and then orally; drainage may be considered	42 to 56 days
Empyema	Drainage followed by parenteral antibiotics	14 to 28 days
Pharyngitis (group A or C streptococci)	Oral penicillin or erythromycin	10 days
Cardiovascular System		
Bacteremia, likely source, no evidence of endocarditis	Parenteral antibiotics, synergistic combinations for shock	14 days
Endocarditis	Parenteral bactericidal antibiotics	28 days or more
CNS Infections		
Meningitis	Parenteral bactericidal antibiotics	14 days
Abscess	Metronidazole, penicillinase-resistant synthetic penicillin, and third-generation cephalosporin	28 days or more
GI Tract		
Dysentery	Oral quinolone	5 to 7 days
Abscess	Parenteral combination antibiotics for aerobic and anaerobic bacteria; consider surgical drainage	14 to 21 days
Peritonitis	Parenteral combination antibiotics for aerobic and anaerobic bacteria; consider surgical intervention if ruptured viscus	14 days
Pseudomembranous colitis	Oral metronidazole or oral vancomycin	10 days
Musculoskeletal System		
Muscle "gas gangrene"	Surgical debridement and parenteral penicillin G	10 to 14 days
Bone	Parenteral and then oral bactericidal antibiotics; consider surgical drainage or debridement	42 to 56 days
Joint		
Gonococcal	Drainage and parenteral bactericidal antibiotics	3 to 7 days
Nongonococcal	Drainage and parenteral bactericidal antibiotics	21 days

organism to resist the normal host's defense mechanisms, (2) the physical location of the infection and its accessibility to therapeutic concentrations of an antimicrobial, (3) the primary activity of the antimicrobial against the organisms, as determined by MIC or MBC, and (4) the frequency of development of resistance of the organism to the drug. Some general guidelines for treatment schedules are given in Table 24–19.

At least 4 to 6 weeks of treatment of osteomyelitis and endocarditis are recommended, since treatment failure or relapse rates rise to unacceptable incidences with shorter periods of therapy (Sande and Scheld, 1980). Conversely, urinary tract infections caused by the same organisms usually can be eradicated within several days of treatment because of very high urinary concentrations of effective drugs (Andriole and Epstein, 1965; O'Grady and Cattle, 1966; Kunin, 1974).

Infections with intracellular pathogens require prolonged therapy. For example, staphylococci are capable of survival intracellularly; this site provides a sanctuary from antibiotic activity. Relapse of staphylococcal infections is common unless treatment is prolonged. The longest durations of treatment are used for mycobacterial infections. *Mycobacterium leprae*'s intracellular location and slow generation time (10 to 15 days) limit the ability of the sulfones to inhibit their replication (Shepard, 1969). Treatment of extrapulmonary tuberculosis must often be continued for 12 to 24 months, depending upon the severity of disease and the sensitivity of the organisms to drugs.

Treatment for infections caused by bacteria that are promptly killed by phagocytosis need not be long, unless endocarditis is present. Pneumococcal pneumonia is a good example of this type of infection. Cures have been reported with a single dose of penicillin (Witt and Hamburger, 1963). However, the usual duration of treatment of pneumococcal pneumonia is a minimum of 5 days or until the patient has been afebrile for at least 3 days. Remember that the recommended duration of therapy is a minimum. These schedules should be considered only guidelines. It is quite possible that antimicrobial therapy might need to be more prolonged.

Factors Responsible for Failure of Treatment

Failure of treatment can result from a number of different factors. In summary, failure can be because

1. Antimicrobial agents that have poor in vitro activity against the infecting organism were selected.
2. Active antimicrobials were not delivered to the site of infection because either an inappropriate route of drug administration was selected, or the wrong dosage was used, or abnormal pharmacokinetic variables in the patients went undetected.
3. The host defenses were inadequate, or the location of the infection (as in endocarditis) was inaccessible.
4. Infections were not treated for a sufficient period to prevent relapse.
5. Serious toxicity necessitated discontinuation of therapy.
6. Antimicrobial resistance by the infecting organism developed.
7. Superinfection occurred.
8. The patient did not comply with the therapeutic regimen.

Much of the potential for failure of treatment can be obviated by basing the initial choice of antimicrobials on principles enumerated in the section on determinants of antimicrobial efficacy (pp. 656–658) and by considering how host defenses can be altered in favor of eradication of the organism. Whenever host defense mechanisms are questionable or inadequate, the physician should try to choose antimicrobials that kill the infecting organism rather than merely inhibiting its growth. The high relapse rate (approximately 50%) seen when patients with endocarditis are treated with bacteriostatic rather than bactericidal drugs is ample testimony to this principle, as are the results from inappropriate use of bacteriostatic agents in patients with severe neutropenia.

Mechanisms of Resistance to Antimicrobials

Organisms may develop resistance to antimicrobials in a number of different ways. Well-recognized mechanisms of bacterial resistance to antibiotics include enzymatic inhibition, changes in permeability in the outer and inner bacterial membranes, alterations in structure or production of targets of the antimicrobials, promotion of efflux pump mechanisms, and selection of auxotrophs that escape drug effects (Moyer et al., 1990). Use of antimicrobials encourages the selection of resistant strains; therefore, indiscriminate use of antimicrobials is inappropriate. It is quite common probably because the consequences of misuse of antibiotics in an individual are easy to attribute to the disease and not the physician. Inappropriate use selects for resistance and promotes infection that will be even more difficult to eradicate with antimicrobials.

The more common mechanisms of resistance associated with failure of the treatment are enzymatic inhibition, alteration in membrane permeability, and alteration in drug targets. The enzymes known as β-lactamases are commonly produced by a variety of bacteria. They are responsible for cleavage of the β-lactam ring, thereby destroying the ability of susceptible β-lactam antibiotics to bind to bacterial penicillin-binding proteins on the inner bacterial membrane (Medeiros, 1984). Other microorganisms inactivate antimicrobials by restricting their entry into the interior of the microbial cell. This mechanism is illustrated by many enterococci that develop resistance to aminoglycosides (Weinstein and Moellering, 1973). The resistance due to lack of drug penetration through the membrane can be overcome by combining aminoglycoside therapy with penicillin. The penicillin facilitates the entry of the aminoglycoside into bacteria (Moellering et al., 1971). Bacteria may be drug-resistant because they modify the target site for antibiotic action or binding. For example, some enterococci resist the action of aminoglycosides at the ribosomal level, despite facilitated entry of the drug by penicillins.

Plasmid-bound antimicrobial resistance factors (R factors), possessed by aerobic gram-negative rods, may mediate resistance by "looking for" enzymes that attach organic groups to the aminoglycoside (adenylation, phosphorylation, or acetylation), thereby blocking the active site(s) of the drug and rendering it inactive (Gale et al., 1972). If organisms contain R factors in the same plasmid, the factors can readily be passed from one species of aerobic gram-negative bacillus to another. This organism-to-organism transfer poses a special threat in the hospital setting, where many patients are receiving antibiotics and the selective pressure of antibiotic therapy favors survival of resistant strains (McGowan, 1983). The problem of superinfection appearing during treatment is often a special example of failure of treatment since the superinfecting organism is often resistant to the original antibiotic.

Monitoring Results of Treatment

The success or failure of treatment should be carefully assessed. Useful end points to follow include the temperature curves, leukocyte counts, elevation of the erythrocyte sedimentation rate during chronic infections such as osteomyelitis, direct demonstration of the extent of tissue injury by radiography, abnormal elevations of concentrations of tissue-derived enzymes in the circulation, and many other tests. Bacteriologic cultures and serologic tests should be repeated periodically. The intervals at which such tests should be obtained depend upon the type, the severity, the site of the infection, the typical course when treatment is successful, and the interval at which most relapses occur. *Principle: Failure of treatment of an infection can be defined as failure to produce a clinical remission of symptoms or as the occurrence of a relapse once treatment is stopped. When treatment does fail, the physician must once again base rational therapy on general principles, including the following:*

1. Reestablishing the microbial cause of infection and determining whether it is caused by the original or a new agent (superinfection)

2. Redetermining the in vitro sensitivity of the isolated organism to the antibiotics

3. Checking blood, urine, or tissue concentrations of antibiotics and their in vitro activity to determine whether they remain adequate in vivo and to confirm that the patient is actually receiving the medication

4. Making certain that treatment failure is not

due to a failure on the part of the physician to identify correctable host factors that contribute to infection (e.g., failure to drain abscesses, remove foreign bodies and necrotic tissues)

5. Excluding the possibility that persisting evidence of inflammation is not due to factors other than the infection (e.g., drug hypersensitivity) and phlebitis from IV catheters

Inappropriate Uses of Antimicrobials

Errors in the treatment of infectious diseases fall into two major categories: omission, in which treatment is indicated but none is given, and commission, in which treatment is given but it is inadequate or inappropriate. From the statistics on the use of antibiotics use in the United States, it is clear that most errors are of commission (see Table 24–20).

Principle: To maximize the benefits/risk ratio of prescribing, constantly reexamine your reasons for treatment and consistently reevaluate your knowledge of the potential hazards of the prescribed drugs.

MANAGEMENT OF SELECTED CLINICAL CONDITIONS

This section is devoted to topics that exemplify important considerations in treatment and prophylaxis with antibiotics. Overviews are provided by discussing selected particular clinical settings and the therapeutic issues they raise. These include rational therapy requiring interference at specific steps in microbial pathogenesis, problems associated with treatment of immunocompromised patients, understanding of pharmacologic features of antimicrobials in order to effect cure, understand-

---

Table 24–20.   ERRORS OF COMMISSION IN ANTIMICROBIAL THERAPY

Errors of Choice
1. Treatment of viral infections with antibiotics
2. Treatment of fever with antimicrobials without clinical evidence and/or microbiologic data to indicate a microbial cause
3. Treatment of infections with drugs that are ineffective in vivo or cannot reach the site of infection
4. Treatment of infections with drugs that are effective in vitro but are not likely to be effective in vivo
5. Treatment with toxic drugs when less toxic drugs would suffice
6. Continued treatment of infections with broad-spectrum or potent antibiotics when a more specific, less-broad-spectrum antimicrobial agent would suffice
7. Treatment with expensive drugs when effective less-expensive drugs are available

Errors in Administration of Antibiotics
1. Wrong dose
2. Wrong route of administration
3. Inappropriate dosage interval
4. Failure to recognize toxicity
5. Failure to modify dosage when elimination pathways are impaired
6. Failure to obtain drug allergy history
7. Changing antibiotics without evidence of antimicrobial treatment failure
8. Changing antibiotics without correcting host factors that contribute to treatment failure (e.g., draining abscesses or debridement of necrotic tissues)

ing of the epidemiologic aspects of infectious disease, and rational preventive measures.

Current Treatment of AIDS

The discovery that the human immunodeficiency virus type 1 (HIV-1) is responsible for the epidemic of acquired immunodeficiency syndrome (AIDS) has resulted in an intensive search for compounds that have antiretroviral activity against HIV and those that can be effective immunoprophylactics. Our current understanding of the HIV life cycle has enabled investigators to isolate compounds that have stage-specific antiviral activity. A rational approach to antiviral therapy requires a basic understanding of the HIV replicative cycle. In this section, the life cycle of HIV, our current clinical experience with agents that have direct antiviral activity against HIV, the effects of combinations, and potential vaccine efficacy are reviewed. Currently, there is still no effective curative treatment for AIDS, and the best advice to persons with high-risk behavior (e.g., illicit use of IV drugs and unprotected sexual activity with partner(s) who might have been exposed to the virus) is to abstain from intimate contact (e.g., with blood products or sexual intercourse) if they want to decrease their chances for acquiring this deadly disease. *Principle: Rational attempts to treat infection often require a basic understanding of microbial pathogenesis.*

Pathogenesis. Infection of a cell by an infectious virion begins with attachment of the virus particle to cell-surface receptors. The HIV attaches to cells by virtue of high-affinity binding of the virion envelope glycoprotein (gp120) to the host cell-surface receptor glycoprotein (CD4). The CD4 receptors are found on certain subpopulations of T lymphocytes, monocytes, and other cells. After binding, the virion penetrates the cell membrane and loses its coat in the cytoplasm, exposing the genomic RNA. The viral RNA is reverse-transcribed to make DNA and a second complementary strand of DNA to form double-stranded DNA. Viral double-stranded DNA can remain in the cytoplasm as circular, unintegrated episomal DNA or be transported to the nucleus, where a complete genomic copy of viral DNA is integrated into the host cell genome. After integration, infection can be latent with no evidence of active viral replication. Active infection involves transcription of mRNA from genomic viral DNA that results in subsequent translation to yield viral structural or regulatory proteins and viral RNA that is packaged into infectious particles. Posttranslational modification of viral proteins occurs later when the viral particles are assembled and released from the host cell.

Compounds Inhibiting Viral Binding. The HIV binds to susceptible cells by viral gp120–CD4 interaction. A soluble form of CD4 protein was synthesized using recombinant technology and found to inhibit HIV infection of T cells in vitro (Smith et al., 1987). In theory, infectious virions would bind to the soluble circulating CD4 protein and fewer virions would remain to bind to and infect lymphocytes bearing CD4 receptors. Phase I clinical trials of soluble recombinant CD4 have demonstrated virtually no toxicity, except for the development of antibodies to CD4. However, its efficacy at the doses given was difficult to ascertain because only a modest decrease in serum p24 antigenemia occurred at the highest dose administered, and there was no significant change in CD4 counts or immune function (Schooley et al., 1990). This soluble form of CD4 has a relatively short half-life, and IV or IM administration was needed to achieve serum CD4 concentrations that had previously been shown to inhibit HIV in vitro. These pharmacokinetic concerns make administration of the soluble CD4 form problematic on a large-scale basis.

Further development has involved construction of a hybrid CD4 protein that combines the amino terminal binding site of CD4 and the Fc portion of IgG heavy chain. This CD4-Ig complex was also found to have in vitro activity against HIV (Capon et al., 1989). Phase I clinical trials are currently ongoing. Another approach that has shown anti-HIV activity in vitro has been to combine CD4 with cellular toxins such as ricin or *Pseudomonas* exotoxin (Chaudhary et al., 1988; Till et al., 1988). Theoretically and in in vitro experiments, these hybrid CD4 proteins can bind to cells expressing viral gp120 on their surface (virally infected cells) and selectively kill these cells by virtue of the incorporated cellular toxin.

There are a number of other agents that appear to interfere with the binding of HIV to host cells, including dextran sulfate, peptide T, and AL721. Dextran sulfate nonspecifically inhibits HIV binding in vitro. This sulfated anionic polysaccharide can attach to host cells; the resulting negative surface charge inhibits HIV binding by charge repulsion (Mitsuya et al., 1988). However, a small trial of low doses of oral dextran sulfate did not show any clinical efficacy (Abrams et al., 1989). Possibly, insufficient drug was orally bioavailable under these conditions.

Peptide T, an octapeptide with four threonine residues, has in vitro activity in blocking HIV binding to susceptible cells (Pert et al., 1986). Further clinical investigation with this compound is ongoing and is too preliminary to make any conclusions about peptide T's clinical utility (Wetterberg et al., 1987). The compound AL721 is a combination of neutral glycerides, phosphatidyl choline, and phosphatidyl ethanolamine in a molar ratio of 7 : 2 : 1 that inhibits HIV infection in vitro. Its mechanism may be that it alters the lipids and cholesterol of cellular membranes, thereby inhibiting HIV penetration into susceptible host cells (Sarin et al., 1985). As yet, there has been no demonstrated in vivo efficacy with this agent (Grieco et al., 1988). *Principle: Despite the desperate nature of a variety of diseases, including AIDS, it is always prudent to have a great deal of skepticism for claims of drug efficacy based on in vitro data alone. Only the clinical studies that follow in vitro findings can define clinical efficacy and toxicity.*

Inhibition of Reverse Transcription

Nucleoside Analogs. Viral reverse transcription is necessary for HIV RNA to be used as a template to produce viral DNA, which can be integrated into the cellular genome. In order for reverse transcription to take place, deoxynucleotides must be added to the 3′ end of the elongating DNA. A 3′-hydroxyl group is present on the sugar moiety of deoxynucleotides that can form a 3′, 5′-phosphodiester bond allowing further addition of nucleotide triphosphates. Several deoxynucleotide analogs have been synthesized that differ from normal deoxynucleotides in that a substitution of the 3′-hydroxyl group of the sugar moiety (deoxyribose) has been replaced with another molecule (e.g., an azido group in the case of AZT). These 3′ substitutions do not allow addition of further nucleotides, and viral chain termination occurs. The abnormal nucleotides also may compete with normal nucleotides in the process of chain elongation. In order for nucleotide analogs to exert their effect, they must be converted to their active triphosphate forms by cellular kinases. Zidovudine (AZT), a 3′-azidothymidine derivative, is currently the only drug used for HIV therapy approved by the FDA for that indication. Originally synthesized in the early 1960s, it was found to have in vitro anti-HIV activity in 1985 (Mitsuya et al., 1985). Several clinical trials have now been completed that evaluated the efficacy of AZT. In brief, they demonstrate (1) prolonged survival in patients with AIDS and AIDS-related complex (ARC), (2) delayed progression of disease in asymptomatic or early ARC patients with CD4 counts $<500/mm^3$, (3) equal efficacy of a large dose (1200–1500 mg/day) versus half that dose (500–600 mg/day), (4) decreased toxicity in patients receiving half-dose AZT, and (5) clinical improvement in children with symptomatic HIV infection (Fischl et al., 1987, 1990; Pizzo et al., 1988; Volberding et al., 1990). Although clinical improvement has been demonstrated in some patients, others exhibit

progression of the disease while on maintenance therapy with AZT.

Current concerns include the recent observation of AZT-resistant clinical isolates, and increased numbers of AIDS patients developing lymphoma after prolonged (>3 years) AZT therapy. In a small series, patients who had received AZT for greater than 6 months were found to have viral isolates that were resistant to AZT in vitro (Larder et al., 1989). Other investigators have made similar observations. It is interesting that AZT-resistant isolates remain sensitive to other dideoxynucleotides, including dideoxyinosine (ddI) (Bach, 1990). Correlation of AZT resistance with progression of disease, the length of administration of AZT, and the dosage of AZT remains to be determined. The observation that patients taking AZT therapy for prolonged periods develop lymphoma in greater frequency than would be expected in the normal population requires further study. Although the finding is disturbing, the lymphoma might represent the natural history of HIV infection in long-term survivors as opposed to a neoplastic consequence of prolonged nucleoside therapy. Further research is obviously needed and will require a controlled study to determine what is causing the lymphoma (see chapters 34, 35, and 41).

Other dideoxynucleoside analogs that have anti-HIV activity in vitro and are currently in phase II trials include ddI and dideoxycytidine (ddC) (Mitsuya and Broder, 1986). Oral ddC can improve CD4 counts and decrease p24 antigenemia in ARC and AIDS patients. However, dose-related toxicity including mucositis and painful peripheral neuropathy have been observed and attributed to the drug (Lambert et al., 1990). Current studies are assessing weekly or monthly alternating AZT and ddC therapy in an attempt to decrease toxicity and resistance to the drug. In a phase I trial, ddI increased CD4 counts and decreased p24 antigenemia. Toxicity included dose-dependent peripheral neuropathy and pancreatitis. Current trials with ddI and ddC as monotherapy have been designed to compare them with AZT in ARC and AIDS patients, in patients who have been on AZT therapy for greater than 1 year, and in patients who are intolerant to AZT. In addition, clinical trials are being conducted to compare combination therapy (such as AZT plus ddI and AZT plus ddC) to single-agent therapy.

Other Inhibitors. Other inhibitors of reverse transcriptase include phosphonoformate (foscarnet), suramin, heteropolymer-23 (HPA-23), and rifabutin. Foscarnet is an analog of pyrophosphate. In vitro studies have shown its inhibitory activity against viral DNA polymerases from cytomegalovirus (CMV) and reverse transcriptase from HIV. In clinical trials, foscarnet was well tolerated and decreased p24 antigenemia (Bergadahl et al., 1988). However, only an IV preparation is available, which makes long-term administration difficult. Other clinical trials involving foscarnet for HIV-associated CMV retinitis are ongoing. Suramin, which has been used as an antiparasitic agent, was fortuitously found to inhibit HIV reverse transcriptase in vitro. However, clinical trials could not demonstrate any clinical or virologic improvement (Cheson et al., 1987). Additional compounds with in vitro inhibitory activity that have been clinically tested but not found to have clear antiviral efficacy include HPA-23 (Moskovitz et al., 1988), a compound containing antimony and tungsten, and the antimycobacterial agent rifabutin (Torseth et al., 1989).

Late-Stage Inhibition. A number of agents interfere with late-life-cycle states of HIV. These include antisense molecules, ribavirin, interferon-α (IFN-α), glucosidase inhibitors, and protease inhibitors. Antisense oligonucleotides are short synthetic sequences of DNA that are complementary to viral RNA sequences. They can bind to viral RNA and inhibit translation and production of protein. These oligonucleotides can pass through cell membranes and when modified by the addition of phosphoramidates or phosphorothioates can resist destruction by host cellular nuclease (Montefiori and Mitchell, 1987; Agrawal et al., 1988). These oligonucleotides have also been shown to be competitive inhibitors of HIV reverse transcriptase (Liu and Owens, 1987).

Ribavirin, a guanosine analog, has demonstrated some anti-HIV effect in vitro, perhaps by inhibiting the guanylation step required for 5′ capping of viral RNA. Results of clinical trials with this agent have not demonstrated any antiviral efficacy (Spector et al., 1989).

Interferon-α, a protein produced by virally infected leukocytes, has anti-HIV activity in vitro (Ho et al., 1985). The exact mechanism of its activity has not been elucidated; however, IFN-α may block final HIV assembly and budding of mature viral particles at the cell surface. It may also have a role in inhibiting protein translation. Clinical trials of IFN-α in HIV-infected patients primarily have involved treatment of Kaposi sarcoma. There is evidence that IFN-α can reduce p24 antigenemia (Lane et al., 1990) and that synergy with AZT exists in vitro (Hartshorn et al., 1987). A clinical trial has shown that AZT administered in combination with IFN-α to AIDS patients with Kaposi sarcoma could be tolerated, but that dose-limiting toxicity was present at higher doses of interferon. Evidence of virologic improvement was observed in some patients (Kovacs et al., 1989).

Prior to viral assembly and release, many viral proteins must be glycosylated. However, more sugars are added than are necessary, and some must be removed prior to release. Cellular glycosidases, primarily α-glycosidase 1, are responsible for cleaving the terminal sugars on the HIV envelop glycoprotein prior to its release. Compounds such as castanospermine and N-butyldeoxynojirimycin (N-butyl DNJ) are cellular glucosidase inhibitors that have demonstrated antiviral activity in vitro (Walker et al., 1987; Gruters et al., 1987). Perhaps inhibition of glucosidase would result in an excess of terminal sugar moieties on the envelope glycoprotein. This could interfere with HIV gp120 binding to the host CD4 molecule, resulting in reduced infectivity of the virus. Clinical trials are currently underway to assess the antiviral efficacy of these compounds.

Finally, other compounds such as tricosanthin (GLQ-223, or compound Q) (McGrath et al., 1989), N-acetylcysteine (NAC) (Roederer et al., 1990), and HIV protease inhibitors (Grinde et al., 1989) have been reported to have anti-HIV activity in vitro. Clinical trials with these agents are currently in progress; until such studies are completed, our knowledge of the clinical efficacy and toxicity of these compounds remains incomplete.

Immunomodulation. In addition to specific agents targeted against HIV, attempts have been made to either restore or augment the host's immune function. Interleukin-2 (IL-2) is a glycoprotein product of T cells. Production of this cytokine results in proliferation of circulating T cells and activation of natural killer (NK) cells. The IV administration of IL-2 to HIV-infected patients had no efficacy, with the exception of some improvement in NK-cell function and T-cell response to antigens (Ernst et al., 1986). Isoprinosine, an immune enhancer, has some mild intrinsic antiviral activity. However, in vitro data have shown that it increases T-cell proliferation and IL-2 production (Fischbach and Talal, 1985). A clinical trial that was recently completed demonstrated delayed progression to AIDS in a select and limited patient population of ARC patients (Pedersen et al., 1990).

Bone marrow transplantation was reported to be effective in one patient who had received concomitant AZT (Holland et al., 1989). Even with the use of the polymerase chain reaction (PCR), HIV could not be detected posttransplantation in this patient. However, the patient developed a malignancy and died a short time after the transplant. Furthermore, the results of bone marrow transplantation on a small series indicate that it is not effective for curing AIDS (Lane et al., 1990).

The use of IV immunoglobulin to treat HIV disease is being explored. Evidence for efficacy in pediatric patients with HIV comes from one small, uncontrolled trial with only a short follow-up. It may have demonstrated a decrease in mortality and concomitant bacterial infections (Calvelli and Rubenstein, 1986). In a trial including adult patients with AIDS, the administration of an enriched p24 immunoglobulin preparation from pooled sera of asymptomatic infected patients demonstrated a decrease in p24 antigenemia and cell-free virus from plasma (Jackson et al., 1988). Finally, experimental treatment modalities such as extracorporeal hyperthermia and photopheresis are currently being explored. *Principle: Procedures that can be feasibly performed* **must** *be evaluated for efficacy as well as drugs need to be before their routine use can be condoned.*

Combination Therapy. Although many individual compounds have demonstrated good in vitro and some in vivo anti-HIV activity when used alone, therapeutic failures are common. The concepts of synergism of antibiotics can be used as a model, and it is reasonable to test the prediction that compounds that inhibit the HIV replicative cycle might exhibit additive or synergistic effects in vitro and in vivo. Combination therapy for HIV disease potentially could affect different stages of viral replication. If these drugs had different toxicities, it might be possible to use lower doses of each individual compound while maintaining antiviral activity, suppressing the emergence of resistant viral strains, or potentiating immunomodulatory effects. Most combination regimens that are being studied involve administering AZT with other compounds. Additive or synergistic in vitro activity with AZT has been observed with acyclovir, IFN-α, CD4, and *N*-butyl-DNJ (Mitsuya and Broder, 1986; Johnson et al., 1989a, 1989b). In vitro synergistic activity has also been observed with ddC and IFN-α (Vogt et al., 1988). The combination of AZT, CD4, and IFN-α shows synergism (Johnson et al., 1990), and AZT in combination with acyclovir may be useful. Although acyclovir has no intrinsic activity against HIV, the herpesviruses may be a cofactor that could potentiate HIV infection. Some clinical improvement was observed when AZT and acyclovir were administered in combination (Surbone et al., 1988). As stated earlier, clinical studies of ddI plus AZT and ddC plus AZT are currently in progress as well as AZT in combination with interferon α and IL-2 and CD4. *Principle: Hypothetical value of therapeutics can be attractive but should not be compelling before evidence of efficacy or toxicity is demonstrated. The need to "do something" in desperate medical settings does not justify hopeful but indiscriminate and potentially dangerous therapeutic decisions.*

Vaccine Strategies. Historically, administration of a vaccine for viral diseases (e.g., polio) has resulted in effective immunity in the host against a specific viral agent. But HIV presents complicated problems in this regard. Many strains of HIV have been isolated, and distinct subtypes can be isolated from a single individual (Saag et al., 1988). Much of the variation is located in a hypervariable region of the envelope glycoprotein (viz., gp160) (Hahn et al., 1985). Neutralizing antibody that is produced during infection with HIV is directed primarily against viral gp120, but the antibody is produced in low concentrations in most patients (Robert-Guroff et al., 1985; Ho et al., 1987). Most of the current efforts at developing a vaccine involve preparations of envelope gp120 or gp160 subunits that are either recombinant, native, or synthetic proteins. These proteins either are administered with an adjuvant to enhance immunogenicity or are inserted into other viruses such as vaccinia that can serve as a vector (Hu et al., 1986). Inactivated whole virus also is being studied as a vaccine with the hope that immunogenicity can be retained despite inactivation. Phase I clinical trials of recombinant gp160 vaccines in HIV-seropositive patients are currently in progress. It will be remarkable if these patients can mount an immune response to the vaccine that will be sufficient to prevent or reverse the disease. Based on our experience with vaccines used in other diseases, the most effective HIV vaccine probably will require administration to individuals prior to their acquisition of the infection. *Principle: Therapeutic options for the patients with AIDS are extremely expensive, complicated, and controversial; they should not be based on limited in vitro data or anecdotal experiences. Management of these patients is best served by participation in national clinical trials that evaluate new experimental therapy for this deadly disease, or providing therapy such as AZT that has been critically proved to be of value for specific subsets of patients.*

Management of the Febrile Neutropenic Patient

Consideration of treatment of the febrile neutropenic patient includes a brief summary of risk factors, organisms responsible for the disease, workup and management of a patient with respect to antimicrobial therapy, and immunoenhancement. Many clinical disease entities can cause a spectrum of immune suppression, and solid and hematologic tumors vary with respect to the degree of immune suppression they produce. We limit this discussion to acute leukemia and the infectious complications that occur following chemotherapy-induced neutropenia.

Risk Factors. Neutropenia is defined as an absolute neutrophil count (ANC) that is less than 1000 cells/μl. As the count falls below 1000/μl, the risk of infection increases (Bodey et al., 1966). Although the degree and rate of fall of neutropenia are important determinants of infection, the duration of profound neutropenia (ANC of < 100 cells/μl) directly predicts the development of infection. Development of infection approaches 100% if profound neutropenia persists for 3 weeks or longer (Bodey et al., 1978). Initial induction of antitumor therapy produces a period of prolonged neutropenia and subjects the patient to the greatest risk of infection. If an infection develops, its successful outcome is determined in large part by recovery of the neutrophil count and not by the choice of antimicrobials. In addition to purely quantitative decreases, neutrophils may have qualitative defects that impair their function. The latter may be the result of premature release of the cells from the marrow secondary to invasion of the marrow by tumor or intrinsic killing defects caused by cytotoxic agents, irradiation, or antimicrobial therapy.

A number of cell lines can be markedly affected by the same insults. Profound lymphopenia results in decreased cell- and antibody-mediated immunity. Other important risk factors for development of infection include disruption of the skin and mucosal barriers secondary to the effects of chemotherapeutic agents or malnutrition, splenectomy, alteration of endogenous microbial flora secondary to antimicrobial prophylaxis or colonization with nosocomial-acquired organisms, the presence of an indwelling catheter, and exposure to health care workers, air, water, food, and supportive equipment found in the hospital (e.g., ventilators, etc.).

Organisms Causing Infection. The types of organisms causing infection have changed over time, largely because of antimicrobial prophylaxis and therapy. Prior to such therapy, the predominant organisms that caused infections were aerobic gram-positive bacteria (e.g., frequently *S. aureus*). With the introduction of effective antistaphylococcal penicillins and cephalosporins and their regular use as empiric therapy in neutropenic patients, the incidence of gram-positive bacterial infections was reduced. However, an increase in gram-negative bacterial infections was subsequently noted, caused by *E. coli*, *Pseudomonas aeruginosa*, and *Klebsiella* species. Because of the high mortality associated with infection caused by these organisms, early intervention with broad-spectrum antibacterial agents at the first sign of fever became routine. This practice has greatly improved survival and led to a decrease in mortality rates for infections caused by these organisms.

Most recently, gram-positive bacterial organisms including *S. aureus* and *S. epidermidis*, viridans streptococci, JK diphtheroid and *Enterococcus* species have again become major pathogens (O'Hanley et al., 1989). This change occurred primarily because of the placement of indwelling IV catheters (Press et al., 1984). In addition, antimicrobial prophylaxis and the reduction in use of specific antistaphylococcal agents as first-line therapy may also have contributed to the change. Fungal organisms such as *Candida* species and *Aspergillus* species have emerged as significant pathogens as well.

Organisms that cause infection in these patients can come from a newly acquired nosocomial pathogen, the patient's endogenous flora, or reactivation of latent organisms such as herpesviruses. The majority of organisms found to cause infection in neutropenic patients were from the patient's flora that was modified by antibiotic treatment (Schimpff et al., 1972). Although some generalizations can be made with respect to which organisms cause infections in neutropenic patients, the clinician should learn about the specific flora found in a given hospital, the organisms that are most frequently isolated from febrile neutropenic patients in that hospital, and the antimicrobial sensitivity and resistance patterns of these organisms. *Principle: Empirical treatment of immunocompromised patients requires that the practitioner know the local epidemiology of infectious diseases, their complications, and the susceptibility patterns for nosocomial pathogens.*

Investigation and Management. A temperature of more than 100°F (38°C) is usually defined as a medically important fever and when observed in neutropenic patients should signal a search for infection. Because of the neutropenia, an inflammatory response may not be evident and fever may be the only clue that infection is present. Infected neutropenic patients with lung infections may have normal chest x-ray films, and they may or may not be able to produce purulent sputum. Infected skin may not show signs of cellulitis or abscess. A careful physical examination can help to define a source of infection. Particular attention should be paid to the retinal fundi and mucocutaneous sites such as the nasooropharynx and perirectal areas—common sites that can reveal evidence of infection. In most patients no obvious source of infection is evident. Therefore appropriate cultures of blood, urine, skin lesions, throat, stool, sputum, or CSF must be obtained. Radiologic examination of the chest, sinuses, and teeth may be helpful in defining a site of infection. Unless the physical examination or x-ray films reveal a specific site of infection to guide specific antimicrobial therapy, the initiation of empirical broad-spectrum antimicrobial therapy must begin as soon as suspicion is serious (Young, 1981).

Empirical Antimicrobial Therapy. Many studies have examined the effects of single-agent versus combination therapy as empirical regimens to treat the febrile neutropenic patient. These studies have provided information on when to initiate therapy for gram-positive bacterial organisms and fungi agents, how to modify therapy and its duration, how to treat the persistently febrile patient, and when adjunct therapy such as granulocyte transfusions or monoclonal antiendotoxin antibody infusion might be of value.

Broad-spectrum combination therapy that includes an antipseudomonal β-lactam antibiotic (e.g., mezlocillin, azlocillin, pipericillin, or ceftazidime) and an aminoglycoside (e.g., gentamicin, or tobramycin) is recommended by many investigators. Because gram-negative bacterial organisms such as *Pseudomonas* species can be associated with rapid mortality, a potentially synergistic combination regimen is attractive. Such combinations provide broader empirical coverage than does therapy with only one agent. Gram-negative coverage and moderate gram-positive coverage is usually required. The choice of which agents to use depends on the most common pathogens and their patterns of antimicrobial resistance in a given hospital.

Aminoglycosides have the potential disadvantage of causing nephrotoxicity and ototoxicity, and concentrations in plasma must be monitored. Aminoglycosides should not be used as monotherapy because of insufficient efficacy (Bodey, 1984). Initial empirical monotherapy with agents such as imipenem, ceftazidime, or ticarcillin-clavulanic acid produces adequate efficacy without the toxicities associated with aminoglycosides (Anaissie et al., 1988). Interpreting the results of these studies is not simple because "adequate clinical response" may not be defined and certainly is different between studies (e.g., some focus on overall clinical outcome or death vs. survival while others note the development of an infection or the necessity to change or add an antimicrobial agent as failure). In many of these studies, no organism was identified, yet response was defined as resolution of fever.

None of the extended-spectrum penicillins or third-generation cephalosporins provide excellent coverage for gram-positive bacteria, especially staphylococci. A major issue in empirical regimens involves the addition of an agent to specifically provide coverage for gram-positive cocci. Although a majority of infections in neutropenic patients are caused by gram-positive organisms, the morbidity and mortality of infection with these organisms is markedly less than those of infections caused by gram-negative bacilli. A recent retrospective review concluded that the addition of vancomycin as an initial empirical agent is not necessary. Although more gram-positive infections were noted in the group of patients who did not receive vancomycin initially, successful treatment of documented infections caused by gram-positive organisms was equal whether vancomycin was instituted initially or delayed (Rubin et al., 1988). However, if the febrile episode is likely the result of an infectious focus by gram-positive organisms (e.g., an infected indwelling IV catheter), then the early empirical use of vancomycin would seem prudent and warranted.

Most investigators agree that since the majority of infections found initially in the febrile neutropenic patient are bacterial, the early use of antifungal agents is not warranted. Most patients respond to empirical antibacterial therapy within a week. By this time several issues may have become clear. The infecting organism may be identified; the neutrophil count may begin to rise; the organism may be identified but the infection may fail to respond; a site of infection may be identified but no organism is identified; or no site of infection may be isolated or organism identified and the patient may still be febrile, possibly indicating fungal infection. If no source or organism is identified, it appears prudent to withhold antifungal treatment until 3 to 7 days of empirical antibacterial therapy has been completed because some patients may have bacterial infections that are slow to respond.

Fungal infections are extremely difficult to diagnose, but initiation of empirical therapy may prevent dissemination. Once the decision is made to initiate empirical antifungal therapy with amphotericin B, the duration of therapy is a matter of some controversy. Some investigators believe that empirical antifungal therapy should be continued until neutropenia resolves. Others continue antifungal therapy based on the clinical response. If a fungal source is identified, a standard course of antifungal treatment would be continued. The experience with the imidazoles or newer triazoles in empirical antifungal therapy is limited. If the patient continues to be febrile and neutropenic despite an antibacterial and antifungal regimen, then the antifungal agent might be discontinued pending reevaluation.

The duration of empirical antibacterial therapy is controversial. If the patient becomes afebrile while receiving an empirical regimen but remains neutropenic, treatment is continued until the patient has been afebrile for several days. If fever returns, then another workup should be initiated and empirical antimicrobial therapy should be resumed. Prolonging antibacterial therapy without identifying a source of infection actually may lead to increased morbidity as resistant organisms or fungal superinfection occur (DiNubile, 1988). Discontinuation of antibacterial agents while the patient is still neutropenic and febrile can result in increased morbidity and mortality, which are primarily related to the development of fungal infections (Pizzo et al., 1982). A subset of patients in whom there is no clinical or laboratory evidence of infection may remain febrile and neutropenic, but such patients should have their antibiotics discontinued (Joshi et al., 1984). Other causes of fever such as the underlying disease or drug fever may be operative in these patients.

The above discussion has revolved around empirical therapy for the neutropenic patient with fever but with no identified site of infection or identified pathogen. After empirical therapy has been initiated, modification of a regimen may be necessary based on subsequent clinical developments. For example, if perianal tenderness, abdominal pain, necrotizing gingivitis, or mucositis occurs, anaerobic organisms may be involved in these clinical conditions, and anaerobic coverage should be added. In general, antimicrobial therapy should not be directed toward anaerobes unless they are cultured from the blood or there is obvious loss of the integrity of the mucosal barrier.

Radiologic evidence of diffuse interstitial pneumonitis may indicate infection with *Pneumocystis carinii* or *Legionella* species. If so, a trial of trimethoprim-sulfamethoxazole or erythromycin, respectively, could be initiated. New pulmonary infiltrates or lesions developing while the patient is receiving antibacterial therapy could indicate pulmonary fungal infection. In such cases, a biopsy (either percutaneous or open) of the pulmonary lesion should be attempted. If the patient is unable to tolerate these procedures, empirical antifungal therapy should be initiated.

Finally, if an organism was found initially but breakthrough bacteremia has occurred, the regimen should be modified to include a antibacterial agent not having cross-resistance.

Prospective studies of the use of granulocyte transfusions have shown improved survival in patients who remained neutropenic and were not adequately responding to antimicrobial therapy (Alavi et al., 1977). However, prophylactic granulocyte transfusions during induction chemotherapy have not shown efficacy. For this therapeutic option to be successful, it is necessary that adequate numbers of transfused granulocytes be administered for at least 4 days (Bodey, 1984). The use of immunoglobulins as adjuvant therapy has benefits only in those with chronic lymphocytic leukemia. Hyperimmune pooled serum containing high titers of antibody to the J5 mutant of *E. coli* has been administered to neutropenic patients without any clear benefit (Ziegler et al., 1982). Clinical trials are in progress to evaluate the efficacy of antiendotoxin antibody preparations in the prevention and treatment of bacterial infections.

Management of Suppurative Bacterial Meningitis

Central nervous system infections, especially suppurative meningitis, frequently are life-threatening and generally constitute medical emergencies that require accurate and prompt treatment. [Portions of this section about meningitis have previously been published (Swartz and O'Hanley, 1987) and permitted by the publisher, American Scientific Medicine, New York.] Fortunately, advances in methods of diagnosis and treatment developed during the past 10 years have significantly improved the prognosis associated with many of these illnesses. New diagnostic methods supplement rather than supplant CSF studies. The CSF studies frequently provide important initial information needed for clinical and microbiologic diagnosis; when not definitive, they serve at least to focus the differential diagnosis. New chemotherapeutic agents, both antibacterial (e.g., the third-generation cephalosporins) and antiviral (e.g., acyclovir), are directly responsible for this improvement. The use of adjunctive therapy with glucocorticoids may lessen some of the pathophysiologic consequences of bacterial meningitis (Tunkel et al., 1990).

This section discusses a number of crucial steps and decisions that must be made by the practitioner in order to provide rational therapy of patients with suppurative bacterial meningitis. Similar decisions must be made by the clinician to rationally treat other infectious diseases. There is always a need for accurate initial diagnosis based on the history and physical exam; confirmation of the diagnosis by use of definitive diagnostic tests; understanding of the epidemiology and natural course of the illness; selection of the best of the available therapeutic options; and choice of appropriate end points of efficacy and toxicity to be followed.

Etiologic Agents. The identity of the bacterial agent in pyogenic meningitis frequently is suspected on the basis of epidemiologic and clinical clues. The first and perhaps the most important clue is a patient's age, since there are striking correlations between the common types of bacterial meningitis and the age groups they afflict. Three fourths of the estimated 25,000 new cases of bacterial meningitis that occur annually in the United States develop in children younger than 12 years (Tauber and Sande, 1984). The principal bacteria responsible for neonatal meningitis are gram-negative bacilli (usually *E. coli* strains bearing the K1 capsular antigen) and group B streptococci (McCracken and Mize, 1976). *Hemophilus influenzae* type b meningitis is the most common form of bacterial meningitis in children and mainly affects those who are 2 months to 3 years of age. The appearance of *H. influenzae* meningitis in adults is so unusual that its presence suggests predisposing anatomic or immunologic defects that have permitted circumvention of the barrier normally provided by serum bactericidal mechanisms. The bacterial agents that most frequently cause bacterial meningitis in adults are *S. pneumoniae* and *N. meningitidis*.

Other bacteria infrequently cause meningitis. *Listeria monocytogenes* is the rare pathogen in the neonate. Its involvement in adult cases has been increasing primarily among those who are immunosuppressed or elderly (Chernik et al., 1973). Isolation of an anaerobic organism from the CSF is rare and strongly suggests intraventricular leakage of a brain abscess or the presence of a parameningeal focus of infection. *Staphylococcus aureus* meningitis is associated with neurosurgical procedures, penetrating cranial trauma, staphylococcal bacteremia and endocarditis, immunosuppressive therapy, and underlying neoplastic disease. Meningitis complicating ventriculoatrial or ventriculoperitoneal shunting procedures is usually caused by *S. aureus* or *S. epidermidis*. Gram-negative bacillary meningitis (caused by *E. coli, Enterobacter, Klebsiella, Proteus, Serratia*, or *Pseudomonas* species) usually is a nosocomial infection and affects neurosurgical, immunosuppressed, and oncologic patients, the elderly, and neonates (Chernik et al., 1973; Nieman and Lorber, 1980; Rahal, 1980).

A specific bacterial agent cannot be identified in 5% to 10% of patients with pyogenic meningitis. Simultaneous mixed meningitis is rare and is found most often in neonates, particularly in association with a neuroectodermal defect, and occasionally in older patients following a penetrating head injury. Therefore, the common rule is that suppurative bacterial meningitis is caused by a single aerobic bacterial pathogen. Broad-spectrum antimicrobials usually are not indicated for this infectious disease. *Principle: The epidemiology of bacterial meningitis, like that of many other infections, is highly age-related. To treat properly, the practitioner must be aware of the common bacterial pathogens associated with suppurative meningitis in each age group.*

Pathogenesis. Pathogenic organisms may enter the meninges in several ways: (1) from the bloodstream during systemic bacteremia, (2) by penetration directly from the upper respiratory tract (skull fracture, congenital dural defect, or eroding sequestrum in mastoid), or from the body surface (neuroectodermal defect), (3) through intracranial passage via nasopharyngeal venules, (4) by direct spread from an adjacent focus of infection (sinusitis or intraventricular leakage of a brain abscess), or (5) by introduction of organisms at the time of a neurosurgical operation. Bacteremia is the most frequent source of infection. Organisms often are demonstrable in the bloodstream in the very early stages of the three most common types of bacterial meningitis beyond the neonatal period: those caused by *H. influenzae, N. meningitidis*, and *S. pneumoniae* (Swartz and Dodge, 1965). Once meningeal infection becomes established, it quickly extends throughout the subarachnoid space. Ventriculitis can be demonstrated at the time of admission in at least 70% of neonates who are diagnosed as having meningitis (McCracken et al., 1980).

Clinical Features. Most cases of *H. influenzae, N. meningitidis*, and *S. pneumoniae* meningitis are preceded by upper respiratory tract infection, otitis media, or pneumonia. The onset is usually sudden and progresses over the course of 24 to 36 hours with fever, generalized headache, vomiting, and stiff neck. Myalgias (particularly in meningococcal disease) and backache are common. Once meningitic signs are evident, the infection progresses rapidly, producing confusion, obtundation, and ultimately coma. Indications of leptomeningeal inflammation (drowsiness, stiff neck, and Kernig and Brudzinski signs) are generally present. The usual manifestations of meningitis may be partially obscured in an elderly person who has underlying congestive heart failure or pneumonia and is obtunded and hypoxic. Similarly, a neonate with meningitis may have decreased appetite, fever, irritability, lassitude, and vomiting but may not always exhibit either stiff neck or bulging fontanelles. Such patients should be examined carefully for meningitic signs; if any question about the presence of meningitis remains in such cases, a lumbar puncture must be performed to obtain CSF for examinations.

Certain clinical conditions are predisposing factors for specific types of bacterial meningitis. The conditions that predispose a person to pneumococcal meningitis include acute otitis media and mastoiditis. These entities precede 30% of cases of meningitis. In adult patients, pneumonia precedes 10% to 25%; nonpenetrating head injury precedes 5% to 10%; CSF rhinorrhea or otorrhea precedes 5%; and in adults, alcoholism and cirrhosis of the liver precede 10% to 25% of cases with pneumococcal meningitis in urban hospitals. Sickle cell anemia, defects in host defenses such as congenital or acquired immunoglobulin deficiencies, asplenic states, and acute sinusitis occasionally precede meningitis.

A number of neurologic findings and complications accompany bacterial meningitis. They include cranial nerve dysfunction (especially third, fourth, sixth, and seventh nerves), focal cerebral signs (hemiparesis, dysphasia, and hemianopsia), focal and generalized seizures, and acute cerebral edema, ultimately leading to death.

The presence of skin lesions may assist the physician in arriving at a diagnosis. A maculopetechial or purpuric rash in a patient with meningitis usually signifies meningococcal infection. Infrequently, petechial and purpuric skin lesions develop in the course of *S. pneumoniae* bacteremia and meningitis, reflecting disseminated intravascular coagulation. Multiple skin lesions almost identical to those observed in patients with meningococcemia occur rarely in patients with acute *S. aureus* endocarditis. Meningitic signs and a CSF neutrophilic pleocytosis also may develop in such patients and are caused by embolic cerebral infarction rather than by bacterial meningitis. The maculopetechial rash of echovirus aseptic meningitis (particularly type 9 that has been responsible for extensive outbreaks) may be mistaken for the rash of meningococcal meningitis. This type of viral meningitis may produce an early and marked CSF neutrophilic pleocytosis. The rash in meningococcal meningitis may involve the face and neck but only after it has already extensively covered other parts of the body; in echovirus type 9 meningeal infection, the rash involves the face and neck early in the course of the exanthem before other parts of the body are significantly involved.

Laboratory Features. The CSF cell count in the majority of patients with untreated bacterial meningitis ranges from 100 to 5000 cells/μl, of which more than 80% are neutrophils. Cell counts of 50,000 cells/μl or higher are occasionally observed in primary bacterial meningitis, but such a marked pleocytosis also suggests the possibility of intraventricular rupture of a cerebral abscess. More than half of patients with bacterial meningitis have glucose concentrations of 40 mg/dl or lower in their CSF (<50%–60% of the simultaneous fasting blood glucose concentration). A normal CSF glucose concentration, however, still is consistent with a diagnosis of bacterial meningitis. The primary importance of the CSF determination of glucose is not in aiding the diagnosis of the typical case of acute pyogenic meningitis (which usually can be diagnosed on the basis of the Gram-stained smear of the CSF and the CSF cell count). Rather, the CSF glucose concentration is most useful in distinguishing chronic meningitides (such as those that are caused by *Listeria*, *Nocardia*, *Actinomyces*, *Cryptococcus*, or *Coccidioides*) marked by hypoglycorrhachia from parameningeal infections and viral aseptic meningitides, which do not lower CSF glucose concentrations (Peacock et al., 1984).

Patients with bacterial meningitis usually have CSF protein concentrations higher than 120 mg/dl (normal is 30–40 mg/dl). Occasionally, values of 1000 mg/dl or greater are observed, suggesting actual or impending subarachnoid block secondary to meningitis.

Definitive diagnosis requires isolation of the causative organism or demonstration of its characteristic antigen. The implicated bacterium can be demonstrated on a CSF Gram-stained smear in about 80% of patients with bacterial meningitis. The bacteria that are most likely to be missed on Gram stain are meningococci and *Listeria* species organisms (Sande and Tierney, 1984). Bacteremia is demonstrable in 80% of patients with *H. influenzae* meningitis, 50% with pneumococcal meningitis, and 30% to 40% with *N. meningitidis* meningitis (Swartz and Dodge, 1965). Cultures of CSF and blood yield enough information to permit determination of the bacterial cause in about 90% of patients with bacterial meningitis. *Principle: Definitive diagnostic studies are mandatory in any life-threatening disease. They confirm the clinical diagnosis, and the data derived from these tests provide rational guidelines for therapy.*

The three most common bacterial meningitides (those caused by *H. influenzae*, *N. meningitidis*, and *S. pneumoniae*) are associated with mean CSF bacterial concentrations ranging from 10^5 to 10^7 organisms per milliliter (Feldman, 1977). This concentration of organisms introduces envelope polysaccharide antigens into the CSF in amounts sufficient to be detectable by counterimmunoelectrophoresis (CIE) and the latex agglutination test. These procedures have been used most extensively in the rapid diagnosis (i.e., 1–2 hours) of *H. influenzae* meningitis. In addition, CIE has been helpful in the rapid diagnosis of pneumococcal and meningococcal (groups A, B, C, and Y) meningitis, and it can be used to detect *E. coli* K1 capsular antigen and group B streptococcal antigen in neonatal meningitis.

The bacterial capsular antigens of the three common etiologic agents in primary bacterial meningitis can be successfully identified in 60% to 80% of cases (Finch and Wilkinson, 1979; McCracken, 1976). The reliability of these immunoprecipitation techniques depends heavily on the activity of the antisera employed. False-positive results occasionally arise from cross-reactions. For example, certain *E. coli* capsular antigens cross-react with antisera to *H. influenzae* type B and group B meningococcal antigens. Because in about 90% of patients with bacterial meningitis the bacterial cause can be established by more traditional microbiologic means, CIE is not essential for diagnosis. It serves as an important adjunct, however, permitting early diagnosis in patients in whom no organisms are seen on smear or in whom cultures remain negative because of prior therapy with antibiotics. Even in cases in which the morphology of the organism is revealed by Gram-stained smears, CIE is useful because it permits definitive identification of the agent.

Radiologic Studies. Roentgenograms of the chest, sinuses, and mastoids should be performed at an appropriate time following institution of antimicrobial therapy for suspected pyogenic meningitis; infections in these areas are frequently associated with meningitis.

When history, clinical setting, or physical findings suggest the presence of a suppurative intracranial collection, such as a brain abscess or subdural empyema, CT scanning should be performed without delay. It is not appropriate or necessary to routinely perform a CT or radionuclide scan to exclude these diagnostic entities when the practitioner is confident of the diagnosis of uncomplicated suppurative meningitis. Meningitis itself induces the following changes on the CT scan: contrast enhancement of the leptomeninges and ventricular lining; widening of the subarachnoid space; and patchy areas of diminished density in the cerebrum from cerebritis and necrosis (Weisberg, 1980; Stovring and Snyder, 1980). In addition, CT scanning may be helpful in evaluating the patient with a prolonged or deteriorating clinical status and in detecting suspected complications, such as sterile subdural collections or empyema, ventricular enlargement secondary to communicating or obstructive hydrocephalus, ventriculitis or ventricular empyema (as revealed by ventricular wall enhancement), or cerebral infarction caused by arteritis or cortical vein thrombophlebitis.

Differential Diagnosis of Suppurative Bacterial Meningitis. Because the clinical features of bacterial meningitis (headache, fever, stiff neck, and obtundation) may be seen in other types of CNS infectious diseases, findings in the CSF are important in the development of an appropriate differential diagnosis. Particular attention should be given to the patient with meningitic signs but an atypical neutrophilic CSF pleocytosis, normal CSF glucose concentrations, or absence of organisms in a Gram-stain smear of the CSF. The differential diagnosis in such cases includes several treatable diseases that require management that is different from that of bacterial pyogenic meningitis. A parameningeal bacterial infection such as an epidural abscess, a subdural empyema, or a brain abscess might be suspected in a patient with these findings who also has a chronic ear, sinus, or lung infection. Isolation of anaerobic organisms from the CSF is highly suggestive of para-

meningeal infection. Anaerobes may enter the CSF via intraventricular leakage of a cerebral abscess, through extension of infection from a focus of osteomyelitis, or from an epidural abscess. Focal cerebral signs may be an indication of a space-occupying intracranial infection; they also may appear during the course of bacterial meningitis as a result of occlusive vascular injury. When focal cerebral signs develop, the history should be reviewed for any neurologic symptoms antedating the onset of the acute meningitis.

Bacterial endocarditis may present with prominent symptoms of meningitis and a pleocytosis in the CSF. This presentation is the result either of frank meningitis caused by pyogenic organisms or of sterile embolic cerebral infarctions produced by normally nonpyogenic organisms, such as *Streptococcus viridans*. Careful auscultation for cardiac murmurs and a search for peripheral signs of endocarditis (petechiae, splenomegaly, or Osler nodes) and echocardiography should be performed.

Most patients with pneumococcal, meningococcal, or *H. influenzae* meningitis become afebrile within 2 to 5 days of the start of appropriate antibiotic therapy. Occasionally, fever continues beyond 8 to 10 days or recurs after having disappeared. Prolonged or recurrent fever accompanied by headache, focal cerebral signs, and obtundation suggests that antimicrobial therapy has been inadequate; another possibility is that a neurologic complication such as cortical vein thrombophlebitis, ventriculitis, ventricular empyema, subdural effusion, or subdural empyema has developed. Reevaluation of the findings in the CSF, including Gram-stain smears and cultures, is essential. Persistent fever in a patient whose clinical course and CSF findings show progressive improvement may be indicative of drug fever.

General Aspects of Antibiotic Treatment. Most antibiotics employed in the therapy of bacterial meningitis, with the exception of chloramphenicol, do not readily penetrate the noninflamed blood–brain barrier. Meningitis enhances the entry of penicillins and some other antimicrobial agents (e.g., vancomycin) into the CSF and allows successful therapy with these drugs provided large parenteral doses are administered. Antibiotics should be administered IV in divided doses at intervals that provide high concentration gradients across the meninges. Dosage should not be decreased when clinical improvement occurs, because the normalization of the blood–brain barrier that accompanies resolution of the infection reduces attainable antibiotic concentrations in the CSF. *Principle: Clinicians should become aware of factors in the dynamics of a disease that affect a therapeutic decision.*

The absence of intrinsic opsonic and bactericidal activity in infected CSF increases the importance of providing bactericidal rather than bacteriostatic agents to treat bacterial meningitis (Simberkoff et al., 1980). Although they are effective in vitro against many species that are capable of causing meningitis, drugs such as clindamycin, erythromycin, and first- and most second-generation cephalosporins (including cefamandole) should never be used in bacterial meningitis. These agents cannot predictably achieve bactericidal concentrations in the CSF. Vancomycin, a microbistatic agent, should also not be routinely used in the treatment of bacterial meningitis. It should be reserved for treatment of methicillin-resistant staphylococcal infections.

Intrathecal therapy is not needed to treat uncomplicated cases of the three most common types of bacterial meningitis, since they can be treated with penicillins and chloramphenicol that enter the CSF in bactericidal quantities. Adjunctive intrathecal therapy with an aminoglycoside is often employed to treat meningitis caused by resistant enteric gram-negative bacilli, *P. aeruginosa*, or enterococci.

The patient's clinical course dictates the frequency needed for examination of the CSF. Repeat examination should be performed 24 to 48 hours after the start of antibiotic therapy if progress seems unsatisfactory or if the cause of the meningitis remains uncertain. Meningococcal meningitis should be treated until the patient remains afebrile for 5 to 7 days. With prompt and satisfactory response to antibiotics, it may not be necessary to repeat the examination of the CSF at the end of the therapy. Patients with *H. influenzae* meningitis should be treated for at least 7 days after they have become afebrile. Again, a follow-up examination of the CSF may not be necessary in patients who show rapid and complete clinical recovery. Patients with pneumococcal meningitis should be treated for 10 to 14 days. Discontinuation of antibiotic therapy is contingent on the presence of fewer than 50 to 75 cells/μl in the CSF, mostly mononuclear cells, on repeat examination. Prolonged therapy is necessary in the presence of an underlying mastoiditis or if the patient has underlying immunosuppression (e.g., neutrophil or B- or T-cell abnormalities or deficiencies).

Specific Antimicrobial Therapy. Bacterial meningitis is a life-threatening medical emergency that requires prompt therapy based on examination of the Gram-stained smear from the sediment of the CSF. A serious but common error in managing a patient with suspected meningitis is to delay performing a diagnostic lumbar puncture and starting antibiotic therapy. If clinical assessment does not suggest the presence of an intracranial mass lesion, lumbar puncture should not be delayed until a head CT scan has been completed. Whether a CT scan is necessary or not, antibiotic therapy should *never* be delayed in cases of suspected bacterial meningitis. This is unfortunately the most common mistake made by practitioners in the treatment of bacterial meningitis. When imaging studies are needed to exclude an intracranial mass before a lumbar puncture is performed, antibiotics should be initiated immediately after blood has been obtained for culture.

The choice of antibiotics depends on the suspected pathogen (Table 24–21) and that which ultimately is isolated (Table 24–22). The scan and the lumbar puncture may be done while the patient is receiving empirical therapy. If a diagnostic lumbar puncture is performed after a mass lesion has been excluded by CT scan and the Gram stain reveals bacterial types not covered by the initial empirical therapy, the regimen can be appropriately altered. Animal models of meningitis suggest that initial empirical therapy will not affect the subsequent results of culture of CSF if the spinal fluid is sampled within 2 to 3 hours of the start of antibiotic therapy (Tauber and Sande, 1984).

Clinical studies suggest that optimal chemotherapy for bacterial meningitis requires the CSF concentration of the antibiotic to be severalfold greater (>10 times) than the MBC for the pathogen measured in vitro. Additional principles that should guide therapy for meningitis include the following: (1) the antibiotic must be capable of killing the pathogen, (2) the pathogen must be shown to be highly susceptible to the selected antibiotic, as measured by quantitative dilution studies (e.g., in vitro CSF killing levels or in vitro MBC tests), (3) because the antibiotic must reach local sites in concentrations sufficient to kill the pathogen, the agent selected must readily penetrate into the infected CSF or, if not, be directly instilled into the CSF by intrathecal or intraventricular injection, and (4) foci of suppurative parameningeal infection must be drained whenever the procedure can be performed without causing serious neurologic damage. The extent to which various antibiotics transport into the CSF during meningitis differs, and the practitioner must know this. In general, concentrations of antibiotic are higher in the CSF of children and neonates than in adults with meningitis.

The presence of local leukocytes, especially neutrophils, is probably necessary for the infected meninges to become permeable to antibiotics. For example, limited experience suggests that vancomycin, which tends to accumulate in the CSF of otherwise healthy adults with bacterial meningitis, does not enter the CSF as well in neutropenic

**Table 24–21. INITIAL ANTIBIOTIC THERAPY FOR
SUPPURATIVE MENINGITIS OF UNKNOWN CAUSE***

PATIENT GROUP	SUSPECTED PATHOGEN	PREFERRED THERAPY ANTIBIOTIC	ALTERNATIVE THERAPY ANTIBIOTIC
Neonate (1 month or younger)	Group B streptococci *E. coli* Listeria	Ampicillin and either gentamicin or cefotaxime	Chloramphenicol and cefotaxime or ampicillin
Child	*H. influenzae* Pneumococci Meningococci	Ampicillin and chloramphenicol	Cefuroxime
Adult	Meningococci Pneumococci	Ampicillin or penicillin G	Chloramphenicol or cefotaxime
Immunocompromised adult (e.g., older than 60, with cirrhosis or neoplastic disease)	*Listeria* *Pseudomonas* Enterobacteriaceae Pneumococci Meningococci	Ampicillin and cefotaxime and gentamicin	Trimethoprim-sulfamethoxazole (TMP-SMX) Cefotaxime
Postcraniotomy patient	Staphylococci *Pseudomonas* Enterobacteriaceae	Nafcillin and cefotaxime and gentamicin	Vancomycin and cefotaxime and gentamicin
	H. influenzae	Cefotaxime or chloramphenicol	Ampicillin
	N. meningitidis	Aqueous penicillin G or cefotaxime	Chloramphenicol
	E. coli, Klebsiella, Proteus, and similar organisms	Gentamicin and cefotaxime	Chloramphenicol
	Pseudomonas	Ceftazidime and gentamicin	—

* Reproduced with permission from Swartz and O'Hanley, 1987.

patients with documented bacterial meningitis. Therefore, serial determinations of the concentration of drug in the CSF or serial studies of CSF bacterial killing should be performed in severely neutropenic patients to document the presence of sufficiently high antibiotic concentrations. Otherwise, serial intrathecal or intraventricular injections of the appropriate antibiotics must be given. The third-generation cephalosprins usually achieve concentrations of CSF that are at least 10 times the MBC against the common Enterobacteriaceae that cause meningitis (e.g., *E. coli, Klebsiella* species, and *Proteus mirabilis*). Such a concentration appears to be needed in order to cure meningitis (Sande, 1981). It is questionable, however, whether these agents, when used alone, can achieve 10-fold MBC concentrations in the CSF against such organisms as *Pseudomonas, Flavobacterium, Enterobacter, Serratia,* and *Acinetobacter* species.

The appearance of penicillinase-producing *H. influenzae* type b strains that are highly resistant to ampicillin (about 10% of isolates in the United States) has required a shift in the focus of initial management of this form of meningitis. Chloramphenicol is now mandatory as empirical therapy for *H. influenzae* meningitis until the isolate has been demonstrated to be susceptible to ampicillin in vitro. There does not appear to be any antagonism between the antibacterial effects of

**Table 24–22. SUGGESTED ANTIBIOTIC THERAPY FOR BACTERIAL MENINGITIS
OF KNOWN CAUSE IN ADULTS**

ORGANISM	PREFERRED THERAPY	ALTERNATIVE THERAPY
S. pneumoniae	Aqueous penicillin G	Either chloramphenicol or cefuroxime
Streptococcus groups A and B	Aqueous penicillin G	Either erythromycin or chloramphenicol
Group D (enterococci)	Aqueous penicillin G and gentamicin	Vancomycin and gentamicin
S. aureus	Nafcillin	Vancomycin
L. monocytogenes	Either aqueous penicillin G or ampicillin	Either chloramphenicol, or tetracycline plus gentamicin

Reproduced with permission from Swartz and O'Hanley, 1987.

chloramphenicol and those of ampicillin against *H. influenzae*. For this reason, and because rare strains of *H. influenzae* resistant to either ampicillin or chloramphenicol alone have been isolated, many pediatricians use both drugs simultaneously until susceptibility testing is performed, and then chloramphenicol is discontinued if the organism is susceptible to ampicillin.

An emerging problem might necessitate a reappraisal of this therapeutic strategy. Some strains of *H. influenzae* have now been found to be resistant to both ampicillin and chloramphenicol. Resistance to ampicillin is caused by production of β-lactamase, whereas resistance to chloramphenicol is associated with production of acetyltransferase (Smith, 1983). Although such resistant strains are currently rare in the United States, epidemiologic data suggest that they may account for as many as 25% of the clinical isolates of *H. influenzae* within the next decade. Therefore, newer third-generation cephalosporins such as cefotaxime might be the agents of choice in the near future because they have been shown to be as effective as standard therapy for *H. influenzae* meningitis in neonates and are not inactivated by bacterial enzymes (Nelson, 1985). *Principle: When a drug is found to produce a very severe adverse effect, physicians correctly use it much more cautiously than if it were less morbid or lethal. But knowing that a drug can produce lethal lesions rarely (e.g., aplastic anemia in 1/40,000 or 1/50,000 cases) should not preclude its appropriate use in settings that are very dangerous and in which its efficacy is unique.*

A patient with *S. aureus* meningitis should be treated with a penicillinase-resistant penicillin such as nafcillin because 80% to 90% of *S. aureus* isolates are resistant to penicillin G.

Enterococcal meningitis requires the use of IV penicillin or ampicillin supplemented by parenterally administered gentamicin. When lumbar puncture reveals an organism that resembles an enterococcus, an immediate intrathecal dose of gentamicin (4–8 mg for an adult) should be considered. Furthermore, if a patient fails to respond promptly to parenteral therapy with penicillin and gentamicin, continued adjunctive intrathecal gentamicin may be given.

The Special Problem of Gram-Negative Bacillary Meningitis. The parenteral antibiotics that have been used in the past to treat gram-negative bacillary meningitis are ampicillin, chloramphenicol, and the aminoglycosides. The results of treatment, however, have been far from satisfactory: mortality has ranged from 30% to 60% (Swartz, 1981; Cherubin et al., 1981). The use of ampicillin as primary therapy for this form of meningitis is limited by the fact that about 30% of strains

of gram-negative bacilli that cause neonatal meningitis, and the majority of isolates from adults with meningitis, are ampicillin-resistant. Chloramphenicol also has drawbacks in addition to its potential toxicity in neonates. Although the MICs of chloramphenicol for many gram-negative bacilli (2–6 μg/ml) are achievable in the CSF, MBCs are generally so much higher (>60 μg/ml) that they are not attainable in the CSF (Rahal and Simberkoff, 1979).

Antagonism of the bactericidal effect of gentamicin by chloramphenicol has been observed in a rabbit model of *P. mirabilis* meningitis (Strausbaugh and Sande, 1978). This combination of antibiotics results in an antibacterial effect comparable to the bacteriostatic effect of chloramphenicol alone against this organism. The significance of this antagonism in the clinical setting is unclear, except in patients with granulocytopenia.

Adjunctive intrathecal antibiotic therapy in the treatment of gram-negative bacillary meningitis came into use for two reasons: (1) parenteral administration of gentamicin and tobramycin yields low (<1 μg/ml) and inconsistent concentrations in the CSF, and (2) patients treated only with systemic agents have a high mortality. The high mortality associated with neonatal gram-negative bacillary meningitis, however, has not been reduced by the addition of lumbar intrathecal administration of gentamicin to parenteral therapy with ampicillin and gentamicin (McCracken and Mize, 1976). Unfortunately, the ventricles are common sites of infection in bacterial meningitis. The undirectional circulation of the CSF inhibits drug entry into the ventricles, and little of the antibiotic introduced intrathecally in the lumbar area reaches the ventricular system. Adjunctive intraventricular administration of gentamicin either via a ventriculostomy reservoir or by percutaneous injection circumvents this obstacle. However, a controlled study of neonates with gram-negative bacillary meningitis demonstrated a higher mortality among infants who received intraventricular gentamicin along with systemic antibiotics (43%) than among those who received systemic antibiotics alone (13%) (McCracken et al., 1980). This finding suggests that intraventricular therapy with gentamicin is harmful in neonates with gram-negative bacillary meningitis. The adjunctive use of lumbar intrathecal aminoglycoside (e.g., gentamicin) was recommended in children and adults with gram-negative bacillary meningitis (other than *H. influenzae* meningitis) because of the high overall mortality associated with this disease when it was treated with parenteral antibiotics alone (Mangi et al., 1977; Rahal, 1980).

The studies discussed above were performed prior to the development of the newer third-generation cephalosporins. Parenteral administration of these drugs unaccompanied by intrathecal use of an antibiotic represents an attractive regimen for successful treatment of gram-negative bacillary meningitis. These cephalosporins are becoming the agents of choice to treat the common gram-negative bacillary meningitides because they can achieve CSF concentrations that exceed by 10-fold the MBC for various bacterial species that commonly cause meningitis. A number of recent clinical trials support their efficacy in the treatment of patients in cases of meningitis that are caused by various bacterial agents and that occur in different age groups (Nelson, 1985).

Several general guidelines have been proposed regarding the use of the newer cephalosporins to treat bacterial meningitis (Neu, 1985): (1) final selection of the antibiotic or antibiotics to treat bacterial meningitis should be based on which drug or drugs have the greatest bactericidal activity for the causative agent, as determined by the MBC; (2) a CSF bactericidal titer test should be performed to demonstrate the value of a selected cephalosporin; (3) for gram-negative bacillary meningitis in adults, one of the newer cephalosporins should be administered parenterally together with an aminoglycoside that is administered both parenterally and intrathecally (this combination is superior to former regimens that employed aminoglycosides and chloramphenicol with or without ampicillin); (4) the newer cephalosporins do not offer any advantage over penicillin G in the treatment of group B streptococcal meningitis; (5) cefotaxime, moxalactam, ceftriaxone, and ceftizoxime appear to be as effective as chloramphenicol or ampicillin in the treatment of *H. influenzae* meningitis; (6) cefotaxime and ceftriaxone appear to be equal to penicillin G or chloramphenicol to treat meningococcal and pneumomococcal meningitides, and either might be considered as a replacement for chloramphenicol in the penicillin-allergic patient; (7) meningitis caused by *Pseudomonas*, *Acinetobacter*, *Enterobacter*, or *Serratia* cannot be successfully treated with third-generation cephalosporins alone; and (8) meningitis caused by *Listeria*, staphylococci, or streptococcal isolates other than group B or *S. pneumoniae* should not be treated with third-generation cephalosporins, because these cephalosporins lack activity against these organisms. Insufficient data are currently available on the use of aztreonam or imipenem in bacterial meningitis.

Treatment of Bacterial Meningitis of Unknown Cause. Empirical treatment should be initiated in patients seriously suspected of having bacterial meningitis if an etiologic agent is not identified on examination of a Gram-stained smear of CSF sediment or if performance of a lumbar puncture must be delayed (because the patient must be transported to another facility or a CT scan must be performed because of a suspected intracranial mass lesion). Treatment is directed at the most likely pathogens based on the age of the patient and available clinical clues (see Table 24-22).

Meningitis in neonates may be caused by a wide range of enteric gram-negative bacilli and gram-positive organisms, such as group B streptococci or *Listeria*. Such a variety of organisms necessitates the use of combined therapy with drugs such as ampicillin and either gentamicin or a third-generation cephalosporin such as cefotaxime. In children, antibacterial therapy is aimed at the three organisms most commonly responsible for childhood bacterial meningitis: *H. influenzae*, *N. meningitidis*, and *S. pneumoniae*. A combination of ampicillin and chloramphenicol is most frequently employed. However, because third-generation cephalosporins have shown clinical efficacy against the common childhood bacterial meningitides, monotherapy using cefotaxime, ceftriaxone, or cefuroxime is now being recommended by some authorities as the preferred or alternative therapy for meningitis of unknown cause in children.

Streptococcus pneumoniae meningitis and *N. meningitidis* meningitis are the meningitides that most commonly affect adults, but the incidence of invasive *H. influenzae* infection in adults is on the rise. Ampicillin, therefore, is the antibiotic of choice to treat bacterial meningitis of unknown cause in the adult because it is effective against *S. pneumoniae* and *N. meningitidis* as well as more than 90% of *H. influenzae* strains. Chloramphenicol is still an appropriate alternative choice for patients who are allergic to penicillin. A third-generation cephalosporin such as cefotaxime or ceftriaxone also can be used as an alternative antibiotic in the empirical therapy for meningitis of unknown cause in adults.

The incidence of uncommon types of meningitis in certain clinical settings has increased, such as meningitis caused by *S. aureus* in post craniotomy patients and meningitis caused by gram-negative bacilli or *Listeria* in patients who are immunocompromised because of advanced age, neoplastic disease, or cirrhosis. Broader initial antibiotic therapy is warranted in the management of patients with these underlying conditions.

Chemoprophylaxis. Meningococcal meningitis is the only type of bacterial meningitis that occurs in epidemic form. Close contacts of an index case (such as other household members, infants in day care centers, or military recruits) are at increased risk for developing meningococcal disease. Casual contacts such as schoolmates do not appear to be at increased risk. Hospital personnel in close patient contact (e.g., during nasotracheal suctioning or mouth-to-mouth resuscitation) are at increased risk, but personnel who come into contact with the patient after institution of respiratory precautions and antibiotic therapy are not.

Chemoprophylaxis is indicated only for close contacts. Sulfonamides, once widely employed in chemoprophylaxis, should no longer be used for that purpose because approximately 25% of meningococcal isolates are now resistant to sulfonamides. Rifampin is the drug of choice to accomplish prophylaxis in close contacts. The recommended dose in adults is either 600 mg orally every 12 hours for 2 days or 600 mg orally every day for 4 days (Ward et al., 1979). About 50% of secondary cases among close contacts occur at least 5 days after onset of the disease in the index case patient. This fact prompts consideration of the use of meningococcal bivalent vaccine (groups A and C) as an adjunct to chemoprophylaxis, to extend protection should chemoprophylaxis be unsuccessful.

Secondary cases of systemic *H. influenzae* type b infections may occur in close household and day care center contacts of an initial case of *H. influenzae* meningitis. The risk for household contacts who are younger than 12 months is 6%; for those younger than 4 years, the risk is 2% (Ward et al., 1979). The risk of severe *H. influenzae* disease among household contacts appears to be 585 times greater than the age-adjusted risk in the general population. A variety of drugs, including ampicillin, trimethoprim-sulfamethoxazole, and cefaclor, have been tested but were ineffective in eradicating nasopharyngeal carriage of *H. influenzae* type b (Overturf, 1982). Rifampin (20 mg/kg daily for 4 days) has been successful in eradicating carriage and appears to be the drug of choice for chemoprophylaxis. Chemoprophylaxis is given to close contacts and the index case. In addition, active immunization of contacts with the polysaccharide vaccine of *H. influenzae* type b may be effective immunoprophylaxis against secondary cases of *H. influenzae* type b disease.

PRINCIPLES OF PROPHYLAXIS

Chemoprophylaxis

Shortly after the sulfonamides and penicillin were proved effective to *treat* infection, they were widely used by physicians to *prevent* infection in situations in which the risk of infection was high. Chemoprophylaxis has had variable success. Antimicrobial administration does not prevent bacterial pulmonary infections in unconscious or artificially ventilated patients or after viral upper respiratory tract infections. Antibiotics do not

prevent urinary tract infections in patients with indwelling Foley catheters. In fact, using antimicrobials in these settings selects for more resistant flora. Despite little evidence of efficacy, excessive use of antimicrobials has continued. Unfortunately, essentially every new class of drug has been used for prophylaxis. Most surveys indicate that using antibiotics for prophylaxis accounts for 25% to 50% of all use of antimicrobials in hospitals (Cruse and Ford, 1973; Gilbert, 1984; Hirschamann and Inui, 1980; Conte et al., 1986). Despite the widespread administration of antibiotics to prevent infection, their use in this way is frequently controversial. Often their use is totally without merit, and potentially dangerous.

Guidelines for Chemoprophylaxis. The term *chemoprophylaxis* implies administration of an antibiotic agent before contamination or infection with bacteria occurs. *Early therapy* denotes immediate or prompt institution of therapy as soon as contamination or infection is recognized. The latter situation is exemplified by beginning antibiotics after bacterial contamination and/or infection has occurred (e.g., GI spillage from a ruptured viscus). Appropriate candidates for chemoprophylaxis to prevent infection include patients who have clinically significant exposure to an infected individual with particular diseases (e.g., invasive meningococcal disease or influenza); patients exposed to environments with a high potential for acquisition of pathogenic microorganisms (e.g., travelers in the developing world who are at risk for bacterial gastroenteritis or malaria); and patients undergoing procedures or surgery that are likely to result in infection (e.g., a dental procedure in a patient with a prosthetic heart valve, or colorectal surgery in an otherwise healthy patient). General principles of antimicrobial prophylaxis that should guide selection of an antimicrobial include the following: (1) benefit must exceed the risks of chemoprophylaxis, (2) the antimicrobial regimen must be effective against the major anticipated pathogen, (3) therapeutic concentrations of an effective chemoprophylactic antimicrobial should be achieved in local tissues at the time of exposure, and (4) prolonged chemoprophylaxis is unwarranted (Garrod, 1975; Griffin, 1983; Gilbert, 1984; Conte et al., 1986).

Chemoprophylaxis with penicillin has been successful in the prevention of β-streptococcal pharyngitis; likewise, prophylaxis with chloroquine or primaquin in the prevention of malaria, with penicillin in the prevention of syphilis and gonorrhea, with amantadine or rimantidine in the prevention of secondary cases of influenza, with rifampin in the prevention of secondary cases of invasive meningococci and *H. influenzae* diseases, with isoniazid in the prevention of systemic tuberculosis, and with trimethoprim-sulfamethoxazole in the prevention of recurrent urinary tract infections due to *E. coli*. Unfortunately, in the vast number of other situations in which antimicrobials are given prophylactically, there is little documentation that efficacy outweighs the risk of drug administration.

Surgical Prophylaxis. Prophylactic treatment of surgical patients undergoing a variety of different procedures has created considerable controversy, especially with regard to prevention of postoperative wound infections (Hurley et al., 1979; Polk et al., 1980; Nichols, 1981, 1982; Gilbert, 1984). Table 24–23 provides generally accepted recommendations regarding those surgical procedures that require antibiotic prophylaxis. Procedures with clean wounds represent the most frequently performed procedures and apply to elective surgical procedures with primary closure and no insertion of a drain through the wound. The wound is nontraumatic and there is no inflammation. There is no break in aseptic technique and the GI, respiratory, and genitourinary tracts are not entered. These procedures require no antibiotic chemoprophylaxis.

Surgical situations that require prophylactic or early therapy are listed in Table 24–23. Host factors associated with increased risk of wound infections, include: old age (>60 years), malnutrition, active infection elsewhere, obesity, the presence of diabetes mellitus, and the use of steroid therapy. Surgical factors that increase the risk of wound infections include: contaminated or dirty wounds, prolonged preoperative hospitalization (i.e., 1 week or more), emergency operations, prolonged (more than 3 hours) surgery, shaving the operation site prior to the procedure, use of an electrosurgical knife, and insertion of drains through the wound at closure.

Numerous studies have evaluated the role of chemoprophylaxis. Table 24–24 summarizes current recommendations concerning when chemoprophylaxis can be beneficial. In general, chemoprophylatic efficacy depends on high antibiotic activity being present at the time of closure and active against the most likely contaminating microorganism(s). Therefore, prophylactic antibiotics should be given preoperatively *or* intraoperatively to achieve maximal concentration of drug at the site of the procedure.

Since staphylococci and coliforms are the most common causes of wound infection, first-generation cephalosporins (e.g., cefazolin) are the most appropriately employed agents for surgical prophylaxis. Second-generation cephalosporins (e.g., cefotetan) should be used when there is concern that anaerobic bacteria, in addition to streptococci and coliforms, may contaminate the wound. Such procedures include surgery on the GI or biliary tracts and gynecologic procedures. Some authorities recommend prophylactic nafcillin or vancomycin for orthopedic or neurosurgical procedures, since the risk of staphylococcal infection is high. There is no role for third-generation cephalosporins in surgical prophylaxis since they have

Table 24–23. SURGICAL INFECTION RATE BY TYPE OF SURGICAL PROCEDURE*†

TYPE OF SURGERY	DEFINITION	APPROXIMATE PERCENTAGE OF ALL OPERATIONS	REPORTED INFECTION RATE (%)	ANTIBIOTIC PROPHYLAXIS RECOMMENDED
Clean	No entry into the respiratory, GI, or GU tracts	75	1–5	No
Clean with insertion of prosthetic material or device	No entry into the respiratory, GI, or GU tracts	1–4	1–5 but high morbidity and mortality	Yes
Clean-contaminated	Unavoidable entry into the respiratory, GI, or GU tracts (e.g., appendectomies, hysterectomies)	14–15	8–15	Yes
Contaminated	Fresh trauma, major break in sterile technique, gross spillage of GI content, entry into infected urinary or biliary tracts	4–5	15–20	Yes
Dirty	Old trauma wounds with devitalized tissue, foreign bodies, fecal contamination	4–5	30–40	Antibiotics are given to treat established infection

* Infection rates listed are the expected infection rates in the absence of antibiotic prophylaxis.
† Reproduced with permission from Gilbert, 1984.

Table 24–24. **EFFICACY OF PREOPERATIVE PROPHYLAXIS IN REDUCING POSTOPERATIVE SURGICAL INFECTIONS AND INCISIONAL INFECTIONS***

Efficacy established for
  Colorectal operation
  High-risk gastroduodenal surgery (gastric ulcer, relief of obstruction, stopping hemorrhage, or patients with achlorhydria)
  Appendectomy (inflamed appendix)
  High-risk biliary surgery (patients older than 70 years, with cholecystitis, undergoing common bile duct explorations or removal of stones, or with jaundice)
  Hysterectomy (vaginal)
  Cesarean section in high-risk patients
  Pulmonary resection
  Vascular grafts of abdomen and lower extremity
  Hip nailing, total hip orthroplasty, open fracture reduction
Possible efficacy for
  Gastric bypass
  Coronary bypass grafting
  Prostatic surgery
  Cardiac pacemaker implantation
Unproven efficacy for
  Low-risk gastroduodenal surgery
  Low-risk cholecystectomy
  Clean neurosurgery procedures without insertion of any prosthesis
  Clean plastic surgery procedures without insertion of any prosthesis
  External ventriculostomy
  Herniorrhaphy, thyroidectomy, mastectomy, tonsillectomy
  Repair of traumatic lacerations

* Reproduced with permission from Conte et al., 1986.

limited coverage of staphylococci and anaerobic bacilli. There are no data to suggest that the rate of postoperative wound infection is lower if antimicrobial therapy is continued after the surgical procedure is completed (Rowlands et al., 1982; Conte et al., 1986). Prolonged use beyond 24 hours leads to the emergence of more resistant bacteria and wound infections caused by antibiotic-resistant microorganisms (Garrod, 1975; Condon, 1975).

Chemoprophylaxis against Endocarditis. Prevention of endocarditis by use of antibiotic(s) before procedures that may cause transient bacteremia has been recommended for patients with selected valvular and congenital cardiac malformations. No controlled trials document the efficacy of such recommendations in preventing *S. viridans* endocarditis after dental or upper respiratory tract procedures, or enterococci endocarditis after GI or genitourinary procedures (Durack, 1990). Prophylaxis for endocarditis is recommended for patients with the following underlying conditions: prosthetic valves, congenital cardiac malformations, surgically constructed systemic–pulmonary shunts, rheumatic and other acquired valvular dysfunction, idiopathic hypertrophic aortic stenosis, previous history of bacterial endocarditis, and mitral valve prolapse with insufficiency. Prophylaxis for endocarditis is not recommended for patients who have undergone previous coronary artery bypass graft surgery or selected atrial secundum septal defects. Chemoprophylaxis is indicated prior to procedures that may lead to a transient bacteremia, such as dental procedures that induce gingival bleeding, tonsillectomy, manipulation or biopsy of the respiratory, GI, or genitourinary tracts, and incision and drainage of infected tissue. The clinician should refer to schedules for endocarditis chemoprophylaxis when selecting the optional regimen (Medical Letter, 1990). In general, penicillin is given to prevent *S. viridans* streptococcal endocarditis, while ampicillin plus gentamicin are given to prevent enterococcal endocarditis. Therapy should not be given until the procedure begins because the peak concentrations of drug should be reached during the procedure. Drug therapy should not be prolonged (not continued for more than one dose after the procedure) so that more resistant organisms will not colonize the affected mucosal surfaces and infect the patient. *Principle: Antimicrobial prophylaxis can prevent and decrease the postoperative incidence of infection in only a select number of clinical conditions. When an antimicrobial is appropriately administered, the choice in timing, agent(s) employed, and duration of chemoprophylaxis are crucial so as to maximize benefit and minimize toxicity. In general, one dose of an agent that kills the most likely pathogen, at* *the time of greatest risk of contamination or exposure, is considered optimal therapy.*

Immunoprophylaxis

Acquired resistance following infection is a part of the natural history of many diseases. Long-lasting immunity is not common to all infections but usually follows most acute viral infections. Resistance to recurrent infection with bacteria and other higher organisms is more variable. Resistance is frequently attended by measurable increases in specific immunoglobulins and reactions mediated by the cellular immune system. The object of immunotherapy is to safely duplicate or exceed the functional resistance in the host that normally follows a natural infection. In contrast to antimicrobial prophylaxis, optimal immunotherapy converts the susceptible individual into a resistant host, permanently protected against the risk of infection without recourse to the repeated use of drugs.

Immunotherapy is the only effective therapy available for most viral infections, since antiviral chemotherapy has not been as well developed as antibacterial chemotherapy. Immunotherapy may be administered passively through the parenteral administration of preformed specific immunoglobulin from human or animal sources. Active immunity can be induced through the use of killed or attenuated agent vaccines, through the administration of subunit chemically defined vaccines, or by giving modified but antigenically active products of an agent in the form of toxoids (Fulginiti, 1973). *Principle: An ounce of prevention is worth a pound of cure: a milliliter of effective vaccine is often of greater value than any subsequent chemotherapeutic intervention.*

Passive Immunization. Each newborn receives the benefits of natural passive immunization through the transplacental transfer of immunoglobulins from the maternal circulation. These immunoglobulins provide the newborn with sufficient protection to avoid infection with a wide variety of agents in the neonatal period. This protection wanes with the half-life of the maternal γ-globulin and has largely disappeared at 2 to 4 months of age (Miller, 1973).

Short-term protection against a wide group of diseases can be conveyed through the parenteral administration of immunoglobulins containing specific antibodies. While past indications for this type of treatment have included prophylaxis or therapy of poliomyelitis, rubella, hepatitis, diphtheria, mumps, pertussis, and rubeola infections, these illnesses are now better managed with active immunization programs. A current list of commonly administered immune globulins is found in Table 24–25. Of these products only botulinum immune serum, tetanus immune globulin, rabies hyperimmune globulin, hepatitis B immune globulin, and human immune globulin for the prophylaxis of hepatitis are commonly used. Vaccinia immune globulin and zoster immune globulin are in short supply and therefore are only available under strict control for high-risk situations.

In the absence of previous immunization, antisera for the prophylaxis or treatment of diphtheria, pertussis, measles, and polio are of some value, but these antisera are not presently widely available. The Centers for Disease Control is a reliable resource for information about immunoprophylaxis in general. The CDC maintains a clearinghouse for those products not commercially available. It also maintains a variety of other hyperimmune sera for use in diseases not commonly seen in the United States, including a number of the more exotic arbovirus and other viral illnesses causing hemorrhagic fever.

Passive immunization is limited in its effectiveness by the half-life of IgG (22–30 days). Thus, a relatively short period of protection is afforded by this approach. All hyperimmune sera and

Table 24–25.   PASSIVE IMMUNOTHERAPY

PREPARATION	USE	SIDE EFFECTS
Hyperimmune trivalent (A, B, E) horse serum	Botulism (treatment)	Hypersensitivity
Hyperimmune horse serum	Diphtheria (treatment)	Hypersensitivity
Hepatitis B immune globulin	Hepatitis B (prophylaxis)	Local reactions
Immune serum	Hepatitis A and B, measles, yellow fever (prophylaxis)	None
Pertussis immune globulin	Pertussis (treatment)	None
Rabies immune globulin	Rabies (prophylaxis and treatment)	None
Tetanus immune globulin	Tetanus (prophylaxis and treatment)	None
Vaccinia immune globulin	Smallpox (prophylaxis)	None
Varicella-zoster immune globulin	Varicella (prophylaxis and treatment)	Local reactions

disease-specific immunoglobulins are in limited supply and are expensive. To be effective, they usually require comparatively large volumes for parenteral administration, and they cause unpleasant local reactions. Allergic reactions may be apparent immediately after injection and may be life-threatening. More commonly, the reactions are of the delayed hypersensitivity or serum sickness type (see chapters 1 and 39). Careful questioning of the patient for a history of allergy to the animal that served as the source for the antiserum and possibly skin testing with the antiserum to be used should be considered before the administration of these agents. If the skin tests are positive, but the need is critical, a carefully administered "desensitization" program may be undertaken using increasing concentrations of the material. Appropriate procedures to accomplish desensitization have been described (Fulginiti, 1973). With the recent availability of human antisera for rabies and tetanus prophylaxis, antisera from animal sources are becoming less frequently required.

Immunologic antagonism of endotoxin in bacterial septic shock by administration of hyperimmune or monoclonal antibodies has been considered and still needs to be proved efficacious in the treatment of septic shock (Wolff, 1973; Parrillo et al., 1990). Antibodies of the IgM and IgG classes that bind to the core lipopolysaccharide moiety of gram-negative bacterial lipopolysaccharide protect against shock induced by a broad spectrum of gram-negative bacteria or their lipopolysaccharides in animal experiments and clinical trials. Patients with septic shock who have naturally occurring antibodies to endotoxin (primarily IgM) appear to have a better prognosis (McCabe et al., 1972). Increased survival among septic patients who received passive anticore (J5 mutant) lipopolysaccharide sera has been observed (Ziegler, 1988). There is considerable controversy as to the benefit of antiendotoxin antibodies (Parrillo et al., 1990). Current clinical trials that employ monoclonal preparations to core lipopolysaccharide should further define the efficacy and toxicity of this approach. *Principle: Passive immunization provides temporary protection for those situations where vaccines either are not available or have not been appropriately administered according to accepted schedules. Since this protection is only temporary, it is necessary to follow it with appropriate active immunization measures if they are available, to ensure long-lasting resistance.*

Active Immunization. Active immunization depends on the host's immune system response to vaccines to provide the protection usually acquired by natural infection. Vaccines may be either living (e.g., contain live virus) or nonliving (e.g., contain dead virus). Live vaccines contain organisms that are attenuated and therefore are capable of only limited replication in a normal host. Vaccinia was the first clinically successful live vaccine. It is a product containing poxvirus that has limited ability to invade the human host but is nevertheless able to produce sufficient local and regional infectivity to ensure that a host response results in the solid resistance of the recipient to subsequent smallpox infection. The resistance was not lifelong, and vaccination had to be repeated approximately every 3 years. The elimination of smallpox worldwide in the 1980s by an effective immunization program is the most dramatic example of how vaccines can be used for the well-being of humankind (Centers for Disease Control, 1985). Since the risk of reaction to smallpox vaccine now outweighs the chance of acquiring the disease, vaccination is recommended only for those involved in smallpox research laboratories. Properties of other commonly used vaccines are listed in Table 24–26.

Living-agent vaccines may be administered either by natural routes (orally) as in oral polio vaccine or by an artificial route (parenterally) as in the presently available live measles vaccine. There is a theoretical advantage in the use of the natural route since there is good evidence that the resultant formation of local antibodies is important in protection from subsequent wild-type infections (Ogra et al., 1968).

Nonliving vaccines may be divided into four groups: (1) suspensions of whole killed agents (e.g., influenza vaccine and typhoid vaccine), (2) suspensions of nonreplicating subparticles of infectious agents (e.g., meningococcal polysaccharide vaccines), (3) modified products of infecting organisms (e.g., tetanus and diphtheria toxoid vaccine), and (4) new subunit vaccines that contain chemically defined reagents (e.g., hepatitis B virus vaccine). The routine schedule for the active immunization of normal infants and children in the United States is presented in Table 24–27. Certain combinations of live vaccines may be given simultaneously, but the close sequential administration of individual live vaccines and immune globulins is not recommended because of evidence of interference with immunogenicity leading to vaccine failure (Stokes et al., 1971).

Evaluation of the Efficacy of Vaccines. Adequate response to immunization is most frequently judged by measuring the development of specific serum immunoglobulins (e.g., antibodies) following a course of administration of vaccine. The concentration of specific immunoglobulin in plasma is usually proportional to the degree of protection from the viral agent. However, the re-

Table 24-26. ROUTINE VACCINES FOR HUMANS

DISEASE	ROUTE	AGENT	AGE APPLICABLE	BASIC OR PRIMARY IMMUNIZATION	NEED FOR BOOSTER	EFFICACY VALUE (%)	ADVERSE REACTIONS OR COMMENT
Diphtheria	Parenteral	Toxoid	2 mo-5 yrs and adults	3 doses over 6 mo	Yes, at 1 and 3 yrs after basic	>90	Mild local reactions
Pertussis	Parenteral	Heat-killed bacteria	2 mo-5 yrs	3 doses over 6 mo	No	~85	Mild local reactions, rare neurologic reactions
Tetanus	Parenteral	Toxoid	2 mo-5 yrs and adults	3 doses over 6 mo	Every 10 yrs	~100	Local pain and rare neurologic reactions due to hypersensitivity
Polio	Oral	Live-attenuated (OVP)	>2 mo	3 doses over 6 mo	Yes, at 1 and 3 yrs after basic	>95	None
Measles	Parenteral	Live-attenuated	>1 yr	1 dose	Probably not	>95	Fever and rash in 15%
Mumps	Parenteral	Life-attenuated	>1 yr	1 dose	None	>95	Local reaction
Rubella	Parenteral	Live-attenuated	Women of childbearing age	1 dose	None	>95	Mild fever, arthralgia, local reactions
Hemophilus infection	Parenteral	Capsular material	>18 mo	1 dose	None	>95	Rare; should be given to all children
Pneumococcal infection	Parenteral	Capsular material	>55 yrs and COPD and immunocompromised patients	1 dose	Probably 10 yrs	>70	Local reactions
Influenza	Parenteral	Formalin-treated virus	>65 yrs and COPD and immunocompromised patients	2 doses over 2 mo	Annually	~60	Fever, malaise, and arthralgia; contraindicated in individuals with hypersensitivity to eggs
Hepatitis B	Parenteral	Surface antigens (protein and lipids)	Health care workers and persons with high risk of contact with blood (e.g., IV drug abuser)	3 doses over 6 mo	Probably not needed	~90	None

Table 24–27. SCHEDULE FOR ACTIVE IMMUNIZATION OF NORMAL INFANTS AND CHILDREN*

AGE	VACCINE OR TOXOID†
2 mo	DTP-1, polio OPV-1
4 mo	DTP-2, polio OPV-2
6 mo	DTP-3, polio OPV-3 (optional; used in hyperendemic regions)
12 mo	Measles,‡ rubella,‡ mumps‡
15 mo	DTP-4, polio OPV-3 (or 4)
18 mo	Hemophilus B conjugate
4–6 yr	DTP-5, polio OPV-4 (or 5)
14–16 yr	Td (and thereafter every 10 years)

* From Centers for Disease Control, 1989.

† DTP = Diphtheria toxoid, tetanus toxoid, pertussis vaccine. Polio OPV = Trivalent oral polio virus vaccine. Td = Tetanus toxoid combined with smaller adult dose of diphtheria antigen.

‡ May be given as combined vaccine.

lation between immunologic response to a vaccine and protection afforded by it to subsequent disease must be documented in field trials. The longevity of the protective response must always be determined to establish the most appropriate interval for revaccination. At its inception, the rubella vaccine program in the United States was targeted for children of primary-school age assuming the "herd immunity" in this group would prevent transmission to young women of childbearing age (Centers for Disease Control, 1987). Herd immunity would in turn protect women of childbearing age from contracting the disease when pregnant, thereby protecting the fetus from the consequences of congenitally acquired rubella infection. The adequacy and duration of the child's immune response to rubella vaccination are unfortunately not sufficient to achieve herd immunity, and maternal immunity wanes at the very time when maximal protection is desirable to protect the fetus (Chang et al., 1970). Therefore, it is now recommended that just prior (3 or more months) to becoming pregnant women receive rubella vaccination, or at least be screened by serologic tests to confirm acquired immunity. *Principle: Vaccination does not guarantee long-term immunity and protection. Host and pathogen exist in a dynamic relationship. In the course of treatment or prophylaxis against infectious diseases, the changes wrought by such therapy may substantially alter the epidemiology of that disease in the individual or in the population as a whole. One must be vigilant to the possibility of variations from "predicted" patterns and adjust one's own responses accordingly.*

Eradication. While the widespread use of antibiotics has had little success in curtailing the prevalence of bacterial infection, and in certain in-

stances has resulted in the appearance of resistant pathogens of potentially greater harm, the success of vaccines in reducing incidence of disease has been remarkable. Lack of success has been largely related to the socioeconomic problems preventing distribution of the vaccine (Horstmann, 1973). When these latter problems have been appropriately solved, eventual eradication of some diseases has become possible. Certain favorable epidemiologic characteristics of smallpox made it an ideal candidate to eradicate. These include the following: (1) humans are the only known host, (2) smallpox is an acute disease with a short incubation period, (3) immunity following infection is relatively long lasting and effective, (4) there is only one antigenic strain of virus, (5) subclinical infections are rare, (6) epidemic patterns are seasonal, and (7) a successful vaccine is available (Hoeprich, 1972). Unfortunately these characteristics are not widely shared by other pathogens. Thus, successful eradication will probably be limited to a small number of diseases. Vaccines that are effective in preventing infectious diseases in individual patients and that possibly could induce herd immunity include tetanus, influenza, polio, measles, mumps, rubella, pertussis, diphtheria, typhoid, meningococcus, yellow fever, pneumococcus, hepatitis B, *H. influenzae* type b, and rabies.

Adverse Effects of Vaccines. Adverse effects of vaccines vary and are often related to the method of preparation of the vaccine (i.e., the cell culture system in which the vaccine has been prepared) (Wilson, 1967). Allergic reactions are too frequently the consequence of inadequate attempts to obtain a detailed history or inattention to the appropriate necessary precautions (e.g., adequate preliminary testing before administration). The clinician is advised to consult local state health officials regarding updated precautions for adverse effects associated with vaccination prior to immunization.

Nonliving vaccine products require a much larger antigenic mass (dose) and more frequent booster injections than do live vaccines to provide adequate levels of protection. This is exemplified by the requirement for multiple boosters of immunization against diphtheria, tetanus, and pertussis, compared with the single administration required for live measles virus vaccine. The larger doses and repeated administration required for nonliving vaccines may lead to higher rates of allergy and other reactions. During the developmental use of at least two killed vaccines (measles vaccine and respiratory syncytial virus vaccine), production of a hypersensitivity state ensued that while not preventing infection produced an exaggerated host response to subsequent natural infections resulting in a clinically unusual and more severe disease than was previously seen (Kapikian et al., 1969).

Although attenuated live-virus vaccines may more effectively mimic natural infection in stimulating host defenses, they can be made in such a way that there is a risk of inadequate attenuation of the virus, or the virus might revert to a less attenuated form. Thus, the full-blown disease may appear following vaccination. Furthermore, since these live-virus vaccines do not go through a process of harsh inactivation before administration, the risk of introducing dangerous adventitious agents into the host is increased. For example, certain animal tumor viruses that contaminated tissue culture support systems in some of the early vaccines were inadvertently introduced into recipients. Fortunately, careful follow-up of cohorts of these recipients has failed to show any increased rates of neoplasia (Shah and Nathanson, 1976).

Accidents related to insufficient attenuation, contamination by adventitious agents, and allergic or hypersensitivity reactions to vaccines have been limited to specific batches or types of vaccine (Wilson, 1967). The probability of recurrence of these adverse effects has been markedly reduced by increasingly rigid guidelines for vaccine production. More frequently, inappropriate administration of live vaccines to compromised hosts, or accidental transmission of the resultant disease to family members with compromised immune functions, has been an adversity caused by vaccines.

The administration of vaccines to pregnant women presents a special problem. In this situation, the probable risk of maternal (and fetal) infection must be balanced against the known adverse effects of vaccination. Adequate immunization against tetanus is essential for both mother and child, and tetanus toxoid immunization is safe during pregnancy. Immunization against poliomyelitis and yellow fever is indicated in pregnant women traveling to epidemic areas. Other live vaccines, including rubella, mumps, and measles, are generally contraindicated during pregnancy because of the risk of infecting the fetus (Levine et al., 1974). *Principle: With the development and introduction of each new vaccine, the physician must balance the seriousness of the disease being prevented against the known and unknown risks involved in widespread use of the product. Prophylaxis with vaccine is warranted only in populations threatened by significant morbidity and mortality from the disease, in whom likely benefits outweigh possible risks.*

Poliomyelitis: A Disease Illustrating the Principles of Immunotherapy. Poliomyelitis is a disease caused by infection with one of three types of poliovirus, a member of the enterovirus group. These viruses are transmitted by both the oral-fecal and respiratory routes, the latter being of lesser importance. Colonization and multiplication of the virus take place in the lymphatic tissue of the oropharynx and bowel. Dissemination occurs thereafter via the regional lymphatics and by viremia. After dissemination, the tissue tropism that allows the poliovirus to multiply within the lower motor neurons of the spinal cord becomes apparent. The injury to these lower motor neurons is responsible for the most devastating clinical manifestations of paralytic polio. Host defenses include the elaboration of local antibody (IgA) in the GI tract and type-specific humoral antibodies that can be detected in the circulation. When present, the latter antibodies indicate that the host is protected against reinfection. There is no cross-protection between the three types of poliovirus.

The clinical manifestations of poliomyelitis appear 1 to 3 weeks after exposure to the virus and appear to be related to age. The overwhelming majority of cases in children are completely asymptomatic. Those persons who do have symptoms usually have a mild fever, headache, some mild GI symptoms, and occasionally a sore throat. In contrast to adolescents and adults, young children rarely have involvement of the CNS. When they develop, neurologic symptoms usually appear from 2 to 6 days after the initial illness. The neurologic involvement is primarily lower motor neuron disease that results in paresis.

Hematologic and biochemical tests usually are within normal limits except for the findings in the CSF, which include an elevation of the leukocyte count (10–500 cells) with polymorphonuclear leukocytes predominating in the first 2 to 4 days and a modest elevation of the concentration of protein. Specific tests that document poliovirus infection include virologic examination of the CSF, respiratory secretions, and feces. These samples should be taken as early as possible in the course of the disease to increase the likelihood of successful isolation of the virus. Paired samples of sera showing a fourfold or greater rise in type-specific antibody against poliovirus are diagnostic of the disease.

There is no acceptable antiviral chemotherapy for an established case of poliomyelitis. Treatment in this instance is entirely supportive and aimed at preventing other infections and reversing or preventing the biochemical or respiratory problems related to the neurologic destruction caused by the disease.

The development and application of polio vaccine provide one of the most successful stories in modern therapeutics (Paul, 1971). Before the introduction of polio vaccine in 1954, recurrent epidemic polio with significant rates of neurologic disease plagued industrialized societies. Nonindustrialized societies usually had their infections during childhood, with very low rates of neurologic disease. As public health measures improved, the oral–fecal spread of polio virus shifted to an older population more prone to neurologic involvement. This natural history has been repeated in developing societies up to the present. With the use of either the Salk killed vaccine (IPV) or the Sabin oral polio vaccine (OPV), this disease has been reduced to rare occurrences in unvaccinated groups (Wehrle, 1967; Schoenberger et al., 1984).

This briefly successful story has had its own problems and setbacks. In 1954, the Salk vaccine from one producer was inadequately inactivated. This resulted in a series of patients who developed paralytic poliomyelitis (Terry, 1962). In a somewhat less publicized incident, it was later shown that certain lots of both Salk and Sabin vaccine were produced and distributed while they still contained varying amounts of viable SV40 virus, a common contaminant of monkey kidney tissue and a virus known to cause tumors in some lower animals. While antibody against this agent was produced in some of the recipients, continuing investigation of cohorts of the populations receiving these contaminated vaccines has shown no demonstrable increase in the occurrence of any tumors in 20 years of follow-up (Shah and Nathanson, 1976).

In recent years, outbreaks of poliomyelitis have been associated with pockets of unvaccinated persons. There have also been individual cases that may have been related to contact with the vaccine itself (Balduzzi and Glasgow, 1967). There is increasing concern in recent years that the gap in herd immunity is developing as a result of complacent public and governmental agencies that fail to immunize indigent children. A society that allows the emergence of susceptible groups of unvaccinated persons to occur may again be visited by this severe disease (Horstmann, 1973; Eichhoff, 1985). So far, the benefits of the vaccine far outweigh its liabilities, and there has been no apparent problem of unusual abnormalities of immune responses in the patients who have received the vaccines.

COMMENTS ON COMMON SPECIFIC AGENTS

This section is devoted to specific clinically relevant points about commonly used antimicrobials. Detailed descriptions of each drug are available in other texts (Gilman et al., 1985; Kucers and Bennett, 1989; Mandell et al., 1990). The major toxicities, dosage adjustments in patients with renal failure, routes of administration, and ability to penetrate into the CSF and urine of these agents already have been mentioned in this chapter.

Penicillin

Penicillin G is an acid that is combined with sodium, potassium, procaine, or benzathine to increase its stability. The latter two are "long-acting" forms. Penicillin G is useful in the treatment of streptococcal infections due to *S. pyogenes* (group A), *S. agalactiae* (group B), *S. pneumoniae*, *S. viridans*, *Corynebacterium diphtheria*, *N. meningitidis*, many strains of *N. gonorrhea*, *Treponema pallidum*, and many anaerobic streptococci, such as peptococcus and peptostreptococcus. In combination with aminoglycosides, any penicillin G compounds can be used to treat enterococci and *L. monocytogenes* infections. These organisms cause many clinical syndromes including cellulitis, pharyngitis, pneumonia, septicemia, endocarditis, meningitis, abscesses in lung, sexually transmitted disease, septic arthritis, and osteomyelitis.

All penicillin-like agents kill susceptible bacteria by interfering with the biosynthesis of the cell wall, eventually lysing the bacteria by autolysis. The penicillins are generally safe except in less than 0.01% of patients who are susceptible to IgE-mediated anaphylaxis (see chapter 39). Other penicillin toxicity is rare unless renal function has been impaired. In patients with renal failure, large doses of penicillin produce neurologic reactions including seizures. One overlooked problem of high concentrations of penicillins in the blood occurs when aminoglycoside concentrations are measured in vitro. The penicillins autolyze aminoglycosides. Prolonged storage of blood containing these antibiotics at room temperature can result in lower-than-real concentrations of aminoglycoside.

Phenoxymethoylpenicillin (penicillin V) is a natural penicillin and is produced by addition of a phenoxyacetic acid during the growth of the organism. It is acid-stable and administered orally. It is useful for minor infections.

Semisynthetic Penicillins. Methicillin, oxacillin, cloxacillin, dicloxocillin, and nafcillin are semisynthetic penicillins that are particularly useful to treat penicillinase-producing staphylococci. They are considered the primary empirical therapy for staphylococcal infections. They kill bacteria in a similar manner to that of penicillin G. Methicillin and nafcillin are the most stable; nafcillin is most used because of its lower incidence of toxicity. In contrast to the other semisynthetic penicillins that are excreted primarily by the kidney, nafcillin is 70% inactivated in the liver. Nafcillin does not usually require adjustment of dose in patients with renal failure. Errors in its administration are commonly made by decreasing the dose of nafcillin in patients with renal failure and continuing high doses in patients with hepatic insufficiency. Depending on subsequent culture results, tailored therapy for staphylococci may include penicillin G (rare) for non-penicillinase-producing strains of staphylococci or vancomycin for nafcillin-resistant staphylococci.

Ampicillin is a semisynthetic penicillin and is unique in that it is active against some gram-negative bacilli that are resistant to penicillin G. Amoxicillin is chemically modified ampicillin. The trihydrate form is administered orally and is much better absorbed than ampicillin, making it the preferred agent for oral administration. Organisms that are susceptible to penicillin G also are susceptible to ampicillin. Ampicillin kills organisms similarly to penicillin G; however, it penetrates into the cell wall better, enabling it to kill many gram-negative bacilli. It is considered appropriate therapy for susceptible *E. coli*, *Klebsiella pneumoniae*, *P. mirabilis*, and species of *Shigella*, *Neisseria gonorrhoeae*, and *N. meningitidis*. The most common error in parenteral ampicillin therapy is administrating it too infrequently. Its relatively short half-life dictates that it should be administered every 4 hours in seriously ill patients. It is especially useful in treating acute and uncomplicated urinary tract infections caused by *E. coli* and/or *Proteus* species. *Hemophilus influenzae* meningitis can be treated with ampicillin if the organisms do not produce β-lactamase.

Carboxypenicillins (carbenicillin, ticarcillin) and ureidopenicillins (mezlocillin, azlocillin, and piperacillin) are semisynthetic penicillins that must be administered parenterally and are particularly useful to treat serious aerobic gram-negative infections of the lung, abdomen, pelvis, muscle, skeleton, and bloodstream. Ureidopenicillins also have activity against many anaerobes, and streptococci, including enterococci. Their primary clinical usefulness relies on their enhanced ability to kill aerobic gram-negative organisms, including species of *E. coli*, *Proteus*, *P. aeruginosa*, other species of *Pseudomonas*, *H. influenzae*, and species of *Klebsiella*. By themselves, these agents usually are sufficient to kill these organisms with the notable exception of *P. aeruginosa*. Serious infections with *Pseudomonas* usually require the synergistic effects of one of the semisynthetic penicillins plus an aminoglycoside. Carbenicillin is no longer used frequently because it contains considerable amounts of sodium. Ureidopenicillins have better bactericidal activity against species of *Pseudomonas* and other gram-negative bacteria. All these agents are susceptible

in varying degrees to inactivation by bacterial β-lactamases, the means of bacterial resistance to these agents.

In an effort to avoid bacterial mechanisms of resistance to penicillins, there has been a considerable effort to develop substances with inhibitory action on β-lactamase. Two — clavulanic acid and sulbactam — are commercially available. Both are known as β-lactamase inhibitors because they bind to conserved regions within the β-lactamase produced by a variety of organisms. The binding alters the structure of the enzyme, thereby preventing it from binding and hydrolyzing the β-lactam of the antibiotic. They have been effectively used in the treatment of non-life-threatening mixed infections (e.g., aspiration pneumonia, diabetic foot ulcers, and intraabdominal and pelvic sepsis). Clavulanic acid is combined with preparations of ticarcillin and amoxicillin, and sulbactam is combined with parenteral ampicillin. These preparations improve the spectrum of activity against most anaerobes, staphylococci, and certain strains of aerobic gram-negative bacteria.

Cephalosporins

Cephalosporins kill bacteria by interfering with synthesis of their cell walls. They are most commonly used in hospitalized patients for prophylaxis because of their broad spectrum of activity. The agents often are inappropriately employed for both prophylaxis and empirical treatment because physicians lack knowledge of their true spectrum of activity.

The cephalosporins are divided into groups based on their spectrum of activity. First-generation cephalosporins are effective against susceptible aerobic gram-positive staphylococci, gram-negative bacteria, and streptococci. They are useful in most cases of surgical prophylaxis and in minor to moderate-severe skin, respiratory, and urinary tract aerobic gram-positive and gram-negative bacterial infections. They have no place in the treatment of mixed infections because they are ineffective against anaerobes. Second-generation cephalosporins have less aerobic gram-positive activity, but enhanced aerobic gram-negative and anaerobic bacterial coverage compared with first-generation cephalosporins. They are most appropriately used to treat mixed infections, including intraabdominal and pelvic sepsis, diabetic foot ulcers, aspiration pneumonia, many abscesses in different anatomic sites, and other polymicrobial infections. In the treatment of mixed anaerobic-aerobic infections, the most common error is the failure to consider surgical intervention (e.g., debridement of dead tissues or a surgical procedure to drain an abscess). The third-generation cephalosporins are even more effective against aerobic gram-negative organisms than their precursors. But they are unreliable against aerobic gram-positive and most anaerobic bacteria. Because of their unique pharmacokinetic properties, they are most useful to treat aerobic gram-negative bacterial meningitis and biliary tract infections. They should not be used as monotherapy to treat mixed infections or as empirical therapy for serious bacterial infections when staphylococci, streptococci, or anaerobes might be the etiologic agents. The overutilization of all cephalosporins has resulted in increased rates of enterococcal superinfections because these microorganisms are not eradicated by this entire class of antibiotic.

Monobactams

Aztreonam is the only currently commercially available monobactam. It kills susceptible microorganisms by binding to penicillin-binding proteins of the bacteria, ultimately interfering with cell wall synthesis. The spectrum of activity of aztreonam is limited, exhibiting activity against only aerobic gram-negative bacteria causing septicemia, pneumonia, osteomyelitis, and urinary tract infections. This agent has little activity against aerobic gram-positive and anaerobic bacteria. Therefore, the drug cannot be used in the majority of infectious syndromes. This relatively safe but expensive agent should be used in patients with gram-negative bacterial infections who have renal insufficiency and require prolonged therapy. The value of this regimen is that aminoglycoside therapy which will further compromise renal function will not have to be initiated in such compromised patients. Another benefit of aztreonam therapy is that it can be administered safely in patients who have anaphylactic reactions to penicillin.

Carbapenems

Carbapenems are a group of β-lactams with a carbapenem nucleus. So far, imipenem is the only available drug in this class. It binds to all the penicillin-binding proteins (PBPs) but preferentially binds to PBP2 and PBP1, which are respectively responsible for maintaining the bacterium's constant diameter and extending its cell wall in any direction. Interference with these bacterial transpeptidases leads to rapid lysis of most anaerobic and aerobic bacteria. Imipenem has the widest spectrum of activity of the currently available β-lactams, and its usage ordinarily should be reserved for multidrug-resistant bacteria. Imipenem may be effective only against extracellular bacteria. It should not be used to treat intracellular pathogens (e.g., *L. monocytogenes*). Because of imipenem's extensive antibacterial effects, it probably is worth remembering that the only bacterial isolates that are not susceptible to imipenem include methicillin-resistant staphylococci, *Streptococcus faecalis*, *Xanthomonas maltophilia*, *P. cepacia*, and rare groups of *Bacteroides* (e.g., *B. ovatus*, *B. disiens*, and *B. thetaiotaomicron*). Imipenem is not recommended for routine monotherapy to treat bacterial infections of the lower respiratory tract, osteomyelitis, bacterial septicemia and endocarditis, or urinary tract, skin, or intraabdominal infections. Imipenem is definitively not recommended to treat bacterial suppurative meningitis until adequate clinical studies justify the practice.

Carbapenem is extensively metabolized by the renal tubular brush border dipeptidase, dehydropeptidase I. A selective competitive antagonist of this enzyme has been identified (viz., cilastatin), and when it is combined with imipenem in a 1:1 ratio, the antibiotic persists in the plasma for prolonged periods. Imipenem rarely produces toxic effects. High doses can produce convulsions in patients who have a prior history of seizure disorders and renal insufficiency. Imipenem can be made safe even in these patients if the rate of administration is slowed and the dose is reduced in proportion to the extent of renal insufficiency.

Aminoglycosides

Aminoglycosides are very potent bactericidal antibiotic agents for susceptible aerobic microorganisms. They kill by inhibiting protein synthesis and to some extent by lysing the cell envelope. All the aminoglycosides including streptomycin, kanamycin, neomycin, gentamicin, amikacin, tobramycin, sisomicin, and netilimicin share common structural features.

Streptomycin is routinely used once a day in combination with other antibiotics to treat mycobacterial infections and selected endocarditides. Neomycin is used topically to treat superficial infections, and also given orally preoperatively for chemoprophylaxis for large-bowel surgery. The other agents are used parenterally to treat bacterial septicemia, bacterial endocarditis, and urinary tract infections.

The physical environment where the aminoglycosides act considerably influences their antibacterial efficacy. Under conditions of low oxygen tension and low pH, and in the midst of extensive proteinaceous debris, aminoglycosides cannot exert antibacterial effects. Such an environment exists in many infectious diseases. In such situations (e.g., pneumonia, abscesses, skin, and skin rupture infections), aminoglycosides should not be used as monotherapy. Likewise, aminoglycosides should not be used as monotherapy to treat osteomyelitis or CNS infections because they do not penetrate well into these tissues.

The major indication for aminoglycosides is in combination with other antibiotics (e.g., β-lactams) to treat serious aerobic bacterial infections. When combined with β-lactams, they are particularly useful for treating aerobic gram-negative septicemia (notably that caused by Enterobacteriaceae) and enterococcal endocarditis. The combination therapy also decreases the rate of bacterial resistance to aminoglycoside by ribosomal mutation and acquisition of aminoglycoside-modifying enzymes. Because gentamicin is less costly than and equally efficacious as tobramycin and amikacin, gentamicin is the preferred aminoglycoside. Amikacin should be reserved to treat bacterial infections that are known to be resistant to gentamicin and tobramycin since it is the most stable aminoglycoside known against bacterial R-plasmid-mediated enzymes. For this reason, amikacin is active against most gentamicin- and tobramycin-resistant gram-negative bacteria. There is concern that extensive usage of amikacin will eventually select for resistant organisms and nullify its current effectiveness. Tobramycin has been recommended by some authorities because its activity against *P. aeruginosa* is greater than that of gentamicin and because it may be less nephrotoxic than other aminoglycosides given parenterally. Despite these recommendations, it is still prudent to use gentamicin if the bacterial isolate is sensitive to this agent.

Regarding nephrotoxicity, a number of points should be kept in mind when deciding when and which aminoglycoside to use. All the aminoglycosides are concentrated in the renal cortex. The proximal tubules are most susceptible to their toxic effects, but glomerular lesions also are part of the nephrotoxicity caused by aminoglycosides. In general, when patients receive these drugs for less than 5 days, nephrotoxic effects are minimal. The nephrotoxicity is more severe in patients with previous renal insufficiency and coexisting prolonged hypovolemia, sodium depletion, and acidosis, and in those who simultaneously are given other agents, including radiocontrast dye, furosemide, hydrocortisone, or indomethacin. Since aminoglycoside nephrotoxicity is related to the dose of the drugs and their concentrations in plasma, monitoring plasma concentrations in clinically unstable patients, or in those who receive prolonged therapy, is mandatory. Based on these drug concentrations, the dose and frequency of administration of aminoglycosides should be modified (see chapters 1, 37, and 38).

Vancomycin

Vancomycin is a high-molecular-weight glycopeptide that is bactericidal for gram-positive microorganisms. It inhibits cell wall synthesis.

Given parenterally, it is the drug of choice for methicillin-resistant staphylococcal infections. It should be used as an alternative for methicillin-sensitive staphylococci if the patient is allergic to penicillin. Based on considerable clinical experience, there is a lack of evidence to use combinations of aminoglycosides or rifampin with parenteral vancomycin to treat staphylococcal infections. However, treatment of serious enterococcal infections with vancomycin requires the bactericidal effects of an aminoglycoside to eradicate the microorganisms outside the urinary tract. Administered orally, vancomycin is poorly absorbed. But the concentration of vancomycin in the GI tract after an oral dose of 125 mg given every 6 hours is sufficient to eradicate — within 5 days of treatment — strains of *C. difficile* responsible for antibiotic-associated colitis.

Vancomycin is excreted by the kidneys in an essentially unchanged form. Vancomycin accumulates in patients with renal failure, and dosage adjustments are required to reduce the chances of adverse effects. Nephrotoxicity attributed to this agent has decreased remarkably because of improvements in the purification procedures in production of this drug.

A "red man's" syndrome characterized by profound hypotension and a maculopapular rash occurs, if the drug is administered too quickly (e.g., less than 30 minutes). If the infusion of vancomycin is prolonged (i.e., one gram infused over at least 60 minutes), the incidence of the red man's syndrome is decreased. Ototoxicity and nephrotoxicity remain well-recognized adverse reactions to vancomycin.

Chloramphenicol

Chloramphenicol exerts its broad antibacterial effects by binding to the 50-S ribosome subunit, inhibiting protein synthesis. Due to its serious toxic profile, which includes aplastic anemia, and gray baby syndrome and the availability of other less toxic but equally effective drugs used for similar indications, chloramphenicol is not extensively used. It nevertheless remains the drug of choice for the treatment of typhoid and paratyphoid fever, life-threatening rickettsial disease, and aerobic and anaerobic gram-negative and gram-positive bacterial infections in patients who have life-threatening allergy to penicillin.

Tetracycline

The molecular structure of tetracyclines includes four benzene rings. They have a broad spectrum of antibacterial activity, and by binding to the 30-S ribosome subunit, they exert their effects by inhibiting protein synthesis. A considerable number of compounds, especially orally active preparations, have been developed. Unfortunately, because of the high prevalence of tetracycline-resistant microorganisms and the availability of alternative effective antibiotics, the tetracyclines' place in therapy has diminished. Tetracyclines remain the drugs of choice to treat brucellosis, which also requires combination with streptomycin. They also are the drugs of choice to treat chlamydial and rickettsial infections and melioidosis. Since resistance to tetracyclines is so prevalent among all species of bacteria, the effectiveness of tetracycline in treating a variety of clinical syndromes cannot be predicted. Major tetracycline toxicity includes nephrotoxicity and hepatotoxicity, especially in the pregnant patient.

Erythromycin

Erythromycin is a macrolide antibiotic that binds to the 50-S subunit of the ribosomes. It kills susceptible bacteria by interfering with their protein synthesis. Erythromycin is active against many aerobic gram-positive bacteria, selected gram-negative bacteria—including species of *Legionella*, *N. meningitidis*, *H. influenzae*, and *Bordetella pertussis*—and nonbacterial species (e.g., *C. trachomatis*, mycoplasma, and certain rickettsial species). There are three available oral preparations of erythromycin: erythromycin stearate, erythromycin ethyl succinate, and erythromycin estolate. The first two preparations do not have intrinsic antibacterial activity until they dissociate or hydrolyze (respectively) to active compounds. They are routinely recommended to be taken orally 1 hour prior to meals so that effective concentrations of drugs in plasma can be consistently achieved. The estolate form is associated with the highest concentrations in plasma.

The parenteral forms of erythromycin include an ethyl succinate form for IM administration and lactobionate or gluceptate forms for use IV. The severity of irritation of veins with erythromycin frequently requires large veins to be catheterized and low concentrations of lidocaine coadministered with the antibiotic to reduce pain. Too-rapid IV infusion of erythromycin results in diffuse cramping and GI discomfort due to contraction of intestinal smooth muscle.

Erythromycin is widely used as an alternative for β-lactam antibiotics in the patient who is allergic to penicillin and requires treatment for non-life-threatening gram-positive bacterial infection. These include streptococcal and pneumococcal systemic infections and staphylococcal skin infections. In more serious infections with these organisms, vancomycin is preferred over erythromycin. Erythromycin has been effective in treating *Legionella* pneumonia and *H. influenzae* respiratory and otitis media infections. It is effectively used as an alternative drug for a variety of sexually transmitted diseases, including gonorrhea, chlamydial infections, syphilis, and chancroid.

Clindamycin

Clindamycin is a chemically modified derivative of lincomycin. It exerts its activity by binding to the 50-S subunit of the bacterial ribosome, inhibiting protein synthesis. Its antibacterial spectrum includes staphylococci, streptococci but not enterococci, many anaerobic gram-positive strains, and most anaerobic gram-negative bacteria. Chloramphenicol, metronidazole, ticarcillin, clavulanic acid, ampicillin, sulbactam, and imipenem are the only other agents that have better activity against anaerobes. Clindamycin is most appropriately used to treat clinical syndromes that involve anaerobic pathogens. Clindamycin is not recommended as a primary agent to treat staphylococcal and streptococcal infections despite its antibacterial activity with these microorganisms.

Clindamycin is extensively eliminated by the liver. Doses should be modified when patients have hepatic insufficiency. The most common serious adverse reaction to clindamycin is pseudomembranous colitis. This effect occurs 2 days to 3 weeks after beginning therapy in 1% to 10% of patients treated with clindamycin. However, as was discussed earlier, this example of superinfection is not unique to the use of clindamycin, since essentially any antibiotic can produce the same condition. The pathogenesis of this syndrome generally involves excretion of the antibiotic in the stool and selection of *C. difficile* in the GI tract. Clinically important *C. difficile* strains elaborate toxins that are cytotoxic to the epithelial muscosal cells, and a pseudomembrane covers the afflicted area. Symptoms of colitis usually include fever, cramping, abdominal pain, and diarrhea. Appropriate management of this syndrome includes sigmoidoscopy or colonoscopy assessment of the stool for the presence of inflammatory cells, detection of the toxin, and culture for *C. difficile* to make the diagnosis. Effective therapy for this superinfection includes oral vancomycin or oral or parenteral metronidazole.

Metronidazole

Metronidazole is a nitroimidazole drug that has anaerobic bacterial and protozoal activity. The drug is postulated to be metabolized within the anaerobe to an active drug that interacts with the anaerobe's DNA to produce cell death. The spectrum of antibacterial activity for metronidazole is confined to most anaerobes. It has essentially no activity against aerobic bacteria. Metronidazole has been effectively used to treat a variety of infectious syndromes, involving anaerobic strains, that include intraabdominal sepsis, genital infections, abscesses, aspiration pneumonia, osteomyelitis, trichomoniasis, amebiasis, and giardiasis. Because of its low resistance rate and cost, metronidazole should be the drug of choice in treatment of anaerobic infections.

Sulfonamides and Trimethoprim

Sulfonamides and trimethoprim are used to treat mild to moderately severe bacterial infections. They exert their antibacterial effects by interfering with the microorganism's folate metabolism, which is essential for purine and ultimately DNA synthesis. There are many sulfonamides available, differing from each other by their duration of action. Sulfadiazine is short-acting (i.e., therefore required every 6–8 hours). Sulfamethoxazole has medium duration of action (i.e., it must be given every 12 hours). Sulfadoxine is ultralong-acting and requires dosage once a week. This agent is readily absorbed from the GI tract.

Trimethoprim frequently is combined with sulfonamides but can be used as a single agent with success equivalent to that expected of sulfonamides used alone. The two agents once had a wide range of antimicrobial activity. However, extensive usage and the rapid development of microbial resistance to these drugs have narrowed their spectrum of activity. Sulfonamide-susceptible microorganisms include staphylococci, many streptococci except *S. faecalis*, many anaerobic gram-positive bacilli, some *L. monocytogenes*, most species of *Nocardia*, the majority of Enterobacteriaceae, many pathogenic species of *Neisseria*, *Xanthomonas maltophilia, H. influenzae*, many other gram-negative anaerobes, strains of *Chlamydia* except *C. psittaci*, some atypical species of mycobacteria, protozoa such as *Toxoplasma gondii* and malaria, and unique fungi such as *P. carinii* when therapy combines pyrimethamine or trimethoprim with sulfonamides.

Trimethoprim is much more active than sulfonamides and has essentially the same spectrum of activity. These agents probably do not exhibit synergistic effects, but the combination is effective to treat urinary tract infections that are caused by a variety of aerobic gram-positive and gram-negative bacteria, otitis media, acute and chronic bronchitis and bacterial pneumonia, venereal diseases (e.g., gonorrhea, chancroid, granuloma venereum, and sometimes *C. trachomatis* infections), typhoid fever from susceptible strains, shigellosis, cholera, brucellosis, nocardiosis, toxoplasmosis, and *P. carinii* pneumonia. Allergic adverse responses are frequent, especially in AIDS patients. They most notably include rashes, drug fever, and bone marrow suppression.

Quinolones

Norfloxacin and ciprofloxacin are the more commonly employed quinolones. They are derivatives of nalidixic acid, which is the prototype compound of this class. In contrast to nalidixic acid, norfloxacin and ciprofloxacin readily penetrate the outer membranes of a large number of gram-negative and selected gram-positive bacteria. These agents exert their antibacterial effects by binding to DNA gyrase, thereby inhibiting replication of bacterial DNA. Microorganisms are killed by quinolones if they continue to synthesize protein. Ultimately, the bacteria cannot divide because of the effects of the quinolone. Resistance develops via chromosomal mutation, especially among enteric flora exposed to subinhibitory concentrations of drug. These drugs are administered orally and are readily absorbed. Norfloxacin is more limited in its distribution within the body than ciprofloxacin. Norfloxacin is used mainly to treat urinary tract infections, whereas ciprofloxacin, in addition to being useful in treating urinary tract infections, also is used to treat bone, respiratory, inner ear, and soft tissue infections.

The quinolones exert their greatest antibacterial effects against susceptible aerobic gram-negative bacteria from the Enterobacteriaceae, including many strains of *P. aeruginosa*. Infections due to these microorganisms are appropriately treated with quinolones. The role of quinolones in the treatment of other gram-negative microorganisms (e.g., *H. influenzae* and *N. gonorrhoeae*) and especially gram-positive aerobic microorganisms (e.g., *S. pneumoniae* and staphylococci) is controversial. Quinolones are not recommended to treat anaerobic infections or monotherapy for serious life-threatening infections or meningitis.

Antituberculosis Drugs

Treatment of mycobacterial infections requires multiple drugs because monotherapy frequently fails. Resistance of *M. tuberculosis* to an antimicrobial agent occurs as a result of spontaneous mutation, at a usual frequency of 1 in 10^5 to 10^6. Mutational resistance to each drug occurs as an independent event, and thus the likelihood of a single organism's being resistant to two drugs is equal to the product of the individual probabilities. Therefore, combined chemotherapy with two or more drugs prevents the emergence of strains resistant to an individual drug. The likelihood of organisms developing resistance is increased if the patient previously has been treated and if the infection was the result of exposure to a resistant strain.

Tuberculocidal drugs are preferred and should be capable of killing both rapidly dividing extracellular organisms and slower dividing intracellular organisms in order to prevent relapse. Isoniazid and rifampin are tuberculocidal in both intra- and extracellular locations and are generally recommended in all patients with mycobacterial infection. Streptomycin is tuberculocidal for extracellular organisms only, while pyrazinamide is tuberculocidal for intracellular organisms. Ethambutol, *p*-aminosalicylic acid, and ethionamide are only tuberculostatic.

The institution of effective chemotherapy results in rapid reversal of infectiousness of mycobacteria within 3 to 7 days. However, the clinical manifestations of disease might persist for prolonged periods. For example, when pulmonary tuberculosis is caused by *M. tuberculosis*, fever and cough should dramatically decrease within 2 weeks. However, a fever may persist for months despite appropriate therapy. Although antimicrobial-resistant mycobacterial strains emerge as an important epidemiologic cause for clinical failure, the major cause of failure of an effective drug regimen for mycobacterial infections is lack of compliance by the patient.

Pulmonary infections with *M. tuberculosis* strains are the most frequent type of mycobacterial infection. They account for more than 90% of all mycobacterial infections. Although with the AIDS epidemic pulmonary infections by atypical strains of mycobacteria have dramatically increased, they are still not as common as infections with *M. tuberculosis*. Hospitalization for initial therapy of tuberculosis is not generally necessary. Effective treatment for pulmonary tuberculosis includes 6- and 9-month regimens. The shorter protocol includes isoniazid and rifampin in therapeutic daily doses for 6 months plus pyrazinamide daily in therapeutic doses for 2 months to treat pulmonary infections. The more prolonged protocol entails isoniazid and rifampin in therapeutic daily doses for 9 months. Ethambutol can be added to either the 6-month or 9-month regimen on an optional basis for 2 months. The patient should be monitored for adverse effects of the drug and efficacy while on therapy. Liver function tests and cell counts and sputum for acid-fast stains should be obtained monthly. Analysis of sputum can be less frequent once acid-fast bacteria have been cleared from the respiratory tract. This usually occurs within 1 to 2 months of initiation of therapy. After a regimen is completed, the patient should be monitored up to 1 year for signs of a relapse. When relapse occurs after the use of isoniazid and rifampin, the mycobacteria are almost always still susceptible to these agents. Further treatment with the same regimen usually is successful. After other regimens, the likelihood of resistance by the organism is greater, and at least two new drugs are required.

The principles of treatment of extrapulmonary tuberculosis generally are the same as for pulmonary tuberculosis. Isoniazid and rifampin remain the primary agents of choice. However, if the infection is immediately life-threatening (e.g., meningitis is present), a total of four tuberculocidal drugs should be employed to cover the possibility of resistance. Also, 18 to 24 months of treatment for extrapulmonary tuberculosis is generally recommended. The exception for such a duration is tuberculosis of lymph nodes, which can be effectively treated with only 9 months of therapy.

Antifungal Drugs

Fungal infections are particularly serious and common among neutropenic, immunocompromised patients who have received prolonged broad-spectrum antibiotics. A number of systemic fungal infections can also afflict otherwise healthy persons (e.g., histoplasmosis, coccidioidomycosis, and paracoccidioidomycosis). Until recently, only amphotericin B was available to treat systemic fungal infection. However, with the rapid development and clinical assessment of azole compounds, a number of these agents are also considered appropriate for treatment of fungal infections.

Amphotericin B is a polyene antibiotic that exerts its antifungal effect by binding to sterol moieties in the membranes of fungi. This causes pores in the cell wall eventually causing leakage of low-molecular-weight cytoplasmic components. This effect, coupled with amphotericin's ability to stimulate granulocytes and T and B cells, ultimately leads to the death of fungi.

Amphotericin B has a wide spectrum of antifungal activity. Susceptible fungi include species of *Candida, Histoplasma capsulatum, Cryptococcus neoformans, Coccidioides immitis, Blastomyces dermatitides, Paracoccidioides brasilensis, Sporathrix schenckii,* and many strains of *Aspergillus.* It is still considered the drug of choice for any life-threatening disseminated fungal disease. This choice may well change with greater experience with the newer azole agents since amphotericin B causes considerable toxicity, most notably anaphylaxis, other allergic reactions, renal insufficiency, and bone marrow suppression.

The newer antifungal agents include ketoconazole, miconazole, itraconazole, and fluconazole. These agents are azoles, and they exert their antifungal activity by inhibiting ergosterol synthesis. Ketoconazole is available in oral form and in normal patients is often erratically absorbed from the GI tract. Achlorhydria caused by any mechanism significantly reduces its absorption. Ketoconazole is metabolized primarily in the liver. To prevent toxicity it must be judiciously employed in patients with hepatic failure or those who receive other drugs that are also metabolized in the liver. A major adverse effect associated ketoconazole includes its affects on the endocrine system (e.g., blunting of cortisol and androgen synthesis and production of gynecomastia). Ketoconazole is particularly effective in treating certain forms of histoplasmosis, coccidioidomycosis, paracoccidioidomycosis, and candidiasis. It is not recommended for treating (1) CNS fungal infections because it penetrates the CSF poorly, or (2) serious life-threatening diseases because GI absorption can be erratic. Miconazole is rarely employed now because of its serious adverse effects and the availability of other agents. However, parenteral miconazole is the drug of choice for infections due to *Pseudoallescheria boydii*. In addition, topical miconazole is frequently used as an effective antimicrobial for vaginal yeast infections.

Itraconazole is administered orally and is well distributed within the body with the exception of penetration into the CSF. Itraconazole should not be used in patients with CNS fungal infections. Its spectrum of activity is similar to that of amphotericin B. Clinical studies to date suggest that is useful to treat selected cases of disseminated candidiasis, histoplasmosis, coccidiomycosis, selected infections with *Aspergillus*, sporotrichosis, blastomycosis, and paracoccidioidomycosis. It has the advantage over amphotericin B of being relatively safe.

Fluconazole is unique among the azoles in that it can penetrate into the CSF in high concentration. Parenteral and oral forms of fluconazole therapy are available. Its spectrum of activity is very similar to that of other azoles and amphotericin B. Limited clinical experience to date suggests that it is the drug of choice for treatment of oroesophageal and mucocutaneous candidiasis and suppressive therapy of cryptococcal meningitis in AIDS patients.

Antiviral Agents

In the last decade, considerable strides have been made developing effective antiviral therapy. A major obstacle in such development has been identifying agents that do not injure host cells but still effectively inhibit viral metabolism and replication. The clinically most important new antiviral agents include acyclovir used to treat herpesviruses, AZT for the HIV agent (see the section on treatment of AIDS), and ganciclovir to treat retinitis caused by cytomegalovirus.

Acyclovir is a purine nucleoside analog. Its antiviral activity is almost exclusive for the herpesviruses (HSV1 and 2, VZV, and EBV). Once acyclovir has penetrated virally infected cells, it is phosphorylated into acyclovir monophosphate by HSV thymidine kinase and sequentially into di-

and triphosphate forms by cellular enzymes. Acyclovir is a potent inhibitor of viral DNA polymerases and also terminates biosynthesis of the strand of viral DNA. Acyclovir distributes widely throughout the body including the CSF. The major route of elimination is via glomerular filtration and tubular secretion. Therefore, dosage adjustment is required in patients with renal dysfunction. Acyclovir is effective in the treatment of a number of infections caused by herpes simplex virus, including mucocutaneous, genital, and encephalitic infections, and varicella-zoster infections.

Ganciclovir (DHPG) is a nucleoside analog. Its antiviral activity is primarily for cytomegalovirus. Once phosphorylated to triphosphate form by cellular enzymes, it interferes with viral replication through competitive inhibition of viral DNA polymerase and also terminates viral DNA synthesis. Ganciclovir is primarily excreted by the kidneys and is well distributed to most organs, including lungs, liver, and the brain. Dosage adjustment is also indicated in patients with renal dysfunction. The primary indication of ganciclovir is for the treatment of cytomegalovirus-associated retinitis in the immunocompromised host. Data on ganciclovir treatment of CMV-associated pneumonitis, encephalitis, and hepatitis remains controversial.

Acknowledgement — The authors want to thank Mary Hanley for her superior secretarial skills and emotional support in the preparation of this chapter.

REFERENCES

Abrams, D. I.; Kuno, S.; and Wong, R.: Oral dextran sulfate (UA001) in treatment of the acquired immunodeficiency syndrome (AIDS) and AIDS-related complex (ARC). Ann. Intern. Med., 110:183–188, 1989.

Adkinson, N.; Swabb, E.; and Sugerman, A.: Immunology of the monobactam aztreonam. Antimicrob. Agents Chemother., 25:93–98, 1984.

Agrawal, S.; Goodchild, J.; and Civeria, M. P.: Oligonucleoside phosphoramidate and phosphorthioates as inhibitors of human immunodeficiency virus. Proc. Natl. Acad. Sci. U.S.A., 85:7079–7083, 1988.

Alavi, J. B.; Root, R. K.; Djerassi, I.; Evans, A. E.; Gluckman, S. J.; Macgregor, R. R.; Guerry, D.; Schrieber, A. D.; Shaw, J. M.; Koch, P.; and Cooper R. A.: A randomized clinical trial of granulocyte transfusions for injection in acute leukemia. N. Engl. J. Med., 296:706–711, 1977.

Anaissie, E.; Rolston, K.; and Bodey, G. P.: Treatment of gram-negative bacteremia in patients with cancer and granulocytopenia. N. Engl. J. Med., 318:1694–1695, 1988.

Andriole, V. T.: Antibiotic synergy in experimental infection with *Pseudomonas*: II. The effect of carbenicillin, cephalothin or cephanone combined with tobramycin or gentamicin. J. Infect. Dis., 129:124–133, 1974.

Andriole, V. T.; and Epstein, F. H.: Prevention of pyelonephritis by water diuresis: Evidence for the role of medullary hypertonicity in promoting renal infection. J. Clin. Invest., 44:73–79, 1965.

Archambaud, M.; Courcoux, P.; Ovin, V.; Chabanon, G.; and Labigne-Roussel, A.: Phenotypic and genotypic assays for the detection and identification of adhesins from pyelonephritic *E. coli*. Ann. Inst. Pasteur Microbiol., 139:557–573, 1988.

Arthur, M.; Johnson, C.; Rubin, R.; Arbeit, R.; Campanelli, R.; Ulman, C.; Steinbach, S.; Agarwal, M.; Wilkinson, R.; and Goldstein, R.: Molecular epidemiology of adhesin and hemolysin virulence factors among uropathogenic *E. coli*. Infect. Immun., 57:303–313, 1989.

Avorn, J.; Soumerai, S.; Taylor, W.; Wessel, M.; Janousek, J.; and Weiner, M.: Reduction of incorrect antibiotic dosing through a structured educational order form. Arch. Intern. Med., 148:1720–1724, 1988.

Avorn, J.; Harvey, K.; Soumerai, S.; Herxheimer, A.; Plumridge, R.; and Bardelay, G.: Information and education as determinants of antibiotic use: Report of task force 5. Rev. Infect. Dis., 9:S286–S296, 1987.

Bach, M. C.: Clinical response to dideoxyinosine in patients with HIV infection resistant to zidovudine. N. Engl. J. Med., 323:275, 1990.

Balduzzi, P.; and Glasgow, L. A.: Paralytic poliomyelitis in a contact of a vaccinated child. N. Engl. J. Med., 276:796–797, 1967.

Barrett-Connor, E.: Bacterial infection and sickle cell anemia: An analysis of 250 infections in 166 patients and a review of the literature. Medicine, 50:97–112, 1971.

Barriere, S.: Cost-containment of antimicrobial therapy. Drug. Intell. Clin. Pharm., 19:278–281, 1985.

Bartlett, J.: Treatment of antibiotic-associated pseudomembranous colitis. Rev. Infect. Dis., 6:235–246, 1984.

Bauer, A. W.; Kirby, W. M. M.; Sherris, J. C.; and Turch, M.: Antibiotic susceptibility testing by a standardized single disk method. Am. J. Clin. Pathol., 45:493–496, 1966.

Beachey, E.: Bacterial adherence: Adhesion-receptor interactions mediating the attachment of bacteria to mucosal surfaces. J. Infect. Dis., 143:325–345, 1981.

Bennett, W. M.: Guide to drug dosage in renal failure. Clin. Pharmacokinet., 15:326–354, 1988.

Bennett, W. M.; Singer, I.; and Coggins, C. H.: A guide to drug therapy in renal failure. J.A.M.A., 230:1544–1553, 1974.

Bentley, R.; and Meganathan, R.: Biosynthesis of vitamin K in bacteria. Microbiol. Rev., 46:241–280, 1982.

Benz, R.; Schmid, A.; Waner, W.; and Goebel, W.: Pore formation by *Escherichia coli* hemolysin: Evidence for an association-disassociation equilibrium of the pore-forming aggregates. Infect. Immunol., 57:887–895, 1989.

Bergadahl, S.; Sonnerborg, A.; Larsson, A.; and Stranegard, O.: Declining levels of p24 antigen in serum during treatment with foscarnet. Lancet, 1:1052, 1988.

Bhakdi, S.; and Tranum-Jensen, J.: Damage to cell membranes by pore-forming bacterial cytolysins. Prog. Allergy, 40:1–43, 1988.

Bhakdi, S.; Mackman, N.; Nicoud, J.; and Holland, I.: *Escherichia coli* hemolysin may damage target cell membranes by generating transmembrane pores. Infect. Immunol., 52:63–69, 1986.

Bodey, G. P.: Antibiotics in patients with neutropenia. Arch. Intern. Med., 144:1845–1851, 1984.

Bodey, G. P.; Rodrigues, V.; Chang, H. Y.; and Narboni, G.: Fever and infection in leukemic patients. A study of 494 consecutive patients. Cancer, 41:1616–1622, 1978.

Bodey, G. P.; Buckley, M.; Sathe, Y. S.; and Freireich, E. J.: Quantitative relationship between circulating leukocytes and infection in patients with acute leukemia. Ann. Intern. Med., 64:328–340, 1966.

Brooks, G.; and York, M.: Cost-effective clinical microbiology and newer tests of importance to the practitioner. In, Current Clinical Topics in Infectious Diseases (Remington, J.; and Swartz, M., eds.). Vol. 7. McGraw-Hill, New York, pp. 157–193, 1986.

Calvelli, T. A.; and Rubenstein, A.: Intravenous gammaglobulin in infant acquired immunodeficiency syndrome. Pediatr. Infect. Dis., 5:S207–S210, 1986.

Capon, D. J.; Chamow, S. M.; Mordenti, J.; Marsters, S. A.; Gregory, T.; Mitsuya, H.; Byrn, R. A.; Lucas, C.; Wurm,

F. M.; Groopman, J. E.; Broder, S.; and Smith, D. H.: Designing CD4 immunoadhesins for AIDS therapy. Nature, 337:525–531, 1989.

Cavalieri, S.; Bohach, G.; and Snyder, J.: *E. coli* alphahemolysin: Characteristics and probable role in pathogenicity. Microbiol. Rev., 48:326–343, 1984.

Centers for Disease Control: Recommendation of the Immunizations Practices Advisory Committee: General recommendation on immunization. M.M.W.R., 38:205–214, 1989.

Centers for Disease Control: Rubella vaccination during pregnancy 1971–1986. M.M.W.R., 36:457–461, 1987.

Centers for Disease Control: Recommendation of the Immunization Practices Advisory Committee: Small pox vaccine. M.M.W.R., 34:341–342, 1985.

Chandra, R.: Nutrition, community, and infection: Present knowledge and future directions. Lancet, 1(8326 part 1):688–691, 1983.

Chang, J.; Des Rosiers, S.; and Weinstein, L.: Clinical and serological studies of an outbreak of rubella in a vaccinated population. N. Engl. J. Med., 283:246–248, 1970.

Chaudhary, V. K.; Mizukami, T.; Fuerst, T. R.; FitzGerald, D. J.; Moss, B.; Pastan, I.; and Berger, E. A.: Selective killing of HIV-infected cells by recombinant CD4-*Pseudomonas* exotoxin hybrid protein. Nature, 335:369–372, 1988.

Chernik, N. L.; Armstrong, D.; and Posner, J. B.: Central nervous system infections in patients with cancer. Medicine (Baltimore), 52:563–581, 1973.

Cherubin, C. E.; Marr, J. S.; Sierra, M. F.; and Becker, S.: *Listeria* and gram-negative bacillary meningitis in New York City, 1972–1979. Am. J. Med., 71:199–209, 1981.

Cheson, B. D.; Levine, A. M.; and Milvan, D.: Suramin therapy in AIDS and related disorders. J.A.M.A., 258:1347–1351, 1987.

Christiansen, L. K.; Hansen, J. M.; and Kristensen, M.: Sulphaphenazole-induced hypoglycemic attacks in tolbutamide-treated diabetics. Lancet, 2:1298–1301, 1963.

Christiansen, P. E.: An epidemic of measles in southern Greenland 1951. Acta. Med. Scand., 144:313–322; 430–449; 450–454, 1952–1953.

Col, N.; and O'Conner, R.: Estimating world-wide current antibiotic usage: Report of task force I. Rev. Infect. Dis., 9: S232–S243, 1987.

Coleman, R.; Rodandi, L.; Kaubisch, S.; Granzella, N.; and O'Hanley, P.: Economic impact of a prospective and continuous parenteral antibiotic control. Am. J. Med., in press, 1990.

Collins, F.: The immunology of tuberculosis. Am. Rev. Respir. Dis., 125:42–49, 1982.

Condon, R. E.: Rational use of prophylactic antibiotics in gastrointestinal surgery. Surg. Clin. North Am., 55:1309–1338, 1975.

Conte, J.; Jacob, L.; and Polk, H.: Antibiotic Prophylaxis in Surgery. J. B. Lippincott, Philadelphia, 1986.

Craig, W. A.; and Kunin, C. M.: Significance of serum protein and tissue binding of antimicrobial agents. Ann. Rev. Med., 27:287–300, 1976.

Craig, W.; Uman, S.; and Shaw, W.: Hospital use of antimicrobial drugs—Survey at 19 hospitals and results of antimicrobial control programs. Ann. Intern. Med., 89:793–798, 1978.

Cruse, P. J. E.; and Foord, R.: A five-year prospective study of 23,649 surgical wounds. Arch. Surg., 107:206–210, 1973.

Darrell, J. H.; Garrod, L. P.; and Waterworth, D. M.: Trimethoprim: Laboratory and clinical studies. J. Clin. Pathol., 21:202–209, 1968.

deShazo, R.; Lopez, M.; and Salvaggio, J.: Use and interpretation of diagnostic immunologic laboratory tests. J.A.M.A., 258:3011–3017, 1987.

DiNubile, M. J.: Stopping antibiotic therapy in neutopenic patients. Ann. Intern. Med., 108:289–292, 1988.

Durack, D.: Prophylaxis of infective endocarditis. In, Principles and Practice of Infectious Diseases (Mandell, G.; Douglas, G.; and Bennett, J., eds.). Churchill Livingstone, New York, pp. 716–721, 1990.

Eichhoff, T.: Immunization: An adult thing to do. J. Infect. Dis., 152:1–8, 1985.

Eisenstein, B.: Interference with mannose binding and epithelial cell adherence of *Escherichia coli* by sublethal concentrations of streptomycin. J. Clin. Invest., 63:1219–1223, 1979.

Ernst, M.; Kern, P.; Flat, H. D.; and Ulmer, A. J.: Effects of systemic in vivo interleukin-2 (Il-2) reconstitution in patients with AIDS and AIDS-related complex (ARC) on phenotypes and functions of peripheral blood mononuclear cells (PBMC). J. Clin. Immunol., 6:170–181, 1986.

Evans, A. S.: Viral Infections of Humans. Plenum Publishing, New York, 1976.

Evans, D. J.; Evans, D. G.; Hohne, C.; Noble, M. A.; Haldane, E. V.; Lior, H.; and Young, L. S.: Hemolysin and K antigens in relation to serotype and hemagglutination type of *E. coli* isolated from extraintestinal infections. J. Clin. Microbiol., 13:171–178, 1981.

Fauci, A. S.; Dale, D. C.; and Balow, J. E.: Glucocorticosteroid therapy: Mechanisms of action and clinical correlations. Ann. Intern. Med., 84:304–315, 1976.

Feldman, W. E.: Relation of concentrations of bacteria and bacterial antigen in cerebrospinal fluid to prognosis in patients with bacterial meningitis. N. Engl. J. Med., 296:433–435, 1977.

Finch, C. A.; and Wilkinson, H. W.: Practical considerations in using counter-immunoelectrophoresis to identify the principal causative agents of bacterial meningitis. J. Clin. Microbiol., 10:519–524, 1979.

Fischbach, M.; and Talal, N.: Ability of isoprinosine to restore interleukin-2 production and T cell proliferation in autoimmune mice. Clin. Exp. Immunol., 61:242–247, 1985.

Fischl, M. A.; Richman, D. D.; Hansen, N.; Collier, A. C.; Carey, J. T.; Para, M. F.; Hardy, W. D.; Dolin, R.; Powderly, W. D.; Allan, J. D.; Wong, B.; Merigan, T. C.; McAuliffe, V. J.; Hyslop, N. E.; Rhame, F. S.; Balfour, H. H. Jr.; Spector, S. A.; Volberding, P.; Pettinelli, C.; Anderson, J.; and the AIDS Clinical Trials Group: The safety and efficacy of zidovudine (AZT) in the treatment of subjects withe mildly symptomatic human immunodeficiency virus type 1, (HIV) infection. Ann. Intern. Med., 112:727–737, 1990.

Fischl, M. A.; Richman, D. D.; Gieico, M. H.; Gottlieb, M. S.; Volberding, P. A.; Laskin, O. L.; Leedem, J. M.; Groopman, J. E.; Mildvan, D.; Schooley, R. T.; Jackson, G. G.; Durack, D. T.; Phil, D.; King, D.; and the AZT Collaborative Working Group: The efficacy of azidothymidine (AZT) in the treatment of patients with AIDS and AIDS-related complex. A double-blind, placebo controlled trial. N. Engl. J. Med., 317:185–191, 1987.

Fowler, J.; and Stamey, T.: Studies of introital colonization in women with recurrent urinary infections: VII. The role of bacterial adherence. J. Urol., 117:472–476, 1977.

Freter, R.: Mechanisms of associate of bacteria with mucosal surfaces. In, Adhesion and Microorganism Pathogenicity (Elliot, K.; O'Connor, M.; and Whelan, J., eds.). Ciba Foundation Symposium 80. Pitman Medical, London, pp. 36–55, 1981.

Fulginiti, V. A.: Active and passive immunization in the control of infectious diseases. In, Immunologic Disorders in Infants and Children (Stiehm, E. R.; and Fulginiti, V. A., eds.). W. B. Saunders, Philadelphia, 1973.

Gale, E. F.; Cundliffe, E.; Reynolds, P. E.; Richmond, M. H.; and Waring, M.: The Molecular Basis of Antibiotic Action. John Wiley & Sons, London, 1972.

Garrod, L. P.: Chemoprophylaxis. Br. Med. J., 2:561–564, 1975.

Gilbert, D.: Current status of antibiotic prophylaxis in surgical patients. Bull. N.Y. Acad. Med., 60:340–357, 1984.

Gilman, A.; Goodman, L.; Rall, T.; and Murad, F. (eds.): The Pharmacological Basis of Therapeutics. Macmillan, New York, 1985.

Giradin, E.; Grau, G.; Doyer, J.; Roux, L.; and Lambert, P.: Tumor necrosis factor and interleukin 1 in the serum of children with severe infectious purpura. N. Engl. J. Med., 319:397–400, 1988.

Gorbach, S. L.; and Bartlett, J. G.: Pseudomembranous en-terocolitis: A review of its diverse forms. J. Infect. Dis., 135:89–104, 1977.

Gorbach, S. L.; and Bartlett, J. G.: Anaerobic infections. N. Engl. J. Med., 290:1177–1184, 1237–1245, 1289–1294, 1974.

Gordon, R.; Thompson, T.; and Carlson, W.: Antimicrobial resistance of shigellae isolated in Michigan. J.A.M.A., 231:1159–1162, 1975.

Grieco, M. H.; Lange, M.; Buimovici-Klein, E.; Reddy, M. M.; England, A.; McKinley, G. F.; Ong, K.; and Metroka, C.: Open study of AL-721 treatment in HIV infected subjects with generalized lymphadenopathy syndrome: An eight week open trial and followup. Antiviral Res., 9:177–190, 1988.

Griffin, W. O.: Current problems in surgery. In, The Prophylactic Use of Antimicrobials in Surgery. Year Book Medical Publishers, Chicago, pp. 70–131, 1983.

Griffiss, J.; and Brandt, B.: Non-epidemic (endemic) meningococcal disease: Pathogenic factors and clinical features. In, Current Clinical Topics in Infectious Diseases (Remington, J.; and Swartz, M., eds.). Vol. 7. McGraw-Hill, New York, pp. 27–50, 1986.

Grinde, B.; Hungnes, O.; and Tjotta, E.: The proteinase inhibitor pepstatin A inhibits formation of reverse transcription in H9 cells with human immunodeficiency virus-1. AIDS Res. Human Retrov., 5:269–274, 1989.

Gruters, R. A.; Neefjes, J. J.; Tersmette, L.; deGoede, R. E.; Tulp, A.; Huisman, H. G.; Miedema, F.; and Ploegh, H. L.: Interference with HIV-induced syncytium formation and viral infectivity by inhibitors of trimming glycosidase. Nature, 350:74–77, 1987.

Hahn, B. H.; Gonda, M. A.; Shaw, G. M.; Popovic, M.; Hoxie, J. A.; Gallo, R. C.; and Wong-Staal, F.: Genomic diversity of the acquired immunodeficiency syndrome virus HTLV III: Different viruses exhibit greatest divergence in their envelope genes. Proc. Natl. Acad. Sci. U.S.A., 82:4813–4817, 1985.

Haley, S.: Extra-charges and prolongation of hospitalization due to nosocomial infections: A prospective interhospital comparison. Am. J. Med., 70:51–58, 1978.

Harada, H.; Ishizaka, A.; Yonemaru, M.; Mallick, A.; Hatherhill, J.; Zheng, H.; Lilly, C.; O'Hanley, P.; and Raffin, T.: Effects of aminophylline and pentoxifylline on multiple organ damage after *Escherichia coli* sepsis. Am. Rev. Respir. Dis., 140:974–980, 1989.

Harber, M.; Topley, N.; and Asscher, A.: Virulence factors of urinary pathogens. Clin. Sci., 70:531–538, 1986.

Hartshorn, K. L.; Vogt, M. W.; Chou, T. C.; Blumburg, R. S.; Byington, R.; Schooley, R. T.; and Hirsch, M. S.: Synergistic inhibition of human immunodeficiency virus in vitro by azidothymidine and recombinant alpha A interferon. Antimicrob. Agents Chemother., 31:168–172, 1987.

Hauser, W.; and Remington, J.: Effects of antibiotics on the immune response. Am. J. Med., 72:711–716, 1982.

Hirschmann, J. V.; and Inui, T. S.: Antimicrobial prophylaxis: A critique of recent trials. Rev. Infect. Dis., 2(1):1–23, 1980.

Ho, D. D.; Sargadharan, M. G.; Hirsch, M. S.; Schooley, R. T.; Rota, T. R.; Kennedy, R. C.; Chanh, T. C.; and Sato, V. L.: Human immunodeficiency virus neutralizing antibodies recognize several conserved domains on the envelope glycoproteins. J. Virol., 61:2024–2028, 1987.

Ho, D. D.; Hartshorn, K. L.; Rota, T. R.; Andrews, C. A.; Kaplan, J. C.; Schooley, R. T.; Hirsch, M. S.; and Infectious Disease Unit, Mass. General Hospital, Harvard Medical School, Boston: Recombinant human interferon alpha A supresses HTLV III replication in vitro. Lancet, 1:602–604, 1985.

Ho, M.: Cytomegalovirus. In, Biology and Infection (Ho, M., ed.). Plenum, New York, 1982.

Hoeprich, P. D.: Immunoprophylaxis of infectious diseases. In, Infectious Diseases (Hoeprich, P. D., ed.). Harper & Row, Hagerstown, Md., Chap. 19, 1972.

Holland, H. K.; Saral, R.; Rossi, J. J.; Donnenberg, A. D.; Burns, W. H.; Berchorner, W. E.; Farzadegan, H.; Jones, R. J.; Quinnan, G. V.; Vogelsang, G. B.; Vriesendorp, H. M.; Wingard, J. R.; Zaia, J. A.; and Santos, G. W.:

Allogeneic bone marrow transplantation, zidovudine and human immunodeficiency virus Type 1 (HIV-1) infection. Ann. Intern. Med., 111:973–981, 1989.

Horstmann, D.: Need for monitoring vaccinated population for immunity levels. Prog. Med. Virol., 16:215–240, 1973.

Horwitz, M.: Adenoviruses. In, Human Viral Diseases (Fields, B.; Melnick, J.; and Chanock, R., eds.). Raven Press, New York, pp. 477–495, 1987.

Hu, S.-L.; Kosowski, S. G.; and Dalrymple, J. M.: Expression of AIDS virus envelope gene in recombinant vaccinia viruses. Nature, 320:537–540, 1986.

Hurley, D. L.; Howard, P.; and Hahn, H. H. II: Perioperative prophylactic antibiotics in abdominal surgery: A review of recent progress. Surg. Clin. North Am., 59:919–933, 1979.

Isberg, R.; Voorhis, D.; and Falkow, S.: Identification of invasin: A protein that allows enteric bacteria to penetrate cultured mammalian cells. Cell, 50:769–778, 1987.

Jackson, G. G.; Perkins, J. T.; Rubenis, M.; Paul, D. A.; Knigge, M.; Despotes, J. C.; Spencer, P.; and Department of Medicine, University of Illinois, College of Medicine, Chicago: Passive immunoneutralisation of human immunodeficiency virus in patients with advanced AIDS. Lancet, 2:647–652, 1988.

Jacobson, E. D.; and Faloon, W. W.: Malabsorptive effects of neomycin in commonly used doses. J.A.M.A., 175:187–190, 1961.

Jadavji, T.; Prober, C.; and Cheung, R.: In vitro interactions between rifampin and ampicillin or chloramphenicol against *Hemophilus influenzae*. Antimicrob. Agents Chemother., 26: 91–96, 1984.

Jawetz, E.: The use of combinations of antimicrobial drugs. Ann. Rev. Pharmacol., 8:151–170, 1968.

Jawetz, E.; Gunnison, J. B.; Speck, R. S.; and Coleman, V. B.: Studies on antibiotic synergism and antagonism: The interference of chloramphenicol with the action of penicillin. Arch. Intern. Med., 87:349–359, 1951.

Jeffrey, L.; and Mahone, C.: A comprehensive system for antimicrobial monitoring and review using a mandatory antimicrobial ordering sheet. Hosp. Pharm., 22:877–883, 1987.

Johnson, V. A.; Barlow, M. A.; Merrill, D. R.; Chou, T. C.; and Hirsch, M. S.: Three-drug synergistic inhibition of HIV-1 replication in vitro by zidovudine, recombinant soluble CD4 and recombinant interferon alpha A. J. Infect. Dis., 161(6): 1059–1067, 1990.

Johnson, V. A.; Barlow, M. A.; Chou, T. C.; Fisher, R. A.; Walker, B. D.; Hirsch, M. S.; Schooley, R. T.; and Infectious Disease Unit, Mass. General Hospital, Boston: Synergistic inhibition of human immunodeficiency virus type 1 (HIV-1) replication in vitro by recombinant soluble CD4 and 3′-azido-3′-deoxythymidine. J. Infect. Dis., 159:837–844, 1989a.

Johnson, V. A.; Walker, B. D.; Barlow, M. A.; Paradis, T. J.; Chou, T. C.; and Hirsch, M. S.: Synergistic inhibition of human immunodeficiency virus type 1 and type 2 replication in vitro by castanospermine and 3′-azido-3′-deoxythymidine. Antimicrob. Agents Chemother., 33:53–57, 1989b.

Joint Commission on Accreditation of Hospitals: Accreditation Manual for Hospitals. Chicago, 1987.

Jordan, G.; and Kawachi, M.: Analysis of serum bactericidal activity in endocarditis, osteomyelitis, and other bacterial infections. Medicine, 60:49–61, 1981.

Joshi, J. H.; Schimpff, S. C.; Tenney, J. H.; Newman, K. A.; and deJongh, C. A.: Can antibacterial therapy be discontinued in persistently febrile granulocytopenic patients? Am. J. Med., 76:450–457, 1984.

Kabins, S. A.: Interactions among antibiotics and other drugs. J.A.M.A., 219:206–212, 1972.

Kapikian, A. Z.; Mitchell, R. H.; Chanock, R. M.; Shvedoff, R. A.; and Stewart, C. E.: An epidemiologic study of altered clinical reactivity to respiratory syncytial (RS) virus infection in children previously vaccinated with an inactivated RS virus vaccine. Am. J. Epidemiol., 89:405–421, 1969.

Kingsburg, D.; and Falkow, S.: Rapid Detection and Identification of Infectious Agents. Academic Press, San Diego, 1985.

Klastersky, J.; Munier-Carpentier, F.; and Prevost, J.: Significance of antimicrobial synergism for the outcome of gram negative sepsis. Am. J. Med. Sci., 273:157–167, 1977.

Kobayashi, G. S.; Cheung, S. C.; Schlesinger, D.; and Medoff, G.: Effects of rifampicin derivatives alone and in combination with amphotericin B against *Histoplasma capsulatum*. Antimicrob. Agents Chemother., 5:16–18, 1974.

Konig, W.; Konig, B.; Scheffer, J.; Hacker, J.; and Goebel, W.: Role of cloned virulence factors from uropathogenic *Escherichia coli* strains in the release of inflammatory mediators from neutrophils and mort cells. Immunology, 67:401–407, 1989.

Kovacs, J. A.; Deyton, L.; and Davey, R.: Combined zidovudine and interferon-α therapy in patients with Kaposi sarcoma and the acquired immunodeficiency syndrome (AIDS). Ann. Intern. Med., 111:280–287, 1989.

Kristiansen, B.: Effect of subminimal inhibitory concentrations of antimicrobial agents on the piliation and adherence of *Neisseria meningitidis*. Antimicrob. Agents Chemother., 24: 731–735, 1983.

Kucers, A.; and Bennett, N. McK. (eds): The Use of Antibiotics. J. B. Lippincott, Philadelphia, 1989.

Kucers, A.; and Bennett, N. McK. (eds): The Use of Antibiotics. A Comprehensive Review with Clinical Emphasis. J. B. Lippincott, Philadelphia, 1975.

Kunin, C. M.: The responsibility of the infectious disease community for the optimal use of antimicrobial agents. J. Infect. Dis., 151:388–398, 1985.

Kunin, C. M.: Detection, Prevention and Management of Urinary Tract Infections, 2nd ed. Lea & Febiger, Philadelphia, 1974.

Kunin, C. M.: Therapeutic implications of serum protein binding of the new semisynthetic penicillins. Antimicrob. Agents Chemother., 1964:1025–1034, 1965.

Kunin, C. M.; and Bugg, A.: Binding of polymyxin antibiotics to tissues: The major determinant of distribution and persistence in the body. J. Infect. Dis., 124:394–400, 1971.

Kunin, C. M.; Tupasi, T.; and Craig, W.: Use of antibiotics: A brief exposition of the problem and some tentative solutions. Ann. Intern. Med., 79:555–560, 1973.

Lambert, J. S.; Seidlin, M.; and Reichman, R. C.: 2′,3′-Dideoxyinosine (ddI) in patients with the acquired immunodeficiency syndrome or AIDS-related complex. N. Engl. J. Med., 322:1333–1340, 1990.

Lane, H. C.; Davey, V.; and Kovacs, J. A.: Interferon α in patients with asymptomatic immunodeficiency virus (HIV) infection. Ann. Intern. Med., 112:805–811, 1990.

Lane, H. C.; Zunich, K. M.; Wilson, W.; et al.: Syngeneic bone marrow transplantation and adoptive transfer of peripheral blood lymphocyte combined with zidovudine in human immunodeficiency virus (HIV) infection. Ann. Intern. Med., 113:512–519, 1990.

Larder, B. A.; Darby, G.; and Richman, D. D.: HIV with reduced sensitivity to zidovudine (AZT) isolated during prolonged therapy. Science, 243:1731–1734, 1989.

Lebow, R.: Hospital cost crisis: Antimicrobial agents and democracy. Am. J. Hosp. Pharm., 73:9–14, 1987.

Lepper, M. H.; and Dowling, H. F.: Treatment of pneumococcic meningitis with penicillin compared with penicillin plus aureomycin. Arch. Intern. Med., 88:489–494, 1951.

Levine, M. M.; Edsall, G.; and Bruce-Schwatt, L. J.: Live-virus vaccine in pregnancy: Risks and recommendations. Lancet, 2:34–38, 1974.

Lindenbaum, J.; Maulitz, R.; and Butler, A.: Inhibition of digoxin absorption by neomycin. Gastroenterology, 71:399–406, 1976.

Liu, D. K.; and Owens, G. F.: Inhibition of viral reverse transcriptase by 2′,5′-oligoadenylates. Biochem. Biophys. Res. Commun., 145:291–297, 1987.

Lundsgaard-Hansen, P.; Senn, A.; Roos, B.; and Waller, U.: Staphyloccic enterocolitis. Report of six cases with two fatalities after intravenous administration of N (pyrrolidinomethyl) tetracycline. J.A.M.A., 173:1008–1013, 1960.

Lyerly, D.; Krwan, H.; and Wilkins, T.: *Clostridium difficile*: Its disease and toxins. Clin. Microbiol. Rev., 1:1–18, 1988.

Maki, D.; and Schunna, A.: A study of antimicrobial misuse in a university hospital. Am. J. Med. Sci., 275:271–281, 1978.

Mandell, G.; Douglas, R. G.; and Bennett, J. (eds.): Principles and Practice of Infectious Diseases. Churchill Livingstone, New York, 1990.

Mandell, L.: The effects of antimicrobial and antineoplastic drugs on the phagocytic and microbicidal function of the polymorphonuclear leucocyte. Rev. Infect. Dis., 4:683–697, 1982.

Mangi, R. J.; Holstein, L. L.; and Andriole, V. T.: Treatment of gram-negative bacillary meningitis with intrathecal gentamicin. Yale J. Biol. Med., 50:31–41, 1977.

Marr, J.; Moffet, H.; and Kunin, C.: Guidelines for improving the use of antimicrobial agents in hospitals: A statement by the Infectious Diseases Society of America. J. Infect. Dis., 157:869–876, 1988.

Maurelli, A.; and Sansonetti, P.: Identification of a chromosomal gene controlling temperature-regulated expression of *Shigella* virulence. Proc. Natl. Acad. Sci. U.S.A., 85:2820–2824, 1988.

McCabe, R.; Brooks, R.; Dorfman, R.; and Remington, J.: Clinical spectrum in 107 cases of toxoplasmic lymphodenopathy. Rev. Infect. Dis., 9:754–761, 1987.

McCabe, W.; Kreger, B.; and Johns, M.: Type-specific and cross-reactive antibodies in gram-negative bacteremia. N. Engl. J. Med., 287:261–267, 1972.

McCracken, G. H. Jr.: Rapid identification of specific etiology in meningitis. J. Pediatr. 88:706–708, 1976.

McCracken, G. H. Jr.; and Mize, S. G.: A controlled study of intrathecal antibiotic therapy in gram-negative enteric meningitis of infancy: Report of the Neonatal Meningitis Cooperative Study Group. J. Pediatr., 89:66–72, 1976.

McCracken, G. H. Jr.; Mize, S. G.; and Threlkeld, N.: Intraventricular gentamicin therapy in gram-negative bacillary meningitis of infancy: Report of the Second Neonatal Meningitis Cooperative Study Group. Lancet, 1:787–791, 1980.

McGowen, J.: Antimicrobial resistance in hospital organisms and its relation to antimicrobial use. Rev. Infect. Dis., 5:1033–1048, 1983.

McGrath, M. S.; Hwang, K. M.; and Caldwell, S. E.: GLQ223: An inhibitor of human immunodeficiency virus replication in acutely and chronically infected cells of lymphocyte and mononuclear cell lineage. Proc. Natl. Acad. Sci. U.S.A., 86: 2844–2848, 1989.

McHenry, M. C.; Gaven, T. L.; Van Omnen, R. A.; and Hawk, W. A.: Therapy with gentamicin for bacteremic infections: Results with 53 patients. J. Infect. Dis., 124(suppl.):S164–S173, 1971.

Mederios, A.: Beta-lactamases. Br. Med. Bull., 40:18–27, 1984.

Medical Letter: Handbook of Antimicrobial Therapy (Abramowicz, M. ed.). The Medical Letter, Inc., New Rochelle, N.Y., 1990.

Merrikin, D. J.; Briant, J.; and Rolinson, G. N.: Effect of protein binding on antibiotic activity in vivo. J. Antimicrob. Chemother., 11:233–238, 1983.

Miller, J.; Mekalanos, J.; and Falkow, S.: Coordinate regulation and sensory transduction in the control of bacterial virulence. Science, 243:916–922, 1989.

Miller, M.: The immunodeficiencies of immaturity. In, Immunologic Disorders in Infants and Children (Steihm, R.; and Fulginitti, V., eds.). W. B. Saunders, Philadelphia, pp. 168–183, 1973.

Minshew, B.; Jorgensen, H.; Counts, G.; and Falkow, S.: Association of hemolysin production, hemagglutination of human erythrocytes, and virulence for chicken embryos of extraintestinal *E. coli* isolates. Infect. Immun., 20:50–54, 1978.

Mitsuya, H.; and Broder, S.: Inhibition of the in vitro infectivity and cytopathic effect of human T-lymphotropic virus type III/lymphadenopathy associated virus (HTLV III/LAV) by 2′,3′dideoxynucleotides. Proc. Natl. Acad. Sci. U.S.A., 83: 1911–1915, 1986.

Mitsuya, H.; Looney, D. J.; Kuno, S.; Ueno, R.; Wong-Staal, F.; and Broder, S.: Dextran sulfate suppression of viruses in the HIV family: Inhibition of virion binding to CD4+ cells. Science, 240:646–649, 1988.

Mitsuya, H.; Weinhold, K. J.; Furman, P. A.; St. Clair, M. H.; Lehrman, S. N.; Gallo, R. C.; Bolognesi, D.; Barry, D. W.; and Broder, S.: 3′-azido-3′-deoxythymidine (BW A509U): An antiviral agent that inhibits the infectivity and cytopathic effect of human T-lymphotropic virus type III/lymphadenopathy associated virus in vitro. Proc. Natl. Acad. Sci. U.S.A., 82:7096–7100, 1985.

Moellering, R.: Use and abuse of antibiotic combinations. R.I. Med. J., 55:341–353, 1972.

Moellering, R. C. Jr.; and Weinberg, A. N.: Studies on antibiotic synergism against enterococci: II. Effect of various antibiotics on the uptake of ^{14}C labelled streptomycin by enterococci. J. Clin. Invest., 50:2580–2584, 1971.

Moellering, R. C. Jr.; Wennerstein, C.; and Weinberg, A. N.: Studies on antibiotic synergism against enterococci: I. Bacteriologic studies. J. Lab. Clin. Med., 77:821–828, 1971.

Moffet, H. L.: Perinatal infections. In, Pediatric Infectious Diseases: A Problem-Oriented Approach (Moffet, H. L., ed.). J. B. Lippincott, Philadelphia, pp. 325–353, 1975.

Montefiori, D. C.; and Mitchell, W. M.: Antiviral activity of mismatched double stranded RNA against human immunodeficiency virus in vitro. Proc. Natl. Acad. Sci. U.S.A., 84: 2985–2989, 1987.

Moskovitz, B. L.; and the HPT-23 Cooperative Study Group: Clinical trials of tolerance of HPA-23 in patients with acquired immunodeficiency syndrome. Antimicrob. Agents Chemother., 32:1300–1303, 1988.

Moyer, K.; Opal, S.; and Mederios, A.: Mechanisms of antibiotic resistance. In, Principles and Practices of Infectious Disease (Mandel, G.; Douglas, G.; and Bennett, J., eds.). Churchill Livingstone, New York, pp. 218–224, 1990.

National Committee for Clinical Laboratory Standards: Methods for Dilution Antimicrobial Susceptibility Test for Bacteria That Grow Aerobically. M7-A2. NCCLS, Villanova, 1990.

Nelson, J. D.: Emerging role of cephalosporins in bacterial meningitis. Am. J. Med., 79(suppl. 2A):47–51, 1985.

Nelson, J. D.: Should ampicillin be abandoned for treatment of *Haemophilus influenzae* disease? J.A.M.A., 229:322–324, 1974.

Nelson, K. E.; Levin, S.; Spies, H. W.; and Lepper, M. H.: Treatment of *Haemophilus influenzae* meningitis: A comparison of chloramphenicol and tetracycline. J. Infect. Dis., 125: 459–465, 1972.

Neu, H. C.: Use of cephalosporins in the treatment of bacterial meningitis. In, Bacterial Meningitis (Sande, M. A.; Smith, A. L.; and Root, R. K., eds.). Churchill Livingstone, New York, pp. 203–238, 1985.

Nicols, R. L.: Techniques known to prevent postoperative wound infection. Infect. Control, 3:34–37, 1982.

Nicols, R. L.: Use of prophylactic antibiotics in surgical practice. Am. J. Med., 70:686–692, 1981.

Nieman, R. E.; and Lorber, B.: Listeriosis in adults: A changing pattern: Report of eight cases and review of the literature, 1968–1978. Rev. Infect. Dis., 2:207–227, 1980.

Nussenzweig, R.: Parasitic disease as a cause of immunosuppression. N. Engl. J. Med., 306:423–424, 1982.

Nyphan, W. L.: Toxicity of drugs in the neonatal period. J. Pediatr., 59:1–20, 1961.

O'Garra, A.; Stapleton, G.; Dhar, V.; Pearce, J.; Schumacher, J.; Rugo, H.; Barbis, D.; Stall, A.; Cupp, J.; Moore, K.; Vieira, P.; Mosmann, T.; Whitmore, A.; Arnold, L.; Haughton, G.; and Howard, M.: Production of cytokines by mouse B cells. B lymphomas and normal B cells produce IL-10. Int. Immunol., 2:821–832, 1990.

O'Grady, F.; and Cattle, W. R.: Kinetics of urinary tract infection: I. The bladder. Br. J. Urol., 38:156–162, 1966.

O'Hanley, P.; Easow, J.; Rugo, H.; and Easow, S.: Infectious disease complications in adult leukemic patients: Five year experience at Stanford University 1982–1986. Am. J. Med., 87:605–613, 1989.

O'Hanley, P.; Low, D.; Romero, I.; Lark, D.; Vosti, K.; Falkow, S.; and Schoolnick, G.: Gal-Gal binding and hemolysin phenotypes and genotypes associated with uropathogenic *E. coli*. N. Engl. J. Med., 313:414–420, 1985a.

O'Hanley, P.; Lark, D.; Falkow, S.; and Schoolnik, G.: Molecular basis of *Escherichia coli* colonization of the upper urinary tract in BALB/c mice. J. Clin. Invest., 75:347–360, 1985b.

Ochs, H.; and Igo, R.: The NBT slide test: A simple screening method for detecting chronic granulomatous disease and female carriers. J. Pediatr., 83:77–86, 1973.

Ogra, P. L.; Karzon, D. T.; Righthand, F.; and MacGillivray, M.: Immunoglobulin responses in serum and secretions after immunization with live and inactivated polio vaccine and natural infection. N. Engl. J. Med., 279:893–900, 1968.

Olling, S.: Sensitivity of gram-negative bacilli to the serum bactericidal activity: A marker of host-parasite relationship in acute and persisting infections. Scand. J. Infect. Dis., 10:1–40, 1972.

Olling, S.; Hanson, L.; Holmgren, J.; Jodel, U.; Lincoln, K.; and Lindberg, U.: The bactericidal effect of normal human serum on *E. coli* strains from animals and from patients with urinary tract infections. Infection, 1:24–36, 1973.

Orskov, F.; and Orskov, I.: Summary of a workshop on the clone concept in the epidemiology, taxonomy, and evaluation of the Enterobacteriaceae and other bacteria. J. Infect. Dis., 148:346–357, 1983.

Orskov, I.; Ferencz, A.; and Orskov, F.: Tamm-Horsfall protein or uromucoid is the normal urinary slime that traps type 1 fimbriated *Escherichia coli*. Lancet, 1:887, 1980.

Overturf, G. D.: Treatment of the child with bacterial meningitis. In, Current Clinical Topics in Infectious Disease (Remington, J. S.; and Swartz, M. N., eds.). Vol. 3. McGraw-Hill, New York, p. 218, 1982.

Parillo, J.; Parker, M.; Natanson, C.; Suffredini, A.; Donner, R.; Cunnion, R.; and Ognibene, F.: Septic shock in humans: Advances in the understanding of pathogenesis, cardiovascular dysfunction, and therapy. Ann. Intern. Med., 113:227–242, 1990.

Parker, R.; and Fossieck, B.: Intravenous followed by oral antimicrobial therapy for staphylococcal endocarditis. Ann. Intern. Med., 93:832–834, 1980.

Paul, J. R.: A History of Poliomyelitis. Yale University Press, New Haven, Conn., Chap. 40, 1971.

Peacock, J. E. Jr.; McGinnis, M. R.; and Cohen, M. S.: Persistent neutrophilic meningitis: Report of four cases and review of the literature. Medicine (Baltimore) 63:379–395, 1984.

Pecha, B.; Low, D.; and O'Hanley, P.: Gal-Gal pili vaccines prevent pyelonephritis by piliated *Escherichia coli* in a murine model: Single-component Gal-Gal pili vaccines prevent pyelonephritis by homologous and heterologous piliated *E. coli* strains. J. Clin. Invest., 83:2102–2108, 1989.

Pedersen, C.; Sandstrom, E.; Peterson, C. S.; Norkrans, G.; Gerstoft, J.; Karlsson, A.; Christensen, K. C.; Hakansson, C.; Pehrson, P. O.; Nielson, J. O.; Jürgensen, H. J.; and the Scandinavian Isoprinosine Study Group: The efficacy of inosine pranobex in preventing the acquired immunodeficiency syndrome in patients with human immunodeficiency virus infection. N. Engl. J. Med., 322:1757–1763, 1990.

Pert, C. B.; Hill, J. M.; Ruff, M. R.; Berman, R. M.; Robey, W. G.; Arthur, L. O.; Ruscetti, F. W.; and Farrar, W. L.: Octapeptides deduced from the neuropeptide receptor like pattern of antigen CD4+ in brain potently inhibit human immunodeficiency virus receptor binding and T cell infectivity. Proc. Natl. Acad. Sci. U.S.A., 83:9254–9258, 1986.

Pizzo, P. A.; Eddy, J.; Falloon, J.; Balis, E. M.; Murphy, R. F.; Moss, H.; Wolters, P.; Brouwers, P.; Jarosinski, P.; Rubin, M.; Broder, S.; Yarchoan, R.; Brunetti, A.; Maha, M.; Nusinoff-Lehrman, S.; and Poplack, D. G.: Effect of continous intravenous infusion of zidovudine (AZT) in children with symptomatic HIV infection. N. Engl. J. Med., 319:889–896, 1988.

Pizzo, P. A.; Robichaud, K. J.; Gill, F. A.; and Witebsky, F. G.: Empiric antibiotic and antifungal therapy for cancer patients with prolonged fever and granulocytopenia. Am. J. Med., 72:101–111, 1982.

Plos, K.; Carter, T.; Hull, S.; Hull, R.; and Svanborg-Eden, C.: Frequency and organization of pap homogenous DNA in relation to clinical origin of uropathogenic *E. coli*. J. Infect. Dis., 161:518–524, 1990.

Polk, H. C. Jr.; Trachtenberg, L. S.; and Finn, M. P.: Antibiotic activity in surgical incisions: The basis of prophylaxis in selected operations. J.A.M.A., 244:1353–1354, 1980.

Press, O. W.; Ramsey, P. G.; Larsen, E. B.; Fefer, A.; and Hickman, R. O.: Hickman catheter infection in patients with malignancies. Medicine, 63:189–200, 1984.

Prober, C.; and Yeager, A.: Use of the serum bactericidal titer to assess the adequacy of oral antibiotic therapy in the treatment of acute hematogenous osteomyelitis. J. Pediatr., 95:131–135, 1979.

Rahal, J. J. Jr.: Diagnosis and management of meningitis due to gram-negative bacilli in adults. In, Current Clinical Topics in Infectious Disease (Remington, J. S., and Swartz, M. N., eds.). Vol. 1. McGraw-Hill, New York, p. 68, 1980.

Rahal, J. J. Jr.; and Simberkoff, M. S.: Bactericidal and bacteriostatic action of chloramphenicol against meningeal pathogens. Antimicrob. Agents Chemother., 16:13–18, 1979.

Relman, D.; and Falkow, S.: A molecular perspective of microbial pathogenicity. In, Principles and Practice of Infectious Diseases (Mardel, G.; Douglas, G.; and Bennett, J., eds.). Churchill Livingstone, New York, pp. 25–32, 1990.

Robert-Guroff, M.; Brown, M.; and Gallo, R. C.: HTLV III-neutralizing antibodies in patients with AIDS and AIDS-related complex. Nature, 316:72–74, 1985.

Roberts, J.; Hardaway, K.; Koack, B.; Fussell, E.; and Baskin, G.: Prevention of pyelonephritis by immunization with P-fimbriae. J. Urol., 131:602–607, 1984.

Robinson, A.; Bartlett, R.; and Mazens, M.: Antimicrobial synergy testing based on antibiotic levels, minimal bactericidal concentration and serum bactericidal activity. Am. J. Clin. Pathol., 84:328–333, 1985.

Roederer, M.; Staal, F. J. T.; and Raju, P.: Cytokine-stimulated human immunodeficiency virus replication is inhibited by *N*-acetyl-L-cysteine. Proc. Natl. Acad. Sci. U.S.A., 87:4884–4888, 1990.

Rose, J.; Chai, H.; and Schentag, J.: Intoxication caused by interaction of chloramphenicol and phenytoin. J.A.M.A., 237:2630–2634, 1977.

Rouse, B.; and Horohov, D.: Immunosuppression in viral infections. Rev. Infect. Dis., 8:850–873, 1986.

Rowlands, B.; Clark, R.; and Richards, D.: Single-dose intraoperative antibiotic prophylaxis in emergency abdominal surgery. Arch. Surg., 177:195–199, 1982.

Rubin, M.; Hathorn, J. W.; Marshall, D.; Gress, J.; Steinberg, S. M.; Pizzo, P. A.; and Pediatric Branch, National Cancer Institute, Bethesda, MD: Gram-positive infections and the use of vancomycin in 550 episodes of fever and neutropenia. Ann. Intern. Med., 108:30–35, 1988.

Ruskin, J.; and Remington, J. S.: Toxoplasmosis in the compromised host. Ann. Intern. Med., 84:193–199, 1976.

Saag, M. S.; Hahn, B. H.; and Gibbons, J.: Extensive variation of human immunodeficiency virus type 1 in vivo. Nature, 334:440–444, 1988.

Sahm, D.; Neuman, M.; Thornsberry, C.; and McGowan, J.: Current concepts and approaches to antimicrobial agent susceptibility testing. Cumitech 25. American Society for Microbiology, Washington D.C., 1988.

Sande, M. A.: Antibiotic therapy of bacterial meningitis: Lessons we've learned. Am. J. Med., 71:507–510, 1981.

Sande, M. A.; and Mandell, G.: Chemotherapy of Microbial Diseases. In, The Pharmacological Basis of Therapeutics (Gilman, A.; Goodman, L.; Rall, T.; and Murad, F., eds.). Macmillan, New York, pp. 1066–1239, 1985.

Sande, M. A.; and Overton, J. W.: In vivo antagonism between gentamicin and chloramphenicol in neutropenic mice. J. Infect. Dis., 128:247–250, 1973.

Sande, M. A.; and Scheld, M.: Combination antibiotic therapy of bacterial endocarditis. Ann. Intern. Med., 92:390–398, 1980.

Sande, M. A.; and Tierney, L. M. Jr.: Meningitis — Medical Staff Conference, San Francisco General Hospital Center and

VA Medical Center, San Francisco. West. J. Med., 140:433–438, 1984.

Sarin, P. S.; Gallo, R. C.; Scheer, D. I.; Crews, F.; and Lippa, A. S.: Effects of a novel compound (AL721) on HTLV III infectivity in vitro. N. Engl. J. Med., 313:1289–1290, 1985.

Saxton, A.; Hassner, A.; and Swabb, E.: Lack of cross-reactivity between aztreonam or monobactam antibiotic, and penicillin in penicillin-allergic subjects. J. Infect. Dis., 149:16–24, 1984.

Schimpff, S. C.; Young, V. M.; Greene, W. H.; Vermuelen, G. D.; Moody, M. R.; and Wiernik, P. H.: Origin of infection in acute nonlymphocytic leukemia: Significance of hospital acquisition of potential pathogens. Ann. Intern. Med., 77:707–714, 1972.

Schoenfield, L. J.: Biliary excretion of antibiotics. N. Engl. J. Med., 284:1213–1214, 1971.

Schoenberger, L.; Kaplan, J.; and Kim-Farley, R.: Control of paralytic poliomyelitis in the United States. Rev. Infect. Dis., 6:424–426, 1984.

Schooley, R. T.; Merigan, T. C.; Gaut, P.; Hirsch, M. S.; Holodniy, M.; Flynn, T.; Liu, S.; Byington, R. E.; Henochowicz, S.; Gubish, E.; Spriggs, D.; Kufe, D.; Schindler, J.; Dawson, A.; Thomas, D.; Hanson, D. G.; Lewtin, B.; Liu, T.; Gulinello, J.; Kennedy, S.; Fisher, R.; and Ho, D. D.: Recombinant soluble CD4 therapy in patients with acquired immunodeficiency syndrome (AIDS) or AIDS-related complex. A phase I/II escalating dose trial. Ann. Intern. Med., 112:247–253, 1990.

Schoolnik, G.; Lark, D.; and O'Hanley, P.: Bacterial adherence and anti-colonization vaccines. In, Current Clinical Topics in Infectious Diseases (Remington, J.; and Swartz, M., eds.). Vol. 6. McGraw-Hill, New York, pp. 85–102, 1985.

Shah, K.; and Nathanson, N.: Human exposure to SV40: Review and comment. Am. J. Epidemiol., 103:1–12, 1976.

Shepard, C. C.: Chemotherapy of leprosy. Ann. Rev. Pharmacol., 9:37–50, 1969.

Simberkoff, M. S.; Moldover, N. H.; and Rahal, J. J. Jr.: Absence of detectable bactericidal and opsonic activities in normal and infected human cerebrospinal fluids: A regional host defense deficiency. J. Lab. Clin. Med., 95:362–372, 1980.

Simon, M.; Zieg, J.; and Silverman, M.: Phase variation: Evaluation of controlling element. Science, 209:1370–1374, 1980.

Smith, A. L.: Antibiotic resistance in Haemophilus influenzae. Pediatr. Infect. Dis., 2:352–355, 1983.

Smith, C.; and Lipsky, J.: Hypoprothrombinemia and platelet dysfunction caused by cephalosporin and axalactam antibiotics. Antimicrob. Agents Chemother., 11:496–501, 1983.

Smith, D. H.; Byrn, R. A.; Marsters, S. A.; Gregory, T.; Groopman, J. E.; Capon, D. J.; and the Department of Molecular Biology, Genentech, Inc., S.S.F., CA: Blocking of HIV-1 infectivity by a soluble form of CD4 antigen. Science, 238:1704–1707, 1987.

Snider, D.: The tuberculin skin test. Am. Rev. Respir. Dis., 125:108–118, 1982.

Spector, S. A.; Kennedy, C.; and McCutchan, J. A.: The antiviral effect of zidovudine and rebarvirin in clinical trials and the use of p24 antigen levels as a virologic marker. J. Infect. Dis., 159:822–827, 1989.

Stamm, W.; Counts, G.; and Running, K.: Diagnosis of coliform infection in acutely dysuric women. N. Engl. J. Med., 307:463–468, 1982.

Steers, E.; Foltz, E. L.; Graves, B. S.; and Riden, J.: An inocula replicating apparatus for routine testing of bacterial susceptibility to antibiotics. Antibiot. Chemother.(Basel), 9:307–311, 1959.

Steigbeigel, R. T.; Greenman, Y. L.; and Remington, J. S.: Antibiotic combinations in the treatment of experimental Staphylococcus aureus infection. J. Infect. Dis., 131:245–251, 1975.

Steigbeigel, R. T.; Johnson, P. K.; and Remington, J. S.: The nitroblue tetrazolium reduction test versus conventional hematology in the diagnosis of bacterial infection. N. Engl. J. Med., 290:235–238, 1974.

Steigbeigel, R. T.; Reed, C.; and Finland, M.: Absorption and excretion of five tetrocycline analogues in normal young men. Am. J. Med. Sci., 25:296–301, 1968.

Steinman, R.; Nogueira, N.; and Witmer, M.: Lymphokine enhances the expression and synthesis of 1a antigens on cultured mouse peritoneal macrophages. J. Exp. Med., 152:1248–1261, 1980.

Stiehm, E. R.; Sztein, M.; and Steeg, P.: Deficient antigen expression on human cord blood monocytes. Reversal with lymphokines. Clin. Immunol. Immunopathol., 30:430–436, 1984.

Stokes, J. Jr.; Weibel, R. E.; Villarejos, V. M.; Arguedas, J. A.; Buynak, E. B.; and Hilleman, M. R.: Trivalent combined measles, mumps, rubella vaccine. J.A.M.A., 218:57–61, 1971.

Stolley, P.; Becker, M.; McEvilla, J.; Lasagna, L.; Gainor, M.; and Sloane, L.: Drug prescribing and use in an American community. Ann. Intern. Med., 76:537–540, 1972.

Stovring, J.; and Snyder, R. D.: Computed tomography in childhood bacterial meningitis. J. Pediatr., 96:820–823, 1980.

Stratton, C.: The usefulness of the serum bactericidal test in orthopedic infections. Orthopedics, 7:1579–1580, 1984.

Strausbaugh, L. J.; and Sande, M. A.: Factors influencing the therapy of experimental Proteus mirabilis meningitis in rabbits. J. Infect. Dis., 137:251, 1978.

Surbone, A.; Yarchoan, R.; McAtee, N.; Blum, M. R.; Maha, M.; Allain, J. P.; Thomas, R. V.; Mitsuya, H.; Lehrman, S. N.; Leuther, M.; Pluda, J. M.; Jacobsen, F. K.; Kessler, H. A.; Myers, C. E.; Broder, S.; Bethesda, MD.; Research Triangle Park, N.C.; Abbot Park, Chicago, IL: Treatment of the acquired immunodeficiency syndrome (AIDS) and AIDS-related complex with a regimen of 3′-azido-2′,3′-dideoxythymidine (azidothymidine or zidovudine) and acyclovir. Ann. Intern. Med., 108:534–540, 1988.

Svanborg-Eden, C.; and deMan, P.: Bacterial occurrence in urinary tract infection. Infect. Dis. Clin. North Am., 1:731–750, 1987.

Swartz, M. N.: Intraventricular use of aminoglycosides in the treatment of gram-negative bacillary meningitis: Conflicting views. J. Infect. Dis., 143:293–296, 1981.

Swartz, M. N.; and Dodge, P. R.: Bacterial meningitis—A review of selected aspects: I. General clinical features, special problems and unusual meningeal reactions mimicking bacterial meningitis. N. Engl. J. Med., 272:725–731, 1965.

Swartz, M. N.; and O'Hanley, P. D.: Central nervous system infections. In, Scientific American Medicine (Rubenstein, E.; and Federman, D., eds.). Vol. 2. Scientific American, New York, pp. 1–43, 1987.

Tam, M.: Culture independent diagnosis of Chlamydia trachomatis using monoclonal antibodies. N. Engl. J. Med., 310:146–151, 1984.

Tauber, M. G.; and Sande, M. A.: Principles in the treatment of bacterial meningitis. Am. J. Med., 76:224–230, 1984.

Terry, L. L.: The Association of Cases of Poliomyelitis with the Use of Type III Oral Poliomyelitis Vaccines: A technical report. U.S. Dept. H.E.W., Sept. 20, 1962.

Thaysen, E. H.; and Eriksen, K. R.: Staphylococcal enteritis following administration of the tetracyclines. Antibiot. Ann., 1955–1956, pp. 867–874.

Till, M. A.; Ghetie, V.; Gregory, T.; Patzer, E. J.; Porter, J. P.; Uhr, J. W.; Capon, D. J.; and Viletta, E. S.: HIV infected cells are killed by rCD4-ricin A chain. Science, 242:1166–1168, 1988.

Torseth, J.; Bhatia, G.; Harkonen, S.; Child, C.; Skinner, M.; Robinson, W. S.; Blaschke, T. F.; and Merigan, T. C.: Evaluation of the antiviral effect of rifabutin in AIDS-related complex. J. Infect. Dis., 159:1115–1118, 1989.

Tracey, K.; Fong, Y.; Hesse, D.; and Cerami, A.: Anti-cachetin/TNF monoclonal antibodies prevent septic shock during lethal bacteremia. Nature, 330:662–664, 1987.

Tramont, E.: General or nonspecific host defense mechanisms. In, Principles and Practice of Infectious Diseases (Mandell, G.; Douglas, G.; and Bennett, J., eds.). Churchill Livingstone, New York, pp. 33–41, 1990.

Tunkel, A.; Wispelwey, B.; and Scheld, M.: Bacterial meningitis: Recent advances in pathophysiology and treatment. Ann. Intern. Med., 112:610–623, 1990.

Tuomanen, E.; Powell, K.; and Marks, M.: Oral chloramphenicol in the treatment of *Haemophilus influenzae* meningitis. J. Pediatr., 99:968–974, 1981.

Turck, M.; and Petersdorf, R.: The epidemiology of nonenteric *E. coli* infections: Prevalence of serological groups. J. Clin. Invest., 41:1760–1765, 1962.

Twomey, J.; Laughter, A.; and Farrow, S.: Hodgkin's disease: An immunodepleting and immunosuppressive disorder. J. Clin. Invest., 56:467–472, 1975.

Vaisanen-Rhen, V.; Elo, J.; Vaisanen, E.; Siitonen, A.; Orskov, I.; Orskov, F.; Svenson, S.; Makela, P.; and Korhonen, T.: P-fimbriated clones among uropathogenic *E. coli* strains. Infect. Immun., 43:149–155, 1984.

Van der Auwera, P.; Meunier-Carpentier, F.; and Kalstersky, J.: Clinical study of combination therapy with oxacillin and rifampin for staphylococcal infections. Rev. Infect. Dis., 5: 515–528, 1983.

Ventur, Y.; Scheffer, J.; Hacker, J.; Goebel, W.; and Konig, W.: Effects of adhesins from mannose-resistant *Escherichia coli* on mediator release from human lymphocytes, manocytes, and basophils and from polymorphonuclear granulocytes. Infect. Immunol., 58:1500–1508, 1990.

Vogt, M. W.; Durno, A. G.; Chou, T. C.; Coleman, L. A.; Paradis, T. J.; Schooley, R. T.; Kaplan, J. C.; and Hirsch, M. S.: Synergistic interaction of 2′,3′-dideoxycytidine and recombinant interferon alpha A on replication of human immunodeficiency virus type 1. J. Infect. Dis., 158:378–385, 1988.

Volberding, P. A.; Lagakos, S. W.; Koch, M. A.; Pettinelli, C.; Myers, M. W.; Booth, D. K.; Balfour, H. H. Jr.; Reichman, R. C.; Bartlett, J. A.; Hirsch, M. S.; Murphy, R. L.; Hardy, W. D.; Soeiro, R.; Fischl, M. N.; Bartlett, J. G.; Merigan, T. C.; Hyslop, N. E.; Richman, D. D.; Valentine, F. T.; Corey, L.; and the AIDS Clinical Trial Group of the National Institute of Allergy and Infectious Diseases: Zidovudine in asymptomatic human immunodeficiency virus infection. A controlled trial in persons with fewer than 500 CD4-positive cells per cubic millimeter. N. Engl. J. Med., 322:941–949, 1990.

Vosti, K.; Goldberg, L.; Monto, G.; and Rantz, L.: Host–parasite interaction in patients with infection due to *E. coli*: I. Serogrouping of *E. coli* from intestinal and extraintestinal sources. J. Clin. Invest., 43:2377–2385, 1964.

Waage, A.; Halstensen, A.; Shalaby, R.; Brandtzaeg, P.; Kierulf, P.; and Espervik, T.: Local production of tumor necrosis factor, interleukin 1, and interleukin 6 in meningococcal meningitis: Relation to the inflammatory response. J. Exp. Med., 170:1859–1867, 1989a.

Waage, A.; Brandtzaeg, P.; Halstensen, A.; Kierulf, P.; and Espervik, T.: The complex pattern of cytokines in serum from patients with meningococcal septic shock. Association between interleukin 6, interleukin 1, and fatal outcome. J. Exp. Med., 169:333–338, 1989b.

Walker, B. D.; Kowalski, M.; Goh, W. C.; Kozarsky, K.; Krieger, M.; Rosen, C.; Rohrschneider, L.; Haseltine, W. A.; and Sodroski, J.: Inhibition of human immunodeficiency virus syncytium formation and virus replication by castanospermine. Proc. Natl. Acad. Sci. U.S.A., 84:8120–8124, 1987.

Ward, J. I.; Fraser, D. W.; Baraff, L. J.; and Plikaytis, B. D.: *Haemophilus influenzae* meningitis: A national study of secondary spread in household contacts. N. Engl. J. Med., 301:122–126, 1979.

Washington, J.: Current problems in antimicrobial susceptibility testing. Diagn. Microbiol. Infect. Dis., 9:135–138, 1988.

Watanakunakorn, C.; and Bakie, C.: Synergism of vancomycin-gentamicin and vancomycin-streptomycin against enterococci. Antimicrob. Agents Chemother., 4:120–124, 1973.

Wehrle, P. F.: Immunization against poliomyelitis. Arch. Environ. Health, 15:485–490, 1967.

Weinstein, A. J.; and Moellering, R. C. Jr.: Penicillin and gentamicin therapy for enterococcal infection. J.A.M.A., 223: 1030–1032, 1973.

Weisberg, L. A.: Cerebral computerized tomography in intracranial inflammatory disorders. Arch. Neurol., 37:137–142, 1980.

Weiss, A. A.; and Falkow, S.: Genetic analysis of phase change in *Bordetella pertussis*. Infect. Immun., 43:263–269, 1984.

Wenneberg, J.; McPhersoon, K.; and Caper, P.: Will payment based on diagnostic related groups control hospital costs? N. Engl. J. Med., 311:295–300, 1984.

Wetterberg, L.; Alexius, B.; Saaf, J.; Sonnerborg, A.; Britton, S.; and Pert, C.: Peptide T in treatment of AIDS. Lancet, 1: 159, 1987.

Wilson, A. G.: The Hazards of Immunization. Vol. 2. Athlone Press, University of London, pp. 7–13, 1967.

Wilson, W.; Jaumin, P.; and Danielson, G.: Prosthetic valve endocarditis. Ann. Intern. Med., 82:751–756, 1975.

Wise, R.: Protein binding of beta-lactams: The effects on activity and pharmacology particularly tissue penetration: II. Studies in man. J. Antimicrob. Chemother., 12:105–111, 1983.

Wise, R.; Gillett, A.; and Cadge, B.: The influence of protein binding upon tissue fluid levels of beta-lactam antibiotics. J. Infect. Dis., 142:77–81, 1980.

Witt, R. L.; and Hamburger, M.: The nature and treatment of pneumococcal pneumonia. Med. Clin. North Am., 47:1257–1270, 1963.

Wolff, S.: Biological effects of bacterial endotoxins in man. J. Infect. Dis., 128:259–264, 1973.

Woodward, R.; Medoff, G.; Smith, M.; and Gray, J.: Antibiotic cost savings from formulary restrictions and physician monitoring in a medical school affiliated hospital. Am. J. Med., 83:817–823, 1987.

Young, L.: Fever and septicemia. In, Clinical Approach to Infection in the Compromised Host (Rubin, R.; and Young, L., eds.). Plenum, New York, pp. 75–122, 1981.

Young, L. Y.; and Koda-Kimble, M. A. (eds.): Applied Therapeutics: The Clinical Use of Drugs, 4th ed., Applied Therapeutics, Vancouver, Washington, 1988.

Yourtee, E.; and Root, R.: Effect of antibiotics on phagocyte-microbe interactions. In, New Dimensions in Antimicrobial Therapy (Root, R.; and Sande, M., eds.). Churchill Livingstone, New York, pp. 243–275, 1984.

Ziegler, E. J.: Protective antibody to endotoxin care: The emperor's new clothes? J. Infect. Dis., 158:286–290, 1988.

Ziegler, E. J.; McCutcheon, J. A.; Fierer, J. A.; Glauser, M. P.; Sadoff, J. C.; Douglas, H.; and Braude, A. I.: Treatment of gram-negative bacteremia and shock with human antiserum to mutant *Escherichia coli*. N. Engl. J. Med., 307: 1254–1260, 1982.

25

Analgesia and Anesthesia

Donald R. Stanski and Michael F. Roizen

CLINICAL PHARMACOLOGY AND ANESTHETIC PRACTICE

The clinical practice of anesthesia involves the use of a broad range of drugs to modify or ablate the response of the body to a wide variety of noxious stimuli. Further increasing the complexity of anesthesia, these stimuli are not equally noxious. Thus, an important part of the practice of anesthesia involves titrating antinociceptive therapies on a moment-to-moment basis with the anticipated strength of the noxious stimulus. The anesthesiologist must choose from a variety of therapeutic options, including reassurance of the patient during an interview; the use of benzodiazepines to relieve anxiety before surgery; the use of benzodiazepines and/or opioids to provide conscious sedation for minor invasive procedures (e.g., endoscopy); the use of potent inhalational anesthetics, IV induction agents, opioids, or local anesthetics to provide unconsciousness, amnesia, and analgesia; the use of muscle relaxants to provide adequate surgical exposure; and the use of diverse drugs to alter autonomic and cardiovascular reflexes, perfusion, and cardiorespiratory homeostasis during surgical procedures. The anesthesiologist is also involved in the therapeutic management of acute and chronic pain syndrome outside the operating room.

Because drug therapy represents the cornerstone of anesthetic practice, principles of rational therapeutics become the scientific basis of anesthetic practice. Since anesthetic drug effects are profound (e.g., unconsciousness with progressive CNS depression, ventilatory depression, muscle paralysis, altered cardiovascular function), observation and quantitation of anesthetic drug effects have helped elucidate many concepts important to clinical pharmacology, especially for dose-response, pharmacokinetic, and pharmacodynamic relations.

It is inappropriate to review in this chapter the broad range of therapeutics encountered in the practice of anesthesia. However, two topics have been chosen that are relevant to the clinician who is not a specialist in anesthetic practice: the rational therapeutic management of acute and chronic pain, and the principles of providing safe and effective conscious sedation for minor invasive procedures.

MANAGEMENT OF ACUTE AND CHRONIC PAIN

The art of life is the art of avoiding pain.
Thomas Jefferson, 1786

Acute and chronic pain are common but have traditionally been poorly treated. Perhaps this lack of successful treatment is caused by the concern of clinicians about side effects or addiction, the narrow therapeutic index of drugs used to treat pain, or the lack of experience with these drugs and the treatment of their adverse effects. But as individuals more skilled in the rational use of such drugs have become involved in care for pain, management of pain has improved (Breslow et al., 1989).

Pain occurs in approximately 40% of patients with cancer and in 60% to 80% of patients with terminal cancer. Pain that requires treatment can occur early in the course of the disease. The incidence of inadequate relief of pain caused by cancer has been estimated to vary from 30% to 80%

in developed countries and up to 90% in undeveloped countries (Foley, 1985; Stjernswärd, 1985). In 1981, chronic noncancer pain cost the United States over $50 billion dollars annually for health care services, loss of productivity, compensation, and related factors (Bonica, 1985). Numerous studies have shown that the great majority of adults and children experiencing acute, postoperative pain receive inadequate relief (Marks and Sacher, 1973; Cohen, 1980; Mather and Mackie, 1983). While there are many reasons for inadequate management of acute and chronic pain by physicians, one component is the less-than-optimal use of clinical pharmacologic concepts in management of pain.

Definition and Classification of Pain

The International Association for the Study of Pain defines pain as "an unpleasant sensory and emotional experience associated with actual or potential tissue damage, or described in terms of such damage" (Merskey, 1986). There are no easily utilized neurophysiologic or chemical tests to measure pain; perhaps stress hormones will be able do so (Breslow et al., 1989). The clinician must frequently accept the patient's report of pain. Pain can be acute or chronic and arises from cutaneous, deep somatic, or visceral structures. Somatic pain tends to be well localized, following the distribution of somatic nerves, and is sharp and definite. Visceral pain is poorly localized, diffuse, dull, vague, and crampy. Somatic pain tends to hurt where the stimulus occurs, whereas visceral pain may be referred to other areas of the body.

Acute pain usually occurs with an intact nervous system and is caused by trauma, surgery, acute medical conditions, or physiologic processes (i.e., labor). Acute pain causes signs of increased autonomic activity such as hypertension, tachycardia, vasoconstriction, sweating, increased ventilation, skeletal muscle spasms, increased GI secretions, decreased intestinal motility, urinary retention, and venous stasis. Acute pain decreases or ceases as the trauma or wound heals or the medical condition resolves.

If severe acute pain persists for a prolonged period, a chronic pain syndrome may develop. Chronic pain has been defined as that pain that persists beyond the expected time of healing or for more than 3 months (Merskey, 1986). Acute and chronic pain may coexist. In the chronic pain state, the sympathoadrenal responses habituate or become exhausted. Vegetative responses, such as sleep disturbances, irritability, loss of appetite, decreased motor activity, and mental depression emerge. Psychologic disturbances can become prominent in chronic pain with limitation of physical, mental, and social activities. A detailed classification of chronic pain, extremely helpful in the diagnosis and treatment of chronic pain, has been developed by the International Association for the Study of Pain (Merskey, 1986). Cancer pain may be acute, chronic, or intermittent. It often has a definable cause associated with occurrence of tumor, its recurrence, or its treatment.

Pathophysiology of Pain

Classic teaching about the neurologic mechanisms of pain describes a spinothalamic tract that relays all messages of pain received from peripheral nerves arising on the contralateral side of the body. Our current knowledge makes this simple model of transmission of pain naive and incomplete. The pathophysiology of pain involves very complex interactions of many different peripheral and CNS structures from the skin surface to the cerebral cortex. The neurophysiologic and neuropharmacologic findings on pain have been extensively reviewed (Yaksh, 1988).

Specific primary afferent nerves, termed nociceptors, signal the presence of noxious stimulation. These receptors are activated by mechanical, thermal, or chemical stimuli. The stimuli are conducted toward the cortex via axons in the spinal cord, brainstem, midbrain, and, finally, higher cortical processing centers. Trauma results in release of potassium and local synthesis of bradykinin and prostaglandins. Substance P, an 11-aminoacid peptide found in small-diameter primary afferents, is transmitted via the nerves to the site of injury. It activates the local vasculature promoting extravasation of fluid into the tissues. Histamine from mast cells and serotonin from platelets are powerful activators of nociceptors. The primary afferent nociceptor not only signals the presence of tissue damage but also plays a direct role in local mechanisms of defense and repair (Yaksh, 1988).

The nerve impulse from the nociceptor travels via primary afferent sensory nerves (unmyelinated C fibers, finely myelinated A-delta fibers) to the spinal cord and enters via the dorsal or ventral nerve roots, which terminate in the ipsilateral dorsal horn of the spinal cord. At this point, neuronal interconnections become extremely complex within the multiple lamina of the dorsal horn cells. Several different endogenous peptides may serve as neurotransmitters at this location. These peptides bind to at least four different types of opioid receptors (mu, kappa, sigma, delta) that have been identified in the spinal cord and brain (Pert and Snyder, 1973). Neurons can interconnect with one another, become part of spinal cord motor neuron reflexes, or modulate connections or reflexes. Second-order neurons carry the nerve impulses via several different routes to higher cortical brain centers via the brainstem and thalamic relays. Modulation of the pain pathways occurs at many different levels of the spinal cord and higher CNS centers. Virtually every pathway carrying nociceptive information is under modulatory control from supraspinal systems (Yaksh, 1988).

The above pathophysiologic discussion is a simplification of current knowledge. It will, however, serve as the basis for understanding the therapeutic options available for the management of pain.

Diagnosis before Treatment

Acute pain is an important signaling mechanism to alert the individual that potential or real damage is occurring and that action needs to be taken to avoid further injury. For example, the pain of a bone fracture leads to voluntary and involuntary immobilization of a fracture site to prevent further damage. Indeed, much of clinical medical diagnosis is based upon the signs and symptoms of acute pain. Prior to initiating therapy for acute or chronic pain, the physician should understand the cause or pathophysiology of the patient's pain. Many therapeutic maneuvers can be performed to decrease pain without using drug therapy. For example, an interview explaining what pain to expect and what treatments are available decreases the perception of pain and the need for drugs (Egbert et al., 1964). Physical immobilization of a fracture decreases or eliminates pain. The use of nasogastric suction can decompress an acutely distended bowel, and emergency radiation therapy can rapidly decrease the pain of severe metastatic bone cancer. Before a physician initiates therapy with drugs, all nonpharmacologic approaches should be considered and implemented when appropriate. While the diagnostic advantage of evaluating a patient with no analgesic present may seem desirable, the administration of analgesic medications does not usually mask diagnostic signs. In a prospective, randomized, blinded study, only 12% of patients presenting with acute pain displayed changes in physical signs, and none had altered diagnosis after administration of analgesics (Zoltie and Cust, 1986). Following proper diagnosis and initiation of treatment, acute pain no longer serves a purpose. *Principle: The decision to withhold drug treatment must be as rational as the decision to use drugs. The clinician should not simply accept warnings to withhold efficacious treatment without knowing the consequences of such actions.*

Overview of Therapeutic Options

Drug therapy with analgesics is only one component of the management of pain. As discussed above, therapy should be directed at the relevant pathophysiology that creates or maintains pain. Local anesthetics can be effectively used for neural blockade to provide relief from acute or chronic pain. Infiltration of a local anesthetic into a surgical wound can provide analgesia at the operative site for many hours. Acute pancreatitis can be treated with epidural, celiac plexus, or splanchnic nerve block. Acute herpes zoster can respond to sympathetic blockade, that is, stellate ganglion block. Nondrug treatments for control of pain include transcutaneous electrical nerve stimulation, neuroaugmentative surgery, cognitive-behavioral methods (e.g., hypnosis, relaxation, biofeedback), and ablative procedures (e.g., neurolytic nerve blocks, ablative surgery). These latter specialized procedures should be performed under the supervision of a physician with specific training in the techniques of managing pain.

While oral, IV, and IM administration are the standard approaches to delivering analgesic drugs, invasive and innovative drug delivery techniques are emerging as important modalities for management of pain. The presence of opioid receptors in the spinal cord enables the epidural, intrathecal, and intraventricular administration of opioids to have significant clinical benefit (Cousins and Mather, 1984; Breslow et al., 1989). Innovative drug delivery will be discussed later. *Principle: A goal of therapy is to make a drug disease- or organ-specific. When devices are used to achieve organ specificity of drug therapy, their relative efficacy and toxicity must be evaluated and compared with more traditional routes of drug administration.*

Classes of Drug Therapy

Therapy for chronic noncancer pain depends upon the cause of the pain; usually nonpharmacologic approaches are tried first. Drug therapy represents the most common approach for the management of acute and chronic pain caused by cancer. There are three classes of analgesic drugs: (1) nonopioid analgesics including aspirin and the nonsteroidal anti-inflammatory drugs (Table 25–1) (NSAIDs), (2) opioid analgesics (Table 25–2), and (3) analgesic adjuvants.

Nonopioid Analgesics. Aspirin, other salicylates, acetaminophen, and the NSAIDs are extensively used to treat mild-to-moderate acute and chronic pain of different causes including postsurgical trauma, arthritis, and cancer (Kantor, 1982). The following generalizations can be made about this group of drugs: (1) it does not produce tolerance, physical, or psychological dependence, (2) there is a "ceiling" on the degree of analgesia obtainable, that is, increasing the dose beyond a certain point does not result in additional relief of pain, (3) the antipyretic, analgesic, and anti-inflammatory effects can vary between drugs, and (4) the presumed mechanism of action is inhibition of the enzyme cyclooxygenase, preventing the formation of prostaglandins (especially PGE_2) (Foley, 1985).

Aspirin or acetylsalicylic acid is one of the oldest oral analgesics available (Table 25–1). Various salicylate salts (choline magnesium trisalicylate) are available and can decrease some of the adverse effects of aspirin (gastric irritation, bleeding, and antiplatelet effects). Acetaminophen is a nonsalicylate with analgesic and antipyretic potency and efficacy similar to that of aspirin. It has few anti-inflammatory effects, does not alter platelet function, and does not affect the gastric mucosa. Its mechanism of action is not dependent upon inhibition of cyclooxygenase.

The NSAIDs are a group of compounds with diverse clinical pharmacokinetics and pharmacodynamics. Numerous NSAIDs have equivalent or possibly better maximal analgesic efficacy than that of aspirin (Kantor, 1982; Beaver, 1988). The onset of analgesia from the NSAIDs is relatively slow (0.5–2 hours) compared with onset after most opioids. This is due in part to the use of the oral route of administration and slow distribution to their peripheral sites of action. The pharmacokinetics of different NSAIDs vary greatly, resulting in different half-lives and dosing intervals. Analgesic response to individual NSAIDs also varies, and none is clearly superior to full doses of aspirin. Thus, if the clinical response to one drug is suboptimal, another NSAID should be considered (Brooks and Day, 1991; medical letter, 1991). *Principle: Understanding the clinical pharmacology of a drug group allows one to optimize care for an individual patient.*

The analgesic efficacy of NSAIDs must be balanced constantly against their common adverse effects: platelet inhibition, GI irritation, and renal insufficiency. The NSAIDs are especially effective in the management of bone pain secondary to tumor metastases (Stambaugh, 1989). The initial effectiveness of NSAIDS for bone pain due to metastases should not lull one into delaying use of narcotics when pain becomes more severe (Hanks, 1985). It is commonly recommended to use morphine with an NSAID, or another drug like hydroxyzine (Hupert et al., 1980) to "spare" the dose of morphine (Foley, 1985). If the half-life of the adjunct is longer than that of the narcotic, sustained analgesia may cause cumulative toxicity of the adjunct. Complex "cocktails" including multiple drugs, such as "Brompton" have redundant and hazardous constituents; they are obsolete (Hanks, 1985). Morphine is a very inexpensive drug (by prescription). An adequate dose

of morphine attenuates pain and prevents its recurrence; patients are comfortable, but not anesthetized. It can be safely titrated, using state of consciousness and respiratory rate, to doses of 500 mg every 4 hours (Hanks and Twycross, 1984).

Until recently, most NSAIDs were available only for oral use because of their limited solubility in traditional vehicles and because they cause significant tissue irritation when given parenterally. When the oral route is not available, the use of NSAIDs for moderate or severe postsurgical pain has been limited. Recently a very potent NSAID, ketorolac, has been approved for parenteral use in the United States. Ketorolac can be used orally, IM, or IV with minimal tissue irritation. Given IM, it has analgesic efficacy equivalent to that of morphine or meperidine in postsurgical patients having moderate to severe pain (O'Hara et al., 1987). The versatility of parenteral administration of ketorolac may allow more extensive utilization of NSAIDs in the management of acute postsurgical pain. *Principle: The clinician usually is well served to look closely for differences between drugs in the same class. Sometimes minor variations of chemical structure can lead to development of a new chemical entity with properties quite different from those of other members of the same class of compounds.* On the other hand, many new analgesics have been heralded with unrealistic enthusiasm and high hopes that did not come to fruition. Ketorolac may or may not be another of these (Buckley and Brogden, 1990).

Opioid Analgesics. There are several categories of opioid analgesics available for the management of pain: (1) morphine-like agonists, (2) mixed agonist-antagonists, and (3) partial agonists (Table 25–2) (Ross and Gilman, 1985; Gal, 1989).

This classification derives from the interaction of these drugs with multiple opioid receptors and the resulting pharmacologic profiles. Morphine is an agonist at both the μ and κ receptors. Activation of these receptors results in analgesia. A mixed agonist-antagonist (pentazocine) can bind to both μ and κ receptors, acting as an agonist on the κ receptor and an antagonist at the μ receptor. This produces analgesia in the nontolerant patient, possibly through the κ-receptor effects, but precipitates withdrawal in the patient tolerant to morphine-like drugs by acting as an antagonist and displacing the morphine-like drugs from the μ receptors. The mixed agonist-antagonists have a ceiling effect with analgesia and respiratory depression. The partial agonist (buprenorphine) has partial pharmacologic activity at the μ receptor but no activity at the κ receptor. The partial

Table 25–1. SELECTED NONOPIOID ANALGESICS: ANALGESIC DOSAGE AND EFFICACY COMPARED WITH ASPIRIN*†

DRUG	PROPRIETARY NAMES (NOT ALL-INCLUSIVE)	AVERAGE ANALGESIC DOSE (P.O.) (MG)	DOSE INTERVAL (HR)	MAXIMAL DAILY DOSE (MG)	ANALGESIC EFFICACY COMPARED WITH ASPIRIN 650 MG	ELIMINATION HALF-LIFE (HR)
Acetaminophen	Numerous	500–1000	4–6	4000	Comparable	2–3
Salicylates						
Aspirin	Numerous	500–1000	4–6	4000	—	0.25
Diflunisal	Dolobid	1000 initial 500 subsequent	8–12	1500	500 mg superior to aspirin, with slower onset and longer duration; an initial dose of 1000 mg significantly shortens time to onset	8–12
Choline magnesium trisalicylate	Trilisate	1000–1500	12	2000–3000	Longer duration of action than aspirin	9–17
NSAIDs						
Propionic Acids						
Ibuprofen	Motrin, Rufen, Nuprin, Advil, Medipren	200–400	4–6	2400	Superior at both doses	2–2.5
Naproxen	Naprosyn	500 initial 250 subsequent	6–8	1250	—	12–15
Naproxen sodium	Anaprox	550 initial 275 subsequent	6–8	1375	275 mg comparable to aspirin, with slower onset and longer duration; 550 mg superior to aspirin	—
Fenoprofen	Nalfon	200	4–6	800	Comparable	2–3
Ketoprofen	Orudis	25–50	6–8	300	Superior at both doses	1.5
Indoleacetic Acids						
Indomethacin	Indocin	25	8–12	100	Comparable	2
Anthranilic Acids						
Mefenamic acid	Ponstel	500 initial 250 subsequent	6	1500	Comparable	2

* Reproduced with permission from *Principles of Analgesic Use in the Treatment of Acute Pain and Chronic Cancer Pain*, 2nd Edition, American Pain Society, Skokie, IL, 1989.

† See text. Not all authors find superior analgesic efficacy.

Table 25-2. OPIOID ANALGESICS COMMONLY USED FOR MODERATE AND SEVERE PAIN[a]

NAME	ROUTE	EQUIANALGESIC DOSE[b] (MG)	PEAK[c] (HR)	DURATION (HR)	ELIMINATION HALF-LIFE (HR)	COMMENTS	PRECAUTIONS
Morphine-like Agonists							
Morphine	IM	10	$\frac{1}{2}$–1	4–6	3–4	Standard of comparison for opioid analgesics	Lower doses for aged patients, impaired ventilation; bronchial asthma; increased intracranial pressure; liver failure
	p.o.	60[d]	$1\frac{1}{2}$–2	4–7			
Meperidine (Demerol)	IM	75	$\frac{1}{2}$–1	4–5	4–6	Slightly shorter acting, used orally for less severe pain	Normeperidine (toxic metabolite) accumulates with repetitive dosing causing CNS excitation; not for patients with impaired renal function or receiving MAO inhibitors[f]
	p.o.	300[e]	1–2	4–6			
Methadone (Dolophine)	IM	10	Like IM morphine	Like IM morphine	12–24	Good oral potency, long plasma half-life	Like morphine; may accumulate with repetitive dosing causing excessive sedation
	p.o.	20	Like p.o. morphine	Like p.o. morphine			
Levorphanol (Levo-Dromoran)	IM	2	Like IM morphine	Like IM morphine	12–16	Like methadone	Like methadone
	p.o.	4	Like p.o. morphine	Like p.o. morphine			
Heroin	IM	5	$\frac{1}{2}$–1	4–5		Slightly shorter acting; biotransformed to active metabolites (e.g., morphine); not available in U.S.	Like morphine
	p.o.	(60)[e]	Like p.o. morphine				
Hydromorphone (Dilaudid)	IM	1.5	Like IM heroin		2–3	Slightly shorter acting	Like morphine
	p.o.	7.5	Like p.o. morphine				
Oxymorphone (Numorphan)	IM	1	Like IM morphine	Like IM morphine		Like morphine	Like morphine
Codeine	IM	130	Like IM morphine		3–6	Like morphine, used orally for less severe pain	Like morphine
	p.o.	200					
Oxycodone	p.o.	30	$\frac{1}{2}$–1	4–6	?	Like morphine, used only for less severe pain	Like morphine

		Dose (mg)[c]		Duration (h)	Comments	
Mixed Agonist-Antagonists						
Pentazocine (Talwin)	IM	60	Like IM morphine	2–3	Used orally for less severe pain; mixed agonist-antagonist; less abuse liability than morphine; included in schedule IV of Controlled Substances Act	May cause psychotomimetic effects; may precipitate withdrawal in opioid-dependent patients; not for myocardial infarction[f]
	p.o.	180[e]	Like p.o. morphine			
Nalbuphine (Nubain)	IM	10	Like IM morphine	5–6	Not available orally; like IM pentazocine but not scheduled	Incidence of psychotomimetic effects lower than with pentazocine
Butorphanol (Stadol)	IM	2	Like IM morphine	3–6	Not available orally like IM nalbuphine	Like IM pentazocine
Partial Agonists						
Buprenorphine (Buprenex)	IM	0.4	Like IM morphine 2–3	3–4	Not available orally; sublingual preparation not yet available in U.S.; less abuse liability than morphine, does not produce psychotomimetic effects	May precipitate withdrawal in opioid-dependent patients
	SL	0.8	5–6			

[a] Modified and reproduced with permission from Inturrisi, 1989.
[b] These doses are recommended starting doses from which the optimal dose for each patient is determined by titration and the maximal dose limited by adverse effects.
[c] Peak time and duration of analgesia are based on mean values and refer to the stated equianalgesic doses in nontolerant patients.
[d] A value of 3 is used when calculating an oral dosage regimen of every 4 hours around the clock.
[e] Not recommended.
[f] Irritating to tissues on repeated administration.

agonist precipitates withdrawal in patients who are physically dependent upon a morphine-like agonist. This withdrawal is believed to be due to the partial agonist's replacing a full morphine-like agonist on the μ receptor. Fewer psychomimetic effects are seen with the partial agonist compared with the mixed agonist-antagonists, possibly due to the lack of κ-receptor interaction.

For at least 2500 years, humans have been using the juice from the seed capsule of the opium poppy (*Papaver somniferum*) to provide relief from pain. Seturner purified one of the constituent alkaloids and named it morphine after Morpheus, the Greek god of dreams. The morphine-like agonists mediate their drug effects via the μ opioid receptors to cause relief of pain, sedation, euphoria, and respiratory depression. They block the transmission of nociceptive signals, activate pain-modulating neurons that project to the spinal cord, and inhibit transmission from primary afferent nociceptors to dorsal horn sensory projection cells (Martin, 1984). The nature of the analgesia induced by all the morphine-like agonists is similar. With increasing doses, the degree of analgesia increases until an anesthetic state is reached. Anesthesiologists are aware that complete respiratory depression occurs before opioid-induced unconsciousness. Such information clearly has not been shared with other specialists. This respiratory depression is caused by decreasing the responsiveness both of medullary chemoreceptors (to CO_2) and of carotid chemoreceptors (to O_2). *Thus, hypercarbia and hypoxia can occur in the conscious patient!* The opioids are distinguished by their time course for onset and duration of analgesia and for their side-effect profile. *Principle: When dose–response curves for efficacy and toxicity have different slopes, then the choice of dose may dramatically alter the benefit/risk ratio.*

Morphine is the standard to which other opioids are compared. The onset of morphine-induced analgesia after IV administration is relatively slow (6–30 minutes) in part because of its limited lipid solubility and slow rate of penetration of the blood–brain barrier. The short terminal elimination half-life of 3 to 4 hours limits the duration of analgesia. Morphine undergoes significant first-pass metabolism; thus, oral doses must be sixfold greater than parenteral doses to achieve the same degree of analgesia (Stanski et al., 1978). Oral, slow-release morphine preparations are available to extend the duration of analgesia. Slow-release morphine preparations are a boon in the management of chronic pain. The dose of the preparation is determined by first using short-acting morphine until a 24-hour dose is determined. When converting to the sustained-release preparation, it is wise to continue a p.r.n.

dose of the short-acting morphine to provide for "crisis" in pain. Additionally, when the patient calls for the p.r.n. dose frequently, it may be timely to increase the dose of the sustained-release preparation. This use is analogous to use of long- and short-acting insulin.

Meperidine is less potent and more lipophilic than morphine. Therefore, meperidine doses are larger than those of morphine, but the onset of analgesia after IV administration of meperidine (3–12 minutes) is more rapid than the onset with morphine. Both drugs have similar but poor (about 15% to 20%) oral bioavailability. Normeperidine (the principal metabolite) is a potent CNS stimulant with a long elimination half-life (14 hours). High doses of meperidine given to patients with renal dysfunction can lead to accumulation of normeperidine and resultant seizures (Kaiko et al., 1983).

The analgesia produced by the IV administration of methadone is similar to that of meperidine. The duration of methadone analgesia is very dose-dependent. With low doses (5–10 mg/70 kg), the duration of analgesia is relatively short (1–2 hours) because the opioid redistributes from the brain to muscle and fat. With increasing doses (10–20 mg/70 kg), the duration of analgesia increases, in part because of the relatively long terminal elimination half-life (6–40 hours). With the careful IV titration of methadone, it is possible to achieve complete pain relief after surgery for 12 to 24 hours (Gourlay et al., 1986). Methadone has a relatively low hepatic clearance and much less first-pass effect than do meperidine or morphine, explaining its high oral bioavailability. Although not stated in the package insert, methadone can be administered by any parenteral route or orally (Gourlay et al., 1986). *Principle: The package insert is a guide to therapy approved by the FDA. There are many medically designated uses of drugs that do not get mentioned or are denied discussion in a package insert. Remember that package inserts are not meant to direct the practice of medicine, as the FDA is restricted by law from doing so.*

In the past, parenteral fentanyl, alfentanil, and sufentanil have not been used extensively for the management of postoperative pain. The duration of analgesia produced with alfentanil, fentanyl, and sufentanil is shorter than that of morphine. This characteristic makes all these opioids extremely useful for intraoperative analgesia, anesthesia, and conscious sedation. Extensive redistribution from the CNS to muscle and fat tissues is a major mechanism for termination of the analgesic effect of these opioids and explains the short duration of clinical effect. With increasing doses to extend the duration of analgesia, the likelihood of excessive respiratory depression at the peak of analgesia also increases. Thus, the use of fentanyl, alfentanil, and sufentanil for short-term analgesia requires appropriate experience and equipment to manage excessive respiratory depression.

Heroin, a widely abused drug, has no unique therapeutic advantages for relief of pain. Heroin produces its analgesia indirectly, being first metabolized to 6-acetylmorphine and morphine. Heroin is really a prodrug with greater lipid solubility than morphine and therefore a more rapid onset of analgesia. The nature and quality of analgesia from heroin is identical to that which can be achieved with morphine (Kiako et al., 1981).

Codeine and propoxyphene are morphine-like agonists that have less analgesic efficacy than the opioids discussed above. With increasing doses, the degree of analgesia becomes limited and undesirable adverse effects emerge. These drugs are almost exclusively used by the oral route to treat mild-to-moderate pain. The analgesic efficacy of propoxyphene is actually less than that of aspirin. Yet propoxyphene still sells well in the United States. What clinical end points could physicians using this drug be following?

Morphine-like agonists produce similar adverse effects: nausea, vomiting (respiratory depression), sedation, and constipation. Tolerance and dependence (physical and psychological) may result with repeated administration. Physical dependence will occur in patients taking opioids over long periods of time (see chapter 27). In the patient who has developed physical dependence, abrupt discontinuation of morphine or administration of an opioid antagonist creates an abstinence syndrome marked by anxiety, irritability, chills and hot flashes, nausea, vomiting, abdominal cramps, piloerection, and insomnia. The time course of the abstinence syndrome parallels the elimination half-life of the opioid; the shorter the elimination half-life, the sooner symptoms occur. With opioids with longer elimination half-lives, symptoms can be delayed several days and are less severe. Physiologic dependence should be distinguished from psychological dependence and addiction. The latter is defined as a pattern of compulsive drug use characterized by a continued craving for an opioid and the need to use it for effects other than relief of pain. The likelihood that the therapeutic use of opioids for management of pain of hospitalized patients will result in opioid dependence or addiction is extremely small (Kanner and Foley, 1981).

The mixed agonist-antagonists (pentazocine, nalbuphine, butorphanol) and the partial agonist buprenorphine have not achieved the clinical utility of the morphinelike agonists. Unacceptable toxicity, especially psychomimetic side effects and sedation, limits their use. They also have a ceiling effect in the analgesia they produce, an undesirable characteristic.

Analgesic Adjuvants. A number of classes of drugs that have not been traditionally categorized as analgesics may either enhance the effects of opioids and aspirinlike drugs or minimize their adverse effects.

Tricyclic antidepressants (amitriptyline, imipramine, desipramine) relieve pain related to chronic neuropathy and postherpetic neuralgia. Analgesic efficacy appears to be independent of the degree of patient depression. Clinical responses to the tricyclic drugs can range from dramatic to partial or no relief. Tricyclic antidepressants block the reuptake of amines (especially serotonin and norepinephrine) in the CNS, which may explain their analgesic effectiveness (Monks and Merskey, 1989).

Anticonvulsants (phenytoin, carbamazepine, sodium valproate) may be effective in brief, lancing pain arising from peripheral nerve syndromes such as trigeminal neuralgia, postherpetic neuralgia, and posttraumatic neuralgias. The mechanism of analgesia from anticonvulsants in these very specific pain syndromes is not known (Swerdlow, 1984).

Antihistamines, specifically hydroxyzine, have analgesic, antiemetic, and sedative activity in addition to antihistaminergic effects. When given IM or orally, hydroxyzine potentiates the analgesic effects of morphine used to treat acute pain and cancer pain. Hydroxyzine provides the equivalent degree of analgesia expected from low doses of IM morphine or meperidine (Stambaugh and Lane, 1983). The mechanism of this analgesic potentiation is not known.

Corticosteroids have specific and nonspecific effects in the management of acute and chronic pain caused by cancer. They can act by lysis of tumors (i.e., lymphoma) and ameliorate painful nerve or spinal cord compression by reducing the edema produced by a tumor (see chapter 23). Corticosteroids are effective in the management of metastatic bone pain (Foley, 1985).

Caffeine increases analgesia when given with aspirin-like drugs or opioids to relieve mild to moderate pain in the postoperative period (Laska et al., 1984). Dextroamphetamine may potentiate the analgesia provided by opiates. It also antagonizes the respiratory depression associated with opioid use (Forrest et al., 1977).

Benzodiazepines may be effective for the management of acute anxiety and muscle spasm causing acute pain. They have no meaningful analgesic effect themselves and can potentiate sedative and respiratory depression induced by the opioids. Although cannabinoids have some analgesic properties in controlled clinical trials, their adverse effects (dysphoria, drowsiness, hypotension, and bradycardia) limit their routine use as an analgesic. Cocaine has local anesthetic properties but no efficacy as an analgesic or adjuvant when used with opiates. Barbiturates have no intrinsic analgesic properties, and their use in the management of pain should be limited to times when amnesia or sedation are desired (see the section on conscious sedation below). *Principle: Treatable signs or symptoms associated with a variety of common diseases offer the opportunity to study useful and dangerous drug interactions. There would have been little logic in combining the drugs that have been found as adjuncts to analgesics if pain were studied only in trauma.*

Principles of Providing Analgesia

Choose the Most Appropriate Drug. For treating chronic pain associated with cancer, the World Health Organization (1986) has established an "analgesic ladder" for the oral use of drugs. Nonopioid analgesics are given initially to achieve maximal analgesia. This may include different NSAIDs at maximal therapeutic doses. If maximal nonopioid analgesia is not adequate, then a "weak" opioid, such as codeine or oxycodone is added. Adjuvant drugs (psychotropics, anticonvulsants) may also be added if indicated. If this sequence does not provide adequate analgesia, then a stronger opioid (morphine, hydromorphone, methadone) is substituted for the weak opioid while the NSAID and adjuvant drugs are continued. The oral opioid dosage is titrated to obtain adequate analgesia. This approach has been tested with substantial success.

Optimize the Route of Administration. Analgesics are most commonly administered orally. The optimal route of administration of analgesics depends on the nature and degree of pain, its clinical cause, and underlying pathophysiology. The oral route becomes less useful in patients with advanced cancer or postoperatively with patients who have had major surgery. The moderate-to-high first-pass metabolism of many of the opioids makes oral dosing less than ideal because bioavailability varies from patient to patient. If oral morphine or meperidine is used, frequent (2–3 hour) dosing prevents rapidly fluctuating blood concentrations and results in more continuous pain relief. The oral dose should be titrated to a desired degree of pain relief over a time period to adjust for the variable rate and extent of oral absorption. The use of slow-release morphine preparations has decreased the interval of dosing necessary via the oral route (Portenoy et al., 1989). Methadone has a lower hepatic clearance than does morphine or meperidine and a longer terminal elimination half-life. This confers some pharmacokinetic advantage in maintaining stable blood concentrations to obtain constant relief of pain. First-pass metabolism is much less pronounced with aspirin and the NSAIDs. Although oral bioavailability is not a major issue with the NSAIDs, oral administration results in peak blood concentrations in 1 to 2 hours, delaying the onset of analgesia.

Intramuscular injection is frequently the route of administration for the opioids. There is ample pharmacokinetic evidence that variable and unpredictable absorption is a major factor in inadequate relief of pain when this route of administration is used (Austin et al., 1980a). Peak concentrations of drug in blood occur 30 to 60 minutes after administration, delaying the onset of analgesia. Additionally, concentrations of drug in blood vary during the traditional 3- to 4-hour administration period, causing patients to cycle between adequate and inadequate relief of pain. The management of pain is improved when the IM route is replaced with other methods of administration.

Intravenous infusion techniques have many pharmacokinetic advantages over the oral or IM routes. The continuous infusion of meperidine can provide constant concentrations of drug in blood (Stapleton et al., 1979). Such constant concentrations above an individual minimum effective concentration can result in complete analgesia for several days in patients who have had major surgical procedures. Similar data are available for the management of chronic cancer pain with continuous infusions (Portenoy et al., 1986). With infusion techniques, opiates with shorter elimination half-lives (morphine) have a kinetic advantage over those with longer elimination half-lives (methadone) because blood concentrations can be more easily titrated. The disadvantage of IV infusion techniques is the continuous need for vascular access, that is, a venous catheter and an appropriate mechanical pumping device. Subcutaneous infusion of morphine obviates the need for vascular access (Coyle et al., 1986; Brenneis et al., 1987).

Patient-controlled analgesia is an adaptation of the IV infusion technique that allows the patient to adjust the administration of the opioid (White, 1988). By means of a pump programmed with a defined "lockout" interval during which drug cannot be dispensed, the patient administers a small IV bolus injection of an opioid. The patient activates the opioid dosing with a hand-held switch; the physician decides on the opioid, bolus dose, and dosing interval. This technique has achieved significant clinical success because it allows the necessary individualization of opioid dosage with direct feedback from the patient. The disadvantages of this technique are the need for constant IV access and the cost of the pumping device.

The transdermal administration of opioids is currently under clinical investigation. Fentanyl, a lipophilic opioid, has been successfully incorporated into rate-controlled transdermal devices. Constant concentrations of fentanyl in blood can be achieved within 12 hours of application of the device and can be maintained for at least 3 days, which can result in a constant degree of analgesia (Caplan et al., 1989). However, because blood concentrations cannot be easily increased or decreased with this method of delivery, supplemental analgesic medication may be necessary in some patients. The attractiveness of transdermal drug administration is its simplicity and noninvasive nature. The disadvantages are the inability to titrate the concentrations of drug in blood over short periods (12–24 hours) to obtain optimal analgesia in all patients, the prolonged absorption of drug from subcutaneous fat deposits after removal of the patch, and the problem of appropriate disposal of a patch that contains large quantities of an addictive substance. The clinical utility of transdermal fentanyl for management of acute and chronic pain requires ongoing investigation.

The epidural and intrathecal routes of administration of opiates are being used more frequently in the management of pain. These routes of administration became clinically useful following the description in the mid-1970s of opioid receptors in the dorsal horn of the spinal cord, and demonstration of behavioral analgesia following the administration of intrathecal morphine in rats (Pert and Snyder, 1973; Yaksh, 1981). The epidural or intrathecal administration of opiates allows small doses to be given very near the site of action, providing excellent analgesia with (theoretically) minimal systemic effects. With epidural administration, drug diffuses into the CSF and spinal cord to exert its effect. Parallel to the movement into the CSF to create desired effects, drug spreads to other tissues near the site of delivery (epidural fat tissue), reaches the blood, and thus can be delivered to other body tissues. The physicochemical properties of an opioid are very important in defining onset and duration of analgesic effects and undesired adverse effects (Cousins and Mather, 1984). Morphine has been extensively administered via the epidural or intrathecal route. Epidurally administered morphine, in single doses of 5 to 10 mg, can provide excellent postoperative analgesia for periods of 12 to 24 hours. Its limited lipid solubility slows the rate of diffusion into the spinal cord and delays the onset of analgesia but also prolongs the duration of analgesic effect. With more lipophilic opioids (meperidine, fentanyl, sufentanil, or methadone), the onset of analgesia is more rapid but duration of analgesia is shorter. The use of an epidural catheter allows the continuous administration of opioid for short-term and long-term management of pain.

Undesirable adverse effects can occur with epidurally administered opiates. Nausea, vomiting, pruritus, and urinary retention have been reported. Respiratory depression also has occurred, possibly due to the rostral migration of morphine in the CSF to the central respiratory centers and/or to systemic absorption into blood with delivery to brain centers. Large clinical studies estimate the risk of severe respiratory depression following epidural morphine to be 1/1000. Some demographic characteristics of patients who may be predisposed to such adverse effects can be identified, but the occurrence of this serious side effect indicates the need for careful surveillance of all patients receiving opioids via this route (Rawal et al., 1987).

Individualize the Dose. A feature common to the use of all opioids for relief of pain is the large variation in the dose needed to provide optimal analgesia. Pharmacokinetic profiles of the opioids vary moderately; clearance and volumes of distribution vary 30% to 50% from patient to patient; even greater variation has been shown for the pharmacodynamic response to these drugs. The relationship between meperidine concentration in blood and degree of pain relief in postsurgical patients is steep, almost a step function (Austin et al., 1980b). The maximum meperidine concentration in blood still associated with severe pain was 0.41 ± 0.17 μg/ml (mean $\pm$ SD), while the point of transition (to some pain or no pain) was 0.46 ± 0.18 μg/ml. A small increase in concentration of meperidine was required to go from poor to complete relief of pain. These investigators also demonstrated that the pharmacodynamic variation was much less within an individual than between individuals. *Principle: Ordinarily drugs with steep dose–response curves are difficult to use, especially if they have a narrow therapeutic index. In some situations, the advantages of the drug may outweigh this relative disadvantage.*

Analgesic dosing techniques that allow individualization of dose and titration to optimal analgesia, as with patient-controlled analgesia or titrated IV infusions, afford the best opportunity for optimal management of pain. These techniques overcome the interpatient pharmacokinetic and pharmacodynamic variability found with the opioids. The traditional, fixed dose given IM (e.g., morphine 10 mg, IM every 4 hours) is a dosing regimen that ignores the existence of pharmacokinetic and pharmacodynamic variability and results in large swings of opioid concentration in blood. These generalized inadequacies explain much of the documented failure to properly control pain in postsurgical patients (Marks and Sacher, 1973).

While between-patient variability is still a problem, other patients tend to require smaller doses of opioids. Intramuscular morphine produces a much longer duration of analgesia in older patients (Kiako, 1980). The contribution of pharmacokinetic versus pharmacodynamic mechanisms for this decreased dose requirement has not been established. *Principle: Age-related changes in dose requirement and proper dose adjustments may precede our knowledge of the precise mechanisms involved.*

Obtain Help When Needed. In the past several years, two concepts have improved the management of pain. One is the development of an in-hospital acute pain service where physicians specialize in the management of pain for postoperative patients (Ready et al., 1988). Such specialized services are usually initiated by anesthesiologists who extend their techniques of pain management from the operating room to the postsurgical wards. By having a small number of highly skilled and knowledgeable physicians manage postoperative pain, it becomes possible to initiate new, innovative, and more invasive methods of pain management (i.e., continuous administration of epidural opioids). For continued success with the implementation of such methods, the education of the patient's physician and the nursing staff of the postsurgical wards is necessary.

The second concept, somewhat older, is the multidisciplinary pain clinic for the management of chronic pain. These clinics involve anesthesiologists, neurologists, neurosurgeons, and psychiatrists along with physical therapists, psychologists, nurse specialists, and social workers. The goal of the clinic for patients with chronic pain is comprehensive assessment followed by therapy for patients who have not achieved optimal management of their pain in a traditional medical environment (Fields, 1987).

CONSCIOUS SEDATION

Conscious sedation is an anesthetic state of amnesia and/or analgesia that allows a patient's cooperation during a diagnostic or therapeutic procedure. During conscious sedation the patient retains the ability to maintain his or her airway, breathe spontaneously, and respond appropriately to verbal commands (NIH Consensus Development Conference, 1986). This degree of CNS depression is highly desirable for various procedures and is used by radiologists, internists, pediatricians, obstetricians, gynecologists, ophthalmologists, family practitioners, surgeons, psychiatrists, dentists, oral surgeons, podiatrists,

and virtually every other physician or provider involved in diagnostic or therapeutic maneuvers (MRI scans, endoscopy, bronchoscopy, removal of a foreign body, cardiac catheterization, PTCA procedures, gastroscopy, laparoscopy, cataract removal, bunionectomy, tooth removal, plastic surgical procedures, electrocardioversion, and electroconvulsive therapies). The recent popularity of a new benzodiazepine, midazolam, and the study of its properties has clarified thinking about the goals of conscious sedation, the choices of drugs available, and the adverse effects of obtaining this therapeutic state.

Goals and Sequelae of Conscious Sedation

Anxiety and fear commonly complicate the performance of diagnostic and therapeutic procedures. In dentistry, anxiety and fear can reduce the efficacy of local anesthetic nerve blocks for noxious stimuli. Thus, one goal of conscious sedation is to relieve anxiety. Such relief is also beneficial in reducing the need for subsequent analgesic medication; statistically significant, psychologically meaningful correlations between measures of states of anxiety and perceptions of the intensity of an acute painful stimulus range from 0.4 to 0.8 and are greatest when the pain comes from an exogenous stimulus (dental surgery, endoscopy) (Dworkin et al., 1978; Levine et al., 1978; Corah et al., 1981; Turner and Chapman, 1982; Turk et al., 1983; Dworkin et al., 1983a and b, 1984). The ability to alter pain threshold by relief of anxiety may be modulated by the endogenous opioid system (Levine et al., 1978).

Additional therapeutic goals of conscious sedation are pain relief and amnesia. Patients who do not experience or remember pain are more likely to agree to be tested or treated in the future. The recent success of midazolam and the former popularity of scopolamine attest to the importance and desirability of amnesia in clinical practice. *Principle: Popularity of a drug may not stem only from marketing techniques. It may teach something about the relative value of the therapeutic goals we are seeking.*

Other goals of conscious sedation include sedation, blockade of unwanted reflexes (such as tachycardia or hypertension caused by endoscope insertion), patient cooperation, and reduction of the risk of pulmonary aspiration. To achieve the above diverse therapeutic goals, a variety of non-pharmacologic and pharmacologic methods have been used (Table 25–3). Many of these methods produce adverse effects, such as loss of protective reflexes, diminished respiratory drive, diminished cardiovascular stability, decreased consciousness, lack of reversibility of effect, impaired psycho-

Table 25–3. METHODS AND AGENTS USED TO ACHIEVE THE GOALS OF CONSCIOUS SEDATION

GOALS OF CONSCIOUS SEDATION	METHODS AND AGENTS
1. Anxiolysis	Patient interview Psychotherapy Sedative hypnotics Narcotics Butyrophenones Phenothiazines Antihistaminics
2. Analgesia	Patient interview Amphetamines Dissociative anesthetics: ketamine Volatile general anesthetics at low dose Nitrous oxide
3. Amnesia	Benzodiazepines Anticholinergics (i.e., sco-polamine) Sedative hypnotics Dissociative anesthetics Phenothiazines Butyrophenones Antihistamines
4. Sedation	Benzodiazepines Sedative hypnotics Dissociative anesthetics: ketamine Antihistamines Butyrophenones Narcotics Volatile general anesthetics Nitrous oxide
5. Patient cooperation	Narcotics Anxiolytics
6. Reduction of risk of aspiration and pneumonia	Antihistamines H_2 blockers Metoclopramide Sodium bicitrate Anticholinergics Butyrophenones

motor function, pain on administration, constipation, urinary retention, and nausea. Although the physician may think that the first five adverse effects are a cause for greater concern, the patient, who may not completely understand the consequences of these adverse effects, may think the last five, and especially nausea, are more troublesome. Others, such as insurance companies investigating auto accidents that occur later in the day, may be concerned more with impaired psychomotor function and increased costs. For example, in Scotland, despite clear instruction to the contrary, 31% of patients went home unescorted. Of the 41% who owned cars, 9% drove themselves home and 73% drove during the 24-hour period after surgery (Ogg, 1972). In Chi-cago, 19% of the patients studied drove within 24 hours of their procedures, despite oral instructions from two different persons prior to the day of surgery, a signed form by which patients agreed to arrange for an escort home, and two sets of instructions on the day of surgery (Lichtor et al., 1990). The role of amnesia and lack of reversibility of psychomotor impairment in causing these actions remains to be determined. *Principle: When multiple goals and adverse effects of a therapy exist, different goals and adverse effects may be more important to the patient than to the physician.* We will use a discussion of the effects of midazolam alone or with other drugs to clarify how the therapeutic principles of clinical pharmacology apply to conscious sedation.

Rational Use of Midazolam for Conscious Sedation

Pharmacokinetic Properties. Midazolam (Versed) has replaced diazepam as the leading drug for conscious sedation. One pharmaceutical manufacturer estimates that midazolam is currently used in more than 70% of all procedures involving conscious sedation. What has caused this replacement for the "tried and true" standard, diazepam (Valium)? Is such use rational?

Midazolam is a water-soluble benzodiazepine with an elimination half-life of 2.5 hours (range, 2.1–3.4 hours) (Greenblatt et al., 1981). The elimination half-life of diazepam is 30 hours (range, 10–50 hours) (Klotz et al., 1976). The metabolites of midazolam are inactive, whereas several of the metabolites of diazepam have pharmacologic properties similar to those of the parent drug. One thus expects midazolam to have a shorter duration of effect. Midazolam was originally marketed for this advantage. In clinical studies, it was more difficult, however, to show that recovery after midazolam was faster than it was after diazepam, and recovery after midazolam was clearly slower than it was after thiopental (Kanto et al., 1982; Korttila, 1984). In studies after dental procedures, oral surgery, and bronchoscopy in which diazepam and midazolam were administered to achieve the same clinical end point of sedation and clinical recovery and psychomotor tests, were similar (Korttila, 1984; Skelly et al., 1984; Korttila and Tarkkanen, 1985). In outpatients who underwent bronchoscopy and received local anesthesia and diazepam (0.2 mg/kg) or midazolam (0.05 or 0.20 mg/kg IV) performance as measured by a visualization test, a perceptual speed test, and a driving-aiming test did not differ between patients 2 hours after administration of drug and was identical to that before sedation (Korttila and Tarkkanen, 1985). Of patients who received 0.1 mg/kg midazolam,

17% were unable to walk a straight line 2 hours after the drug was administered, in contrast to 100% of patients able to walk a straight line who received either 0.05 mg/kg midazolam or 0.1 mg/kg diazepam. The amnestic properties of midazolam, however, may be four (not two) times as great as those of diazepam. In a test of recovery characteristics after 0.1 to 0.3 mg/kg diazepam or 0.05 to 0.15 mg/kg midazolam, no differences could be found (White et al., 1988). Nevertheless the results of psychomotor tests as measures of recovery characteristics must be viewed with caution. Are clinical correlates of visual reaction time, aiming-driving skills, or perceptual tests relevant to life situations? *Principle: The tests of therapeutic end points need to be based on actual end points or some very accurate substitute (surrogate) for those end points.*

There is slightly better subtle psychomotor performance after midazolam than after diazepam when volunteers who were allowed food were tested 4 hours after administration of the drug (Nuotto et al., 1989). This effect 4 hours later may reflect an enterohepatic circulation for diazepam not seen with midazolam. Food may increase diazepam concentrations in blood because diazepam is excreted in bile and reabsorbed from the intestine, although the actual mechanism for this phenomenon is not clear. Change in serum concentrations of diazepam has been associated with recurrence of fatigue (Linnoila et al., 1975). Thus there is a slight advantage for midazolam in this regard.

Although the terminal elimination half-life of midazolam is much shorter than that of diazepam because of more rapid hepatic metabolism, elimination half-life does not determine the termination of clinical effects after a single dose of either drug. Because both drugs are moderately lipophilic with large volumes of distribution, their rate of redistribution from the CNS to peripheral tissues (muscle or fat) is the major factor in terminating the drug effect (see chapter 1). The rate and extent of redistribution for midazolam and diazepam are relatively similar. The long, slow, terminal elimination half-life of diazepam only becomes relevant in decreasing concentrations in blood several hours after a single dose. With long-term, multiple dosing, the terminal elimination half-life assumes increasing relevance in terminating the drug effect.

Pharmaceutic Properties. A clearer advantage of midazolam over diazepam is that midazolam is not associated with thrombophlebitis or pain on injection. In studies of patients who received diazepam IV, 39% suffered from thrombophlebitis (Hegarty and Dundee, 1977; Pagano et al., 1978). That midazolam does not produce pain on injection or subsequent thrombophlebitis may be due to the vehicle in which it is delivered. Midazolam is more water-soluble; diazepam is solubilized in propylene glycol. *Principle: The vehicle for the active ingredient, and not the active ingredient itself, may confer either beneficial or adverse properties to a particular formulation.*

Achieving Amnesia. Both sedation and amnesia are reliably achieved with midazolam, perhaps better than they are with diazepam in doses equivalent for disturbing psychomotor function. The effectiveness of midazolam as a sedative and amnesic agent has been shown by investigators using blinded observers, patient's self-report measures, and a range of doses (Reinhart et al., 1985; Barclay et al., 1985; Korttila and Tarkkanen, 1985; van Wijhe et al., 1985; Barker et al., 1986; Forrest et al., 1987; Bianchi et al., 1988; Boldy et al., 1988; Brouillette et al., 1989). Two hours after insertion of a bronchoscope, 67% of patients who received diazepam (0.2 mg/kg) versus 36% of patients who received midazolam (0.05 mg/kg) and 75% who received midazolam (0.1 mg/kg) did not remember insertion of the bronchoscope. The following day only 22%, 52%, and 8%, respectively, of the patients remembered bronchoscopy (Korttila and Tarkkanen, 1985). When diazepam and midazolam were titrated to slurring of speech, 63% and 53% of midazolam-sedated patients reported total amnesia for colonoscopy and endoscopy procedures, respectively, versus 20% and 23% of diazepam-sedated patients (Brouillette et al., 1989). Others have found either no difference or advantage with midazolam for providing amnesia. Thus, the main advantages with midazolam may be that thrombophlebitis is avoided and amnesia is produced.

Reduction in Anxiety. Reduction in anxiety, however, which correlates with faster return to work and fewer hospital days, appears better with diazepam than it does with midazolam. One difficulty with these studies is that all appear to have been done only with placebo control. Little mention is made of the effect and quality of preprocedure information. In several studies, providing the patient with information before a procedure appears to be more anxiolytic than administration of any medication. Classic studies showed that enhanced physician–patient rapport, developed by encouragement and instruction of patients, was as good as pentobarbital for sedation and relief of anxiety and significantly reduced postoperative pain and decreased hospital stay by an average of 2.7 days for 97 patients undergoing abdominal surgery (Egbert et al., 1963, 1964). Similar studies for cholecystectomy patients (Johnson et al., 1978), for cardiac surgery patients (Anderson, 1987), and for spinal surgery patients (Lawlis et al., 1985) have demonstrated anxiolysis from both interview and relaxation training. Whether midazolam or diazepam is as good as or better than an interview is not known. *Principle: It is easier to demonstrate benefit when the control group receives an inactive placebo. However, the drug being evaluated should be at least as good as or better than currently available techniques and drugs.*

Midazolam Use in Older Patients. Age has a pronounced effect on midazolam dose requirement. The dose of midazolam required to produce adequate sedation for a 20-year-old patient, 0.15 mg/kg IV, declines approximately 15% per decade, so that 0.03 mg/kg would be appropriate for a 90-year-old patient (Dundee et al., 1985; Bell et al., 1987). This decrease in dose requirement is greater than the decrease for diazepam, 10% per decade (Reidenberg et al., 1978). *Principle: Do not assume similarities in dose decrements with age among drugs of the same class.*

The safe clinical use of IV midazolum involves careful titration of the dose to clinical end points of sedation. Peak clinical effects occur 2 to 4 minutes after slow IV administration. Thus, one must wait the appropriate period of time before additional doses of midazolam are given. Failure to observe this principle will result in an increased risk of overdosage and excessive CNS depression. Most clinicians give midazolam in combination with a narcotic; such a combination intensifies the decrease in vascular resistance, venodilation, and respiratory depression associated with midazolam (Massaut et al., 1983; Heikkilä et al., 1984). Cardiovascular and respiratory changes with midazolam are additive to those of a narcotic and frequent enough to warrant continuous monitoring of blood pressure and oxygen saturation in all patients undergoing conscious sedation (Kraut, 1985; Lieberman et al., 1985; Rodrigo and Rosenquist, 1988; Hovagim et al., 1989). Such monitoring is now a standard of the American Society of Anesthesiologists and a de facto standard of oral surgeons and gastroenterologists.

Reports of serious adverse sequelae with midazolam have virtually ceased. Thus, improvements in monitoring technology now allow us to prescribe drugs in a way that allow greater patient safety. *Principle: Information obtained from adverse incident reports can lay the foundation for principles of practice that allow a drug to be used more safely. New monitoring technology may make possible the safer use of existing drugs.*

While many other drugs can be used for conscious sedation, a review of these is beyond the scope of this chapter (see Lichtor, 1990, for an excellent review). The properties of a drug that clinicians consider important (for example, patient acceptance of a drug that is not painful on injection, or the desirability of a drug that produces amnesia) and the procedure for administering a drug safely (for example, by continuously monitoring oxygen saturation) are important clinical pharmacologic lessons that have been derived from study of the treatment of pain and the use of conscious sedation techniques.

REFERENCES

Anderson, E. A.: Preoperative preparation for cardiac surgery facilitates recovery, reduces psychological distress, and reduces the incidence of acute postoperative hypertension. J. Consult. Clin. Psychol., 55:513–520, 1987.

Austin, K. L.; Stapleton, J. V.; and Mather, L. E.: Multiple intramuscular injections: A major source of variability of meperidine in man. Pain, 8:47–62, 1980a.

Austin, K. L.; Stapleton, J. V.; and Mather, L. E.: Relationship between blood meperidine concentrations and analgesic response: A preliminary report. Anesthesiology, 53:460–466, 1980b.

Barclay, J. K.; Hunter, K. M.; and McMillan, W.: Midazolam and diazepam compared as sedatives for outpatient surgery under local analgesia. Oral Surg. Oral Med. Oral Pathol., 59:349–355, 1985.

Barker, I.; Butchart, D. G. M.; Gibson, J.; Lawson, J. I. M.; and MacKenzie, N.: I.V. sedation for conservative dentistry. A comparison of midazolam and diazepam. Br. J. Anaesth., 58:371–377, 1986.

Beaver, W. T.: Impact of non-narcotic analgesics in pain management. Am. J. Med., 84:3–15, 1988.

Bell, G. D.; Spickett, G. P.; Reeve, P. A.; Morden, A.; and Logan, R. F.: Intravenous midazolam for upper gastrointestinal endoscopy: A study of 800 consecutive cases relating dose to age and sex of patient. Br. J. Clin. Pharmacol., 23:241–243, 1987.

Bianchi Porro, G.; Baroni, S.; Parente, F.; and Lazzaroni, M.: Midazolam versus diazepam as premedication for upper gastrointestinal endoscopy: A randomized, double-blind, crossover study. Gastrointest. Endosc., 34:252–254, 1988.

Boldy, D. A.; Lever, L. R.; Unwin, P. R.; Spencer, P. A.; and Hoare, A. M.: Sedation for endoscopy: Midazolam or diazepam and pethidine? Br. J. Anaesth., 61:698–701, 1988.

Bonica, J. J.: Treatment of cancer pain: Current status and future needs. In, Advances in Pain Research and Therapy (Fields, H. L.; Dubner, R.; Cervero, F., eds.). Vol. 9. Proceedings of the Fourth World Congress on Pain, Seattle. Raven Press, New York, pp. 589–616, 1985.

Brenneis, C.; Michaud, M.; Bruera, E.; and MacDonald, R. N.: Local toxicity during the subcutaneous infusion of narcotics (SCIN): Cancer Nurs., 10(4):172–176, 1987.

Breslow, M. J.; Jordan, D. A.; Christopherson, R.; Rosenfeld, B.; Miller, C. F.; Hanley, D. F.; Beattie, C.; Traystman, R. J.; and Rogers, M. C.: Epidural morphine decreases postoperative hypertension by attenuating sympathetic nervous system hyperactivity. J.A.M.A., 261:3577–3581, 1989.

Brouillette, D. E.; Leventhal, R.; Kumar, S.; Berman, D.; Kajani, M; Yoo, Y. K.; Carra, J.; and Tarter, R.: Midazolam versus diazepam for combined esophagogastroduodenoscopy and colonoscopy. Dig. Dis. Sci., 34:1265–1271, 1989.

Buckley, M. M.-T.; and Brogden, R. N.: Ketorolac: A review of its pharmacodynamic and pharmacokinetic properties, and therapeutic potential. Drugs, 39(1):86–109, 1990.

Caplan, R.; Ready, L.; Oden, R.; Matsen, F. A.; Nessly, M. L.; and Olsson, G. L.: Transdermal fentanyl for postoperative pain management. J.A.M.A., 261:1036–1039, 1989.

Cohen, F. L.: Postsurgical pain relief: Patient's status and nurses' medication choices. Pain, 9:265–274, 1980.

Corah, N. L.; Gale, E. N.; Pace, L. F.; and Seyrek, S. K.: Relaxation and musical programming as means of reducing psychological stress during dental procedures. J. Am. Dent. Assoc., 103:232-234, 1981.

Cousins, M. J.; and Mather, L. E.: Intrathecal and epidural administration of opiates. Anesthesiology, 61:276-310, 1984.

Coyle, N.; Mauskop, A.; Maggard, J.; and Foley, K. M.: Continuous subcutaneous infusions of opiates in cancer patients with pain. Oncol. Nurs. Forum., 13(4):53-57, 1986.

Dundee, J. W.; Halliday, N. J.; Loughran, P. G.; and Harper, K. W.: The influence of age on the onset of anaesthesia with midazolam. Anaesthesia, 40:441-443, 1985.

Dworkin, S. F.; Chen, A. C. N.; Schubert, M. M.; and Clark, D. W.: Cognitive modification of pain: Information in combination with N₂O. Pain, 19:339-351, 1984.

Dworkin, S. F.; Chen, A. C. N.; LeResche, L.; and Clark, D. W.: Cognitive reversal of expected nitrous oxide analgesia for acute pain. Anesth. Analg., 62:1073-1077, 1983a.

Dworkin, S. F.; Chen, A. C. N.; Schubert, M. M.; and Clark, D. W.: Analgesic effects of nitrous oxide with controlled painful stimulation. J. Am. Dent. Assoc., 107:581-585, 1983b.

Dworkin, S. F.; Ference, T. P.; and Giddon, D. R.: Behavioral Science and Dental Practice. C. V. Mosby, St. Louis, 1978.

Egbert, L. D.; Battit, G. E.; Welch, C. E.; and Bartlett, M. K.: Reduction of postoperative pain by encouragement and instruction of patients. J.A.M.A., 270:825-827, 1964.

Egbert, L. D.; Battit, G. E.; Turndorf, H.; and Beecher, H. K.: The value of the preoperative visit by an anesthetist. J.A.M.A., 185:553-555, 1963.

Fields, H. L.: Pain. McGraw-Hill, New York, pp. 335-345, 1987.

Foley, K. M.: The treatment of cancer pain. N. Engl. J. Med., 313:84-95, 1985.

Forrest, P.; Galletly, D. C.; and Yee, P.: Placebo controlled comparison of midazolam, triazolam and diazepam as oral premedicants for outpatient anaesthesia. Anaesth. Intensive Care, 15:296-304, 1987.

Forrest, W. H.; Brown, B. W.; Brown, C. R.; Defalque, R.; Gold, M.; Gordon, H. E.; James, K. E.; Katz, J.; Mahler, D. L.; Schroff, P.; and Teutsch, G.: Dextroamphetamine with morphine for treatment of postoperative pain. N. Engl. J. Med., 296:712-715, 1977.

Gal, T. J.: Naloxone reversal of buprenorphine-induced respiratory depression. Clin. Pharmacol. Ther., 45:66-71, 1989.

Gourlay, G. K.; Willlis, R. J.; and Lamberty, J.: A double-blind comparison of the efficacy of methadone and morphine in postoperative pain control. Anesthesiology, 64:322-327, 1986.

Greenblatt, D. J.; Locniskar, A.; Ochs, H. R.; and Lauven, P. M.: Automated gas chromatography for studies of midazolam pharmacokinetics. Anesthesiology, 55:176-179, 1981.

Hanks, G. W.: Drug treatments for relief of pain due to bone metastases. J. R. Soc. Med., 78(suppl. 9):26-30, 1985.

Hanks, G. W.; and Twycross, R. G.: Pain, the physiological antagonist of opioid analgesics. Lancet, 1(8392):1477-1478, 1984.

Hegarty, J. E.; and Dundee, J. W.: Sequelae after the intravenous injection of three benzodiazepines—diazepam, lorazepam and flunitrazepam. Br. Med. J., 2:1384-1385, 1977.

Heikkilä, H.; Jalonen, J.; Arola, M.; Kanto, J.; and Laadsonen, V.: Midazolam as adjunct to high-dose fentanyl anaesthesia for coronary artery bypass grafting operation. Acta Anaesthesiol. Scand., 28:683-689, 1984.

Hovagim, A. R.; Vitkun, S. A.; Manecke, G. R.; and Reiner, R.: Arterial oxygen denaturation in adult dental patients receiving conscious sedation. J. Oral Maxillofac. Surg., 47: 936-939, 1989.

Hupert, C.; Yacoub, M.; and Turgeon, L. R.: Effect of hydroxyzine on morphine analgesia for the treatment of postoperative pain. Anesth. Analg., 59:690-696, 1980.

Inturrisi, C. E.: Clinical pharmacology of opioid analgesics. Anesthesiol. Clin. North Am., 7:33-49, 1989.

Johnson, J. E.; Rice, V. H.; Fulters, S. S.; and Endress, M. P.: Sensory information: Instruction in a coping strategy and recovery from surgery. Res. Nurs. Health, 1:3-17, 1978.

Kanner, R. M.; and Foley, K. M.: Patterns of narcotic drug use in a cancer pain clinic. Ann. N.Y. Acad. Sci., 362:161-172, 1981.

Kanto, J.; Sjovall, S.; and Vuori, A.: Effects of different kinds of premedication on the induction properties of midazolam. Br. J. Anaesth., 54:507-511, 1982.

Kantor, T. G.: The control of pain by nonsteroidal anti-inflammatory drugs. Med. Clin. North Am., 66:1053-1059, 1982.

Kiako, R. F.: Age and morphine analgesia in cancer patients with postoperative pain. Clin. Pharmacol. Ther., 28:823-826, 1980.

Kiako, R. F.; Foley, K. M.; Grabinski, P. Y.; Heidrich, G.; Rogers, A. G.; Inturrisi, C. E.; and Reidenberg, M. M.: Central nervous system excitatory effects of meperidine in cancer patients. Ann. Neurol., 13:180-185, 1983.

Kiako, R. F; Wallenstein, S. L.; Rogers, A. G.; Grabinski, P. Y.; and Houde, R. W.: Analgesic and mood effects of heroin and morphine in cancer patients with postoperative pain. N. Engl. J. Med., 304:1501-1505, 1981.

Klotz, U.; Antonin, K. H.; and Bieck, P. R.: Pharmacokinetics and plasma binding of diazepam in man, dog, rabbit, guinea pig and rat. J. Pharmacol. Exp. Ther., 199:67-73, 1976.

Korttila, K.: Clinical effectiveness and untoward effects of new agents and techniques used in intravenous sedation. J. Dent. Res., 63:848-852, 1984.

Korttila, K.; and Tarkkanen, J.: Comparison of diazepam and midazolam for sedation during local anesthesia for bronchoscopy. Br. J. Anaesth., 57:581-586, 1985.

Kraut, R. A.: Continuous transcutaneous O₂ and CO₂ monitoring during conscious sedation for oral surgery. J. Oral Maxillofac. Surg., 43:489-492, 1985.

Laska, E. M.; Sunshine, A.; Mueller, F.; Elvers, W. B.; Siegel, C.; and Rubin, A.: Caffeine as an analgesic adjuvant. J.A.M.A., 251:1711-1718, 1984.

Lawlis, G. F.; Selby, D.; Hinnant, D.; and McCoy, C. E.: Reduction of postoperative pain parameters by presurgical relaxation instructions for spinal pain patients. Spine, 10: 649-651, 1985.

Levine, J. D.; Gordon, N. C.; and Fields, H. L.: The mechanism of placebo analgesia. Lancet, 2:654-657, 1978.

Lichtor, J. L.: Psychological preparation and preoperative premedication. In, Anesthesia, 3rd ed. (Miller, R. D., ed.). Churchill Livingstone, New York, pp. 895-928, 1990.

Lichtor, J. L.; Sah, J.; Apfelbaum, J.; Zacny, J.; and Coalson, D.: Some patients may drink or drive after ambulatory surgery (abstract). Anesthesiology, 73:A1083, 1990.

Lieberman, D. A.; Wuerker, C. K.; and Katon, R. M.: Cardiopulmonary risk of esophagogastroduodenoscopy. Role of endoscope diameter and systemic sedation. Gastroenterology, 88:468-472, 1985.

Linnoila, M.; Kortilla, K.; and Mattila, M. J.: Effect of food and repeated injections on serum diazepam levels. Acta Pharmacol. Toxicol., 36:181-186, 1975.

Marks, R. M.; and Sacher, E. J.: Undertreatment of medical patients with narcotic analgesics. Ann. Intern. Med., 78:173-181, 1973.

Martin, W. R.: Pharmacology of opiates. Pharmacol. Rev., 35: 283-323, 1984.

Massaut, J.; d'Hollander, A.; Barvais, L.; and Dubois-Primo, J.: Hemodynamic effects of midazolam in the anaesthetized patient with coronary artery disease. Acta Anaesthesiol. Scand., 27:299-302, 1983.

Mather, L. E.; and Mackie, J.: The incidence of postoperative pain in children. Pain, 15:271-282, 1983.

Merskey, H. (ed.): Classification of chronic pain. Description of chronic pain syndromes and definitions of pain terms. Pain, 3(suppl.):S195-S199, 1986.

Monks, R.; and Merskey, H.: Psychotropic drugs. In, Textbook of Pain, 2nd ed. (Wall, P. D.; and Melzack, R., eds.). Churchill Livingstone, New York, pp. 702–721, 1989.

NIH Consensus Development Conference: In, Anesthesia and Sedation in the Dental Office (Dionne, R. A.; and Laskin, D. M., eds.). Elsevier, New York, pp. 161–170, 1986.

Nuotto, E.; Korttila, K.; Lichtor, L.; Ostman, P.; and Rupani, G.: Sedative effects and recovery after different doses of intravenous midazolam and diazepam (abstract). Anesth. Analg., 68:S214, 1989.

O'Hara, D. A.; Fragen, R. J.; Kinzer, M.; and Pemberton, D.: Ketorolac tromethamine as compared with morphine sulfate for treatment of postoperative pain. Clin. Pharmacol. Ther., 41:556–561, 1987.

Ogg, T. W.: An assessment of postoperative outpatient cases. Br. Med. J., 4:573–576, 1972.

Pagano, R. R.; Graham, C. W.; Galligan, M.; Conner, J. T.; and Katz, R. L.: Histopathology of veins after intravenous lorazepam and RO 21-3981. Can. Anaesth. Soc. J., 25:50–52, 1978.

Pert, C. B.; and Snyder, S. H.: Opiate receptors: Demonstration in nervous tissue. Science, 179:1011–1014, 1973.

Portenoy, R. K.; Maldonado, M.; Fitzmartin, R.; Kiako, R.; and Kanner, R.: Controlled-release morphine sulfate: Analgesic efficacy and side effects of a 100 mg. tablet in cancer pain patients. Cancer, 63:2284–2288, 1989.

Portenoy, R. K.; Moulin, D. E.; Rogers, A.; Inturrisi, C. I.; and Foley, K. M.: IV infusion of opiates for cancer pain: Clinical review and guidelines for use. Cancer Treat. Rep., 70:575–581, 1986.

Rawal, N.; Arner, S.; Gustafsson, L. L.; and Allvin, R.: Present state of extradural and intrathecal opioid analgesia in Sweden. A nationwide follow-up study. Br. J. Anaesth., 59:791–799, 1987.

Ready, L. B.; Oden, R.; Chadwick H. S.; Benedetti, C.; Rooke, G. A.; Caplan, R.; and Wild, L. M.: Development of an anesthesiology-based postoperative pain management service. Anesthesiology, 68:100–106, 1988.

Reidenberg, M. M.; Levy, M.; Warner, H.; Coutinho, C. B.; Schwartz, M. A.; Yu, G.; and Cheripko, J.: Relationship between diazepam dose, plasma level, age, and central nervous system depression. Clin. Pharmacol. Ther., 23:371–374, 1978.

Reinhart, K.; Dallinger-Stiller, G.; Dennhardt, R.; Heinemeyer, G.; and Eyrich, K: Comparison of midazolam, diazepam and placebo I. M. as premedication for regional anesthesia. A randomized double-blind study. Br. J. Anaesth., 57:294–299, 1985.

Rodrigo, M. R.; and Rosenquist, J. B.: Effect of conscious sedation with midazolam on oxygen saturation. J. Oral Maxillofac. Surg., 46:746–750, 1988.

Ross, E. M.; and Gilman, A. G.: Pharmacodynamics: Mechanisms of drug action and the relationship between drug concentration and effect. In, Goodman and Gilman's The Pharmacological Basis of Therapeutics, 7th ed. (Gilman, A. G.; Goodman, L. S.; Rall, T. W.; Murad, F., eds.). Macmillan, New York, pp. 35–48, 1985.

Skelly, A. M.; Boscoe, M. J.; Dawling, S.; and Adams, A. P.: A comparison of diazepam and midazolam as sedatives for minor oral surgery. Eur. J. Anaesthesiol., 1:253–267, 1984.

Stambaugh, J. E.: The use of nonsteroidal anti-inflammatory drugs in chronic bone pain. Orthop. Rev., 18:54–60, 1989.

Stambaugh, J. E.; and Lane, C.: Analgesic efficacy and pharmacokinetic evaluation of meperidine and hydroxyzine, alone and in combination. Cancer Inves., 1:111–117, 1983.

Stanski, D. R.; Greenblatt, D. J.; and Lowenstein, E.: Kinetics of intravenous and intramuscular morphine. Clin. Pharmacol. Ther., 24:52–59, 1978.

Stapleton, J. V.; Austin, K. L.; and Mather, L. E.: A pharmacokinetic approach to postoperative pain: Continuous infusions of pethidine. Anaesth. Intensive Care, 7:25–32, 1979.

Stjernswärd, J.: Cancer pain relief: An important global public health issue. In, Advances in Pain Research and Therapy (Fields, H. L.; Dubner, R.; Cervero, F., eds.). Vol. 9. Proceedings of the Fourth World Congress on Pain, Seattle. Raven Press, New York, pp. 555–558, 1985.

Swerdlow, M.: Anticonvulsant drugs and chronic pain. Clin. Neuropharmacol., 7:51–82, 1984.

Turk, D.; Meichenbaum, D.; and Genest, M.: Pain and Behavioral Medicine. Guilford Press, New York, 1983.

Turner, J. A.; and Chapman, C. R.: Psychological interventions for chronic pain: A critical review: I. Relaxation training and biofeedback. Pain, 12:1–21, 1982.

van Wijhe, M.; de Voogt-Frenkel, E.; and Stijnen, T.: Midazolam versus fentanyl/droperidol and placebo as intramuscular premedicant. Acta Anaesthesiol. Scand., 29:409–414, 1985.

White, P. F.: Use of patient-controlled analgesia for management of acute pain. J.A.M.A., 259:243–247, 1988.

White, P. F.; Vasconez, L. O.; Mathes, S. A.; Way, W. L.; and Wender, L. A.: Comparison of midazolam and diazepam for sedation during plastic surgery. Plast. Reconstr. Surg., 81:703–712, 1988.

World Health Organization: Cancer Pain Relief. WHO, Geneva, 1986.

Yaksh, T. L.: Neurologic mechanisms of pain. In, Neural Blockade in Clinical Anesthesia and Management of Pain, 2nd ed. (Cousins, M. J.; and Bridenbaugh, P. O., eds.). J. B. Lippincott, Philadelphia, pp. 791–844, 1988.

Yaksh, T. L.: Spinal opiate analgesia: Characteristics and principles of action. Pain, 11:293–346, 1981.

Zoltie, N.; and Cust, M. P.: Analgesia in the acute abdomen. Ann. R. Coll. Surg. Engl., 68:209–210, 1986.

26

Treatment in the Intensive Care Unit

Deborah J. Cook and Ronald G. Pearl

A major challenge to physicians working in the intensive care unit (ICU) setting is safe, rapid, and efficacious treatment of life-threatening pathophysiologic processes. The multidisciplinary interventional approach to the critically ill patient has important implications for pharmacotherapy.

The ICU differs from general medical or surgical wards in several ways. The patients are more often critically ill with multisystem organ failure, which may affect absorption, metabolism, and elimination of drugs. In addition, therapy with multiple drugs is common in the ICU. Table 26–1 describes several characteristics of critically ill patients and examples of associated pharmacologic problems.

Critically ill patients often have decreased tissue perfusion that may cause delayed or unpredictable absorption of drugs administered by the subcutaneous or IM route. Decreased GI motility may reduce the availability of orally administered drugs. Most ICU patients have increased total body water; this may increase the volume of distribution of a number of drugs and results in the need for higher loading doses of some medications such as aminoglycosides (Summer et al., 1983; Chelluri and Jastremski, 1987).

Organ failure may significantly alter the metabolism or excretion of drugs. Hepatic dysfunction,

for example, may cause a prolonged duration of action of benzodiazepines or may potentiate the problem of hepatic encephalopathy. The impaired elimination of drugs in patients with renal insufficiency can cause accumulation of active drug metabolites such as N-acetylprocainamide. Chronic β-adrenergic receptor stimulation in the critically ill causes down-regulation of these β receptors, which may be responsible for the tolerance to epinephrine observed with chronic administration. In addition, acid–base disturbances in the critically ill patient may cause insensitivity to catecholamines. Hypokalemia and other electrolyte disturbances may potentiate digitalis toxicity. Hypoalbuminemia can increase the effect of free, unbound drug in the circulation. Critically ill patients with CNS disease may show increased sensitivity to certain drugs, such as cimetidine. Patients with normal coagulation may develop a thrombocytopathy associated with the use of synthetic penicillin derivatives. Finally, therapy with multiple drugs can predispose to a number of recognized or unrecognized drug interactions, such as the decreased clearance of lidocaine seen in patients treated with cimetidine. Although these pharmacologic problems may be similar to those seen in general medical or surgical patients, their magnitude and frequency is increased in the ICU

Table 26–1. EXAMPLES OF CHARACTERISTICS OF CRITICALLY ILL PATIENTS AND ASSOCIATED PHARMACOLOGIC PROBLEMS

ICU CHARACTERISTIC	PHARMACOLOGIC PROBLEM	EXAMPLE
Decreased tissue perfusion	Delayed or variable drug absorption of subcutaneously or IM administered drugs	Unpredictable response to subcutaneous insulin in shock
Decreased GI motility	Decreased drug availability	Decreased efficacy of oral furosemide
Increased total body water	Increased volume of distribution	Need for higher aminoglycoside loading doses
Hepatic dysfunction	Impaired drug metabolism Increased sensitivity to drug	Prolonged duration of action of benzodiazepines Potentiation of hepatic encephalopathy with opiates
Renal insufficiency	Decreased drug elimination	Accumulation of procainamide and N-acetylprocainamide in renal failure
Chronic adrenergic receptor stimulation	Down-regulation of β receptors	Tolerance to epinephrine during chronic administration
Metabolic dysfunction	Acid–base abnormalities	Insensitivity to catecholamines in acidosis
Electrolyte disturbance	Hypokalemia	Potentiation of digitalis toxicity
Hypoalbuminemia	Decreased protein binding and increased free-drug fraction	Increased effect of unbound (free) dilantin
Central nervous system disease	Increased sensitivity to drug	Altered mental status with use of cimetidine
Bleeding diatheses	Acquired platelet dysfunction	Thrombocytopathy associated with ticarcillin
Multiple drugs	Drug interactions	Decrease in lidocaine clearance by cimetidine by inhibiting cytochrome P450 system

population. Also, critically ill patients may be less able to tolerate some of these adverse effects because of diminished physiologic reserve.

Invasive physiologic monitoring is available to the physician caring for the critically ill patient. Since the advent of the flow-directed pulmonary artery catheter (Swan et al., 1970), bedside hemodynamic monitoring has become routine in ICUs. Several studies have demonstrated the inadequacy of clinical hemodynamic assessment for estimating hemodynamic variables during resuscitation. Eisenberg and colleagues (Eisenberg et al., 1984) examined 94 ICU patients to determine the accuracy of clinical assessment compared with measurement by pulmonary artery catheterization. Clinical assessment correctly predicted central venous pressure, cardiac index, systemic vascular resistance, and pulmonary artery wedge pressure (PAWP) in only 55%, 51%, 44%, and 30% of cases, respectively. In a similar study, a team consisting of an attending physician, critical care fellow, resident, intern, and medical student predicted right atrial pressure, cardiac index, and PAWP correctly only 40% of the time (Connors

et al., 1983). The rationale for pulmonary artery catheterization is that by monitoring PAWP and cardiac output, physicians may evaluate a patient's hemodynamic status and the effects of interventions, thereby adjusting therapy accordingly.

Data obtained from pulmonary artery catheterization have limitations. For example, varying left ventricular compliance in critically ill patients means that PAWP may bear little relation to left ventricular end-diastolic volume (Calvin et al., 1981). Factors such as equipment malfunction and misinterpretation of data may limit the potential benefit of information obtained. A randomized trial to address the question of whether pulmonary artery catheterization changes ICU morbidity or mortality has yet to be performed (Guyatt et al., 1986). Nevertheless, invasive hemodynamic monitoring gives the physician a rational approach to fluid and vasoactive therapy in the ICU and is heavily relied upon by many clinicians in the management of patients with cardiovascular instability.

In addition to hemodynamic monitoring, the

ICU environment allows careful observation of respiratory status through the use of oxygen saturation monitors, end-tidal CO_2 monitors, and assessment of pulmonary function in mechanically ventilated patients. Arterial catheters allow frequent arterial blood-gas analysis and continuous monitoring of blood pressure. Intracranial pressure monitors and frequent neurologic examinations are used to assess patients with CNS disease associated with increased intracranial pressure. Foley catheters usually are inserted in the critically ill patient to monitor hourly urine output and to ensure accurate urine collections for creatinine clearance tests.

In summary, the ICU environment is unique in that invasive monitoring of the critically ill patient provides an opportunity for ongoing physiologic evaluation and immediate feedback as to the effects of therapeutic interventions.

In many cases, drugs administered in the ICU can be titrated to the desired physiologic end point, balancing the pharmacokinetic properties (dose versus blood concentration) and pharmacodynamic properties (blood concentration versus drug effect). *Principle: Meticulous prescribing habits are necessary when administering drugs to the critically ill, who often present with rapidly evolving pathologic conditions, unstable hemodynamics, and a high incidence of organ system failure. Restricting the use of drugs in the ICU to those clearly necessary, adjusting doses according to established guidelines, limiting the duration of therapy, measuring serum concentration of drug where indicated, and monitoring for signs of toxicity are important general principles for physicians working in the ICU setting to follow and for those who do not work in that environment to understand.*

This chapter discusses some common clinical conditions in the critically ill patient and will highlight their pharmacologic management.

SHOCK

Circulatory shock is a clinical syndrome of inadequate tissue perfusion characterized by anaerobic metabolism, organ dysfunction, and lactic acidosis. The clinical presentation of shock varies with the cause of the shock syndrome, the effects of compensatory mechanisms, and previous levels of organ function. The management of shock requires recognition and treatment of the underlying cause of shock and of the abnormal hemodynamic pathophysiology.

Although there are many different causes of shock, there are three basic categories: hypovolemic, hyperdynamic (septic), and cardiogenic shock. These three categories share some common clinical and metabolic features. Moreover, some ICU patients may exhibit characteristics of more than one category of shock. For example, the patient with anaphylaxis may demonstrate clinical signs of hypovolemic, hyperdynamic, and cardiogenic shock. The following section will describe the etiology and pathophysiology of the three shock syndromes.

Etiology and Pathophysiology of Shock

Hypovolemic Shock. Relative or absolute depletion of intravascular volume decreases venous return, thereby decreasing ventricular filling and cardiac output. The cause of hypovolemic shock can be classified as hemorrhagic or nonhemorrhagic (Table 26-2).

The vital organs most often affected by shock are the brain and kidneys. The brain is able to autoregulate its perfusion despite wide changes in cerebral perfusion pressure (CPP) [CPP = mean arterial pressure (MAP) − intracranial pressure (ICP)] until blood pressure falls below 60 to 70 mm Hg (Lassen, 1959). However, the minimum blood pressure to maintain cerebral autoregulation is higher in patients with chronic hypertension. The clinical manifestations of cerebral hypoperfusion range from mild changes in mental status to confusion or coma.

Renal autoregulation remains intact between a MAP of 70 to 180 mm Hg. Significant hypotension decreases renal perfusion and may result in acute renal failure (see chapter 11). Renin, produced as a result of juxtaglomerular hypoperfusion, is a major renal afferent arteriolar constrictor. In the presence of renin, angiotensinogen is converted to angiotensin I, which blocks renin release in a negative-feedback loop. Angiotensin II, produced by the action of angiotensin-converting enzyme (ACE) on angiotensin I, is a potent vasoconstrictor with a major site of action on the efferent arteriole. In mild states of hypoperfusion, glomerular filtration is maintained by renin-induced afferent arteriolar constriction and angiotensin II–induced efferent arteriolar constriction. The vascular theory of acute renal failure maintains that reduced renal blood flow is the principal mechanism for acute renal failure in shock. One possible cause of decreased renal blood flow is afferent renal arteriolar constriction due to sympathetic stimulation and the effect of prostaglandins. Failure of renal reperfusion following resuscitation may occur as a result of endothelial cell swelling.

Clinically, the patient in hypovolemic shock often is cool, clammy, pale, hypotensive, and tachypneic, showing signs of organ hypoperfusion (such as confusion or oliguria).

Table 26–2. ETIOLOGY OF THE THREE MAJOR SYNDROMES OF SHOCK

A. Hypovolemic shock
  1. Hemorrhagic
    a. GI bleeding
    b. Internal bleeding
      (1) Aortic aneurysm
      (2) Fracture of a long bone
      (3) Blunt trauma
      (4) Retroperitoneal bleeding
  2. Nonhemorrhagic
    a. GI losses
      (1) Vomiting
      (2) Diarrhea
    b. Renal losses
      (1) Diuretics
      (2) Salt-wasting nephropathy
      (3) Diabetes insipidus
    c. Fluid redistribution
      (1) Ascites
      (2) Effusions
      (3) Fistulas
      (4) Burns
      (5) Pancreatitis
B. Cardiogenic shock
  1. Impaired contractility
    a. Myocardial infarction
    b. Cardiomyopathy
    c. Myocarditis
  2. Valvular disease
    a. Mitral regurgitation
    b. Mitral stenosis
    c. Aortic regurgitation
    d. Aortic stenosis
  3. Arrhythmias
  4. Extrinsic factors
    a. Pericardial tamponade
    b. Tension pneumothorax
    c. Pulmonary emboli
    d. Constrictive pericarditis
  5. Pharmacologic
    a. β-Blockers
    b. Calcium blockers
    c. Chemotherapeutics (doxorubicin)
    d. Antiarrhythmics (quinidine)
C. Hyperdynamic shock
  1. Bacteremia
  2. Fungemia
  3. Viremia
  4. Release of vasoactive substance
    a. Toxins
    b. Complement
    c. Kinins
    d. Prostaglandins

Cardiogenic Shock. Decreased myocardial contractility results in decreased cardiac output, accompanied by an increase in preload and vascular resistance. Clinically, the patient in cardiogenic shock appears similar to the patient in hypovolemic shock—hypotensive, tachycardic, cold, clammy, and showing signs of organ hypoperfusion. Hypotension may decrease coronary perfusion, worsen cardiac dysfunction, and predispose to arrhythmias. As ventricular end-diastolic pressure rises, cardiac failure may ensue. Therefore, additional manifestations of cardiogenic shock can include a dyskinetic apical beat, a third or fourth heart sound, a murmur of mitral regurgitation secondary to papillary muscle dysfunction, increased jugular venous pressure, tachypnea, rales, and/or respiratory failure. The cause of cardiogenic shock is related to primary myocardial, pericardial, or valvular dysfunction (Table 26–2).

Hyperdynamic Shock (Septic Shock). Hyperdynamic shock usually is initiated by a fall in vascular resistance. Since blood pressure = cardiac output × systemic vascular resistance, the ability to maintain perfusion is dependent upon the ability of the heart to maintain cardiac output. This in turn is dependent upon adequate preload and contractility (see chapter 4). In hyperdynamic shock, decreased preload may result from vasodilatation or an increase in capillary permeability, secondary to release of bacterial toxins, bradykinin, prostaglandins, tumor necrosis factor, complement, endorphins, and/or histamine (Shine, 1980). Reduced myocardial contractility is not an uncommon sequela of hyperdynamic shock and is likely multifactorial, contributed to by myocardial depressant factors (Lefer, 1978), myocardial ischemia, β-receptor down-regulation, increased peripheral vascular resistance, abnormal myocardial metabolism, and/or myocardial edema (McGuire and Pearl, 1990). The patient in early septic shock often appears warm, normotensive, and well perfused with bounding pulses. When cardiac output falls and peripheral resistance rises, the appearance of cardiogenic or hypovolemic sepsis develops. The etiology of hyperdynamic shock includes bacteremia, fungemia, or viremia, and the release of vasoactive substances from infection or anaphylaxis (Table 26–2).

Management of Shock – General Principles

The initial approach to any critically ill patient is to establish a patent airway, provide ventilation if necessary, and ensure adequate hemodynamics. Because the respiratory muscles receive a disproportionate share of the cardiac output during shock, assisted ventilation is useful to allow redistribution of blood flow, minimize oxygen consumption, and control acidosis. In hypovolemic and hyperdynamic shock, relative or absolute intravascular depletion is almost always present; volume expansion is thus the cornerstone of therapy. In cardiogenic shock, a further increase in intravascular volume may be valuable in selected patients.

The end points of administration for volume should be a satisfactory cardiac output and urine output, and reversal of metabolic acidosis. Subsequent management begins with assessing whether problems exist with preload, afterload, or contractility, exemplified by classic hypovolemic, septic, or cardiogenic shock.

Treatment of Hypovolemic Shock. The general approach to hypovolemic shock is rapid restoration of intravascular volume and correction of the underlying cause. While volume is being replaced, vasoactive therapy may be required. The choice of fluids for resuscitation is discussed in the section on supportive therapy below.

Assessing the adequacy of replacement therapy often requires both a measure of volume status (CVP [central venous pressure] and PAWP) and a measure of cardiac performance [MAP, cardiac output (CO), and urine output]. Information provided by pulmonary artery catheters may guide fluid and vasoactive therapy in hypovolemic shock.

Treatment of Cardiogenic Shock. If the patient in cardiogenic shock has not developed pulmonary edema, *volume should be administered.* However, care must be exercised in patients with coronary ischemia because increases in left ventricular end-diastolic pressure (LVEDP) may significantly reduce coronary perfusion pressure (CPP) (CPP = diastolic arterial pressure − LVEDP). Pulmonary edema can be precipitated by infusion of volume, and hemodynamic parameters should be monitored carefully in this situation.

The failing ventricle in cardiogenic shock is very sensitive to increased afterload. Therefore, to maintain an adequate cardiac output, therapy is often directed at decreasing systemic vascular resistance. The main goal of afterload reduction is achieving adequate cardiac output (3–5 l/min) and MAP (60–70 mm Hg). When vasodilators are used to increase cardiac output in the setting of heart failure, the dose should be titrated to achieve a systemic vascular resistance in the low-normal range (700–900 dyne·sec·cm^{-5}). If vasodilators are titrated to blood pressure only, the result may be inadequate reduction in systemic vascular resistance.

Afterload reduction initially may be accomplished with a short-acting vasodilator such as sodium nitroprusside that causes both venous and arterial dilatation. The effect of venodilatation may be a decrease in preload. Therefore, treatment with sodium nitroprusside should include ongoing assessment of the adequacy of preload

(pulmonary artery diastolic pressure and PAWP). When vasodilators are used for afterload reduction in patients with cardiogenic shock, administration of volume often is necessary.

Obtaining and maintaining optimal hemodynamics in cardiogenic shock may require both inotropic and vasodilator therapy. Two drugs can be used; epinephrine is often administered together with sodium nitroprusside, for example. Alternatively, dobutamine, a β_1-adrenergic agonist with mild β_2 properties, or amrinone, a phosphodiesterase inhibitor, can be used individually. These drugs alone increase cardiac output and promote afterload reduction in the setting of cardiogenic shock.

Treatment of Hyperdynamic Shock. Replacing intravascular volume, correcting metabolic acidosis, and treating the underlying cause (i.e., antibiotics, surgical drainage) are important in the management of patients in septic shock. The rationale for further therapy depends on the hemodynamic status of the patient in septic shock. Initial evaluation of a patient with sepsis usually reveals a low systemic vascular resistance and a high cardiac output. In early stages, blood pressure may be only slightly decreased. In later stages, both systemic vascular resistance and blood pressure may be low, while cardiac output may be relatively depressed. Therefore, both vasoconstrictor drugs and inotropes may be used in this setting.

An example of a useful algorithm for the management of hyperdynamic shock is displayed in Fig. 26–1. Clinical judgment and hour-to-hour assessment of hemodynamic status often is necessary in managing this problem. If preload is low (PAWP < 15 mm Hg), volume expansion is indicated. If preload is high, but cardiac output is low (< 10 l/min), inotropes may be useful. If cardiac output is high (> 10 l/min) but preload is low, administration of volume is indicated. The major decision in the face of high cardiac output (> 10 l/min) and high PAWP (> 15 mm Hg) with persistent hypotension is the use of inotropes versus vasopressors. If blood pressure remains low despite optimal preload, there are two options: inotropic agents to increase cardiac output or vasopressor agents to increase peripheral resistance. Vasopressor agents may successfully elevate decreased vascular resistance but can result in severe vasoconstriction in some vascular beds (mesenteric and renal), thereby restoring blood pressure at the expense of ischemia to vital organs. Inotropic therapy may, on the other hand, further augment cardiac output and theoretically increase blood flow to all vascular beds. However, inotropic agents may be proarrhythmic and exacerbate myocardial ischemia. The decision to use any of

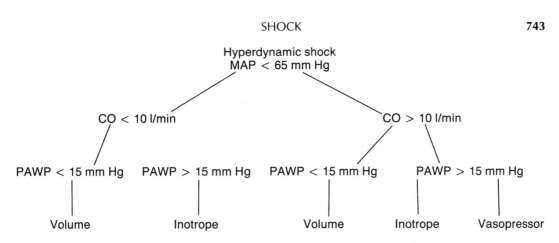

Fig. 26-1. An approach to the management of hyperdynamic shock.

these agents is based on a thorough understanding of the patient's hemodynamic status and careful evaluation of the hemodynamic response.

Adjunctive Therapy for Septic Shock

The use of high-dose IV steroids in septic shock was shown in one early study to improve survival (Schumer, 1976). But the study was criticized because various doses of two glucocorticoids were employed and the fluid resuscitation may have been suboptimal. Sprung and colleagues found that methylprednisolone 30 mg/kg or dexamethasone 6 mg/kg, repeated 4 hours later if shock persisted, was associated with reversal of shock and lower short-term, but not long-term, mortality (Sprung et al., 1984).

The Veterans Administration Systemic Sepsis Cooperative Study Group (Veterans Administration, 1987) conducted a multicenter randomized double-blind placebo-controlled trial of early treatment with short-term methylprednisolone in 223 patients with clinical signs of systemic sepsis. There was no difference in 14-day mortality between the groups, although resolution of secondary infection within 14 days was significantly higher in the placebo group. In a similarly designed study of 382 patients in septic shock, no significant differences were found in the prevention of shock, reversal of shock, or overall mortality (Bone et al., 1987). In the subgroups of patients with elevated concentrations of serum creatinine (>2 mg/dl) at enrollment, *14-day mortality was significantly higher in those receiving methylprednisolone. In addition, among patients treated with steroids, significantly more deaths were related to secondary infection. Principle: When therapy is largely empiric, the physician must carefully define therapeutic goals so that his or her therapeutic judgment can be carefully compared with alternative therapies. There is nothing worse in therapeutics than to continue a tradition of treatment, largely based on prejudice, whose toxicity could easily be attributed to the disease being treated.*

To determine the effect of steroid therapy on the outcome of adult respiratory distress syndrome (ARDS) in septic patients, a randomized trial of methylprednisolone versus mannitol placebo was performed (Luce et al., 1988). The results indicated that steroids neither prevent ARDS nor reduce mortality.

These studies argue strongly against the use of high-dose corticosteroids as adjunctive therapy for septic shock. Similarly, steroids are relatively contraindicated in cardiogenic shock because they potentially impair myocardial healing and predispose to myocardial rupture (Roberto et al., 1976).

On the other hand, glucocorticoids are appropriate for the treatment of shock associated with adrenal insufficiency and hypothyroidism. Patients with fulminant meningococcemia and associated hemorrhagic adrenal disease (the Waterhouse-Friderichsen syndrome), also may benefit from steroid therapy. Patients with an impaired pituitary–adrenal axis, including those receiving steroids regularly, should receive stress-dose steroids (100 mg of hydrocortisone every 8 hours, or the equivalent) during resuscitation.

The use of naloxone in septic shock was prompted from results of animal models that demonstrated reversal of hypotension. Uncontrolled studies in humans have failed to show a favorable outcome in patients with late septic shock (Rock et al., 1985; Bonnet et al., 1985). A prospective randomized controlled trial of naloxone in early hyperdynamic septic shock showed that naloxone caused an overall increase in MAP, whereas no change was noted in the placebo group. However, the difference between naloxone and placebo groups was not statistically significant, nor was there any effect on survival (Safani et al., 1989). Reported adverse effects of naloxone include pulmonary edema, cardiac failure, and seizure activity (Rock et al., 1985). *Principle: Observational epidemiologic and uncontrolled studies cannot be used in an unqualified way to study efficacy when the indication for the drug is a confounding variable in the outcome of the study. Clinicians understandably will hope for the best from a new therapy and attribute complications to a disease if they can. Beware of the statement that the patient did poorly "in spite of therapy." The outcome could well have been because of therapy!*

Plasma fibronectin is a glycoprotein with nonspecific opsonic activity that may play a protective role against capillary microembolism in multiple organ system failure. The association of sepsis with low concentration of fibronectin in plasma, and the ability to replenish stores either with cryoprecipitate or purified fibronectin, has provoked considerable interest and controversy in the area of fibronectin therapy to decrease mortality of sepsis. Results of a metaanalysis of the six published trials yield a common odds ratio of 0.97 [95% confidence interval (CI) = 0.58–1.61] (Cook et al., 1989). These results do not show a significant effect favoring treatment (see chapters 34, 35 and 41).

The NSAIDs prevent the synthesis of prostaglandins by inhibiting the cyclooxygenase pathway of arachidonic acid metabolism. Prostaglandins depress release of norepinephrine; therefore, blockade of prostaglandin synthesis should enhance release of norepinephrine (Kopin, 1977). This may explain the reduced mortality in the rat model of septic shock (Ball et al., 1986). Studies in humans are ongoing. Prostaglandins also play an important role in renal autoregulation. Therefore, interference with prostaglandin synthesis by NSAIDs may potentiate acute renal failure in some patients. Don't be surprised if uncontrolled studies of NSAIDS attribute renal failure to the disease.

Recent advances in molecular biology have increased the profile of immunotherapy as potential treatment for septic shock. In a randomized controlled trial, human antiserum against *Escherichia coli* lipopolysaccharide core antigen was administered to bacteremic patients (Ziegler et al., 1982). Mortality was reduced in the profoundly septic subset of patients. When given prophylactically to patients who underwent abdominal surgery and traumatized patients, in a randomized controlled clinical trial (Baumgartner et al., 1985), there was no benefit in prevention of gram-negative infections; the overall mortality and mortality due to sepsis were reduced. Trials involving anti-LPS immunoglobulin to decrease mortality in sepsis are pending. In baboons, antic-

achectin monoclonal antibodies have successfully prevented gram-negative sepsis (Tracey et al., 1987). Thus, immunotherapy appears to have promise and has been approved for use in humans. *Principle: Be sure to distinguish hypothetical from proven efficacy of a therapy. All too frequently, the hypothesis generated by a controlled experiment in an animal or an uncontrolled observation in humans becomes "truth" without testing, particularly when the indication is in a desperate setting.*

VASOACTIVE DRUG THERAPY IN SHOCK

The following sections discuss the pharmacologic agents often used by the intensivist for the management of circulatory failure.

Catecholamines

Catecholamines are autacoids and neurotransmitters. Catecholamines have hydroxyl groups on the third and fourth carbon positions of a benzene ring; this 3,4-dihydroxybenzene is called a *catechol.*

The endogenous catecholamine response to disease usually is manifested by elevations in plasma norepinephrine and epinephrine concentrations. However, the body may respond to stress states insufficiently because of inadequate release of catecholamines or because of decreased tissue responses as a consequence of desensitization. Also, acidosis diminishes cardiovascular responsiveness to exogenously administered catecholamines. Alkalosis blunts the vasoconstrictor effect of catecholamines yet enhances the action of vasodilator amines and may decrease release of endogenous catecholamine (Barton et al., 1982).

Endogenous and synthetic catecholamines are important in the response to and recovery from serious illness or injury (Chernow et al., 1982). Exogenous catecholamines used in the treatment of the critically ill patient will be discussed here. Table 26–3 summarizes the selectivity of different catecholamines for α-adrenergic, β-adrenergic and dopaminergic receptors.

Dopamine. Dopamine is the immediate precursor of norepinephrine in the catecholamine synthetic pathway. When administered exogenously, dopamine has direct and indirect sympathomimetic effects. It may directly stimulate α, β, and dopamine receptors and also may be converted to norepinephrine. Exogenous dopamine also may have indirect effects by releasing norepinephrine from sympathetic nerves.

The cardiovascular effects of dopamine are dose-dependent and are mediated by three different adrenergic receptors. At low doses (infusion rates of 0.5–2.0 μg/kg per minute), dopamine

Table 26–3.   SELECTIVITY OF CATECHOLAMINES FOR ADRENERGIC RECEPTORS

AGENTS	α_1	α_2	β_1	β_2	DOPAMINE
Dopamine*	0 to + + + +	+ +	+ + to + + + +	+ +	+ + + +
Dobutamine*	0 to +	0	+ + + +	+ +	0
Epinephrine*	+ + + +	+ + + +	+ + +	0	0
Norepinephrine*	+ + + +	+ + +	+ + +	0	0
Isoproterenol	0	0	+ + + +	+ + + +	0
Ephedrine	+ +	0	+ + +	+ +	0
Phenylephrine	+ + + +	0	0	0	0

* Variable dose-dependent effects.

stimulates dopaminergic receptors to produce renal and splanchnic arteriolar vasodilatation (Goldberg, 1974). It may increase cardiac output and MAP through stimulation of β_1 receptors (McNay et al., 1965). At infusion rates of 2 to 10 μg/kg per minute, dopamine acts primarily on β_1 receptors (with some residual dopaminergic activity from 2 to 5 μg/kg per minute) to increase myocardial contractility and cardiac output. Infusion rates of 10 to 20 μg/kg per minute activate both β_1 and α receptors. At maximal doses, the α effect predominates to cause vasoconstriction in most vascular beds (Herbert and Tinker, 1980). At these high doses, the beneficial effect of dopamine on renal blood flow is eliminated (Goldberg et al., 1977). The chronotropic activity of dopamine is less than that of isoproterenol, but high doses may be arrhythmogenic. Dopamine also has minimal (rarely clinically significant) β_2 vasodilating effects.

Dopamine is frequently the drug of choice in the treatment of shock, especially in patients with oliguria and/or decreased peripheral vascular resistance. When peripheral vascular resistance is high, dopamine may be effectively combined with a vasodilator such as sodium nitroprusside, in order to increase cardiac output.

Individual variation in sensitivity to dopamine may be important, with increases in heart rate and blood pressure noted at doses of 2 to 5 μg/kg per minute in some patients. Moreover, the endogenous release of norepinephrine is stimulated at infusion rates >5 μg/kg per minute. Therefore, predicting the hemodynamic effects of dopamine infusions is difficult (Jarnberg et al., 1981). Therapy with dopamine requires regular evaluation of hemodynamic parameters to assess efficacy.

In the absence of pulmonary hypertension, dopamine increases pulmonary blood flow with little change in mean pulmonary artery pressure or PAWP. However, in patients with pulmonary hypertension, infusion of dopamine may lead to increases in mean pulmonary artery pressure (Holloway et al., 1975). Through venoconstriction, dopamine may lead to an increase in PAWP in some situations (Jardin et al., 1979).

Stimulation of dopaminergic receptors is accompanied by an increase in glomerular filtration rate and sodium excretion (Hilberman et al., 1984). Although renal blood flow may be redistributed to the juxtaglomerular nephrons, the dopamine-induced increase in urine flow and natriuresis likely is due in part to inhibition of aldosterone secretion (Noth et al., 1980).

The half-life of IV dopamine is approximately 1 minute. Dopamine is metabolized by both catechol O-methyltransferase and monoamine oxidase enzyme systems. Alkalinity inactivates dopamine. Therefore bicarbonate should not be administered into an IV line through which dopamine is being infused. *Principle: Serious direct drug interactions do not often show themselves in the bottle. If they are not considered (as in this case), it is easy to see why the drug would be considered useless! Unfortunately, a disappointed experience in therapy can linger in the clinician's mind and the value (benefit) of this drug may well be denied to subsequent patients for the wrong reasons!*

Dobutamine. Dobutamine is a synthetic catecholamine with a biochemical structure similar to that of isoproterenol. Unlike dopamine, dobutamine does not increase release of norepinephrine. It is predominantly a direct β_1 receptor agonist, with only weak α and β_2 activity.

The selective β_1-adrenergic action of dobutamine increases myocardial contractility with little change in heart rate, MAP, or systemic vascular resistance. Dobutamine is useful to treat heart failure because it has minimal chronotropic effects compared with isoproterenol, it rarely causes the arrhythmias associated with epinephrine and dopamine, and it does not cause the peripheral vasoconstriction seen with norepinephrine. A peripheral vasodilating effect through stimulation of β_2 receptors may limit the use of this agent if cardiac output cannot be increased enough to overcome low systemic vascular resistance (Robie and Goldberg, 1975). When both β_1 and dopaminergic effects are desirable (e.g., the hypotensive oliguric patient), combination therapy with dobutamine and dopamine is appropriate.

Dobutamine may decrease an elevated PAWP secondary to improved stroke volume and thereby reduce myocardial oxygen consumption by decreasing left ventricular wall tension. As described with dopamine, increased pulmonary blood flow associated with increased cardiac output may increase intrapulmonary shunting (Jardin et al., 1979, 1981).

Dobutamine has no selective vascular effects on the renal or splanchnic beds. Nevertheless, patients with shock who respond to dobutamine may have increased urine output secondary to augmented cardiac output (Leier et al., 1977).

Positive inotropic effects are observed with doses of 0.5 μg/kg per minute, though the usual dosage range is 2.5 to 10.0 μg/kg per minute. The elimination half-life of dobutamine is approximately 2 minutes, and elimination follows first-order kinetics. Dobutamine is metabolized by catechol O-methyltransferase followed by glucuronide transformation in the liver, with most of the drug excreted in the urine and bile.

Epinephrine. Epinephrine is synthesized from norepinephrine predominantly in the adrenal medulla. With preganglionic sympathetic stimulation, the chromaffin cells of the adrenal medulla release their contents (mainly epinephrine and small amounts of norepinephrine and dopamine) into the circulation.

The cardiac effects of epinephrine are mediated through β receptors. Epinephrine has potent inotropic and chronotropic effects, increasing heart rate, stroke volume, cardiac output, and oxygen consumption. Epinephrine accelerates transmission through the sinoatrial node and decreases the refractory period, thereby predisposing to arrhythmias. At doses of 2 to 10 μg/min (25–120 ng/kg per minute), these β-adrenergic effects predominate (Clutter et al., 1980). In addition, vasodilatation occurs in the skeletal muscle bed via activation of β_2 receptors. At doses above 10 μg/min (>120 ng/kg per minute), α-receptor stimulation results in generalized vasoconstriction (Clutter et al., 1980).

The direct effect of epinephrine on the juxtaglomerular apparatus of the kidney stimulates renin secretion, which increases blood pressure through the combined renin–angiotensin and α-adrenergic effects. Epinephrine therefore acts directly and indirectly as a potent renal vasoconstrictor and, accordingly, is often used together with "renally protective" doses of dopamine.

As one of the stress autacoids, epinephrine has important metabolic effects, including lipolysis, glycolysis, and gluconeogenesis. The net result is an increase in the concentration of plasma glucose, free fatty acids, glycerol, lactate, and β-hydroxybutyrate.

Editor's Note: Many of the drugs described in this chapter can be used for an individual in doses that will result in truly selective effects. In this chapter ranges of doses are given that have selective effects attributed to them; but these ranges are approximate and may not be applicable to a given patient. Since the ICU environment allows unusually good feedback and monitoring of these cardiovascular drug effects, use such data as frequently as possible to adjust doses for the individual patient.

Norepinephrine. Norepinephrine is the neurotransmitter of the postganglionic sympathetic nerves. It also is released from the adrenal medulla. In low doses (<2 μg/min, or <30 ng/kg per minute), norepinephrine stimulates β_1-adrenergic receptors. At usual clinical doses of >3 μg/min (>50 ng/kg per minute), its prominent clinical effect appears to be vasoconstriction secondary to α-adrenergic stimulation (Zaritsky and Chernow, 1983).

Norepinephrine increases blood pressure, with the systolic blood pressure increasing disproportionately more than the diastolic. The heart rate usually is reflexly slowed by baroreceptor stimulation, and cardiac output is unchanged or slightly decreased. The potent venoconstrictor effects of norepinephrine increase venous return. Norepinephrine greatly increases myocardial oxygen demand by increasing afterload and preload and by its chronotropic and inotropic actions. When using vasopressors, it is important to maintain adequate filling pressures, as prolonged vasoconstriction may result in progressive loss of intravascular volume and a true decrease in preload. This may result in *pressor amine dependence* upon withdrawal of the drug (Botticelli et al., 1965).

Norepinephrine may increase pulmonary vascular resistance through vasoconstriction. Caution has been advised in using this drug in patients with pulmonary hypertension (O'Neill et al., 1978). Norepinephrine is also a potent constrictor of the renal arteries and splanchnic beds; high doses or prolonged administration may result in acute renal failure, mesenteric ischemia, and hypoperfusion of the extremities. Combination therapy using vasoactive agents with different actions often can maximize the therapeutic benefits while minimizing undesirable effects. Evidence from animals suggests that infusion of norepinephrine alone or in combination with low-dose dopamine produces similar increases in mean arterial pressure, but that the addition of dopamine results in significantly higher renal blood flow and lower renal vascular resistance (Schafer et al., 1985). In some centers, when norepinephrine is used to treat shock, low-dose dopamine is also administered to prevent excessive renal vasoconstriction and thereby diminish the risk of renal ischemia. The half-life of IV norepinephrine is approximately 2.5 minutes. It is cleared by enzymatic degradation in the liver and kidney as well as by uptake into the sympathetic nerve endings of effector organs. Increased serum concentrations of glucose, β-hydroxybutyrate, and acetoacetate may occur with IV infusions.

Isoproterenol. Isoproterenol, a catecholamine structurally similar to epinephrine, produces β_1 and β_2 adrenergic stimulation. Isoproterenol is a potent inotropic and chronotropic agent that markedly increases myocardial contractility, heart rate, and oxygen consumption. With adequate preload, systolic blood pressure is increased secondary to increased cardiac output, and diastolic blood pressure is reduced because of vasodilatation. Vasodilatation often limits the role of the drug in treating shock because much of the increase in cardiac output goes to the cutaneous and skeletal muscle beds. Proportionally less blood flows to the renal and splanchnic circulation. Isoproterenol generally is used for its chronotropic effects in the treatment of hypotension associated with bradycardia or heart block.

Relaxation of bronchial smooth muscle through β_2 stimulation with isoproterenol may increase the diameter of the airway in asthmatic patients (Widdicombe, 1975). Isoproterenol directly reduces pulmonary vascular resistance and may be of use in the acute and chronic management of pulmonary hypertension (Mentzer et al., 1976). However, potentiation of arrhythmias may preclude the use of isoproterenol in many situations.

Noncatecholamine Sympathomimetic Agents

Sympathomimetic agents include catecholamines and other drugs that mimic their action. The basic structure of a catecholamine includes 3,4-dihydroxybenzene. That is absent in the noncatecholamine sympathomimetic agents. Examples of noncatecholamine sympathomimetic drugs include phenylephrine, ephedrine, metaraminol, and methoxamine. While some noncatecholamine sympathomimetics exert their effect directly on adrenergic receptors, many work indirectly, through stimulating release of norepinephrine from sympathetic nerve terminals. Noncatecholamine sympathomimetic agents have a long history in clinical medicine but largely have been replaced by more potent and selective drugs (Zaritsky and Chernow, 1983).

Phenylephrine. Phenylephrine (Neo-Synephrine) is structurally similar to epinephrine and is a potent direct-acting α-adrenergic agonist. Phenyl-

ephrine increases systolic, diastolic, and mean arterial pressure by vasoconstriction that may lead to reflex bradycardia. Phenylephrine has little direct effect on contractility, so arrhythmias are infrequent, but cardiac output may decrease because of a marked increase in systemic vascular resistance. The associated increased oxygen demand may cause myocardial ischemia (Yamazaki et al., 1982). However, positive inotropic responses to selective α-adrenoreceptor agonists have been documented (Williamson and Broadley, 1987). The α-adrenoreceptor-mediated positive inotropic effect differs from the response to β-adrenoreceptor stimulation in that it develops relatively slowly, causes a prolongation of contraction, and is not associated with changes in cyclic AMP or cyclic GMP (Scholz et al., 1986). Administration of phenylephrine also may decrease cutaneous, renal, and splanchnic blood flow because of vasoconstriction.

The dose of phenylephrine is variable because it is titrated to the desired response. One should start at 10 to 20 μg/min with an IV infusion. It may also be injected over a short time interval at a dose of 10 to 100 μg IV in hypotensive emergencies.

Phenylephrine may be useful in hyperdynamic septic shock with low systemic vascular resistance, or other hypotensive states when cardiac output is not impaired [i.e., hypotension after carotid endarterectomy surgery (Yamazaki et al., 1982)].

Ephedrine. Ephedrine has both a direct effect on α- and β-adrenergic receptors and indirect effects mediating stimulation of release of norepinephrine. The cardiovascular effect of ephedrine is increased systolic blood pressure and a modest inotropic response. Ephedrine diminishes renal and splanchnic blood flow and increases coronary, cerebral, and skeletal muscle circulation (Zaritsky and Chernow, 1983).

Bolus infusion of ephedrine is useful for treating the hypotension related to both decreased systemic vascular resistance and decreased cardiac output. For example, when hypotension is associated with spinal anesthesia, ephedrine is a useful drug to increase blood pressure without impairing cardiac output. Ephedrine is rarely used in continuous infusions. Tachyphylaxis may develop with long-term administration of ephedrine due to depletion of stores of norepinephrine from peripheral receptor sites. Toxic effects are similar to those seen with epinephrine use.

Metaraminol. The effects of metaraminol (Aramine) are similar to those of norepinephrine, though less potent and longer-acting (Herbert and Tinker, 1980). It is both a direct- and an indirect-acting sympathomimetic. Metaraminol increases systolic and diastolic blood pressure by vasoconstriction that may result in bradycardia and decreased cardiac output. The drug increases myocardial wall tension and oxygen demand and decreases cerebral and renal blood flow. Since the actions of metaraminol are partly indirect, its effect may be diminished in patients with depleted stores of catecholamine.

As a slow IV infusion of 0.4 mg/min, metaraminol may be titrated to the desired effect. Metaraminol is used primarily in the emergency treatment of hypotension. The indications for its use are similar to those for ephedrine.

Methoxamine. Methoxamine (Vasoxyl) has similar effects to those of phenylephrine as an almost pure α-adrenergic agonist. Methoxamine elevates systolic, diastolic, and mean arterial pressure. Although it has little direct myocardial effect, it can cause reflex bradycardia and depress cardiac output. Methoxamine also reduces cerebral, renal, and limb blood flow.

Intravenous doses of 3 to 5 mg are used to treat hypotension.

Phosphodiesterase Inhibitors

Amrinone. Amrinone is a nonglycoside, nonadrenergic agent with positive inotropic and vasodilating properties. Amrinone inhibits cAMP phosphodiesterase (Endoh et al., 1982). Whether this action explains all the pharmacologic effects of the drug is not clear.

Intravenous administration of amrinone in patients with heart failure increases cardiac output and reduces PAWP and systemic vascular resistance. Heart rate and systemic blood pressure are rarely affected, although at high doses, a chronotropic effect and decrease in mean arterial pressure may occur (Colucci et al., 1986). The hemodynamic effects of amrinone are similar to those of a combination of dobutamine and nitroprusside. *Principle: A single drug with multiple mechanisms leading to a desired response has value over administration of multiple drugs that can be combined to give the same effects as long as the proportion of effects from the single agent is reproducible and is within desirable ranges.*

Intravenous amrinone was approved for use in 1984 for the short-term treatment of refractory congestive heart failure. Most clinical trials evaluating cardiac index, left ventricular end-diastolic pressure and pulmonary capillary wedge pressure have favorably compared patients receiving amrinone, digoxin, and diuretics with patients receiving digoxin and diuretics alone (Ward et al., 1983). Improvement in exercise tolerance can also be achieved with amrinone administration (Siskind et al., 1981); however, drug withdrawal usually precipitates rapid clinical deterioration and loss of this benefit (Ward et al., 1983).

Few studies have compared amrinone with other inotropic agents. A trial evaluating amrinone (10 μg/kg per minute) and dobutamine (11.8 μg/kg per minute) showed that although initial hemodynamics were better with dobutamine, the effects of amrinone were maintained over 24 hours, whereas tolerance to the effects of dobutamine were evident over 8 hours (Klein et al., 1981).

The initial dose of IV amrinone is usually 0.75 mg/kg infused over several minutes. Maintenance infusion is started at 5 to 10 μg/kg per minute, titrated according to hemodynamic response. There is considerable variation in the half-life of amrinone. In healthy subjects, the half-life is 2.5 hours, but in patients with heart failure, it may exceed 12 hours (Edelson et al., 1981).

With IV use, a 2% incidence of hepatotoxicity and thrombocytopenia have been reported (Bottorff et al., 1985). Life-threatening thrombocytopenia appears to be dose-related. Oral amrinone has been withdrawn from use because of thrombocytopenia and GI and CNS side effects.

Milrinone. Milrinone, which is biochemically and pharmacologically similar to amrinone, is a phosphodiesterase inhibitor that is 20 times more potent than amrinone (Baim et al., 1983).

The oral bioavailability of milrinone is 75% to 85% in patients with congestive heart failure and 92% in healthy volunteers (Hasegawa, 1986). Peak plasma concentrations occur within 1 to 2 hours; the duration of action is 3 to 6 hours. Milrinone is renally excreted. Initial doses are 2.5 to 5.0 mg orally every 6 hours. This dose can be increased to 50 mg/day if necessary. Hemodynamic effects of IV milrinone last only 60 to 90 minutes after administration.

Like amrinone, milrinone has positive inotropic and vasodilating effects. Short-term administration of milrinone consistently increases cardiac index and lowers pulmonary capillary wedge pressure and systemic vascular resistance in patients with congestive heart failure (Hasegawa, 1986). These beneficial hemodynamic effects occur when therapy with digitalis, diuretics, and vasodilators is continued. However, the short-term hemodynamic benefits of milrinone are not necessarily followed by sustained responses to oral milrinone. Like amrinone, milrinone has not been shown to improve the natural progression of chronic congestive heart failure or to impact on mortality.

Digitalis Glycosides

Digitalis glycosides (the most commonly used digoxin), inhibit the sodium-potassium-activated adenosine triphosphatase (Na^+, K^+-ATPase) pump that actively transports sodium across the myocardial cell membrane. Digoxin is a weak inotrope that augments calcium influx, resulting in enhanced myocardial contractility. Long-term administration improves left ventricular function in heart failure (Arnold et al., 1980).

In the absence of heart failure, digitalis constricts arterioles and veins. However, in the patient with congestive heart failure, this increase in afterload is overshadowed by the increase in cardiac output. The best results of digitalis therapy in shock are therefore in patients with congestive heart failure. However, the risk of arrhythmias due to digitalis toxicity, electrolyte imbalance (particularly hypokalemia), and acid-base disturbances has minimized use as an inotrope in the acute care setting. Administration of digoxin in the ICU is usually restricted to the management of supraventricular arrhythmias (see chapter 6).

Vasodilators

Vasodilatation can be produced by three mechanisms: (1) direct relaxation of smooth muscle, (2) α-adrenergic receptor blockade, and (3) ganglionic blockade. The commonly used vasodilators may be categorized by their relative effects on the arterial versus venous system. The following discussion will focus on the vasodilators used most frequently in the ICU.

Sodium Nitroprusside. Sodium nitroprusside produces balanced venous and arterial vasodilatation. Because of its rapid onset of action and the rapidly reversible effects upon discontinuation of therapy, the drug is well suited to clinical situations where titratable minute-to-minute vasodilatation is required. The venodilatation induced by this drug may cause relative hypovolemia and hypotension that is usually reversible with administration of volume. Severe hypotension, an extension of its pharmacologic effects, is its major adverse effect.

Knowledge of the metabolism of sodium nitroprusside is important to understand. Nitroprusside binds promptly to hemoglobin as Fe^{2+} that is oxidized to Fe^{3+}, forming methemoglobin and an unstable nitroprusside radical. This radical quickly breaks down and releases five cyanide ions. One of the five cyanide groups combines with methemoglobin to form cyanomethemoglobin. The remaining four cyanide groups are converted to thiocyanate in the liver and kidneys by the rhodenase enzyme system in the presence of thiosulfate and cyanocobalamin (Smith and Kruszyna, 1976). Thiocyanate is then excreted in the urine.

The toxicity associated with sodium nitroprusside administration can be categorized as acute or chronic. Acute toxicity is believed to be secondary to incomplete cyanide conversion. Cyanide inactivates the intracellular cytochrome oxidase system producing anaerobic metabolism and lactic acidosis. One rate-limiting step in detoxification of cyanide is the supply of rhodanese. The enzyme may be deficient in such rare conditions as Leber optic atrophy or tobacco amblyopia (Cohn and Burke, 1979). In addition, variable thiosulfate levels may explain different concentrations of cyanide in the plasma of patients with the same infusion rates of sodium nitroprusside (Vesey and Cole, 1985).

Long-term administration of sodium nitroprusside may cause toxicity as a result of accumulation of thiocyanate. Accumulation of thiocyanate causes fatigue, nausea, anorexia, miosis, psychosis, and convulsions. Toxicity begins to occur at plasma thiocyanate concentrations of 5 to 10 mg/dl.

Monitoring thiocyanate and/or cyanide concentrations is prudent in patients receiving this drug for more than 72 hours. The monitoring is especially important in patients with impairment of renal function (see chapter 11). The recommended dose range of sodium nitroprusside is 0 to 5 μg/kg per minute, toxicity being a concern at infusion rates of >10 μg/kg per minute or 3 mg/kg per day (Rieves, 1984).

The goals of prevention or treatment of cyanide toxicity are to decrease cyanide binding to cytochrome c and to remove cyanide from the blood. Several antidotes have been suggested for the treatment of suspected cyanide poisoning. Sodium nitrite reacts with hemoglobin to form methemoglobin, which competes with cytochrome oxidase for the cyanide ion. Administration of thiosulfate, which serves as a sulfur donor, may facilitate the conversion of cyanide to thiocyanate. Another means of decreasing the blood cyanide concentration is based on the combination of hydroxycobalamin (vitamin B_{12}) with cyanide to form cyanocobalamin. In a study of prophylaxis (Cottrell et al., 1978), 14 patients were randomized to receive nitroprusside alone or in combination with hydroxycobalamin. Red cell and plasma cyanide concentrations were significantly lower in the latter group.

Occasionally, hypoxia may develop during infusion of sodium nitroprusside in patients with lung disease. This is thought to be due to reversal of hypoxemia and alveolar hypoxic pulmonary vasoconstriction of the pulmonary circulation.

Hydralazine. Hydralazine is a direct-acting arterial dilator with a delayed onset of action (10–30 minutes) and a prolonged duration of action (4–24 hours). The drug is metabolized in part by acetylation, the rate of which is genetically determined; slow acetylators achieve higher plasma levels of hydralazine than do fast acetylators.

Since the hypotensive effect correlates with concentrations of the parent drug in plasma, slow acetylators generally require smaller doses of the drug than do fast acetylators. Hydralazine usually is administered as repeated IV or oral doses of 2.5 to 20 mg. However, it also may be administered as an infusion (Sladen and Rosenthal, 1979). Hydralazine is commonly used to treat hypertension during pregnancy and preeclampsia.

A common adverse effect of hydralazine is reflex tachycardia in response to decreased systemic vascular resistance. Because coronary perfusion pressure is a function of diastolic pressure and diastolic time, this cardiac response to the drug may increase coronary ischemia. Coadministration of a β-adrenergic receptor antagonist with hydralazine usually blunts these unwanted effects. Long-term administration of hydralazine may be associated with a peripheral neuropathy, a positive anti-nuclear antibody test, and a lupus-like syndrome (see chapters 2 and 11).

Trimethaphan Camsylate (Arfonad). This balanced vasodilator works through ganglionic blockade, leading to loss of sympathetic tone and relaxation of vascular smooth muscle. The net hemodynamic effect is to decrease preload, afterload, and blood pressure. When sympathetic tone is high, ganglionic blockade may result in bradycardia. If parasympathetic tone predominates, infusion of trimethaphan may result in tachycardia.

Trimethaphan is very useful in the setting of dissecting aortic aneurysm, which mandates urgent institution of medical therapy. Initial treatment often consists of sodium nitroprusside, which alone may increase the velocity of ventricular contraction, and a β-adrenergic receptor blocker such as propranolol. If β-blocker therapy is contraindicated, or a single agent is preferred, trimethaphan 1 to 2 mg/min is useful. Administration of this ganglionic blocking agent alone may obviate the problem of the undesirable inotropic and chronotropic response that may be associated with sodium nitroprusside (DeSanctis et al., 1987).

The usual dose of trimethaphan is up to 10 μg/kg per minute. However, tachyphylaxis may develop with chronic use of this agent. The use of trimethaphan is sometimes limited by adverse effects of ganglionic blockade, including urinary retention, paralytic ileus, and decreased visual accommodation. Since sodium nitroprusside has a slightly shorter duration of action, trimethaphan is primarily used when a contraindication exists to sodium nitroprusside. For example, the use of nitroprusside, nitroglycerin, and hydralazine is associated with increased intracranial pressure in patients with decreased intracranial compliance. Trimethaphan, however, appears to be the safest

of the vasodilators and may therefore be the agent of choice in hypertensive patients with raised intracranial pressure (Turner et al., 1977). Trimethaphan also is useful in some patients when it is combined with sodium nitroprusside to block the hyperdynamic response that may be associated with administration of sodium nitroprusside. Vasodilatation induced by sodium nitroprusside may stimulate baroreceptors to reflexly increase sympathetic tone, making blood pressure very difficult to control. This increase in afterload may be offset by concomitant treatment with the ganglion blocker.

Nitroglycerin. Nitroglycerin is predominantly a venodilator when IV doses range up to 1.5 μg/kg per minute. At higher doses, nitroglycerin also produces arterial dilatation. As a result of these actions, systemic vascular resistance (afterload) and left ventricular end-diastolic volume (preload) are reduced, favorably altering two determinants of myocardial oxygen consumption (chapter 4). In patients with pulmonary edema, nitroglycerin reduces PAWP with little effect on cardiac output or blood pressure. In hypovolemic patients, however, cardiac output and blood pressure may markedly decrease during administration of nitroglycerin. As with sodium nitroprusside, the use of IV nitroglycerin should be guided by adequate hemodynamic monitoring. In addition to the effects of nitroglycerin on the systemic circulation, beneficial dilatation of the coronary and pulmonary circulations (Pearl et al., 1983) can occur (Greenberg et al., 1975).

Intravenous nitroglycerin is used in the ICU for the management of active cardiac ischemia and congestive heart failure, or prophylactically in patients with known coronary artery disease.

Supportive Therapy

β-Adrenergic Receptor Antagonists

Labetalol (Trandate). Labetalol is a competitive antagonist of α_1-, β_1-, and β_2-adrenergic receptors. Labetalol is a nonselective β-adrenergic blocker, 1.5 to 18 times less potent than propranolol (Carter, 1983). In humans, the effective β-to-α blocking activity is approximately 7 : 1. The half-life is 1.5 to 2 hours.

Hemodynamic effects of IV administration include reduced blood pressure, heart rate, and peripheral resistance, with little effect on cardiac output or stroke volume. Labetalol may have advantages over pure β-adrenergic blocking drugs in that the α blockade may ablate the bradycardic effects of the β blockade and may increase the antihypertensive effect of the drug (Wallin and O'Neill, 1983).

In open and controlled trials, labetalol has been

used effectively to treat moderate and severe hypertension, as well as hypertensive emergencies. The most frequent adverse effects include orthostatic hypotension, headache, and GI symptoms. Labetalol appears not to diminish renal plasma flow, or glomerular filtration rate, in contrast to pure β-adrenergic receptor blockers. The concomitant α blockade may play a role in preventing undesirable alternatives in renal hemodynamics (Wallin and O'Neill, 1983).

Esmolol (Breriblock).   Esmolol is a β-receptor antagonist with a relatively short half-life of 9 to 10 minutes. Esmolol is particularly useful in the critical care setting, where administration by continuous IV infusion permits controlled, readily reversible β-receptor blockade (Benfield and Sorkin, 1987).

Esmolol is rapidly metabolized by red cell esterase to form an inactive metabolite. Pharmacokinetics are not significantly affected by renal impairment or hepatic dysfunction. Its hemodynamic and electrophysiologic effects are similar to those of other β-receptor antagonists. Esmolol exhibits neither intrinsic sympathomimetic activity nor significant membrane-stabilizing activity.

Clinical studies indicate that esmolol is safe and effective in reducing heart rate in patients with supraventricular tachycardias (comparing favorably with propranolol) and in treating tachycardia associated with acute myocardial infarction and unstable angina. Esmolol is also useful in attenuating the hemodynamic responses to stressful stimuli intraoperatively, and in treating postoperative hypertension (Turlapaty et al., 1987).

Fluids and Electrolytes.   In addition to treating the underlying causes of shock and choosing appropriate inotropic or vasopressor therapy, the physician in the ICU must decide on the optimal fluid for resuscitation. Packed red blood cells or fresh-frozen plasma should be administered to correct significant anemia or coagulopathy, respectively. However, the use of blood products for the sole purpose of expansion of plasma volume is uncommon now because of growing concerns about the transmission of infections such as hepatitis C and the human immunodeficiency virus.

Volume resuscitation may be achieved with either colloid (albumin, hetastarch, and pentastarch) or crystalloid administration. In humans, albumin provides approximately 80% of the intravascular colloid osmotic pressure (COP). A 5% albumin solution has a COP of about 20 mm Hg and an average molecular weight of 69,000. In the normal state, the capillary membrane is relatively impermeable to albumin. Consequently, the hemodynamic improvement after infusion of a 5% albumin solution may persist for 24 to 36 hours (Rothschild et al., 1955). Hetastarch is a synthetic colloid with an *average* molecular weight of 69,000. Particle sizes range from molecular weights of 10,000 to 1 million. The COP of a 6% solution of hetastarch is 32 mm Hg. Plasma clearance of hetastarch is complex. The largest particles are phagocytosed by the reticuloendothelial system; average-size particles are degraded in the liver and then excreted in the stool or urine; and the low-molecular-weight substances are either excreted in the urine or penetrate the vascular membrane to enter the interstitial space (Thompson, 1978). Approximately 90% of the dose of hetastarch is eliminated from the body with a half-life of 17 days. In clinical use, hetastarch expands the intravascular volume for 24 to 36 hours, with approximately 40% of the plasma expansion still present at 24 hours. Despite modest effects on the coagulation profile of patients receiving hetastarch, a randomized trial comparing albumin and hetastarch in septic shock failed to demonstrate any differences in the prothrombin time, partial thromboplastin time, platelet count, or incidence of bleeding (Falk et al., 1988). Pentastarch, a new lower-molecular-weight hydroxyethyl starch derivative, has an initial intravascular half-life of only 2.5 hours and is more rapidly hydrolyzed and excreted than hetastarch. The lower-molecular-weight and higher-concentration formula (10%) of pentastarch may result in a greater degree of expansion of plasma volume than that of hetastarch, although the duration of action is shorter (Mischler et al., 1983). In a randomized clinical trial comparing pentastarch and albumin for volume expansion after cardiac surgery, hemodynamic, respiratory, and hematologic function were similar, as was mean serum colloid osmotic pressure (London et al., 1989). Although pentastarch is used for leukopheresis, it has not yet been approved for use as a volume expander.

Results of the prospective trials comparing the efficacy of colloid or crystalloid resuscitation, their effect on the COP–wedge pressure gradient, and the development of pulmonary edema are conflicting (Stein et al., 1974; Lucas et al., 1978; Weaver et al., 1978; Boutros et al., 1979; Virgilo et al., 1979; Moss et al., 1981; Shires et al., 1983; Pearl et al., 1988; Ley et al., 1990). The decision to use colloid, crystalloid, or a combination of the two in resuscitation has been reviewed (Shine et al., 1980). To summarize, cardiac function and hemodynamic stability may be restored with adequate amounts of either type of fluid. In general, colloid therapy requires approximately one third the volume of crystalloid for an equivalent volume expansion (Shoemaker, 1976; Shoemaker and Hauser, 1979).

Because the aim of the management of shock is

to maximize oxygen transport to the tissues, the arterial PaO_2 is maintained at 70 to 80 mm Hg using a concentration of oxygen below 60%, and positive end-expiratory pressure. Concentrations of oxygen greater than 60% may cause absorption atelectasis, thereby worsening pulmonary function. However, oxygen administration will not increase tissue oxygenation in the absence of adequate preload and myocardial performance (oxygen transport = arterial O_2 content × cardiac output).

Anaerobic glycolysis in shock causes metabolic lactic acidosis, which reduces the effectiveness of endogenous catecholamines and sympathomimetic drugs. Correction to a pH of 7.30 to 7.35 may be appropriate in septic shock. In the intubated patient, alveolar hyperventilation may be used to compensate for metabolic acidosis. However, appropriate therapy often is the administration of sodium bicarbonate. Lactate buffers are not recommended in view of their relatively weak alkalinizing activity and because lactate is metabolized aerobically to bicarbonate only in the absence of tissue hypoxia. Caution must be advised against vigorous bicarbonate therapy. Alkalemia may decrease catecholamine responsiveness and shift the oxygen dissociation curve to the left, decreasing tissue oxygen delivery. Ionized hypocalcemia is also associated with alkalemia, which may result in decreased cardiac output and blood pressure. Alkalemia may increase carbon dioxide production and also cause respiratory acidosis. There may have been more to the statement that patients died in pH balance than meets the eye!

GASTROINTESTINAL HEMORRHAGE DUE TO STRESS ULCERATION

Incidence, Risk Factors, and Approach to Prophylaxis

Minor upper GI bleeding due to stress ulceration is common in seriously ill hospitalized patients (Shuman et al., 1987). The reported incidence of bleeding is dependent upon the method by which stress ulcers are defined. Almost all trauma or burn patients have endoscopic evidence of stress ulcers, although only 2% to 3% of patients have overt bleeding (Shuman et al., 1987). Moreover, the incidence of overt bleeding appears to be decreasing in the last decade, possibly due to improved hemodynamic management, attention to nutrition, and treatment of coagulopathy in the critically ill.

The pathogenesis of stress ulceration involves disruption of gastric mucosal integrity. Hypotension and systemic acidosis decrease gastric blood flow, resulting in impaired turnover of gastric epithelium, loss of the protective mucous and bicarbonate barrier, and back diffusion of hydrogen

ions across the gastric mucosa (Gottlieb et al., 1986). Serious hemorrhage due to these lesions, although unusual, is accompanied by a high degree of morbidity and mortality (Schuster et al., 1984). Several risk factors for bleeding have been identified, including sepsis, renal failure, trauma, burns, respiratory failure, and coagulopathy. Regression analysis has determined that prolonged mechanical ventilation and the presence of coagulopathy are the two most highly ranked risk factors for bleeding (Schuster et al., 1984).

Prophylactic therapy against stress ulceration has focused on cytoprotection (with sucralfate) and reduction in the rate of synthesis of gastric acid with histamine-receptor antagonists or neutralization of acid with antacids. All these agents are efficacious in preventing GI hemorrhage in the critically ill compared with placebo or control groups. In a recent review, the data from 16 randomized trials of prophylaxis for stress ulcer involving 2133 patients were combined and categorized according to the criteria used for the diagnosis of bleeding (either occult or overt bleeding) (Shuman et al., 1987). When the results of all trials using all bleeding end points were combined, antacids appeared to have a prophylactic advantage over cimetidine. However, when considering only overt bleeding, antacids and cimetidine were equally effective and both were significantly more effective than placebo. This has been corroborated in a subsequent metaanalysis (Lacroix et al., 1989).

Oral prostaglandin E_1 and E_2 also have been studied in three clinical trials. One study comparing prostaglandins with antacids showed a significant reduction in overt bleeding due to the prostaglandins (Skillman et al., 1984). However, subsequent studies failed to show a difference when compared with placebo (Van Essen et al., 1985) or antacids (Zinner et al., 1989). Pirenzipine is an anticholinergic that specifically blocks muscarinic receptors, effectively blocking gastric acid secretion and preventing stress ulceration; it is used widely in Europe for prophylaxis.

The positive results of randomized trials in the prophylaxis of stress ulcer have led to recommendations that prophylaxis be administered to a large proportion of critically ill patients (Weigelt et al., 1981; Zinner et al., 1981; Friedman et al., 1982; Pinilla et al., 1985). As such, control of gastric pH has been described as standard practice in ICUs in North America and Europe (Borrero et al., 1986; Noseworthy et al., 1987).

In evaluating prophylaxis against GI bleeding, many trials have included occult bleeding (positive guaiac tests of either gastric contents or stool) in their definition of bleeding. Results of guaiac slide testing often are insensitive and nonspecific (Norfleet et al., 1980; Layne et al., 1981). It is likely that occult bleeding, even in the absence of prophylactic therapy, rarely progresses to overt bleeding (Pinilla et al., 1985) and may not be clinically important (Weigelt et al., 1981; Kingsley, 1985; Zinner et al., 1989).

In contrast, some studies have defined bleeding as only overt (such as hematemesis). The profile of a patient with overt bleeding may range from a transiently bloody nasogastric aspirate to hypovolemic shock. Accordingly, there may be only a small proportion of critically ill patients who actually develop clinically important bleeding due to stress ulceration. However, there are no trials that evaluate prophylactic agents with regard to the end point of clinically significant bleeding.

Adverse effects of stress-bleeding prophylaxis are infrequent, but potentially important. Histamine H_2 receptors in the myocardium mediate the positive inotropic and chronotropic effects of histamine. Rapid infusion of H_2-receptor antagonists may therefore rarely be associated with bradycardia, decreased cardiac output, and asystole. Although most of the cases of mental confusion reported with histamine-receptor antagonists have been described with cimetidine, all such agents cross the blood–brain barrier and have this potential. Elderly patients and those with renal failure or liver failure are particularly susceptible to CNS toxicity. Cimetidine inhibits the cytochrome P450 system in the liver, impairing elimination of numerous drugs that are commonly used in the ICU such as aminophylline. Antacid administration may be associated with diarrhea, metabolic alkalosis, and hypophosphatemia.

Role of Gastric pH in Nosocomial Pneumonia

In the critically ill patient, the normally sterile acidic gastric environment may be altered by drugs used for prophylaxis of stress ulcer; the result is a marked growth of intragastric gramnegative bacteria. Several studies have documented the time sequence of intragastric and subsequent tracheal colonization in patients receiving antacids or histamin-receptor antagonists (duMoulin et al., 1982; Goularte et al., 1986; Donowitz et al., 1986). Aspiration of colonizing organisms in these secretions is believed to be the principal mechanism whereby pathogenic organisms reach the tracheobronchial tree and cause nosocomial pneumonia.

Although most published trials for prophylaxis of stress ulcer have employed histamine-receptor antagonists or antacids, recent studies have favorably evaluated the cytoprotective agent sucralfate, a basic aluminum salt that does not materially affect gastric pH. The latter is a potentially important characteristic of sucralfate in light of the possible role of gastric pH in the development of nosocomial pneumonia. In the trials comparing sucralfate with pH-altering drugs which evaluate the outcome of nosocomial pneumonia, the common odds ratio is 0.55 (0.28–1.06) (Cook et al., 1991). This indicates a trend toward a reduced rate of pneumonia with the prophylactic use of sucralfate as compared with pH-altering drugs (approximately a 45% risk reduction with the use of sucralfate) (Driks et al., 1987; Laggner et al., 1989; Tryba, 1987; Ryan et al., 1990). However, methodologic deficiencies, small sample sizes, and the failure to examine the effects of antacids and H_2-receptor antagonists separately make a large prospective randomized trial necessary to confirm or refute these findings.

ACUTE RENAL FAILURE IN THE CRITICALLY ILL

Acute renal failure (ARF) occurs commonly in critically ill patients, with an associated mortality of 17% to 44% in nonoliguric patients and 50% to 87% in oliguric patients (Anderson et al., 1977; Frankel et al., 1983; Bullock et al., 1985). Acute renal failure is defined as a reduction in renal function resulting in the accumulation of nitrogenous wastes. Urine output of < 100 ml/day usually is classified as anuria, while output of 100 to 500 ml/day is classified as oliguria (see chapter 11).

However, nonoliguric persons currently constitute the majority of patients with ARF (Myers et al., 1980). It is generally accepted that nonoliguric ARF is associated with lower morbidity (better acid–base control and electrolyte stability) and mortality than oliguric failure. The higher incidence of nonoliguric ARF as opposed to oliguric ARF in the last decade may reflect advances in cardiovascular management (volume expansion, afterload reduction, dopamine and diuretic therapy) that have potentially favorable effects on renal function.

Etiology of ARF

The causes of ARF may be divided into prerenal, renal, and postrenal categories. In general, prerenal ARF is due to reduced renal perfusion, secondary to volume depletion or reduced cardiac output. Intrinsic renal failure usually is secondary to postischemic acute tubular necrosis, nephrotoxins, or glomerular lesions. Postrenal ARF is most often due to mechanical outlet obstruction. This schematic approach based on history and physical examination, along with ancillary laboratory tests of urine sediment and blood chemistry, will aid the physician in determining the cause and subsequent management of ARF (see chapter 11).

Drug-induced ARF may represent 5% of all

cases of ARF (Mann et al., 1986). The kidneys receive 20% to 25% of the resting cardiac output; reabsorption and secretion of drugs expose the parenchyma to high concentrations of solutes that may cause renal tubular toxicity. In patients with preexisting renal disease and a decreased number of functioning nephrons, exposure of the remaining nephrons to high concentrations of drugs, especially in the face of hypovolemia, may potentiate the nephrotoxic insult. Thus, the onset of ARF in the critically ill should always herald reevaluation of a patient's medication profile to assess the need for, and to adjust the dose of, drugs when necessary. However, administration of the same loading dose of drug to patients with renal failure is important because the longer half-life prolongs the time to reach an effective steady-state concentration.

Prevention and Treatment of ARF in the ICU

Therapy for ARF consists of preventive measures, supportive care, and attempts at improving renal function. Specific supportive goals include maintenance of adequate renal blood flow and urine output, achieving normal fluid and electrolyte balance, removal of metabolic waste products, and minimizing further nephrotoxic insults. The following discussion will focus on controlled human studies in the prevention or treatment of ARF in the critically ill.

Mannitol.   Mannitol is a six-carbon alcohol osmotic diuretic (see chapter 11). Proposed mechanisms for the beneficial effects of mannitol on renal function include improved renal blood flow, increased filtration pressure, tubular flushing, and reduced swelling of damaged cells. There are no published controlled trials of the use of mannitol in established renal failure. Uncontrolled trials have documented increased urine flow rates but no consistent improvement in creatinine clearance.

Several controlled trials of mannitol given to prevent ARF have been conducted in patients undergoing cardiopulmonary bypass surgery (Etheredge et al., 1963; Ridgen et al., 1984), aortic aneurysmectomy (Barry et al., 1961; Mueller, 1966), renal transplantation (Weimer et al., 1983), IV pyelography (Anto et al., 1981), amphotericin B therapy (Bullock et al., 1976), and operations in jaundiced patients (Dawson, 1965). Overall, these studies show either improved urine output, an attenuated decrease in creatinine clearance compared with control groups, or, in one study (Weimer et al., 1983), a decrease in requirements for dialysis. *No significant deleterious effects on renal function, adverse reactions, or differences in survival have been reported. However, pulmo-nary edema and acute hyperosmolarity are complications sometimes associated with infusion of mannitol.*

Diuretics.   The loop diuretics, including furosemide, ethacrynic acid, and bumetanide, exert their major effect at the loop of Henle, causing a sodium diuresis (see chapter 11). The proposed beneficial effects of these agents in ARF include increased regional blood flow, improved filtration, and flushing of cellular debris from the tubules. Although ethacrynic acid induces diuresis in acute tubular necrosis, reports of ototoxicity have limited its use. Bumetanide has not been studied extensively in ARF. Controlled trials of furosemide in established renal failure have documented improved urine output but generally no consistent difference in creatinine clearance, dialysis requirements, or mortality (Cantarovich et al., 1973; Kleinknecht et al., 1976; Powell et al., 1980).

Following bolus injection of furosemide, a prompt and vigorous diuresis usually ensues. However, this diuretic response is often transient and diminishes within 4 to 6 hours (Rupp, 1974). To obviate the problem of hypotension often associated with bolus administration, continuous infusion of loop diuretics may be useful in patients with hemodynamic instability when a gentle, sustained diuresis is desired. The diuretic effect of furosemide by bolus injection and by continuous infusion was studied in 18 cardiac surgery patients. Nine were randomly assigned to receive 0.3 mg/kg of furosemide as a bolus, at time 0, and 6 hours later. Nine were administered a constant infusion of 0.05 mg/kg per hour for 12 hours. There were no differences in creatinine clearance, urinary sodium, urinary potassium, or urine volume excreted. However, the diuresis during continuous infusion was less variable than after bolus injection and was sustained throughout the infusion period (Copeland et al., 1983). Although continuous infusion may be useful in some patients, it may not provide the vigorous diuresis required in other situations.

Dopamine.   Dopamine may improve renal function by increasing cardiac output and by causing direct renal arteriolar vasodilatation through dopaminergic receptors, and by inhibiting tubular solute resorption. In one study, the effect of dopamine on enhancing sodium excretion was independent of its effect on augmenting cardiac output (Hilberman et al., 1984). The combination of dopamine and furosemide in oliguric ARF refractory to furosemide or mannitol alone can result in conversion of oliguric to nonoliguric ARF (Lindner et al., 1979; Henderson et al., 1980; Graziani et al., 1982). Dopamine, in doses of 1 to 5 μg/kg per minute, is commonly used prophylactically and in the treatment of acute renal failure. There are no randomized controlled trials that definitively support its use.

In summary, the evaluation of the efficacy of treatment in ARF is hampered by the variable definitions of ARF, the lack of randomized controlled trials, and the focus on urine output rather than a physiologic end point or survival in clinical studies. Nevertheless, mannitol, furosemide, and dopamine may convert oliguric to nonoliguric renal failure in 30% to 50% of cases (Mann et al., 1986).

PHARMACOLOGIC TREATMENT OF BLEEDING DISORDERS IN THE ICU

Up to 40% of critically ill patients ultimately develop at least one bleeding episode during their ICU admission (Brown et al., 1988). Anticoagulant or antimicrobial therapy, renal failure, sepsis, malnutrition, mechanical ventilation, and surgical procedures all are associated with bleeding in the ICU. The following discussion focuses on newer medical therapy for two specific bleeding disorders common in the ICU. For the management of other coagulopathies, the reader is referred to chapter 22.

Postoperative Bleeding

Excessive postsurgical bleeding may be related to both vascular trauma and inherited or acquired defects of hemostasis. Cardiopulmonary bypass may result in thrombocytopenia, a thrombocytopathy, reduced concentrations and function of coagulation factors, fibrinolysis, hypothermia, circulating heparin, or excessive protamine. Clearly, replacing blood products (packed red cells, platelets, fresh-frozen plasma, and cryoprecipitate), when appropriate, is the mainstay of treatment.

However, defective platelet function is thought to be an important factor contributing to the tendency for bleeding in cardiac surgery patients. Desmopressin acetate (DDAVP) is a synthetic vasopressin analog that may shorten the bleeding time in mild hemophilia, von Willebrand disease, uremia, and aspirin ingestion. The mechanism of action is related to an increase in the concentration of von Willebrand factor, especially the high-molecular-weight multimers. Two comparative trials in adults undergoing cardiac surgery (Salzman et al., 1986; Czer et al., 1987) and one in patients undergoing spinal fusion (Kobrinsky et al., 1987) demonstrated that DDAVP reduced operative and postoperative blood loss. A fourth study reported a decrease in bleeding during cardiac operations (Rocha et al., 1988). Another found that DDAVP did not reduce operative or postoperative blood loss (Hackmann et al., 1989). One explanation relates to patient selection; DDAVP appears to be without benefit in patients with adequate hemostasis, in whom bleeding is mild. However, it may be useful in patients with excessive bleeding.

Uremic Coagulopathy

A prolonged bleeding time, normal coagulation tests, and a thrombocytopathy are the hallmarks of the coagulopathy associated with uremia. Hemodialysis does not completely correct the platelet abnormality (Remuzzi et al., 1978). Chronic administration of human recombinant erythropoietin, although used to correct the anemia of renal failure, also shortens the bleeding time and corrects the thrombocytopathy (Moia et al., 1987). Transfusion of red blood cells to achieve a hematocrit of 26% to 30% also may be hemostatically effective in uremic patients with prolonged bleeding times (Livio et al., 1982; Fernandez et al., 1985). Infusion of cryoprecipitate (rich in factor VIII and fibrinogen) corrects the bleeding time in uremia within 4 to 12 hours, with an effect lasting 24 to 36 hours (Janson et al., 1980).

In a double-blind randomized controlled trial, DDAVP has been shown to significantly reduce bleeding time in uremic patients, 1 to 4 hours after administration (Mannucci et al., 1983). This temporary restoration of hemostasis makes DDAVP treatment useful before procedures in the uremic critically ill patient. In a similar study, infusion of conjugated estrogens (0.6 mg/kg) for 5 days or longer also shortened the bleeding time in patients with renal failure (Liu et al., 1984; Livio et al., 1986). Although the mechanism is unknown, the effect is detectable 6 hours after the first infusion, reaching a maximum between 5 and 7 days, lasting for up to 14 days. Therefore, conjugated estrogens offer the therapeutic advantage of a longer duration of action when an immediate hemostatic effect is not essential.

SEDATION IN THE CRITICALLY ILL PATIENT

Sedative drugs are among the most frequently prescribed medications in the ICU, with approximately 40% of patients regularly receiving one or more agents (Farina et al., 1981). The cause of agitation and altered mental status in the critically ill patient usually is multifactorial and includes pain, intubation, sensory deprivation or overstimulation, insomnia, "ICU psychosis," and paralysis with incomplete sedation. The metabolic, infectious, neurologic, or pharmacologic features of a patient's illness also may contribute to an altered mental status.

Nonpharmacologic approaches to treating agitation in the critically ill include treatment of the underlying condition, adequate analgesia, reassurance and orientation, establishment of a normal sleep–wake cycle, and maintenance of appropriate auditory and visual stimulation. Pharmacologic intervention should be considered when agitation prevents adequate mechanical ventilation, when the patient is a risk to him- or herself or staff, and when induction of sleep is desired. The ideal level of sedation in critically ill patients has been described as that in which the patient appears comfortable and free from pain but will rouse easily if required (Hopkinson and Freeman, 1988).

Sedative-Hypnotics in the ICU

The ideal sedative for the critically ill patient would have a rapid onset and predictable duration of action, a wide therapeutic index, amnestic properties, an elimination unaltered by hepatic or renal disease, inactive metabolites, and minimal respiratory suppression or hemodynamic effects. Unfortunately, no single agent has all these characteristics. Tolerance develops to many drugs used for sedation in the ICU. Withdrawal from the effect of sedative drugs also may pose a management problem.

Opiate Agonists.   Opiate receptor agonists, including meperidine, dilaudid, morphine, and fentanyl are used commonly in the ICU for analgesia, sedation, and to reduce the discomfort of endotracheal intubation. The most frequent adverse effects include hypotension, respiratory depression, and GI hypomotility. These adverse effects are usually reversible with the antagonist naloxone. Opiates are administered most effectively by IV, IM, or epidurally.

The problems of tolerance, hemodynamic instability, and depressed levels of consciousness often seen with IV sedatives may be obviated by continuous infusion of epidural narcotics. Epidural opiates can give potent long-lasting analgesia without sensory, sympathetic, or motor block. However, epidural administration of opiates is not an effective way to provide sedation. This technique has been used for the management of acute and chronic pain and for the relief of pain in ICU patients (Rawal and Tandon, 1985). Respiratory suppression appears to be less problematic with epidural narcotics than with IV narcotics.

Benzodiazepines.   Benzodiazepines are used extensively in the ICU setting and produce anxiolysis, sedation, amnesia, and muscle relaxation. Their mechanism of action is through potentiation of neuronal inhibition mediated by GABA. Intravenous agents available include chlordiazepoxide, diazepam, lorazepam and midazolam, which have a variable duration of action and number of active metabolites (Table 26-4; chapter 13). Adverse effects include hypotension, respiratory depression, and elevated liver function tests. Paradoxical excitation and drug interactions, particularly potentiation of other psychoactive drugs, may complicate their use.

Continuous IV infusion of these agents, particularly midazolam (elimination half-life of 1–4 hours), provides a relatively stable, reversible sedative effect (Freeman and Hopkinson, 1988). In a group of postoperative cardiac surgery patients treated with a midazolam infusion, the drug was rapidly eliminated, did not prolong the ICU stay, and was found to decrease the total narcotic dosage required compared with standard therapy (Westphal et al., 1987).

Continuous infusion of opioids supplemented by a benzodiazepine is a common method of sedation in the ICU (Gast et al., 1984). Neither fentanyl nor diazepam, when given alone, produces important hemodynamic suppression (Bird et al., 1984); however, administration of diazepam to patients anesthetized with fentanyl can cause profound decreases in blood pressure, systemic vas-

Table 26–4. BENZODIAZEPINES AVAILABLE FOR IV USE IN THE CRITICALLY ILL

DRUG	ONSET OF ACTION AFTER IV ADMINISTRATION (MINUTES)	DURATION OF ACTION (HOURS)	$T_{1/2}$ (HOURS)	METABOLITES (HALF-LIFE, HOURS)
Chlordiazepoxide	1–5	0.25–1	5–30	Demoxepam (15–95) Desmethyldiazepam (5–45) Oxazepam (15–200)
Diazepam	1–5	0.25–1	20–50	Oxazepam (4–12) Desmethyldiazepam (5–45) 3-Hydroxydiazepam (15–200)
Lorazepam	1–5	12–24	10–20	–
Midazolam	1–5	0.25–1	1–4	Hydroxymethylmidazolam (1–2)

cular resistance, and cardiac output, possibly due to effects on sympathetic nervous system activity (Tomicheck et al., 1983). Adequate sedation and analgesia may be achieved by the combination of continuous IV fentanyl and the benzodiazepine midazolam (whose short half-life of 2 hours makes it attractive for sedation by infusion). Widespread adoption of this regimen in many centers reflects the current paucity of satisfactory methods of safe sedation in the critically ill.

Phenothiazines and Butyrophenones. The phenothiazine-butyrophenone group of drugs also are used in the ICU as sedatives, antiemetics and anxiolytics and to control underlying psychiatric disease. Hypotension, extrapyramidal adverse effects, and a propensity to lower the seizure threshold may limit the use of these agents. The increase in renal blood flow and glomerular filtration rate does not appear to be reduced by the antidopaminergic effect of butyrophenones in the dog model (Armstrong et al., 1986).

Propofol. A relatively new short-acting anesthetic, propofol (2,6-diisopropylphenol), is an effective sedative when given by infusion to mechanically ventilated patients (Newman et al., 1987). In a study in post–cardiac surgery patients, infusion of propofol was associated with earlier extubation than midazolam (Grounds et al., 1987).

In summary, disadvantages of sedation in the critically ill patient include adverse effects of the drug or metabolite, possible drug interactions (as has been described with benzodiazepines and opiate agonists (McDonald et al., 1986), drug dependence, and the sequelae of immobilization, such as deep venous thrombosis, decubitus ulcers, and contractures.

Sedation is required by the vast majority of ICU patients at some point during their admission. A simple, safe sedative regimen is a necessity in the ICU. The agent of choice depends upon the desired effect and underlying medical status of the patient.

PHARMACOLOGY IN NEONATAL AND PEDIATRIC ICUs

The major objective of intensive care for infants and children is to provide maximum surveillance and support of organ systems during acute life-threatening illness (Downs et al., 1972). Although the principles of intensive care for infants and children are similar to those for adult intensive care, the age spectrum from infancy through adolescence requires that the pediatric intensive care staff have particular expertise in fetal development, as well as neonatal and pediatric physiology, pharmacology, and psychology. This subject is considered in more detail in chapter 30.

Fewer children than adults are admitted to ICUs with chronic or degenerative disorders. An exception is the presence of respiratory failure that may necessitate prolonged ventilation in the critically ill pediatric patient. Recent randomized trials in premature infants with hyaline membrane disease have demonstrated improved gas exchange and a decreased need for short-term ventilatory support with the use of bovine surfactant. However, in one trial, the number of infants requiring assisted ventilation for longer than 30 days was the same in the treatment and placebo group (Kwong et al., 1985; Jobe and Michiko, 1987).

The influence of developmental factors on pharmacokinetics and pharmacodynamics in children may be amplified by critical illness, multiple system organ failure, and administration of other drugs. In treating critically ill pediatric patients, knowledge of basic pharmacologic principles must be supplemented by a detailed knowledge of specific drugs and their use in children (see chapter 30).

Pharmacodynamic differences between adults and children may be considered in the context of adverse effects and therapeutic effects in children. For example, dopamine antagonists such as metoclopramide, haloperidol, and chlorpromazine, which are used frequently in the ICU, appear to cause more acute dystonic reactions in children and adolescents than in adults (Bateman et al., 1983). In contrast, aminoglycoside ototoxicity and nephrotoxicity probably are less common in infants and children than in adults (Heimann, 1983; McCracken, 1986). Reduced responsiveness to catecholamines in the young has been documented extensively in animals, although systematic age-related differences in catecholamine pharmacokinetics or pharmacodynamics have not been demonstrated in humans (Notterman, 1988).

Pharmacokinetics (including absorption, distribution, biotransformation and excretion of drugs) also may vary between children and adults. Although some differences exist, most drugs are absorbed equally well in the newborn and in the adult. However, in premature infants, GI transit time is prolonged, peristalsis is erratic, and membrane permeability may be decreased. If intestinal transit is rapid, poorly soluble drugs or those requiring a long time for dissolution are poorly absorbed. However, digoxin, administered in an alcohol solution, as it is most commonly given to neonates, appears to be reasonably well absorbed under a variety of pathophysiologic conditions (Larese and Mirkin, 1974).

The volume of drug distribution also is different in children compared with adults. Volume of distribution determines the concentration of drug at a specific receptor site and is affected by body composition. A higher percentage of body weight is water in premature and full-term infants (85% and 75%, respectively) than in adults (60%). This may explain the altered dosing of some drugs in newborns compared with older children and adults. Premature infants also have a lower percentage body fat (1%) than the full-term infant (15%). Therefore, organs that take up lipophilic drugs in adults and children may not exhibit the same affinity for these compounds as in infants (see chapters 30, 37, and 38).

Plasma protein binding of drugs is an important factor in the distribution and rate of removal of a drug. Drug–protein binding may be less in the neonate than in the adult when phenytoin, quinidine, and furosemide are administered. In treating children with phenytoin, the free-drug concentration, rather than total concentration, should be monitored. Drugs may also displace bound molecules from albumin in infancy; an example of this is the displacement of bilirubin by sulfonamides, which may result in CNS deposition of bilirubin.

Biotransformation of many drugs may be slower in children. At birth, the cytochrome P450 content of the liver is only about a quarter of that in adults. Conjugation of drugs also may be slowed, predisposing to drug accumulation. During early development, a dramatic acceleration in the transformation rates of many compounds occurs, such that disposition rates that are less than 30% of adult values in the newborn become severalfold greater than adult values by the end of the first year of life (Morselli et al., 1980). A consequence of the decreased drug metabolism in infants is that many drugs such as phenobarbital, acetaminophen, and theophylline have prolonged plasma half-lives and an increased duration of action.

Renal function in neonates is significantly reduced compared with that in older patients. Glomerular filtration at birth is approximately 30% to 40% of adult function. Glomerular filtration, tubular secretion, and reabsorption all mature at different rates. Drugs eliminated by the kidney, such as salicylates, thiazides, penicillin, and aminoglycosides, may have prolonged half-lives in the neonate.

Therefore, the pediatric ICU physician must be aware of developmental physiology, the alteration of pharmacotherapy in disease states, and the pharmacokinetic and pharmacodynamic principles involved in managing critically ill infants and neonates.

SUMMARY

A pharmacology unique to the practice of critical care medicine has recently evolved. With the growth in the number of ICUs, the complexity of patient problems, and the wide variety of drugs available to the ICU clinician, pharmacotherapy in the critically ill patient often is a challenge. Pharmacokinetics and pharmacodynamics may be abnormal in the face of organ dysfunction. Therefore, appropriate monitoring of hemodynamics or drug concentrations is often necessary in order to guide therapy. Medication profiles should be reviewed daily in the ICU. Physicians should be aware of both the therapeutic and the toxic effects of each drug administered. The number of drugs in the critically ill should be minimized and drug–drug interactions should be actively sought.

Pharmacotherapy is a complex science in the ICU setting. Optimal pharmacotherapy requires a thorough understanding of both clinical pharmacology and abnormal pathophysiology in the critically ill patient.

REFERENCES

Anderson, R. J.; Linas, S. L.; Berns, A. S.; Henrich, W. L.; Miller, T. R.; Gabow, P. A.; and Schrier, R. W.: Nonoliguric acute renal failure. N. Engl. J. Med., 138:950–955, 1977.

Anto, H. R.; Chou, S. Y.; Porush, J. G.; and Shapiro, W. B.: Infusion intravenous pyelography and renal function. Effects of hypertonic mannitol in patients with chronic renal insufficiency. Arch. Intern. Med., 141:1652–1656, 1981.

Armstrong, D. K.; Dasta, J. F.; Reilley, T. E.; and Tallman, R. D.: Effect of haloperidol on dopamine-induced increase in renal blood flow. Drug Intell. Clin. Pharmacol., 20:543–546, 1986.

Arnold, S. B.; Byrd, R. C.; and Meister, W.: Long-term digitalis therapy improves left ventricular function in heart failure. N. Engl. J. Med., 303:443–448, 1980.

Baim, D. S.; McDowell, A. V.; Cherniles, J.; Monrad, E. S.; Parker, J. A.; Edelson, J.; Braunwald, E.; and Grossman, W.: Evaluation of a new bipyridine inotropic agent—milrinone—in patients with severe congestive heart failure. N. Eng. J. Med., 309(13):748–756, 1983.

Ball, H. A.; Cook, J. A.; Wise, W. C.; and Haluska, P. V.: Role of thromboxane, prostaglandins and leukotrienes in endotoxic and septic shock. Intensive Care Med., 12(3):116–126, 1986.

Barry, K. G.; Cohen, A.; Knochel, J. P.; Whelan, T. J. Jr.; Beisel, W. P.; Vargas, C. A.; and LeBlanc, P. C. Jr.: Mannitol infusion: II. The prevention of acute functional renal failure during resection of an aneurysm of the abdominal aorta. N. Engl. J. Med., 264:967–971, 1961.

Barton, M.; Lake, C. R.; Rainey, T. G.; and Chernow, B.: Is catecholamine release pH mediated? Crit. Care Med., 10:751–753, 1982.

Bateman, D. N.; Craft, A. W.; Nicholson, E.; and Pearson, A. D.: Dystonic reactions and the pharmacokinetics of metoclopramide in children. Br. J. Clin. Pharmacol., 15:557–559, 1983.

Baumgartner, J.-D.; McCutchon, J. A.; van Melle, G.; Vogt, M.; Luethy, R.; Glauser, M. P.; Ziegler, E. J.; Klauber, M. R.; Muehlen, E.; and Chiolero, R.: Prevention of gram-negative shock and death in surgical patients by antibody to endotoxin core glycolipid. Lancet, 2:59–63, 1985.

Benfield, P.; and Sorkin, E. M.: Esmolol: A preliminary review of its pharmacodynamic and pharmacokinetic properties, and therapeutic efficacy. Drugs, 33:392–412, 1987.

Bird, T. M.; Edbrooke, D. L.; Newby, D. M.; and Hebron, B. S.: Intravenous sedation for the intubated and spontaneously breathing patient in the intensive care unit. Acta Anaesthesiol. Scan., 28:640–643, 1984.

Bone, R. C.; Fisher, C. J.; Clemmer, T. P.; Slotman, G. J.; Metz, C. A.; and Balk, R. A.: A controlled clinical trial of high-dose methylprednisolone in the treatment of severe sepsis and septic shock. N. Engl. J. Med., 317:653–658, 1987.

Bonnet, F.; Billaine, J.; Lhoste F.; Mankikian, B.; Kerdelhue, B.; and Rapin, M.: Naloxone therapy of human septic shock. Crit. Care Med., 13:972–975, 1985.

Borrero, E.; Ciervo, J.; and Chang, J. B.: Antacid versus sucralfate in preventing acute gastrointestinal tract bleeding in abdominal aortic surgery. Arch. Surg., 121:810–812, 1986.

Botticelli, J. T.; Tsagaris, T. J.; and Lange, R. L.: Mechanisms of pressor amine dependence. Am. J. Cardiol., 16:847–858, 1965.

Bottorff, M. B.; Rutledge, D. R.; and Pieper, J. A.: Evaluation of intravenous amrinone: The first of a new class of positive inotropic agents with vasodilator properties. Pharmacotherapy, 5(5):227–236, 1985.

Boutros, A. R.; Ruess, R.; Olson, L.; Hoyt, J. L.; and Baker, W. H.: Comparison of hemodynamic pulmonary and renal effects of three types of fluids after major surgical procedures on the abdominal aorta. Crit. Care Med., 7:9–13, 1979.

Brown, R. B.; Klar, J.; Teres, D.; Lemeshow, S.; and Sands, M.: Prospective study of clinical bleeding in intensive care unit patients. Crit. Care Med., 16(12):1171–1176, 1988.

Bullock, M. L.; Umen, A. J.; Finkelstein, M.; and Keane, W. F.: The assessment of risk factors in 462 patients with acute renal failure. Am. J. Kidney Dis., 5:97–103, 1985.

Bullock, W. E.; Luke R. G.; Nuttal, C. E.; and Bhathena, D.: Can mannitol reduce amphotericin B nephrotoxicity? Double blind study and description of a new vascular lesion in kidneys. Antimicrob. Agents Chemother., 10:555–563, 1976.

Calvin, J. E.; Driedger, A. A.; and Sibbald, W. J.: Does the pulmonary capillary wedge pressure predict left ventricular preload in critically ill patients? Crit. Care Med., 9:4347–442, 1981.

Cantarovich, F.; Galli C.; Benedetti, L.; Chena, C.; Castro, L.; Correa, C.; Perez-Loredo, J.; Fernandez, J. C.; Locatelli, A.; and Tizado, J.: High dose furosemide in established acute renal failure. Br. Med. J., 4:449–450, 1973.

Carter, B. L.: Labetalol. Drug Intell. Clin. Pharmacol., 17: 704–712, 1983.

Chelluri, L.; and Jastremski, S.: Inadequacy of standard aminoglycoside loading doses in acutely ill patients. Crit. Care Med., 15:1143–1145, 1987.

Chernow, B.; Rainey, T. G.; and Lake, C. R.: Endogenous and exogenous catecholamines in critical care medicine. Crit. Care Med., 10:409–416, 1982.

Clutter, W. E.; Bier, D. M.; Shah, S. D.; and Cryer, P.: Epinephrine plasma metabolic clearance rates and physiologic thresholds for metabolic and hemodynamic actions in man. J. Clin. Invest., 66:94–101, 1980.

Cohn, J. N.; and Burke, L. P.: Nitroprusside. Ann. Intern. Med., 91:752–575, 1979.

Colucci, W. S.; Wright, R. F.; and Braunwald, E.: New positive inotropic agents in the treatment of congestive heart failure. N. Engl. J. Med., 314(6):349–338, 1986.

Connors, A. F.; McCaffree, D. R.; and Gray, B. A.: Evaluation of right heart catheterization in the critically ill patient without acute myocardial infarction. N. Engl. J. Med., 308: 263–267, 1983.

Cook, D. J.; Laine, L. A.; Guyatt, G. H.; and Raffin, T. A.: Nosocomial pneumonia and the role of gastric pH—A meta-analysis. Chest, 100:7–13, 1991.

Cook, D. J.; Grossman, J.; Teres, E.; and Oxman, A. D.: Does fibronectin reduce mortality in sepsis? A meta-analysis. J. Intens. Care Med., 4:265–271, 1989.

Copeland, J. G.; Campbell, D. W.; Plachetka, J. R.; Salomon, N. W.; and Larson, D. F.: Diuresis with continuous infusion of furosemide after cardiac surgery. Am. J. Surg., 146:796–799, 1983.

Cottrell, J. E.; Casthely, P.; and Brodie, J. D.: Prevention of nitroprusside-induced cyanide toxicity with hydroxycobalamin. N. Engl. J. Med., 298(15):809–811, 1978.

Czer, L. S. C.; Bateman, T. M.; and Gray, R. J.: Treatment of severe platelet dysfunction on hemorrhage after cardiopulmonary bypass: Reduction in blood product usage with desmopressin. J. Am Coll. Cardiol., 9:1139–1147, 1987.

Dawson, J. L.: Post-operative renal function in obstructive jaundice: Effect of mannitol diuresis. Br. Med. J., 1:82–86, 1965.

DeSanctis, R. W.; Doroghazi, R. M.; Austin, W. G.; and Buckley, M. J.: Aortic dissection. N. Engl. J. Med., 317(17):1060–1067, 1987.

Donowitz, G. L.; Page, M. C.; Mileur, B. L.; and Guenthner, S. H.: Alteration of normal gastric flora in critical care patients receiving antacid and cimetidine therapy. Infect. Control, 7:23–26,1986.

Downs, J. J.; Fulgencio T.; and Raphaelly, R. C.: Acute respiratory failure in infants and children. Pediatr. Clin. North Am., 19:423–440, 1972.

Driks, M. R.; Craven, D. E.; Celli, B. R.; Manning, M.; Burke, R. A.; Garvin, G. M.; Kunches, L. M.; Farber, H. W.; Wedel, S. A.; and McCabe, W. R.: Nosocomial pneumonia in intubated patients given sucralfate as compared with antacids or histamine type 2 blockers. N. Engl. J. Med., 317(22): 1376–1382, 1987.

duMoulin, G. C.; Paterson, D. G.; Hedley-Whyte, J.; and Lisbon, A.: Aspiration of gastric bacteria in antacid-treated patients: A frequent cause of post-operative colonization of the airway. Lancet, 1:242–245, 1982.

Edelson, J.; LeJemtel, T. H.; Alousi, A. A.; Biddlecome, C. H.; Maskin, C. S.; and Sonnenblick, E. H.: Relationship between amrinone plasma concentration and cardiac index. Clin. Pharmacol. Ther., 29:723–728, 1981.

Eisenberg, P. R.; Jaffe, A. S.; and Schuster, D. P.: Clinical evaluation compared to pulmonary artery catheterization in the hemodynamic assessment of critically ill patients. Crit. Care Med., 12:549–553, 1984.

Endoh, M.; Yamashita, S.; and Taira, N.: Positive inotropic effect of amrinone in relation to cyclic nucleotide metabolism in the canine ventricular muscle. J. Pharmacol. Exp. Ther., 221:775–783, 1982.

Etheredge, E. E.; Levitin, H.; Nakamura, K.; and Glenn, W. W. L.: Effect of mannitol on renal function during open heart surgery. Ann. Surg., 161:53–62, 1963.

Falk, J. L.; Rackow, E. C.; Astiz, M. E.; and Weil, M. H.: Effects of hetastarch and albumin on coagulation in patients with septic shock. J. Clin. Pharmacol., 28:412–415, 1988.

Farina, M. L.; Levati, A.; and Tognoni, G.: A multicentre study of ICU drug utilization. Intens. Care Med., 7:125–131, 1981.

Fernandez, F.; Goudable C.; Sie, P.; Ton-That, H.; Durand, D.; Suc, J. M.; and Boneu, B.: Low hematocrit and prolonged bleeding time in uremic patients: Effect of red cell transfusions. Br. J. Hematol., 59:139–148, 1985.

Frankel, M. C.; Weinstein, A. M.; and Stenzel K. H.: Prognostic patterns in acute renal failure: The New York Hospital, 1981–1982. Clin. Exp. Dial. Apheresis, 7:145–167, 1983.

Freeman, J. W.; and Hopkinson, R. B.: Therapeutic progress in intensive care sedation and analgesia: Part II. Drug selection. J. Clin. Pharmacol. Ther., 13:41–51, 1988.

Friedman, C. J.; Oblinger, M. J.; Surrat, P. M.; Bowers, J.; Goldberg, S. K.; Sperling, M. H.; and Blitzer, A. H.: Prophylaxis of upper gastrointestinal hemorrhage in patients requiring mechanical ventilation. Crit. Care Med., 10:316–319, 1982.

Gast, P. H.; Fisher, A.; and Sear, J. W.: Intensive care sedation now. Lancet, 2:863–864, 1984.

Goldberg, L. I.: Dopamine. Clinical uses of an endogenous catecholamine. N. Engl. J. Med., 291:707–710, 1974.

Goldberg, L. I.; Hsuh, Y.; and Resnekov, L.: Newer catecholamines for treatment of heart failure and shock. Prog. Cardiovasc. Dis., 19:327–340, 1977.

Gottlieb, J. E.; Menashe, P. I.; and Cruz, E.: Gastrointestinal complications in critically ill patients: The intensivist's overview. Am. J. Gastroenterol., 81(4):227–238, 1986.

Goulart, T. A.; Lichtenberg, D. A.; and Craven, D. E.: Gastric colonization in patients receiving antacids and mechanical ventilation: A mechanism for pharyngeal colonization. Am. J. Infect. Control., 14:88, 1986.

Graziani, G.; Cantaluppi, A.; Casati, S.; Citerrio, A.; Scala-mogna, A.; Arnoldi, A.; Silenzio, R.; Brancaccio, D.; and Ponticelli, C.: Dopamine and furosemide therapy in acute renal failure. Proc. Eur. Dial. Transplant Assoc., 19:319–324, 1982.

Greenberg, H.; Dwyer, E. M.; Jameson, E. G.; and Pinkernell, B. H.: Effects of nitroglycerin on the major determinants of myocardial oxygen consumption: An angiographic and hemodynamic assessment. Am. J. Cardiol., 36:426–432, 1975.

Grounds, R. M.; Lalor, J. M.; Lumley, J.; and Morgan, M.: Propofol infusion for sedation in the intensive care unit: Preliminary report. Br. Med. J., 294:397–400, 1987.

Guyatt, G. H.; Tugwell, P.; Feeny, D. H.; Drummond, M. F.; and Haynes, R. B.: The role of before–after studies of therapeutic impact in the evaluation of diagnostic technologies. J. Chron. Dis., 39:295–304, 1986.

Hackmann, T.; Gascoyne, R. D.; and Naiman, S. C.: A trial of desmopressin (1-desamino-8-D-arginine vasopressin) to reduce blood loss in uncomplicated cardiac surgery. N. Engl. J. Med., 321(21):1437–1443, 1989.

Hasegawa, G. R.: Milrinone, a new agent for the treatment of congestive heart failure. Clin. Pharmacol., 5:201–205, 1986.

Heimann, G.: Renal toxicity of aminoglycosides in the neonatal period. Pediatr. Pharmacol., 3:251–257, 1983.

Henderson, I. S.; Beattie, T. J.; and Kennedy, A. C.: Dopamine hydrochloride in oliguric states. Lancet, 2:827–829, 1980.

Herbert, P.; and Tinker, J.: Inotropic drugs in acute circulatory failure. Intensive Care Med., 6:101–111, 1980.

Hilberman, M.; Maseda, J.; Stinson, E. B.; Derby, G. C.; Spencer, R. J.; Miller, D. C.; Oyer, P. E.; and Myers, B. D.: The diuretic properties of dopamine in patients after open heart operation. Anesthesiology, 61:489–494, 1984.

Holloway, E. L.; Palumbo, R. A.; and Harrison, D. C.: Acute circulatory effects of dopamine in patients with pulmonary hypertension. Br. Heart J., 37:482–485, 1975.

Hopkinson, R. B.; and Freeman, J. W.: Therapeutic progress-review XXX. Therapeutic progress in intensive care: Sedation and analgesia. Part I – Principles. J. Clin. Pharm. Ther., 13:33–40, 1988.

Janson, P. A.; Jubelirer, S. J.; Weinstein, M. J.; and Deykin, D.: Treatment of the bleeding tendency in uremia with cryoprecipitate. N. Engl. J. Med., 303:1318–1322, 1980.

Jardin, F.; Sportiche, M.; Bazil, M.; Bourokba, A.; and Margairaz, A.: Dobutamine: A hemodynamic evaluation in septic shock. Crit. Care Med., 9:329–332, 1981.

Jardin, F.; Gurdjian, F.; Desfords, P.; and Margalraz, A.: Effect of dopamine on intrapulmonary shunt fraction and oxygen transport in severe sepsis with circulatory and respiratory failure. Crit. Care Med., 7:273–277, 1979.

Jarnberg, P. O.; Bengtsson, L.; Ekstrand, J.; and Hamberger, B.: Dopamine infusion in man: Plasma catecholamine levels and pharmacokinetics. Acta. Anaesthesiol. Scand., 25:328–331, 1981.

Jobe, A.; and Michiko, I.: Surfactant for treatment of respiratory distress syndrome. Am. Rev. Resp. Dis., 136:1256–1275, 1987.

Kingsley, A. N.: Prophylaxis for acute stress ulcers: Antacids or cimetidine. Am. Surg., 51(9):545–547, 1985.

Klein, N. A.; Siskind, S. J.; Frishman, W. H.; Sonnenblick, E. H.; and LeJemtel, T. H.: Hemodynamic comparison of intravenous amrinone and dobutamine in patients with chronic congestive heart failure. Am. J. Cardiol., 48:170–175, 1981.

Kleinknecht, D.; Ganeval, D.; Gonzallez-Duque, L. A.; and Fermanian, J.: Furosemide in acute oliguric renal failure. A controlled trial. Nephron, 17:51–58, 1976.

Kobrinsky, N. L.; Letts, R. M.; Patel, L. R.; Israels, E. D.; Monson, R. C.; Schwartz, N.; and Cheang, M. S.: 1-Desamino-8-D-arginine vasopressin (desmopressin) decreases operative blood loss in patients having Harrington rod spinal fusion surgery. Ann. Intern. Med., 107:446–450, 1987.

Kopin, I. J.: Catecholamine metabolism and the biochemical assessment of sympathetic activity. Clin. Endocrinol. Metab., 6:525–549, 1977.

Kwong, M. S.; Egan, E. A.; Notter, R. H.; and Shapiro D. L.: Double-blind clinical trial of calf lung surfactant extract for the prevention of hyaline membrane disease in extremely premature infants. Pediatrics, 76:585–592, 1985.

Lacroix, J.; Infante-Rivard, C.; Jenicek, M.; and Gauthier, M.: Prophylaxis of upper gastrointestinal bleeding in intensive care units: A meta-analysis. Crit. Care Med., 17(9):862–869, 1989.

Laggner, A. N.; Lenz, K.; Base, W.; Drume, W.; Schneeweiss, B.; and Grimm, G.: Prevention of upper gastrointestinal bleeding in long term ventilated patients: sucralfate versus ranitidine. Am. J. Med., 86(suppl. 6A):81–84, 1989.

Larese, R. J.; and Mirkin, B. L.: Kinetics of digoxin absorption and relation of serum levels to cardiac arrhythmias in children. Clin. Pharmacol. Ther., 15:387–396, 1974.

Lassen, N. A.: Cerebral blood flow and oxygen consumption in man. Physiol. Rev., 39:183, 1959.

Layne, E. A.; Mellow, M. H.; and Lipman, T. O.: Insensitivity of guaiac slide tests for detection of blood in gastric juice. Ann. Intern. Med., 94:774–776, 1981.

Lefer, A. M.: Properties of cardioinhibitory factors produced in shock. Fed. Proc., 37:2734–2740, 1978.

Leier, C. V.; Weber, J.; and Bush, C. A.: The cardiovascular effects of the continuous infusion of dobutamine in patients with severe cardiac failure. Circulation, 56:468–472, 1977.

Ley, S. J.; Miller, K.; Skov, P.; and Preisig, P.: Crystalloid versus colloid fluid therapy after cardiac surgery. Heart Lung, 19(1):31–40, 1990.

Lindner, A.; Cutler, R. E.; Goodman, W. G.; Pansing, A. A.; and Knester, R.: Synergism of dopamine plus furosemide in preventing acute renal failure in the dog. Kidney Int., 16:158–166, 1979.

Livio, M.; Mannucci, P. M.; Vigano, G.; Mingardi, G.; Lombardi, R.; Mecca G.; and Remuzzi, G.: Conjugated estrogens for the management of bleeding associated with renal failure. N. Engl. J. Med., 315(12):731–735, 1986.

Livio, M.; Marchesi, D.; Remuzzi, D.; Gotti, E.; Mecca, G.; and deGaetano, G.: Uremic bleeding: Role of anemia and beneficial effects of red cell transfusions. Lancet, 2:1013–1015, 1982.

Liu, Y. K.; Kosfeld, R. E.; and Marcum, S. G.: Treatment of uremic bleeding with conjugated estrogen. Lancet, 2:887–890, 1984.

London, M. J.; Ho, J. S.; Triedman, J. K.; Verrier, E. D.; Levin, J.; Merrick, S. H.; Hanley, F. L.; Browner, W. S.; and Mangano, D. T.: A randomized clinical trial of 10% pentastarch (low molecular weight hydroxyethyl starch) versus 5% albumin for plasma volume expansion after cardiac operations. J. Thorac. Cardiovasc. Surg., 97(5):786–797, 1989.

Lucas, C. E.; Weaver, D.; Higgins, R. F.; Ledgewood, A. M.; Johnson, S. D.; and Bouwman, D. L.: Effects of albumin versus nonalbumin resuscitation on plasma volume and renal excretory function. J. Trauma, 18:564–570, 1978.

Luce, J. M.; Montgomery, A. B.; and Marks, J. D.: Ineffectiveness of high dose methylprednisolone in preventing parenchymal lung injury and improving mortality in patients with septic shock. Am. Rev. Respir. Dis., 138:62–68, 1988.

Mann, H. J.; Fuhs, D. W.; and Hemstrom, C. A.: Acute renal failure. Drug Intell. Clin. Pharm., 20:421–438, 1986.

Mannucci, P. M.; Remuzzi, G.; Pusineri, F.; Lombardi, R.; Valsecchi, C.; Mecca, G.; and Zimmerman, T. S.: Deamino-8-D-arginine vasopressin shortens the bleeding time in uremia. N. Engl. J. Med., 308(1):8–12, 1983.

McCracken, G. H.: Aminoglycoside toxicity in infants and children. Am. J. Med., 80:172, 1986.

McDonald, C. F.; Thomson, S. A.; Scott, N. C.; Grant, I. W. B.; and Crompton, G. K.: Benzodiazepine-opiate antagonism – A problem in intensive care therapy. Intens. Care Med., 12:39–42, 1986.

McGuire, G. P.; and Pearl, R. G.: Sepsis and the trauma patient. Overview of trauma, anesthesia and critical care. Crit. Care Clin., 6(1):121–146, 1990.

McNay, J. L.; McDonald, R. H.; and Boldberg, L.: Direct renal vasodilatation produced by dopamine in the dog. Circ. Res., 16:510, 1965.

Mentzer, R. M.; Alegre, C. A.; and Nolan, S. P.: The effects of dopamine and isoproterenol on the pulmonary circulation. J. Thorac. Cardiovasc. Surg., 71:807–814, 1976.

Mischler, J. M.; Hester, J. P.; Heustis, D. W.; Rock, G. A.; and Stravs, R. G.: Dosage and scheduling regimens for erythrocyte-sedimenting macromolecules. J. Clin. Apheresis, 1:130–143, 1983.

Moia, M.; Vizzotto, L.; Cattaneo, M.; Mannucci, P. M.; Casati, S.; and Ponticelli, C.: Improvement in the hemostatic defect on uremia after treatment with recombinant human erythropoietin. Lancet, 2:1227–1229, 1987.

Morselli, P. L.; Franco-Morselli, R.; and Bossi, L.: Clinical pharmacokinetics in newborns and infants. Clin. Pharmacokinet., 5:485–527, 1980.

Moss, G. S.; Lowe, R. J.; Jilek, J.; and Levine, H. D.: Colloid or crystalloid in the resuscitation of hemorrhagic shock: A controlled clinical trial. Surgery, 89:434–438, 1981.

Mueller, C. B.: Mechanism and use of mannitol diuresis in major surgery and in trauma. South Med. J., 59:408–410, 1966.

Myers, B. D.; Carrie, B. J.; Yee, R. R.; Hilberman, M.; and Michaels, A. S.: Pathophysiology of hemodynamically mediated acute renal failure in man. Kidney Int., 18:495–504, 1980.

Newman, L. H.; McDonald, J. C.; Wallace, G. M.; and Ledingham, I. M.: Propofol infusion for sedation in intensive care. Anaesthesia, 42:927–937, 1987.

Norfleet, R. G.; Rhodes, R. A.; and Saviage, K.: False positive "Hemoccult" reaction with cimetidine. N. Engl. J. Med., 302:467, 1980.

Noseworthy, T. R. W.; Shustack, A.; Johnston, R. G.; Anderson, B. J.; Konopad, E.; and Grace, M.: A randomized clinical trial comparing ranitidine and antacids in critically ill patients. Crit. Care Med., 15(9):817–819, 1987.

Noth, R. H.; McCallum, R. W.; Contino, C.; and Havelick, J.: Tonic dopaminergic suppression of plasma aldosterone. J. Clin. Endocrinol. Metab., 51:64–69, 1980.

Notterman, D. A.: Pediatric pharmacotherapy. In, The Pharmacologic Approach to the Critically Ill Patient (Chernow, B., ed.). Williams & Wilkins, Baltimore, pp. 131–155, 1988.

O'Neill, M. J.; Pennock, J. L.; Seaton, J. F.; Dortimer, A. C.; Waldhausen, J. A.; and Harrison, T. S.: Regional endogenous catecholamine concentration in pulmonary hypertension. Surgery, 84:140–146, 1978.

Pearl, R. G.; Halperin, B. D.; Mihm, F. G.; and Rosenthal, M. H.: Pulmonary effects of crystalloid and colloid resuscitation from hemorrhagic shock in the presence of oleic acid–induced pulmonary capillary injury in the dog. Anesthesiology, 68:12–20, 1988.

Pearl, R. G.; Rosenthal, M. H.; Schroeder, J. S.; and Ashton, J. P. A.: Acute hemodynamic effects of nitroglycerin in pulmonary hypertension. Ann. Intern. Med., 99:9–13, 1983.

Pinilla, J. C.; Oleniuk, F. H.; Reed, D.; Malik, B.; and Laveity, W. H.: Does antacid prophylaxis prevent upper gastrointestinal bleeding in critically ill patients? Crit. Care Med., 13:646–650, 1985.

Powell, H. R.; McCredie D. A.; and Rotenberg, E.: Response to furosemide in acute renal failure: Dissociation of renin and diuretic responses. Clin. Nephrol., 14:55–59, 1980.

Rawal, N.; and Tandon, B.: Epidural and intrathecal morphine in intensive care units. Intensive Care Med., 11:129–133, 1985.

Remuzzi, G.; Livio, M.; Marchiaro, G.; Mecca, G.; and de Gaetano, G.: Bleeding in renal failure: Altered platelet function in renal failure only partially corrected by hemodialysis. Nephron, 22:347–353, 1978.

Ridgen, S. P.; Dillon, M. J.; Kind, P. R. N.; De Leval, M.; Stark, J.; and Barratt, T. M.: The beneficial effect of mannitol on postoperative renal function in children undergoing

cardiopulmonary bypass surgery. Clin. Nephrol., 21:148–151, 1984.

Rieves, D.: Importance of symptoms in recognizing nitroprusside toxicity. South. Med. J., 77:1035–1037, 1984.

Roberto, R.; DeMillo, V.; and Sobel, B. E.: Deleterious effects of methylprednisolone in patients with myocardial infarction. Circulation, 53(suppl. 1):204, 1976.

Robie, N. W.; and Goldberg, L. I.: Comparative systemic and regional hemodynamic effects of dopamine and dobutamine. Am. Heart J., 90:340–345,1975.

Rocha, E.; Llorens, R.; Paramo, J. A.; Arcas, R.; Cuesta, B.; and Trenor, A. M.: Does desmopressin acetate reduce blood loss after surgery in patients in cardiopulmonary bypass? Circulation, 77:1319–1323, 1988.

Rock, P.; Silverman, H.; Plump, D.; Kecala, Z.; Smith, P.; Michael, J. R.; and Summer, W.: Efficacy and safety of naloxone in septic shock. Crit. Care Med., 13:28–33, 1985.

Rothschild, M. A.; Bowman, A.; Yalow, R. S.; and Berson, S. A.: Tissue distribution of I^{131}-labelled human serum albumin following intravenous administration. J. Clin. Invest., 34:1354–1358, 1955.

Rupp, W.: Pharmacokinetics and pharmacodynamics of Lasix. Scott. Med. J., 19:5–13, 1974.

Ryan, P.; Dawson, J.; Teres, D.; and Navab, F.: Continuous infusion of cimetidine versus sucralfate: Incidence of pneumonia and bleeding compared. Crit. Care Med., 18(4)(suppl): S253, 1990.

Safani, M.; Blair, J.; Ross, D.; Waki, R.; Li, C.; and Libby, G.: Prospective, controlled, randomized trial of naloxone infusion in early hyperdynamic septic shock. Crit. Care Med., 17:1004–1009, 1989.

Salzman, E. W.; Weinstein, M. J.; Weintrau, R. M.; Ware, J. A.; Thurer, R. L.; Robertson, L.; Donovan, A.; Gaffney, T.; Bertelle, V.; Troll, J.; Smith, M.; and Chute, L. E.: Treatment with desmopressin acetate to reduce blood loss after cardiac surgery. N. Engl. J. Med., 314(22):1402–1406, 1986.

Schafer, G. L.; Fink, M. P.; and Parrillo, J. E.: Norepinephrine alone versus norepinephrine plus low dose dopamine: Enhanced renal blood flow with combination pressor therapy. Crit. Care Med., 13:492–496, 1985.

Schumer, W.: Steroids in the treatment of clinical septic shock. Ann. Surg., 184:333–341, 1976.

Scholz, H.; Bruckner, R.; Mugge, A.; and Reupcke, C.: Myocardial alpha-adrenoceptors and positive inotropy. J. Mol. Cell Cardiol., 18(suppl. 5):79–87, 1986.

Schuster, D. P.; Rowley, H.; Feinstein, S.; McGue, M. K.; and Zuckerman, G. R.: Prospective evaluation of the risk of upper gastrointestinal bleeding after admission to a medical intensive care unit. Am. J. Med., 76:623–630, 1984.

Shine, K. I.; Kuhn, M.; Young, L.; and Tillisch, J. H.: Aspects of the management of shock. Ann. Intern. Med., 93:223–234, 1980.

Shires, G. T. III; Peitzman, A. B.; Albert, S. A.; Illner, H.; Silane, M. F.; Perry, M. O.; and Shires, G. T.: Response of extravascular lung water to intraoperative fluids. Ann. Surg., 197:515–519, 1983.

Shoemaker, W. C.: Comparison of the relative effectiveness of whole blood transfusions and various types of fluid therapy in resuscitation. Crit. Care Med., 4:71–78, 1976.

Shoemaker, W. C.; and Hauser, C. J.: Critique of crystalloid versus colloid therapy in shock lung. Crit. Care Med., 7:117–124, 1979.

Shuman, R. B.; Schuster, D. P.; and Zuckerman, G. R.: Prophylactic therapy for stress ulcer bleeding: A reappraisal. Ann. Intern. Med., 106:562–567, 1987.

Siskind, S. J.; Sonnenblick, E. H.; Forman, R.; Scheuer, J.; and LeJemtel, T. H.: Acute substantial benefit of inotropic therapy with amrinone on exercise hemodynamics and metabolism in severe congestive heart failure. Circulation, 64:966–973, 1981.

Skillman, J. J.; Lisbon, A.; Long, P. C.; and Silen, W.: 15(R)-15-methyl prostaglandin E_2 does not prevent gastrointestinal bleeding in seriously ill patients. Am. J. Surg., 147:451–455, 1984.

Sladen, R. N.; and Rosenthal, M. H.: Specific afterload reduction with parenteral hydralazine following cardiac surgery. J. Thorac. Cardiovasc. Surg., 72:195–202, 1979.

Smith, R.; and Kruszyna, H.: Toxicity of some inorganic antihypertensive anions. Fed. Proc., 35:69–72, 1976.

Sprung, C. L.; Caralis, P. V.; Marcial, E. H.; Pierce, M.; Gelbard, M. A.; Long, W. M.; Duncan, R. C.; Terdler, M. D.; and Karpf, M.: The effects of high dose corticosteroids in patients with septic shock: A prospective, controlled study. N. Engl. J. Med., 311(18):1137–1143, 1984.

Stein, L.; Beraud, J.; Cavanilles, J.; da Luz, P.; Weil, M. H.; and Shubin, H.: Pulmonary edema during fluid infusion in the absence of heart failure. J.A.M.A., 229:65–68, 1974.

Summer, W. R.; Michael, J. R.; and Lipsky, J. L.: Initial aminoglycoside levels in the critically ill. Crit. Care Med., 11: 948–950, 1983.

Swan, H. J. C.; Ganz, W.; Forrester, J.; Marcus, H.; Diamond, G.; and Chonette, D.: Catheterization of the heart in man with the use of a flow directed balloon tipped catheter. N. Engl. J. Med., 283:447–451, 1970.

Tomicheck, R. C.; Rosow, C. E.; Philbin, D. M.; Moss, J.; Teplick, R. S.; and Schneider, R. C.: Diazepam-fentanyl interaction—Hemodynamic and hormonal effects in coronary artery surgery. Anesth. Analg., 62:881–824, 1983.

Thompson, W. L.: Hydroxyethyl starch. In, Blood Substitutes and Plasma Expanders (Jamieson, G. A.; and Tibo, eds.). Alan R. Liss, New York pp. 283–292, 1978.

Tracey, K. J.; Fong, Y.; Hesse, D. G.; Manogue, K. R.; Lee, A. T.; Kuo, G. C.; Lowry, S. F.; and Cerami, A.: Anticachectin/tumour necrosis factor monoclonal antibodies prevent septic shock during lethal bacteremia. Nature, 330:662–664, 1987.

Tryba, M.: Risk of acute stress bleeding and nosocomial pneumonia in ventilated intensive care patients: sucralfate versus antacids. Am. J. Med., 83(suppl. 3B):117–124, 1987.

Turlapaty, P.; Laddu, A.; Murthy, S.; Singh, B.; and Lee, R.: Esmolol: A tritratable short-acting intravenous beta blocker for acute critical care settings. Am. Heart. J., 114(4):866–885, 1987.

Turner, J. M.; Powell, D.; Gibson, R. M.; and McDowall, D. G.: Intracranial pressure changes in neurosurgical patients during hypotension induced by sodium nitroprusside or trimethaphan. Br. J. Anaesth., 49:419–425, 1977.

Van Essen, H. A.; Van Blankenstein, M.; Wilson, P.; Vandenberg, B.; and Bruining, H. A.: Intragastic prostaglandin E₂ and the prevention of gastrointestinal hemorrhage in ICU patients. Crit. Care Med., 13(11):957–960, 1985.

Vesey, C. J.; and Cole, P. V.: Blood cyanide and thiocyanate concentrations produced by long-term therapy with sodium nitroprusside. Br. J. Anaesth., 57:148–155, 1985.

The Veterans Administration Systemic Sepsis Cooperative Study Group: Effect of high dose glucocorticoid therapy on mortality in patients with clinical signs of systemic sepsis. N. Engl. J. Med., 317:659–665, 1987.

Virgilio, R. W.; Rice, C. L.; Smith, D. E.; James, D. R.; Zarins, C. K.; Hobelmann, C. F.; and Peters, R. M.: Crystalloid versus colloid resuscitation. Is one better? A randomized clinical study. Surgery, 85:129–139, 1979.

Wallin, J. D.; and O'Neill, W. M.: Labetalol: Current research and therapeutic status. Arch. Intern. Med., 143:485–490, 1983.

Ward, A.; Brogden, R. N.; Heel, R. C.; Speight, T. M.; and Avery, G. S.: Amrinone: A preliminary review of its pharmacologic properties and therapeutic use. Drugs, 26:468–502, 1983.

Weaver, D. W.; Ledgerwood, A. M.; Lucas C. E.; Higgins, R.; Bouwman, D. L.; and Johnson, S. D.: Pulmonary effects of albumin resuscitation for severe hypovolemic shock. Surgery, 113:387–392, 1978.

Weigelt, L. A.; Aurbakken, C. M.; Gewertz, B. L.; and Snyder, W. H. III: Cimetidine versus antacid in prophylaxis for stress ulceration. Arch. Surg., 116:597–601, 1981.

Weimer, W.; Geerlings, W.; Bijnen, A. B.; Obertop, H.; van Urk, H.; Lameijer, L. D.; Wolf, E. D.; and Jeekel, J.: A controlled study of the effect of mannitol on immediate renal function after cadaver donor kidney transplantation. Transplantation, 35:99–101, 1983.

Westphal, L. M.; Cheung, E. Y.; White, P. F.; Sladen, R. N.; Rosenthall, M. H.; and Sung, M. L.: Use of midazolam infusion for sedation following cardiac surgery. Anesthesiology, 67:257–262, 1987.

Widdicombe, J. G.: Action of catecholamines on bronchial smooth muscle. In, Handbook of Physiology: Endocrinology Section VII, Volume 6, Chapter 32 (Blaskhko, H.; Sayers, G.; and Smith, D. A., eds.). American Physiology Society, Washington, D.C., pp. 507–513, 1975.

Williamson, K. L.; and Broadley, K. J.: Characterization of the alpha-adrenoreceptors mediating positive inotropy of rat left atria by use of selective agonists and antagonists. Pharmacodynamics, 285:181–198, 1987.

Yamazaki, T.; Shimada, Y.; Taenaker, N.; Oshumi, H.; Takezawa, J.; and Yoshiya, I.: Circulatory responses to afterload with phenylephrine in hyperdynamic sepsis. Crit. Care Med., 10:432–435, 1982.

Zaritsky, A. L.; and Chernow, B.: Catecholamines, sympathomimetics. In, The Pharmacologic Approach to the Critically Ill Patient (Chernow, B.; Lake, C. R., eds.). Williams & Wilkins, Baltimore, pp. 481–549, 1983.

Ziegler, E. J.; McCutchan, J. A.; Fierer, J.; Glauser, M. P.; Sadoff, J. C.; Douglas, H.; and Braude, A. I.: Treatment of gram negative bacteremia and shock with human antiserum to a mutant Escherichia coli. N. Engl. J. Med., 307:1225–1230, 1982.

Zinner, M. J.; Rypins, E. B.; Martin, L. R.; Jonasson, O.; Hoover, E. L.; Swab, E. A.; and Fakouhi, T. D.: Misoprostol versus antacid titration for preventing stress ulcers in postoperative surgical ICU patients. Ann. Surg., 210(5):590–595, 1989.

Zinner, M. J.; Zuidema, G. D.; Smith, P. L.; and Mignosa, M.: The prevention of upper gastrointestinal tract bleeding in patients in an intensive care unit. Surg. Gynecol. Obstet., 153:214–220, 1981.

27

Substance Abuse: Dependence and Treatment

Neal L. Benowitz

GENERAL CONSIDERATIONS: THERAPEUTIC ISSUES IN SUBSTANCE ABUSERS

At this stage in the book it should be clear that drugs alter body functions. While for the most part drugs are used to treat or prevent medical illness, those that have psychoactivity or other desirable effects may also be consumed for these effects in the absence of illness. The self-administration of drugs that alter mood is commonplace around the world and exemplified by the nearly ubiquitous consumption of caffeine in coffee, tea, or soft drinks.

Most drugs that are abused are abused primarily for their psychoactive effects. An exception is androgenic steroids that are used to enhance muscle mass and athletic performance. Most of this chapter will focus on the abuse of psychoactive drugs; androgenic steroids will be discussed in the concluding section of the chapter.

Pharmacologic processes in common to most drugs of abuse include rapid delivery of the drug from the dose form to the brain, psychoactivity

associated with the presence of the drug in the brain, neuroadaptation or the development of tolerance, and the development of withdrawal symptoms after regular use of a drug is discontinued.

Four therapeutic issues arise in treating substance abusers: intoxication, withdrawal syndromes, dependence-addiction, and medical complications.

Intoxication

With acute intoxication, most drugs of abuse can produce marked disturbances of CNS function and in many cases cardiovascular function; both can be life-threatening. Some drugs of abuse are associated with syndromes of subacute or chronic intoxication that may involve both CNS and systemic effects of the drug. An example is chronic abuse of cocaine with paranoid schizophrenia and cachexia.

Withdrawal Syndromes

After sustained exposure to a drug of abuse, particularly when there has been considerable

Table 27-1. AMERICAN PSYCHIATRIC ASSOCIATION (DSM-III-R) DIAGNOSTIC CRITERIA FOR PSYCHOACTIVE SUBSTANCE DEPENDENCE*

A. At least three of the following:
   1. Substance often taken in larger amounts or over a longer period than the person intended.
   2. Persistent desire or one or more unsuccessful efforts to cut down or control substance abuse.
   3. A great deal of time spent in activities necessary to get the substance (e.g., theft), taking the substance (e.g., chain smoking), or recovering from its effects.
   4. Frequent intoxication or withdrawal symptoms when expected to fulfill major role obligations at work, school, or home (e.g., does not go to work because hung over, goes to school or work "high," intoxication while taking care of his or her children), or when substance use is physically hazardous (e.g., drives when intoxicated).
   5. Important social, occupational, or recreational activities given up or reduced because of substance abuse.
   6. Continued substance use despite knowledge of having a persistent or recurrent social, psychological, or physical problem that is caused or exacerbated by the use of the substance (e.g., keeps using heroin despite family arguments about it, cocaine-induced depression, or having an ulcer made worse by drinking).
   7. Marked tolerance; need for markedly increased amounts of the substance (i.e., at least a 50% increase) in order to achieve intoxication or desired effect, or markedly diminished effect with continued use of the same amount.
   Note: The following items may not apply to cannabis, hallucinogens, or phencyclidine (PCP):
   8. Characteristic withdrawal symptoms.
   9. Substance often taken to relieve or avoid withdrawal symptoms.
B. Some symptoms of the disturbance have persisted for at least 1 month, or have occurred repeatedly over a longer period of time.

* From the DSM-III-R, 1987.

neuroadaptation, withdrawal of that drug may produce signs and symptoms that are highly disruptive or even life-threatening. In general, these *withdrawal symptoms are opposite to the effects of the drug that were initially sought by the user and to which tolerance had developed.* Withdrawal syndromes can be severe and challenging management problems, such as occurs with withdrawal from alcohol and sedative drugs, or may be subtle but play a critical role in maintaining addiction, such as with withdrawal from cocaine or nicotine.

Dependence-Addiction

Drug dependence has been defined by the World Health Association as "a behavioral pattern in which the use of a psychoactive drug is given sharply higher priority over other behaviors which once had significantly higher value" (Edwards et al., 1982). In other words, the drug has come to control behavior to an extent that is considered detrimental to the individual or to society. Specific criteria for drug dependence have been presented by the American Psychiatric Association (DSM-III-R, 1987) and in a recent Surgeon General's report: *The Health Consequences of Smoking—Nicotine Addiction* (Tables 27-1 and 27-2). Some clarification of terms is necessary. Drug addiction was at one time used to refer to drugs that produced clear physical dependence (i.e., symptoms of abstinence when use of the drug was discontinued) and produced damage not only to the individual but also to society. A proto-

typical drug of this sort was heroin. Drug addiction was distinguished from habituation in which there was thought to be psychologic dependence but no physical dependence and no damage to society. Examples of this class of drugs included cocaine and nicotine. However, subsequent investigation into the human pharmacology of these drugs revealed that the behavioral characteristics and strengths of drug use were similar, that physical dependence could be observed for most or all of these drugs, and that social damage accompanies individual damage. As a result, the distinction has been dropped. In this chapter, drug dependence and drug addiction are taken to be scientifically equivalent.

Table 27-2. CRITERIA FOR DRUG DEPENDENCE*

Primary Criteria
   Highly controlled or compulsive use
   Psychoactive effects
   Drug-reinforced behavior

Additional Criteria
   Addictive behavior often involves
      Stereotypical patterns of use
      Use despite harmful effects
      Relapse following abstinence
      Recurrent drug cravings
   Dependence-producing drugs often produce
      Tolerance
      Physical dependence
      Pleasant (euphoriant) effects

* From the Department of Health and Human Services, 1988.

Tolerance is referred to in various definitions of drug dependence. Tolerance indicates that a given dose of a drug produces less of an effect than that produced by the same dose on an earlier exposure and/or that larger doses are required to achieve the same effect. Tolerance can develop by several mechanisms. For the most part, tolerance to psychoactive drugs is pharmacodynamic tolerance, occurring as a consequence of changes in receptor function, activation of homeostatic mechanisms, and/or alterations of neural responsiveness. Other mechanisms that may contribute are metabolic tolerance, in which the rate of metabolism is accelerated with chronic use (for example, for alcohol or barbiturates), and behavioral tolerance, in which a person learns to compensate for a drug-induced impairment in a specific behavioral context.

For some drugs of abuse, such as for cigarettes, addiction is a major therapeutic issue faced by most practicing physicians. For other drugs, such as heroin, alcohol, and cocaine, addiction is a problem that is often dealt with secondarily to treatment of drug intoxication, drug withdrawal, or medical complications, but, in fact, addiction may be the underlying pharmacologic problem.

Medical Complications of Drug Abuse

In addition to the problems related to the pharmacology of the drugs as described above, drug abuse is associated with many medical complications. For example, cigarette smoking is responsible for 350,000 deaths per year that represent one of every six deaths in the United States (Department of Health and Human Services, 1989). These deaths are primarily from cancer, coronary artery disease, and chronic obstructive lung disease, but the pharmacologic culprit is tobacco or nicotine. Alcoholism is associated with many deaths from automobile accidents as well as alcoholic liver disease. Intravenous drug abuse, primarily heroin and cocaine, are associated with the spread of viral infections such as hepatitis B and AIDS and with bacterial infections that produce endocarditis, osteomyelitis, and local abscesses. Cocaine and other stimulants also produce injury to specific organs, such as myocardial infarction or stroke, as extensions of their primary pharmacologic actions. This chapter will focus on pharmacologic aspects of drug abuse.

PRINCIPLES OF TREATMENT OF SUBSTANCE ABUSE

Rational therapy of problems of drug abuse requires understanding of pharmacology and pathophysiology. Each of the therapeutic issues will be addressed.

Intoxication

Management of intoxication requires an understanding of the pharmacology of the offending drug. Intoxication with narcotics, alcohol, and sedative hypnotic drugs produces death primarily by respiratory depression. The mainstay of therapy is supportive care, such as assisted ventilation and cardiovascular resuscitation, as for any critically ill patient (see chapter 28). In some cases, specific antidotes, that is, receptor antagonists, are available. These include naloxone for narcotics and flumazenil for benzodiazepines. The use of these agents will be discussed later.

Intoxication with a stimulant drug such as with cocaine characteristically produces a picture of a sympathetic neural storm with hypertension, tachyarrhythmias, seizures, hyperthermia, and sometimes acute psychosis. Although no antidotes are available, treatment can be selected to reverse specific pharmacologic actions of the intoxicating drug. Treatment of intoxication by cocaine, for example, might include sympathetic blocking drugs to correct hypertension and arrhythmias. Other aspects of supportive care such as anticonvulsants, sedatives, and cooling are employed as needed (see chapter 28).

Withdrawal Syndromes

Syndromes of drug withdrawal represent the unopposed consequences of drug-induced neuroadaptation. That is, the brain has adapted to the effects of a drug to normalize brain function in the presence of the drug (associated with the development of tolerance), but in the absence of the drug the adaptive responses become maladaptive. The maladaptive response is often the opposite of the adaptive response. For example, excitation and agitation tend to occur during withdrawal from alcohol or other sedative drugs.

The extent and rate of development of tolerance depend on the concentrations of the drug and the duration of its presence in the brain. The higher the dose of the drug and the greater the half-life of the drug in the brain, the greater the extent of adaptation and the greater the magnitude of the potential withdrawal syndrome. Conversely, the faster a drug exits from the brain, the greater the magnitude of the withdrawal syndrome (Fig. 27–1).

The pharmacologic approaches to management of syndromes of drug withdrawal include treatment with an agonist drug that has a long half-life. Examples are methadone and diazepam for heroin and alcohol withdrawal, respectively. Patients may be stabilized on the appropriate dose of the substitute agonist; then the replacement therapy is gradually tapered. If tapering is done slowly enough, there is time for deadaptation,

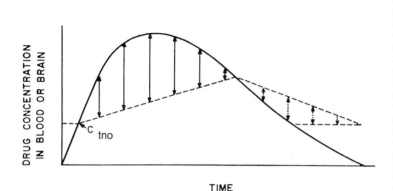

Fig. 27-1. Model for acute tolerance and withdrawal. The solid line indicates concentrations of a drug over time. The dashed line indicates the threshold concentration for drug effect, where C_{tno} is the threshold in the absence of prior exposure to the drug. The arrows indicate the magnitude of the effect of the drug. When the concentration of drug exceeds C_{tno}, neuroadaptation results in a rise in the threshold concentration and a lessening of the drug effect at any given concentration. When the concentration of drug falls below the threshold, deadaptation begins. The dashed arrows indicate the severity of the unresolved reaction (from Kalant et al., 1971, with permission).

and withdrawal symptoms are minimized. Of course, other aspects of supportive care such as nutritional and electrolyte therapy, management of seizures, and so forth, may also be necessary, depending on the patient and the type of addiction. In some cases, withdrawal syndromes may be primarily behavioral, such as the profound depression that may follow the use of a stimulant drug. An important concern with such patients is suicide, and an optimal therapy needs to address the potential for self-inflicted injury. ***Principle: As in the therapy of any serious disease, aim at the most morbid or mortal determinant even if it is not simply or specifically manageable.***

Addiction

Drug addiction is a complex process, involving an interplay of pharmacology, learned or conditioned factors, personality, and social setting. The elements will be briefly described, with the use of addiction to tobacco as an example. The pharmacologic reasons for drug use can be considered as enhancement (alteration) of mood or functioning. Drugs may directly enhance mood or may do so by relieving negative consequences of prior drug use, that is, the relief of withdrawal symptoms.

Pharmacologic actions of nicotine are involved in tobacco addiction in several ways: smokers report positive effects such as pleasure, arousal, and relaxation (Benowitz, 1988). Smoking may improve attention and reaction time and improve performance on certain tasks. Smokers may also experience the relief of aversive emotional states, including the reduction of anxiety or stress, relief from hunger and prevention of weight gain, and relief from symptoms of withdrawal from nicotine. Whether the positive rewards, that is, enhanced performance and mood after smoking, are due to relief of symptoms of abstinence or to an intrinsic enhancement effect of nicotine is unclear.

Taking a drug is a behavior that is strengthened (reinforced) by the consequences of the behavior, that is, the pharmacologic action of the drug, as discussed above. At the same time, the drug abuser begins to associate specific moods or situations or environmental factors with the rewarding effects of the drug. The association between such cues and anticipated drug effects and the resulting urge to use the drug is referred to as conditioning.

Cigarette smoking provides a nice example. People often smoke cigarettes in specific situations such as after a meal, along with a cup of coffee or an alcoholic beverage, or along with friends who smoke. The association between smoking and these other events repeated many times results in the environmental situation's becoming a powerful cue for the urge to smoke. Likewise, aspects of the drug-taking process, such as the manipulation of smoking materials, or the taste, smell, or feel of smoke in the throat, become associated with the pleasurable effects of smoking. Even unpleasant moods can become conditioned cues for smoking. For example, a smoker may learn that not having a cigarette provokes irritability (one of the common symptoms of the nicotine abstinence syndrome). Smoking a cigarette relieves the withdrawal symptom. After repeated experiences of this sort, the smoker may come to regard irritability from any source (such as stress or frustration) to be a cue for smoking. Although conditioning becomes an important element of drug addiction, it must be remembered that conditioning develops only because of the pairing of the pharmacologic actions of the drug with behaviors. Conditioning loses its power without the presence of an active drug. Hence, no one smokes nicotine-free cigarettes. *Principle: There are important analogies between withdrawal from addictive drugs and some toxicities of conventional drugs. When withdrawal produces the opposite effects from what was wanted in the first place, it is easy to understand the temptation for the patient and sometimes the therapist to give more drug. If one aspect of toxicity of some drugs is to mimic the indication for the drug in the first place (arrhythmias caused by antiarrhythmic agents; congestive heart failure caused by inotropic agents; infection caused by antibiotics, etc.), it is easy to see why giving more drug would be considered. In each case, yielding to the temptation to give more drug courts real trouble!*

Conditioning is a major factor that causes relapse to drug use after a period of cessation. It must be addressed as a component of behavioral therapy of drug addiction. *Principle: All too often as clinicians we focus on the drugs that can be used to counter problems caused by drugs to the exclusion of proper use of nonpharmacologic adjunctive measures that are key determinants of the efficacy of the antidote.*

Other factors in drug addiction include personality and social setting. Not every person experiments with drugs, and not everyone who experiments becomes addicted. Personality factors such as rebelliousness, risk-taking, and possibly affective disorders appear to increase the likelihood of addiction to drugs. There are no clear guidelines linking specific personalities with substance abuse. Interactions between drug abuse and a patient's personality need to be examined to design optimal treatment. Personal imagery may contribute to drug abuse, as seen, for example, in cigarette smoking by adolescents who view smoking as adult, sophisticated behavior or a behavior linked with physical attractiveness (such as the advertising image of slim, attractive women). Finally, sociologic factors may be determinants of substance abuse risk and drug-use patterns. Drug-taking behavior within a family or among friends is a strong motivator and reinforcer of drug use.

An understanding of the complexity of factors motivating drug addiction is essential to successful therapy. To optimally treat drug addiction, one may need to address both pharmacologic and behavioral processes. Pharmacologic treatments that have proved most successful have been substitution therapies in which the drug or a pharmacologically similar drug is provided by the physician in controlled doses to relieve the symptoms of drug withdrawal. Examples include nicotine chewing gum and methadone for cigarette smoking and heroin addiction, respectively. Other pharmacologic approaches may include aversive therapies such as disulfiram for alcoholism and receptor antagonist therapy such as naltrexone for addiction to heroin. However, drug addictions are not cured by pharmacologic agents. Substitution therapy of one drug or another is not the desired end point of therapy. A drug-free state on a long-term (years) basis in a patient who has a reasonable degree of peace of mind is the goal of treatment. Alcoholic or other drug-addicted patients may have no problem "stopping" for a short time (days to months), but they do have trouble "quitting."

Behavioral therapy is critical to the successful treatment of drug dependence. Behavioral therapies may address an individual's reasons for abusing a drug (i.e., personality factors, conditioned factors, etc.), may attempt to develop alternative lifestyles that do not include drug use, and/or may use social supports to induce and maintain cessation of drug use. Examples of behavioral therapies include individual or group psychotherapy, coping skills training to deal with urges to use drugs and ways to manage stress without the use of drugs, and development of social system supports, either within the family or among peers in voluntary groups, such as Alcoholics Anonymous (Alcoholics Anonymous, 1976, 1988). For addicted persons of low socioeconomic background with whom unemployment is a major problem, occupational training may be an important element of rehabilitation. A review of behavioral therapies for drug addiction is beyond the scope of this chapter. In general, multicomponent treatments addressing both behavioral and pharmacologic aspects of drug addiction are probably most effective.

Whatever the basis for addictive behavior is, there is no known "cure" at present, but adequate control of the behavior can be obtained with a variety of nonpharmacologic means, some probably more effective than others (Vaillant, 1983; Whitfield, 1988). A "personality" problem could lead to an ingestive addiction, and the converse may be true; this is a moot point. Psychiatric problems may coexist in patients with addictive behavior (Kranzler and Liebowitz, 1988). Whatever the cause may be, there can be no certainty about the diagnosis or opportunity for nonpharmacologic therapy to be effective until a drug-free state is attained and maintained for a long time, measured in months to years (DeSoto et al., 1985; Goldman, 1986; Kranzler and Liebowits, 1988; Schuckit et al., 1990).

Either the underlying problems that led to the ingestive addiction must be resolved or an adequate substitute for the psychologic effects of the ingested substance must be found for prolonged recovery in a reasonably peaceful patient to result. Let no one doubt that alcoholic and drug-addicted patients have will power. Consider the extremes of behavior to which they will go to obtain their substance of choice, despite full knowledge of the adverse effects of continued or renewed ingestion! Abstinence alone is a very painful (anxious, hostile, negative, depressed) state for the patient and all others in his or her environment, and is therefore rarely effective.

Stress reduction or substitute behaviors that permit sufficient serenity to allow long-term sobriety could include aversive techniques, physical exercise, intellectual means, "emotional" therapy, or "spiritual" endeavors. Aversive techniques (association of a painful or noxious stimulus with ingestion of the substance) are poorly studied and not tolerated for long, and long-term successes are probably fewer than 50% (Council on Scientific Affairs, 1987b). It is not practicable to run a marathon every day to obtain an endorphin-mediated "high" to forestall ingestion. Intellectual self-knowledge and a reasonable knowledge of the pharmacology of the substance involved does not prevent 10% of physicians from becoming addicted (Herrington et al., 1982; Southgate, 1986).

Treatment of drug abuse is often frustrating for physicians because of the poor success rate and the high rates of relapse among patients who briefly quit using a drug. As is true for other behavioral disorders, such as obesity, failed attempts to quit and relapse should be anticipated and dealt with in a supportive manner. For example, cigarette smokers typically require multiple attempts before they successfully quit. The physician can continue to remind the patient of the hazards of smoking and to try to rekindle motivation for another attempt to quit, while at the same time analyzing prior failures to develop alternative treatments for the next try.

Finally, primary prevention of drug addiction probably is the most effective approach to the drug addiction problem. Primary prevention such as in schools and other community-based antidrug programs benefits from the support and active participation of knowledgeable physicians. A relatively recent development in attempting to prevent drug abuse is work-site urine drug testing. The idea is that if a worker knows employment will be terminated if drugs are found in his or her urine, then drug abuse will be deterred. The practice has been controversial because of technical problems in performing and interpreting urine drug tests and because of invasion of personal privacy, particularly when there is no correlation between the results of the urine test and performance of work (Council on Scientific Affairs, 1987a). Nonetheless, the practice seems to be growing, and the reader is referred to recent reviews for more detailed information (Osterloh and Becker, 1990).

NICOTINE AND TOBACCO ADDICTION

Pharmacology

Tobacco contains thousands of chemicals. Nicotine is the chemical responsible for most of the pharmacologic actions of tobacco and for addiction (Benowitz, 1988). Tobacco contains (S)-nicotine, which binds to acetylcholine receptors at autonomic ganglia, the adrenal medulla, neuromuscular junctions, and the brain. Stimulation of nicotinic receptors in the brain, primarily acting on presynaptic sites, results in the activation of several CNS neurotransmitter systems. Nicotine also enhances systemic and local vascular release of catecholamines and causes release of vasopressin, cortisol, and β-endorphins.

The primary CNS effects of nicotine in smokers are arousal, relaxation (particularly in stressful situations), and enhancement of mood, attention, and reaction time, with improvement in performance of some behavioral tasks. Some or all of these effects may result from the relief of withdrawal symptoms in addicted smokers rather than a direct enhancing effect on the brain. Nicotine also suppresses appetite and increases metabolic rate, resulting in lower body weight in smokers compared with nonsmokers.

Smoking and nicotine also have sympathomimetic actions, producing brief increases in blood pressure, heart rate, and cardiac output, with cutaneous vasoconstriction. Nicotine causes muscle relaxation by stimulating discharge of the Renshaw cells and/or pulmonary afferent nerves, with inhibition of activity of motor neurons.

In most smokers, cessation of smoking results in the development of a withdrawal syndrome including restlessness, irritability, anxiety, drowsiness, frequent wakening from sleep, and confusion and/or impaired concentration. Some performance measures such as reaction time and attention may be impaired. Abstinent smokers also gain weight. The symptoms reach their maximum intensity at 24 to 48 hours after cessation and then gradually diminish over a period of a few weeks. That nicotine itself is responsible for the withdrawal symptoms is supported by the appearance of similar symptoms with sudden withdrawal from the use of chewing tobacco, snuff, or nicotine gum, and the relief of these symptoms by nicotine itself.

Pharmacokinetics and Metabolism

Nicotine in tobacco smoke is absorbed rapidly through the lungs. Nicotine is a weak base; absorption through mucous membranes depends on pH. Chewing tobacco, snuff, and nicotine gum are buffered at an alkaline pH to facilitate absorption through the buccal mucosa. Smoking is an effective form of drug administration in that the drug enters the circulation rapidly through the lungs and moves into the brain within seconds. Thus, high concentrations of the drug may be delivered to the brain very rapidly after a puff, which enhances the reinforcing properties of the drug. The smoking process also allows precise dose titration so that the smoker may obtain desired effects. It is not surprising that a number of substances of abuse, including marijuana, cocaine, opiates, phencyclidine, and organic solvents, are abused by the inhalational route because access to the brain is so direct. *Principle: Direct access to the brain via an inhalation route, plus the fact that the route allows a drug to escape the first-pass effect, makes deliberate use of this route of administration very attractive for drugs with high partition coefficients that are used for their effects in the CNS. Be alert to developments along these lines.*

Nicotine is rapidly and extensively metabolized by the liver, primarily to cotinine. The metabolite cotinine is widely used as a quantitative marker for exposure to nicotine and could be potentially useful as a diagnostic test for use of tobacco and compliance to a regimen for withdrawal from nicotine. The half-life of nicotine averages 2 to 3 hours. Thus, although there is considerable peak-to-trough oscillation in blood levels from cigarette to cigarette consistent with a half-life of 2 to 3 hours, nicotine accumulates in the body over 6 to 9 hours of regular smoking. Thus, smoking results not in intermittent and transient exposure to nicotine but in an exposure that lasts 24 hours a day. Persistence of nicotine in the brain results in changes in nicotinic receptors in the brain, and changes in receptor numbers or function are presumably the substrate for the syndrome of withdrawal from nicotine.

Pharmacodynamics

Two issues are particularly relevant to understanding the pharmacodynamics of nicotine. First, there is a complex dose–response relationship, so that low doses may stimulate while higher doses depress neural systems. For example, low doses of nicotine produce central or peripheral nervous system stimulation with arousal and an increase in heart rate and blood pressure, while nicotine intoxication produces ganglionic blockade and other effects resulting in bradycardia, hypotension, and depressed mental status. A second issue is the development of tolerance. Smokers know that tolerance develops to the dysphoria, nausea, and vomiting that often occur after one's first cigarette. Tolerance to subjective effects and acceleration of heart rate develop within the day in regular smokers. Thus, even within a single day, because of development of tolerance, the positive rewards of smoking diminish and smoking may become motivated more by relief of withdrawal symptoms.

Drug Interactions

Drug Metabolism. Cigarette smoking may interact with medications through effects on drug metabolism or pharmacodynamics. Smoking is well known to accelerate the metabolism of many drugs. Because there are more than 3000 components in cigarette smoke, it is difficult to know which ones are responsible for changes in drug metabolism. One likely group of chemicals is the polycyclic aromatic hydrocarbons. In animals, polycyclic aromatic hydrocarbons accelerate the metabolism of drugs by cytochrome P448 enzymes, in contrast to the effects of phenobarbital, which affects cytochrome P450 enzymes. Consequently, cigarette smoking and phenobarbital affect different drugs and different metabolic pathways.

Drugs whose metabolism is accelerated by cigarette smoking are listed in Table 27–3. An interaction of particular concern is that of cigarette smoking with theophylline. Smokers require, on average, a 50% larger than normal maintenance dose of theophylline because of a comparable increase in theophylline clearance. In a large survey, theophylline toxicity was found to be less common in cigarette smokers, a finding consistent with accelerated metabolism (Pfeifer and Greenblatt, 1978). Within 7 days of the beginning of abstinence from tobacco, the clearance of theophylline declines by an average of 35% (Lee et al., 1987). Thus, when smokers stop smoking, as, for example, during hospitalization for acute illness, the doses of theophylline may need

Table 27–3.   DRUGS WHOSE METABOLISM IS ACCELERATED AND DRUGS WHOSE METABOLISM IS UNCHANGED BY CIGARETTE SMOKING*

ACCELERATED METABOLISM	MINIMAL OR NO CHANGE IN METABOLISM
Antipyrine	Chlordiazepoxide
Caffeine	Codeine
Desmethyldiazepam	Dexamethasone
Flecainide	Diazepam†
Imipramine	Ethanol
Lidocaine	Lorazepam
Oxazepam	Meperidine
Pentazocine	Nortriptyline
Phenacetin	Oral contraceptives
Propranolol	Phenytoin
Theophylline	Pindolol
	Prednisolone
	Prednisone
	Quinidine
	Warfarin

* Adapted from Jusko, 1984.
† Metabolism of active metabolite is accelerated.

reduction to avoid the development of theophylline toxicity (see chapters 1, 7, and 40).

Drugs with a high degree of presystemic metabolism may be particularly affected by cigarette smoking. For such drugs, accelerated metabolism may result in a substantial decrease in bioavailability, which could result in subtherapeutic concentrations in blood. Examples of such interactions resulted in lower concentrations of propranolol in blood in the β Blocker Heart Attack Trial and reduced analgesic efficacy of pentazocine in cigarette smokers (Vaughan et al., 1976; Walle et al., 1985).

Pharmacodynamic Interactions. Several pharmacodynamic interactions arise from the hemodynamic effects of nicotine in cigarette smoke. For example, by reducing the blood flow to the skin and subcutaneous tissue, cigarette smoking may slow the absorption of insulin from subcutaneous sites. After one smokes a single cigarette, the diastolic blood pressure increases more after treatment with propranolol, a nonselective β blocker, than it does after treatment with placebo or atenolol, a cardioselective β blocker (Trap-Jensen et al., 1979). Presumably these effects are explained by the fact that nicotine releases epinephrine while propranolol blocks the β_2-mediated vasodilation, but not the α-adrenergic vasoconstriction. In patients with angina pectoris, the frequency of angina and the duration of exercise before the development of chest pain or electrocardiographic changes are improved by β blockers or nifedipine less when smoking than they are when not smoking (Deanfield et al., 1984). In the Medical Research Council Hypertension Trial, propranolol was less effective than was a thiazide diuretic in decreasing blood pressure and reducing the risk of stroke in smokers, whereas the drugs were equally effective in nonsmokers (Dollery and Brennan, 1988). Cigarette smoking and oral contraceptives may interact synergistically to increase the risk of stroke and premature myocardial infarction in women (Shapiro et al., 1979). Cigarettes appear to enhance the procoagulant effect of estrogens. For this reason, oral contraceptives are relatively contraindicated in women who smoke cigarettes.

Cigarette smokers experience less sedation than do nonsmokers from several drugs that act on the CNS, including diazepam, chlordiazepoxide, and chlorpromazine (Swett, 1974). Smoking probably acts by producing arousal of the CNS rather than by accelerating metabolism and reducing the brain levels of these drugs. The efficacy of analgesics such as propoxyphene may be reduced in cigarette smokers, even in the absence of pharmacokinetic interactions (Boston Collaborative Drug Surveillance Program, 1973). Cigarette smoking

is a major risk factor for the recurrence of peptic ulcer disease and the failure of treatment with antacids or H_2 blockers (Kikendall et al., 1984). *Principle: There may be more reasons to attempt to stop or at least reduce the use of addictive drugs that are unnecessary for therapeutics than simply to avoid their direct toxicities. The effects that they have on other diseases or the efficacy of therapy for those diseases may create separate legitimate goals for therapy. In such a setting, reducing the use of addictive drugs, even if complete cessation is not possible, may help with the incidence, severity, or manageability of other diseases!*

Clinical and Therapeutic Issues

Nicotine Intoxication. Acute intoxication with nicotine is uncommon in cigarette smokers but has been well described after accidental or suicidal exposure to nicotine containing pesticides or occupational exposure to tobacco leaves. Intoxication with nicotine results in nausea, vomiting, pallor, weakness, dizziness, lightheadedness, and sweating. More severe intoxication may result in hypotension, bradycardia, seizures, and respiratory arrest. Some of the peripheral manifestations such as bradycardia and hypotension appear to be mediated by release of acetylcholine and can be reversed by atropine. Theoretically, mecamylamine, a nicotinic (and ganglionic) antagonist that can penetrate the CNS, would reverse all aspects of nicotine toxicity; however, the medication (once used to treat hypertension) is now obsolete and is not readily available.

Addiction to Tobacco. Addiction to tobacco is best treated with behavioral therapies using pharmacologic therapy as an adjunct. The most successful pharmacologic therapy is nicotine chewing gum (Hughes and Miller, 1984). Nicotine gum chewing can generate blood levels of nicotine that are adequate to suppress symptoms of withdrawal from nicotine, thereby facilitating concurrent behavioral therapy. Because absorption of nicotine from gum is gradual, peak concentrations in the blood and brain are much lower and the rate of rise much slower than are those with smoking, and there is little of the arousal or euphoria that is expected from smoking a cigarette. Accordingly, the desire to smoke a cigarette, especially in stressful situations, may not be diminished by nicotine gum.

Nicotine gum is most effectively used after a smoker has quit smoking. In most trials, nicotine gum is used as part of a comprehensive program that includes behavioral therapy, as reported in smoking cessation centers. Nicotine gum enhances the success rate (for example, 27% for nicotine gum versus 18% for placebo) (Lam et al., 1987). However, in general medical practice, the gum is much less successful. This is probably because patients are less motivated and the physician or the health care workers are less experienced and spend less time with the patients. Part of the problem appears to be inadequate instructions from physicians on the use of gum (Cummings et al., 1988). In a recent trial conducted in smoking clinics, 4-mg nicotine gum was found to be more effective than 2-mg gum in highly dependent smokers, and this rate of effectiveness was found comparable to that obtained with 2-mg gum in smokers with a medium or low level of dependence (Tonnesen et al., 1988). Other trials find that nicotine gum is especially efficacious compared with placebo in highly dependent smokers (Blondal, 1989). The results of these studies suggest that, for optimal results, the dose of nicotine replacement may need to be individualized according to the severity of dependence. *Principle: Premarketing testing for efficacy of a drug is made under clinically stringent conditions. If the rates of efficacy in the field are less than those expected from the results of premarketing testing, look for factors in the ordinary management of the disease that limit the utility of the drug to less than its tested potential.*

In a practical approach to the use of nicotine gum, the rationale and expected results of the therapy should be discussed with the patient. An agreement should be made about when the patient will stop smoking. The gum is prescribed for use immediately after the patient stops. Instructions are given to chew the gum for 20 to 30 minutes whenever the urge to smoke arises, up to a maximum of 30 pieces per day. Patients should be told that the effects of nicotine from the gum develop gradually and will not provide the rapid satisfaction of a cigarette, but will reduce withdrawal symptoms and make it easier to quit.

Most people chew 10 to 15 pieces of gum per day. Chewing too few may result in inadequate doses of nicotine or therapeutic failure. Frequent office and telephone or letter follow-ups should be planned to provide ongoing information and support. The gum is typically used for 3 months, with gradual tapering once the patient feels secure in his or her ability not to smoke. Using the gum for too short a period also may contribute to therapeutic failure. Some people become dependent on nicotine gum; 13% to 38% of the patients treated continue to use the gum for 1 or more years despite advice to stop. We have no information on the health benefit of stopping smoking but continuing to use nicotine.

The use in the U.S. and parts of Europe of skin patches that deliver nicotine theoretically could provide nicotine to the patient in a manner quite different from nicotine gum. Whether these differences in pharmacokinetics of nicotine translate into alternate rates of efficacy or toxicity remains to be studied. So does the possibility of therapeutically using nicotine for other of its pharmacologic properties besides addiction.

Alternative approaches to replacement of nicotine that are currently under investigation include nicotine nasal spray and nicotine aerosols.

Other pharmacologic therapies may include the use of receptor antagonists (such as mecamylamine) or nonreceptor antagonists (such as clonidine). Mecamylamine reduces the satisfaction and other effects of cigarette smoking. In short-term trials it had the effect of making smokers smoke more, however, presumably to overcome the effects of blockade. Mecamylamine has been administered for up to 6 weeks in an open trial as an adjunct to treatment to help smokers stop smoking, but it will probably not be useful for most patients because of the potential complications of ganglionic blockade that include orthostatic hypotension, ileus, and urinary retention. Clonidine reduces the intensity of both the craving for tobacco and the symptoms of tobacco withdrawal, presumably by acting on the α_2-adrenergic receptors of the CNS. In one recent trial, clonidine treatment for 6 weeks was found to be more effective than placebo as an aid to smoking cessation, although the benefit was seen only in women (Glassman et al., 1988). Other trials have found no benefit, and an assessment of the utility and safety of clonidine for routine treatment awaits the results of recent large clinical trials. *Principle: When individual drugs with different mechanisms of action each are partially efficacious for an indication, look next for the effects of combinations.*

ETHANOL

Pharmacology

Ethanol acts on cell membranes, resulting in their fluidization. By effects on the local lipid environment, ethanol affects proteins that constitute receptors or enzyme systems, affects release of neurotransmitter, controls intracellular respiration, and affects cationic ion channels (Charness et al., 1989). Activation of γ-aminobutyric acid (GABA) stimulated chloride channels are a likely site for the ethanol-induced intoxication effect. Particular neural pathways seem to be essential for the reinforcing and neurologic effects of ethanol. Noradrenergic, dopaminergic, endogenous opioid, and serotonergic sites have been implicated in mediating the pleasurable effects of ethanol (Koob and Bloom, 1988).

Tolerance develops rapidly to the effects of ethanol. Mechanisms of tolerance include a theoretical "stiffening" of membranes so that ethanol results in less fluidization. Chronic ethanol use may also increase the number of excitatory postsynaptic receptors. Other studies show substantial tolerance to some but not all effects of ethanol and show environmental influences on tolerance, indicating that tolerance to specific neural pathways may also be involved.

Clinically, ethanol is a CNS depressant, although at lower doses there may be behavioral stimulation owing either to direct effects of the drug or to disinhibition. At moderate doses, the effect of ethanol is usually perceived as pleasurable. But higher doses produce CNS depression progressively affecting greater areas of the CNS (Table 27-4). These effects are described more fully in the section on alcohol intoxication.

Pharmacokinetics and Metabolism

The usual drink (one cocktail, 4-oz glass of wine, or 12-oz beer in the United States) contains 10 to 15 g of ethanol. Ethanol is well absorbed through the GI tract and is primarily metabolized by the liver. Metabolism is primarily by the cytoplasmic enzyme alcohol dehydrogenase (ADH), with a minor component being metabolized via liver microsomes (Fig. 27-2). Recently, the presence of ADH in the intestinal tract with evidence of intestinal first-pass metabolism of ethanol has been described (Frezza et al., 1990). The extent of first-pass metabolism seems to be greater in men than it is in women, with the result that women achieve higher concentrations of alcohol in blood with similar body weight–adjusted doses.

The major product of metabolism of alcohol is acetaldehyde, which in turn is metabolized by aldehyde dehydrogenase. A genetic deficiency in aldehyde dehydrogenase resulting in excess accumulation of acetaldehyde may explain flushing in some Orientals and other people, and not surprisingly because of the discomfort it engenders may be associated with a low risk of alcoholism (Suwacki and Ohara, 1985).

Table 27-4.   CLINICAL EFFECTS OF ETHANOL AT VARIOUS BLOOD CONCENTRATIONS

BLOOD ETHANOL CONCENTRATIONS (MG/DL)	CLINICAL EFFECTS
30–100	Mild euphoria, talkativeness Decreased inhibitions Impaired attention, judgment Mild incoordination, nystagmus
100–200	Emotional instability (excitement; withdrawal) Impaired memory, reaction time Loss of critical judgment Conjunctival hyperemia Ataxia, nystagmus, dysarthria Hypalgesia
200–300	Confusion, disorientation, dizziness Disturbed perception, sensation Diplopia, dilated pupils Marked ataxia, dysarthria
300–400	Apathy, stupor Decreased response to stimuli Vomiting, incontinence Inability to stand or walk
Over 400	Unconsciousness, coma Anesthesia Decreased or abolished reflexes Hypothermia Hypoventilation Hypotension Death (respiratory arrest)

After absorption, alcohol is distributed in body water with a volume of distribution of about 0.6 l/kg. Elimination of ethanol follows mostly zero-order kinetics, that is, the rate of elimination, about 7 to 10 g/h, is independent of concentration of the ethanol in blood. For a typical adult, blood alcohol concentration declines at a rate of 15 mg/dl per hour, a calculation that is widely used in forensic medicine to back-extrapolate to alcohol concentrations in blood at earlier times,

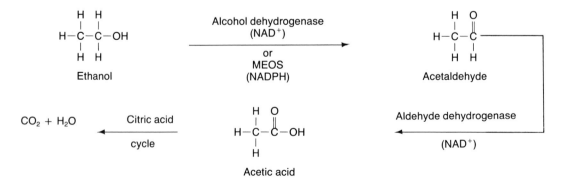

Fig. 27-2.   Metabolism of ethanol. MEOS = microsomal enzyme oxidizing system.

such as at the time of an automobile accident. The rate of alcohol metabolism is considerably faster in chronic alcoholics.

Pharmacodynamics

The primary acute effects of alcohol are on the CNS. The relationship between blood alcohol concentration and effects is summarized in Table 27–4. The relationship is influenced by the degree of tolerance that is present and by the rate of rise of alcohol in the blood and brain. Thus, the degree of ethanol intoxication is greater when levels are rising than it is when it is falling. Ethanol also relaxes smooth muscle, resulting in vasodilation and reduction of uterine contractility, the latter effect having historically been used to control premature labor. While alcohol can acutely vasodilate and reduce blood pressure, chronic consumption of alcohol is associated with elevation of blood pressure. The mechanisms are not clear.

With regular consumption of ethanol, considerable tolerance develops to its CNS effects. Thus, a chronic alcoholic may function normally at a blood alcohol concentration of 500 mg/dl, a concentration that could cause death in a nonalcoholic.

Drug Interactions

Chronic consumption of alcohol is associated with accelerated hepatic microsomal metabolism of a number of drugs, including warfarin and hypoglycemic sulfonylureas, although acute alcohol intoxication may inhibit drug metabolism. The most important interactions with ethanol involve excessive sedation when ethanol is used with sedative hypnotic drugs, antidepressants, neuroleptic drugs, sedating antihistamines, or narcotics. This combination is of particular concern when motor skills such as driving an automobile or operating machinery are required. Alcohol may also potentiate the effects of hypoglycemic drugs and enhance the risk of aspirin-induced gastritis. The alcohol–disulfiram interaction is described below.

Clinical and Therapeutic Issues

Acute Intoxication. The dose-dependent progression of neural depression, as listed in Table 27–4, can be viewed as similar to that observed for anesthetics. At lower concentrations, inhibitory polysynaptic influences are inhibited, resulting in cortical disinhibition with the associated changes in mood and cognitive function. At greater levels of intoxication, neural activity is depressed, resulting in cerebellar dysfunction, delirium, or coma. Death may ensue from respiratory depression. Death has occurred at blood alcohol concentrations as low as 400 mg/dl, while

survival at concentrations greater than 700 mg/dl also has been described.

Hypoglycemia may be a cause of coma in alcoholic patients. Since alcohol blocks gluconeogenesis, the combination of alcohol consumption (even at moderate levels) plus fasting may lead to hypoglycemia and loss of consciousness. Children, or people with chronic liver disease, are particularly susceptible to alcohol-induced hypoglycemia.

The treatment of an alcohol-intoxicated patient is primarily supportive, with specific attention placed on maintaining a patent airway, assisting ventilation if necessary, and treatment of hypoglycemia (see chapter 28). Intravenous fructose can increase the rate of ethanol metabolism by about 25%; however, since patients do quite well with supportive care and because fructose is potentially toxic, such treatment is not recommended.

Alcohol Withdrawal. The severity of symptoms of alcohol withdrawal is related to the amount and the duration of prior consumption of alcohol. Alcohol withdrawal symptoms occur not only after abrupt cessation of use but may be seen even with reduction in the daily level of intake of alcohol.

The clinical manifestations of alcohol withdrawal are shown in Table 27–5. Minor or early symptoms are typically observed for up to 48 hours after cessation of consumption of alcohol, with a peak intensity observed at 24 hours. Minor withdrawal typically presents with one or more of three signs: tremulousness, hallucinations, and seizures. Major or late withdrawal typically

Table 27–5. CLINICAL FEATURES OF ALCOHOL WITHDRAWAL

MINOR (EARLY WITHDRAWAL)	MAJOR (LATE WITHDRAWAL)
Tremulousness	Delirium tremors
Coarse action tremor	Extreme agitation
Irritability, restlessness	Appears frightened,
Anxiety, agitation	confused
Insomnia	Hallucinations
Anorexia, vomiting	Disorientation
Diaphoresis	Disordered sensory per-
Tachycardia	ception
Mild hypertension	Marked autonomic hy-
Hallucinosis	peractivity
Visual most common	Dilated pupils
Patient remains ori-	Tachycardia
ented	Hypertension
Seizures	Fever
Grand mal	
Multiple seizures	
common	

occurs from 1 to 6 days after the cessation of drinking and is characterized by profound agitation, insomnia, hallucinations or delusions, tremor, hypertension, tachycardia, and hyperthermia. Because disorientation and confusion are commonly present, the syndrome is referred to as delirium tremens. This syndrome carries substantial morbidity and mortality owing primarily to concurrent infection, pancreatitis, trauma, or heart disease. Cardiac arrhythmias are common and may be the cause of sudden death.

Seizures generally occur from 6 to 30 hours after cessation of drinking, with a peak occurrence from 12 to 24 hours. Of note is that seizures and other manifestations of withdrawal from alcohol can be delayed in onset by the administration of sedative hypnotic or anesthetic drugs, as is often the case when alcoholic patients are admitted to the hospital for trauma or elective surgery. Usually seizures are self-limited, but status epilepticus occasionally develops. One recent study suggests that seizures commonly occur during drinking and that the probability of seizures is in proportion to amount of alcohol consumption and not to abstinence (Ng et al., 1988). These data suggest that alcohol may have a direct cortical effect to induce seizures.

The primary objectives of treatment of withdrawal from alcohol are relief of symptoms, prevention or treatment of more serious complications, and preparation for long-term rehabilitation. Hospitalization is necessary on medical grounds for a minority of patients undergoing alcohol withdrawal (Whitfield et al., 1978; Naranjo et al., 1983). The need for inpatient therapy for the usual 28-day programs of initial detoxification is open to question since the 1-year abstinence rate for the program without follow-up care is in the range of 10% to 40% (Anderson, 1978; Pickens et al., 1985; Stockwell et al., 1986; Holden, 1987; Hayashida et al., 1989).

Management of more severe alcohol withdrawal consists of supportive care and specific pharmacotherapy. Supportive care includes administration of glucose, hydration, correction of electrolyte abnormalities, adequate nutrition, and appropriate reassurance. Thiamine is routinely given to prevent the development of Wernicke encephalopathy (which may be precipitated by IV glucose) (see chapter 10). For mild alcohol withdrawal, supportive care may be sufficient. For more severe withdrawal, pharmacotherapy is indicated.

Pharmacotherapy is designed to replace alcohol with a sedative drug that can then be tapered in a controlled manner. A number of sedative drugs have been evaluated (Sellers and Kalant, 1976). Benzodiazepines are the drugs of choice because they are effective and less toxic than are the alternatives: phenothiazines, barbiturates, or paralde-

hyde. All benzodiazepines appear to be effective. A logical approach is to load a patient with a long-acting benzodiazepine such as diazepam or chlordiazepoxide until sedation is achieved, and then to taper at 25% to 50% per day. Because of long half-lives of these drugs and their metabolites, the levels of drug in the body will decline gradually (even in the absence of tapering) to provide a gradual withdrawal with relatively few symptoms of abstinence over many days.

A typical drug regimen is diazepam, 20 mg IV or p.o., or chlordiazepoxide, 100 mg p.o., each hour until the patient is mildly sedated. Commonly, 40 to 80 mg of diazepam or equivalent doses of chlordiazepoxide are required, although in some cases enormous doses (1000 mg or more IV diazepam) may be required for sedation (Woo and Greenblatt, 1979). Following initial loading, no more diazepam may be required, as its concentration declines with a half-life of 40 to 50 hours, or longer in patients with cirrhosis.

In patients with severe cirrhosis, who metabolize the long-acting benzodiazepines very slowly and may, particularly with prior hepatic encephalopathy, be extraordinarily sensitive to the sedative effects of benzodiazepines, it is preferable to administer shorter-acting benzodiazepines to treat alcohol withdrawal. Some benzodiazepines like lorazepam and oxazepam are metabolized primarily by conjugation, and their metabolism is not impaired in the presence of alcoholic cirrhosis.

Alcohol-induced hallucinations may be better controlled with haloperidol, 0.5 to 2.0 mg every 2 hours, although benzodiazepines may also be administered to provide some protection against convulsions (Kaim et al., 1969). Seizures usually respond to diazepam. It has been common to follow this with a loading dose of phenytoin (1000 mg IV); however, a recent placebo-controlled trial found no effect of phenytoin treatment after an alcohol withdrawal seizure on the risk of later, recurrent seizures (Alldredge et al., 1989). In alcoholic patients with their first seizure or those presenting with focal seizures, a workup for structural lesions should be performed. Seizures in alcoholic patients do not usually indicate epilepsy and do not require prolonged anticonvulsive therapy.

β Blockers or clonidine reduce adrenergic manifestations of withdrawal from alcohol such as hypertension, tachycardia, and tremor. A recent study indicates that atenolol reduces alcohol withdrawal symptoms and slightly shortens the hospital stay for patients with mild withdrawal (Kraus et al., 1985). However, β blockers and clonidine are potentially toxic; the β blockers may aggravate asthma or chronic lung disease, and both can precipitate hypotension or cardiac failure, particularly in patients with more severe withdrawal. On balance the modest benefits seem to be outweighed by the considerable and potentially life-threatening risks, so the routine use of these drugs that antagonize the sympathetic elements of withdrawal from alcohol is not encouraged.

Alcoholism. Considering lifetime prevalence, alcohol abuse-dependence is the most common among psychiatric diagnoses, affecting 11% to 16% of the U.S. population (Robins et al., 1984). Alcoholism results in disability and premature death both from its medical complications and by promoting accidents. While alcoholism has been defined in various ways, the most useful definition for the physician is based on the development of significant social or health problems related to alcohol use. Social problems may include marital difficulties, job loss, abuse of spouse or children, and drunk-driving arrests. Medical complications include alcoholic liver disease, pancreatitis, cardiomyopathy, neurologic disorders, or an alcohol withdrawal syndrome that may first appear when a person is hospitalized for some unrelated medical problem. Biochemical tests that suggest alcohol abuse include elevation of uric acid concentrations, mean corpuscular volume, and/or concentrations of liver enzymes in the blood, particularly γ-glutamyltransferase (GGT) and serum aspartate aminotransferase (AST).

The treatment of alcoholism begins with recognition of the problem. Some people will stop or limit their drinking when abuse becomes apparent, such as after counseling by a physician. Various forms of psychiatric, psychologic, or sociologic approaches afford some relief for many alcoholic patients (Stinson et al., 1979; Goldman, 1986). Patients should be encouraged to ask potential therapists about the therapist's interest in addictive disorders and his or her success in managing such patients before embarking on a long and expensive program of individual therapy. Most communities have alcoholism treatment programs. Prolonged abstinence (more than 1 year) is facilitated by participation in groups such as Alcoholics Anonymous (A.A.) (Vaillant et al., 1983; Collins et al., 1985). These groups provide intellectual, emotional, and spiritual guidance to the recovering. Many members of A.A. choose to attend meetings several times weekly, for life. A group of recovering physicians ranked A.A. as the most influential of the modalities contributing to their recovery, more so than they did 3 months of transitional residence, counseling, family commitments, monitoring by their peers, and the desire to return to work (Galanter et al., 1990). Alcoholics Anonymous has been likened to "cults and zealous self-help movements" (Galanter, 1990). This comparison is unwarranted as A.A. does not advocate any particular religion, and its 12th step encourages people to "practice these principles in all our affairs," that is, the world

outside A.A. (Alcoholics Anonymous, 1976, 1988). The service is easily available (see the white pages of a telephone book) and free. A detailed review of alcohol treatment programs and other forms of behavioral therapy is beyond the scope of this chapter.

Medications *do not play a major role in the treatment of alcoholism*, and, in fact, sedative hypnotic drugs should be avoided, if possible, as there is a substantial risk of additional abuse of these drugs. ***Principle: There is true pathos in the clinician who feels that there is no treatment but that found in the use of drugs, devices, or procedures. This is especially poignant when nonmedical structures have provided the proof that nonpharmacologic alternatives work.***

Disulfiram (Antabuse) may be used as an adjunct to treating alcoholism. Disulfiram chelates metal ions that are cofactors for enzymes such as ADH and dopamine β-hydroxylase (DBH). After consumption of alcohol, inhibition of ADH results in accumulation of acetaldehyde with symptoms of flushing, headache, nausea, vomiting, and hypotension. Inhibition of DBH, the enzyme responsible for conversion of dopamine to norepinephrine, may result in impaired cardiovascular reflexes that contribute to the development of hypotension. The disulfiram–alcohol reaction may be quite severe; fatalities have occurred. As the effects of alcohol in the presence of disulfiram are aversive, alcoholic patients taking the drug avoid drinking alcohol. Patients must also be counseled about other sources of ethanol including mouthwashes, cough syrups, and cold preparations. Disulfiram is taken daily (usual dose 250 mg). Psychologically, taking the daily dose of disulfiram represents a commitment not to drink and is especially useful for the impulsive drinker. Therapy is maintained for a period up to 1 year, during which behavioral therapy is ongoing.

Serious adverse effects of disulfiram in addition to the alcohol–disulfiram reactions include optic neuritis, peripheral neuropathy, seizures, and hepatitis. Aggravation of chronic psychosis is a side effect of interest in that a mechanism may be inhibition of DBH with a resultant increase in dopamine in the brain. A recent trial in a large group of alcoholic veterans suggests that disulfiram is not very effective for most alcoholic patients (Fuller et al., 1986). In light of its toxicity and low level of efficacy, disulfiram should be reserved for alcoholic patients who are impulsive, highly motivated drinkers.

SEDATIVE-HYPNOTICS

Pharmacology

The sedative-hypnotic drugs of most clinical importance are the barbiturates and benzodiazepines. Barbiturates and benzodiazepines potentiate the actions of the inhibitory neurotransmitter GABA (Eldefrawi and Eldefrawi, 1987), which exerts its effects by increasing chloride ion conductance through the neuronal membrane chloride channel. Barbiturates may act by enhancing the binding of GABA to its receptor site on the membrane, possibly by decreasing the rate of dissociation of GABA from its receptor. In high concentrations, barbiturates may depress calcium-dependent action potentials and enhance chloride conduction in the absence of GABA. Barbiturates act throughout the brain but affect polysynaptic transmission and the reticular activating system at relatively low concentrations, so these sites are most sensitive to the actions of barbiturates.

The action of benzodiazepines appears to be mediated by a receptor on the $GABA_A$–chloride ionophore complex that is distributed on postsynaptic neurons in the CNS. By increasing chloride flux, GABA hyperpolarizes cell membranes and inhibits neuronal firing. Benzodiazepines potentiate the effects of GABA on the chloride flux and thereby enhance the inhibitory neurotransmitter effects of GABA.

Long-term treatment with benzodiazepines in animals is associated with down-regulation of brain binding that is associated with the development of behavioral tolerance (Miller et al., 1987a). Conversely, discontinuation of benzodiazepines is associated with up-regulation of receptor binding and function of the GABA-receptor complex (Miller et al., 1987b).

The pharmacokinetics, metabolism, and drug interactions of sedative-hypnotics are described in chapters 12 and 13.

Pharmacodynamics

With increasing concentrations of sedative drugs, there is a progression of signs and symptoms in overdose as summarized in Table 27–6. As was the case for ethanol, tolerance develops rapidly to the depressant effects of sedative hypnotic drugs.

Clinical and Therapeutic Issues

Acute Intoxication. Sedative-hypnotic drugs are commonly abused and often involved in intentional drug intoxications. Although barbiturates and benzodiazepines are the most important drugs in this class, other drugs that are occasionally abused include chloral hydrate, ethchlorvynol, glutethimide, meprobamate, methaqualone, and methyprylon. For the most part, therapeutic considerations for the latter group resemble those for barbiturates.

Ingestion of excessive quantities of barbiturates results in a progressive metabolic encephalopathy

Table 27–6.   SEDATIVE-HYPNOTIC DRUG INTOXICATION

INTOXICATION LEVEL	CLINICAL SYMPTOMS
Mild	Sedation
	Disorientation
	Slurred speech
	Ataxia
	Nystagmus
Moderate*	Coma; arousal by painful stimulation
	Depressed or absent deep tendon reflexes
	Slow respiration
	Absent oculocephalic reflexes
	Intact pupillary light reflex
Severe	Coma; unarousable
	Absent corenal, gag, and deep tendon reflexes
	Absent oculocephalic reflexes
	Intact pupillary light reflex
	Hypothermia
	Respiratory depression; apnea
	Hypotension; shock

* May observe in the early phase of intoxication in occasional patients a state of neuromuscular hyperexcitability with increased muscle tone, hyperactive reflexes, ankle clonus, and/or decerebrate posturing.

and coma. The signs and symptoms of barbiturate intoxication are summarized in Table 27–6. Intoxication with other sedative-hypnotic drugs produces a similar picture with a few distinctions. Benzodiazepine intoxication is less likely to be associated with respiratory depression or hypotension, unless there is a coingestion of other sedative drugs or alcohol, or after the drug is absorbed extremely rapidly (as occurs with respiratory arrest following IV diazepam or midazolam or oral triazolam).

The time course of sedative-hypnotic drug intoxication depends on the pharmacokinetics of the particular drug. For intermediate-acting barbiturates such as pentobarbital, secobarbital, or amobarbital, and many of the benzodiazepines, intoxication usually resolves within 48 hours. Long-acting barbiturates such as phenobarbital, benzodiazepines such as flurazepam, or ethchlorvynol (the latter of which exhibits dose-dependent metabolism) are associated with prolonged coma that may persist as long as 5 to 7 days. Glutethimide has associated waxing and waning of consciousness, due either to its anticholinergic effects producing intermittent bowel activity and absorption or to enterohepatic recirculation of an active metabolite (see chapter 28).

The management of overdoses of sedative drugs centers on respiratory and cardiovascular support (see chapter 28). Most patients supported with appropriate, nonspecific intensive care recover fully even in the face of prolonged coma. Occasionally it is desirable to shorten the course of coma in a patient with pulmonary edema, respiratory tract infection, severe hypotension, or other life-threatening medical illness. This may be done for certain drugs by hemodialysis (chloral hydrate, phenobarbital) or hemoperfusion (phenobarbital, short-acting barbiturates, ethchlorvynol). Repeated doses of oral charcoal accelerate the elimination of phenobarbital by interrupting enteroenteric recirculation but in one study did not shorten the duration of phenobarbital-induced coma (Pond et al., 1984). In that study, patients awakened at a similar time after acute intoxication even though the blood concentrations of drug were lower in the group receiving charcoal treatment. Most likely this is because tolerance had developed to the high concentration of barbiturate in the untreated group.

A specific antagonist to benzodiazepines has recently been developed. Its role in the management of intoxication is not yet defined. Flumazenil binds to benzodiazepine receptors, stabilizes the receptors, and thereby reverses sedation and coma caused by benzodiazeopines. Clinical trials in patients with mixed overdoses involving benzodiazepines showed significant improvement in coma scores within 5 minutes when treated patients were compared with placebo controls (O'Sullivan and Wade, 1987). The dose was titrated into 0.2- to 0.3-mg increments to a total of 1 mg IV over approximately 5 minutes. A major hazard in using flumazenil is precipitation of acute withdrawal from benzodiazepine, including seizures. The duration of action of flumazenil is relatively short (half-life 60–90 minutes) compared with the duration of action of many of the benzodiazepines; repeated doses may be necessary to maintain stable reversal of intoxication. Of concern is the possibility that intoxication with benzodiazepine will be reversed with flumazenil, then the patient will be left unattended, the flumazenil will be eliminated more quickly than the benzodiazepine, and the patient will decompensate and suffer respiratory arrest. For this reason, even with the availability of an antagonist, it is necessary to manage serious benzodiazepine overdoses with careful consistent observation and intensive supportive care. *Principle: When the half-life or duration of action of an antidote (antagonist) is considerably shorter than that of the agent causing toxicity, dosing becomes crucial to prevent the morbidity of swings in and out of toxicity. Consider the use of antagonists of opiates, and cholinergic agonists as additional examples of this principle.*

Sedative-Hypnotic Drug Withdrawal. Habitual use of sedative-hypnotic drugs is associated with the development of tolerance. When use of these drugs suddenly ceases, a withdrawal syndrome similar to that of alcohol withdrawal ensues. In general, patients with serious withdrawal syndromes have a history of taking three or more times the usual sedative dose daily for longer than 1 month. However, milder syndromes of abstinence may occur after cessation of usual therapeutic doses (Busto et al., 1986).

The clinical manifestations are similar to those described for alcohol withdrawal, although the incidence of seizures may be higher after withdrawal from high doses of barbiturates (Fraser et al., 1958). Most patients experience anxiety, irritability, agitation, tremor, muscle twitching, insomnia, anorexia, and/or weakness during abstinence. Many develop generalized seizures with or without a subsequent state of delirium. Some patients develop an acute psychosis or delirium without seizures. The time course of withdrawal symptoms depends on the pharmacokinetics of the drug involved. Following cessation of pentobarbital, secobarbital, or amobarbital (half-lives 20 to 24 hours), symptoms usually begin within 8 to 12 hours. The time to peak is 2 to 3 days, and symptoms persist for 6 to 7 days. For phenobarbital and diazepam, with half-lives of 50 to 100 hours or more, symptoms of withdrawal tend to develop 5 to 7 days after cessation of drug use and may persist for several weeks. In general, the severity of abstinence symptoms is greater after cessation of short-half-life than after cessation of long-half-life drugs, consistent with the idea that the brain has more time to adapt to changing drug effects when the rate of decline of the concentration of the drug is gradual. *Principle: In general, signs of withdrawal of potent drugs, whether they act on the CNS or peripheral organs, are more likely to occur with short-acting rather than they are with long-acting drugs. The principal rationale behind "tapering" the doses of such drugs with short half-lives rests on this observation. Consider examples of antihypertensives.*

Severe withdrawal symptoms from barbiturates are most commonly seen in patients who abuse many drugs simultaneously (polydrug abusers). In contrast, withdrawal symptoms from benzodiazepines are most commonly seen in patients who are being treated for chronic psychiatric disturbances or anxiety. Once again a drug can cause toxicity that mimics the original signs and symptoms that signaled reason for its use. The anxiety and agitation seen during withdrawal from benzodiazepines may resemble the original condition for which the drug was taken, thereby unfortunately reinforcing chronic use of even more drug. Some patients develop considerable apprehension about the idea of withdrawal from benzodiazepines and may develop anxiety on that basis alone (pseudowithdrawal) (Roy-Byrne and Hommer, 1988).

Treating withdrawal signs and symptoms from sedative-hypnotics requires replacement with a sedative-hypnotic drug, followed by subsequent gradual tapering of the dose. Many approaches have been described (Roy-Byrne and Hommer, 1988). Selection of long-acting drugs such as phenobarbital for barbiturate and diazepam for benzodiazepine dependence is reasonable and effective in managing the syndrome (Robinson et al., 1981; Harrison et al., 1984). Typically, such schedules involve loading with a long-acting sedative-hypnotic drug until the symptoms of withdrawal are controlled. Then the patient is stabilized on this dose for a few days, and later the replacement drug is withdrawn at a rate of 10% of the dose every few days until it is totally discontinued.

Sedative-Hypnotic Drug Addiction. Sedative-hypnotic drugs are among the most widely prescribed medications. More than 15% of Americans use these drugs in any year (Harrison et al., 1984). The majority of addicted patients are receiving these drugs (particularly benzodiazepines) by prescription for treatment of anxiety or insomnia; then they become psychologically and/or physically dependent. A minority of persons addicted to these drugs (primarily barbiturates and other nonbenzodiazepine sedatives) obtain the drugs illegally for "recreational" use. They are most often polydrug abusers.

Benzodiazepines are the most widely abused sedative-hypnotic drugs and will be discussed as a prototype for that class of drugs. Benzodiazepines possess the typical features of an abusable drug: they are behaviorally reinforcing, both in relief of anxiety and, in some people, in producing pleasure; tolerance to the depressant effects (although not so much to anxiolytic effects) develops rapidly; and physical dependence accompanies prolonged use. People who have previously abused alcohol or other sedative drugs are at higher risk for abusing sedative drugs again (Busto, 1986; Woods et al., 1988). Evidence of inappropriate drug-taking behavior includes escalation of the dose, obtaining prescriptions from multiple physicians, or taking the drug for reasons other than that for which it was prescribed.

One of the primary issues in treatment of benzodiazepine dependence is safely and effectively reducing doses or inducing abstinence. As discussed previously, cessation of use of sedatives may elicit anxiety that resembles the original problem for which the sedatives were prescribed. The physician should be alert for evidence of sedative drug abuse, and all patients on these drugs should anticipate some degree of physical dependence. When sedative-hypnotics are discontinued, the dose should be gradually reduced to minimize the severity of withdrawal symptoms (DuPont, 1990). A schedule of discontinuation over 6 to 12 weeks is reasonable, but sometimes reduction may need to be even more gradual. Usually dose reduction can be accomplished using the same benzodiazepine a person has been taking, but when that approach fails, switching from a short-acting to a long-acting drug, such as for example from lorazepam to diazepam, may make drug withdrawal less disruptive. The use of antidepressants such as desipramine or fluoxetine may be a useful adjunct to benzodiazepine withdrawal, particularly in patients with panic disorders or depression. In all patients receiving sedative-hypnotic drugs for prolonged periods of time, the risks of dependence should be discussed, and the risks weighed against the benefits. In particular, a patient should be advised that an increase in anxiety during withdrawal may not mean a return of previous symptoms, that a period of temporary discomfort may be followed by substantial improvement, and that the patient will do better in the long term without medication.

OPIATES

Pharmacology

The pharmacology, pharmacokinetics, metabolism, and pharmacodynamics of opiates are described in chapter 25.

Clinical and Therapeutic Issues

Intoxication. Many different opiates are used for analgesia and/or are abused. A detailed discussion of pharmacologic characteristics of the particular drugs in this class is beyond the scope of this chapter. Instead, opiates will be discussed as a class, with reference to particular drugs when relevant to diagnosis or management.

Opiate intoxication occurs relatively frequently in drug abusers who have either misjudged their dose or are suicidal. But intoxication also occurs during therapeutic use in patients with pain. Clinical features of opiate intoxication are summarized in Table 27–7. The usual cause of death from opiate intoxication is respiratory arrest that may occur within a minute of IV injection. After IM or subcutaneous dosing with narcotics such as morphine, respiratory depression peaks 30 to 60 minutes after injection; the interval from dose to peak effect may even be longer after oral dosing. There appears to be a delay between peak concentrations in plasma and peak depression of respiration. The delay is presumably due to a delay of entry of morphine into the brain. After IM, subcutaneous, or oral dosing, a progression of intoxi-

Table 27-7. CLINICAL FEATURES OF OPIATE INTOXICATION AND WITHDRAWAL

Intoxication
Stupor or coma
Symmetric, pinpoint, reactive pupils
Hypothermia
Bradycardia
Hypotension
Skin cool, moist
Hypoventilation (respiratory slowing, irregular breathing, apnea)
Pulmonary edema
Seizures (meperidine, propoxyphene, morphine)
Reversal with naloxone

Withdrawal
Anxiety, restlessness
Insomnia
Chills, hot flashes
Myalgias, arthralgias
Nausea, anorexia
Abdominal cramping
Vomiting, diarrhea
Yawning
Dilated pupils
Tachycardia, hypertension (mild)
Hyperthermia (mild), diaphoresis, lacrimation, rhinorrhea
Piloerection
Spontaneous ejaculation

cation from sedation and slowing of respiratory rate to coma and respiratory arrest can be expected. Respiratory depression from opiates may be enhanced when patients are receiving barbiturates or other sedative-hypnotics, phenothiazines (including prochlorperazine), or drugs with neuromuscular blocking activity (Reier and Johnstone, 1970).

Particular opiates may produce specific manifestations in addition to those described in Table 27-7. Chronic therapy with meperidine, either in high doses or in patients with chronic renal failure, may result in neuromuscular excitability, including myoclonic jerks and convulsions, believed to be due to accumulation of the metabolite normeperidine (Armstrong and Bersten, 1986). Propoxyphene intoxication is associated with seizures, diabetes insipidus, and cardiovascular collapse due to myocardial depression, the latter thought to be caused by the metabolite norpropoxyphene (Lawson and Northridge, 1987). Methadone produces a typical picture of opiate intoxication, but because of its long half-life, intoxication may be prolonged for a day or longer.

Most signs and symptoms of opiate intoxication are reversed by naloxone. This reversal is an important element in both diagnosing and treating opiate intoxication. Some intoxications, however, such as with propoxyphene, may require extremely large doses (more than 10 mg) of naloxone for reversal, and even then reversal may be incomplete. Some manifestations of intoxication such as seizures may respond poorly or not at all to naloxone. Naloxone in high doses (usually 5 to 10 mg or more) may also have arousal effects in patients with alcohol or benzodiazepine intoxication, and in some patients with stroke. Management of opiate intoxication should be directed toward maintaining a patent airway and adequate ventilation. Naloxone, 0.4 to 2 mg IV, may be administered to reverse opiate intoxication. However, the patient must still be observed for several hours as the effects of naloxone (2-3 hours) may be briefer than are the effects of many narcotics. Thus late, recurrent intoxication may ensue. In patients with intoxications caused by long-acting opiates such as methadone, continuous infusions or repeated boluses of naloxone may be administered. Pulmonary edema due to intoxication with narcotics probably is a result of increased pulmonary capillary permeability and may take several days to resolve. Severe hypoxemia due to pulmonary edema may require positive pressure mechanical ventilation.

Withdrawal from Opiates. Prolonged use of opiates leads to tolerance and, after cessation of use, a withdrawal syndrome. Tolerance is selective and expresses itself by a high level of tolerance to the effects of opiates that cause nausea, sedation, and respiratory depression, but relatively little tolerance to the pupillary constriction or constipation caused by the drugs. The severity of the withdrawal syndrome depends on the prior daily dose of opiates. It is generally more severe in opiate abusers than it is in patients taking opiates for analgesia. Withdrawal symptoms can occur following administration of naloxone even after a single dose of morphine (Heighman et al., 1989). Opiate withdrawal is not life-threatening but is associated with severe psychological and moderate physical distress. The clinical features of the withdrawal syndrome range from a mild, flulike illness to a multisystem disorder, as described in Table 27-7.

The onset of withdrawal symptoms typically occurs 8 to 16 hours after cessation of the use of heroin or morphine. Autonomic disturbances and myalgias tend to appear first. By 36 hours, severe restlessness, piloerection, lacrimation, abdominal cramps, and diarrhea become more prominent. Symptoms reach their peak intensity at 48 to 72 hours, and then resolve over 7 to 10 days. Abstinence symptoms after ceasing to use methadone develop more gradually, with an onset of 36 to 72 hours that peaks at about 6 days. The signs tend to be less severe than are those with heroin.

Treatment of opiate withdrawal includes specific replacement of the opiates and supportive care. Most addicted patients can undergo withdrawal in a supportive environment without medication, experiencing a syndrome resembling influenza. However, the severity of withdrawal can be reduced by medications. The most commonly used replacement medication is methadone, usually dosed at 20 to 40 mg/day by mouth as required to make the patient comfortable. After 2 or 3 days of stabilization, the dose can be gradually tapered over 1 to 3 weeks. Detoxification per se is not very effective in promoting long-term abstinence; attempts should be made to enter the patient into a longer-term treatment program, such as a methadone maintenance clinic or Narcotics Anonymous.

Clonidine in high doses produces opiate-like effects. In therapeutic doses it has been used to manage symptoms of opiate withdrawal (Gold et al., 1980). Typically, clonidine is initiated at 0.1 to 0.2 mg every 8 hours. Then the dose is increased as needed to 0.8 to 1.2 mg/day. Subsequently, clonidine is tapered over 10 to 14 days. The main side effects are drowsiness and hypotension. Nonspecific treatment for opiate withdrawal includes the use of benzodiazepines or chloral hydrate for anxiety and sleep and prochlorperazine for GI symptoms. Propoxyphene and/or NSAIDs may be useful for the treatment of myalgias. It is somewhat ironic that propoxyphene, originally touted as an analgesic without addictive properties, turns out to have little if any analgesic effects, is addictive, and has legitimacy as an opiate substitute for the same reasons that methadone is useful.

Buprenorphine, a mixed opiate agonist-antagonist, has recently been shown to be effective for outpatient detoxification of persons addicted to heroin (Bickel et al., 1988). A potential advantage of buprenorphine over methadone is that there is less withdrawal discomfort after cessation of buprenorphine than there is after cessation of methadone. Medical patients who abuse narcotics usually have chronic pain. Such patients often abuse sedative drugs as well. Health care personnel in particular seem to be at higher risk for abusing opiates because of their ready access to the drug.

Opiate Addiction. Illicit use of heroin remains a major health care issue, particularly in light of the association between IV drug abuse and the transmission of AIDS. Narcotics may also be consumed by other routes including smoking, snorting (intranasal), and ingesting orally (opiates other than heroin). Many people who abuse heroin are from lower socioeconomic classes and minorities. All these factors must be addressed in developing treatment regimens. Middle-class persons addicted to opiates, while they may be physically dependent, are better able to function in society and to escape their addiction. An example was seen in Viet Nam veterans who had a high prevalence of heroin addiction in Viet Nam, presumably in response to stress, boredom, and ready availability of heroin, but stopped heroin use as soon as they returned to their communities (Robins et al., 1975).

The principles of treatment of opiate addiction contain all the elements used to manage other addictions. Behavioral therapy including group therapy, social skills training, and occupational rehabilitation often is combined with pharmacologic therapy. The primary pharmacologic therapy involves substitution with the long-acting narcotic methadone, which may be maintained for months or years while rehabilitation is ongoing. Typically, the initial dose of methadone is titrated on the basis of control of withdrawal symptoms while avoiding intoxication. For detoxification, the dose is tapered gradually over 21 days. For maintenance, the dose of methadone may be increased to a level (usually 40 to 100 mg/day) that keeps the patient comfortable and reduces the desire to abuse illicit narcotics. In high doses, methadone produces sufficient cross-tolerance that there is little effect of IV heroin. Therefore, a decreased craving for heroin results. There is a report that there is a better outcome, that is, reduction of IV drug abuse, with a trough concentration of methadone in plasma of greater than 200 ng/ml (Holmstrand et al., 1978). Coadministration of phenytoin, rifampin, or barbiturates may accelerate drug metabolism, precipitating withdrawal symptoms and/or requiring higher doses for methadone maintenance. Another long-acting opiate, levomethadyl acetate (L-acetylmethadol, LAAM), can be dosed 3 days a week and is also used for maintenance in some programs (Ling et al., 1976). The management of pain in patients on opiate maintenance therapy is often regarded as problematic. It should be remembered that with chronic therapy, tolerance develops to the analgesic effects of opiates. Therefore, the usual doses of narcotics may be administered above the maintenance dose of the opiate. Mixed agonist-antagonist narcotics, such as pentazocine, butorphanol, nalbuphine, and buprenorphine, should be avoided in people on methadone or LAAM maintenance, as these drugs may precipitate severe withdrawal symptoms.

A long-acting narcotic antagonist, naltrexone, is also available for the treatment of narcotic addiction. As a receptor antagonist, naltrexone blocks the pleasurable effects of heroin. This would be expected to discourage continued drug abuse (O'Brien, 1984). Patients must, of course, be fully detoxified from narcotics before beginning antagonist therapy. Naltrexone has not achieved widespread acceptance among addicted persons, but, like disulfiram in alcoholics, naltrexone may be useful for motivated patients who are participating in rehabilitation programs. Recovering physicians and other health care professionals who have continued access to narcotics, for example, may respond well to naltrexone treatment (Ling and Wesson, 1984).

Many persons addicted to heroin have a history of psychiatric disorders, especially depression, that may predate the addiction (Khantzian and Treece, 1985). Current research is focusing on antidepressant drug therapy as an adjunct to methadone maintenance and detoxification therapies for those addicted to heroin.

COCAINE

Pharmacology

Cocaine abuse is one of the most frequent causes of drug-induced toxicity (Gawin and Ellinwood, 1988; Litovitz et al., 1988). Cocaine has become relatively inexpensive and is widely available for IV, intranasal, and inhalational (smoked) use. Crack cocaine (chunks of solid cocaine base) is most commonly smoked because the free base is more volatile than is the hydrochloride salt, the latter of which decomposes with heating.

The mechanism of action of cocaine resembles that of amphetamines and related drugs. The major neurochemical actions include (1) blockade of neuronal uptake of catecholamines, (2) CNS stimulation with release of dopamine and systemic activation of the sympathetic nervous system, (3) release and/or blockade of uptake of serotonin, and (4) a local anesthetic effect, due to blockade of the fast sodium channel. The receptors for cocaine in the brain appear to be the catecholamine transporter. Blockade of the dopamine transporter has been linked with the euphoric actions of cocaine (Wyatt et al., 1988). Cocaine use produces euphoria, mental stimulation, and generalized sympathetic nervous system activation. The rewarding effects and many of the toxic effects of cocaine can be blocked by dopamine antagonists, consistent with the idea that dopamine release is critical to cocaine's action. With chronic exposure in animals, there is depletion of brain catecholamines with increased receptor sensitivity to their presence.

Pharmacokinetics and Metabolism

Cocaine is readily absorbed from a variety of sites, including mucous membranes and the GI tract. It is hydrolyzed by plasma and liver cholinesterase to ecgonine methyl ester, and it undergoes nonenzymatic hydrolysis to benzoylecgo-

nine. In addition, a small amount of cocaine is N-demethylated to norcocaine. The plasma half-life of cocaine averages 60 to 90 minutes after IV administration but is longer, up to several hours, after snorting or oral administration. The latter presumably is due to continued absorption across mucous membranes or from the GI tract. Urine screens for cocaine primarily detect the metabolite benzoylecgonine, which has a much longer half-life (8 hours) than does the parent cocaine.

Pharmacodynamics

Tolerance develops quickly and completely to the euphoric and other subjective effects of cocaine. Tolerance develops only incompletely to the cardiovascular effects of cocaine (Ambre et al., 1988). Thus, a situation may evolve in which cocaine is repeatedly used to seek the cocaine high with the consequence being progressive cardiovascular toxicity. *Principle: Often, drugs that produce tolerance to their CNS effects continue to affect other tissues. As doses rise to stimulate the CNS, severe morbidity and even mortality result as a consequence of the dose–response toxicity on peripheral tissues. Consider alcohol, barbiturates, and opiates as examples of such drugs.*

Drug Interactions

The most important concern for drug interactions with cocaine involves blockade of catecholamine uptake, resulting in enhanced sensitivity to catecholamines. For example, when epinephrine is coadministered with cocaine, excessive hypertension may result. Since cocaine results in release of catecholamines, including epinephrine that has both α- and β-adrenergic agonist activity, administration of a nonspecific β blocker such as propranolol may result in unopposed α-adrenergic activity, enhancement of vasoconstriction, and aggravation of hypertension (Ramoska and Sacchetti, 1985). Cocaine is metabolized in part by cholinesterases, and people with genetic differences of pseudocholinesterase activity (who are abnormally sensitive to succinylcholine) may eliminate cocaine more slowly (Jatlow et al., 1979). Patients receiving cholinesterase inhibitors, such as pyridostigmine for treatment of myasthenia gravis, *may be* more sensitive to the effects of cocaine.

Clinical and Therapeutic Issues

Intoxication. The clinical picture of intoxication with cocaine is summarized in Table 27–8. Psychiatric disturbances are particularly common emergency department presentations of abusers of cocaine. Acute intoxication often presents with an acute anxiety state, panic attack, or agitated

**Table 27-8.   MANIFESTATIONS OF
INTOXICATION WITH COCAINE
AND OTHER STIMULANT DRUGS**

BEHAVIORAL OR PSYCHIATRIC	AUTONOMIC OR NEUROMUSCULAR
Euphoria	Tachycardia†
Hyperactivity, irritability*	Hypertension
Insomnia	Hyperthermia
Mood lability	Dilated pupils
Anorexia	Tremulousness*
Anxiety, agitation	Seizures
Suspiciousness, aggressiveness	Respiratory arrest
Psychosis (often paranoid)	Cardiovascular collapse
Delirium (agitated)	
Stupor	
Coma	

* Particularly neonatal intoxication.
† Except phenylpropanolamine and other primarily α-adrenergic agonists, which produce reflex bradycardia.

delirium. Because cocaine has a relatively short half-life, acute intoxication usually resolves within 6 hours. Chronic intoxication may present as paranoid psychosis, indistinguishable from paranoid schizophrenia, and may last for many days. Neonatal intoxication has been reported both immediately after birth and during breast-feeding by a cocaine-using mother (see chapter 29). Typical features are irritability, tremulousness, tachycardia, and tachypnea, although seizures also have been reported. A number of complications that may be life-threatening have been reported with cocaine intoxication (see Table 27-8). The most significant of those involves excessive sympathetic neural stimulation and includes severe hypertension that may be complicated by stroke or dissecting aortic aneurysm, cardiac arrhythmias that may include ventricular fibrillation, and sudden death. In addition, the vasoconstriction can lead to ischemia of the heart, kidney, and GI tract. The other major complications involve the CNS (Table 27-9). The most important ones are headache that may be due to hypertension or to a migraine-like mechanism, seizures, and stroke.

Withdrawal. Abstinence after habitual use of cocaine can be associated with neuropsychiatric symptoms (Gawin and Kleber, 1986). A cocaine "crash," a state of profound exhaustion, sometimes accompanied by anxiety, depression, and a craving for cocaine is described. Decreased energy, anhedonia, and hypersomnolence ensue and may last for weeks or months. An intense desire for cocaine to ameliorate the severity of the abstinence syndrome commonly leads to relapse, thus sustaining addiction. Suicidal ideation is common in the cocaine abstinence state.

Cocaine Addiction. Compulsive use of cocaine appears to be motivated both by a craving for the cocaine-induced high (psychological dependence) and by relief of the postcocaine depression (physical dependence). Addiction to stimulants such as amphetamines may be motivated more by physical dependence.

Because the drug was expensive, cocaine abuse in the 1970s and 1980s primarily occurred among young, middle-class people. More recently, cocaine is much more widely available and is increasingly abused by people of lower socioeconomic classes. Cocaine is commonly abused along with other drugs, particularly alcohol and opiates.

While cocaine addiction is well recognized, there is little systematic research on its treatment. The goal of treatment is to achieve and maintain abstinence. Minimizing the discomfort of withdrawal and the associated craving for cocaine have been the major foci of pharmacologic therapy to date. Current research is evaluating the use

**Table 27-9.   MEDICAL COMPLICATIONS OF
COCAINE INTOXICATION**

Cardiovascular
  Hypertension
    Intracranial hemorrhage
    Aortic dissection or rupture
  Arrhythmias
    Sinus tachycardia
    Supraventricular tachycardia
    Ventricular tachyarrhythmias
  Organ ischemia
    Myocardial ischemia and infarction
    Renal infarction
    Intestinal infarction
    Limb ischemia
  Myocarditis
  Shock
Central Nervous System
  Headache
  Seizures
  Transient focal neurologic deficits
  Stroke
    Subarachnoid hemorrhage
    Intracranial hemorrhage
    Cerebral infarction
    Embolic (endocarditis)
  Toxic encephalopathy or coma
  Neurologic complications
Respiratory
  Pneumomediastinum
  Pneumothorax
  Pulmonary edema
  Respiratory arrest
Metabolic and other
  Hyperthermia
  Rhabdomyolysis
  Wound botulism
  Tetanus

of a variety of drugs including tricyclic antidepressants, bromocriptine, buprenorphine, and carbamazepine as potential pharmacologic adjuncts to treatment. The rationale for use of tricyclic antidepressants was to manage the severe depression that follows cocaine withdrawal; tricyclic antidepressants may also, by blocking catecholamine uptake, stabilize adrenergic and dopaminergic receptors. In open trials, desipramine appeared effective in reducing cocaine use and craving, but controlled clinical trials have been less encouraging (Kosten et al., 1987). Bromocriptine, a dopamine agonist, and amantadine, which releases dopamine from neurons, have been evaluated in an attempt to modify the dopamine depletion state that is speculated to cause drug craving and cocaine withdrawal symptoms. These drugs appear to reduce symptoms of cocaine withdrawal, although their effects on drug use are less well established (Tennant and Sagherian, 1987).

Buprenorphine has been shown to decrease cocaine self-administration in monkeys and has been of considerable interest for treatment of combined opioid-cocaine addiction (Kosten et al., 1989).

Carbamazepine was considered as a potential therapy because of the findings in animals that repeated administration of cocaine may "kindle" seizures, and that these seizures may somehow be related to the desire for human use of cocaine. Clinical trials of carbamazepine are ongoing. Substitution therapy with stimulants such as methylphenidate have also been tried but have not been particularly successful (Gawin and Kleber, 1985).

The physician treating patients who have discontinued use of cocaine should counsel the patient about the depression that follows cessation of use and the likelihood of recurrent intense craving to use the drug for several months.

MARIJUANA

Marijuana is commonly abused and is abused along with almost every other drug. The drug consists of the dried leaves and stems of the *Cannabis sativa* plant. The primary psychoactive chemical is Δ-9-tetrahydrocannabinol (THC). The biochemical basis of THC action is not well understood. The THC is extremely lipid-soluble and has a half-life of several days, representing slow release from adipose and other tissues. THC is extensively metabolized by the liver to a number of metabolites.

Marijuana is primarily smoked in cigarettes (joints) or pipes but may also be taken orally and sometimes cooked in foods (such as marijuana brownies). Marijuana produces euphoria, relaxation, alteration of time sense, depersonalization, and ultimately sleepiness. Short-term memory is impaired, and the ability to execute multiple sequential tasks is impaired. Physiologic effects include tachycardia, tremulousness, and conjunctival injection. Orthostatic hypotension occasionally occurs due to inhibition of sympathetic nervous reflexes (Benowitz and Jones, 1975). THC (also called dronabinol) has antiemetic qualities, for which it is occasionally employed as an adjunct to cancer chemotherapy (Carey et al., 1983). Analogs of THC, such as nabilone, also have been used for this indication (Ward and Holmes, 1985).

The primary clinical problems with marijuana are acute intoxication and an increased risk of accidents with automobiles and other machinery. Smoking large quantities of marijuana, or smaller quantities of marijuana with high percentages of THC, or taking THC or analogs as a medication, particularly by novices, may result in panic reactions or even acute psychosis. At very high doses, visual hallucinations occur. Sedation, impaired reaction time, and impaired driving skills are common effects.

Treatment of THC intoxication primarily involves reassurance and supportive care. The use of benzodiazepines may be useful in managing panic reactions.

ANABOLIC STEROIDS

While this chapter primarily discusses abuse of psychoactive drugs, the abuse of anabolic steroids is also discussed because it presents a substance abuse problem of current public health concern. Anabolic steroid abuse is an example of drug abuse that is primarily reinforced by the anticipated physical effects rather than psychological effects of the drug. These hormones are used by athletes to increase muscle mass and strength. Although the evidence that the steroids actually enhance athletic performance is weak (Hallagan et al., 1989), anabolic steroid use is very commonplace, both in professional sports and in college and even high school athletics. The prototype anabolic steroid is testosterone. It has both androgenic and anabolic effects; the androgenic effects are relatively undesirable for athletes. Synthetic hormones such as ethylestrenol, methandrostenolone, methanedienone, nandralone, oxandrolone, oxymetholone, stanozolol, testosterone cypionate, and others have reduced androgenic/anabolic potency ratios compared with testosterone.

Anabolic steroids are thought to enhance muscle mass in three ways: (1) protein synthesis is increased owing to binding of steroids to DNA with increased transcription of RNA and enhanced protein synthesis, (2) the catabolic effects of glucocorticoid release by stress are blocked, and (3) a state of euphoria and diminished fatigue, and possibly more aggressive behavior that promotes more intensive weight training, may result. Although not a primary reason for abuse, the euphoric effects of high doses of anabolic steroids could contribute to persistent abuse or dependence (Kashkin and Kleber, 1989).

The doses of anabolic steroids used by athletes are 10 to 100 times higher than are those prescribed for medical indications. The various steroids are often used in combination, such as an oral and an injectable, and are commonly used in cycles of a couple of months or so, alternating with intervals with no use or low-dose steroids, with complete cessation 1 or 2 months prior to competition at which the urine will be tested.

There are several toxicities that are of concern attendant on high-dose androgenic steroid use (Council on Scientific Affairs, 1988; Hallagan et al., 1989). Psychiatric disturbances including mental changes, manic depressive illness, and paranoid psychosis have been described. Liver disease, particularly peliosis hepatitis, cholestasis, and hepatomas have been associated with chronic medicinal use of androgenic steroids and have been a concern in athletes as well. Anabolic steroids may increase low-density lipoprotein and decrease high-density lipoprotein cholesterol concentrations and increase blood pressure, all of which could increase the risk of coronary heart disease. Reproductive concerns include oligospermia and testicular atrophy in men and menstrual abnormalities in women. The development of gynecomastia in men and masculinization in women may also be seen. The major role of the physician in treating the abuse of androgenic steroids involves a recognition of use and counseling. Perhaps most important is the involvement of the physician as a community resource to describe the potential hazards of androgenic steroid use.

REFERENCES

Alcoholics Anonymous, 3rd ed. A.A. World Services, New York, 1976.

Alcoholics Anonymous 12 Steps and 12 Traditions. A.A. World Services, New York, 1988.

Alldredge, B. K.; Lowenstein, D. H.; and Simon, R. P.: Placebo-controlled trial of intravenous diphenylhydantoin for short-term treatment of alcohol withdrawal seizures. Am. J. Med., 87:645–648, 1989.

Ambre, J. J.; Belknap, S. M.; Nelson, J.; Ruo, T. I.; Shin, S.-G.; and Atkinson, A. J. Jr.: Acute tolerance to cocaine in humans. Clin. Pharmacol. Ther., 44:1–8, 1988.

Anderson, M.: Treatment in an alcoholism and drug addiction unit. N. Zealand Med. J., 88:233–237, 1978.

Armstrong, P. J.; and Bersten, A.: Normeperidine toxicity. Anesth. Analg., 65:536–538, 1986.

Benowitz, N. L.: Pharmacologic aspects of cigarette smoking and nicotine addiction. N. Engl. J. Med., 319:1318–1330, 1988.

Benowitz, N. L.; and Jones, R. T.: Cardiovascular effects of prolonged delta-9-tetrahydrocannabinol ingestion. Clin. Pharmacol. Ther., 18:287–297, 1975

Bickel, W. K.; Stitzer, M. L.; Bigelow, G. E.; Liebson, I. A.; Jasinski, D. R.; and Johnson, R. E.: A clinical trial of buprenorphine: Comparison with methadone in the detoxification of heroin addicts. Clin. Pharmacol. Ther., 43:72–78, 1988.

Blondal, T.: Controlled trial of nicotine polacrilex gum with supportive measures. Arch. Intern. Med., 149:1818–1821, 1989.

Boston Collaborative Drug Surveillance Program: Decreased clinical efficacy of propoxyphene in cigarette smokers. Clin. Pharmacol. Ther., 14:259–263, 1973.

Busto, U.: Patterns of benzodiazepine abuse and dependence. Br. J. Addict., 81:94–97, 1986.

Busto, U.; Sellers, E. M.; Naranjo, C. A.; Cappell, H.; Sanchez-Craig, M.; and Sykora, K.: Withdrawal reaction after long-term therapeutic use of benzodiazepines. N. Engl. J. Med., 315:854–859, 1986.

Carey, M. P.; Burish, T. G.; and Brenner, D. E.: Delta-9-tetrahydrocannabinol in cancer chemotherapy: Research problems and issues. Ann. Intern. Med., 99:106–114, 1983.

Charness, M. E.; Simon, R. P.; and Greenberg, D. A.: Ethanol and the nervous system. N. Engl. J. Med., 321:442–454, 1989.

Collins, G. B.; Janesz, J. W.; Byerly-Thorpe, J.; and Manzeo, J.: Hospital sponsored chemical dependency self-help groups. Hosp. Community Psychiatry, 36:1315–1316, 1985.

Council on Scientific Affairs: Drug abuse in athletes. Anabolic steroids and human growth hormone. J.A.M.A., 259:1703–1705, 1988.

Council on Scientific Affairs: Scientific issues in drug testing. J.A.M.A., 257:3110–3114, 1987a.

Council on Scientific Affairs: Aversion therapy. J.A.M.A., 258:2562–2566, 1987b.

Cummings, S. R.; Hansen, B.; Richard, R. J.; Stein, M. J.; and Coates, T. J.: Internists and nicotine gum. J.A.M.A., 260:1565–1569, 1988.

Deanfield, J.; Wright, C.; Krikler, S.; Ribeiro, P.; and Fox, K.: Cigarette smoking and the treatment of angina with propranolol, atenolol, and nifedipine. N. Engl. J. Med., 310:951–954, 1984.

Department of Health and Human Services, Public Health Service: The Health Consequences of Smoking: Nicotine Addiction. A Report of the Surgeon General. DHHS publication No. (CDC) 88-8406. U.S. Government Printing Office, Washington, DC, 1988.

De Soto, C. B.; O'Donnell, W. E.; Allred, L. J.; and Lopes, C. E.: Symptomatology in alcoholics at various stages of abstinence. Alcoholism: Clin. Exp. Res., 9(6):505–512, 1985.

Diagnostic and Statistical Manual of Mental Disorders 3rd ed. rev. (DSM-III-R). American Psychiatric Association, Washington, D.C., pp. 167–168, 1987.

Dollery, C.; and Brennan, P. J.: The Medical Research Council Hypertension Trial: The smoking patient. Am. Heart J., 115:276–281, 1988.

DuPont, R. L.: A physician's guide to discontinuing benzodiazepine therapy. West. J. Med., 152:600–603, 1990.

Edwards, G.; Arif, A.; and Hodgson, R.: Nomenclature and classification of drug- and alcohol-related problems: A shortened version of a WHO memorandum. Br. J. Addict., 77:3–20, 1982.

Eldefrawi, A. T.; and Eldefrawi, M. E.: Receptors for γ-aminobutyric acid and voltage-dependent chloride channels as targets for drugs and toxicants. F.A.S.E.B. J., 1:262–271, 1987.

Fraser, H. F.; Wikler, A.; Essig, C. F.; and Isbell, H.: Degree of physical dependence induced by secobarbital or pentobarbital. J.A.M.A., 166:126–129, 1958.

Frezza, M.; diPadova, C.; Pozzato, G.; Terpin, M.; Baraona, E.; and Lieber, C. S.: High blood alcohol levels in women. N. Engl. J. Med., 322:95–99, 1990.

Fuller, R. K.; Branchey, L.; Brightwell, D. R.; Derman, R. M.; Emrick, C. D.; Iber, F. L.; James, K. T.; Lacoursiere, R. B.; Lee, K. K.; Lowenstam, I.; Maany, I.; Neiderhiser, D.;

Nocks, J. J.; and Shaw, S.: Disulfiram treatment of alcoholism: A Veterans Administration cooperative study. J.A.M.A., 256:1449–1455, 1986.

Galanter, M.: Cults and zealous self-help movements: A psychiatric perspective. Am. J. Psychiatry, 147:543–551, 1990.

Galanter, M.; Talbott, D.; Gallegos, K.; and Rubenston, E.: Combined Alcoholics Anonymous and professional care for addicted physicians. Am. J. Psychiatry, 147:64–68, 1990.

Gawin, F. H.; and Ellinwood, E. H. Jr.: Cocaine and other stimulants: Actions, abuse, and treatment. N. Engl. J. Med., 318:1173–1182, 1988.

Gawin, F. H.; and Kleber, H. D.: Abstinence symptomatology and psychiatric diagnosis in cocaine abusers. Arch. Gen. Psychiatry, 43:107–113, 1986.

Gawin, F. H.; and Kleber, H. D.: Methylphenidate treatment of cocaine abusers without ADD. Am. J. Drug Alcohol Abuse, 11:193–197, 1985.

Glassman, A. H.; Stetner, F.; Walsh, B. T.; Raizman, P. S.; Fleiss, J. L.; Cooper, T. B.; and Covey, L. S.: Heavy smokers, smoking cessation, and clonidine: Results of a double-blind, randomized trial. J.A.M.A., 259:2863–2866, 1988.

Gold, M. S.; Pottash, A. C.; Sweeney, D. R.; and Kleber, H. D.: Opiate withdrawal using clonidine. J.A.M.A., 243:343–346, 1980.

Goldman, M. S.: Neuropsychological recovery in alcoholics: Endogenous and exogenous processes. Alcoholism: Clin. Exp. Res., 10:136–144, 1986.

Hallagan, J. B.; Hallagan, L. F.; and Snyder, M. B.: Anabolic-androgenic steroid use by athletes. N. Engl. J. Med., 321:1042–1046, 1989.

Harrison, M.; Busto, U.; Naranjo, C. A.; Kaplan, H. L.; and Sellers, E. M.: Diazepam tapering in detoxification for high-dose benzodiazepine abuse. Clin. Pharmacol. Ther., 36:527–532, 1984.

Hayashida, M.; Alterman, A. I.; McLellan, A. T.; O'Brien, C. P.; Purtill, J. J.; Volpicelli, J. R.; Raphaelson, A. H.; and Hall, C. P.: Comparative effectiveness and costs of inpatient and outpatient detoxification of patients with mild-to-moderate alcohol withdrawal syndrome (special article). N. Engl. J. Med., 320(6):358–365, 1989.

Heighman, S. J.; Stitzer, M. L.; Bigelow, G. E.; and Liebson, I. A.: Acute opioid physical dependence in postaddict humans: Naloxone effects after brief morphine exposure. J. Pharmacol. Exp. Ther., 248:127–134, 1989.

Herrington, R. E.; Benzer, D. G.; Jacobsen, G. R.; and Hawkins, M. K.: Treating substance-use disorders among physicians. J.A.M.A., 247:2253–2257, 1982.

Holden, C.: Is alcoholism treatment effective? Science, 236:20–22, 1987.

Holmstrand, J.; Anggard, M. D.; and Gunne, L.: Methadone maintenance: Plasma levels and therapeutic outcome. Clin. Pharmacol. Ther., 23:175–180, 1978.

Hughes, J. R.; and Miller, S. A.: Nicotine gum to help stop smoking. J.A.M.A., 252:2855–2858, 1984.

Jatlow, P.; Barash, P. G.; Van Dyke, C.; Radding, J.; and Byck, R.: Cocaine and succinylcholine sensitivity: A new caution. Anesth. Analg., 58:235–238, 1979.

Jusko, W. J.: Smoking effects in pharmacokinetics. In, Pharmacokinetic Basis for Drug Treatment (Benet, L. Z.; Massoud, N.; Gambertoglio, J. G., eds.). Raven Press, New York, 1984, pp. 311–320.

Kaim, S. C.; Klett, C. J.; and Rothfeld, B.: Treatment of the acute alcohol withdrawal state: A comparison of four drugs. Am. J. Psychiatry, 125:1640–1646, 1969.

Kalant, H.; LeBlanc, A. E.; and Gibbins, R. J.: Tolerance to, and dependence on, some non-opiate psychotropic drugs. Pharmacol. Rev., 23:135–191, 1971.

Kashkin, K. B.; and Kleber, H. D.: Hooked on hormones? An anabolic steroid addiction hypothesis. J.A.M.A., 262:3166–3170, 1989.

Khantzian, E. J.; and Treece, C.: DSM-III psychiatric diagnosis of narcotic addicts: Recent findings. Arch. Gen. Psychiatry, 42:1067–1071, 1985.

Kikendall, J. W.; Evaul, J.; and Johnson, L. F.: Effect of cigarette smoking on gastrointestinal physiology and non-neoplastic digestive disease. J. Clin. Gastroenterol., 6:65–79, 1984.

Koob, G. F.; and Bloom, F. E.: Cellular and molecular mechanisms of drug dependence. Science, 242:715–723, 1988.

Kosten, T. R.; Kleber, H. D.; and Morgan, C.: Role of opioid antagonists in treating intravenous cocaine abuse. Life Sci., 44:887–892, 1989.

Kosten, T. R.; Schuman, B.; Wright, D.; Carney, M. K.; and Gawin, F. W.: A preliminary study of desipramine in the treatment of cocaine abuse in methadone maintenance programs. J. Clin. Psychiatry, 48:442–444, 1987.

Kranzler, H. R.; and Liebowtiz, N. R.: Anxiety and depression in substance abuse: Clinical implications. Med. Clin. North Am., 72:867–885, 1988.

Kraus, M. L.; Gottlieb, L. D.; Horwitz, R. I.; and Anscher, M.: Randomized clinical trial of atenolol in patients with alcohol withdrawal. N. Engl. J. Med., 313:905–909, 1985.

Lam, W.; Sze, P. C.; Sacks, H. S.; and Chalmers, T. C.: Meta-analysis of randomised controlled trials of nicotine chewing gum. Lancet, 2:27–30, 1987.

Lawson, A. A. H.; and Northridge, D. B.: Dextropropoxyphene overdose. Epidemiology, clinical presentation and management. Med. Toxicol., 2:430–444, 1987.

Lee, B. L.; Benowitz, N. L.; and Jacob, P. III: Cigarette abstinence, nicotine gum, and theophylline disposition. Ann. Intern. Med., 106:553–555, 1987.

Ling, W.; and Wesson, D. R.: Naltrexone treatment for addicted health care professionals: A collaborative private practice experience. J. Clin. Psychiatry, 45:46–48, 1984.

Ling, W.; Charuvastra, V. C.; Kaim, S. C.; and Klett, C. J.: Methadryl acetate and methadone as maintenance treatments for heroin addicts. Arch. Gen. Psychiatry, 33:709–720, 1976.

Litovitz, T. L.; Schmitz, B. F.; Matyunas, N.; and Martin, T. G.: 1987 annual report of the American Association of Poison Control Centers national data collection systems. Am. J. Emerg. Med., 6:479–515, 1988.

Miller, L. G.; Greenblatt, D. J.; Barnhill, J. G.; and Shader, R. I.: Chronic benzodiazepine administration: I. Tolerance is associated with benzodiazepine receptor downregulation and decreased γ-aminobutyric acid$_A$ receptor function. J. Pharmacol. Exp. Ther., 246:170–176, 1987a.

Miller, L. G.; Greenblatt, D. J.; Roy, R. B.; Summer, W. R.; and Shader, R. I.: Chronic benzodiazepine administration: II. Discontinuation syndrome is associated with upregulation of γ-aminobutyric acid$_A$ receptor complex binding and function. J. Pharmacol. Exp. Ther., 246:177–182, 1987b.

Naranjo, C. A.; Sellers, E. M.; Chater, K.; Iversen, P.; Roach, C.; and Sykora, K.: Non-pharmacologic intervention in acute alcohol withdrawal. Clin. Pharmacol. Ther., 34:214–219, 1983.

Ng, S. K. C.; Hauser, W. A.; Brust, J. C. M.; and Susser, M.: Alcohol consumption and withdrawal in new-onset seizures. N. Engl. J. Med., 319:666–673, 1988.

O'Brien, C. P.: A new approach to the management of opioid dependence: Naltrexone. J. Clin. Psychiatry, 45:57–58, 1984.

O'Sullivan, G. F.; and Wade, D. N.: Flumazenil in the management of acute drug overdosage with benzodiazepines and other agents. Clin. Pharmacol. Ther., 42:254–259, 1987.

Osterloh, J. O.; and Becker, C. E.: Chemical dependency and drug testing in the workplace. West. J. Med., 152:506–513, 1990.

Pfeifer, H. F.; and Greenblatt, D. J.: Clinical toxicity of theophylline in relation to cigarette smoking: A report from the Boston Collaborative Drug Surveillance Program. Chest, 73:455–459, 1978.

Pickens, R. W.; Hatsukami, D. K.; Spicer, J. W.; and Svikis, D. S.: Relapse of alcohol abusers. Alcoholism: Clin. Exp. Res., 9:244–246, 1985.

Pond, S. M.; Olson, K. R.; Osterloh, J. O.; and Tong, T. G.: Randomized study of the treatment of phenobarbital overdose with repeated doses of serial charcoal. J.A.M.A., 251:3104–3108, 1984.

Ramoska, E.; and Sacchetti, A. D.: Propranolol-induced hypertension in treatment of cocaine intoxication. Ann. Emerg. Med., 14:1112–1113, 1985.

Reier, C. E.; and Johnstone, R. E.: Respiratory depression: Narcotic versus narcotic-tranquilizer combinations. Anesth. Analg., 49:119–124, 1970.

Robins, L. N.; Helzer, J. E.; Weissman, M. M.; Orvaschel, H.; Gruenberg, E.; Burke, J. D. Jr.; and Regier, D. A.: Lifetime prevalence of specific psychiatric disorders in three sites. Arch. Gen. Psychiatry, 1984, 41, 949–958.

Robins, L. N.; Helzer, J. E.; and Davis, D. H.: Narcotic use in Southeast Asia and afterward. Arch. Gen. Psychiatry, 32: 955–961, 1975.

Robinson, G. M.; Sellers, E. M.; and Janecek, E.: Barbiturate and hypnosedative withdrawal by multiple oral phenobarbital loading dose technique. Clin. Pharmacol. Ther., 30:71–76, 1981.

Roy-Byrne, P. P.; and Hommer, D.: Benzodiazepine withdrawal: Overview and implications for the treatment of anxiety. Am. J. Med., 84:1041–1052, 1988.

Schuckit, M. A.; Irwin, M.; and Brown, S. A.: The history of anxiety symptoms among 171 primary alcoholics. J. Stud. Alcohol, 51(1):34–41, 1990.

Sellers, E. M.; and Kalant, H.: Alcohol intoxication and withdrawal. N. Engl. J. Med., 294:757–762, 1976.

Shapiro, S.; Stone, D.; Rosenberg, L.; Kaufman, D. W.; Stolley, P. D.; and Miettinen, O. S.: Oral-contraceptive use in relation to myocardial infarction. Lancet, 1:743–747, 1979.

Southgate, M. T.: Prevalance of alcohol and other drug problems among physicians. J.A.M.A., 39:127–144, 1985.

Stinson, D. J.; Smith, W. G.; Amidjaya, I.; and Kaplan, J.: Systems of care and treatment outcomes for alcoholic patients. Arch. Gen. Psychiatry, 36:535–539, 1979.

Stockwell, T.; Bolt, E.; and Hooper, J.: Detoxification from alcohol at home managed by general practitioners. Br. Med. J., 292:733–735, 1986.

Suwacki, H.; and Ohara, H.: Alcohol-induced facial flushing and drinking behavior in Japanese men. J. Stud. Alcohol, 116:196–198, 1985.

Swett, C. Jr.: Drowsiness due to chlorpromazine in relation to cigarette smoking: A report from the Boston Collaborative Drug Surveillance Program. Arch. Gen. Psychiatry, 31:211–214, 1974.

Tennant, F. S.; and Sagherian, A. A.: Double-blind comparison of amantadine and bromocriptine for ambulatory withdrawal from cocaine dependence. Arch. Intern. Med., 147: 109–112, 1987.

Tonnesen, P.; Fryd, V.; Hansen, M.; Helsted, J.; Gunnersen, A. B.; Forchammer, H.; and Stockner, M.: Effect of nicotine chewing gum in combination with group counseling on the cessation of smoking. N. Engl. J. Med., 318:15–18, 1988.

Trap-Jensen, J.; Carlsen, J. E.; Svendsen, T. L.; and Christensen, N. J.: Cardiovascular and adrenergic effects of cigarette smoking during immediate non-selective and selective beta adrenoceptor blockade in humans. Eur. J. Clin. Invest., 9: 181–183, 1979.

Vaillant, G. E.: The National History of Alcoholism. Harvard University Press, Cambridge, 1983.

Vaillant, G. E.; William, C.; Cyrus, C.; Milofsky, E. S.; Kipp, J.; Wulsin, V. W.; and Mogielnicki, N. P.: Prospective study of alcoholism treatment. Am. J. Med., 75:455–464, 1983.

Vaughan, D. P.; Beckett, A. H.; and Robbie, D. S.: The influence of smoking on the intersubject variation in pentazocine elimination. Br. J. Clin. Pharmacol., 3:279–283, 1976.

Walle, T.; Byington, R. P.; Furberg, C. D.; McIntyre, K. M.; and Vokonas, P. S.: Biologic determinants of propranolol disposition: Results from 1308 patients in Beta-Blocker Heart Attack Trial. Clin. Pharmacol. Ther., 38:509–518. 1985.

Ward, A.; and Holmes, B.: Nabilone. A preliminary review of its pharmacological properties and therapeutic use. Drugs, 30:127–144, 1985.

Whitfield, C. L.: Advances in alcoholism and chemical dependence. Am. J. Med., 85:465, 1988.

Whitfield, C. L.; Thompson, G.; Lamb, A.; Spencer, V.; Pfeifer, M.; and Browning-Ferrando, M.: Detoxification of 1,024 patients without psychoactive drugs. J.A.M.A., 239: 1409–1410, 1978.

Woo, E.; and Greenblatt, D. J.: Massive benzodiazepine requirements during acute alcohol withdrawal. Am. J. Psychiatry, 136:821–823, 1979.

Woods, J. H.; Katz, J. L.; and Winger, G.: Use and abuse of benzodiazepines. J.A.M.A., 260:3476–3480, 1988.

Wyatt, R. J.; Karoum, F.; and Suddath, R.: The role of dopamine in cocaine use and abuse. Psychiatry Ann., 18:531–534, 1988.

28

Management of Poisoning

Stanley Nattel

Poisoning is an important clinical problem, both in terms of the resulting mortality and morbidity of individual patients and also as a consequence of the medical resources required to care for this group of patients. Poisoning may occur in three general ways: accidental, intentional, or iatrogenic. Accidental ingestion occurs most commonly in children. Intentional overdosage, often with suicidal intent, is the most common cause of poisoning in adults. While the overall number of accidental poisonings is much greater, intentional overdoses have a higher case mortality rate. For example, the American Association of Poison Control Centers (AAPCC) reported that the number of accidental poisonings monitored by their National Data Collection System in 1987 (1,037,549) was approximately 10 times the number of intentional poisonings (105,491) (Litovitz et al., 1988). Nevertheless, the number of deaths due to intentional overdoses was about 5 times as great (304; 288 per 100,000) as for accidental poisonings (66; 6 per 100,000). Iatrogenic "poisoning" includes the vast array of adverse drug reactions, many of which are preventable without compromising the development of efficacy from the drug. The extent of adverse drug reactions is difficult to ascertain, but this category may be even more important than the other two, particularly among the elderly (Lancet Editorial Board, 1988). The subject of adverse drug reactions and their prevention is dealt with in chapter 39. This chapter will focus on the management of self-poisoning, whether accidental or intentional.

Clinical poisoning may result from a wide variety of compounds (Litovitz et al., 1988). The agents most commonly implicated in lethal poisonings are listed in Table 28-1. While the 15 compounds with the highest case fatality rates accounted for less than 10% of the intoxications reported by the AAPCC in 1987, they were responsible for over 80% of deaths (Litovitz et al., 1988). Attention to the treatment of poisoning with such compounds is particularly important. This chapter will deal with general principles applicable to overdoses in general and will attempt to indicate the instances in which specific approaches to a given intoxication are necessary. Finally, the management of six specific types of poisoning will be discussed in detail to illustrate the application of principles previously discussed.

DIAGNOSIS

Recognition of Drug Overdose

There are two key issues in the diagnosis of poisoning. The first is the recognition of intoxication as the cause of a patient's clinical presentation. An obtunded patient brought in by his or her family with a suicide note and an empty pill bottle does not usually present a diagnostic challenge. On the other hand, many patients suffering from drug intoxications present without any clear history of drug ingestion or suicidal intent. Families may be adamant that their loved one had no access to medications and/or would never have taken an overdose. In such cases, the correct identification of poisoning as the underlying problem depends on the physician's alertness to this possi-

Table 28-1.   INTOXICATIONS AND MORTALITY RATE BY CATEGORY OF AGENT*

DRUG	NUMBER		PERCENTAGE		
	INGEST.	DEATHS	INGEST.	DEATHS	CASE FAT.
Antiarrhythmics	746	10	0.07	2.52	1.340
Cocaine	2445	27	0.22	6.80	1.104
Calcium antagonists	1835	18	0.16	4.53	0.981
Cyanide	322	3	0.03	0.76	0.932
Tricyclic antidepressants	11752	97	1.05	24.43	0.825
Digitalis	1399	11	0.13	2.77	0.786
Narcotics	3404	22	0.30	5.54	0.646
Carbon monoxide	4908	28	0.42	7.05	0.570
Methanol	1601	6	0.14	1.51	0.375
Theophylline	4712	15	0.42	3.78	0.318
Amphetamines	3883	11	0.35	2.77	0.283
Aspirin	14629	36	1.31	9.07	0.246
Lithium	1636	4	0.15	1.01	0.244
Glycols	4543	11	0.41	2.77	0.242
Sedative-hypnotics	36851	48	3.30	12.09	0.130
Ethanol	16440	16	1.47	4.03	0.097
Acetaminophen	66634	35	5.97	8.82	0.053
Hydrocarbons	46186	13	4.14	3.27	0.028
Insecticides	37856	6	3.39	1.51	0.016
Cleaning substances	114888	14	10.29	3.53	0.012

* Ingest. = ingestions; Case fat. = case fatality rate (percentage of ingestions of a given compound associated with death). Percentage of ingestions and deaths is the percentage of the total number of ingestions (1,166,940) and deaths (397) in the report in which a given agent is implicated. Because of multiple drug overdoses, more than one compound may be associated with a given case. Results shown are based on analysis of data from the 1987 annual report of the American Association of Poison Control Centers National Data Collection System (Litovitz et al., 1988).

bility. A number of typical clinical presentations of drug overdoses are listed in Table 28-2. When a patient presents with some of these findings and no alternate diagnosis has been clearly established, the possibility of drug overdose should always be considered until excluded by an appropriate test.

Drug overdose is an important cause of unexplained CNS depression. Characteristic findings include symmetrically depressed reflexes along

Table 28-2.   CHARACTERISTIC PRESENTATIONS OF POISONING

	PRESENTATION	AGENTS (PRODUCTS)
Syndrome		
General CNS depression	Drowsiness, stupor, coma, respiratory depression (signs generally symmetric)	Sedative-hypnotics, antipsychotics, narcotics, ethanol, salicylates (severe toxicity)
CNS excitation	Psychosis, tachycardia, seizures	Cocaine, amphetamines, theophylline, phencyclidine
Unexplained metabolic acidosis	Hyperventilation, features specific to each agent	Methanol, ethylene glycol, salicylates
Cardiac electrotoxicity	Unexplained arrhythmias, cardiac conduction disturbances	Antiarrhythmic drugs, digitalis, tricyclic antidepressants
Cardiac depression	Bradycardia, hypotension, AV block	Calcium antagonists, β blockers (rarely)
Anticholinergic toxicity	Dry mouth, delirium, CNS depression, tachycardia, dilated pupils	Antihistamines, tricyclic antidepressants, belladonna alkaloids
Mode		
Acid or alkali ingestion	Dysphagia, substernal and abdominal pain, oral burns, vomiting, drooling	Toilet bowl cleaners, drain cleaners, car battery acids
Hydrocarbon ingestion	CNS depression, pulmonary toxicity	Gasoline, kerosene, thinners, pine oil, furniture polish

with stupor or coma. Ocular reflexes typically are the last to be lost; CNS depressant drugs can result in complete areflexia and even a flat electroencephalogram, mimicking a brainstem vascular catastrophe. Similarly, the other syndromes listed in Table 28-2 can be mistaken for a variety of acute illnesses, including status epilepticus, shock, acute myocardial infarction, acute psychoses, cardiogenic pulmonary edema, and infectious pneumonias.

A valuable tool in diagnosing and following the course of many drug overdoses is a quantitative assay of drug concentrations in plasma. While not available for all potential intoxicants, drug assays can be obtained in a timely way for most. When the diagnosis of poisoning is clear and the treatment of choice is general supportive therapy, plasma concentration measurements may offer little more than a good prediction as to when the crisis will be over. On the other hand, when the diagnosis in uncertain or when knowledge of plasma drug concentration is necessary to guide treatment, quantitative assays may be very important. *Principle: The physician's natural fascination with the intricacies of the pharmacology of a poison and the possible ways of removing it should not overshadow his or her attention to the details of supportive care that can be less dramatic but more efficacious.*

Definition of the Intoxicating Agent

For some types of poisoning, identification of the specific agent(s) involved may not be critical. Intoxication with CNS depressants is often managed by general supportive measures. Knowledge of the compound(s) responsible is useful to provide realistic expectations of the time course of recovery and is important for compounds that have other important pharmacologic actions (e.g. salicylates, antidepressants). On the other hand, for many other types of overdoses, prompt recognition of the offending agent and the institution of specific treatment are critical if serious sequelae are to be prevented. A careful physical examination and routine laboratory testing (serum electrolyte concentrations, arterial blood-gas analysis, electrocardiogram (ECG), chest x-ray films) can provide important clues to the diagnosis of specific overdoses. Selected findings of potential significance are listed in Table 28-3.

Role of Laboratory Techniques to Detect and Quantify Poisons

If a specific intoxicant is suspected on the basis of the general clinical assessment, confirmation by analytic techniques generally is useful. Measurements of concentrations in plasma are particularly important for therapeutic decision making in the case of potentially dangerous intoxications that require specific therapies with intrinsic risks and/or substantial costs. Examples of such poisonings in which analytic techniques are important to guide therapy include salicylate, phenobarbital, lithium, methanol, ethylene glycol, and theophylline (decisions regarding hemodialysis or hemoperfusion), acetaminophen (*N*-acetylcysteine therapy), and massive digitalis (potential use of Fab antibodies) intoxications.

The value of broad-spectrum toxicologic screens is controversial. Disadvantages of such screens include the limited panel of drugs that they can detect, potential confusion resulting from the qualitative detection of a compound that is a minor component in a multiple-drug overdose, and the undue reliance of physicians on such screens at the expense of a careful physical examination and analysis of general laboratory data. A recent retrospective analysis suggested that *the results of toxicologic screens altered the management in only 3 of 209 cases* (Brett, 1988). In none of these cases was the change in treatment resulting from toxicologic analysis crucial to the outcome. Furthermore, there may be important differences in the results of toxicologic screens performed in different laboratories on the same samples (Ingelfinger et al., 1981). Misleading information may therefore result from incomplete, erroneous, or inaccurate screens. The most valuable form of toxicologic analysis is directed toward the quantitative assessment of specific suspected agents or groups of compounds, while broad-based, qualitative approaches have limited value.

TREATMENT OF POISONING: GENERAL ASPECTS OF THERAPY

Supportive Care

The single most important aspect of treating poisoned patients is the provision of adequate supportive care. The most important advance in the management of drug overdoses was the replacement of CNS stimulants by the use of protected airways, mechanical ventilation (when necessary), and support of the circulation (Henderson and Merrill, 1966). This approach, developed initially in Scandinavia, resulted in a dramatic reduction in mortality rate. Since the adoption of this approach, there has been no significant change in the mortality rate of drug intoxications despite all the subsequent therapeutic developments (e.g., forced diuresis, hemodialysis, hemoperfusion, activated charcoal therapy). *Principle: The single most important determinant of the outcome of poisoning is the provision of good supportive care. The value of any intervention must be weighed critically, particularly if it can prejudice the provision of supportive care.* With the exception of a few intoxications that

Table 28–3.   FINDINGS SUGGESTIVE OF SPECIFIC POISONINGS

SIGNS	ASSOCIATED WITH:
1. CNS	
a. Ataxia	Ethanol, phenytoin, barbiturates, hallucinogens, heavy metals
b. Seizures, muscle twitching	Cocaine, amphetamines, sedative-hypnotic withdrawal (including ethanol), organophosphates, cyanide, strychnine, salicylates, tricyclic antidepressants, isoniazid, phencyclidine, antipsychotics, theophylline
c. Rigidity, dystonias, muscle tremor	Antipsychotic drugs, phenothiazine antiemetics
d. Drowsiness, coma, respiratory depression	Sedative-hypnotics, antipsychotics, narcotics, ethanol, salicylates, antidepressants
e. Muscle weakness	Botulism, heavy metals
2. Eyes	
a. Pupillary constriction	Narcotics, organophosphates (cholinesterase inhibition), mushrooms (muscarinic), propoxyphene
b. Pupillary dilation	CNS stimulants (amphetamines, cocaine), anticholinergics (antihistamines, tricyclic antidepressants, etc.), glutethimide, LSD
c. Nystagmus	Phenytoin, sedative hypnotics
d. Impaired vision	Methanol, organophosphates, botulism
3. Mouth	
a. Salivation	Cholinergic enhancers (organophosphates, some mushrooms), corrosives, strychnine, arsenic, mercury
b. Dryness	Anticholinergics, amphetamines, narcotics
c. Discolored gums	Lead, mercury, arsenic
4. Cardiovascular system	
a. Bradycardia	Digitalis, narcotics, calcium antagonists, β blockers
b. Tachycardia	Anticholinergics (tricyclic antidepressants, antihistamines, etc), CNS stimulants (amphetamines, cocaine, etc), theophylline
c. Hypotension	Calcium antagonists, sedative-hypnotics, phenothiazines
d. Conduction disturbances, arrhythmias	Tricyclic antidepressants, digitalis, antiarrhythmic drugs, cocaine
5. Respiratory system	
a. Tachypnea	Agents causing acidosis (salicylates, methanol), pulmonary edema (hydrocarbons, narcotics), CNS stimulants
b. Pulmonary edema	Narcotics, hydrocarbons, salicylates, aspiration with any overdose
6. Gastrointestinal	
a. Nausea, vomiting	Corrosives, salicylates, theophylline, acetaminophen, heavy metals, boric acid
b. Diarrhea	Organophosphates, colchicine, arsenic, iron, mushrooms (muscarinic), boric acid
7. Skin	
a. Needle marks	Narcotics, amphetamines, cocaine
b. Sweating	Amphetamines, cocaine, LSD, barbiturates, cholinergic agents (organophosphates, mushrooms)
c. Purpura	Snake and spider toxins, salicylates
d. Bullae	Barbiturates, carbon monoxide
e. Jaundice	Carbon tetrachloride, arsenic, castor bean, acetaminophen (delayed), mushrooms (delayed)
f. Red, flushed	Anticholinergics, ethanol, carbon monoxide, cyanide

require a specific therapeutic approach (see Table 28–4), good supportive care alone will ensure a positive outcome in most patients. Even when a specific approach to a given intoxicant is necessary, good general supportive care is an essential component of management. *Principle: Remember to treat the patient, not the poison.*

Supportive care involves the maintenance of vital bodily functions in a physiologic state until the intoxicant(s) is(are) eliminated. Central nervous system depression causes death by cessation of breathing. This can be prevented by tracheal intubation and mechanical ventilation prior to respiratory arrest. If the gag reflex is absent or severely depressed, intubation and mechanical ventilation are generally indicated. It is inappropriate to wait for severe respiratory failure before instituting ventilatory support. Other factors that may be suppressing CNS function, such as hypoglycemia, acid–base, electrolyte, and other metabolic abnormalities, should be excluded by the appropriate test and treated promptly if present. *Principle: Most CNS depressant drugs have no intrinsic toxicity; they cause death by suppressing breathing or (rarely) causing severe hypotension. If a patient intoxicated with a CNS depressant agent*

Table 28-4. INTOXICATIONS WITH A SPECIFIC THERAPEUTIC APPROACH

SPECIFIC APPROACH NECESSARY	SPECIFIC APPROACH OF VALUE
Cyanide (nitrites, thiosulfates)	Antiarrhythmics (sodium bicar-
Carbon monoxide (oxygen)	bonate)
Methanol (ethanol, hemodialysis)	Antidepressants (alkalinization for
Ethylene glycol (ethanol, hemodialysis)	arrhythmias)
Salicylates (dialysis when severe)	Narcotics (naloxone)
Acetaminophen (*N*-acetylcysteine)	Phenobarbital (hemodialysis)
Lithium (dialysis when severe)	
Digitalis (Fab's for worst cases)	
Organophosphates (pralidoxime, atropine)	
Isoniazid (pyridoxine)	
Metals (chelators)	
Snakebites (antivenins)	
Theophylline (hemoperfusion when severe)	

arrives in the hospital breathing and with an adequate blood pressure, proper supportive management should ensure recovery.

The nervous system also is essential for regulation of blood pressure. Severe CNS depression often results in hypotension. In addition, drugs can cause hypotension by a direct vasodilating action (calcium antagonists, ethanol, vasodilator antihypertensives) or by causing fluid depletion (salicylates, diuretics). Adequate volume expansion is the most important intervention in the hypotensive patient. Central hemodynamic monitoring with a central venous pressure line or a Swan-Ganz catheter are useful to guide volume expansion. Measurement of pulmonary capillary wedge pressure as an index of left ventricular filling is necessary in patients with left ventricular disease, and in the presence of pulmonary edema with a possible cardiogenic component. Equal amounts of colloid and crystalloid solutions generally should be used. The exclusive use of crystalloids (such as physiologic saline solution) may expand the interstitial water compartment excessively and cause peripheral and/or pulmonary edema. Severe or resistant hypotension may reflect acute blood loss, and occult hemorrhage (GI, retroperitoneal bleeding, aneurysms) should be excluded. The hemoglobin concentration (or hematocrit) should be monitored, and red blood cells should be used for volume expansion if these indices suggest bleeding.

If hypotension is severe and fails to respond to volume expansion, adrenergic agonists may be necessary, particularly if there is clinical evidence of diminished blood flow to kidneys, heart, or brain. Hypotension in the presence of adequate tissue perfusion does not necessarily require pharmacologic intervention. The detailed pharmacology of these compounds and their use is covered elsewhere in this textbook (chapters 2–6) and will not be discussed here. A few points specific to poisoning will be made. Some intoxicants compete with adrenergic agonists for their receptors and may importantly alter the resulting response. For example, some antipsychotic agents and antidepressants block α receptors and inhibit the α-adrenergic component of the response to agents with mixed α- and β-receptor-stimulating activity, such as dopamine and epinephrine (Baldessarini, 1985). Because of the vasodilating effect of peripheral β_2 stimulation, mixed α-β stimulants may not be very effective in treating hypotension due to such intoxicants. Compounds with more specific α-agonist activity such as norepinephrine or even phenylephrine may be needed. Patients requiring adrenergic stimulation should have central hemodynamic monitoring and continuous recording of their arterial pressure. Measurement of cardiac output by thermodilution and calculation of hemodynamic variables (cardiac index, systemic vascular resistance, and stroke work index) can be valuable in the rational adjustment of hemodynamic therapy. β-Adrenergic stimulation primarily acts to increase cardiac output, while α stimulation increases peripheral vascular resistance. The arterial pressure is not a "magic number" to be treated in and of itself. Attention to indices of tissue perfusion, including urine output (in the absence of renal failure and diuretics), arterial pH, and mental status (if there is no drug-induced CNS depression) is important. A low pressure may be perfectly acceptable if there are no signs of tissue hypoperfusion.

Sustained seizure activity should be suppressed with IV diazepam and/or phenytoin, because persistent seizures can directly cause brain damage. A search for the cause of seizures should be undertaken, looking for electrolyte abnormalities, intracranial pathologic lesions, and specific intoxicants that may cause seizures (see Table 28–3) and may require specific therapy (Table 28–4). Cardiac arrhythmias should be treated if they interfere with hemodynamic function. This is often the case for sustained tachyarrhythmias (other than sinus tachycardia), but ectopic complexes per se generally do not require therapy. ***Principle: Drugs should be used carefully in the treatment of poisoning and only when there are specific indications for their administration. Avoid treating one poison with another poison.***

Metabolic, acid–base, and electrolyte variables should be monitored and any abnormalities appropriately managed. Acute renal failure may result from prolonged hypotension or from rhabdomyolosis (amphetamines and cocaine), can complicate fluid and electrolyte management, and may require dialysis. Acute hepatic dysfunction (carbon tetrachloride, acetaminophen) requires specific therapy. A urinary catheter is necessary in stuporous or comatose patients, and precautions are necessary to avoid bladder infection and secondary sepsis. Vigilance is necessary for the prompt recognition and treatment of secondary conditions that can complicate therapy, such as aspiration pneumonia, pneumonia from other causes, septicemia, and gastroduodenal erosions, ulcers, and hemorrhage. Careful nursing care is needed to prevent aspiration, nerve trauma, bedsores, corneal injury (in comatose patients), and excessive retention of bronchial secretions.

Decreasing the Quantity of Drug Absorbed

Three types of procedures are widely used to decrease GI absorption of orally ingested poisons: induced emesis, GI lavage, and the instillation of activated charcoal.

Induction of Emesis. Emesis usually is induced with syrup of ipecac, whose active moieties, the alkaloids emetine and cephaeline, induce vomiting by acting at receptor sites in both the CNS and GI tract (Habib and Harkiss, 1969). Vomiting occurs after an average of 18 minutes, but may require up to 30 minutes (Meester, 1985). In experimental animals, administration of ipecac at the time of an experimental overdose results in recovery of 30% to 60% of the dose ingested with recovery decreasing to 15% to 30% when ipecac is administered 1 hour after the overdose (Arnold et al., 1959; Corby et al., 1967; Abdallah and Tye, 1967). Early administration of ipecac to children poisoned with acetaminophen decreased subsequent concentrations of drug in plasma relative to values expected based on the dose taken, particularly when the emetic was given at home soon after ingestion (Amitai et al., 1987). On the other hand, older children or adults with overdoses present to the hospital an average of 3.3 hours after ingestion, a time when relatively little of the intoxicant is left in the stomach (Kulig et al., 1985). The induction of emesis can result in disastrous aspiration in patients with depressed

ability to protect their airway because of CNS depression. *Ipecac should never be given to patients with an impaired gag reflex.* Even in the presence of an adequate gag reflex at the time of ipecac administration, continued drug absorption can result in inadequate airway protection at the onset of vomiting because of the latency of ipecac's action. A variety of unusual complications, including Mallory-Weiss tears of the esophagus, also may occur (Robertson, 1979; Tandberg et al., 1981; Timberlake, 1984; Wolowdiuk et al., 1984). Ipecac occasionally fails to produce vomiting and should then be removed by nasogastric aspiration because of a risk of GI irritation and cardiac toxicity. Apomorphine also has been used to induce vomiting, since it acts more quickly than does ipecac; however its use has been largely abandoned because of risks of CNS depression and hypotension (Ellenhorn and Barceloux, 1988).

Gastric Lavage. Gastric lavage requires the insertion of a wide-bore orogastric tube, with repetitive gastric washes until the returns are clear. Perhaps because of the large tube that is needed, lavage has a relatively large number of associated complications. A complication rate of 3% has been cited, including aspiration pneumonia, esophageal damage, and cardiorespiratory arrest (Matthew et al., 1966). In a recent study, ECG changes were seen during lavage in 42% of patients, and decreases in arterial oxygen pressure were frequently noted (Thompson et al., 1987). Drug materials may form compactions too large to be removed by lavage, and a recent trial found that lavage did not alter the absorption of ampicillin following an experimental overdose in volunteers (Tenenbein et al., 1987). Gastric lavage recovered more than two therapeutic doses of CNS-depressant poisons in only one sixth of a series of clinical poisonings (Comstock et al., 1982). Lavage is contraindicated by an absent gag reflex unless a cuffed endotracheal tube is in place to protect the airway.

Activated Charcoal. The use of activated charcoal has been gaining increasing favor. Activated charcoal in the form of a slurry can be taken orally or via a nasogastric tube, with an initial dose of 50 g, sometimes followed by additional doses of 17 to 50 g every 4 hours. A cathartic is coadministered to prevent the constipation frequently produced by charcoal. Activated charcoal is able to adsorb large quantities of a wide variety of agents (Lancet Editorial Board, 1987). Furthermore, multiple-dose charcoal at 4-hour intervals is capable of reducing the half-life and increasing the clearance of IV administered agents such as theophylline and phenobarbital (Berg et al., 1982; Kulig et al., 1987). Enterohepatic recirculation does not appear to be involved in the latter effect, and it has been suggested that adsorption of drug to charcoal in the gut produces a continuous gradient favoring the movement of free drug from the blood into the GI tract, a process that has been termed *gastrointestinal dialysis* (Levy, 1982). Acceleration of elimination may also accelerate recovery from the overdose (Goldberg and Berlinger, 1982).

In the ampicillin-overdose model cited above, the instillation of activated charcoal was superior to both induced emesis and gastric lavage in reducing drug absorption (Tenenbein et al., 1987). One additional clinical study suggested that instillation of charcoal alone is superior to the induction of vomiting (Curtis et al., 1984). Induction of emesis or gastric lavage may provide little additional benefit over a single dose of activated charcoal (Kulig et al., 1985). Only in comatose patients presenting within 1 hour of ingestion was there apparent benefit from lavage (Kulig et al., 1985). A reviewer concluded that the administration of activated charcoal "is indicated in almost all serious overdoses except caustic agents, some heavy metals, and aliphatic hydrocarbons" (Jones et al., 1987).

In spite of the current enthusiasm for the use of charcoal, some notes of caution are in order. While activated charcoal can prevent absorption and favor elimination of a wide variety of agents, it has yet to be shown to alter the clinical outcome of a series of intoxications in a controlled trial. One small randomized trial compared multiple-dose charcoal with single-dose administration in the management of phenobarbital overdoses (Pond et al., 1984). While the drug's half-life was reduced by multidose charcoal from 93 to 36 hours, the duration of mechanical ventilation and of total hospitalization were unchanged. Activated charcoal must pass beyond the pylorus to be effective and is of little value in patients with severe vomiting (Kulig et al., 1987). While it is said to be very safe, activated charcoal usually requires the administration or moderate volumes of fluid via a nasogastric tube, with attendant interference with airway protection and a risk of aspiration (Pollack et al., 1981; Lancet Editorial Board, 1987; Jones et al., 1987). Furthermore, charcoal can interfere with the absorption of agents needed for therapy, such as *N*-acetylcysteine in acetaminophen overdoses (Ekins et al., 1987). Therefore, before giving activated charcoal to all patients with poisoning, one should remember the excellent results achieved by good supportive therapy alone. Controlled clinical trials of activated charcoal therapy in patients with specific types of overdoses would be very helpful in clarifying its clinical value.

Summary and Conclusions Regarding Drug Absorption in Poisoning. The induction of vomiting may be useful if it can be performed soon after the ingestion of an intoxicant (within about 30 minutes). It is contraindicated in the presence of a depressed gag reflex or overdoses with hydrocarbons and caustic substances. When activated charcoal is to be used, ipecac should be avoided because charcoal is ineffective in the presence of vomiting. The weight of evidence at the moment balances against the use of gastric lavage as a routine procedure in the treatment of poisoning. Activated charcoal may be valuable in preventing the absorption and possibly (as multiple-dose therapy) enhancing the elimination of a broad range of compounds and is probably the procedure of choice to prevent GI absorption of poisons ingested more than 30 minutes prior to presentation. Clarification of its precise role in the management of poisonings, in both single- and multiple-dose forms, awaits the performance of carefully conducted clinical trials.

All interventions to decrease drug absorption are associated with a risk of inducing aspiration and are contraindicated if the airway cannot be inadequately protected. Endotracheal intubation is not entirely protective against pulmonary aspiration, and prolonged combined gastric and endotracheal intubation is associated with an increased risk of tracheoesophageal fistulas. Just as for other interventions, the potential value of reducing GI drug absorption must be viewed in the context of the success of simple supportive therapy, and the risks of these procedures must be accordingly weighed against the potential benefit in each individual case. *Principle: In therapy as well as in the treatment of overdose, respect for the patient's physiology and its role in effecting new homeostasis must enter into clinical pharmacologic strategies.*

Enhancing Drug Elimination

Poisons normally are eliminated by hepatic biotransformation, renal excretion, or a combination of these mechanisms. It is intuitively appealing to increase the rate of drug elimination, either by enhancing intrinsic mechanisms (forced diuresis) or by extrinsic processes (hemodialysis, hemoperfusion).

Forced Diuresis. Administering large volumes of fluid can greatly increase urinary volume. Clearance of some drugs that are eliminated primarily by the kidney also may be enhanced, but the changes in drug elimination are much smaller than are those in urinary flow. While the physician may feel much better seeing profuse amounts of urine being produced, it is doubtful whether the patient's condition will be much improved. Manipulation of urinary pH can produce important changes in the elimination rate of a drug. By "trapping" drug in the nondiffusible, ionized form in the urine, alkalinization (for an acidic drug) or acidification (for a basic one) prevents back-diffusion into peritubular capillaries and increases renal excretion. Effective alteration of urinary pH may require substantial quantities of IV alkalinizing or acidifying agents and careful monitoring of systemic pH, urine pH, and plasma electrolytes. Forced diuresis necessitates the administration of large volumes of fluid, with a need for careful (and often central catheter) monitoring of the hemodynamic status.

The risks of forced diuresis include producing pulmonary edema, changing systemic pH and electrolyte balance with their attendant pathologic conditions, and initiating complications due to central hemodynamic monitoring procedures. These consequences clearly are prejudicial to the goals of providing good supportive care. Given the excellent results of supportive care alone, it is difficult to justify forced diuresis in overdoses of mild to moderate severity. When increased drug elimination is essential for a severe overdose, extracorporeal techniques (hemodialysis and hemoperfusion) are more effective than, and probably at least as safe as, forced diuresis.

Hemodialysis and Hemoperfusion. Hemodialysis and hemoperfusion can achieve significant clearance rates for a wide range of toxins (Cutler et al., 1987; Winchester, 1989). Hemodialysis involves the equilibration of the patient's blood with a physiologic dialysis solution across a semipermeable membrane. Hemoperfusion uses microencapsulated granules of activated charcoal that provide an enormous effective adsorption surface area (Chang, 1969). They are contained in a hemoperfusion cannister and used to clear blood of toxins. While hemodialysis devices have an effective dialysis surface limited to several square meters, hemoperfusion units have adsorbent surface areas of several thousand square meters (Garella, 1988).

The value of an extracorporeal technique for a given toxin is not necessarily reflected by its capacity to clear the drug from plasma. If a compound has a very large volume of distribution, reflecting extensive tissue stores, a relatively small fraction of the total body load of drug is available to be removed from the plasma. For example, while the plasma may be rapidly cleared of drugs such as tricyclic antidepressants, haloperidol, and methaqualone, resulting in apparent improvement during dialysis, a relatively small amount of these agents is removed during a standard 4-hour dialysis or hemoperfusion session. When the ses-

sion is terminated, rapid redistribution of the drug from extensive tissue stores into the plasma returns the patient to his or her previous state. Furthermore, some agents, like the toxic herbicide paraquat, bind tightly to their receptor sites explaining the inefficacy of dialysis in preventing or diminishing toxicity (Okonen et al., 1976; Vale et al., 1977; Garella, 1988).

Extracorporeal drug-removal techniques can be risky. The need for vascular access sites and the requirement of systemic anticoagulation to prevent clotting in the extracorporeal circuit can result in complications. Fluid and electrolyte abnormalities can occur during hemodialysis, as can hypotension due to the blood volume removed into the extracorporeal circuit (especially for dialysis). Hemoperfusion results in a small but measurable decrease in platelet count. A subtle risk of all extracorporeal drug removal techniques is that they tend to become viewed as the "treatment of the overdose" and distract attention from the details of careful supportive care that often are more important.

In view of the excellent results obtained in most patients with overdose by supportive care alone, the decision to use an extracorporeal drug removal technique must be taken very carefully on the basis of clinical findings such as the presence of difficult-to-manage hypotension. There are, however, specific overdoses in which dialysis or hemoperfusion are extremely important. The success of supportive therapy is limited to compounds whose toxic effects on vital organs are dose-dependent and reversible and can be compensated by appropriate management. In the case of agents that can cause irreversible tissue damage, simply supporting the patient as the drug is eliminated may not suffice. If such a compound can be removed in significant quantities by dialysis or hemoperfusion, these techniques can be very valuable. Examples of poisons that may fit the above description (and depending on the severity of poisoning) include methanol, ethylene glycol, salicylates, and theophylline.

TREATMENT OF SPECIFIC POISONINGS

Approach to Understanding the Treatment of Specific Overdoses

The answers to a number of key questions determine the management of specific intoxications.

1. **How does this compound produce morbidity or mortality?** That is, what are the pathophysiologic mechanisms by which excess quantities of this compound adversely affect the patient?

2. **What are the indices that best predict the likelihood of complications?** These are the indicators of the severity and risk of the overdose.

3. **What interventions can be used to prevent drug-induced adverse events?** Such interventions may include supporting or substituting for the function of an organ reversibly depressed by the drug, interfering with the pathophysiologic mechanisms by which the drug causes toxicity, and/or maneuvers that reduce the effect of the drug by preventing its absorption or enhancing its elimination. The efficacy of the latter maneuvers depends on the closeness of the relationship between drug load and serious complications, and the extent to which such maneuvers can limit the drug load. *Principle: For all cases of poisoning, general supportive measures are very important. In a few types of poisonings, specific therapies are available that favorably modify the course of the illness.*

The management of a number of specific overdoses will now be discussed in the context of the approach outlined above.

CNS Depressants

Included in this category are the barbiturates, nonbarbiturate sedative-hypnotics, benzodiazepines, narcotics, and other compounds to the extent that their toxicity is due to CNS depression (e.g., antipsychotics, antihistamines, antidepressants, etc.).

1. These compounds produce morbidity and mortality predominantly by causing CNS depression. They have no intrinsically irreversible toxic actions. Therefore, if the consequences of CNS depression can be managed while the patient eliminates the drug, no adverse sequelae should result. The most important vital system directly controlled by the CNS is the respiratory system, and respiratory arrest is far and away the most common cause of death due to overdoses of CNS depressants. Fortunately, respiratory depression is readily managed in the hospital by mechanical ventilation. Most deaths due to overdoses of CNS depressants result from respiratory arrest and irreversible hypoxic damage to the brain prior to the patient's receiving medical attention. Other potential causes of adverse effects include aspiration of gastric contents because of an inadequate gag reflex, and hypotension related to both depressed cardiac function and peripheral vasodilation.

2. The index best predicting the likelihood of complications is the patient's clinical state upon arrival in hospital. If the patient has had a period of frank respiratory arrest or severe respiratory depression, the prognosis is guarded. On the other hand, if the patient has breathed spontaneously until the time of his or her arrival at the emergency room and his or her arterial blood-gas concentrations are within the physiologic range, serious complications are very unlikely if good supportive care is given. A depressed gag reflex indicates impairment of protection of the airways, and an attendant risk of aspiration. Furthermore, depression of brainstem reflexes such as the gag reflex suggests an important likelihood of present or imminent depression of respiratory centers in the brainstem. Clinical signs are much more useful indices of the severity of the overdose than are the dose ingested by history (often unreliable) or concentrations of drug in plasma (Chazan and Garrella, 1971; Goodman et al., 1976; Ingelfinger et al., 1981). Consideration of patient factors may enhance the utility of plasma concentrations (McCarron et al., 1982). Moreover, plasma concentrations may provide useful information in assessing the course of an overdose: failure to see improvement despite substantial reductions in concentrations of drug may indicate irreversible brain damage.

3. The most important interventions in preventing complications are those associated with the provision of good supportive care. If the gag reflex is impaired, the patient should be intubated. Mechanical ventilation (or assisted ventilation) is required if ventilatory failure is present. If very close monitoring of ventilatory function is not possible, prophylactic ventilation may be advisable, since undetected ventilatory failure can produce irreversible brain damage within minutes. Other supportive measures should be applied as outlined above in the section on general aspects of therapy.

Procedures to decrease gastric absorption have a limited role to play, as discussed above. Repeated doses of activated charcoal reduce the half-life of phenobarbital considerably (Berg et al., 1982; Goldberg and Berlinger, 1982). Whether this alters the outcome of phenobarbital overdoses is uncertain (Pond et al., 1984). Similar considerations apply to the removal of CNS depressant drugs by dialysis or hemoperfusion. While the clearance of some compounds (particularly intermediate- and long-acting barbiturates) is significantly enhanced by these measures (Cutler et al., 1987), it is debatable whether their benefits outweigh their risks. The primary determinant of outcome, the patient's state upon presentation, is not changed by enhancing elimination of drug. The value of extracorporeal procedures depends on the balance between an improved ability to provide supportive care because the duration of the overdose is shortened and the negative consequences of the need for arterial and venous access anticoagulation and the complications of the procedure.

Prior to the 1950s, nonspecific CNS stimulants were widely used as antidotes for CNS-depressant drugs. They have been universally replaced by

supportive therapy. The specific narcotic antagonist naloxone may be very useful in managing
overdoses with narcotic drugs. Because most narcotics have a longer half-life than naloxone, bolus
administration of the latter can result in a fluctuating clinical status necessitating multiple doses
and close monitoring. Alternatively, if an initial
dose produces substantial improvement, a maintenance infusion of 0.4 to 0.8 mg/hour can be
used until the respiratory-depressant effect of the
narcotic has been eliminated (Ellenhorn and Barceloux, 1988). All patients with CNS depression
due to presumed drug overdose should receive a
bolus of glucose after a blood sample has been
obtained for measurement of blood glucose, because of the possibility of hypoglycemia as an
alternative or ancillary diagnosis.

The administration of physostigmine has been
advocated as antidotal therapy for anticholinergic
overdoses. Physostigmine's arousing action is not
specific for any one type of overdose, and because
of its potential adverse effects, the use of physostigmine as an antidote for tricyclic antidepressant overdoses is not recommended (Newton,
1975; Nattel et al., 1979).

Cyclic Antidepressants

Intoxications with cyclic antidepressants consistently account for a substantial proportion of
lethal poisonings (e.g., see Table 28–1). The importance of this problem is likely related to the
frequency and intensity of suicide attempts in depressed patients and the significant pharmacologic toxicity of those compounds. Included in
this category are the tricyclic agents amitriptyline,
imipramine, and their derivatives, as well as
newer agents such as doxepin, maprotiline (a tetracyclic compound), amoxapine, nomifensine,
and trazodone.

1. Morbidity and mortality caused by the cyclic
antidepressants results from two pharmacologic
actions: CNS depression and cardiovascular toxicity. The consequences and nature of CNS depression caused by antidepressants are similar to
those for the general category of CNS depressants
discussed above, with the exception that antidepressants are more likely to cause seizures. Cardiotoxicity is a serious potential consequence of
antidepressant overdoses. Ventricular tachyarrhythmias are associated with severe slowing of
intraventricular conduction resulting from drug-
induced blockade of sodium channels and are presumably due to facilitation of ventricular reentry
(Nattel et al., 1984) (see chapter 6). Sinus tachycardia results from anticholinergic actions that
occur at much lower concentrations of drug than
do those producing ventricular arrhythmias (Nattel et al., 1984). The anticholinergic effects play

a permissive role in ventricular arrhythmias by
enhancing rate-dependent sodium-channel blockade (Nattel, 1985). Newer antidepressants like
amoxepine and nomifensine seem to have considerably less cardiotoxicity, although this appears
not to be the case for maprotiline (Knudsen and
Heath, 1984; Coccaro and Siever, 1985).

2. The indices predicting the likelihood of complications are indicators of CNS and respiratory
depression (as discussed above), and signs of cardiotoxicity. Ventricular tachyarrhythmias and
prolongation of the QRS interval on the ECG are
suggestive of clinically important cardiotoxicity.
Clinically significant overdoses generally prolong
the QRS duration to > 0.10 second, although values in this range also can be seen on a chronic
basis in otherwise normal persons (Biggs et al.,
1977). Perhaps because of their anticholinergic
action, which decreases GI motility, antidepressants can be absorbed slowly, and instances have
been reported of serious arrhythmias after an
asymptomatic latent period (Callaham, 1982).
Extensive retrospective reviews did not identify
patients with apparently mild antidepressant toxicity who later developed serious cardiac arrhythmias (Greenland and Howe, 1981; Pentel and
Sioris, 1981; Goldberg et al., 1985). In a retrospective analysis of 18 lethal overdoses with cyclic antidepressants, half the patients had minimal signs
of toxicity upon presentation; however, major
toxic signs developed within 2 hours in all patients
(Callaham and Kassel, 1985).

3. As for all overdoses that produce CNS
depression, the prevention of complications depends on good supportive care and on the management of cardiovascular complications. Sodium bicarbonate effectively reverses slowing
of ventricular conduction and the arrhythmias
caused by tricyclic antidepressants (Brown, 1976).
A considerable portion of the benefit of administration of sodium bicarbonate appears to be due
to alkalinization. Hyperventilation-induced respiratory alkalosis also may reverse cyclic antidepressant cardiotoxicity (Kingston, 1979; Nattel
and Mittleman, 1984). There is some evidence
that the sodium moiety of sodium bicarbonate
may also contribute to its efficacy (Pentel and
Benowitz, 1984; Sasyniuk and Jhamandas, 1984).
Lidocaine also can reverse antidepressant-induced
ventricular arrhythmias, but higher than usual
concentrations appear to be necessary (Nattel and
Mittleman, 1984). Administration of phenytoin
in an animal model increased the severity of ventricular arrhythmias caused by amitriptyline, indicating that sodium-channel blocking drugs probably have little role to play in treating arrhythmias
caused by cyclic antidepressants (Pentel et al.,
1981).

Plasma clearance rates of tricyclic antidepressants induced by hemoperfusion are substantial. Extracorporeal removal initially was highly touted as a potentially important treatment of overdose. In fact, in the 1986 AAPCC review, 28 cases of cyclic antidepressant overdose were treated by dialysis or hemoperfusion, compared with 26 for salicylates (Litovitz and Veltri, 1988). However, because of their extensive tissue distribution, cyclic antidepressants are present in very small quantities in the plasma, and hemoperfusion can be expected to remove only about 50 mg of a 2500-mg tricyclic overdose during a 4-hour session (Garella, 1988). Extracorporeal techniques therefore have little role to play in cyclic antidepressant poisoning in the absence of concomitant renal failure.

The cholinesterase inhibitor physostigmine has been advocated as an antidote to the CNS-depressant anticholinergic effects of cyclic antidepressants. Physostigmine increases the incidence of seizures and death in mice intoxicated with cyclic antidepressants and can cause bradyarrhythmias, excessive secretions, and seizures in humans (Newton, 1975; Vance et al., 1977). Its role in the treatment of cyclic antidepressant poisoning is therefore not recommended.

Salicylates

Most salicylate overdoses are due to the ingestion of aspirin, although poisonings with methyl salicylate (oil of wintergreen) occur and can be quite serious because of a high salicylate content per volume. With the increased use of childproof containers, acute salicylate intoxication is less of a problem in the pediatric population than it once was. Chronic salicylate intoxication generally is more serious than is acute poisoning.

Causes of morbidity and mortality produced by salicylate include adverse effects on the CNS, and fluid and electrolyte imbalances. In a retrospective analysis of nine lethal salicylate overdoses at the Montreal General Hospital, all patients had altered CNS function (delirium, stupor, coma, or seizures) on presentation, while serum electrolyte concentrations, acid–base status, and salicylate concentrations varied widely among patients (Nattel, unpublished data). While blood salicylate concentrations varied widely at the time of death among rats poisoned with salicylate, brain salicylate concentrations were remarkably consistent (Hill, 1973). Central nervous system toxicity seems, therefore, to be critically involved in salicylate-induced lethality. The mechanism of salicylate-induced cerebral dysfunction is unclear, but salicylates cause hypoglycemia in the CNS in the presence of normal blood sugar concentrations (Thurston et al., 1970). Uncoupling of oxidative phosphorylation could account for many

of the toxic effects of salicylate, including cerebral hypoglycemia, an increased respiratory quotient, and respiratory alkalosis (due to metabolic dysfunction of respiratory control centers), hyperpyrexia, and lactic acidosis (Smith and Jeffrey, 1956).

A variety of other factors may play a contributory role to the adverse consequences of salicylate poisoning. Salicylates produce complex acid–base abnormalities, including both respiratory alkalosis and metabolic acidosis. Respiratory alkalosis probably is due to the direct effects of salicylate on the brain centers controlling breathing. Metabolic acidosis is associated with an increased anion gap, with contributions from stimulated production of lactate and increased productions of ketones (Smith and Jeffrey, 1956; Gabow et al., 1978). Only a fraction of the anion gap can be explained by salicylate ion per se. Other drugs taken along with salicylates in multiple-drug overdoses can complicate the picture by inducing respiratory acidosis (CNS depression) or by causing a normal anion gap metabolic acidosis (Gabow et al., 1978). In Gabow's series, all patients with severe acidemia had ingested other drugs that caused respiratory depression.

Salicylate excess not only causes nausea and vomiting as a result of gastric irritation but also can produce hyperpyrexia with fevers as high as 105°F. The insensible fluid loss resulting from fever and hyperventilation combined with the liquids lost in vomiting may produce important hypovolemia. Fluid loss also may result in hyponatremia and hypokalemia, with respiratory alkalosis tending to enhance excretion of potassium via the kidney. High fever may require vigorous treatment with cooling blankets. Salicylate overdoses may be associated with noncardiogenic pulmonary edema. There is some evidence that salicylate may have a direct toxic effect on pulmonary endothelium, resulting in extravasation of fluid (Walters et al., 1983). In some cases, iatrogenic fluid overload in an effort to cause a forced diuresis may play an important role. Aspirin (but not salicylic acid) inhibits platelet adhesiveness, even at therapeutic doses, and salicylates can reduce the hepatic synthesis of vitamin K–dependent clotting factors. These effects are rarely sufficient to cause clinical bleeding.

The most important indicator of risk in salicylate poisoning probably is the CNS status. In the absence of other intoxicants, impaired cerebral function (delirium, stupor, coma, or seizures) indicates an overdose with substantially increased risk of death. Salicylate concentrations in serum are useful to index the potential severity of the overdose, particularly if the concentrations are related to the time since ingestion and clinical signs (Done, 1978). Systemic acidemia is very deleterious and must be treated vigorously (Proudfoot, 1969). Salicylate is an acid with a pK_a of 3 and is very highly ionized at physiologic pH. The nonionized form is free to cross membranes, and its concentration is decreased by alkalosis and increased by acidosis. Local acidosis favors egress of salicylate, while alkalosis results in trapping of salicylate in a compartment. Systemic acidosis results in redistribution of salicylate from the blood into the relatively more alkaline CNS, resulting in greater brain concentrations, more CNS toxicity, and a higher mortality rate (Hill, 1971).

Interventions to prevent complications include meticulous attention to the fluid, acid–base, and electrolyte disorders described above. If signs of CNS toxicity are present and blood salicylate concentrations are in a range consistent with a severe overdose, enhancement of salicylate elimination is indicated (Done, 1978). A single salicylate determination may be inadequate to evaluate the severity of an overdose because salicylate delays gastric emptying, because concretions of pills may form (resulting in slow GI release), or because of the ingestion of enteric-coated formulations that are absorbed slowly. Repeated determinations of concentrations in serum are necessary to exclude sustained absorption. When absorption is sustained, measures to decrease it (as discussed above) may be particularly important. Activated charcoal binds salicylate well, and repeated doses may both reduce absorption and enhance elimination of salicylate (Hillman and Prescott, 1985).

Therapeutic concentrations of salicylate are eliminated by hepatic biotransformation to a variety or metabolites (Levy et al., 1972). These pathways become saturated at concentrations in the toxic range as a result of poisoning, resulting in nonlinear accumulation of drug and slowed elimination (Levy et al., 1972). Renal clearance of salicylate is heavily dependent on urinary pH and is greatly increased when the urine is alkalinized (Prescott et al., 1982). Urinary alkalinization by the systemic administration of sodium bicarbonate is therefore desirable, both to enhance urinary excretion of salicylate and to limit CNS salicylate concentrations by keeping the serum slightly alkaline. In practice, salicylate poisoning often causes aciduria, and very large quantities of sodium bicarbonate may be necessary to alkalinize the urine in severe overdoses (Robin et al., 1959; Done, 1965). The consequent risks of volume overload and acid–base and electrolyte abnormalities are not trivial. Acetazolamide inhibits renal carbonic anhydrase and allows effective urinary alkalinization but can produce systemic acidosis, which is highly undesirable. In an animal model, acetazolamide substantially *increased* the lethality of salicylate overdoses (Hill, 1971). The safe use of acetazolamide requires very close monitoring

of systemic acid–base and electrolyte status and has been largely abandoned in favor of sodium bicarbonate administration. In view of the attendant risks of fluid overload and electrolyte imbalance, it usually is advisable to proceed to extracorporeal removal of salicylate if urinary alkalinization proves difficult in the face of a serious overdose.

Salicylate is readily removed by both hemodialysis and hemoperfusion (Cutler et al., 1987; Garella, 1988; Winchester, 1989). Hemodialysis is generally preferred, because it also may improve the fluid and electrolyte imbalances that frequently accompany severe salicylate poisoning. Hemodialysis should always be considered when there are signs of cerebral effects of salicylates such as altered mental states or severe hyperpyrexia. *Principle: Clearance of a poison from the body is not the only determinant of whether an intervention is working. If redistribution of the remaining drug concentrates it in critically dangerous sites, the results might be dangerous and, although in a sense predictable, not always obvious to the physician.*

Acetaminophen

Because of the fear of Reye syndrome, acetaminophen has largely replaced aspirin in pediatric therapy. Its use as a mild analgesic-antipyretic also has increased in adults because of the gastric irritation and other adverse effects that aspirin can produce. Before the introduction of an effective antidote, hepatic necrosis and death were among the consequences of acetaminophen poisoning. While the likelihood of these complications has been greatly reduced by the advent of effective therapy, acetaminophen remains an important cause of death due to drug overdoses (Table 28–1).

Acetaminophen produces one major toxic effect — hepatic necrosis. The lesion results from conversion of the drug into highly reactive intermediate metabolites via the cytochrome P450 system (Rollins et al., 1979). At therapeutic doses of acetaminophen, most is conjugated with sulfate and glucuronide, and the small quantities of reactive intermediate formed are rapidly reduced by hepatic glutathione (Mitchell et al., 1974). Acetaminophen poisoning saturates the conjugation systems and results in the production of intermediates that exhaust the capacity of the glutathione system, bind covalently to hepatic macromolecules, and cause tissue necrosis (Mitchell et al., 1974; Corcoran et al., 1980). Rarely, acetaminophen causes acute renal failure by a similar mechanism (McMurtry et al., 1978; Cobden et al., 1982; Curry et al., 1982; Gabriel, 1982).

The natural history of severe acetaminophen

poisoning consists of early nonspecific GI symptoms (anorexia, nausea, and vomiting). This generally is followed by a 2- to 3-day asymptomatic period. Signs of liver damage begin to appear 2 to 4 days after the overdose, and death from fulminant hepatic necrosis can occur between 4 and 18 days after ingestion.

The best indicator of the likelihood of hepatic toxicity due to acetaminophen is the concentration of acetaminophen in serum. Since there is a relatively asymptomatic period of several days prior to the onset of hepatotoxicity, clinical findings are of little value in predicting the risk of complications. Concentrations of drug in serum have to be interpreted in the light of the time lapse since ingestion. Nomograms are available that indicate the risk of toxicity as a function of drug concentration in blood (Rumack et al., 1981). Acetaminophen has a half-life of about 4 hours, and the concentrations in plasma associated with a >60% risk of severe toxicity (transaminase levels >1000 IU/l) are 200, 100, 50 and 25 mg/l at 4, 8, 12, and 16 hours, respectively, after ingestion (Rumack et al., 1981). Plasma concentrations greater than 300 mg/l at 4 hours are associated with a 90% risk of hepatic encephalopathy and about a 10% mortality if untreated. Concentrations in plasma that are under 120 mg/l at 4 hours are unlikely to produce any toxic effects (Prescott et al., 1971).

The prevention of hepatotoxicity can be achieved by the antidote, N-acetylcysteine. Acetylcyteine is a reducing agent capable of entering hepatocytes and reducing acetaminophen metabolites, either directly or by reducing previously oxidized glutathione. The drug is better tolerated and more effective than the previously used reducing agents, methionine and cysteamine (Prescott et al., 1979). The critical factor determining outcome in treated patients with acetaminophen poisoning is the time between ingestion and treatment (Prescott, 1981). Severe hepatic toxicity was seen in only one patient (2%) of those receiving acetylcysteine within 10 hours of ingestion, and none in patients treated within 8 hours (Prescott, 1981). This contrasts with an 85% incidence of severe liver damage in patients receiving antidote therapy 15 to 24 hours after ingestion, and an 89% incidence in patients treated prior to the advent of effective antidotes (Prescott, 1981).

Given the great efficacy of early therapy with antidote and the critical role of time from ingestion to initiation of therapy, acetylcysteine should be started as soon as possible. A blood sample for assay of acetaminophen should be obtained as soon as the poisoning is suspected. Depending on the time required for the assay to be performed and reported, it may be desirable to begin therapy prior to obtaining the result, particularly if there is a reliable history of the ingestion of over 7.5 g (or 140 mg/kg) of acetaminophen. In all cases falling into the group with "probable risk" according to concentrations in plasma, acetylcysteine therapy should be begun immediately after the results of the drug assay are known (Rumack et al., 1981). Where the IV formulation of acetylcysteine is available (e.g., in Canada and the United Kingdom), it should be used in preference, particularly early after acetaminophen ingestion when nausea and vomiting tend to be prominent. If only oral acetylcysteine is available, administration by nasogastric tube may be necessary to allow adequate absorption. N-Acetylcysteine generally is innocuous, but several cases of associated bronchospasm and one case of lethal hypotension and cyanosis have been reported (Lancet Note, 1984).

Cocaine

With the increasing use of cocaine as a drug of abuse, deaths due to cocaine are becoming more frequent. The toxicology of cocaine is complicated by the wide range of pharmacologically active impurities that can contaminate "street" cocaine. These include local anesthetics (procaine, lidocaine, tetracaine, benzocaine), CNS stimulants (amphetamine, caffeine, theophylline, strychnine), hallucinogens (phencyclidine, marijuana, LSD), opioids (heroin, codeine), and depressants such as ethanol (Ellenhorn and Barceloux, 1988). In addition, there are a wide range of cocaine substitutes available on the streets (Siegel, 1980).

Cocaine produces serious morbidity and mortality by actions on the brain and the cardiovascular system. The two primary mechanisms involved are blockade of catecholamine uptake and local anesthetic action (Muscholl, 1961; Ritchie and Greene, 1985). Increased catecholamine effects due to blockade of uptake result in rostral–caudal CNS stimulation, with restlessness and euphoria progressing to tremulousness, hyperreflexia, and seizures as the drug's effects increase. Coma and respiratory depression may occur, possibly as a result of local anesthetic action on the brain. Tachycardia and hypertension result from stimulation of hypothalamic cardiovascular control centers, combined with decreased local neuronal noradrenaline reuptake in the heart and blood vessels. Cardiac arrhythmias result from an excess of adrenergic stimulation, sodium-channel blockade, and acute myocardial ischemia (Weidmann, 1955). Acute myocardial infarction within hours after use of cocaine is not rare and can occur in young patients with normal coronary arteries (Isner et al., 1986). Contributing factors may include arterial spasm due to cocaine's well-known vasoconstricting action (possibly due to high local noradrenaline concentrations), increased myocardial oxygen need resulting from tachycardia and hypertension, and thrombogenic properties. Autopsies among patients with cocaine-related deaths show an increased prevalence of focal myocarditis without an increased prevalence of coronary atherosclerotic lesions (Virmani et al., 1988). On the other hand, sudden death associated with cocaine abuse is frequently associated with significant coronary atherosclerosis (Mittleman and Wetli, 1987).

As in overdoses that cause CNS depression, the best predictor of clinical outcome in cocaine overdoses is the patient's state at the time of arrival at hospital. Most deaths due to cocaine intoxication occur within the first few minutes after exposure (Ellenhorn and Barceloux, 1988). Exceptions to this rule are patients who die when condoms or balloons filled with cocaine rupture in their GI tract, or patients who swallow solid crystalline free-base cocaine ("rock") that may require hours to be fully absorbed. A syndrome of cocaine-induced rhabdomyolysis has been described (Roth et al., 1988). One third of these patients developed acute renal failure, and almost half of the patients with renal failure died. Other complications included severe liver damage and disseminated intravascular coagulation (DIC). DIC occurred in just over half the patients with renal failure and was associated with a mortality rate of over 80%. The mechanism by which cocaine poisoning causes rhabdomyolysis is unknown.

The complications of cocaine overdose are managed by supportive therapy. Cocaine-induced seizures respond well to IV diazepam, while phenobarbital and phenytoin may be less effective in preventing them (Jonsson et al., 1983; Ritchie and Greene, 1985). In dogs exposed to lethal doses of cocaine, seizures and hyperpyrexia are central to the mechanism of death, and both can be prevented by administering IV diazepam (Catravas and Waters, 1981). Should CNS depression and hypotension occur, they should be treated supportively as described above. Cardiac arrhythmias caused by cocaine may respond to β-adrenergic-receptor blockers, and studies in animals suggest the potential value for calcium-channel blockers (Nahas et al., 1985; Cregler and Mark, 1986; Billman and Hoskins, 1988).

Hypertension is usually transient in patients with cocaine overdoses. But severe persistent hypertension should be managed as described in chapter 2. Propranolol may increase blood pressure in the face of high circulating catecholamine concentrations by blocking only β_2-mediated vasodilation and leaving α-adrenergic actions unopposed. Such a response has been noted in cocaine overdose (Ramoska and Sacchetti, 1985). Hyper-

pyrexia may require the use of ice baths or a hypothermic blanket. The acute agitation of mild overdoses or the early or late phases of more severe intoxications may require sedation.

Methanol and Ethylene Glycol

Methanol is produced by the distillation of fermented wood ("wood alcohol"), and is erroneously ingested as a substitute for ethanol. Ethylene glycol commonly is present in antifreezes and is ingested either as an alcohol substitute or in suicide attempts.

These compounds produce their major toxic effects by being converted by the liver into toxic metabolites. Since their toxic actions require biotransformation of the progenitor, there is a lag between the time of the overdose and the appearance of symptoms. Methanol is less intoxicating than is ethanol. A typical history is one of ingestion of an unclearly labeled product said to be alcohol, a disappointing lack of inebriation, and then the onset of neurologic and visual symptoms. Ethylene glycol has intoxicating properties similar to those of ethanol, and the initial "high" often is followed by a latent phase before the onset of symptoms. Methanol's toxicity is due to the elaboration of the metabolites formaldehyde and formic acid, with formic acid being more important because of the short biologic half-life of formaldehyde (McMartin et al., 1980). Ethylene glycol's toxicity results from conversion to glycolic acid and to a much lesser extent oxalic acid (Clay and Murphy, 1977; Gabow et al., 1986). Both intoxications are characterized by an increased anion gap metabolic acidosis. The acidosis results from acidic metabolites and to a lesser extent from formation of lactic acid due to altered cellular metabolism (Gabow et al., 1986; Jacobson and McMartin, 1986).

Methanol's toxicity is directed toward the CNS and the eyes. The CNS symptoms range from headache, vertigo, and confusion to coma and convulsions in severe cases. Blurred vision and photophobia may be accompanied by fixed, dilated pupils, retinal edema, and hyperemia of the optic disks. Ethylene glycol's toxicity is directed at the CNS, the cardiovascular system, and the kidneys. Nausea and vomiting often are early symptoms. The CNS depression generally precedes cardiovascular and renal complications and may be severe enough to cause coma and seizures. Heart failure, sometimes associated with hypertension, and acute tubular necrosis can occur in severe overdoses. The characteristic course of symptoms is said to be triphasic, with CNS manifestations appearing in the first 12 hours, followed by cardiovascular and then renal toxicity (Friedman et al., 1962; Parry and Wallach, 1974).

Oxalate crystals are typically, but not invariably, present in the urine (Turk et al., 1986).

Indicators of the likelihood of complications include the severity of the metabolic acidosis, the concentrations of the ingested drug and its metabolites in plasma, and clinical signs of toxicity. Concentrations of the poison in plasma are useful, particularly when they are correlated with the time since ingestion. Remember though that the toxicity is due to metabolites and not to the parent compound. The severity of the acidosis correlates better with the outcome than do concentrations of the intoxicant in plasma, perhaps because the former is directly related to concentrations of the toxic metabolites (Bennett et al., 1953). Methanol and ethylene glycol are metabolized by alcohol dehydrogenase, the enzyme that ordinarily metabolizes ethanol. Consequently, ethanol competes very strongly with methanol and ethylene glycol for alcohol dehydrogenase. Coingestion of ethanol with these intoxicants reduces the toxicity for a given dose of methanol or ethylene glycol and may greatly reduce the complications resulting from any given plasma concentration of these poisons. The presence of any significant clinical complication, such as visual symptoms, CNS changes, renal failure, and crystalluria, indicate a severe intoxication.

The main treatment modalities include administration of ethanol to prevent the formation of toxic metabolites, and hemodialysis for severe overdoses. Ethanol may be more important and should be administered at the appropriate dose to maintain blood ethanol concentrations of 100 to 150 mg/dl (McCoy et al., 1979). This concentration of ethanol will markedly inhibit the rate of metabolism of either methanol of ethylene glycol since, for example, ethanol is many times more potent than methanol in binding to alcohol dehydrogenase. Since ethanol inhibits the metabolism of these substances, it greatly prolongs their half-life, and several days may be required for the plasma concentrations of the methanol or ethylene glycol to substantially decline. Ethanol should be administered to any patient with a strongly suspected intoxication with these agents while awaiting the results of blood concentration measurements, and to all patients with a concentration greater than 20 mg/l of toxin, with systemic acidosis, or with clinical symptoms suggestive of complications. Dialysis is effective in removing both toxic metabolites and the parent compound, is clearly superior to hemoperfusion, and appears to reduce the complication rate of methanol overdoses (Gonda et al., 1978; Whalen et al., 1979; McCoy et al., 1979; McMartin et al., 1980). Indications for dialysis include methanol concentrations greater than 50 mg/dl in plasma, acidosis that is resistant to therapy, or any complications

of the poisoning. Since dialysis also removes ethanol, the latter must be added to the dialysis bath at a concentration of 100 mg/dl, or its maintenance dose must be increased.

The specific overdoses discussed above are intended to illustrate the considerations needed to develop a rational approach to managing poisonings. Space limitations do not allow a discussion of the specific therapy of all potential poisonings. For a more extensive treatment, the reader is referred to textbooks (Gossel and Bricker, 1984; Ellenhorn and Barceloux, 1988).

In summary:

1. **Treat the patient, then his or her poison.** Conservative therapy to control symptoms common to many drugs may be enough to permit survival. Do not let the patient die of respiratory arrest or shock while you are on the telephone to a poison control center.

2. **If possible, find out what has been ingested.** This provides a guide to the severity of poisoning and to any unique features of the intoxication that may warrant specific monitoring or therapy.

3. **Attempt to establish the severity of the intoxication and, after consideration of factors such as concurrent diseases of the liver or kidney, decide whether or not the drug can and/or should be removed.**

4. **Read the clinical literature on poisoning with the suspected drug or drugs with great care to acquire and analyze all data needed to make therapeutic decisions.**

REFERENCES

Abdallah, A. H.; and Tye, A.: A comparison of the efficacy of emetic drugs and stomach lavage. Am. J. Dis. Child., 113: 571–575, 1967.

Amitai, Y.; Mitchell, A. A.; McGuigan, M. A.; and Lovejoy, F. H. Jr.: Ipecac-induced emesis and reduction of plasma concentrations of drugs following accidental overdose in children. Pediatrics, 80:364–367, 1987.

Arnold, F. J.; Hodges, J. B.; and Barta, R. A. Jr.: Evaluation of the efficacy of lavage and induced emesis in treatment of salicylate poisoning. Pediatrics, 23:286–301, 1959.

Baldessarini, R. J.: Drugs and the treatment of psychiatric disorders. In Goodman Gilman, A.; Goodman, L. S.; Rall, T. W.; and Murad, F. (eds): Goodman and Gilman's The Pharmacological Basis of Therapeutics, 7th ed. Macmillan, New York, pp. 387–445, 1985.

Bennett, Y. L.; Cary, F. H.; Mitchell, G. L.; and Cooper, M. N.: Acute methyl alcohol poisoning: A review based on experiences in an outbreak of 323 cases. Medicine, 32:431–463, 1953.

Berg, M. J.; Berlinger, W. G.; Goldberg, M. J.; Spector, R.; and Johnson, G. F.: Acceleration of the body clearance of phenobarbital by oral activated charcoal. N. Engl. J. Med., 307:642–644, 1982.

Biggs, J. T.; Spiker, D. G.; Petit, J. M.; and Ziegler, V. E.: Tricyclic antidepressant overdose. J.A.M.A., 238:135–138, 1977.

Billman, G. E.; and Hoskins, R. S.: Cocaine-induced ventricular fibrillation: Protection afforded by the calcium antagonist verapamil. F.A.S.E.B. J., 2:2990–2995, 1988.

Brett, A. S.: Implications of discordance between clinical impression and toxicology analysis in drug overdose. Arch. Intern. Med., 148:437–441, 1988.

Brown, T. C. K.: Sodium bicarbonate treatment for tricyclic antidepressant arrhythmias in children. Med. J. Aust., 2:380–382, 1976.

Callaham, M.: Admission criteria for tricyclic antidepressant ingestion. West. J. Med., 137:425–429, 1982.

Callaham, M.; and Kassel, D.: Epidemiology of fatal tricyclic antidepressant ingestion: Implications for management. Ann. Emerg. Med., 14:1–9, 1985.

Catravas, J. D.; and Waters, I. W.: Acute cocaine intoxication in the conscious dog: Studies on the mechanism of lethality. J. Pharmacol. Exp. Ther., 217:350–356, 1981.

Chang, T. M. S.: Removal of exogenous toxins by microencapsulated adsorbent. Can. J. Physiol. Pharmacol., 47:1043–1045, 1969.

Chazan, J. A.; and Garella, S.: Glutethimide intoxication. Arch. Intern. Med., 128:215–219, 1971.

Clay, K. L.; and Murphy, R. C.: On the metabolic acidosis of ethylene glycol intoxication. Toxicol. Appl. Pharmacol., 39:39–49, 1977.

Cobden, I.; Record, C. O.; Ward, M. K.; and Kerr, D. N. S.: Paracetamol-induced acute renal failure in the absence of fulminant liver damage. Br. Med. J., 284:21–22, 1982.

Coccaro, E. F.; and Siever, L. J.: Second generation antidepressants: A comparative review. J. Clin. Pharmacol., 25:241–260, 1985.

Comstock, E. G.; Boisaubin, E. V.; Comstock, B. S.; and Faulkner, T. P.: Assessment of the efficacy of activated charcoal following gastric lavage in acute drug emergencies. Clin. Toxicol., 19:149–165, 1982.

Corby, D. G.; Lisciandro, R. C.; Lehman, R. H.; and Decker, W. J.: The efficiency of methods used to evacuate the stomach after acute ingestions. Pediatrics, 40:871–874, 1967.

Corcoran, G. B.; Mitchell, J. R.; Vaishnav, Y. N.; and Horning, E. C.: Evidence that acetaminophen and N-hydroxyacetaminophen form a common arylating intermediate, N-acetyl-p-benzoquinoneimine. Mol. Pharmacol., 18:536–542, 1980.

Cregler, L. L.; and Mark, H.: Medical complications of cocaine abuse. N. Engl. J. Med., 315:1495–1500, 1986.

Curry, R. W.; Robinson, J. D.; and Sughrue, M. J.: Acute renal failure after acetaminophen ingestion. J.A.M.A., 247:1012–1014, 1982.

Curtis, R. A.; Barone, J.; and Giacona, N.: Efficacy of ipecac and activated charcoal/cathartic: Prevention of salicylate absorption in a simulated overdose. Arch. Intern. Med., 144:48–52, 1984.

Cutler, R. E.; Forland, S. C.; St. John Hammond, P. G.; and Evans, J. R.: Extracorporeal removal of drugs and poisons by hemodialysis and hemoperfusion. Ann. Rev. Pharmacol. Toxicol., 27:169–191, 1987.

Done, A. K.: Aspirin overdosage: Incidence, diagnosis, and management. Pediatrics, 62:890–897, 1978.

Done, A. K.: Salicylate poisoning. J.A.M.A., 192:100–102, 1965.

Ekins, B. R.; Ford, D. C.; Thompson, M. I. B.; Bridges, R. R.; Rollins, D. E.; and Jenkins, R. D.: The effect of activated charcoal on N-acetylcysteine absorption in normal subjects. Am. J. Emerg. Med., 5:483–487, 1987.

Ellenhorn, M. J.; and Barceloux, D. G.: Medical Toxicology—Diagnosis and Treatment of Human Poisoning. Elsevier Publishing, New York, 1988.

Friedman, E. A.; Greenberg, J. B.; Merrill, J. P.; and Dammin, G. J.: Consequences of ethylene glycol poisoning. Am. J. Med., 32:891–902, 1962.

Gabow, P. A.; Clay, K.; Sullivan, J. B.; and Lepoff, R.: Organic acids in ethylene glycol intoxication. Ann. Intern. Med., 105:16–20, 1986.

Gabow, P. A.; Anderson, R. J.; Potts, D. E.; and Schrier, R. W.: Acid-base disturbances in the salicylate-intoxicated adult. Arch. Intern. Med., 138:1481–1484, 1978.

Gabriel, R.: Paracetamol-induced acute renal failure in the absence of fulminant liver damage. Br. Med. J., 284:505–506, 1982.

Garella, S.: Extracorporeal techniques in the treatment of exogenous intoxications. Kidney Int., 33:735–754, 1988.

Goldberg, M. J.; and Berlinger, W. G.: Treatment of phenobarbital overdose with activated charcoal. J.A.M.A., 247:2400–2401, 1982.

Goldberg, R. J.; Capone, R. J.; and Hunt, J. D.: Cardiac complications following tricyclic antidepressant overdose. J.A.M.A., 254:1772–1775, 1985.

Gonda, A.; Gault, H.; Churchill, D.; and Hollomby, D.: Hemodialysis for methanol intoxication. Am. J. Med., 64:749–758, 1978.

Goodman, J. M.; Bischel, M. D.; Wagers, P. W.; and Barbour, B. H.: Barbiturate intoxication. Morbidity and mortality. West. J. Med., 124:179–186, 1976.

Gossel, T. A.; and Bricker, J. D.: The Principles of Clinical Toxicology. Raven Press, New York, 1984.

Greenland P.; and Howe, T. A.: Cardiac monitoring in tricyclic antidepressant overdose. Heart Lung, 10:856–859, 1981.

Habib, M. S.; and Harkiss, K. J.: Quantitative determination of emetine and cephaëline in ipecacuanha root. J. Pharm. Pharmacol., 21:57S–59S, 1969.

Henderson, I. W.; and Merrill, J. P.: Treatment of barbiturate intoxication. Ann. Intern. Med., 64:876–890, 1966.

Hill, J. B.: Salicylate intoxication. N. Engl. J. Med., 288:1110–1113, 1973.

Hill, J. B.: Experimental salicylate poisoning: Observations on the effects of altering blood pH on tissue and plasma salicylate concentrations. Pediatrics, 47:658–664, 1971.

Hillman, R. J.; and Prescott, L. F.: Treatment of salicylate poisoning with repeated oral charcoal. Br. Med. J., 291:1472, 1985.

Ingelfinger, J. A.; Isakson, G.; Shine, D.; Costello, C. E.; and Goldman, P.: Reliability of the toxic screen in drug overdose. Clin. Pharmacol. Ther., 29:570–575, 1981.

Isner, J. M.; Estes, N. A. M. III; Thompson, P. D.; Costanzo-Nordin, M. R.; Subramanian, R.; Miller, G.; Katsas, G.; Sweeney, K.; and Sturner, W. Q.: Acute cardiac events temporally related to cocaine abuse. N. Engl. J. Med., 315:1438–1443, 1986.

Jacobsen, D.; and McMartin, K. E.: Methanol and ethylene glycol poisonings: Mechanism of toxicity, clinical course, diagnosis, and treatment. Med. Toxicol., 1:309–334, 1986.

Jones, J.; McMullen, M. J.; Dougherty, J.; and Cannon, L.: Repetitive doses of activated charcoal in the treatment of poisoning. Am. J. Emerg. Med., 5:305–311, 1987.

Jonsson, S.; O'Meara, M.; and Young, J. B.: Acute cocaine poisoning. Am. J. Med., 75:1061–1064, 1983.

Kingston, M. E.: Hyperventilation in tricyclic antidepressant poisoning. Crit. Care Med., 7:550–551, 1979.

Knudsen, K.; and Heath, A.: Effects of self poisoning with maprotiline. Br. Med. J., 288:601–603, 1984.

Kulig, K. W.; Bar-Or, D.; and Rumack, B. H.: Intravenous theophylline poisoning and multiple-dose charcoal in an animal model. Ann. Emerg. Med., 16:842–846, 1987.

Kulig, K.; Bar-Or, D.; Cantrill, S. V.; Rosen, P.; and Rumak, B. H.: Management of acutely poisoned patients without gastric emptying. Ann. Emerg. Med., 14:562–567, 1985.

Lancet Editorial Board: Repeated oral activated charcoal in acute poisoning. Lancet, 1:1013–1015, 1987.

Lancet Editorial Board: Need we poison the elderly so often? Lancet, 2:20–22, 1988.

Lancet Note: Death after N-acetylcysteine. Lancet, 1:1421, 1984.

Levy, G.: Gastrointestinal clearance of drugs with activated charcoal. N. Engl. J. Med., 307:676–678, 1982.

Levy, G.; Tsuchiya, T.; and Amsel, L. P.: Limited capacity for salicyl phenolic glucuronide formation and its effect on the kinetics of salicylate elimination in man. Clin. Pharmacol. Ther., 13:258–268, 1972.

Litovitz, T.; and Veltri, J. C.: The role of hemoperfusion and hemodialysis in toxicology. Am. J. Emerg. Med., 6:80, 1988.

Litovitz, T. L.; Schmitz, B. F.; Matyunas, N.; and Martin, T. G.: 1987 Annual report of the American Association of Poison Control Centers National Data Collection System. Am. J. Emerg. Med., 6:479–544, 1988.

McCarron, M. M.; Schulze, B. W.; Walberg, C. B.; Thompson, G. A.; and Ansari, A.: Short-acting barbiturate overdosage. J.A.M.A., 248:55–61, 1982.

McCoy, H. G.; Cipolle, R. J.; Ehlers, S. M.; Sawchuk, R. J.; and Zaske, D. E.: Severe methanol poisoning. Application of a pharmacokinetic model for ethanol therapy and hemodialysis. Am. J. Med., 67:804–807, 1979.

McMartin, K. E.; Ambre, J. J.; and Tephly, T. R.: Methanol poisoning in human subjects. Am. J. Med., 68:414–418, 1980.

McMurtry, R. J.; Snodgrass, W. R.; and Mitchell, J. R.: Renal necrosis, glutathione depletion, and covalent binding after acetaminophen. Toxicol. Appl. Pharmacol., 46:87–100, 1978.

Matthew, H.; Mackintosh, T. F.; Tompsett, S. L.; and Cameron, J. C.: Gastric aspiration and lavage in acute poisoning. Br. Med. J., 1:1333–1337, 1966.

Meester, W. D.: Emesis and lavage. Vet. Hum. Toxicol., 22:225–234,1985.

Mitchell, J. R.; Thorgeirsson, S. S.; Potter, W. Z.; Jollow, D. J.; and Keiser, H.: Acetaminophen-induced hepatic injury: Protective role of glutathione in man and rationale for therapy. Clin. Pharmacol. Ther., 16:676–684, 1974.

Mittleman, R. E.; and Wetli, C. V.: Cocaine and sudden "natural" death. J. Forensic. Sci., 32:11–19, 1987.

Muscholl, E.: Effect of cocaine and related drugs on the uptake of noradrenaline by heart and spleen. Br. J. Pharmacol., 16:352–359, 1961.

Nahas, G.; Trouvé, R.; Demus, J. F.; and von Sitbon, M.: A calcium-channel blocker as antidote to the cardiac effects of cocaine intoxication. N. Engl. J. Med., 313:519–520, 1985.

Nattel, S.: Frequency-dependent effects of amitriptyline on ventricular conduction and cardiac rhythm in dogs. Circulation, 72:898–906, 1985.

Nattel, S.; and Mittleman M.: Treatment of ventricular tachyarrhythmias resulting from amitriptyline toxicity in dogs. J. Pharmacol. Exp. Ther., 231:430–435, 1984.

Nattel, S.; Keable, H.; and Sasyniuk, B. I.: Experimental amitriptyline intoxication: Electrophysiologic manifestations and management. J. Cardiovasc. Pharmacol., 6:83–89, 1984.

Nattel, S.; Bayne, L.; and Ruedy, J.: Physostigmine in coma due to drug overdose. Clin. Pharmacol. Ther., 25:96–102, 1979.

Newton, R. B.: Physostigmine salicylate in the treatment of tricyclic antidepressant overdosage. J.A.M.A., 231:941–943, 1975.

Okonen, A.; Hofman, A.; and Henningsen, B.: Efficacy of gut lavage, hemodialysis, and hemoperfusion in the therapy of paraquat or diquat intoxication. Arch. Toxicol., 36:43–51, 1976.

Parry, M. F.; and Wallach, R.: Ethylene glycol poisoning. Am. J. Med., 57:143–150, 1974.

Pentel, P.; and Benowitz, N.: Efficacy and mechanism of action of sodium bicarbonate in the treatment of desipramine toxicity in rats. J. Pharmacol. Exp. Ther., 230:12–19, 1984.

Pentel, P.; and Sioris, L.: Incidence of late arrhythmias following tricyclic antidepressant overdose. Clin. Toxicol., 18:543–548, 1981.

Pollack, M. M.; Dunbar, B. S.; Holbrook, P. R.; and Fields, A. I.: Aspiration of activated charcoal and gastric contents. Ann. Emerg. Med., 10:528–529, 1981.

Pond, S. M.; Olson, K. R.; Osterloh, J. D.; and Tong, T. G.: Randomized study of the treatment of phenobarbital overdose with repeated doses of activated charcoal. J.A.M.A., 251:3104–3108, 1984.

Prescott, L. F.: Treatment of severe acetaminophen poisoning with intravenous acetylcysteine. Arch. Intern. Med., 141:386–389, 1981.

Prescott, L. F.; Balali-Mood, M.; Critchley, J. A. J. H.; Johnstone, A. F.; and Proudfoot, A. T.: Diuresis or urinary alkalinisation for salicylate poisoning? Br. Med. J., 285:1383–1386, 1982.

Prescott, L. F.; Illingworth, R. N.; Critchley, J. A. J. H.; Stewart, M. J.; Adam, R. D.; and Proudfoot, A. T.: Intravenous N-acetylcysteine: The treatment of choice for paracetamol poisoning. Br. Med. J., 2:1097–1100, 1979.

Prescott, L. F.; Wright, N.; Roscoe, P.; and Brown, S. S.: Plasma-paracetamol half-life and hepatic necrosis in patients with paracetamol overdosage. Lancet, 1:519–522, 1971.

Proudfoot, A. T.; and Brown, S. S.: Acidaemia and salicylate poisoning in adults. Br. Med. J., 2:547–550, 1969.

Ramoska, E.; and Sacchetti, A. D.: Propranolol-induced hypertension in treatment of cocaine intoxication. Ann. Emerg. Med., 14:1112–1113, 1985.

Ritchie, J. M.; and Greene N. M.: Local anesthetics. In Goodman Gilman, A.; Goodman, L. S.; Rall, T. W.; and Murad, F. (eds): Goodman and Gilman's The Pharmacological Basis of Therapeutics, 7th ed. Macmillan, New York, pp. 302–321, 1985.

Robertson, W. O.: Syrup of ipecac associated fatality: A case report. Vet. Hum. Toxicol., 21:87–89, 1979.

Robin, E. D.; Davis, R. P.; and Rees, S. B.: Salicylate intoxication with special reference to the development of hypokalemia. Am. J. Med., 26:869–882, 1959.

Rollins, D. E.; von Bahr, C.; Glaumann, H.; Moldéus, P.; and Rane, A.: Acetaminophen: Potentially toxic metabolite formed by human fetal and adult liver microsomes and isolated fetal liver cells. Science, 205:1414–1416, 1979.

Roth, D.; Alarcon, F. J.; Fernandez, J. A.; Preston, R. A.; and Bourgoignie, J. J.: Acute rhabdomyolysis associated with cocaine intoxication. N. Engl. J. Med., 319:673–677, 1988.

Rumack, B. H.; Peterson, R. C.; Koch, G. G.; and Amara, I. A.: Acetaminophen overdose. Arch. Intern. Med., 141:380–385, 1981.

Sasyniuk, B. I.; and Jhamandas, V.: Mechanism of reversal of toxic effects of amitriptyline on cardiac Purkinje fibers by sodium bicarbonate. J. Pharmacol. Exp. Ther., 231:387–394, 1984.

Siegel, R. K.: Cocaine substitutes. N. Engl. J. Med., 302:817–818, 1980.

Smith, M. J. H.; and Jeffrey, S. W.: The effects of salicylate on oxygen consumption and carbohydrate metabolism in the isolated rat diaphragm. Biochem. J., 63:524–528, 1956.

Tandberg, D.; Liechty, E. J.; and Fishbein, D.: Mallory-Weiss syndrome: An unusual complication of ipecac-induced emesis. Ann. Emerg. Med., 10:521–523, 1981.

Tenenbein, M.; Cohen, S.; and Sitar, D. S.: Efficacy of ipecac-induced emesis, orogastric lavage, and activated charcoal for acute drug overdose. Ann. Emerg. Med., 16:838–841, 1987.

Thompson, A. M.; Robins, J. B.; and Prescott, L. F.: Changes in cardiorespiratory function during gastric lavage for drug overdose. Hum. Toxicol., 6:215–218, 1987.

Thurston, J. H.; Pollock, P. G.; Warren, S. K.; and Jones, E. M.: Reduced brain glucose with normal plasma glucose in salicylate poisoning. J. Clin. Invest., 49:2139–2145, 1970.

Timberlake, G. A.: Ipecac as a cause of the Mallory-Weiss syndrome. South. Med. J., 77:804–805, 1984.

Turk, J.; Morrell, L.; and Avioli, L. V.: Ethylene glycol intoxication. Arch. Intern. Med., 146:1601–1603, 1986.

Vale, J. A.; Crome, P.; Volans, G. N.; Widdop, B.; and Goulding, R.: The treatment of paraquat poisoning using oral sorbents and charcoal haemoperfusion. Acta Pharmacol. Toxicol., 4l(suppl. 2):109–117, 1977.

Vance, M. A.; Ross, S. M.; Millington, W. R.; and Blumberg, J. B.: Potentiation of tricyclic antidepressant toxicity by physostigmine in mice. Clin. Toxicol., 11:413–421, 1977.

Virmani, R.; Robinowitz, M.; Smialek, J. E.; and Smyth, D. F.: Cardiovascular effects of cocaine: An autopsy study of 40 patients. Am. Heart J., 115:1068–1076, 1988.

Walters, J. S.; Woodring, J. H.; Stelling, C. B.; and Rosenbaum, H. D.: Salicylate-induced pulmonary edema. Radiology, 146:289–293, 1983.

Weidmann, S.: Effects of calcium ions and local anaesthetics on electrical properties of Purkinje fibres. J. Physiol., 129: 568–582, 1955.

Whalen, J. E.; Richards, C. J.; and Ambre, J.: Inadequate removal of methanol and formate using the sorbent based regeneration hemodialysis delivery system. Clin. Nephrol., 11:318–321, 1979.

Winchester, J. F.: Poisoning: Is the role of the nephrologist diminishing? Am. J. Kidney Dis., 13:171–183, 1989.

Wolowdiuk, O. J.; McMicken, D. B.; and O'Brien, P.: Pneumomediastinum and retropneumoperitoneum: An unusual complication of syrup of ipecac-induced emesis. Ann. Emerg. Med., 13:1148–1151, 1984.

29

Drugs in Special Patient Groups: Pregnancy and Nursing

Peter C. Rubin

Chapter Outline

Epidemiology of Drug Use During Pregnancy
  Drugs in the First Trimester
  Case Reports
  Case Studies
  Epidemiologic Studies
  Anticonvulsants
  Drugs Given after the First Trimester
  Behavioral Teratology
  Late Morphologic Effects
Influence of Pregnancy on Drug Dose
    Requirements

Pharmacokinetics During Pregnancy
Drug Metabolism by the Placenta
Therapeutic Drug Monitoring During
  Pregnancy
Using Drugs During Pregnancy—Practical
  Considerations
The Clinical Pharmacology Consultation:
  General Approach
Principles of Pharmacologic Management
  of a Medical Condition During
  Pregnancy: Epilepsy

Three decades ago the simultaneous publication of two case reports suggested that thalidomide, a sedative that had been claimed to be safer than other drugs of its type, seemed to cause serious birth defects when taken during the first trimester of pregnancy (Lenz, 1961; McBride, 1961). Confirmation of this observation came rapidly from all countries in which thalidomide had been used, and it was clear that a disaster of major proportions and considerable implications had occurred (Mellin and Katzenstein, 1962). The thalidomide tragedy had ramifications that extended far beyond the limited issue of drug-induced fetal abnormality. This event had political, social, and legal implications that were far-reaching. Present-day research into the use of drugs in pregnancy is carried out under "thalidomide's long shadow" (Anonymous, 1976). Developments in the clinical pharmacology of pregnancy have been slow because of the general fear that a drug given during pregnancy may have disastrous and unforeseeable consequences for the unborn baby. This fear naturally has greatly limited *experimental* research on drugs used in pregnancy. But we are left with inadequate anecdotal information on which we base decisions. For example, despite the fact that hypertension is one of the most common complications of pregnancy, there have only been two placebo-controlled studies to evaluate the role of drug treatment: a remarkable contrast to the study of drugs in hypertension in the nonobstetric practice. Yet conditions that require drug treatment, or for which drug treatment may be beneficial, occur frequently during pregnancy: in addition to hypertension examples include epilepsy, asthma, and bacterial infections. The physician wishing to treat one of these conditions must make a decision that like other decisions balances risk and benefit, but unlike the situation with other populations for whom analogous decisions are made, reliable data on neither risk nor benefit in pregnancy are available. While no one argues for immoral experiments to gather the necessary data, we do lament the absence of application of observational techniques to link medically important events with drugs taken by pregnant women. The purpose of this chapter is to bring together information concerning drug use in pregnancy and to discuss general approaches to the clinical pharmacology of pregnancy.

EPIDEMIOLOGY OF DRUG USE DURING PREGNANCY

Six studies of reasonable size and data ascertainment will be described here. There have been several small studies (some involving fewer than 100 patients). These are excluded on the grounds that the sample size is probably inadequate to draw conclusions about the wider populations. The six larger studies themselves vary considerably in methodology and the population being studied, although they were all carried out in either the United States or in the United Kingdom. Five of the six studies were prompted directly or indirectly by the thalidomide tragedy, but the largest, the Collaborative Perinatal Project, was begun before the thalidomide tragedy (Heinonen et al., 1977). This study involved 50,282 pregnancies, with data collected before the outcome of pregnancy was known. Chronologically the next study was carried out among 3072 patients attending Kaiser Permanente clinics as the thalidomide story was developing (Peckham and King, 1963). The information was collected from medical records. Just after this study another survey on 911 women was carried out in Edinburgh with data being collected by interview at the end of pregnancy and cross-checking with prescriptions that had been taken to the local pharmacies (Forfar and Nelson, 1973). Ten years later a study of 2528 Medicaid recipients was performed in Nashville with details being obtained from pharmacists' records of prescriptions (Brocklebank et al., 1978). Another study based on Medicaid claims was carried out in Michigan among 18,886 women who were delivered of a live infant (Piper et al., 1987).

Finally a prospective survey of drug use during pregnancy was performed from 1982 to 1984 in Glasgow, where drug-taking histories were taken from 2765 women at each attendance of the antenatal clinic (Rubin et al., 1986). Information on a random 10% subset was cross-checked with general practitioner records. Overall drug use in pregnancy from these various studies is shown in Fig. 29–1, and more detailed information with regard to specific drug groups is shown in Fig. 29–2. With the exception of our most recent study from Glasgow, there is a surprising degree of consistency with regard to drug use during pregnancy over the 3 decades and in patients from considerably different circumstances. *Principle: The totals of observations on the effects of drugs on pregnancy and the fetus are depressingly few. Fewer than 100,000 patients (total) were studied in the groups mentioned above. Since many of the total were not taking the same drugs or combinations during the same periods of pregnancy, we cannot be confident about the incidence data of even major morbidity or unanticipated efficacy that is less frequent than 1/5000 (trimester drug is used) (see chapters 34, 35, and 41).*

Somewhere between one third and two thirds of all pregnant women will take at least one drug during the pregnancy (excluding dietary supplements and excluding drugs taken at the time of delivery). The lower proportion of women taking drugs during pregnancy in the Glasgow study was likely to be a result of special circumstances at that time. A drug called Bendectin (Debendox in the United Kingdom) was the subject of considerable interest in the news media, and the drug was actually withdrawn by the manufacturers halfway

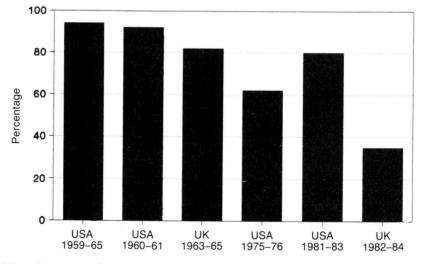

Fig. 29–1. Percentage of pregnant women taking a drug during pregnancy in the United States or United Kingdom at different times during a 25-year period. Iron and vitamin supplements are excluded from the data.

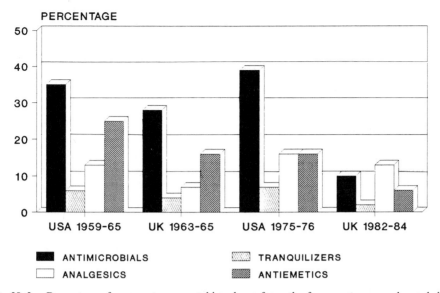

Fig. 29-2. Percentage of pregnant women taking drugs from the four most commonly used drug groups as determined in separate studies in the United States and United Kingdom over a 25-year period.

through the Glasgow study because of fears that it may be teratogenic. This matter will be considered later in the chapter, but it seems reasonable to assume that the highly negative publicity being given to drug use in pregnancy at the time of the study decreased drug consumption by pregnant women. Indeed, preliminary data from a World Health Organization survey into drug use in pregnancy in 10 countries suggest that the proportion of women taking at least one drug during pregnancy in the last few years has once again risen to over 60% (Matheson et al., 1989). Clearly in a review of the 100 most used drugs in the United States, many of those high on the list are used most frequently during pregnancy.

The Glasgow study attempted to identify any group that was more or less likely to either be prescribed a drug or use an OTC preparation, but no clear pattern emerged. There was no significant difference in any kind of drug use with regard to social class; additionally, whether or not a woman smoked or drank alcohol regularly did not seem to influence her use of medications. In the very different Medicaid population of Michigan it appeared that black mothers had higher rates of exposure to a variety of drugs, including analgesics, ampicillin, and vaginal preparations (Rubin et al., 1986). However, it seems possible that these women also had a higher incidence of disease, although the study design could not confirm this possibility.

These studies demonstrate that drug use during pregnancy is common; the Glasgow study found

that the 34.8% of women who took a medication used 154 different drugs from 35 drug groups. Therefore, while there is public concern about the possible adverse effects of drug use in pregnancy, the fact remains that drugs are widely used, and much more systematically gathered information about the consequences of prescribing in pregnancy is needed.

In considering the risk of medications during pregnancy, it is important to emphasize that pregnancy is divided into distinctly different periods that may have important implications for evaluating the impact of a particular drug. For example, the first trimester of pregnancy is the period of organogenesis, and concern about fetal malformations is paramount; on the other hand, near term the physician needs to be concerned with the potential effects of a drug on the baby's breathing rather than on teratogenicity.

Drugs in the First Trimester

Teratogenicity. Derived from the ancient Greek word *teratos* ("monster"), the word *teratogen* refers to a substance that leads to the birth of a baby who is malformed. Fetal malformation is a fact of reproductive life. In developed countries, somewhere in the region of 2% of all pregnancies end with the birth of a baby who has some kind of anatomic abnormality. In most of these cases it is impossible to identify any external agent that could have been responsible. This background incidence of fetal abnormality is crucially important in the interpretation of reports suggesting that a particular drug led to a particular abnormality.

Before discussing drug-induced teratogenicity in more detail, it is necessary to address two issues that are highly relevant to this question.

Placental Transfer of Drug. In order for a drug to cause harm in this context it must cross the placenta and be present in fetal tissue. Many studies have addressed the pharmacokinetics of placental transfer, and there are several good reviews in this area (Waddell and Marlowe, 1981; Kraver et al., 1988). Unfortunately most studies have emphasized the rate of placental transfer following a single IV injection. While useful pharmacokinetic models have been established to describe the different situations that can occur depending on, for example, lipid solubility of a drug or maternal protein binding and metabolism, the rate of placental transfer is not of prime importance in most cases of drug exposure. Almost all cases in which drug exposure can lead to fetal abnormality concern not a single administration of a drug but a course of drug treatment over days or longer.

Consequently, the pertinent question is not how quickly the drug crosses the placenta but whether it will cross at all in the long run. Currently available data suggest that almost all drugs actually do cross the placenta after multiple doses irrespective of their pharmacokinetic characteristics. The only major exception encountered in clinical practice is heparin, a large and polar molecule that does not reach measurable concentrations on the fetal side of the circulation. In the case of all other drugs studied, placental transfer occurs, although it should be emphasized that most of these investigations have been carried out in the third trimester. Probably it is appropriate to extrapolate these findings to the first trimester, but there is relatively little direct information.

As indicated above, in most cases the pharmacokinetic profile of a drug seems not to be important with regard to passage across the placenta. For example, atenolol, a hydrophilic drug with poor lipid solubility, was not considered likely to cross the placenta, in contrast to its more lipophilic counterpart, propranolol. However, studies have not confirmed this speculation; indeed, atenolol reaches high concentrations in cord blood (Rubin et al., 1983). For practical purposes the prescribing physician should therefore assume that any candidate drug will cross the placenta.

Period of Organogenesis. Between approximately 18 and 55 days following conception, the human fetus undergoes organogenesis, in which major anatomic structures are created (Fig. 29–3). A drug can cause a structural abnormality only if given during this period since, for example, it is not possible to cause a neural tube defect after closure of the neural tube has taken place. This simple and seemingly self-evident principle is widely overlooked but is a very important concept in both understanding drug-induced teratogenicity and in advising women who may have been or could be exposed to a potential teratogen whether drug or viral infection.

Identifying Drug Teratogens. It took 10,000 episodes of phocomelia before thalidomide was identified as a teratogen. Yet the discovery was considered efficient. In spite of the fact that the type of abnormality (phocomelia) is very unusual and that thalidomide caused this defect in a high percentage of exposures, more people than necessary suffered. Clearly if surveillance had been more systematic, many fewer would have needed to be deformed by the drug (see chapters 34, 35, and 41). This combination of rarity of an event and sudden increase in frequency of the drug-induced event is very unusual. For most drugs the certainty of whether or not a drug is or can be teratogenic is elusive. The uncertainty could be considerably reduced if available observational methodology were systematically applied to event monitoring of drugs taken by women in the childbearing ages. *Principle: The absence of toxicity data about drugs used during pregnancy does not preclude such toxicity.*

Animal studies of drug effects in pregnancy are of dubious value despite the fact that they are widely performed and, indeed, in many countries must be performed during the development of a new drug. However, such studies are generally unhelpful for two reasons. First, any link between toxic effects in a rat and the consequences of therapeutic administration in a pregnant woman is tenuous at best, but many studies offer a target for observational focus in women. A further problem with animal studies is that there is considerable species variation (Szabo and Brent, 1974; Elia et al., 1987). Thalidomide is a teratogen only in primates. There are many additional examples of major differences between animals and humans. For example, lithium given to rats in the dose of 200 mg/kg produces no fetal abnormality; 300 mg/kg increases the incidence of cleft palate to 6%, while 45 mg/kg causes a 30% increase in cleft palate (Szabo, 1970). However, in the human, lithium appears to cause cardiac abnormalities at doses far below the 200 mg/kg used in rat studies. An absence of teratogenic effect in an animal therefore cannot be taken to assume safety in the human.

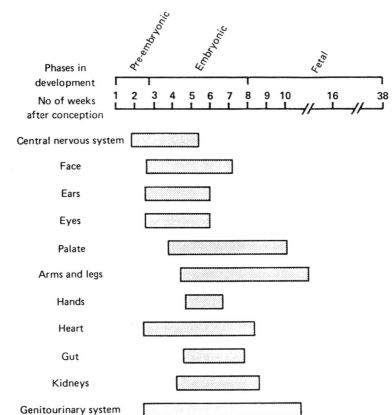

Fig. 29-3. Period of human organogenesis. (Reproduced courtesy of Dr. Martin Whittle, Queen Mother's Hospital, Glasgow, and British Medical Journal.)

In the absence of suitable laboratory models of teratogenicity of drugs in humans, studies aimed at identifying drug teratogens must be performed in the human. Such studies are generally of three types and are discussed in greater detail in two excellent references (Cordero and Oakley, 1983; Goldberg and Golbus, 1986).

Case Reports

Reports of individual patients taking a drug can have enormous value in drawing attention to a possible association that later can be confirmed or refuted by other investigators. Case reports first drew attention to the fact that thalidomide (Lenz, 1961; McBride, 1961) and warfarin (Kerber et al., 1968) were teratogenic. But case reports can be misleading, as demonstrated by suggestions that Bendectin (Debendox) caused a limb-reduction defect. The Bendectin saga demonstrated the most misleading power of "the well-chosen" anecdote.

When a woman has a baby with an abnormality and when that woman also took a drug during the first trimester, it is inevitable that an association between the drug and the abnormality will be drawn, particularly by the woman herself. But the association only should be a hypothesis. There is at least a 2% incidence of fetal abnormalities whether or not a drug is used. The first association cannot exclude the chance relationship. The case against Bendectin was pursued not only to the highest courts in the United States but also through television and newspapers in several countries, where emotive pictures of deformed children had their inevitable effect of effectively removing the drug from ethical obstetric practice. However, almost all the scientifically credible cohort studies involving Bendectin would suggest that the drug is not a teratogen, the relative risk being 0.89 with 95% confidence limits of 0.7 and 1.04 (MacMahon, 1981). In addition several case control studies have been performed that found no association between Bendectin and fetal abnormality (Orme, 1985; Anonymous, 1984). The case against Bendectin was never proved either scientifically or in the courts, yet to protect themselves from the undeserved public pressure the manufacturers withdrew the drug in 1983, after it had been given to approximately 3 million pregnant women. *Principle: When the medical profession does not discipline itself by monitoring the effects of its tools (drugs, devices, or procedures), it risks losing those tools for inappropriate reasons only after the population has been put at risk but to no ultimate advantage* (Melmon, 1990).

Case Studies

This sort of report involves several patients who have received a particular drug and in whom a similar malformation has been seen in the offspring. The fetal hydantoin syndrome (Hanson and Smith, 1975) and teratogenicity of isotretinoin (Rosa, 1983) both came to light by using this observational methodology.

Epidemiologic Studies

This type of study has already been alluded to with regard to Bendectin and tends to be of two major types. A cohort study aims to compare the outcome of pregnancy in two groups — one of whom was exposed to the agent of interest and the other of whom was not exposed. A case control study begins with a fetal abnormality and compares this group of pregnancies with a matched pregnancy population that had a normal outcome. The study assesses exposure to the agent of interest in each group. Studies of this type, particularly prospective cohort studies, are expensive and time-consuming since large numbers of patients may be required to detect a relatively subtle teratogenic effect. For example, the association between diethylstilbestrol (DES) and vaginal adenocarcinoma strongly suggested the drug effect in case control studies. About 100,000 exposed women would be necessary to confirm this relationship prospectively (Cordero and Oakley,

1983). Therefore, the confirmatory study has not been done but for medical purposes is not needed. *Principle: The requirements that allow a drug on the market or change its indication in a package insert are very different from those needed to optimize the use of the drug.*

Teratogenic Drugs. The physician must know which drugs *are likely to cause harm* when given during pregnancy. Table 29–1 lists those drugs in common clinical use for which a teratogenic effect has been demonstrated. The drugs in this list are those for which evidence is either conclusive or highly suggestive. Not included in this list are drugs that are used infrequently during pregnancy or drugs for which a teratogenic effect may occur but for which the evidence is lacking. In other words, drugs not on this list may later be found to be teratogenic. The short list establishes certain high risk when using these drugs. The list does not include the likely risk of fetal abnormality following exposure in the first trimester. The omission is deliberate and will be discussed further in relation to each drug. However, for all the drugs listed, with the possible exception of retinoic acid, the risk probably does not exceed 10% (i.e., 10 in 100 pregnancies will be affected). In other words in 90% of pregnant women, the same drug will not negatively impact the fetus. Different effects of high-risk drugs in different women must be considered and will be discussed.

Anticonvulsants

The role of anticonvulsant drugs in producing fetal abnormality illustrates the difficulties of drawing conclusions about drug effects in this

Table 29–1.   COMMONLY USED DRUGS THAT HAVE DEMONSTRATED TERATOGENICITY IN HUMANS

DRUG	EFFECT	PRENATAL DIAGNOSIS
Lithium	Cardiac defects (Ebstein complex)	Feasible
Warfarin	Chondrodysplasia punctata	Unlikely
	Facial anomalies	Unlikely
	Severe anomalies of the CNS	Unlikely
Phenytoin	Craniofacial	Feasible
	Limb	Feasible
	Growth deficiencies	Feasible
Sodium valproate	CNS	Feasible
Carbamazepine	Craniofacial	Feasible
	Fingernail	Feasible
Sex hormones	Cardiac defects	Feasible
	Multiple anomalies	Feasible
Retinoic acids	Craniofacial	Feasible
	Cardiac	Feasible
	CNS	Feasible

area of clinical pharmacology. The suggestion that there is a "fetal hydantoin" syndrome was first made in a report of several cases in 1975 (Hanson and Smith, 1975). The syndrome comprises poor growth and development with various structural abnormalities, including hypoplasia of the nail, hypertelorism, microcephaly, cleft lip or palate, and various other less frequent abnormalities. The original case reports suggested an 11% incidence of the syndrome. The fetal hydantoin syndrome has been both confirmed and refuted in the years since this original report.

One of the most persuasive studies to cast doubt on the existence of a specific syndrome related to administration of phenytoin comes from the Collaborative Perinatal Project in the United States (Shapiro et al., 1976). This study found that the malformation rate among children born to epileptic mothers was 10.5% compared with 6.4% in the remainder of the population ($p <$ 0.01). The difference still held when only major malformations were considered (6.6% in epileptic pregnancies vs. 2.7% in normals). However, there was no significant difference in fetal abnormality according to the drug used. In addition, certain malformations, such as cleft palate, were more common not only in the children of epileptic mothers but also in the children of epileptic fathers. These data have been interpreted as indicating that it is epilepsy, rather than its treatment, that is responsible for fetal abnormality. The evidence from several studies is that the rate of fetal malformations in the offspring of epileptic mothers is around 10%, but what is not clear is whether the syndrome is a consequence of the epilepsy itself, the result of a common genetic determining factor in either parent, or the result of the drug alone or when used in combination with all these different influences. To dissect out the contribution of different factors is difficult because so often the drug and the disease are inseparable. For example, data have been reported by another group indicating that the frequency of fetal malformation increases with the number of anticonvulsant drugs used (Lindout et al., 1984). However, it is reasonable to assume that more severely epileptic women require a greater number of drugs. So it is possible that the increase in birth defects was the result of more severe disease rather than the drugs. An interesting study to help disclose the direct effects of the anticonvulsants on the fetus would be a survey of outcomes of pregnancy in mothers taking the drugs for indications other than pregnancy (e.g., treatment of an arrhythmia).

The issues surrounding anticonvulsant drug teratogenicity are far from resolved, but in recent years there have been some interesting findings that point clearly to a genetic determinant that causes fetal abnormality in epileptic pregnancies. However, whether this genetic factor operates separately from, or in conjunction with, pharmacologic factors is unknown.

An interesting study of 62 families with fetal exposure to phenytoin in two or more pregnancies recently has been reported (Van Dyke et al., 1988). Ten mothers who had a baby with some of the physical features of the hydantoin syndrome went on to have a subsequent pregnancy during which phenytoin was taken again. Nine of these ten pregnancies produced a baby having features of the fetal hydantoin syndrome. In contrast, 52 mothers who had an unaffected baby at the end of their first pregnancy went on to a subsequent pregnancy while still taking phenytoin, and only five of these pregnancies produced a baby showing the characteristics of the fetal hydantoin syndrome. This difference between the two groups was highly significant. However, whether the mothers would have had abnormal babies even if phenytoin had not been given cannot be determined from this study. Another recent report describes the features of fetal hydantoin syndrome occurring in only one of dizygotic twins of different paternity. These results again point strongly to a genetic factor that determines the syndrome (Phenlan et al., 1982).

Further recent developments add interesting pieces to solve the puzzle. Carbamazepine often has been proposed as the safest anticonvulsant for use in pregnancy. But a retrospective and prospective study now has shown that this drug too is associated with fetal abnormalities, including hypoplasia of the fingernail, poor growth, and developmental delay, very similar to the fetal hydantoin syndrome (Jones et al., 1989). This report is particularly interesting because carbamazepine and phenytoin are metabolized to similar reactive, electrophilic compounds called arene oxides. These unstable intermediate compounds bind to fetal macromolecules in the rat and have been implicated in this animal species in the production of malformations (Martz et al., 1977). Arene oxides are themselves metabolized by epoxide hydrolase. Perhaps a genetic defect in epoxide hydrolase activity could be associated with phenytoin-induced teratogenicity (Spielberg, 1982). The effects of phenytoin metabolites generated by a murine hepatic microsomal drug-metabolizing system on lymphocytes from children with and without the features of the fetal hydantoin syndrome have been studied (Strickler et al., 1985). Fourteen of 24 children studied had a significant increase in cell death associated with the phenytoin metabolites, and each of these children had one parent in whom excessive cell death also was shown. A significant correlation between this "positive" lymphocyte in vitro challenge and the occurrence of major birth defects has been established.

A separate approach to this question has looked directly at epoxide hydrolase activity (Buehler, 1987). When the heteropaternal discordant twins referred to above were studied, a clear difference in enzyme activity was found between the two children (Phenlan et al., 1982). A preliminary study suggests that it is possible to predict which children will or will not have features of the fetal hydantoin syndrome on the basis of epoxide hydrolase activity measured in skin fibroblasts. The activity is decreased in about 50% of normal affected children. If confirmed in other studies, this finding would permit the prediction of susceptibility to the fetal hydantoin syndrome and could also pave the way to dissecting out the relative contributions of drug and genetics on disease in producing abnormalities in the fetus.

Two other factors should be mentioned in the context of anticonvulsant drugs and fetal abnormality. Anticonvulsants lower serum folate concentrations, and folate deficiency has long been suspected (but never proved) to be involved in causing fetal abnormality. It is therefore noteworthy that in 125 women with epilepsy no association was found between serum folate concentration and the outcome of pregnancy even though this study included both women with very low folate concentrations and pregnancies that ended in the birth of a baby having features of the fetal hydantoin syndrome (Hillesmaa et al., 1983).

Finally, although not strictly a teratogenic effect, the impaired intellectual activity that has been associated with epilepsy and anticonvulsant drugs could also be a consequence of the disease rather than the drug. One report has demonstrated abnormalities of the fetal heart rate during a grand mal seizure (Hillesmaa et al., 1985), and it is quite possible that poorly controlled epilepsy could be associated with fetal cerebral hypoxia. *Principle: Understanding the mechanism of a drug effect often leads to appropriate strategies to detect the same effect in what otherwise could be considered unrelated drugs. The understanding also can be critical in choosing alternative drugs used for the same indication that would not contribute to similar events.*

Selection of Anticonvulsant. Even though there is still uncertainty as to whether anticonvulsants are teratogenic, is there one anticonvulsant that is preferable to any other when considering the management of epilepsy in a woman who may become pregnant? Advice has been given in this regard (Anonymous, 1981; Saunders, 1989). In each case the advice has been rapidly superseded by new events. In the early 1980s, sodium valproate was recommended as the drug of choice

for female epileptic patients since by this time phenytoin had acquired a reputation of being teratogenic. Hardly had this recommendation been made than the first reports began to appear suggesting that sodium valproate was associated with a neural tube defect (Editorial, 1988). Carbamazepine then took up the mantle of the drug of choice for epilepsy in the woman. But it too has been implicated as a teratogen. Consequently, at this point and after discussion with the patient, physicians should use the drug that is most effective and most acceptable to the woman concerned. On the basis of current information, there seems no compelling reason to select one particular drug on the grounds that it is less teratogenic than any other. Perhaps we should test the efficacy of phenobarbitone as an anticonvulsant in those susceptible to pregnancy!

Anticonvulsants and Coagulation. A neonatal coagulation defect can follow the use of anticonvulsant drugs during pregnancy. Studies of coagulation in 16 neonates born to epileptic mothers taking either a barbiturate or phenytoin revealed abnormalities in eight of the babies (Mountain et al., 1970). The coagulation defect is similar to that seen in vitamin K deficiency and is characterized by prolonged prothrombin time, long activated partial thromblastin time, and low concentrations of factors II, VII, IX, and X. Furthermore, significantly high concentrations of protein induced by the absence of vitamin K (PIVKA) have been found in the blood of epileptic patients taking a variety of medications (Davies et al., 1985) and in mother–infant pairs following the use of anticonvulsant therapy during pregnancy (Argent et al., 1986). Interestingly, the mother's coagulation profile can be normal even when her baby has severe coagulation defects (Mountain et al., 1970). The drug-induced bleeding in neonates occurs earlier than is usual in the classic hemorrhagic disease of the newborn. The bleeding appears within 24 hours of birth, and it can be serious when it involves unusual sites, such as the pleural and abdominal cavities. To prevent the hemorrhage, vitamin K, 20 mg daily, should be given to the mother for 2 weeks before delivery (Delaby et al., 1982).

Barbiturates taken by the mother can produce a number of effects in the neonate. Neonatal behavior can be affected either by sedation caused by the drug or withdrawal symptoms as the drug is eliminated. Protein binding and drug clearance in the neonate probably are the major determinants of the type of symptoms experienced (Kuhnz et al., 1988). Those who have an unusually high free fraction of phenobarbitone in plasma have a tendency to become sedated, while those in whom the clearance of phenobarbitone is unusually rapid have a tendency to show symptoms of withdrawal from the drug.

A potential toxic effect of sodium valproate has been suggested by two (and only two) case reports that described liver failure in the offspring of women who had received the drug throughout pregnancy (Felding and Rane, 1984; Legius et al., 1987). The clinical significance of this observation is not known, and at most the effect must be rare since many thousands of exposures of pregnant women to valproate have occurred. Nonetheless sodium valproate has hepatoxic effects in the adult, and it would not be surprising to see the same effect in neonates.

Lithium. Strongly suggestive evidence indicates that lithium taken during the first trimester can lead to Ebstein anomaly. The extent of the risk is unclear. The first suggestion that lithium could have this effect came from the register of lithium babies that was established in Scandinavia to try to achieve early identification of fetal abnormalities. Among 118 babies reported to the registry by the early 1970s, six had congenital cardiovascular defects including two cases of Ebstein anomaly (Schou et al., 1973b). This report was soon followed by another describing two further cases of Ebstein anomaly following use of lithium in early pregnancy (Nora et al., 1974). Given that Ebstein anomaly is a rare malformation, such an occurrence seemed unlikely to have been the result of chance alone. A subsequent and separate study confirmed the excess of cardiovascular malformations in babies whose mothers used lithium. This cohort study provides an estimate of risk. Among 350 babies who had been exposed to lithium in the first trimester, six had heart defects compared with an expected frequency of 2.1 (Kallen and Tandberg, 1983). Interestingly, none of these cardiac defects was of the Ebstein type. This study suggests that use of lithium is associated with a 1.7% risk of cardiac abnormality compared with 0.6% in the general population—a threefold increase while using the drug. Thus, the risk of Ebstein anomaly seems to be a good deal less than the risk of cardiac abnormalities in general. When unpublished data from the lithium register are used, the risk specifically of Ebstein anomaly is 1 case per 1000 exposures—a 20-fold increase over that of the general population (Elia et al., 1987).

Lithium clearly is a human teratogen, particularly on the cardiovascular system. However, the drug also is an effective agent in managing bipolar depressive illness. The decision whether the drug should be continued during the first trimester should be made individually with the various risks and benefits assessed and shared with the patient in each case (see chapter 13).

Warfarin. Warfarin causes chondrodysplasia punctata that involves bone and cartilage abnormalities (Becker et al., 1975; Shaul et al., 1975). In addition, the drug is associated with microcephaly, asplenia, and diaphragmatic hernia (Hall et al., 1980). When the drug is taken in late pregnancy, it can produce intracerebral microhemorrhages in the fetus (Shaul and Hall, 1977). The incidence of congenital abnormalities is no clearer with warfarin than it is with the other drugs discussed in this section.

In 22 pregnancies in which warfarin was used in the first trimester (because the patient had an artificial heart valve) there were 8 spontaneous abortions. This study did not show cases of chondrodysplasia punctata or microcephaly (Chen et al., 1982a). On the other hand, from 49 pregnancies in which warfarin was given during the first trimester for the same indication, there were 9 spontaneous abortions, 1 stillbirth, and 10 cases of classic warfarin embryopathy (Iturbe-Alessio et al., 1986). In this series the risk of an anomaly with the fetus was about 25%. Few would argue with the proposal that warfarin is contraindicated in the first trimester unless there is an overwhelming indication, which ordinarily would be contained to the presence of an artificial heart valve (Oakley, 1983).

Retinoic Acids. These vitamin A analogs have been used since the early 1980s to treat severe cystic acne and some other chronic dermatoses. From the onset of their availability on the market, these drugs were strongly suspected to be teratogenic. They were contraindicated in pregnancy but nonetheless inadvertently used by some pregnant women (Rosa, 1983). They caused a number of major malformations, including craniofacial, cardiac, thymic, and CNS abnormalities. The relative risk has been reported as 25 with 95% confidence interval of 11.4 to 57.5 (Lammer et al., 1985).

As was indicated earlier, many more drugs in relatively common clinical use could be teratogenic. We simply do not have relevant information about the risks attending their use. An example of the kind of information that is produced and which must be assessed is given by two reports of a very rare defect in skull ossification in the babies of mothers who conceived while taking an ACE inhibitor (Anonymous, 1989). This type of spontaneous defect is exceedingly rare. The circumstantial evidence in the two reports associating the defect with the same group of drugs raises suspicions but does not prove the hypothesis. In the context of inadequate information, the physician often has to make a therapeutic decision. There are other antihypertensive drugs for which a similar hypothesis is not raised. The physician should consider their use but be equally concerned about the consequences. *Principle: The risk of drug use during pregnancy often is completely unknown. In such settings the physician must be very clear on the need for the drug; he or she must use reasonable criteria to estimate efficacy in order to minimize both the dose and the duration of treatment. If possible most drugs should be even more scrupulously avoided in early pregnancy than during later pregnancy— much more scrupulously avoided than in men with the comparable indication.*

Drugs Given after the First Trimester

The risk of anatomic defects in the fetus recedes after the first trimester. For the remainder of pregnancy, the fetus undergoes growth and development. The impact of drugs given after the first trimester moves from structural to physiologic effects. In addition, the long-term use of some agents can have adverse effects on the mother that, if not unique to pregnancy, are at least exaggerated by the gravid state.

Heparin. Heparin during pregnancy threatens the mother rather than the fetus. Osteoporosis is a recognized complication of long-term (many years) administration of heparin (Griffith et al., 1965). The risk of osteoporosis seems to be relatively small if less than 10,000 units is used per day. However, multiple vertebral compression fractures have been described in a pregnant woman receiving 10,000 units twice daily throughout pregnancy (Wise and Hall, 1980). The effect of heparin therapy in pregnancy has been studied systematically by radiologic assessment of the thoracolumbar spine, femur, and hands following delivery (De Swiet et al., 1983). Women in this study were given heparin 10,000 units twice daily either for 6 weeks preceding delivery or for a period exceeding 20 weeks. Demineralization of bone was assessed by measuring the ratio of the metacarpal cortical area to the total area and that of the phalangeal cortical area to the total area. Patients receiving long-term heparin therapy showed significant cortical thinning that appeared to be dose-dependent.

The use of anticoagulants during pregnancy demonstrates the dilemma of assessing benefits versus risks. In women who have artificial heart valves, the risk of valve thrombosis if anticoagulation is not used places the life of the mother at unacceptable risk (Oakley, 1983; Iturbe-Alessio et al., 1986). On the other hand, the use of warfarin may lead to severe fetal damage, and the use of heparin in doses adequate to achieve anticoagulation may lead to vertebral compression fractures. With the data we have at hand it may be sensible

to use as low a dose of heparin as possible during early pregnancy and switch to lowest possible useful doses of warfarin in later pregnancy. Obviously this is not a recommendation of the authors or editors but simply presentation of a strategy that can be considered and shared with a patient as the physician makes a contract for therapy (see chapter 33).

Methyldopa. While it is correct to highlight the risks of using drugs during pregnancy, the physician should not overlook the circumstances under which the benefits of treatment appear quite substantially to outweigh the risks. Such is illustrated in a small number of studies that have been performed in the field of therapy of hypertension during pregnancy. The first large controlled study of antihypertensive treatment in pregnancy was carried out in Oxford in the 1970s. Methyldopa was compared with no treatment in an open prospective study in women who mainly had essential hypertension (Redman et al., 1976). The drug control of hypertension significantly improved fetal outcome mainly by reducing the number of midtrimester fetal deaths. Nine pregnancy losses in the control group (including four midtrimester fetal deaths) compared with one in the treated group ($p < 0.02$). The well-known adverse effects of methyldopa, including sedation and postural hypotension, led to 15% of the women being withdrawn (Redman et al., 1977), but no adverse effects were demonstrated on the fetus either immediately following delivery or at long-term follow-up (see the section on behavioral teratology below).

β-Adrenergic-Receptor Antagonists. The use of β-receptor antagonists during pregnancy generated considerable controversy during the 1970s and early 1980s. A number of reports claimed that these drugs caused intrauterine growth retardation and neonatal complications such as hypoglycemia, hypotension, bradycardia, and even death (Rubin, 1981). These reports well exemplify the difficulty of drawing rational conclusions about the use of drugs during pregnancy. Most involved either individual cases or retrospective study by chart review, sometimes many years after the index pregnancy (Rubin, 1981). Since the β-adrenergic antagonists were new, they likely most often were reserved for treating the most severe hypertension. It was difficult to separate the effects of the disease from the effects of the drugs. Encouraged by the results of the methyldopa study cited above, but noting that there had been a high rate of discontinuation of therapy because of adverse effects, atenolol was studied during pregnancy in a prospective and systematic manner (Rubin et al., 1983). This was the first placebo-controlled study done on hypertensive pregnant women, indicating the reluctance of physicians to undertake rigorous studies in this population. After a pilot study was carried out with atenolol in essential hypertension (Rubin et al., 1982), 120 women with pregnancy induced hypertension who had been admitted for treatment with bed rest were additionally treated with either atenolol or placebo. Atenolol lowered their blood pressure significantly more and longer than did placebo (Fig. 29–4). At the time of this study it had been a widely held belief that bed rest itself lowers blood pressure in pregnant patients with hypertension (Chamberlain et al., 1978). A further important difference between the two groups was that six babies from the placebo group required ventilation for idiopathic respiratory distress syndrome compared with none in the group treated with atenolol. The preterm delivery that gave rise to the respiratory distress resulted partly from poor controls of the mother's blood pressure, which prompted obstetricians to expedite delivery, but mainly from a higher incidence of spontaneous preterm labor in the group treated with placebo (Rubin et al., 1984). With the exception of efficacy in favor of treatment, the only other significant difference between the babies from the two groups was a reduced heart rate in the atenolol babies that lasted 24 hours. The bradycardia was not clinically important. The blood pressure and blood glucose concentrations in the two groups of babies were the same throughout the early neonatal period. In addition, there was no significant difference in either neonatal or placental weight between the two groups. Therefore, the adverse effects attributed to β blockers in case reports were not substantiated in a prospective, randomized, double-blind, and placebo-controlled study.

But nothing is simple and without risks. An additional study indicates that atenolol can retard growth under certain circumstances (Butters et al., 1990). This study (placebo-controlled and double-blind) was concerned with the management of essential hypertension during pregnancy; consequently, women received atenolol for a considerably longer time than in the trial just discussed. A pilot study using atenolol to treat essential hypertension in pregnancy that had progressed 28 weeks or longer (Rubin et al., 1982) had shown good control of blood pressure and no adverse consequences. In particular the median weight of the babies from treated mothers was within 2 standard deviations of the normal gestational mean. The more recent study treated mothers as early as 12 weeks into the pregnancy and found that babies from the atenolol-treated group were significantly smaller than those from the placebo group (2.62 ± 0.7 kg vs. 3.48 ± 0.48 kg; $p < 0.05$). Similar differences were found in placental weight. Thus, not only with regard to teratogenicity but also with regard to growth and development, the same drug can have different effects depending on the time of pregnancy at which it is administered. The mechanism of the effect of atenolol on growth is unclear but may be related to a fall in placental lactogen in the atenolol group (Reynolds et al., 1984). Fortunately, the low-weight atenolol babies did not differ from those of the placebo group in weight at 1 year postpartum (Butters et al., 1990).

Inhibitors of Prostaglandin Synthesis. Aspirin and indomethacin have been associated with characteristic but different adverse effects during pregnancy. Aspirin frequently is taken during pregnancy (Fig. 29–2) and influences hemostasis in the neonate. In one study hemorrhagic phe-

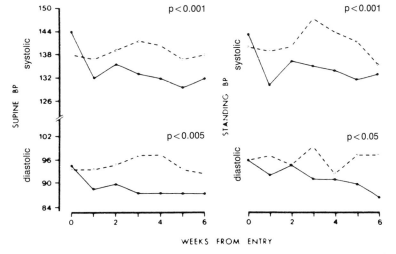

Fig. 29–4. Average blood pressure from point of entry into double-blind trial following administration of placebo (---) or atenolol (—). Data are presented in this way, rather than in terms of gestation, because women were entered and delivered at different times. Reproduced by permission of The Lancet.

nomena were seen in 3 of 14 neonates whose mothers had taken aspirin compared with 1 of 17 control infants (Bleyer and Breckenridge, 1970). More recently this observation has been confirmed and refined (Stuart et al., 1982). In the latter study, ingestion of aspirin by the mother was monitored by measuring platelet malondialdehyde formation. This measurement gives an accurate estimate of when the last dose of aspirin was taken. The case control study found that 1 of 34 control maternal-neonatal pairs had hemostatic abnormalities. In 10 maternal-neonatal pairs in which the mother had taken aspirin within 5 days of delivery, 6 of the mothers and 9 of the infants had bleeding problems. In contrast, when aspirin was taken 6 to 10 days before delivery, no bleeding tendencies were found in 7 maternal-neonatal pairs. The total dose of aspirin taken ranged between 5 and 10 g. The manifestation of hemostatic abnormalities included petechiae, hematuria, cephalhematoma, subconjunctival hemorrhage, and bleeding from the site of circumcision. A prudent conclusion from the two studies is to recommend acetaminophen (paracetamol) when a mild analgesic is needed during pregnancy. This drug has not (yet?) been implicated in any adverse consequences. In addition, if aspirin has been consumed within 5 days of delivery, the physician should look carefully for bleeding problems in the baby.

Possibly even before Heymann and Rudolph defined a role for bradykinin and prostaglandins in the patency of the ductus arteriosus, concern has been expressed that indomethacin could prematurely close the ductus (Manchester et al., 1976). The drug does have this effect. The two most likely circumstances in which indomethacin is administered during pregnancy are to treat moderately severe rheumatoid arthritis (Byron, 1987) or for a tocolytic agent (Moise et al., 1988). Focusing on the latter indication, 13 patients with premature labor between 2 and 31 weeks of gestation received indomethacin in doses up to 175 mg/day for a maximum of 3 days (Moise et al., 1988). Echocardiographic study revealed constriction of the ductus in 7 of 14 cases (one woman had twins). Tricuspid regurgitation was also identified in 3 cases. The ductal constriction could occur as early as 9.5 hours following the first administration of indomethacin. The constriction reversed in all cases within 24 hours of discontinuing the drug. The results of the study confirm that indomethacin can cause closure of the ductus, and it would seem unwise to proceed to use the drug for other than the shortest terms without careful evaluation of the fetal ductus by echocardiography. *Principle: Frequently, understanding the pharmacology of a drug and pathogenesis of a disease or biologic setting allows prediction or observation of a drug effect. Often such prediction is the cornerstone of a new indication or contraindication for using the drug.*

Drugs and Breast Feeding. Drugs are given to a majority of breast-feeding women; the most widely used are iron, mild analgesics, antibiotics, laxatives, and hypnotics (Klebanoff and Berendes, 1988). The major concern when a drug is given to a nursing mother is whether harm may come to her baby. There has been very little systematic research in this area. Most information about passing drugs or metabolites from mother to baby comes from anecdotal observations. A much greater body of information has been generated with regard to pharmacokinetic factors that can influence the passage of drug into breast milk. While interesting, this is clearly less important than pharmacodynamic and clinical data.

Milk is produced and secreted in alveolar cells, from which it is expelled by contractile myoepithelial cells into the duct system. The milk itself comprises fat globules in an isotonic aqueous solution containing protein and various nutrients. Drugs enter breast milk by passive diffusion; the rate and extent of transfer depends on the drug's physicochemical properties. Breast milk is more acidic than plasma, and drugs that typically pass readily into milk are weak bases that are lipid-soluble and do not bind to protein very well. The clinical pharmacokinetics of drug passage into human breast milk has been reviewed in detail (Atkinson et al., 1988).

Even when drugs pass readily into breast milk, dilution has already occurred in the rest of the mother's body and often means that the dose of drug received by the baby is very low, even when considered on a per-weight basis. The dilution probably explains the lack of pharmacologic effects of the drug in the baby after the mother uses drugs listed in Table 29–2. In other cases, anecdotal reports suggest that harm may be

Table 29–2.   DRUGS THAT HAVE A GOOD SAFETY RECORD WHEN GIVEN TO NURSING MOTHERS*

Nonnarcotic analgesics
Penicillins
Cephalosporins
Methyldopa
β-receptor antagonists
Bronchodilators (inhaled)
Phenytoin
Carbamazepine
Sodium valproate

* This list is not intended to be comprehensive. Further details are found in Briggs et al., 1986.

Table 29–3. SOME COMMONLY USED DRUGS THAT MAY CAUSE ADVERSE EFFECTS IN A BREAST-FED INFANT*

Laxatives (diarrhea)

Amiodarone (possible effects on neonatal thyroid function)

Indomethacin (neonatal convulsions)

Barbiturates (drowsiness)

Benzodiazepines (drowsiness; failure to thrive with continued use)

Lithium (hypotonia, lethargy, cyanosis)

Carbimazole (neonatal hypothyroidism)

Methimazole (neonatal hypothyroidism)

* This list is not intended to be comprehensive. Further details are found in Briggs et al., 1986.

caused to the baby if particular drugs are used by a nursing mother (Table 29–3). Particular mention should be made of oral contraceptives. Once the milk supply has been established, there is no evidence that these drugs have any material influence on the quality or quantity of milk. Data with regard to long-term safety for the breast-fed infant are inadequate.

Behavioral Teratology

Most studies in human teratology have concerned themselves with morphologic observations made near the time of delivery. The possibilities that a drug taken during pregnancy could affect the growth and development of a child have been investigated to a far lesser extent. There are practical reasons for this imbalance in favor of morphologic observations.

Pediatric follow-up studies are difficult to carry out. Families move and can be difficult to trace without concerted effort; however, useful information on late teratologic effects is unlikely to be forthcoming until children approach school age. Another factor that makes follow-up studies difficult is that the more subtle the drug effect, the more difficult the study. For example, assessing physical growth and development (e.g., height, weight, etc.) is relatively straightforward. But assessing psychomotor development retarded, for example, by alcohol consumption by the mother is far more complicated since it requires a detailed and labor-intensive battery of investigations. In addition, psychomotor testing must be carefully controlled because of the strong influence that social and environmental factors have on these variables. The type of psychomotor test used also changes with increasing age of the child as he or she moves from nonverbal to verbal communication. For these reasons and more, the number of studies in the area of behavioral teratology has been small and the quality somewhat variable. This field has been reviewed in Gal and Sharpless (1984). For a detailed review of the many animal

studies performed with psychotherapeutic medications, see Elia et al., 1987.

Anticonvulsants. Several studies have reported the possible effects on the intellectual development of the child when the mother is treated with anticonvulsant therapy. The results are inconclusive (Gal and Sharpless, 1984). A common weakness of a number of these studies has been the lack of a genuine control group of untreated maternal epileptic patients. Even when this criterion has been applied, the results are contradictory. One study in which children exposed to phenytoin in utero were compared with a control group from untreated epileptic mothers came to the conclusion that phenytoin is a risk factor for mental deficiency in the child (Hanson et al., 1976). In contrast, a much larger study from the Collaborative Perinatal Project found no difference in mental and motor scores at 8 months or intelligent quotient (IQ) scores at 4 years in children exposed to phenytoin or phenobarbitone in utero versus those from epileptic mothers who were untreated (Shapiro et al., 1976). A third recent prospective study involved all the children of epileptic mothers born in a single hospital in Finland during a 5-year period (Gaily et al., 1988). In this study, 148 children from epileptic mothers and 105 children from normal pregnancies were compared at 5.5 years of age. Intelligence was assessed by both verbal and nonverbal methods. Among the 148 children in the epilepsy group, 131 had received an anticonvulsant, of which phenytoin was the most common (103 exposures). Mental deficiency was found in two children from the epilepsy group and none from the control group. However, in each of the two retarded children it was difficult to identify a clear association with the anticonvulsant used (carbamazepine in one case and phenytoin in the other) since one child had a family history of mental retardation and the other came from a pregnancy complicated not only by poorly controlled epilepsy but also by alcohol abuse. This study also failed to find any relationship between low intelligence and concentration of anticonvulsant drug in maternal plasma.

The most appropriate conclusion to be drawn from these studies is that anticonvulsant therapy during pregnancy does not appear to influence mental development in the offspring.

Neuroleptic Drugs During Pregnancy. When rats are exposed in utero either to dopamine-receptor antagonists or to drugs that deplete presynaptic stores of dopamine, the brain dopamine receptors in the offspring are persistently reduced (Rosengarten and Friedhoff, 1979). The possibility that drugs that influence dopamine stores or receptors could have a long-term effect when given during human pregnancy has been investigated by the Collaborative Perinatal Project (Platt et al., 1989). Three different types of drug were studied: 239 cases involved antipsychotic neuroleptics such as chlorpromazine; 45 cases involved prochlorperazine, which was usually administered as an antiemetic; and 180 cases involved dopamine-depleting drugs such as reserpine. Motor development was measured in the newborn and again at 8 months, 4 years, and 7 years.

Children whose parents had received an antipsychotic neuroleptic demonstrated abnormal motor activity in the neonatal period. But the anomaly probably was the result of residual drug rather than a long-term permanent effect. The children of parents who had received prochlorperazine for more than 2 months during pregnancy demonstrated abnormalities of fine motor movement at 8 months of age. The most substantial differences, however, were found in the children of parents who had taken a dopamine-depleting drug. Abnormalities of both fine and gross motor movement at 8 months of age and unusual motor movements and postural adjustments at 7 years of age were found in these children (Platt et al., 1989). Because of the nature of the study it is difficult to identify whether there was a particular period of gestation when drug exposure was most likely to produce late effects. For this reason the investigators emphasized that by including all exposures to the relevant drugs they may have underestimated the risk when the drug was given at particular stages of gestation.

Antihypertensive Drugs

Methyldopa. The randomized and prospective assessment of methyldopa compared with no treatment in the management of hypertension during pregnancy referred to earlier (Redman et al., 1977) included a detailed and comprehensive pediatric follow-up at 4 years (Ounsted et al., 1980) and 7.5 years (Cockburn et al., 1982). The follow-up was remarkably complete, with 195 (97%) of the live-born children successfully located and studied at 7.5 years. Both physical and psychomotor development were assessed by a wide range of tests. At 4 years of age, the boys in the treated group had a slightly smaller head circumference than those in the untreated group. But there was no relationship between head circumference and developmental score. The children from the treated group tended to have higher scores across a wide range of motor and intellectual tests compared with the untreated hypertensive group. At 7.5 years of age, the frequency of problems of health, physical and mental handicap, sight, hearing, and behavior was the same in the children from both groups. Boys whose

mothers had been entered into the treatment group between 1 and 20 weeks gestation had marginally smaller head circumference than those from the untreated group, but at 4 years there was no detectable difference in intelligence.

The primary conclusion of this very careful study is that methyldopa appears to be a safe drug to be used during pregnancy, but it may be preferable to avoid methyldopa between 1 and 20 weeks gestation if possible.

Atenolol. The placebo-controlled trial of atenolol in pregnancy-induced hypertension referred to above also included a pediatric follow-up of 1 year (Reynolds et al., 1984). In addition to physical measurements of growth, the children also had a Denver Developmental Screening test at 3, 8, and 12 months of age. There was no difference between the groups in physical indices. Differences on the Denver Developmental Screen were found only in babies from a placebo group, two of whom were graded as doubtful at 8 months but were normal at 12 months, and one of whom was clearly abnormal at all stages. This baby appeared to have suffered from brain damage, probably associated with spontaneous preterm labor. The conclusion so far is that atenolol used in pregnancy-induced hypertension in the third trimester appears to confer no adverse effects at 1 year of age.

Aspirin. There is considerable interest in the use of low-dose aspirin for the prevention of both preeclampsia and intrauterine growth retardation (Beaufils et al., 1985; Wallenberg et al., 1986). Large prospective studies to assess the role of aspirin currently are being undertaken by both the Medical Research Council in Britain and the National Institutes of Health in the United States. If the use of aspirin becomes widespread in pregnancy, it is clearly important to know if it has any long-term adverse effects. While there is some information available regarding this question, it is of limited relevance to the current trials with aspirin since the dose of aspirin was higher and the duration of use much shorter in previously reported studies. The two studies reported so far have come to opposing conclusions. Both looked at aspirin use during the first 20 weeks of pregnancy with regard to assessment of IQ at 4 years of age. One study found significant reduction in IQ in association with aspirin use during the first 20 weeks of pregnancy (Streissguth et al., 1987). The other study based on the Collaborative Perinatal Project found that the IQ of children exposed to aspirin was significantly greater than that of children whose mothers had not taken aspirin during the relevant stage of pregnancy. Hopefully both the large prospective assessments of low-dose aspirin that are currently being undertaken will include a careful and detailed pediatric follow-up to help address this important question.

Late Morphologic Effects

In addition to late effects on behavioral development, drugs used during pregnancy also can produce morphologic changes. Late morphologic and physiologic effects have been described following the use of DES during early pregnancy. That drug was once thought but never demonstrated to prevent several obstetric complications including miscarriage. Vaginal carcinoma in the female offspring and infertility in the male offspring are among several consequences of giving DES in the first trimester of pregnancy (NCI DES Summary, 1983). A very worrying aspect of the consequences of using this drug is that the effects often are not seen until the late teenage years. This raises a specter that has clear implications: a drug should be given during pregnancy only if the likely benefits are clear and well established, and those engaged in research on drugs in pregnancy should wherever possible follow the offspring into later life. Both these objectives, and particularly the latter, have been and will continue to be difficult to achieve.

INFLUENCE OF PREGNANCY ON DRUG DOSE REQUIREMENTS

The overwhelming emphasis of studies of the clinical pharmacology of pregnancy has involved what the drug could do to the pregnancy and its outcome. Understandable and important though this subject is, there is another side to the coin that is less well studied but of considerable value in demonstrating clinical pharmacologic principles and in prescribing. Pregnancy influences both drug disposition and effect.

Pregnancy is accompanied by many physiologic changes that could influence pharmacokinetics and pharmacodynamics. The transit time in the gut is prolonged (Parry et al., 1970). Plasma proteins undergo substantial changes. For example, the concentration of albumin decreases, whereas the concentration of α_1 acid glycoprotein increases (Studd et al., 1970). The amount of both body water and fat increase (Hytten and Leitch, 1971). By the third trimester, renal blood flow has almost doubled compared with prepregnancy values (Dunlop, 1976). On the other hand, liver blood flow does not change (Munnell and Taylor, 1947). Certain metabolic pathways in the liver may increase during pregnancy, an inference that has been drawn from the increased urinary excretion of D-glucaric acid (Davis et al., 1973). Further physiologic changes of pregnancy that could influence drug disposition and effect include increases in cardiac output (De Swiet, 1989),

changes in blood pressure that reach a minimum during the second trimester and rise as term approaches (MacGuillivray et al., 1969), reduction in the vascular sensitivity to infused angiotensin II (MacDonald, 1973), increases in renal tubular sodium reabsorption (Lindheimer and Katz, 1973), and hyperventilation resulting in a compensated respiratory alkalosis (Greenberger and Patterson, 1985).

Pharmacokinetics During Pregnancy

Detailed clinical pharmacokinetic studies allowing conclusions to be drawn about possible alterations in drug disposition during pregnancy are relatively few. There have been a good deal of opportunistic observations involving measurement of single steady-state drug concentrations in women taking oral therapy, and several of these studies have been reviewed (Cummings, 1983; Perucca, 1987). Studies featuring the IV administration of drug that allows calculation of drug clearance are few.

Systemic Clearance of Drugs During Pregnancy. By far the most clinically important pharmacokinetic changes to occur during pregnancy involve the metabolic clearance of anticonvulsants. Many reports describe a reduction in the concentration of phenytoin (Eadie et al., 1977; Lander et al., 1977; Landon and Kirkley, 1979; Dam et al., 1979), phenobarbitone (Dam et al., 1979; Rating et al., 1982), carbamazepine (Dam et al., 1979; Niebyl et al., 1979), and sodium valproate (Nau et al., 1981) in plasma during pregnancy. Most studies agree that anticonvulsant concentrations fall progressively during pregnancy reaching their lowest levels in the third trimester and then rising again over a few weeks postpartum (Nau et al., 1982). The reason for this decreased concentration of drug could be a reduction in oral bioavailability, an increase in volume of distribution, an increase in systemic clearance, or some combination of these. In order to obtain definitive data on anticonvulsant pharmacokinetics during pregnancy, IV and oral formulations must be used, preferably in the same women during and following pregnancy. Completely rigorous studies have not been performed. However, the available data do suggest that by far the most important factor leading to these changes in drug concentration is an increase in systemic clearance of the drug from the body.

One study describes the pharmacokinetic data of phenytoin following IV administration in five women who presented with epilepsy during pregnancy. After their initial IV dose, they were given oral therapy (Lander et al., 1984). The oral bioavailability was in the region of 90%, making it unlikely that a marked reduction in bioavailability contributes to the alterations in plasma concentrations. Systemic clearance of phenytoin in two studies was approximately double to triple that typically seen in nonpregnant patients. Further evidence supporting increased clearance as an important factor in the decreased concentration of anticonvulsant drugs seen during pregnancy is provided by the observation that falls in the plasma concentrations of carbamazepine are associated with a decreased ratio of parent drug to the 10, 11-epoxide metabolite in plasma (Perucca, 1987). While the evidence is limited, likely increases in systemic clearance of anticonvulsants are substantial and clinically important during pregnancy.

Clearance of all drugs by the liver is not dramatically changed during pregnancy. The clearance of both labetalol and propranolol in the third trimester of pregnancy were unchanged by pregnancy. This finding is perhaps not unexpected since both drugs are cleared at a rate that approximates liver blood flow, which is itself unchanged by pregnancy (Munnell and Taylor, 1947). The difference between the clearance of phenytoin and propranolol may well reflect the difference between "capacity-limited" and "flow-limited" drug clearance.

In view of the fact that renal blood flow increases substantially during pregnancy, we expect and find that drugs eliminated by this route show alterations in their clearance. Lithium (Schou et al., 1973a) and ampicillin (Philipson, 1977) are among relatively commonly used drugs whose clearance is increased up to 100% during pregnancy. Further information on pharmacokinetics during pregnancy is available in review articles by Cummings (1983) and Perucca (1987).

Protein Binding of Drugs During Pregnancy. In view of the fall in the concentration of albumin in plasma during pregnancy, we should expect and have found that binding of several drugs including phenytoin (Ruprah et al., 1980; Chen et al., 1982b), phenobarbitone (Chen et al., 1982b), sodium valproate (Perucca et al., 1981), and diazepam (Perucca et al., 1981) is reduced. The mechanism of decreased protein binding has not been fully elucidated. The relationship between the free-drug fraction and concentration of albumin (Perucca et al., 1981; Chen et al., 1982b) is inverse but does not necessarily indicate cause and effect. Possibly other endogenous substances contribute to the reduction in drug protein binding. In the case of diazepam, there is no correlation between binding and concentration of albumin.

Drug Metabolism by the Placenta

The placenta contains enzymes relevant to all the major metabolic pathways for drugs and receives a substantial blood supply (Juchau, 1980). For this reason it is theoretically possible that the placenta could contribute to systemic clearance of drugs. However, so far the contribution of the placenta to drug metabolism actually is found to be very small and clinically unimportant (Juchau, 1980; Prach and Rubin, 1988).

Therapeutic Drug Monitoring During Pregnancy

Several studies that demonstrated a reduction in the concentration of anticonvulsants in plasma during pregnancy also detected an increase in seizure frequency in these women. Therapeutic drug monitoring has been routine practice in the management of epilepsy for many years (see chapters 12, 37, and 38). Although the therapeutic range for many drugs is imprecise, nonetheless the management of conditions such as epilepsy during pregnancy provides one of the clearest settings to use measurements of drug concentrations as a guide to therapeutic decision making. Provided the relevant medical condition has been well controlled prior to the onset of pregnancy, it is generally helpful to use the plasma concentrations obtained prior to the pregnancy as a guide to subsequent management. If the drug's concentration falls with advancing gestation, then the dose should be increased accordingly. Drugs that are highly protein-bound, and for which an increased free fraction has been demonstrated during pregnancy, need special consideration when interpreting the therapeutic range during pregnancy. In most laboratories the total drug concentration (bound plus free) is provided to the clinician. Since the free fraction of drugs such as phenytoin and sodium valproate increase by up to 20% during pregnancy, the therapeutic range should be revised downward in pregnant women. This problem in interpretation is avoided if free-drug concentrations (rather than total) are measured. An alternative approach to obtaining concentrations that reflect free drug for the anticonvulsants is to measure the concentration in saliva. At least in the case of phenytoin, the salivary concentration correlates well with the unbound concentration of phenytoin in plasma (Knott et al., 1986). However, in spite of these considerations, the clinical necessity for measuring free drug in plasma or salivary concentrations of anticonvulsants has yet to be established because the therapeutic range of these drugs is not precisely defined.

The application of any therapeutic range for pregnancy based on responses in nonpregnant patients makes the a priori assumption that a given concentration of drug will have the same effect in pregnancy as in the nonpregnant state. In view of the many physiologic changes referred to at the beginning of this section, that assumption may not be justified. In other words, it is possible that a given drug concentration may have different effects in pregnant than in nonpregnant women.

The Influence of Pregnancy on Drug Action. The effort in investigation of possible pharmacodynamic changes in pregnancy has been small. Such studies require that measurements of drug concentration and drug effect be obtained simultaneously. One such study has been carried out with propranolol in 12 women with pregnancy-induced hypertension. The study followed the pharmacokinetics and pharmacodynamics of IV administration of the drug during the third trimester and again 2 or 3 months postpartum (Rubin et al., 1987). Because some of the pharmacologic effects of propranolol can be easily measured, there is little if any immediate clinical value in measuring its concentration–effect relationships (see chapters 2 and 6). On the other hand, the very ease with which propranolol's effect on heart rate can be measured made it an attractive drug to test the hypothesis that pregnancy can alter the action of a drug. Drug effect was modeled as a function of concentration by a method that allows for the fact that response to a drug may be out of phase with its concentration in plasma. A hypothetical effect compartment was assumed (Sheiner et al., 1979). Pregnancy did not alter the pharmacokinetics of propranolol, but its concentration–effect relationship was indeed changed. During pregnancy, propranolol reduced the heart rate by 0.1 ± 0.23 beats/min per ng/ml compared with 0.39 ± 0.19 beats/min per ng/ml in the same women postpartum. This difference was significant and was not influenced either by blood pressure or by pretreatment heart rate. These data were corroborated in a study that described a greater reduction in exercise-induced tachycardia by metoprolol during pregnancy compared with postpartum (Hogstedt, 1986). The mechanism by which β-receptor antagonists exert a greater effect during pregnancy is unclear. However, the change in heart rate and in the concentration of noradrenaline in plasma in response to both tilting and isometric stress is diminished during pregnancy (Barron et al., 1986; Parry et al., 1970). Perhaps a change in the ratio of antagonist to endogenous agonist is a possible explanation for propranolol's altered pharmacodynamics during pregnancy.

The principle underlying these observations with β-receptor agonists is important. The physiologic alterations of pregnancy are not likely to be contained to altering the pharmacodynamics of propranolol alone.

USING DRUGS DURING PREGNANCY— PRACTICAL CONSIDERATIONS
The Clinical Pharmacology Consultation: General Approach

The ideal time to give advice concerning the risks and benefits of drug use during pregnancy is at a preconception counseling clinic. Unfortunately, the majority of requests for information come after the pregnancy has begun, usually after an exposure that occurred when neither the patient nor her physician considered the existence of pregnancy.

An approach to this problem is outlined in Fig. 29-5. First and most important the physician should take a careful clinical history to establish which drug(s) the patient took and precisely when exposure to these drugs occurred. Then the time of gestation for each exposure can be determined as accurately as possible by dating the gestation using a combination of menstrual history and examination with ultrasound. Then the risk of teratogenicity from the drug can be determined using available reference sources (see bibliography). This simple approach works. Drug exposure can frequently be established to have been at a time when the patient was not pregnant or if pregnant beyond the period of organogenesis. Often one can develop some confidence that the drug used is unlikely to be teratogenic. Then one should sensibly reassure the patient *but* state clearly that up to 2% of all pregnancies end with some kind of fetal abnormality in the absence of drugs or other known circumstances. This advice is important because without it, should the particular pregnancy (by chance alone) produce an abnormal baby, the patient's inevitable conclusion would be that the drug was responsible.

Should it appear that exposure to a teratogen occurred at a critical phase of gestation, then the situation is potentially much more serious and difficult. The type of abnormality expected should be ascertained and detailed ultrasound scanning performed on at least two occasions between 18 and 22 weeks. If an abnormality is detected, the subsequent management depends partly on its severity and partly on the attitude of the patient. Many of the more common abnormalities (e.g. cleft palate or minor neural tube defect) can be corrected at birth. A pediatric surgeon should be involved at this early stage to discuss the likelihood of successful treatment at birth or later in childhood. However, if the defect is

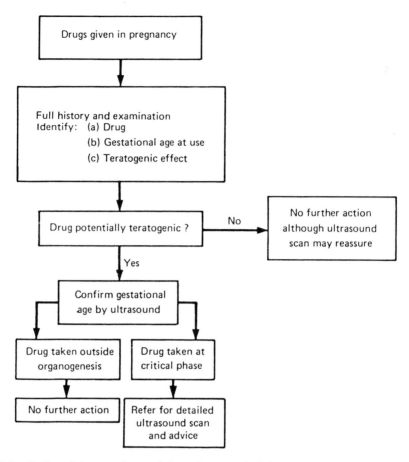

Fig. 29–5. Outline of the procedure to follow when consulted about the use of a drug during pregnancy (reproduced by permission of Dr. Martin Whittle, Queen Mother's Hospital, Glasgow, and British Medical Journal).

severe, the possibility of termination of pregnancy should be discussed carefully with the patient and her partner.

Principles of Pharmacologic Management of a Medical Condition During Pregnancy: Epilepsy

Many of the clinical pharmacologic principles relevant to the use of drugs in pregnancy are illustrated by the management of an epileptic patient.

Prepregnancy Counseling. Much value can be achieved before pregnancy begins, and the optimum time to begin addressing the questions raised by the use of anticonvulsants is when the patient begins to contemplate pregnancy. The risks and benefits of treatment can be carefully considered in a relatively dispassionate manner. The risks of untreated epilepsy include maternal

death, and this must be made absolutely clear to the patient. On the other hand, anticonvulsants carry a teratogenic risk, although this probably does not exceed 10% of exposures.

Second, the need for treatment can be established: there is no better way to avoid drug-induced teratogenicity than by not giving the drug. If the patient meets the usual medical criteria for withdrawing therapy, then her treatment could be slowly discontinued.

If treatment must be continued, then optimal control should be achieved, ideally with monotherapy, before the pregnancy begins.

Pregnancy. During pregnancy, drug concentrations should be monitored monthly. The aim is to maintain the concentration known to be associated with good control in that patient before pregnancy while allowing for the protein binding changes referred to above. If the concentration of drug in plasma decreases, the dose of the drug should be appropriately increased.

Women taking medication during pregnancy should have a detailed ultrasound scan at 18 to 22 weeks gestation in order to identify any fetal abnormality, and if necessary, appropriate action should be taken as detailed above.

At the end of pregnancy, vitamin K (20 mg daily) should be given for 2 weeks in order to prevent the coagulation abnormalities of the neonate whose mother has needed the drug.

Puerperium. Breast feeding is safe with the three most commonly used acute convulsant drugs: phenytoin, sodium valproate, and carbamazepine. Breast feeding should be avoided in women receiving phenobarbitone.

Drug concentrations should be monitored every 2 weeks until it is clear how quickly the pharmacokinetics of the drug are returning to prepregnant values. The dose should be adjusted accordingly. Prepregnancy dose requirements usually can be resumed by 6 weeks postpartum.

SUGGESTED READING

Briggs, G. G.; Freeman, R. K.; and Yaffe, S. J. (eds.): Drugs in Pregnancy and Lactation, 3rd ed. Williams & Wilkins, Baltimore, 1990.

De Swiet, M. (ed.): Medical Disorders in Obstetric Practice, 2nd ed. Blackwell Scientific Publications, Oxford, 1989.

Rubin, P. C. (ed.): Prescribing in Pregnancy. BMA, London, 1987.

REFERENCES

Anonymous, 1989: Are ACE inhibitors safe in pregnancy? Lancet, 2:482–483, 1989.

Anonymous, 1984: Debendox is not thalidomide. Lancet, 2: 205–206, 1984.

Anonymous, 1981: Teratogenic risks of antiepileptic drugs. Br. Med. J., 283:515–516, 1981.

Anonymous, 1976: Thalidomide's long shadow. Br. Med. J., 2: 1155–1156, 1976.

Argent, A. C.; Rothberg, A. D.; and Pienaar, N.: Precursor prothrombin status in 2 mother-infant pairs following gestational anticonvulsant therapy. Pediatr. Pharmacol., 4(J3T7): 183–187, 1986.

Atkinson, H. C.; Begg, E. J.; and Darlow, B. A.: Drugs in human milk: Clinical pharmacokinetic considerations. Clin. Pharmacokinet., 14:217–240, 1988.

Barron, W. M.; Mujais, S. K.; Zinaman, M.; Bravo, E. L.; and Lindheimer, M. D.: Plasma catecholamine responses to physiologic stimuli in normal human pregnancy. Am. J. Obstet. Gynecol., 154:80–84, 1986.

Beaufils, M.; Uzan, S.; Donsimoni, R.; and Colau, J. C.: Prevention of pre-eclampsia by early antiplatelet therapy. Lancet, 1:840–842, 1985.

Becker, M. H.; Genieser, N. B.; and Feingold, M.: Chondrodysplasia punctata: Is maternal warfarin therapy a factor? Am. J. Dis. Child., 129:356–359, 1975.

Bleyer, W. A.; and Breckenridge, R. T.: Studies on the detection of adverse drug reactions in the newborn: II. The effects of prenatal aspirin on newborn hemostasis. Rev. Esp. Estomatol., 213:2049–2053, 1970.

Briggs, G. G.; Freeman, R. K.; and Yaffe, S. J. (eds.): Drugs in Pregnancy and Lactation, 3rd ed. Williams & Wilkins, Baltimore, 1990.

Brocklebank, J. C.; Ray, W. A.; Federspiel, C. F.; and Schaffner, W.: Drug prescribing during pregnancy: A controlled study of Tennessee Medicaid recipients. Am. J. Obstet. Gynecol., 132(3):235–244, 1978.

Buehler, B. A.: Epoxide hydrolase activity in fibroblasts: Correlation with clinical features of the fetal hydantoin syndrome. Proc. Greenwood Genet. Cent., 6:117–118, 1987.

Butters, L.; Kennedy, S.; and Rubin, P.: Atenolol in essential hypertension during pregnancy. Br. Med. J., 301:587–589, 1990.

Byron, M. A.: Treatment of rheumatic diseases. In, Prescribing in Pregnancy (Rubin, P. C., ed.). BMA, London, 1987.

Chamberlain, G. V. P.; Lewis, P. J.; DeSwiet, M.; and Bulpitt, C. J.: How obstetricians manage hypertension in pregnancy. Br. Med. J., 1:626–629, 1978.

Chen, W. W. C.; Chan, C. S.; Lee, P. R.; and Wang, V. C. W.: Pregnancy in patients with prosthetic heart valves: An experience with 45 pregnancies. Q. J. Med., 51:358–365, 1982a.

Chen, S. S.; Perucca, E.; Lee, J. M.; and Richens, A.: Serum protein binding and free concentration of phenytoin and phenobarbitone in pregnancy. Br. J. Clin. Pharmacol., 13:547–554, 1982b.

Cockburn, J.; Moar, V. A.; Ounsted, M.; and Redman, C. W. G.: Final report of study on hypertension during pregnancy: The effects of specific treatment of the growth and development of the children. Lancet, 1:647–649, 1982.

Cordero, J. F.; and Oakley, G. P.: Drug exposure during pregnancy: Some epidemiologic considerations. Clin. Obstet. Gynecol., 26(2):418–428, 1983.

Cummings, A. J.: A survey of pharmacokinetic data from pregnant women. Clin. Pharmacokinet., 8:344–354, 1983.

Dam, H.; Christiansen, J.; Munck, O.; and Mygind, K. I.: Antiepileptic drugs: Metabolism in pregnancy. Clin. Pharmacokinet., 4:53–62, 1979.

Davies, V. A.; Rothberg, A. D.; Argent, A. C.; Atkinson, P. M.; Staub, H.; and Pienaar, N. L.: Precursor prothrombin status in patients receiving anticonvulsant drugs. Lancet, 1:126–129, 1985.

Davis, M.; Simmons, C. J.; Dordini, B.; Maxwell, J. D.; and Williams, R.: Induction of hepatic enzymes during normal pregnancy. J. Obstet Gynaecol. Br. Commonw., 80:690–694, 1973.

Deblay, M. F.; Vert, P.; Andre, M.; and Marchal, F.: Transplacental vitamin K prevents haemorrhagic disease of infant of epileptic mother. Lancet, 1:1247, 1982.

De Swiet, M.: Heart disease in pregnancy. In, Medical Disorders in Obstetric Practice (De Swiet, M., ed.). Blackwell Scientific, Oxford, 1989, pp. 116–148.

De Swiet, M.; Dorrington Ward, P.; Fidler, J.; Horsman, A.; Katz, D.; Letsky, E.; Peacock, M.; and Wise, P. H.: Prolonged therapy in pregnancy causes bone demineralization. Br. J. Obstet. Gynaecol., 90:1129–1134, 1983.

Dunlop, W.: Investigations into the influence of posture on renal plasma flow and glomerular filtration rate during late pregnancy. Br. J. Obstet. Gynaec., 83:17–23, 1976.

Eadie, M. J.; Lander, C. M.; and Tyrer, J. H.: Plasma drug level monitoring in pregnancy. Clin. Pharmacokinet., 2:427–436, 1977.

Editorial: Valproate, spina bifida and birth defect registries. Lancet, 2:1040–1045, 1988.

Elia, J.; Katz, I. R.; and Simpson, G. M.: Teratogenicity of psychotherapeutic medications. Psychopharmacol. Bull., 23(4):531–586, 1987.

Felding, I.; and Rane, A.: Congenital liver damage after treatment of mother with valproic acid and phenytoin? Acta Paediatr. Scand., 73:565–568, 1984.

Forfar, J. O.; and Nelson, M. M.: Epidemiology of drugs taken by pregnant women: Drugs that may affect the fetus adversely. Clin. Pharmacol. Ther., 14:632–642, 1973.

Gaily, E.; Kantola-Sorsa, E.; and Granstrom, M.-L.: Intelligence of children of epileptic mothers. J. Paediatr., 113(4): 677–684, 1988.

Gal, P.; and Sharpless, M. K.: Fetal drug exposure – behavioural teratogenesis. Drug. Intell. Clin. Pharm., 18:186–201, 1984.

Goldberg, J. D.; and Golbus, M. S.: The value of case reports in human teratology. Am. J. Obstet. Gynecol., 154(3):469–482, 1986.

Greenberger, P. A.; and Patterson, R.: Management of asthma during pregnancy. N. Engl. J. Med., 312:897–902, 1985.

Griffith, G. C.; Nichols, G.; Asher, J. D.; and Flanagan, B.: Heparin osteoporosis. J.A.M.A., 193(2):85–88, 1965.

Hall, J. G.; Pauli, R. M.; and Wilson, K. M.: Maternal and fetal sequelae of anticoagulation during pregnancy. Am. J. Med., 68:122–140, 1980.

Hanson, J. W.; Myrianthopoulos, N. C.; Sedgewick Harvey, M. A.; and Smith, D. W.: Risks to the offspring of women treated with hydantoin anticonvulsants, with emphasis on the fetal hydantoin syndrome. J. Paediatr., 89:662–668, 1976.

Hanson, J. W.; and Smith, D. W.: The fetal hydantoin syndrome. J. Pediatr., 87:285–290, 1975.

Heinonen, O. P.; Slone, D.; and Shapiro, S.: Birth Defects and Drugs in Pregnancy. Publishing Sciences Group, Littleton, Mass., 1977.

Hillesmaa, V. K.; Bardy, A.; and Teramo, K.: Obstetric outcome in women with epilepsy. Am. J. Obstet. Gynaecol., 152(5):499–503, 1985.

Hillesmaa, V. K.; Teramo, K.; Granstrom, M. L.; and Bardy, A. H.: Serum folate concentrations during pregnancy in women with epilepsy: Relation to antiepileptic drug concentrations, number of seizures, and fetal outcome. Br. Med. J., 287:577–579, 1983.

Hogstedt, S.: Ph.D. thesis, Hypertension in pregnancy: an epidemiological, clinical and experimental study with special reference to metoprolol treatment. Uppsala University, Sweden 1986.

Hytten, F. E.; and Leitch, I.: The Physiology of Human Pregnancy. Blackwell Scientific Publications, Oxford, 1971.

Iturbe-Alessio, I.; DelCarmen Fonseca, M.; Mutchinik, O.; Santos, M. A.; Zajarias, A.; and Salazar, E.: N. Engl. J. Med., 315(22):1390–1393, 1986.

Jones, K. L.; Lacro, R. V.; Johnson, K. A.; and Adams, J.: Pattern of malformations in the children of women treated with carbamazepine during pregnancy. N. Engl. J. Med., 320:1661–1666, 1989.

Juchau, M. R.: Drug biotransformation in the placenta. Pharmacol. Ther., 8:501–524, 1980.

Kallen, B.; and Tandberg, A.: Lithium and pregnancy. A cohort study on manic-depressive women. Acta Psychiatr. Scand., 68:134–136, 1983.

Kerber, I. J.; Warr, O. S.; and Richardson, C.: Pregnancy in a patient with a prosthetic mitral valve, associated with a fetal anomaly attributed to warfarin sodium. J.A.M.A., 203:223–225, 1968.

Klebanoff, M. A.; and Berendes, H. W.: Aspirin exposure during the first 20 weeks of gestation and IQ at four years of age. Teratology, 37:249–255, 1988.

Knott, C.; Williams, C. P.; and Reynolds, F.: Phenytoin kinetics during pregnancy and the puerperium. Br. J. Obstet. Gynaecol., 93:1030–1037, 1986.

Kraver, B.; Kraver, F.; and Hytten, F.: Drug Prescribing in Pregnancy. Churchill Livingstone, New York, 1988.

Kuhnz, W.; Koch, S.; Helge, H.; and Nau, H.: Primidone and phenobarbital during lactation period in epileptic women: Total and free drug serum levels in the nursed infants and their effects on neonatal behaviour. Dev. Pharmacol. Ther., 11:147–154, 1988.

Lammer, E. J.; Chen, D. T.; Hoar, R. M.; Agnish, N. D.; Benke, P. J.; Braun, J. T.; Curry, C. J.; Fernhoff, P. M.; Grix, A. W.; Lott, I. T.; Richard, J. M.; and Sun, S. C.: Retinoic acid embryopathy. N. Engl. J. Med., 313(14):837–841, 1985.

Lander, C. M.; Smith, M. T.; Chalk, J. B.; de Wytt, C.; Symoniw, P.; Livingstone, I.; and Eadie, M. J.: Bioavailability and pharmacokinetics of phenytoin during pregnancy. Eur. J. Clin. Pharmacol., 27:105–110, 1984.

Lander, C. M.; Edwards, V. C.; Eadie, M. J.; and Tyrer, J. H.: Plasma anticonvulsant concentrations during pregnancy. Neurology, 27:128–131, 1977.

Landon, M. J.; and Kirkley, M.: Metabolism of diphenylhydantoin during pregnancy. Br. J. Obstet. Gynaecol., 86:125–132, 1979.

Legius, E.; Jaeken, J.; and Eggermont, E.: Sodium valproate, pregnancy and infantile fatal liver failure. Lancet, 2:1518–1519, 1987.

Lenz, W.: Kindliche Missbildungen nach Medikament-Einnahme während der Gravidität. Dtsch. Med. Wochenschr., 86:2555, 1961.

Lindheimer, M. D.; and Katz, A. I.: Sodium and diuretics in pregnancy. N. Engl. J. Med., 288:891–894, 1973.

Lindout, D.; Hoppener, J. E. A.; and Meinardi, H.: Teratogenicity of antiepileptic drug combinations with special emphasis on expoxidation (of carbamazepine). Epilepsia, 25(1):77–83, 1984.

MacDonald, P. C.: A study of angiotensin II pressure response throughout primigravid pregnancy. J. Clin. Invest., 52:2682–2689, 1973.

MacGuillivray, I.; Rose, G. A.; and Roe, B.: Blood pressure survey in pregnancy. Clin. Sci., 37:395–407, 1969.

MacMahon, B.: More on Bendectin. J.A.M.A., 246:371–372, 1981.

Manchester, D.; Margolis, H. S.; and Sheldon, R. E.: Possible association between maternal indomethacin therapy and primary pulmonary hypertension of the newborn. Am. J. Obstet. Gynecol., 126:467–469, 1976.

Martz, F.; Failinger, C.; and Blake, D. A.: Phenytoin teratogenesis: Correlation between embryopathic effect and covalent binding of putative arene oxide metabolite in gestational tissue. J. Pharmacol. Exp. Ther., 203:231–239, 1977.

Matheson, I.; Soderman, P.; and the Collaborative Group on Drug Use in Pregnancy. Drug use in pregnancy: Preliminary results from Norway and Sweden. Eur. J. Clin. Pharmacol., 36:A111, 1989.

McBride, W. G.: Thalidomide and congenital abnormalities. Lancet, 2:1358, 1961.

Mellin, G. W.; and Katzenstein M.: The saga of thalidomide. N. Engl. J. Med., 267:1184–1192; 1238; 1244; 1962.

Melmon, K. L.: Attitudinal factors that influence the utilization of modern evaluative methods. In, Modern Methods of Clinical Investigation. Vol. 1, Medical Innovation at the Crossroads. Institute of Medicine Committee on Technological Innovations. National Academy Press, Washington, D.C., pp. 135–145, 1990.

Moise, K. J.; Huhta, J. C.; Sharif, D. S.; Ou, C.-N.; and Kirshon, B.: Wasserstrum, N.; and Cano, L.: Indomethacin in the treatment of premature labor: Effects on the fetal ductus arteriosus. N. Engl. J. Med., 319(6):327–331, 1988.

Mountain, K. R.; Hirsh, J.; and Gallus, A. S.: Neonatal coagulation defect due to anticonvulsant drug treatment in pregnancy. Lancet, 1:265–268, 1970.

Munnell, E. W.; and Taylor, H. C.: Liver blood flow in pregnancy – Hepatic vein catheterisation. J. Clin. Invest., 26:952–956, 1947.

Nau, H.; Kuhnz, W.; Egger, H.-J.; Rating, D.; and Helge, H.: Anticonvulsants during pregnancy and lactation. Transplacental, maternal and neonatal pharmacokinetics. Clin. Pharmacokinet., 7:508–543, 1982.

Nau, H.; Rating, D.; Koch, S.; Hauser, I.; and Helge, H.: Valproic acid and its metabolites. J. Pharmacol. Exp. Ther., 219:768–777, 1981.

NCI DES Summary: Prenatal diethylstilbestrol (DES) exposure. Clin. Pediatr., 22:139–143, 1983.

Niebyl, J. R.; Blake, D. A.; Freeman, J. M.; and Luff, R. D.: Carbamazepine levels in pregnancy and lactation. Obstet. Gynaecol., 53:139–140, 1979.

Nora, J. J.; Nora, A. H.; and Toews, W. H.: Lithium, Ebstein's anomaly, and other congenital heart defects. Lancet, 1:594–595, 1974.

Oakley, C.: Pregnancy in patients with prosthetic heart valves. Br. Med. J., 286:1680–1681, 1983.

Orme, M. L.: The debendox saga. Br. Med. J., 291:918–919, 1985.

Ounsted, M. K.; Moar, V. A.; Good, F. J.; and Redman, C. W. G.: Hypertension during pregnancy with and without specific treatment; the development of the children at the age of four years. Br. J. Obstet. Gynaecol., 87:19–24, 1980.

Parry, E.; Shields, R.; and Turnbull, A. C.: Transit time in the small intestine in pregnancy. J. Obstet. Gynaecol. Br. Commonw., 77:900–901, 1970.

Peckham, C. H.; and King, R. W.: A study of intercurrent conditions observed during pregnancy. Am. J. Obstet. Gynecol., 87:609–620, 1963.

Perucca, E.: Drug metabolism in pregnancy, infancy and childhood. Pharmacol. Ther., 34:129–143, 1987.

Perucca E.; Ruprah, M.; and Richens, A.: Altered drug binding to serum proteins in pregnancy. J.R. Soc. Med., 74:422–426, 1981.

Phenlan, M. C.; Pellock, J. M.; and Nance, W. E.: Discordant expression of fetal hydantoin syndrome in heteropaternal dizygotic twins. N. Engl. J. Med., 307(2):99–101, 1982.

Philipson, A.: Pharmacokinetics of ampicillin during pregnancy. J. Infect. Dis., 136:370–376, 1977.

Piper, J. M.; Baum, C.; and Kennedy, D. L.: Prescription drug use before and during pregnancy in a Medicaid population. Am. J. Obstet. Gynecol., 157:148–156, 1987.

Platt, J. E.; Friedhoff, A. J.; Broman, S. H.; Bond, R.; and Laskas, E.: Effects of prenatal neuroleptic drug exposure on motor performance in children. Hum. Psychopharmacol., 4: 205–213, 1989.

Prach, A. T.; and Rubin, P. C.: Fetoplacental drug clearance in the rabbit: Studies with trimazosin and tolmesoxide. Xenobiotica, 18(8):967–972, 1988.

Rating, D.; Nau, H.; Jager-Roman, E.; Schmidt, D.; and Helgt, H.: Teratogenic and pharmacokinetic studies of primidone during pregnancy and in the offspring of epileptic women. Acta Paediatr. Scand., 71:301–311, 1982.

Redman, C. W. G.; Beilin, L. J.; and Bonnar, J.: Treatment of hypertension in pregnancy with methyldopa: Blood pressure control and side effects. Br. J. Obstet. Gynaecol., 84:419–426, 1977.

Redman, C. W. G.; Beilin, L. J.; Bonnar, J.; and Ounsted, M. K.: Fetal outcome in trial of antihypertensive treatment in pregnancy. Lancet, 2:754–756, 1976.

Reynolds, B.; Butters, L.; Evans, T.; and Rubin, P. C.: First year of life after the use of atenolol in pregnancy associated hypertension. Arch. Dis. Child., 59:1061–1063, 1984.

Rosa, F. W.: Teratogenicity of isotretinoin. Lancet, 2:513, 1983.

Rosengarten, H.; and Friedhoff, A. J.: Enduring changes in dopamine receptor cells of pups from drug administration to pregnant and nursing rats. Science, 203:1133–1135, 1979.

Rubin, P. C.: Beta-Blockers in Pregnancy. N. Engl. J. Med., 305:1323–1326, 1981.

Rubin, P. C.; Butters, L.; McCabe, R.; and Kelman, A.: The influence of pregnancy on drug action: Concentration–effect modelling with propranolol. Clin. Sci., 73:47–52, 1987.

Rubin, P. C.; Craig, G. F.; Gavin, K.; and Sumner, D.: Prospective survey of use of therapeutic drugs, alcohol, and cigarettes during pregnancy. Br. Med. J., 292:81–83, 1986.

Rubin, P. C.; Butters, L.; Clark, D.; Sumner, D.; Belfield, A.; Pledger, D.; Low, R. A. L.; and Reid, J. L.: Obstetric aspects of the use in pregnancy-associated hypertension of the β-adrenoceptor antagonist atenolol. Am. J. Obstet. Gynaecol., 150(4):389–392, 1984.

Rubin, P. C.; Butters, L.; Reynolds, B.; Evans, J.; Sumner, D.; Low, R. A.; and Reid, J. L.: Atenolol elimination in the neonate. Br. J. Clin. Pharmacol., 16:659–662, 1983.

Rubin, P. C.; Butters, L.; Low, R. A.; and Reid, J. L.: Atenolol in the treatment of essential hypertension during pregnancy. Br. J. Clin. Pharmacol., 14:279–281, 1982.

Ruprah, M.; Perucca, E.; and Richens, A.: Decreased serum protein binding of phenytoin in late pregnancy. Lancet, 2: 316–317, 1980.

Saunders, M.: Epilepsy in women of childbearing age. Br. Med. J., 299:581, 1989.

Schou, M.; Amdisen, A.; and Steenstrup, O. R.: Lithium and pregnancy: II. Hazards to women given lithium during pregnancy and delivery. Br. Med. J., 2:137–138, 1973a.

Schou, M.; Goldfield, M. D.; Weinstein, M. R.; and Villeneuve, A.: Lithium and pregnancy: I. Report from the register of lithium babies. Br. Med. J., 2:135–136, 1973b.

Shapiro, S.; Slone, D.; Hartz, S. C.; Rosenberg, L.; Siskind, V.; Monson, R. R.; Mitchell, A. A.; and Heinonen, O. P.: Anticonvulsants and parental epilepsy in the development of birth defects. Lancet, 1:272–275, 1976.

Shaul, W. L.; and Hall, J. G.: Multiple congenital anomalies associated with oral anticoagulants. Am. J. Obstet. Gynecol., 127:191–198, 1977.

Shaul, W. L.; Emery, H.; and Hall, J. G.: Chondrodysplasia punctata and maternal warfarin use during pregnancy. Am. J. Dis. Child., 129:360–362, 1975.

Sheiner, L. B.; Stanski, D. R.; Vozel, S.; Miller, R. D.; and Ham, J.: Simultaneous modeling of pharmacokinetics and pharmacodynamics: Application to *d*-tubocurarine. Clin. Pharmacol., 25:358–371, 1979.

Spielberg, S. P.: Pharmacokinetics and the fetus. N. Engl. J. Med., 307(2):115–116, 1982.

Streissguth, A. P.; Treder, R. P.; Barr, H. M.; Shepard, T. H.; Bleyer, W. A.; Sampson, P. D.; and Martin, D. C.: Aspirin and acetaminophen use by pregnant women and subsequent child IQ and attention decrements. Teratoloty, 35:211–219, 1987.

Strickler, S. M.; Dansky, L. V.; Miller, A. M.; Seni, M.-H.; Andermann, E.; and Spielberg, S. P.: Genetic predisposition to phenytoin-induced birth defects. Lancet, 2:746–749, 1985.

Stuart, M. J.; Gross, S. J.; Elrad, H.; and Graeber, J. E.: Effects of acetylsalicylic-acid ingestion on maternal and neonatal hemostasis. N. Engl. J. Med., 307(15):909–912, 1982.

Studd, J. W. W.; Starke, C. M.; and Blainey, J. D.: Serum protein changes in the parturient mother, fetus and newborn infant. J. Obstet. Gynaecol. Br. Commonw., 77:511–517, 1970.

Szabo, K. T.: Teratogenic effects of lithium carbonate in the fetal mouse. Nature, 225:73–75, 1970.

Szabo, K. T.; and Brent, R.: Species differences in experimental teratogenesis by tranquillising agents. Lancet, 1:565, 1974.

Van Dyke, D. C.; Hodge, S. E.; Heide, F.; and Hill, L. R.: Family studies in fetal phenytoin exposure. J. of Paediatrics, 113:301–306, 1988.

Waddell, W. J.; and Marlowe, C.: Transfer of drugs across the placenta. Pharmacol. Ther., 14:375–390, 1981.

Wallenburg, H. C.; Dekker, G. A.; Makovitz, J. W.; Rotmans, P.: Low-dose aspirin prevents pregnancy induced hypertension and pre-eclampsia in angiotensin sensitive primigravidae. Lancet, 1:1–3, 1986.

Wise, P. H.; and Hall, A. J.: Heparin-induced osteopenia in pregnancy. Br. Med. J., 2:110–111, 1980.

30

Drugs in Special Patient Groups: Neonates and Children

Wayne R. Snodgrass

Chapter Outline

Extreme Importance of Clinical Drug Trials in Infants and Children
Pharmacokinetic Principles of Drug Therapy in Children
  Use of Drugs in Ambulatory Children
  Use of Drugs in Hospitalized Children
  Drug Distribution, Metabolism, and Elimination in Children
  Drug Excretion into Breast Milk
  Pharmacogenetics and Polymorphisms of Drug Metabolism
Compliance with Prescribed Therapy
Adverse Drug Reactions and Interactions in Children

Teratology and Drug Effects on the Fetus
Selected Therapeutic Problems in Pediatric Patients
  Neonatal Abstinence Syndrome or Substance Abuse in Children
  Sedation and Analgesia in Children
  Ocular Drug Administration in Children
  Pediatric Total Parenteral Nutrition
  Cardiopulmonary Resuscitation in Children
Summary
Sources of Pediatric Drug Information

Pediatric clinical pharmacology as a discipline provides some of the most exciting yet difficult challenges in all of medicine. Rapid and marked age-related physiologic changes beginning in the newborn and continuing throughout childhood including onset of puberty demand an approach to therapy of infants and children that is dynamic yet ever-cautious and distinct from that in adults.

Significant changes in distribution of body water including shifting of extracellular to intracellular body water ratios have a significant effect on drug distribution of some agents within the first few days of life. One example is the marked change in volume of distribution of gentamicin, ranging from 0.8 l/kg on the first day of life in a 28-week-gestation premature infant to 0.2 l/kg on the first day of life in a full-term newborn (Dodge et al., 1991a). Such a change has enormous implications for dosing to achieve adequate plasma and tissue concentrations in these patients.

Rapid and unpredictable age-related changes in drug metabolism and elimination occur in the first few months of life with a magnitude unlike that of any drug therapy phenomena found in adult medicine. For example, there is the marked change in furosemide's serum half-life in premature infants, dropping from 15 to 20 hours at 1 week of life to less than 1 hour only 3 months later in those infants with chronic bronchopulmonary dysplasia (Peterson et al., 1980). The mechanism involves both maturation of renal excretion and increased liver conjugative drug metabolism (Snodgrass et al., 1983).

Similar data are known for phenytoin, with an apparent half-life initially prolonged and then markedly shortened to sometimes less than 5 hours in the first few months of life only to lengthen later again in early childhood (Chiba et al., 1980; Dodson, 1980; Blain et al., 1981; Albani and Wernicke, 1983; Bourgeois and Dodson, 1983; Whelan et al., 1983). Theophylline is yet another example of marked dispositional changes in children, with increases in clearance progressing onward from birth such that by approximately 18 months of age the most rapid clearance of theophylline in life on a weight basis occurs, only to decrease over the next few years to adult values (Aranda et al., 1976; Leung et al., 1977; Rangsithienchai et al., 1977; Simons and Simons, 1978; Rosen et al., 1979; Nassif et al., 1981; Weinberger et al., 1981; Grygiel et al., 1983; Tserng et al., 1983; Kubo et al., 1986; Dothey et al., 1989). *Principle: The child represents a condition of remarkably unstable pharmacokinetics. Whether physiologically or pathologically in-*

duced, such states require well-chosen quantitative surrogate or definite therapeutic end points that can be frequently and accurately monitored in order to adjust therapy appropriately. Failing availability of such end points, frequent and well-chosen timing of monitoring of concentrations of drug in plasma (particularly when the drug has a narrow therapeutic index) allows optimization of the dose (see chapters 37 and 38).

EXTREME IMPORTANCE OF CLINICAL DRUG TRIALS IN INFANTS AND CHILDREN

The difficult challenges in pediatric clinical pharmacology are increased by the many obstacles that prevent more rational and timely accumulation of important, often critical data regarding drug handling and response in children. These obstacles include (1) a lack of requirement by the federal government in the United States that at least certain drugs likely to be used in infants and children be studied in this population prior to or shortly after marketing for use in adults, (2) continued concern, often unfounded, regarding informed consent for participation in clinical trials of drugs in infants and children, and (3) a lack of funding not only for clinical trials of certain drugs and/or drug classes in pediatrics but also, as in all clinical pharmacology (but much more serious in pediatrics), a lack of funding for viable and stable training programs for physician fellow trainees that specifically would produce more pediatric clinical pharmacologists. The existence of fewer than a dozen full-time academic pediatric clinical pharmacologists in the United States is woefully inadequate. In the only international survey of its type, just 10 pediatric clinical pharmacology training programs actively training physician fellows were identified, of which two programs are no longer in existence (Koren and MacLeod, 1989).

It is ironic that pediatric clinical pharmacologic studies are not required currently in the United States. The two major federal legislative actions in 1938 and 1962 that markedly expanded the Food and Drug Administration's regulatory authority, with its current impact on the approach that the pharmaceutic industry must take to market a drug, both arose as a response to primarily pediatric therapeutic disasters. Several dozen children died from ethylene glycol poisoning due to use of ethylene glycol as a solvent vehicle for sulfanilamide. This led to the 1938 amendment. The teratogenic tragedy caused by thalidomide led to the 1962 amendment. Yet, despite these lessons, clinical trials of drugs in infants and children are still not required. Prohibiting controlled experiments necessitates uncontrolled experiments, because sick children must have treatment (Mrongovius and Seyberth, 1980; Furlow, 1980).

The information gap in pediatric drug therapy is emphasized by the fact that less than 10% of the drugs listed in the 1990 *Physicians' Desk Reference* (*PDR*) contain an approval for use in children.

PHARMACOKINETIC PRINCIPLES OF DRUG THERAPY IN CHILDREN

Use of Drugs in Ambulatory Children

This section describes pharmacokinetic principles that are particularly important in children. Chapters 1 and 37 contain a more comprehensive discussion of pharmacokinetics.

A large portion of pediatric practice takes place in an outpatient setting. Pediatricians average 0.9 outpatient drugs prescribed per patient contact compared with 1.1 drugs per patient contact for all physicians combined (Kennedy and Forbes, 1982). Antibiotics are the most commonly prescribed outpatient medication; 95% of children receive or are prescribed medication by prescription before their fifth birthday; children receive an average of 8.5 courses of prescription medication and 5.5 different medications in their first 5 years, with the greatest number of prescription medications being given between 7 and 12 months of age (Fosarelli et al., 1987). By comparison, nonprescription over-the-counter (OTC) medications were given to 97.5% of children within 6 months of hospitalization and 35% of children within 1 week of hospitalization (Bryant and Mason, 1983). Interestingly, drug histories taken by nurses (would physicians do any better?) upon hospital admission showed that only 17% of children were using nonprescription drugs compared with 35% elicited by a questionnaire (Bryant and Mason, 1983). *Principle: Drug histories must be carefully and thoroughly taken to ensure a best possible identification of all agents, including nonprescription drugs, to which a patient is exposed.*

Outpatient drug therapy in infants and children encompasses a large variety of diagnoses and diseases. One common pediatric diagnosis, upper respiratory infection (URI, or the common cold), usually of a viral origin, illustrates the frequent lack of a pediatric scientific data base upon which to base therapeutic decisions.

So-called cough and cold preparations, that is, usually antihistamines and decongestants (sympathomimetics) often in combination preparations, are prescribed frequently for a URI. With essentially no published pharmacokinetic data in children and with little or no scientifically validated published objective measures of pharmacodynamic response that are widely used,

Table 30-1.   STANDARD PEDIATRIC DOSING UNITS (SPDUs)*

SPDU	AGE	WEIGHT	
		(LB)	(KG)
0.5	<4 months	6–11	2.5– 5.4
1	4–11 months	12–17	5.5– 7.9
1.5	12–23 months	18–23	8.0–10.9
2	2– 3 years	24–35	11.0–15.9
3	4– 5 years	36–47	16.0–21.9
4	6– 8 years	48–59	22.0–26.9
5	9–10 years	60–71	27.0–31.9
6	11 years	72–95	32.0–43.9
8	12 years & over	96 and over	44.0 and over

* Reproduced with permission from Temple, unpublished 1985.

the pediatrician and family practitioner rely on clinical judgment and patient's or parent's subjective reports to assess therapeutic response.

One rational proposal for dosing of OTC products in children attempts to simplify the current wide variety of dose volumes and relate dosing to weight (Temple, 1985, unpublished). This approach uses the concept of a *standard pediatric dosing unit* (SPDU) to allow adjustment of dose over the pediatric age ranges of less than 1 year to 12 years, such that less variable doses, based on weight, would be administered. The SPDU based on boy-girl averages for the 50th percentile weights for age was chosen to be one eighth of the standard adult dose. In addition, eight age- and weight-based dosing increments or incremental age periods were chosen (see Table 30–1). The SPDUs can be chosen for common OTC drugs (see Table 30–2). This approach to dosing OTC products in children, if products were appropriately reformulated where necessary for concentration of drug per volume of liquid or amount of drug per tablet, can be shown to result in less variability in dose received on a weight basis compared with current labeling. However, this approach does not obviate the need for specific age-related pharmacodynamic and pharmacokinetic data in children.

Another proposed approach uses length-based (height) dosing (Lubitz et al., 1988; Broselow, 1989, unpublished). A multicolored cloth tape measure, developed using growth chart data derived from the National Center for Health Statistics (NCHS), provides a length-based estimate of weight. The specific color zone for a child's length determines which dose unit group is appropriate for that child (see Table 30–3). Length-based dosing avoids overdosing obese pediatric patients compared with calculating doses by weight. The 10th and 90th percentiles of weight determined from length describe lean and obese children, respectively, but normally proportioned children may be in the 10th and 90th percentiles of

weight determined by age (Broselow, 1989, unpublished). Consideration of the variability of weight estimated from age versus the variability of weight estimated from length shows that estimating weight by length is more accurate than estimating weight by age. From 12 months to 12 years, the average variability in estimating weight from age using NCHS growth charts is about 40%; by contrast, the average variability in estimating weight from length is about 25%.

Dosing by body surface area upon initial consideration would appear to be the most accurate method for drugs that are distributed in extracellular water (ECW). The explanation is that total body water and ECW are better correlated with body surface area than they are with body weight. Drugs that are distributed in the extracellular space must be given in a higher dose per kilogram of body weight in small children than they are in adults because of the greater amount of ECW in infants and children. If not, similar concentrations of drug at receptor sites would not be reached (Boreus, 1982). This is true of most drugs and is the basis for the statement that dosing based on surface area is more accurate than dosing based on body weight. However, in underweight or obese children or those with genetically different drug metabolism or for drugs not dis-

Table 30-2.   STANDARD PEDIATRIC DOSING UNITS FOR SOME COMMON OTC INGREDIENTS*†

DRUG	SPDU (MG)
Acetaminophen	80
Chlorpheniramine	0.5
Dextromethorphan	2.5
Pseudoephedrine	7.5

* Reproduced with permission from Temple, unpublished 1985.

† Based on FDA proposed monograph adult doses of these drugs.

Table 30–3. SUGGESTED ZONES FOR LENGTH-BASED DOSING*

DOSE UNITS	DOSE (MG)	LENGTH RANGE (CM)	AVERAGE WEIGHT FOR LENGTH (KG)†	AGE	COLOR‡
0.5	40	51–59	3.5–5.3	Newborn–3 mo	Red
1	80	59–69	5.3–8.1	3–7 mo	Orange
1.5	120	69–83	8.1–11.3	7–19 mo	Yellow
2	160	83–105	11.3–16.3	19–48 mo	Green
3	240	105–123	16.3–23.2	48 mo–7.5 yr	Blue
4	320	123–135	23.2–29.8	7.5–9.5 yr	Violet
5	400	135–	29.8–	9.5 yr	Black

* Reproduced with permission from Broselow, unpublished 1989.
† 50th percentile weight for length.
‡ Recommended color scheme to use with length-based dosing zones.

tributed primarily in body water, dosing by surface area may not lead to predictable therapeutic responses. Charts and nomograms for plotting surface area from known height and weight often are not readily available and require additional time and effort that does not appear to many pediatricians to make a difference in therapeutic outcome. There simply is no strong evidence that dosing by surface area is a better method for many drugs. Noncompliance and individual variations in drug metabolism may be more significant factors than variations in surface area. Essentially no pediatric data are available that evaluate the effect on therapeutic outcome of dosing drugs by surface area versus body weight (Maxwell, 1989). *Principle: The applicability of any shortcut for calculating drug therapy must be verified before the shortcut is used. No regulatory agency is responsible for how we use drugs, only whether they will be available for us to use. Know whether the advice you use in drug therapy is glib or scholarly.*

One traditional exception to using weight rather than surface area to calculate dosage is in children with cancer, in whom the dosage of many antitumor agents is calculated on the basis of surface area. Even here, an important point may be missed. In a child significantly underweight due to cancer but with a normal height, a surface area dosage regimen derived from weight alone (Lowe's method) would be less likely to lead to toxicity than a surface area dosage regimen

based on both weight and height (Dubois's method) (Maxwell, 1989). The formulas are as follows:

Lowe:

$$\text{Surface area (m}^2) = K \times \sqrt[3]{\text{weight (kg)}^2}$$

where $K = 0.103$ for neonates and 0.1 for young children.

Dubois:

$$\text{Surface area (cm}^2) = [\text{weight (kg)}^{0.425}] \times [\text{height (cm)}^{0.725}] \times [71.84]$$

Table 30–4 shows that the weight-only method (Lowe) gives about a 10% lower estimate of surface area (Maxwell, 1989).

Use of Drugs in Hospitalized Children

There is relatively little information about the type and frequency of therapeutic drug usage in hospitalized infants and children. The Boston Collaborative Drug Surveillance Program provides some information on inpatient pediatric therapeutic drug usage (Jick et al., 1972). These may be the only prospectively collected data of this type in children. These data come from 361 infants and children admitted 403 times. The most common diagnoses reflect infectious disorders and respiratory tract disease (see Table 30–5). The most common indications for therapy

Table 30–4. COMPARISON OF SURFACE AREAS OF A 10-YEAR-OLD BOY BY DUBOIS'S OR LOWE'S FORMULAS*†

BUILD	HEIGHT (CM)	WEIGHT (KG)	SA (DB) (M²)	SA (L) (M²)	VARIANCE (%)
Thin	136	23	0.92	0.81	12.0
Average	136	30	1.06	0.96	10.4
Fat	136	40	1.28	1.16	10.3

* Data from Maxwell, 1989.
†DB = Dubois's formula = height and weight; L = Lowe's formula = weight alone; SA = surface area.
Note: $1.0 \text{ m}^2 = 10,000 \text{ cm}^2$.

Table 30-5.   MOST FREQUENT DISCHARGE DIAGNOSES AMONG 361 PEDIATRIC PATIENTS*

DIAGNOSIS	NUMBER	PERCENT
Otitis media	34	9.4
Seizures	24	6.7
Upper respiratory tract infection	24	6.7
Pneumonia	21	5.8
Congenital heart disease	21	5.8
Renal disease (except urinary tract infection)	18	5.0
Lymphatic leukemia	18	5.0
Asthma	17	4.7
Gastroenteritis	16	4.4
Meningitis	12	3.3
Urinary tract infection	11	3.0

* Data from Jick et al., 1972.

Table 30-7.   MOST COMMON INDICATIONS FOR THERAPY: ADULT HOSPITALS*

INDICATION	NUMBER OF DRUG EXPOSURES	PERCENT DRUG EXPOSURES
Constipation	4899	9.2
Insomnia	4778	9.0
Dehydration/electrolyte depletion	4465	8.4
Pain	4461	8.4
Infection	3983	7.5
Fluid retention	3726	7.0
Vitamin depletion	2547	4.8
Bronchospasm	2432	4.8
Anxiety	2092	4.0

* Data from Jick et al., 1972.

are shown in Table 30-6. More often, children are admitted for one single diagnosis compared to adults, who frequently have more than one diagnosis (see Table 30-7). This results in a different pattern of therapy for children compared with adults.

The drugs most frequently prescribed to infants and children are listed in Table 30-8. The information from this study is somewhat outdated, for example, streptomycin is now no longer used to any significant extent in pediatrics. Also, the relative ranking of drugs frequently used in current practice is different, for example, oral and parenteral penicillin are now used much less for inpatients, but IV ceftriaxone and cefuroxime are used frequently. However, Table 30-8 illustrates the types of drugs used in children hospitalized in the late 1960s and early 1970s, allows comparison of inpatient drug usage in adults during a similar time period (see Table 30-7), and provides a basis for comparison with current inpatient pediatric

Table 30-6.   MOST COMMON INDICATIONS FOR THERAPY: PEDIATRIC HOSPITAL*

INDICATION	NUMBER OF DRUG EXPOSURES	PERCENT DRUG EXPOSURES
Infection	236	13.5
Respiratory problems	181	10.4
Dehydration or electrolyte depletion	123	7.2
Hematologic problems	102	5.8
Leukemia	63	3.6
Seizures	54	3.1
Gastrointestinal upsets	49	2.8
Pain	46	2.7
Hormone replacement	20	1.3
Tumors	8	0.4

* Data from Jick et al., 1972.

drug usage for which comparable data are unavailable.

A detailed retrospective survey of drug use in over 4000 hospitalized children documented the significantly greater usage in children, compared with adults, of antimicrobial drugs, anticonvulsants, atropine, antihistamines, and decongestants and the significantly less frequent use of cardioactive agents, diuretics, sedative-hypnotics, and tranquilizers (Moreland et al., 1978). Anesthetic agents, electrolyte solutions, and insulin use were not evaluated nor was drug use in infants less than 4 weeks of age. Another study of 45 children hospitalized 66 times during the first 5 years of life stated that 65.6% of medications given were anesthetic or sedative agents used during surgery, cardiac catheterization, or bronchoscopy, with children receiving an average of 3.2 anesthetic or sedative agents per procedure (Fosarelli et al., 1987).

A report of drug use in newborn intensive care units from a survey utilizing mail-out questionnaires with a return rate of 23% suggests that a wide variety of drugs as well as approaches to use of drugs occurs in this population (Russell and McKenzie, 1983). Particular concern emerged for an estimated 10% incidence of IV phlebitis in newborns, especially that due to calcium gluconate infusions, an essential therapy in most premature infants.

Due to the slow infusion rates of fluids required in small infants—for example, 4 ml/h in a 1.0-kg premature infant provides maintenance fluid requirements of 100 ml/kg per 24 hours—unanticipated highly significant delays in delivery time of the dose of a drug given IV may occur and have indeed been documented (Gould and Roberts, 1979). Pediatric drug dose volumes may vary from 0.06–1.0 ml for a 1.0-kg infant to 1.4–50 ml for a 50-kg child, based on about 30 of the most commonly prescribed parenteral drugs in pediat-

**Table 30-8. MOST COMMONLY PRESCRIBED DRUGS
AMONG 361 PEDIATRIC PATIENTS***

DRUG	PERCENT OF PATIENT EXPOSURES	PERCENT OF ALL DRUG EXPOSURES	ADVERSE REACTIONS (%)
Prednisone	14	2.8	4.1
Phenobarbital	13	2.8	10.4
Oral penicillin	10	2.2	2.7
Streptomycin	10	2.1	—
Pseudoephedrine	10	2.1	—
Guaifenesin	9	2.0	—
Aspirin	9	1.9	9.1
Parenteral penicillin	9	1.9	6.1
Ampicillin	9	1.9	15.1
Brompheniramine with phenylephrine	9	1.8	—

* Data from Jick et al, 1972.

rics. Figure 30–1 shows the marked delay of 190 to 200 minutes to complete infusion of gentamicin in an infant receiving drug at an infusion rate of 3 ml/hour given at a Y site in the infusion apparatus. Drug dose delivery time to the patient varies with both the infusion rate and the volume in which the drug dose is contained, as shown in Fig. 30–2 (Leff and Roberts, 1981). With the very slow IV rates necessary in some infants, there is both a delay in the time for the drug dose to begin to reach the patient and a prolonged time for the complete dose to be infused. The delay for drug to begin to reach the patient can shift significantly the time that a peak serum drug concentration is reached after the drug is administered into the IV tubing. *Principle: Lack of knowledge of the actual time of drug delivery to the patient can result in obtaining blood samples at times other than the expected peak or trough time points. Subsequent calculation will be more than useless.*

Detailed study of intraluminal tubing diameter, IV flow rate, and tubing length shows that intraluminal tubing diameter has the greatest influence on drug delivery time (Kubajak et al., 1988). Fig-

ure 30–3 shows that drug delivery time can be as long as 140 minutes in a tubing of only 24-in length with an intraluminal diameter of 0.12 in when the flow rate is only 5 ml/h, a not uncommon rate in small infants. Use of small-bore tubing at the distal end of the line between the drug-injection site and the patient minimizes this problem. Drugs with a high specific gravity may settle in a dependent loop portion of tubing and possibly layer against the inner wall of the infusion line, an area with minimal flow in laminar flow movement (Rajchgot et al., 1981).

In critical care situations in children less than 3 years old, for example, shock or respiratory or cardiac arrest, small collapsed veins are difficult to cannulate rapidly. This has lead to a resurgence of interest in the intraosseous route of administration of fluids and emergency drugs and the inhalation route via the endotracheal tube (ET) for drug administration (Spivey, 1987; Zimmerman, 1989). An intraosseous needle or a 16- or 18-gauge spinal needle is inserted directly into the anterior tibia about 2 to 3 cm below the tibial tuberosity. A crunching or popping sound usually

Fig. 30–1. Infusion profile for gentamicin delivery from a Y-site injection IV system. Infusion rates: ●——● 3 ml/hour; ○ - - - ○ 10 ml/hour; △ · · · △ 25 ml/hour; ▲ — · — ·▲ 100 ml/hour. Reproduced with permission from Gould, T.; and Roberts, R. J.: Therapeutic problems arising from the use of the intravenous route for drug administration. J. Pediatr., 95:465–471, 1979.

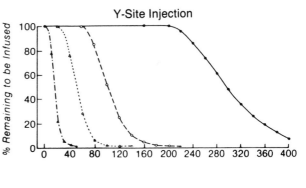

Time (Minutes)

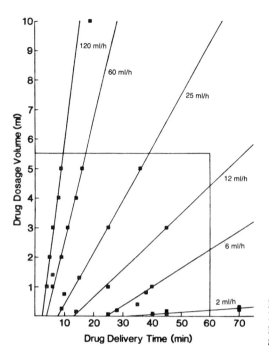

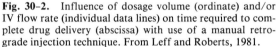

Fig. 30-2. Influence of dosage volume (ordinate) and/or IV flow rate (individual data lines) on time required to complete drug delivery (abscissa) with use of a manual retrograde injection technique. From Leff and Roberts, 1981.

indicates entry into the bone marrow space. Fluid should flow freely by gravity if entry into the bone marrow space is successful. Initial resuscitation fluids of 10 to 40 ml/kg or more for circulatory shock may be given via the intraosseous route. The intraosseous route, although posing an increased risk for subsequent osteomyelitis, may be life-saving in allowing rapid delivery of adequate fluids for resuscitation. The inhalation route of drug administration is as rapid or more so than is IV dosing. Only about 7 seconds elapse for inhaled cocaine to reach the brain, whereas

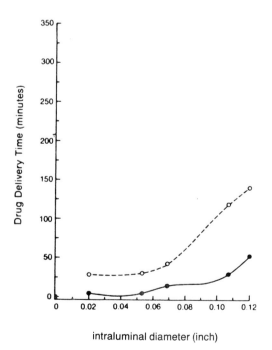

Fig. 30-3. Time required for complete drug delivery with various intraluminal diameters and infusion of 5 (broken line) or 25 (solid line) ml/hour. From Kubajak, C.A.; Leff, R. O.; and Roberts, R. J.: Influence of physical characteristics of intravenous systems on drug delivery. Dev. Pharmacol. Therap., 11:189-195, 1988. Reproduced with permission from S. Karger AG, Basel.

about a 15-second delay occurs for antecubital vein–injected cocaine to reach the brain. The mnemonic LANE can be used to remember drugs that can be given via the ET tube: lidocaine, atropine, naloxone, and epinephrine (Bromage and Robson, 1961; Roberts et al., 1979; Greenberg et al., 1982; Tandberg and Abercrombie, 1982; Powers and Donowitz, 1984). Essentially no published data document efficacy or pharmacokinetics of drugs given to infants or children by the inhalation or intraosseous routes.

Rectal drug administration in pediatrics has traditionally been limited to a few agents such as acetaminophen or aspirin. Because of concern that erratic and incomplete absorption may occur, the rectal route has not been extensively used. More recent data suggest that rectal administration of drugs in infants and young children may be more reliable and desirable than was previously appreciated (Saint-Maurice et al., 1986). Acetaminophen administered rectally in children gives efficacy equal to that of oral administration, but with a delayed absorption and onset of effect; conflicting data exist regarding absorption rate and bioavailability from polyethylene glycol versus triglyceride vehicle base (Keinanen et al., 1977; Vernon et al., 1979; Cullen et al., 1989). Minimal published data exist to document efficacy and/or pharmacokinetics of most all other drugs that might be given rectally to infants and children.

Intramuscular injection of drugs continues to be used in infants and children. Erratic absorption means that IM injection of drugs such as ampicillin, possibly many or most cephalosporins, diazepam, digoxin, phenytoin, and quinidine should be avoided (Greenblatt and Koch-Weser, 1976). A complication rate of about 0.4% from IM injections includes uncommonly described quadriceps muscle contracture and fibrosis (McCloskey and Chung, 1977). Muscle damage appears dependent on volume, pH, chemical composition, and how quickly the injected material diffuses from the site. Nerve damage is determined by the specific injection site and mechanical trauma. Other complications include abscesses, tissue necrosis, atrophy, periostitis, gangrene, IM hemorrhage, skin pigmentation, scars, and cysts (Bergeson et al., 1982). The anterolateral thigh remains the most accepted site for IM injection in infants and in children under 2 years of age. Gluteus maximus injections present a less desirable site because of the proximity of the sciatic nerve; possibly less hazardous may be ventrogluteal injections (Bergeson et al., 1982). Computed tomograph scans suggest that most gluteus maximus injections actually enter subcutaneous fat rather than muscle (Cockshott et al., 1982). Repeated IM injections of hydroxyzine or promethazine may produce fever with or without signs of local tissue injury (Semel, 1986). *Principle: Intramuscular administration of drugs has a variety of implications for efficacy as well as local adverse reactions; use of this route of drug administration in infants and children requires careful consideration.*

Inhalation of drugs for treatment of reactive airway disease (e.g., asthma) in infants and children is an important route of drug administration. Albuterol or fenoterol (the latter is not available in the United States), both β_2 agonists, and beclomethasone or budesonide (the latter not available in the United States), both glucocorticoid steroids, and more recently ipratropium, an anticholinergic drug, are or may be employed as inhalation agents in children (see chapter 7). The devices for delivering these drugs include nebulizers, metered dose inhalers (MDIs), powder inhalers, and spacers (e.g., Nebuhaler or Aerochamber). Nebulizers provide continuous flow output of a stream of aerosol, require an electric power source, and are relatively expensive. The MDI devices are powered by a propellant such as freon, are relatively small, and can be carried in a pocket or purse, but require coordination of inhaled breath with firing of the device to deliver a dose. Spacers or pear-shaped spacers are MDIs with a volume of space inserted between the MDI and the mouth and require inspiratory effort from the patient to open a one-way valve from the spacer into the mouth. Powder inhalers are similar to MDIs but do not contain any propellent and require inspiratory effort from the patient (see chapter 7).

Few well-designed studies on the efficacy, safety, and pharmacodynamics of drug administration by the inhalation route to infants and children are available. Inhalation therapy has been used in adults for many years (Graeser and Rowe, 1935). Pharmacokinetic studies in adults of drugs administered by inhalation have been done (Davies, 1975). Reliability and accuracy of particle size and dose output are of paramount importance in pediatrics. For adults, the "ideal" aerosol MDI is stated to put out particles with a mass median aerodynamic diameter (MMAD) of 7.5 μm with a monodispersed, not polydispersed, distribution that would achieve a maximum theoretical tracheobronchial deposition of 25% of dose (Bouchikhi et al., 1988). However, these theoretical criteria have not yet been achieved in any commercial MDI, and they apply only to adults (an assumed inspired volume of 1500 ml and inspiratory time of 2 seconds). Bioavailability of MDIs may vary significantly and result in inadequate clinical response (Chhabra, 1987). Dose output must be measured directly and cannot be estimated from weight loss of the MDI after each administration (O'Callaghan et al., 1989). For nebulizers, similar differences exist and may have clinical significance, as has been shown for pentamidine nebulization in patients with AIDS (O'Doherty et al., 1988). The pear-shaped spacer device (e.g., Nebuhaler of 750-ml volume or Aerochamber of 100-ml volume) with a one-way valve allows larger drug-containing particles to settle out before inhalation of smaller (1 to 5 μm) particles that reach and stay in the lower respiratory tract. Radiotracer techniques (in adults; no pediatric data are known) show that about 20% of a dose reaches the lungs with use of the pear-shaped spacer compared with less than 9% without a spacer when only an MDI is used (Newman et al., 1984). Data in infants and children show that pear-shaped spacer devices are effective and can be used in younger children including those as young as 6 months with appropriate modification of equipment and instruction of parents or other caretakers (Freelander and VanAsperen, 1984; Benoist et al., 1988; Croft, 1989; Conner et al., 1989; Bisgaard and Ohlsson, 1989). One study of the inhalation route in infants deserves particular mention because it is double-blind and placebo-controlled (Conner et al., 1989). Children above age 7 years who can coordinate actuation and inhalation prefer a multidose powder inhaler (e.g., Turbuhaler) to a pressurized MDI (Fuglsang and Pedersen, 1989). Safe home use of nebulizers is possible in children (Zimo et al., 1989). The output of the small-particle aerosol generator (SPAG) unit widely used to deliver ribavirin in the treatment of respiratory syncytial virus (RSV) pneumonia in infants remains stable for prolonged periods of time and delivers smaller particles, that is, about 10%, that are 1 μm diameter and 30% that are 3 μm, so more of these particles survive and travel through a mechanical ventilator circuit and an endotracheal tube to reach the lower airways (Newth and Clark, 1989). *Principle: New delivery devices have dramatically improved the ability to provide adequate inhalation doses of drugs to infants and children. Nonetheless, proper instruction in use and continued monitoring of the patient's progress are necessary.*

A problem involving oral administration of drugs to some infants is that they have such short GI transit times and rapid passage of resin forms (sustained-release) that unabsorbed drug is excreted rectally; this is known to occur for theophylline resin forms in some young infants. Occasionally this phenomenon coupled with an unusually rapid theophylline clearance results in the inability to achieve adequate absorption almost regardless of the amount of the resin form dose. In such situations, pediatricians may resort to use of more frequent dosing of standard liquid

preparations in addition to or in lieu of use of the resin form. Obviously, in these circumstances, frequent and close monitoring of the patient's response to therapy and serum drug concentration measurements are important.

Drug Distribution, Metabolism, and Elimination in Children

Excellent reviews of pharmacokinetics applied to infants and children are available (Morselli et al., 1980; Yaffe, 1980; Boreus, 1982; Maxwell, 1984; Roberts, 1984; MacLeod and Radde, 1985). One simplified approach to pharmacokinetics that some physicians find clinically helpful is utilization of the following formulas:

$$\text{Loading dose (mg/kg)} = V_d(\text{l/kg})$$
$$\times \text{ desired } C_p \text{ (mg/l)}$$

$$\text{Maintenance dose (mg/kg·h)} = Cl(\text{l/h·kg})$$
$$\times \text{ desired } C_p(\text{mg/l})$$

See chapters 1 and 37 for additional explanation of these concepts.

The maintenance dose calculation is for first-order-kinetics drugs; first-order kinetics generally apply to most commonly used drugs except phenytoin, aspirin, and ethanol (these latter three drugs have zero-order kinetics). For adults, volume of distribution and clearance for many drugs are listed in appendix I. Unfortunately, no similar listing of pharmacokinetic information useful in pediatric therapeutics exists, primarily because of the lack of published data. These formulas provide a general approach to dosing and may be useful as a starting point for dosing in some patients. However, disease processes and other factors may significantly alter an individual patient's pharmacokinetic parameters. Repeated assessment of the patient's response to therapy and serum drug level monitoring may be needed. *Principle: Individualization of the dosing regimen is especially important in infants and children because of age-related developmental changes, differing disease processes, and often lack of specific age-appropriate pediatric pharmacokinetic data.*

Major developments in pharmacokinetic theory including Bayesian and stochastic control theory and pharmacokinetic programs such as the ADAPT or NONMEM programs that can be run on a personal computer have yet to be applied in any significant way to the pediatric age group (Sheiner and Beal, 1982; Jelliffe, 1986). See chapters 37 and 38 for a description of these methods.

For drugs cleared from the body primarily by metabolism in the liver, newborns generally have slow metabolism in the first few days to several

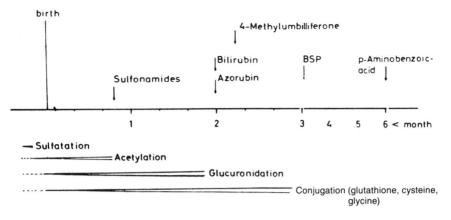

Fig. 30–4. The sequence of maturation of different metabolic liver functions. Reproduced with permission from Gladtke and Heimann, 1975.

weeks, depending on the particular metabolic pathway involved. Bromsulfophthalein (BSP) can be used to measure a component of the liver's capacity to metabolize some types of drugs. The BSP is conjugated with glutathione (GSH) and the conjugate is excreted into the bile. Thus, BSP serves as a test of GSH conjugation, an important detoxification pathway for many chemicals. The uptake of BSP into liver reaches values found in older children and adults at about age 3 months (Gladtke and Heimann, 1975); however, conjugation and secretion mature later, although detailed age-related data are not available. Bilirubin undergoes glucuronidation; its elimination half-life in newborns is prolonged nearly fivefold and reaches adult values by about 2 months of age (Gladtke and Heimann, 1975). Glucuronidation may mature at different rates for different drugs and may be altered by disease processes in infants (Snodgrass and Whitfield, 1983). Glucuronidation of acetaminophen does not reach adult values until about age 12 years (Miller et al., 1976). Glycine conjugation, measured by *p*-aminoben-

zoic acid (PABA) conjugation with glycine, minimal at birth, rapidly increases to normal adult values by about 3 months of age (Gladtke and Heimann, 1975). Acetylation may develop at an earlier age since PABA is acetylated in the newborn. Sulfation may be present at birth, as sulfate conjugates of steroids are present in newborn urine (Gladtke and Heimann, 1975). Figure 30–4 depicts one estimated sequence of maturation of some drug metabolism pathways in human infants. Age-related changes in these drug metabolism pathways must be studied in infants and children in order to attempt rational prediction of liver-dependent drug elimination.

For drugs cleared from the body by renal excretion, both glomerular filtration and tubular secretion require days to months after birth to reach adult values. Using elimination half-life of test substances or drugs instead of surface area or body weight for estimates of filtration or secretion may be preferable because of the difficulties in using the latter parameters as previously described. Kidney weight, extracellular fluid

Fig. 30–5. Total body water (TBW) and extracellular water (ECW), expressed as percentage of body weight, in fetuses, children, and adults. Reproduced with permission from Boreus, 1982.

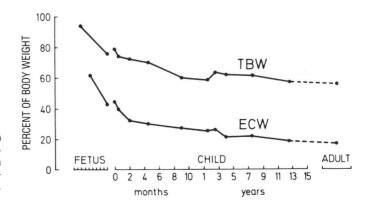

ml H₂O retained

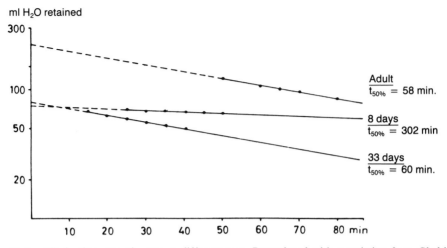

Fig. 30–6. Elimination rate of water at different ages. Reproduced with permission from Gladtke and Heimann, 1975.

volume, and basal metabolic rate are proportional to body surface area. For these reasons, values of renal function often are expressed as a function of body surface area. However, surface area–based comparisons may be misleading. Infants and children have a higher water content in their tissues than do adults for both total body water and extracellular water (see Fig. 30–5). If an infant and an adult are given a water load, comparison of the volumes excreted on the basis of volume of body water (42 liters in the adult) is more meaningful than it is on the basis of body surface area (1.73 m²). Even this comparison does not take into account the difference in the ability of an infant to respond to a water load (Boreus, 1982). At age 8 days, the elimination half-life of water is prolonged fivefold compared with that of adults (see Fig. 30–6).

Glomerular filtration measured by inulin clearance reaches adult values after 3 months of age if

clearance is related to body surface area, but after 10 days of age if clearance is calculated on the basis of weight (see Fig. 30–7). Dextran clearance in neonates is minimal but ultimately increases to 90% of inulin clearance (Gladtke and Heimann, 1975). Thiosulfate is more than 80% glomerularly filtered and is eliminated nearly three times slower in newborns than in older children (see Fig. 30–8). Iothalamate clearance to estimate the glomerular filtration rate (GFR) may be a more readily applied method in patients (Dodge et al., 1991b).

Tubular secretion takes longer to mature than does glomerular filtration. Phenol red dye, a weak acid with a tubular secretion of 94% (but no glomerular filtration), has an elimination half-life about four times longer in the newborn than it does in older children (see Fig. 30–8). *p*-Aminohippuric acid (PAH), which undergoes both glomerular filtration and tubular secretion, has an elimination half-life more than four times longer

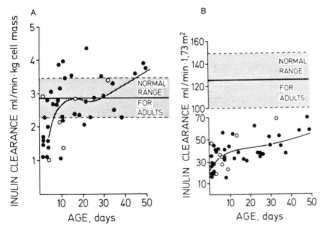

Fig. 30–7. The rate of development of glomerular filtration (inulin clearance) in humans expressed on the basis of (A) weight and (B) body surface area; ○ = female infant, ● = male infant. Reproduced with permission from Boreus, 1982.

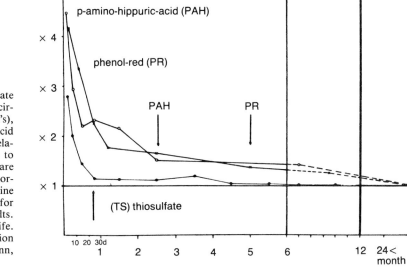

Fig. 30–8. Elimination rate of thiosulfate (TS; closed circles), phenol red (PR; x's), and *p*-aminohippuric acid (PAH; open circles) in relation to age. Arrows: Up to this time the differences are significant compared to normal. The ×1 horizontal line represents normal value for older children and adults. EHL = elimination half-life. Reproduced with permission from Gladtke and Heimann, 1975.

in the newborn than it does in older children (Fig. 30–8). Phenol red requires about 5 to 6 months to reach adult half-life values; PAH requires about 2 to 3 months to reach adult half-life values (Gladtke and Heimann, 1975). Table 30–9 shows age-related development of GFR and tubular excretion (Boreus, 1982).

Tubular reabsorption can be pH-dependent. Urine pH may alter drug excretion by the phenomenon of ion trapping. In older infants who sleep less in the daytime, the biphasic urinary pH pattern (more acidic urine pH at night) lengthens the half-life of sulfisoxazole from about 3.5 hours (daytime) to about 6.5 hours (nighttime) (Krauer, 1975). This effect (ion trapping) depends on whether a drug is an acid or a base and what its pK_a value is.

Little known is the fact that tubular excretion can be "induced," apparently similar to induction of liver drug metabolism. Penicillin can increase tubular transport of PAH. Children ages 7 to 10 years have increased PAH output in urine and a 20% to 30% shortening of PAH half-life if they are pretreated with PAH itself or with sulfonamides (Boreus, 1982). Newborn infants given ampicillin have a shortened plasma half-life of PAH; and ampicillin is reported to shorten its own half-life in newborn infants, an effect thought not to be due to physiologic maturation of kidney tubular excretion (Boreus, 1982). After birth, the sudden new load of organic anions coming from a milk diet may stimulate maturation of tubular excretion in infants. *Principle: Developmental changes in renal drug excretion have not been studied adequately in children, making predictions about the effect of age in infants in renal drug excretion very difficult.*

Free-drug concentration and plasma protein

Table 30–9.   FUNCTIONAL DEVELOPMENT OF THE HUMAN KIDNEY*

AGE	KIDNEY WEIGHT (G)	GFR (ML/MIN/1.73 M^2)	MAXIMAL TUBULAR EXCRETION CAPACITY TMPAH (MG/MIN/1.73 M^2)
Newborn	22–24	38.5	16.0
2 months	27–30	70.2	49.6
6 months	37–43	110.7	46.0
8 months	55–61	110.0	60.6
12–19 months	69–74	117.5	61.6
3 years	91–94	127.0	73.7
9 years	139–141	127.0	73.7
12 years	143–178	127.0	73.7
Adults	257–323	127.0	79.8

* Reproduced with permission from Boreus, 1982.
GFR = glomerular filtration rate.

Table 30-10. DRUGS WITH LOWER PLASMA PROTEIN BINDING IN SERUM FROM THE UMBILICAL CORD THAN IN SERUM FROM ADULTS*

Ampicillin	Lidocaine
Benzylpenicillin	Nafcillin
Bupivacaine	Phenobarbital
Diazepam	Phenytoin
Digoxin	Salicylates
Desmethylimipramine	Sulfamethoxypyrazine
Imipramine	

* Data from Rane, 1980.

drug binding may be important considerations in the pharmacokinetics of some drugs used in infants and children (see chapters 1 and 37 for general discussions of plasma protein binding). Albumin from newborn infants displays quantitatively decreased binding for some drugs, reaching adult values by about 10 to 12 months of age (Pruitt and Dayton, 1971; Kurz et al., 1977). Plasma protein binding of selected drugs known to be diminished in infants compared with adults is shown in Table 30-10 (Rane, 1980). α_1-Acid glycoprotein concentration is low in umbilical cord blood, resulting in low protein binding of certain basic drugs (Piafsky and Woolner, 1982). Neonatal serum may contain free fatty acids that can significantly displace certain drugs from albumin, in addition to which the displacement by fatty acids may not always be similar for different drugs even when bound to the same ligand-binding site of albumin (Kiem et al., 1984). In uremia, endogenous 2-hydroxybenzoylglycine displaces drugs from albumin (Lichtenwalner et al., 1983). Drug binding by plasma protein alters drug distribution as illustrated in Table 30-11 (Boreus, 1982). A large fraction of drug bound to plasma protein does not necessarily mean that the protein (e.g.,

Table 30-11. TOTAL AMOUNT OF DRUG (BOUND + UNBOUND) IN PLASMA AND OUTSIDE PLASMA AT DIFFERENT DEGREES OF PLASMA PROTEIN BINDING (ADULTS)*

BINDING TO PLASMA PROTEIN(%)	DRUG IN PLASMA (% OF TOTAL AMOUNT IN BODY)	DRUG OUTSIDE PLASMA (% OF TOTAL AMOUNT IN BODY)
0	6.7	93.3
50	12	88
60	15	85
70	19	81
80	26	74
90	42	58
95	59	41
98	78	22
99	88	12
100	100	0

* Data from Boreus, 1982.

albumin or α_1 acid glycoprotein) is saturated and that no more binding can occur. An estimate of binding saturation can be made from the product of the binding site concentration times the affinity of binding; for highly bound drugs, three general types of saturation or binding capacity can be described as shown in Table 30-12 (Tillement et al., 1984). One might speculate that binding capacity as shown in Table 30-12 for adult human plasma would be less in plasma from infants and children, but no similar pediatric data are known. Free or unbound drug concentration usually is the important parameter when attempting to make judgments regarding relationship to pharmacodynamic effects (Greenblatt et al., 1982) (see chapter 37).

What is the clinical significance of drug plasma protein binding in pediatrics? A low protein binding in plasma with an increased tissue distribution is the rule rather than the exception in neonatal pharmacokinetics and also in special situations such as malnourished children with kwashiorkor, who have markedly decreased binding of some drugs. With regard to pharmacodynamic effect or risk of toxicity, for most drugs there is a sufficiently stable relationship between unbound and total drug plasma concentrations so that measurement of total drug concentration is adequate for clinical purposes. However, in situations in which changes in plasma protein binding occur, it becomes important to measure the ratio of free to unbound drug (Rowland, 1980; Boreus, 1982). Examples include addition of another drug to the therapeutic regimen that may displace a drug already being used, or development of uremia or excessive circulating free fatty acids, that is, liver or kidney disease (see chapters 8, 9, 11, and 40).

Pharmacokinetic studies in children utilizing stereoisomers where appropriate or incorporating nonradioactive stable isotope methodology are quite limited. Elegant studies of caffeine metabolism in children utilizing stable isotope labeling and breath test analysis demonstrate the importance and feasibility of this approach, including the fact that relatively noninvasive methods can be developed (Lambert et al., 1983). Other uses of stable isotopes in pediatric pharmacology exist (Pons, 1987), but most use in children has been in studies of general metabolism and nutrition (Watkins et al., 1973; Roberts et al., 1986; Yudkoff et al., 1987; Chapman et al., 1990). Age-related differences in drug-receptor responses are not described to any major extent; use of stereoisomers coupled with measurements of pharmacodynamic response might provide valuable information relevant to this important pediatric therapeutic issue. For example, why do infants with severe croup (laryngotracheobronchitis) occasionally become "nonresponsive" to frequently

Table 30–12.   DRUG DISTRIBUTION AS A RESULT OF ITS RELATIVE BINDING CAPACITIES IN ADULT PLASMA AND TISSUES*

	BINDING CAPACITY†		
	PLASMA > TISSUES	INTERMEDIATE	TISSUES > PLASMA
Drugs	Types I, II‡	Propranolol	Phenothiazines
Plasma binding (%)	>90	>90	>80
NK (plasma)	>50	3.8	>10
Apparent volume of distribution (l/kg)	0.1–0.5	3.6	>20

* Data from Tillement et al., 1984.
† The binding capacity is expressed as NK, the product of binding site concentration multiplied by the affinity constant. The apparent volume of distribution is an index of the extent of drug diffusion in tissues.
‡ Types I and II drugs are acidic, almost totally ionized at plasma pH, and highly bound to albumin, e.g., warfarin and clofibrate.

repeated doses of nebulized racemic epinephrine (Westley et al., 1978)? Would an optically active isomer minimize this problem? Why is the refractoriness reversed in many instances by use of corticosteroids (James, 1969; Leipzig et al., 1979; Bass et al., 1980)? Perhaps corticosteroids alter the availability, sensitivity, or responsiveness of the receptors for catecholamines, an interesting, but untested hypothesis.

The important role that pharmacokinetics can play in pediatrics is illustrated by the drug tolazoline. Tolazoline, used nearly 20 years in pediatrics before pharmacokinetic data in infants were available (Cotton, 1965; Monin et al., 1982; Ward et al., 1986), is a drug with multiple effects (α blockade, histamine agonist, and histamine release) and is cleared primarily by the kidneys in young infants. Because of its major toxicity (hypotension, oliguria, gastric bleeding, and death) the drug has been used as a last resort in the treatment of persistent fetal circulation (PFC), also called persistent pulmonary hypertension of the newborn (PPHN), a severe and often fatal disorder, in an effort to decrease resistance to flow in the pulmonary artery. Traditional maintenance dosing of 1.0 mg/kg per hour, arrived at empirically, results in continued accumulation of drug, ultimately yielding serum tolazoline concentrations that are frequently 10 times more elevated than serum concentrations now known to be effective. Such markedly elevated serum tolazoline concentrations undoubtedly provide at least part if not most of the explanation of why this drug has exhibited such toxicity in its past use in infants. Clearly, 20 years should not have elapsed before resources were available to study the pediatric clinical pharmacology of this drug.

Drug Excretion into Breast Milk

Drug excretion in human milk is an increasingly important concern of both the parents and the physician. A healthy trend in the United States toward increased breast feeding of infants is occurring. Lack of data or minimal data still retards thorough evaluation of the risk to the infant of most drugs excreted through breast milk. Principles of excretion of drugs in breast milk that provide accurate prediction of which drugs are excreted, and to what quantitative extent, simply do not exist at the present time. Several excellent reviews are available (Berlin, 1980; Wilson, 1983; Bennett, 1988) (see chapter 29). A recent statement by the Committee On Drugs of the American Academy of Pediatrics (Roberts et al., 1989) contains information useful to making the decision to alter breast feeding for specific drugs. Drugs that are contraindicated during breast feeding include bromocriptine, cocaine, cyclophosphamide, cyclosporine, doxorubicin, ergotamine, lithium, methotrexate, phencyclidine, and phenindione. Drugs (radiopharmaceuticals) that require temporary cessation of breast feeding include gallium 67, indium 111, iodine 125, iodine 131, radioactive sodium, and technetium-99m.

Pharmacogenetics and Polymorphisms of Drug Metabolism

When data are available for infants and children, they probably will show, like adults, pharmacogenetic variability in metabolism of certain drugs. Few pediatric studies are available documenting these processes. Exciting new data strongly suggest that genetic differences in metabolism of sulfonamides relate to predisposition to erythema multiforme in children (Shear et al., 1986). Similarly, acetylator phenotype differences are well known to be associated with adverse reactions to sulfasalazine (Das, 1973). More recent data demonstrate the utility in children of simultaneous administration of dextromethorphan (for oxidation phenotyping) and caffeine (minor metabolites for acetylation phenotyping) for the study of drug polymorphisms (Evans et al., 1989). Future study of these processes in children potentially offer the possibility of predicting those individuals with increased susceptibility to certain drug reactions. Malignant hyperthermia, glucose 6-phosphate dehydrogenase deficiency, and cholinesterase deficiency are just a few areas in need of further study in children (see chapter 32).

COMPLIANCE WITH PRESCRIBED THERAPY

Noncompliance is a significant problem in pediatrics just as it is in adult medicine (see chapter 33). Noncompliance in the pediatric age group has been reported to vary from about 34% to as high as 84% (Mattar and Yaffe, 1974). About 21% of adolescents are reported noncompliant with anticonvulsant therapy; about 28% of asthmatic children are reported noncompliant with recommended theophylline treatment; and about 34% of adolescents are reported noncompliant with oral contraceptive therapy after 3 months (Weinstein and Cuskey, 1985; Friedman et al., 1986; Emans et al., 1987; Lantos, 1989; Donnelly et al., 1989). Compliance with antitumor therapy in pediatric cancer patients decreases over time from about 80% at 2 weeks to about 60% at 20 to 50 weeks (Tebbi et al., 1986). We have documented over 30% noncompliance with single daily dosing of 6-mercaptopurine in children in remission with leukemia (no detectable drug in serum) (Snodgrass et al., 1984). About 17% of parents are reported to refuse immunizations for their children (Guest et al., 1986). A 43% noncompliance rate was reported among children with renal transplants (Beck et al., 1980). In India, 10% of the parents refused admission of their children into the hospital when this was recommended, and about 7% more took their children out of the hospital against medical advice (Ahmad et al., 1985; Lantos, 1989).

Reasons for noncompliance range from simple forgetfulness or carelessness to the extreme of malicious neglect. Lack of understanding of the need for treatment, inability to afford the cost of medication, and lack of belief that treatment is necessary, are also involved. Compliance is related to the patient's or parent's perception of the seriousness of the illness and the degree of effort required by the recommended treatment or attractiveness of the treatment (Gordis et al., 1969).

Compliance can be improved. Remediable problems include inadequate information provided to the parent or patient, failure to motivate or encourage the parent, and practical difficulties of drug administration at home to young children including the taste and flavoring of liquid medications (Yaffe et al., 1977). Taking time to establish rapport with the parent, to explain the nature of the illness, and to give thorough and precise instructions for carrying out the treatment including the names and purposes of the drug or drugs prescribed and specific instructions regarding dosage (e.g., dose volume if a liquid) are all actions that enhance compliance (Yaffe et al., 1977;

Becker et al., 1981). Another specific action to enhance compliance is to provide written material that contains prescription or drug information (Gibbs et al., 1989). Individual patient medication sheets for specific drugs used commonly in pediatrics are available from the American Academy of Pediatrics (American Academy of Pediatrics, Publication Department, Box 927, Elk Grove Village, IL 60009).

One randomized clinical trial involving otitis media in children documented about a 5% and a 10% improvement in compliance and resolution of infection, respectively, by the simple physician action of obtaining a verbal commitment from the parent or patient (Kulik and Carlino, 1987). The physician asked half the patients or parents, "Will you promise me that you will give (or take) all the doses?" Another randomized trial documented the efficacy of a continuing medical education tutorial (two sessions, a total of 5 hours) in increasing pediatrician's compliance-enhancing practices (Maiman et al., 1988). Another study shows that the degree to which adult patients (and one might presume parents) independently volunteer information, as well as answer physician questions during the office visit, explains over half the variance in compliance with a new medication (Rost et al., 1989). *Principle: Ignoring simple logical and proven steps to enhance therapeutic compliance can lead to poor therapeutic outcomes.*

Objective methods to assess compliance have not been applied widely to the pediatric population. Recent data in adults clearly document the unreliability of return tablet counts as a measure of compliance (Pullar et al., 1989). An innovative approach reports the use of stable isotope water, that is, deuterium oxide, added to liquid medications for the purpose of assessing compliance (Rodewald et al., 1989). One can objectively distinguish acute, short-term noncompliance from chronic, longer-term noncompliance by measurement of the concentration ratio of parent drug to metabolite in a randomly obtained urine or serum sample when the metabolite has a longer half-life than does the parent drug (Douidar et al., 1989). Then, computer kinetic simulation allows estimates of the time of the last dose knowing the measured drug/metabolite ratio.

Noncompliance may seriously alter the outcome and interpretation of clinical trials of drugs, especially those in which several treatments are simultaneously studied (Brittain and Wittes, 1989). Some clinical trials may not detect noncompliance. Even modest degrees of noncompliance may considerably diminish the power of multiple-treatment clinical trials to detect treatment effects.

Costs of drugs and how the clinical settings in

which drugs are used in children affect such costs have not been well studied. For outpatients, the costs of drugs may influence compliance with treatment. One useful source of wholesale costs of drugs to the retail pharmacist in the United States is the *Redbook* (*The Annual Pharmacists' Reference: Drug Topics Redbook*, Oradell, N.J., Medical Economics Co., 1990). However, for inpatients, the time to prepare and deliver the drug dose often are a majority of the full cost of each drug dose given. For example, for cefazolin, the materials cost for drug administration ranged from $0.24 to $0.61 per dose, but the total cost (nursing and pharmacy labor included) ranged from $4.42 to $5.87 per dose (Smith and Amen, 1989). As new developments, including more complicated therapies, recombinant technology therapeutic products, and rising salaries for ancillary personnel occur, these costs will rise further. Certain new advances, for example, use of a more lung-selective β_2-receptor adrenergic agonist (i.e., albuterol), although the specific drug is more costly, sometimes result in an overall savings because of lower total drug-use costs and lower physician, emergency room, and hospital-use costs (Tierce et al., 1989) (see chapter 7).

ADVERSE DRUG REACTIONS AND INTERACTIONS IN CHILDREN

Recent data document that pediatric adverse drug reactions account for only a small portion of admissions to children's hospitals. Of over 10,000 infants and children studied, about 0.2% of neonatal intensive care unit admissions, about 22% of admissions of children with cancer, and about 2% of admissions to the general pediatric ward were due to adverse drug reactions (Mitchell et al., 1988). Deaths due to adverse drug reactions in children are rare, about 3/10,000 pediatric admissions, compared with 20/10,000 admissions for adults (Mitchell et al., 1988). However, life-threatening reactions are stated to occur in 3.6% of all hospitalized children compared with 4.7% of adults (Bleyer, 1973). Two causes of adverse drug reactions constitute the large majority of these reactions in children: those related to excessive drug concentration and those related to acute hypersensitivity. Older data based on autopsy histologic criteria for an adverse drug reaction suggest that the liver was the most frequently involved organ and that most of the reactions to therapeutic dosing occurred in the first month of life (Mullick et al., 1973). In a study of adverse drug reactions occurring after admission to a hospital (*n* = 1669), nearly 17% of pediatric patients had an adverse drug reaction (Mitchell et al., 1979). In a study of adverse drug reactions in pediatric outpatients, involving more than 3000

children and more than 4000 separate courses of therapy, most reactions were antibiotic-associated GI complaints and rashes, and a variety of effects due to CNS stimulation from bronchodilators; in general, adverse drug reactions did not commonly occur in general pediatric outpatients, but about 50% were estimated to be preventable (Kramer et al., 1985). *Principle: Adverse drug reactions clearly are to be avoided if possible, but sometimes it is not possible to avoid them if you truly need efficacy. When considering adverse reactions, consider their avoidability in the precise context of the efficacy you seek.*

Other factors contribute importantly to the risk of adverse drug reactions and drug interactions in pediatrics. Nondrug constituents in nebulizers for inhalation pose a risk. Osmolality must be appropriate; hypotonic or hypertonic solutions for nebulization may produce bronchoconstriction. Excessive acidity of nebulized solutions may increase airway resistance. Preservatives such as sodium metabisulfite (releases sulfur dioxide), benzalkonium chloride, and ethylenediaminetetraacetic acid (EDTA) may cause bronchoconstriction (Beasley et al., 1988). Tenfold errors in drug dose calculations occur with unfortunate frequency, especially in the neonatal intensive care unit, because of the small volumes of drugs involved (Koren et al., 1986). Conversion to SI units for dosing and for interpretation of drug serum concentrations as well as performing pharmacokinetic calculations poses an additional risk for dose-related adverse drug reactions (Roberts et al., 1987).

Although adverse drug reactions in children, especially life-threatening ones, are not common, they are critical. *Principle: Pediatric adverse drug reactions may be life-threatening, even if rare. The physician must continually be alert to the possibility of such reactions in children.* Perhaps wider attempts to apply the principles of nonexperimental assessment of excess risk would be helpful in the earlier recognition of adverse drug reactions in children (Miettinen and Caro, 1989). A more detailed discussion of adverse drug reactions and interactions is presented in chapters 39 and 40.

Teratology and Drug Effects on the Fetus

The tragedy caused by thalidomide focused attention on the unique risks that drugs may pose to infants and children. More recent data have documented the high frequency of ethanol's teratogenicity, that is, the fetal alcohol syndrome, and the high risk of teratogenicity with the two drugs etretinate and isotretinoin (Accutane). In the case of etretinate, this agent may be the first very long lasting human teratogen. Women have delivered malformed infants even when the interval between the last dose and conception was nearly 1 year (Lammer, 1988). In West Germany, it is required by law that 2 years of posttherapy contraception be given following the use of etretinate in women of childbearing age (Rinck et al., 1989). Thus, a continued high index of suspicion is needed for the risk of teratogenicity from a variety of agents (Shepard, 1989) (see chapter 29 for a more extensive discussion of teratology).

SELECTED THERAPEUTIC PROBLEMS IN PEDIATRIC PATIENTS

Neonatal Abstinence Syndrome or Substance Abuse in Children

Maternal drug abuse results in significant exposure of infants to these chemicals in utero during critical periods of brain development. As many as 10% of all pregnant women have used cocaine or marijuana during pregnancy, highlighting the magnitude of this problem in the United States (Fried et al., 1983; Lee, 1986). Drug abuse withdrawal is the most frequent drug abuse problem for newborn infants. The neonatal abstinence syndrome usually consists of symptoms of CNS irritability (e.g., drug withdrawal seizures), GI signs (e.g., vomiting, diarrhea), respiratory difficulty [e.g., higher risk for sudden infant death syndrome (SIDS); decreased sensitivity to carbon dioxide], and autonomic nervous system signs (e.g., increased skin sweating, increased skin color mottling, increased body temperature instability) (Zelson et al., 1971, 1973; Kandall et al., 1976; Herzlinger et al., 1977; Chavez et al., 1979; Olsen and Lees, 1980; Finnegan, 1985; Van Baar et al., 1989).

Neonatal drug withdrawal from cocaine includes behavioral effects, a higher risk of SIDS, and probable teratogenicity (cocaine has a nitroxide free-radical toxic metabolite that may cause teratogenicity). Cerebral infarction in the infant in utero from maternal abuse, and infant seizures from breast feeding by a mother abusing cocaine are reported toxicities in infants (Chasnoff et al., 1985; Chasnoff, 1986; Bingol, 1987; Chaney, 1988; Chasnoff et al., 1989). Marijuana causes intrauterine growth retardation, birth defects, and abnormal neurologic findings in infants born to mothers abusing cannabis (Qazi et al., 1985). High-dose marijuana abuse has been reported to produce cortical atrophy in adults (Campbell et al., 1971); consequently, brain and behavioral abnormalities can be predicted for infants exposed in utero. Thus, when abused by the mother during pregnancy, the major drugs of abuse pose extremely serious risks of short-term and long-term toxicities for newborn infants. The extent of the long-term toxicities remains to be fully elucidated.

Various scoring systems have been proposed to assist in the evaluation of neonatal withdrawal (Finnegan et al., 1975; Lipsitz, 1975). Table 30-13 shows one scoring system that physicians and nurses can use serially in the individual infant. A score greater than 8 may be an indication for therapy (Finnegan et al., 1975). Table 30-14 suggests starting doses for therapy with a diluted alcoholic morphine solution when specifically treating narcotic withdrawal (not sedative-hypnotic withdrawal) in children.

Substance abuse (including nicotine) by children and adolescents continues to be a truly devastating problem. One in 20 high school seniors reports drinking alcohol daily; nearly 50% of male high school seniors and 30% of female seniors report drinking excessively at least once every 2 weeks (Sanders et al., 1987). Multiple approaches are needed to attempt to reduce alcohol use by teenagers. One specific proposal is to ban all advertising for alcohol-containing products. Anabolic steroid abuse among teenagers and young adults produces multiple serious toxicities including behavior abnormalities and probable cardiovascular disease (Salva and Bacon, 1989).

Sedation and Analgesia in Children

Therapeutic sedation and analgesia in infants and children constitutes an area in great need of further productive study. A virtual lack of prospective, controlled, double-blind clinical trials provides little foundation for therapy other than anecdotal experience.

A few concepts exist to serve as guidelines for future studies:

1. Choose specifically or know exactly what your goal of therapy is (Do you want sedation only, analgesia only, or both?).
2. Choose drugs for use and for study for which prior data in adults suggest the best possible benefit/risk ratio.
3. Use agents based on rational pharmacologic principles.

Generations of pediatricians have been trained to use the so-called lytic cocktail (which has a variety of other names, including DPT cocktail, cardiac cocktail, pediatric cocktail, and procedure cocktail), an irrational mixture of two phenothiazines and a narcotic (the latter having a convulsant-producing metabolite) that consists of meperidine, promethazine, and chlorpromazine. This combination is used widely for premedication for procedures in pediatrics. However, more rational alternatives exist (Snodgrass and Dodge, 1989).

Table 30-13. NEONATAL ABSTINENCE SCORE*

NAME _____

DATE _____

SIGNS AND SYMPTOMS	SCORE	DATE	TIME 2	6	10	2	6	10	COMMENTS	DATE	TIME 2	6	10	2	6	10	COMMENTS
High Pitched Cry	2																
Continuous High Pitched Cry	3																
Sleeps Less Than 1 Hour After Feed	3																
Sleeps Less Than 2 Hours After Feed	2																
Sleeps Less Than 3 Hours After Feed	1																
Hyperactive Moro Reflex	2																
Markedly Hyperactive Moro Reflex	3																
Mild Tremors When Disturbed	1																
Marked Tremors When Disturbed	2																
Mild Tremors When Undisturbed	3																
Marked Tremors When Undisturbed	4																
Increased Muscle Tone	2																
Generalized Convulsion	5																
Frantic Sucking of Fists	1																
Poor Feeding	2																
Regurgitation	2																
Projectile Vomiting	3																
Loose Stools	2																
Watery Stools	3																
Dehydration	2																
Frequent Yawning	1																
Sneezing	1																
Nasal Stuffiness	1																
Sweating	1																
Mottling	1																
Fever – Less Than 101°	1																
Fever – Greater Than 101°	2																
Respiratory Rate Over 60/min.	1																
Respiratory Rate >60 With Retractions	2																
Excoriation of Nose	1																
Excoriation of Knees	1																
Excoriation of Toes	1																
Total Hourly Score (Sum Over 4 Hours)																	

* From Finnegan et al., 1975.

843

Table 30–14. AMOUNT OF DILUTED (25-FOLD) TINCTURE OF OPIUM (MORPHINE IN ETHANOL) PER DOSE (IN ml) FOUR TIMES DAILY ACCORDING TO ABSTINENCE SCORE*†

	SCORE				
WEIGHT (G)	>8	8–10	11–13	14–16	>17
900–1300	0.04	0.06	0.13	0.25	0.31
1301–1800	0.07	0.10	0.20	0.40	0.50
1801–2200	0.10	0.14	0.27	0.55	0.69
2201–2700	0.12	0.18	0.35	0.70	0.98
2701–3200	0.13	0.20	0.40	0.80	1.00
3201–3600	0.15	0.23	0.47	0.95	1.18
3601–4100	0.18	0.27	0.55	1.10	1.37
4101–4500	0.20	0.30	0.60	1.20	1.50

* Data from Finnegan et al., 1975.
† Opium tincture = 1% morphine (10 mg/ml) solution (19% ethanol). This must be diluted 25-fold to equal a final concentration of 0.4 mg/ml of morphine.

Newer sedatives with a greater margin of safety and an amnesia-inducing effect (desirable in many situations) have been used in infants and children. One example is midazolam, a short-acting benzodiazepine (Diament and Stanley, 1988; Silvasi et al., 1988). For analgesia, morphine (or possibly nalbuphine with comparatively fewer adverse hemodynamic effects) is desirable for many of the more common clinical problems (Way et al., 1964; Dahlstrom et al., 1979; Miser et al., 1980; Glenski et al., 1984; Westerling, 1985; Nahata et al., 1985; Koren et al., 1985; Schechter et al., 1986; Attia et al., 1986; Lynn and Slattery, 1987; Greene et al., 1987; Olkkola et al., 1988).

Ocular Drug Administration in Children

Dilation of the pupils, especially in the premature infant, is often done to examine the fundi for evidence of retinopathy of prematurity. Systemic hypertension is a well-documented risk following topical application of older used formulations of high-concentration (10%) eye drops such as phenylephrine. Current use of 2.5% phenylephrine drops has minimal risk of systemic hypertension. Tropicamide eye drops (a short-acting tertiary amine antimuscarinic anticholinergic) in 0.5% or 1.0% concentration also appear to be safe. A smaller drop size, for example, 8-μl versus a 30-μl total volume, one drop instilled in each eye, achieves equal efficacy for dilation. Serum phenylephrine concentrations following an 8-μl versus a 30-μl volume drop size of 2.5% phenylephrine were 0.97 and 1.9 μg/l, respectively (Lynch et al., 1987).

Dose considerations of past usage are informative. If a 1.0-kg infant received 6 drops of 2.5% phenylephrine of 50 μl each, the total dose would be 7.5 mg/kg. This dose is equivalent to a 15-fold overdose if the same drug had been administered systemically (Merritt and Kraybill, 1981)! *Usually more than 90% of a topical eye drop dose in solu-*

tion is systemically absorbed in infants because the infant usually is in a supine position and does not lose eye drop solution onto the skin of the face.

Recent advances include the use of smaller drop size to more closely approximate the tear film volume of 10 μl and cul-de-sac volume of 30 μl and the use of nasolacrimal occlusion for 5 minutes. Clinical trials suggest certain combinations are useful such as a solution with final concentrations of phenylephrine 2.5% plus tropicamide 0.5% (Caputo and Schnitzer, 1978) or tropicamide 0.25% plus hydroxyamphetamine 1.0% (Larkin et al., 1989). Future research in infants and children is needed to determine the optimal drug–drug combination, dose, dose–volume relation, vehicle, and dose schedule for various purposes such as pupil dilation, antibiotic or antiviral eye infection therapy, and the less common glaucoma in a child (Borromeo-McGrail et al., 1973; Patton and Robinson, 1976; Laor et al., 1977; Mapstone, 1977; Fraunfelder and Hanna, 1977; Korczyn et al., 1978; Scruggs et al., 1978; Nagataki and Mishima, 1980; Shell, 1982; Zimmerman et al., 1984; Palmer, 1986; Schulman et al., 1986; LaRoche, 1987; Van Der Spek, 1987; Khurana et al., 1988; Roarty and Keltner, 1990).

Pediatric Total Parenteral Nutrition

Lack of data prevents discussion of known drug–nutrient interactions in infants and children. Total parenteral nutrition (TPN) is used widely in hospitalized infants and children. Data published from studies in adults clearly provide evidence that nutrition amount and type may alter drug effects (Campbell and Hayes, 1974; Pantuck et al., 1984; Blumberg, 1986; Anderson, 1988) (see chapter 10). Data from infants and animals also show that TPN as currently used may produce liver injury that may be predicted to alter drug metabolism (Black et al., 1981; Berger et al., 1985; Bhatia et al., 1990). Hypocalcemia and hyperkalemia also occur frequently in infants receiving TPN. To some extent these undesired occurrences may be viewed as a dosing problem to which application of principles of clinical pharmacology may be helpful. Carbohydrate intolerance occurs more frequently in infants treated with parenteral antibiotics compared with infants not given antibiotics (all were receiving oral formula or human milk feedings), 76% versus 8%, respectively (Bhatia et al., 1986).

Cardiopulmonary Resuscitation in Children

Controlled clinical trials of drug therapy during cardiopulmonary arrest by the very nature of the clinical setting are nearly impossible to carry out. However, animal studies and clinical experience now provide some guidelines to therapy. Routes of administration, mentioned earlier, include IV, endotracheal, and intraosseous. Agents such as epinephrine, sodium bicarbonate, atropine, lidocaine, naloxone, normal saline, 50% dextrose in water, and calcium gluconate all can be given by the intraosseous and IV routes. A few drugs—lidocaine, atropine, naloxone, and epinephrine (mnemonic, LANE), and probably others—can be given by the endotracheal route (Prete et al., 1987; Spivey, 1987; Zimmerman, 1989; Orlowski et al., 1990). Recent data clearly document the value of monitoring end-tidal carbon dioxide during cardiopulmonary resuscitation to assess cardiac output (Falk et al., 1988).

SUMMARY

Therapeutic drug use in infants and children still is not often on a firm scientific basis primarily because of lack of therapeutic clinical trials in children. A clear need exists for further controlled clinical trials of most drugs used in children and for these studies to be based on sound scientific, physiologic, and pharmacologic principles. Perhaps a study group for pediatric clinical pharmacology studies, similar to the study groups (consortiums, networks) organized in clinical oncology, should be developed to perform multicenter clinical trials that otherwise could not be performed. Such a proposal deserves serious consideration as a potential mechanism to decrease the prevalence of the "therapeutic orphan" status of children.

The "detail man" continues to be a source of drug "information" to physicians. Concern has been expressed that continuous exposure of residents to medical advertising will influence their prescribing habits and that this may pose conflicts with the professional obligation to do the best for the patient (Ferguson, 1989; Hall, 1989). In one study based on a structured interview with 124 physicians, nearly 60% named commercial sources of information as most influential in their first decision to prescribe an antianxiety drug (Peay and Peay, 1988). It is incumbent upon the physician to use the highest quality sources of drug information reasonably available to him or her.

SOURCES OF PEDIATRIC DRUG INFORMATION

Because of lack of data there are no specific large compendia devoted entirely to pediatric drug therapy. However, there are a few excellent textbooks, handbooks, and newsletters that are useful:

Bennett, D. R. (ed.): Drug Evaluations, 6th ed. American Medical Association, Chicago, 1986. Although not a pediatric reference, this text probably should be used more often than the *PDR*. It provides comparative information that assists in the decision of what treatment or drug to use for a variety of clinical conditions.

Boreus, L. O.: Principles of Pediatric Pharmacology. Churchill Livingstone, New York, 1982. In-depth, well-written, and particularly useful for those interested in clinical pharmacology.

DiGregorio, G. J.; Barbiers, E. J.; and Fahl, J. C.: Handbook of Commonly Prescribed Pediatric Drugs. Medical Surveillance, P. O. Box 1629, West Chester, PA, 1985. Useful for finding drug doses.

Gellis, S. S.; and Kagan, B. M. (eds.): Current Pediatric Therapy, 12th ed. W. B. Saunders, Philadelphia, 1986. A useful reference source. A good supplement to *Drug Evaluations* listed above.

MacLeod, S. M.; and Radde, I. C.: Textbook of Pediatric Clinical Pharmacology. PSG Publishing, Littleton, Mass., 1985. A comprehensive and useful textbook. Includes information on children beyond infancy.

Maxwell, G. M.: Principles of Pediatric Pharmacology. Oxford University Press, New York, 1984. Well-written; particularly useful for those interested in clinical pharmacology.

Morselli, P. L.; Garattini, S.; and Sereni, F.: Basic and Therapeutic Aspects of Perinatal Pharmacology. Raven Press, New York, 1975. Contains much useful fundamental information. Excellent for an in-depth background.

Nelson, J. D.: Pocketbook of Pediatric Antimicrobial Therapy. Available from John D. Nelson, M.D., Department of Pediatrics, University of Texas Southwestern Medical School, Dallas, TX, 1989. Very useful for antibiotic therapeutics in children.

Pagliaro, L. A.; and Pagliaro, A. M. (eds.): Problems in Pediatric Drug Therapy, 2nd ed. Drug Intelligence Publications, Hamilton, Ill., 1987. A well-organized and useful handbook containing a variety of tables and data. Especially useful for obtaining drug doses not listed in other sources and human breast milk drug excretion data.

Roberts, R. J.: Drug Therapy in Infants. W. B. Saunders, Philadelphia, 1984. An excellent and one of the most useful textbooks on pediatric therapy. Oriented primarily toward therapy in infants.

Rowe, P. C. (ed.): Harriet Lane Handbook, 11th ed. Year Book Medical Publishers, Chicago, 1987. Widely used; jam-packed with information.

Shirkey, H. C.: Pediatric Dosage Handbook. American Pharmaceutical Association, Washington, D.C., 1980. Useful for dosing information, including less commonly used drugs.

Shirkey, H. C. (ed.): Pediatric Therapy, 4th ed., C. V. Mosby, St. Louis, 1972. Contains information that is still useful including practical ideas not found elsewhere.

Stile, I. L.; Hegyi, T.; and Hiatt, I. M.: Drugs Used with Neonates and During Pregnancy. Medical Economics Co., Oradell, N.J., 1984. Provides good background information. A useful resource.

Yaffe, S. J. (ed.): Pediatric Pharmacology. Grune & Stratton, New York, 1980. Multiauthored; several chapters on specific topics are especially good.

REFERENCES

Ahmad, S. H.; Sharma, S. K.; and Siddiqui, A. Q.: Parental refusal of medical care. Indian J. Pediatr., 22:835–839, 1985.

Albani, M.; and Wernicke, I.: Oral phenytoin in infancy: Dose requirement, absorption, and elimination. Pediatr. Pharmacol., 3:229–236, 1983.

Anderson, K. E.: Influence of diet and nutrition on clinical pharmacokinetics. Clin. Pharmacokinet., 14:325–346, 1988.

Aranda, J. V.; Sitar, D. S.; Parsons, W. D.; Loughnan, P. M.; and Neims, A. H.: Pharmacokinetic aspects of theophylline in premature newborns. N. Engl. J. Med., 295:413–416, 1976.

Attia, J.; Ecoffey, C.; Sandouk, P.; Gross, J. B.; and Samii, K.: Epidural morphine in children: Pharmacokinetics and CO_2 sensitivity. Anesthesiology, 65:590–594, 1986.

Bass, J. W.; Bruhn, F. W.; and Merritt, W. T.: Corticosteroids and racemic epinephrine with IPPB in the treatment of croup. J. Pediatr., 94:173–174, 1980.

Beasley, R.; Rafferty, P.; and Holgate, S. T.: Adverse reactions to the non-drug constituents of nebulizer solutions. Brit. J. Clin. Pharmacol., 25:283–287, 1988.

Beck, D. E.; Fennell, R. S.; and Yost, R. L.: Evaluation of an educational program on compliance with medication regimens in pediatric patients with renal transplants. J. Pediatr., 96:1094–1097, 1980.

Becker, M. H.; and Maiman, L. A.: Patient compliance. In, Drug Therapeutics: Concepts for Physicians (Melmon, K. L., ed.). Elsevier, New York, pp. 65–79, 1981.

Bennett, P. N. (ed.): Drugs and Human Lactation. Elsevier Science, New York, 1988.

Benoist, M. R.; Rufin, P.; DeBlic, J.; and Scheinmann, P.: Nebuhaler in young asthmatic children. Arch. Dis. Child., 63:997, 1988.

Berger, H. M.; DenOuden, A. L.; and Calame, J. J.: Pathogenesis of liver damage during parenteral nutrition: Is lipofuscin a clue? Arch. Dis. Child., 60:774–776, 1985.

Bergeson, P. S.; Singer, S. A.; and Kaplan, A. M.: Intramuscular injections in children. Pediatrics, 70:944–948, 1982.

Berlin, C. M.: The excretion of drugs in human milk. In, Yaffe, S. (ed.). Drug And Chemical Risks to the Fetus and Newborn. Alan R. Liss, New York, pp. 115–127, 1980.

Bhatia, J.; Moslen, M. T.; Haque, A. K.; Rassin, D. K.; McMillan, S.; McCleery, R.; and Kaphalia, L.: Altered hepatic function in rats after light exposure of parenteral nutrients. Clin. Res., 38:44A, 1990.

Bhatia, J.; Prihoda, A. R.; and Richardson, C. J.: Parenteral antibiotics and carbohydrate intolerance in term neonates. Am. J. Dis. Child., 140:111–113, 1986.

Bingol, N.: Teratogenicity of cocaine in humans. J. Pediatr., 110:93–96, 1987.

Bisgaard, H.; and Ohlsson, S.: PEP (positive expiratory pressure)-spacer: An adaptation for administration of MDI (metered dose inhalation) to infants. Allergy, 44:363–364, 1989.

Black, D. D.; Suttle, E. A.; Whitington, P. F.; Whitington, G. L.; and Korones, S. D.: The effect of short-term parenteral nutrition on hepatic function in the human neonate: A prospective randomized study demonstrating alteration of hepatic canalicular function. J. Pediatr., 99:445–449, 1981.

Blain, P. G.; Mucklow, J. C.; Bacon, C. J.; and Rawlins, M. D.: Pharmacokinetics of phenytoin in children. Br. J. Clin. Pharmacol., 12:659–661, 1981.

Bleyer, W. A.: Surveillance of pediatric adverse drug reactions:

A neglected health care program. Pediatrics, 67:308–309, 1973.

Blumberg, J. B.: Clinical significance of drug-nutrient interactions. Trend. Pharmacol. Sci., 7:33–35, 1986.

Boreus, L. O.: Principles of Pediatric Pharmacology. Churchill Livingstone, New York, 1982.

Borromeo-McGrail, V.; Bordiuk, J. M.; and Keitel, H.: Systemic hypertension following ocular administration of 10% phenylephrine in the neonate. Pediatrics, 51:1032–1036, 1973.

Bouchikhi, A.; Becquemin, M. H.; Bignon, J.; Roy, M.; and Teillac, A.: Particle size study of nine metered dose inhalers, and their deposition probabilities in the airways. Eur. Respir. J., 1:547–552, 1988.

Bourgeois, B. F. D.; and Dodson, W. E.: Phenytoin elimination in newborns. Neurology, 33:173–178, 1983.

Brittain, E.; and Wittes, J.: Factorial designs in clinical trials: The effects of non-compliance and subadditivity. Stat. Med., 8:161–171, 1989.

Bromage, P. R.; and Robson, J. G.: Concentrations of lignocaine (lidocaine) in the blood after intravenous, intramuscular, epidural, and endotracheal administration. Anaesthesia, 16:461–478, 1961.

Broselow, J. B.: Length-based OTC drug dosaging in children. Unpublished, 1989.

Bryant, B. G.; and Mason, H. L.: Nonprescription drug use among hospitalized pediatric patients. Am. J. Hosp. Pharm., 40:1669–1673, 1983.

Campbell, T. C.; and Hayes, J. R.: Role of nutrition in the drug-metabolizing enzyme system. Pharmacol. Rev., 26:171–197, 1974.

Campbell, A. M. G.; Evans, M.; Thomson, J. L. G.; and Williams, M. J.: Cerebral atrophy in young cannabis smokers. Lancet, 2:1219–1225, 1971.

Caputo, A. R.; and Schnitzer, R. E.: Systemic response to mydriatic eye drops in neonates: Mydriatics in neonates. J. Pediatr. Ophthalmol. Strabis., 15:109–122, 1978.

Chaney, N. E.: Cocaine convulsions in a breast-feeding baby. J. Pediatr., 112:134–135, 1988.

Chapman, T. E.; Berger, R.; Reyngoud, D. J.; and Okken, A. (eds.): Stable Isotopes in Pediatric Nutritional and Metabolic Research. Intercept, Andover, Hants, England, 1990.

Chasnoff, I. J.: Perinatal cerebral infarction and maternal cocaine use. J. Pediatr., 108:456–459, 1986.

Chasnoff, I. J.; Hunt, C. E.; Kletter, R.; and Kaplan, D.: Prenatal cocaine exposure is associated with respiratory pattern abnormalities. Am. J. Dis. Child., 143:583–587, 1989.

Chasnoff, I. J.; Burns, W. J.; Schnoll, S. H.; and Burns, K. A.: Cocaine use in pregnancy. N. Engl. J. Med., 313:666–669, 1985.

Chavez, C. J.; Ostrea, E. M.; Stryker, J. C.; and Smialek, Z.: Sudden infant death syndrome among infants of drug-dependent mothers. J. Pediatr., 95:407–409, 1979.

Chhabra, S. K.: Differing bioavailability of salbutamol metered-dose inhalers. J. Asthma, 24:215–218, 1987.

Chiba, K.; Ishizaki, T.; Miura, H.; and Minaganua, K.: Michaelis-Menton pharmacokinetics of diphenylhydantoin and application in the pediatric age group. J. Pediatr., 96:479–482, 1980.

Cockshott, W. P.; Thompson, G. T.; Howlett, L. J.; and Seeley, E. T.: Intramuscular or intralipomatous injections? N. Engl. J. Med., 307:356–358, 1982.

Conner, W. T.; Dolovich, M. B.; Frame, R. A.; and Newhouse, M. T.: Reliable salbutamol (albuterol) administration in 6- to 36-month old children by means of a metered dose inhaler and aerochamber with mask. Pediatr. Pulmonol., 6:263–267, 1989.

Cotton, E. F.: The use of priscoline (tolazoline) in the treatment of the hypoperfusion syndrome. Pediatrics, 36:149, 1965.

Croft, R. D.: Two year old asthmatics can learn to operate a tube spacer by copying their mothers. Arch. Dis. Child., 64:742–743, 1989.

Cullen, S.; Kenny, D.; Ward, O. C.; and Sabra, K.: Paracetamol (acetaminophen) suppositories: A comparative study. Arch. Dis. Child., 64:1504–1505, 1989.

Dahlstrom, B.; Bolme, P.; Feychting, H.; Noack, G.; and Paalzow, L.: Morphine kinetics in children. Clin. Pharmacol. Ther., 26:354–365, 1979.

Das, K. M.: Adverse reactions during salicylazosulfapyridine therapy and the relation with drug metabolism and acetylator phenotype. N. Engl. J. Med., 289:491–495, 1973.

Davies, D. S.: Pharmacokinetics of inhaled substances. Postgrad. Med. J., 51 (suppl. 7):69–75, 1975.

Diament, M. J.; and Stanley, P.: The use of midazolam for sedation of infants and children. Am. J. Roentgenol., 150:377–378, 1988.

Dodge, W. F.; Jelliffe, R. W.; Richardson, C. J.; McCleary, R. A.; Hokanson, J. A.; and Snodgrass, W. R.: Gentamicin population pharmacokinetic models for low birth weight infants using a new nonparametric method. Clin. Pharmacol. Ther., 50:25–31, 1991a.

Dodge, W. F.; Jelliffe, R. W.; LaGrone, L.; Hokanson, J. A.; Snodgrass, W. R.; and Brouhard, B. H.: Simple accurate GFR (glomerular filtration rate) measurement: Pharmacokinetically predicted iothalamate clearance. Submitted, 1991b.

Dodson, W. E.: Phenytoin kinetics in children. Clin. Pharmacol. Ther., 23:704–707, 1980.

Donnelly, J. E.; Donnelly, W. J.; and Thong, Y. H.: Inadequate parental understanding of asthma medications. Ann. Allergy, 62:337–341, 1989.

Dothey, C. I.; Tserng, K. Y.; Kaw, S.; and King, K. C.: Maturational changes of theophylline pharmacokinetics in preterm infants. Clin. Pharmacol. Ther., 45:461–468, 1989.

Douidar, S. M.; Dodge, W. F.; and Snodgrass, W. R.: Acute versus chronic noncompliance: Baseline control study in children given sulfisoxazole. Pediatr. Res., 25:66A, 1989.

Emans, S. J.; Grace, E.; and Woods, E. R.: Adolescents' compliance with the use of oral contraceptives. J.A.M.A., 257:3377–3381, 1987.

Evans, W. E.; Relling, M. V.; Petros, W. P.; Meyer, W. H.; Mirro, J.; and Crom, W. R.: Dextromethorphan and caffeine as probes for simultaneous determination of debrisoquin-oxidation and N-acetylation phenotypes in children. Clin. Pharmacol. Ther., 45:568–573, 1989.

Falk, J. L.; Rackow, E. C.; and Weil, M. H.: End-tidal carbon dioxide concentration during cardiopulmonary resuscitation. N. Engl. J. Med., 318:607–611, 1988.

Ferguson, R. P.: Training the resident to meet the detail men. J.A.M.A., 261:992–993, 1989.

Finnegan, L. P.: Effects of maternal opiate abuse on the newborn. Fed. Proc., 44:2315–1218, 1985.

Finnegan, L. P.; Kron, R. E.; Connaughton, J. F.; and Emich, J. P.: A scoring system for evaluation and treatment of the neonatal abstinence syndrome: A new clinical and research tool. In, Basic and Therapeutic Aspects of Perinatal Pharmacology (Morselli, P. L.; Garattini, S.; and Sereni, F., eds.). Raven Press, New York, pp. 139–153, 1975.

Fosarelli, P.; Wilson, M.; and DeAngelis, C.: Prescription medications in infancy and early childhood. Am. J. Dis. Child., 141:772–775, 1987.

Fraunfelder, F. T.; and Hanna, C.: Trends in topical ocular medication. In, Symposium on Ocular Therapy (Leopold, I. H.; and Burns, R. P., eds.), vol. 10. John Wiley & Sons, New York, pp. 85–98, 1977.

Freelander, M.; and VanAsperen, P. P.: Nebuhaler versus nebulizer in children with acute asthma. Br. Med. J., 288:1873–1874, 1984.

Fried, P. A.; Buckingham, M.; and VonKulmiz, P.: Marihuana use during pregnancy and perinatal risk factors. Am. J. Obstet. Gynecol., 146:992–994, 1983.

Friedman, I. M.; Litt, I. F.; and King, D. R.: Compliance with anticonvulsant therapy by epileptic youth. J. Adolesc. Health Care, 7:12–17, 1986.

Fuglsang, G.; and Pedersen, S.: Comparison of a new multidose powder inhaler with a pressurized aerosol in children with asthma. Pediatr. Pulmonol., 7:112–115, 1989.

Furlow, T. G.: Consent for minors to participate in nontherapeutic research. In, Legal Medicine (Wecht, C. H., ed.). W. B. Saunders, Philadelphia, pp. 261–273, 1980.

Gibbs, S.; Waters, W. E.; and George, C. F.: The benefits of prescription information leaflets. Br. J. Clin. Pharmacol., 27:723–739, 1989.

Gladtke, E.; and Heimann, G.: The rate of development of elimination functions in kidney and liver of young infants. In, Basic and Therapeutic Aspects of Perinatal Pharmacology (Morselli, P. L.; Garattini, S.; and Sereni, F., eds.). Raven Press, New York, pp. 393–403, 1975.

Glenski, J. A.; Warner, M. A.; Dawson, B.; and Kaufman, B.: Postoperative use of epidurally administered morphine in children and adolescents. Mayo Clin. Proc., 59:530–533, 1984.

Gordis, L.; Markowitz, M.; and Lilenfeld, A.: Why patients don't follow medical advice: A study of children on long-term antistreptococcal prophylaxis. J. Pediatr., 75:957–968, 1969.

Gould, T.; and Roberts, R. J.: Therapeutic problems arising from the use of the intravenous route for drug administration. J. Pediatr., 95:465–471, 1979.

Graeser, J. B.; and Rowe, A. H.: Inhalation of epinephrine for the relief of asthmatic symptoms. J. Allergy, 6:415–420, 1935.

Greenberg, M. I.; Mayeda, D. V.; Chrzanowski, R.; Brumwell, D.; Baskin, S. I.; and Roberts, J. R.: Endotracheal administration of atropine sulfate. Ann. Emerg. Med., 11:546–548, 1982.

Greenblatt, D. J.; and Koch-Weser, J.: Intramuscular injection of drugs. N. Engl. J. Med., 295:542–546, 1976.

Greenblatt, D. J.; Sellers, E. M.; and Koch-Weser, J.: Importance of protein binding for the interpretation of serum or plasma drug concentrations. J. Clin. Pharmacol., 22:259–263, 1982.

Greene, R. F.; Miser, A. W.; Lester, C. M.; Balis, F. M.; and Poplack, D. G.: Cerebrospinal fluid and plasma pharmacokinetics of morphine infusions in pediatric cancer patients and rhesus monkeys. Pain, 30:339–348, 1987.

Grygiel, J. J.; Ward, H.; Ogborne, M.; Goldin, A.; and Birkett, D. J.: Relationships between plasma theophylline clearance, liver volume and body weight in children and adults. Eur. J. Clin. Pharmacol., 24:529–532, 1983.

Guest, M.; Horn, J.; and Archer, L. N. J.: Why some parents refuse pertussis immunization. Practitioner, 230:210, 1986.

Hall, J. F.: Training the resident to meet the detail man. J.A.M.A., 262:900–901, 1989.

Herzlinger, R. A.; Kandall, S. R.; and Vaughan, H. G.: Neonatal seizures associated with narcotic withdrawal. J. Pediatr., 91:638–641, 1977.

James, J. A.: Dexamethasone in croup. Am. J. Dis. Child., 117:511–513, 1969.

Jelliffe, R. W.: Clinical applications of pharmacokinetics and control theory: Planning, monitoring, and adjusting dosage regimens. In, Selected Topics in Clinical Pharmacology (Maronde, R., ed.). Springer-Verlag, New York, pp. 26–82, 1986.

Jick, H.; Slone, D.; Shapiro, S.; and Lawson, D. H.: Drug surveillance. Problems and challenges. Pediatr. Clin. North Am., 19:117–129, 1972.

Kandall, S. R.; Albin, S.; Lowinson, J.; Berle, B.; Eidelman, A. I.; and Gartner, L. M.: Differential effects of maternal heroin and methadone use on birth weight. Pediatrics, 58:681–685, 1976.

Keinanen, S.; Hietula, M.; Simila, S.; and Kouvalainen, K.: Antipyretic therapy. Comparison of rectal and oral paracetamol (acetaminophen). Eur. J. Clin. Pharmacol., 12:77–80, 1977.

Kennedy, D.; and Forbes, M.: Drug therapy for ambulatory pediatric patients in 1979. Pediatrics, 70:26–29, 1982.

Khurana, A. K.; Ahluwalia, B. K.; and Rajan, C.: Status of cyclopentolate as a cycloplegic in children: A comparison with atropine and homatropine. Acta Ophthalmol., 66:721–724, 1988.

Kiem, E.; Fehske, K. J.; and Muller, W. E.: Competition between drugs and nutrients for specific ligand binding sites on human serum albumin. World Rev. Nutr. Diet., 43:179–182, 1984.

Korczyn, A. D.; Laor, N.; and Nemet, P.: Autonomic pupillary activity in infants. Metab. Ophthalmol., 2:391–394, 1978.

Koren, G.; and MacLeod, S. M.: The state of pediatric clinical pharmacology: An international survey of training programs. Clin. Pharmacol. Ther., 46:489–493, 1989.

Koren, G.; Barzilay, Z.; and Greenwald, M.: Tenfold errors in administration of drug doses: A neglected iatrogenic disease in pediatrics. Pediatrics, 77:848–849, 1986.

Koren, G.; Butt, W.; Chinyanga, H.; Soldin, S.; Tan, Y. K.; and Pape, K.: Postoperative morphine infusion in newborn infants: Assessment of disposition characteristics and safety. J. Pediatr., 107:963–967, 1985.

Kramer, M. S.; Hutchinson, T. A.; Flegel, K. M.; Naimark, L.; Contardi, R.; and Leduc, D. G.: Adverse drug reactions in general pediatrics outpatients. J. Pediatr., 106:305–310, 1985.

Krauer, B.: The development of diurnal variation in drug kinetics in the human infant. In, Basic and Therapeutic Aspects of Perinatal Pharmacology (Morselli, P. L.; Garattini, S.; and Sereni, F., eds.). Raven Press, New York, pp. 347–356, 1975.

Kubajak, C. A.; Leff, R. D.; and Roberts, R. J.: Influence of physical characteristics of intravenous systems on drug delivery. Dev. Pharmacol. Ther., 11:189–195, 1988.

Kubo, M.; Odajima, Y.; Ishizaki, T.; Kanagawa, S.; Yamaguchi, M.; and Nagai, T.: Intraindividual changes in theophylline clearance during constant aminophylline infusion in children with acute asthma. J. Pediatr., 108:1011–1015, 1986.

Kulik, J. A.; and Carlino, P.: The effect of verbal commitment and treatment choice on medication compliance in a pediatric setting. J. Behav. Med., 10:367–376, 1987.

Kurz, H.; Mauser-Ganshorn, A.; and Stickel, H. H.: Differences in the binding of drugs to plasma proteins from newborn and adult man. Eur. J. Clin. Pharmacol., 11:463–467, 1977.

Lambert, G. H.; Kotake, A. N.; and Schoeller, D.: The CO_2 breath tests as monitors of the cytochrome P450 dependent mixed function monooxygenase system. In, Developmental Pharmacology (MacLeod, S. M.; Okey, A. B.; and Spielberg, S. P., eds.). Alan R. Liss, New York, pp. 119–145, 1983.

Lammer, E. J.: Embryopathy in an infant conceived one year after termination of maternal etretinate. Lancet, 2:1080–1081, 1988.

Lantos, J. D.: Treatment refusal, noncompliance, and the pediatrician's responsibilities. Pediatr. Ann., 18:255–260, 1989.

Laor, N.; Korczyn, A. D.; and Nemet, P.: Sympathetic pupillary activity in infants. Pediatrics, 59:195–198, 1977.

Larkin, K. M.; Charap, A.; Cheetham, J. K.; and Frank, J.: Ideal concentration of tropicamide with hydroxyamphetamine 1% for routine pupillary dilation. Ann. Ophthalmol., 21:340–344, 1989.

LaRoche, G. R.: Safety of ocular drugs in pediatrics. Ophthalmology, 94:202–203, 1987.

Lee, M. I.: As many as 10% of gravidas may be using cocaine. Pediatr. News, 20:64, 1986.

Leff, R. D.; and Roberts, R. J.: Methods for intravenous drug administration in the pediatric patient. J. Pediatr., 98:631–635, 1981.

Leipzig, B.; Oski, F. A.; Cummings, C. W.; Stockman, J. A.; and Swender, P.: A prospective randomized study to determine the efficacy of steroids in treatment of croup. J. Pediatr., 94:194–197, 1979.

Leung, P.; Kalisker, A.; and Bell, T. D.: Variation in theophylline clearance rate with time in chronic childhood asthma. J. Allergy Clin. Immunol., 59:440–444, 1977.

Lichtenwalner, D. M.; Suh, B.; and Lichtenwalner, M. R.: Isolation and chemical characterization of 2-hydroxybenzoylglycine as a drug binding inhibitor in uremia. J. Clin. Invest., 71:1289–1296, 1983.

Lipsitz, P. J.: A proposed narcotic withdrawal score for use with newborn infants. Clin. Pediatr., 14:592–594, 1975.

Lubitz, D. S.; Seidel, J. S.; and Chameides, L.: A rapid method for estimating weight and resuscitation drug dosages from length in the pediatric age group. Ann. Emerg. Med., 17:576–581, 1988.

Lynch, M. G.; Brown, R. H.; Goode, S. M.; Schoenwald, R. D.; and Chien, D. S.: Reduction of phenylephrine drop size in infants achieves equal dilation with decreased systemic absorption. Arch. Ophthalmol., 105:1364–1365, 1987.

Lynn, A. M.; and Slattery, J. T.: Morphine pharmacokinetics in early infancy. Anesthesiology, 66:136–139, 1987.

Mattar, M. E.; and Yaffe, S. J.: Compliance of pediatric patients with therapeutic regimens. Postgrad. Med., 56:181–188, 1974.

MacLeod, S. M.; and Radde, I. C. (eds.): Textbook of Pediatric Clinical Pharmacology. PSG Publishing, Littleton, Mass., 1985.

Maiman, L. A.; Becker, M. H.; Liptak, G. S.; Nazarian, L. F.; and Rounds, K. A.: Improving pediatricians' compliance-enhancing practices. A randomized trial. Am. J. Dis. Child., 142:773–779, 1988.

Mapstone, R.: Dilating dangerous pupils. Br. J. Ophthalmol., 61:517–524, 1977.

Maxwell, G. M.: Pediatric drug dosing. Bodyweight versus surface area. Drugs, 37:113–115, 1989.

Maxwell, G. M.: Principles of Pediatric Pharmacology. Oxford University Press, New York, 1984.

McCloskey, J. R.; and Chung, S. M. K.: Quadriceps contracture as a result of multiple intramuscular injections. Am. J. Dis. Child., 131:416–417, 1977.

Merritt, J. C.; and Kraybill, E. N.: Effect of mydriatics on blood pressure in premature infants. J. Pediatr. Ophthalmol. Strabis., 18:42–46, 1981.

Miettinen, O. S.; and Caro, J. J.: Principles of nonexperimental assessment of excess risk, with special reference to adverse drug reactions. J. Clin. Epidemiol., 42:325–331, 1989.

Miller, R. P.; Roberts, R. J.; and Fischer, L. J.: Acetaminophen elimination kinetics in neonates, children, and adults. Clin. Pharmacol. Ther., 19:284–294, 1976.

Miser, A. W.; Miser, J. S.; and Clark, B. S.: Continuous intravenous infusion of morphine sulfate for control of severe pain in children with terminal malignancy. J. Pediatr., 96:930–932, 1980.

Mitchell, A. A.; Lacouture, P. G.; Sheehan, J. E.; Kauffman, R. E.; and Shapiro, S.: Adverse drug reactions in children leading to hospital admission. Pediatrics, 82:24–29, 1988.

Mitchell, A. A.; Goldman, P.; Shapiro, S.; and Slone, D.: Drug utilization and reported adverse reactions in hospitalized children. Am. J. Epidemiol., 110:196–204, 1979.

Monin, P.; Vert, P.; and Morselli, P. L.: A pharmacodynamic and pharmacokinetic study of tolazoline in the neonate. Dev. Pharmacol. Ther., 4(suppl. 1):124–128, 1982.

Moreland, T.; Rylance, G.; and Christopher, L.: Patterns of drug prescribing for children in hospitals. Eur. J. Clin. Pharmacol., 14:39–46, 1978.

Morselli, P. L.; Franco-Morselli, R.; and Bossi, L.: Clinical pharmacokinetics in newborns and infants. Clin. Pharmacokinet., 5:485–527, 1980.

Mrongovius, R.; and Seyberth, H. W.: Medical, ethical and legal aspects of clinical trials in pediatrics. Eur. J. Clin. Pharmacol., 18:121–127, 1980.

Mullick, F. G.; Drake, R. M.; and Irey, N. S.: Adverse reactions to drugs: A clinicopathologic survey of 200 infants and children. J. Pediatr., 82:506–510, 1973.

Nagataki, S.; and Mishima, S.: Pharmacokinetics of instilled drugs in the human eye. Int. Ophthalmol. Clin., 20:33–49, 1980.

Nahata, M. C.; Miser, A. W.; Miser, J. S.; and Reuning, R. H.: Variation in morphine pharmacokinetics in children with cancer. Dev. Pharmacol. Ther., 8:182–188, 1985.

Nassif, E. G.; Weingerger, M. M.; Shannon, D.; Guiang, S. F.; Hendeles, L.; Jimenez, D.; and Ekwo, E.: Theophylline disposition in infancy. J. Pediatr., 98:158–160, 1981.

Newman, S. P.; Millar, A. B.; Lennard-Jones, T. R.; Moren, F.; and Clarke, S. W.: Improvement of pressurized aerosol deposition with nebuhaler spacer device. Thorax, 39:935–941, 1984.

Newth, C. J.; and Clark, A. R.: In vitro performance of the small particle aerosol generator (SPAG-2). Pediatr. Pulmonol., 7:183–188, 1989.

O'Callaghan, C.; Clarke, A. R.; and Milner, A. D.: Inaccurate calculation of drug output from nebulizers. Eur. J. Pediatr., 148:473–474, 1989.

O'Doherty, M. J.; Thomas, S.; Page, C.; Barlow, D.; Bradbeer, C.; Nunan, T. O.; and Bateman, N. T.: Differences in relative efficiency of nebulizers for pentamidine administration. Lancet, 2:1283–1286, 1988.

Olkkola, K. T.; Maunuksela, E. L.; Korpela, R.; and Rosenberg, P. H.: Kinetics and dynamics of postoperative intravenous morphine in children. Clin. Pharmacol. Ther., 44:128–136, 1988.

Olsen, G. D.; and Lees, M. H.: Ventilatory response to carbon dioxide of infants following chronic prenatal methadone exposure. J. Pediatr., 96:983–989, 1980.

Orlowski, J. P.; Porembka, D. T.; Gallagher, J. M.; Lockrem, J. D.; and VanLente, F.: Comparison study of intraosseous, central intravenous, and peripheral intravenous infusions in emergency drugs. Am. J. Dis. Child., 144:112–117, 1990.

Palmer, E. A.: How safe are ocular drugs in pediatrics? Ophthalmology, 93:1038–1040, 1986.

Pantuck, E. J.; Pantuck, C. B.; Weissman, C.; Askanazi, J.; and Conney, A. H.: Effects of parenteral nutritional regimens on oxidative drug metabolism. Anesthesiology, 60:534–536, 1984.

Patton, T. F.; and Robinson, J. R.: Pediatric dosing considerations in ophthalmology. J. Pediatr. Ophthalmol., 13:171–178, 1976.

Peay, M. Y.; and Peay, E. R.: The role of commercial sources in the adoption of a new drug. Soc. Sci. Med., 26:1183–1189, 1988.

Peterson, R. G.; Simmons, M. A.; Rumack, B. H.; Levine, R. L.; and Brooks, J. G.: Pharmacology of furosemide in the premature newborn infant. J. Pediatr., 97:139–143, 1980.

Piafsky, K. M.; and Woolner, E. A.: The binding of basic drugs to alpha-1-acid glycoprotein in cord serum. J. Pediatr., 110:820–822, 1982.

Pons, G.: Stable isotopes and mass spectrometry. Use in clinical pharmacology in children. Therapie, 42:457–461, 1987.

Powers, R. D.; and Donowitz, L. G.: Endotracheal administration of emergency medications. South. Med. J., 77:340–346, 1984.

Prete, M. R.; Hannan, C. J.; and Burkle, F. M.: Plasma atropine concentrations via intravenous, endotracheal, and intraosseous administration. Am. J. Emerg. Med., 5:101–104, 1987.

Pruitt, A. W.; and Dayton, P. G.: A comparison of the binding of drugs to adult and cord plasma. Eur. J. Clin. Pharmacol., 4:59–62, 1971.

Pullar, T.; Kumar, S.; Tindall, H.; and Feely, M.: Time to stop counting the tablets? Clin. Pharmacol. Ther., 46:163–168, 1989.

Qazi, Q. H.; Mariano, E.; Milman, D. H.; Beller, E.; and Crombleholme, W.: Abnormalities in offspring associated with prenatal marihuana exposure. Dev. Pharmacol. Ther., 8:141–148, 1985.

Rajchgot, P.; Radde, I. C.; and MacLeod, S. M.: Influence of specific gravity on intravenous drug delivery. J. Pediatr., 99:658–661, 1981.

Rane, A.: Basic principles of drug disposition and action in infants and children. In, Pediatric Pharmacology, Therapeutic Principles in Practice (Yaffe, S. J., ed.). Grune & Stratton, New York, pp. 7–28, 1980.

Rangsithienchai, P.; and Newcomb, R. W.: Aminophylline therapy in children: Guidelines for dosage. J. Pediatr., 91:325–330, 1977.

Rinck, G.; Gollnick, H.; and Orfanos, C. E.: Duration of contraception after etretinate. Lancet, 1:845–846, 1989.

Roarty, J. D.; and Keltner, J. L.: Normal pupil size and anisocoria in newborn infants. Arch. Ophthalmol., 108:94–95, 1990.

Roberts, J. R.; Greenberg, M. I.; and Baskin, S. I.: Endotracheal epinephrine in cardiorespiratory collapse. J. Am. Coll. Emerg. Physicians, 8:515–519, 1979.

Roberts, R. J.: Drug Therapy in Infants. Pharmacologic Principles and Clinical Experience. W. B. Saunders, Philadelphia, 1984.

Roberts, R. J.; Blumer, J. L.; Gorman, R. L.; Lambert, G. H.; Rumack, B. H.; and Snodgrass, W. R.: Transfer of drugs and other chemicals into human milk. Pediatrics, 84:924–936, 1989.

Roberts, R. J.; Mirkin, B. L.; and Rumack, B. H.: SI units and pediatric therapeutics. J. Pediatr., 110:494–495, 1987.

Roberts, S. B.; Coward, W. A.; Schlingenseipen, K. H.; Nohria, V.; and Lucas, A.: Comparison of the doubly labeled water (2-H_2,18-O) method with indirect calorimetry and a nutrient-balance study for simultaneous determination of energy expenditure, water intake, and metabolizable energy intake in preterm infants. Am. J. Clin. Nutr., 44:315–322, 1986.

Rodewald, L. E.; Maiman, L. A.; Foye, H. R.; Borch, R. F.; and Forbes, G. B.: Deuterium oxide as a tracer for measurement of compliance in pediatric clinical drug trials. J. Pediatr., 114:885–891, 1989.

Rosen, J. P.; Danish, M.; Ragni, M. C.; Saccar, C. L.; Yaffe, S. J.; and Lecks, H. I.: Theophylline pharmacokinetics in the young infant. Pediatrics, 64:248–251, 1979.

Rost, K.; Carter, W.; and Inui, T.: Introduction of information during the initial medical visit: Consequences for patient follow-through with physician recommendations for medication. Soc. Sci. Med., 28:315–321, 1989.

Rowland, M.: Plasma protein binding and therapeutic drug monitoring. Ther. Drug Monit., 2:29–37, 1980.

Russell, W. L.; and McKenzie, M. W.: Drug usage in newborn intensive care units. Hosp. Formul., 18:625–638, 1983.

Saint-Maurice, C.; Meistelman, C.; Rey, E.; Esteve, C.; DeLauture, D.; and Olive, G.: The pharmacokinetics of rectal midazolam for premedication in children. Anesthesiology, 65:536–538, 1986.

Salva, P. S.; and Bacon, G. E.: Parents and steroid use by non-athletes. Pediatrics, 84:940–941, 1989.

Sanders, J. M.; Brookman, R. R.; Brown, R. C.; Greene, J. W.; McAnarney, E. R.; and Schonberg, S. K.: Alcohol use and abuse: A pediatric concern. Pediatrics, 79:450–453, 1987.

Schechter, N. L.; Allen, D. A.; and Hanson, K.: Status of pediatric pain control: A comparison of hospital analgesic usage in children and adults. Pediatrics, 77:11–15, 1986.

Schulman, J.; Peyman, G. A.; Fiscella, R.; Greenberg, D.; Horton, M. B.; and DeMiranda, P.: Intraocular acyclovir levels after subconjunctival and topical administration. Br. J. Ophthalmol., 70:138–140, 1986.

Scruggs, J.; Wallace, T.; and Hanna, C.: Route of absorption of drug and ointment after application to the eye. Ann. Ophthalmol., 10:267–271, 1978.

Semel, J. D.: Fever associated with repeated intramuscular injections of analgesics. Rev. Infect. Dis., 8:68–72, 1986.

Shear, N. H.; Spielberg, S. P.; and Kalow, W.: Differences in metabolism of sulfonamides predisposing to idiosyncratic toxicity. Ann. Intern. Med., 105:179–184, 1986.

Sheiner, L. B.; and Beal, S. L.: Bayesian individualization of pharmacokinetics: Simple implementation and comparison with non-Bayesian methods. J. Pharm. Sci., 71:1344–1348, 1982.

Shell, J. W.: Pharmacokinetics of topically applied ophthalmic drugs. Surv. Ophthalmol., 26:207–218, 1982.

Shepard, T. H.: Catalog of Teratogenic Agents. Johns Hopkins University Press, Baltimore, 1989.

Silvasi, D. L.; Rosen, D. A.; and Rosen, K. R.: Continuous intravenous midazolam infusion for sedation in the pediatric intensive care unit. Anesth. Analg., 67:286–288, 1988.

Simons, F. E. R.; and Simons, K. J.: Pharmacokinetics of theophylline in infancy. J. Clin. Pharmacol., 18:472–476, 1978.

Smith, C. F.; and Amen, R. J.: Comparing the costs of i.v. drug delivery systems. Am. J. Nurs., 89:500–501, 1989.

Snodgrass, W. R.; and Dodge, W. F.: Lytic/dpt cocktail: Time for rational and safe alternatives. Pediatr. Clin. North Am., 36:1285–1291, 1989.

Snodgrass, W. R.; and Whitfield, S.: Furosemide biotransformation in a premature infant: Urinary excretion of furosemide and its glucuronide metabolite. In, Developmental Pharmacology (MacLeod, S. M.; Okey, A. B.; and Spielberg, S. P., eds.). Alan R. Liss, New York, pp. 413–416, 1983.

Snodgrass, W. R.; Smith, S. D.; Trueworthy, R.; Vats, T. S.; Klopovich, P.; and Kisker, S.: Pediatric clinical pharmacology of 6-mercaptopurine: Lack of compliance as a factor in leukemia relapse. Proc. Am. Soc. Clin. Oncol., 3:204, 1984.

Spivey, W. H.: Intraosseous infusions. J. Pediatr., 111:639–643, 1987.

Tandberg, D.; and Abercrombie, D.: Treatment of heroin overdose with endotracheal naloxone. Ann. Emerg. Med., 11:443–445, 1982.

Tebbi, C. K.; Cummings, M.; and Sevon, M. A.: Compliance of pediatric and adolescent cancer patients. Cancer, 58:1179–1184, 1986.

Temple, A. R.: A rational approach to the dosing of nonprescription medications in the pediatric patient. Unpublished, 1985.

Tierce, J. C.; Meller, W.; Berlow, B.; and Gerth, W. C.: Assessing the cost of albuterol inhalers in the Michigan and California medicaid programs: A total cost-of-care approach. Clin. Ther., 11:53–61, 1989.

Tillement, J. P.; Houin, G.; Zini, R.; Urien, S.; Albengres, E.; Barre, J.; Lecomte, M.; D'Athis, P.; and Sebille, B.: The binding of drugs to blood plasma macromolecules: Recent advances and therapeutic significance. Adv. Drug Res., 13:59–94, 1984.

Tserng, K. Y.; Takieddine, F. N.; and King, K. C.: Developmental aspects of theophylline metabolism in premature infants. Clin. Pharmacol. Ther., 33:522–528, 1983.

Van Baar, A. L.; Fleury, P.; Soepatmi, S.; Ultee, C. A.; and Wesselman, P. J. M.: Neonatal behavior after drug dependent pregnancy. Arch. Dis. Child., 64:235–240, 1989.

Van Der Spek, A. F. L.: Cyanosis and cardiovascular depression in a neonate: Complications of halothane anesthesia or phenylephrine eyedrops? Can. J. Ophthalmol., 22:37–39, 1987.

Vernon, S.; Bacon, C.; and Weightman, D.: Rectal paracetamol (acetaminophen) in small children. Arch. Dis. Child., 54:469–479, 1979.

Ward, R. M.; Daniel, C. H.; Kendig, J. W.; and Wood, M. A.: Oliguria and tolazoline pharmacokinetics in the newborn. Pediatrics, 77:307–315, 1986.

Watkins, J. B.; Ingall, D.; Szczepanik, P.; Klein, P. D.; and Lester, R.: Bile-salt metabolism in the newborn. Measurement of pool size and synthesis by stable isotope technic. N. Engl. J. Med., 288:431–434, 1973.

Way, W. L.; Costley, E. C.; and Way, E. L.: Respiratory sensitivity of the newborn infant to meperidine and morphine. Clin. Pharmacol. Ther., 6:454–461, 1964.

Weinberger, M.; Hendeles, L.; Wong, L.; and Vaughan, L.: Relationship of formulation and dosing interval to fluctuation of serum theophylline concentration in children with chronic asthma. J. Pediatr., 99:145–152, 1981.

Weinstein, A. G.; and Cuskey, W.: Theophylline compliance in asthmatic children. Ann. Allergy, 54:19–24, 1985.

Westerling, D.: Rectally administered morphine: Plasma concentrations in children premedicated with morphine in hydrogel and in solution. Acta Anesthesiol. Scand., 29:653–656, 1985.

Westley, C. R.; Cotton, E. K.; and Brooks, J. G.: Nebulized racemic epinephrine by IPPB for the treatment of croup. A double-blind study. Am. J. Dis. Child., 132:484–487, 1978.

Whelan, H. T.; Hendeles, L.; Haberkern, C. M.; and Neims, A. H.: High intravenous phenytoin dosage requirement in a newborn infant. Neurology, 33:106–108, 1983.

Wilson, J. T.: Determinants and consequences of drug excretion in breast milk. Drug Metab. Rev., 14:619–652, 1983.

Yaffe, S. J. (ed.): Pediatric Pharmacology: Therapeutic Principles in Practice. Grune & Stratton, New York, 1980.

Yaffe, S. J.; Mattar, M.; and Markello, J. R.: Pediatric compliance: The physician's responsibilities. Drug Ther., 1:47–53, 1977.

Yudkoff, M.; Nissim, I.; McNellis, W.; and Polin, R.: Albumin synthesis in premature infants: Determination of turnover with 15-N-glycine. Pediatr. Res., 21:49–53, 1987.

Zelson, C.; Rubio, E.; and Wasserman, E.: Neonatal narcotic addiction: 10 year observation. Pediatrics, 48:178–189, 1971.

Zelson, C.; Lee, S. J.; and Casalino, M.: Neonatal narcotic addiction. Comparative effects of maternal intake of heroin and methadone. N. Engl. J. Med., 289:1216–1220, 1973.

Zimmerman, J. J.: History and current applications of intravenous therapy in children. Pediatr. Emerg. Care, 5:120–127, 1989.

Zimmerman, T. J.; Kooner, K. S.; Kandarakis, A. S.; and Ziegler, L. P.: Improving the therapeutic index of topically applied ocular drugs. Arch. Ophthalmol., 102:551–553, 1984.

Zimo, D. A.; Gaspar, M.; and Akhter, J.: The efficacy and safety of home nebulizer therapy for children with asthma. Am. J. Dis. Child., 143:208–211, 1989.

31

Drugs in Special Patient Groups: The Elderly

Robert E. Vestal, Stephen C. Montamat, and Christopher P. Nielson

---

Chapter Outline

Epidemiology of Drug Use in the Elderly
  Patterns of Drug Use and Drug Prescribing
  Adverse Drug Reactions in the Elderly
  Compliance in the Elderly
Pharmacokinetics in the Elderly
  Drug Absorption in the Elderly
  Drug Distribution in the Elderly
  Drug Metabolism in the Elderly
  Renal Excretion of Drugs in the Elderly

Nutrition, Environmental Factors, and
  Drug Interactions
Drug Therapy and Pharmacodynamics
  Analgesics
  Anticoagulants
  Cardiovascular Drugs
  Psychotropic Drugs
  Drug–Disease Interactions
  Guidelines for Geriatric Prescribing

The elderly constitute a particularly heterogeneous patient group since physiologic aging does not necessarily parallel chronologic aging and on account of the accumulation of the effects of disease processes. Even in the absence of recognized pathologic conditions, and despite similar ages, some individuals seem to be physiologically older or younger than others. For example, renal function, which on average declines with age (Rowe et al., 1976), may be normal or markedly impaired in a particular individual in the absence of clinically apparent renal disease (Lindeman et al., 1985). In contrast to childhood growth and development, which occurs in a relatively predictable manner, the processes of aging in various organ systems may begin as early as the fourth decade and can proceed at different rates from person to person. In addition, geriatric patients (those >65 years old) often suffer from multiple diseases that in combination with age-related changes in physiology create severe therapeutic challenges. Efforts to separate the effects of age per se from those of underlying disease have prompted investigators to study the disposition and action of drugs in groups of *healthy* elderly subjects in comparison with groups of healthy younger subjects. Studies of this sort do not address the possible differing effects of disease on drug action in elderly compared with younger patients. Also, such studies generally are cross-sectional rather than longitudinal in design; they only provide information about age *differences* as opposed to *changes* with age or the effects of *aging* (Rowe, 1977). Since disease-related pathologic conditions often play a major role in determining the fate and action of drugs, the clinician must use information on the effects of old age on the fate and action of drugs to guide therapeutic decisions in a particularly thoughtful manner. We address this problem by reviewing what is known about geriatric clinical pharmacology and identifying principles that can be applied to the practical management of geriatric patients. The reader also is referred to several reviews of this subject (Schmucker, 1985; Nielson et al., 1987; Schmucker, 1979; Montamat et al., 1989; Tsujimoto et al., 1989a and 1989b; Vestal and Cusack, 1990).

EPIDEMIOLOGY OF DRUG USE IN THE ELDERLY

The growing importance of geriatric clinical pharmacology is in part a consequence of demographic trends. The proportion of elderly persons in the populations of developed countries has been rising steadily over the past several decades. This is due to a combination of a falling birth rate coupled with economic, social, and medical factors that promote longevity. Although 12% of the population in the United States was over 65 years of age, this older age group consumed approximately 30% of all drugs prescribed in this country (Baum et al., 1981). In 1986 elderly patients accounted for 25% of all visits to physicians and 32% of all drug mentions, which are defined as drugs prescribed, recommended, or administered in a medical setting by a representative panel of over 2000 physicians (Food and Drug Administration, 1987). By comparison, in 1974 elderly patients represented only 24% of all drug mentions.

Patterns of Drug Use and Drug Prescribing

Data on the patterns of drug use by ambulatory persons over age 65 years in the United States are provided in two large studies. The Dunedin Program in Florida, which screens approximately 3000 ambulatory elderly persons on an annual basis for undetected medical illness, reported that over a 5-year period 93% of this population took at least one medication. The mean drug use increased from 3.2 to 3.7 medications per patient during the same period of observation (Hale et al., 1987). Women consumed more drugs than men, and drug use increased with age. Antihypertensives, nonnarcotic analgesics, antiarthritics, vitamins, and cathartics were the most common therapeutic agents. Similar observations have been made in the Iowa 65 + Rural Health Study (Helling et al., 1987). Compared with 13% of persons aged 65 to 69 years, only 7% of individuals 85 years or older did not use any drugs. Cardiovascular drugs (55%), CNS agents (11%), and analgesics (9%) were the most common categories of prescription drugs. Analgesics (40%), vitamins and nutritional supplements (33%), and GI agents including laxatives (22%) were the most common categories of over-the-counter (OTC) drugs. The mean number of drugs per respondent was 2.9. A comparison of the most frequently used prescription drugs in the general North American population and in the elderly who are enrolled in the Pharmaceutical Assistance Contract for the Elderly, which is administered by the Pennsylvania Department of Aging (Snedden and Cadieux, 1988), is shown in Table 31-1.

There are few studies that evaluate the appropriateness of prescribing. In one study, doses of cimetidine, flurazepam, and digoxin were analyzed on a milligram per kilogram basis. Patients weighing 50 kg or less received doses that were 31% to 46% higher than the group mean, and 70% to 88% higher than for patients weighing more than 90 kg (Campion et al., 1987). Despite a decline in body weight with age, doses in older patients were not proportionately decreased. The

Table 31-1. COMPARISON OF MOST FREQUENTLY PRESCRIBED DRUGS DURING 1989 IN NORTH AMERICA AND IN THE LARGEST PHARMACEUTICAL ASSISTANCE PROGRAM FOR THE ELDERLY IN THE UNITED STATES

RANK	MOST FREQUENTLY PRESCRIBED DRUGS IN NORTH AMERICA*	MOST FREQUENTLY PRESCRIBED DRUGS IN THE ELDERLY†‡
1	Amoxicillin	Hydrochlorothiazide-triamterine (Dyazide, Maxide, etc.)
2	Furosemide (Lasix)	• Potassium chloride (Slow K, Micro K, etc.)
3	Acetaminophen–codeine phosphate (Tylenol w/codeine)	• Diltiazem (Cardizem)
4	Digoxin (Lanoxin)	• Dipyridamole (Persantine)
5	Prednisone	Furosemide (Lasix)
6	Ibuprofen (Motrin)	Ranitidine (Zantac)
7	Cefaclor (Ceclor)	• Nitroglycerin (topical)
8	Naproxen (Naprosyn)	Captopril (Capoten)
9	Aspirin	• Nifedipine (Procardia)
10	Ranitidine (Zantac)	• Insulin
11	Hydrochlorothiazide-Triamterine (Dyazide)	Digoxin (Lanoxin)
12	Theophylline (TheoDur)	• Verapamil (Calan, Isoptin)
13	Ampicillin	• Enalopril (Vasotec)
14	Acetaminophen (Tylenol)	Atenolol (Tenormin)
15	Diltiazem (Cardizem)	Alprazolam (Xanax)
16	Alprazolam (Xanax)	• Diclofenac (Voltaren)
17	Captopril (Capoten)	• Propoxyphene napsylate–Acetaminophen (Davocet-N)
18	Conjugated estrogens (Premarin)	• Propranolol (Inderal)
19	Atenolol (Tenormin)	• Glyburide (Micronase)
20	Hydrochlorothiazide	• Metoprolol (Lopressor)

* From a 1989 compilation of the 100 most frequently used prescription drugs in North America (IMS America, Ltd., Plymouth Meeting, Pa.).

† From 1989 claims records of the Pennsylvania Pharmaceutical Assistance Contract for the Elderly (PACE) program (personal communication, Janeen Duchane and Thomas M. Snedden, PACE Program, Department of Aging, Commonwealth of Pennsylvania).

‡ • = Drug not on list of most frequently prescribed drugs in North America.

Table 31–2.   CHEMICAL ENTITIES MOST FREQUENTLY DISPENSED IN HOSPITALS AND TOP DIAGNOSIS-RELATED GROUPS AND DIAGNOSES IN HOSPITALS IN 1987 FOR PATIENTS AGED 64 YEARS AND OLDER*

CHEMICAL ENTITIES DISPENSED TO HOSPITALIZED ELDERLY		DIAGNOSES IN HOSPITALIZED ELDERLY PATIENTS		
RANK	CHEMICAL ENTITY	RANK	DRG DESCRIPTION†	ICD-9-CM DIAGNOSIS
1	Furosemide	1	Heart failure and shock	Cardiac dysrhythmias
2	Acetaminophen	2	Specific cerebrovascular disorder except TIA	Essential hypertension
3	Potassium chloride			
4	Heparin	3	Angina pectoris	Other forms of chronic ischemic heart disease
5	Nitroglycerin			
6	Aluminum or magnesium hydroxide(s)	4	Simple pneumonia and pleurisy, >17 years w/complication and/or comorbidity	Diabetes mellitus
7	Digoxin			
8	Ranitidine	5	Esophagitis, gastroenteritis, and misc. digestive disorders, >17 years, w/complication and/or comorbidity	Heart failure
9	Meperidine			
10	Cefazolin			
11	Docusate compounds			
12	Triazolam	6	Major joint and limb reattachment procedures	Disorders of fluid, electrolyte, and acid–base balance
13	Lidocaine			
14	Bisacodyl	7	Cardiac arrhythmia and conduction disorders w/complication and/or comorbidity	Other disorders of urethra and urinary tract
15	Diazepam			
16	Aspirin			
17	Morphine	8	Nutritional and misc. metabolic disorders, >17 years, w/complication and/or comorbidity	Chronic airway obstruction
18	Hydroxyzine			
19	Dipyridamole			
20	Nifedipine			
		9	Other factors influencing health states	Bacterial infection
		10	Bronchitis and asthma, >17 years, w/complication and/or comorbidity	General symptoms

* From IHS Hospital Pharmacy Data Base, International Health Services, Ltd., Acton, Mass. (Food and Drug Administration, 1988).
† DRG = diagnosis-related group.

risk of excessive dosage is further exacerbated by impaired elimination of many drugs in the elderly. Since low body weight and advanced age are both risk factors for adverse drug reactions, available data suggest that current prescribing practices do not reflect the need to reduce doses in low-weight elderly patients. *Principle: Commonly used drug doses may be excessive in some elderly patients and must be reduced to achieve the desired therapeutic effect without adverse effects.*

Studies of prescribing patterns in hospitals have concentrated mainly on adverse drug reactions with limited attention devoted to the effects of patient age on the number and types of drugs prescribed and whether efficacy was attained (Nolan and O'Malley, 1988a). In the United Kingdom and in Scandinavia, the average number of drugs per elderly inpatient ranges from 2.5 to 6.3, with most older patients receiving five drugs. Table 31-2 shows the 20 most frequently dispensed drugs and the top 10 diagnosis-related groups (DRGs) and ICD-9-CM diagnoses for patients aged 64 years and older hospitalized in the United States in 1987. Although evaluation of the appropriateness of prescribing is difficult, in at least one study the number of drugs prescribed was not considered to be inappropriate (Gosney and Tallis, 1984). *Principle: Although multiple drugs may be justifiable because of multiple indications in geriatric patients, the prescriber must frequently reevaluate the need for multiple medications and be alert to the increased risk of drug interactions in patients taking multiple drugs.*

In general, the data on prescribing for the elderly in chronic care facilities are scanty (Nolan and O'Malley, 1988a). Studies suffer from small sample sizes and failure to report important variables such as mean age, the male/female ratio, the size of the nursing home, and types of health care providers employed. The average patient receives from 1.5 to 7.1 medications, with a large fraction (about three drugs per patient, or 40% of all prescriptions) administered on an "as needed" basis; this group of "prn drugs" consists mainly of sedatives, hypnotics, analgesics, and laxatives.

Psychoactive drugs are widely used in chronic care facilities. A study of antipsychotic drugs prescribed for Medicaid patients in Tennessee revealed that among nursing home patients, CNS drugs were the most frequently prescribed medications (74% of patients). Only 36% of the ambulatory comparison group received CNS drugs. Alarmingly, nursing home patients often received drugs from multiple categories of CNS drugs: 34% from two or more different categories, 9% from three or more, and 1.6% from four or more (Ray et al., 1980). And 60% of Medicaid recipients in Illinois nursing homes received at least one psychotropic medication in 1984 (Buck, 1988). A recent study conducted in chronic care facilities in Massachusetts concluded that psychoactive drugs are widely used with little medical supervision or understanding by staff members of their possible adverse effects or interactions (Avorn et al., 1989). *Principle: When specific end points of drug therapy are not sought, there is no way to optimize dosage, minimize irrational combinations, or reduce the incidence of adverse reactions.*

Adverse Drug Reactions in the Elderly

Studies from the United States, Ireland, and Israel indicate that the incidence of adverse drug reactions in hospitalized patients over 60 years old, or as a course for hospitalization in this age group is 10% to 25%. This rate is two- or threefold greater than that in patients less than 30 years of age (Seidl et al., 1966; Hurwitz, 1969; Levy et al., 1980). Demographic factors that correlate with the likelihood of adverse drug reactions include advanced age, female gender, small body size, hepatic or renal insufficiency, multiple-drug therapy, and previous drug reactions (Jue and Vestal, 1984). In addition, the physiologic response to a standard therapeutic drug concentration and the homeostatic response to a pharmacologically induced stress may be altered in the elderly (Fig. 31-1). The importance of age as a determinant of predisposition to adverse reactions, however, is controversial (Nolan and O'Malley, 1988b). The incidence of adverse drug reactions increased with age in only 5 of 12 studies that evaluated age as a variable. Of five studies in outpatients, only two showed an increased incidence with age. Two showed no effect, and one showed a U-shaped relationship between adverse drug reactions and age. Among four studies of hospital admissions due to adverse drug reactions, two showed an increase with age and two showed no effect. Basically there is little to say that age per se predisposes to adverse reactions to drugs.

Although some epidemiologic data suggest that elderly patients are at increased risk for adverse drug reactions, the magnitude and the cause of this association are difficult to evaluate because many of the studies have either methodologic or interpretive weaknesses (Klein et al., 1981; Jue and Vestal, 1984; Nolan and O'Malley, 1988b; Gurwitz and Avorn, 1991). A recent study of drug-associated hospital admissions in patients ranging in age from 50 to 94 years attempted to address some of these deficiencies (Grymonpre et al., 1988). Of 863 eligible admissions during a 4-month period, 19% exhibited at least one drug-related adverse event at the time of hospitalization. The risk of an adverse event was related to the number of diseases prior to admission and the number of drugs used, but not to age. Underrecognition of adverse effects in and by geriatric patients also is a factor to be considered (Klein et al., 1984). The true relationship between age and adverse drug reactions will not be established until additional studies are performed that control for severity of disease, prevalence of drug use, and type of drug consumed as well as age. *Principle: Although an elderly patient's physiology and medical condition may predispose to the risk of one or more adverse drug reactions, inappropriate therapeutic intervention by the physician or another health care provider often may be the most important factor.*

Compliance in the Elderly

Compliance or adherence to drug therapy frequently is a critical factor in the successful management of acute and chronic illness. Between 25% and 50% of outpatients fail to take medication as prescribed (Blackwell, 1972). Estimates for elderly patients are similar (Morrow et al., 1988). Lack of a clear understanding of a regimen often is a greater problem than willful failure to follow instructions. However, one study found that for about 40% of elderly patients there was a discrepancy between the use of a drug and the prescription directions. In these instances of nonadherence, 90% of cases were due to underuse, of which nearly 75% was intentional (Cooper et al., 1982). The intentionally nonadherent were more likely to use two or more pharmacies and to receive prescriptions from two or more physicians. *Principle: Do not assume that your patients are taking the drugs that you prescribe or that you are the only person who is prescribing their drugs.*

Case History.

A 69-year-old woman presented to her local physician with complaints of abdominal pain, fatigue, and dark stools. Her medications included an NSAID for treatment of pain due to osteoarthritis. The evaluation of this patient led to an esophagogastroduodenoscopy that revealed a duodenal ulcer. She was placed on an H₂ antagonist, and she was instructed to return after 6 weeks for a repeat endoscopy. Four weeks later, the patient

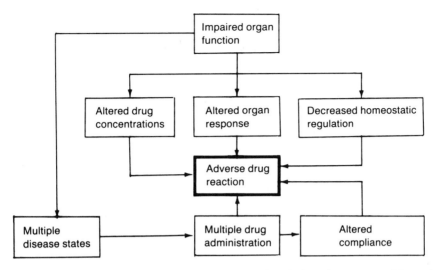

Fig. 31–1. Factors contributing to adverse drug reactions in elderly patients. From Nielson, C. P.; Cusack, B. J.; and Vestal, R. E.: Geriatric clinical pharmacology and therapeutics. In Speight, T. M., (ed.): Avery's Drug Treatment: Principles and Practice of Clinical Pharmacology and Therapeutics, 3rd ed. AIDS Health Science Press, Aukland, pp. 160–193, 1987. Reproduced with permission.

was brought to the emergency room for hematemesis and hypotension that required immediate resuscitative measures. When she was asked about her medications, she said that she had discontinued her ulcer medication after 10 days of therapy since her abdominal pain had resolved.

Comment: Studies of compliance with drug therapy in the elderly have shown divergent results, depending on the type of therapy and the amount of drugs taken. Factors that lead to poor compliance may be more common in the elderly, such as cognitive impairment, hearing and visual deficits, social isolation, and inadequate finances. The predominant form of noncompliance is underadherence, or taking too little medication, as is the case in this patient. Underadherence may be intentional for a variety of reasons, including the patient's attempt to reduce adverse effects. Clear communication between the patient and the health professional is probably the most important factor to address. Simplifying drug regimens and attaining aids for drug administration are also important.

One way to enhance compliance is to reduce the number of medications that patients have to take each day. In patients over age 65, the rate of nonadherence more than doubles when more than three drugs are prescribed, whereas for patients under age 65, the rates of nonadherence to prescribed drug therapy are similar when one, two, three, or more drugs are prescribed (Bergman and Wilholm, 1981). Additional hindrances to compliance include tamper-resistant (Sherman, 1985) and child-resistant (Keram and Williams, 1988) packaging that elderly persons may have difficulty using.

Despite the prevalence of nonadherence among elderly patients, objective measures indicate that they do as well as or better than younger patients. In several studies the highest compliance rate was found in patients over age 70 (Weintraub et al., 1973; Weintraub, 1981). Compliance was high (80%–90%) in all age categories, including those over age 80, in the preliminary phase of a large multicenter clinical trial on the treatment of systolic hypertension in the elderly (Black et al., 1987). While the efficacy of antihypertensive therapy is established and can be understood by patients, the value of various other remedies for the maladies of old age, such as Gerovital, vitamin C, and vitamin E, which are faithfully taken by some individuals, has not been determined. ***Principle: There are many ironies in drug therapy, not the least being that compliance may not necessarily be related to the value of therapy.***

Noncompliance does not always result in adverse consequences. Some patients alter prescribed therapy, usually decreasing the prescribed dose or omitting their medication, in order to minimize toxic effects (Weintraub, 1976). About 10% of patients taking digoxin were judged to be intelligently noncompliant (Weintraub et al., 1973). Research is needed to determine the prevalence of and the factors that characterize intelligent noncompliance and how the physician should recognize and utilize them. ***Principle: Many factors that are important determinants of*** *compliance must be recognized and accounted for to accomplish therapeutic efficacy with the least toxicity.*

PHARMACOKINETICS IN THE ELDERLY

The major pharmacokinetic characteristics of any drug—absorption, distribution, metabolism, and elimination—are potentially modified by aging since there are important physiologic changes that occur with "normal" aging. The general principles of pharmacokinetics are presented in chapter 1 and a more detailed description is in chapter 36. Many of these changes are independent of the multiple diseases so often present in geriatric patients. By influencing drug disposition, these age-related changes might be expected to alter the response to drugs which may explain why older patients seem to be more susceptible to both the therapeutic and the toxic effects of many drugs. Except for drugs eliminated predominantly by renal excretion, it is not possible to generalize on the type, magnitude, or importance of age-related differences in pharmacokinetics. Conflicting data in the literature for various drugs may be attributed to small numbers of subjects studied, to differences in selection criteria for subjects, and to differences in the design of protocols. Apparent age-related differences in drug disposition are multifactorial and influenced by environmental, genetic, physiologic, and pathologic factors, many of which are summarized in Table 31–3.

Drug Absorption in the Elderly

Elderly persons exhibit several alterations in GI function that might result in impaired or delayed absorption of drug (Table 31–3). Basal and peak gastric acid production has been reported to decline with age (Baron, 1963). The resultant increased gastric pH may alter the lipid solubility or dissolution of some drugs and reduce absorption. However, the net effect of alterations in gastric pH is unpredictable; for example, a higher gastric pH may hasten gastric emptying, leading to a drug's reaching absorptive sites in the small intestine more rapidly. In a small study, absorption of tetracycline by elderly patients with achlorhydria (which decreases the dissolution of the drug) was similar to that of young healthy controls (Kramer et al., 1978). Gastric emptying and motility determine the rate of delivery of a drug to the small intestine, where absorption of most drugs occurs by passive diffusion. An age-related decrease in the rate of gastric emptying has been reported

Table 31–3. FACTORS AFFECTING DRUG DISPOSITION IN THE GERIATRIC PATIENT*

PHARMACOKINETIC PARAMETER	AGE-RELATED PHYSIOLOGIC CHANGE	PATHOLOGIC CONDITION	THERAPEUTIC AND ENVIRONMENTAL FACTOR
Absorption	Increased gastric pH Decreased absorptive surface Decreased splanchnic blood flow Decreased GI motility	Achlorhydria Diarrhea Postgastrectomy Malabsorption syndromes Pancreatitis	Antacids Anticholinergics Cholestyramine Drug interactions Food or meals
Distribution	Decreased cardiac output Decreased total body water Decreased lean body mass Decreased serum albumin concentration Increased α_1 acid glycoprotein concentration Increased proportion of body fat	Congestive heart failure Dehydration Edema or ascites Hepatic failure Malnutrition Renal failure	Drug interactions Protein-binding displacement
Metabolism	Decreased hepatic mass Decreased hepatic blood flow	Congestive heart failure Fever Hepatic insufficiency Malignancy Malnutrition Thyroid disease Viral infection or immunization	Dietary composition Drug interactions Insecticides Tobacco (smoking)
Excretion	Decreased renal blood flow Decreased glomerular filtration rate Decreased tubular secretion	Hypovolemia Renal insufficiency	Drug interactions

* Adapted from Vestal and Dawson, 1985. Reproduced with permission.

(Evans et al., 1981; Moore et al., 1983), but the rate of acetaminophen absorption, which correlates with the rate of gastric emptying (Heading et al., 1973), does not differ with age (Divoll et al., 1982a). Drugs that decrease GI motility, such as narcotic analgesics and antidepressants, might be expected to impair drug absorption to a greater extent in the elderly than in the young. This has not been investigated but should be "looked for." Based on microscopic examination of biopsy material from the upper jejunum of well-nourished elderly and young control patients without malabsorption, mucosal surface area was found to be decreased by 20% in the older age group (Warren et al., 1978). The clinical significance of this observation is unknown but doubtful in view of the fact that very few drugs demonstrate delayed or reduced absorption after oral administration in elderly patients (Cusack and Vestal, 1986). In contrast, the active transport of calcium, iron, thiamine, and vitamin B_{12} declines with age (Bhanthumnavin and Schuster, 1977). Methyldopa and levodopa are both absorbed by active transport via an amino acid transport mechanism. The effect of age on the absorption of methyldopa has not been studied, but there is evidence for increased rather than decreased absorption of levodopa in the elderly (Evans et al., 1980; Evans et al., 1981). *Principle: Although the physiologic rationale for an altered drug response may have been demonstrated, therapeutic actions should be guided by careful clinical trials or actual clinical experience, since the results of these investigations may be difficult to predict in advance.*

The transdermal route of drug delivery has several advantages over conventional oral therapy that make it attractive for use in geriatric patients (Ridout et al., 1988). Unfortunately, little is known about percutaneous drug absorption as a function of age. The evidence pointing to possible alterations in the barrier function of skin is inconclusive (Roskos et al., 1986).

The bioavailability of drugs depends on both absorption and presystemic (first-pass) metabolism by the wall of the GI tract and the liver (see chapters 1 and 37). The bioavailability of drugs such as lidocaine (Cusack et al., 1985), propranolol (Castleden and George, 1979; Vestal et al., 1979a) and labetalol (Kelly et al., 1982) that have high intrinsic clearance by the liver is greater in elderly patients, reflecting less presystemic metabolism in this age group. On the other hand, the opposite findings have been made for prazosin (Rubin et al., 1981). Therefore, one cannot generalize regarding the effect of age on bioavailability of high-clearance drugs. Presystemic metabolism of low-clearance drugs, such as theophylline, is negligible. Any alteration in bioavailability would have to be caused by an age-related difference in absorption. Since age does not seem to alter absorption to a clinically important extent, it is no surprise to find that the bioavailability of theophylline, and probably most other low-clearance drugs, does not change with age (Vestal et al., 1987). *Principle: Agents that have high intrinsic clearance by the liver may exhibit increased bioavailability in the elderly. Unfortunately, the specific age-related effect on bioavailability must be determined by clinical trial for each drug, and for that matter, for each patient.*

Drug Distribution in the Elderly

Body composition is one of the most important factors that may produce altered distribution of drugs in elderly patients (Table 31–3). Total body water, both in absolute terms and as a percentage of body weight (Edelman and Leibman, 1959; Shock et al., 1963; Vestal et al., 1975), is decreased by 10% to 15% between ages 20 and 80. However, body composition may be population-dependent (Shock et al., 1963; Norris et al., 1963). Lean body mass in proportion to total body weight also is diminished with age because of a relative increase in body fat (Novak, 1972). Comparing the age groups 18 to 25 and 65 to 85 years, body fat increases from 18% to 36% of body weight in men and from 33% to 45% in women. In very elderly persons, however, the proportion of fat tends to be decreased (Norris et al., 1963). The age differences in total body water and body fat mean that lean body mass as a proportion of total body weight is decreased in the elderly. To what extent these changes are due to aging, rather than physical inactivity in the elderly, remains an area of active investigation.

Hydrophilic drugs that are distributed mainly in body water or lean body mass should have higher concentrations in blood in the elderly when the dose is based on total body weight or surface area. In line with this prediction, the volume of distribution of water-soluble drugs is smaller in the elderly, with increased initial concentrations in plasma. This has been directly demonstrated for ethanol (Vestal et al., 1977); consequently, equivalent concentrations of ethanol in the blood of elderly persons will be achieved by a dose that is 10% to 15% less than that in younger persons. Other examples include digoxin (Cusack et al., 1979), antipyrine (Vestal et al., 1975), and cimetidine (Redolfi et al., 1979). Notable exceptions include pancuronium and tobramycin, which have unchanged volumes of distribution in elderly patients (McLeod et al., 1979; Bauer and Blouin, 1981).

Conversely, highly lipophilic drugs tend to have larger volumes of distribution in older persons because of increased proportions of body fat.

This may account in part for the age-related increase in the volume of distribution of thiopental found in some, but not all studies, and for similar observations with some of the benzodiazepines (Klotz et al., 1975; Shull et al., 1976; Shader et al., 1977; Christensen et al., 1981; Jung et al., 1982; Greenblatt et al., 1982; Homer and Stanski, 1985). *Principle: Because lean body mass decreases and body fat increases in the elderly, in general the volumes of distribution for water-soluble drugs decrease and those for lipid-soluble drugs increase. These changes in volumes of distribution can lead to higher or lower plasma concentrations following administration of standard loading doses of drugs in these groups.*

Since free-drug concentration in plasma is an important determinant of distribution and elimination of the drug, alterations in the binding of drugs to plasma proteins, red blood cells, and other tissues might be considered important causes of altered pharmacokinetics in aged patients. Many basic drugs have a higher affinity for α_1 acid glycoprotein than acidic drugs, but acidic drugs generally have a higher affinity for albumin. Although quite variable, the concentrations of α_1 acid glycoprotein tend to increase with age (Abernethy and Kerzner, 1984). The binding of some basic drugs, such as lidocaine and disopyramide, is increased in the elderly, but this change probably does not have as much clinical importance as the increase that typically occurs in patients with acute myocardial infarction (LeLorier et al., 1977; Routledge et al., 1980). Serum albumin concentrations may be decreased by as much as 10% to 20% in old age, but chronic disease and immobility are probably more important determinants of albumin synthesis (Woodford-Williams et al., 1964; Greenblatt, 1979; Adir et al., 1982). The authors of a report showing only a 0.054 g/dl per decade decline in serum albumin concentration concluded that the age-related decline in healthy individuals is far less than previously described and that hypoalbuminemia is not a simple consequence of normal aging (Campion et al., 1988). Nevertheless, some studies have shown changes in the protein binding of acidic drugs that are potentially quite important in elderly subjects. The mean concentration of unbound (free) naproxen in plasma in the elderly is twice that in the young (Upton et al., 1984). The relation between the free-drug level and drug efficacy or toxicity has not been established in this case, but the possibility that the dose of naproxen in advanced age should be substantially decreased is raised by these findings.

An age-related increase in the unbound fraction by more than 50% occurs for only a few drugs, such as acetazolamide, etomidate, valproate, diflunisal, salicylate, and naproxen (Wallace and Verbeek, 1987). The net effect of changes in protein binding is complicated, but an altered pattern of elimination of drugs with low intrinsic clearance and high (greater than 90%) protein binding (Table 31-4) can result. For example, higher-than-ordinary total plasma clearance of phenytoin in elderly subjects is invoked as an explanation of the low binding in plasma after a single dose (Hayes et al., 1975). With chronic dosing, however, unbound concentrations of drugs tend to "renormalize" as a result of the enhanced availability of unbound drug for elimination by the liver and kidney (see chapter 1). For drugs with a low therapeutic ratio, such as phenytoin, measurement of the plasma free-drug concentration may be helpful in guiding therapy in complicated cases. *Principle: Individualization of drug therapy is often best accomplished by a combination of close attention to clinical response and determination of plasma drug concentrations, including free concentrations of drug in plasma when necessary.*

Drug Metabolism in the Elderly

Biochemical Studies. Since it is difficult to study hepatic drug metabolism in humans, nonhuman primates and rodents have been used as experimental models. In rodents, after maturity hepatic drug metabolism declines with increasing age (Schmucker, 1979; Schmucker, 1985; Vestal and Dawson, 1985; Birnbaum, 1987; Vestal and Cusack, 1990). The age-dependent decrement in catalytic efficiency of the hepatic microsomal mixed-function system may be attributed to one or more of the following factors: (1) decline in membrane fluidity as a result of changes in lipid composition of hepatic microsomes, (2) alterations of the enzymes or heme proteins, (3) loss of smooth endoplasmic reticulum membrane and microsomal mixed-function oxidase system constituents, and (4) decrease in the cytochrome P450 concentration and NADPH–cytochrome c reductase activity with age. In addition, the profile of cytochrome P450 isozymes may be related to age, gender, and diet (Kamataki et al., 1985; Schmucker et al., 1991). The reported age-related changes in conjugation reactions have been variable without a consistent pattern.

Unfortunately, data obtained from inbred rodents cannot be extrapolated to either nonhuman primates or humans. For example, total cytochrome P450 content, NADPH–cytochrome c reductase activity, and metabolism of benzo[a]pyrene in microsomes isolated from livers of female pigtailed macaque monkeys ranging in age from 2 to 21 years did not differ with age (Sutter et al., 1985). Neither age- nor sex-related changes in the concentration of microsomal protein or

Table 31–4. PHARMACOKINETIC CLASSIFICATION OF DRUGS ELIMINATED PRIMARILY BY HEPATIC METABOLISM*

CLASS	DRUG	EXTRACTION RATIO	% BOUND
Flow-limited	Lidocaine	0.83	45–80†
	Meperidine	0.60–0.95	60
	Morphine	0.50–0.75	35
	Nortriptyline	0.50	95
	Pentazocine	0.80	—
	Propoxyphene	0.95	—
	Propranolol	0.60–0.80	93
Capacity-limited, binding-sensitive	Chlorpromazine	0.22	91–99†
	Clindamycin	0.23	94
	Diazepam	0.03	98
	Digitoxin	0.005	97
	Phenytoin	0.03	90
	Quinidine	0.27	82
	Tolbutamide	0.02	98
	Warfarin	0.003	99
Capacity-limited, binding-insensitive	Acetaminophen	0.43	< 5
	Amylobarbital	0.03	61
	Antipyrine	0.07	10
	Chloramphenicol	0.28	60–80†
	Hexobarbital	0.16	—
	Theophylline	0.09	59
	Thiopental	0.28	72

* Adapted from Blaschke, T. F.: Protein binding and kinetics of drugs in liver diseases. Clin Pharmacokinet., 2:32–44, 1977. Reproduced with permission.
† Concentration-dependent.

the content of cytochrome P450 were found in the rhesus monkey, and the specific activity of NADPH–cytochrome c reductase increased rather than decreased with age (Maloney et al., 1986). Data on the effects of aging on conjugation reactions in nonhuman primates are not available. *Principle: Interspecies differences in hepatic drug metabolism often preclude extrapolation from animal models to humans. Confirmation of the suspicion of drug-induced effects can come only from clinical trials.*

Data on the effect of age on in vitro drug metabolism in human tissues are sparse. One study of liver biopsy samples from 40 men and 30 women ranging in age from 16 to 76 years with suspected liver disease failed to identify correlations between age or sex and cytochrome P450 content, or the activities of cytochrome c reductase and aryl hydrocarbon hydroxylase (Brodie et al., 1981). However, only 30 of the biopsies were normal, and the study was not primarily designed to investigate the effects of age on microsomal drug metabolism. Likewise, there were no significant relationships between age or smoking and microsomal protein content, aldrin epoxidation, 7-ethoxycoumarin-*O*-deethylation, epoxide hydrolase activity, or reduced glutathione activity in normal biopsies from men and women ranging in age from 18 to 83 years (Woodhouse et al., 1984).

In that study potential age differences may have been obscured by small sample sizes. Neither study provides information on the content or activity of isozymes of cytochrome P450. Thus, the results with human liver microsomes generally are consistent with those obtained with microsomes from nonhuman primates; based on presently available biochemical data, intrinsic hepatic drug-metabolizing enzyme activity has not been found to differ significantly with increasing age in humans.

A recent report, however, provides the most extensive and comprehensive data to date (Schmucker et al., 1990). Liver samples from 54 donors who ranged in age from 9 to 89 years did not show any effect of age or gender on the concentration of microsomal protein, the specific activity of NADPH-cytochrome c reductase, the carbon monoxide-binding capacity of microsomal cytochrome P450, or the relative microsomal concentrations of three isozymes of cytochrome P450.

Clinical Studies. Age-related decreases in liver size and liver blood flow may account for the age-related differences in clearance of some drugs (Woodhouse and Wynne, 1988). Hepatic clearance of drugs depends on the activity of the enzymes responsible for biotransformation and on hepatic blood flow, which determines the rate of delivery of the drug to the liver. In the case of drugs with low intrinsic clearance (drugs that are metabolized relatively slowly by the liver), clearance is proportional to the rate of hepatic metabolism (see chapter 37). Autopsy studies indicate that liver weight falls about 18% to 25% between the ages of 20 and 80 years (Boyd, 1933; Calloway et al., 1965). Ultrasound studies demonstrate decreases in liver volume ranging from 17% to 32% across the age span (Swift et al., 1978; Bach et al., 1981; Marchesini et al., 1988; Wynne et al., 1989). Since hepatic mass decreases with age in absolute terms, as well as in proportion to total body weight, the clearance of drugs with low intrinsic clearance (extraction ratios <0.3; see Table 31–4) would be expected to be decreased.

Antipyrine, a drug with low intrinsic clearance, has been used extensively as a model substrate for studies of oxidative drug metabolism in humans. Most studies using antipyrine have shown decreased plasma clearance and a longer half-life in older subjects (O'Malley et al., 1971; Vestal et al., 1975; Swift et al., 1978; Wood et al., 1979; Bach et al., 1981). The effect of age is less pronounced in women than in men (Greenblatt et al., 1982; Greenblatt et al., 1988). Biologic variation among subjects and the presence of other factors, such as smoking, overshadow the effect of age (Vestal et al., 1975; Wood et al., 1979). Data also suggest that the clearance of antipyrine correlates with the age-related decline in liver volume (Swift et al., 1978; Bach et al., 1981). Additional factors that may influence the apparent rates at which the drug is eliminated include concurrent drug intake, diet, illness, cigarette smoking, and alcohol use. *Principle: Even if an age-related "change" in the metabolism of a drug has been demonstrated, its clinical importance may be completely dwarfed by individual variations in other important factors.*

For drugs that exhibit high intrinsic clearance (drugs with a very rapid rate of metabolism), the rate of extraction by the liver is high (extraction ratio >0.7; see Table 31–4) and hepatic blood flow is rate-limiting for their metabolism. Indocyanine green and propranolol are compounds that are avidly extracted by the liver. Estimates of liver blood flow from an analysis of the clearance of indocyanine green, as well as the simultaneous IV and oral kinetics of propranolol, are consistent with a 25% to 35% reduction in liver blood flow between ages 30 and 75 (Wood et al., 1979; Vestal et al., 1979a; Wynne et al., 1989).

As previously stated, old age is associated with a reduction in the presystemic metabolism of propranolol and labetalol, both of which have high extraction ratios. Accordingly, the bioavailability of these drugs is increased with age (Castleden

and George, 1979; Kelly et al., 1982). For the same reasons, although data are incomplete, other drugs with high rates of hepatic extraction (e.g., calcium-entry blockers, tricyclic antidepressants, and most major tranquilizers) should be administered cautiously in elderly patients as lower doses may be sufficient for expected effects and toxicity.

In addition to a physiologic classification of drug metabolism based upon extraction ratios, biotransformation reactions are classified into either phase I (oxidation, reduction, and hydrolysis) or phase II (glucuronidation, acetylation, and sulfation) (see chapter 1). Microsomal and nonmicrosomal enzymes are involved in both phases. The activities of phase I pathways are reduced or unchanged in the elderly, whereas phase II pathways generally are unaffected. Chlordiazepoxide, diazepam, clorazepate, and prazepam, all of which undergo oxidative metabolism (phase I reactions) to active metabolites, exhibit decreased clearance and prolonged half-life of elimination in elderly patients (Bellantuono et al., 1980). In contrast, oxazepam, lorazepam, and temazepam are eliminated by conjugation (phase II) reactions and their clearance is not reduced in old age. This means that cumulative or prolonged sedative effects are less likely with the latter group of benzodiazepines. *Principle: An understanding of how a drug is metabolized can assist the clinician in making therapeutic choices that will minimize the possibility of adverse effects.*

In addition to certain disease states (Table 31–3), the intrinsic genetic characteristics of the patient for whom a drug is prescribed may be the most important determinant of its rate of clearance (see chapter 35). For example, there is a positive association between age and the development of the slow-acetylator phenotype (Iselius and Evans, 1982; Gachályi et al., 1984; Paulsen and Nilsson, 1985; Pontiroli et al., 1985; Kergueris et al., 1986). Slow-acetylator phenotype is associated with increased susceptibility to the development of bladder cancer during chronic exposure (often industrial) to arylamines and hydrazines (Cartwright et al., 1982). The extensive debrisoquin hydroxylation phenotype has been reported to be more common in patients with bronchogenic carcinoma than in age- and sex-matched controls (Ayesh et al., 1984), but only one study has investigated the relationship between this phenotype and age, and no change was found with age (Steiner et al., 1988). The importance of this kind of information is that individuals with genetically determined enhancement or impairment of certain biotransformation pathways may be particularly susceptible to drug-induced toxicity or lack of therapeutic efficacy. Examples include encainide, procainamide, and phenytoin (Kutt et al., 1964; Woosley et al., 1978; Roden et al., 1980). Although at present we do not routinely obtain pharmacogenetic phenotypes in our patients, this may become the standard of practice in the future. The importance of determining the phenotype should at least come to mind when an elderly patient shows unusual dose responses to these drugs. Once the phenotype is established in a family, further treatment of other family members can be tempered by knowledge of the phenotype. Stereoselective drug metabolism also is becoming increasingly important in understanding drug action and toxicity. A recent study showed that the clearance of L-hexobarbital is doubled in young compared with elderly subjects, although no psychomotor differences were observed. This inconsistency probably is explained by the similar clearance of D-hexobarbital, the more active enantiomer, in young and elderly subjects (Chandler et al., 1988).

Renal Excretion of Drugs in the Elderly

The most consistent effect of age on pharmacokinetics is the age-related reduction in the rate of elimination of drugs by the kidney. Both glomerular and tubular functions are affected. The glomerular filtration rate (GFR) as measured by inulin or creatinine clearance may fall as much as 50%, with an average decline of about 35% between ages 20 and 90 (Rowe et al., 1976). However, interindividual variation is considerable, and some healthy individuals show only a very small decline, no decline, or even a slight increase in GFR during aging (Lindeman et al., 1985). Renal plasma flow declines approximately 1.9% per year (Bender, 1965). In contrast to intrinsic hepatic drug metabolism, for which the effects of old age are less certain and probably less important than the effects of disease and interindividual variation, the possibility of diminished renal function in elderly patients is a frequent clinical issue in drug dosing. Creatinine clearance can be used along with concentrations of drug in plasma in adjusting doses and dosage schedules of drugs that are primarily excreted by the kidney. In general, drugs that are significantly excreted by the kidney can be assumed to have diminished clearance of plasma from the elderly in proportion to the decrease in creatinine clearance. Drugs with predominant renal elimination and potentially serious toxic effects in the elderly include aminoglycosides, amantadine, lithium, digoxin, procainamide, chlorpropamide, cimetidine, and some NSAIDs (Table 31–5). Also, drugs with potentially toxic metabolites that are excreted by the kidney, such as meperidine, are potentially hazardous in patients with markedly impaired renal

Table 31–5. DRUGS WITH DECREASED RENAL ELIMINATION IN OLD AGE*

N-Acetylprocainamide	Gentamicin
Amantadine	Hydrochlorothiazide
Amikacin	Lithium
Ampicillin	Pancuronium
Atenolol	Penicillin
Ceftriaxone	Phenobarbital
Cephradine	Procainamide
Chlorpropamide	Ranitidine
Cibenzoline	Solalol
Cimetidine	Sulfamethiazole
Digoxin	Tetracycline
Doxycycline	Tobramycin
Furosemide	Triamterene

* Adapted from Cusack, B. J.; and Vestal, R. E.: Clinical pharmacology: Special considerations in the elderly. In Calkins, E.; Davis, P. J.; and Ford, A. B., (eds.): Practice of Geriatric Medicine. W. B. Saunders Co., Philadelphia, pp. 115–134, 1986. Reproduced with permission.

function (see chapter 1). If renal function is normal (> 80 ml/min per 1.73 m^2), age-related differences in pharmacokinetics are unlikely, as shown for amikacin, gentamicin, and tobramycin (Bauer and Blouin, 1981, 1982, 1983). Since 24-hour urine collections are often not feasible, there are many formulas and nomograms available to help estimate clearance values (Cl_{creat}). The equation of Cockcroft and Gault (1976) is one of the most widely used:

$$Cl_{creat} \text{ (ml/min)} = \frac{(140 - \text{age}) \times \text{weight (kg)}}{72 \times C_{p, creatinine} \text{ (mg/dl)}}$$

The result should be multiplied by 0.85 for women. This formula has been validated in ambulatory and hospitalized patients, but for reasons that are not known, it may not be accurate in nursing home patients (Drusano et al., 1988). *Principle: Estimates of creatinine clearance are only an aid to help calculate initial dose requirements of drugs primarily eliminated by the kidneys. Drug concentrations should be monitored when drugs with a low therapeutic index are used (see chapter 37).*

Case History.

A 75-year-old white man with a history of stable angina was brought to the emergency room complaining of chest pain and shortness of breath. His pulse was irregularly irregular with an apical pulse rate of 126 over 1 minute. Blood pressure was 120/84, and an electrocardiogram revealed atrial fibrillation without evidence for acute ischemia. Measurement of the arterial blood gas concentration revealed mild hypoxia, and blood chemistry tests were normal for the laboratory (BUN, 24 mg/dl; creatinine, 1.1 mg/dl). The patient (55 kg) was given a 1-mg IV loading dose of digoxin over the next 24 hours, followed by a maintenance oral dose of 0.25 mg/day. His heart rate responded with a decrease to 90 beats per minute by the next day. His chest pain was relieved by topical nitroglycerin, which was continued. By the third day of hospitalization, the patient was ambulating comfortably with a heart rate of 82 beats per minute after walking 100 feet briskly. Repeat electrocardiogram showed the patient to have spontaneously converted to normal sinus rhythm. The patient was discharged on the fourth day after admission. Five days later, the patient was brought into the emergency room by family members. The patient complained of nausea and vomiting for 2 days. He was lethargic and disoriented, and on examination his abdomen was found to be diffusely tender without rebound tenderness. The serum digoxin concentration was 2.7 ng/ml at this time.

Comment: Alterations in the disposition of certain drugs in elderly patients require appropriate alterations in dosage, and health care providers should be well aware of the commonly used drugs that tend to be handled differently in aged compared with younger patients. The administration of digoxin illustrates several principles of pharmacokinetics in geriatric patients. The distribution of digoxin is dependent on lean body mass, which decreases in relation to total body mass with age. Therefore, loading doses should be proportionately lower in elderly patients. Maintenance doses also require adjustment since digoxin is predominantly excreted by the kidney, which undergoes age-related decline in glomerular filtration. In this patient, the Cockcroft-Gault equation predicts a creatinine clearance of 45 ml/min, clearly indicating the need for more than a 50% reduction in maintenance dose. The maintenance dose that he was actually given was therefore too high; drug accumulation occurred after the patient left the hospital, resulting in digoxin toxicity. The judicious use of measuring plasma drug levels can be helpful for some drugs, such as digoxin.

Nutrition, Environmental Factors, and Drug Interactions

Nutritional status of the very elderly persons often is marginal. Dietary composition is an important environmental determinant of drug metabolism and drug toxicity (Campbell and Hayes, 1974), and overt protein-calorie malnutrition is associated with impaired drug metabolism in undernourished children and adults (Krishnaswamy, 1978). Elderly persons, including those in nursing homes, are at increased risk of malnutrition. The reduced rate of elimination of antipyrine in a group of elderly persons with vitamin C defi-

ciency was increased after supplementation with vitamin C, but in another study changes in the amounts of dietary ascorbic acid did not affect caffeine metabolism (Smithard and Langman, 1977, 1978; Trang et al., 1982). The possible effects of so-called megadose vitamin therapy on drug kinetics have not been studied, although high doses of several vitamins and minerals can cause toxicity in their own right.

Hepatic microsomal enzyme activity is induced by cigarette smoking (Jusko, 1980; Vestal and Wood, 1980). Although most studies have shown that induction of antipyrine metabolism by smoking is impaired in older persons, the response is variable (Vestal et al., 1975; Wood et al., 1979; Mucklow and Fraser, 1980). The induction of propranolol's metabolism is restricted to young and middle-aged adults (Vestal et al., 1979a). In contrast, theophylline clearance is enhanced in both young adult and elderly smokers (Vestal et al., 1987; Crowley et al., 1988). Therefore, routinely decreasing the dosage of metabolized drugs simply on the basis of age may result in inadequate therapeutic efficacy in elderly smokers. **Principle: Cigarette smoking is likely to accelerate the oxidation and increase the dose requirement of drugs that are metabolized by the liver. Therapeutic monitoring will help guide dose adjustments in patients who smoke, regardless of age.**

Case History 1.

A 72-year-old man presented to his physician complaining of dysuria and urinary frequency. He had no fever or flank pain. His medications included nitrates and a calcium-entry blocker for coronary artery disease. He was also taking an oral anticoagulant (warfarin) for 8 weeks due to a deep venous thrombosis that occurred during hospitalization after coronary bypass surgery. Physical examination was unremarkable, including a firm, nontender prostate. A urinalysis showed pyuria. The prothrombin time was 18 (1.5 times control, or 3.0 international normalized ratio, INR). The patient was begun on a 10-day course of trimethoprim-sulfamethoxazole, and he was released to return home. Five days later, the patient called his physician complaining of bleeding gums after brushing his teeth. His prothrombin time was remeasured and was found to be 34 (2.8 times control, 7.0 INR).

Case History 2.

A 67-year-old man with chronic bronchitis came to the emergency clinic complaining of dyspnea and a productive cough. The patient's medications included a nebulized β-adrenergic agonist and theophylline. He was afebrile, and his chest exam revealed only upper airway rhonchi. An arterial blood-gas test was unremarkable when compared with previous measurements, and his chest x-ray film showed no infiltrates. The plasma theophylline concentration was 15 µg/ml. The patient was given a prescription for an antibiotic, ciprofloxacin, to take for 10 days. The patient returned to the clinic after 1 week complaining of nausea and vomiting. At this time, his plasma theophylline concentration was 29 µg/ml.

Case History 3.

A 79-year-old woman with hypertension was seen in a routine office visit. Her hypertension had been well controlled with a thiazide diuretic, with blood pressures of about 140/70. At this visit, her blood pressure was found to be 170/90. This degree of blood pressure elevation was recorded on two other occasions during the following week. She had recently been complaining of nasal congestion but had bought an OTC cold preparation with relief of these symptoms. The physician asked the patient to bring all her medications to the office, and he found that the OTC medication contained phenylpropanolamine. This medication was discontinued with return of the patient's blood pressure to normotensive readings.

Comment: Although there are few studies investigating the incidence of drug–drug interactions with respect to age, it is generally considered that elderly patients are more likely to encounter drug interactions. Therefore, the surveillance for possible drug interactions should be particularly vigilant in elderly patients taking multiple medications. For example, in Case 1 the addition of any new medication to a regimen that includes an oral anticoagulant should be done with caution. Sulfonamides are known to enhance warfarin activity by decreasing its metabolism and displacing it from binding sites. In Case 2, a new drug (ciprofloxacin) was added that impairs the metabolism of a drug that was already part of the patient's treatment regimen (theophylline). The mechanism for this pharmacokinetic interaction is inhibition of P450 microsomal–mediated metabolism (Wijnands et al., 1986; Thomson et al., 1987). Finally, in Case 3, a common sympathomimetic relief of nasal congestion interfered with blood pressure control in a hypertensive patient.

As previously discussed, elderly persons are commonly assumed to have an increased risk of sustaining unintended drug–drug interactions. Nevertheless, studies that have investigated this possibility are few (Table 31–6). Although the response to induction of hepatic oxidative drug metabolism as a function of age is variable, the response to enzyme inhibition by cimetidine appears to be uniformly similar in young and elderly persons and suggests that the risk of drug toxicity is unchanged in this age group (Divoll et al., 1982c; Feeley et al., 1984; Vestal et al., 1987; Adebayo and Coker, 1987). However, to the extent that elderly patients receive more drugs to begin with (including warfarin or diazepam), equal enzyme inhibition by cimetidine is more likely to lead to a clinically important drug interaction in an elderly than in a younger patient.

DRUG THERAPY AND PHARMACODYNAMICS

Pharmacodynamics, the study of the pharmacologic and therapeutic effects of drugs, has been investigated less extensively in elderly persons than has pharmacokinetics. Since the effect of age on the sensitivity to drugs varies with the drug studied and the response measured, generalizations are again difficult. Valid studies of drug sensitivity require measurement of concentrations of drug in plasma, because differences in pharmacokinetics with increasing age may increase or

Table 31–6. EFFECT OF AGE ON INDUCTION AND INHIBITION OF HEPATIC DRUG METABOLISM IN HUMANS*

INTERACTING DRUG	MARKER DRUG SUBSTRATE	EFFECT IN OLD VS. YOUNG SUBJECTS	REFERENCE
Inducer			
Dichloralphenazone	Antipyrine	Decreased	Salem et al., 1978
Dichloralphenazone	Quinine	Decreased	Salem et al., 1978
Glutethimide	Antipyrine	Same or increased	Pearson and Roberts, 1984
Phenytoin	Theophylline	Same	Crowley et al., 1988
Rifampin	Antipyrine	Decreased	Twum-Barima et al., 1984
Rifampin	Propranolol	Same or increased	Herman et al., 1986
Inhibitor			
Cimetidine	Antipyrine	Same	Divoll et al., 1982c
Cimetidine	Desmethyldiazepam	Same	Divoll et al., 1982c
Cimetidine	Theophylline	Same	Feely et al., 1984; Vestal et al., 1987; Adebayo and Coker, 1987

* Adapted from Vestal and Cusack, 1990. Reproduced with permission from Academic Press.

decrease differences in response to the drug. Only a few areas of drug therapy have been evaluated in this manner (Table 31-7). Four broad classes of drugs will be discussed along with drug–disease interactions as illustrative examples.

Analgesics

Elderly patients frequently receive analgesics and anti-inflammatory agents with analgesic properties. Both morphine and meperidine are associated with decreased rates of plasma clearance in older persons (Holmberg et al., 1982; Owen et al., 1983). Total pain relief and the duration of relief achieved with morphine and pentazocine were greater in older than in younger patients (Bellville et al., 1971; Kaiko, 1980), consistent with a lower dose requirement. Some studies have shown impaired hepatic metabolism of acetaminophen in elderly persons (Divoll et al., 1982b), but dose adjustments are not necessary.

The use of NSAIDs requires close monitoring in elderly patients. These drugs increase the risk of complications such as hyperkalemia or renal failure [particularly when these drugs are used in treating gout (Blackshear et al., 1983)] and death from GI hemorrhage (Griffin et al., 1988). *Principle: Excessive use of analgesics, particularly NSAIDs, is a major cause of adverse drug reactions. Efficacy in relation to risk should be carefully evaluated in each individual, but even more so in elderly patients.*

Anticoagulants

When warfarin is prescribed to elderly patients, the effects of age on dose requirements (O'Malley et al., 1977; Reidenberg, 1987) and the risk of bleeding (Coon and Willis, 1974; Gurwitz et al., 1988) are controversial. One study has shown greater inhibition of synthesis of vitamin K–dependent clotting factors at similar plasma concentrations of warfarin in plasma of older as opposed to younger patients (Shepherd et al., 1977). Increased caution should be exercised when prescribing warfarin to elderly patients, with careful titration of the dose according to the prothrombin time. The coadministration of drugs that may inhibit the metabolism of warfarin (e.g., cimetidine) or displace warfarin from binding sites on plasma proteins (chlorpropamide) must be done carefully. Although age per se is not a contraindication to oral anticoagulant therapy, clinical conditions such as gait abnormalities, recurrent falls, poor medical compliance, peptic ulcer disease, and alcoholism predispose to complications. Although one study found an increased risk of bleeding with heparin in elderly women (Jick et al., 1968), the relationship between plasma heparin concentration and anticoagulant effect does not change with increasing age (Whitfield et al., 1982). Thus, heparin dose probably does not require an adjustment based on age. *Principle: Risk of adverse effects from anticoagulants may be increased and therapy in the elderly should be closely monitored.*

Cardiovascular Drugs

The high prevalence of cardiac and peripheral vascular disorders results in extensive use of cardiovascular drugs in the elderly. The clinical benefit of digoxin therapy for heart failure with sinus rhythm is controversial. Since the distribution of digoxin is related to lean body mass (Cusack et al., 1979), loading doses should be proportionately lower in the elderly. Also, because the glomerular filtration rate is a major determinant of the clearance of digoxin, the maintenance dose should be adjusted based on renal function.

Diuretics are used to treat hypertension and congestive heart failure. The response to furosemide is decreased in the elderly (Andreasen et al., 1984; Chaudhry et al., 1984), but the clinical importance of this observation has not been established. With all diuretics, the elderly are vulnerable to fluid and electrolyte disorders, including volume depletion, hypokalemia, hyponatremia, and hypomagnesemia.

The reduced clearance and prolonged elimination half-life in the elderly of antiarrhythmic agents, such as quinidine, procainamide, and N-acetylprocainamide, together with a low therapeutic index for these drugs, put the elderly at higher risk for toxicity than younger patients. Monitoring concentrations of antiarrhythmic drugs in the plasma of elderly patients is essential. Age-related changes in the kinetics of IV lidocaine are minor, but adverse reactions are frequent in the elderly (Cusack et al., 1985). Common side effects of lidocaine toxicity include confusion, paresthesias, respiratory depression, hypotension, and seizures.

Calcium-entry blockers have been evaluated in elderly patients with hypertension. The EC_{50} of verapamil on PR-interval prolongation was higher after acute IV dosage, indicating less sensitivity to its acute effects on cardiac conduction in the elderly (Abernethy et al., 1986). There was a trend toward a greater decrease in blood pressure and heart rate in the older patients; this may be explained by an increased sensitivity to the negative inotropic and vasodilator effects of verapamil as well as diminished baroreceptor function. In another study the acute administration of diltiazem also resulted in greater prolongation of the PR interval in young than in elderly subjects (Montamat and Abernethy, 1989). *Principle: There are multiple adverse drug effects to which the elderly*

Table 31–7. PHARMACODYNAMICS AND AGING*

DRUG	PLASMA CONC. MEASURED	EFFECT ON INCREASING AGE	EFFECT MEASURED	REFERENCE
Alfentanil	Yes	↑	EEG spectral edge frequency	Scott and Stanski, 1987
Antidepressants†	No	↔	Systolic time intervals	Burkhardt et al., 1978
Chlormethiazole	Yes	↑	Choice reaction time, flicker-fusion threshold, postural sway	Hockings et al., 1982
Coumarins‡	No	↑	Prothrombin time	Husted and Andreasen, 1977
Deslanoside	No	↔	Systolic time intervals	Cokkinos et al., 1980
Diazepam	Yes	↑	Sedation for endoscopy	Giles et al., 1978
Diazepam	Yes	↑	Sedation for cardioversion	Reidenberg et al., 1978
Diazepam	No	↑	Postural sway	Swift et al., 1980
Dichloralphenazone	Yes	↑	Postural sway	Hockings et al., 1982
Diltiazem	Yes	↑	Acute antihypertensive effect	Schwartz and Abernethy, 1987
Diltiazem	Yes	↓	PR-interval prolongation	Montamat et al., 1989
Diphenhydramine	Yes	↔	Psychomotor function	Berlinger et al., 1982
Enalapril	Yes	↑	Acute antihypertension effect	Ajayi et al., 1986
Furosemide	Yes	↓	Latency and size of peak diuretic response	Andreasen et al., 1984
Furosemide	No	↓	Latency and size of peak diuretic response	Chaudhry et al., 1984
Fentanyl	Yes	↑	EEG spectral edge frequency	Scott and Stanski, 1987
Heparin	Yes	↔	Activated partial thromboplastin time	Whitfield et al., 1982
Isoproterenol	No	↓	Chronotropic effect	Bertel et al., 1980
Isoproterenol	No	↓	Chronotropic effect	Klein et al., 1986
Isoproterenol	No	↓	Forearm blood flow, chronotropic effect, renin output response	Van Brummelen et al., 1981
Isoproterenol	No	↓	Dorsal hand vein dilation	Pan et al., 1986
Isoproterenol	No	↓	Chronotropic effect	Vestal et al., 1979b
Levodopa	No	?↑	Dose limitation due to side effects	Grad et al., 1974
Morphine	No	↑	Analgesic effect	Bellville et al., 1971
Morphine	No	↑	Extent and duration of pain relief	Kaiko, 1980
Nitrazepam	Yes	↑	Psychomotor function, sedation	Castleden et al., 1977
Nitroglycerin	No	↔	Dorsal hand vein dilation	Pan et al., 1986
Pancuronium	Yes	↔	Depression of muscle twitch tension	Rupp et al., 1987
Pentazocine	No	↑	Analgesic effect	Bellville et al., 1971
Propranolol	Yes	↓	Chronotropic effect	Vestal et al., 1979b
Temazepam	Yes	↑	Postural sway, flicker-fusion threshold, choice-reaction time, sedation	Swift et al., 1981
Thiopental	Yes	↔	EEG spectral edge frequency	Stanski and Maitre, 1990
Timolol	No	↔	Chronotropic effect	Klein et al., 1986
Tolbutamide	No	↓	Hypoglycemic effect	Swerdloff et al., 1967
Verapamil	Yes	↑	Acute peak antihypertensive effect	Abernethy et al., 1986
Warfarin	No	↑	Thrombotest	O'Malley et al., 1977
Warfarin	Yes	↑	Prothrombin time, clotting factor synthesis	Shepherd et al., 1977
Warfarin§	No	↑	Prothrombin time	Routledge et al., 1979

* Adapted from Cusack, B. J.; and Vestal, R. E.: Clinical pharmacology: Special considerations in the elderly. In Calkins, E.; Davis, P. J.; and Ford, A. B., (eds.): Practice of Geriatric Medicine. W. B. Saunders Co., Philadelphia, pp. 115–134, 1986. Reproduced with permission.
† Including amitriptyline, trimipramine, imipramine, maprotiline, and mianserin.
‡ Including warfarin, phenoprocoumarin, bishydroxycoumarin.
§ Only in patients treated for thromboembolic disease and coronary artery disease and not in patients with peripheral vascular disease or valvular heart disease.

may be particularly susceptible because of impaired homeostatic responses, but pharmacodynamic effects are not easily predicted.

Among cardiovascular drugs, those acting on β-adrenergic receptors have received the most intensive investigation. Several studies have confirmed that elderly patients are less sensitive than are young patients to the chronotropic effects of isoproterenol (Vestal et al., 1979b; Bertel et al., 1980; Van Brummelen et al., 1981; Klein et al., 1986). The results of other studies are less consistent. Although some reports indicate that effects of age on β-adrenergic receptor stimulation are β_1-cardioselective, the β_2-mediated relaxation of forearm and dorsal hand veins induced by isoproterenol declines with age (Van Brummelen et al., 1981; Kendall et al., 1982; Pan et al., 1986; Klein et al., 1988). The responsiveness of the hand vein to phenylephrine, an α-adrenergic agonist, and nitroglycerin, a nonspecific vasodilator, did not differ with age (Pan et al., 1986). Also, in contrast to the nonselective β-adrenergic antagonist propranolol, the effect of timolol, a newer nonselective β-adrenergic blocking agent, does not differ with age (Vestal et al., 1979b; Klein et al., 1986).

In an effort to define the mechanism for the age differences in β-adrenergic responsiveness, many studies have investigated adrenergic responsiveness in lymphocytes or neutrophils isolated from persons of different ages. Possibilities include a decreased number of high-affinity receptors, a decreased affinity of receptors for agonist, an impairment in the activity of adenylate cyclase, or a reduction in the cAMP-dependent activity of protein kinase. Although β-receptor density and affinity for antagonist on human lymphocytes are not altered in old age, lower concentrations of cAMP and adenylate cyclase activity after β-adrenergic stimulation have been found in lymphocyte preparations from elderly compared with young subjects (Abrass and Scarpace, 1981; Scarpace, 1986). The EC_{50} of isoproterenol for stimulation of cAMP production and receptor affinity for agonists are decreased in association with a reduction in the ability to form the high-affinity state for agonists (Feldman et al., 1984; Montamat and Davies, 1989). These results suggest an age-related alteration in the interaction between the β-adrenergic receptor and the stimulator GTP-binding protein that couples the receptor to adenylate cyclase. However, others have failed to confirm this finding of altered affinity states (Zahniser et al., 1988). Studies of the function of α-adrenergic receptors have revealed no change or a decrease in the number and affinity of receptors with age (Buckley et al., 1986; Supiano et al., 1987). Despite all the research on aging

and adrenergic pharmacology, individual variation precludes reliable dose predictions. Therefore, the clinician must titrate dosage according to response in each patient.

Psychotropic Drugs

Psychotropic drugs are often inappropriately prescribed for elderly patients (Ray et al., 1980; Campion et al., 1987; Avorn et al., 1989). The choice among neuroleptic agents that can be beneficial in the treatment of psychosis, paranoid illnesses, and agitation associated with dementia depends on the syndrome being treated and the patient's other clinical problems. Since the response to such agents can be variable, the initial dose should be small and carefully titrated upward. Elderly patients are particularly vulnerable to adverse effects from these agents, including delirium, extrapyramidal symptoms, arrhythmias, and postural hypotension. The incidence of tardive dyskinesia is higher and more likely to be irreversible in the elderly (Smith and Baldessarini, 1980; Waddington and Youssef, 1985). Acute dystonic reactions may be more common in younger patients, but the frequency of choreiform side effects increases with age (Moleman et al., 1986). Most psychotropics and numerous other drugs can cause cognitive impairment in elderly patients (Table 31-8).

Table 31-8. DRUGS THAT CAUSE DELIRIUM OR COGNITIVE IMPAIRMENT IN THE ELDERLY*

Drugs that produce central anticholinergic effects
Anticholinergic drugs (e.g., propantheline)
Tricyclic antidepressants or trazodone
Phenothiazines (e.g., thioridazine)
Other antipsychotic drugs (e.g., haloperidol, loxapine)
Opiate analgesics (e.g., meperidine, morphine)
Disopyramide

Other drugs that can also cause confusion
Alcohol
Amantadine
Benzodiazepines (e.g., diazepam, triazolam)
β Blockers (e.g., propranolol)
Bromocriptine
Cimetidine
Corticosteroids (e.g., prednisone)
Digoxin
Levodopa
Lithium
NSAIDs
Penicillin (high doses)
Phenobarbital
Phenytoin, primidone
Quinidine

* Reproduced with permission from Cusack, 1989.

Because of age-related alterations in hepatic demethylation, the metabolism of many antidepressant agents, particularly tertiary amines such as amitriptyline and imipramine and their metabolites, is impaired in elderly patients (Kitanaka et al., 1982; Abernethy et al., 1985). Older patients treated with these agents are prone to side effects that include postural hypotension, urinary retention, and sedation. Initial doses should be small and preferably given at bedtime. Among the more serious complications, falls that lead to hip fracture have been associated with increasing dosages and prolonged half-lives of psychotropic drugs, including antidepressants and benzodiazepines (Ray et al., 1987).

Elderly persons appear to be more sensitive than young persons to the acute effects of benzodiazepines on the CNS. Sedation is induced by diazepam at lower doses and lower plasma concentrations (Giles et al., 1978; Reidenberg et al., 1978) in elderly patients. Although the pharmacokinetics were unchanged, elderly patients also have been observed to be more sensitive to nitrazepam (Castleden et al., 1977). The toxicity of flurazepam is increased in elderly patients who receive standard adult doses (Greenblatt et al., 1977), and despite apparent development of tolerance after multiple-dose therapy (Greenblatt et al., 1981), dosage reductions are recommended. Not all studies show age differences, however. Caution must be exercised in interpreting the results of studies showing no difference between young and elderly subjects. For example, a study showing that the effects of temazepam and chlormethiazole do not differ with age has been criticized on the grounds that the techniques for measuring drug effects were not sufficiently sensitive, the sample size was too small, and the study design and data analysis were suboptimal (Briggs et al., 1980; Oswald and Adam, 1980; Swift et al., 1980). *Principle: Although we rely upon clinical research to provide information about the effects of age on pharmacokinetics and pharmacodynamics, the interpretation of the results depends upon the appropriateness of the study design, the nature of the study population, and the quality of the methodology.*

Case History.
A 79-year-old woman was scheduled for endoscopy of the upper GI tract for evaluation of abdominal pain that was characteristic for peptic ulcer. She was otherwise in good health, and her medications included only an occasional OTC laxative. The patient was quite anxious about the procedure. Upon arrival to the endoscopy suite, she was given 2 mg of diazepam IV. After 5 minutes, the patient remained alert and anxious. An additional 5 mg of diazepam was administered. The remainder of the endoscopy was performed without difficulty. Several minutes after the procedure was completed, the patient was found to be cyanotic with labored respirations and required ventilation with an oxygenated resuscitation bag. She was transferred to the intensive care unit, where she began breathing spontaneously. Arterial-blood-gas tests revealed a PO_2 of 52 on a 40% O_2 face mask. Chest x-ray examination was subsequently consistent with an aspiration pneumonia.

Comment: Independent of possible changes in drug kinetics, older patients may be more or less sensitive than younger patients to certain drugs even when similar concentrations occur at the drug's site of action. Elderly patients appear to be more sensitive to the sedating effects of benzodiazepines. Therefore, these drugs should be initiated at lower doses than used for younger patients and titrated slowly for safe and appropriate sedation. Also, agents with a favorable pharmacokinetic profile, for example, rapid onset and relatively brief duration, should be chosen. Thus, a short-acting benzodiazepine such as midazolam might be preferable. Other classes of drugs that should be titrated carefully on the basis of pharmacodynamic studies in elderly patients are narcotic analgesics, oral anticoagulants, and antihypertensive agents. On the basis of clinical experience, some other classes of drugs should probably be started at lower doses in elderly persons, including tricyclic antidepressants and antipsychotic agents.

DRUG–DISEASE INTERACTIONS

Certain diseases may alter the disposition or effect of a drug (Table 31–9). Elderly patients often have more than one disease. Congestive heart failure or chronic liver disease, conditions that are associated with diminished hepatic blood flow, may lead to the accumulation of drugs such as lidocaine and imipramine in the plasma; normally, these drugs are highly extracted by the liver, thus increasing the risk of toxicity. Hyperthyroidism has an age-dependent inducing effect on the disposition of propranolol (Feely et al., 1981). Although age-related reductions in the dosage of warfarin may be required in patients treated for coronary artery disease or venous thromboembolism, this appears not to be necessary in those treated for peripheral vascular or valvular heart disease (Routledge et al., 1979). *Principle: Aging and pathologic conditions may interact in logical or unpredictable ways to complicate therapeutic decisions. Careful selection of therapeutic agents and close clinical and*

Table 31–9.   IMPORTANT DRUG–DISEASE INTERACTIONS IN GERIATRIC PATIENTS*

UNDERLYING DISEASE	DRUGS	ADVERSE EFFECT
Dementia	Psychotropic drugs, levodopa, antiepileptic agents	Increased confusion, delirium
Glaucoma	Drugs with antimuscarinic side effects	Acute glaucoma
Congestive heart failure	β-Blockers, verapamil	Acute cardiac decomposition
Cardiac conduction disorders	Tricyclic antidepressants	Heart block
Hypertension	NSAIDs	Increase in blood pressure
Peripheral vascular disease	β-Blockers	Intermittent claudication
Chronic obstructive pulmonary disease	β-Blockers	Bronchoconstriction
	Opiate agents	Respiratory depression
Chronic renal impairment	NSAIDs, contrast agents, aminoglycosides	Acute renal failure
Diabetes mellitus	Diuretics, prednisone	Hyperglycemia
Prostatic hypertrophy	Drugs with antimuscarinic side effects	Urinary retention
Depression	β-Blockers, centrally acting antihypertensives, alcohol, benzodiazepines, steroids	Precipitation or exacerbation of depression
Hypokalemia	Digoxin	Cardiac arrhythmias
Peptic ulcer disease	NSAIDs, anticoagulants	Gastrointestinal hemorrhage

* Reproduced with permission from Cusack, 1989.

Table 31–10.   PRINCIPLES OF GERIATRIC PRESCRIBING*

Evaluate the need for drug therapy
    Not all diseases afflicting the elderly require drug treatment
    Avoid drugs if possible, but do not withhold because of age drugs that might enhance quality of life
    Strive for a diagnosis before treatment
Take a careful history of habits and drug use
    Patients often seek advice and receive prescriptions from several physicians
    Knowledge of existing therapy, both prescribed and nonprescribed, helps anticipate potential drug interactions
    Smoking, alcohol, and caffeine may affect drug response and need to be taken into account
Know the pharmacology of the drug prescribed
    Use a few drugs well
    Awareness of age-related alterations in drug disposition and drug response is helpful
In general, begin therapy with relatively small doses in the elderly
    The standard dose is often too large for elderly patients
    Although the effect of age on hepatic drug metabolism is less predictable, it is known that renal excretion of drugs and their active metabolites tends to decline
    The elderly are particularly sensitive to drugs affecting CNS function
Titrate drug dosage with patient response
    Establish reasonable therapeutic end points
    Adjust dosage until end points are reached or side effects prevent further increases
    Use an adequate dose; this is particularly important in the treatment of pain associated with malignancy
    Sometimes combination therapy is appropriate and effective
Simplify the therapeutic regimen and encourage compliance
    Try to avoid intermittent schedules; once- or twice-daily dosage is ideal
    Label drug containers clearly; when appropriate, specify standard containers instead of containers with locking caps
    Give careful instructions to both the patient and a relative or friend
    Explain why the drug is being prescribed
    Suggest the use of a medication calendar or diary
    Encourage the return or destruction of old medications
    Supervision of drug therapy by a neighbor, relative, friend, or visiting nurse may be desirable or necessary
Regularly review the treatment plan, and discontinue drugs no longer needed
Remember that drugs may cause new problems or exacerbate chronic problems

* From Vestal, R. E.: Clinical pharmacology. In Hazzard, W. R.; Andres, R.; Bierman, E. L.; and Blass, J. P., (eds.): Principles of Geriatric Medicine and Gerontology, 2nd ed. McGraw-Hill, New York, pp. 201–211, 1990. Reproduced with permission of the publisher.

laboratory assessment of the response to therapy are essential.

Case History.

A 72-year-old man visited his physician complaining of difficulty sleeping. His medical problems included mild chronic obstructive pulmonary disease, stable angina, and benign prostate hypertrophy. The patient was taking many medications, and he was apt to take OTC medications frequently for minor complaints. He was not satisfied with the nonpharmacologic methods that had been used to improve his sleep disorder, and he demanded a sleeping pill from his physician. The physician decided to prescribe diphenhydramine to help initiate sleep in the patient. While the patient was pleased with the effects of diphenhydramine on his sleep, he noticed that he now had to arise several times a night to urinate rather than his usual once-nightly voiding pattern. He was referred to a urologist, whose exam revealed an unchanged, but hypertrophied prostate. A postvoid residual urinary volume was now 250 ml, increased from 30 ml on a prior examination. The patient was scheduled for transurethral resection of the prostate.

Comment: Common clinical presentations in the elderly, such as incontinence, falls, and impaired cognition, may actually be mimicked by the adverse effects of commonly prescribed or OTC medications. Drugs with anticholinergic effects, such as diphenhydramine, are used often in the elderly population without regard to their potential for interactions with physiologic or pathologic organ changes that occur in the aged individual. Possible adverse consequences of agents with anticholinergic activity are delirium, dry mouth, provocation of glaucoma, and constipation, as well as urinary retention. Other drugs can aggravate impaired homeostasis found in the elderly. For example, diuretics may worsen impaired blood pressure regulation, leading to postural hypotension, or they may cause hyponatremia in an elderly patient with diminished renal diluting capacity. Patients who have impairment that may be exacerbated by drug therapy should be monitored closely if alternative therapies are not available. It is frequently vital to detect these problems; for example, in this case the patient was subjected to a potentially unnecessary prostatic resection.

GUIDELINES FOR GERIATRIC PRESCRIBING

The general principles of rationally prescribing for geriatric patients do not differ in any essential way from those that apply to patients of any age (Table 31–10). Nevertheless, because of multiple diseases, the need for multiple medications, the potential for altered drug response, and the increased occurrence of unwanted drug effects, the physician must be especially cautious and monitor therapy particularly carefully. Because of these factors, variability of drug response is much greater in elderly populations. In addition, impaired homeostatic mechanisms in these patients may increase the risk and severity of drug-induced toxicity. *Principle: While rational therapeutics in the elderly does not raise unique issues, the need for caution, thoughtfulness, and vigilance by the physician is magnified.*

The primary goal of drug therapy in the elderly is to relieve symptoms and enhance the quality of life. Often the cure of disease is not possible. Nevertheless, the alleviation of symptoms can involve simple measures and may not require the use of drugs. When drugs are needed, increased knowledge of the action of drugs in the elderly and improved communication between patient and physician can improve the overall care of the elderly.

REFERENCES

Abernethy, D. R.; and Kerzner, L.: Age effects on alpha-1-acid glycoprotein concentration and imipramine plasma protein binding. J. Am. Geriatr. Soc., 32:705–708, 1984.

Abernethy, D. R.; Schwartz, J. B.; Todd, E. L.; Luchi, R.; and Snow, E.: Verapamil pharmacodynamics and disposition in young and elderly hypertensive patients. Altered electrocardiographic and hypotensive response. Ann. Intern. Med., 105:329–336, 1986.

Abernethy, D. R.; Greenblatt, D. J.; and Shader, R. I.: Imipramine and desipramine disposition in the elderly. J. Pharmacol. Exp. Ther., 232:183–188, 1985.

Abrass, I. B.; and Scarpace, P. J.: Human lymphocyte beta-adrenergic receptors are unaltered with age. J. Gerontol., 36:298–301, 1981.

Adebayo, G. I.; and Coker, H. A. B.: Cimetidine inhibition of theophylline elimination: The influence of adult age and the time course. Biopharm. Drug Dispos., 8:149–158, 1987.

Adir, J.; Miller, A. K.; and Vestal, R. E.: Effects of total plasma concentration and age on tolbutamide plasma protein binding. Clin. Pharmacol. Ther., 31:488–493, 1982.

Ajayi, A. A.; Hockings, N.; and Reid, J. L.: Age and the pharmacodynamics of angiotensin converting enzyme inhibitors enalapril and enalaprilat. Br. J. Clin. Pharmacol., 21:349–357, 1986.

Andreasen, F.; Hansen, V.; Husted, S. E.; Mogensen, C. E.; and Pedersen, E. B.: The influence of age on renal and extrarenal effects of frusemide. Br. J. Clin. Pharmacol., 18:65–74, 1984.

Avorn, J.; Dreyer, P.; Connelly, K.; and Soumerai, S. B.: Use of psychoactive medication and the quality of care in rest homes. N. Engl. J. Med., 320:227–232, 1989.

Ayesh, R.; Idle, J. R.; Ritchie, J. C.; Crothers, M. J.; and Hetzel, M. R.: Metabolic oxidation phenotypes as markers for susceptibility to lung cancer. Nature, 312:169–170, 1984.

Bach, B.; Hansen, J. M.; Kampmann, J. P.; Rasmussen, S. M.; and Skovsted, L.: Disposition of antipyrine and phenytoin correlated with age and liver volume in man. Clin. Pharmacokinet., 6:389–396, 1981.

Baron, J. H.: Studies of basal and peak acid output with an augmented histamine test. Gut, 4:243–253, 1963.

Bauer, L. A.; and Blouin, R. A.: Influence of age on amikacin pharmacokinetics in patients with normal renal function.

Comparison with gentamicin and tobramycin. Eur. J. Clin. Pharmacol., 24:639–642, 1983.

Bauer, L. A.; and Blouin, R. A.: Gentamicin pharmacokinetics: The effect of age in patients with normal renal function. J. Am. Geriatr. Soc., 30:309–311, 1982.

Bauer, L. A.; and Blouin, R. A.: Influence of age on tobramycin in pharmacokinetics in patients with normal renal function. Antimicrob. Agents Chemother., 9:587–589, 1981.

Baum, C.; Kennedy, D. L.; Forbes, M. B.; and Jones, J. K.: Drug use in the United States in 1981. J.A.M.A., 251:1293–1297, 1981.

Bellantuono, C.; Reggi, V.; Tognoni, G.; and Garattini, S.: Benzodiazepines: Clinical pharmacology and therapeutic use. Drugs, 19:195–219, 1980.

Bellville, J. W.; Forrest, W. H.; Miller, E.; and Brown, B. W.: Influence of age on pain relief from analgesics. A study of postoperative patients. J.A.M.A., 217:1835–1841, 1971.

Bender, A. D.: The effect of increasing age on the distribution of peripheral blood flow in man. J. Am. Geriatr. Soc., 13:192–198, 1965.

Bergman, U.; and Wilholm, B. E.: Patient medication on admission to a medical clinic. Eur. J. Clin. Pharmacol., 20:185–191, 1981.

Berlinger, W. J.; Goldberg, M. J.; Spector, R.; Chiang, C.-K.; and Ghoneim, M. M.: Diphenhydramine: Kinetics and psychomotor effects in elderly women. Clin. Pharmacol. Ther., 32:387–391, 1982.

Bertel, O.; Bühler, F. R.; Kiowski, W.; and Lutold, B. E.: Decreased beta-adrenoceptor responsiveness as related to age, blood pressure, and plasma catecholamines in patients with essential hypertension. Hypertension, 2:130–138, 1980.

Bhanthumnavin, K.; and Schuster, M. M.: Aging and gastrointestinal function. In, Handbook of the Biology of Aging (Finch, C. E.; and Hayflick, L., eds.). Van Nostrand Reinhold, New York, 1977, pp. 709–723.

Birnbaum, L. S.: Age-related changes in carcinogen metabolism. J. Am. Geriatr. Soc., 35:51–60, 1987.

Black, D. M.; Brand, R. J.; Greenlick, M.; Hughes, G.; and Smith, J.: Compliance to treatment for hypertension in elderly patients: The SHEP pilot study. J. Gerontol., 42:552–557, 1987.

Blackshear, J. L.; Davidman, M.; and Stillman, M. T.: Identification of risk for renal insufficiency for nonsteroidal antiinflammatory drugs. Arch. Intern. Med., 143:1130–1134, 1983.

Blackwell, B.: The drug defaulter. Clin. Pharmacol. Ther., 13:841–848, 1972.

Blaschke, T. F.: Protein binding and kinetics of drugs in liver diseases. Clin. Pharmacokinet., 2:32–44, 1977.

Boyd, E.: Normal variability in weight of the adult human liver and spleen. Arch. Pathol., 16:350–372, 1933.

Briggs, R. S.; Castleden, C. M.; and Kraft, C. A.: Improved hypnotic treatment using chlormethiazole and temazepam. Br. Med. J., 280:601–604, 1980.

Brodie, M. J.; Boobis, A. R.; Bulpitt, C. J.; and Davies, D. S.: Influence of liver disease and environmental factors on hepatic monooxygenase activity in vitro. Eur. J. Clin. Pharmacol., 20:39–46, 1981.

Buck, J. A.: Psychotropic drug practice in nursing homes. J. Am. Geriatr. Soc., 36:409–418, 1988.

Buckley, C.; Curtin, D.; Walsh, T.; and O'Malley, K.: Ageing and platelet α_2-adrenoceptors. Br. J. Clin. Pharmacol., 21:721–722, 1986.

Burkhardt, D.; Raeder, E.; and Muller, V.: Cardiovascular effects of tricyclic and tetracyclic antidepressants. J.A.M.A., 239:213–216, 1978.

Calloway, N. O.; Foley, C. F.; and Lagerbloom, P.: Uncertainties in geriatric data: II. Organ size. J. Am. Geriatr. Soc., 13:20–28, 1965.

Campbell, T. C.; and Hayes, J. R.: Role of nutrition in the drug-metabolizing enzyme system. Pharmacol. Rev., 26:171–197, 1974.

Campion, E. W.; deLabry, L. O.; and Glynn, R. J.: The effect of age on serum albumin in healthy males: Report from the normative aging study. J. Gerontol., 43:M18–M20, 1988.

Campion, E. W.; Avorn, J.; Reder, V. A.; and Olins, N. J.: Overmedication of the low-weight elderly. Arch. Intern. Med., 147:945–947, 1987.

Cartwright, R. A.; Glashan, R. W.; Rogers, H. J.; Ahmad, R. A.; Barham-Hall, D.; Higgins, E.; and Khan, M. A.: Role of N-acetyltransferase phenotypes in bladder carcinogenesis. Lancet, 2:842–845, 1982.

Castleden, C. M.; and George, C. F.: The effect of ageing on the hepatic clearance of propranolol. Br. J. Clin. Pharmacol., 7:49–54, 1979.

Castleden, C. M.; George, C. F.; Marcer, D.; and Hallett, C.: Increased sensitivity to nitrazepam in old age. Br. Med. J., 1:10–12, 1977.

Chandler, M. H. H.; Scott, S. R.; and Blouin, R. A.: Age-associated stereoselective alterations in hexobarbital metabolism. Clin. Pharmacol. Ther., 43:436–441, 1988.

Chaudhry, A. Y.; Bing, R. F.; Castelden, C. M.; Swales, J. D.; and Napier, C. J.: The effect of aging on the response to furosemide in normal subjects. Eur. J. Clin. Pharmacol., 27:303–306, 1984.

Christensen, J. H.; Andreasen, F.; and Jansen, J. A.: Influence of age and sex on the pharmacokinetics of thiopentone. Br. J. Anaesth., 53:1189–1195, 1981.

Cockcroft, D. W.; and Gault, M. H.: Prediction of creatinine clearance from serum creatinine. Nephron, 16:31–41, 1976.

Cokkinos, D. V.; Tsartsalis, G. D.; Heimonas, E. T.; and Gardikas, C. D.: Comparison of inotropic action of digitalis and isoproterenol in younger and older individuals. Am. Heart J., 100:801–806, 1980.

Coon, W. W.; and Willis, P. W.: Hemorrhagic complications of anticoagulant therapy. Arch. Intern. Med., 133:386–392, 1974.

Cooper, P. S.; Love, D. W.; and Raffoul, P. R.: Intentional prescription nonadherence (noncompliance) by the elderly. J. Am. Geriatr. Soc., 30:329–333, 1982.

Crowley, J. J.; Cusack, B. J.; Jue, S. G.; Koup, J. R.; Park, B. K.; and Vestal, R. E.: Aging and drug interactions: II. Effect of phenytoin and smoking on the oxidation of theophylline and cortisol in healthy men. J. Pharmacol. Exp. Ther., 245:513–523, 1988.

Cusack, B. J.: Polypharmacy and clinical pharmacology. In, Geriatrics Review Syllabus: A Core Curriculum in Geriatric Medicine (Beck, J. C., ed.). American Geriatrics Society, New York, pp. 127–136, 1989.

Cusack, B. J.; and Vestal, R. E.: Clinical pharmacology: Special considerations in the elderly. In, Practice of Geriatric Medicine (Calkins, E.; Davis, P. J.; and Ford, A. B., eds.). W. B. Saunders, Philadelphia, pp. 115–134, 1986.

Cusack, B.; O'Malley, K.; Lavan, J.; Noel, J.; and Kelly, J. G.: Protein binding and disposition of lidocaine in the elderly. Eur. J. Clin. Pharmacol., 29:232–329, 1985.

Cusack, B.; Kelly, J.; O'Malley, K.; Noel, J.; Lavan, J.; and Horgan, J.: Digoxin in the elderly: Pharmacokinetic consequences of old age. Clin. Pharmacol. Ther., 25:772–776, 1979.

Divoll, M.; Ameer, B.; Abernethy, D. R.; and Greenblatt, D. J.: Age does not alter acetaminophen absorption. J. Am. Geriatr. Soc., 30:240–244, 1982a.

Divoll, M.; Abernethy, D. R.; Ameer, B.; and Greenblatt, D. J.: Acetaminophen kinetics in the elderly. Clin. Pharmacol. Ther., 31:151–156, 1982b.

Divoll, M.; Greenblatt, D. J.; Abernethy, D. R.; and Shader, R. I.: Cimetidine impairs clearance of antipyrine and desmethyldiazepam in the elderly. J. Am. Geriatr. Soc., 30:684–689, 1982c.

Drusano, G. L.; Munice, H. L. Jr.; Hoopes, J. M.; Damron, D. J.; and Warren, J. W.: Commonly used methods of estimating creatinine clearance are inadequate for elderly debilitated nursing home patients. J. Am. Geriatr. Soc., 36:437–441, 1988.

Edelman, I. S.; and Leibman, J.: Anatomy of body water and electrolytes. Am. J. Med., 27:256–277, 1959.

Evans, M. A.; Triggs, E. J.; Cheung, M.; Broe, G. A.; and Creasey, H.: Gastric emptying rate in the elderly: Implications for drug therapy. J. Am. Geriatr. Soc., 29:201-205, 1981.

Evans, M. A.; Triggs, E. J.; Broe, G. A.; and Saines, N.: Systemic availability of orally administered L-dopa in the elderly parkinsonian patient. Eur. J. Clin. Pharmacol., 17:215-221, 1980.

Feely, J.; Pereira, L.; Guy, E.; and Hockings, N.: Factors affecting the response to inhibition of drug metabolism by cimetidine—Dose response and sensitivity of elderly and induced subjects. Br. J. Clin. Pharmacol., 17:77-81, 1984.

Feely, J.; Crooks, J.; and Stevenson, I. H.: The influence of age, smoking and hyperthyroidism on plasma propranolol steady state concentration. Br. J. Clin. Pharmacol., 12:73-78, 1981.

Feldman, R. D.; Limbird, L. E.; Nadeau, J.; Robertson, D.; and Wood, A. J. J.: Alterations in leukocyte β-receptor affinity with aging—A potential explanation for altered β-adrenergic sensitivity in the elderly. N. Engl. J. Med., 310:815-819, 1984.

Food and Drug Administration: Drug Utilization in the U.S.—1987: Ninth Annual Review. Publication No. PB89-143325. National Technical Information Service, U.S. Department of Commerce, Springfield, Va., December 1988.

Food and Drug Administration: Drug Utilization in the U.S.—1987: Eighth Annual Review. Publication No. PB88-146527. National Technical Information Service, U.S. Department of Commerce, Springfield, Va., December 1987.

Gachályi, B.; Vas, A.; Hajós, P.; and Káldo, A.: Acetylator phenotypes: Effect of age. Eur. J. Clin. Pharmacol., 26:43-45, 1984.

Giles, H. G.; MacLeod, S. M.; Wright, J. R.; and Sellers, E. M.: Influence of age and previous use on diazepam dosage required for endoscopy. Can. Med. Assoc. J., 118:513-514, 1978.

Gosney, M.; and Tallis, R.: Prescription of contraindicated and interacting drugs in elderly patients admitted to hospital. Lancet, 2:564-567, 1984.

Grad, B.; Wener, J.; Rosenberg, G.; and Wener, S. W.: Effects of levadopa therapy in patients with Parkinson's disease: Statistical evidence for reduced tolerance to levodopa in the elderly. J. Am. Geriatr. Soc., 22:489-494, 1974.

Greenblatt, D. J.: Reduced serum albumin concentration in the elderly: Report from the Boston Collaborative Drug Surveillance Program. J. Am. Geriatr. Soc., 27:301-312, 1979.

Greenblatt, D. J.; Divoll, M.; Harmatz, J. S.; and Shader, R. I.: Antipyrine absorption and disposition in the elderly. Pharmacology, 36:125-133, 1988.

Greenblatt, D. J.; Divoll, M.; Abernethy, D. R.; Harmatz, J. S.; and Shader, R. I.: Antipyrine kinetics in the elderly: Prediction of age-related changes in benzodiazepine oxidizing capacity. J. Pharmacol. Exp. Ther., 220:120-126, 1982.

Greenblatt, D. J.; Divoll, M.; Harmatz, J. S.; MacLaughlin, D. S.; and Shader, R. I.: Kinetics and clinical effects of flurazepam in young and elderly noninsomniacs. Clin. Pharmacol. Ther., 30:475-486, 1981.

Greenblatt, D. J.; Allen, M. D.; and Shader, R. I.: Toxicity of high-dose flurazepam in the elderly. Clin. Pharmacol. Ther., 21:355-361, 1977.

Griffin, M. R.; Ray, W. A.; and Schaffner, W.: Nonsteroidal anti-inflammatory drug use and death from peptic ulcer in elderly persons. Ann. Intern. Med., 109:359-363, 1988.

Grymonpre, R. E.; Mitenko, P. A.; Sitar, D. S.; Aoki, F. Y.; and Montgomery, P. R.: Drug-associated hospital admissions in older medical patients. J. Am. Geriatr. Soc., 36:1092-1098, 1988.

Gurwitz, J. H.; and Avorn, J.: The ambiguous relation between aging and adverse drug reactions. Ann. Intern. Med., 114:956-966, 1991.

Gurwitz, J. H.; Goldberg, R. J.; Holden, A.; Knapic, N.; and Ansell, J.: Age-related risks of long-term oral anticoagulant therapy. Arch. Intern. Med., 148:1733-1736, 1988.

Hale, W. E.; May, F. E.; Marks, R. G.; and Stewart, R. B.: Drug use in an ambulatory elderly population: A five-year update. Drug Intell. Clin. Pharmacol., 21:530-535, 1987.

Hayes, M. J.; Langman, M. J. S.; and Short, A. H.: Changes in drug metabolism with increasing age: 2. Phenytoin clearance and protein binding. Br. J. Clin. Pharmacol., 2:73-79, 1975.

Heading, R. C.; Nimmo, J.; and Prescott, L. R.: The dependence of paracetamol absorption on the rate of gastric emptying. Br. J. Pharmacol., 47:415-421, 1973.

Helling, D. K.; Lemke, J. H.; Semla, T. P.; Wallace, R. B.; Lipson, D. P.; and Cornoni-Huntley, J.: Medication use characteristics in the elderly: The Iowa 65+ rural health study. J. Am. Geriatr. Soc., 35:4-12, 1987.

Herman, R. J.; Biolliaz, J.; Shaheen, O.; Wood, A. J. J.; and Wilkinson, G. R.: Induction of propranolol metabolism by rifampin in the elderly (abstract 274). Abstracts I. III World Conference on Clinical Pharmacology & Therapeutics, Stockholm, Sweden. Gotab, Stockholm, p. 102, 1986.

Hockings, N.; Stevenson, I. H.; and Swift, G. C.: Hypnotic response in the elderly—Single dose effects of chlormethiazole and dichoralphenazone. Br. J. Clin. Pharmacol., 14:143P, 1982.

Holmberg, L.; Odar-Cederlöf, I.; Borêus, L. O.; Heyner, L.; and Ehrnebo, M.: Comparative disposition of pethidine and norpethidine in old and young patients. Eur. J. Clin. Pharmacol., 22:175-179, 1982.

Homer, T. D.; and Stanski, D. R.: The effect of increasing age on thiopental disposition and anesthetic requirement. Anesthesiology, 62:714-724, 1985.

Hurwitz, N.: Predisposing factors in adverse reactions to drugs. Br. Med. J., 1:536-539, 1969.

Husted, S.; and Andreasen, F.: The influence of age on the response to anticoagulants. Br. J. Clin. Pharmacol., 4:559-565, 1977.

Iselius, L.; and Evans, D. A. P.: Formal genetics of isoniazid metabolism in man. Clin. Pharmacokinet., 8:541-544, 1982.

Jick, H.; Slone, D.; Borda, I. T.; and Shapiro, S.: Efficacy and toxicity of heparin in relation to age and sex. N. Engl. J. Med., 279:284-286, 1968.

Jue, S. G.; and Vestal, R. E.: Adverse drug reactions in the elderly: A critical review. In, Medicine in Old Age—Clinical Pharmacology and Drug Therapy (O'Malley, K., ed.). Churchill Livingstone, Edinburgh, pp. 52-70, 1984.

Jung, D.; Mayershohn, M.; Perrier, D.; Calkins, J.; and Saunders, R.: Thiopental disposition as a function of age in female patients undergoing surgery. Anesthesiology, 56:263-268, 1982.

Jusko, W. J.: Role of tobacco smoking in pharmacokinetics. J. Pharmacokinet. Biopharm., 6:7-39, 1980.

Kaiko, R. F.: Age and morphine analgesia in cancer patients with postoperative pain. Clin. Pharmacol. Ther., 28:823-826, 1980.

Kamataki, T.; Maeda, K.; Shimada, M.; Kitani, K.; Nagai, T.; and Kato, R.: Age-related alterations in the activities of drug-metabolizing enzymes and contents of sex-specific forms of cytochrome P-450 in liver microsomes from male and female rats. J. Pharmacol. Exp. Ther., 233:222-228, 1985.

Kelly, J. G.; McGarry, K.; O'Malley, K.; and O'Brien, E. T.: Bioavailability of labetalol increases with age. Br. J. Clin. Pharmacol., 14:304-305, 1982.

Kendall, M. J.; Woods, K. L.; Wilkins, M. R.; and Worthington, D. J.: Responsiveness to β-adrenergic receptor stimulation: The effects of age are cardioselective. Br. J. Clin. Pharmacol., 14:821-826, 1982.

Keram, S.; and Williams, M. E.: Quantifying the ease or difficulty older persons experience in opening medication containers. J. Am. Geriatr. Soc., 36:198-201, 1988.

Kergueris, M. F.; Bourin, M.; and Larousse, C.: Pharmacokinetics of isoniazid: Influence of age. Eur. J. Clin. Pharmacol., 30:335-340, 1986.

Kitanaka, I.; Ross, R. J.; Cutler, N. R.; Zavadil, A. P. III; and Potter, W. Z.: Altered hydroxydesipramine concentrations in elderly depressed patients. Clin. Pharmacol. Ther., 31:51-55, 1982.

Klein, C.; Hiatt, W. R.; Gerber, J. G.; and Nies, A. S.: Age does not alter human vascular and nonvascular β_2-adrenergic responses to isoproterenol. Clin. Pharmacol. Ther., 44:573–578, 1988.

Klein, C.; Gerber, J. G.; Gal, J.; and Nies, A. S.: Beta-adrenergic receptors in the elderly are not less sensitive to timolol. Clin. Pharmacol. Ther., 40:161–164, 1986.

Klein, L. E.; German, P. S.; Levine, D. M.; Feroli, E. R.; and Ardery, J.: Medication problems among outpatients. A study with emphasis on the elderly. Arch. Intern. Med., 144:1185–1188, 1984.

Klein, L. E.; German, P. S.; and Levine, D. M.: Adverse drug reactions among the elderly: A reassessment. J. Am. Geriatr. Soc., 29:525–530, 1981.

Klotz, U.; Avant, G. R.; Hoyumpa, A.; Schhenker, S.; and Wilkinson, G. R.: The effects of age and liver disease on the disposition and elimination of diazepam in adult man. J. Clin. Invest., 55:347–359, 1975.

Kramer, P. A.; Chapron, D. J.; Benson, J.; and Mercik, S. A.: Tetracycline absorption in elderly patients with achlorhydria. Clin. Pharmacol. Ther., 23:467–472, 1978.

Krishnaswamy, K.: Drug metabolism and pharmacokinetics in malnutrition. Clin. Pharmacokinet., 3:216–240, 1978.

Kutt, H.; Wolk, M.; and McDowell, F.: Insufficient parahydroxylation as a cause of dephenylhydantoin toxicity. Neurology (Minneapolis), 14:542–548, 1964.

LeLorier, J.; Grenon, D.; and Latour, Y.: Pharmacokinetics of lidocaine after prolonged intravenous infusions in uncomplicated myocardial infarction. Ann. Intern. Med., 87:700–702, 1977.

Levy, M.; Kewitz, H.; Altwein, W.; Hillebrand, J.; and Eliakim, M.: Hospital admissions due to adverse drug reactions: A comparative study from Jerusalem and Berlin. Eur. J. Clin. Pharmacol., 17:25–31, 1980.

Lindeman, R. D.; Tobin, J.; and Shock, N. W.: Longitudinal studies on the rate of decline in renal function with age. J. Am. Geriatr. Soc., 33:278–285, 1985.

Maloney, A. G.; Schmucker, D. L.; Vessey, D. S.; and Wang, R. K.: The effects of aging on the hepatic microsomal mixed-function oxidase system of male and female monkeys. Hepatology, 6:282–287, 1986.

Marchesini, G.; Bua, V.; Brunori, A.; Bianchi, G.; Pisi, P.; Fabbri, A.; Zoli, M.; and Pisi, E.: Galactose elimination capacity and liver volume in aging man. Hepatology, 8:1079–1083, 1988.

McLeod, K.; Hull, C. J.; and Watson, M. J.: Effects of ageing on the pharmacokinetics of pancuronium. Br. J. Anaesth., 50:435–438, 1979.

Moleman, P.; Janzen, G.; von Bargen, B. A.; Kappers, E. J.; Pepplinkhuizen, L.; and Schmitz, P. I. M.: Relationship between age and incidence of parkinsonism in psychiatric patients treated with haloperidol. Am. J. Psychiatry, 143:232–234, 1986.

Montamat, S. C.; and Abernethy, D. R.: Calcium antagonists in geriatric patients: Diltiazem in elderly hypertensives. Clin. Pharmacol. Ther., 450:682–691, 1989.

Montamat, S. C.; and Davies, A. O.: Physiological response to isoproterenol and coupling of beta-adrenergic receptors in young and elderly human subjects. J. Gerontol., 44:M100–M105, 1989.

Montamat, S. C.; Cusack, B. J.; and Vestal, R. E.: Management of drug therapy in the elderly. N. Engl. J. Med., 321:303–309, 1989.

Moore, J. G.; Tweedy, C.; Christian, P. E.; and Datz, F. L.: Effect of age on gastric emptying of liquid-solid meals in man. Dig. Dis. Sci., 28:340–344, 1983.

Morrow, D.; Leirer, V.; and Sheikh, J.: Adherence and medication instructions: Review and recommendations. J. Am. Geriatr. Soc., 36:1147–1160, 1988.

Mucklow, J. C.; and Fraser, H. S.: The effects of age and smoking upon antipyrine metabolism. Br. J. Clin. Pharmacol., 9:612–614, 1980.

Nielson, C. P.; Cusack, B. J.; and Vestal, R. E.: Geriatric clinical pharmacology and therapeutics. In, Avery's Drug Treatment: Principles and Practice of Clinical Pharmacology and Therapeutics, 3rd ed. (Speight, T. M., ed.). ADIS Press, Aukland, pp. 160–193, 1987.

Nolan, L.; and O'Malley, K.: Prescribing for the elderly: I. Sensitivity of the elderly to adverse drug reactions. J. Am. Geriatr. Soc., 36:142–149, 1988a.

Nolan, L.; and O'Malley, K.: Prescribing for the elderly: II. Prescribing patterns: Differences due to age. J. Am. Geriatr. Soc., 36:245–254, 1988b.

Norris, A. H.; Lundy, T.; and Shock, N. W.: Trends in selected indices of body composition in men between the ages of 30 and 80 years. Ann. N. Y. Acad. Sci., 110:623–639, 1963.

Novak, L. P.: Aging, total body potassium, fat-free mass, and cell mass in males and females between the ages of 18 and 85 years. J. Gerontol., 27:438–443, 1972.

O'Malley, K.; Stevenson, I. H.; Ward, C. A.; Wood, A. J. J.; and Crooks, J.: Determinants of anticoagulant control in patients receiving warfarin. Br. J. Clin. Pharmacol., 4:309–314, 1977.

O'Malley, K.; Crooks, J.; Duke, E.; and Stevenson, I. H.: Effect of age and sex on human drug metabolism. Br. Med. J., 3:607–609, 1971.

Oswald, I.; and Adam, K.: Chlormethiazole and temazepam (letter). Br. Med. J., 280:860–861, 1980.

Owen, J. A.; Sitar, D. S.; Berger, L.; Brownell, L.; Duke, P. C.; and Mitenko, P. A.: Age-related morphine kinetics. Clin. Pharmacol. Ther., 34:364–368, 1983.

Pan, H. Y.-M.; Hoffman, B. B.; Pershe, R. A.; and Blaschke, T. F.: Decline in beta adrenergic receptor-mediated vascular relaxation with aging in man. J. Pharmacol. Exp. Ther., 239:801–807, 1986.

Paulsen, O.; and Nilsson, L. G.: Distribution of acetylator phenotype in relation to age and sex in Swedish patients. Eur. J. Clin. Pharmacol., 28:311–315, 1985.

Pearson, M. W.; and Roberts, C. J. C.: Drug induction of hepatic enzymes in the elderly. Age Ageing, 13:313–316, 1984.

Pontiroli, A. E.; De Pasqua, A.; Bonisolli, L.; and Pozza, G.: Ageing and acetylator phenotype as determined by administration of sulphadimidine. Eur. J. Clin. Pharmacol., 28:485–486, 1985.

Ray, W. A.; Griffin, M. R.; Schaffner, W.; Baugh, D. K.; and Melton, L. J. III: Psychotropic drug use and the risk of hip fracture. N. Engl. J. Med., 316:363–369, 1987.

Ray, W. A.; Federspiel, C. F.; and Schaffner, W.: A study of antipsychotic use in nursing homes: Epidemiologic evidence suggesting misuse. Am. J. Public Health, 70:485–491, 1980.

Redolfi, A.; Borgogelli, E.; and Lokola, E.: Blood level of cimetidine in relation to age. Eur. J. Clin. Pharmacol., 15:257–261, 1979.

Reidenberg, M. M.: Drug therapy in the elderly: The problem from the point of view of a clinical pharmacologist. Clin. Pharmacol. Ther., 42:677–680, 1987.

Reidenberg, M. M.; Levy, M.; Warner, H.; Coutinho, C. B.; Schwartz, M. A.; Yu, G.; and Cheripko, J.: Relationship between diazepam dose, plasma level, age, and central nervous system depression. Clin. Pharmacol. Ther., 23:371–374, 1978.

Ridout, G.; Santus, G. C.; and Guy, R. H.: Pharmacokinetic considerations in the use of newer transdermal formulations. Clin. Pharmacokinet., 15:114–131, 1988.

Roden, D. M.; Reele, S. B.; Higgens, S. B.; Mayol, R. F.; Gammans, R. E.; Oates, J. A.; and Woosley, R. L.: Total suppression of ventricular arrhythmias by encainide. Pharmacokinetic and electrocardiographic characteristics. N. Engl. J. Med., 302:877–882, 1980.

Roskos, K. V.; Guy, R. H.; and Maibach, H. I.: Percutaneous absorption in the aged. Dermatol. Clin., 4:455–465, 1986.

Routledge, P. A.; Stargel, W. W.; Wagner, G. S.; and Shand, D. G.: Increased alpha-1-acid glycoprotein and lidocaine disposition in myocardial infarction. Ann. Intern. Med., 93:701–704, 1980.

Routledge, P. A.; Chapman, P. H.; Davis, D. M.; and Rawlins, M. D.: Pharmacokinetics and pharmacodynamics of warfarin at steady state. Br. J. Clin. Pharmacol., 8:243–247, 1979.

Rowe, J. W.: Clinical research on aging: Strategies and directions. N. Engl. J. Med., 297:1332–1336, 1977.

Rowe, J. W.; Andres, R.; Tobin, J. D.; Norris, A. H.; and Shock, N. W.: The effect of age on creatinine clearance in man: A cross-sectional and longitudinal study. J. Gerontol., 31:155–163, 1976.

Rubin, P. C.; Scott, P. J. W.; and Reid, J. L.: Prazosin disposition in young and elderly subjects. Br. J. Clin. Pharmacol., 12:401–404, 1981.

Rupp, S. M.; Castagnoli, K. P.; Fisher, D. M.; and Miller, R. D.: Pancuronium and vecuronium pharmacokinetics and pharmacodynamics in younger and elderly adults. Anesthesiology, 67:45–49, 1987.

Salem, S. A. M.; Rajjayabun, P.; Shepherd, A. M. M.; and Stevenson, I. H.: Reduced induction of drug metabolism in the elderly. Age Ageing, 7:68–73, 1978.

Scarpace, P. J.: Decreased β-adrenergic responsiveness during senescence. Federation Proc., Fed. Am. Soc. Exp. Biol., 45:51–54, 1986.

Schmucker, D. L.: Aging and drug disposition: An update. Pharmacol. Rev., 37:133–148, 1985.

Schmucker, D. L.: Age-related changes in drug disposition. Pharmacol. Rev., 30:445–456, 1979.

Schmucker, D. L.; Wang, R. K.; Snyder, D.; Strobel, H.; and Marti, U.: Caloric restriction affects liver microsomal monooxygenases differentially in aging male rats. J. Gerontol., 46:1323–1327, 1991.

Schmucker, D. L.; Woodhouse, K. W.; Wang, R. K.; Wynne, H.; James, O. F.; McManus, M.; and Kremers, P.: Effects of age and gender on in vitro properties of human liver microsomal monooxygenases. Clin. Pharmacol. Ther., 48:365–374, 1990.

Schwartz, J. B.; and Abernethy, D. R.: Responses to intravenous and oral diltiazem in elderly and younger patients with systemic hypertension. Am. J. Cardiol., 59:1111–1117, 1987.

Scott, J. C.; and Stanski, D. R.: Decreased fentanyl and alfentanil dose requirements with age. A simultaneous pharmacokinetic and pharmacodynamic evaluation. J. Pharmacol. Exp. Ther., 240:159–166, 1987.

Seidl, L. G.; Thornton, G. F.; Smith, J. W.; and Cluff, L. E.: Studies on the epidemiology of adverse drug reactions: III. Reactions in patients on a general medical service. Bull. Johns Hopkins Hosp., 119:299–315, 1966.

Shader, R. I.; Greenblatt, D. J.; Harmatz, J. S.; Franke, K.; and Koch-Weser, J.: Absorption and disposition of chlordiazepoxide in young and elderly male volunteers. J. Clin. Pharmacol., 17:709–718, 1977.

Shepherd, A. M.; Hewick, D. S.; Moreland, T. A.; and Stevenson, I. H.: Age as a determinant of sensitivity to warfarin. Br. J. Clin. Pharmacol., 4:315–320, 1977.

Sherman, F. T.: Tamper-resistant packaging: Is it elder-resistant, too? J. Am. Geriatr. Soc., 33:136–141, 1985.

Shock, N. W.; Watkin, D. M.; Yiengst, B. S.; Norris, A. H.; Gaffney, G. W.; Gregerman, R. E.; and Falzone, J. A.: Age differences in the water content of the body as related to basal oxygen consumption in males. J. Gerontol., 18:1–8, 1963.

Shull, H. J.; Wilkinson, G. R.; Johnson, R.; and Schenker, S.: Normal disposition of oxazepam in acute viral hepatitis and cirrhosis. Ann. Intern. Med., 84:420–425, 1976.

Smith, J. M.; and Baldessarini, R. J.: Changes in prevalence, severity, and recovery in tardive dyskinesia with age. Arch. Gen. Psychiatry, 37:1368–1373, 1980.

Smithard, D. J.; and Langman, M. J. S.: The effect of vitamin supplementation upon antipyrine metabolism in the elderly. Br. J. Clin. Pharmacol., 5:181–185, 1978.

Smithard, D. J.; and Langman, M. J. S.: Drug metabolism in the elderly. Br. Med. J., 3:520–521, 1977.

Snedden, T. M.; and Cadieux, R.: State preserves PACE program for elderly. Penn. Med., 91:44, 46, 1988.

Stanski, D. R.; and Maitre, P. O.: Population of pharmacokinetics and pharmacodynamics of thiopental: The effect of age revisited. Anesthesiology, 72:412–422, 1990.

Steiner, E.; Bertilsson, L.; Säwe, J.; Bertling, I.; and Sjöqvist, F.: Polymorphic debrisoquin hydroxylation in 757 Swedish subjects. Clin. Pharmacol. Ther., 44:431–435, 1988.

Supiano, M. A.; Linares, O. A.; Halter, J. B.; Reno, K. M.; and Rosen, S. G.: Functional uncoupling of the platelet α₂-adrenergic receptor-adenylate cyclase complex in the elderly. J. Clin. Endocrin. Metab., 64:1160–1164, 1987.

Sutter, M. A.; Wood, W. G.; Williamson, L. S.; Strong, R.; Pickham, K.; and Richardson, A.: Comparison of the hepatic mixed function oxidase system of young, adult, and old non-human (Macaca nemestrina). Biochem. Pharmacol., 34:2983–2987, 1985.

Swerdloff, R. S.; Pozefsky, T.; Tobin, J. D.; and Andres, R.: Influence of age on the intravenous tolbutamide response test. Diabetes, 16:161–170, 1967.

Swift, C. G.; Haythorne, J. M.; Clarke, P.; and Stevenson, I. H.: The effect of ageing on measured responses to single doses of oral temazepam. Br. J. Clin. Pharmacol., 11:413P–414P, 1981.

Swift, C. G.; Haythorne, J. M.; Clarke, P.; and Stevenson, I. H.: Chlormethiazole and temazepam (letter). Br. Med. J., 280:1322, 1980.

Swift, C. G.; Homeida, M.; Halliwell, M.; and Roberts, C. J. C.: Antipyrine disposition and liver size in the elderly. Eur. J. Clin. Pharmacol., 14:149–152, 1978.

Thomson, A. M.; Thomson, G. D.; Hepburn, M.; and Whiting, B.: A clinically significant interaction between ciprofloxacin and theophylline. Eur. J. Clin. Pharmacol., 33:435–436, 1987.

Trang, J. M.; Blanchard, J.; Conrad, K. A.; and Harrison, G. G.: The effect of vitamin C on the pharmacokinetics of caffeine in elderly men. Am. J. Clin. Nutr., 35:487–494, 1982.

Tsujimoto, G.; Hashimoto, K.; and Hoffman, B. B.: Pharmacokinetic and pharmacodynamic principles of drug therapy in old age. Part I. Int. J. Clin. Pharmacol. Ther. Toxicol., 27:13–26, 1989a.

Tsujimoto, G.; Hashimoto, K.; and Hoffman, B. B.: Pharmacokinetic and pharmacodynamic principles of drug therapy in old age. Part II. Int. J. Clin. Pharmacol. Ther. Toxicol., 27:102–116, 1989b.

Twum-Barima, Y.; Finnigan, T.; Habsh, A. I.; Cape, R. D. T.; and Carruthers, S. G.: Impaired enzyme induction by rifampicin in the elderly. Br. J. Clin. Pharmacol., 17:595–597, 1984.

Upton, R. A.; Williams, R. L.; Kelly, J.; and Jones, R. M.: Naproxen pharmacokinetics in the elderly. Br. J. Clin. Pharmacol., 18:207–214, 1984.

Van Brummelen, P.; Bühler, F. R.; Kiowski, W.; and Amann, F. W.: Age-related decrease in cardiac and peripheral vascular responsiveness to isoprenaline: Studies in normal subjects. Clin. Sci., 60:571–577, 1981.

Vestal, R. E.: Clinical pharmacology. In, Principles of Geriatric Medicine and Gerontology, 2nd ed. (Hazzard, W. R.; Andres, R.; Bierman, E. L.; and Blass, J. P., eds.). McGraw-Hill, New York, pp. 201–211, 1990.

Vestal, R. E.; and Cusack, B. J.: Pharmacology and aging. In, Handbook of the Biology of Aging, 3rd ed. (Schneider, E. L.; and Rowe, J. W., eds.). Academic Press, San Diego, pp. 349–383, 1990.

Vestal, R. E.; and Dawson, G. W.: Pharmacology and aging. In, Handbook of the Biology of Aging, 2nd ed. (Finch, C. E.; and Schneider, E. L., eds.). Van Nostrand Reinhold, New York, pp. 744–819, 1985.

Vestal, R. E.; and Wood, A. J. J.: Influence of age and smoking on drug kinetics in man: Studies using model compounds. Clin. Pharmacokinet., 5:309–319, 1980.

Vestal, R. E.; Cusack, B. J.; Mercer, G. D.; Dawson, G. W.; and Park, B. K.: Aging and drug interactions: I. Effect of cimetidine and smoking on the oxidation of theophylline and cortisol in healthy men. J. Pharmacol. Exp. Ther., 241:488–500, 1987.

Vestal, R. E.; Wood, A. J. J.; Branch, R. A.; Shand, D. G.; and Wilkinson, G. R.: Effects of age and cigarette smoking on propranolol disposition. Clin. Pharmacol. Ther., 26:8–15, 1979a.

Vestal, R. E.; Wood, A. J. J.; and Shand, D. G.: Reduced β-adrenoceptor sensitivity in the elderly. Clin. Pharmacol. Ther., 26:181–186, 1979b.

Vestal, R. E.; McGuire, E. A.; Tobin, J. D.; Andres, R.; Norris, A. H.; and Mezey, E.: Aging and ethanol metabolism. Clin. Pharmacol. Ther., 21:343–3542, 1977.

Vestal, R. E.; Norris, A. H.; Tobin, J. D.; Cohen, B. H.; Shock, N. W.; and Andres, R.: Antipyrine metabolism in man: Influence of age, alcohol, caffeine and smoking. Clin. Pharmacol. Ther., 5:309–319, 1975.

Waddington, J. L.; and Youssef, H. A.: Late onset involuntary movements in chronic schizophrenia: Age-related vulnerability to "tardive" dyskinesia independent of extent of neuroleptic medication. Ir. Med. J., 78:143–146, 1985.

Wallace, S. M.; and Verbeek, R. K.: Plasma protein binding of drugs in the elderly. Clin. Pharmacokinet., 12:41–72, 1987.

Warren, P. M.; Pepperman, M. A.; and Montgomery, R. D.: Age changes in small-intestinal mucosa. Lancet, 2:849–850, 1978.

Weintraub, M.: Intelligent noncompliance with special emphasis on the elderly. Contemp. Pharm. Pract., 4:8–11, 1981.

Weintraub, M.: Intelligent and capricious noncompliance. In, Patient Compliance (Lasagna, L., ed.). Futura, Mt. Kisco, pp. 39–47, 1976.

Weintraub, M.; Au, W. Y. W.; and Lasagna, L.: Compliance as a determinant of serum digoxin concentration. J.A.M.A., 244:481–485, 1973.

Whitfield, L. R.; Schentag, J. J.; and Levy, G.: Relationship between concentration and anticoagulant effect of heparin in plasma of hospitalized patients: Magnitude of predictability of interindividual differences. Clin. Pharmacol. Ther., 32:503–516, 1982.

Wijnands, W. J. A.; Vree, T. B.; and van Herwaarden, C. L. A.: The influence of quinolone derivatives on theophylline clearance. Br. J. Clin. Pharmacol., 22:677–683, 1986.

Wood, A. J. J.; Vestal, R. E.; Wilkinson, G. R.; Branch, R. A.; and Shand, D. G.: Effect of aging and cigarette smoking on antipyrine and indocyanine green elimination. Clin. Pharmacol. Ther., 26:16–20, 1979.

Woodford-Williams, E.; Alvarez, A. S.; Webster, D.; Landless, B.; and Dixon, M. P.: Serum protein patterns in "normal" and pathological aging. Gerontologia, 10:86–99, 1964/65.

Woodhouse, K. W.; Mutch, E.; Williams, F. M.; Rawlins, M. D.; and James, O. F. W.: The effect of age on pathways of drug metabolism in human liver. Age Ageing, 13:328–334, 1984.

Woodhouse, K. W.; and Wynne, H. A.: Age-related changes in liver size and hepatic blood flow: The influence of drug metabolism in the elderly. Clin. Pharmacokinet., 15:287–294, 1988.

Woosley, R. L.; Drayer, D. E.; Reidenberg, M. M.; Nies, A. S.; Carr, K.; and Oates, J. A.: Effect of acetylator phenotype on the rate at which procainamide induces antinuclear antibodies and the lupus syndrome. N. Engl. J. Med., 298:1157–1159, 1978.

Wynne, H. A.; Cope, L. H.; Mutch, E.; Rawlins, M. D.; Woodhouse, K. W.; and James, O. F. W.: The effect of age upon liver volume and apparent liver blood flow in healthy man. Hepatology, 9:297–301, 1989.

Zahniser, N. R.; Parker, D. C.; Bier-Laning, C. M.; Milelr, J. A.; Gerber, J. G.; and Nies, A. S.: Comparison between the effects of aging on antagonist and agonist interactions with beta-adrenergic receptors on human mononuclear and polymorphonuclear leukocyte membranes. J. Gerontol., 43:M151–M157, 1988.

Drugs in Special Patient Groups: Clinical Importance of Genetics in Drug Effects

Urs A. Meyer

GENERAL CONCEPTS

History of Pharmacogenetics

The study of genetically determined variations in drug response, commonly referred to as *pharmacogenetics*, is a relatively new field of clinical investigation. In 1957, Motulsky emphasized that certain adverse reactions to drugs are due to genetically determined variations in enzyme activity (Motulsky, 1957). Pseudocholinesterase variants became associated with suxamethonium sensitivity, and inherited abnormalities in red cell glutathione metabolism were identified as causes of primaquine sensitivity. At about the same time genetic differences in the acetylation of isoniazid were discovered. In 1959, Vogel first proposed the term *pharmacogenetics*, and in 1962, Kalow wrote the first monograph on the subject (Vogel, 1959; Kalow, 1962).

In the last 30 years more than a hundred additional examples of strikingly *exaggerated responses to drugs*, *novel drug effects*, or *lack of effectiveness of drugs* as a manifestation of inherited individual traits have been observed (for reviews, see Nebert, 1981; Vesell, 1984; Kalow, Goedde and Agarwal, 1986; Ayesh and Smith, 1989; Meyer et al., 1989).

The field of pharmacogenetics was stimulated in the 1970s when Vesell and his colleagues demonstrated that plasma half-lives of many drugs are less divergent in monozygotic than in dizygotic twin pairs (for review, see Vesell, 1990). The implication was that *multifactorial inheritance*, or multiple genes, may determine individual drug metabolism (*multigenic* inheritance). More recently, common genetic polymorphisms of drug metabolism such as the debrisoquine-sparteine polymorphism, the mephenytoin polymorphism, and the acetylation polymorphism have received much attention because they affect the metabolism of numerous clinically useful drugs and concern a sizable proportion of patients.

The objectives of research in pharmacogenetics are (1) the identification of genetically controlled variations in drug response, (2) the study of the molecular mechanisms causing these variations, (3) the evaluation of their clinical significance, and (4) the development of simple methods by which susceptible individuals can be recognized before the drug is administered. The "new genetics," with its emphasis on molecular structure and function of genes, a by-product of developments in recombinant DNA technology, has been increasingly applied to problems in pharmacogenetics (Meyer, 1990b). These techniques have already revealed a number of mechanisms of pharmacogenetic variation at the level of the gene (Meyer et al., 1989; LaDu, 1989; Luzzatto and Metha, 1989). It is likely that much will be learned about the variations in human genes causing pharmacogenetic traits in the near future. Indeed, many of these conditions can already be diagnosed in small samples of genomic DNA. *Principle: Understanding the mechanisms of genetic variation in drug*

*effects is key to applying pharmacogenetic princi-
ples to result in greater efficacy and fewer adverse
reactions of numerous drugs. When the molecular
mechanism of a genetic variation is known, simple tests utilizing genomic DNA can frequently
identify patients at risk.*

A relatively recent addition to the discipline of
pharmacogenetics is the field of *ecogenetics*,
which is concerned with the dynamic interactions
between genotype and environmental agents such
as industrial chemicals, pollutants, plant and
food components, insecticides, pesticides, and so
forth. They include interindividual differences in
ethanol sensitivity, sensitivity to milk because of
lactase deficiency, induction of pulmonary emphysema in patients with α_1-antitrypsin deficiency, and many other interactions between the environment and the genetic makeup of the individual
(Omenn and Gelboin, 1984).

Interethnic differences in reactions to drugs
and chemicals, sometimes called pharmacoan-
thropology, represent another area of recent interest. Interethnic differences may be produced
by different environments as well as by different
genetic backgrounds (Kalow et al., 1986; Nei,
1987). These racial or ethnic differences in drug
kinetics and dynamics, although assumed to occur for a long time, have only recently been the
subject of detailed epidemiologic and mechanistic
investigations.

Definitions

The basic tenets of pharmacogenetics are relatively simple. The genetic endowment of the individual, phenotypically expressed in protein structure, configuration, and concentration, may alter
drug action in multiple ways. A drug entering the
body interacts with numerous enzymes and other
proteins. Nearly all drugs undergo enzymatically
controlled transformations during their passage
through the liver and other organs (see chapters
1 and 37). They react with plasma and tissue
proteins by various processes, pass thorough
membranes, and interact with drug-receptor sites.
Theoretically, genetic mutations that alter the
quantity or quality of any of these proteins could
lead to a recognizable disturbance in *drug pharmacokinetics* or *drug–cell interactions* (see chapters 37 and 40). For instance, common inherited
deficiencies in enzymes of drug metabolism can
retard inactivation and consequent excretion of
drugs, resulting in toxic concentrations with usual
doses. Structural differences in serum proteins
could presumably change binding affinities and
alter the ratios of bound to free drug. Similarly,
aberrant gene products at the site of a drug's action in organs, tissues, or cells may confer increased or decreased responsiveness to usual ther-

apeutic concentrations of a drug. The plausibility
of these basic concepts is supported by a number
of detailed investigations of inherited variants involving the fate or action of drugs in the organism.

In some persons, *unexpected*, *novel*, or *unusual*
reactions to drugs may be inherited without the
hereditary defect's being directly associated with
the pharmacokinetic behavior or with the unusual
response of organs, tissues, or cells to a particular
drug. In fact, pharmacogenetics had its initial
impact on medicine predominantly through the
discovery of such unexpected alterations in drug
response. The prototype of this phenomenon is
represented by the syndrome of drug-induced
hemolytic anemia in persons genetically deficient
in glucose-6-phosphate dehydrogenase in their
erythrocytes, discussed later in this chapter. The
pathogenesis of unusual drug effects in hereditary
disorders frequently is not understood, but the
affected patients and their relatives may require
special consideration when given drugs. Some inherited metabolic diseases are uncovered or dramatically precipitated by the administration of
drugs, the unusual drug response serving as a phenotypic marker of the genetic disease. *Principle:
Unexpected or quantitatively unusual responses
of an individual to a drug may be a signal to
investigate the genetic or environmental source of
the variation in the patient and his or her family.*

The basic principles of genetic influences
on drug action may be summarized as follows:
(1) Genetic factors influence drug action by affecting pharmacokinetic and/or pharmacodynamic properties of the agent. Clinically, this may
result in an alteration of the intensity and the
duration of the expected "normal" effect of a
drug. (2) Unexpected, uncommon, or "abnormal"
effects of drugs may be associated with certain
genetically transmitted disorders. Under these circumstances the modified drug response may have
both diagnostic and therapeutic implications.
*Principle: When some patients do not obtain the
expected drug effect or instead show serious toxicity or unusual effects after taking the "standard
and safe" dose of a drug, genetic variability or an
inherited metabolic defect may be the explanation.*

Separation of Genetic and
Environmental Factors

A key issue in research on variation in drug
response is the differentiation of genetic and environmental factors. Obviously, the interaction of
genetic and environmental influences may be difficult to disentangle in an individual patient. Variations in drug response, whether controlled by
genes, environmental factors, or both, may occur

at sites of absorption, distribution, protein binding, drug–cell interaction, metabolism, and excretion. Moreover, several independent variables may modulate more than one of these discrete processes.

Only when one of the numerous interactions of a drug in the body with the product of one aberrant gene assumes decisive importance for drug action can we expect its easy recognition and its transmission by classic Mendelian inheritance, that is, as an autosomal dominant or recessive or X-linked recessive trait. A Mendelian, or *monogenic*, trait often divides a population into two or three distinct groups. Under these circumstances, the frequency distribution of a given parameter of drug response or drug reaction in a sample population shows discontinuous variation, or a multimodal distribution of drug response, each subpopulation corresponding to a different phenotype. This is the case for most classic examples of pharmacogenetic conditions, for example, the slow metabolism of isoniazid or the prolonged apnea after administration of succinylcholine, as discussed in detail below. Family studies easily reveal the mode of inheritance of the inherited variant in these disorders.

More often, since drug action depends on numerous events, each presumably controlled by different gene products, several pairs of genes may interact with environmental factors to result in a particular variation in drug effect. This is called *multifactorial, or polygenic, inheritance* and is more difficult to detect and to distinguish from environmental factors. Thus, when sample populations are tested for characteristics controlled by multiple genes, the resulting distribution curve often does not segregate pharmacogenetic subpopulations. Rather, the interaction of the multiple environmental and genetic factors results in an apparently statistically normal, unimodal, or continuous, distribution of drug response. In this case careful studies of families still may disclose genetic control of the suspected pharmacogenetic trait. For instance, three independent studies of different families have demonstrated predominant genetic control of the plasma pharmacokinetics of bishydroxcoumarin, phenylbutazone, and nortriptyline, although the distribution of concentrations of drug in plasma after standard doses in sample populations was unrevealing (Motulsky, 1964; Whittaker and Evans, 1970; Asberg et al., 1971). However, even pedigree studies involving several generations frequently do not uncover the polygenic contribution to an observed variation, because, by necessity, subjects of different age, sex, and environment are compared. This results in a large "nongenetic" contribution to variation and hides the genetic components of variation.

An important and strikingly simple method to distinguish between hereditary and environmental components of variability is the comparison of small series of mono- and dizygotic twins in whom the variation within pairs can be analyzed by established statistical methods (Galton, 1875; Vesell, 1990). The rationale of the twin method is that for traits controlled primarily by environmental factors, intratwin differences are of similar magnitude in monozygotic and dizygotic twins, while for traits controlled predominantly by genetic factors, there is virtually no intratwin difference in monozygotic twins. In these studies, the contribution of heredity to large individual variation in a chosen parameter of drug response can be expressed quantitatively as *heredity coefficient*, permitting a range of values from 0 to 1, from *negligible hereditary contribution* to *virtually complete hereditary influence*. However, the study methods using twins do not permit a distinction between modes of Mendelian or polygenic inheritance. Recent extensive application of the "twin method" has demonstrated important genetic factors in the pharmacokinetic behavior of a large number of commonly used drugs. Drugs so far investigated by the twin method, usually by administration of a single oral dose, include amylobarbitone, antipyrine, dicoumarol, ethanol, halothane, nortriptyline, phenylbutazone, phenytoin, sodium salicylate, and tolbutamide (for review, see Vesell, 1990). For all these agents, determination of the plasma half-life or other kinetic parameters revealed much greater similarity between identical than between fraternal twins. Most of these studies were done in healthy, otherwise nonmedicated subjects, and drugs were chosen that depend on metabolism to polar metabolites before they are eliminated. In clinical practice, major influences on pharmacokinetics are obviously introduced by disease-related and environmental factors that modify the underlying genetically controlled rate of drug metabolism or its induction. The twin method also has major limitations and problems, which have to be considered (Neel et al., 1954; Vesell, 1990). *Principle: Because of genetic control, the basic capacity of a healthy individual to eliminate a drug is stable and reproducible, while environmental influences and the effects of disease often rapidly change.*

Genetic Polymorphisms and the Diversity of Human Genes

The concept of genetic polymorphism arose from the finding that many phenotypic traits such as blood groups, histocompatibility antigens (HLA system), and enzyme variants exist in the population in frequencies that could not be maintained by spontaneous mutations. A genetic polymorphism is defined as a Mendelian, or monogenic, trait that exists in the population in at least two phenotypes (and presumably at least two genotypes), neither of which is rare, that is, neither of which occurs with a frequency of less than 1% to 2% (Vogel and Motulsky, 1986). The definition of a phenotype frequency of more than 1% as *common* or *polymorphic* is arbitrary and does not specify if the rare phenotype is of heterozygous or homozygous genotype for the variant allele. The evolutionary impact of the phenomenon of genetic polymorphism is that there is variability built into the population so that a change in the environment (e.g., exposure to chemicals, nutritional components, etc.) can elicit a change in the structure of the population, increasing its chance of survival. Genetically, these polymorphisms are due to multiple alleles at one (or more than one) gene locus and are characterized by a high frequency of heterozygotes in the population.

By using gene frequency data, Nei (1987) has evaluated the extent of genetic polymorphism in different human populations: in all three major human races, white, black, and Asian, about 50% of structural loci are polymorphic at the electrophoretic level. If one assumes that the human genome has about 50,000 structural genes, this indicates that human populations are polymorphic at about 25,000 loci. Estimates of heterozygosity show that an "average" individual is heterozygous at about 14% of structural gene loci. At the DNA level, two randomly chosen alleles seem to have on the average three nucleotide differences, but most of these do not result in amino acid changes. The human genome is known to consist of about 3×10^9 pairs of nucleotides; therefore, if the nucleotide diversity is 0.003, an average person is heterozygous at about nine million nucleotide sites. *Principle: Genetic polymorphisms in enzymes and other proteins are the rule rather than the exception, and genetic diversity is a large source of interindividual, interethnic, and racial differences in drug response.*

SPECIFIC PHARMACOGENETIC PHENOMENA

Inherited Variations Affecting Pharmacokinetics of Drugs

Genetic Polymorphisms of Drug Metabolism: Overview. Genetic polymorphisms of drug-metabolizing enzymes give rise to distinct subgroups in the populations that differ in their ability to perform a certain drug biotransformation reaction. Individuals with deficient metabolism of a certain drug are called *poor metabolizers* or *PM phenotypes* compared with the "normal" *extensive metabolizer* or *EM phenotype*. A list of

genetic polymorphisms of drug-metabolizing enzymes is given in Table 32-1. These polymorphisms were discovered by the incidental observation that some patients or volunteers experienced unpleasant and disturbing adverse effects when standard recommended doses of these drugs were administered.

In addition to the polymorphisms listed in Table 32-1, genetic polymorphisms are known for the hydrolysis of paraoxon (Mueller et al., 1983) and the *N*-glucosidation of amobarbital (Tang et al., 1983, Tang, 1990); the clinical relevance of these deficiencies, however, is small. Genetic polymorphisms also have been demonstrated for the oxidative metabolism of antipyrine (Penno and Vesell, 1983) and theophylline (Miller et al., 1985), and for enzymes other than catechol *O*-methyltransferase (COMT) such as thiol methyltransferase and thiopurine methyltransferase involved in methylconjugation of drugs such as captopril, D-penicillamine, 6-mercaptopurine, 6-thioguanine, and azathioprine (Weinshilboum, 1989). However, confirmation of the presence of a classic genetic polymorphism (e.g., monogenic inheritance, frequency of the rarer of two phenotypes of > 1%) or the association of these polymorphisms with clinical problems has not been conclusively established. An existing genetic polymorphism may be difficult to uncover if additional environmental factors influence the affected enzyme or increase the overall metabolism of the substrate by other enzymes.

What Makes a Polymorphism Clinically Relevant. Whether a polymorphism has relevance for drug therapy mainly depends on the characteristics of the drug that is metabolized by the polymorphic enzyme. *First*, the quantitative role of the polymorphic enzyme in the overall elimination (clearance) of the drug has to be assessed. Does the polymorphic pathway result in a major difference in the clearance of the drug in the two phenotypes? Thus cosegregation of a particular drug metabolism pathway affected by the debrisoquine polymorphism may produce only marginal overall phenotype differences as is the case for propranolol (4-hydroxylation, Ward et al., 1989), or result in a six- to sevenfold difference in total plasma clearance between EMs and PMs, as for desipramine (Brøsen et al., 1986) and perphenazine (Dahl-Puustinen et al., 1989). In addition, the formation and elimination of an *active metabolite* via the polymorphic enzyme and its potency relative to the parent drug have to be considered, as for instance with encainide and propafenone, as discussed later in this chapter. *Second*, pharmacokinetic differences between phenotypes are only relevant if the drug in question has a narrow therapeutic range, that is, a

Table 32–1. GENETIC POLYMORPHISMS OF DRUG-METABOLIZING ENZYMES

DESIGNATION	ARCHETYPAL EXAMPLES	OTHER DRUG SUBSTRATES	INCIDENCE OF "POOR METABOLIZERS" IN WHITES (%)	ENZYME INVOLVED	REFERENCE
Debrisoquine-sparteine polymorphism	Debrisoquine, sparteine, bufuralol	Antidepressants, antiarrhythmics, β-adrenergic-receptor blocking drugs, codeine, dextromethorphan, neuroleptics	5–10	Cytochrome P450IID6	Mahgoub et al., 1977 Eichelbaum et al., 1979
Mephenytoin polymorphism	Mephenytoin	Mephobarbital, hexobarbital, diazepam, omeprazol	4 (Japanese, Chinese, 15–20)	Cytochrome P450IIC?	Küpfer et al., 1984
Acetylation polymorphism	Isoniazid, sulphadiazine	Isoniazid, hydralazine, phenelzine, procainamide, dapsone, sulfamethazine, sulfapyridine	40–70 (Japanese 10–20)	N-Acetyltransferase (NAT$_2$)	Hughes et al., 1954
Sulfoxidation polymorphism	S-Carboxymethyl-L-Cysteine	D-Penicillamine (?), aurothiomalate (?)	30	Cysteine oxidase?	Mitchell et al., 1984
Polymorphism of methylconjugation	Catecholamines	L-Dopa, methyldopa	25–30	Catechol O-methyltransferase (COMT)	Weinshilboum, 1989

879

small therapeutic index. Thus, for many β-adrenergic receptor antagonists, plasma concentrations considerably above ideal therapeutic concentrations may not result in markedly increased subjective or objective adverse effects. *Third*, an important issue is whether the dose is individually adjusted on the basis of evaluation of the therapeutic effect. For example, this is routinely done for antihypertensive drugs—interphenotype differences in kinetics are thereby automatically corrected by the physician generally without knowing that there is pharmacokinetic variation.

It is obvious from these considerations, recently summarized by Brøsen and Gram (1989) and Eichelbaum and Gross (1990), that the drug-related criteria that make a genetic polymorphism relevant are similar to those for drug concentration monitoring (see chapter 38). Indeed, genetic polymorphism can be considered a special form of interindividual variability in which a single phenotyping or genotyping test can identify the predisposition of patients at the extremes. *Finally*, the clinical relevance also is dependent on whether the drug is widely used by many physicians (e.g., the tricyclic antidepressants) or is only occasionally used by a clinical specialist.

Studies have emphasized the therapeutic importance of the PM phenotype. However, whereas the PM patient may be at higher risk to develop adverse effects, the other extreme, the EM patient, may not respond to standard doses because of his or her highly efficient metabolism of the active drug. Patients who require relatively large doses of tricyclic antidepressants to achieve concentrations considered therapeutic have been described by Bertilsson et al. (1988). If adverse reactions to a drug are not caused by the parent drug but by a metabolite, the EM phenotype may predispose to these reactions, as postulated for the proarrhythmic effect of encainide (see chapter 6). The EM phenotype may also confer a higher risk for developing drug–drug *interactions*, as exemplified by the numerous drugs substrates and inhibitors of cytochrome P450IID6, the target of the debrisoquine-sparteine polymorphism (see Tables 32–2 and 32–3).

The sometimes voiced opinion that genetic polymorphisms of drug metabolism are of little or no clinical relevance is mostly due to the fact that many physicians are not aware of this source of variation and are reluctant to accept that, for certain drugs, genetic factors are important and should be incorporated in their dosage considerations. Unawareness of these common variabilities will continue to result in undertreatment of EMs and overtreatment of PMs. A substantial number of patients will be affected. *Principle: The clinical relevance of a genetic polymorphism of drug metabolism depends on the relative importance of the affected metabolic pathway to the overall elimination of the drug, or the therapeutic index of the drug, and on the question of whether the variability in drug response can be easily monitored clinically. The identification of patients at the extremes of variation (e.g., rapid and slow metabolizers) before treatment can serve to predict dose requirements and prevent therapeutic failure or toxicity.*

Table 32–2. PHARMACOKINETIC AND CLINICAL CONSEQUENCES OF POLYMORPHIC DRUG METABOLISM IN POOR (PM) AND EXTENSIVE (EM) METABOLIZERS*

KINETIC CONSEQUENCES			
PM INDIVIDUALS	EM INDIVIDUALS	CLINICAL CONSEQUENCES	EXAMPLES
1. Reduced first-pass metabolism, increased oral bioavailability, and elevated plasma levels		Exaggerated drug response, potential drug toxicity	Debrisoquine, phenformin
2. Reduced overall metabolic clearance, prolonged half-life, drug accumulation		Prolonged drug effect, drug toxicity, exaggerated drug response, drug toxicity	Perhexiline, thioridazine, isoniazid, sulfapyridine
3. Alternative pathway of metabolism		Formation of toxic metabolites	Phenacetin (encainide)
4. Failure to generate active metabolite		Altered concentration/ effect relationship between EM and PM	Encainide, propafenone, codeine (analgesic effect)
	1. Multiple substrates and inhibitors competing at active site of enzyme	Drug interactions	Quinidine, propafenone, flecainide, metoprolol, etc.

* Modified from Evans, 1986; Ayesh and Smith, 1989; Brøsen and Gram, 1989; Eichelbaum and Gross, 1990.

Table 32–3. PHARMACOKINETIC CONSEQUENCES FOR SELECTED DRUGS METABOLIZED UNDER THE CONTROL OF THE DEBRISOQUINE-SPARTEINE POLYMORPHISM

PHARMACOKINETIC CONSEQUENCES FOR PMS	DRUG	REFERENCE
1. Reduced first-pass metabolism, increased oral bioavailability, increased plasma levels, reduced metabolic clearance	*β-Adrenergic blockers*	
	Metoprolol	Lennard et al., 1983
	Timolol	Lewis et al., 1985
	Antiarrhythmics	
	N-Propylajmaline	Zekorn et al., 1985
	Flecainide	Beckmann et al., 1988
	Mexiletine	Broly et al., 1990
	Tricyclic antidepressants	
	Nortriptyline	Bertilsson et al., 1980
	Desipramine	Brøsen et al., 1986
		Balant-Gorgia et al., 1986
	Clomipramine	
	Neuroleptics	
	Perphenazine	Dahl-Puustinen et al., 1989
	Thioridazine	von Bahr et al., 1989
	Miscellaneous	
	Debrisoquine	for review, see Eichelbaum and
	4-Hydroxyamphetamine	Gross, 1990; Brøsen and
	Phenformin	Gram, 1989.
	Amiflamine	
	Perhexiline	
	Dextromethorphan	
	Guanoxan	
	Indoramin	
	Methoxyphenamine	
2. Accumulation of parent drug and failure to produce active metabolite	Encainide (*O*-desmethylencainide)	Wang et al., 1984
	Propafenone (5-OH-propafenone)	Siddoway et al., 1987
	Codeine (morphine)	Sindrup et al., 1990
3. Accumulation of active metabolite	Imipramine (desipramine)	Brøsen et al., 1986
4. Accumulation of parent drug and of active metabolite	Amitriptyline (nortriptyline)	Mellström et al., 1983

Polymorphic Oxidation of Debrisoquine, Sparteine, and Other Drugs

Discovery, Incidence, and Molecular Aspects. The existence of a genetic polymorphism causing variable metabolism of the two drugs debrisoquine and sparteine became apparent from independent studies in England and Germany (Mahgoub et al., 1977; Eichelbaum et al., 1979) (see Table 32–1). The 4-Hydroxylation of debrisoquine and the formation of 2- and 5-dehydrosparteine from sparteine were impaired or nearly absent in 5% to 10% of Europeans and North Americans. The mean incidence of PMs in Europe is 7.7% ± 2.2% (SD) in a total of 5005 persons tested (Alvan et al., 1990). The frequency of the PM phenotype appears to be similar in other white populations, but markedly lower (~ 1%) in Asians (for review, see Meyer et al., 1990).

The clinical importance of this polymorphism was initially questioned, because the drugs lead-

ing to its discovery were soon either obsolete or of small distribution. However, it soon became known that many other drugs are inefficiently metabolized in PM subjects, including important antiarrhythmics such as N-propylajmaline, flecainide, propafenone, and mexiletine; antidepressants such as imipramine, nortriptyline, and clomipramine; neuroleptics such as perphenazine and thioridazine; antianginals (perhexiline); and opioids (dextromethorphan, codeine). Moreover, a large number of β-adrenergic receptor antagonists are influenced in their elimination by this polymorphism (Brøsen and Gram, 1989; Meyer et al., 1989; Eichelbaum and Gross, 1990) (see Table 32–3).

The PM phenotype is inherited as an autosomal recessive trait; the PMs are homozygous for an autosomal recessive gene. Studies in the author's laboratory have revealed that this gene codes for a cytochrome P450 isozyme, P450IID6, that is absent in the liver of most PMs (for review, see

Meyer et al., 1990). The P450IID6 cDNA and gene (*CYP2D6*) have been characterized (Gonzalez et al., 1988; Kimura et al., 1989). Moreover, by a combination of restriction analysis (Skoda et al., 1988) and cloning of mutant alleles of this gene from genomic DNA of PM individuals (Kagimoto et al., 1990), at least five different mutant alleles of the *CYP2D6* gene on chromosome 22 have been established, and all can cause absence of the P450IID6 protein in the liver and consequently the development of the PM phenotype (Meyer et al., 1990; Kagimoto et al., 1990). A simple method for genotyping PMs with a small sample of genomic DNA based on specific amplification of parts of mutant *CYP2D6* genes has been developed (Heim and Meyer, 1990). This approach may ultimately replace the presently used phenotype determination by the administration of test drugs such as debrisoquine, sparteine, or dextromethorphan followed by collection of urine and determination of the ratio between parent drug and its metabolite(s). A PM individual is defined by these tests as one in whom the urinary metabolic ratio is >20 for sparteine (Eichelbaum et al., 1986), >12.6 for debrisoquine (Evans et al., 1980), or >0.3 for dextromethorphan (Schmid et al., 1985). The phenotyping by urinary metabolic ratio has limitations because of adverse drug reactions, drug interactions, and the confounding effects of liver and kidney disease.

Clinical Consequences of the Debrisoquine-Sparteine Polymorphism. For some of the numerous substrates of cytochrome P450IID6, the polymorphic oxidation has therapeutic consequences (see Tables 32–2 and 32–3). This concerns antiarrhythmics, antidepressants, neuroleptics, and opioids. For these drugs, knowledge of the phenotype can markedly help to "forecast" the individual dose range required for optimal therapy.

ANTIARRHYTHMIC DRUGS. For most antiarrhythmic drugs a relationship between the suppression of arrhythmias and concentration of drug in plasma has been established (see chapter 6). A serious problem is the adverse proarrhythmic effect associated with these drugs that occurs more frequently at high concentrations of parent drug or of active metabolites. The metabolism of several antiarrhythmic and antianginal drugs cosegregates with the debrisoquine-sparteine polymorphism, notably the metabolism of flecainide, encainide, propafenone, *N*-propylajmaline, and perhexiline. *Principle: If a specialist (e.g., a cardiologist) becomes too focused on his or her expertise in the specialty, phenomena that occur in his or her patients and are not understood often are relegated to the unknown rather than to another specialty interest. The clinician must strive to know when and how to ask for help with therapeutic as well as diagnostic decisions.*

FLECAINIDE. Recently available data from the multicenter Cardiac Arrhythmia Suppression Trial (CAST) demonstrated an excess mortality among patients with nonsustained ventricular arrhythmias who were treated with encainide and flecainide after myocardial infarctions (CAST, 1989). The polymorphic metabolism of these drugs apparently was not considered in the interpretation of these results, which have major consequences for the future use of these agents. Elimination of flecainide is dependent both upon hepatic metabolism and renal excretion. Pronounced differences in plasma half-life and metabolic clearance between EM and PM individuals have been observed (Mikus et al., 1989; Gross et al., 1990). The implications are that the plasma steady-state concentrations of flecainide are achieved only after 4 days of therapy (e.g., on 100 mg flecainide t.i.d.) in PMs but after 2 days in EMs. On the other hand, concentrations of flecainide in serum reach therapeutic ranges more rapidly in PMs. However, in PM subjects with normal renal function and urinary pH, the clearly higher steady-state concentration of flecainide may still be within the therapeutic range (Gross et al., 1990).

These data apply to healthy young volunteers. The majority of patients receiving antiarrhythmic treatment are advanced in age. As renal function diminishes with age, the contribution of metabolism to overall elimination of flecainide is expected to progressively increase. Elderly PMs and those with other causes of impaired renal function are thus at greater risk of developing flecainide toxicity, because decreased renal clearance magnifies the effect of "poor" metabolism, leading to potentially fatal accumulation of drug. Phenotyping or genotyping patients with renal disease for the debrisoquine-sparteine polymorphism prior to initiating flecainide therapy would alert the physician to the need for reducing the dosage even further than anticipated on the basis of creatinine clearance. This may then prevent some fatal sustained ventricular tachycardias that are reported to be associated predominantly with excessively high flecainide concentrations in plasma (Beckmann et al., 1988).

ENCAINIDE. Polymorphic hepatic metabolism and the subsequent variable production of a highly active (and potentially toxic) metabolite must also be considered in the interpretation of the dose–response relationship with this agent (for review, see Woosley et al., 1988). PMs form only trace amounts of the active metabolite *O*-desmethylencainide (ODE), which is further metabolized to 3-methoxy-*O*-desmethylencainide (MODE), also an active antiarrhythmic agent. As a consequence during chronic therapy, the plasma concentrations of encainide observed in PMs are far greater than those in EMs. However, these high concentrations of parent drug are associated with an adequate therapeutic response and also apparently not associated with a higher incidence of adverse effects in PM patients. This has to be realized when interpreting plasma concentrations for therapeutic monitoring. Encainide provides an example of a drug for which in PMs high concentrations of parent drug are required to achieve the required response, whereas in EMs the more active metabolites are the major determinants of efficacy and toxicity. ***Principle: Characteristics of patients may be key determinants of the dominant mechanisms of drug effects.***

PROPAFENONE. Propafenone is metabolized in the liver to the active metabolites 5-hydroxypropafenone and *N*-desalkylpropafenone. Formation of 5-hydroxypropafenone is markedly impaired in PMs, resulting in very low or absent concentrations of this active metabolite (for review, see Funck-Brentano et al., 1990). Whereas EMs exhibit a substantial first-pass hepatic metabolism, PMs have a marked decrease in presystemic elimination with consequent higher oral bioavailability and a very prolonged elimination half-life (12–32 vs. 2–10 hours). The doses required to suppress arrhythmias are similar in patients of the two phenotypes, because the decreased formation of 5-hydroxypropafenone in PMs is compensated by increased propafenone concentrations. However, the incidence of neurologic adverse effects (visual blurring, dizziness) is significantly higher in PM patients. Propafenone is administered as a racemate, and both enantiomers have similar activity at sodium channels. However, the S enantiomer has weak β-adrenergic receptor antagonist properties. Although there is no pronounced enantioselectivity of metabolism between the two phenotypes, the high steady-state concentration of both enantiomers in PMs allows the S enantiomer to reach concentrations at which blockade of β-adrenergic receptors can be substantial. This presumably accounts for the striking increase in CNS side effects in PMs. Moreover, in PM patients with compromised cardiac function, β-adrenergic receptor blockade can be life-threatening.

The metabolism of *N*-propylajmalin (Zekorn et al., 1985), of perhexiline (Cooper et al., 1984), and of mexiletine (Broly et al., 1990) also cosegregates with those of debrisoquine and sparteine. In fact, patients developing peripheral neuropathy or hepatotoxicity on antianginal therapy with perhexiline predominantly are of the PM phenotype; one of the reasons that this drug is no longer generally used is on account of this problem. The clinical significance of the polymorphic metabolism of *N*-propylajmaline and mexiletine has not yet been adequately evaluated.

β-ADRENERGIC ANTAGONISTS. A number of drugs in this group are subject to polymorphic metabolism of the debrisoquine type. This topic has recently been reviewed by Lennard (1989). Phenotype differences are documented in particular for metoprolol and timolol, with which the PM phenotype is associated with increased plasma drug concentrations, a prolongation of elimination half-life, and more sustained β-receptor antagonism. Only a minor pathway of the metabolism of propranolol, 4-hydroxylation, appears to be affected, and no differences in disposition between the two phenotypes are observed for propranolol. Of interest is the enantioselectivity, both of metabolism and receptor interaction, for these compounds, which are given as racemers (with the exception of timolol). For instance, the β-adrenergic antagonism of metoprolol resides almost exclusively with the S enantiomer, whereas the metabolism by the polymorphic enzyme favors the R enantiomer. Loss of stereoselective metabolism in PMs thus shifts the concentration-effect relationship of the total concentration to the right because there is a relative increase of the (R)-metoprolol. The PMs indeed appear to require higher total concentrations compared with EMs to achieve the same β-receptor antagonism. It would be expected that PMs also are at higher risk to develop dose-dependent adverse effects and that β_1 selectivity of some of these agents is lost at high concentrations, resulting in additional β_2 blockade. However, the clinical relevance of the PM phenotype for the use of polymorphically metabolized β-adrenergic receptor antagonist is not established; indeed it has been questioned (Clark et al., 1984).

Prospective studies of long-term treatment with these agents are not available. Also these drugs have a relatively large therapeutic index, and the dose frequently is individually adjusted according to clinical signs of β-receptor antagonism, and this should compensate for the kinetic effects of the PM phenotype. Nevertheless, a considerable fraction of patients has unpleasant side effects from these drugs. A prospective study to assess polymorphic metabolism would be desirable.

PHENOTHIAZINES. Recent evidence indicates that the metabolism of a number of neuroleptic drugs cosegregates with that of debrisoquine (see chapter 13). Several of these agents were found to be competitive inhibitors of cytochrome P450IID6 in vitro in human liver microsomes (Otton et al., 1984; Fonné-Pfister and Meyer, 1988). Moreover, the urinary metabolic ratio of sparteine or debrisoquine was markedly increased during neuroleptic therapy (Syvählahti et al., 1986; Gram et al., 1989). The metabolism of only three of these drugs has been studied. Both perphenazine (Dahl-Puustinen et al., 1989) and thioridazine (von Bahr et al., 1989) are polymorphically metabolized, whereas haloperidol, although a potent competitive inhibitor of the polymorphic enzyme, is not metabolized by P450IID6 (Gram et al., 1989). The clinical importance of the polymorphic metabolism of these psychotropic drugs awaits to be investigated. The potential of these drugs to cause interactions with other substrates of P450IID6, particularly tricyclic antidepressants, has been known for a long time. Table 32–4 lists some of the known interactions of chlorpromazine, haloperidol, thioridazine, and fluphenazine with substrates of P450IID6.

ANTIDEPRESSANTS. The metabolism of amitriptyline, clomipramine, desipramine, imipramine, and nortriptyline is influenced by the debrisoquine-sparteine polymorphism to various degrees (for review, see Brøsen et al., 1986; Brøsen and Gram, 1989). For these agents, there are clearly two patient groups that pose clinical problems. The PMs of debrisoquine-sparteine and the "slow EM" individuals often develop elevated plasma concentrations of drug in plasma while taking recommended doses of tricyclic antidepressants. The other group are the rapid EMs, who do not respond to the drug because the drug concentrations are by far too low. At least 20% to 30% of patients belong to these two risk groups. Although adverse effects that presumably occur more frequently in PMs are rarely life-threatening, they usually are so unpleasant that they cause problems with compliance. Moreover, toxic reactions may be misinterpreted as symptoms of depression and lead to erroneous further increases in the dose. Obviously, prospective and well-designed trials are needed to evaluate the value of phenotyping or genotyping depressive patients in selecting the starting dose to enhance therapeutic efficacy and prevent toxicity. These concepts have

recently been reviewed by Brøsen and Gram (1989).

OPIOIDS. Both dextromethorphan and codeine O-demethylation are catalyzed by polymorphic P450IID6 (Schmid et al., 1985; Dayer et al., 1988). Whereas dextromethorphan has few adverse effects and little addiction potential, the clinical significance of its longer half-life and higher plasma concentration in PMs has not been established. In fact, because of its worldwide availability and safety, it is recommended as a test compound to phenotype for the debrisoquine-sparteine polymorphism.

The polymorphic O-demethylation of codeine is, however, of clinical importance when this drug is given as an analgesic. Approximately 10% of codeine is O-demethylated to morphine, and it is this pathway that is deficient in PMs. Since the analgesic effect of codeine apparently is dependent on its transformation to morphine, PMs therefore receive no analgesic effect, as has been recently demonstrated (Sindrup et al., 1989). Moreover, competitive inhibitors of P450IID6 such as quinidine given concomitantly with codeine in EMs abolishes the analgesic effect. Codeine is frequently recommended as a drug of first choice for treatment of chronic severe pain. The physician must appreciate that no analgesic effect is to be expected in the 5% to 10% of patients who are of the PM phenotype, or who are extensive metabolizers during continued treatment with a potent inhibitor of P450IID6 (see Table 32–4).

DRUG-DRUG INTERACTIONS. The demonstration of competitive and noncompetitive inhibition by cosubstrates and other drugs of cytochrome P450IID6 in human liver microsomes has opened

Table 32–4. INHIBITORS OF HUMAN P450IID6

INHIBITOR	SUBSTRATE OF P450IID6 WHOSE METABOLISM IS INHIBITED IN VIVO	REFERENCE
Quinidine	Metoprolol	Leeman et al., 1986
	Sparteine	Brinn et al., 1986
	Debrisoquine	Brøsen et al., 1987
	Desipramine	Steiner et al., 1988
	Codeine	Desmeules et al., 1989
Propafenone	Debrisoquine	Siddoway et al., 1987
		Wagner et al., 1987
	Metoprolol	
Flecainide	Dextromethorphan	Haefely et al., 1990
Chlorpromazine	Nortriptyline	
Haloperidol	Imipramine	Gram et al., 1989
	Sparteine	
Thioridazine	Desipramine	Hirschowitz et al., 1983
		Syvählahti et al., 1986
	Debrisoquine	
Fluphenazine	Imipramine	Siris et al., 1982

a rational approach to predicting drug–drug interaction (Fonné-Pfister and Meyer, 1988; reviewed by Brøsen, 1990). Several of these interactions subsequently have been shown to occur in vivo at therapeutic doses of these drugs (see Table 32–4). Thus, the strong in vitro inhibitors quinidine, propafenone, fluphenazine, haloperidol, chlorpromazine, thioridazine, and paroxetine have the potential to inhibit the metabolism of substrates of P450IID6 in EMs. One of the clinically most relevant interactions is the inhibitory effect of neuroleptics on tricyclic antidepressants, first reported to occur in 1972 (Gram and Overo, 1972; Brøsen, 1990). These types of interactions clearly are clinically important and a source of faulty interpretation of phenotyping tests.

CONCLUSIONS. The debrisoquine-sparteine polymorphism of drug metabolism is an important stable determinant of interindividual variation in the kinetics, effects, and adverse reactions of several clinically useful drugs. When the changes in kinetics are clinically significant, a simple phenotyping or genotyping test, performed once in a patient's lifetime, can predict the dose requirements and prevent overdosage in PMs and treatment failures and interactions in EMs. This applies in particular to some antiarrhythmic drugs, phenothiazines, tricyclic antidepressants, and codeine.

Genetic Polymorphism of Mephenytoin Oxidation.

A genetic polymorphism of another cytochrome P450 isozyme was revealed by the discovery of deficient 4′-hydroxylation of mephenytoin, a now rarely used anticonvulsant drug (Küpfer et al., 1984). The deficiency is restricted to one of the two major metabolic pathways of mephenytoin disposition, namely stereoselective hydroxylation of (S)-mephenytoin in the p-phenyl position to 4′-OH-mephenytoin. The other main reaction, N-demethylation of (R)-mephenytoin to 5-phenyl-5-ethylhydantoin (PEH, Nirvanol) remains unaffected (Küpfer et al., 1984). This deficiency occurs with a frequency of 2% to 5% in whites, but with a much higher frequency (15% to 23%) in Japanese and Chinese subjects (for review, see Wilkinson et al., 1989). The molecular mechanism of deficient mephenytoin hydroxylation is not known, except that it concerns a deficiency of one of the P450 isozymes of the P450IIC subfamily (Ged et al., 1988; Meier and Meyer, 1987).

Individuals of the PM phenotype are predisposed to suffer from the central adverse effects of mephenytoin, for example, sedation after administration of a single dose of 100 mg for phenotyping purposes. Additional substrates for the enzyme metabolizing (S)-mephenytoin to 4′-OH-mephenytoin have been suspected by in vitro inhibition studies, and some of these have been confirmed by cosegregation in populations. Thus the metabolism of the N-demethylated metabolite of mephenytoin, nirvanol; the metabolism of mephobarbital, and hexobarbital; the side-chain oxidation of propanolol; and the metabolism of diazepam and desmethyldiazepam (Bertilsson et al., 1989) cosegregate with the 4′-hydroxylation of (S)-mephenytoin (for review, see Wilkinson et al., 1989). More recent studies also suggest that the metabolism of the proton-pump inhibitor omeprazol (Andersson et al., 1990) and of the antimalarial drug proguanyl (Helsby et al., 1990) cosegregate with polymorphic mephenytoin metabolism. The clinical consequences of impaired mephenytoin hydroxylation have not been evaluated. There is some evidence that the frequency of adverse effects of mephobarbital and hexobarbital may be higher in poor metabolizers of mephenytoin. The effect of polymorphic diazepam metabolism also appears to be small because of the wide therapeutic range and index of this drug.

N-Acetylation Pharmacogenetics

Discovery, Incidence, and Molecular Aspects. The acetylation polymorphism probably is the best known classic example of a genetic defect in drug metabolism. It was observed over a quarter of a century ago with the advent of isoniazid therapy for tuberculosis (Hughes et al., 1954). Patients could be classified as *rapid (fast)* or *slow* eliminators of isoniazid, and family studies revealed that the ability to eliminate isoniazid was determined by two alleles at a single autosomal gene locus, slow acetylators being homozygous for a recessive allele (Evans et al., 1960). The polymorphism of N-acetylation has recently been reviewed by Weber (1987), Evans (1989), and Meyer et al. (1989).

The proportions of rapid acetylators (RAs) and slow acetylators (SAs) vary remarkably in different ethnic and/or geographic populations. For example, the percentage of slow acetylators among Canadian Eskimos is 5%, whereas it rises to 83% among Egyptians and 90% among Moroccans (for review, see Weber, 1987; Evans, 1989). Most populations in Europe and North America have an approximately equal number of RAs and SAs. Numerous subsequent studies have demonstrated that the acetylation polymorphism affects the metabolism of a wide variety of other arylamine and hydrazine drugs and numerous foreign chemicals. These include the drugs sulfamethazine (SMZ) and several other sulfonamides, hydralazine, procainamide, dapsone, p-aminobenzoic acid (PABA), phenelzine, and aminoglutethimide. The polymorphism also involves the metabolism of caffeine, clonazepam, and nitrazepam as well as the potential arylamine carcinogens benzidine, 2-aminofluorene, and β-naphthylamine. Initial phenotyping procedures with isoniazid were later replaced by testing with sulfamethazine or dapsone. More recently, a simple phenotyping procedure using caffeine as a test substance has been developed by Grant et al. (1984) and further refined by Tang et al. (1987).

The molecular mechanism of polymorphic N-acetylation has only recently been studied. A cytosolic N-acetyltransferase (NAT2) was identified as the polymorphic enzyme in livers of RAs and found in markedly decreased amounts in livers of SAs in the author's laboratory (Grant et al., 1990). We found the gene for this enzyme to be localized on chromosome 8 (Blum et al., 1990), and several mutant alleles of this locus have been identified to date to be associated with the SA phenotype. The identification of these mutations on these alleles will soon elucidate the molecular mechanism of deficient NAT and serve to develop genotyping tests for this polymorphism.

Clinical Importance. The acetylator polymorphism has a number of consequences for drug efficacy and the occurrence of adverse effects that are summarized in Table 32–5 (for review, see Weber, 1987; Evans, 1989). With isoniazid, hydralazine, and salicylazosulfapyridine, clinical phenomena are known that are clearly associated with the acetylator phenotype. None of these are major clinical problems, however, and the phenotyping test is rarely used in clinical practice. In restricted use of the drugs affected, marked differences in the frequency of the two phenotypes

in different populations and other sources of variability make it difficult to recognize the clinical importance of this polymorphism.

Peripheral Neuropathy. Patients who slowly inactivate isoniazid are more likely to accumulate isoniazid to toxic concentrations and to develop peripheral neuropathy (Hughes et al., 1954; Devadatta et al., 1960). Conversely, rapid acetylators of isoniazid or other drugs that are metabolized by the same enzyme might have to be given unusually high doses to reliably obtain efficacy. Since the neuropathy caused by isoniazid is regularly prevented by the common simultaneous prophylactic administration of pyridoxine, a drug that can be used safely in large amounts, prevention of neuropathy does not necessarily require identification of the acetylator phenotype of the patient as long as malnutrition is corrected or pyridoxine is "routinely" coadministered with isoniazid.

Phenytoin–Isoniazid Interaction. Of greater clinical significance is the increased occurrence of serious phenytoin toxicity in slow acetylators of isoniazid when these drugs are given simultaneously (Kutt et al., 1970). Concentrations of phenytoin in plasma are increased and phenytoin toxicity is greater in the slowest acetylators who have the highest concentration of isoniazid in plasma. Isoniazid noncompetitively inhibits the microsomal p-hydroxylation of phenytoin. Although the exact mechanism of this inhibition and of the consequent interaction of the two drugs remains obscure, it is clearly aggravated by the genetic variant of slow acetylation of isoniazid. It thus

Table 32–5. PHENOTYPE-ASSOCIATED CLINICAL RESPONSES AND ADVERSE REACTION IN SLOW AND RAPID ACETYLATORS*

DRUG	PHENOTYPE	CLINICAL PHENOMENON	REFERENCE
Isoniazid	Slow	More prone to develop peripheral neuropathy on conventional doses and if therapy is not supplemented with pyridoxine	Devadatta et al., 1960
	Slow	More prone to phenytoin adverse effects when simultaneously treated with isoniazid	Kutt et al., 1970
	Slow	Non-Orientals are more prone to elevation of transaminase and bilirubin concentrations if treated with isoniazid and rifampicin	For review, see Evans, 1989
	Rapid	In Japanese and Chinese subjects hepatotoxic effects of isoniazid more common	For review, see Evans, 1989
	Rapid	Less favorable results of treating tuberculosis with once-weekly isoniazid	Madras study, 1970
Hydralazine	Slow	More prone to develop antinuclear antibodies and systemic lupus erythematosus-like syndrome	Uetrecht and Woosley, 1981
	Rapid	Requirement of higher doses to control hypertension	Zacest and Koch-Weser, 1972
Salicylazosulfapyridine	Slow	Increased incidence of hematologic and GI adverse reactions	Schröder and Evans, 1972

* Modified from Evans, 1989.

represents an interesting example of the role of genetic factors in the pathogenesis of a drug–drug interaction.

Isoniazid Efficacy. Interestingly, despite altered kinetics of isoniazid, in the treatment of tuberculosis no significant difference in the clinical effectiveness of isoniazid has been identified in SAs. This impression is based on experiments with patients on long-term treatment with daily or twice-weekly doses of isoniazid. However in all the once-weekly regimens, the RAs responded less favorably than the SAs (Madras Study, 1970). Therefore, phenotyping before once-weekly regimens and consequent changes in dosage are recommended.

Isoniazid Hepatitis. The RAs have been postulated to have susceptibility to isoniazid-induced liver damage (Mitchell et al., 1976). But conflicting and complex biochemical and epidemiologic data do not support this general hypothesis. Probably, when isoniazid is given alone, SAs are more at risk to develop hepatotoxicity than RAs in white and black populations. With regimens that contain both isoniazid and rifampicin, the incidence of hepatoxicity is greater in SAs in white populations, whereas in Orientals RAs more frequently develop biochemical (but not clinical) signs of liver toxicity (for review, see Evans, 1989).

Other Phenomena. Other phenomena associated with slow and rapid acetylation are the higher doses of hydralazine required to control blood pressure of RAs (Zacest and Koch-Weser, 1972). It is well documented that drug-induced lupus erythematosus is overwhelmingly a disease of SAs (Uetrecht and Woosley, 1981). Sulfapyridine arises from *salicylazosulfapyridine* in the gut by attack of the azo linkage by bacterial enzymes. Sulfapyridine then is absorbed and acetylated. The serum sulfapyridine concentration is higher in SAs treated with salicylazosulfapyridine, and the adverse effects of sulfapyridine occur earlier and more frequently in these patients (Schröder and Evans, 1972). Phenotyping before treatment or close monitoring of sulfapyridine concentrations are recommended in most of these studies. The situations in which phenotyping for acetylator status may be advantageous are listed in Table 32–6.

In addition to increased adverse reactions in SAs treated with drugs whose elimination is primarily determined by acetylation, there are a number of as yet poorly understood associations of acetylator phenotype with drug induced and spontaneous diseases (for review, see Weber, 1987; Evans 1989). Thus, there is a statistical association between cancer of the bladder and the SA phenotype in workers exposed to amine carcinogens, presumably because carcinogenic

Table 32–6. WHEN ONE SHOULD DETERMINE THE ACETYLATOR PHENOTYPE IN CLINICAL PRACTICE

1. Simultaneous therapy with phenytoin and isoniazid
2. Before treating tuberculosis with once-weekly regimen
3. Before treating hypertension with high dose of hydralazine
4. Before treating inflammatory bowel diseases with salicylazosulfapyridine
5. Potential exposure to carcinogenic amines known to cause bladder cancer

amines are substrates for *N*-acetyltransferase. The greatly increased prevalence of SAs in Gilbert disease, the association of the RA phenotype with diabetes, the possible association of the RA phenotype with breast cancer and of the SA phenotype with leprosy, and the earlier age of onset of thyrotoxicosis in SAs have recently been reviewed (Evans, 1989). These associations remain mechanistically unexplained. However, the recent cloning of the human gene for polymorphic *N*-acetyltransferase may clarify some of these associations (Blum et al., 1990).

Other Polymorphisms of Potential Clinical Importance. *Methyl conjugation* is an important pathway in the metabolism of many drugs. Individual variations in the activities of three methyltransferases, COMT, thiopurine methyltransferase (TPMT), and thiol methyltransferase (TMT), have only been studied in the last few years (Weinshilboum, 1989). A genetic polymorphism of COMT activity was first discovered in erythrocytes and apparently reflects the activity in other tissues, including the liver. About 20% to 30% of whites are homozygous for the low-activity gene and have low COMT activity. The COMT activity determines the proportion of L-dopa and methyldopa being converted to 3-*O*-methyl metabolites. The TPMT is involved in the metabolism of 6-mercaptopurine, 6-thioguanine, azathioprine, and the TMT in the metabolism of captopril and D-penicillamine, respectively (Weinshilboum, 1989). However, the clinical importance of the genetic variability in these two enzymes is speculative at present.

Sulfoxidation of the mucolytic agent *S*-carboxymethyl-L-cysteine (carboxycysteine) appears to be deficient as an inherited recessive trait in about 30% of the white population (see chapter 7) (Mitchell et al., 1984; Mitchell and Waring, 1989). Adverse effects to the sulfur-containing drugs D-penicillamine and aurothiomalate are more pronounced in poor sulfoxidizers (Emery et al., 1984; Ayesh et al., 1987). However, several laboratories have been unable to reproduce the reported phenotyping procedures.

Rare Genetic Phenotypes

Sensitivity to Succinylcholine. The inherited sensitivity to the muscle relaxant drug succinylcholine is one of the most thoroughly studied examples of a pharmacogenetic disorder. Shortly after the introduction of succinylcholine as an adjunct to anesthesia, a small number of patients were discovered who had prolonged apnea following the administration of a single dose of this drug. A familial occurrence of this increased sensitivity to succinylcholine was soon disclosed (Kalow and Genest, 1957). Sensitivity to succinylcholine appears to be inherited as an autosomal recessive trait. Succinylcholine is normally hydrolyzed in the serum by a cholinesterase, often referred to as pseudocholinesterase. In normal persons, this enzyme rapidly converts succinylcholine to succinylmonocholine, allowing very little of the parent compound to reach myoneural receptor sites. In patients with either an unexpected sensitivity to the drug or an abnormal resistance to its effects, different variant forms of the enzyme with altered qualitative or quantitative properties have been detected (LaDu, 1989). In the most common variant conferring low activity, so-called atypical pseudocholinesterase, the enzyme has a lower affinity for choline ester substrates, including dibucaine, and therefore is less susceptible to inhibition by dibucaine; this fact and inhibition by other chemicals, for example, sodium fluoride, have been widely used for the characterization of atypical pseudocholinesterases. A total of 10 rare and common variants of the enzyme have been described, and some of the mutations have now been characterized at the DNA level (LaDu, 1989). In general, 0% to 1% of whites may be homozygous for a low-activity variant. Deficient pseudocholinesterase variants are extremely rare in Asians and blacks.

Clinical Importance of Succinylcholine Sensitivity. Patients who are homozygous for the "atypical," "fluoride-resistant," or "silent" genes show prolonged paralysis when they are given the usual dose of succinylcholine. For them, artificial respiration may be required for several hours before the drug's effect subsides. Whenever unusual responses to succinylcholine occur, the patient and relatives should be subjected to the in vitro tests developed to classify variants of cholinesterase or to the recently developed DNA analysis. This will result in the prevention of future exposures for sensitive individuals or application of the drug with increased caution.

An interesting approach to the therapy of prolonged apnea in persons with atypical pseudocholinesterase has been proposed (Goedde and Altland, 1971). Injection of purified normal cholinesterase before and after administration of suc-cinylcholine shortened the period of apnea in sensitive individuals. This is one of the few examples of the apparently successful treatment of an inborn error of metabolism by replacement of the deficient enzyme. Although a number of other drugs such as procaine and aspirin are metabolized by hydrolysis of ester linkages, the clinical significance of cholinesterase variants or esterase deficiency seems so far to be restricted to succinylcholine hydrolysis.

Rare Inherited Variation in the Metabolism of Phenytoin, Phenacetin, and Warfarin. Several families have been reported with a genetically determined limited ability to metabolize phenytoin (Kutt, 1971; review by Inaba, 1990). The propositus in each of these families developed toxic symptoms when given the usual dose of the drug. A few patients have been observed who metabolized phenytoin unusually rapidly. Consequently phenytoin at its usual doses had no efficacy. No studies have been performed on the families of these patients (Kutt et al., 1966). Phenytoin, like a variety of other drugs, induces its own metabolism when it is repeatedly administered. Whether slow and rapid metabolism of phenytoin reflects the state of genetically controlled induction of microsomal enzymes or is related to a defective component of the drug oxidation system is not known. Abnormal metabolism of phenacetin to toxic metabolites that cause hemolysis and methemoglobinemia was observed in two sisters (Shahidi, 1968). Phenobarbital apparently increased the production of the toxic metabolite. A patient with extreme sensitivity to warfarin had a markedly delayed disappearance of bishydroxycoumarin from plasma, and his family history suggested the possibility of an inherited sensitivity to coumarin anticoagulants (Solomon, 1968). On the other hand, relative resistance to the anticoagulant effect of warfarin has been described in several subjects who seem to metabolize the drug rapidly (Lewis et al., 1967). Whether genetic factors are solely responsible for these differences is not known.

Inherited Variations in Drug Effects Independent of Pharmacokinetics

A number of genetic disorders or enzyme defects confer to their carriers modifications in response to drugs, without the biochemical defect's being directly associated with the pharmacokinetics of the offending drug (Table 32–7). Hereditary resistance to coumarin anticoagulants is the classic example of an alteration in the intensity of a response to a drug, while glucose-6-phosphate dehydrogenase (G-6-PD) deficiency is the prototype of a genetic disorder that predisposes its oth-

Table 32-7. MONOGENIC POLYMORPHISMS AND RARE VARIANTS OF PHARMACOLOGIC RESPONSE

INHERITED CONDITION	MUTANT ENZYME OR PROTEIN	INCIDENCE	INHERITANCE	DRUGS	CLINICAL PROBLEM
		Polymorphisms			
Defects in erythrocyte enzymes	Glucose-6-phosphate dehydrogenase	10% of world population, frequent in tropical and subtropical countries	X-linked	Analgesics, sulfonamides, antimalaria drugs, etc.	Hemolysis
Glaucoma	Unknown	5% of U.S. population	Autosomal recessive	Corticosteroids	Scotomas
		Rare Conditions			
Warfarin resistance	Unknown	2 white families	Autosomal dominant	Warfarin	Decreased effect of warfarin
Unstable hemoglobins	Hb H, Hb Zurich, Hb M, etc.	Multiple very rare variants described	Autosomal dominant	Sulfonamides, nitrites, etc.	Methemoglobinemia
Hepatic porphyria	Enzymes of heme biosynthesis	1/10,000 to 1/50,000	Autosomal dominant	Barbiturates, phenytoin, inducers of cytochrome P450	Exacerbation of neuropsychiatric symptoms
Defects in erythrocyte enzymes	GSH reductase, GSH peroxidase*	Very rare	Autosomal dominant	Sulfonamides, chloroquine, etc.	Hemolysis
Malignant hyperthermia with muscle rigidity	Unknown Ca^{2+}-binding protein or channel	1 in 15,000	Autosomal dominant	Halothane, succinylcholine	Hyperthermia, hyperrigidity

* GSH = glutathione.

889

erwise healthy carriers to an abnormal, novel response to drugs, that is, drug-induced hemolysis. In addition to the inherent therapeutic implications of these abnormal drug responses, an additional aspect involves the diagnostic importance of drugs in patients with genetic disorders. Drugs prove to be excellent tools at times for the discovery of hitherto-unsuspected hereditary defects.

Hereditary Warfarin Resistance. Variation in the hypoprothrombinemic response to coumarin anticoagulant drugs in humans is continuous and has a unimodal frequency distribution in heterogenous populations. Family and twin studies have established that the pharmacokinetics of this drug effect apparently is under polygenic control (Vesell and Page, 1968). Since the action of coumarin anticoagulants is easily and routinely monitored, individual adjustment of dose to variation in response usually poses no major problem. In contrast to these inherited influences on the "normal" variation in the pharmacokinetics of coumarin anticoagulants, an unusual hereditary resistance to the action of these drugs may be due to an alteration in drug–receptor interaction.

Two unrelated kindreds in whom a striking resistance to warfarin was inherited as a Mendelian autosomal dominant have been reported (O'Reilly, 1974). A large single dose of warfarin administered orally or IV to the propositus resulted in the expected concentrations in plasma and pharmacokinetic parameters; however, virtually no hypoprothrombinemic response occurred. The dosage requirement for the drug to finally induce an anticoagulant effect was approximately 20 times the usual dose. In addition to this striking resistance to the anticoagulant drug, the propositi and some of their relatives required less vitamin K to reverse hypoprothrombinemia but had higher-than-normal requirements for the vitamin when it was deleted from the diet. An alteration of the receptors for vitamin K and warfarin are suspected, although the molecular basis for this abnormality is not yet fully understood.

G-6-PD Deficiency and Drug-Induced Hemolytic Anemia. Since the discovery of primaquine-induced hemolytic anemia in blacks and its relationship to a genetically transmitted deficiency in erythrocyte G-6-PD, a large number of inherited enzyme defects in erythrocyte metabolism have been described. These abnormalities mostly involve enzymes in either the pentose phosphate pathway or in the metabolism of glutathione (GSH). By far the most common of these abnormalities is G-6-PD deficiency, an X-linked genetic trait. In fact, deficiency of G-6-PD is one of the most prevalent inherited enzyme defects in humans, probably affecting over 400 million

people throughout the world (for review, see Luzzatto and Metha, 1989). The enzyme G-6-PD catalyzes the initial step in the hexose monophosphate oxidation pathway of carbohydrate metabolism, causing reduction of NADP to NADPH. Since mature human erythrocytes lack the oxidative enzymes of the Krebs cycle, the hexose monophosphate shunt pathway is of particular importance in erythrocytes in generating NADPH. The NADPH is required by red cell GSH reductase to maintain GSH in its reduced form. Many oxidant drugs, but also infection and nutritional factors such as components of Fava beans, apparently increase the concentration of H_2O_2 in red cells and exceed the capacity of GSH peroxidase to covert H_2O_2 to H_2O, a reaction requiring NADPH. The higher demand for NADPH cannot be met in subjects with severe G-6-PD deficiency, and consequently erythrocyte integrity is disrupted and hemolysis occurs.

Numerous drugs and other compounds are capable of precipitating hemolysis in individuals with G-6-PD deficiency. Over 300 distinct variants of G-6-PD have been reported. They are distinguishable from one another by their kinetic characteristics, electrophoretic mobilities, and substrate specificities. Most of the G-6-PD variants are caused by structural gene mutations, that is, by single amino acid substitutions. The G-6-PD gene has been cloned and the primary structure of the protein deduced (Persico et al., 1981), and DNA probes for the common mutations are available. Racial and geographic differences in G-6-PD deficiency are marked.

Clinical Importance of G-6-PD Deficiency. Some variants are associated with severe, others with only mild or no reduction in erythrocyte G-6-PD activity. Frequently, the severity of the "red cell G-6-PD deficiency" (i.e., the activity of G-6-PD in vitro) and chronic hemolytic manifestations or susceptibility to drug-induced hemolysis do not correlate well. This problem can be partially resolved by assaying the enzyme under simulated physiologic conditions, taking into consideration the physiologic concentrations of the substrate, the coenzymes, and various metabolites that affect G-6-PD activity.

People with G-6-PD deficiency should be counseled against ingesting drugs that can cause hemolysis. If hemolysis occurs while taking a drug, its discontinuation depends on the severity of hemolysis, the patient's need for the drug in spite of hemolysis, and the availability of alternative drugs. The component of Fava beans causing hemolysis in G-6-PD deficiency is the glucoside divicine and its aglycone isouramile (Arese, 1982). The widespread distribution of genetic variants of G-6-PD is due to the relative resistance of G-6-PD-deficient erythrocytes to *Plasmodium falciparum.* This explains the high incidence of deficient G-6-PD in population of areas where malaria was or is endemic.

Other Enzyme Defects and Molecular Disorders of Pharmacogenetic Interest. Numerous additional examples of the modification of drug action by genetic disorders have been documented (Nebert, 1981; Kalow, et al., 1986) (see Table 32–7). Rare inherited variations in the structure of hemoglobin, such as hemoglobin H and hemoglobin Zurich or hemoglobin M, may predispose a patient to unexpected drug effects, such as hemolysis after sulfonamide therapy or methemoglobinemia after nitrite ingestion (Bunn and Forget, 1986).

Acute neuropsychiatric attacks in patients with inherited hepatic porphyrias (intermittent acute porphyria, hereditary coproporphyria, variegate porphyria) are frequently precipitated by average doses of various drugs, particularly by barbiturates, anticonvulsants, griseofulvin, and steroids. Hereditary hepatic porphyrias are characterized by a disturbance of hepatic heme biosynthesis. The primary genetic lesion in intermittent acute porphyria is a partial deficiency of porphobilinogen deaminase that results in increased inducibility of hepatic δ-aminolevulinic acid synthetase, the rate-limiting enzyme of the pathway. Hereditary coproporphyria and variegate porphyria are caused by partial defects in enzymes more distal in the pathway (Meyer, 1990). Drugs that precipitate porphyria are inducers of hepatic cytochrome P450, the terminal oxidase in microsomal drug metabolism. In the presence of a partial block in heme synthesis, the drug-mediated induction of this hemoprotein apparently results in an exaggerated response of δ-aminolevulinic acid synthetase, causing massive accumulation of the porphyrin precursors δ-aminolevulinic acid and porphobilinogen, the putative neurotoxic agents.

There are numerous additional examples of unusual or undesired drug effects in patients with rare hereditary disorders; neither the metabolic or molecular defect nor the mechanism of the abnormal drug response can be explained in most of these. They include conditions such as the hereditary malignant hyperthermia associated with anesthesia, in which the defect is suspected to be related to a defective Ca^{2+}-release channel of the sarcoplasmic reticulum (McLennan et al., 1990). The reader is referred to recent reviews, symposia, and conferences on these and other rare conditions or traits that confer a potential risk to unusual drug effects.

Editor's Note: The remarkable contrast between the third and the second editions of this text is most pronounced in this chapter. Descriptions of rare anomalies in drug effects caused by genetic differences between patients have been replaced by the ability to detect the presence and substantive contribution of polymorphism that accounts for common differences in patient response to an increasing number of commonly used drugs. The wise clinician will keep an eye on this area of investigation for even more progress in the next decade.

REFERENCES

Alvan, G.; Bechtel, P.; and Iselins, L.: The hydroxylation polymorphisms of debrisoquine and mephenytoin in European populations. Eur. J. Clin. Pharmacol., 39:533–537, 1990.

Arese, P.: Favism – A natural model for the study of hemolytic mechanisms. Rev. Pure Appl. Pharmacol. Sci., 3:123–183, 1982.

Andersson, T.; Regard, C.-G.; Dahl-Puustinen, M.-L.; and Bertilsson, L.: Slow omeprazole metabolites are also poor *S*-mephenytoin hydroxylators. Ther. Drug Monit., 12(4):415–416, 1990.

Åsberg, M.; Evans, D. A. P.; and Sjoqvist, F.: Genetic control of nortriptyline kinetics in man. J. Med. Genet., 8:129–135, 1971.

Ayesh, R.; and Smith, R. L.: Genetic polymorphism in human toxicology. In, Recent Advances in Clinical Pharmacology and Toxicology (Turner, P.; and Volans, G. N.; eds.). Churchill Livingstone, New York, pp. 137–157, 1989.

Ayesh, R.; Mitchell, S. C.; Waring, R. H.; Withrington, C. H.; Seifert, M. H.; and Smith, R. L.: Sodium aurothiomalate toxicity and sulfoxidation capacity in rheumatoid arthritic patients. Br. J. Rheumatol., 26:197–201, 1987.

Balant-Gorgia, A. E.; Balant, L. P.; Genet, C.; Dayer, P.; Aeschlimann, J. M.; and Garonne, G.: Importance of oxidative polymorphism and levopromazine treatment on the steady-state blood concentration of clomipramine and its major metabolites. Eur. J. Clin. Pharmacol., 31:449–455, 1986.

Beckmann, J.; Hertrampf, R.; Gundert-Remy, U.; Mikus, G.; Gross, A. S.; and Eichelbaum, M.: Is there a genetic factor in flecainide toxicity? Br. Med. J., 297:1326, 1988.

Bertilsson, L.; Henthorn, T. K.; Sanch, E.; Tybring, G.; Säwe, J.; and Villén, T.: Importance of genetic factors in the regulation of diazepam metabolism: Relationship to *S*-mephenytoin, but not debrisoquine hydroxylation phenotype. Clin. Pharmacol. Ther., 45:348–355, 1989.

Bertilsson, L.; Aberg-Wistedt, A.; Dumont, E.; and Lundström, J.: Rapid conjugation in an extremely rapid hydroxylator of debrisoquine: A case report supporting a coregulation of certain phase I and II metabolic reaction. Ther. Drug Monit., 10:242–244, 1988.

Bertilsson, L.; Eichelbaum, M.; Mellström, B.; Säwe, J.; Schulz, H.-U.; and Sjöqvist, F.: Nortriptyline and antipyrine clearance in relation to debrisoquine hydroxylation in man. Life Sci., 27:1673–1677, 1980.

Blum, M.; Grant, D. M.; McBride, W.; Heim, M.; and Meyer, U. A.: Human arylamine *N*-acetyltransferase genes: Isolation, chromosomal localization, and functional expression. DNA Cell Biol., 9:193–203, 1990.

Brinn, R.; Brøsen, K.; Gram, L. F.; Haghfelt, T.; and Otton, S. V.: Sparteine oxidation is practically abolished in quinidine-treated patients. Br. J. Clin. Pharmacol., 22:194–197, 1986.

Broly, F.; Libersa, C.; Lhermitte, M.; and Dupuis, B.: Inhibitory studies of mexiletine and dextrometorphan oxidation in human liver microsomes. Biochem. Pharmacol., 39:1045–1053, 1990.

Brøsen, K.: Recent developments in hepatic drug oxidation. Clin. Pharmacokinet., 18:220–239, 1990.

Brøsen, K.; and Gram, L. F.: Clinical significance of the sparteine/debrisoquine oxidation polymorphism. Eur. J. Clin. Pharmacol., 36:537–547, 1989.

Brøsen, K.; Otton, S. V.; and Gram, L. F.: Imipramine demethylation and hydroxylation: Impact of the sparteine oxidation phentoype. Clin. Pharmacol. Ther., 40:543–549, 1986.

Brøsen, K.; Gram, L. F.; Haghfelt, T.; and Bertilsson, L.: Extensive metabolizers of debrisoquine become poor metabolizers during quinidine treatment. Pharmacol. Toxicol., 60: 312–314, 1987.

Bunn, H. F.; and Forget, B. G.: Hemoglobin: Molecular, Genetic and Clinical Aspects. W. B. Saunders, Philadelphia, 1986.

CAST, The Cardiac Arrhythmic Suppression Trial (CAST) Investigators: Preliminary report: Effect of encainide and flecainide on mortality in a randomized trial of arrhythmia suppression after myocardial infarction. N. Engl. J. Med., 321:406–412, 1989.

Clark, D. W. J.; Morgan, A. K. W.; and Waal-Manning, H.: Adverse effects from metoprolol are not generally associated with oxidation status. Br. J. Clin. Pharmacol., 18:965–966, 1984.

Cooper, R. G.; Evans, D. A. P.; and Whibley, E. J.: Polymorphic hydroxylation of perhexiline maleate in man. J. Med. Genet., 21:27–33, 1984.

Dahl-Puustinen, M. J.; Lidén, A.; Alm, C.; Nordin, C.; and Bertilsson, L.: Disposition of perphenazine is related to polymorphic debrisoquine hydroxylation in human beings. Clin. Pharmacol. Ther., 46:78–81, 1989.

Dayer, P.; Desmeules, J.; Leemann, T.; and Striberni, R.: Bioactivation of the narcotic drug codeine in human lives is mediated by the polymorphic monooxygenase catalyzing debrisoquine 4-hydroxylation (cytochrome P450 dbl/bufI). Biochem. Biophys. Res. Comm., 152:411–416, 1988.

Devadatta, S.; Gangadharam, P. R. J.; Andrews, R. H.; Fox, W.; Ramakrishnan, C. V.; Selkon, J. B.; and Vela, S.: Peripheral neuritis due to isoniazid. Bull. W.H.O., 23:587–598, 1960.

Eichelbaum, M.; and Gross, A. S.: The genetic polymorphism of debrisoquine/sparteine metabolism—clinical aspects. Pharmacol. Ther., 46:377–394, 1990.

Eichelbaum, M.; Reetz, K.-P.; Schmidt, E. K.; and Zekorn, C.: The genetic polymorphism of sparteine metabolism. Xenobiotica, 16:465–481, 1986.

Eichelbaum, M.; Spannbrucker, N.; Steincke, B.; and Dengler, J. J.: Defective N-oxidation of sparteine in man: A new pharmacogenetic defect. Eur. J. Clin. Pharmacol., 16:183–187, 1979.

Emery, P.; Panayi, G. S.; Huston, G.; Welsh, K. I.; Mitchell, S. C.; Shah, R. R.; Idle, J. R.; Smith, R. L.; and Waring, R. H.: D-Penicillamine induced toxicity in rheumatoid arthritis: The role of sulfoxidation status and HLA-DR3. J. Rheumatol., 11:626–632, 1984.

Evans, D. A. P.: N-Acetyltransferase. Pharmacol. Ther., 42: 157–234, 1989.

Evans, D. A. P.: Therapy. In, Ethnic Differences in Reactions to Drugs and Xenobiotics (Kalow, W.; Aoedde, H. W.; and Agarwal, D. P.; eds.). Alan R. Liss, New York, pp. 491–526, 1986.

Evans, D. A. P.; Mahgoub, A.; Sloan, T. P.; Idle, J. R.; and Smith, R. L.: A family and population study of the genetic polymorphism of debrisoquine oxidation in a white British population. J. Med. Genet., 17:102–105, 1980.

Evans, D. A. P.; Manley, F. A.; and McKusick, V. A.: Genetic control of isoniazid metabolism in man. Br. Med. J., 2:485–491, 1960.

Fonné-Pfister, R.; and Meyer, U. A.: Xenobiotic and endobiotic inhibitors of cytochrome P450db1 function, the target of the debrisoquine/sparteine type polymorphism. Biochem. Pharmacol., 37:3829–3835, 1988.

Funck-Brentano, C.; Kroemer, H. K.; Lee, J. T.; and Roden, D. M.: Drug therapy—Propafenone. N. Engl. J. Med., 322: 518–525, 1990.

Galton, F.: The history of twins as a criterion of the relative powers of nature and nurture. J. Br. Anthropol. Inst., 5:391, 1875.

Ged, C.; Umbenhauer, D. R.; Bellew, T. M.; Bork, R. W.;

Shrivastava, P. K.; Shinriki, N.; Lloyd, R. S.; and Guengerich, F. P.: Characterization of cDNAs, mRNAs, and proteins related to human liver microsomal cytochrome P450 (S)-mephenytoin 4′-hydroxylase. Biochemistry, 27:6929–6940, 1988.

Goedde, H. W.; and Altland, K.: Suxamethonium sensitivity. Ann. N. Y. Acad. Sci., 179:695–703, 1971.

Gonzalez, F. J.; Skoda, R. C.; Kimura, S.; Umeno, M.; Zanger, U. M.; Nebert, D. W.; Gelboin, H. V.; Hardwick, J. P.; and Meyer, U. A.: Characterization of the common genetic defect in humans deficient in debrisoquine metabolism. Nature, 331:442–446, 1988.

Gram, L. F.; and Overø, K. F.: Drug interaction: Inhibitory effect of neuroleptics on metabolism of tricyclic antidepressants in man. Br. Med. J., 1:463–465, 1972.

Gram, L. F.; Debruyne, D.; Caillard, V.; Boulenger, J. P.; Lacotte, J.; Moulin, M.; and Zarifian, E.: Substantial rise in sparteine metabolic ratio during haloperidol treatment. Br. J. Clin. Pharmacol., 27:272–275, 1989.

Grant, D.; Mörike, K.; Eichelbaum, M.; and Meyer, U. A.: Acetylation pharmacogenetics. The slow acetylator phenotype is caused by decreased or absent arylamine N-acetyltransferase in human liver. J. Clin. Invest., 85:968–972, 1990.

Grant, D. M.; Tang, B. K.; and Kalow, W.: A simple test for acetylator phenotype using caffeine. Br. J. Clin. Pharmacol., 17:459–464, 1984.

Gross, A. S.; Mikus, G.; Fischer, C.; and Eichelbaum, M.: Polymorphic flecainide disposition under conditions of uncontrolled urinary flow and pH. Eur. J. Clin. Pharmacol., 40:155–162, 1991.

Haefely, W. E.; Bargetzi, M. J.; Follath, F.; and Meyer, U. A.: Potent inhibition of cytochrome P450IID6 by flecainide in vitro and in vivo. J. Cardiovasc. Pharmacol., 15:776–779, 1990.

Heim, M.; and Meyer, U. A.: Genotyping of poor metabolizers of debrisoquine by allele-specific PCR amplification. Lancet, 336:529–532, 1990.

Helsby, N. A.; Ward, S. A.; Howells, R. E.; and Breckenridge, A. M.: In vitro metabolism of the biguanide antimalarials in human liver microsomes: Evidence for a role of the mephenytoin hydroxylase (P450MP) enzyme. Br. J. Clin. Pharmacol., 30:287–291, 1990.

Hirschowitz, J.; Bennet, J. A.; Semian, F. P.; and Garber, D.: Thioridazine effect on desipramine plasma levels. J. Clin. Psychopharmacol., 3:376–379, 1983.

Hughes, H. B.; Biehl, J. P.; Jones, A. P.; and Schmidt, L. H.: Metabolism of isoniazid in man as related to the occurrence of peripheral isoniazid neuritis. Am. Rev. Respir. Dis., 70: 266–273, 1954.

Inaba, T.: Phenytoin: Pharmacogenetic polymorphism of 4′-hydroxylation. Pharmacol. Ther., 46:341–347, 1990.

Kagimoto, M.; Heim, M.; Kagimoto, K.; Zeugin, T.; and Meyer, U. A.: Multiple mutations of the human cytochrome P450IID6 gene (CYP2D6) in poor metabolizers of debrisoquine: Study of the functional significance of individual mutations by expression of chimeric genes. J. Biol. Chem., 265: 17209–17214, 1990.

Kalow, W.: Pharmacogenetics: Heredity and the Response to Drugs. W. B. Saunders, Philadelphia, 1962.

Kalow, W.; and Genest, K.: A method for the detection of atypical forms of human serum cholinesterase. Can. J. Biochem. Physiol., 35:339–346, 1957.

Kalow, W.; Goedde, H. W.; and Agarwal, D. P. (eds): Ethnic Differences in Reactions to Drugs and Xenobiotics. Alan R. Liss, New York, 1986.

Kimura, S.; Umeno, M.; Skoda, R. C.; Gelboin, H. V.; Meyer, U. A.; and Gonzalez, F. J.: The human debrisoquine 4-hydroxylase (CYP2D) locus: Sequence and identification of the polymorphic CYP2D6 gene, a related gene and a pseudogene. Am. J. Hum. Gen., 45:889–904, 1989.

Küpfer, A.; Desmond, P.; Patwardhan, R.; Schenker, S.; and Branch, R. A.: Mephenytoin hydroxylation deficiency: Kinetics after repeated doses. Clin. Pharmacol. Ther., 35:33–39, 1984.

Kutt, H.: Biochemical and genetic factors regulating dilantin metabolism in man. Ann. N.Y. Acad. Sci., 179:704–722, 1971.

Kutt, H.; Brennan, R.; Dehejia, H.; and Verebely, K.: Diphenylhydantoin intoxication: A complication of isoniazid therapy. Am. Rev. Respir. Dis., 101:377–384, 1970.

Kutt, H.; Haynes, J.; and McDowell, F.: Some causes of ineffectiveness of diphenylhydantoin. Arch. Neurol., 14:489–492, 1966.

LaDu, B. N.: Identification of human serum cholinsterase variants using the polymerase chain reaction amplification technique. Trends Pharmacol. Sci., 10:309–319, 1989.

Leeman, T.; Dayer, P.; and Meyer, U. A.: Single-dose quinidine treatment inhibits metropolol oxidation in extensive metabolizers. Eur. J. Clin. Pharmacol., 29:739–741, 1986.

Lennard, M. S.: The polymorphic oxidation of beta-adrenoceptor antagonists. Pharmacol. Ther., 41:461–477, 1989.

Lennard, M. S.; Tucker, G. T.; Silas, J. H.; Freestone, S.; Ramsay, L. E.; and Woods, H. F.: Differential stereoselective metabolism of metoprolol in extensive and poor debrisoquine metabolizers. Clin. Pharmacol. Ther., 34:732–737, 1983.

Lewis, R. V.; Lennard, M. S.; Jackson, P. R.; Tucker, G. T.; Ramsay, L. E.; and Woods, H. F.: Timolol and atenolol: Relationship between oxidation phenotype, pharmacokinetics and pharmacodynamics. Br. J. Clin. Pharmacol., 19:329–333, 1985.

Lewis, R. J.; Spivack, M.; and Spaet, T. H.: Warfarin resistance. Am. J. Med., 42:620–624, 1967.

Luzzatto, L.; and Metha, A.: Glucose-6-phosphate dehydrogenase deficiency. In, The Metabolic Basis of Inherited Disease (Scriver, C. R.; Beandet, A. L.; Sly, W. S.; Valle, D.; eds.). McGraw-Hill, New York, pp. 2237–2265, 1989.

Madras Study: Tuberculosis Chemotherapy Centre. A controlled comparison of a twice-weekly and three once weekly regimens in the initial treatment of pulmonary tuberculosis. Bull. W.H.O., 43:143, 1970.

Mahgoub, A.; Idle, J. R.; Dring, L. G.; Lancester, R.; and Smith, R. L.: Polymorphic hydroxylation of debrisoquine in man. Lancet, 1:584–586, 1977.

McLennan, D. H.; Duff, C.; Zorzato, F.; Fujii, J.; Phillips, M.; Korneluk, R. G.; Frodis, W.; Britt, B. A.; and Worton, R. G.: Ryanodine receptor gene is a candidate for predisposition to malignant hyperthermia. Nature, 343:559–561, 1990.

Meier, U. T.; and Meyer, U. A.: Genetic polymorphism of human cytochrome P450 (S)-mephenytoin 4-hydroxylase. Studies with human autoantibodies suggest a functionally altered cytochrome P450 isozyme as cause of the genetic deficiency. Biochemistry, 26:8466–8474, 1987.

Mellström, B.; Bertilsson, L.; Lou, Y.-C.; Säwe, J.; and Sjöqvist, F.: Amitriptyline metabolism: Relationship to polymorphic debrisoquine hydroxylation. Clin. Pharmacol. Ther., 34:516–520, 1983.

Meyer, U. A.: Porphyrias. In, Harrison's Principles of Internal Medicine, 12th ed. (Wilson, J. D.; Braunwald, E.; Isselbacher, K. J.; Petersdorf, R. G.; Martin, J. B.; Fauci, A. S.; and Root, R. J.; eds.). McGraw-Hill, New York, pp. 1829–1834, 1991.

Meyer, U. A.: Molecular genetics and the future of pharmacogenetics. Pharmacol. Ther., 46:349–355, 1990b.

Meyer, U. A.; Skoda, R. C.; and Zanger, U. M.: The genetic polymorphism of debrisoquine/sparteine metabolism — Molecular mechanism. Pharmacol. Ther., 46:297–308, 1990.

Meyer, U. A.; Zanger, U. M.; Grant, D.; and Blum, M.: Genetic polymorphisms of drug metabolism. In, Advances in Drug Research (Testa, B., ed.). Vol. 19. Academic Press, London, pp. 197–241, 1989.

Mikus, G.; Gross, A. S.; Beckmann, J.; Hertrampf, R.; Gundert-Remy, U.; and Eichelbaum, M.: The influence of the sparteine/debrisoquine phenotype on the disposition of flecainide. Clin. Pharmacol. Ther., 45:562–567, 1989.

Miller, C. A.; Slusher, L. E.; and Vesell, E. S.: Polymorphism of theophylline metabolism in man. J. Clin. Invest., 75:1415–1425, 1985.

Mitchell, J. R.; Zimmerman, H. J.; Ishak, K. G.; Thorgeirsson, U. P.; Tibrell, J. A.; Snodgrass, W. R.; and Nelson, S. D.: Isoniazid liver injury: Clinical spectrum, pathology and probable pathogenesis. Ann. Intern. Med., 84:181–192, 1976.

Mitchell, S. C.; and Waring, R. H.: The deficiency of sulfoxidation of S-carboxymethyl-L-cysteine. Pharmacol. Ther., 43:237–249, 1989.

Mitchell, S. C.; Waring, R. H.; Haley, C. S.; Idle, J. R.; and Smith R. L.: Genetic aspects of the polymodally distributed sulfoxidation of S-carboxymethyl-L-cysteine in man. Br. J. Clin. Pharmacol., 18:507–521, 1984.

Motulsky, A. G.: Pharmacogenetics. Prog. Med. Genet., 3:49–74, 1964.

Motulsky, A.: Drug reactions, enzymes and biochemical genetics. J.A.M.A., 165:835–837, 1957.

Mueller, R. F.; Hornung, S.; Furlong, C. E.; Anderson, J.; Giblett, E. R.; and Motulsky, A. G.: Plasma paraoxonase polymorphism: A new enzyme assay population, family, biochemical and linkage studies. Am. J. Hum. Genet., 35:393–408, 1983.

Nebert, D. W.: Clinical pharmacology. Possible clinical importance of genetic differences in drug metabolism. Br. Med. J., 283:537–542, 1981.

Neel, J. V.; and Schull, W. J.: Human Heredity. The University of Chicago Press, Chicago, 1954.

Nei, M.: Molecular Evolutionary Genetics. Columbia University Press, New York, 1987.

Omenn, G. S.; and Gelboin, H. V. (eds): Banbury Report 16, Genetic Variability in Responses to Chemical Exposure. Cold Spring Harbor Laboratory, New York, 1984.

O'Reilly, R. A.: The pharmacodynamics of the oral anticoagulant drugs. Prog. Hemost. Thromb., 2:175–213, 1974.

Otton, S. V.; Inaba, T.; and Kalow, W.: Competitive inhibition of sparteine oxidation in human liver by β-adrenoceptor antagonists and other cardiovascular drugs. Life Sci., 34:73–80, 1984.

Penno, M. B.; and Vesell, E. S.: Monogenic control of variations in antipyrine metabolite formation: New polymorphism of hepatic drug oxidation. J. Clin. Invest., 71:1698–1709, 1983.

Persico, M. G.; Toniolo, D.; Nobile, C.; D'Urso, M.; and Luzzatto, L.: cDNA sequences of human glucose-6-phosphate dehydrogenase cloned in pBR 322. Nature, 294:778–780, 1981.

Schmid, B.; Bircher, J.; Preisig, R.; and Küpfer, A.: Polymorphic dextrometorphan metabolism: Cosegregation of oxidative O-demethylation with debrisoquine hydroxylation. Clin. Pharmacol. Ther., 38:618–624, 1985.

Schröder, H.; and Evans, D. A. P.: Acetylator phenotype and adverse effects of sulphasalazine in healthy subjects. Gut, 13:278–284, 1972.

Shahidi, N. T.: Acetophenetidin-induced methemoglobinemia. Ann. N.Y. Acad. Sci., 151:822–832, 1968.

Siddoway, L. A.; Thompson, K. A.; McAllister, B.; Wang, T.; Wilkinson, G. R.; Roden, D. M.; and Woosley, R. L.: Polymorphism of propafenone metabolism and disposition in man: Clinical and pharmacokinetic consequences. Circulation, 4:785–791, 1987.

Sindrup, S. H.; Brøsen, K.; Bjerring, P.; Arendt-Nielsen, L.; Larsen, U.; Angelo, H. R.; and Gram, L. F.: Codeine increases pain thresholds to copper vapor laser stimuli in extensive but not poor metabolizers of sparteine. Clin. Pharmacol. Ther., 48:686–693, 1990.

Siris, S. G.; Cooper, T. B.; Rifbain, A. E.; Brenner, R.; and Liebermann, J. A.: Plasma imipramine concentration in patients receiving concomitant fluphenazine decanoate. Am. J. Psychiatry, 139:104–106, 1982.

Skoda, R. C.; Gonzalez, F. J.; Demierre, A.; and Meyer, U. A.: Two mutant alleles of the human cytochrome P450db1 gene (P450IID1) associated with genetically deficient metabolism of debrisoquine and other drugs. Proc. Natl. Acad. Sci. U.S.A., 85:5240–5243, 1988.

Solomon, H. M.: Variations in metabolism of coumarin anticoagulant drugs. Ann. N.Y. Acad. Sci., 151:932–935, 1968.

Steiner, E.; Dumont, E.; Spina, E.; and Dahlqvist, R.: Inhibition of desipramine 2-hydroxylation by quinidine and quinine. Clin. Pharmacol. Ther., 43:577–581, 1988.

Syvählahti, E. K. G.; Lindberg, R.; Kallio, J.; and de Vocht, M.: Inhibitory effects of neuroleptics on debrisoquine oxidation in man. Br. J. Clin. Pharmacol., 22:89–92, 1986.

Tang, B. K.: Drug glucosidation. Pharmacol. Ther., 46:53–56, 1990.

Tang, B. K.; Kadar, D.; and Kalow, M. D.: An alternative test for acetylator phenotyping with caffeine. Clin. Pharmacol. Ther., 42:509–513, 1987.

Tang, B. K.; Kalow, W.; Inaba, T.; and Kadar, D.: Variation in amobarbital metabolism: Evaluation of a simplified population study. Clin. Pharmacol. Ther., 34:202–206, 1983.

Uetrecht, J. P.; and Woosley, R. L.: Acetylator phenotype and lupus erythemetosus. Clin. Pharmacokinet., 6:118–134, 1981.

Vesell, E. S.: Pharmacogenetic perspectives gained from twin and family studies. Pharmacol. Ther., 41:535–552, 1990.

Vesell, E. S.: Pharmacogenetic perspectives: Genes, drugs and disease. Hepatology, 4:959–965, 1984.

Vesell, E. S.; and Page, J. G.: Genetic control of dicumarol levels in man. J. Clin. Invest., 47:2657–2663, 1968.

Vogel, F.: Moderne Probleme der Humangenetik. Ergebn. Inn. Med. Kinderheilkd., 12:52–125, 1959.

Vogel, F.; and Motulsky, A. G.: Human Genetics Problems and Approaches. Springer, New York, p. 435, 1986.

von Bahr, C.; Guengerich, F. P.; Movin, G.; and Nordin, C.: The use of human liver banks in pharmacogenetic research.

In, Clinical Pharmacology in Psychiatry (Dahl, S. G.; and Gram, L. F.; eds.). Psychopharmacology Series 7. Springer, Heidelberg, pp. 163–171, 1989.

Wagner, F.; Kalusche, D.; Trenk, D.; Jähnchen, E.; and Roskamm, H.: Drug interaction between propafenone and metoprolol. Br. J. Clin. Pharmacol., 2:213–220, 1987.

Wang, T.; Roden, D. M.; Wolfenden, H. T.; Woosley, R. L.; Wood, A. J. J.; and Wilkinson, G. R.: Influence of genetic polymorphism on the metabolism and disposition of encainide in man. J. Pharmacol. Exp. Ther., 228:605–611, 1984.

Ward, S. A.; Walle, T.; Walle, K.; Wilkinson, G. R.; and Branch, R. A.: Propranolol's metabolism is determined by both mephenytoin and debrisoquine hydroxylase activities. Clin. Pharmacol. Ther., 45:72–79, 1989.

Weber, W. W.: The Acetylator Genes and Drug Response. Oxford University Press, New York, 1987.

Weinshilboum, R.: Methyltransferase pharmacogenetics. Pharmacol. Ther., 43:77–90, 1989.

Whittaker, J. A.; and Evans, D. A. P.: Genetic control of phenylbutazone metabolism in man. Br. Med. J., 4:323–28, 1970.

Wilkinson, G. R.; Guengerich, F. P.; and Branch, R. A.: Genetic polymorphism of S-mephenytoin hydroxylation. Pharmacol. Ther., 43:53–76, 1989.

Woosley, R. L.; Wood, A. J. J.; and Roden, D. M.: Drug therapy—Encainide. N. Engl. J. Med., 318:1107–1115, 1988.

Zacest, R.; and Koch-Weser, J.: Relation of hydralazine plasma concentration to dosage and hypotensive action. Clin. Pharmacol. Ther., 13:420–425, 1972.

Zekorn, C.; Achtert, G.; Hausleiter, H. J.; Moon, C. H.; and Eichelbaum, M.: Pharmacokinetics of N-propylajmaline in relation to polymorphic sparteine oxidation. Klin. Wochenschr., 63:1180–1186, 1985.

33

Prescriptions

Terrence F. Blaschke

There are considerable data about drug utilization and broad general agreement that prescription and nonprescription drugs are often misused and overused (chapter 1). The explanation is not simply that physicians have not been properly educated in how to use drugs; in part, suboptimal use of drugs results because prescribing is part of the important and poorly understood interpersonal relationship between the patient and the physician. Patients seeking medical attention have certain expectations, even though they may not be consciously recognized or acknowledged by either the patients or their physicians. The physician has traditionally used the act of writing a prescription to signal to the patient that the encounter is over. Yet these are but two facets of a complex relationship that carries with it a number of implicit assumptions and agreements between the patient and the physician.

The first objective of this chapter is to analyze the nature of the physician–patient relationship as it applies to therapeutics with the hope that this will improve the dialogue and understanding between patient and physician. An important concept in this relationship is that the often brief encounter between a patient and physician leads to the establishment of a patient–physician *contract*, an unwritten relationship that ultimately contributes to the success or failure of therapy.

THE CONTRACT BETWEEN PATIENT AND PHYSICIAN

Effective treatment is based not only on the proper application of clinical pharmacologic principles to therapeutic decisions but also upon effective communication between patient and physician by verbal and nonverbal means. A primary goal of the initial interaction between patient and physician should be the development of a *therapeutic contract*. The key to the success of this unwritten contract is *mutual* trust. Past experiences of both the physician and the patient significantly influence each other's trust. The physician-patient contract is a collaboration, and if either the physician or the patient fails to contribute, the probability of a successful therapeutic outcome is greatly reduced.

Physicians rarely choose their patients. Patients seek medical attention and choose physicians for complex reasons. Both have expectations of their encounter that may be unrealistic. Early in the encounter the physician must begin to try to understand the nature of the patient's medical experiences and needs, a process that will form the basis of initial and continuing trust. Ideally, the physician and the patient will define a collaboration in which the patient takes responsibility for curing his or her own illness or reducing his or her own symptoms with the assistance of the physician. However, the acceptance of responsibility by the patient cannot automatically be assumed and must be explicitly discussed during the negotiations. During the course of the therapeutic contract the basic agreements made between the parties are maintained by continuing dialogue.

The establishment of the therapeutic contract is influenced by the setting, consisting not only of the physical environment but also the expectations of the persons involved. The physician must attempt to understand the patient's expectations as well as to define, for the patient, his or her own expectations of therapy. If the physician is not clear about his or her overall goal of treatment or the reason for writing a specific prescription (e.g., distinguishing between treating the disease or simply alleviating symptoms), transmission of a proper set of expectations to the patient will not be possible. If the physician fails to understand the patient's expectations, he or she may fail to satisfy them and will surely fail if they are unrealistic. If either the physician's or the patient's expectations are not fulfilled, mutual trust will be lost.

Two specific issues regarding the physicians's role in the therapeutic contract deserve further emphasis: control and answering questions. Patients frequently request specific treatments, and if they do not receive the expected treatment, they may go to another physician (Schwartz et al., 1989). Controlling behavior occurs with all aspects of medical care, including therapeutics. Whenever patients attempt to play the role of the physician, the physician should determine the reason for a specific request. It may be that the patient was previously given a drug and believes that it works, or that he or she wants a particular drug as an affirmation or denial of a specific disease. The physician should be concerned about the patient's concept of his or her illness because it will be a major determinant of what therapeutic approach the patient will accept or resist. Although it is permissible to assign certain aspects of therapy to the patient, the physician should determine the role of the participants in the therapeutic contract. Physicians must, however, be sensitive to the needs and fears of the patient.

In answering questions, the physician should recognize differences in the amount of information desired by the patient. This may be reflected in how the patient asks questions and how he or she perceives the role of the physician. In discussing treatment, the physician must individualize the amount of information provided to the patient. Patients vary considerably in terms of their need for information and their need to control a situation. Negotiations establish the appropriate division of control necessary for an effective and successful therapeutic contract. Physicians must be aware that *how* instructions are given may also be an important determinant of therapeutic success. Hurried or interrupted instructions can also influence trust and therapeutic outcome.

PLACEBOS AND THE PLACEBO EFFECT

The issues of control and answering questions are intertwined with the use of placebos. The Latin verb *placebo* means "I shall please," and a

placebo is defined as "any therapeutic procedure (or that component of any therapeutic procedure) which is objectively without specific activity for the disease being treated" (Shapiro, 1964). The placebo effect is "the psychological, physiological or psychophysiological effect of any medication or procedure given without therapeutic intent, which is independent or minimally related to the pharmacologic effects of the medication or to the specific effects of the procedure, and which operates through a psychological mechanism" (Shapiro, 1959). Although it seems self-evident that physicians should try to avoid therapy that is "without specific activity," the decision about whether or not placebos are justified in clinical practice or even some clinical trials is not clear-cut. The appropriate analysis of many clinical trials depends on determining placebo effects, one source of substantial variability that confounds the measurement of true drug effects. In clinical practice, many therapeutic contracts are closely intertwined with placebos and placebo effects. For these reasons, it is essential that physicians understand the concepts and principles governing placebos and placebo effects and, when appropriate, use them correctly. Ethical concerns in the use of placebos also deserve consideration.

Although placebos are usually thought of as pills or injections that simulate administration of an active drug, many interventions or procedures can elicit positive or negative placebo effects. The "pure" placebo drug is a substance that could have no conceivable pharmacologic effect on the patient, while an "impure" placebo has potential pharmacologic effects, though not necessarily any specific activity for the condition under treatment. Examples of the latter are administration of vitamin B_{12} or iron in the absence of anemia, or use of antibiotics to treat viral infections. Most therapeutic and diagnostic procedures, from simple blood drawing to cardiac catheterization, undoubtedly have considerable placebo effects. The physician and his or her associates are also important instruments of placebo effects through their appearance, attitudes, and communications with patients.

Documentation and Mechanism of the Placebo Effect

The placebo effect has been studied extensively and observed in a wide variety of conditions. Almost 40 years ago Beecher (1955) investigated placebo therapy in 1082 patients with conditions as varied as postoperative wound pain, cough, mood disturbances, angina, headache, and the common cold, and observed that satisfactory relief was obtained in 35% of these patients. Since then, many other diseases and symptoms have been added to the list. Paradoxically, as more potent and effective drugs have been developed, the placebo effect may have become even more powerful because of a generally increased faith in the value of drugs by both the patient and the physician.

Despite widespread use of placebos, the mechanism(s) underlying placebo effects are poorly understood. Whatever the mechanism, there are two requirements that are necessary if placebo effects are to be sought and achieved. First, the disease process itself or its symptoms must be capable of variable intensity, both over time and in different patients. In most situations, the powerful resilience of the human body can result in improvement of symptoms, and at times, even remissions or cures of usually progressive or fatal illnesses. It is this resilience that is enhanced by the use of placebos in about a third of all patients. In other settings where resilience has already failed, such as cardiac arrest or severe acidosis, placebos have no possible role.

Second, significant placebo effects are seen only when there is a physician–patient contract, actual or implied. While self-medication with over-the-counter (OTC) drugs may have some placebo effect, the patient's perception of the physician as a "healer" is a powerful stimulus to the placebo effect, whether it is a positive or a negative one.

This is likely related to the psychoanalytic concept of transference that can be a dynamic part of the physician–patient relationship. According to this concept, patients may transfer emotions directed at objects (including people) in their past environment onto current objects. Translated into the therapeutic situation, the good or bad results of previous experiences with drugs or physicians may be a determinant of present therapeutic success. Purely psychological stimuli from the past can influence behavior and even autonomic responses. For example, gastric acid secretion or heart rate may be affected by stimuli of which the patient is unaware at the conscious level (Katkin and Murray, 1968). Placebo responses occur much more frequently when the end point of therapy is a change in behavior (as in psychiatric treatment), subjective sensations, or pain, all of which can be influenced by patients' prior experiences and their attitudes toward those experiences. Placebo effects are also more likely when the condition under treatment is under autonomic control, such as gastric acidity, bronchoconstriction, sexual potency, or blood pressure. In general, increased anxiety and stressful situations favor placebo effects; normal control subjects are probably less likely to have placebo effects than are sick patients, who may be more ready to manifest transference or operant conditioning responses. Placebo responses are less common in protracted diseases with unremitting courses (Lesse, 1962).

Despite the above generalizations, it is still difficult to predict which patients will respond to placebo medications. Contrary to common beliefs, the "hypersuggestible" hysterical personality does not predispose to positive or negative placebo responses (Lesse, 1962), nor are women more likely than men to respond to a placebo (Trouton, 1957). Lasagna and co-workers (1954), in a carefully designed study of the placebo response in patients with postoperative pain, showed that it was impossible for an observer to determine by conversation or examination, even retrospectively, whether any given patient might manifest a placebo response. When consistent "placebo reactors" (14% of the population studied) and "nonreactors" (31%) were subjected to psychological testing, certain characteristics of both groups could be defined. The reactor group was more outgoing, more dependent on outside stimulation from the environment for emotional satisfaction, more favorably disposed to hospitalization, more concerned with visceral or pelvic complaints, somewhat more anxious, and less mature than the nonreactor group. Interestingly, the nonreactor group appeared to respond less well to active analgesic therapy, raising the possibility of classifying patients as reactors or nonreactors based on their sensitivity to active compounds; this approach has not been prospectively tested.

If a true personality type typical of the placebo reactor exists, it must be expressed to some degree in all patients since the mechanisms responsible for the placebo effect are probably operative in everyone. Occasionally a consistent placebo reactor on one day may be a nonreactor on another day; physicians may also vary in their susceptibility to produce and detect placebo effects. Perhaps the most significant clinical principle about the placebo reaction is that a positive reaction to placebo does not mean that the condition being treated is "only psychological" and not "real," nor does a negative reaction to placebo imply that the condition *is* "real." In considering placebo therapy or placebo effects, physicians should focus on the disease process and the patients' environmental and emotional stresses, rather than attempting to pigeonhole personalities.

Placebos and Toxicity

While it is obvious that adverse reactions and undesirable effects can occur with impure placebos, even pure placebos can produce adverse effects; dermatitis medicamentosa and angioneurotic edema have resulted from placebo therapy (Wolf and Pinsky, 1954). More subtle but equally important negative effects must occur when the physician himself or herself transmits, verbally or otherwise, his or her own feelings of uncertainty, doubt, or mistrust to the patient. Another possible and very important adverse effect of placebo use is the overlooking of a condition for which specific and effective treatment might be available. Placebos should never be used diagnostically, as the presence or absence of a placebo response does not differentiate between organic and psychological disorders and can only confuse and potentially delay more appropriate diagnostic tests and therapeutic maneuvers. Placebo administration also carries with it the great danger that if the patient discovers that a placebo was prescribed, he or she may feel deceived. In such cases, that physician or a subsequent physician may fail to establish a therapeutic contract.

Use of Placebos in Clinical Trials

The AIDS epidemic has once again strongly focused attention on the role of placebo medications in clinical trials. Placebo effects are seen in almost any therapeutic setting, even in progressive diseases such as AIDS, due to the "resilience"-of patients as discussed earlier. Therefore, random assignment to treatment with placebo is mandatory if no treatment has been demonstrated to have genuine benefit, in order to estimate the true effect of a new therapy accurately. With few exceptions, such as a disease that is uniformly and rapidly fatal such as human rabies, historical controls are inadequate because of variations in the effect of supportive care and time itself on the natural history and time course of the disease. The *absence* of a placebo group, when no other therapy has been shown to have genuine benefit, may delay the introduction of effective treatments developed subsequently because of the necessity of comparing these newer treatments to possibly ineffective therapies, thus increasing the baseline noise (variability), complexity, and therefore the cost and duration of the study. Also, the use of a placebo group is important to determine accurately the true toxicity of the drug being tested. There is another difficulty with trials that do not use a placebo. If the new agent is effective but less so than the standard agent, it might be discarded (appropriately or inappropriately) because of the results of a study that does not compare its effect with those of a placebo.

On the other hand, it is usually inappropriate and unethical to use placebos in a clinical trial for treating important disease if another mode of therapy has already been shown to have genuine benefit. In this situation, patients receiving placebo are being deprived of available therapy, and the real question of whether the new therapy is superior to the best existing therapy cannot be answered by such a design.

In some trials the use of a "pure" placebo may be difficult because the active compound produces symptoms or signs that may be detectable by the patient, the physician, or both. The single- or double-blind design of the experiment is lost, and the bias of the patient and physician affects the outcome of the trial, potentially invalidating it entirely. Impure placebos are sometimes necessary to avoid this problem. Other appropriate uses of placebos in clinical trials are to define and remove from a trial those patients who are placebo reactors, using the remaining patients to quantitate more clearly the difference between a known active compound and a test compound, or to determine medication noncompliers who can subsequently be excluded from the comparative trial, greatly reducing sample size requirements. The latter approach, with an impure placebo containing riboflavin, was used during the early Veterans Administration Cooperative Study Group antihypertensive drug trials (1967). The recent development of another approach to estimating compliance in clinical trials using specially designed medication dispensers may reduce problems in analysis of clinical trial data associated with the detection of placebos by patients and noncompliance in either the active or the placebo group.

Ethics of Placebo Administration

Whether placebo administration is morally justifiable in any therapeutic situation is a fundamental question. Bok (1974) argues strongly that the deception involved in the therapeutic use of placebos is intrinsically dangerous, because "deceptive practices, by their very nature, tend to escape the normal restraints of accountability and so can spread more easily. . . . There are ever stronger pressures — from drug companies, patients eager for cures and busy physicians — for more medication, whether it is needed or not." There is a real danger that liberal use of pure or impure placebos encourages other forms of deception in medicine. The trust between patient and physician, so critical to the success of the therapeutic contract, could also be threatened. More obvious breeches of the professional ethics and responsibilities of the physician are the use of placebos as an appealing substitute for the difficult task of diagnosis ("take two aspirin and call me in the morning"), as a mechanism for dealing with a difficult and demanding patient, or for providing financial or emotional rewards to the physician.

Therapeutic Use of Placebos

Because the use of placebos poses a fundamental threat to professional ethics and to the patient–physician relationship, the use of placebos *must* be limited. There are very few appropriate indications for the use of a placebo: one is when a placebo has long-term efficacy and is safer than is the use of other active agents, as has been suggested in the treatment of mild depression (Overall et al., 1962). An argument can also be made for using a placebo in a very small subset of patients who cannot be convinced that no specific drug is available, require something tangible that they can define as treatment, and will clearly continue to seek other physicians until one who will provide impure placebos is found. Furthermore, the rational use of a placebo requires that the physician follow his or her patient for evidence of therapeutic benefit or toxicity. As with any other therapeutic intervention, lack of efficacy or development of toxicity (negative placebo effects when administering a pure placebo) are indications for discontinuation of placebo therapy.

While the use of a placebo is rarely justified, the physician can often improve the therapeutic outcome by means of clear, direct communication with the patient in the course of negotiating the therapeutic contract. As indicated earlier in this chapter, the ability of the physician to produce placebo effects, through communication, is sometimes more important than the use of drugs or placebos themselves; this was nicely shown in a study of postoperative analgesia (Egbert et al., 1964). In this study preoperative patients were divided into two groups. One group had a routine preoperative visit and preoperative medication appropriate to the planned surgery. The second group had more extensive contact with the anesthesiologist, who discussed the nature, causes, and course of normal postoperative pain (chapter 25). Though both groups underwent comparable elective intraabdominal procedures, the group with greater contact with the anesthesiologist required almost 50% less analgesic medication than did the other group and were sent home an average of 2.7 days earlier by their surgeons, who were not aware of the study. Clear, direct communication between patient and physician is a critical requirement of the therapeutic contract and is essential when drugs are prescribed, since the patient's understanding of disease and treatment may influence both compliance with and efficacy of drug therapy. *Principle: No drug can substitute for planned and careful communication between physician and patient.*

COST–BENEFIT ANALYSIS AND THERAPEUTICS

An essential component of all therapeutic decisions, both qualitative and quantitative, is a thoughtful weighing of costs and benefits (cost–benefit assessment). In medicine in general, cost–benefit analyses for any diagnostic or therapeutic decisions are complex. They often require information that is unavailable or of questionable reliability and assigning "values" to possible outcomes under circumstances in which the values assigned by the patient and the physician may differ markedly. Again, the quality of the communication between patient and physician in establishing the therapeutic contract determines how accurately the physician understands how the patient values various outcomes, allowing the physician to incorporate the patient's values into the cost–benefit assessment.

In terms of medical information currently available, there are at best only a few situations that lend themselves to carrying out a formal cost–benefit analysis using a decision tree approach and sensitivity analysis. Some elegant examples of such approaches are illustrated by cost–benefit analyses applied to the management of renovascular hypertension, acute renal failure, anticoagulation in atrial fibrillation, and the treatment of Hodgkin disease. This approach has found more application in assessing diagnostic procedures than in assessing therapeutic plans (Kassirer et al., 1987), perhaps because there are surprisingly little hard data available concerning probabilities of various therapeutic outcomes. Recognition of this paucity of "hard data" has led to the growth of the field of *outcomes research*.

When information is limited, an alternative strategy must be used to maximize efficacy and minimize harm in the face of uncertainty. A first consideration is the actual disease-specific cost–benefit information available in the medical literature about a given therapeutic approach. If very little or no such information exists, or if the information is irrelevant to the particular patient for whom the assessment must be made, no proper cost–benefit analysis is possible. Therapy in such situations should be carried out only in the setting of clinical investigation, which will allow this therapeutic experience to contribute to the science of therapeutics. In some circumstances, an N of 1 therapeutic trial might be considered (see chapter 36).

Physicians should not be motivated primarily by an eagerness to treat and should not generally base therapy predominantly on theoretic considerations or on past personal experiences with "similar" patients. Conversely, fear of toxicity from a therapeutic program should not result in the denial of appropriate or adequate therapy that is indicated. For example, although there are excellent data documenting the value of achieving adequate peak concentrations of aminoglycoside antibiotics in the treatment of gram-negative bacillary sepsis or pneumonia (Noone et al., 1974;

Moore et al., 1987), there are also considerable data to indicate that underdosing in such situations is common, possibly because of concerns about the potential nephrotoxicity of aminoglycosides, even though the lesion is almost always reversible (Luft, 1984).

No physician, no matter how busy his or her practice or how careful in his or her documentation, can accumulate enough *personal* therapeutic experience to use this as the basis for most subsequent therapeutic decisions regarding individual patients. The physician is responsible, however, for trying to determine how closely his or her individual patient matches the patient population in the literature upon which the physician is basing the therapeutic plan for the individual (see chapter 41). Coupled with this matching process is the following very important concept, emphasized in chapter 1: *Principle: Every therapeutic contract and every prescription is the beginning of an experiment that requires that the physician have end points (efficacy, toxicity) in mind at the beginning and reassess the patient during the course of treatment.*

WRITING PRESCRIPTIONS

Although the first result of writing a prescription may be to indicate that the visit is over, this little-taught action is intended to set into motion behavior that is critical to the success of the therapeutic contract. As mentioned, the manner and setting in which the physician carries out this action, and the verbal and nonverbal communication that accompanies the physician's handing the prescription to the patient, can have considerable impact. The focus here, however, is the practical and technical aspects of prescription writing, the goal of which is to ensure that the pharmacist accurately interprets the intentions of the physician.

Because mistakes in filling prescriptions can have disastrous consequences, written prescriptions have followed a traditional format that minimizes errors. A basic rule is that only one prescription, which may be for a multicomponent formulation, should be written on each prescription order blank. The format of a sample prescription, shown in Fig. 33–1, contains the following minimum elements.

1. **The Date.** This is important for record keeping and because prescriptions for certain drugs are not valid beyond a specified period.

2. **Patient Identification.** The full name and address and the age or, preferably, the birthdate of the patient. These ensure proper handling and labeling of the medication and identification of the patient. This information also assists in monitoring for possible dosage errors, especially in the pediatric or geriatric patient.

3. **The Superscription.** On most blank order forms, this is preprinted using the symbol Rx (recipe, or "take"). If the superscription is absent, the physician should introduce his or her prescribed drug with this symbol.

4. **The Inscription.** Immediately below the superscription, this area contains the name, unit dose, and exact formulation of the drug to be dispensed. Only the officially approved generic name or brand name should be used. Abbreviations should be avoided, since many drugs have similar spellings and sound alike when spoken (Teplitsky, 1975). The names of drugs should be capitalized. When a generic product combination, such as triamterene and hydrochlorothiazide, is prescribed, the name and amount of each component should be written on separate lines directly

Date:	September 1, 1991
Address:	William Smith, Jr. 2115 Main Street LaCrosse, WI 12345
Birthdate:	DOB: 6/11/17
Superscription:	*Rx:*
Inscription:	Levodopa, 100 mg Carbidopa, 25 mg
Subscription:	Dispense 100 combination tablets in non childproof container
Signa:	Label Take two tablets orally with breakfast, lunch, and dinner. Take with food.
Refill:	Refill 4 times.
Prescriber's Signature:	Anne Blake, M.D. 1 Medical Plaza Drive Milwaukee, WI 54321 DEA No. AB1357902

Fig. 33–1. Format of a sample prescription.

underneath one another. Amounts should always be written in the metric system using arabic numerals.

5. **The Subscription (#).** This area provides directions to the pharmacist about the quantity of medication to provide to the patient, along with any specific instructions about the formulation, such as compounding instructions for extemporaneous (not preformulated or precompounded) prescriptions. Prescriptions may be written for any amount of medication, subject to legal and storage limits for some drug classes. Cost, convenience, and safety are factors in determining the appropriate quantity. The mental state of the patient and the potency of the drug should be considered. If a patient is depressed and potentially suicidal, a single prescription should not be written for a quantity that would be lethal if taken all at once. For conditions of limited duration, only enough drug to treat the illness should be prescribed, and patients should be instructed to discard any unused medication. Medication sharing is common, especially among the elderly, and accidental poisonings and suicides occur with stockpiled drugs. The choice of medication container is sometimes worth specifying, especially in older patients who may have difficulty in opening childproof or tamperproof pill containers and as a result transfer their medications to unlabeled or improperly labeled containers.

6. **The Signa.** *Signa* is Latin for "label," and in the past this section was introduced by the abbreviated *Sig.* It consists of the directions for the patient that will become printed instructions on the container. Write these instructions in proper English grammar, avoiding Latin or other abbreviations (such as *q.i.d.*, *q.o.d.*, etc.), which are easily misinterpreted and which must, in any case, be retranslated into English or some other language familiar to the patient. The label instructions tell the patient the amount of drug to take, the frequency and possibly the precise times of day that the medication is to be taken, and the route of administration. Sometimes, other instructions such as "Shake well before using," "Take with food," a dilution, or a caution such as "Use only externally" are included here.

Certain conventions are useful and help minimize patient error. The first word of the instructions should indicate the route of administration (e.g., "Take" for oral, "Apply" for topical, "Insert" for rectal, and "Place" or "Instill" for conjunctival, nasal, or external auditory canal administration). The indication for the medication may also be included such as "for relief of pain" or "for itching." Expressions such as "Take as directed" should be avoided. If instructions are complex or lengthy, they should be written out for the patient on a separate instruction sheet.

The importance of clear directions to the patient on how to take prescription medications cannot be overemphasized, and the instructions on the medication container itself, even when they are accurate, are rarely adequate (Stewart and Caranasos, 1989). *Principle: Even the best therapeutic approach will fail if the patient does not comply with the drug regimen or unintentionally takes it incorrectly.*

7. **Refill Information.** Physicians should consider and indicate their desire with regard to refills for each prescription written, even when several prescriptions are written at the same time. Refill instructions must comply with federal and state laws; federal law, for example, forbids refilling schedule III and IV drugs more than five times, and the prescription order is invalid 6 months after the date of issue. Schedule II drugs cannot be refilled; if more of the drug is needed, a new prescription must be written. Other factors such as suicide risk or abuse potential must also be considered here, as with the quantity of each prescription.

8. **Prescriber's Identification.** When all of the above are completed to the satisfaction of the physician, he or she should sign the order form in indelible pen with his or her name followed by the appropriate professional degree (e.g., M.D., D.O., D.D.S.). For schedule II drugs, the physician's address and Drug Enforcement Administration (DEA) registration number must also appear on the form. Other legal requirements for the prescription order form can vary from state to state, and country to country. It is always useful for the physician to provide his or her printed name, address, and phone number, to facilitate communication between the pharmacist and the prescriber. When the prescription is written by a housestaff physician on behalf of an attending physician, it is useful to provide the name of the physician of record as well.

Commonly, physicians have prescription blanks on which their name, address, telephone number, and DEA registration number have been preprinted. Keeping an exact or carbon copy of each prescription is advisable since many physicians do not transcribe such details into the patient visit note. Preprinted prescriptions, containing proprietary names and containing blanks to be filled in, should not be used as they fundamentally interfere with the thought processes that should be a part of every therapeutic decision. However, the use of preprinted forms for complicated orders or prescriptions, such as those for parenteral nutrition or cancer chemotherapy, may greatly improve the accuracy and clarity of such prescriptions (Thorn et al., 1989).

An excellent time to negotiate the responsibilities of the patient and the physician in the therapeutic contract between them is after the prescriptions are written and before the encounter is concluded. The patient must understand the physician's impression of the illness and the associated prognosis. If drugs are prescribed, the physician should explain how the medication is expected to alter the natural history or the symptoms of the illness. Patients frequently discontinue medications such as penicillin for streptococcal pharyngitis because they have not been told why the medication needs to be taken after the symptoms subside (Bergman and Werner, 1963). Patients may discontinue drug therapy at the first sign of a minor adverse effect if they have not been advised that certain effects are common and are not to be feared. Patients should be warned about dangerous adverse effects and told that they should be immediately reported to the physician (e.g., sore throat with a potentially myelosuppressive drug). Special care should be taken to give instructions related to excessive dosages. Patients should be carefully questioned about preexisting symptoms so that useful drugs are not needlessly discontinued when they complain of these symptoms for the first time in subsequent visits. Patients with long-term illnesses requiring chronic therapy, especially if it is prophylactic or suppressive, need careful explanation of the rationale for treatment.

Lack of explanation about the reasons for therapy is a major cause of noncompliance and therapeutic failures (Mazzullo et al., 1974; Larrat et al., 1990). The dialogue between patient and physician should be viewed as a process of information gathering, instruction, and motivation for both parties as they begin a therapeutic contract. If desired, the physician can also give the patient a preprinted information sheet about the drugs just prescribed. In the United States, such sheets are readily available for the most common drugs from a variety of sources (e.g., the *U.S. Pharmacopeial Convention*, the *AMA, Facts and Comparisons*, etc.).

PATIENT COMPLIANCE WITH TREATMENT PLANS

Closely intertwined with the writing of a prescription and the therapeutic contract is patient compliance with the prescribed medication regimen as well as other aspects of the treatment plan. A prescription commonly incorporates a rather involved set of instructions, making the patient responsible for self-administration of a specific drug in the correct dose, at the proper time(s) of day, and for a certain duration of therapy. When this responsibility is extended to several drugs, the complexity becomes formidable, and some deviation from perfect compliance is likely inevitable.

For example, a hypertensive patient taking two medications 4 times daily and one 3 times daily is responsible for 11 individual drug administrations per day. It is tempting to think that compliance is inversely related to the complexity of a drug regimen, and that noncompliance can be minimized by designing a simple drug regimen.

The causes of noncompliance are multifactorial (Larrat et al., 1990), and, despite beliefs to the contrary, physicians are generally unable to estimate compliance in individual patients using subjective appraisal of the patient's "character." Just as physician estimates are often faulty, patient reports of compliance must be viewed with a critical eye. Patients generally exaggerate their true intake of prescription drugs. In a study of a 10-day oral penicillin regimen for streptococcal pharyngitis in which the drug was to be given by the parent to the child, 83% of parents claimed that no dose had been missed during the 10 days of therapy. However, pill counts and urine assay for penicillin activity revealed that 55% of patients had stopped medication by the third day, 70% by the sixth day, and 85% by the ninth day (Bergman and Werner, 1963). Admission of noncompliance may be more truthful: in one group of depressed patients admitting noncompliance, the noncompliance was confirmed in almost 90% of the reported instances (Park and Lipman, 1964).

Consequences of Imperfect Compliance

Recognizing that perfect compliance is virtually impossible to achieve, it is useful to think of the consequences of less-than-perfect compliance in terms of "adequate" and "inadequate" compliance. Adequate compliance has occurred when the patient takes the medication and manifests drug-related benefit or toxicity. Adequate compliance allows the physician to assess the utility of treatment and make subsequent therapeutic decisions in a rational manner. Minor and sometimes even major departures from perfect compliance may be inconsequential, either because the full prescribed dose is not necessary for efficacy or because the therapy is inappropriate or ineffective for the condition being treated.

Inadequate compliance has occurred when not enough drug is taken to manifest either drug-related benefit or toxicity. The result of inadequate compliance is not only that the treatment regimen cannot possibly succeed but also that the physician, if he or she is unaware of inadequate compliance, cannot accurately assess the utility of therapy. This is a significant obstacle to rational therapeutic management since the physician may conclude that therapy has failed or that the diagnosis is in error. If the patient is then subjected to additional diagnostic tests or a more toxic therapy, the patient has been exposed to unnecessary risk. Another risk for the inadequately compliant patient is hospitalization (Maronde et al., 1989). If the patient has been partially but inadequately compliant and has, as a result, been prescribed a higher-than-needed dose of a drug with a narrow therapeutic ratio, enforced compliance in hospital may result in toxicity. Examples of this problem are seen frequently when patients receiving digitalis or insulin, or those with "refractory" hypertension are hospitalized. *Principle: Use of a supervised environment may reveal noncompliance rather than refractoriness to therapy as a reason for therapeutic failure.*

Compliance and Clinical Research

Partial compliance or noncompliance among test subjects in a clinical trial is of considerable importance in planning, conducting, and analyzing clinical trials. *Inadequate compliance*, as defined above, has the consequence of diluting drug effects in the treatment groups of a clinical trial and reducing the statistical power of a study. If inadequate compliance is unrecognized or its extent underestimated, incorrect qualitative or quantitative conclusions invariably ensue. At the minimum, the true difference (whether it is a positive or a negative difference) between various treatment groups or between treatment groups and control groups will be underestimated. When the true difference is small, sample size is marginal, or variability in response is large, even modest degrees of unrecognized, inadequate compliance may lead to the incorrect conclusion that there is no difference between the treatments. If such inadequate compliance is recognized, the results of such a study can be appropriately interpreted.

A costly and unfortunate example of this was seen in the University Group Diabetes Program (1970). This large multicenter project involved over 1000 patients and spanned 15 years. The fact that only about 25% of patients adequately complied with their initially assigned regimen was a major cause of the inability to draw clear conclusions from this expensive study addressing important therapeutic questions in the management of diabetes (Feinstein, 1976). In the Veterans Administration Cooperative Hypertension Study (1967), which has had a major influence in attitudes about the management of hypertension, compliance was assessed prior to enrollment by using an impure placebo containing riboflavin in the preliminary phase. Subjects who were noncompliant were dropped from the subsequent study. They made up almost 50% of potential candidates for the trial. Although these two examples are over 20 years old and well described

in the literature, the problem has not disappeared and has not been effectively resolved. In recent years, large-scale clinical trials in patients with acquired immunodeficiency syndrome (AIDS) or with asymptomatic human immunodeficiency virus (HIV) infection have been difficult to interpret because compliance was not measured and had to be inferred indirectly. Given the difficulties in subjectively determining which subjects will be inadequate compliers and recognizing the serious costs, both scientific and economic, of inadequate compliance, assessment of compliance should be and is becoming an important design consideration in clinical trials.

The ability to quantify patient compliance with reasonable accuracy using medication monitors (see below) has created the possibility of novel designs and new types of analyses of data derived from clinical trials. For example, uncontrollable variability in compliance, which occurs to some degree despite all efforts to minimize it, might be used to advantage. At the most fundamental level, the presence of a dose–response relationship is central to demonstrating that a drug has some activity (whether it is efficacy or toxicity). There may be further value in understanding the shape of dose–response curve for a drug in a population. It might reveal, hypothetically, that 90% of patients taking only 30% of the intended dose of a drug in a clinical trial demonstrated a full response while the full response rate in those taking the full intended dose was only 95%. With such data, the conclusion should then be that the correct dose of the drug should be only a third of that previously thought necessary. This could not have been recognized without the compliance measurement. Since monitoring devices also record the time and frequency of dosing, this information might theoretically be used to generate information about minimum effective doses and maximal dosing intervals still producing efficacy. As yet, these uses of electronic monitoring devices have not been validated. *Principle: Postmarketing surveillance has so far been the main site for determining a dose–response curve in the population at risk.*

Assessment of Patient Compliance

Given the limitations of subjective methods of estimating compliance and the importance of compliance to the success of a therapeutic contract or a clinical trial, one might ask what objective methods can be used for estimating compliance, and what the advantages and disadvantages of each are.

Medication Counts. Counting the number of pills or ounces of medication remaining after a given time and subtracting this from the original quantity prescribed offers an objective estimate of the quantity of medication used by the patient that can be compared with the intended intake. It is a simple and practical approach that a physician can use in the office or when the patient is admitted to the hospital and has been found to agree generally with estimates of compliance based on more sophisticated (and more expensive) measurements of drug in blood or urine (Roth et al., 1970). The obvious limitation is that actual intake is not measured and the method is subject to "pill dumping."

Measurement of Drug in Biologic Fluids. One approach to validating actual ingestion of a given drug is to look for the presence of the drug or a metabolite in blood or urine using an appropriate assay. This is frequently the justification used for making such a determination, but this approach is much less exact than is generally appreciated. It also is subject to significant misinterpretation if pharmacokinetic principles are not well understood (see chapters 1, 37, and 38). Interindividual differences in bioavailability and clearance influence the quantitative relationship between the amount actually ingested and the plasma concentration profile during a dosing interval. The concentration of a drug, measured at a single point in time during a dosing regimen, is affected by the time interval since ingestion of the last dose and by the number of doses taken during a finite time just prior to the sample. In essence, measurement of concentrations of drug in blood or urine can, at best, reflect semiquantitatively the amount of drug ingested in the time interval just before sampling. This time interval is roughly equal to about three half-lives of the drug.

Thus for drugs such as digoxin, with long half-lives and modest interindividual variation in kinetics, the measurement of concentration of drug may provide a reasonably reliable estimate of patient compliance (Weintraub et al., 1973). For drugs with short half-lives, measurement of drug concentrations is less helpful and potentially misleading, since some patients may comply with their medication only in the short interval prior to a visit to their physician (a phenomenon that has been called the "toothbrush effect") and have concentrations of drug consistent with full compliance. The timing of taking the sample relative to the last dose is very critical. Further disadvantages are the relatively high cost of some drug assays and the lack of availability of routine assays for many commonly used drugs.

A variant of direct measurement of the drug of interest in blood or urine is to use "inert markers" given with the drug. This approach was applied with the use of riboflavin in the VA hypertension trial. The method is subject to the same limitations as the measurement of the drug itself, except that often the assay for the marker is simple and inexpensive. This method may be of particular value when no assay for the drug of interest is available.

Electronic Medication Monitors. Devices that can be used to determine when drugs are removed from a medication dispenser are available. One of the early devices used a radiation source in the dispenser. Recently, the availability of microswitches, integrated circuits, and memories on a microchip have allowed relatively inexpensive electronic medication dispensers to be developed. They can record and store events such as the opening and closing of the container or the tilting of an eyedropper bottle. This information can be recovered and subsequently analyzed, tabulated, and displayed in a variety of formats (Cramer et al., 1989). The advantage of these devices is that actual times of dosing are recorded and can easily be recovered and displayed. A major limitation is that the microprocessor records the opening and closing of the device, rather than actual ingestion of the drug. Therefore, like pill counts, the data could be confounded by pill dumping or by removal of less or more than one dose with a single opening. Studies published thus far suggest that these limitations are not significant. These devices accurately and quantitatively reflect true compliance. The cost of the devices and the necessary ancillary equipment for recovering the data from the dispenser are still beyond what most physicians or patients are willing to invest. While interest in this technology is currently highest in the field of clinical trials, it has very significant potential in clinical practice, where it could play an important role in the ongoing dialogue that is a necessary component of the therapeutic contract between patient and physician.

USING DRUGS FOR NONAPPROVED INDICATIONS

As a result of its enabling legislation in 1906 and subsequent amendments in 1938 and 1962, the Food and Drug Administration (FDA) in the United States is charged with evaluating the safety and efficacy of drugs using data submitted to the agency by the pharmaceutical sponsor. However, the FDA is specifically restrained from controlling or interfering with the use of drugs or practice of medicine by physicians (see chapters 1, 34, 35, and 41). Companies submit data from Phase I–III clinical trials to the FDA in the form of a New Drug Application (NDA) claiming efficacy and safety in the treatment of one or more specified conditions. The FDA responds to these claims by approving or disapproving the NDA or by requesting additional information.

As part of the NDA approval process, the labeling of the drug, in the form of the "package insert," is negotiated between the company and the FDA. This labeling can list only those conditions for which the drug has been officially approved by the FDA. A key fact in the labeling of a drug is that the FDA can react only to data that is submitted to it and not to data that is published in the literature but *not* submitted to the agency. As a result, much of the data about the efficacy and toxicity of a drug that is accumulated after a drug is approved for marketing is never formally submitted to the FDA, never reviewed by the agency, and never becomes part of the package insert.

As discussed in greater detail in chapters 34 and 41, the limited numbers of patients and conditions studied prior to submission of an NDA significantly limits the amount of information available about a drug at the time of approval for marketing. A considerable amount of important information about a drug, including new indications, contraindications, unexpected toxicity and efficacy, and optimal dosing regimens in various special patient groups, becomes available only after many more patients have been exposed to the drug than is possible during premarketing trials (Strom and Melmon, 1979). If drugs are to be used appropriately, the physician must be knowledgeable about the limitations of the package insert and aware of the possible nonapproved indications for the use of a drug.

There is a subtle but very important distinction between nonapproved *uses* and nonapproved *indications*. The term *indication* carries with it the implication that, although not formally reviewed and approved by the FDA, the data available in the literature are sufficient to support a claim for efficacy and the indication is, therefore, generally accepted by the medical community. As such, the failure to use a drug for a nonapproved medical indication could, under some circumstances, constitute malpractice. In contrast, there are many other examples in which drugs are used to treat conditions for which the drug has not been approved and in which clear evidence of efficacy is lacking in the medical literature. There may be valid reasons for a lack of data supporting efficacy, even though the nonapproved use of the drug is indicated for a given condition. One of the most common examples is the use of a drug from a general class of drugs in which not all the members have been shown to be efficacious for a given condition but in which the pharmacologic similarities among the members of the drug class would be anticipated to result in efficacy. A well-known example is the use of many β-adrenergic receptor antagonists for either hypertension or angina, when individual drugs may have received approval for one indication but not the other. The advantage, in this situation, is the possibility of evaluating the efficacy in each individual patient, which is often not possible for other nonapproved uses of drugs (see chapter 36). For example, the use of a NSAID as a substitute for aspirin in the prevention of embolization in patients with atrial fibrillation might have some pharmacologic rationale in a patient unable to tolerate aspirin, but there are no data to support this use and only limited means of evaluating efficacy in the individual patient. Because this particular problem is uncommon and the outcome of therapy is difficult to evaluate, it is very unlikely that data will ever be generated to support or refute this particular use of the NSAID. Unfortunately, many nonapproved uses are based on substantially weaker evidence, such as individual case reports, or on purely theoretical considerations (see Fig. 41–1). While the use of drugs for such nonapproved indications cannot generally be condoned, it is neither illegal nor uncommon.

If the official package insert negotiated between the manufacturer and the FDA cannot be considered as the complete source of information about the appropriate indications for the use of a drug (Herxheimer, 1987), where can this information be found? While the medical literature is the original source of most new data relevant to drugs after they have been marketed, it is extremely difficult for practicing physicians to use journals as a source of new or comparative information about drug therapy. Over 1500 medical journals are published regularly in the United States alone; of those two to three dozen with circulations in excess of 70,000, the great majority are supported entirely by industry and are sent without charge to physicians. They cannot be considered free of bias. The profusion of information is daunting, and recent studies have shown that physicians obtain much of their information about drugs and indications from the intense activities of the marketing branch of the pharmaceutical industry (Avorn et al., 1982) and from the *Physicians' Desk Reference* (*PDR*). The latter is provided without charge to virtually all physicians in the United States. It is primarily a compilation of the package inserts for drugs with all the attendant limitations just noted. It contains no comparative data on adverse effects, efficacy, or cost.

There are several inexpensive, unbiased sources of clinical information about drugs that are preferable to the industry-supported *PDR*. They recognize that the physician's use of a drug is not limited to the indications approved by the FDA.

AMA Drug Evaluations, compiled by the American Medical Association Department of

Drugs in cooperation with the American Society for Clinical Pharmacology and Therapeutics, includes general information on the clinical use of individual drugs as well as the use of drugs in special situations. The advice it contains represents a consensus of a panel of experts. Previously published every few years, this information resource is changing over to a loose-leaf, updatable version that will also be available electronically. *Facts and Comparisons*, published by a division of J. B. Lippincott Company, is organized by drug classes and contains information in a relatively standard format that incorporates FDA-approved information supplemented with current data from the literature. A useful feature of this publication is its listing of available preparations along with a "cost index" relating the average wholesale price for equivalent quantities of identical or similar drugs and formulations. Other useful sources are *The U.S. Pharmacopeia Dispensing Information*, and the *American Hospital Formulary Service* published by the American Society of Hospital Pharmacists.

A concern that arises from the current practice of allowing drugs to be used for nonapproved indications is whether such a policy encourages pharmaceutical companies to claim safety and efficacy for the most easily documented condition when they file an NDA for a new drug. If the drug also happens to be a member of a class of drugs with approved or nonapproved indications in a variety of other conditions, the company may hope to take advantage of pharmacologic similarities to broaden the indications. Although the pharmaceutical sponsor may not legally promote the drug directly for these other indications, the promotion is subtle, automatic, and real. Another potential result of discouraging or delaying additional clinical testing for other indications is that important differences in efficacy or toxicity may not be recognized if assumptions are made about similarities among drugs in a sometimes arbitrary or artificial definition of drug "classes." A look at the significant differences in efficacy and toxicity between so-called β blockers or calcium-channel blockers serves to emphasize this point that has been made repeatedly throughout this book.

GENERIC DRUGS AND DRUG SUBSTITUTION

Once the patent protection for an FDA-approved drug expires, *generic* products may become available. A generic drug formulation is one that contains the same therapeutically active chemical ingredient as the brand-name product marketed by the drug's developer, usually in similar dose amounts and dosage forms (e.g., capsules, tablets). The Drug Price Competition and

Patent Term Restoration Act, enacted in 1984, is intended primarily to simplify and expedite the approval of generic drugs, and, largely because of a desire to reduce the cost of drugs to the consumer (and state-supported health programs), generic substitution is permitted or even mandated in many states unless specifically prohibited by the prescribing physician. These actions are based on the assumption that relatively simple and limited testing can be used to identify generic drug formulations that are therapeutically equivalent to the brand-name product marketed by the pharmaceutical company that developed the drug and that these formulations will be less expensive. These assumptions, however, are not universally accepted, and the debate has been further intensified by charges that FDA review of applications for approval of generic formulations and supervision of their manufacturing has been flawed. For a more extensive discussion of this topic, see the reviews by Schwartz (1985) and Strom (1987). This section will focus on the pharmacologic issues that should be considered by the physician in deciding how to prescribe a drug available generically.

Two fundamental facts bear on the prescribing issue. One is that current FDA statistical guidelines permit the bioavailability of a generic product to differ by as much as 30% from the brand-name product, although for some drugs with narrow therapeutic ratios (e.g., warfarin) a 10% maximum difference is required. Moreover, these bioequivalence studies are normally single-dose studies carried out in relatively small numbers of young healthy volunteers using crossover designs. Patient factors that could influence bioavailability, such as concurrent illnesses and other drugs, or differences that would only be apparent with multiple-dose administration would not be detected with this design. The second fact is that the FDA has insufficient resources to monitor the pharmaceutic industry and ensure that all firms follow good manufacturing practices that minimize lot-to-lot variability. A consequence of these facts is that if patients receive different generic or brand products during a chronically administered course of a drug, the amount of drug to which the patient's target tissues are exposed with time may vary by about twofold or more. However, either most drugs have a wide therapeutic ratio and are usually given in doses in excess of those required to achieve the desired therapeutic effect (e.g., many antibiotics) or their dosage, using any chosen product, can be titrated to achieve the desired clinical effect (e.g., analgesics, anti-inflammatory agents, psychoactive drugs). Therefore, from a practical clinical viewpoint, variability of this magnitude is relevant primarily for chronically administered drugs having a narrow therapeutic ratio, such as antiarrhythmic drugs, cardiac glycosides, anticonvulsants, antidepressants, and anticoagulants.

To encourage physicians to prescribe generically and to assist them in determining which drugs are not likely to have bioequivalence problems, the FDA has published a series of monographs entitled *Approved Prescription Drug Products with Therapeutic Equivalence Evaluations* (1985). Although there is disagreement with some of the FDA bioequivalence evaluation methods, such information is helpful to physicians considering whether to prescribe a particular drug generically or to permit generic substitution by the pharmacist. When using a drug with a narrow therapeutic ratio, although the physician may choose to prescribe a less expensive generic equivalent, if available, he or she must always individualize the dose for the patient using the same product that will be employed during long-term therapy. Once the dose has been titrated, substitution to another product should be explicitly avoided; this may require the physician to communicate directly with the pharmacist responsible for providing refills and to explain to the patient the need for obtaining the drug from a single source. If substitution of another brand name or generic equivalent is necessary, the physician must monitor the patient for possible loss of efficacy or toxicity. Measurements of drug concentrations in serum or plasma are available for many drugs having narrow therapeutic ratios. A steady-state measurement of drug concentration should be obtained whenever there is a change in the product used, especially when the drug is being administered as prophylaxis against infrequent but potentially serious events, such as cardiac arrhythmias or seizures. In the event of apparent loss of efficacy during chronic therapy, a change in product bioavailability should be considered as a possible explanation, although noncompliance is a more likely explanation. Again, if available, measurement of concentrations of drug in serum may help in working up this therapeutic problem. Unexpectedly low concentrations could represent either poor bioavailability or poor compliance, while concentrations within the therapeutic range suggest loss of efficacy due to change in the patient.

It is often difficult for the physician to determine whether there will be significant cost savings to the patient or the insurance provider if a prescription is filled with a generic product as opposed to a specific product whose brand name is familiar to the physician. *Facts and Comparisons*, mentioned earlier, is indexed by both generic and brand names, lists drug products with identical formulations, and gives the name of the manufacturer; it also provides a cost index, which is a ratio of the average *wholesale* prices for equivalent quantities of a drug. While this type of information may alert the physician to potentially large differences in the cost of various generic equivalents, the actual cost of the drug to the patient is determined by many factors, including the profit margin of the source used to fill the prescription as well as the price charged by the manufacturer. Not only is it appropriate to discuss prescription costs with the patient, but such exchanges may improve the physician–patient relationship by demonstrating the physician's interest in financial matters that are frequently of concern to the patient and may broaden the dialogue in this important area. If, as discussed above, the therapeutic ratio and chronicity of treatment favor the use of a particular drug product, this should be explained to the patient. On the other hand, when prescribing drugs for which modest differences in bioavailability are unlikely to affect efficacy or toxicity, the physician should permit substitution of the least expensive generic equivalent.

NONPRESCRIPTION DRUGS

Nonprescription, or OTC, drugs are medications that can be obtained without a prescription. The fact that nonprescription drugs can be obtained without consultation with a physician may seem to imply that they have little significant pharmacologic activity and that the physician need not be concerned about their use. Both implications are certainly false. Nonprescription drugs represent an important part of the therapeutic armamentarium available to patients as well as to physicians. If a physician is not aware of the use of such drugs by his or her patient or does not recommend them when indicated, an important part of the therapeutic contract will have been neglected.

Nonprescription drugs are a multibillion dollar industry in the United States. Recognizing that they can have significant therapeutic or toxic activity, one might ask why nonprescription drugs exist at all, and why they differ from country to country. The answer relates to access, economics, and individual liberties. The history of nonprescription drugs in the United States can be traced back to the mid-1850s, when the majority of health care was provided not by physicians but by lay practitioners, and when most remedies or medicines were concocted and administered in the home. Following the Civil War, the preparation of remedies in the home was replaced by the purchase of patent medicines. By 1905, the market for patent medicines was immense, well over $100 million per year, and the profits were enormous. The patent medicine makers were the first American manufacturers to use advertising in order to establish a national market and spent as much as $400,000 advertising a single product. Between about 1890 and 1920, however, an intense economic and political struggle (including the passage of the Pure Food and Drug Act of 1906), along with a change in public preferences away from home medical care to professional care, resulted in a marked decline in the public's demand for and use of patent medicines.

The public's fear and mistrust of hospitals and physicians was replaced by concerns about the dangers of self-treatment and greater confidence in the medical profession. Coincidentally there was a sharp increase in the sale of prescription drugs. Patent medicines, which were no longer able to compete with prescription drugs, were replaced by a wide variety of OTC products aimed primarily at providing symptomatic relief for minor problems and complementing rather than competing with medical services provided by physicians (Caplan, 1989).

Currently, the trend toward self care, an increasing role for the patient in maintaining his or her own health, and the reclassification of many drugs formerly available only by prescription to OTC status has increased the nonprescription drug market. It now amounts to over $4 billion, or more than $15 for every person in the United States per year. However, accurate statistics on the individual use of nonprescription drugs are scarce. Surveys suggest that a high percentage of Americans use nonprescription drugs. These drugs constitute 70% of the initial therapy of episodes of illness (Knapp and Knapp, 1972).

Given this background, the significance of nonprescription drugs to the therapeutic contract between patient and physician must now be put into context. Some questions that need to be addressed are: What kinds of nonprescription drugs are used? Who uses them? How does their use relate to prescription drug use or to the seeking of professional care? Not surprisingly, data indicate that both prescription and nonprescription drug use are more common in elderly persons. In a study among ambulatory elderly patients in mainly rural areas of northeastern New York state, 81% reported that they were taking at least one prescription or nonprescription medication (Stoller, 1988). About half of those surveyed reported taking nonprescription medications in the past month. Among these, the average number of nonprescription medications was 1.5 per person. The most frequently used nonprescription medications were analgesics, taken by 39% of respondents; laxatives, taken by 17%; vitamins, taken by 5%; antacids, taken by 4%; and cough or cold preparations, taken by about 2%. The Health Insurance Experiment of the Rand Corporation (Leibowitz, 1989) found fairly infrequent purchase of nonprescription drugs by noninstitutionalized individuals under age 65, who averaged just under one purchase per person per year (Leibowitz et al., 1985). Analgesics and cold remedies accounted for about 25% of the purchases, while antacids, bronchodilators, and diuretics, commonly associated with more chronic illnesses, also accounted for about 25% of purchases. Both Stoller and Leibowitz attempted to analyze the factors explaining the use of nonprescription drugs and its impact on the use of prescription drugs and the seeking of professional health care. Both reached the same general conclusions that nonprescription drugs are not used as a substitute for prescription medications or for obtaining professional medical care for illnesses perceived as serious by the patient.

There are a number of factors that seem to influence the use of nonprescription medications. Elderly persons and women are the most frequent users of nonprescription drugs. Patients with higher educational levels, less time available for physician visits, or less access to professional medical care are more likely to use nonprescription medications, as are patients who are socially isolated or who have chronic illnesses. The factor that has the greatest influence on the use of nonprescription medications is the number of recent symptoms, while both symptoms and the frequency of visits to the physician influence the number of prescription medications (Stoller, 1988). The use of nonprescription and prescription drugs is correlated, partly because less healthy individuals use more of both types of drugs. Interestingly, as the cost to the patient of prescription and nonprescription drugs increases, fewer of each type are purchased per capita (Leibowitz, 1989). These two careful studies suggest that nonprescription drugs are used primarily for symptomatic relief, and not as substitutes for prescription drugs or visits to the physician except when access to professional care is limited and then only for nonthreatening symptoms.

Despite the widespread use of nonprescription drugs, the incidence and frequency of serious toxicity from these agents is very low. Fear of *dramatic* increases in nephrotoxicity with the reclassification of NSAIDs such as ibuprofen, making them available on a nonprescription basis, has not been warranted, although deterioration of renal function may occur in patients with certain preexisting clinical conditions such as congestive heart failure, cirrhosis, and renal insufficiency (Murray and Brater, 1990). The most common adverse reaction to nonprescription drugs undoubtedly is GI bleeding due to acetylsalicylic acid. As with adverse reactions to prescription drugs, most unwanted reactions to nonprescription drugs are predictable, mechanism-based, and dose-related effects that are due to drug use in improper settings, excessive doses, or interactions with other prescription or nonprescription drugs.

The attitudes and responsibilities of physicians with regard to nonprescription drugs determines whether this type of drug has a positive or a negative impact on the therapeutic contract. In a study of prescribing behavior for anti-inflammatory drugs in two VA hospitals, although physicians believed that aspirin was equally as effective as proprietary nonsteroidals in treating musculoskeletal complaints, had a similar frequency of adverse effects, and was considerably less expensive, they used prescription nonsteroidals almost six times as often as aspirin (Epstein et al., 1984). These authors concluded that physician attitudes about the importance of such issues as costs and placebo effects play a more important role in drug selection than factual information about the alternative drugs themselves.

Physicians should recognize the legitimate role of nonprescription medications in the current environment in which sophisticated and busy patients play a greater role in their own health care decisions. In this regard, an important initial activity at the time of the first encounter with a new patient is to obtain a complete drug history from the patient. The history should include nonprescription drugs and should be updated at each subsequent visit. This history may provide useful insights about the patient's attitudes about drugs and expectations of medical care, as well as providing an opportunity to discuss the proper indications and use of nonprescription medications. This history is also important in avoiding potential interactions with prescribed medications. Moreover, as drugs formerly available only by prescription are changed to nonprescription status, physicians should consider using the nonprescription equivalent, which is usually considerably less expensive. *Principle: The dialogue between patient and physician regarding the indication, proper use, and potential side effects of the nonprescription drug should be no different than if the physician had written a prescription. In an era when cost considerations are greater than ever before, nonprescription drugs should be considered, when appropriate, as alternatives to prescription medications.*

REFERENCES

Approved Prescription Drug Products with Therapeutic Equivalence Evaluations, 6th ed. Department of Health and Human Services, Public Health Service, Food and Drug Administration, Center for Drugs and Biologics, Rockville, Md., 1985.

Avorn, J.; Chen, M.; and Hartley, R.: Scientific versus commercial sources of influence on the prescribing behavior of physicians. Am. J. Med., 73:4–8, 1982.

Beecher, H. K.: The powerful placebo. J.A.M.A., 159:1602–1606, 1955.

Bergman, A. B.; and Werner, R. J.: Failure of children to receive penicillin by mouth. N. Engl. J. Med., 268:1334–1338, 1963.

Bok, S.: The ethics of giving placebos. Sci. Am., 231:17–23, 1974.

Caplan, R. L.: The commodification of American health care. Soc. Sci. Med., 28:1139–1148, 1989.

Cramer, J. A.; Mattson, R. H.; Prevey, M. L.; Scheyer, R. D.; and Ouellette, V. L.: How often is medication taken as prescribed? A novel assessment technique. J.A.M.A., 261:3273–3277, 1989.

Egbert, L. D.; Battit, G. E.; Welch, C. E.; and Bartlett, M. K.: Reduction of postoperative pain by encouragement and instruction of patients. A study of physician-patient rapport. N. Engl. J. Med., 270:825–827, 1964.

Epstein, A. M.; Read, J. L.; and Winickoff, R.: Physician beliefs, attitude and prescribing behavior for anti-inflammatory drugs. Am. J. Med., 77:313–318, 1984.

Feinstein, A. R.: Clinical biostatistics: XXXV. The persistent clinical failures and fallacies of the UGDP study. Clin. Pharmacol. Ther., 19:78–93, 1976.

Herxheimer, A.: Basic information that prescribers are not getting about drugs. Lancet, 1:31–32, 1987.

Kassirer, J. P.; Moskowitz, A. J.; Lau, J.; and Pauker, S. G.: Decision analysis: A progress report. Ann. Intern. Med., 106:275–291, 1987.

Katkin, E. S.; and Murray, E. W.: Instrumental conditioning of autonomically mediated behavior: Theoretical and methodological issues. Psychol. Bull., 70:52–68, 1968.

Knapp, D. A.; and Knapp, D. E.: Decision-making and self medication: Preliminary findings. Am. J. Hosp. Pharm., 29:1004–1012, 1972.

Larrat, E. P.; Taubman, A. H.; and Willey, C.: Compliance-related problems in the ambulatory population. Am. Pharm., NS30:18–23, 1990.

Lasagna, L.; Mosteller, F.; von Felsinger, J. M.; and Beecher, H. K.: A study of the placebo response. Am. J. Med., 16:770–779, 1954.

Leibowitz, A.: Substitution between prescribed and over-the-counter medications. Med. Care, 27:85–94, 1989.

Leibowitz, A.; Manning, W. G. Jr.; and Newhouse, J. P.: The demand for prescription drugs as a function of cost sharing. Soc. Sci. Med., 21(10):1063–1069, 1985.

Lesse, S.: Placebo reactions in psychotherapy. Dis. Nerv. Syst., 23:313–319, 1962.

Luft, F. C.: Clinical significance of renal changes engendered by aminoglycosides in man. Br. Soc. Antimicrob. Chemo., 13(suppl. A):23–28, 1984.

Maronde, R. F.; Chan, L. S.; Larsen, F. J.; Strandberg, L. R.; Laventurier, M. F.; and Sullivan, S. R.: Underutilization of antihypertensive drugs and associated hospitalization. Med. Care, 27:1159–1166, 1989.

Mazzullo, J.; Cohn, K.; Lasagna, L.; and Griner, P.: Variation in interpretation of prescription instructions. J.A.M.A., 227:929–931, 1974.

Moore, R. D.; Lietman, P. S.; and Smith, C. R.: Clinical response to aminoglycoside therapy: Importance of the ratio of peak concentrations to minimal inhibitory concentration. J. Infect. Dis., 155:93–99, 1987.

Murray, M. D.; and Brater, D. C.: Adverse effects of nonsteroidal anti-inflammatory drugs on renal function (editorial). Ann. Intern. Med., 112:559–560, 1990.

Noone, P.; Parsons, T. M. C.; Pattison, J. R.; Slack, R. C. B.; Garfield-Davies, D.; and Hughes, K.: Experience in monitoring gentamicin therapy during treatment of serious gram negative sepsis. Br. Med. J., 1:447–481, 1974.

Overall, J. E.; Hollister, L. E.; Pokorny, A. D.; Casey, J. F.;

and Katz, G.: Drug therapy in depressions. Controlled evaluation of imipramine, isocarboxazide, dextroamphetamine-amobarbital, and placebo. Clin. Pharmacol. Ther., 3:16–22, 1962.

Park, L. C.; and Lipman, R. S.: A comparison of patient dosage deviation reports with pill counts. Psychopharmacologia, 6:299–302, 1964.

Roth, H. P.; Caron, H. S.; and Bartholomeau, P.: Measuring intake of a prescribed drug, a bottle count and a tracer technique compared. Clin. Pharmacol. Ther., 11:228–237, 1970.

Schwartz, L. L.: The debate over substitution policy. Its evolution and scientific bases. Am. J. Med., 79(suppl. 2B):38–44, 1985.

Schwartz, R. K.; Soumerai, S. B.; and Avorn, J.: Physician motivations for nonscientific drug prescribing. Soc. Sci. Med., 28:577–582, 1989.

Shapiro, A. K.: Factors contributing to the placebo effect. Their implications for psychotherapy. Am. J. Psychother., 18(suppl. 1):73–88, 1964.

Shapiro, A. K.: The placebo effect in the history of medical treatment: Implications for psychiatry. Am. J. Psychiatry, 116:298–304, 1959.

Stewart, R. B.; and Caranasos, G. J.: Medication compliance in the elderly. Med. Clin. North Am., 73:1551–1563, 1989.

Stoller, E. P.: Prescribed and over-the-counter medicine use by the ambulatory elderly. Med. Care, 26:1149–1157, 1988.

Strom, B. L.: Generic drug substitution revisited. N. Engl. J. Med., 316:1456–1462, 1987.

Strom, B. L.; and Melmon, K. L.: Can post-marketing surveillance help to effect optimal drug therapy? J.A.M.A., 242: 2420–2423, 1979.

Teplitsky, B.: Caution! 1,000 drugs whose names look-alike or sound-alike. Pharm. Times, 41:75–79, 1975.

Thorn, D. B.; Sexton, M. G.; Lemay, A. P.; Sarigianis, J. S.; Melita, D. D.; and Gustafson, N. J.: Effect of a cancer chemotherapy prescription form on prescription completeness. Am. J. Hosp. Pharm., 46:1802–1806, 1989.

Trouton, D. S.: Placebos and their psychological effects. J. Ment. Sci., 103:344–354, 1957.

University Group Diabetes Program: A study of the effects of hypoglycemic agents on vascular complications in patients with adult-onset diabetes: I. Design, methods and baseline characteristics. Diabetes, 19(suppl. 2):747–783, 1970.

Veterans Administration Cooperative Study Group on Antihypertensive Agents: Effects of treatment on morbidity in hypertension: Results in patients with diastolic blood pressure averaging 115–129 mmHg. J.A.M.A., 202:1028–1034, 1967.

Weintraub, M.; Au, W. Y.; and Lasagna, L.: Compliance as a determinant of serum digoxin concentration. J.A.M.A., 224: 481–485, 1973.

Wolf, S.; and Pinsky, R. H.: Effects of placebo administration and occurrence of toxic reactions. J.A.M.A., 155:339–341, 1954.

34

Drug Discovery and Development

Richard D. Mamelok

The discovery and development of a drug is a many-step process. The activity requires that multiple skills and various experts be focused on a single goal: producing a useful therapeutic agent. The history of how skills from academia and industry have been melded to produce new drugs is simply fascinating. Equally impressive is the apparent delicate balance that must be maintained if the relationship is to flourish (Swann, 1988). The early discovery process, the initial realization that a particular chemical might have medical utility, can have many wellsprings. Important drugs have been discovered by carefully planned, highly logical interventions in a well-defined biochemical pathway, or by serendipity, or by the screening (the more diversified the better) of a large number of chemical entities for a preconceived desirable pharmacologic effect. Recounting the logical approaches that led, for example, to purine analogs as antimetabolic drugs (Elion, 1989) or to the discovery of β-adrenergic antagonists or of H_2 antagonists is to recount scientific intellect and technology transfer at the Nobel Prize level. Examples of the serendipitous discovery of drugs illustrate the potential power of recognizing the unexpected and how to take advantage of it.

From discovery of a new chemical entity (NCE) to marketing often takes a decade or longer (Lasagna, 1979). The cost of establishing the evidence that allows a new drug to become available to patients ranges from tens of millions of dollars to over one hundred million dollars (Lasagna, 1979; Chakrin and Byron, 1987). Over time, the cost seems to be rapidly rising.

What evidence is required to show that a drug is safe and effective? What decisions need to be made during development of a drug in order to decide to persevere or to discontinue development of an NCE? What information is required to make such decisions? There are no absolute answers to any of these questions. The purpose of this chapter is to provide some insight into the problems grappled with by basic scientists, toxicologists, pharmaceutical chemists, clinical investigators, governmental regulators, and clinicians in deciding how to make use of a new chemical entity or a new drug.

DRUG DISCOVERY AND PRECLINICAL DEVELOPMENT

Drug discovery is the portion of drug development in which NCEs are sought for a particular in vitro or in vivo biologic activity. A biologic target is chosen and compounds are tested to see how they interact with the target. The biologic target could be a particular biochemical reaction that is thought to be important in causing a pathologic process; it could be a receptor, a microorganism, or a more macroscopic effect such as inhibiting an inflammatory reaction or lowering blood pressure. The target, at this stage, is not human.

The choice of an initial target system depends on the depth of our understanding of the pathogenesis of a particular disease for which treatment is sought. For example, if one wanted to discover a drug to treat infection caused by a specific bacterium, the killing of that bacterium in vitro would be a logical initial test of the possible efficacy of the NCE. Such a specific target, highly predictive of activity against the organism wherever it is encountered, is possible only because we have a very detailed and basic understanding of what a bacterial infection is. Contrast bacterial infection with rheumatoid arthritis, in which the basic pathogenetic mechanisms are not known.

In the latter case, a number of actions could be appropriate candidates for initial screening of compounds, including inhibition of synthetic enzymes for prostaglandins or cytokines, inhibition of helper T-lymphocyte activation, or even specific binding to the MHC II locus on lymphocytes. While a compound having any such activity might be useful to patients with rheumatoid arthritis, the predictability of success is less than it would be for antibiotics against a particular infectious organism. Moreover, few, if any, new drugs will cure rheumatoid arthritis. Symptomatic relief or possibly a slowing of progression may be the best result of research that one can hope for with today's understanding of the disease.

The screening of compounds for biologic activity requires several steps, usually in progressively complex systems. Early in the discovery process, the goal is to screen a large number of compounds in order to identify those with highest activity and potency toward a particular target. Often hundreds of chemical entities are so screened. Of those, several may be tested further. In the example of a bacterial infection, the disease can be induced in a susceptible animal and the ability of the investigational drug to cure the infection can be observed. In the case of rheumatoid arthritis, the drug can be given to an animal in which arthritis has been induced by administering a foreign substance to the joint. The induced arthritis is not rheumatoid arthritis, but rather an arthritis that shares some, but certainly not most, of the *attributes* of rheumatoid arthritis. An approximation of a human disease in an animal is called a *model* of the disease. In the examples of bacterial infection and rheumatoid arthritis, the animal model for infection actually is the same infection as in the human disease for which treatment is desired, whereas for rheumatoid arthritis the model is much less like the human disease and the drug's effects in the model may be much less applicable to humans. Models are extensively used in pharmaceutic development, but to the degree that they are imprecise reflections of human diseases, they are variably reliable in predicting efficacy in humans even though the efficacy is seen in the model. Conversely, an absence of effect in the model does not preclude value in humans. The frequency with which useful compounds are discarded because of their failure to affect a particular animal model is not known, since negative results in models almost always lead to discontinuation of the development process before testing occurs in humans. *Principle: The effects of drugs in humans are precious and often unique. Full analysis of events drugs can cause is a major way of revealing benefits that were not expected at the time of marketing.*

Bacterial infections are not the only diseases in which a good understanding of the pathophysiology has lead to effective and rather specific therapies. Therapeutically successful drugs that were designed to react with specifically identified molecular targets now are numerous. These include β-adrenergic antagonists, histamine H_2 antagonists, tissue-derived plasminogen activator, and inhibitors of enzymes such as angiotensin-converting enzyme (ACE) and HMG-CoA reductase, the rate-limiting enzyme in the synthesis of cholesterol. Undoubtedly, as diseases are better understood at the molecular level, more specific, but not necessarily more effective, therapies will ensue. Generally speaking, the discovery of disease-specific drugs is heavily dependent on the understanding of basic molecular mechanisms of that disease. The recent application of molecular biologic techniques to isolate and synthesize a wide variety of endogenous, biologically active molecules has increased the interaction between the discovery of drugs and the discovery of molecular pathogenetic mechanisms (Hood, 1988; Halperin, 1988; Mario, 1988).

In some settings, instead of screening many compounds to see their effect in a model of a disease, a specific molecule, known to participate in biologic processes, is screened for use in a variety of diseases. This screening philosophy operates even if the test substance has no known activity in the pathologic process of interest. For example, interferons have been tested in a variety of viral infections and cancers. While interferons are important in modulating immune reactions to such diseases, whether they play a central role in immunity has not been established. Nevertheless, the feasibility of testing such endogenous, biologically active compounds in a spectrum of diseases might lead to new (possibly simultaneous) discoveries in the pathogenesis and therapy of those diseases. *Principle: The unexpected effects of drugs often helps to extend knowledge of the pharmacology of the drug and the pathogenesis of the disease it affects.*

The purpose of "drug discovery" is to identify chemicals that have a high chance of providing therapeutic benefit. Once such a compound is identified, a series of investigations in animals and humans takes place to demonstrate that the compound is efficacious and that it is safe enough for use in people. This phase of investigation is known as *development*. Most drugs that are discovered and go into development do not evolve into marketed medicines. The reasons for the high rate of failure include unacceptable toxicity; lack of efficacy; and problems with developing an acceptable way to deliver the drug to a patient.

The steps required to develop a chemical as a drug are straightforward. In addition to establishing that the NCE has a desired pharmacologic effect in animals, its other pharmacologic effects must be determined. Understanding the full pharmacologic profile of the NCE allows prediction of what to anticipate in humans. Discovery of an undesired effect may terminate further development. For example, if a potential antihypertensive drug causes a fall in blood pressure but also produces extreme sedation, the drug is not likely to be acceptable to patients. Another purpose of pharmacologic testing is to define the dose–response relationship of the drug. The lowest dose (on a basis of weight of drug per weight of animal, e.g., mg/kg) that causes a discernible pharmacologic effect must be determined. This is established in several species of animal in order to establish the safe dose that can be used to initiate testing in humans. The shape (steepness) of the dose–response curve also is useful in design of the first studies in humans. If the dose–response curve is steep, the drug may be difficult to give to humans without producing extreme effects. If the curve is shallow, the dose can be progressively increased to carefully establish the tolerated dose range.

Knowing the metabolic profile of a drug in several species points toward the methods of search for and discovery of metabolites in humans. Major metabolites should be tested for their pharmacologic or toxicologic activity and then sought during testing in humans. However, before a drug is given to humans, it is very difficult to know which animal species will most mimic the metabolic profile that will be seen in humans.

The distribution of drug throughout an animal's body also is determined using radiolabeled drug. This information can alert investigators to look for effects that relate to organs where large concentrations of the drug may reside in humans.

Toxicologic testing in animals helps to focus observation when the drug is given to humans. The toxicologist also can determine the mutagenic, carcinogenic, and teratogenic potential the drug might have. Almost always, IV administration is used in animal testing because using that route ensures that the drug will reach the systemic circulation. Depending on what the eventual route of administration in humans is likely to be, other routes also are tested. Very large doses are given during toxicologic studies in animals. The premise is that large doses will exaggerate effects and reduce variability in results due to individual and species differences in susceptibility to a given toxic effect. High doses also are used in order to compensate for the observation that small mammals usually tolerate doses higher than humans do. As in the case of the metabolic studies, humans may be uniquely susceptible to a given effect, and animal studies will not reveal this.

Toxicologic testing is done in animals for periods that often are shorter than those that eventually will be used in humans for chronic therapies. Since small mammals have a life cycle that is considerably shorter than humans', we assume that the time it takes for many reactions to occur during chronic administration of drug also will be shortened (Gogerty, 1987). Toxicologic studies will not detect allergic or other idiosyncratic reactions that might occur in humans, nor will they predict symptomatic or subjective experiences that might be produced in people.

The duration of toxicologic studies varies. Usually single, very high dose studies are done first. Later, studies of progressively longer duration are used. The longest studies usually are 2 years of daily dosing in order to detect carcinogenic effects in rodents. Exceptions to this are human recombinant peptides and proteins, because nonhuman species develop antibodies to these. Thus, long-term delivery is not feasible.

Drug development involves physical and chemical research, in addition to the obvious, biologic research. Economically feasible synthetic production processes have to be designed. Strict manufacturing procedures are followed to ensure consistency in purity of the chemical, regardless of the batch. In addition, the drug must be formulated as a final product. Formulation is the process of inserting the active drug into a vehicle that allows practical storage and administration. Milligram or microgram quantities of a pure drug could not be administered accurately. Thus, the drug must be mixed either in solution or in a matrix of solid, pharmacologically inert materials (excipient) that can be formed into a capsule or tablet. Solid-dose forms must dissolve adequately in the GI tract, and the excipient component must not interact with the NCE. In addition, the drug product must be chemically stable to ensure that it will not rapidly degrade during storage. The time past which a substantial percentage of the drug will deteriorate must be well described. This time yields the *expiration date* for drugs.

CLINICAL DEVELOPMENT OF A NEW CHEMICAL ENTITY

Understanding the spectrum of a drug's pharmacologic effects in humans is the basis for clinicians designing the most effective use of the drug in patients. Experiments designed to discover pharmacologic effects in patients have their underpinnings in the experimental data obtained from animals. Such testing in humans, as much as possible, duplicates the testing in animals. Of course certain procedures cannot be carried out in people, and, in such instances, data from animals must be used alone.

When experiments in animals confirm that a drug has a desired set of potentially efficacious effects and that excessively dangerous toxicologic effects occur at doses substantially higher than those that could produce efficacy, testing in humans can be justified. There are three major objectives in testing in humans. The first is to determine whether the pharmacologic effects seen in humans confirm predictions derived from data from animals. When effects in the two species are equivalent, further development in humans may proceed. If a potentially beneficial but unexpected effect is observed in humans, further animal testing may be required before additional studies proceed in humans. The second objective is to show that the pharmacologic actions lead to therapeutically useful effects. The third objective is to demonstrate that the drug is safe enough to be used in humans. Safety is considered in the context of the measured beneficial effects. Tests in humans classically are divided into at least three phases (I–III) (Fig. 34–1).

Phase I Testing

In order to make testing in humans as safe as possible, the first doses, chosen with data from animals in mind, are small enough so that no effects are expected. Usually a small number of people, generally healthy volunteers, are observed after they are given a single small dose. If this dose is tolerated, successively higher doses are administered to determine the range of doses that are well tolerated. The escalation of dose is progressive and often is carried out until a limiting adverse event occurs. For example, either a potential antihypertensive agent may cause an excessive drop in blood pressure or the adverse event may be unrelated to the desired primary pharmacologic effect.

The low-dose challenges are then followed by studies in which higher doses are given over sev-

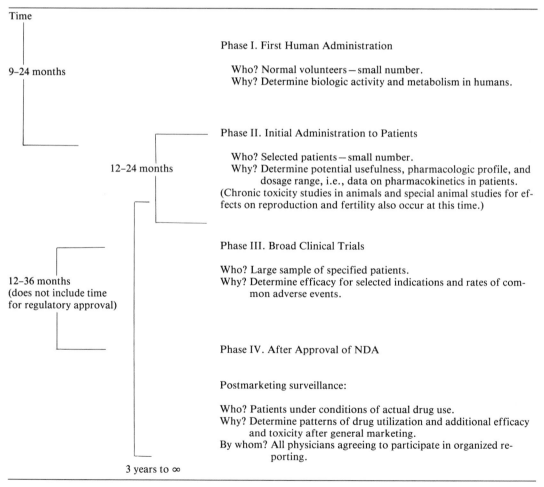

Fig. 34–1. Drug development in humans. Adapted from Melmon and Morrelli, 1978.
Permission granted by editor.

eral weeks. Generally, test doses in phase I are given to normal subjects. This practice is appropriate when the drug's expected effects are likely to be transient and easily tolerated. For instance, hemodynamically active drugs intended for patients with congestive heart failure may be safely administered to healthy subjects who can tolerate rapid or large hemodynamic changes better than patients with compromised cardiovascular systems. But when the drug's expected effect is likely to be dangerous even when it is efficacious, testing in normal people is not ethically acceptable. For instance, antineoplastic agents are too dangerous to give to anyone except to patients who could possibly benefit from the drug, or at least who would not be exposed to much excessive risk relative to the risk of their disease. In spite of the fact that phase I testing in normal people has turned out to be extraordinarily safe, the ethics of performing these tests on normal people is legitimately debated. A drug being developed to treat heart failure may have dose–response curves or even qualitative effects in patients with congestive heart failure that differ enough from those seen in healthy subjects to render results in healthy subjects of little value. No matter how safe the early administration of an NCE to normals is, it seems sensible to test for early effects of drugs in the patient population that has something to gain from the experiment.

Pharmacokinetic and metabolic studies also are carried out in humans. Identifying metabolites in humans that were not detected in animals is very important. Such metabolites might require additional animal testing for their pharmacologic, toxicologic, and carcinogenic activity. Knowledge of the major pathways for elimination of the drug, whether hepatic or renal, will be useful to predict necessary adjustments of dose that may be required in patients with hepatic or renal disease. Knowledge of the distribution, clearance, and half-life, coupled to information on the relationship of the concentration of the drug in plasma to its pharmacologic effect, can help in designing appropriate dosing regimens for definitive testing of efficacy.

Types of Clinical Trials: Phases II and III

The keystone to any drug development program and the gold standard of experimentation with drugs in humans is the controlled clinical trial. These trials are designed to test whether a drug is efficacious; they essentially are a test of the null hypothesis.

The null hypothesis assumes there is no difference between two treatments, A and B. If B is highly effective compared with A (penicillin vs. placebo for pneumococcal meningitis), a very small study, or even use of historical controls, will reject the null hypothesis in both statistically *significant*, *clinically important* terms. If B is marginally effective compared with A [β-adrenergic blockade to prevent sudden death during the year post myocardial infarction reduces sudden death rate by 50% (from *5%* to *2.5%*)], a large sample is needed to show a statistically *significant* difference. Whether or not this difference is *clinically important* enough to warrant the risks of therapy in many who would not benefit (97.5% of tested subjects) is another matter. Statistical design tells us how many patients we must study to find a given degree of difference between A and B with a mathematical probability of, for example, 95%, $p = .05$; 99%, $p = .01$; or 99.9%, $p = 001$. *Principle: Keep your eye on the "doughnuts" (clinical goals) and not on the "holes,"* **p** = *.000001.*

Several important conditions must be met in the design of such trials. The end points to be measured to determine efficacy must be clearly defined. Careful consideration must be given to the definition of therapeutic efficacy. For example, if a drug is purported to lower cholesterol concentrations, is it medically appropriate and adequate to show that the drug simply lowers cholesterol concentrations, or should the experiment be designed to prove or disprove that it *also* prevents myocardial infarction? Should an antihypertensive be shown merely to lower blood pressure, or should prevention of the morbid consequences of hypertension, such as stroke and renal failure, be the end points of the experiment? The general question is whether achievement of a so-called surrogate end point is adequate to establish efficacy, or whether some more obviously clinically beneficial end point should be demonstrated before a drug is marketed. For a cholesterol-lowering agent, the actual goal of therapy (end point) is to prevent atherosclerosis and its consequences. We treat hypertension not simply to lower blood pressure, but to prevent its consequences, stroke, and renal and heart failure. The lower plasma cholesterol concentration and the lower blood pressure are surrogate (not ultimate) end points of benefit.

It is usually quicker, and sometimes the only feasible method, to use a surrogate end point to show that a drug is efficacious. It may be slower or impossible to show an effect on a more definitive end point. Whether one is satisfied that a surrogate end point is adequate to establish efficacy is determined by several considerations, such as how closely changes in the surrogate end point are linked to causing changes in the definitive end point; how much risk is associated with the therapy (the more risk the surer one wants to be that the definitive end point is affected); and what other therapies are available to treat the targeted disease. If alternative therapies already are available for the same indication, the physician has a right to ask for increasingly definitive evidence of effects on the medical objective before giving the drug. *Principle: Drug development resembles Bismark's description of politics in this regard: it is the art of the possible.*

The choice of controls is crucial in a controlled clinical trial. The most rigorous and most widely used control is the concurrent control. A concurrent control ideally consists of a group that is exactly like the group being given the active drug. The concurrent control group is observed simultaneously with the group given the experimental drug.

Most concurrently controlled trials are *double-blind* and *randomized*. Randomization ensures that each subject in the trial had an equal chance of being assigned to either the treatment or the control group. This attribute is essential for the proper application of statistical tests that will be used to assess the results. Double-blind means that neither the subjects in the trial nor the observers making the measurements, which will be used to measure efficacy, know who is taking which treatment. Both the response of a subject and the perceptions of an observer will be influenced if they know which treatment is being administered. While blinding is desired and usually attempted, it is not always feasibly maintained. Sometimes, pharmacologic or toxic effects allow a patient or an investigator to determine the nature of the treatment.

In order for a trial to be blinded, the control group must also be given a treatment. Otherwise everyone would immediately know who was in the control group. The control group must take something that looks like, and in the case of oral administration tastes like, or in the case of an injection feels like the active treatment. The nature of the control substance can be either placebo, a substance without specific pharmacologic effects, or an active control, such as another drug used for the same indication. Placebo controls are an absolute standard (see chapter 33). From the results of a placebo-controlled trial one can infer whether the active treatment is efficacious or even harmful relative to no treatment. Comparisons of efficacy can be made relative to an active control. However, when no placebo is included and drug A is not as efficacious as drug B, one cannot differentiate between no efficacy or just less efficacy than drug B. If drug A has some efficacy, it could still be useful in those patients who show insufficient or no response to B, or who are allergic to B. Discovering marginal utility requires a placebo control. If a placebo group is added to a trial so that drug A, drug B, and placebo are

tested, then comparisons can be made between both active drugs and placebo. In the development of a new drug, actively controlled trials in the absence of a placebo are used when a proven treatment exists for the targeted disease and it is dangerous for patients to be removed from the established treatment for the period of time required to conduct the clinical trial. The investigational drug can be substituted for the standard treatment being used for the active control if there is enough evidence from animal studies that the experimental drug is very similar to the standard therapy in terms of its mechanism(s) of action. However, if the experimental drug has a new mechanism of action and is unproved for the same therapeutic benefit as the standard treatment, then it may not be possible to discontinue the standard treatment in any trial. In that case, a clinical trial might consist of the following treatments:

Treatment I: standard treatment +
experimental treatment
Treatment II: standard treatment + placebo

For such a trial to show that the experimental treatment is efficacious, the new treatment would have to provide benefit beyond the standard treatment. Unless this added benefit is very substantial, a very large number of patients are needed in the trial to validate the difference statistically. A large study may not always be feasible, particularly if the disease under study is rare.

It might not be possible to demonstrate the added efficacy provided by the experimental drug. In such a case, a useful alternative to standard therapy could be wrongly discarded. Although this dilemma is not easy to solve, sometimes there are ways to circumvent the problem. For example, if the mechanism of the disease is very well understood, then one could argue that the experimental drug has such a high chance of working that it could be substituted for the standard treatment. This setting is rare. Sometimes a trend suggesting that the experimental drug is efficacious can be found in patients who are not substantially helped by the standard treatment. Discovery of such a trend could justify another trial comparing the two drugs without the need to compare the new therapy to placebo.

In addition to efficacy, the safety of a new drug has to be evaluated in clinical trials in humans. Information on adverse events associated with taking a drug is collected in the course of every clinical trial. Both objective evidence, such as changes in physical condition or laboratory data, and subjective complaints are obtained from patients and normal subjects.

The rigor with which these data are evaluated

is limited. Data on safety come from a variety of trials, not all controlled. Thus, it is not possible to be certain which adverse effects are due to the drug. This problem is especially difficult when the disease being treated causes many events that might be mistaken for drug-induced events. Conversely, an event caused by a drug may be ascribed to the disease being treated. A important example of this latter problem is that most drugs that diminish the frequency of cardiac arrhythmias also can increase the frequency of arrhythmias in susceptible patients.

The number of people treated with a new drug in experimental programs before a drug is approved is relatively small. The range in studies is about 500 to 3000 people (Strom et al., 1984). Thus, only events that commonly are caused by the drug can be detected. Table 34–1 gives estimates of how many people are needed in studies to detect events caused by a drug at given incidence rates and with given relative risks. Medically important events often occur at rates of less than 1 in 10,000 with relative risks that are much less than 2 (see chapter 39). Two characteristics of an adverse event caused by a drug determine how readily the adverse event can be ascribed to the drug with some reasonable assurance. The first is the frequency with which the drug causes the event; the second is the frequency with which the event occurs spontaneously in the absence of the drug. The required number of patients exposed to a drug in order to detect a drug-induced event increases as the following ratio decreases:

$$\frac{\text{Frequency of drug-induced event}}{\text{Frequency by which event occurs spontaneously}}$$

For example, as shown in Table 34–1, in order to have a 90% chance of detecting a drug-induced adverse event that occurs spontaneously in 1 in 1000 people of the control group, about 31,000 patients need to be studied in the experimental group to detect an event that occurs with a frequency of 2/1000 in the drug-treated group. For an event that occurs with a frequency of 5/1000

in the drug-treated group, about 3900 patients would have to be studied in the experimental group.

Another factor that determines how difficult it will be to correctly ascribe an event to a drug is the time of onset of the event relative to the time of administration of the drug. If the drug-related event is slow to manifest, recognizing that the event could be related to therapy is difficult.

No drug is absolutely safe. Like all other things in life, taking drugs involves some risk (see chapter 35). Ideally, safety and efficacy must be evaluated together in order to decide if a drug is efficacious enough to justify the risk. For example, more risk is acceptable in a drug that has the potential of curing a fatal disease than in a drug to treat the common cold. Regulatory agencies are very aware of the need for balancing efficacy versus toxicity. The Food and Drug Act in the United States does not define safety and efficacy. These decisions ultimately are made by the regulators and the medical profession.

Regulatory Functions and Drug Development

In virtually all countries, no drug can be sold to the general population before a governmentally sponsored regulatory review of its safety and efficacy has taken place. This review may be followed by approval for sale. The philosophies and practices of regulatory agencies vary from country to country and are constantly evolving. Most of the remarks in this chapter relate to the Food and Drug Administration (FDA) of the United States in the 1980s.

The FDA can approve a drug for general use if adequately controlled clinical trials show it is "safe and effective." As mentioned above, the judgment regarding safety and efficacy is a relative one. Higher risks become more acceptable (1) as the seriousness of the disease being treated increases, (2) as the evidence for efficacy becomes stronger, (3) when efficacy is defined as decreasing disability or mortality due to the disease (as opposed to an effect on a surrogate end point that has not been definitively linked to progressive

Table 34–1. REQUIRED SAMPLE SIZE*

INCIDENCE IN CONTROL GROUP	RELATIVE RISK TO BE DETECTED		
	1.25	2.0	5.0
0.0001	3.8×10^6	3.2×10^5	3.9×10^4
0.001	3.8×10^5	3.1×10^4	3.9×10^3
0.01	3.7×10^4	3.1×10^3	3.8×10^2

* Type I error = 0.05; type II error = 0.1 (power = 90%). The sample size is the number of subjects that would have to be studied in each of the control and experimental groups (Adapted from Strom, 1989).

morbidity or mortality), (4) when several clinical trials show the same beneficial effect, and (5) when no other treatment exists that offers the same therapeutic advantage as the drug being considered for approval. As in the cases of safety and efficacy, the term *adequately controlled clinical trials* also is subject to interpretation. In most cases, *adequately controlled* means randomized, double-blind, and with concurrent controls. However, sometimes a randomized, double-blind trial is not required. When the disease is rare, there may not be enough patients to make a statistically valid, randomized, concurrently controlled trial feasible. In those cases, historical controls may be necessary. Some diseases have an inexorable and predictable course. Reversal of that course by a drug, even in the absence of a control, might convince regulators and physicians that a drug is effective. Examples include the rapid reversal of pneumococcal pneumonia by penicillin, or the reversal of opiate-induced coma by naloxone. Such clinical situations are rare; an expert's "belief" that they exist often raises more debate than agreement. As a rule, the need for concurrent controls is respected and should be a high priority of most studies.

The approval process involves multiple steps. After information about a drug has been collected in animals, a sponsor (usually a pharmaceutical company) desiring to investigate a drug in humans must submit an application to the FDA seeking approval to start clinical trials in humans. The application is called an Investigational New Drug application (IND). The application must convince the FDA that the drug has a reasonable chance of being effective, that toxicologic data suggest that the drug should not cause undue harm, that the physical-chemical characteristics of the drug are well described, and that the process to produce the drug is reproducible and results in a sufficiently pure preparation. Once an IND is approved, clinical testing may begin.

Throughout the world, clinical testing classically proceeds in three general phases. Phase I includes initial dosing to establish the range of doses that humans can tolerate. Some information on the drug's pharmacokinetic profile and metabolism is determined. Phase II includes work to define the pharmacologic effects in humans and also includes small clinical trials to determine if the drug is likely to show efficacy in large definitive trials. Phase III includes large clinical trials designed to investigate whether the drug is efficacious and safe. The majority of drugs that enter phases I and II do not go to phase III, either because a toxic effect appears that was not anticipated before the study or because the pharmacologic promise hinted at by animal studies did not

materialize in early clinical testing. In addition, when a drug enters phase I testing, generally not all the long-term animal toxicology has been completed. Findings in these long-term toxicology trials occasionally preclude administering the drug to people for protracted periods.

When phase III trials are completed and the sponsor believes that efficacy and safety have been adequately demonstrated, the sponsor compiles all the data to support that assertion in the form of a New Drug Application (NDA). After the FDA reviews this information, it can approve the drug for general use or deny approval. *Principle: The Food, Drug and Cosmetic Act and its amendments require the agency to approve or disapprove marketing of a drug. They do not require that every medically important event caused by the drug, or that the best and optimal uses and indication for the drug, be known. The act was wise and theoretically allows a product with proven efficacy to reach the market in a reasonable time. The rest of the information developed about the drug requires its use in the field. Observations of the results of the drug's use are the profession's and not the FDA's responsibility.*

What is it that the FDA actually is able to approve? What is the authority of the FDA? When an NDA is filed, it is filed for a specific indication. An indication can be a symptom such as relief of pain or it can be for a disease such as hypertension or congestive heart failure. An indication can be modified or restricted, such as "the relief of moderate or moderately severe pain" or as "adjunctive therapy in the management of heart failure in patients not responding to diuretics or digitalis." Evidence in an NDA must support the use of a drug for such a particular indication. When approving a drug, the FDA regulates what claims can be made for a drug by the company that will sell it. Regulation of such claims is through two mechanisms. The first is the package insert that is provided to physicians and is published in the *Physicians' Desk Reference* (*PDR*). This package insert, sometimes referred to as the "label," provides information on the chemical composition of the drug, description of some of the preclinical and clinical data known about the drug, approved indication or indications, contraindications (situations in which the drug should not be used), adverse events associated with the drug, dosing instructions, and advice on potential problems that could be associated with use of the drug. The other mechanism by which FDA regulates claims about a drug is by regulating advertisements for it. Only approved indications can be advertised, and advertised claims must be based on supporting data that has been reviewed by the FDA.

The FDA legally cannot regulate *how* a drug actually is used by physicians. Such regulation would "interfere with the practice of medicine," and the agency is expressly forbidden from this function by the Food and Drug Act. No physician is bound by any law to follow instructions in the drug's label. If a physician believes that a particular drug should, would, or could be useful for a particular patient with a particular disease, prescribing that drug for that disease may be legitimate and expected, even if FDA has not approved such a use. The physician should be acting on solid information gathered from clinical trials that either have not been reviewed by FDA or that might not have been submitted to FDA, but nevertheless are quite valuable in helping to make medical decisions. Alternatively, the basis for "off label" use of a drug could be solid physiologic and pharmacologic principles and logic that predict the drug's possible efficacy for a particular disease. In the absence of evidence to support or refute such a use directly, the physician should proceed and evaluate the experience very much like an experiment in which $N = 1$ (chapter 36). Finally, it even is "legal" for a poorly informed physician to use a drug inappropriately, although it may constitute malpractice. The FDA has no authority over such practices of medicine. Thus, by law, when the FDA approves a drug for any indication, one may use the drug in any way a physician sees fit.

During the first few years after a drug is released, it may be used in a variety of plausible ways. Whether the use was "judicious" or not becomes clear only with extensive experience. Propranolol was initially "labeled" for idiopathic subaortic hypertrophic sternosis, arrhythmias, and pheochromocytoma. Its "unlabeled" use in angina pectoris and essential hypertension was, in retrospect, logical and correct. Some of the other *published* uses have also withstood the test of time and trials, but many have not (Morrelli, 1973). *Principle: There is no foolproof way to know when to use a new drug. Osler's adage "The physician is advised not to be the first to adopt the new remedy nor the last to discard the old" has the merit of wisdom. Introduction of pharmacologically unique and innovative drugs is rare. Few patients will be seriously deprived if a physician awaits published evidence of efficacy before adopting a new drug.*

Society and the regulatory agency appropriately give the physician wide latitude in the use of a drug, device, or procedure. Society has a right to access drugs when the potential for important efficacy is established and can be put into preliminary perspective with the drug's toxicity. However, both efficacy and safety are preliminarily defined by the premarketing data. Furthermore, the setting of experiments done for regulatory purposes rarely mimics "field" circumstances of using drugs in practice.

POSTMARKETING ASSESSMENTS OF DRUG EFFECTS

Recently, an increasing amount of attention has been paid to more completely collecting data about drug-related events that occur once the product is released for marketing. In addition, debate is active regarding the best ways to evaluate such data in order to obtain more and better information on both unanticipated (or at least unestablished) adverse and beneficial events due to drugs. The overall activity of collecting data about drugs that are available to the general population is known as *postmarketing surveillance*. A perceived advantage of postmarketing surveillance is that it studies how drugs are used in "the real world" (Strom and Melmon, 1979, 1989; Strom, 1989). Populations that are almost never studied in premarketing studies, such as pregnant women, children, and the unborn, inevitably get exposed to many drugs in normal medical practice. Postmarketing surveillance may be the only ethical way to look for pharmacologic or toxicologic effects in these populations.

The clinical evaluation of a drug prior to its release is limited for several reasons. First, the patients treated are highly screened. They must meet certain criteria to enter clinical trials. These criteria are established primarily to reduce intersubject variability, making experimental observations interpretable. In addition, certain criteria are set to increase safety to the patients in the trial. Patients in trials usually are observed much more intensively than ordinary patients in clinical practice. Concomitant therapies often are eliminated, decreasing the chance for drug interactions. The presence of concomitant diseases is also established as a criterion for being excluded from the study. Knowledge gained from clinical trials is dictated by the hypothesis being tested and the design of experiments that test the hypothesis. If efficacy for a particular indication is not tested in the trial, the efficacy of the drug for that indication will not be discovered, even if the drug, in fact, were useful for the untested indication. As mentioned above, the limited size of the patient population tested to support the approval of a drug limits the possibility of discovering uncommon adverse events. *Principle: If society has a right to access to drugs with important efficacy, it also has a right to expect that the profession will follow up on its obligation to monitor and use data that can be accumulated after the drug is marketed. It would disappoint the patients and the profession to realize how truly little of the important medical consequences is known about an NCE at the time it becomes a salable product. What should be more important to all of us is how lax we are in detecting available data that could optimize our use of drug products.*

After approval, most drugs will be used in millions of people, and in a variety of ways. Those patients will not be "typical" of the patients used in clinical trials. Patients given the drug after its approval will not be monitored as closely as patients in a premarketing clinical trial. They will have more concurrent diseases; they may be taking more concomitant medications; they may be younger or older or of a different sex; and they may be pregnant, nonambulatory, and so forth. Because of the sensible limitation on the size of the preapproval clinical trials, it is possible that new serious adverse events or new beneficial effects will occur that could not be detected sooner because they occur too infrequently or because they depend on a particular set of circumstances, such as in the setting of concomitant therapy with another drug or of a concurrent disease that was not studied in the preapproval studies.

The patients that receive a drug in its general use could be a vast source of new information regarding the drug's effects. Mechanisms are in place around the world to collect data on drugs once they reach the marketplace. In the United States, adverse events thought to be due to a drug are reported to FDA by physicians on a voluntary basis. While this has led to discoveries of previously unrecognized adverse events, it is almost certain that this system is not optimal, efficient, or even cost-effective.

Methods are available to capture such information by postmarketing surveillance so that therapy can be improved. Postmarketing surveillance can be performed by patients, practicing or academic physicians, pharmacists, pharmaceutical companies, or governmental agencies (Strom and Melmon, 1979; Rawlins, 1988; Strom, 1989). Ideally, such a system could confirm unproven, though anticipated, efficacy and toxicity. A good system of postmarketing surveillance also could detect unanticipated efficacy and toxicity. Postmarketing surveillance can report events from the field, monitor large patient data bases, or work by a combination of these approaches. In the United States, a major issue is who should sponsor and financially support such an effort. Thus far only sporadic efforts have been undertaken by academics and by pharmaceutical companies. There is no generally accepted systematic program in place in the United States as there are in some European countries. Interested parties such as practicing physicians, patients, pharmaceutical companies, and the government are subject to various combinations of ethical, financial, and scientific incentives and disincentives to support a universal system of postmarketing surveillance. At present, no agreement has been reached as to the desirability or the methodology to be used in such a system (Lortie, 1986; Edlavitch, 1988).

Some have proposed that a rigorous, consistently applied application of epidemiologic techniques to postmarketing surveillance could shorten the premarket development of a drug. That is, the elapsed time from the first experiments in humans to regulatory approval could be reduced. Whether or not this proposal is valid, developing useful information about unanticipated drug effects certainly should optimize the use of the drug and define its most appropriate market much faster than is done today. In order to expose more patients to a drug to increase the sensitivity for discovering toxicity in phase III clinical trials, phase III may be prolonged beyond the point presently needed solely to demonstrate efficacy (Strom and Melmon, 1979). A good system of postmarketing surveillance could efficiently and more completely detect adverse events and make these known to physicians. Whether the risks in allowing earlier public access to drugs would be outweighed by the benefit of distributing the proven efficacy to more patients more quickly is not known, and it would vary from case to case. By monitoring the effects of a drug in representative patients in all the settings in which it is actually used, data could also accrue that would establish more optimal uses of drugs.

Drug development is a scientifically rigorous, costly, and time-consuming process. While the general principles of experimentally proving a drug's efficacy are widely accepted, there is much discussion regarding alternative methods to gather convincing evidence for efficacy and safety. The acceptance of any method always includes value judgments regarding the balance of safety and efficacy and regarding how certain one needs to be that a perceived effect is real. Because there is no absolute correctness in those judgments, debates will continue and these approaches will continue to evolve.

REFERENCES

Chakrin, L.; and Byron, D. A.: Lab's labor lost? R&D in an era of change. Pharmaceut. Executive, 30–34, July 1987.
Edlavitch, S. A.: Postmarketing surveillance methodologies. Drug Intell. Clin. Pharm., 22:68–78, 1988.
Elion, G. B.: The purine pathway to chemotherapy. Science, 244:41–47, 1989.
Gogerty, J. H.: Preclinical Research Evaluation in New Drug Approval Processes (Guarino, R. A., ed.). Marcel Dekker, New York, pp. 25–54, 1987.
Halperin, J. A.: Challenge, opportunity, promise, and risk: The pharmaceutical industry moving toward the 21st century. Drug Info. J., 22:25–32, 1988.

Hood, L.: Biotechnology and medicine of the future. J.A.M.A., 259:1837–1844, 1988.

Lasagna, L.: Toxicological barriers to providing better drugs. Arch. Toxicol., 43:27–33, 1979.

Lortie, F. M.: Postmarketing surveillance of adverse drug reactions: Problems and solutions. Can. Med. Assoc. J., 135:27–32, 1986.

Mario, E.: A vision of the pharmaceutical industry in the year 2000. Pharm. Tech., 23–25, April, 1988.

Melmon, K. L.: Attitudinal factors that influence the utilization of modern evaluative methods. In, Medical Innovation at the Crossroads (Geljins, A. C., ed.). Vol. 1. Committee on Technological Innovation of Medicine, Institute of Medicine, The National Academy Press, Washington, D.C., pp. 136–146, 1990.

Melmon, K. L.; and Morrelli, H. K. (eds.): Clinical Pharmacology: Basic Principles in Therapeutics, 2nd ed. (Melmon, K. L.; and Morrelli, H. F.; eds.). Macmillan, New York, 1978.

Morrelli, H. K.: Propranolol. Ann. Intern. Med., 78:913–917, 1973.

Rawlins, M. D.: Spontaneous reporting of adverse drug reactions: II. Uses. Br. J. Clin. Pharmacol., 26:7–11, 1988.

Strom, B. L. (ed.): Pharmacoepidemiology. Churchill Livingstone, New York, 1989.

Strom, B. L.; and Melmon, K. L.: The use of pharmacoepidemiology to study beneficial drug effects. In, Pharmacoepidemiology (Strom, B. L., ed.). Churchill Livingstone, New York, 1989, 307–324.

Strom, B. L.; and Melmon, K. L.: Can postmarketing surveillance help to effect optimal drug therapy? J.A.M.A., 242: 2420–2423, 1979.

Strom B. L.; Miettinen, O. S.; and Melmon, K. L.: Postmarketing studies of drug efficacy: How? Am. J. Med., 77:703–708, 1984.

Swann, J. P.: Academic Scientists and the Pharmaceutical Industry. Johns Hopkins University Press, Baltimore, Maryland, 1988.

35

Risk in Taking Drugs

Hugh Tilson

Selecting the right medication—pharmacotherapeutic decision making—may be thought of as a choice among potential treatment agents based upon the balance of likely benefits to likely risks in the individual patient. Every physician knows that the purpose of medication is to gain the beneficial effect associated with that drug for a specific patient. Likewise, every physician knows that an inevitable concomitant of chemical effects of a medicine is the occurrence of adverse effects. The evolution of the field of drug development has resulted in better and better-targeted interventions that can more selectively alter specific cellular or chemical mechanisms to achieve specific desired biologic effects. Nevertheless, only exceptionally is the mechanism so specific that it influences the course of progress of a single disease or cellular process to the exclusion of all others. When other components of the organism are affected, the result is drug effects other than, or in addition to, those sought. They are called side effects. Some of these may be beneficial, neutral, or minor in effect. Major episodes of serious medication-attributable morbidity or mortality stand out clearly as signals of the need to survey for unexpected actions of marketed drugs (Geiling and Carmon, 1938; McBride, 1961; Lenz, 1962; Taussig, 1962; Best, 1967; Markush and Siegel, 1969; Herbst et al., 1971; Ziel and Finkle, 1975; Kono, 1980; U.S. Congress, 1983; and Stern et al., 1984). On balance, medicines are "re-markably non-toxic" (Jick, 1974). Consideration of the possibility of significant adverse side effects of medicines is a critical element in the risk–benefit equation. The decision to proceed with a particular therapy should entail a highly sophisticated understanding of drug risk: What do we really know about the likelihood of adverse events in association with exposure to this product in this person?

LIMITS OF KNOWLEDGE WHEN A NEW DRUG IS APPROVED

When a New Drug Application (NDA) is reviewed for approval by the Food and Drug Administration (FDA), evidence from an elaborate and complex program of clinical trials must show that the drug is efficacious, at least for the one clinical use for which it has been tested (see chapter 34). The requirement that efficacy be demonstrated according to the rules of statistical analysis and probability theory in at least two properly controlled clinical trials has spurred the science of clinical drug development in a number of countries. Detailed clinical management, extensive clinical laboratory supporting information, and documentation of thorough clinical observations have produced rich data bases. Paper submissions for NDAs have filled entire tractor trailer trucks for delivery to the FDA (Janssen, 1981).

Although the same can be said about documentation of safety, the implications of the safety experience data in the NDA are very different from those concerning efficacy. Preclinical animal and laboratory testing are applied to protect against introduction of highly toxic substances into humans. Still, such screens are incomplete predictors of the safety of a new chemical entity. The ultimate test of safety must be in humans. Because of the elegance of the modern clinical trial and the richness of resulting data, the per-patient prices of drug development have greatly increased. It is not unusual to hear about the "$10,000 patient" in a clinical trial. Therefore, the economic and scientific pressures are directed toward restricting the numbers of patients in a clinical trial to those required for documentation of efficacy with adequate statistical power. Documentation of safety is driven by the same economics. Safety documentation for an NDA is frequently limited to 2000 or so patients—those 1000 or so enrolled in the pivotal trials (Idanpaan-Heikkila, 1983) and 1000 or so patients enrolled in nonpivotal studies. Thus, when adverse experience patterns of a newly approved medication are described, for example in the product label, they can only be expected to reflect those experiences that occur frequently enough to be detected in a sample of 1000 to 3000 patients at most, that is, at a frequency of 1/1000 to 1/300 or greater. If truly serious or life-threatening adverse effects were occurring at that frequency, then it is the rare drug indeed that would not already have fallen by the wayside in the drug development process. Yet, in a sample of up to 3000 patients, there is no way to be sure that we know about the 1/10,000 fatal anaphylaxis or Stevens-Johnson syndrome that may accompany the use of a drug in a population. Only a population experience—possible only outside and after the drug development process—could answer such a question.

Furthermore, the process of drug development is highly focused in a series of other ways that restrict the generalizability of the safety information developed during the preapproval period. In order to maximize the resolution power of a clinical trial to detect efficacy, certain patients are excluded, such as those who have multiple concomitant illnesses, take multiple concomitant medications, have compromised metabolic systems, or are very young, very old, or women of childbearing age. Clinical trials are also time-limited.

Society needs and deserves useful, new medicines as quickly as science and due caution (including regulatory review) will permit. Likewise, the research-intensive pharmaceutic company, investing an average of more than $200 million for each new drug approved, wants to begin to re-cover its costs in the marketplace (DiMasi, 1990). There is no way a 2-year follow-up program can document the effects of 5 years of chronic use or latent effects occurring after a 10-year period. All these issues are simply not knowable at the time a drug is first approved (i.e., released for marketing) and, therefore, cannot be reflected in the safety statements available to physicians at the time a new drug is introduced into general use. In selecting such a new agent, it is critical that the therapist incorporate the factor of uncertainty into the implicit benefit–risk assessment in any therapeutic decision.

Fast-Track Drug Approvals in the United States

The decade of the 1980s witnessed a phenomenon that has further changed the balance of what is known at the time of approval of a new medicine and what can only eventually be known about it. Impatient and desperate over an acute incidence of acquired immunodeficiency syndrome (AIDS), a vocal public demanded that new medicines showing promise against AIDS be expedited through a regulatory process that typically requires several years of negotiation, review, and requests for further information.

The FDA replied by instituting fast-track provisions that ensured both rapid review and broader availability of a putative life-saving drug. The drug could be made available while the review was underway, as early as completion of a single definitive trial that showed strong evidence of efficacy with numbers of patients adequate to provide some minimal assurances of safety (Palca, 1989).

Under this mechanism, called the *treatment IND*, an experimental drug can be as widely available as supplies and circumstances permit through physicians who agree to participate (USDHHS, 1987). It brings the physician more directly into contact with the drug development process than ever before. Such involvement ensures both the patient's fully informed consent and an agreement by the treating physician adequately to monitor and promptly report safety aspects of the drug in clinical experience. The first such treatment IND—concerning the anti-AIDS drug, gancyclovir (Retrovir)—distributed the drug to more than 4800 AIDS patients who had had *Pneumocystis carinii* pneumonia. Sufficient data were collected to verify that the findings of an initial study involving only 282 persons held true in a larger population without any unexpected toxicities. This finding permitted the new drug to be marketed with a safety data base in excess of 5000 treated persons (Creagh-Kirk et al., 1986; Wastila and Lasagna, 1990).

EPIDEMIOLOGIC INTELLIGENCE

The Role and Limitations of the Spontaneous Reporting System

Following marketing of a new drug, information about its safety is gained as therapeutic experience unfolds. With larger populations of patients being treated under different circumstances and for different periods of time from those in premarketing clinical trials, new adverse experiences will inevitably arise (USGAO, 1990). In the United States, the official method of learning about these is the spontaneous voluntary adverse reactions reporting system of the FDA (USDHHS, 1985). Physicians and other treating professionals are requested to voluntarily register with the FDA any adverse experience that they encounter during the course of drug therapy. In 1989, more than 60,000 such reports were registered. However, by far the vast majority of these reports are registered indirectly, that is, primarily through product inquiries and complaints initially lodged with the drug's manufacturers.

In the United States, more than 85% of the spontaneous voluntary adverse reaction reports from clinical practice reach the FDA through the pathway of an initial voluntary report by the practitioner to the industry and a subsequent mandatory company report to the FDA (Faich et al., 1987). A second and growing source of these reports via the manufacturer is the drug information specialist in industry. When a practitioner requests a reprint regarding adverse effects of a drug, the information specialist responds not solely with the requested information but also with a query about the episode. The practitioner provides details of the actual patient case that precipitated the request (Tilson et al., 1990).

It is estimated that fewer than 1 in 1000 of all serious adverse experiences occurring in clinical practice ever come to the attention of anyone either in the FDA or in a position to further report them to the FDA (Griffin and Weber, 1986). How could this be?

Fundamental to a system of voluntary reports is the concept of attribution — causal reasoning that links particular exposure to a particular medicine with a particular adverse experience in a particular patient. In order for an adverse experience to become the object of an adverse drug reaction report, someone in a position to report it must have the idea that there may be a causal association. The barriers to making such associations are considerable and well documented (Venning, 1983a, 1983b, 1983c, 1983d, 1988). Nonetheless, when an adverse event occurs in a patient in such a way that the physician, pharmacist, nurse, or other member of the treating team feels that one or another of the medications that person is taking may have caused it, a workup of the individual case is important.

The simple reflex assumption that if an event occurred the drug may have caused it may be plausible and may render an expedient, practical therapeutic decision (e.g., stop the drug). But in the long run, such an approach may do the patient a triple disservice. First, changing therapeutic regimens involves exposure to new and different risks and/or the potential for lessened efficacy or interrupted therapy. Second, blaming the drug may divert attention from other more important and also potentially remediable causes. Third, for the patient, that drug is ever thereafter regarded as "one that I am allergic to."

Attribution algorithms that may be useful to the therapist in deciding the likelihood that a certain drug in a certain patient may have caused a certain event are numerous and have been described elsewhere in this text (see chapters 1 and 34) (Karch and Lasagna, 1977; Kramer et al., 1979; Naranjo et al., 1981). They are to be recommended to the therapist in the situation in which a medication may need to be withdrawn. When there is residual doubt and the stakes are great, there is every reason to withdraw a medicine if suitable alternative therapy is available or if the suspected reaction or adverse effect is worse than the disease being treated.

Whenever the therapist's index of suspicion is such that the event is attributed to exposure to drug, the therapist should take action not only at the patient level, but also at the public level: report this drug–event association through the spontaneous voluntary adverse reactions report system in the United States, the yellow card system in the United Kingdom, or other similar systems. The information that the system needs to have reported is not unlike the information needed to make the therapeutic decision at the bedside: dose, duration, and timing of drug exposure (and of all concomitant and antecedent drug exposures); timing and nature of the events that were deemed adverse; plausible alternative explanations for those events (e.g., could they just be complications of the underlying disease or the result of some intercurrent third cause); response to removal of the drug (*dechallenge*); and, on occasion, response to *rechallenge*.

Any system that must rely upon professional recognition of possible association and/or attribution and reporting by busy practitioners will have problems. Most adverse drug reactions are clinically and often pathologically identical to their naturally occurring disease counterparts. A headache is a headache. Thus, to make the link, the physician must have an awareness of the existence of the complaint, the entire profile of the patient's medication, the plausibility of a drug cause, and the likelihood of alternative explanations. This state of affairs offers the invitation to misattribution in both directions — "blaming" a drug that did not cause and failing to recognize a drug that did cause the problem.

There are profound limits to a national epidemiologic intelligence system that relies solely upon spontaneous reporting. Society's unawareness translates directly to the lack of awareness on the part of some prescribing physicians of their opportunity and responsibility to improve things. Studies of the spontaneous adverse drug reactions reporting system suggest that most physicians most of the time do not report the adverse experiences they observe. The extent of underreporting clearly varies from time to time, practice to practice, drug to drug, and certainly physician to physician (Milstien et al., 1986). In a survey of practices in Maryland, more than 40% of physicians reported that they had never heard of the spontaneous voluntary adverse drug reactions reporting system; only 37% said that they had seen an adverse reaction in their practice during the past year (although it is implausible that any had failed to see an adverse experience several times each week) (Rogers, 1987, 1990). Asked why they had failed to report, answers included concern over being harassed by the industry or regulatory authority for further data, and the assumption that the adverse event was already well known and therefore did not need to be reported. The latter answer ignores the point that it is critical to monitor and understand changes in the current frequency of an adverse event if one is to make prescribing decisions that are up-to-date.

Nowhere does the problem of monitoring adverse drug reactions become both more complex and more important than in the outpatient setting. Here, where hundreds of thousands of persons may receive a newly approved medicine in the first year, the alert physician, seeing and inquiring about an unusual clinical experience, can provide the necessary first or confirmatory signal of a rare but unacceptable adverse event. Particularly if such events mimic problems otherwise seen in practice, their association with the drug being used may not be apparent. And, if they are rare, each event is likely to be seen by any individual treating physician only once, if at all, during the early years of marketing. Therefore, both a high index of suspicion and a lively interaction with the reporting system (industry and/or regulatory authority) are especially important.

In this regard, a renewed interest in adverse experience monitoring in the hospital environment in the 1990s is also likely to bring the treating physician directly into contact with the reporting system. Under the voluntary accreditation requirements of the Joint Commission on Accred-

itation of Health Care Organizations (JCAHO), all accredited hospitals are required to have a system that monitors and manages adverse experiences in association with medication (JCAHO, 1988). In the first instance, the adverse experience monitoring system of the hospital provides consultation to the individual therapist trying to decide what to do in a patient who may be having a reaction. In the second, these experiences are summarized, pooled, and reported back for overall institutional monitoring, particularly to detect institution-specific problems such as medication errors. But the truly responsible organization also reports (as required) on a regular basis to the nation's system. The emergence of drug information units in hospitals and in the pharmaceutical industry, staffed by professional pharmacists who can provide each other consultation and reporting, is building toward a nationwide network of colleagues. This network will enhance early awareness of possible unusual clusters of adverse events that might signal a new drug-related problem (Grasela and Schentag, 1987).

The system of spontaneous voluntary adverse drug reaction reporting is the single most powerful source of warning signs, especially of rare adverse drug reactions, drawing as it does from the entire universe of treatment experience. However, underreporting, selective reporting, and misinterpretation of adverse clinical experiences as possible adverse reactions render the system an inappropriate source of data from which to draw conclusions about true rates of adverse experiences in general clinical practice, much less to compare such rates (Avorn, 1990b; Juergens, 1990).

Monitoring Literature

Generally, as experience with a drug unfolds, multiple publications relating to the medication arise. These articles describe (1) further formal clinical trials, especially concerning indications other than those in the initial approval, (2) case series, especially "interesting" sorts of patients or clinical settings, and (3) individual case reports, sometimes in the form of letters to the editor, depicting unusual clinical outcomes that are frequently thought to be adverse drug experiences. The monitoring and reporting of the accumulated experience in the literature is required of the manufacturer under FDA regulations.

Every serious adverse experience is reported immediately to the FDA by the manufacturer if it is unexpected (i.e., unlabeled). All important published experiences are summarized annually. Journals are full of letters to the editor and brief clinical notes relating to specific clinical experiences. These constitute the published side of the spontaneous voluntary adverse drug reactions reporting system. As with reports submitted spontaneously to manufacturers and/or the regulatory authority, reports submitted spontaneously to journals suffer from the same sorts of biases, both errors of omission (most adverse effects never reach the printed page) and commission (authors wishing to call attention to interesting or potentially important problems with new medicines may rush to print with incompletely conceived observations). Cases in the published literature—however potentially useful they might seem for establishing an association between a drug and adverse effect(s)—must not be used for direct comparison. First, there is enormous variation in the extent with which information needed by the reader to understand what may have happened in the individual case is included in the published report. Lack of attention to clinical detail reinforces the diminished utility of many published reports. Second, there is a tendency, particularly in the publish-or-perish world of academia, to write up one's experience again and again, "accumulating experience." Third, the reader must be aware that the case in which "nothing happened" or the case series in which the rates of problems were low often is not published. In addition, all the other problems with the spontaneous voluntary adverse reactions reporting systems already described apply no less here.

Prescription-Event Monitoring

Over the past decade, major improvements have been made in the extent and reliability, and thus the utility, of approaches building upon spontaneous reporting. Perhaps the most sophisticated and effective of these is the prescription-event monitoring (PEM) system founded by W. H. W. Inman, professor of pharmacoepidemiology and director of the Drug Safety Research Unit (DSRU), now a trust in Southampton, England (Inman, 1981). In the United Kingdom, physicians voluntarily report adverse experiences much as is done in the United States. But in the United Kingdom, the regulatory authority receives from the physician a simple, small yellow reporting form, called the *yellow card*. With this system, Great Britain has achieved one of the highest per-physician reporting rates in the world and has thus provided early signals of important drug-related problems. However, the limitations of spontaneous reporting already described also apply to the yellow card system. Thus, to estimate accurately the number of exposures and the most extensive sampling of the number of adverse events possible, Inman developed a system that actively solicits reporting of adverse events from clinical practice.

In the United Kingdom, all outpatient prescription medicines are reimbursed by the National Health Service financing scheme. They are paid by the Prescription Pricing Authority (PPA). Thus in theory, it is possible (and Inman by dint of excellent diplomacy and a highly respected career in public service has succeeded) to obtain copies of these prescriptions from the PPA for essentially all instances in which a new medicine is prescribed. Cohorts of 10,000 or 20,000 new users of important new medicines in the United Kingdom can be assembled early after their approval for marketing. Data from these prescriptions are entered into an automated system that locates each specific patient in a specific physician's practice and, having done so, generates a "green card"—a form addressed to the physician to indicate that the system has become aware that the physician has prescribed a medicine under surveillance to a specific named patient. The physician is requested to report *all* important medical events in the specific patient on the form. The events include items of medical importance even if they do not appear to be drug-related (e.g., a broken leg). If the events occur in the specified interval subsequent to the receipt of the prescription, they are reviewed and the card is returned to the DSRU.

These data are then entered into the automated data base that is systematically searched by Inman and his associates for unusual patterns of important, potentially drug-attributable, events. The findings of these searches have provided a few signals of potential problems with new medicines (Rawson et al., 1990). However, Professor Inman himself emphasizes that the far greater contribution of PEM is that for virtually all newly marketed medicines in the United Kingdom, if serious problems were occurring, they were occurring at rates less than those that would have been detected in cohorts of this size using methods of this type.

A similar PEM program in the United States has been developed by one pharmaceutic manufacturer, the Upjohn Company. This program, the Medication Monitoring Program, has enlisted the help of a nationwide network of collaborating community pharmacies (Borden and Lee, 1982). When receiving a prescription for medication under surveillance, the pharmacist provides the patient with a standard invitation to participate in the surveillance with that patient's informed consent. If the patient concurs in writing, that patient is registered in the follow-up program and receives periodic telephone inquiries regarding all important medical events at intervals appropriate to the groups of medications under surveillance (Luscombe, 1985).

In summary, spontaneous reports—direct reports from physicians to manufacturers, regulatory authority, or the published literature—are vital to the protection of the public health, but also have limited value. Such reports permit society to draw from the aggregate experience of hundreds of thousands of prescribers and millions of prescription event associations. Even with vast underreporting, they represent the most powerful and sensitive tool available for detecting drug-induced problems. However, the tool must not be misused. Such spontaneous reports draw from widely varying experiences that occur with widely varying frequencies. The extent of overreporting and underreporting is unknown. What is known is that there is so much unquantifiable variation that the calculation of a "rate"—in which the frequency of reports might be used as the numerator and the estimated population used as the denominator—is almost never appropriate. Likewise, the comparison of misbegotten rates—e.g., for regulatory or therapeutic decision making—although almost irresistibly tempting, is a practice to be assiduously avoided. An example of this is the experience with the anti-inflammatory medicines. The nonsteroidal anti-inflammatory drugs (NSAIDs) (see chapters 8, 12, 19, and 20) in the otherwise healthy nonulcer patient are thought to be associated with a certain, albeit rather low, risk of precipitating GI bleeding that may sometimes be life-threatening. The extent, frequency, and severity of such bleeds is important for the physician to understand when attempting to choose among drugs in this class. However, the prescriber who understands the reporting system also will be aware that drugs marketed more recently, in the face of increased awareness of a particular adverse effect, are subject to more reporting of that effect. Therefore, more reports of adverse experiences and particularly more reports of GI bleeds with newer agents than older ones will appear even if the "true" rates of these events are the same as or even lower than those occurring with use of the older agents. The appearance of a single published article about an interesting adverse event with a new drug may be associated with a flurry of spontaneous reports ("me too" reports), whereas exactly the same event in association with an older drug might not be of such great interest and would not result in similar reports. Recognizing the vagaries of spontaneous reporting, the epidemiologist, attempting to help the clinician, helps most by calling attention to the need for proper epidemiologic study.

The Concept of Acceptable Risk

Each time a therapeutic decision maker chooses a course of therapy, the likelihood of benefits must be balanced against the chance and severity of risks. If a new drug is accompanied by a low level (e.g., 1 in every 100,000 encounters) of a severe adverse experience that, however infrequent, renders that drug less acceptable in view of its marginal benefits, the prescriber will think twice before recommending its use. However, if no other efficacious intervention is available, or if the patient is intolerant to alternative therapies, and if the condition is not self-limiting and/or has serious long-term consequences, then the risk of exposing a patient to such an adverse effect may be worthwhile. It is in such a multidimensional decision matrix that the physician often must make a therapeutic decision (Lane and Hutchinson, 1987).

The only way that the existence of the rare, but potentially "unacceptable" problem will be known is through the unfolding of the therapeutic experience in the early years following marketing. *With predictability, for every million treatments, an event that occurs once in 100,000 treatments will appear roughly 10 times.* Perhaps one of these may have been reported to the manufacturer or directly to the regulatory authority. Thus, after several million treatments, enough reports may have been registered to signal a potential problem.

The appropriate response to such a signal depends upon the nature of the adverse experience, its apparent frequency, and its apparent acceptability in light of the therapeutic benefit from the use of the drug, keeping in mind the availability of suitable therapeutic alternatives. Thus, a rare anaphylactic event might be "acceptable" in an antibiotic (e.g., penicillin), but it would be unacceptable with a specific NSAID (Strom et al., 1987).

An alternative way of thinking about this concept recognizes that no risk is ever really "acceptable" in the societal sense. However, as we await the development of better interventions, we must tolerate a certain level of risk.

The Concept of Acceptable Uncertainty

There always will be a certain amount of uncertainty in the estimation of drug risks. Some problems inevitably will be missed by the spontaneous adverse reactions reporting epidemiologic intelligence system. Rare problems frequently (perhaps usually) will be unknown at the time of marketing. The only proper method for quantitating the true risk is the scientific, large, often long-term epidemiologic study. However, as will be demonstrated below, such studies are often costly and methodologically difficult or even impossible to conduct. The decision to undertake such a study (if feasible) is based upon the extent to which society is willing to tolerate not knowing the exact risk.

Progressively, over the past decade, society has taken the position that it wants such studies— postmarketing surveillance. The decision is particularly strong in situations in which a new drug will be used by large numbers of people and/or taken over long periods of time (Grahame-Smith, 1986). The extent to which not knowing the risk would be acceptable would vary directly with the extent to which society felt the need for the new product and, more explicitly, with the inherent risks and severity of the underlying illnesses themselves and the relative lack of satisfactory therapies.

The Epidemiologic Approach to Drug Safety

The only proper means for assessing the actual rate with which adverse experiences are occurring in association with use of medical products is the structured, epidemiologic, population-based study, often referred to as a postmarketing surveillance study. While a history of solid research into drug safety issues clearly antedates it, structured epidemiologic research has become an inseparable and prominent part of the drug safety armamentarium since the publication of the report of the Joint Commission on Prescription Drug Use (JCPDU) (the Melmon Commission) (JCPDU, 1980). The report reviewed our understanding of adverse drug experience and portrayed the limitations of information potentially and actually available from clinical trials, published literature, and spontaneous voluntary adverse reactions reports. The JCPDU recommended a uniform approach to understanding drug safety following marketing. The approach included all the above components, and, recognizing their limitations, a program of structured epidemiologic postmarketing surveillance studies.

Classic Epidemiologic Approaches. The traditional epidemiologic study has made enormous contributions to our understanding of the safety and impact of pharmaceuticals on the population. Epidemiologic (i.e., nonexperimental, observational) methods have been applied to supplement the data from clinical trials and anecdotal reports, particularly when experimentation was either impractical or infeasible. The need for large numbers of patients followed over longer periods than clinical experimentation would permit contributes to this infeasibility. In its classic form, such a study involves "hands-on" methods, that is, finding treated and untreated populations, recruiting them into the study and their physicians into collaboration, obtaining data by interview or abstracting records, and assembling data. Early studies of the safety of oral contraceptives embodied such approaches (Vessey et al., 1976, 1981, 1987).

How Sure Is Sure Enough? There is no magic number for the denominator of the risk fraction, at which point collecting larger samples is no longer necessary. Looking at a treatment population of 1000, one can be relatively certain that the absence of a significant adverse event suggests that one is not occurring more frequently than 1/350. Looking at 9000 to 10,000 recipients, the absence of a significant finding suggests that if it occurs at all, an adverse drug event must occur rather rarely, that is, less frequently than 1/3000. To be much more certain of finding a rare event if it exists, one needs to move the decimal point one space to the right—i.e., monitor 10 times more patients. Experts reviewing goals for a postmarketing epidemiologic study that would answer society's demand for reasonable safety assurance suggest that 10,000 to 20,000 persons be monitored. That would rule out rates of 1/3000 to 1/6000 for adverse experiences that might be important for both public policy and medical practice.

Editors' Note: Remember that unanticipated but finally recognized adverse responses to drugs considered medically important range from 1/5000 to 1/10,000 (Venning, 1983, 1987).

Obviously, the required size of a program of postmarketing surveillance would also be determined by the extent to which even a relatively rare but severe adverse experience would make the risk/benefit ratio for a specific agent intolerable. Other considerations include the severity of the underlying disease (the more severe, the more one is willing to accept side effects as a consequence of a necessary therapy); the presence of other satisfactory alternatives (the more alternatives, the less risk one is willing to take with the additional therapy); side effects in existing alternatives (the more toxicity in other drugs, for example, among anticancer agents, the more one is willing to accept toxicity for a marginal benefit); and, of course, the extent of the additional benefit (the more other drugs fall short of the ideal therapeutic impact, the more one would accept additional toxicity for a drug with clear therapeutic superiority).

How Long Is Long Enough? Related to the question of size of a postmarketing study is that of duration. The absence of such problems as acute toxicity or frequent adverse effects shortly after exposure to the drug does not indicate a lack of effects that occur only upon long-term, cumulative dosing (e.g., digoxin toxicity in renal compromise) or with long latency (e.g., liver failure or neoplasia occurring months or years after cessation of therapy). Although theoretical concepts about the likelihood of such events may be helpful in making the decision to conduct such a long-term study (e.g., the absence of significant animal toxicity in preapproval toxicology studies and/or in animal models or in vitro models for mutagenicity), the only true study of humankind is the human being, and the only method of observing a period of long latency is a study of long duration.

However, very long term follow-up, particularly of large cohorts, is almost impossible. With notable exceptions (e.g., the Framingham study), losses to follow-up in enrolled cohorts create imponderable questions regarding the representativeness of the population remaining under surveillance over time. Further, the labor intensity of studying long-term cohorts creates enormous costs for such studies.

An alternative to the expensive, prospectively enrolled population study or cohort study is the more-resource-efficient case control study (Ibrahim, 1979). The cohort study begins with the exposed population and has, as its method, the intuitively reasonable prospective follow-up of an exposed group and one or more comparison groups. In contrast, the case control study is counterintuitive. It starts with the outcome (e.g., cancer) and looks backward to assess the extent to which exposure to one or more possible causative agents can be detected historically in the disease group to a greater extent than would have been expected from the experience in one or more appropriate comparison populations. The studies are more resource-efficient than large prospective population studies in that they do not require long-term case holding. On the other hand, they too are fraught with methodologic problems, most notably recall bias (patients are hard-pressed to remember what happened to them last week, much less 10 or 20 years prior) and selection bias (which individuals really constitute appropriate controls, exactly the same in every way as the cases except that they did not happen to have cancer?) (Mitchell et al., 1986). Case control studies are not useful for developing hypotheses concerning a new unexpected outcome, because one must start with a postulated disease outcome to have a "case" at all (Lawson, 1988). Because of the substantial problems — costs, lag time, and methodologic difficulties — ad hoc postmarketing epidemiologic studies of medications have not enjoyed popularity and were not widely used prior to the 1980s. When they had been tried, the value of their results was often contested, particularly for the purpose of discovery of rare but important adverse experiences eventually incorporated into the product label (Rossi et al., 1983).

The physician assessing the risk/benefit ratio has been required to base that judgment upon the anecdotal and often seriously biased information of spontaneous voluntary adverse reaction reports, the highly refined (and perhaps inappropri-

ate) findings from small numbers of patients in clinical trials, and "best professional judgment." Such judgment is based on extensive knowledge, intuition, and, of course, personal first-hand experience. However, experience in this case is definitely not the best teacher. Specifically, rare events happen rarely. As an example, consider the very rare Stevens-Johnson syndrome that occurs in association with the use of an antibiotic at a rate of 1/300,000 treatments. If a physician sees one patient with Stevens-Johnson syndrome, the next time that antibiotic is considered, in the absence of proper population data and reasonable comparatives of the same risks and/or similar risks across other antibiotic choices, the physician probably will shy away from the use of it, even though the odds of a second 1/300,000 chance ever occurring in that physician's practice lifetime approach zero. If you rely strongly on personal experience, the opposite also is true. Because you have not seen a serious but rare reaction does not mean you should ignore the potential for that reaction when choosing a drug. *Principle: The physician who leans very heavily on personal experience for therapeutic decisions will not prescribe drugs properly.*

Case Series Monitoring. The first systematic assessment of rates of adverse experiences in association with multiple exposures to drugs that compared and contrasted the experiences among recipients of drugs in the same pharmacologic class was performed by Hershel Jick. His intensive inpatient monitoring program (Boston Collaborative Drug Surveillance Program) has extended over the past 25 years (Jick et al., 1970; Jick, 1977, Miller and Greenblatt, 1976). In this program, every medication prescribed in the inpatient medical and/or surgical services of a series of collaborating hospitals was recorded and all subsequent medical events were ascertained (Danielson et al., 1982). Thus, both the timing and the frequency of events could be traced to exposure to drug and, controlling for those things that would have been expected within the underlying condition, so could unusual frequencies of adverse events that likely were causally associated with specific drugs. This remarkable effort resulted in documented and quantitated adverse effects of many drugs, as well as the absence of such effects in many more (Miller and Greenblatt, 1976). The approach proved very useful in determining the frequency of relatively common adverse experiences (occurring at rates $> 1/500$), but the collaborators determined that such a system, in order to erect cohorts of exposed populations at numbers large enough to detect rarer events (e.g., 1/5000 exposures) or to monitor new medication, would be prohibitively expensive and/or protracted. Over the long periods required for prospective monitoring, secular trends such as incidence of disease, drug utilization, and development of new or concomitant therapies would make the earlier exposure data not comparable to that occurring decades later. The Boston experience indicated that such traditional methods were felt to have become prohibitively expensive and too confounded to warrant continuation. By the early 1980s, further cohort collection was abandoned. Several other noteworthy examples of prospective monitoring in inpatients marked the early history of the field, including those at Johns Hopkins (Seidl et al., 1966) and Shands Hospital (Cluff et al., 1964) in the United States and at hospitals from Switzerland (Zoppi et al., 1982) to New Zealand (Smidt and McQueen, 1972).

Case Control Surveillance. A refinement of the labor-intensive case history follow-up system of the Boston Collaborative Drug Surveillance Program is the so-called case control surveillance system conducted by the Slone Epidemiology Unit (formerly Drug Epidemiology Unit) of Boston University (Slone et al., 1977). Under this method, systematic ongoing collection of comprehensive drug histories is undertaken for persons hospitalized with diseases thought a priori to be likely to have been caused by drugs. This collection provides a ready bank of such cases to enable rapid testing of problem signals generated elsewhere, for example, from spontaneous reports. Through the use of well-trained, consistently active nurse monitors and careful questionnaire design, this ongoing approach minimizes problems inherent in all hands-on case control methodologies (Slone et al., 1966; Mitchell et al., 1986).

THE NEED FOR BETTER SURVEILLANCE OF MARKETED DRUGS

In considering the state of definition of risk, the Joint Commission on Prescription Drug Use (JCPDU, 1980) recommended:

1. A systematic and comprehensive system of postmarketing drug surveillance should be developed in the United States.
2. Such a system should be able to detect important adverse drug reactions that occur more frequently than once per 1000 uses of a drug, to develop methods to detect less frequent reactions, and to evaluate the beneficial effects of drugs as used in ordinary practice. New methods will have to be developed for the study of delayed drug effects, including both therapeutic and adverse effects. *[Editor's Note: The JCPDU realized that event rates of 1/10,000 would likely be approachable by available techniques. In the appendixes*

to the report they sought to persuade colleagues that that level of detection should be a national goal.]
3. An integral function of the postmarketing system should be to report the uses and effects of both new and old prescription drugs.
4. Recognizing the progress that the FDA has made in the area of postmarketing drug surveillance, the commission recommended that postmarketing surveillance should be a priority program of the FDA and that the FDA should continue to strengthen its program in this area.

A fifth and final recommendation of the commission — that a private nonprofit center for drug surveillance should be established — never was implemented. However, the first four recommendations, so basic and yet so far-reaching, have received widespread recognition and have formed the basis for a burgeoning field of pharmacoepidemiology. The field did not possess this name in 1980. Pharmacoepidemiology couples the observational tools and methods of epidemiology (including epidemiologic intelligence and the structured cohort and case control methods) with the problems of pharmaceuticals. However, to gain impetus and overcome some of the methodologic and economic problems of its traditional use, the field needed not simply a new name but also a new partner, one that had not been available before the last decade, namely, the development of the large automated multipurpose data base.

The fundamental ingredient in the recipe of the Melmon Commission report was this rapidly emerging capacity. During the 1970s, particularly in the United States, large prepaid medical plans, health maintenance organizations (HMOs), and many of the large third-party insurance programs (e.g., Blue Cross/Blue Shield and, notably, Medicare) had instituted administrative efficiency provisions as part of a nationwide emphasis on cost containment and an organizational emphasis upon competitive pricing of services. Early in the decade, the monitoring of hospital discharge patterns through the use of automated data bases with encoded discharge diagnoses was becoming customary. Thus, hundreds of hospitals were participating in an automated data system of the Commission for Professional Hospital Accreditation (CPHA) (Jick, 1979). Under these arrangements, every discharge diagnosis for every person admitted to the hospital would be entered into a large automated data base along with a patient identifier. In the HMOs, this patient identifier frequently was the patient's membership number, because it also was in the third-party reimbursement systems. These data were as useful for claims payment and premium justification to the plans as they were for service planning for the institutions themselves.

By the mid-1970s, a consensus emerged in modern pharmacy circles about the benefit of automation, particularly for cost-efficient management of the pharmacies supporting HMOs. A single computer entry of prescription information was used for computer-assisted patient profiling, to generate dispensing labels, for computer-driven inventory and stocking control, and for "billing" to a patient master account. To accomplish these, a unifying number, generally again the patient's plan membership number, was used as the common denominator for development of the data base.

Professor Jick, the developer of the Boston Collaborative Drug Surveillance Program, recognized and harnessed the potential of automated data bases by linking the individual patient pharmaceutic exposure data in the pharmacy data base with the discharge diagnostic data base. Automated, multipurpose, record-linkage studies of medication-associated medical effects were thus born, extending the concept of manual record linkage from Oxford (Skegg and Doll, 1981). The prototype of such a system is the data base of the Group Health Cooperative of Puget Sound. This HMO, with 330,000 persons enrolled, has kept automated hospital diagnosis data in a patient-specific data base since the early 1970s as well as fully automated pharmacy information systems, again coded to individual patients since 1976 (Jick, 1985; Stergachis, 1988). Thus, accumulated over the past 15 years, 4 1/2 million person years of clinical experience can be retrieved for drug–disease associational studies. And, more germane, *such longitudinal data bases provide the possibility for defining cohorts of persons using drugs over longer periods of time.* Such cohorts are useful for ascertainment of possible chronic effects and long-term follow-up of these same populations (as long as they stay enrolled in the HMO) for identification of possible late effects (e.g., if a drug administered 10 years before is suspected of possible carcinogenicity). A further advantage to monitoring in an HMO, such as Group Health Cooperative of Puget Sound, is that provisions can be made to render the data base "anonymized" such that it may be used by external resources and investigators (as is the case with the Boston Collaborative Drug Surveillance Program) without direct access to the identity of any individual patient. Yet, using "scrambling and descrambling" techniques for such patient tracking, it is also possible for people directly involved in the health care setting to identify specific individuals and, where important, explore directly the medical record or, if necessary, make direct inquiry to develop important information that might not be available in the data base.

The data base of the Group Health Cooperative of Puget Sound, as developed and applied under the leadership of the Boston Cooperative Drug Surveillance Program, met the criteria laid out by the JCPDU for a resource that can rapidly assemble data on an entire population within reasonable costs. Thus, the opportunity for a new generation of postmarketing surveillance opened. Developing at the same time were data resources in other HMOs or group practice settings, particularly those of the Kaiser Permanente Health Plans in Oregon, northern California, and more recently across the United States (Friedman, 1989). Though these plans were slower to automate their pharmacies, the development of their useful data resources is now well underway. It is estimated that early in the 1990s, drug exposure- and hospital discharge–linked data will be available for populations in excess of 4 million persons in Kaiser Permanente health plans alone. Whether they can be used for drug surveillance remains to be determined. At any rate, we have come to know what we need and what we can expect from data bases used for pharmacoepidemiologic purposes (see Table 35–1).

Similar data bases have been developed that permit capture of administrative data from third-party payment systems. The best established and most epidemiologically useful one is that of the Province of Saskatchewan in Canada (West, 1988; Downey and Strand, 1989). Through this data base all hospital discharge summary data have been available on computer since 1972; all pharmacy data linked to the same unique patient identifying number have been available since 1976; and a series of other public health data bases (births, deaths, cancer registries) linked or linkable through patient number or coded algorithms is available. In the United Kingdom (in

Table 35–1. ATTRIBUTES OF AN IDEAL MULTIPURPOSE DATA BASE FOR PHARMACOEPIDEMIOLOGY VS. WHAT IS REASONABLE TO EXPECT

IDEAL	ADEQUATE OR USUAL

• Comprehensive medical data
  All prescriptions
  All diagnoses
  All major life events
	• Most transactions
	  Outpatient prescriptions
	  Hospital diagnoses
	  Births and deaths (including cause)

• Population-based	• Most people
• Fully linked	• Single unique patient ID Family codes
• Longitudinal and continuous	• Continuous from start date — membership turnover can be detected
• Validated	• Medical records available or patient interview is possible

Tayside, Scotland), a similarly promising project, Medication Events Monitoring (MEMO), takes advantage of automation of hospital diagnoses (Crombie et al., 1984). Though MEMO currently requires manual linkage with available printed prescriptions, automation of prescription records and creation of a multipurpose linked data base is planned.

In the United States, the largest of comparable data bases are those providing administrative support to medical payment programs for the medically indigent under Medicaid. Data from several state Medicaid programs have been made available to individual researchers in Tennessee and California (Ray and Griffin, 1989), New Jersey (Avorn, 1990a), Maine (Walker, personal communication, 1991), Michigan, Minnesota, Florida, and others (Carson et al., 1987; Strom and Carson, 1989; Avorn, 1990; and others). The ground-breaking work of the contract firm Health Information Designs to develop the Medicaid-derived data base COMPASS (Computerized On-line Medicaid Pharmaceutical Analysis and Surveillance System) (Strom et al., 1985b), under contract to the FDA (Calren et al., 1981), helped to translate the policy recommendations of the JCPDU into action. Through this contract, longitudinal, linked data concerning cohorts of millions of Medicaid recipients permitted investigation of the association between drug exposure and disease outcome (as billed in hospital payments) and made these data available on line for the FDA as well as university researchers. This is currently enabling agency, academic, and industry scientists to make systematic population checks, for example, to verify cautionary signals from spontaneous reports of events serious enough to result in hospitalization in association with drug-exposed cohorts, and to do so at a small fraction of the costs of a traditional epidemiologic approach. A recent report from the FDA (Faich, 1989) listed more than 40 policy decisions made by the agency over the prior 5 years that rested entirely or in major part upon such data.

The Ideal Data Base

Consumers of information from the large, multipurpose data bases will need a sophisticated understanding of the strengths and limitations of each resource. Each of the data bases, erected for purposes other than drug epidemiology, contains information on some but not all vital parts of the "ideal" data set for an epidemiologic study (see Table 35–1).

What would such an ideal data set look like? For an epidemiologic study of the impact of a medication in a population, it would be important to know all instances of prescription; all "major" medical events (at the very least, all hospitalizations) by accurately coded diagnosis (i.e., all discharge diagnoses); all important demographic data (including age, race, sex, marital status, occupational status, and family size); major vital statistics (at least births and deaths, and if death, cause and date); and important information about aspects of life and lifestyle that may influence the association between drug exposure and morbid outcome (e.g., smoking behavior, alcohol intake, substance abuse). If one or more of these critical elements are missing, however, the data bases still may be useful, particularly if supplemented with other information. Thus, if an association between drug exposure and excess frequency of hospital diagnoses that appear plausibly related to drug is found, and data from the death certificate were not included in the data base, a link to state medical examiners might be arranged, as has been done by the Boston Collaborative Drug Surveillance Program working with the Group Health Cooperative data set. Of course, insofar as lifestyle data or more subtle medical diagnostic information may be necessary, special arrangements would need to be made for follow-up with physicians or patients themselves. Under certain circumstances, these inquiries already have been demonstrated to be possible, but they bring with them additional costs, intervention into the practice setting, and many of the biases and problems of previous hands-on approaches.

The quality of outpatient data in the large multipurpose linked data sets is in general dubious. There are several reasons for this. In automated medical record settings where outpatient data are recorded, most often physicians' shorthand gets in the way of complete recording of events necessary to understand associations between drug and disease. In fact, some of the most easily omitted record entries (e.g., the reason a drug was stopped) might be the most important for pharmacoepidemiology. In outpatient billing data, generally only one diagnosis is required (if any), and often this one is likely to be that which is most easily recalled, is most expedient, or on balance achieves the higher reimbursement rate. However, with *proper access to the ambulatory medical record for validation and/or automated laboratory, diagnostic, and procedural data for cross-diagnostic corroboration, computer-linked ambulatory data are more frequently found to be useful in substantiating, reinforcing, and extending the diagnostic information from hospital data sets in multipurpose linked data sets.*

A final critical element in the linked multipurpose data base is the quality of the "link" itself. The ideal is an unduplicated, continuous patient identification number that can be linked (e.g., by extra digits) to all family members. But, of course, people move in and out (of geographic or categorical eligibility), get married and divorced, have multiple children from different marriages, and so forth. What is critical is to ensure that the computer is programmed to recognize such tenuous links.

Inpatient Monitoring

A development similar to that in the prepaid health care sector has more recently occurred within hospitals themselves. In addition to the automated monitoring of discharge diagnoses for hospital management purposes that occurred during the 1980s, the automation of hospital pharmacy systems has been realized, as well as automation of other hospital support services, including laboratory reporting and admissions and demographic activities. The state of this automation varies from hospital to hospital and is evolving rapidly. However, even at the beginning of the 1990s, the feasibility and usefulness of linking automated hospital pharmacy data with patient-specific automated hospital diagnosis data have been demonstrated (Platt et al., 1988; Burke et al., 1989). In such schemes, every time a physician orders a medication for any patient, that patient's drugs are "billed" to the patient's account in a way that allows their specific identification. Similar to the HMO experience, all discharge diagnoses are also linked to the same patient number, as are the data from the admitting office. Thus, it is possible to characterize a population receiving one of a series of drugs requiring monitoring and to document all important diagnoses for comparison. For monitoring the short-term effects that may have been missed in clinical trials early in the life of a newly marketed product, these automated data bases have enormous promise. Because the patients are in the hospital, the ability to rapidly assemble populations of recipients of a monitored medication is accompanied by the availability of medical records complete with nursing as well as medical progress notes — often a very rich source of information regarding adverse experiences that might not be reflected in hospital discharge diagnoses. These same records are available for exploration of possible explanatory or confounding variables in the event that an association between drug exposure and an excess of certain problems is observed.

The linked automated multipurpose data base has fulfilled the promise of the JCPDU. Because "all" the data are in the computer for administrative reasons, there are no data-collection or data-entry costs associated with research. Indeed, it is a wonderful, serendipitous spinoff that the data have proved so useful. All data regarding pre-scriptions are entered without any hypotheses or research interests. The computer remembers them all, with no problem of recall bias. The same is true of medical events. Because most important medical events are in the computer for administrative reasons, there is no need to ask the physician to draw an association between exposure and event for it to be registered. All the physician needs to do is practice good medicine and record keeping and the search for excess frequencies of important medical events that may be "caused" by the drugs can be accomplished independently, eliminating the biases and intellectual barriers of reporters and the cost-inefficient use of busy practitioners' time. This "objective" approach is especially useful when the adverse event is one that occurs spontaneously and frequently in clinical practice without drugs, so that the physician might not even consider the role of a drug (e.g., in pancreatitis); when the physician treating the event is unaware that the patient was taking the medication (e.g., the internist prescribes the cataract causer, but the ophthalmologist observes the cataract); or when the event is separated widely over time from the exposure (e.g., a congenital defect observed by the pediatrician who was not the mother's physician, or neoplasia observed several generations of physicians after the exposure).

AUTOMATED MEDICAL RECORDS

One promising development in the computing side of pharmacoepidemiology useful to clinician and researcher alike is the automated medical record system. The fully automated medical record — that is, the truly paperless practice — remains a vision of the future. However, many such practices exist in the United States (e.g., the Regenstrief Institute in Indianapolis and the Harvard Community Health Plan in Boston) and in Europe (e.g., the computer-assisted practice networks in the United Kingdom, particularly VAMP and AAH Meditel). They give a glimpse of this future. In such systems, the decision to prescribe a medication results in a single computer entry that is then "routed" to the patient's permanent medical record, various drug-interaction algorithms, and an automated patient medication inventory. Automatically generated prescription linkage to plan pharmacies is not far away. In these, the benefits of automation for computer-generated dispensing labels, inventory control, and patient profiling are clear. Likewise, in the automated medical record, every diagnosis and clinical finding, including adverse events that may be occurring in association with prescriptions, will be documented. Early efforts at attempting to link drug exposure with such adverse events (e.g., Hershel Jick with VAMP in the

United Kingdom and Richard Platt with Harvard Community Health Plan in Boston) suggest that this resource will yield a very rich background of information regarding events in outpatient medical practice as well as association between medication exposure and major medical events such as hospitalization.

Such data are already most promising, particularly for tracing events that might not be so serious as to precipitate a hospitalization. The practitioner still has to remember that the quality of the data coming out is only as good as the quality of the data going in. The quality of automated outpatient medical records is no better than the quality of outpatient medical records in general.

Limitations of Developments

Pharmacoepidemiology has brought substantial progress to the development of methods to produce good, affordable data on drug safety for the prescriber. However, there also are substantial limitations that must be understood if these resources are to benefit society—that is, to help prescribers know what they need to know as quickly and as accurately as necessary in order to factor such information into the therapeutic decision. Specifically, concerning all data bases, a computer can only hold those data the system provides to it. Thus, only coded hospital discharge diagnoses are entered into the computer—diagnoses deemed by the treating physician to be important enough to have been listed on a discharge summary. Many subtle but medically important conclusions lie fallow in the medical record.

Another limitation involves questions relating to drug exposure. Only medicines that are prescribed can be monitored. Therefore, nonprescribed (for example, many of the OTC) medicines do not appear in the data bases. If the plan in which the drug–disease association is being reviewed chooses not to include that medication in the formulary (perhaps because the drug is a new chemical entity, early in its postapproval phases, and the plan's physicians are therapeutically conservative, or when the formulary committee or other drug decision-making group feels that there are suitable and cheaper alternatives), then a new medication may not be used in the plan, and it therefore cannot be monitored. To date, the majority of HMO plans most useful for pharmacoepidemiology have not automated their medication distribution systems within hospitals, thus (paradoxically) swinging the pendulum from a time in the early days of hands-on epidemiology with intensive inpatient monitoring to a time when inpatient drug exposure may be the most difficult to monitor. Help is on the way in this

arena with the emerging automated hospital systems.

Limiting the usefulness of these resources yet further is the mobility of the population served. Mobility is particularly a problem in "high turnover" plans such as Medicaid. There is a lack of generalizability in some of the populations—relative underrepresentation of minorities, the chronically ill, and the elderly in the HMOs; relative overrepresentation of women and small children in Medicaid; and disproportionate contribution to the experience in the data base of people who do not move on because they are chronically ill. These are important drawbacks to the study of the most representative populations.

Validity problems with diagnostic data in Medicaid were demonstrated in a quality assessment funded by the FDA (Lessler and Harris, 1984). This report reinforced the growing awareness of researchers that careful validation of data from such diagnostic data bases is needed prior to drawing conclusions about associations between drug and disease. Yet because of the public welfare nature of the Medicaid program and the perceived sensitivity of privacy issues, such as access to records, availability of medical records to validate automated data has been difficult to ensure. This contrasts with the situation in HMOs. Depending on the question to be asked, even the medical record represents an inadequate instrument for proper research. This is particularly true in lack of information on important or potential confounding variables, such as smoking and use of alcohol. When validity requires such data, the traditional hands-on approach must be used (Shapiro, 1989), though linked data may complement such research (Strom and Carson, 1989; Jick and Walker, 1989; Faich and Stadel, 1989).

Two further important factors that prevent society from achieving the full benefits of pharmacoepidemiology are the limit of availability of qualified researchers—those who generate the data—and limited epidemiologic training of practitioners, policymakers, and the public at large—those who must deal appropriately with the data. The pharmacoepidemiologic era demands very sophisticated approaches and very complicated and extensive computer data sets, requiring skills often not available even at the most competent academic, industrial, or commercial pharmacology or epidemiology research unit. We face a serious technology lag in which such skills must be taught and mastered. The dangers of idle, unskilled use of powerful tools, such as the automated linked data set, cannot be overemphasized. Society lacks systems to protect itself against bad science. For example, once a possible excess rate of a problem in association with the use of a drug is found, the true epidemiologic work has only just begun. While this is a problem with all epidemiology, not simply the new pharmacoepidemiology, it is especially acute in a situation in which large, automated, multipurpose data bases permit "fishing" expeditions in which the investigator "trolls" for all associations between exposure and outcome irrespective of any plausible cause. In traditional research settings, the researcher was required to think through possible causal associations in advance of hypothesis. Now, the data are all already entered in a grand national social experiment.

For example, if a new NSAID that was nonirritating to the GI mucosa were to be introduced, physicians probably would switch their NSAID-intolerant prior bleeders to the new drug. The data base would show an increased frequency of GI problems associated with the new drug, probably even GI bleeds in this GI bleed–prone population, even though much less frequent bleeding was seen than would have been had they used an old NSAID. This *confounding by indication* is a classic epidemiologic trap, one that could probably (though not necessarily) have been carefully addressed by the baseline data questionnaire in a traditional epidemiologic study. Once the computer finds the association, though it lacks underlying data about the patient's initial medical condition, there will doubtless be a substantial delay before such research can be done. On the other hand, the signal once generated develops a life of its own. The solution to this quandary lies in part in careful conduct of such studies by thoughtful and thorough investigators.

Regarding Efficacy

The emphasis of this chapter is upon safety. The focus has been on the contributions of epidemiologic studies, and in particular large automated data bases, toward refining estimates of drug safety and developing new and heretofore unavailable information on large populations over a long period. At times, the field has been faulted for accentuating the negative. There are important positive applications of the same data. For example, if longitudinal data can be linked for an individual person and generalized to broad populations of persons with similar experiences, for the first time we will have ready access to population-based "natural history" data relating to most diseases, even relatively rare ones. Therefore, when the question is asked about the expectation of survival or recurrence or continued or repeated institutionalization for specific diseases, the practitioner, rather than having to rely on expert judgment or an ad hoc case series at the local medical school, will be able to turn to the large data bases and obtain a current "state of the practice" assessment of the natural history of important concomitant and subsequent medical events.

A special area of interest relating to linked data bases may contribute to a better understanding of the positive impact of therapeutic interventions and perhaps even efficacy (Melmon, 1990; 1991). To guard against biases, a cardinal rule of science holds that when testing for the efficacy of new medicines, the randomized, blinded, controlled clinical trial is needed, preferably with placebo control or at very least with active medication control. When exposed groups are not randomized, the anticipation of therapeutic benefit that underlies the choice of one drug versus another cannot be documented but clearly could have an impact upon the likelihood of a beneficial outcome. Furthermore, expecting that a patient will do well on an efficacious drug is likely to prejudice the reviewer who determines how well the person does. However, these and other concerns to the contrary notwithstanding, the data from large epidemiologic data sets may inform us about efficacy in clinical practice (Strom et al., 1984; Strom et al., 1985a). Certainly, continued prescription of a medication is a sign that whether correct or not, the treating community and the population being treated find the intervention acceptable. Understanding patterns of therapy—which interventions are selected for which diseases with what frequency, and with what frequency and pattern patients are switched to other interventions—now has become relatively affordable and is highly useful in helping us to understand current practices irrespective of documentation that they make a difference (Piper et al., 1987).

Some situations simply preclude randomized clinical trials, either for practical reasons (e.g., in very rare diseases or apparently lifesaving situations) or for ethical reasons (e.g., in women who may become pregnant during the trial). In such cases, the measurement of clinical outcomes that are beneficial, in addition to the documentation of absence of untoward medical events, may be the only way to know whether a drug has impact in this population. Similarly, as epidemiologic studies are at their best when they are monitoring adverse events that could not have been predicted by the intervention and the practitioner doing the intervening, so too, totally unexpected therapeutic outcomes that are beneficial may emerge from such epidemiologic studies. The discovery that the incidence of myocardial infarction was reduced in persons who were chronic aspirin recipients was reported early in such multipurpose studies (see Table 35–2) (Jick and Miettinen, 1976).

The vast body of research in this field finds, time after time, that if serious unexpected side effects are happening, they must be occurring less

Table 35–2. **EXAMPLES OF EPIDEMIOLOGIC STUDIES THAT REVEALED UNEXPECTED EFFECTS OF MEDICATIONS**

TYPE OF SURVEILLANCE	DRUG	EFFECT DETECTED
• Epidemiologic intelligence or spontaneous reports	Zimelidine	Guillain-Barré
	Suprofen	Flank pain
• Classic approaches		
Cohort studies	Oral contraceptives	Thromboembolism
	Aspirin	Prevention of myocardial infarction
Case control studies	A number of drugs	Agranulocytosis
		Cancer
• Systematic approaches		
Intensive inpatient monitoring	Ampicillin	Rash
Case control surveillance	Estrogens	Breast cancer
Prescription event monitoring	Innovase	Cough
• Multipurpose data bases	Accutane	Birth defects
	NSAIDS	GI bleeding
	Thiazide	Hip fracture
	Estrogens	Endometrial cancer

frequently than 1/3000 to 1/10,000 uses of the medicine, depending upon the size of the follow-up study. The size of such a study is, of course, determined by practical, medical, and economic constraints. The studies certainly provide perspective that the anecdotal or spontaneous adverse reaction report simply cannot do. Thus, the Boston Collaborative Drug Surveillance Program alone has reported over 100 such studies using the large automated data base with Group Health Cooperative of Puget Sound (Cohen, 1986); Medicaid researchers have conducted dozens more, and yet more are under way (Strom and Carson, 1989). The FDA recently reported over 40 instances in the past 5 years in which it has turned to the large automated data bases to clarify the situation particularly with regard to a possible adverse effect suggested by one or more spontaneous reports (Faich, 1990). Recently, for example, a cluster of cases of sudden death was reported in association with use of human insulin. The FDA and several manufacturers responded by turning to the various data bases at their disposal in North America and England. They examined the association, controlling for variables likely to be associated with sudden death, such as age and coexisting heart disease, and found that the differences in death rates disappeared: the signal was a false alarm.

Some epidemiologic studies have contributed to the discovery of important adverse effects, and their correlates lead to major therapeutic recommendations. Spontaneous voluntary adverse reactions reports (epidemiologic intelligence) have repeatedly resulted in signals that could not possibly be false alarms and that have resulted in early termination of marketing and/or major revisions in medical practices relating to specific medica-

tions. Society learned to respect the adverse potential of chloramphenicol when aplastic anemia became apparent. Indeed, medical practice has only gradually put the adverse effects of chloramphenicol into perspective with its benefits over the intervening 20 years. Recently, zimelidine was removed from the market in Sweden following spontaneous reports of Guillain-Barré syndrome (Fagius et al., 1985). Similarly, in the United States, an "epidemic" of flank pain, otherwise unexplained, resulted in removal of suprofan from the market (Rossi et al., 1988).

Classic epidemiologic approaches have likewise made their positive contributions. Large hands-on cohort studies confirmed and quantified the association of thromboembolism with oral contraceptives (Markush and Siegel, 1969) and subsequently clarified and quantified risk factors for coronary occlusion and stroke (Porter et al., 1985). More recently, such approaches have helped to clarify the association between aspirin use and Reye syndrome (Hurwitz et al., 1985). On the affirmative side, a cohort study showed a reduction in the incidence of myocardial infarction among chronic aspirin users (Jick and Miettinen, 1976).

Case control studies have been used on many occasions to test and quantitate associations between specific outcomes and excess drug exposures in order to calculate relative risks, including the risk ratios of various antibiotics and analgesics with agranulocytosis (Jick and Vessey, 1978; International Agranulocytosis and Aplastic Anemia Study, 1986).

The systematic approaches to hands-on epidemiology also have resulted in important findings. The intensive inpatient monitoring programs of the Boston Collaborative Drug Surveillance Program and others already mentioned have found and quantitated numerous associations, such as rash with ampicillin, and allopurinol–ampicillin interaction. Case control surveillance has clarified the association between estrogens and cancers, and PEM detected and warned against respiratory problems ("cough") with innovase (Inman et al., 1988).

The multipurpose data base, already a great producer of large numbers of affordable, feasible, and powerful studies that have found the absence of associations, has also found its share of current associations, including the likelihood of birth defects with the use of isotretinoin during pregnancy (Faich, 1990); frequency, nature, severity, and drug-specific risk rates of upper GI bleeding in association with NSAIDs (Beard et al., 1987; Bortnichak and Sachs, 1986a; Guess et al., 1988); negative association of hip fracture with thiazide diuretics (Ray et al., 1989); and positive association between hip fracture and psychotropic drugs (Ray et al., 1987); and quantitation of the risk of endometrial cancer with the use of estrogen, including a dramatic secular trend when these use patterns and doses change (Jick et al., 1980).

To summarize, data from the automated multipurpose linked data bases are a powerful new resource from which to provide rapid, useful hypotheses related to possible drug effects; of considerable importance in medical decision making and public policy. Studies can confirm and assess the relative frequency of signals of potentially major harm in association with a drug use (see Table 35–2 for examples). This development has materially changed the availability and quality of information for prescribing clinicians. The data are particularly useful in that they permit proper comparison across different drugs used for the same indication.

The products of this resource have only begun to be available to the physician to assist in medical benefit–risk assessments, but the importance is clear. Today, the physician relies on the theoretical possibility of association between treatment and possible adverse events or waits for the results of the more elegant traditional study. By the end of the 1990s the physician will have available for any widely used new medicine data that will enable direct comparison of risks of similar severity by frequency as low as 1/10,000 therapeutic courses.

UNDERSTANDING RISKS: THE CHALLENGES AHEAD

Ten years after the report of the JCPDU, the progress has been substantial. But that progress also lays out the agenda for the decade ahead.

Spontaneous Reporting

Reporting of adverse reactions by treating physicians will continue to be the point of departure for any safety surveillance system. By drawing from the experience of the entire population, we will learn about relatively rare events. However, physician reporting has not improved much, if any, over the past decade. Efforts to improve physician participation in spontaneous voluntary adverse reactions reporting have been launched (e.g., under contract from the FDA to the states of Maryland, Rhode Island, and Mississippi). After initially encouraging results, the rates, without frequent reinforcement, tended to decline. Furthermore, it is not clear that the "right" reactions are being reported, that the system is capable of follow-up of these reports to validate impressions, or that the benefits of the system are worth the extra costs and inefficiencies on the part of already-overburdened state public health departments and clinicians (Scott et al., 1990). Efforts to encourage physician participation in spontaneous reporting will always be needed but should be balanced against the inherent limitations of the system and the marginal value of further refining it.

Improved reporting in the published literature, likewise, certainly is needed. Editors must more rigorously ensure that data necessary for the understanding of an adverse experience are included in letters to the editor or other brief reports in which a possible drug–disease association is flagged. At a minimum, information regarding dose and dates of exposure, exposure to other important alternative causes, timing of events, nature of events, and response to the challenge and rechallenge of therapy should be required. And no editor should accept such a report unless the author attests to having already reported it directly to someone who is in a position to do something about it—the industry or the regulatory authority. More reporting physicians, whether reporting to their peers in print or their colleagues through spontaneous reports to industry or directly to the FDA, are needed, and all need to be more thoughtful about what they report. Hospitals, as a source of spontaneous adverse reactions reports, are sorely underutilized. Recent recognition of the importance of systems for monitoring adverse drug reactions in hospitals has prompted changes in the requirements of the JCAHO.

Improved Capacity for Structured Studies

For the new field of pharmacoepidemiology, the work ahead is substantial and vitally needed. Although the United States currently has large, automated, multipurpose data sets describing health care delivery in over 5 million persons, more such data sets are needed if we are to know as much as we need to know as quickly as we would like to know it. As more HMOs automate their data, attention must be given to the necessary prerequisites for research applications of these data. Not only will this rigor not drive up costs, but it will materially contribute to social usefulness. Better, more rapid, and more complete mechanisms are needed for medical record retrieval and other documentation activities for data derived from claims payment programs outside HMOs. Good practice standards must be developed for appropriate uses of (and safeguards regarding) these important data sets. More training is needed for more skilled researchers. And a better social support system is needed for financing the ongoing efforts of important data resources and research institutions. While not of direct concern to the practicing clinician, these aspects of the field nevertheless should be understood. For example, with inadequate data base resources, populations smaller than those which would be ideal are monitored. Thus, large-scale epidemiologic studies are only able to report the actual experience in the actual exposed populations in actual monitored populations. Furthermore, chance occurrences may be found and epidemiologic clusters occur by chance alone from time to time. An association once found in one data base needs to be confirmed in the second. The absence of the second data base leaves the prescriber with a confusing signal—a definite maybe. Further, the inadequate financial support to the core function of these research resources often leads researchers to plumb questions for which a commercial sponsor could be found but not to tackle questions that may be more important and relevant and urgently needed by the clinician. Also, playing to a commercial sponsor can distract attention from spontaneous monitoring (Inman, 1990).

Initiatives to Help Move the Postmarketing Surveillance Sector Forward

In the 1980s several powerful multinational efforts helped to translate the promise of pharmacoepidemiology into daily practical reality. Particularly noteworthy were the creation of an International Working Group on Pharmacoepidemiology, the Risk Assessment of Drugs—Analysis and Response (known as RADAR) initiative, and the formation of International Society for Pharmacoepidemiology. The RADAR initiative, started under the aegis of the Ciba Geigy Corporation, has convened representatives from the pharmaceutical world to focus on the dual problem of assessing the medication-associated risks

and translating them in plain talk to all those who need to understand them. Among products of these deliberations have been the creation of several national working groups on risk assessment and risk communication; a fledgling effort at the development of an international foundation to help to fund many of the much needed efforts, particularly to provide core support to emerging large multipurpose data bases and disease or drug registries; and an international working group of epidemiologists in the pharmaceutical industry (EPI) (Tilson and Bruppacher, 1990). One of the strongest recommendations of the EPI working group was that a multidisciplinary, multisector, multinational forum was needed for full airing of the problems and progress in this emerging field (Tilson et al., 1990).

Pharmacoepidemiology for the Clinician

Today's therapeutic decision maker needs to know everything about safety that his or her predecessors knew. The objective remains the same: to assess the likelihood of significant benefit for the patient compared with the same adjusted likelihood for alternative interventions, including no medication at all. What has changed is the requirement to understand the nature, quality, and extent of the data on efficacy and safety upon which these decisions are made.

Absence of data does not mean absence of problems. To put into perspective the absence of a signal from the spontaneous voluntary adverse reactions reporting system, the prescriber needs to consider the likelihood that such an event, were it occurring in association with therapy, would be recognized and reported. Also, the importance of this signal "nonsignal" needs to be understood by having more information about the denominator—the extent of the population experience against which one can assess just how rare a benefit or risk would need to be to escape such detection.

Finally, the clinician must prepare to assimilate pharmacoepidemiology by demanding better understanding of the extent to which the risks associated with a medication choice are truly known; by actively encouraging and participating in efforts to reduce the residual uncertainty; and by insisting on better application of that knowledge in therapeutic decision making (see chapter 41).

The focus of this chapter has been on the ways in which safety data are generated to help the physician make a medication choice and understand not only the inventory of likely adverse effects and frequencies of each but also the extent to which the data supporting these descriptions is solid. The need for better confirmed and more useful and more timely data is clear. Equally clear should be the worth of such efforts—they make an important difference. From time to time, researchers in this field get discouraged, regulators get criticized, and politicians get nervous, all because the primary product of pharmacoepidemiology is "negative results." But new and better drugs are truly needed; the purpose of these epidemiologic endeavors is not to cause new and needed drugs to be removed from or restricted in the market unnecessarily or to find things that are not there. This is one body of science in which the absence of findings is socially useful.

REFERENCES

Avorn, J.: Medicaid-based pharmacoepidemiology: Claims and counterclaims. Epidemiology, 1:98–100, 1990a.

Avorn, J.: Reporting drug side effects: Signals and noise. J.A.M.A., 263(13):1823, 1990b.

Beard, J.; Walker, A. M.; Perera, D. R.; and Jick, H.: Nonsteroidal anti-inflammatory drugs and hospitalization for gastroesophageal bleeding in the elderly. Arch. Intern. Med., 147:1621–1623, 1987.

Best, W. R.: Chloramphenicol-associated blood dyscrasias. A review of cases submitted to the American Medical Association Registry. J.A.M.A., 201:181–188, 1967.

Borden, E. K.; and Lee, J. G.: A methodologic study of postmarketing drug evaluation using a pharmacy-based approach. J. Chronic Dis., 35:803–816, 1982.

Bortnichak, E. A.; and Sachs, R. M.: Piroxicam in recent epidemiologic studies. Am. J. Med., 81(suppl. 5B):44–48, 1986.

Burke, J. P.; Platt, R.; and Tilson, H. H.: Expanding roles of hospital epidemiology: Pharmacoepidemiology. Infect. Control Hosp. Epidemiol., 10:253–254, 1989.

Calren, S.; Nalley, P.; Gregory, G., et al.: The Evaluability Assessment of the Developing Experiment in Postmarketing Surveillance of Prescription Drugs. NBS-GCR-ETIP-81-96. Experimental Technology Incentives Program, Washington, D.C., 1981.

Carson, J. L.; Strom, B. L.; Morse, M. L.; West, S. L.; Soper, K. A.; Stolley, P. D.; and Jones, J. K.: The relative gastrointestinal toxicity of the non-steroidal anti-inflammatory drugs. Arch. Intern. Med., 147:1054–1059, 1987.

Cluff, L. E.; Thronton, G. F.; and Seidl, L. G.: Studies on the epidemiology of adverse drug reactions: I. Methods of surveillance. J.A.M.A., 188:976–983, 1964.

Cohen, M. R.: A compilation of abstracts and index published by the Boston Collaborative Drug Surveillance Program 1966–1985. Hosp. Pharm., 21:497, 1986.

Creagh-Kirk, T.; Doi, P.; Andrews, E.; Nusinoff-Lehrman, S.; Tilson, H.; Hoth, D.; and Barry, D. W.: Survival experience among persons with AIDS receiving zidovudine: Follow-up of patients in a compassionate plea program. J.A.M.A., 260: 3009–3015, 1986.

Crombie, I. K.; Brown, S. V.; and Hamley, J. G.: Postmarketing drug surveillance by record linkage in Tayside. J. Epidemiol. Community Health, 38:226–231, 1984.

Danielson, D. A.; Porter J. B.; Dinan, B. J.; O'Connor, P. C.; Lawson, D. H.; Kellaway, G. S. M.; and Jick H.: Drug monitoring of surgical patients. J.A.M.A., 248:1482–1485, 1982.

DiMasi, J.: FDC Reports, CSDD Study. Chevy Chase, Md, The Pink Sheet, 1990.

Downey, W.; and Strand, L.: Current status of the Saskatchewan Drug Plan. In, Pharmacoepidemiology (Edlavitch, S., ed.). Proceedings of the Third International Conference on Pharmacoepidemiology, Minneapolis, 1987. Lewis Publishers, Ann Arbor, 1989.

Fagius, J.; Osteman, P. O.; Siden, A.; and Wilholm, B.-E.: Guillain-Barré syndrome following zimelidine treatment. J. Neurol. Neurosurg. Psychiatry, 48:65–69, 1985.

Faich, G. A.: FDA contribution (presentation). DIA Annual Meeting, San Francisco, June, 1990.

Faich, G. A.: Record linkage for postmarketing surveillance. Clin. Pharmacol. Ther., 49:479–480, 1989.

Faich, G. A.; and Stadel, B. V.: The future of automated record linkage for postmarketing surveillance: A response to Shapiro. Clin. Pharmacol. Ther., 46:387–389, 1989.

Faich, G. A.; Milstien, J. B.; Anello, C.; and Baum, C.: Sources of spontaneous adverse drug reaction reports received by pharmaceutical manufacturers. Drug Info. J., 21: 251–255, 1987.

Friedman, G. P.: Kaiser Permanente Medical Care Program: Northern California and Other Regions. In, Pharmacoepidemiology (Strom, B. L., ed.). New York: Churchill Livingstone, pp. 161–172, 1989.

Geiling, E. M. K.; and Carmon, P. R.: Pathologic effects of elixir of sulfanilamides (diethylene glycol) poisoning. J.A.M.A., 111:919–926, 1938.

Grahame-Smith, D. G.: Report of the Adverse Reaction Working Party to the Committee on Safety of Medicines. Department of Health and Social Security, London, 1986.

Grasela, T. H.; and Schentag, J. J.: A clinical pharmacy-oriented drug surveillance network: I. Program description. Drug Intell. Clin. Pharm., 21:902–908, 1987.

Griffin, J. P.; and Weber, J. C. P.: Voluntary systems of adverse reaction reporting. Acute Poisoning Rev., 5:23–55, 1986.

Guess, H. A.; West, R.; Strand, L. M.; Helston, P.; Lydick, E. G.; Bergman, U.; and Wolski, K.: Fatal upper gastrointestinal hemorrhage or perforation among users and nonusers of nonsteroidal anti-inflammatory drugs in Saskatchewan, Canada, 1983. J. Clin. Epidemiol., 41:35–45, 1988.

Herbst, A. L.; Ulfelder, H.; and Poskanzer, D. C.: Adenocarcinoma of the vagina: Association of material stilbestrol therapy with tumor appearance in young women. N. Engl. J. Med., 284:878–881, 1971.

Hurwitz, E. S.; Barrett, M. J.; Bregman, D.; Gunn, W. J.; Schonberger, L. B.; Fairweather, W. R.; Drage, J. S.; LaMontagne, J. R.; Keslow, R. A.; Burlington, D. B.; Quinnan, G. V.; Parker, R. A.; Phillips, K.; Pinsky, P.; Dayton, D.; and Dowdle, W. R.: Public Health Service Study on Reye's syndrome and medication. Report of the pilot phase. N. Engl. J. Med., 313:849–857, 1985.

Ibrahim, M. A. (ed.): Case-control study: Consensus and controversy. J. Chronic Dis., 32:1, 1979.

Idanpaan-Heikkila, J.: A review of safety information obtained from phases I, II and III clinical investigations of sixteen selected drugs. Food and Drug Administration, Center for Drug and Biologics, Rockville, Md, 1983.

Inman, W. H. W.: Postmarketing surveillance of adverse drug reactions in general practice: II. Prescription-event monitoring at the University of Southampton. Br. Med. J., 282:1216–1217, 1981.

Inman, W. H. W.; Rawson, N. S. D.; Wilton, L. V.; Pearce, G. L.; and Speirs, C. J.: Post-marketing surveillance of analapril: I. Results of prescription-event monitoring. Br. Med. J., 297:826–829, 1988.

International Agranulocytosis and Aplastic Anemia Study: Risks of agranulocytosis and aplastic anemia: A first report of their relation to drug use with special reference to analgesics. J.A.M.A., 256:1749–1757, 1986.

Janssen, W. F.: Outline of the history of US drug regulation and labeling. Food, Drug, Cosmetic Law J., August, Vol 36: 420–441, 1981.

Jick, H.: Use of automated data bases to study drug effects after marketing. Pharmacotherapy, 5:278–279, 1985.

Jick, H.: The Commission on Professional and Hospital Activities—Professional activity study. Am. J. Epidemiol., 109: 625–627, 1979.

Jick, H.: The discovery of drug-induced illness. N. Engl. J. Med., 296:481–485, 1977.

Jick, H.; and Miettinen, O. S.: Regular aspirin use and myocardial infarction. Br. Med. J., 1:1057, 1976.

Jick, H.: Drugs—remarkably nontoxic. N. Engl. J. Med., 291: 824–828, 1974.

Jick, H.; and Vessey, M.: Case-control studies in the evaluation of the drug-induced illness. Am. J. Epidemiol., 107:1–7, 1978.

Jick, H.; and Walker, A. M.: Uninformed criticism of automated record linkage. Clin. Pharmacol. Ther., 46:478–479, 1989.

Jick, H.; Miettinen, O. S.; Shapiro, S.; Lewis, G. P.; Suskind, V.; and Slone, D.: Comprehensive drug surveillance. J.A.M.A., 213:1455–1460, 1970.

Jick, H.; Walker, A. M.; Watkins, R. N.; Diewart, D. C.; Hunter, J. R.; Danford, A.; Madsen, S.; Dinan, B. J.; and Rothman, K. J.: Replacement estrogens and breast cancer. Am. J. Epidemiol., 112(6):586–594, 1980.

Joint Commission for Accreditation of Health Care Organizations (JCAHO): The Definition and Review of All Significant Untoward Drug Reactions. Accreditation Manual for Hospitals, Vol. 129. 1988.

Joint Commission on Prescription Drug Use (JCPDU): Final Report. Joint Commission on Prescription Drug Use. Washington, D.C., 1980.

Juergens, J.: Controversies in adverse drug reaction reporting. Am. J. Hosp. Pharm., 47:76–77, 1990.

Karch, F. E.; and Lasagna, L.: Toward the operational identification of adverse drug reactions. Clin. Pharmacol. Ther., 21:247–254, 1977.

Kono, R.: Trends and lessons of SMON research. In, Drug-Induced Sufferings (Soda, T., ed.). Excerpta Medica, Princeton, p. 11, 1980.

Kramer, M. S.; Leventhal, J. M.; Hutchinson, T. A.; and Feinstein, A. R.: An algorithm for the operational assessment of adverse drug reactions. J.A.M.A., 242:623–632, 1979.

Lane, D. A.; and Hutchinson, T. A.: The notion of "acceptable risk." The role of utility in drug management. J. Chronic Dis., 40:621–625, 1987.

Lawson, D. H.: Scientific problems in collecting and analyzing safety data in nonexperimental studies. Drug Info. J., 22:11–18, 1988.

Lenz, W.: Thalidomide and congenital abnormalities. Lancet, 1:45, 1962.

Lessler, J. T.; and Harris, B. S. H.: Medicaid Data as a Source for Post Marketing Surveillance Information. Final Report. Research Triangle Institute, Research Triangle Park, N.C., 1984.

Luscombe, F. A.: Methodologic issues in pharmacy-based post-marketing surveillance. Drug Info. J., 19:269–274, 1985.

Markush, R. E.; and Seigel, D. G.: Oral contraceptives and mortality trends from thromboembolism in the United States. Am. J. Public Health, 59:418–434, 1969.

McBride, W. G.: Thalidomide and congenital abnormalities. Lancet, 2:1358, 1961.

Melmon, K. L.: Attitudinal factors that influence the utilization of modern evaluative methods. In, Medical Innovations at the Crossroads: Volume I. Modern Methods of Clinical Investigation. National Academy Press, 1990, pp. 135–146.

Melmon, K. L.: The Joint Commission on Prescription Drug Use: A ten year retrospective. Post Marketing Surveillance, 5(1):1–12, 1991.

Miller, R. R.; and Greenblatt, D. J.: Drug Effects in Hospitalized Patients. John Wiley & Sons, New York, 1976.

Milstien, J. B.; Faich, G. A.; Hsu, J. P.; Knapp, D. E.; Baum, C.; and Dries, M. W.: Factors affecting physician reporting of adverse drug reactions. Drug Info. J., 20:157–164, 1986.

Mitchell, A. A.; Cottler, L. B.; and Shapiro, S.: Effect of questionnaire design on recall of drug exposure in pregnancy. Am. J. Epidemiol., 123:670–676, 1986.

Naranjo, C.; Busto, E. M.; Seller, P.; Sandor, P.; Ruiz, I.; Roberts, E. A.; Janecek, E.; Domecq, L.; and Greenblatt, D. J.: A method for estimating the probability of adverse drug reactions. Clin. Pharmacol. Ther., 30:239–245, 1981.

Palca, J.: AIDS drug trials enter new age. Science, 246:19–21, 1989.

Piper, J. M.; Baum, C.; and Kennedy, D. L.: Prescription drug use before and during pregnancy in a Medicaid population. Am. J. Obstet. Gynecol., 157:148–156, 1987.

Platt, R.; Stryker, W. S.; and Komaroff, A. L.: Pharmacoepidemiology in hospitals using automated data systems. Am. J. Prev. Med., 4(suppl. 2):39–42, 1988.

Porter, J. B.; Hunter, J. R.; Jick, H.; and Stergachi, S.: Oral contraceptives and nonfatal vascular disease. Obstet. Gynecol., 66:1–4, 1985.

Rawson, N. S.; Pearce, G. L.; and Inman, W. H. W.: Prescription event monitoring: Methodology and recent progress. J. Clin. Epidemiol., 43:509–522, 1990.

Ray, W. A.; and Griffin, M. R.: The use of Medicaid data for pharmacoepidemiology. Am. J. Epidemiol., 129:837–849, 1989.

Ray, W. A.; Griffin, M. R.; Downey, W.; and Melton, L. J. III: Long-term use of thiazide diuretics and risk of hip fracture. Lancet, 1:687–690, 1989.

Ray, W. A.; Griffin, M. R.; Schaffner, W.; Baugh, D. K.; and Melton, L. J. III: Psychotropic drug use and the risk of hip fracture. N. Engl. J. Med., 316:363–369, 1987.

Rogers, A. S.: FDA sponsored project to promote physician reporting of adverse drug events in Maryland 1985–1988. Clin. Res. Practice and Drug Regulatory, 8:29–43, 1990.

Rogers, A. S.: Adverse drug events: Identification and attribution. Drug Intell. Clin. Pharm., 21:915–920, 1987.

Rossi, A. C.; Bosco, L.; Faich, G. A.; Tanner, A.; and Temple, R.: The importance of adverse reaction reporting by physicians: Suprofen and the flank pain syndrome. J.A.M.A., 259:1203–1204, 1988.

Rossi, A. C.; Knapp, D. E.; Anello, C.; O'Neill, R. T.; Graham, C. F.; Mendelis, P. S.; and Stanley, G. R.: Discovery of adverse drug reactions: A comparison of selected phase IV studies with spontaneous reporting methods. J.A.M.A., 249:2226–2228, 1983.

Scott, H. D.; Thacher-Renshaw, A.; Rosenbaum, S. E.; Waters, W. J. Jr.; Green, M.; Andrews, L. G.; and Faich, G. A.: Physician reporting of adverse drug reactions. J.A.M.A., 263(13):1785–1794, 1990.

Seidl, L. G.; Thorton, G. F.; and Smith, J. W.: Studies on the epidemiology of adverse drug reactions: III. Reactions in patients on a general medical service. Bull. Hopkins Hosp., 119:299–315, 1966.

Shapiro, S.: The role of automated record linkage in the post-marketing surveillance of drug safety. A critique. Clin. Pharmacol. Ther., 46:371–386, 1989.

Shimizu, N.; Tanaka, V.; Joncs, J.; and Taylor, D. (eds.): Improving Drug Safety: The Assessment, Management and Communication of the Therapeutic Benefits and Risks of Pharmaceutical Products. Pharma. International, Tokyo, Japan, 1990.

Skegg, D. C. G.; and Doll, R.: Record linkage for drug monitoring. J. Epidemiol. Community Health, 35:25–31, 1981.

Slone, D.; Shapiro, S.; and Miettinen, O. S.: Case-control surveillance of serious illnesses attributable to ambulatory drug use. In, Epidemiological Evaluation of Drugs (Colombo, F.; Shapiro, S.; Slone, D.; Tognoni, G.; eds.). PSG Publishing, Littleton, Mass., 1977, pp. 59–82.

Slone, D.; Jick, H.; Borda, I.; Chalmers, T. C.; Feineib, M.; Muench, H.; Lipworth, L.; Bellotti, C.; and Gilman, B.: Drug surveillance utilizing nurse monitors. Lancet, 2:901–902, 1966.

Smidt, N.; and McQueen, E. G.: Adverse reactions to drugs: A comprehensive hospital inpatient survey. NZ Med. J., 76:397–401, 1972.

Stergachis, A.: Record linkage studies for postmarketing drug surveillance: Data quality and validity considerations. Drug Intell. Clin. Pharm., 22:157–161, 1988.

Stern, R. S.; Rosa, F.; and Baum, C.: Isotretinoin and pregnancy. J. Am. Acad. Dermatol., 10:851–854, 1984.

Strom, B. L.; and Carson, J. L.: Automated databases used for pharmacoepidemiology research. Clin. Pharmacol. Ther., 46:390–394, 1989.

Strom, B. L.; Carson, J. L.; Morse, M. L.; West, S. L.; and Soper, K. A.: The effect of indication on hypersensitivity reactions with zomiperac sodium and other nonsteroidal antiinflammatory drugs. Arthritis Rheum., 30:1142–1148, 1987.

Strom, B. L.; Melmon, K. L.; and Miettinen, O. S.: Post-marketing studies of drug efficacy: Why? Am. J. Med., 78: 475–480, 1985a.

Strom, B. L.; Carson, J. L.; Morse, M. L.; and Leroy, A. A.: The computerized online medicaid analysis and surveillance system: A new resource for post-marketing drug surveillance. Clin. Pharmacol. Ther., 38:359–364, 1985b.

Strom, B. L.; Miettinen, O. S.; and Melmon, K. L.: Post-marketing studies of drug efficacy: How? Am. J. Med., 77: 703–708, 1984.

Taussig, H. B.: A study of the German outbreak of phocomelia. J.A.M.A., 180:1106–1114, 1962.

Tilson, H. H.; and Bruppacher, R.: A Working Group on Epidemiology in the Pharmaceutical Industry (EPI) A new force for the field. J. Clin. Res. Pharmacoepidemiol., 4:91–97, 1990.

Tilson, H. H.; Collins, G. E.; and Simpson, R.: Post-marketing Experience with Drug Products. Information Sources in Pharmaceuticals (Pickering, W. R., ed.). Bowker-Sour, London, 1990, pp. 242–262.

U.S. Congress, Committee on Government Operations: Deficiencies in FDA's regulation of the new drug "Oraflex." House Report, 98:511:1, 1983.

U.S. Department of Health and Human Services (USDHHS): Investigational new drug, antibiotic, and biological drug product regulations; Section 312.42, Treatment Use and Sale. Fed. Reg., Vol. 22:19466–19477, May 22, 1987.

U.S. Department of Health and Human Services (USDHHS): New drug, antibiotic, regulations; Section 314.80, postmarketing reporting of adverse drug experiences. Fed. Reg., Vol. 50(30):7452–7519, 1985.

U.S. Government Accounting Office: FDA Drug Review: Post-approved Risks 1976–1985 (PEMD-90-15). USGAO, Gaithersburg, Md., 1990.

Venning, G. R.: Identification of adverse reactions to new drugs: I. What have been the important adverse reactions since thalidomide? Br. Med. J., 286:199–202, 1988.

Venning, G. R.: Identification of adverse reactions to new drugs: II. How were 18 important adverse reactions discovered and with what delays? Br. Med. J., 286:289–292, 1983a.

Venning, G. R.: Identification of adverse reactions to new drugs: II (continued). How were 18 important adverse reactions discovered and with what delays? Br. Med. J., 286:365–368, 1983b.

Venning, G. R.: Identification of adverse reactions to new drugs: III. Alerting processes and early warning system. Br. Med. J., 286:458–460, 1983c.

Venning, G. R.: Identification of adverse reactions to new drugs: IV. Verification of suspected adverse reactions. Br. Med. J., 286:544–547, 1983d.

Vessey, M. P.; Metcalfe, A.; Wells, C.; McPherson, K.; Westhoff, C.; and Yates, D.: Ovarian neoplasms, functional ovarian cysts, and oral contraceptives. Br. Med. J., 294:1518–1520, 1987.

Vessey, M. P.; McPherson, K.; and Doll, R.: Breast cancer and oral contraceptives: Findings in Oxford-Family Planning Association contraceptive study. Br. Med. J., 282:2093–2094, 1981.

Vessey, M. P.; Doll, R.; Peto, R.; Johnson, B.; and Wiggins, P.: A long-term follow-up study of women using different methods of contraception—An interim report. J. Biosoc. Sci., 8:373–427, 1976.

Wastila, L.; and Lasagna, L.: The history of zidovudine (AZT). J. Clin. Res. Pharmacoep., 4:25–37, 1990.

West, R.: Saskatchewan Health data bases—A developing resource. Progress in pharmacoepidemiology. Am. J. Prev. Med., 46(2) (suppl.):25–27, 1988.

Ziel, H. K.; and Finkle, W. D.: Increased risk of endometrial carcinoma among users of conjugated estrogens. N. Engl. J. Med., 293:1167–1170, 1975.

Zoppi, M.; Török, M.; Stoller-Güleryüz, D.; Winzenried, P.; Marthy, H.; Hess, T.; Stucki, P.; Bickel, M. H.; Stocker, F.; and Hoigné, R.: Adverse drug reactions as probable causes of death. Results of the Comprehensive Hospital Drug Monitoring, Berne (CHDMB). Swiss Med. J., 112:1808–1810, 1982.

The Clinician's Actions When $N = 1$

Gordon Guyatt and David Sackett

CONCEPT OF $N = 1$ RANDOMIZED CONTROL TRIAL

The title of this chapter bears reflection. Clinical trials by physician-scientists are done on groups of patients. The letter N has been designated as the symbol for sample size; $N = 30$ means that there were 30 subjects involved in the trial. Clinicians, however, do not treat groups of patients. Rather, they treat individuals. In this sense, the clinician's N is always 1. Implied in this statement is that the clinician's goal always should be to find the best treatment for the patient he or she faces. How can the clinician best meet this goal?

Forty years ago, relatively uncontrolled observations suggesting therapeutic benefit from a drug were accepted as valid evidence. Since that time, it has become clear that uncontrolled observations can be misleading. A sophisticated methodology incorporating strategies to avoid misleading results has been adopted. The key elements of this strategy include randomization (to ensure comparable patients receiving experimental and alternative treatments), double masking or double blinding (to reduce the likelihood of bias in measurement, or in administering concomitant treatment), reliable and valid measurement of outcomes, and the use of statistics to help arrive at the appropriate conclusion regarding strength of inference. Studies that use these strategies are likely to yield far more accurate conclusions about appropriate treatment strategies than are those at the other extreme, an individual clinician's conclusions based on his or her own experience with a drug.

Clinicians face many situations in which the best course of action is dictated by conclusions from randomized trials that apply to groups of patients. Examples include studies of drugs that are given to increase longevity, or to prevent or delay events that occur only once, or infrequently, in the life of patients (stroke, myocardial infarction, exacerbation of inflammatory bowel disease). In these situations the clinician will not be able to determine if an individual patient is one destined to benefit from a drug. Treatment for the individual must then be based on results derived from a large group of (hopefully) similar people.

General Meaning

However, there are other situations (the characteristics of which we will describe in some detail) in which it is possible to determine the individual patient's response to a drug. In this situation, the results of randomized trials are still a good starting point for choosing the best therapy. Of course, the relevant trial may never have been done, or the patient at hand may be so different from those who participated in the trial (older or younger, sicker or less sick) that generalizing from the results of the trial may be questionable. Even if a relevant trial with a comparable patient population has been done, one can be sure that the responses were not uniform. The thrust of this book is to reemphasize that given a particular antianginal, antihypertensive, antiparkinsonian, antiasthmatic (and so on) agent, different patients respond differently. Even if patients as a group benefit from a drug, there are likely to be individuals who do not. Since no drug is free of adverse effects or potential toxicity (or of expense), the nonresponders are subject to risk or at least cost without benefit.

These considerations suggest that a policy of treating all patients with a particular presentation in a uniform pattern will not lead to optimal treatment for all patients. How can clinicians deal with this problem? One option is to conduct the time-honored "trial of therapy" in which the patient is given a treatment and the subsequent clinical course determines whether the treatment is judged effective and continued. Unfortunately, many factors may mislead physicians conducting conventional therapeutic trials.They include the placebo effect, the natural history of the illness, the expectations that the clinician and patient have about the effect of treatment, and the desire of the patient and the clinician not to disappoint one another.

To avoid these pitfalls, trials of therapy would have to be conducted with safeguards that permit both the natural, untreated course of the disorder to be observed and keep both patients and their clinicians "blind" to when active treatment was being administered. These are the safeguards that are routine in large-scale randomized control trials (RCTs) involving dozens or hundreds of patients. We will describe an approach to transferring these safeguards to the evaluation of therapy in the individual patient, an approach we call a single-patient randomized trial, or *N of 1 RCT*.

The *N* of 1 RCT is an example of a *single-subject experiment*. Such experiments are an established research method in psychology (Kratchwill, 1978; Kazdin, 1982; Barlow and Hersen, 1984). This strategy has only recently has been applied in medical practice (Guyatt et al., 1986a; Guyatt et al., 1988). The goal of this chapter is to provide sufficient detail to allow clinicians to plan and execute their own *N* of 1 RCTs.

Although there are many ways of conducting *N* of 1 RCTs, the method we have found most widely applicable can be summarized as follows:

1. A clinician and patient agree to test a therapy (hereafter called the *experimental therapy*) for its ability to improve or control the symptoms, signs, or other manifestations (hereafter called the *treatment targets*) of the patient's ailment.

2. The patient then undergoes *pairs* of treatment *periods* organized so that one period of each pair applies the experimental therapy and the other period applies either an alternative treatment or placebo (Fig. 36-1). The order of these two periods within each pair is randomized by a coin toss or other method that ensures that each period has an equal chance of applying the experimental or alternative therapy.

3. Whenever possible, both the clinician and the patient are "blind" to the treatment being given during any period.

4. The treatment *targets* are monitored (often through the use of a patient diary) to document the effect of the treatment currently being applied.

5. Pairs of treatment periods are replicated until the clinician and patient are convinced that the experimental therapy is effective, is harmful, or has no effect on treatment targets.

Editor's Challenge

The need to envision all patient–drug encounters as experiments and therefore the requirement that all regimens should be individualized has been stressed throughout this book. The authors of this chapter have given succinct formal reasoning why this need to individualize arises. Other chapters in the book have pointed out where individualization of drug therapy usually can be accomplished with relatively simple steps. Ordinarily, objectively measured signs of efficacy

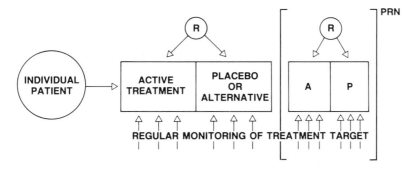

Fig. 36-1. A basic design for *N* of 1 randomized control trial. Circled R indicates that the order of placebo and active periods in each pair is determined by random allocation. Bracketed pair with "PRN" indicates that, beyond the first pair of treatment periods, as many additional pairs of treatment periods as necessary are conducted until patient and physician are convinced of the efficacy, or lack of efficacy, of the trial medication. A = active drug; P = placebo or alternative drug.

without excessive toxicity constitute enough data for the physician to be satisfied that therapy is at least adequate. Furthermore, when concerns about compliance become important to determine whether a drug is working or the disease is spontaneously regressing to the mean (normalizing), measures of pharmacologic effects of drugs that are independent of efficacy can be used as an objective guide. For example, if a hypertensive patient is taking a β-adrenergic antagonist and has his or her blood pressure reduced, but the pulse rate at rest and after measured exercise persists at pretreatment levels, it would be hard to attribute the positive change in the disease to cardiac effects of those drugs. Conversely if the blood pressure does not drop but the pulse rates do, then the drug is being taken and is exerting pharmacologic effects but is not sufficiently efficacious. Thus, the therapist will have to "experiment" with another drug. The effects of therapeutic decisions when N = 1 probably most often can be assessed using this more informal pattern of analysis. However, there are times when an answer about how therapy is progressing is very difficult to evaluate with this informal approach. The formal approach represented in this chapter is fairly new, and represents an evaluative scheme that can be applied in difficult settings of therapy.

COMPONENTS OF AN *N* OF 1 RANDOMIZED CONTROL TRIAL

The remainder of this chapter will describe an *N* of 1 randomized trial in detail. To aid in its implementation, each step will address a question that must be answered before proceeding to the next step (summarized in Table 36–1).

Is an N of 1 Randomized Control Trial Indicated for This Patient?

Because *N* of 1 RCTs are unnecessary for some ailments (such as self-limited illnesses) and unsuited for some treatments (such as operations), it is important to determine, at the outset, whether an *N* of 1 RCT really is indicated for the patient and treatment in question. If an *N* of 1 RCT is appropriate, the answers to each of the following questions should be yes.

Is the Effectiveness of the Treatment Really in Doubt?   One or several randomized clinical trials may have shown that the treatment is highly effective. If one is unsure whether such trials have been undertaken, efficient strategies for searching the medical literature are available (Haynes et al., 1986a–1986e; McKibbon et al., 1986). However, if a substantial proportion of subjects in such tri-

Table 36–1.   GUIDELINES FOR *N* OF 1 RANDOMIZED TRIALS

1. Is an *N* of 1 randomized control trial indicated for this patient?
   a. Is the effectiveness of the treatment really in doubt?
   b. Will the treatment, if effective, be continued long-term?
   c. Is the patient eager to collaborate in designing and carrying out an *N* of 1 RCT?
2. Is an *N* of 1 randomized control trial feasible in this patient?
   a. Does the treatment have a rapid onset?
   b. Does the treatment cease to act soon after it is discontinued?
   c. Is an optimal treatment duration feasible?
   d. Can clinically relevant targets be measured?
   e. Can sensible criteria for stopping the trial be established?
   f. Should an unmasked run-in period be conducted?
3. Is an *N* of 1 randomized control trial feasible in my practice setting?
   a. Is there a pharmacist who can help me?
   b. Are strategies for the interpretation of the trial data in place?

als have proved unresponsive, an *N* of 1 RCT may be appropriate.

Alternatively, a patient may have exhibited such a dramatic response to the treatment that both clinician and patient are convinced that it works. *N* of 1 trials really are not necessary in such cases and are best reserved for situations in which

1. Neither the clinician nor the patient is confident that a treatment is really providing benefit.
2. The clinician is uncertain whether a treatment that has not yet been started will work in a particular patient.
3. The patient insists on taking a treatment that the clinician thinks is useless or potentially harmful (and mere words won't change the patient's mind).
4. A patient has symptoms that both the clinician and patient suspect but are not certain are due to the side effects of the medications.
5. Neither the clinician nor the patient is confident of the optimal dose of a medication or replacement therapy.

Will the Treatment, if Effective, Be Continued Long-Term?   If the underlying condition is self-limited and treatment will be continued only over the short term, an *N* of 1 RCT may not be worthwhile. *N* of 1 studies are most useful when conditions are chronic and maintenance therapy is likely to be prolonged.

Is the Patient Eager to Collaborate in Designing and Carrying Out an *N* of 1 Randomized Control Trial?   *N* of 1 RCTs are indicated only when patients can fully understand the nature of the experiment and are enthusiastic about participating. By its nature, the *N* of 1 RCT is a cooperative venture between clinician and patient.

Is an N of 1 Randomized Control Trial Feasible in This Patient?

The clinician may wish to determine the efficacy of treatment in an individual patient but the ailment, or the treatment, may not lend itself to the *N* of 1 approach. Once again, we shall approach the issue with a series of questions; for the *N* of 1 approach to be feasible, the answer to each must be yes.

Does the Treatment Have a Rapid Onset? *N* of 1 RCTs are much easier to do when a treatment, if effective, begins to act within hours. Although it may be possible to do *N* of 1 RCTs with drugs that have longer latency for the development of signs of efficacy (such as gold or penicillamine in rheumatoid arthritis, or tricyclics for depression) the requirement for very long treatment periods before the effect can be evaluated (e.g., estrogens in prevention of major bone fractures in postmenopausal women) may become prohibitive.

Does the Treatment Cease to Act Soon after It Is Discontinued? Treatments whose effects abruptly cease when they are withdrawn are most suitable for *N* of 1 RCTs. (Obviously, evaluation of vaccines could not be done this way.) If the treatment continues to act long after it is stopped, a prolonged "washout period" may be necessary. If this washout period is longer than a few days, the feasibility of the trial is compromised. Similarly, treatments that have the potential to "cure" the underlying condition, or at least lead to a permanent change in the treatment target, are not suitable for *N* of 1 RCTs.

Is an Optimal Duration of Treatment Feasible? Although short periods of treatment boost the feasibility of *N* of 1 studies, they may need to be long to be valid. For example, if active therapy takes a few days to reach full effect and a few days to cease acting once stopped, treatment periods of sufficient duration to avoid distortion from these delayed peak effects and washouts are required. Thus, our *N* of 1 RCTs of theophylline in asthma use treatment periods of at least 10 days: 3 days to allow the drug to reach steady state or wash out, and 7 days thereafter to monitor the patient's response to treatment.

Second, since many *N* of 1 RCTs test a treatment's ability to prevent or blunt attacks or exacerbations of disease (such as migraines or seizures),

each treatment period must be long enough to include an attack or exacerbation. A rough rule of thumb, called the *inverse rule of 3*, tells us: if an event occurs, on average, once every *x* days, we need to observe 3*x* days to be 95% confident of observing at least one event. Applying this rule in a patient with Familial Mediterranean Fever with attacks, on average, once every 2 weeks, calls for treatment periods at least 6 weeks long.

Finally, the clinician may not want the patient to take responsibility for crossing over from one treatment period to the next, or may need to examine the patient at the end of each period. Thus, the clinician's office schedule, and patient travel considerations, may dictate the length of each period of treatment.

Can Clinically Relevant Target(s) of Treatment Be Measured? The targets of treatment, or outcome measures, usually go beyond a set of physical signs (the rigidity and tremor of parkinsonism; the jugular venous distension and the S3, S4, and pulmonary crackles of congestive heart failure), a laboratory test (erythrocyte sedimentation rate, and concentration of blood sugar, uric acid, and serum creatinine), or a measure of patient performance (recordings of peak flow, or score on a 6-minute walk test). Each of these is only an indirect measure of the patient's prognosis and quality of life.

In most situations, it is not only possible but preferable to measure the patient's symptoms directly, their feelings of well-being, or their quality of life. Principles of measurement of quality of life can be applied in a simple fashion to *N* of 1 RCTs (Guyatt et al., 1985; Kirshner and Guyatt, 1985; Guyatt et al., 1986b). To begin with, one asks patients to identify the most troubling symptoms or problems they experience and then decides which of these symptoms or problems are likely to respond to the experimental treatment. Second, this responsive subset of symptoms or problems forms the basis of a self-administered patient diary or questionnaire.

For example, a patient with chronic limitation of airflow identified his problem as shortness of breath while walking up stairs, bending, or vacuuming. A patient with fibrositis (to whom we shall return later) identified fatigue, aches and pains, morning stiffness, and sleep disturbance as problems that should become the treatment targets for her illness.

The questionnaire to record the patient's symptoms can be presented using a number of formats (Fig. 36–2). A daily diary is best for some; for others a weekly summary may be better. For some targets, patients can quantify their symptoms using a visual analog scale, a straight line the ends of which present the extremes of the target being

Fig. 36-2.   **DATA COLLECTION FORM**

N OF 1 RANDOMIZED CONTROL TRIAL—DATA SHEET 1

PHYSICIAN: DAN SAUDER

PATIENT: _____

SEX: 1) MALE   2) FEMALE   DATE OF BIRTH _____ _____ _____

DIAGNOSIS: _____

OCCUPATION: _____

PRESENT MEDICATIONS: _____

TRIAL MEDICATION: KETANSERIN   DOSE:

DURATION OF STUDY PERIODS: 2 WEEKS

OUTCOMES: SYMPTOM RATINGS

INFORMED CONSENT OBTAINED (PLEASE SIGN): _____

ANSWERS TO SYMPTOM QUESTIONS, PAIR 1, PERIOD 1:

1. How many episodes of the Raynaud's phenomenon did you have in the last week?

First Week (to be completed on _____ _____) _____

Second Week (to be completed on _____ _____) _____

2. On average, in comparison to your usual episodes, how long were the attacks?

a. Very long; as long as or longer than they have ever been
b. Very long; almost as long as they have ever been
c. Longer than usual
d. About as long as usual
e. Not as long as usual
f. Not nearly as long as usual
g. Very short; as brief as or briefer than they have ever been

Write in the best number for each week.

First Week (to be completed on _____ _____) _____

Second Week (to be completed on _____ _____) _____

3. On average, in comparison to your usual episodes, how severe were the attacks?

a. Very bad; as severe as or more severe than they have ever been
b. Very bad; almost as severe as they have ever been
c. More severe than usual
d. About as severe as usual
e. Not as severe as usual
f. Not nearly as severe as usual
g. Very mild; as mild as or milder than they have ever been

Write in the best number for each week.

First Week (to be completed on _____ _____) _____

Second Week (to be completed on _____ _____) _____

---

measured (no shortness of breath, extreme shortness of breath). For other targets and patients, graded descriptions from none to severe symptoms (No shortness of breath, A little shortness of breath, Moderate shortness of breath . . . Extreme shortness of breath) are sometimes easier. Constructing simple symptom questionnaires is not difficult and allows the patient and the clinician to collaborate in the quantification of patient symptoms upon which the analysis of the *N* of 1 RCT often relies.

Whatever formats are chosen for measuring treatment targets, our experience has taught us that patients should rate each of them at least twice during each study period. The identifying patient information and the ratings on the treatment targets often can be combined onto one page; Fig. 36-2 displays such a form for an *N* of 1 RCT examining the effectiveness of a new drug, ketanserin, in Raynaud phenomenon. More detailed guides for constructing the sort of simple questionnaires required for *N* of 1 RCTs are available (Sudman and Bradburn, 1982; Woodward and Chambers, 1983).

A final point concerning measurement of a patient's symptoms is that side effects should also receive attention. A patient diary or questionnaire can be used to measure nausea, GI disturbances, dizziness, or other common side effects along with symptoms of the primary condition. In *N* of 1 RCTs designed to determine if medication side effects are responsible for a patient's symptoms (for example, whether a patient's fatigue is caused by an antihypertensive agent), side effects become the primary treatment targets.

Can Sensible Criteria for Stopping the Trial Be Established?   There are advantages to not specifying the number of pairs of treatment periods in advance. Under these circumstances the clinician and patient can stop anytime they are convinced that the experimental treatment ought to be stopped or continued indefinitely. Thus, if there is a dramatic improvement in the treatment target between the two periods of the first pair, both clinician and patient may want to stop the trial immediately. On the other hand, if there continues to be a minimal difference between the two periods of each pair, both clinician and the patient may need three, four, or even five or more pairs before confidently concluding that the treatment is or is not effective.

On the other hand, if one wishes to conduct a formal statistical analysis of data from the *N* of 1 RCT, the analysis will be considerably strengthened if the number of pairs is specified in advance. This issue is discussed further in the section concerning strategies for interpretation of *N* of 1 RCTs.

Whether or not one specifies the number of treatment periods in advance, it is advisable to conduct at least two pairs of treatment periods before breaking the code. Too many conclusions drawn after a single pair will be either false-positive judgments (that the treatment is effective when it isn't) or false-negative judgments (that the treatment is not effective when it is). Indeed, we recommend that clinicians resist the temptation and refrain from breaking the code until they are quite certain they are ready to terminate the study.

Should an Unmasked Run-in Period Be Conducted?   A preliminary run-in period on active therapy, during which both the physician and patient know that active therapy is being received, could save a lot of time. After all, if there is no hint of response during such an open trial, or if intolerable side effects occur, an *N* of 1 RCT may be fruitless or impossible. For example, we prepared for a double-blind *N* of 1 RCT of methylphenidate in a child with hyperactivity only to find a dramatic increase in agitation over the first 2 days of the first study period (during which the patient was receiving the active drug) mandating an abrupt termination of the study. Finally, an open run-in may be used to determine the optimal dose of the medication.

Is an N *of 1 Randomized Control Trial Feasible in My Practice Setting?*

Clinicians may answer yes to the preceding questions and still be unsure about how to proceed. In this section of the paper we describe the mechanisms that will ensure the feasibility of an *N* of 1 RCT in a given practice.

Is There a Pharmacist Who Can Help Me?   Conducting an *N* of 1 RCT that incorporates all the aforementioned safeguards against bias and misinterpretation requires collaboration between the clinician and a pharmacist or pharmacy service. Preparation of placebos identical to the active medication in appearance, taste, and texture is required. Occasionally, pharmaceutical firms can supply such placebos. More often, however, you will want your local pharmacist to repackage the active medication; if it comes in pill form, it can be crushed and repackaged in capsule form. Identical-appearing placebo capsules can be filled with lactose. While somewhat time-consuming, preparation of placebos is not technically difficult. Our own average cost for preparing medication for *N* of 1 studies in which placebos have not been available from the pharmaceutical company has been $125.

The pharmacist is also charged with preparing the randomization schedule (which requires nothing more than a coin toss for each pair of treatment periods). This allows the clinician, along with the patient, to remain blind to allocation. The pharmacist also may be helpful in planning the design of the trial. Information regarding the time to onset of action and the washout period may be provided, helping with decisions about the duration of study periods. The pharmacist can help monitor compliance and drug absorption. Both pill counts and measuring serum drug concentrations at the end of each treatment period can help establish that the patient conscientiously takes the study medication throughout the trial.

Are Strategies for the Interpretation of the Trial Data in Place?   Once you carefully gather data on the treatment targets in your *N* of 1 trial, how will you interpret them? One approach is to simply plot the data and examine the results by visual inspection. Evaluation of results by visual inspection has a long and distinguished record in the psychology literature concerning single-subject designs and is strongly advocated by some practitioners of single-subject studies (Kratchwill, 1978; Kazdin, 1982; Barlow and Hersen, 1984). Visual inspection is simple and easy. Its major disadvantage is that it is open to viewer or observer bias.

An alternative approach to analysis of data

from N of 1 RCTs is to utilize a statistical test of significance. The simplest test would be based on the likelihood of a patient's preferring active treatment in each pair of treatment periods. This situation is analogous to the likelihood of heads coming up repeatedly on a series of coin tosses. For example the likelihood of the patient's preferring active treatment to placebo during three consecutive pairs if the treatment was ineffective would be $\frac{1}{2} \times \frac{1}{2} \times \frac{1}{2} = \frac{1}{8}$ or 0.125. The disadvantage of this approach (which is called the sign test) (Conover, 1971) is that it lacks power: five pairs must be conducted before there is any chance of reaching conventional levels of statistical significance.

A second statistical strategy is to use Student's t test. The t test offers increased power because not only the direction but also the strength of the treatment effect in each pair is taken into account. The disadvantage of the t test is that it makes additional assumptions about the data that may not be valid. The assumption of greatest concern is that observations are independent of one another, that is, that a patient is equally likely to feel good or bad on a particular day irrespective of whether he or she felt good or bad the day before. The term used to describe data that are not independent is *autocorrelation*. While some autocorrelation is likely to exist in many N of 1 RCTs, the impact of the autocorrelation can be reduced if one uses the average of all measurements in a given period in the statistical analysis, rather than the individual observations. Furthermore, the paired design of the N of 1 RCT that we recommend further reduces the impact of any autocorrelation that exists.

If any statistical test is going to be used to interpret the data, the clinician faces another potential problem: if the clinician and patient use the results from the studies to determine when to stop the trial, the true p value may be inflated above the nominal p value. Therefore, we once again recommend that if a statistical test is planned, the number of periods be determined before the study begins.

To conduct a paired t test, a single score is derived for each pair by subtracting the mean score of the placebo period from the mean score for the active period. These difference scores constitute the data for the paired t; the number of degrees of freedom is simply the number of pairs minus 1. Statistical packages that will allow quick calculation of the p value are available for any programmable pocket calculator or microcomputer.

An example of the results of an N of 1 RCT is presented in Table 36–2. In this trial the effectiveness of amitriptyline in a dose of 10 mg at bedtime for a patient with fibrositis (referred to earlier) was tested. Each week, the patient rated the severity of a number of symptoms, including fatigue, aches and pains, and sleep disturbance, each on a seven-point scale in which a higher score represented better function. The treatment periods were 4 weeks, and three pairs were undertaken. The mean scores for each of the 24 weeks of the study are presented in Table 36–2.

The first step in analyzing the results of the study is to calculate the mean score for each period (presented in the last column of Table 36–2). In each pair the score favored the active treatment. The sign test tells us that the probability of this result occurring by chance if the treatment was ineffective is $\frac{1}{2} \times \frac{1}{2} \times \frac{1}{2} = \frac{1}{8}$ (or $p = .125$)!!

However, this analysis ignores the magnitude and consistency of the difference between active and placebo treatments. A paired t test takes these factors into account. We did our t test using a Hewlett-Packard HV 41C with a Stat Pac, but any programmable hand calculator or microcomputer with a simple statistical package would have served as well. All that is required is to punch in the pairs of results: 4.68 and 4.22; 5.01 and 4.07; 5.04 and 4.18. The calculator tells us that the t

Table 36–2.   RESULTS OF AN N OF 1 RANDOMIZED CONTROL TRIAL IN A PATIENT WITH FIBROSITIS

TREATMENT*	SEVERITY SCORE				
	WEEK 1	WEEK 2	WEEK 3	WEEK 4	MEAN SCORE
Pair 1					
Active	4.43	4.86	4.71	4.71	4.68
Placebo	4.43	4.00	4.14	4.29	4.22
Pair 2					
Active	4.57	4.89	5.29	5.29	5.01
Placebo	3.86	4.00	4.29	4.14	4.07
Pair 3					
Active	4.29	5.00	5.43	5.43	5.04
Placebo	3.71	4.14	4.43	4.43	4.18

* The active drug was amitriptyline hydrochloride. Higher scores represent better function.

value is 5.07 and there are two degrees of freedom; the associated p value is .037. This analysis makes us considerably more confident that the consistent difference in favor of active drug is unlikely to have occurred by chance.

Clinicians and statisticians may remain uncomfortable with the suggested approach to analysis of data from N of 1 RCTs. The use of N of 1 RCTs to improve patient care does not depend on the statistical analysis of the results. *Principle: Even if statistical analysis is not used in the interpretation of the trial, the strategies of randomization, double blinding, replication, and quantifying outcomes, when accompanied by careful visual inspection of the data, still allow a much more rigorous assessment of effectiveness of treatment than is possible in conventional clinical practice.*

ETHICS OF SUCH CLINICAL TRIALS

Is the conduct of an N of 1 RCT a clinical or a research undertaking? If the former, is it the sort of clinical procedure, analogous to an invasive diagnostic test, that requires written informed consent? We would argue that the N of 1 RCT can, and should be, a part of routine clinical practice. But, like all medical innovations, it may require a period of experimentation and study before being accepted by clinicians and by ethics committees.

Nevertheless, a number of ethical issues are important. We believe that patients should be fully informed of the nature of the study in which they are participating, and there should be no element of deception in the use of placebos as part of the study. Written informed consent should be obtained. Patients should be aware that they can terminate the trial at any time without jeopardizing their care or their relationship with their physician. Finally, follow-up should be close enough to prevent any important deleterious consequences of institution or withdrawal of therapy.

Can N of 1 Randomized Control Trials Really Become a Part of Clinical Practice?

We have conducted over 50 N of 1 RCTs, each one designed to improve the care being delivered to an individual patient. Patients have suffered from a wide variety of conditions, including chronic airflow limitation, asthma, fibrositis, arthritis, syncope, anxiety, insomnia, and angina pectoris. In general, these trials have been very successful in sorting out whether or not the treatment was effective. In approximately a third, the ultimate treatment differed from that which would have been given had the trial not been conducted. In most of these, medication that would

otherwise have been given over the long term was discontinued.

While confirming the potential of N of 1 RCTs, conduct of these trials also has highlighted the time and effort required. It is unlikely that full implementation of N of 1 RCTs will become a major part of clinical practice. Clinicians can, however, incorporate many of the key principles of N of 1 RCTs into their practice without adopting the full rigor of the approach presented here. Medication can be repeatedly withdrawn and reintroduced in an open or unmasked fashion. Symptoms and physical findings can be carefully quantified. However, without the additional feature of double blinding, both the placebo effect and physician and patient expectations can still bias the results.

In summary, the N of 1 approach clearly has potential for improving the quality of medical care and the judicious use of expensive and potentially toxic medication in patients with chronic disease. Using the guidelines offered here, we believe that clinicians will find the conduct of N of 1 RCTs feasible, highly informative, and fun.

REFERENCES

Barlow, D. H.; and Hersen M.: Single Case Experimental Designs: Strategies for Studying Behavior Change, 2nd ed. Pergamon Press, New York, p. 419, 1984.

Conover, W. J.: Practical Nonparametric Statistics. John Wiley & Sons, New York, pp. 121–126, 1971.

Guyatt, G. H.; Sackett, D. L.; Adachi, J. D.; Roberts, R.; Chong, J.; Rosenbloom, D.; and Keller, J.: A clinician's guide for conducting randomized trials in individual patients. Can. Med. Assoc. J., 139:497–503, 1988.

Guyatt, G. H.; Sackett, D.; Taylor, D. W.; Chong, J.; Roberts, R.; and Pugsley, S.: Determining optimal therapy—Randomized trials in individual patients. N. Engl. J. Med., 314:889–892, 1986a.

Guyatt, G. H.; Bombardier, C.; and Tugwell, P. X.: Measuring disease-specific quality of life in clinical trials, Can. Med. Assoc. J., 134:889–895, 1986b.

Guyatt, G. H.; Berman, L. B.; Townsend, M.; and Taylor, D. W.: Should study subjects see their previous responses? J. Chron. Dis., 38:1003–1007, 1985.

Haynes, R. B.; McKibbon, K. A.; Fitzgerald, D.; Guyatt, G. H.; Walter, C. J.; and Sackett, D. L.: How to keep up with the medical literature: I. Why try to keep up and how to get started. Ann. Intern. Med., 105:149–153, 1986a.

Haynes, R. B.; McKibbon, K. A.; Fitzgerald, D.; Guyatt, G. H.; Walker, C. J.; and Sackett, D. L.: How to keep up with the medical literature: II. Deciding which journals to read regularly. Ann. Intern. Med., 105:309–312, 1986b.

Haynes, R. B.; McKibbon, K. A.; Fitzgerald, D.; Guyatt, G. H.; Walker, C. J.; and Sackett, D. L.: How to keep up with the medical literature: III. Expanding the volume of literature that you read regularly. Ann. Intern. Med., 105:474–478, 1986c.

Haynes, R. B.; McKibbon, K. A.; Fitzgerald, D.; Guyatt, G. H.; Walker, C. J.; and Sackett, D. L.: How to keep up with the medical literature: IV. Using the literature to solve clinical problems. Ann. Intern. Med., 105:636–640, 1986d.

Haynes, R. B.; McKibbon, K. A.; Fitzgerald, D.; Guyatt, G. H.; Walker, C. J.; and Sackett, D. L.: How to keep up with the medical literature: V. Personal computer access to the medical literature. Ann. Intern. Med., 105:810–824, 1986e.

Kazdin, A. E.: Single-Case Research Designs: Methods for Clinical and Applied Settings. Oxford University Press, New York, p. 368, 1982.

Kirshner, B.; and Guyatt, G. H.: A methodological framework for assessing health indices. J. Chron. Dis., 38:27–36, 1985.

Kratchwill, T. R. (ed.): Single Subject Research: Strategies for Evaluating Change. Academic Press, Orlando, Fla., p. 316, 1978.

McKibbon, K. A.; Haynes, R. B.; Fitzgerald, D.; Guyatt, G. H.; Walker, C. J.; and Sackett, D. L.: How to keep up with the medical literature: VI. How to store and retrieve articles worth keeping. Ann. Intern. Med., 105:978–984, 1986.

Sudman, S.; and Bradburn, N. M.: Asking Questions: A Practical Guide to Questionnaire Design. Jossey-Bass, San Francisco, 1982.

Woodward, C. A.; and Chambers, L.W: Guide to Questionnaire Construction and Question Writing. Canadian Public Health Association, Ottawa, 1983.

37

Clinical Pharmacokinetics and Pharmacodynamics: The Quantitative Basis for Therapeutics

Nick Holford

As has been emphasized repeatedly in this book, rational therapeutics requires two steps: the qualitative choice of an appropriate medicine and the quantitative prescription of the dose and frequency of administration. This chapter and the following are concerned with describing the basis for the second step.

Note: Quantitative clinical pharmacology involves the manipulation of numbers. Explanation of the principles underlying the manipulation commonly requires the use of some algebra and even elementary calculus. No other field of medicine accessible to the general practitioner requires these skills today, and many readers will be unwilling to risk exploration of the subject because of these prerequisites. Remember, however, that these skills were required for entry to medical school. You had them once, and now is the time to take advantage of your knowledge. The effort will be worth it to you and your patients.

PHARMACODYNAMICS AND PHARMACOKINETICS

A map of the basis of therapeutics is shown in Fig. 37–1. The fundamental goal of the physician is to produce a desired effect by giving the right drug in the right dose. The pharmacologic effect is determined by the concentration at the site of action. In turn the concentration is determined by the dose. Pharmacodynamics encompasses the principles connecting concentration with effect; pharmacokinetics deals with the principles connecting dose with concentration. Pharmacodynamics generally addresses time-independent phenomena, whereas pharmacokinetics mainly is concerned with describing time dependence. To dissect therapeutics into those areas is a valuable conceptual device separating those that are dose- and time-dependent from these that primarily are concentration driven and representative of the pharmacokinetic steady state.

Why Quantitative Models Are Important

The nature and time course of drug action are complex. They are based on the interaction of drug molecules with tissues throughout the body. A complete description of what is currently understood about the action of a familiar drug such as digoxin would draw heavily on large areas of anatomy, physiology, biochemistry, and molecular biology. Simplification is required in order to focus on the essential factors that can be identified in individual patients and thus influence the choice of a drug. The simple representation of the essential parts of the complex whole is a *model*.

Models take many forms; graphic and mathematical types lend themselves to clinical phar-

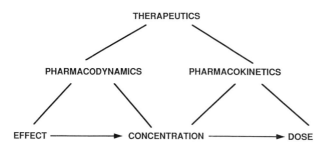

THERAPEUTICS

PHARMACODYNAMICS   PHARMACOKINETICS

EFFECT ——————→ CONCENTRATION ——————→ DOSE

Fig. 37-1. The therapeutic triangle: The object of therapeutics is to achieve a desired effect, which is determined by a target concentration at the site of action. The level and time course of concentration is in turn determined by the dose. The arrows indicate the sequence of rational steps involved in choosing a suitable dose.

macology. Models are useful when they achieve simplification without loss of association with essential features of real phenomena. They can be extended as the need arises to take account of more detailed processes. When models fail to predict important observations, they open our eyes to our ignorance. If we can figure out why the discrepancy exists through thought and experiment, we are advancing scientific knowledge. The next revision of the model poises us for further advances.

Parameters and Variables

Because emphasis in this chapter is on the use of models, it is important to get a clear idea of the structural components of a model. Quantitative models, usually expressed in the symbolic algebraic form of an equation, consist of dependent and independent variables and constants known as parameters. The dependent variable (usually the left-hand side of an equation) is predicted by different values of the independent variables (on the right-hand side) modified by suitable parameters that we will see are the customizable parts that represent an individual.

Common medical usage has expanded the meaning of parameter to include all variables including those that are observable (dependent) or controllable (independent). For example, the phrase *monitoring the patient's vital parameters* often is used to mean observations of variations in blood pressure and heart and respiratory rate. In the context of the structure of a model, however, *parameters* should be viewed as *constants* at least within the context and relevant time scale of the model. For example, sex and weight may determine the size of a drug's volume of distribution (a parameter of the pharmacokinetic model). As a human being grows and develops, the volume of distribution of a drug will change and is therefore not truly constant. However, the volume of distribution can usually be considered to be constant over a period of days or weeks when it is used to predict loading doses and half-life.

PHARMACOKINETIC MODELS

Several alternative and equivalent representations of drug disposition can be used to describe the relationship between dose and concentration and can be modified to account for the passage of time. In the early days of pharmacokinetics, emphasis was placed on half-life (and the closely related elimination rate constant) to describe the time course of drug concentration. Now we usually think of clearance and volume of distribution as the essential parameters of pharmacokinetic processes because of the close mapping of these parameters onto identifiable functional and structural features of the body. We also recognize that half-life is entirely dependent upon clearance and volume of distribution. When the physiologic and anatomic correlates of drug movement are not apparent, it may then be necessary to resort to a simpler, but less informative, model based on drug half-life alone.

The clearance and volume of distribution model of pharmacokinetics can be described in several ways. It may be constructed physically from a glass beaker filled with water (to explain volume of distribution) with the addition of a tap as a water source to keep the water level constant (to indicate stable physiology) and a pump to extract water from the beaker (to explain clearance).

A convenient model for the body in pharmacokinetic terms is the bathtub model (Fig. 37-2). This will be used to define precisely the meaning of volume of distribution and clearance and extended to introduce more complex pharmacokinetic models and their parameters. One should be careful to note that the metaphor for drug in the bathtub is sometimes the water itself and sometimes a substance dissolved in the water.

Volume of Distribution

The simple bathtub model is an example of a one-compartment pharmacokinetic model. For many purposes the body is well represented by this model. The physical volume of water in the bath represents a physical volume in the body (e.g., total body water, or extracellular water, or

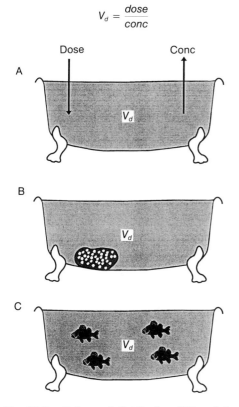

$$V_d = \frac{dose}{conc}$$

A

B

C

Fig. 37-2. Volume of distribution (V_d) and the bathtub model of pharmacokinetics. **a)** Closed drain. The concentration in the water is determined by the physical volume and the dose of drug. **b)** Sponge in the tub. Drug is absorbed by the sponge so that the concentration in the water is lower than without the sponge. The apparent volume of distribution is larger than the actual physical volume. **c)** Red herrings. Drug is attached to the red herrings, which are small enough to be included in the sample of bath water. The measured concentration includes that bound to the red herrings and is therefore higher than the bath water value. The apparent volume is smaller than the physical volume.

even plasma water). The apparent volume of distribution frequently may approximate a physical volume. For example, theophylline, a water-soluble, small, un-ionized molecule has an apparent volume of distribution close to that of total body water (0.5 l/kg). Gentamicin, a water-soluble, larger, ionized molecule is excluded (largely) from cells and has an apparent volume of distribution similar to that of extracellular water (0.25 l/kg). But note that digoxin, quite a large molecule, has an apparent volume of 7 l/kg, several times larger than the physical volume of the body. Warfarin, a water-soluble, small, un-ionized molecule, which might be expected to distribute like

theophylline, unexpectedly appears to have a volume of only 0.1 l/kg. How can these numbers be explained?

The bathtub model shows how to determine the apparent volume of distribution in a human being. One injects a known dose of drug into the bathtub water, stirs until the drug is distributed uniformly, and then removes a sample of water and measures the concentration. If the bathtub drain is closed (or relatively small so that little water is lost before sampling), the apparent volume of distribution can be calculated from the following:

$$\text{Concentration} = \frac{dose}{volume}$$

or

$$\text{Volume} = \frac{dose}{concentration}$$

The same thing could be done with a human subject, but now we must wait for the drug to be mixed in the blood (1–2 minutes) and then distributed to the tissues (several minutes to hours or even days, depending on the drug).

In the case of the bathtub model, we would expect the apparent volume to correspond very closely with the physical volume. This is a reasonable approximation to the behavior of theophylline, which penetrates into cells and reaches distribution equilibrium 15 to 30 minutes after an IV loading infusion.

Now imagine there is a sponge in the bathtub that the drug binds to with high affinity (Fig. 37-2B). Given the same dose, the concentration of drug in water must necessarily be lower because the drug is attached to the sponge and is no longer in the water; when the apparent volume of distribution is calculated, it will appear to be larger than the physical volume. Digoxin is thought to exert its clinical effects by binding to and inhibiting Na^+, K^+ = ATPase. This enzyme is ubiquitous but is especially highly concentrated in the brain, liver, kidneys, and muscle. The extensive binding of digoxin to the enzyme is analogous to the binding of drug to the sponge in the bathtub model. Because the concentration of digoxin in the plasma is low, the apparent volume of distribution is high, about 7 l/kg. Elderly and chronically ill persons have less muscle mass per kilograms than young healthy adults. People with chronic renal failure often have small kidneys. It should come as no surprise that these individuals have smaller apparent volumes of distribution for digoxin.

Drugs commonly bind to plasma proteins,

which are included in the sample of blood removed for measurement of the concentrations of drug. Nearly all drug assays denature these proteins and thus liberate the bound drug during preparation of the sample. Therefore, the concentration that is measured reflects both the concentration of drug that was bound to plasma proteins (C_b) and unbound drug (C_u) in plasma. The effect of this may be appreciated by imagining that there are little fish swimming around in the bathtub (Fig. 37–2C). For reasons that will become clear later, the fish usually are identifiable as a variety of red herring. Red herring sometimes have a high affinity for drugs, so that if they are included in a sample of bath water the total concentration of drug (C_{tot}) in the sample will be higher than in the pure water itself. The mathematical model for volume now predicts that the apparent volume of distribution will be smaller (with or without a sponge in the tub) if it is calculated from total concentration. Warfarin provides a clear example of this phenomenon. Total drug concentration of warfarin consists of about 99% bound, mainly to albumin, leaving only 1% unbound. Although its physical properties indicate that the drug should penetrate cells, its apparent volume of distribution is less than the extracellular fluid volume and approaches the distribution volume of albumin (0.1 l/kg). Plasma proteins are the equivalent of the red herring swimming in the bathtub. For most pharmacokinetic situations, they do not influence the concentration of active, excretable, unbound drug but only make it more difficult to interpret measured concentrations of total drug (C_{tot}).

Clearance

We expect water to be eliminated from the bathtub through the drain. The most obvious property of a drain is its size. For any particular height of water in the bathtub, the flow rate of water out of the tub will be determined by the size of the drain:

Flow rate out = water height × drain size

Drug concentration is analogous to water height as the driving force, while clearance is the exact analog of the size of the drain (Fig. 37–3). The drain itself most commonly is the kidney or liver, that is, the physiologic organs involved in elimination of drugs. The above equation can be rewritten using terms more appropriate to pharmacokinetics:

Rate of elimination = drug concentration
                          × clearance

or

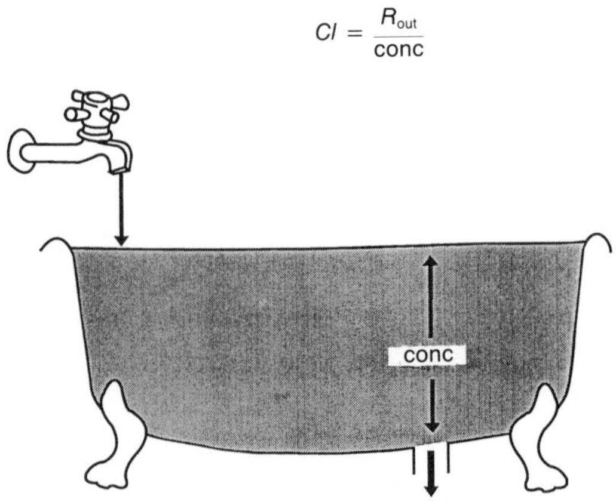

$$Cl = \frac{R_{out}}{conc}$$

Fig. 37–3. Drug clearance. The drain size represents clearance, and the water from the tap represents input of drug. The height of the water is the analog of concentration of the drug.

$$Clearance = \frac{rate\ of\ elimination}{drug\ concentration}$$

Under the special case that drug concentration in plasma is constant (steady-state concentration) because drug ingestion exactly equals elimination, then

$$Clearance = \frac{rate\ of\ drug\ input}{steady\text{-}state\ concentration}$$

Clearance can therefore be defined as the factor that determines the relationship between drug excretion rate and drug concentration. This definition of clearance is more useful in clinical pharmacology than the traditional "volume of plasma from which drug is completely cleared per unit time" because drug excretion and concentration are directly observable.

Plasma Protein Binding

It is useful, but not usual, to start with the assumption that plasma protein binding has no important effects on the disposition of drugs in clinical practice.

If plasma protein binding had an important effect on pharmacokinetics, then it would be expected that there would be detectable differences in the time course of drug concentration if one were to measure unbound concentrations under different circumstances of plasma protein binding. In practice, no such difference is detectable because changes in the amount of drug bound to plasma protein that are observable are relatively small in relation to the total amount of drug in the body.

Because it is technically easier to measure *total* drug concentration (C_{tot}, comprising both bound and unbound components), most estimates of the volume of distribution (V_d) and clearance (Cl) are defined in terms of total drug concentration. Note that both Cl and V_d involve concentration in their quantitative definition so that a change in the source of the concentration measurement will inevitably change the calculated value. Commonly observed changes in the extent of plasma protein binding can cause large apparent changes in volume of distribution and clearance based on total drug concentration (C_{tot}), but little or no change occurs in these values if unbound concentrations (C_u) are used.

An understanding of the role of protein binding is important, however, when attempting to interpret measured concentrations of drug in the course of therapeutic drug monitoring. For instance, phenytoin is about 90% bound to plasma protein (mainly albumin). If the concentration of albumin is low, for example, because of liver disease or the nephrotic syndrome, then total drug concentration will be correspondingly lower even if unbound concentrations are the same as in a person with normal concentrations of plasma proteins. Suppose the concentration of albumin is half of normal and the measured total phenytoin concentration (C_{tot}) is 5 mg/l; then one should mentally double the measured concentration to 10 mg/l in order to compare it with expected values. Lidocaine provides another example of a problem in interpreting total drug concentrations as measured. The plasma concentration of α_1 acid glycoprotein (AAG) rises after myocardial infarction as part of the acute-phase response. Since lidocaine binds avidly to AAG, the concentration of lidocaine in plasma rises after myocardial infarction. In the absence of evidence of toxicity, it would be reasonable not to reduce the dose in spite of the rising concentrations because the unbound, pharmacologically active concentration is not likely to be changing much (Routledge, 1986).

Concentration-Dependent Clearance

The definition of clearance given above is in terms of drug concentration and the corresponding elimination rate. For most drugs, clearance is independent of concentration, that is, it can be considered a constant (at least in the short term) in an individual in the absence of changes in medical condition or drug–drug interactions. However, several drugs do not have clearance that is independent of concentration. The primary explanation for this is that their elimination involves a saturable metabolic pathway. A common example of such a drug is ethanol, which is eliminated mainly by hepatic metabolism through alcohol

dehydrogenase. This enzyme has a maximum elimination capacity of about 8 g/h in a 70-kg person. A typical can of beer contains 10 g of ethanol, so it is easy to appreciate that the elimination capacity is readily approached. The liver reaches 50% of its capacity to eliminate ethanol at a blood concentration of 80 mg/l, which is well below common legal driving limit concentrations of 1000 mg/l (Holford, 1987).

The relationship between the elimination rate for ethanol and its concentration in blood can be expressed as before by

$$\text{Rate of elimination} = \text{drug concentration} \times \text{clearance}$$

However, the fact that the clearance of ethanol is dependent on its concentration requires the following extension of this relationship:

$$\text{Rate of elimination} = C_B \times \frac{V_{max}}{K_m + C_B}$$

where V_{max} is the elimination capacity (i.e., maximum possible rate of elimination) and K_m is the Michaelis-Menten constant defining the concentration of blood (C_B) at which the rate of elimination is 50% of V_{max}.

Note that this is exactly equivalent to defining clearance as

$$\text{Clearance} = \frac{V_{max}}{K_m + C_B}$$

For this reason, ethanol is defined as having concentration-dependent clearance. Synonyms for this concept are saturable elimination, dose-dependent elimination, nonlinear elimination, and Michaelis-Menten elimination.

In terms of the bathtub model of drug elimination described above, it may be helpful to think of concentration-dependent clearance as the equivalent of an apparent decrease in drain size due to turbulent flow created by high water pressures (Fig. 37–4).

Other drugs that have clinically important concentration-dependent clearance are phenytoin, propranolol, and aspirin. Most clinically used drugs that are extensively metabolized have K_m's that are large compared with the concentrations in plasma; consequently, their clearances can be approximated by V_{max}/K_m, a relationship that is independent of concentration. An important point about drugs having clearances that are concentration-dependent is that a small increase in dose may lead to a large increase in drug concentration as elimination becomes saturated.

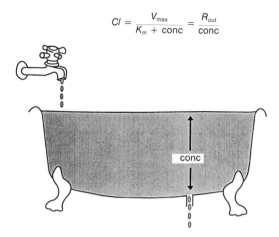

$$Cl = \frac{V_{max}}{K_m + conc} = \frac{R_{out}}{conc}$$

Fig. 37–4. Concentration-dependent clearance. When flow rates are high, turbulent flow through the drain means the flow rate is no longer proportional to the height of water. This is equivalent to concentration-dependent clearance.

Flow-Dependent Clearance

A second important factor that may influence clearance is blood flow in the organ of elimination. If an organ can completely remove all the drug in the blood that passes through it, the theoretical maximum elimination rate that it can achieve is determined by the blood flow and the concentration of drug in blood (C_B):

Maximum organ elimination rate
$$= \text{drug delivery rate}$$
$$= C_B \times \text{blood flow}$$

Using the definition of clearance given above, it follows that the clearance of the drug is identical to the blood flow to the organ of elimination.

Because extraction usually is less than complete, a more general expression is

Organ elimination rate $= C_B \times$ blood flow
$$\times \text{ extraction ratio}$$

The extraction ratio is defined as the fraction of drug entering the organ that is removed while flowing through the organ. This leads to a physiologic definition of clearance by an organ (Wilkinson and Shand, 1975):

Organ clearance $=$ blood flow
$$\times \text{ extraction ratio}$$

The extraction ratio is itself determined by blood flow and the ability of the organ to clear drug. This ability is known as *intrinsic* clearance and is equivalent to the organ clearance if the delivery rate of drug ($C_B \times$ blood flow) is not a limiting factor. The concept of intrinsic clearance is illustrated using the bathtub model in Fig. 37–5. Some useful relationships among blood flow, organ and intrinsic clearance and extraction ratio are

$$\text{Extraction ratio} = \frac{\text{organ clearance}}{\text{flow}}$$

$$= \frac{\text{intrinsic clearance}}{\text{flow} + \text{intrinsic clearance}}$$

Since we generally assume that only unbound drug is available for extraction, it usually is desirable to think of intrinsic clearance with reference to the unbound concentration of drug, that is, intrinsic clearance$_u$. In this case the flow must be adjusted to that equivalent flow of unbound drug

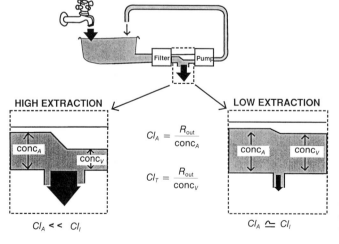

HIGH EXTRACTION

$$Cl_A = \frac{R_{out}}{conc_A}$$

$$Cl_T = \frac{R_{out}}{conc_V}$$

LOW EXTRACTION

$Cl_A \ll Cl_I$

$Cl_A \simeq Cl_I$

Fig. 37–5. Intrinsic clearance. If water is pumped past the drain, then the average height of water above the drain will be influenced by the relative size of the pump (blood flow) and the drain (intrinsic clearance). Conc$_A$ is the concentration entering the organ and Conc$_V$ is the concentration leaving it. Cl_A is the apparent clearance calculated from the Conc$_A$—this is organ clearance. Cl_I is the intrinsic clearance calculated from Conc$_V$.

that would achieve the same delivery rate. If fu is the fraction of unbound drug in the blood (i.e., not bound to plasma proteins or sequestered in blood cells), then the flow of unbound drug is obtained from blood flow divided by fu, that is,

Extraction ratio

$$= \frac{\text{intrinsic clearance}_u}{(\text{blood flow}/fu) + \text{intrinsic clearance}_u}$$

This leads to the following model for organ clearance:

Organ clearance

$$= \frac{\text{Blood flow} \times \text{intrinsic clearance}_u}{(\text{blood flow}/fu) + \text{intrinsic clearance}_u}$$

If blood flow/fu is small in relation to intrinsic clearance$_u$, then it can be ignored in the denominator of the definition of extraction ratio so that the extraction ratio approaches 1 and organ clearance approaches blood flow. On the other hand if intrinsic clearance$_u$ is small in relation to blood flow/fu, then the extraction ratio approaches zero and the organ clearance approaches intrinsic clearance$_u$/fu.

Drugs with a large intrinsic clearance have high extraction ratios, and organ clearance is influenced by blood flow, while those with small intrinsic clearances have low extraction ratios, and organ clearance is relatively independent of blood flow.

Lidocaine is a good example of a drug with a high extraction ratio. Liver blood flow is about 90 l/h (1500 ml/min), and hepatic clearance of lidocaine is about 54 l/h (900 ml/min). Its extraction ratio is 54/90, that is, 60%. Patients with heart failure have reduced hepatic blood flow and consequently reduced hepatic clearance, leading to a reduced IV dose requirement to achieve similar concentrations of drug in blood.

On the other hand, hepatic clearance of theophylline is only about 5 l/h (80 ml/min). Its extraction ratio is only 5/90, that is, 6%. Its clearance would not be expected to be affected by changes in liver blood flow.

However, it is well known that heart failure reduces clearance of theophylline (typically by 50%) meaning that theophylline's intrinsic clearance must be affected. This is most likely caused by limited delivery of factors required for drug metabolism (e.g., oxygen), which is a consequence of reduced blood flow and reduced arterial oxygen concentration.

The fraction of lidocaine that is bound to plasma proteins usually increases after myocardial infarction, which means that at any particular unbound concentration, the delivery rate of lidocaine to the liver is increased because the total concentration in blood is increased. Given the high extraction ratio for lidocaine, it would be expected that the elimination rate would increase and thus lead to a lower unbound concentration. Measurements of unbound lidocaine after myocardial infarction do not confirm this predicted fall in unbound concentration as plasma protein binding increases (Routledge, 1986). This may be because metabolites of lidocaine inhibit lidocaine metabolism and decrease its intrinsic clearance.

Multicompartment Models

The course of concentration of drug over time can usually be described adequately by a model of the body similar to the bathtub model used earlier. This simple model ignores the time needed for mixing the drug in the bloodstream and distributing it throughout the tissues. A common approach to the description of these distributional processes is to envision the body as consisting of more than one compartment (see chapter 1). The central compartment is characterized by a volume of distribution that includes plasma. There are one or more additional compartments, each of which has two parameters—a volume of distribution and a distribution clearance—that determine the kinetics of drug transfer between each peripheral compartment and the central compartment. The sum of all the compartment volumes is known as the steady-state apparent volume of distribution. Given a certain total amount of drug in the body, it is the apparent volume of the body that would account for the measured concentration in the central compartment after the distribution steady state had been reached. The removal of drug from the system is characterized by an elimination clearance that usually is assumed to be from the central compartment.

Figure 37-6 shows a model of a two-compartment system that consists of two beakers containing water. Drug is injected into one of the beakers (the central compartment), and its concentration is affected by distribution and elimination. Distribution clearance is determined by the flow rate of a pump that circulates water between the beakers. It is analogous to blood flowing to the various organs of the body. Elimination clearance is produced by the flow of water pumped into, and draining from, the central compartment. This is analogous to elimination of a drug by glomerular filtration. The time course of concentration of a drug in the central compartment beaker has two phases—an initial rapid decline determined mainly by the redistribution of drug into the second beaker, and a second slower phase due to drug elimination in the water flowing through the first beaker.

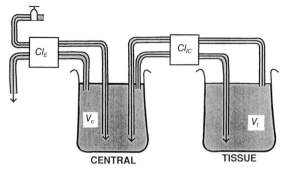

Fig. 37–6. A two-compartment pharmacokinetic model can be simulated with two pumps and two beakers containing water. One pump flushes water through one beaker while another recycles water between the two beakers. The volumes of water in each beaker correspond to the central (V_c) and tissue (V_t) volumes of distribution. The flow rates of each pump correspond to elimination (Cl_E) and distribution (intercompartment) clearances (Cl_{IC}).

Physiologic Models

Models of pharmacokinetics have been devised that combine features of a multicompartment model and established knowledge of anatomy and physiology. The simplest of these has already been described – the organ clearance model. The identifiable physiologic component in this model is organ blood flow. This model of organ clearance can be substituted for elimination clearance in a compartmental-type model. An alternative to compartmental models, which are defined by apparent volumes and distribution (intercompartment) clearances, is a model based on the actual volumes of organs and tissues in the body and blood flows connecting the organs and tissues. Such models should be useful in predicting changes in blood or organ concentrations arising from changes in blood flow (e.g., during heart failure), or when the sizes of organs change (e.g., changes as a child grows to be an adult or scaling from small animals to humans). However, full-fledged physiologic models have had limited application because of the difficulty of obtaining reliable estimates of blood flows in various tissues and concentrations of drugs in these tissues.

Pharmacodynamic Models

The relationship between concentrations and effect of drug usually is founded on the expected binding properties of a drug at a receptor site. In its simplest form, binding at a receptor site is determined by the affinity of the drug for the receptor and the concentration of binding sites (B_{max}). Affinity usually is defined in terms of an equilibrium dissociation constant (K_D). Note that K_D is inversely proportional to affinity but is, however, expressed in readily understood units of concentration of drug. For example, a drug with a K_D of 2 $\mu g/l$ would have five times the affinity of a drug with a K_D of 10 $\mu g/l$. This parameter says nothing about the effect of the drug; it only defines the concentration of drug expected to occupy 50% of available receptor sites:

$$\text{Bound drug} = \frac{B_{max} \times \text{conc}}{K_D + \text{conc}}$$

The relationship between binding and effect of a drug can be derived by assuming that the effect is proportional to the extent of binding (i.e., receptor occupancy). Because there usually are several steps in the chain of events between receptor activation and expression of a drug effect by an agonist, the resulting effect usually is not linearly related to occupancy. Nevertheless, a simple model, useful for many drugs, relates concentration to effect in an analogous way to that relating concentration to binding:

$$\text{Effect} = \frac{E_{max} \times \text{conc}}{EC_{50} + \text{conc}}$$

The maximum effect (E_{max}) is related to the maximum binding (B_{max}) by a proportionality constant known as the intrinsic activity. The concentration producing 50% of maximum response (EC_{50}) is nearly always less than the K_D. The ratio EC_{50}/K_D is the fraction of receptor sites that must be occupied to produce 50% of E_{max}. When this fraction is less than 1, it is sometimes said that "spare receptors" exist. However, this is an inexact conceptual model because the apparent number of spare receptors depends upon the efficacy with which a drug activates the receptor (a drug property) and is therefore not a characteristic of the biologic response mechanism or tissue itself. The phenomenon of apparently spare receptors is better explained by the nonlinear occupancy relationship arising from the chain of events between binding and expression of drug effect (Kenakin, 1987).

Figure 37–7 illustrates the relationship between concentration and effect for the E_{max} model using values typical for the action of theophylline on forced expiratory volume in an asthmatic patient. The EC_{50} is 10 mg/l (Holford and Sheiner, 1981).

Contrasting the relative predictions of the E_{max} model with accumulation of drug using a one-

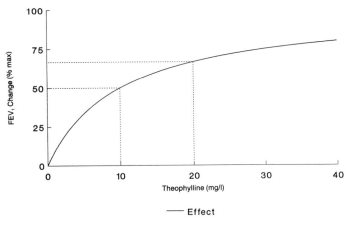

Fig. 37–7. The predictions of the E_{max} pharmacodynamic model are shown using values typical of theophylline effects in stable asthmatics. Half the maximum improvement in forced expiratory volume in 1 second (FEV_1) is expected at 10 mg/l. Doubling concentration to 20 mg/l will only achieve a further 17% improvement.

compartment pharmacokinetic model describing continuous drug infusion is useful. After 1 half-life, the plasma concentration is 50% of the eventual steady-state concentration. At 2 half-lives, the concentration increases to 75%, and after 4 half-lives to over 90% of the eventual steady-state concentration. In contrast, the E_{max} model predicts that a threefold increase in concentration over the EC_{50} is needed to achieve 75% and a ninefold increase is needed to achieve 90% of the maximum response (see chapter 7).

TIME COURSE OF DRUG ACTION

The interaction between the time course of drug concentration defined by a one-compartment pharmacokinetic model and the consequent drug effect determined by an E_{max} pharmacodynamic model is illustrated in Fig. 37–8. Some useful values from Fig. 37–8 are shown in Table 37–1.

Time is expressed in terms of the drug elimination half-life, and concentration as multiples of the EC_{50}. Between concentrations producing 80% and 20% of the maximum response, the disappearance of drug effect is approximately linear (about 15% is lost over each half-life). When the

effect reaches 20% of maximum, the drug-effect time course is approximately exponential, that is, the effect is nearly halved at each half-life. The disappearance of drug effect is very slow, only a few percent with each half-life, when effects are greater than 90% of maximum.

The combination of these basic pharmacokinetic and pharmacodynamic models provides an explanation for the seemingly puzzling observation that a drug with a short elimination half-life can be effective over dosing intervals that are many times longer than its half-life. β-Adrenoceptor antagonists can be given in doses that reach concentrations that are many times their EC_{50}. Suppose a concentration of propranolol blocks 50% of receptors at 10 ng/ml. If the peak concentration after a single dose is 320 ng/ml and the half-life is 4 hours, then β blockade will vary from 97% to 33% over a 24-hour period. Drug concentration will change by a factor of more than 60, but effects will vary by less than a factor of 3.

Cumulative Effects of Drugs

The therapeutic effects of drugs are not always related to their immediate pharmacologic

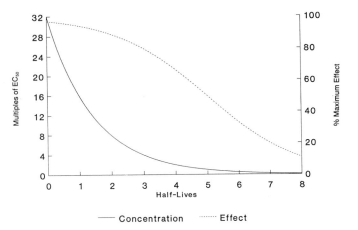

Fig. 37–8. The time course of drug concentration predicted by a one-compartment pharmacokinetic model (solid lines) and the drug effect predicted by an E_{max} pharmacodynamic model (dotted lines). Between 80% and 20% of maximum response the time course of drug effect is approximately linearly related to time while drug concentrations are declining exponentially. The time course of effect becomes exponential only at effects less than 20% of E_{max}.

Table 37–1. RELATIONSHIP BETWEEN DRUG CONCENTRATION AND EFFECT*

TIME (HALF-LIVES)	DRUG CONCENTRATION (EC_{50}'S)	DRUG EFFECT (% MAXIMUM)
0	32	97
1	16	94
2	8	89
3	4	80
4	2	67
5	1	50
6	0.5	33
7	0.25	20
8	0.125	11
9	0.0625	6
10	0.03125	3

* The time course of drug concentration and effect predicted by a one-compartment model for elimination and an E_{max} model for effect. Time is expressed as drug half-lives, and concentrations are multiples of the EC_{50}.

actions. For example, angiotensin-converting enzyme (ACE) inhibitors lower the blood pressure initially by causing a rapid decrease in angiotensin II, which acts directly on blood vessels; in addition, the drug has a slower effect probably due to establishment of a new salt and water balance. This slower effect will be determined by the cumulative effect of ACE inhibition and effects such as reduced angiotensin II stimulation of aldosterone synthesis. In this situation, the eventual antihypertensive effect of an ACE inhibitor may be predicted better by the average inhibition of ACE over a dosing interval than by its time course during the day. Figure 37–9 shows how drug concentration and extent of ACE inhibition can vary widely over a 24-hour interval yet achieve a 50% average reduction in ACE activity. The average reduction in ACE activity over several days probably determines the overall antihypertensive effect rather than the pattern of plasma ACE activity in a 24-hour period.

Steep Concentration-Effect Curves

The simple E_{max} pharmacodynamic model predicts that a 16-fold change in concentration is required to increase effect from 20% to 80% of maximum. Some drugs have much steeper concentration-response curves. Many cardiac antiarrhythmic agents fall into this category, to the extent that a twofold change in concentration may mean the difference between no effect and complete suppression of an arrhythmia. In contrast to the antiarrhythmic effects, the electrocardiographic effects of these drugs show a linear relationship between concentration and effect. These phenomena are illustrated in Figure 37–10.

Many arrhythmias are thought to be generated by reentrant circuits (Hondeghem and Mason 1989) (see chapter 6). These circuits can exist only within a certain range of electrophysiologic properties. When repolarization is delayed beyond a certain critical value, the reentry circuit cannot be sustained and the arrhythmia suddenly ends. The linear increase in QT interval observable for sodium-channel blocking agents (e.g., quinidine) is expected to have corresponding changes in repolarization time of individual cardiac cells involved in an arrhythmogenic reentry circuit. A quinidine plasma concentration of 2 mg/l may produce a 66-msec increase in QT interval but does not have an appreciable effect on the reentry circuit. Doubling the quinidine concentration to 4 mg/l prolongs the QT interval by 132 msec. If the corresponding delay in repolarization is incompatible with reentry, then the arrhythmia ceases. The sharp transition of the reentry circuit will be manifested as a steep concentration-effect curve.

Steep concentration effect curves can be described by a modification to the E_{max} model. Because the resulting curves are S-shaped, this model is commonly known as the sigmoid E_{max} model.

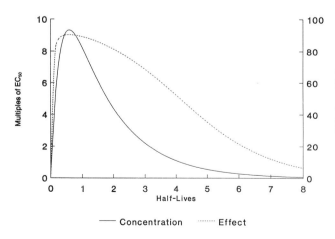

— Concentration   ······· Effect

Fig. 37–9. The predicted time course of an oral dose of ACE inhibitor concentration (solid lines) and its effect (dotted lines) on plasma ACE activity. Although the extent of inhibition varies over the dosing interval, the average ACE inhibition is 50% of the baseline value. Eventual antihypertensive effects may be more closely related to average ACE inhibition than the time course of ACE inhibition in plasma or tissues.

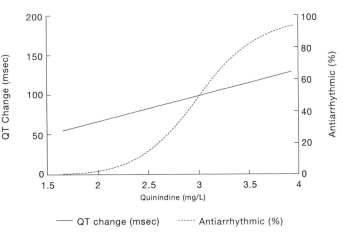

Fig. 37-10. The linear relationship between change in QT interval and the concentration of the antiarrhythmic drug predicts a 33-msec increase for each mg/l increase in concentration (—). A 50% inhibition of arrhythmia frequency occurs at 3 mg/l, yet little inhibition exists at 2 mg/l and almost complete abolition is produced at 4 mg/l (----). The steep concentration-effect relationship to the frequency of the arrhythmia may be explained by interruption of a reentry mechanism by a critical change in repolarization corresponding to a QT interval of 100 msec occurring at 3 mg/l.

$$\text{Effect} = \frac{E_{max} \times \text{conc}^N}{EC_{50}^N + \text{conc}^N}$$

The exponent N is an empirical parameter that controls the steepness of the curve. The simple E_{max} model corresponds to a situation in which $N = 1$. The curve in Fig. 37-10 was produced with an N of 10. Shallow concentration-effect curves are predicted when N is less than 1.

Hysteresis

Peak drug effects commonly lag behind peak concentrations of the drug in plasma, a phenomenon known as hysteresis. A frequently cited cause for such delayed effects is the time needed for a drug to penetrate to its site of action, a consequence of distribution predictable from a multicompartment pharmacokinetic model. The time course of the effects of digoxin on the heart after rapid IV administration clearly lags behind plasma concentrations. Figure 37-11 shows the predicted time course of concentrations of digoxin in plasma using a two-compartment pharmacokinetic model after injection of a bolus of 1 mg. The central compartment volume of distribution is 50 liters and distribution clearance is 25 l/h. The tissue compartment has a volume of 450 liters, and elimination clearance is 9 l/h. The initial concentration of 20 ng/ml falls rapidly as drug is redistributed. The concentration of digoxin in the tissue compartment peaks at about 6 hours and falls slowly in parallel with plasma concentration.

The half-time for equilibration of concentrations of digoxin between the central and tissue compartments can be calculated from the distribution clearance and the tissue compartment volume.

$$t_{1/2} \text{ redistribution} = \frac{0.7 \times 450\,\text{l}}{25\,\text{l/h}}$$

$$= 12.5 \text{ hours}$$

(Note that 0.7 is an approximation to the natural logarithm of 2.) If the effect of digoxin were lin-

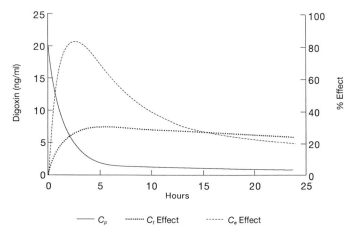

Fig. 37-11. The time course of drug concentration in the plasma (—) predicted by a two-compartment pharmacokinetic model. The time course of drug effects determined by the kinetics of drug in the two tissue compartments (.....) and (----) is shown. This example is typical of observations of concentrations of digoxin in plasma and its cardiac effects after a 1-mg IV bolus.

early proportional to the drug's concentration in tissues, then the peak cardiac effects of digoxin would be expected at the time of maximum concentration in the tissue compartment. However, observations of the effects of digoxin show a peak occurring somewhat earlier and a more rapid fall in effect after the peak. This can be explained by proposing a hypothetical compartment for digoxin that equilibrates more quickly with concentrations in plasma in the central compartment. If the half-time for equilibration is 3 hours, then the predicted time course of concentration of digoxin in the effect compartment and the corresponding effects are shown by the third curve in Fig. 37–11. The model for these predictions is defined by a set of differential equations:

$$V_c \frac{dC_p}{dt} = (Cl_{\text{dist}} \times C_t) \qquad \text{Equation for } C_p$$
$$- (Cl_e \times C_p)$$

$$V_t \frac{dC_t}{dt} = (Cl_{\text{dist}} C_p \times C_p) \qquad \text{Equation for } C_t$$
$$- (Cl_{\text{dist}} \times C_t)$$

$$\frac{dC_e}{dt} = (K_{\text{eq}} \times C_p) \qquad \text{Equation for } C_e$$
$$- (K_{\text{eq}} \times C_e)$$

The concentration of drug in the central compartment or plasma (C_p) is determined by the volume of the central compartment (V_c), the elimination clearance (Cl_e the distribution clearance (Cl_{dist}), and the concentration of digoxin in the tissue compartment (C_t). The concentration of digoxin in the tissue compartment (C_t) is determined by C_t, C_p, Cl_{dist}, and the volume of the tissue compartment (V_t). The concentration of digoxin in the effect compartment (C_e) is determined by C_e, C_p, and an equilibration rate constant (K_{eq}). Notice that there is no connection between the effect compartment and the plasma compartment in terms of mass balance. It is as if the effect compartment observes plasma concentration without influencing it. While the net transfer of drug from plasma to site of effect and back again exists in reality, the amount of drug involved is assumed to be insignificant in comparison with the amount in the central and tissue compartments because the time course of plasma concentration is adequately described by the central and tissue compartments alone.

The equilibration rate constant is related to the equilibration half-time according to $T_{1/2 \text{ equilibration}} = 0.7/K_{\text{eq}}$. If digoxin plasma concentration were increased from zero to 2 ng/ml and kept constant, then the concentration in the effect compartment would reach 1 ng/ml after 3 hours and more than

90% of the steady-state value of 2 ng/ml after 12 hours. The high initial concentration and rapid fall in concentration of digoxin in plasma accounts for the peak effect time between 2 and 3 hours after an IV bolus.

The physiologic interpretation of the equilibration half-time may be quite complex. When the time course of concentration of drug in the effect compartment is similar to the expected time course of drug concentration predicted in the effect tissue on pharmacokinetic grounds, it is reasonable to interpret the equilibration half-time as the result of drug distribution. In this case, factors that change the rate of distribution (e.g., tissue blood flow) would be expected to directly influence the half-time of equilibration. The interpretation of the digoxin equilibration half-time may not be so simple. Digoxin is thought to act by inhibiting a Na^+, K^+-ATPase at the cardiac muscle cell surface. The rate of distribution of digoxin to this extracellular site should be similar to those of other drugs acting at the cardiac cell surface. The equilibration half-time of quinidine is only a few minutes, which is compatible with the time taken for distribution from plasma to cardiac cells. This suggests that the longer delay observed for digoxin effects may arise from an additional cause. After inhibition of Na^+, K^+-ATPase, sodium balance in the cell changes, leading to a higher intracellular concentration of sodium. Subsequent to this the sodium–calcium exchange mechanism operates more slowly and calcium accumulates within the cell. The delay in onset of effect of digoxin may be explained partly by the kinetics of its distribution to the cell surface, but a more important component may be the kinetics of sodium and calcium within the cardiac cell.

The change in prothrombin ratio produced by warfarin provides a more simply understood mechanism of delay in the apparent onset of drug action. The effect of warfarin on prothrombin ratio lags several days behind changes in concentration of warfarin in plasma. Warfarin indirectly inhibits the hepatic synthesis of coagulation factors II, VII, IX, and X by blocking the recycling process that converts vitamin K epoxide back to active vitamin K. The inhibition of synthesis is rapid and closely linked to concentrations of warfarin in plasma. Once synthesis is inhibited, the concentrations of these coagulation factors in plasma decrease with a time course determined by their half-lives. The average half-life of the prothrombin complex of coagulation factors is about 14 hours. After changes in concentrations of warfarin in plasma, several days must elapse before the corresponding steady-state concentrations of coagulation factors is reached (Holford, 1986). This is illustrated in Figure 37–12.

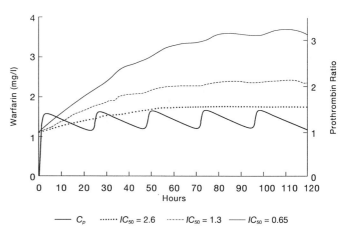

Fig. 37–12. The use of a loading and a maintenance dose of warfarin achieves the desired target concentration (C_p) rapidly (———). Effects on the prothrombin ratio (PR) are delayed because of the time needed to eliminate coagulation factors that were formed before therapy was adequate. The target effect of a PR of 2.0 takes about 3 days to develop when the IC_{50} for warfarin is 1.3 mg/l. A higher PR is reached in the same time if the IC_{50} is 0.65 mg/l and a lower PR if the IC_{50} is 2.6 mg/l.

A physiologic pharmacokinetic-pharmacodynamic model for these predictions of warfarin effect can be defined by the following differential equation:

$$\frac{dP}{dt} = (\text{Syn} \times PD(\text{W})) - (K_p \times P)$$

where P is concentration of the prothrombin complex concentration, K_p is the average elimination rate constant for the prothrombin complex, and $PD(\text{W})$ is a pharmacodynamic model for the effect of warfarin (W) on the synthesis rate of the prothrombin complex (Syn). A suitable model for warfarin is based on an inhibitory form of the E_{max} model:

$$PD(\text{W}) = 1 - \frac{\text{W}}{\text{W} + \text{IC}_{50}}$$

where IC_{50} is the concentration of warfarin producing 50% inhibition.

A rational approach to the initiation of warfarin therapy is to give a loading dose that will achieve concentrations similar to those seen on the usual maintenance dose. Because warfarin has a half-life of a day and a half, it ordinarily would take a week to reach steady-state concentrations. The combination of a loading dose (15 mg) and maintenance dose (5 mg/day) rapidly achieves the target concentration that produces a 50% inhibition of synthesis of the prothrombin complex (1.3 mg/l). This is associated with a prothrombin ratio of 2.0, which is reached on day 3 of treatment. The time course of warfarin effects might be described equally well by an effect compartment model, but a model based on known physiology explains the observations in a more insightful and understandable manner.

Proteresis

Less commonly, peak drug effects precede peak plasma concentrations, a phenomenon known as *proteresis*. This situation may arise if the effects of a drug are more closely linked to concentrations in arterial blood but concentrations of drug are determined in venous blood. Because the time course of concentrations in venous plasma lags behind concentrations in arterial blood, it will appear that drug effects precede the appearance of drug in the venous blood. Proteresis also may arise if tolerance to the drug develops during exposure to it. Among other mechanisms, tolerance may be caused by accumulation of a metabolite that is a direct inhibitor of the drug effect or by the activity of a physiologic reflex system designed to maintain homeostasis (Sheiner, 1989).

UNION OF PHARMACOKINETICS AND PHARMACODYNAMICS: THE TARGET CONCENTRATION STRATEGY

There are two distinct stages in deciding on the particular dose of a drug that should be given to achieve a desired effect. The first stage uses any available prior knowledge of the pharmacokinetics and pharmacodynamics of the drug. This will typically involve taking into account the size of the patient and factors such as renal function, which may modify clearance, and drug or disease interactions that may influence the EC_{50}. The second stage comes when the drug has been given to the patient and observations are available of the effects achieved (desirable and undesirable), and in some cases the concentration of drug in plasma may also be known. This second stage allows more precise individualization of dose of the drug that can be based on improved understanding of the pharmacodynamic and pharmacokinetic parameters in that patient.

Both these stages can be incorporated in a general strategy for rational therapeutics based on a target concentration strategy (Sheiner and Tozer, 1978). This strategy follows naturally from the division of the problem into its pharmacokinetic and pharmacodynamic components. First a desired effect is identified. Pharmacodynamic knowledge is then used to derive what concentration is likely to achieve the desired effect. In the current state of incomplete knowledge about pharmacodynamics, we usually assume that the time course of concentration is not a determinant of the desired effect. Therefore, a single-target concentration can be selected. Pharmacokinetic principles can now be applied to calculate the first (loading dose) and any subsequent dose sizes along with a dosing interval (maintenance dose regimen).

When concentrations of drug are measured by clinical laboratories, the laboratory usually provides a so-called therapeutic range. Provision of these data is often motivated by a desire for completeness so that the concentrations of drug in a laboratory handbook can be listed alongside endogenous substances such as sodium and glucose that have a definable "normal range." Because the normal concentration of a drug is zero, it is not possible to apply the usual methods applicable to endogenous substances to define a range for concentrations of drug. A conceptually better approach to understanding drug concentrations is to define the concentration that is most commonly associated with the desired therapeutic end point. This lends itself naturally to defining a starting point for a target concentration in an individual.

REFERENCES

Holford, N. H. G.: The clinical pharmacokinetics of ethanol. Clin. Pharmacokinet., 13:273–292, 1987.

Holford, N. H. G.: Clinical pharmacokinetics and pharmacodynamics of warfarin. Understanding the dose-effect relationship. Clin. Pharmacokinet., 11:483–504, 1986.

Holford, N. H. G.; and Sheiner, L. B.: Understanding the dose-effect relationship: Clinical application of pharmacokinetic-pharmacodynamic models. Clin. Pharmacokinet., 6:429–453, 1981.

Hondeghem, L. M.; and Mason, J. W.: Agents used in cardiac arrhythmias. In, Basic and Clinical Pharmacology, 4th ed. (Katzung, B. G.; ed.). Lange, Palo Alto, pp. 165–182, 1989.

Kenakin, T. P.: Pharmacologic Analysis of Drug-Receptor Interaction. Raven Press, New York, 1987.

Routledge, P. A.: The plasma protein binding of basic drugs. Br. J. Clin. Pharmacol., 22:499–506, 1986.

Sheiner, L. B.: Clinical pharmacology and the choice between theory and empiricism. Clin. Pharmacol. Ther., 46:605–615, 1989.

Sheiner, L. B.; and Tozer, T. N.: Clinical pharmacokinetics: The use of plasma concentrations of drugs. In, Clinical Pharmacology. Basic Principles of Therapeutics, 2nd Ed. (Melmon, K. L.; and Morrelli, H. F.; eds.). Macmillan, New York, pp. 71–109, 1978.

Wilkinson, G. R.; and Shand, D. G.: Commentary: A physiological approach to hepatic clearance. Clin. Pharmacol. Ther., 18:377–390, 1975.

38

Variability and Control Strategies in Quantitative Therapeutics

Brian Whiting

WHAT IS VARIABILITY?

There is a well-recognized degree of unpredictability about therapeutic outcome. The desired response may be achieved, but alternative end points are lack of response and/or unacceptable toxicity. Careful observation of the patient over time is required to reveal whether therapy has been successful and whether some quantitative or qualitative adjustment is called for. The relationship between quantitative adjustment of therapy and the observation time necessary to see the effects of such adjustment vary remarkably depending on the clinical circumstances and the drug or drugs involved. The time is, for example, relatively short and the adjustment crucial during administration of anaesthesia; it can be relatively long and the adjustment less critical when rheumatoid arthritis is being treated.

Two objectives may be worth considering, the direct objective of the desired response and the indirect (or surrogate) objective of a concentration of drug in plasma. A close relationship between concentration of drug in plasma and response to the drug has been demonstrated for many drugs and provides a good rationale for therapeutic drug monitoring. When such a relationship exists, although response can be (partly) explained by concentration of drug in plasma, drug therapy results in a range of concentrations and a range of responses when an individual, or a group of individuals, is considered. This range represents the uncertainty in quantitative drug therapy caused by all sources of variability that exist within and between patients. The skill with which this uncertainty is handled has a strong bearing on the outcome of drug therapy.

An approach to this uncertainty must therefore be formulated. A range of concentrations or responses is the net effect of many underlying processes, each of which makes its own contribution to the outcome and each of which also is subject to variability. In statistical terms, therefore, the net effect of a drug administration—the spread of observed concentrations or responses—can be thought of as the joint probability of several underlying variable processes. These must be clearly identified, understood, and properly responded to.

This leads us to the interesting point of defining a hierarchy of variabilities. For example, an important component contributing to the range of concentrations achieved in a group of patients will be the clearance of a drug. The variability in clearance to some extent generates the range of concentrations and therefore different responses in different people. But what causes the variability in clearance? The answer to this rests on an understanding of the various pathophysiologic mechanisms that help determine clearance of a drug, including glomerular filtration, activity of cytochrome P450, or left ventricular ejection. Each of these factors, in turn, is influenced by other, perhaps more fundamental factors such as alterations in pH or electrolyte status. The understanding of variability as far as drug therapy is concerned is therefore a matter of understanding the complex relationships between physiology, biochemistry, pathology, pharmacology, and clinical medicine—the essence of clinical pharmacology.

Clearance is only one component of variability that is relatively high in the hierarchy of perturbing factors. The other components at this level are volume of distribution and the mechanisms responsible for absorption of a drug. Moreover, if there is a clear relationship between concentration of drug in plasma and response (effect), then an important component of the variability in response will be due to pharmacologic factors such as those that may modify drug receptors and possible coupling of their effects. All pathophysiologic and pharmacologic sources of variability will be confounded by experimental and/or observer error, likely to be relatively small in the case of measurements of drug concentration but potentially increasing considerably when responses, particularly in the routine clinical context, are involved.

Components of Variability

We may formalize variability, expressing it in traditional clinical pharmacologic terms. The two major components are

1. Pharmacokinetic
2. Pharmacodynamic

Pharmacokinetic Variability. Pharmacokinetic variability is best understood by relating it to models that explain the relationship between drug dose and resulting plasma concentration. The simplest model is that which defines the steady-state plasma concentration (C_{pss}) thus:

$$C_{pss} = \frac{\text{dose rate}}{\text{clearance}}$$

For a given dose rate (ignoring possible variability in bioavailability), the range of possible steady-state concentrations is determined by the variability in clearance. The steady-state equation can therefore be rewritten as a statistical statement:

$$C_{pss} \text{ (range)} = \frac{\text{dose rate}}{\overline{Cl} \pm \text{SD}}$$

where $\pm$ SD introduces the idea that the clearance is not a single number but is (in this case) normally distributed with a range of values described by a mean clearance ($\overline{Cl}$) and standard deviation. Experimental (assay) error must be introduced because it will always magnify variability to some extent. If the variability simply is additive, the equation will be modified thus:

$$C_{pss} \text{ (range)} = \frac{\text{dose rate}}{\overline{Cl} \pm \text{SD}} + \epsilon$$

where ϵ can be regarded as a source of random variability, again characterized by a normal distribution with a mean of zero and a standard devia-

tion that reflects the coefficient of variation of the drug assay. Finally, uncertainty in dose rate should be introduced to account for realistic differences in bioavailability, and perhaps more important, ambiguities in compliance, lumped together in the term $\overline{F}$.

The final steady-state equation can therefore take the form

$$C_{pss} \text{ (range)} = \frac{(\overline{F} \pm \text{SD}) \times \text{dose rate}}{\overline{Cl} \pm \text{SD}} + \epsilon$$

Interestingly enough, the variabilities implicit in $\overline{F}$, $\overline{Cl}$, and the actual measurement of drug concentration do not necessarily combine to produce a range of concentrations (C_{pss} values in this case) that is normally distributed. Indeed, the range of values associated with $\overline{F}$ and $\overline{Cl}$ may not themselves be normally or even unimodally distributed. They may, for example, be lognormally distributed so that the variability can be described as proportional (constant coefficient of variation) rather than as simply additive.

More complex pharmacokinetic models can be treated in the same way to determine the likely range of concentrations that will be associated with any particular dosage regimen over specified periods of time. Moreover, if a link between pharmacokinetic variables (such as clearance) and identifiable patient factors such as age, weight, sex, and renal or hepatic function can be identified, then these links can be used as "explanatory" variables.

Returning to the steady-state equation, if clearance is simply proportional to weight, then this fact can be introduced as follows:

$$C_{pss} \text{ (range)} = \frac{(\overline{F} \pm \text{SD}) \times \text{dose rate}}{(\overline{P} \pm \text{SD}) \times \text{weight}} + \epsilon$$

Here, clearance is a linear function of weight, thus:

$$\text{Clearance} = P \times \text{weight}$$

but still is subject to variability because of the persisting uncertainty in the relationship between clearance and weight, expressed by $\overline{P} \pm \text{SD}$. The variability in clearance is, however, reduced because weight now serves to explain (some of the) differences in clearance (see Fig. 38–1).

More complex pharmacokinetic models contain other pharmacokinetic variables such as volume(s) of distribution and terms defining absorption processes. All these variables possibly may be expressed in terms of a number of pathophysiologic factors. The goal to be borne in mind is to be able to predict concentrations of drug in plasma in

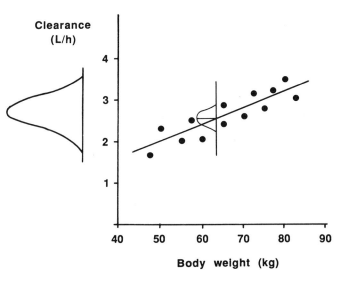

Fig. 38-1. The influence of a covariate (in this case body weight) as an explanatory variable. The total variability in clearance is represented by the bell-shaped curve adjacent to the *Y* axis. The relationship between clearance and body weight is revealed by the data (•) and by the straight line that describes these data. The smaller bell-shaped curve superimposed on this line shows the reduction in variability that has been achieved by explaining clearance in terms of body weight.

individuals given a proposed dosage regimen and as much pharmacokinetic and clinical information as possible. For example, if all the components contributing to the pharmacokinetic variability of theophylline are taken into account and these are applied to an equation that predicts steady-state concentrations, then the distribution of concentrations (expressed here as the mean and 68% confidence interval) will be similar to that shown in Fig. 38-2. At 12 hours, for example, the 68% confidence interval ranges from 4.5 to 17.6 mg/l, with a mean of 11.1 mg/l. This is in many ways disappointing when it is considered that all a priori information on the variability of the pharmacokinetics of theophylline has been used to construct this diagram. But the results serve to illustrate the difficulty of obtaining ade-

quate, relevant, and meaningful information that is sufficient to approach our goal with some drugs.

Pharmacodynamic Variability. The same approach can be applied to consideration of pharmacodynamic variability. Two choices present themselves. Drug response can be viewed in terms of a range of either doses or concentrations. The fundamental relationships between dose, concentration, and response can be expressed diagrammatically as in Fig. 38-3.

The relationship can simplify to linking dose directly to concentration. Subtraction of the pharmacokinetic component inevitably leads to a relationship that contains much more variability. Nevertheless, the form of the PD and PD′

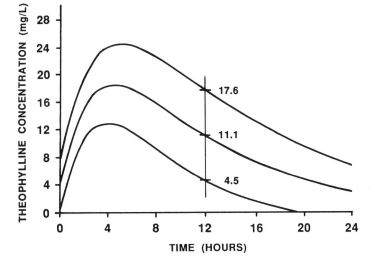

Fig. 38-2. Spread in theophylline concentrations associated with population pharmacokinetic parameter estimates. In this simulation, the dosage interval is 24 hours. The 68% confidence interval at 12 hours is 4.5 to 17.6 mg/l. Note that, in general, therapeutic concentrations lie between 8 and 20 mg/l.

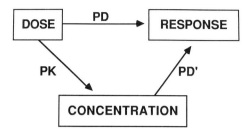

Fig. 38-3. The interrelationships between drug dose, concentration, and response. PD is the direct dose–response relationship; PK is the pharmacokinetic link between dose and concentration; and PD′ is the pharmacodynamic link between concentration and response.

relationships in Fig. 38–3 are the same as presented earlier in this chapter. In the most general sense, the E_{max} model can be written as

$$E = \frac{E_{max} \times dose}{ED_{50} + dose} \quad \text{for the PD relationship}$$

and

$$E = \frac{E_{max} \times concentration}{EC_{50} + concentration} \quad \begin{array}{l}\text{for the PD}'\\ \text{relationship}\end{array}$$

When a group of patients is considered, the parameters of these relationships (E_{max}, ED_{50}, and EC_{50}) take on statistical characteristics with, for example, mean values and standard deviations, and the variability in E is also confounded by error in measurement.

There may be some advantage in focusing on the PD′ relationship because it is devoid of pharmacokinetic variability and therefore expresses variability intrinsic to pharmacodynamics. This focus does have the drawback, however, that unless "steady-state" concentrations are considered as the independent variable, response usually will be out of phase to a greater or lesser extent with concentration (see chapter 37). This introduces further complexities into the relationship.

While pharmacokinetic variability has been explored in some detail and useful relationships with identifiable factors in patients have been determined, this has not been accomplished to the same extent with variability in pharmacodynamics. Whereas many relationships between kinetic variables such as clearance, volume of distribution, and pathophysiologic factors have been proposed, and subsequently experimentally confirmed or refuted, the sources of pharmacodynamic variability (conveniently expressed by PD′ in Fig. 38–3) are more elusive, residing at the level of cellular and molecular pharmacology.

The Expression of Variability

From a therapeutic point of view, the kinds of variability discussed so far are unfortunate. A great deal of effort has gone into trying to understand the mechanisms that underlie variability. Only thus can it be minimized in specific identifiable subgroups and individual patients. For example, in a group of patients with obstructive airway disease, clearance of theophylline may vary from 1 to 5 l/h, based on a mean clearance of 3 l/h and a standard deviation of approximately ±1.5 l/h (coefficient of variation approximately 50%). Knowledge of a patient's body weight, however, will immediately reduce the uncertainty about clearance because theophylline clearance is proportional to body weight, thus:

Theophylline clearance (in l/h)
= (0.04 l/h per kg)(body weight in kg)

There will still be some uncertainty about the clearance in a given individual, but the variability has been reduced by the introduction of body weight as an important explanation of variability. This is illustrated in Fig. 38–1.

Moreover, other factors may be entered into the equation to further reduce variability. The confidence with which these factors are known is highly dependent on the available clinical data. For example, other factors influencing clearance of theophylline include smoking, acute respiratory failure, cirrhosis of the liver, and the co-administration of cimetidine. Each of these factors, singly or in combination, moves the value of clearance away from the value determined by body weight. Therefore, any individual can be placed in a particular subgroup depending on the presence of each variable. The lack of precision in determining these relationships, however, still generates the uncertainty in concentration values illustrated in Fig. 38–2. This is passed on into the PD relationship to create analogous uncertainty in response to the drug.

The Quantitation of Variability

A number of analytic methods have been used to estimate the parameters that express the variability described above. These range from stepwise multiple linear regression to analysis of variance techniques based on the nonlinear regression functions that describe relationships between pharmacokinetics and pharmacodynamics.

The principal aim always is to estimate the characteristics of the distributions of the relevant parameters. This is most efficiently done by clearly specifying the nature of these distributions in model form. In other words, if the starting point is a set of pharmacokinetic data (basically, a set of concentration of drug in plasma versus time points) from a group of individuals (hereinafter referred to as a *population*), then the questions that must be addressed include

1. What pharmacokinetic model would be most suitable for these data (i.e., which model would "fit" best) if it could be applied to each individual in turn? (Note here that in typical population studies, there often are very few points per individual, certainly not enough to justify a traditional nonlinear least-squares-fitting approach.)

2. Can the pharmacokinetic parameters included in this model (clearance, volume of distribution, etc.) be linked to identifiable patient factors (age, weight, sex, etc.)?

3. What statistical model(s) can be proposed that will explain the variability in the pharmacokinetic parameters? In other words, what is the nature of the distribution that underlies the variability?

4. What statistical model(s) can be proposed that will explain all other variability, principally error in assays and spontaneous fluctuations of pharmacokinetics within individuals?

A simple example should help to illustrate, why these questions are useful. Suppose a drug is given by single-bolus IV injection to a number of patients. Two to three blood samples are withdrawn from each patient at various times after the injection. Assuming that the decline in concentrations can be modeled as a single exponential (answer to question 1), then the samples should be "spread out" to obtain as much information as possible about the *intercept* (concentration at time zero) and *slope* (first-order elimination rate constant) of the exponential process. If all the points from all the subjects were plotted on the same graph, the range of concentrations would then be a reflection of the underlying variability in the kinetic parameters.

Now suppose that there is a good reason to believe that the clearance of this drug is closely related to renal function (creatinine clearance, Cl_{creat}) and that the volume of distribution is related to body weight (BW) (answers to questions 2). Two simple linear models that express these ideas are

$$\text{Clearance} = \Theta_1 + \Theta_2 \times Cl_{creat}$$

$$\text{Volume of distribution} = \Theta_3 \times \text{BW}$$

where Θ_1, Θ_2, and Θ_3 are the mean values of the parameters linking Cl and V to creatinine clearance and weight, respectively. Bearing in mind that the two parameters of this pharmacokinetic

model are clearance and volume of distribution and that the primary task now is to estimate the way in which these are distributed in the group (population) of patients, ideas about the nature of their distributions must be specified in statistical terms to provide an answer to question 3. For example, if the concept is that these parameters are normally distributed, then this idea can be expressed as follows:

$$Cl_j = (\Theta_1 + \Theta_2 \times CrCl_j) + \eta_{Clj}$$

$$V_j = \Theta_3 \times \text{BW}_j + \eta_{Vj}$$

where the drug clearance and volume of distribution for the jth individual are denoted by Cl_j and V_j and the η_{Clj} and η_{Vj} are distributed normally (in this case) with a mean of zero. The variance of η_{Cl} and η_V are the variances of Cl and V respectively.

Finally, question 4 must be addressed in terms of the nature of the assay error and any other errors not taken account of by the η's specified above. If, for example, we assume that each measurement is subject to a small random error that is independent of each concentration, then this variability can be specified as follows:

$$c_{ij} = c^*_{ij} + \epsilon_{ij}$$

where c_{ij} is the ith concentration measurement ($i = 1, 2, 3$, etc.) in the jth individual, c^*_{ij} is the corresponding concentration predicted by the chosen pharmacokinetic and statistical models (in answer to questions 1, 2, and 3), and ϵ_{ij} is normally distributed with a mean of zero and a variance primarily reflecting assay error. The full pharmacostatistical model can then be written

$$c_{ij} = \frac{\text{DOSE}_j}{\Theta_3 \times \text{BW}_j + \eta_{Vj}} e^{-\frac{(\Theta_1 + \Theta_2 \times CrCl_j) + \eta_{Clj}}{\Theta_3 \times \text{BW}_j + \eta_{Vj}} t_{ij}} + \epsilon_{ij}$$

where DOSE_j is the dose given to the jth individual whose body weight is BW_j and creatinine clearance is $CrCl_j$, and t_{ij} is the sampling time relevant to c_{ij}. In this example, therefore, there are six *population pharmacokinetic parameters*, Θ_1, Θ_2, Θ_3, the variances (or SDs) of Cl and V, and the residual variance, largely attributable to experimental error. While estimation of these parameters is a relatively complex task, it can be performed with suitable software, for example, the NONMEM (*Non*linear *M*ixed *E*ffects *M*odel) system (Beal and Sheiner, 1979–1989). The great advantage of this system over most other methods is that the raw concentration-versus-time data from all subjects are analyzed simultaneously to estimate all parameters without any intermediate steps. The effects of including or excluding pathophysiologic factors that might influence clearance and/or volume of distribution can be tested statistically, but success or failure in this type of analysis depends very much on the quality and quantity of available data. It stands to reason that if a relationship between, for example, clearance and age is postulated, there must be a wide enough age range to justify a test of this relationship. The design of studies that can yield the best estimates of population pharmacokinetic parameters still is a matter for further research.

Although exactly the same concepts can be applied to pharmacodynamic data, experience from this is much more limited. Sheiner et al. (1989) have discussed experimental designs that might facilitate the estimation of population pharmacodynamic parameters such as ED_{50} and EC_{50} and their variances and have shown that this is feasible using the NONMEM system. Success is critically dependent, however, on the implementation of a dose escalation design in which all subjects are given the opportunity of experiencing set increments in dose to the point of overall therapeutic success or maximal individual tolerance to the drug. All subjects, therefore, contribute more or less data to support the underlying dose (or concentration)–response relationship. The aspect of repeated measures of this design is essential if there is to be a satisfactory discrimination between inter- and intrasubject pharmacodynamic variability.

UTILITY OF POPULATION PHARMACOKINETIC AND PHARMACODYNAMIC DATA

Pharmacokinetic Data

Pharmacokinetic data on a variety of drugs from a number of sources have been analyzed by the NONMEM system. The analysis provides the kind of population information discussed above. These data have been of two main types: routine and experimental.

Routine implies that no particular attention has been paid to issues of experimental design. These data have arisen largely as a result of monitoring routine therapeutic situations. Nevertheless, in some cases extra samples have been obtained in an attempt to improve the information content of the data. *Experimental* implies that an effort has been made to collect samples at specific, predetermined times, usually according to a protocol.

The objective of the analysis of data gathered during routine treatment of patients is to exploit the information about variability exhibited by a typical population of patients. In the postmarketing phase of drug use, this variability is likely to be at its maximum. Data that are gathered entirely during routine care, however, may not necessarily yield as much information as data collected according to some form of protocol. Planning data collection prospectively, even when the subjects are patients undergoing routine clinical care, has real value.

Data from experiments are ideally collected during development of a drug. Their analysis yields accurate population information that can be used to maximize efficacy and limit toxicity during treatment in the postmarketing phase of drug use. The input of patients during phase II and III premarketing studies eventually should ensure a high degree of heterogeneity in the patient base. If these studies have included a (prospective) population pharmacokinetic component (say three or four deliberately timed samples per subject), then our objectives for such study should be fulfilled. Each subject (patient) provides a very small fraction of the total information on which the analysis is based. Carelessness in recording and/or measurement of drug or effects leads to errors that compromise the ability to accurately define the population pharmacokinetic parameters in terms of their means and variances. Unwanted "noise" in the data tends to magnify one or other sources of variance and obscures underlying important kinetic-pathophysiologic relationships.

Successful studies and population pharmacokinetic analyses have been performed with a number of drugs that have been the subject of extensive review (for examples, see Whiting et al., 1986, 1990). Diverse groups of drugs have been studied, ranging from those traditionally associated with therapeutic drug monitoring (digoxin, phenytoin, theophylline, gentamicin, procainamide, lidocaine) to those that were studied in the premarketing phase of drug development [for example, lisinopril (Thomson et al., 1989), and bisoprolol (Grevel et al., 1989)]. In most instances, the influence of one or more identifiable patient factors on clearance and/or volume of distribution was determined. This information can be written in terms of equations or used to construct nomograms.

Bearing in mind that population pharmacokinetics seeks to explain the uncertainty in plasma concentration data in terms of characteristics of patients, the question must be asked: How much is gained if a population equation or nomogram is applied to a particular patient? From the discussion developed above, we learned that the incorporation of covariate information (age, weight, smoking habits, etc.) reduces uncertainty so that there is a shift from the *population mean* toward a value more representative of the particular patient. Nevertheless, even when all covariate information is taken into account, the net uncertainty still may be relatively large, as is illustrated in Fig. 38–2. This implies that in general, population equations or nomograms only represent starting points for therapeutic decisions. Further refinements of quantitative therapeutic decisions that more precisely characterize the individual's pharmacokinetics may be necessary.

As an example, we will examine what has been achieved with the analysis of routinely gathered data on concentrations of phenytoin in plasma. The nonlinear pharmacokinetics of phenytoin makes this drug an ideal candidate given the drug requires careful therapeutic control in view of its relatively narrow therapeutic index. In one of the first population pharmacokinetic studies, the average values of the Michaelis-Menten parameters, V_{max} and K_m, were obtained from routinely gathered clinical pharmacokinetic data (Sheiner and Beal, 1980). The mean V_{max} was 7.22 mg/kg per day, with an interindividual coefficient of variation (CV) of 24%. The mean K_m was 4.44 mg/l with an interindividual CV of 54% (no covariate information was obtained). Grasela et al., (1983) carried out a more comprehensive analysis of routinely gathered data on phenytoin obtained from a heterogeneous population, including Japanese, Europeans, and children. These "extra" factors allowed more questions to be asked about the relationships between patient characteristics and V_{max} and/or K_m. There had been some debate previously about the relationship between age and/or weight and V_{max}; the analysis of this large data set demonstrated that the best estimate of V_{max} could be obtained from the equation

$$V_{max} \text{ (mg/day)} = 32 \times \text{(weight)}^{0.6}$$

The coefficient of variation associated with this relationship was 20% for Europeans and 11% for Japanese.

Unlike the results of the first study, Grasela found that, on average, K_m values were determined by age and by race. Young people (less than 15 years) had smaller values than older people (greater than 15 years). The average K_m value in the young was 3.2 mg/l (Europeans) and 2.2 mg/l (Japanese). In the older group, average values of K_m were 5.7 mg/l (Europeans) and 3.8 mg/l (Japanese). These explanatory factors did not, however, reduce the K_m variability in this somewhat larger (and different) population; the coefficient of variation remained at approximately 50%.

These population studies, therefore, have helped explain the kinetics of phenytoin in terms of body weight, age, and race. However, a large degree of the variability, especially in K_m, remains unexplained. Proper control of phenytoin therapy

(as far as the nonlinear dose–concentration relationship is concerned) therefore depends on further measures that will more confidently identify values of V_{max} and K_m in individuals.

The same conclusions can be arrived at for most other drugs studied in this way. For drugs displaying linear kinetics, the end point will be relationships between pathophysiologic variables and clearance and/or volume(s) of distribution and their associated variances. In practically all cases for which fine tuning of dose is required to achieve specific target concentrations, the degree of unexplained variability is such that further refinement of the relevant pharmacokinetics for the individual patient is required. This is achieved by the simple expedient of measuring one or more drug concentrations in the patient and viewing these as being generated by a (relatively) unique set of pharmacokinetic parameters.

Within the routine clinical context, this set of parameters cannot be estimated by traditional means, but advantage is taken of the information that has been gained from population pharmacokinetic studies. The assumption is that the patient of interest has a set of parameters that lies within the previously determined population distribution and that the measurement(s) of concentration can be used to reveal this set of parameters. In statistical terms, the a priori population distribution is transformed into a patient-specific a posteriori distribution. This is achieved computationally by a combination of Bayes theorem and maximum likelihood estimation (Sheiner et al., 1979; Peck et al., 1980; Sheiner and Beal, 1982). Briefly, if the pharmacokinetic equation(s) appropriate to a patient's drug and dosage administration can be specified, then the expected values of the concentration measurements (Y_E) can be computed. The maximum likelihood estimates (MLEs) of the parameters are then the set that minimizes the negative log likelihood function M thus:

$$M = \sum_{i=1}^{K} \frac{(\Theta_i - \overline{\Theta}_i)^2}{\sigma_i^2} + \sum_{j=1}^{n} \frac{(Y_j - Y_{Ej})^2}{\sigma^2_{Yj}}$$

where Θ_i represents each pharmacokinetic parameter, the value of which is estimated during the computation, $\overline{\Theta}_i$ is the corresponding mean population value and σ_i^2 is its variance, Y_j represents each concentration measurement, subject to an error specified by σ^2_{Yj}, and Y_{Ej} is the corresponding expected value, computed from estimates of Θ_i as the computation proceeds. The method assumes that each parameter is normally distributed in the population and that each measurement is subject to a normally distributed random error. A number of other methods exist for estimating pharmacokinetic parameters from relatively sparse routine data in clinical practice, but experience has shown that the Bayesian approach is the most statistically robust and relatively precise method (Burton et al., 1985; Vozeh and Steimer, 1985). In general terms, the method is outlined in Fig. 38–4.

The starting point is a set of population parameter estimates that characterize the a priori distribution. These parameters enter into one or more pharmacokinetic equations that define the concentration-versus-time profile(s) relevant to the dosage history. One or more concentration measurements Y_j from an individual then are used to obtain a revised, a posteriori distribution of the set of parameters. This is now the conditional probability distribution for the set of parameters and the set of measurements. The revised set of (Bayesian) parameters will now reflect the individual rather than the population; this to a greater or lesser extent, shifts these values to ones with reduced standard deviations. A successful outcome is measured in terms of the confidence with which a patient's pharmacokinetic parameters are now known. If a particular dosage regimen is specified, this in turn can be translated into the confidence with which concentrations can be predicted. Bearing in mind the spread of concentrations that may be associated with population information only (Fig. 38–2), a dramatic reduction in the spread can be achieved if one (or more) concentration measurements is analyzed in the Bayesian context. Figure 38–5 shows that whereas the 68% confidence interval ranged from 4.5 to 17.6 mg/l, one measurement (in this case taken at 22 hours) reduced the confidence interval to a range of 9.2 to 12.4 mg/l.

This is of considerable use in making adjustments in the dosage required in a given patient. Indeed, the Bayesian method has been applied to many clinical circumstances in which target concentrations must be achieved with a fair degree of precision. Examples of drugs requiring this kind of control include aminoglycoside antibiotics, digoxin, theophylline, phenytoin, lithium, and cyclosporin. A number of microcomputer-based systems have been developed for Bayesian parameter estimation (e.g., Kelman et al., 1982; Jelliffe, 1989). These have created an extremely useful facility for handling and interpretation of drug concentration data in routine clinical pharmacokinetic (therapeutic drug monitoring) laboratories.

The Bayesian concept also can be graphically represented (Vozeh et al., 1981). Examination of Figs. 38–6 through 38–9 reveals the advantage of the Bayesian method. The Michaelis-Menten equation appropriate for phenytoin can be written in the following steady-state form:

$$C_{pss} = \frac{DR \times K_m}{V_{max} - DR}$$

where C_{pss} is the steady-state phenytoin concentration in plasma measured at dose rate DR. This equation can be rearranged (Winter and Tozer, 1986) to give a straight line relationship, thus:

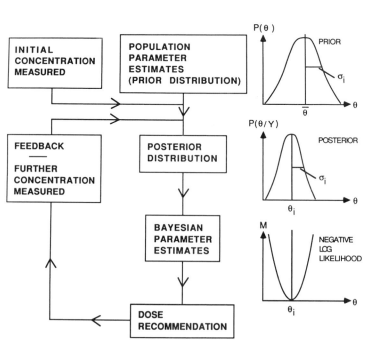

Fig. 38–4. Bayesian parameter estimation. Information from the a priori distribution ($\overline{\Theta}$, σ_i) and an initial concentration measurement is used to obtain the revised a posteriori distribution that yields MLEs of the parameters (Θ_i). These are then used to make a dose recommendation. Further concentration measurements can be used to further refine the a posteriori distribution through feedback of this additional information (from Kelman, A.W.; Whiting, B.; and Bryson, S.M.: OPT: A package of computer programs for parameter estimation in clinical pharmacokinetics. Br. J. Clin. Pharmacol., 14:247–256, 1982, reprinted with permission).

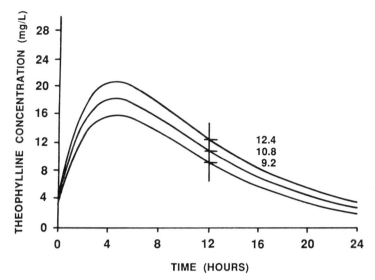

Fig. 38-5. Reduced spread in predicted theophylline concentrations after Bayesian parameter estimation. (Compare with Fig. 38-2.) The 68% confidence interval at 12 hours is now 9.2 to 12.4 mg/l.

$$V_{max} = DR + \frac{DR}{C_{pss}} \times K_m$$

where V_{max} and K_m are now treated as variables and a plot of V_{max} against K_m values for a given DR, C_{pss} pair will have a Y intercept of DR and an X intercept of $-C_{pss}$, as in Fig. 38-6.

This would, of itself, be of no value if V_{max} and K_m were unknown. Given a measured C_{pss} for a given dose rate DR, the line joining C_{pss} and DR extrapolated into the V_{max}, K_m region would have a continuous set of values for V_{max} and K_m, defined by the extrapolated line. A line drawn

through a second (different) DR, C_{pss} pair in the same patient would intersect at that patient's coordinate for V_{max}, K_m. But a more interesting approach is to superimpose population pharmacokinetic information about V_{max} and K_m onto the graph (Fig. 38-7).

Here, the contour (or *orbit*) plot describes the probability with which values of V_{max}, K_m occur jointly in the population (the outcome of a NONMEM analysis, Sheiner and Beal, 1980). The graph is now much more informative as it ascribes different probabilities to V_{max}, K_m coordinates throughout the V_{max}, K_m region. The

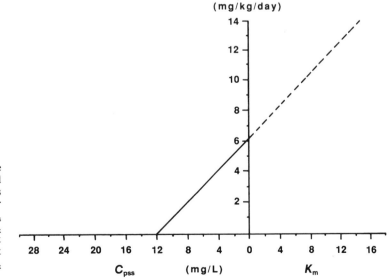

Fig. 38-6. Graph of dose rate (DR) against C_{pss} extrapolated into the V_{max}, K_m region. In this example, DR was 6 mg/kg per day and the corresponding C_{pss} was 12 mg/l. The values of V_{max} and K_m unique to this patient cannot be determined. Note that the Y axis shares DR and V_{max} values (same units).

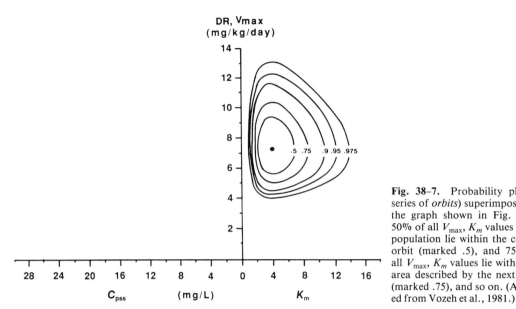

Fig. 38-7. Probability plot (a series of *orbits*) superimposed on the graph shown in Fig. 38-6: 50% of all V_{max}, K_m values in the population lie within the central orbit (marked .5), and 75% of all V_{max}, K_m values lie within the area described by the next orbit (marked .75), and so on. (Adapted from Vozeh et al., 1981.)

line joining DR, C_{pss} and extrapolated into this region can now be seen in the context of the a priori population information because the latter now shows where V_{max}, K_m coordinates (for the individual patient) are most likely along this line (Fig. 38-8).

The midpoint of the line crossing the innermost orbit through which the line passes gives the coordinate of the most likely values for V_{max} and K_m for that patient. Information unique to the patient has therefore been used to refine more general information previously acquired from a simi-

lar population of patients. Further control over treatment can then be exercised by drawing a line from the most likely V_{max}, K_m coordinate to the (new) desired C_{pss} and reading off the new dose rate on the Y axis (Fig. 38-9).

Pharmacodynamic Data

Most, if not all, attempts to control drug therapy have focused on the measurement of a concentration of drug in plasma as the control variable. The Bayesian method has proved to be the

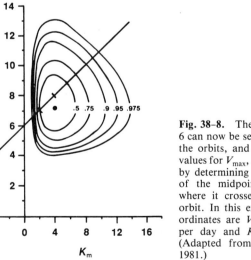

Fig. 38-8. The line in Fig. 38-6 can now be seen in relation to the orbits, and the most likely values for V_{max}, K_m can be found by determining the coordinates of the midpoint of this line where it crosses its innermost orbit. In this example, the coordinates are V_{max} = 8 mg/kg per day and K_m = 3.8 mg/l. (Adapted from Vozeh et al., 1981.)

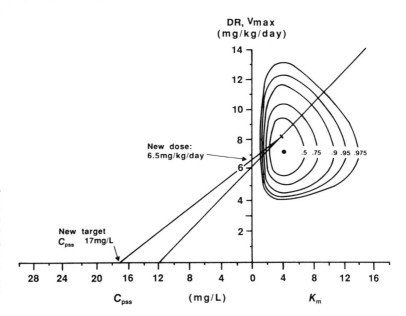

Fig. 38-9. Determination of the dose of phenytoin required to achieve a new C_{pss}, in this example, 17 mg/l. A (second) line is drawn from the patient's V_{max}, K_m coordinate to the desired C_{pss}. This cuts the Y axis at the new dose, in this example, 6.5 mg/kg per day. (Adapted from Vozeh et al., 1981.)

most statistically robust and reliable method in practice. Drug response data should be amenable to similar treatment if meaningful responses can be measured in an efficient way. The response data could then be used to extend traditional clinical pharmacokinetic practice so that not only could a posteriori pharmacokinetic parameter distributions be estimated but also analogous a posteriori pharmacodynamic parameter distributions. The concept could be further extended to include measurements of adverse drug effects so that a utility function (Sheiner and Melmon, 1978) could be computed. The maximum of the utility function specifies a target concentration on an individual patient basis (Kelman and Whiting, 1988). This concentration of drug in plasma rep-

resents the point at which the most therapeutic benefit for the least harm would be achieved. However, although this seems to be a very attractive concept, it is very difficult to put into practice because of the number of assumptions involved and the errors that apparently cannot be avoided. Success would depend on

1. The correct pharmacodynamic models for both beneficial and adverse drug responses
2. Good estimates of population pharmacodynamic parameters
3. Meaningful and accurate measurements of response
4. A careful assessment of adverse effects
5. Good compliance with drug therapy (as is

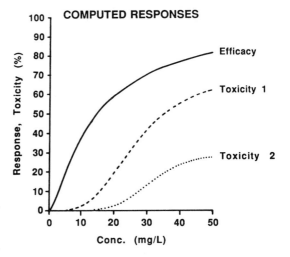

Fig. 38-10. Bayesian estimates of one beneficial and two toxic responses as a function of concentration. Each curve has a form determined by the sigmoid E_{max} (Hill) equation. Different weights were assigned to the two "toxicities" because they were not of equal importance. The ratio of weights was 0.7 : 0.3 for toxicities 1 and 2, respectively. The weight for the beneficial effect was 1.0 (from Whiting and Kelman, 1988, reprinted with permission).

assumed in all pharmacokinetic and/or pharmacodynamic data interpretation)

If these conditions were met, then individual concentration–response curves could be constructed from Bayesian estimates of the relevant pharmacodynamic parameters as is illustrated in Fig. 38–10. These curves would represent the refinement of population curves achieved with appropriate measurements of response and toxicity made at one, or more, concentrations. The utility curve (see Fig. 38–11) is then calculated by subtracting all toxicity from beneficial response values at equivalent concentrations; that is, it is the difference between response and toxicity curves.

There are clinical situations in which such a degree of control would be of considerable advantage, notably where there is almost overlap of therapeutic and toxic concentrations. Cyclosporin treatment in transplantation exemplifies this situation in which a fine balance between avoidance of rejection of the transplanted organ and cyclosporin toxicity must be achieved.

Considerable expertise now exists in both clinical pharmacokinetics and pharmacodynamics. The interpretation of drug concentration measurements in plasma can go a long way to enhancing the control of drug therapy by specifying particular dosage regimens that will achieve target concentrations. This control theoretically can be tightened further by incorporating parallel information on response and toxicity. The accurate quantitative clinical assessment of these two important variables is a challenge for the future.

REFERENCES

Beal, S. L.; and Sheiner, L. B.: NONMEM User's Guide, Parts I to VI. Division of Clinical Pharmacology, University of California, San Francisco, 1979–1989.

Burton, M. E.; Vasko, M. R.; and Brater, D. C.: Comparison of drug dosing methods. Clin. Pharmacokinet., 10:1–37, 1985.

Grasela, T. H.; Sheiner, L. B.; Rambeck, B.; Boegigh, H. E.; Dunlop, A.; Mullen, P. W.; Wadsworth, J.; Richens, A.; Ishizaki, T.; Chiba, K.; Miura, H.; Minagawa, K.; Blain, P. G.; Mucklow, J. C.; Bacon, C. T.; and Rawlins, M.: Steady-state pharmacokinetics of phenytoin from routinely collected patient data. Clin. Pharmacokinet., 8:355–364, 1983.

Grevel, G.; Thomas, P.; and Whiting, B.: Population pharmacokinetic analysis of bisoprolol. Clin. Pharmacokinet., 17: 53–63, 1989.

Jelliffe, R. W.: USC*PACK PC and ADAPT PC clinical research programs. University of Southern California School of Medicine, Los Angeles, 1989.

Kelman, A. W.; and Whiting, B.: A Bayesian approach to the utility of drug therapy. Biomed. Meas. Inf. Contr., 2:170–175, 1988.

Kelman, A. W.; Whiting, B.; and Bryson, S. M.: OPT: A package of computer programs for parameter estimation in clinical pharmacokinetics. Br. J. Clin. Pharmacol., 14:247–256, 1982.

Peck, C. C.; Brown, W. D.; Sheiner, L. B.; and Schuster, B. C.: A microcomputer drug (theophylline) dosing program which assists and teaches physicians. In, Proceedings of the 4th Annual Conference on Computers in Medical Care (O'Neill, J. T., ed.). Vol. 2. pp. 988–991, 1980.

Sheiner, L. B.; and Beal, S. L.: Bayesian individualization of pharmacokinetics: Simple implementation and comparison with non-Bayesian methods. J. Pharm. Sci., 71:1344–1348, 1982.

Sheiner, L. B.; and Beal, S. L.: Evaluation of methods for estimating population pharmacokinetic parameters: I. Michaelis-Menten Model: Routine clinical pharmacokinetic data. J. Pharmacokinet. Biopharmacol., 8:553–571, 1980.

Sheiner, L. B.; and Melmon, K. L.: The utility function of antihypertensive therapy. Ann. N.Y. Acad. Sci., 304:112–122, 1978.

Sheiner, L. B.; Beal, S. L.; and Sambol, N. C.: Study designs for dose ranging. Clin. Pharmacol. Ther., 46:63–77, 1989.

Sheiner, L. B.; Beal, S.; Rosenberg, B.; and Marathe, V. V.: Forecasting individual pharmacokinetics. Clin. Pharmacol. Ther., 26:294–305, 1979.

Thomson, A. H.; Kelly, J. G.; and Whiting, B.: Lisinopril population pharmacokinetics in elderly and renal disease patients with hypertension. Br. J. Clin. Pharmacol., 27:57–65, 1989.

Vozeh, S.; and Steimer, J. L.: Feedback control methods for drug dosage optimisation. Concepts, classification and clinical application. Clin. Pharmacokinet., 10:457–476, 1985.

Vozeh, S.; Muir, K. T.; Sheiner, L. B.; and Follath, F.: Predicting individual phenytoin dosage. J. Pharmacokinet. Biopharmacol., 9:131–146, 1981.

Whiting, B.; Grevel, J.; and Kelman, A. W.: In, Comprehensive Medicinal Chemistry (Taylor, J. B., ed.). Vol. 5. Pergamon Press, Elmsford, N.Y., pp. 297–304, 1990.

Whiting, B.; Kelman, A. W.; and Grevel, J.: Population pharmacokinetics: Theory and clinical application. Clin. Pharmacokinet., 11:387–401, 1986.

Winter, M. E.; and Tozer, T. N.: Phenytoin. In, Applied Pharmacokinetics, 2nd ed. (Evans, W. E.; Schentag, J. J.; and Jusko, W. J.; eds.). Applied Therapeutics, pp. 506–507, 1986.

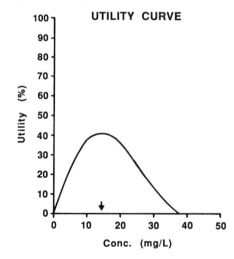

Fig. 38–11. The utility function derived from the curves shown in Fig. 38–10. The concentration associated with the maximum of this function is 15 mg/l (from Whiting and Kelman, 1988, reprinted with permission).

39

Adverse Drug Reactions

Frederic S. Glazener

Drugs can be remarkably powerful in modifying even the most sophisticated homeostatic mechanisms. In doing so, one must consider risk whenever biochemical and physiologic processes are modulated. Drugs that produce adverse effects that occur less often than 1 in 10,000 times the drug is given present elusive signals in spite of the fact that these events can be profoundly significant (Allan, 1976). Well-gathered, highly representative information about the adverse effects of drugs helps physicians use drugs in spite of their hazard.

With the increased development of novel drugs, there has been a rise in the potential for adverse drug effects. While the pharmacologic effects of novel molecules may be more powerful or efficacious than those of their predecessors, in general there is no reason to believe that they will prove to be safer. It is unfortunate, but not surprising, that toxicity frequently occurs in patients in whom a particular drug was inappropriately prescribed in the first place (Palmer, 1969; Stolley and Lasagna, 1969; Lennard et al., 1970; and Venulet, 1975).

DEFINITION OF ADVERSE DRUG REACTIONS

A useful working definition of adverse drug reaction is the following: an adverse drug reaction is any drug-induced noxious change in a patient's condition that occurs at normal dosages and that (1) requires treatment, (2) indicates decrease or cessation of therapy with the drug, or (3) suggests that future therapy with the drug poses an unusual risk to the patient (Koch-Weser, 1968; Koch-Weser et al., 1969; Blaschke, 1986).

The term usually excludes nontherapeutic overdosage (accidental exposure or attempted suicide) or failure of the drug to have its intended effect (excludes lack of efficacy). However, for reporting purposes, the Food and Drug Administration (FDA) in the United States includes adverse events occurring from (1) overdosage, either accidental or intentional, (2) drug abuse, (3) withdrawal of drug, and (4) any significant adverse events occurring from failure of expected pharmacologic action. Serious or unexpected adverse drug reactions should be reported to the drug's manufacturer as well as to the FDA (as described in chapter 35). Not discussed in this section are the adverse reactions to the agents used in drug formulation. An in-depth guide to reactions associated with excipients and a reminder of their importance to the problem of adverse drug reactions has been published recently by Weiner and Bernstein (1989).

INCIDENCE OF ADVERSE DRUG REACTIONS

Clinically important adverse drug reactions are underappreciated and underreported by physicians. Schimmel (1964) noted that 20% of patients admitted to a medical teaching hospital experienced one or more untoward episodes during an 8-month period. Steel et al. (1981) reported that at least 19% of patients on a general medical service of a tertiary-care hospital had a drug-related illness. In 2% of all patients, and more than 5% of those hospitalized with complications, the iatrogenic illness was believed to be contributory to the patients' deaths. Jick (1974) reported an adverse drug reaction either caused the hospital admission or strongly influenced it in 3% to 7% of the patients studied by the Boston Collaborative Drug Surveillance Project. In hospital, there was a 5% incidence of drug reactions; of these 10% were major. The death rate from drug effects was 3 per 1000 patients, or 0.3%. Jick made no attempt to determine what percentage of deaths were avoidable without compromising the therapeutic effects of using the drug. There are limited data concerning the incidence of adverse drug reactions in the ambulatory setting. Available figures vary over the range of 3% to 41% but with variations of the criteria and methodology used. About 20% of adverse reactions require withdrawal of the offending drug, with serious adverse reactions occurring in a lesser percentage (Blaschke, 1986).

Lacking in most studies is information about drugs other than the assumed toxic agent being taken by the patient. The degree of the patient's compliance with the treatment program and whether excipients rather than the active drug could have been playing a role simply are not retrievable (Lockey, 1971; Michaelson, 1973; Weiner and Bernstein, 1989). Patient variables such as age, sex, disease, genetic factors, geographic factors, and drug-related factors such as type of drug, dosage, bioavailability, route of administration, and duration of therapy can affect the incidence and severity of drug toxicity. It is not known to what extent faulty prescribing practices or mistakes in patient compliance contribute to adverse drug reactions. The clinician should always question whether the medication the patient is taking may be responsible for an untoward (or for that matter any unexpected efficacious) response. Just because the reaction has not been ascribed previously to the particular drug does not mean that the suspected drug is not at fault.

Adverse drug reactions are more frequently encountered at the extremes of age. In the neonate, the liver and kidney enzymes necessary for drug metabolism and elimination have not yet become optimally functional and clearance of many drugs is less than in adults (chapter 30). In the elderly, changes in liver and kidney function may decrease drug elimination (chapter 31). Pharmacokinetic and pharmacodynamic alterations in children and the elderly that might contribute to adverse drug effects are described in chapters 30 and 31. In fact, genetic polymorphisms seem very likely explanations for a number of positive and adverse responses to drugs in the adult (chapter 32).

From several series, women are reported to have a higher percentage of adverse drug reactions than men, about 60% to 40%. Though women may more frequently obtain medical attention and medications than men, there are definite periods during a woman's lifetime when there is alteration of the pharmacokinetics of drugs: menarche, pregnancy and delivery, lactation, and menopause (Wilson, 1984). Thus, women may be at a higher risk than men for experiencing drug reactions.

Patients with a past history of reactions to medications are more apt to experience adverse drug reactions. In a New Zealand hospital study reported by Smidt and McQueen (1972), 28% of those patients who had an adverse drug reaction had experienced an adverse reaction previously. A history of allergic disease is also associated with an increased risk of reactions. Adverse responses are not entirely unexpected since careful questioning usually reveals prior exposure to the drug. There may be a genetically determined propensity to form considerably larger amounts of IgE with an increased liability to anaphylatic-type reactions.

There is an increased incidence of adverse reactions when multiple medications are given. This may in part explain the more numerous untoward reactions encountered by the elderly. The average number of drugs received by both hospitalized and ambulatory elderly patients ranges from 2.8 to 8.3 from various studies (Kondo and Blaschke, 1989). There are many potential interactions between drugs and diseases that can lead to greater potential for adverse effects. For example, diseases involving the liver or kidneys may modify drug elimination that can lead to the accumulation of parent drug or toxic metabolites. Alternatively, diseases may modify physiologic reserve that can predispose to adverse drug effects. For example, in a patient with preexisting congestive heart failure, a drug that injures the heart will likely have greater effects than in a person with a normal cardiovascular system.

Genetic factors may be very important in predisposing to adverse drug effects. These may include polymorphisms in drug metabolism as well as other metabolic variants (see chapter 32). For example, there are patients who are at increased risk of suffering hemolytic episodes associated with drugs that alter redox potential and produce oxidative stresses of the red blood cells that may be due to sex-linked deficiency of glucose-6-phosphate dehydrogenase. In these persons, cells are incapable of sufficiently rapid regeneration of NADPH (Bloom et al., 1983). Primaquine has been the prototype of such drugs, but there are more than 50 drugs and substances known to be capable of inciting hemolysis. In addition to antimalarials, the list includes sulfones, sulfonamides, nitrofurans, antipyretics, analgesics, vitamin K preparations, fava beans, and other vegetables (Webster, 1985).

The route of administration can alter the bioavailability of drugs, for example, the poor absorption of medications from IM sites during a period of shock, the unreliable absorption of phenytoin after IM administration due to its high pH and in situ precipitation, and poor antibody response to hepatitis B vaccine when given in the gluteal muscles compared with a deltoid site (Kostenbauder et al., 1975; Pead et al., 1985; Ukena et al., 1985). Topical medication, such as an acetylcholinesterase inhibitor or a β-adrenergic antagonist, instilled into the eye for treatment for glaucoma may have systemic absorption by entry into the lacrimal duct with drainage into the nasal cavity and ultimately the GI tract (Gibaldi, 1984). There may be enough systemic absorption to cause increased intestinal peristalsis and abdominal cramps from the first agent or exacerbation of asthma and/or alteration of heart rate or AV nodal conduction from the latter. Absorption from the mucous membranes of the nasopharynx can be considerable and enhanced by membrane engorgement or associated nasal polyps. The active ingredients in long-acting nasal sprays or nasal drops are oxymetazoline or xylometazoline. These sympathomimetic agents are peripheral α_1 agonists at the usual dosage with vasoconstriction of nasal mucous membranes and at times a severe degree of elevation of both the systolic and the diastolic blood pressure. There is an increased risk factor due to the sustained period of hypertension. With increased frequency of dosing, the plasma concentration of these agents is such that they cross the blood–brain barrier in sufficient amount to produce the effect of CNS α_2 agonists with diminution of sympathetic outflow from the CNS. This can cause bradycardia, hypotension, near syncope, falls with injuries, and consideration of cardiac pacemaker placement if one is not cognizant of these adverse effects of the long-acting nasal decongestants (Glazener et al., 1983). The large surface area of the alveoli, the rich blood supply of the lungs, and the high permeability of the alveolar epithelium make the lungs remarkably efficient organs for drug absorption and ensure the rapid uptake of drugs given by inhalation. Anesthetic agents are the most important examples of drugs routinely given by this route. Several illicit drugs are also absorbed following inhalation (Gibaldi, 1984). Bronchodilators such as sympathomimetics and adrenocorticosteroids that affect pulmonary function are frequently administered by this route. Between 1961 and 1966 increased sales of pressurized aerosols of sympathomimetics in England and Wales corresponded with an increase in mortality due to asthma, with the increase greatest in children 10 to 14 years of age. Since March 1967 there has been a sharp decline in deaths due to asthma along with a reduction of the use of pressurized aerosols (Inman and Adelsteen, 1969).

There was consideration that the propellant might be at fault. Early information from the British Thoracic Association's confidential inquiry into asthma deaths has indicated that, in general, patients die from asthma rather than its treatment. When excessive use of bronchodilators has occasionally coincided with asthma deaths, it is likely that this indicates the need of further treatment with other drugs such as corticosteroids and is not itself the cause of death (Stewart et al., 1981) (chapter 7).

RECOGNIZING ADVERSE DRUG REACTIONS

There are no general methods that allow a physician to demonstrate easily the causal relationship between medication being taken by the patient and an untoward event. Karch and Lasagna (1975, 1977) suggest some general criteria that are helpful in an effort to establish that an adverse effect is caused by a drug the patient is taking:

1. Is the temporal sequence from the administration of the drug to the onset of the untoward event appropriate?
2. Is the untoward event in keeping with a known pharmacologic effect or adverse effect of the drug?
3. Is the patient's illness or nonpharmacologic therapy sufficient to account for the event?
4. What happens when the drug is discontinued?
5. What happens when the patient resumes the drug, either accidentally or intentionally?

No clinically useful drug is devoid of toxicity. The lack of adequate treatments for many diseases makes it imperative that new drugs, despite their attendant hazards, continue to be introduced into research and practice. Consequently, physicians must accept a commitment to understand the effects of drugs in disease, the predisposing factors to drug reactions, and the effects of disease on drugs in order to use them as safely as possible. Adverse drug reactions may not be recognized if physicians assume that pharmacologic therapy is always beneficial (Melville, 1984; Blaschke et al., 1985). It is just as important for clinicians to recognize the presence of an adverse drug reaction as it is to diagnose a serious disease. Although this may be difficult, it is very important since prompt withdrawal of the drug may be essential for recovery from the drug-induced illness and to prevent a potential recurrence (McQueen, 1987). Though the testing procedures prior to the introduction of a new drug are expensive and often lengthy, this cannot guarantee efficacy of the drug in all situations in which it is indicated, and it must be remembered that considerable numbers of adverse effects will not be discovered until the drug has been used by many thousands of patients. Chapters 34, 35, and 41 describe in detail the use of clinical trials, and postmarketing surveillance of pharmacotherapy in the detection of adverse drug reactions.

TYPES OF ADVERSE DRUG EFFECTS

Drug-induced adverse effects may be classified into two general groups: those that are intrinsic and those that are idiosyncratic. A third and unusual type of drug reaction may occur exclusively as a consequence of discontinuing the use of a drug. An inverse reaction is the withdrawal or rebound response after the abrupt interruption of therapy. This is an unusual reaction in that it occurs in the absence of the provocative agent. Common examples are withdrawal symptoms after narcotic analgesia (chapters 9, 13, 25, and 27); sympathetic overactivity and severe hypertension, which may occur after suddenly stopping clonidine therapy (chapter 2); adrenal insufficiency precipitated by the abrupt cessation of adrenal corticosteroid therapy (chapters 18 and 19); and the delirium, confusion, agitation, and seizures that may occur after discontinuing CNS depressants such as alcohol, benzodiazepines, or barbiturates. Intrinsic adverse drug effects are direct extensions of the pharmacologic actions of either the drug or its metabolites. These adverse effects are primarily dependent upon the inherent chemical properties of the drug and are generally concentration- or dose-dependent. Intrinsic adverse effects may constitute 70% to 80% of drug reactions and are often predictable and thus preventable in many instances.

One prototype of investigation that has established a mechanism of drug toxicity due to a reactive intermediate is that which has helped us to understand the cause of toxicity by acetaminophen (Tylenol). Acetaminophen is a relatively safe drug when it is used in standard doses that produce analgesia. However, when large overdoses have been taken, fatal hepatic necrosis has resulted. The toxic effect of the drug did not correlate with its concentration in plasma or in the liver, suggesting that a metabolite was responsible for the disease. In fact, animals pretreated with drugs (e.g., phenobarbital or 3-methylcholanthrene) that induced hepatic microsomal mixed-function oxidase activity (Fig. 39–1) more readily developed the toxicity after being given smaller doses; and as might be expected when animals are pretreated with inhibitors (e.g., piperamyl butoxide or cobaltous chloride) of the hepatic microsomal enzyme system, the toxicity was prevented, but not reversed once it had started: the inhibitors or inducers of the hepatic microsomal enzyme

system did not alter the bioavailability of the native drug. When the drug was labeled, its metabolites were found covalently linked to the areas of hepatic tissue that were destroyed; a reactive arylating agent had been produced. Furthermore, the amount of covalent binding was increased by the enzyme inducers but inhibited by the enzyme inhibitors.

One curious feature of the studies was the observation that covalent binding did not commence until about 60% of the native drug had been excreted from the body. This finding was to be explained, and in the process of the explanation, a clinically and therapeutically important observation was made. The investigators found that as long as glutathione (GSH) was in the liver, the acetaminophen metabolites were conjugated to GSH and excreted as a mercapturic acid (Fig. 39–2). When the supply of GSH was exhausted, the toxic intermediates were free to bind to nuclear macromolecules and subsequently produced cell death. If drugs were used to modulate availability of GSH before the animal was given acetaminophen, their effects were predictable.

Pretreatment with GSH itself or its precursor cysteine decreased the toxicity of acetaminophen; pretreatment with depletors of GSH (e.g., with diethylmaleate) potentiated the drug's toxicity (Mitchell et al., 1974).

Thus two potential pathways were elucidated that might be perturbed to modify the natural course of acetaminophen toxicity in humans: alter P450 activity or modify availability of GSH. Some evidence indicated that people were at higher risk of toxicity if they had taken phenobarbital before large doses of acetaminophen. However, an inhibitor of P450 activity, desipramine, did little to the syndrome, perhaps because it was too rapidly cleared (Vesell et al., 1972). Nevertheless, glutathione-like nucleophiles that can penetrate the hepatocyte, for example, cysteine, cysteamine, and dimercaprol (Mitchell et al., 1973a, 1973b, 1974), prevented the acetaminophen-induced hepatic necrosis, and cysteamine has been successfully used in some patients with overdose of acetaminophen (Prescott et al., 1974.) *Does one need a more convincing example of the pragmatic importance of understanding the biochemical mechanisms of drug action?*

The toxic metabolite has been identified as *N*-acetyl-*p*-benzoquinoneimine, one of the products of metabolism of acetaminophen by the cytochrome P450 mixed-function oxidase system. This reactive metabolite normally is rapidly detoxified by glutathione in the liver. In overdose, production of the toxic metabolite exceeds GSH capacity and the metabolite reacts directly with hepatic macromolecules, causing liver injury. Renal metabolism is such that kidney injury may

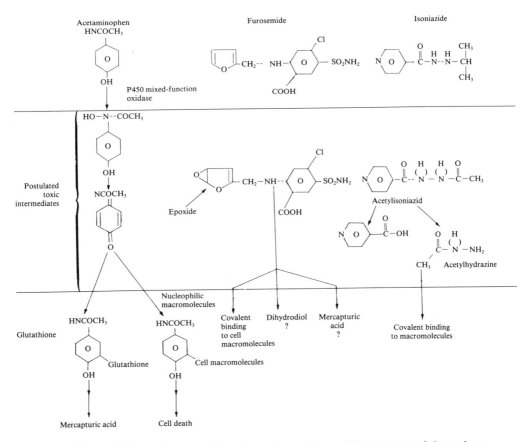

Fig. 39–1. The probable reactive metabolic intermediates of three different types of drug whose toxicity is likely to be based on covalent binding of the metabolites to cells where they are made. Note that in the case of acetaminophen, modulation of toxicity might be accomplished by modifying P450 activity or the availability of glutathione.

occur by the same mechanism. *N*-Acetylcysteine given during the optimal period after ingestion of acetaminophen is an effective antidote. As a sulfhydryl donor, it facilitates GSH synthesis and may aid also in sulfate conjugation. Smilkstein et al. (1988) review the efficacy of oral *N*-acetylcysteine in the treatment of acetaminophen overdosage for the period 1976 to 1985.

Idiosyncratic adverse effects are of major concern as they are difficult to predict and may not be discovered until the drug has been used in many patients. These reactions are generally host-dependent, seemingly dose-independent, difficult to reproduce in animals, and comparatively uncommon. Some reactions are associated with congenital enzyme deficiencies in the host, such as the lack of glucose-6-phosphate dehydrogenase with increased vulnerability of erythrocytes to oxidative injury by several drugs. Other untoward reactions have a hypersensitivity (immunologic) basis.

Hypersensitivity Reactions

Drug allergies can be extremely varied in their clinical presentations, and some can be life-threatening. Clinical manifestations may include anaphylaxis, asthma, dermatitis, fever, granulocytopenia, hemolytic anemia, hepatitis, lupus erythematosus-like syndrome, nephritis, pneumonitis, thrombocytopenia, and vasculitis. Often several of these reactions may occur at the same time. How intrinsically nonimmunogenic small organic molecules cause allergic reactions is not well known. Pohl and others (1988) point out that most of what is known about the immune system has been derived from model studies with molecules that are intrinsically immunogenic rather than from investigations in which drugs have been administered to animals or humans.

Drug Hypersensitivity. Usually for an organic molecule to be recognized as nonself and to in-

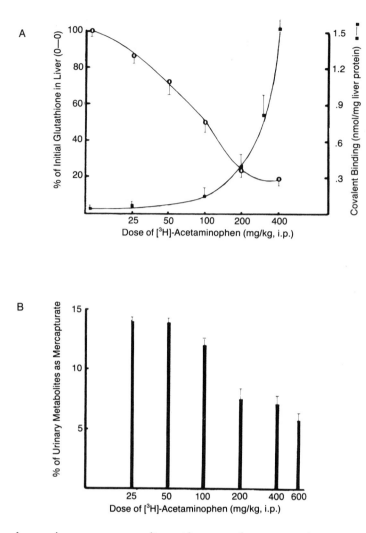

Fig. 39-2. Relationship in vivo between the concentration of GSH in the liver, the formation of an acetaminophen–glutathione conjugate (measured in urine as acetaminophen–mercapturic acid), and covalent binding of an acetaminophen metabolite to liver proteins. Several doses of [^{3}H]acetaminophen were administered intraperitoneally to hamsters, and GSH concentrations and covalent binding of radiolabeled material were determined 3 hours later. An additional group of hamsters were treated similarly, and urinary metabolites were collected for 24 hours. (From Mitchell et al., 1975.)

duce an immune response, it must have a molecular mass of at least 1000 daltons, which is larger than most drugs. Though there may be some exceptions, it is believed that small nonimmunogenic organic molecules, or haptens, must become covalently bound to an endogenous carrier macromolecule to form a drug–carrier conjugate. Drug–carrier conjugates may be formed if the drug or its decomposition products produced during manufacturing are chemically reactive, or if the drug is activated into reactive status in the body by biotransformation or by photoactivation of the drug in the skin to create reactive molecules to form drug–carrier conjugates. The drug–carrier conjugate can then become an immunogen and elicit a specific antibody (humoral) response or a specific T-lymphocyte (cellular) response or both (Melmon and Morrelli, 1978; Lien, 1987a; Pohl et al., 1988). The hapten conjugate and antibody interaction must take place in the proper

setting to cause tissue injury. The inflammatory process that develops expresses that reaction. These multiple steps are under separate genetic control (McDevitt and Benacerraf, 1969; Benacerraf, 1981). An important feature of this group of toxicities that makes them difficult to study in both humans and animals is their relatively low frequency of occurrence.

The classification of Gell and Coombs into four types of hypersensitivity reactions is commonly used and continues to assimilate newer mechanisms that have been described. Type I hypersensitivity reactions are of the immediate-type, anaphylactic, or IgE-mediated hypersensitivity reactions. Reactions result from the release of pharmacologically active substances such as histamine, leukotrienes, prostaglandins, platelet-activating factor, and eosinophilic chemotactic factor from IgE-sensitized basophils and mast cells after contact with specific antigen. Clinical conditions in which type I reactions play a function include systemic anaphylaxis, reactions to stinging insects, allergic extrinsic asthma, seasonal allergic rhinitis, some cases of urticaria, and some reactions to foods and drugs. Type II hypersensitivity reactions represent cytotoxic hypersensitivity, antibody-dependent cytotoxicity, or cytolytic complement-dependent cytotoxicity. Clinical examples of cell injury in which antibody reacts with antigenic components of a cell are Coombs-positive hemolytic anemia, antibody-induced thrombocytopenia, leukopenia, pemphigus, pemphigoid, Goodpasture's syndrome, and pernicious anemia. Type III hypersensitivity reactions result from the deposition of soluble circulating antigen–antibody (immune) complexes in vessels or tissue. Some clinical conditions in which immune complexes are considered to have operational purpose are serum sickness due to serum, drugs, or viral hepatitis antigen; systemic lupus erythematosus; rheumatoid arthritis; polyarteritis; chronic membranoproliferative glomerulonephritis; and other systemic reactions. Drug- or serum-induced serum sickness, and some forms of renal disease, is IgE-mediated and believed to precede the type III reaction. The local Arthus reaction and experimental serum sickness are model laboratory examples of type III effect. Type IV reactions are cell-mediated, delayed, or tuberculin-type hypersensitivity reactions. They are caused by sensitized lymphocytes (T cells) after contact with antigen. Delayed hypersensitivity differs from other hypersensitivity reactions since it is not mediated by antibody but by sensitized lymphocytes. With peripheral blood leukocytes or with an extract of these cells (transfer factor), but not with serum, the transfer of delayed hypersensitivity from sensitized to normal persons can be shown. Clinical conditions in which type IV reactions are considered to be involved include contact dermatitis, allograft rejection, some forms of drug sensitivity, and thyroiditis. Patch tests are used to identify allergens causing a contact dermatitis, but testing is not done until the dermatitis has cleared so as to avoid an exacerbation.

There are several clinical criteria that help in the diagnosis of allergic reactions to a drug: (1) The reactions usually occur only after prior exposure; however, often the patient is unaware of previous exposure to a specific drug. (2) Reactions occur only after 8 to 9 days from the first exposure, suggesting that a period of sensitization is required. (3) Reactions appear to be dose-independent. (4) Reactions are often accompanied by tissue and blood eosinophilia and fever. (5) The symptoms usually subside promptly after the drug is discontinued unless a drug-induced autoimmune reaction has been initiated. (6) On rechallenge with the drug, the patient should show the same pathologic involvement. (7) Definitive proof that a toxicity has an allergic basis requires that the reaction be produced in animals with a thorough study of the immunologic process. This has not been done with drugs that must be altered metabolically in order to elicit an untoward response (Theofilopoulos and Dixon, 1979; Smith et al., 1980; Condemi, 1987).

Hypersensitivity to a drug is dependent on many factors. The drug or its metabolites must be antigenic or capable of acting as a hapten in order to stimulate antibody production (Lien, 1987a, b; Pohl et al., 1988). Then the antibody–haptene conjugate or antibody–antigen interaction must take place in the proper setting to cause a type of tissue injury. Then an inflammatory process develops that expresses the reaction. Each step of the process — formation of the complete immunogen, induction of antibody synthesis, and expression of the antibody–antigen reaction — is under separate genetic control (Benacerraf, 1981). Despite the exposure of many people to drugs of many varieties, hypersensitivity reactions account for only 6% to 10% of all drug reactions (Borda et al., 1968), and relatively few drugs cause hypersensitivity.

Penicillin Allergy. A detailed analysis of penicillin allergy is useful as one of the best-defined models of hypersensitivity reactions. The penicillin preparation (Stewart, 1967; Kovotzer and Haddad, 1970; Stewart and McGovern, 1970) and its route and rate of administration may determine the type of antibody produced and, therefore, the type of reaction. The age of the patient at the time the dose is given (2% of patients ages 17–30 have positive skin tests to penicillin, but 7% at ages 31–45 and 10% at ages 46–60 have positive tests for IgE) and the dose he or she receives may also be determinants of the degree of response to a given stimulus and the type of response that will develop. Exposure to a drug may not be obvious (e.g., a patient taking a vaccine containing penicillin or drinking milk from cows treated for mastitis with penicillin). Although physicians may carefully seek evidence of previous exposure or reaction, the information may not be available from the patient or his or her records. For example, the indiscriminate and inappropriate use of penicillin, sometimes without the knowledge of the patient, often makes an accurate account of previous drug exposure impossible. However, reactions to penicillin are likely to occur in patients who have previously reacted to penicillin or other drugs and in patients who are atopic (Sogn, 1984).

The apparent overall prevalence of hypersensitivity response to penicillin is about 2%. Responses are clinically (and pathogenetically, see below) divided into *immediate* (occurring within a few minutes of administration of the drug), *accelerated* (occurring within hours), or *late* (occurring days after the patient has been given the drug). The syndromes that can be seen in each category are listed in Table 39–1. Any combination, sequence of appearance, or severity of each manifestation can be seen in any given patient. The pattern of response is not even easily predicted in patients with a well-established past history of sensitivity to penicillin. About 1.4% of the 2% overall reactions are expressed as the *late* type, with 0.3% being *accelerated* and 0.3% being *immediate*. One in 2500 patients exposed to penicillin therapy develops anaphylaxis, and 1 in 100,000 dies (Smith et al., 1980). About 600 deaths due to penicillin anaphylaxis occur annually in the United States. All these data must be taken as estimates and only estimates, but they do help the therapist to rationally approach the problem of hypersensitivity. For instance, it is reasonable to conclude that penicillin is generally safe for most who receive it, that most hypersensitivity reactions are not life-threatening, but that it would be highly desirable to be able to predict which patients are going to be at high risk of lethality before they take the drug (Parker, 1975). This ability has been developed over the last decade and a half but does not appear to be optimally exploited. *Principle: Quantitative estimates of efficacy and toxicity of pharmacologic agents can be used to establish acceptable behavior patterns in using the drug in spite of personal experience with it.*

The physician who never uses penicillin on any patient because he or she has "seen" an anaphylactic reaction that appears to create unnecessary suffering is as thoughtless as the physician who uses it casually because he or she has "never had any problems" with it.

The antibodies produced by penicillin appear specific for different aspects of the chemistry of the penicillin, that is, at least three types of IgE antibody can be made (Table 39–1). One is to the benzylpenicilloyl moiety (BPO), a frequent antigen and so-called major determinant; one is to penicilloate; and one is to the other chemicals related to penicillin that are often responsible for antigenicity, that is, the so-called minor determinants (Tsuji et al., 1975; Yamana et al., 1975). Although each of these antibodies can be a distinctly different molecule, the antibody combining site recognizes the whole molecule and can, in part, be carrier-specific. Thus, it is not surprising to find cross-reactivity to a variety of the chemicals that have the penicillin structure in common (Adkinson et al., 1971). Cross-reactivity among the natural and semisynthetic penicillins is believed due to their common 6-aminopenicillanic acid and nucleus and sensitizing derivatives. Cross-reactivity to cephalosporins may occur in 3% to 5% of patients with allergy to penicillin. When the allergic reactions to either group of antimicrobial agents has been of the immediate type, there should be particular concern in using the alternate drug (Sheffer and Pennoyer, 1984; Parry, 1987; Wright and Wilkowske, 1987).

Immediate hypersensitivity is clearly *caused* by the IgE molecule; there may be some types of *immediate* reactions that might be mediated by IgG. Some combinations of IgM plus other anti-

Table 39–1.   SYNDROMES CAUSED BY ANTIGENIC EFFECTS OF PENICILLIN

TYPE	LIKELY CAUSATIVE ANTIBODY	CLINICAL MANIFESTATION
Intermediate (2–30 minutes)	IgE (?IgG)	Anaphylaxis—diffuse or organ-specific (e.g. cardiac) Asthma, urticaria Laryngeal edema (occurs 1 : 100 in comparison with anaphylaxis)
Accelerated (1–72 hours)	?IgG	Urticaria, laryngeal edema, asthma Local inflammatory reactions

Late (more than 72 hours)	IgM and other antibodies	Commonly
		  Urticaria
		    Exanthem
		    Fever
		    Arthralgia
		  Hemolysis
		    Granulocytopenia
		    Interstitial nephritis
		    Eosinophilia
		Rarely
		  Acute renal insufficiency
		  Thrombocytopenia

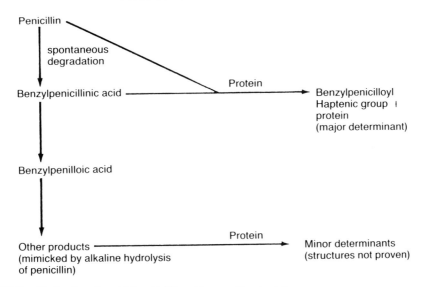

Fig. 39-3. Mechanisms by which penicillin achieves antigenic status.

bodies may account for *late* hypersensitivity reactions, and IgG may contribute to the *accelerated* response (Table 39-1). The skin tests we will discuss usually detect tissue-fixed (skin) IgE and thus have proved useful in screening for those patients who are not likely to have *immediate* types of reactions to either the major or minor antigenic determinants of the penicillin molecule.

Degradation of the penicillin molecule to a reactive proimmunogen can proceed without enzymatic intervention. This event with penicillin is in marked contrast to most other drugs, which must undergo enzymatic degradation (usually in the liver) before they become antigenic or before they conjugate with endogenous protein to form complete antigens. This difference in active versus spontaneous degradation may be the reason that hypersensitivity reactions to penicillin do not express themselves in the liver. That is, isoniazid, for instance, is degraded in the liver, where the antigen or reactive metabolic intermediate may express its effects as clinically important hepatitis. The steps in development of the antigenicity of penicillin are illustrated in Fig. 39-3.

The skin-sensitizing (IgE) antibodies in penicillin allergy are most commonly developed to the penicilloyl metabolite of penicillin ("major" determinant). The IgE is thought to be responsible for anaphylactic reactions and may also be produced in response to the unaltered drug or to another metabolite (e.g., penaldate, penicilloate, or penicillamine) (Levine, 1966; Turk and Baker, 1968). Both IgM and IgG antibodies may be produced after exposure of patients to penicillin and are usually specific for the penicilloyl metabolite (major determinant).

The "minor" determinants (unaltered drug or other drug metabolites) may be responsible for disastrous allergic reactions, and the nomenclature (major and minor determinants) is misleading. Better terms might be *frequent* and *infrequent* determinants of antigenicity. There are many possible determinants of antigenicity after administration of penicillin (Table 39-2).

Although IgE antibodies may cause immediate anaphylactic reactions, the significance of IgM and IgG antibodies is less clear. The IgG antibodies may act as blocking antibodies to prevent or modify the course of reactions in patients who are skin-test-sensitive to antigen but who develop skin rashes rather than anaphylaxis on exposure to the allergen. In some patients, the concentration of IgG falls during the acute allergic reaction and rises during the recovery period.

Hemagglutinating antibodies (IgG) are usually specific for the penicilloyl determinant, but these antibodies may be found in 60% to 100% of populations, if sensitive methods for their detection are used. Although patients with a history of allergy have higher concentrations of IgG than normal persons, it is not known if these antibodies are responsible for most reactions. In addition, lymphocytes from patients allergic to penicillin are more rapidly transformed by penicillin in vitro than are those taken from normal persons. This observation suggests that some lymphocytes have been "sensitized" to components of the penicillins (Gimenez-Camarasa et al., 1975; Reidenberg and Caccese, 1975). These lymphocytes, on contact with the antigen, release a substance that causes blood monocytes to migrate across endothelial linings of vessels, become converted to

Table 39–2.   DETERMINANTS OF ANTIGENICITY AFTER ADMINISTRATION OF PENICILLIN

	ANTIBODY		
	IGM	IGG	IGE (REAGIN, OR SKIN-SENSITIZING ANTIBODY)
Svedberg sedimentation	19 S	7 S	
Aggutination of penicillin-incubated erythrocytes			
Saline	+ + +	+	
Serum	+ + +	+ + +	
Antigenic determinants	Major ?Minor	Major ?Minor	Major and minor
Role	?Exanthems	Blocking hemolysis	Immediate anaphlaxis, urticaria

macrophages, and destroy tissues by release of lysosomal enzymes. This hypothesis may explain those allergic reactions to penicillin that stimulate serum sicknesses.

Skin tests have been developed to predict the propensity of a given individual to react dangerously to therapeutic doses of penicillin. These tests are very useful in detecting such patients (Levine and Zolov, 1969; Adkinson et al., 1971). The basis of the efficacy of the test is to link alkaline hydrolysate of penicillin (for minor determinants) or the benzylpenicilloyl metabolite (for major determinants) to a carrier (the safest is a polymer of lysine). The conjugate is injected into the skin. When the IgE is fixed to histamine-containing cells (mast cells or basophils), the conjugate produces histamine release in the area of injection, and the characteristic effects of histamine appear in 15 to 20 minutes if the IgE antibody is present. When the test is used, those without IgE do not react; they safely accept therapeutic amounts of drug without serious reactions. If the skin tests show a reaction, therapeutic doses of penicillin will predictably produce some manifestations of an immediate reaction even if the patient is "protected" by preadministration of antihistamines and/or some small doses of penicillin used to "desensitize" him or her (see below). The test has been used for more than 25 years; the predictive capabilities have been verified; and its safety is assured if the instructions are carefully followed. Although there is a commercially available preparation of benzyl penicilloyl polylsine (PPL; Pre-Pen), for skin testing for allergy to the major determinant of penicillin, there is no commercially available preparation of minor determinants in the United States because the costs of what might be considered unnecessary preclinical testing are too great for most commercial pharmaceutic manufacturers to seriously consider (Solley et al., 1982). *Principle: Therapists are remiss if they expect and act as if federal regulatory agents should do their thinking for them. Drugs not available are not necessarily harmful, and those available are not necessarily safe.*

Skin testing with unmodified penicillin is efficacious but is associated with an unacceptable incidence of severe reactions. The safety of the PPL or minor determinants linked to polylysine is predicated on the lack of immunogenicity of these conjugates. That is based on the fact that very few lysines are unconjugated to the derivative of penicillin. Therefore, they are unable (in guinea pigs and presumably in humans) to activate T cells that are necessary to initiate production of antibodies. If more than one lysine in the polylysine sequence were left unconjugated, they would be able to activate the T cells and presumably would then be antigenic (able to elicit both antibody responses and antigen-induced antibody reactions) or at least immunogenic and therefore able to elicit production of antibody. Both are undesirable and constitute the mechanisms by which other penicillin preparations cause unfortunate reactions in reactive patients. Basophil degranulation tests and passive transfer of IgE to monkeys are research procedures and are impracticable for clinical use.

Skin testing for IgE may reveal positive tests of PPL, penicillin, or both. Seventeen studies of a total of 2332 patients with a history of allergy who were skin-tested with PPL antigen showed positive responses to PPL in 17% to 91%, most groups reporting 40% to 60%. These investigators tested 22,462 individuals with no history of penicillin allergy and found positive reactions in 0% to 10% (Table 39–3).

In seven studies (410 patients) comparing skin tests with PPL and penicillin in patients with a positive history of reaction, a higher percentage of positive reactions was obtained with PPL than with penicillin (50% vs. 25%).

Although the initial experience with PPL minor, or infrequent, antigen indicated that anaphylactic reactions were much more common when the patient had a positive skin test to the minor determinant antigens, some patients have positive skin tests to PPL alone and develop anaphylactic reactions when penicillin is given (Rosenblum, 1968). When the skin test is positive, penicillin should not be used when appropriate alternative antibiotics are available. If penicillin must be used, desensitization (producing, in essence, multiple but small and controllable reactions) should precede full-scale therapy.

Desensitization may be effective, utilizing several possible mechanisms. Since 85% of patients with IgM and IgG antibodies to penicillin are not reactive to appropriate skin testing, a large number of patients given small doses of penicillin to minimize the reaction would never have reacted anyway. Some patients have IgG-blocking antibodies that absorb the antigen to an extent and by this mechanism limit any potential reaction. Actual immunologic desensitization can be obtained in some patients. The small doses of drug liberate small amounts of histamine to produce minor or subclinical reactions. As the IgE titer decreases, the skin test becomes negative and the patient can tolerate large doses of drug.

The following recommendations for use of penicillin (slightly modified) have been proposed by a committee of the World Health Organization:

1. Always have an emergency kit available for treatment of allergic reactions.

2. Always obtain an exact history of the patient's previous contact with penicillin, previous penicillin reactions, and allergic diathesis. In infants less than 3 months old, ask about penicillin allergy in the mother.

3. Do not give penicillin to patients with a previous history of reactions; indications for administration of penicillin are severely restricted in patients with an allergic diathesis.

Editor's Note: This is a disputable point in certain infections such as subacute bacterial endocarditis. Remember too that if a patient develops hemolysis when penicillin is being used to treat subacute or acute bacterial endocarditis, the hematocrit may not return to normal despite the efficacy of the drug (Kerr et al., 1972). If a rise in hematocrit is the therapist's criterion for efficacy, he or she may discontinue the drug without knowing that it is useful.

4. If possible, refer patients with suspected penicillin allergy to a center capable of performing both skin tests and immunologic tests to provide the patient with objective diagnosis and permanent records.

5. Always tell the patient that he or she is going to receive penicillin.

Table 39–3. **ANTIBODY TITERS IN BLOOD AFTER PENICILLIN ADMINISTRATION: NONREACTORS VS. REACTORS***

ANTIBODY PRODUCED	PERCENTAGE OF PATIENTS WITH ANTIBODY PRODUCED		
A. NONREACTORS	NO RECENT TREATMENT (112 PATIENTS)	TREATMENT WITH MODERATE DOSES (103 PATIENTS)	TREATMENT WITH HIGH DOSES (12 PATIENTS)
None	3	0	0
IgM	77	61	92
IgG plus IgM	17	30	8
IgE plus IgG and IgM	3	8	0
Major and minor determinants plus IgG and IgM	0	1	0

	PERCENTAGE OF PATIENTS WITH ANTIBODY TITERS WHO DEVELOPED:				
B. REACTORS (7 TO 14 DAYS AFTER INITIATION OF TREATMENT)	IMMEDIATE REACTIONS (12 PATIENTS)	ACCELERATED REACTIONS (10 PATIENTS)	LATE URTICARIA (11 PATIENTS)	URTICARIA PLUS ARTHRALGIA (16 PATIENTS)	SKIN RASH (15 PATIENTS)
IgM	0	0	0	0	58
IgM (high titiers)	0	0	0	0	32
IgE plus IgG and IgM	0	60	91	0	5
Minor determinant plus IgM	42	0	0	56	0
Minor determinant plus IgG and IgM	16	0	0	25	0
Minor determinant plus IgE, IgG, and IgM	42	40	9	19	5

* Data for this table were compiled from Parker et al., 1962; Brown et al., 1964; Levine, 1966; Voss et al., 1966; and Idsoe et al., 1968. Available data do not permit calculation of the frequency of reactions, which is reported to vary from 0.7% to 10% in various studies. Among the reactions, anaphylaxis may occur in about 0.0015% to 0.004%, with a fatality rate of 0.00015% to 0.0002%.

6. Do not use penicillins topically.

7. Avoid the use of penicillinase-resistant penicillins unless there is a known infection with penicillinase-producing staphylococci. Owing to the cross-sensitivity of the semisynthetic penicillins (all have the 6-aminopenicillanic acid nucleus), there is no security in changing to one of these drugs. Although less frequent, cross-reactions may also occur with cephalosporins.

8. To avoid contamination, use disposable equipment for penicillins when possible.

9. Observe all patients receiving penicillin for at least one half hour after injection. The therapist is well advised to look for subtle but clinically important manifestations of penicillin allergy whenever a minor manifestation of allergy presents itself. A patient with a mild exanthem may not impress the clinician enough to have him or her discontinue important therapy with penicillin. However, the exanthem may herald less obvious Coombs-positive hemolytic anemia associated with high titer of IgG, the beginnings of interstitial nephritis that could proceed to death but be heralded only by asymptomatic microscopic hematuria in a patient with a delayed positive skin test, or the beginnings of the rare complication of agranulocytosis. If any of these dangerous signs accompany the use of penicillin, the drug must be stopped.

Principle: When the pathogenetic factors of minor and major problems that can be produced by drugs are similar to the factors of major problems, then the minor aberration can be used to signal the need for concern of major trouble. That observation is a sweet use of adversity.

In summary, (1) When seeking possible reactors, a history might be helpful, but a negative history should not exclude further testing with agents incapable of stimulating production of causative antibody. Penicillin scratch or conjunctival tests can be dangerous, as they can cause severe reactions and stimulate antibody production. (2) When hypersensitivity is present but the drug must be used, small doses given at frequent intervals may minimize the effects of hypersensitivity. However, if the drug is again indicated after a drugless interval, the desensitizing procedure must be repeated. (3) Because we are unwittingly exposed to many drugs, as in foods, the incidence of hypersensitivity may increase. (4) A therapist must always be ready to treat the most severe forms of hypersensitivity, and antidotes must always be considered before administering dangerous drugs.

The pathogenesis of hypersensitivity is similar for a number of drugs that stimulate antibody production and result in tissue-damaging antigen-antibody reactions. The sequence of events is identical to that seen in an acute inflammatory response elicited by other antigen–antibody interactions, with or without complement, and is dependent on local tissue response or response of the formed elements in blood. The morphologic changes in the microvasculature are characteristic of the acute inflammatory lesion, and similar therapeutic maneuvers aimed at preventing or reversing the acute disease are effective in many varieties of hypersensitivity. These observations oversimplify the events in hypersensitivity responses associated with drugs; minor but important variations occur. These variations are important when therapy of a specific event is considered. For example, if the complement system is unimportant in the development of a reaction to penicillin, there is no purpose in trying to prevent its activation by using anticomplement drugs. However, once a host of reactions has been initiated by different drugs, a number of therapeutic agents with broad anti-inflammatory, bronchodilating, or antihistaminic actions might be useful (Sheffer, 1966).

The manifestations of hypersensitivity depend on the drug's dose and distribution and on host genetic and other factors, including the distribution, quantity, and quality of the antibody. After administration of penicillin, urticaria, maculopapular rashes, local reactions, angioedema, anaphylaxis, and fever can occur, simultaneously or in some sequence.

Unusual syndromes have been described that are probably due to the distribution of the drug and the manifestations of hypersensitivity. The Stevens-Johnson syndrome is characterized by lesions in various mucous membranes and is classically caused by phenolphthalein and a variety of other drugs such a sulfonamides. There is no difference between the pathogenesis of this syndrome and that caused by other drugs that induce hypersensitivity. Some antigen–antibody-dependent reactions (e.g., photoallergic phenomena) require more than the drug for manifestations of sensitivity (Haber and Levine, 1969). Some reactions that look like hypersensitivity are not so and do not depend on antigen–antibody reactions; they apparently produce similar chemicals and morphlogic changes in tissues and resemble those seen with hypersensitivity.

Radiographic Contrast Media. Intravascular radiographic contrast media may also cause reactions characterized by the release of histamine and serotonin and by the activation of cascade systems including complement, fibrinolysin, and kinins. The clinical manifestations are similar to those of a classic allergic response, but IgE seemingly is not involved. Hyperosmolality and alkalinity are responsible for most of the undesirable physiologic and chemotoxic effects associated with these agents. However, some researchers believe there is an antigen–antibody response. Others believe that the reactions are more properly termed anaphylactoid and that they are induced by other mechanisms that may involve some of the same reaction pathways. Hypertonic contrast media may cause endothelial disruptions with the release of active chemical substances or transmitters (Swanson et al., 1986; Morris and Fischer, 1986). From conventional 1.5 (3/2) ionic contrast media, severe reactions occur in from 1/1000 to 1/2000 patients. Fatal reactions have been variously reported at 1/10,000 to 1/93,000 exposures. Patients with allergic histories have a two to four times increased risk for an adverse reaction. The risk may be increased fivefold with a documented history of asthma (Greenberger, 1984). Persons with a history of a previous reaction to contrast media are at greater risk, with 15% to 35% having adverse reactions on repeat intravascular administration of contrast material.

Greenberger (1984) proposed a pretreatment program for patients with a high risk of reaction with the following medications: prednisone, 50 mg, 13, 7, and 1 hour before the procedure; diphenhydramine, 50 mg, by mouth or IM, 1 hour before the procedure; and ephedrine, 25 mg, by mouth, 1 hour before the procedure. The latter was withheld if there was arrhythmia, angina, or other contraindications. In spite of this pretreatment, six mild reactions (3.1%) occurred in 192 high-risk procedures. However, a significant reduction in reaction rate was achieved with three drugs during intravascular procedures.

New ratio-3 agents have been developed with an increased ratio (6/2) of iodine to osmotic particles. While retaining the same iodine content, osmolality of the agents is 50% reduced, but they are still significantly hyperosmolar compared with blood. Some of the ratio-3 agents have the cation replaced by nonionizing polyhydroxyl alkyl groups that confer water solubility with reduced alkalinity and with apparent reduction in chemotoxicity. Though it is believed that the new molecules will significantly reduce the incidence of adverse reactions, the available data are incomplete. A 10- to 20-fold increase in cost of the new contrast agents compared with conventional contrast media has been a restriction on the wide clinical use of the former.

Other Drugs. In susceptible persons, aspirin and other NSAIDs may cause anaphylaxis by modification of the function of mast cells or other unidentified mechanisms independent of IgE. The azo dye tartrazine yellow no. 5, opiates, metabisulfites, and physical exertion itself may occasionally cause non-IgE-mediated anaphylaxis. An estimated incidence of tartrazine sensitivity is 1 in 10,000 (Drug and Therapeutics Bulletin, 1980). The cross-reactivity with aspirin has been questioned by the Food Advisory Committee (1987). In considering the reports of tartrazine, the Food Advisory Committee (1987) reported that similar evidence of intolerance might well be obtained for a variety of natural food ingredients if as many studies were conducted on them as on tartrazine. The committee considered that tartrazine posed no more problems than other colors or food ingredients and recommended that the continued use of tartrazine in food is acceptable (the committee did not say the use of tartrazine was safe, however). The use of tartrazine in medicines appears to be diminishing, and in some countries its presence is declared on the label.

SELECTED ADVERSE EFFECTS ON SELECTED ORGAN SYSTEMS

The following examples of adverse drug reactions involving selected, specific organ systems are intended to be illustrative examples of adverse reactions and not by any means an exhaustive list of possible adverse effects of drugs. These are representative of relatively frequent problems in clinical pharmacology as encountered over the past years from consult requests originating from the wards and intensive care units and from inquiries by community physicians at Stanford and on morning work rounds and report with the medical house staff. The manifestation of adverse effects of medications by many patients are often subtle and could easily be ascribed to other causes by the inexperienced or less inquiring observer. From time to time, even seasoned physicians in the various subspecialty areas fail to appreciate some of the uncommon adverse effects of drugs they commonly use. As noted earlier, clinically important drug reactions are underrecognized and underreported. The prescribing physician must always try to keep an open mind and a quizzical attitude toward his or her own prescribing practice. If the response to a particular program of treatment is not the anticipated one, the prescriber should always asks himself or herself, "Why not? And why couldn't this be attributed to a drug?" There are no patterns in the way adverse responses appear. The end of the list of new adverse effects is nowhere in sight. In a number of areas of this book, adverse reactions also are focused on particular organ systems where they are emphasized (particularly, see chapters 2, 9–25, 28–32, 40, and 41).

Dermatologic Toxicity

Cutaneous reactions induced by drugs can occur as solitary manifestations or be part of a more serious systemic involvement with renal, hepatic, pulmonary, or hematologic toxicity (chapter 21). Although skin disorders may be seemingly minor, drug-induced skin reactions may precede or be premonitory of more serious adverse involvement of other vital organs in susceptible patients. Drugs most frequently associated with allergic skin reactions are the penicillins, sulfonamides, and blood products (Reid et al., 1989).

Patients may have exaggerated injury after exposure to sun when they are taking sun-sensitizing medications such as the phenothiazines or tetracycline. At times a generalized erythroderma may be due to a solubilizing agent or stabilizer rather than the active drug, such as reactions to the ethanolamine component of aminophylline or topical preparations (Nierenberg and Glazener, 1982). Bisacodyl and phenolphthalein are the primary diphenylmethane laxatives that may induce allergic reactions including fixed drug eruptions and Stevens-Johnson syndrome (Brunton, 1985). Exfoliative dermatitis, characterized by redness, scaling, and thickening of the entire skin surface, and toxic epidermal neurolysis manifested by peeling of the epidermis in sheets leaving widespread denuded areas may be fatal. Patients should be hospitalized. Close medical observations and experienced nursing care are essential. Suspected medications should be stopped immediately, and essential systemic medications should be changed to ones of a different chemical group. Exfoliative dermatitis can usually be managed with the use of topical treatment. Patients with toxic epidermal necrolysis should be isolated to minimize exogenous infections and treated similarly to patients with severe burns. The skin and denuded areas should be protected from trauma and infection and fluid and electrolyte losses should be replaced. Systemic corticosteroids often are used to treat exfoliative dermatitis and toxic epidermal necrolysis.

The most common form of vasculitis in the skin is cutaneous necrotizing vasculitis involving primarily small postcapillary venules of the skin and characterized as leukocytoclastic vasculitis. This is manifest clinically as palpable purpura with the most common site of involvement being the lower extremities, particularly the feet and ankles. Pathologically, sites of cutaneous vasculitis show endothelial cell edema and necrosis, hemorrhage, fibrin deposition, a neutrophil-rich infiltrate, and leukocytoclasis. Hypersensitivity to various agents is the presumed cause of cutaneous necrotizing vasculitis, but in about half of the cases no inciting agent is found. Drugs are responsible for the majority of the remaining cases. The most commonly implicated drugs are antibacterials including penicillins and sulfonamides, diuretics, NSAIDs, and anticonvulsant agents. The incidence of associated systemic involvement has been variously estimated to be as follows: arthralgia and arthritis, 40%; renal, 12.5% to 63%, with the most common finding being asymptomatic hematuria or proteinuria; and neurologic, with both motor and sensory peripheral neuropathy, 5% to l0%; GI involvement occurs in those with the Henoch-Schönlein variant; pulmonary findings may be clinically quiescent but show changes on the chest x-ray film (Swerlick and Lawley, 1989).

Ototoxicity

Many drugs as well as industrial chemicals and solvents are associated with impaired auditory or vestibular function that at times may be irreversible. Dizziness, tinnitus, and hearing loss were discovered in the late 1800s in association with the use of aspirin and quinine. Beginning with streptomycin in the 1940s, ototoxicity has become an important clinical problem. Indeed, it has been suggested that over 130 drugs and chemicals have been associated with ototoxicity. The major classes are basic aminoglycosides and other antibiotics, antimalarials, anti-inflammatory drugs, antineoplastic agents, diuretics, some topical agents, and heavy metals (Lien et al., 1983; Koegel, 1985; Rybak, 1986). The Boston Collaboration Drug Surveillance Program reported the frequency of drug-induced deafness in patients in the United States to be 3 per 1000, and 1.6 per 1000 is cited by Lien (1987b). The most frequently implicated drugs were aspirin and the aminoglycoside antibiotics.

The likelihood of ototoxicity is markedly increased in patients with impaired renal function, in elderly persons, and is associated with a high dose or large total dose of an ototoxic drug, or if there has been a prior course or the concurrent use of another ototoxic drug (Jackson and Arcieri, 1971). Though the damage may involve vestibular and/or cochlear mechanisms, cochlear dysfunction is considerably more incapacitating. Varying with the drugs involved and the mechanisms of action, inner ear deafness may be preceded by tinnitus, diplacusis, or the sense of fullness in the ear (Bernstein and Weiss, 1967; Porter and Jick, 1977).

Aminoglycosides. In humans, aminoglycoside-induced cochlear ototoxicity involves progressive loss of the hair cells in the organ of Corti. Hair cells in the basal turn of the cochlea are affected first with destruction progressing toward the apex. This is in keeping with clinical experience since the basal region responds to high frequency sounds and the apex to sounds of low frequency. Streptomycin primarily affects the vestibular system, and neomycin, kanamycin, and amikacin are primarily toxic to the cochlea. Gentamicin and tobramycin show both vestibular and cochlear toxicity with vestibular toxicity occurring more frequently (Brummett and Fox, 1989a; Pratt and Fekety, 1986). Loss of hearing has occurred due to the systemic absorption of the neomycin solution used to irrigate surgical wounds or used in the dressings of severe burns. Audiometric testing as well as electronystagmography can determine subclinical changes in eighth cranial nerve functions. Cochlear dysfunctions usually affects these frequencies above 4000 Hz. Serial audiometric testing has been recommended for patients on extended periods of treatment with the aminoglycosides in the attempt to avoid irreversible cochlear toxicity in the frequencies used in the conversational range. However, testing requires a degree of patient cooperation that is often not feasible in patients ill enough to require treatment with this group of drugs. Since the therapeutic index with these drugs is narrow, serum concentrations of the aminoglycosides should be monitored. The use of aminoglycosides is described in chapter 24. Monitoring concentrations of drug in plasma can help to avoid toxicity. Peak serum concentrations should be determined 30 minutes after completion of IV infusion or 1 hour after IM injection. Trough values should be determined just prior to the next dose. Edson and Terrell (1987) give recommended dosages and serum concentrations for the various aminoglycosides based on normal renal function. Dosage adjustments based on age and impaired renal function are discussed by Van Scoy and Wilson (1987). Additional dosing guidelines are to be found in Bennett, 1990, and Bennett et al., 1991.

Vancomycin. A major toxicity associated with the use of vancomycin is ototoxicity that may develop when the peak serum concentrations exceed 30 mg/l (Hermans and Wilhelm, 1987). The distribution phase of vancomycin is complex. The peak concentrations in serum should be obtained 2 hours after an IV infusion is completed (Levine, 1987). Toxicity occurs more frequently when the patient has impaired renal function and during the concurrent use of other ototoxic drugs. When ototoxicity occurs, the drug should be discontinued to prevent further hearing loss. In fact, hearing loss may improve after vancomycin has been stopped. Tinnitus and vertigo have also been reported and usually are reversible if the drug is discontinued.

Erythromycin. Bilateral sensorineural hearing loss may be encountered during the use of erythromycin (usually after IV administration at a daily dosage of 4 g or more). Though some patients who develope ototoxicity have renal impairment, the majority have normal renal function. Hepatic insufficiency also may increase the risk of ototoxicity (Brittain, 1987). Erythromycin-induced tinnitus and hearing loss are reversible. Though recovery generally begins within 24 hours of discontinuing the drug, nearly complete recovery may take 1 to 2 weeks, and several months are required for total recovery (Haydon et al., 1984; Schweitzer and Olson, 1984; Koegel, 1985; Brittain, 1987; Wilson and Cockerill, 1987; Brummett and Fox, 1989b).

Diuretics. Hearing loss that may be reversible but on occasion has been irreversible, has occurred in patients receiving the loop diuretics ethacrynic acid and furosemide (chapter 11). These agents have been shown to produce a dose-related, reversible reduction in endocochlear potential in animals. Edema of the stria vascularis, loss of outer hair cells in the basal turn of the cochlea, and cystic degeneration of the hair cells in the ampulla of the posterior canal and in the macula of the saccule have been noted (Arnold et al., 1981; Rybak, 1982; Rybak, 1986). Hearing loss more often occurs in patients with impaired renal function and is associated with the rapid IV administration of the drug; at times there is concomitant use of other ototoxic medication. Permanent deafness has been reported up to 6 months after treatment with relatively small repeated doses of furosemide. Reversible deafness has occurred with the use of large oral doses in patients with the nephrotic syndrome. The uremic patient is considered to be at special risk, and monitoring of the hearing during treatment with loop diuretics has been advised. The neonate is considered vulnerable since the clearance of furosemide is significantly prolonged in such patients (chapter 30). To minimize the risk of ototoxicity when the loop diuretics are used, rapid bolus injection should be avoided, especially in the patient with renal impairment. For example, uremic patients who received furosemide at the rate of 25 mg/minute developed ototoxicity, whereas, those whose dosage rate was 5.6 mg/minute or less remained free of symptoms (Bosher, 1977). The use of loop diuretics should be avoided as much as possible in premature infants and neonates. If possible, loop diuretics should be avoided in patients receiving other ototoxic drugs such as aminoglycosides (Bosher, 1977; Gallagher and Jones, 1979; Arnold et al., 1981; Rybak, 1982; Brummett, 1982).

Salicylates. Although salicylate-induced ototoxicity has been known since the late 1800s, the mechanism for hearing loss, tinnitus, and vertigo is undiscovered. In those with normal hearing, tinnitus associated with salicylate administration first occurs over a broad range (20–50 mg/100 ml of plasma concentrations). Consequently, tinnitus cannot be relied upon to predict plasma salicylate concentrations above the usual therapeutic range (Mongan et al., 1973). Salicylate-induced deafness and tinnitus are almost always reversible within a few days after the medication is discontinued (Porter and Jick, 1977).

Quinine, Quinidine, and Chloroquine. Quinine, used to ameliorate nocturnal leg cramps in the elderly, may induce vertigo, tinnitus, and hearing loss. Although the ototoxic symptoms usually resolve rapidly upon withdrawal of the drug, some patients are left with irreversible tinnitus and hearing loss (Koegel, 1985). Women who have attempted to induce abortion by taking a large dose of quinine may give birth to infants who are congenitally deaf (Drug and Therapeutics Bulletin, 1983). Tinnitus, vertigo, and infrequently reversible, mild hearing loss may occur with usual doses of quinidine (Rosketh and Storstein, 1963). Tinnitus and hearing loss can be caused by chloroquine. The hearing loss may not become apparent until some time after the drug has been discontinued, is usually associated with high dosage for an extended period of time, and is generally irreversible (Toone, 1965).

Cisplatin. Ototoxicity caused by cisplatin produces tinnitus and hearing loss in the high-frequency range, 4000 to 8000 Hz (chapter 23). It tends to be more frequent and severe following repeated doses, may be more conspicuous in children, and can be unilateral or bilateral. Patients followed up to 18 months after discovery of hearing loss have not shown any evidence of reversibility. Patients who receive cisplatin as a bolus seem to have a significantly greater incidence of hearing loss compared with those who receive the drug as a slow infusion (Chapman, 1982; Wiemann and Calabresi, 1985; Koegel, 1985).

Miscellaneous Ototoxic Agents. Regional perfusion with nitrogen mustard (mechlorethamine) may cause vestibular symptoms and sometimes hearing loss (Ballantyne, 1976). Quaternary ammonium compounds such as benzalkonium, chlorhexidine, and benzathonium chloride should not be used for skin preparation prior to surgery on or in the region about the ear, especially for repair of a perforated tympanic membrane, as total and permanent deafness has been reported (Bicknell, 1971). Povidone iodine also can have an ototoxic effect if applied to the area of the round window.

Ocular Toxicity

The eyes are responsive to influences from both systemic and topical medications that may cause varied complications. These adverse effects include blurred vision, disturbances of color vision, scotomata, degeneration of the retina, and other untoward effects on the cornea, sclera, lens, optic nerve, and extraocular muscles. The adverse effects of some drugs can be predicted and occur soon after therapy has begun; other drugs produce adverse effects on the eye that cannot be predicted and that occur only after long-term administration. Fortunately, many of the adverse ocular effects are transient, but some may cause severe visual damage that is irreversible. Patients who are being considered for long-term systemically administered medication, especially new drugs, should have careful ophthalmologic screening before starting the drug and during the course of therapy (Lien, 1987b; Abel and Leopold, 1987).

Multiple factors are involved in the production of ocular adverse effects by a drug. The ease with which a drug passes into the general circulation and into the eye determines its potential to directly affect the eye. Toxic concentrations of drugs may be reached in some instances by high systemic dosage over short periods and in others by prolonged use. Not only may the eye be affected as the drugs are administered (orally, parenterally, or topically), but toxic levels may accumulate slowly and continuously even after administration is discontinued and in situations when the metabolism and elimination of drugs are altered by the presence of severe liver and/or renal disease (see below). Individual idiosyncrasy may be responsible at times for ocular side effects; at other times the untoward responses are genetically determined (Willetts, 1969). In prescribing drugs for long-time use (e.g., digitalis glycosides, antimalarials, phenothiazines, and corticosteroids), the physician must be aware of potential diverse effects on the eye.

Digitalis Glycosides. Ocular effects of systemically administered drugs have been observed for many years. Withering, in 1785, wrote that "foxglove when given in large and quickly repeated doses occasions sickness, vomiting, giddiness, confused vision, objects appearing green or yellow" (White, 1965). The incidence of ocular manifestations in patients with digitalis toxicity has been estimated to be as high as 25%. In approximately 10% of patients, the ocular complaints may occur prior to other symptoms of toxicity; however, usually adverse ocular effects appear simultaneously with or later than the other signs of cardiac toxicity. These ocular manifestations may present in ways unknown to Withering. For example, we have seen an elderly man for his conduction abnormality discovered on a routine preoperative ECG. His concentration of digoxin in plasma was elevated. His only complaint was that he was troubled by excessive yellow coloration when watching television. This was not corrected by a home visit and adjustment of his television set by a TV repair technician! Subsequently, it has been our practice to ask patients taking digitalis glycosides if they have been experiencing any difficulty with the color of their TV programs. Blurred vision and disturbed color vision are the most common ocular symptoms of digitalis toxicity. Objects may appear yellow (xanthopsia) or green; less commonly they appear red, brown, blue, or white ("snowy vision"). Photophobia and scintillating scotomata may occur, as does alteration of visual acuity. Xanthopsia may occur with administration of chlorothiazide and other drugs (Post, 1960).

Ocular muscle palsies, retrobulbar neuritis, and alteration of pupil size also may be associated with digitalis toxicity. Patients who have visual complaints while receiving digitalis should be examined for the presence of central scotomata. These may indicate retrobulbar neuritis or be due to toxic effects on the retinal receptor cells. Digitalis may cause an elevation of the cone dark-adaptation threshold. Even formed visual hallucinations have been reported as a consequence of digoxin toxicity (Volpe and Soave, 1979).

Phenothiazine Derivatives and Quinolines. Certain of the phenothiazines and quinolines may adversely affect the retina and other ocular structures (Applebaum, 1963; Rab, 1969). Adverse effects have been reported for the 4-aminoquinolines (chloroquine and hydroxychloroquine), but there is no evidence that the 8-aminoquinolines (primaquine) cause ocular problems. Those phenothiazine derivatives with piperidine side chains such as thioridazine have a higher risk of inducing retinal toxicity than other phenothiazines (Applebaum, 1963). There have been relatively fewer cases reported for those with aliphatic side chains, while those with a piperazine group do not seem to exert direct ocular toxicity. The phenothiazines as a group can also cause cataract formation, mostly of an anterior polar variety (Prien et al., 1970; Crombie, 1981). The phenothiazine-induced retinopathy may be related to both dose and duration. The retinopathy may present either acutely with sudden loss of vision associated with retinal edema and hyperemia of the optic disc or slowly with chronic, fine pigmentation scattered in the central area of the fundus, extending peripherally, but sparing the macula. There may be chronic central and paracentral scotomata (Spiteri and James, 1983).

The phenothiazines can accumulate in the pigment cells, particularly in the melanin fraction. The risk of ocular toxicity may be dose- and time-dependent. In most cases, this complication occurs after patients have received 600 to 800 mg

of thioridazine daily. Pigmentary retinal changes have also been described following the use of prochlorperazine and chlorpromazine (Applebaum, 1963).

Chloroquine, Hydroxychloroquine, and Quinine. The incidence of chloroquine keratopathy is high. Corneal deposits appear in about 30% to 70% of treated patients starting after 1 to 2 months of treatment at full therapeutic doses. Chloroquine keratopathy is not related to chloroquine retinopathy; it is often asymptomatic, and visual changes occur in less than 50% of those with corneal deposits. The keratopathy is usually completely reversible after stopping treatment. Chloroquine-induced retinal changes can lead to progressive loss of vision. For the long-term therapy of rheumatoid arthritis, the dose of chloroquine probably should not exceed 4.0 mg/kg daily and of hydroxychloroquine should not exceed 6.5 mg/kg daily. The toxic threshold for retinopathy may be 5.1 mg/kg daily for chloroquine and 7.8 mg/kg per day for hydroxychloroquine (Mackenzie, 1983). Maculopathy with impaired vision was present in 2% of 95 patients with rheumatoid arthritis who had taken a total dose of less than 100 g of chloroquine; in about 7% of 93 who had taken 101 to 300 g; in about 10% of 59 who had taken 301 to 600 g; and in 17% of 23 who had taken more than 600 g. An additional disturbing feature is the possibility of *retinopathy developing several years after chloroquine therapy had been discontinued* (Elman et al., 1976; Ehrenfeld et al., 1986). *Principle: Adverse reactions cover a gamut of pathologic lesions, many of them quite consequential to the patient. The fact that some severe reactions can be quite delayed after drugs are discontinued (e.g., aplastic anemia and retinopathy) and that many cannot be reversed by discontinuing a drug simply means that a drug* **must be indicated** *before it is used!*

Transient, total blindness has been associated with the parenteral administration of quinine for malaria. At a peak plasma quinine concentration of 90 nmol/ml, one patient was blinded and deafened but recovered over the subsequent 3 days (Migasena, 1984). Sudden loss of vision also was reported in a 63-year-old woman following the ingestion of 39 g of quinine. Vision slowly improved over 2 months, but the visual fields remained restricted, and the color and night vision remained defective (Fong et al., 1984).

In addition to chloroquine, hydroxychloroquine, and the phenothiazines, drugs that have been associated with corneal deposits include amiodarone and lovastatin. Photophobia and amblyopia have been reported with zidovudine.

Ethambutol, Ethionamide, and Chloramphenicol. The major toxicity of ethambutol is optic neuritis that is dose-related. It is infrequent at a dose of 15 mg/kg per day (Goldberger, 1988). The dosage should be reduced when the glomerular filtration rate is less than 30 to 50 ml/minute (Bennett et al., 1991). Symptoms of retrobulbar neuritis include decreased visual acquity, scotomata, and defective red-green vision. Ethionamide is a derivative of isonicotinic acid, and optic neuritis occurs infrequently with its use. Optic neuritis has occurred with prolonged therapy with chloramphenicol (Citron, 1969; Goldberger, 1988).

Miscellaneous Drugs. Ocular manifestations have been reported in association with the use of transdermal scopolamine patches including anisocoria and a fixed dilated pupil (Verdier and Kennerdell, 1982; Bienia, 1983). Narrow-angle glaucoma has been precipitated by scopolamine (Fraunfelder, 1982). Roder et al. (1989) described five cases of mydriasis induced by use of a transdermal scopolamine delivery system with anisocoria and narrow-angle glaucoma in four patients. Mydriatics, both anticholinergics and sympathomimetic amines, may cause an eye with a shallow or narrow angle to abruptly shut off the drainage of intraocular fluid, causing a rapid increase in intraocular pressure, resulting in acute closed (or narrow)-angle glaucoma. The phenothiazines and tricyclic antidepressants, because of their anticholinergic effects, also may precipitate closed-angle glaucoma. Topical ophthalmic corticosteroid preparations may produce open-angle glaucoma due to increases in outflow resistance of the aqueous humor attributed to the hydration of mucopolysaccharides in the trabecular network (Oppelt et al., 1969; Reid et al., 1976).

Since the eye is exposed to light, photosensitive drugs when present may have the potential of contributing to toxic effects, though definite proof is lacking. Some potential examples include sulfonamides, carbamazepine, tricyclic antidepressants, psoralens, and phenothiazines. Patients taking these drugs should protect their eyes from exposure to sunshine or ultraviolet light (Bron, 1979; Stempel and Stempel, 1973). *Principle: When drug action or toxicity can be attributed to a chemical property of a drug, the clinician should consider similar consequences when using any drug with the same chemical properties. He or she may be wrong, but the patient cannot help but gain from such thoughtfulness.*

Miotic agents, such as diisopropyl fluorophosphate and echothiophate, especially anticholinesterase drugs for the treatment of glaucoma, are known to cause lenticular opacities. The causal role of pilocarpine in cataract formation has been questioned since many patients have retained clear lenses after using this drug for several years. Corticosteroids used systemically for the treatment of rheumatoid arthritis have caused irreversible posterior subcapsular cataracts. The lens opacity appears to be dependent on both the dosage and the duration of treatment (Shaffer and Hetherington, 1966; Williamson et al., 1969). Anticancer agents such as busulfan, methotrexate, and nitrogen mustards also have been known to cause cataracts.

Nephrotoxicity

Many drugs have been demonstrated to cause renal dysfunction (chapter 11). Certain drugs are especially likely to cause renal injury, and renal function should be monitored during their use (Table 39–4). In the following discussion, selected examples are given.

Analgesic Nephropathy. Zollinger and Spühler (1950) originally described an association between the chronic ingestion of large doses of analgesics and the development of papillary necrosis and interstitial nephritis. Although initially thought to be caused only by phenacetin, all simple analgesics including aspirin, acetaminophen, antipyrine, aminopyrine, and phenacetin have been implicated. Chronic analgesic abuse, in addition to causing papillary necrosis, has been reported to cause a high incidence of transitional cell carcinoma of the renal pelvis and bladder carcinoma (Küng, 1976; Prescott, 1982). More recently an association with retroperitoneal fibrosis has been reported (Critchley et al., 1985). Symptoms of papillary necrosis include nocturia, flank pain, hematuria, and fever and can be confused with nephrolithiasis.

A salt-losing nephropathy may also occur. Analgesic nephropathy is an important but not always recognized cause of renal failure. In the United States it is estimated that in 20% of patients with chronic interstitial disease, analgesic abuse is the cause. If the analgesic habit is given up, useful renal function returns in about 50% of those cases. Analgesic nephropathy is not a frequent complication of patients with rheumatoid arthritis under treatment with salicylates. However, the use of compound analgesics probably should be avoided (Cove-Smith and Knapp, 1978).

NSAIDs. The most common adverse renal effect associated with the use of NSAIDs is prostaglandin-dependent reversible renal insufficiency (chapter 11). It is characterized clinically by a fall in urine output, weight gain, rapidly rising serum concentrations of BUN and creatinine, and in some cases elevated concentrations of potassium in serum. Generally clinical improvement ensues within 24 to 72 hours after the drug is discontinued. Elderly patients with volume depletion,

Table 39–4. DRUG-INDUCED KIDNEY DISEASE

DISEASE	CAUSATIVE AGENT
Prerenal Azotemia	ACE inhibitors NSAIDs Cyclosporin Interleukin-2
Acute Tubular Necrosis	Acetaminophen Aminoglycoside antibiotics Amphotericin B Cephalosporins Cisplatin Methoxyflurane Mithramycin Radiocontrast agents Tetracycline
Intratubular Obstruction	Acyclovir Methotrexate Sulfonamides
Nephrolithiasis	Allopurinol Carbonic anhydrase inhibitors Triamterene
Acute Interstitial Nephritis	Allopurinol Ampicillin, methicillin, other β-Lactams Cimetidine Diuretics NSAIDs p-Aminosalicyclic acid Phenytoin Rifampin Sulfonamides

Chronic Interstitial Nephritis	Analgesics:
	  Acetaminophen
	  Aspirin
	  Phenacetin
	  NSAIDs
	Cyclosporin
	Lithium
	Methyl-CCNU

congestive heart failure, cirrhosis, and preexisting renal disease are at greatest risk for this adverse effect. The NSAIDs may also cause interstitial nephritis and the nephrotic syndrome. Additional syndromes, well documented but relatively rare, are hyporeninemic hypoaldosteronism and inappropriate antidiuretic hormone action (Stillman et al., 1984) (chapter 11).

Acute Interstitial Nephritis. The major cause of acute interstitial nephritis is drugs. Though numerous agents can produce this syndrome, the most frequent offenders are penicillins, especially methicillin, sulfonamides, rifampin, cimetidine, allopurinol, diuretics, and NSAIDs (Adler et al., 1986). Usually one can obtain a history of more than 10 days of therapy prior to onset of symptoms (consisting of maculopapular rash, fever, eosinophilia, hematuria, proteinuria, and eosinophiluria). The onset of acute interstitial nephritis may be sudden and accompanied by oliguria. Up to one third of patients can have enough compromise in glomerular filtration rate to require dialysis (Adler et al., 1986).

Antimicrobial Agents. From 10% to 20% of patients being treated with aminoglycoside antibiotics show impairment of renal function. These polybasic antibiotics have relatively high urine/blood ratios. The likelihood of renal injury is accentuated by the concomitant use of another potentially nephrotoxic agent or if there is preexisting impairment of kidney function. These drugs cause necrosis of the proximal tubular epithelium resulting in slowly progressive nonoliguric renal failure that becomes apparent about 7 days after the initiation of therapy. Increased excretion of brush border antigens and β_2-microglobulin occur. Peak and trough concentrations of the aminoglycosides in serum should be monitored to prevent these complications (Pancoast, 1988). Therapeutic efficacy correlates best with peak levels; and though trough values are not perfect predictors of renal toxicity, they provide helpful guidelines (Meyer, 1986).

Nephrotoxicity appears to be most closely related to the length of time that trough concentrations are above 2 μg/ml for gentamicin and tobramycin and greater than 10 μg/ml for amikacin and kanamycin. The initial toxic result usually is expressed as nonoliguric renal failure that can be reversed if the drug is discontinued. Reversal may take weeks to months to occur. Continued administration of the drug may lead to oliguric renal shutdown.

While receiving therapy, the patient's serum creatinine values should be followed every 2 to 3 days. Adjustment in dosage should then be made if creatinine values increase. Although rises in the serum creatinine concentrations are often late and not particularly sensitive predicators of decline in renal function, such changes in the serum creatinine value remain the only useful indicator of impending renal toxicity. In general, clinicians being very cautious in their dosing of the aminoglycosides to avoid toxicity, tend to underdose to a significant degree and leave their patients vulnerable to therapeutic failure (Pancoast, 1988).

Amphotericin B. Nephrotoxicity is the most serious adverse effect of amphotericin B therapy.

The site of toxicity is the renal tubules, where the drug is believed to cause a lytic action on the cholesterol-rich liposomal membranes. The usual adverse effects include urinary abnormalities, hyposthenuria, azotemia, hypokalemia, renal tubular acidosis, and nephrocalcinosis. Hyaline and granular casts and pyuria are commonly found. Hypokalemia may be particularly profound in patients also receiving carbenicillin or ticarcillin. Toxicity may be related to the total dose of amphotericin B. Quantities less than 600 mg produce few abnormalities, but doses in excess of 3 g produce renal toxicity in up to 80% of patients. When the creatinine concentration exceeds 3 mg/dl or the BUN concentration 50 mg/dl, discontinuation or alternate-day therapy is advised (Bodey, 1988).

Although renal toxicity is generally reversible, prolonged therapy with large doses or several therapeutic courses can result in irreversible renal damage. In an attempt to reduce nephrotoxicity, amphotericin has been incorporated into liposome carriers. Administration of this complex resulted in marked reduction of nephrotoxicity in mice as well as in experimental clinical trials, due to alternations in the interaction of the polyene molecule with mammalian cell membranes. Amphotericin apparently does not transfer from liposomes to mammalian cells but does transfer effectively from donor liposomes to fungal cell walls, maintaining toxicity for fungi (Lopez-Berestein, 1986).

The incidence of acute nephrotoxicity caused by vancomycin is not clear. Faber and Moellering (1983) estimated that 5% of patients treated with vancomycin alone showed signs of renal impairment, but 35% of patients receiving vancomycin concurrently with an aminoglycoside were affected, suggesting that these antibiotics may act synergistically in producing renal dysfunction. Because an adverse interaction between the aminoglycosides and vancomycin may exist, close monitoring of renal function and serum concentrations of both drugs is necessary (Levine, 1987; Hewlett et al., 1988).

Cisplatin. The use of cisplatin is limited by dose-related nephrotoxicity produced by a poorly defined mechanism. In humans the lesions are predominately in the distal tubules and collecting duct. The lesions lead to acute tubular necrosis. Some studies indicate early involvement of the proximal tubules (Fillastre et al., 1988). Hypomagnesemia was found in more than 50% of the patients and, in many, persisted for as long as 20 months. Cisplatin probably should not be used if the glomerular filtration rate is less than 50 ml/min. Continuous infusions seem to be less toxic than bolus administration of the drug (Ries and Klastersky, 1986; Fillastre et al., 1988).

Other Cancer Therapeutic Drugs. Other cancer therapeutic drugs produce nephrotoxicity, each by a different mechanism. Methotrexate causes intrarenal obstruction by the intraluminal precipitation of methotrexate and its metabolite, 7-hydroxymethotrexate. Adequate hydration and alkalinization of the urine help to prevent this problem. Mithramycin can result in both acute and chronic tubular injury, even when given in the doses used to treat hypercalcemia. It can also induce a hemolytic uremic syndrome with renal abnormalities. Lomustine (CCNU) given over 1 to 2 years can produce chronic interstitial nephritis. The nephrotoxicity is dose-related. Streptozotocin-induced tubular injury can result in the Fanconi syndrome and rarely in acute renal failure (Ries and Klastersky, 1986).

Cyclosporine. Renal toxicity is a major problem with cyclosporine. Cyclosporine is a renal arteriolar vasoconstrictor and may accentuate other ischemic insults to produce acute renal failure. This risk may be increased when the drug is parenterally administered. More gradual elevations in serum creatinine concentrations appear to be hemodynamically mediated and usually respond to a reduction in dosage. Chronic interstitial fibrosis develops by an uncertain mechanism after prolonged therapy. Cyclosporine can produce hyperkalemia, elevate blood pressure, and induce a hemolytic uremic syndrome. Toxicity correlates loosely with trough concentrations of the drug. The narrow therapeutic index, marked individual variability in clearance, low and variable bioavailability, and a large number of drug interactions make cyclosporine an obvious candidate for therapeutic drug monitoring (see chapters 37 and 38). Some confusion arises regarding whether to use serum, plasma, or whole blood for analysis and whether to use high-performance liquid chromatography (HPLC) or radioimmunoassay (RIA) as the analytic method (Kahan, 1986; Cal et al., 1988).

Radiocontrast-Induced Nephropathy. Acute renal insufficiency has been reported following the administration of radiocontrast agents by oral, IV, and intraarterial routes. Increased use of angiography, computed tomography, and IV pyelography has increased the incidence of acute renal failure secondary to contrast material. The diagnosis should be suspected when an acute deterioration in renal function occurs within 24 to 48 hours after use of a contrast agent and when alternative explanations have been excluded. A persistent abnormal nephrogram and a low fractional excretion of sodium are typical concomitants of the complication. Risk factors include preexisting renal insufficiency with a serum creatinine concentration greater than 3.0 mg/dl, history of prior contrast-induced acute renal failure, the use of large doses of contrast medium, age greater than 60, presence of diabetes mellitus, dehydration, and/or multiple myeloma. A good state of hydration and the use of mannitol just prior to or immediately after injection of the dye may be of prophylactic value. Newer contrast agents that are nonionic, have lower osmolality, and have reduced alkalinity are now available. Whether or not these agents will prove to be less nephrotoxic than the standard cationic dyes is not yet clear (Berkseth and Kjellstrand, 1984; Swanson et al., 1986; LaDelfa and Melmon, 1989).

Additional Forms of Kidney Damage. Additional, drug-induced responses of the kidneys have been described. Methotrexate, the sulfonamides, and large doses of acyclovir can precipitate in the renal tubules. By somewhat different mechanisms, triamterene, allopurinol, and acetazolamide may cause renal stones. Systemic vasculitis and associated glomerular changes have occurred with the use of penicillin, sulfonamides, allopurinol, thiazides, and amphetamines. In addition to streptozotocin and 5-azacytidine, degradation products of outdated tetracycline can produce proximal tubular damage (Fanconi syndrome). Retroperitoneal fibrosis and secondary obstructive uropathy have been caused by methylsergide. A similar clinical syndrome has been due to ergot alkaloids. Lithium and methoxyflurane cause nephrogenic diabetes insipidus (Singer et al., 1972; Ettinger et al., 1980).

Hemopoietic Toxicity

The hemopoietic system is notably vulnerable to the toxic effects of drugs. These may be expressed against formed elements of the blood or the bone marrow. Several drugs are regularly associated with idiosyncratic reactions in susceptible persons. For the most part, the reactions are due either to decreased production or increased destruction of blood elements. Bleeding disturbances and coagulation disorders are often caused by drugs. A large number of drugs associated with or presumed to be associated with hematologic disorders have been summarized by Verstrete and Boogaerts (1987) and Girdwood (1976).

Drugs and Platelet and Coagulation Defects. Because aspirin inhibits platelet function, it should be avoided in patients receiving oral anticoagulants (chapters 19, 20, and 25). Aspirin decreases platelet aggregation by blocking the synthesis of thromboxane A_2 and the releasing of ADP, mediators of the second phase of platelet aggregation. The results may be serious in the neonate patients who have coagulation defects, or those who are taking anticoagulants or undergoing surgery. The acetylation of platelets by aspirin occurs in the bone marrow before the platelets are released from the marrow. The functional abnormality persists for the lifetime of that particular group of platelets. (The normal half-life of platelets is around 5 days.) Carbenicillin and ticarcillin cause platelet dysfunction and prolong bleeding time, increasing the risk of clinically significant hemorrhage in patients with uremia or who have undergone surgery. Large doses of penicillin G and valproic acid also may modify platelet function (von Voss et al., 1976; Stuart, 1980). Cephalosporins possessing an N-methylthiotetrazole side chain, moxalactam, cefoperazone, cefotetan, and cefamandole have been reported to cause hypoprothrombinemia with episodes of clinically significant bleeding. The mechanism is stated to be inhibition of the γ carboxylation of glutamic acid that is the vitamin K–dependent step in prothrombin synthesis. Cephalosporins without the N-methylthiotetrazole side chain do not produce this effect (Bechtold et al., 1984).

Aplastic Anemia. Drug-induced aplastic anemia is unpredictable. The clinical manifestations are severe and often fatal. At least half of all cases are associated with the use of drugs. The most frequently implicated are chloramphenicol, phenylbutazone, oxyphenbutazone, sulfonamides, and gold. Inhaled solvents, especially benzene, other organic chemicals, and insecticides have also been implicated (Williams et al., 1973). Chloramphenicol accounts for the greatest number of cases, and two types of hematotoxicity have been delineated (Yunis, 1988). The more common is the dose-related, reversible bone marrow suppression affecting primarily the erythroid series and usually occurring when concentrations of chloramphenicol in serum reach 25 μg/ml or higher. Rarer is the devastating complication of bone marrow aplasia characterized by pancytopenia that can occur at any dose and frequently has a fatal outcome due to hemorrhage or infection. Reversible marrow suppression seems due to mitochondrial injury (Yunis, 1988). Concentrations as low as 10 μg/ml in plasma can be associated with profound chloramphenicol-induced inhibition of mitochondrial protein synthesis in bone marrow. In vitro reversibility has been demonstrated at the mitochondrial level with restoration of protein synthesis after the drug is removed. The biochemical basis for the erythroid sensitivity to chloramphenicol remains uncertain. Inhibited synthesis of ferrochelatase, a mitochondrial membrane–associated enzyme, and consequent block in heme synthesis has been proposed as a contributing factor.

Aplastic anemia from chloramphenicol is rare, occurring in 1/10,000 to 1/40,000 exposed persons with a risk when given by any route and with no relation to dose or duration of therapy. A genetically determined predisposition of chloramphenicol-induced aplastic anemia has been suggested by the occurrence of this complication in identical twins (chapter 32). The rarity and unpredictability of the complication and the lack of a suitable experimental model have impeded studies of its pathogenic mechanism. Yunis et al. (1980) hypothesized that the p-NO$_2$ group of chloramphenicol is the structural feature underlying aplastic anemia from chloramphenicol. The p-NO$_2$ group undergoes nitroreduction, producing nitroso and hydroxylamine, toxic intermediates that cause stem cell damage. Thiaphenicol, which lacks the p-NO$_2$ group, is not associated with an increased incidence of aplastic anemia. With an increasing number of comparably effective broad-spectrum antibiotics now available, the risks of prescribing chloramphenicol may be beginning to outweigh the benefits of the drug in most clinical settings (Franke and Neu, 1987; Yunis, 1988). On the other hand, if the drug is well or uniquely suited for specific important efficacy, the frequency of its toxicity is low and its use may well be worth the limited risk.

Thrombocytopenia. Drugs can cause thrombocytopenia by increasing platelet destruction or by bone marrow suppression (Miescher, 1973). Such hypersensitivity or allergic thrombocytopenia can be caused by a large number of drugs. These patients are thought to have drug-related antibodies of both IgG and IgM classes that are involved in the destruction of the platelets. Thrombocytopenia can appear within a few hours following administration of a drug that causes thrombocytopenia in patients who had taken the drug previously. An acute syndrome generally develops with petechiae, often initially more prominent on the lower extremities, and bleeding from the mucous membranes. Because the half-life of the platelet is so short, the thrombocytopenia shows signs of beginning to subside within several hours or up to a few days after the offending drug has been withdrawn.

Two mechanisms are believed to be involved in inducing the thrombocytopenia. Either the drug may be bound to the platelet membrane and the antibody directed against the drug–membrane complex with subsequent activation of complement-induced injury to the platelet, or circulating drug–antibody may complex with the platelets, playing a more or less passive role in the destruction. Immune complexes are phagocytized by platelets, and subsequently the platelets release some of their components. The resulting "release reaction" may cause intravascular platelet aggre-gation and thrombocytopenia. Systemic symptoms may accompany the immune complex thrombocytopenia. The latter mechanism is involved when rifampin, thiazides, thiouracils, quinine, and quinidine cause the problem (Joist, 1985).

Transient, mild thrombocytopenia occurs in about 25% of patients receiving heparin. This is believed to result from heparin-induced platelet aggregation but may be accompanied by a paradoxical decrease of the anticoagulant effect. Severe thrombocytopenia follows the formation of heparin-dependent antiplatelet antibodies. Usually the reaction is delayed until the 8th to the 12th day of therapy. It is characterized by recurrent thrombotic disease and loss of the anticoagulant effect. A platelet count as low as 5000/mm^3, elevated fibrin split products, and adequate megakaryocytes in the bone marrow are seen. Improvement of the thrombocytopenia occurs after heparin is stopped. Patients with such heparin-induced thrombocytopenia may have received heparin prepared from bovine lung rather than pork intestine (O'Reilly, 1985). An immunoglobulin directed against an antigen common to several properties of heparin has been detected in the plasma of heparinized patients with thrombocytopenia (Trowbridge et al., 1978).

Agranulocytosis. Contrasted with drug-induced aplastic anemia, in which some cases may appear after the drug has been discontinued, drug-induced agranulocytosis occurs during treatment with the drug. In this context, agranulocytosis is a diagnosis that refers to patients with neutrophil counts of less than 200/mm^3 or total white blood cell counts of less than 500/mm^3. Agranulocytosis may result from bone marrow depression or increased peripheral destruction of white blood cells. Agranulocytosis may occur as a component of drug-induced aplastic anemia or as an adverse drug effect without accompanying anemia or thrombocytopenia. A number of drugs can produce either aplastic anemia or agranulocytosis. Drug-induced agranulocytosis is more common than aplastic anemia but less common than thrombocytopenia (DeGrunchy, 1975). Even though agranulocytosis usually is reversible following withdrawal of the causative drug, there is still about a 20% associated mortality (Wilson and Mielke, 1983).

Several mechanisms may lead to agranulocytosis (Pisciotta, 1978). They include peripheral damage through an immune mechanism, direct damage to marrow cells, and production of antinuclear antibodies or a drug-induced lupus syndrome. Representative drugs for each type include sulfonamides, acetaminophen, chlorpropamide, and propylthiouracil for the first; phenothiazines and tricyclic antidepressants for the second type; and procainamide, isoniazid, and phenytoin for the latter type. The agranulocytosis due to marrow depression often is due to the phenothiazine group of drugs. Though chlorpromazine has been implicated most often, thioridazine and other members of this class have been at fault (Shaw et al., 1964). The onset is generally after a period of 3 to 6 weeks of cumulative dosing.

Constitutional symptoms may occur at the onset of agranulocytosis prior to signs of infection, especially of the immunologic type, and are believed to be due to the rapid intravascular destruction of granulocytes. Leukocyte antibodies may be demonstrated in the blood for a limited time after administration of the implicated drug, and there may be history of a previous course of the drug. *Principle: When prescribing a drug that may cause agranulocytosis, physicians should describe the risk and symptoms to patients so that the problem will be recognized quickly if it occurs.*

Recovery is to be anticipated after the drug is stopped, but the future exposure to even very small amounts of the drug will precipitate a recurrence. See chapters 22 and 24 for discussion of aplastic anemia caused by drugs.

Cardiotoxicity

Both acute and chronic cardiotoxicities are produced by the anthracyclines. In fact, the therapeutic potential of doxorubicin and other anthracycline drugs is limited by cardiotoxicity. The mechanism of the toxicity is not fully understood. Theories of the mechanism of anthracycline toxicity include the overloading of myocytes with calcium, the production of free radicals, and the cardiotoxicity of the C-13 hydroxy metabolites of doxorubicin (Mushlin and Olson, 1988.) Acute toxicity is characterized by the ECG changes of nonspecific ST-T wave abnormalities, lengthening of the QRS complexes, low voltage, dysrhythmias, myocarditis, and transient cardiac dysfunction. Acute toxicity may infrequently cause disturbances of cardiac rhythm and sudden death during or shortly after the infusion of doxorubicin (Mushlin and Olson, 1988). Chronic toxicity, linked to the cumulative dose of drug, is a more common problem that may lead to a fatal congestive cardiomyopathy. Gated radionuclide angiography often reveals diastolic dysfunction following doses of doxorubicin below those that produce systolic dysfunction (Mushlin and Olsen, 1988). Right ventricular endomyocardial biopsies provide a sensitive means of detecting myocardial injury and help determine whether patients are able to tolerate additional doses of anthracyclines.

Limiting the total dose of doxorubicin is the best way to prevent cardiomyopathy. Epidemiologic data from the 1970s advised that the total cumulative doses of doxorubicin should be limited to 550 mg/m^2 (Bristow et al., 1978). At this dose, congestive heart failure developed in 10% of patients; failure developed in 30% at higher doses. The incidence of failure is 1% to 5% at cumulative doses less than 500 mg/m^2. Risk factors for developing the cardiomyopathy include age below 10 and over 40 years, the presence of preexisting cardiac disease, hypertension, liver dysfunction, prior or concurrent radiation therapy, and previous treatment with other anthracyclines or cyclophosphamide. Cardiotoxicity may be somewhat limited by using slow infusions designed to minimize peak concentrations of drug in plasma for any given dosage of anthracycline (Legha et al., 1982).

Cyclophosphamide. Cyclophosphamide in large doses (greater than 180 mg/kg) may cause cardiac failure through direct damage to the heart (Applebaum et al., 1976). Cardiotoxicity has been observed in some patients receiving doses of cyclophosphamide ranging from 120 to 270 mg/kg given over a few days, usually as a part of a multidrug antineoplastic regimen. In a few instances, severe and fatal heart failure may develop with histologic study revealing hemorrhagic myocarditis.

Phenothiazines. The phenothiazines, and particularly thioridazine, produce repolarization changes in the ECG. The most common electrocardiographic findings are prolongation of the QT$_c$ interval, ST-T wave changes, and flattening and notching of the T waves. With higher doses, T-wave inversion may occur as well as the appearance of prominent U waves. These patients are vulnerable for torsades de pointes–type ventricular tachyrhythmia that may be prefibrillatory (Giles and Modlin, 1968) (chapter 6).

Other Types of Drugs. Several other types of drugs may cause serious adverse effects on the heart. Overdosage of tricyclic antidepressants may cause severe disturbances in ventricular rhythm (see chapter 6) (Thorstrand, 1976). Lithium can produce ECG changes similar to those of the phenothiazines and may also cause interstitial myocarditis (Len Tseng, 1971) (chapters 2 and 6). Emetine is the alkaloid obtained from ipecacuanha (ipecac) and has been used as a direct amebicide since 1912. Both emetine and its analog dehydroemetine are being replaced by less toxic amebicides of the nitroimidazole class. Emetine is known to have cardiotoxic effects (Murphy et al., 1974). Syrup of ipecac is a useful household emetic available in 0.5 and 1 fluid oz sizes that can be purchased without prescription. Overdose in young children can produce toxic effects on the heart because of its emetine content (Allport, 1959). There are reports of the chronic abuse of ipecac to induce vomiting by persons with eating disorders. Cardiotoxicity and myopathy have occurred and may be the result of the accumulation of emetine (Harris, 1983; Palmer and Guay, 1985).

Myocarditis Due to Hypersensitivity to Drugs. Hypersensitivity myocarditis, an inflammatory disease of the myocardium, may occur because of drug allergy. Hypersensitivity myocarditis is rarely recognized as a clinical entity; most cases have been discovered unexpectedly at autopsy. The initial reports of apparent hypersensitivity myocarditis coincided with the introduction of the sulfonamides (French and Weller, 1942). Other drugs associated with this entity include penicillins, α-methyldopa, phenylbutazone, streptomycin, sulfonylureas, and tetracycline. When cardiac symptoms or electrocardiographic abnormalities occur in a setting consistent with drug allergy, hypersensitivity myocarditis should be considered. Endomyocardial biopsy may help confirm the diagnosis. Discontinuance of the drug responsible for the reaction and the use of corticosteroids and immunosuppressive therapy are advised (Taliercio et al., 1985; Fenoglio and Wagner, 1989).

Hepatotoxicity

Drugs in common use can cause liver toxicity that can mimic almost every naturally occurring liver disease in humans (Dickinson et al., 1981; Black, 1989; Lewis, 1989; Lewis and Zimmerman, 1989) (chapter 9). Though hepatic injury represents a relatively small proportion of all adverse drug effects, drugs are responsible for 2% to 5% of hospital admissions for jaundice in the United States and for about 10% of hospitalized patients with "acute hepatitis" in Europe (Lewis and Zimmerman, 1989). Drugs such as halothane, acetaminophen, and phenytoin are an important cause of fulminant liver failure. Many agents cause asymptomatic liver injury detected only by abnormal liver function tests. The estimated prevalence of asymptomatic disease as well as overt hepatitis varies from agent to agent and usually is less common in children compared with adults. Conspicuous exceptions are valproic acid and injury from salicylate. Most of the cases of drug-induced liver disease result from unexpected reactions to a therapeutic dose of a drug and considerably less often as a predictable sequel to the intrinsic toxicity of the particular agent (Lewis and Zimmerman, 1989).

When any patient with liver disease is evaluated, every medication that has been taken over the past 3 months must be known. Occupational toxins and other causes such as viral hepatitis must be excluded. Severity is increased if the drug is continued after symptoms develop or serum transaminase concentrations rise. Early and accurate diagnosis of a drug-induced hepatic reaction depends on the early suspicion by the physician of a possible drug-related cause. Discontinuing a hepatotoxic agent early significantly reduces or eliminates the injury. Should a hepatotoxic drug be continued, chronic liver disease or cirrhosis may result. The clinical history is crucial because the diagnosis can seldom be made on the basis of the histologic findings from liver biopsy alone. Recent or ongoing exposure to the suspected drug, the profile of liver function abnormalities, the histologic injury pattern most often associated with a particular drug, and the presence or absence of associated signs and symptoms that may or may not accompany injury with the suspected drug basically support a presemptive diagnosis. When the response to removal of the offending drug is less than conclusive, a challenge dose may afford definitive means of diagnosing drug injury. Rechallenge is generally unnecessary if an alternative therapeutic agent is available for the clinical situation. Rechallenge testing may be warranted in situations in which no equally efficacious substitute agent is available and continuation of therapy is mandatory (Lewis, 1989).

Acute hepatic injury may be cytotoxic (overt damage to hepatocytes), cholestatic (arrested bile flow), or mixed (features of both cytotoxic and cholestatic injury). Chronic injury from drugs includes chronic necroinflammatory disease, chronic steatosis, chronic cholestasis, granulomatous disease, vascular injury, cirrhosis, and several types of liver tumors (Mullick, 1987). Hepatotoxicity from drugs may be either predictable or idiosyncratic. Predictable injury resulting in hepatocellular necrosis is dose-related, usually reproducible in animals, and due to the intrinsic toxicity of a drug or its metabolite produced in the liver. Examples include overdoses with inorganic iron or acetaminophen. Idiosyncratic reactions are unpredictable. In these cases, the reaction generally does not directly relate to drug dose and may occur due to hypersensitivity with the usual clinical correlates. In other patients, there is no evidence of hypersensitivity and the underlying metabolic or genetic differences placing these persons at risk may be obscure. These differences in the biologic pathways of drug toxification or detoxification are genetically determined (chapter 30). Chronic alcohol ingestion and the concomitant use of rifampin may increase the hepatic toxicity of isoniazid (Lewis and Zimmerman, 1989).

The complexity of determining the mechanism of toxic drug effects on the liver is well illustrated by halothane-induced liver injury. Halothane hepatotoxicity has been suggested to be immune-mediated. On the other hand, the hepatotoxicity may occur in experimental animals by the conversion of halothane to a radical metabolite by inducing the cytochrome P450 system. This may be another explanation for the pivotal role of multiple exposures. Oxidative biotransformation yields a metabolite that binds to the hepatocyte membrane and alters its antigenic character. In a low-oxygen environment, biotransformation yields a free-radical metabolite capable of producing necrosis. Consequently, halothane hepatotoxicity could be due to a combination of toxic metabolites and immunologic factors (Cousins et al., 1985).

Cytochrome P450 enzymes, a complex family under genetic control, modify drugs oxidatively or reductively, producing two principal types of toxic metabolites: electrophiles and free radicals. *Electrophiles* are reactive metabolites that act as alkylating or arylating agents that covalently bind to nucleophilic sites. The principal nucleophilic site is the thiol group of GSH, which with glutathione *S*-alkyltransferases serves as a major protective substance in binding these toxins. The toxic metabolites of acetaminophen and bromobenzene have a GSH threshold, and only when the concentration of cellular GSH falls to a low level does toxicity occur (Kaplowitz et al., 1986). *Free radicals*, metabolites with an unpaired electron, are produced by oxidative or reductive reactions of cytochrome P450. These free radicals can bind covalently to proteins and unsaturated fatty acids of cell membranes (lipid peroxidation) and cause membrane damage. The end result is hepatocyte death related to the failure to pump calcium from the cytosol and to depressed mitochondrial function.

Oxygen Radicals. A third type of toxic reaction involving redox-cycling compounds has been recognized in studies of experimental hepatotoxicity. These redox-cycling compounds, such as nitrofurantoin, doxorubicin, and paraquat have a chemical structure that permits the acceptance of an unpaired extra electron to form a free radical. This free radical reacts directly with oxygen to form a superoxide anion (O_2^-) and regeneration of the parent drug. Toxicity is caused by these metabolites of oxygen. Liver injury from nitrofurantoin may be caused in part by this mechanism (Kaplowitz et al., 1986).

Pulmonary Toxicity

Adverse pulmonary reactions to drugs should be considered when the cause of a respiratory illness is not clear (Table 39–5). The nature of the pulmonary reaction may range from asthma to pulmonary infiltrates. More than 20 different noncytotoxic agents were associated with pulmonary reactions (Cooper et al., 1986b) (Table 39–6). Clinical syndromes are heterogeneous and

Table 39–5.   PULMONARY SYNDROMES CAUSED BY DRUGS

SYNDROME	CAUSATIVE AGENT
Hypersensitivity Lung Disease	Ampicillin
	Carbamazepine
	Chlorpropamide
	Cromolyn
	Dantrolene
	Hydralazine
	Imipramine
	Isoniazid
	Mecamylamine
	Mephenesin carbamate
	Methylphenidate
	Nitrofurantoin
	p-Aminosalicylic acid
	Penicillin
	Phenytoin
	Sulfadiazine
	Sulfasalazine
	Bleomycin
	Methotrexate
	Procarbazine
Drug-Induced Lupus with Potential for Lung Involvement	Chlorpromazine
	Ethosuximide
	Griseofulvin
	Gold salts
	Hydralazine
	Isoniazid
	Lithium carbonate
	Mephenytoin
	Methyldopa
	Nitrofurantoin
	Oral contraceptives
	Penicillin
	Penicillamine
	Phenylbutazone
	Phenytoin
	Prazosin
	Procainamide
	Propylthiouracil
	Quinidine
	Sulfonamides
	Trimethadione
Noncardiac Pulmonary Edema	*Opioid Overdose*
	Heroin
	Methadone
	Propoxyphene
	Sedatives
	Chlordiazepoxide
	Ethchlorvynol
	Hydrochlorthiazide
	Lidocaine
	Salicylates
	Tocolytic drugs
	Ritodrine
	Terbutaline
	Sequela of neuroleptic malignant syndrome
	Phenothiazines
	Butyrophonones
	Thioxanthenes

Table 39-6.   CYTOTOXIC DRUG-INDUCED PULMONARY PARENCHYMAL DISEASE

DRUG	MECHANISM OF LUNG INJURY	INCIDENCE AND RISK FACTORS	CLINICAL FINDINGS	FINDINGS ON CHEST X-RAY FILM	HISTOPATHOLOGIC FINDINGS	TREATMENT	OUTCOME
Cytotoxic Antibiotics							
Bleomycin	Reactive oxygen metabolites	From 2% to 40%. Cumulating dose; O_2 therapy; radiotherapy; other chemotherapy	Hypersensitivity; lung disease; interstitial pneumonitis; pulmonary fibrosis	Bibasilar reticular pattern; multiple small nodules	Endothelial cell damage; type I pneumocyte necrosis; fibroblast proliferation	Stop drug; corticosteroids for acute hypersensitivity reaction; no controlled human studies	May develop chronic progressive pulmonary fibrosis
Mitomycin	Unknown—has alkylating effect	From 3% to 12%. Risk factors not well established; radiotherapy; O_2 therapy	Acute or gradual restrictive ventilatory defect; reduction in D_{Lco}; rare microangiopathic hemolytic anemia	X-ray film may be normal; diffuse or acinarreticular pattern; may show nodularity	Endothelial damage; type I pneumocyte necrosis; collagen deposition and fibrogen-fibrin deposits	Stop drug; early administration of corticosteroids may alter prognosis	Reported mortality of about 50%
Nitrosoureas							
Carmustine	Formation of electrophilic series; reduction of stores of glutathione-oxidant injury	From 20% to 30%. Total dose of cyclophosphamide important	Dyspnea; cough; basal rales; restrictive ventilatory defect	X-ray film may be normal; bibasilar reticular pattern most common	Dysplastic pneumocytes; proliferation of fibroblasts; fibrosis without inflammatory cells	Stop drug; many patients are already receiving corticosteroids and their value is questionable	Progressive pulmonary toxicity; mortality as high as 90%
Lomostine (CCNU) Semustine (methyl-CCNU)			Similar to carmustine; pulmonary toxicity; decreased D_{Lco}		Similar to carmustine; pulmonary toxicity; interstitial infiltration of mononuclear cells		

Alkylating Agents

Busulfan	Sensitivity to alkylating effects on epithelial cells	Symptomatic, 4%; asymptomatic, 46%. Radiotherapy; other cytotoxic drugs	Cough; dyspnea; fever; pulmonary rales. Toxicity may occur first some time after drug is discontinued. Restrictive ventilatory defect; decreased D_{LCO}	Chest x-ray film rarely normal; basilar reticular pattern or acinar infiltrates; pleural effusion may be present	Dysplastic pneumocytes; proliferation of fibroblasts; fibrosis; mononuclear cell infiltration	Stop drug; trial of corticosteroids; supportive measures; there are no defined therapies	Prognosis is poor; mean survival after diagnosis is 5 months
Cyclophosphamide	Alkylation of cellular DNA; redox reaction of metabolites; hypersensitivity reaction	Low incidence, below 1%. High concentration of inspired O_2	Fever; cough; dyspnea; restrictive ventilatory defect; decreased D_{LCO}	Basilar reticular pattern; at times noncardiac pulmonary edema	Endothelial swelling; pneumocyte dysplasia; fibroblast proliferation; lymphocyte and histiocyte infiltration	Stop drug; corticosteroids have no effect on mortality	Variable prognosis; about 60% of patients recover
Chlorambucil	Alkylating effect with cross-linking of DNA molecules	Low incidence since first report in 1967	Fever; anorexia; restrictive ventilatory defect; decreased D_{LCO}	X-ray film may be normal; diffuse basilar reticular pattern	Pneumocyte dysplasia; extensive fibrosis; scattered interstitial mononuclear infiltrate	Stop drug; may progress despite corticosteroid therapy	Variable; about 50% of patients recover
Melphalan	Alkylating properties	Low incidence of symptomatic disease; subclinical disease may be significant	Fever; cough; dyspnea; malaise; basilar rales; markedly reduced D_{LCO}	Diffuse reticular pattern; modular and acinar shadows may occur	Atypical alveolar pneumocytes; fibrosis; bronchiolar epithelial proliferation; endothelial changes have not been reported	Stop drug; corticosteroids not of proven value	Variable; mortality about 50%

(continued)

1003

Table 39-6. CYTOTOXIC DRUG–INDUCED PULMONARY PARENCHYMAL DISEASE *(continued)*

DRUG	MECHANISM OF LUNG INJURY	INCIDENCE AND RISK FACTORS	CLINICAL FINDINGS	FINDINGS ON CHEST X-RAY FILM	HISTOPATHOLOGIC FINDINGS	TREATMENT	OUTCOME
Antimetabolites							
Methotrexate	Hypersensitivity reaction; direct toxic effect may also be involved	Uncertain, probably about 8%. Frequency of administration; use with cyclophosphamide	Acute or chronic onset; fever; malaise; eosinophilia; restrictive ventilatory defect; impaired D_{LCO}	X-ray film may be normal; diffuse reticular pattern; pleural effusion may be present	Atypical pneumocytes; inflammatory cells; fibrosis; diffuse edema with hyaline membrane formation	Stop drug; corticosteroids may hasten recovery; alternative therapy should be selected	Favorable; mortality about 1%
Azathioprine and 6-mercaptopurine			Acute restrictive lung disease			Stop drug; alternate immunosuppressive therapy; corticosteroids	Favorable
Cytosine-arabinoside			Acute respiratory failure	Diffuse infiltrates; pulmonary edema	Pulmonary infiltrates; pulmonary edema	Stop drug; supportive therapy	Variable; may be unfavorable
Other Cytotoxic Drugs							
Procarbazine	Hypersensitivity reaction; pulmonary edema		Hypersensitivity pneumonitis; pulmonary edema; fever; eosinophilia		Scattered eosinophils; mononuclear cell infiltration; fibrosis	Stop drug; supportive measures; corticosteroids may be of value	Probably favorable
Vinca alkaloids Vinblastine Vindesine Vincristine	Unknown—may be due to combined therapy with mitomycin		Dyspnea; bronchospasm; acute diffuse pulmonary infiltrates and respiratory failure		Dysplasia of alveolar lining cells; fibrosis; interstitial and alveolar influx of inflammatory cells	Stop drug; assisted ventilatory support; corticosteroids may be of value	Prognosis is poor if pulmonary infiltrates develop
Podophyllotixin derivatives Etoposide (VP-16) Teniposide (VM-26)	Unknown—may be due in part to prior carmustine therapy			Acinar and reticular infiltrates	Hyaline membrane formation; marked interstitial mononuclear and histiocytic infiltration	Stop drug; supportive therapy	Unclear; unfavorable with associated pulmonary infection

1004

Table 39–7. NONCYTOTOXIC DRUG-INDUCED PULMONARY PARENCHYMAL DISEASE

DRUG	MECHANISM OF LUNG INJURY	INCIDENCE AND RISK FACTORS	CLINICAL FINDINGS	FINDINGS ON CHEST X-RAY FILM	HISTOPATHOLOGIC FINDINGS	TREATMENT	OUTCOME
Nitrofurantoin	Hypersensitivity; production of oxygen radicals	More than 500 cases since 1961; age; extensive use of drug	Acute and chronic forms; fever; dyspnea; ventilatory defect; impaired $D_{L_{CO}}$	Acute: diffuse bibasilar and acinal infiltrates Chronic: infiltrates; may also have pleural effusion	Pulmonary vasculitis; interstitial and alveolar cellular infiltration; eosinophilia; granuloma formation; fibrosis	Stop drug; corticosteroids of questionable value	Acute: good; low mortality Chronic: fair; mortality about 10%
Sulfasalazine	Hypersensitivity	Unclear; salicylate and/or sulfonamide allergy may predispose to adverse reaction	Hypersensitivity reaction; fibrosing alveolitis; bronchiolitis obliterans; obstructive ventilatory pattern	Bilateral acinar infiltrates	Alveolitis; interstitial infiltration with eosinophils; fibrosis; bronchiolitis obliterans	Stop drug; corticosteroids may hasten recovery	Variable but generally good prognosis
Amphotericin B	Mechanism of pulmonary toxicity associated with leukocyte transfusions is not well understood; damage to transfused leukocytes or direct pulmonary tissue damage	About 60% in patients receiving both modes of therapy	Fever; chills; dyspnea; hypoxemia; hemoptysis	Diffuse interstitial infiltrates	Lung biopsy; diffuse intraalveolar hemorrhage; edema; without infection	Stop drug; supportive care; assisted ventilation may be needed	Prognosis poor; 50% need assisted ventilation; mortality about 35%

(continued)

1005

Table 39-7. NONCYTOTOXIC DRUG–INDUCED PULMONARY PARENCHYMAL DISEASE *(continued)*

DRUG	MECHANISM OF LUNG INJURY	INCIDENCE AND RISK FACTORS	CLINICAL FINDINGS	FINDINGS ON CHEST X-RAY FILM	HISTOPATHOLOGIC FINDINGS	TREATMENT	OUTCOME
Amiodarone	May be multifactorial; acquired lysosomal storage disease; immunologic mechanism	Numerous reports of pulmonary damage; 1% to 6%; toxicity partially related to maintenance dose	Delayed onset; dyspnea; cough; fever; reduced D_{LCO}	Diffuse reticular and patchy acinar infiltrates; pleural thickening; pleural effusions	Intraalveolar foamy macrophages; septal thickening; hyperplasia; type II pneumocytes	Stop drug; role of corticosteroids is unclear; these agents will not completely protect against toxic effects	Variable; reversal may occur; the lung injury may be progressive
Penicillamine	Unclear; altered collagen metabolism; epithelial toxicity; hypersensitivity	Low incidence of pulmonary injury; risk factors are unclear	Acute hypersensitivity reaction; subacute alveolitis or bronchiolitis; pulmonary renal syndrome	Similar to those of idiopathetic alveolitis; bronchiolitis or Goodpasture syndrome	Obliterated small airways; dysplastic pneumocytes; fibroblast proliferation and alveolar hemorrhage	Stop drug; supportive therapy; no apparent help by corticosteroids	Variable; but generally unfavorable
Gold salts	Unclear; proposed release of lymphokines; monocyte chemotactic factors; macrophage inhibitory factors	Incidence less than 1%; risk factors are unclear	Hypersensitivity lung disease or chronic pneumonitis/fibrosis	Diffuse retriculonodular infiltrates; restrictive ventilatory defect; decreased D_{LCO}	Interstitial and alveolar infiltration with histiocytes; plasma cells and lymphocytes; electron-dense deposits of macrophages in interstitium	Stop drug; role of chelating agents or corticosteroids uncertain	Low mortality; 50% of patients have residual pulmonary dysfunction

D_{LCO} = Pulmonary function test-diffusing capacity of the lung for carbon dioxide.

include pneumonitis-fibrosis, bronchiolitis obliterans, hypersensitivity lung disease, and noncardiogenic pulmonary edema.

Cytotoxic drugs may also cause severe pulmonary disease. Risk factors predisposing to development of pulmonary toxicity caused by different categories of cytotoxic agents include total cumulative dose, age of the patient, prior or concurrent radiation therapy, oxygen therapy, and other cytotoxic drug therapy. Bleomycin-induced pulmonary damage has become a model for interstitial pneumonitis and pulmonary fibrosis. Whether administered subcutaneously, intraperitoneally, or IV, bleomycin induces pulmonary fibrosis in many animal species including humans (chapter 23). Bleomycin may have adverse effects on the lungs by generating reactive oxygen metabolites (Cooper et al., 1986a). In humans no control studies have evaluated systematically the efficacy of corticosteroids. There have been anecdotal reports of hastened resolution of pulmonary abnormalities following such therapy.

Mitomycin is an alkylating agent that had been in use for several years before the report of its producing pulmonary toxicity. Its mechanism of adverse reaction may be included in the drug's alkylating properties. The nitrosoureas have both alkylating and carbamoylating properties. They produce interstitial pulmonary fibrosis seemingly related to the total dose administered and to the length of survival of the patient. The prognosis of progressive fibrosis is poor. Alkylating agents, busulfan, cyclophosphamide, and melphalan all are associated with poor prognosis once symptomatic pulmonary involvement begins (Table 39-7). Generally treatment with methotrexate, azathioprine, 6-mercaptopurine, and procarbazine are somewhat less likely to cause the pulmonary lesions (Cooper et al., 1986a).

Pulmonary damage associated with cytotoxic drugs is a clinically significant problem. With the improving prognosis for many patients with treated malignancies and the increased need to use these agents, the incidence of drug-induced pulmonary disease may escalate. A critical problem in cytotoxic drug-induced pulmonary disease is determining how to treat or prevent pulmonary toxicity while sustaining tumor toxicity. No one has yet come up with a solution.

Summary Principle: Adverse reactions occur in every physician's practice. Physicians' recognition depends on their knowledge of the pharmacology of the drugs they use and on their willingness to recognize that they may cause reactions despite their good intentions. Unless all the pharmacologic effects of a drug that are known are appreciated, new symptoms may be falsely ascribed to extension or complications of the disease rather than to drug toxicity or reaction. Our success in preventing adverse reactions is critically dependent on our capacity for and interest in acquiring and using valid information.

SUGGESTED READING

1. Kastrup, E. K. (ed.): Drug Facts and Comparisons, 1990 ed. Facts and Comparisons Division of J. B. Lippencott, St. Louis.
2. Reuben, B. G.; and Wittcoff, H. A.: Pharmaceutical Chemicals in Perspective, John Wiley & Sons, New York, 1989.
3. Reynolds, J. E. F. (ed.): Martindale; The Extra Pharmacopoeia, 29th ed. The Pharmaceutical Press, London, 1989.

REFERENCES

Abel, R.; and Leopold, I. H.: Drug-induced ocular diseases. In, Avery's Drug Treatment, 3rd ed. (Speight, T. M., ed.). Adis Press, Hong Kong, pp. 409–417, 1987.

Adkinson, N. F. Jr.; Thompson, W. L.; Maddrey, W. C.; and Lichenstein, L. M.: Routine use of penicillin skin testing on an in-patient service. N. Engl. J. Med., 285:22–24, 1971.

Adler, S. G.; Cohen, A. H.; and Border, W. A.: Hypersensitivity phenomena and the kidney: Role of drugs and environmental agents. Am. J. Kidney Dis., 5:75–96, 1986.

Allan, F. M. (ed.).: Assessing drug reactions—adverse and beneficial. In, Philosophy and Technology of Drug Assessment, Vol. 7. The Interdisciplinary Communications Program. The Smithsonian Institution, Washington, D.C., 1976.

Allport, R. B.: Ipecac is not innocuous. Am. J. Dis. Children, 98:786–787, 1959.

Applebaum, A.: Ophthalmoscopic study of patients under treatment with thioridazine. Arch. Ophthalmol., 69:578–580, 1963.

Applebaum, F. R.; Strauchen, J. A.; Graw, R. G. Jr.; Savage, D. D.; Kent, K. M.; Ferrans, V. J.; and Herzig, G. P.: Acute lethal carditis caused by high-dose combination chemotherapy: A unique clinical and pathological entity. Lancet, 1:58–62, 1976.

Arnold, W.; Nadol, J. B.; and Weidauer, H.: Ultrastructural histopathology in a case of human ototoxicity due to loop diuretics. Acta Otolaryngol., 91:399–414, 1981.

Ballantyne, J. C.: Ototoxicity. J. Laryngol. Otol., 8(suppl.): 9–12, 1983.

Bechtold, H.; 'Andrassy, K.; Jänchen, E.; Koderisch, J.; Koderisch, H.; Weilmann, L. S.; Sonntag, H.-G.; and Ritz, E.: Evidence for impaired vitamin K_1 metabolism in patients treated with N-methyl-thiotetrazole cephalosporins. Thromb. Haemost., 51:358–361, 1984.

Benacerraf, B.: Role of MHC gene products in immune regulation. Science, 212:1229–1238, 1981.

Bennett, W. M.: Drug therapy in renal failure. In, Scientific American Medicine (Rubenstein, E., ed.). Scientific American, New York, 10(II):A3–A35, 1990.

Bennett, W. M.; Arnoff, G. R.; Golper, T. A.; Morrison, G.; Singer, I.; and Brater, D. C.: Drug Prescribing in Renal Failure, 2nd ed. American College of Physicians, Philadelphia, 1991.

Berkseth, R. O.; and Kjellstrand, C. M.: Radiologic contrast-induced nephropathy. Med. Clin. North. Am., 68:351–370, 1984.

Bernstein, J. M.; and Weiss, A. D.: Further observations on salicylate ototoxicity. J. Laryngol. Otol., 81:915–925, 1967.

Bicknell, P. G.: Sensorineural deafness following myringoplasty operations. J. Laryngol. Otol., 85:957–961, 1971.

Bienia, R. A.; Smith, M.; and Pellegrino, T.: Scopolamine skin-disks and anisocoria. Ann. Intern. Med., 99:572–573, 1983.

Black, M.: Chronic drug-induced hepatotoxicity: Clinical aspects. In, Current Perspectives in Hepatology (Seeff, L. B.; and Lewis, J. H.; eds.). Plenum Medical Book, New York, pp. 243–251, 1989.

Blaschke, T. F.: Pharmacokinetics and pharmacoepidemiology. In, Scientific American Medicine (Rubenstein, E., ed.). Scientific American, New York, pp. 1–12, 1986.

Blaschke, T. F.; Nies, A. S.; and Mamelok, R. D.: Principles of therapeutics. In, Goodman and Gilman's The Pharmacologic Basis of Therapeutics, 7th ed. (Gilman, A. G.; Goodman, L. S.; Rall, T. W.; and Murad, F.; eds.). MacMillan, New York, pp. 49–65, 1985.

Bloom, K. E.; Brewer, G. J.; Magon, A. M.; and Weterstroem, N.: Microsomal incubation test of potentially hemolytic drugs for glucose-6-phosphate dehydrogenase deficiency. Clin. Pharmcol. Ther., 33:403–409, 1983.

Bodey, G. P.: Topical and systemic antifungal agents. Med. Clin. North Am., 72:637–659, 1988.

Borda, I. T.; Slone, D.; and Jick, H.: Assessment of adverse reactions within a drug surveillance program. J.A.M.A., 205:99–101, 1968.

Bosher, S. K.: Ethacrynic ototoxicity as a general model in cochlear pathology. Adv. Otorhinolaryngol., 22:81–99, 1977.

Bristow, M. R.; Mason, J. W.; Billingham, M. E.; and Daniels, J. R.: Doxorubicin cardiomyopathy: Evaluation by phonocardiography, endomyocarial biopsy and cardial catherization. Ann. Intern. Med., 88:168–175, 1978.

Brittain, D. C.: Erythromycin. Med. Clin. North. Am., 71:1147–1154, 1987.

Bron, A. J.: Mechanisms of ocular toxicity. In, Drug Toxicity (Gorrod, J. W., ed.). Taylor & Francis, London, pp. 229–253, 1979.

Brown, B. B.; Price, E. V.; and Moore, M. B.: Penicilloyl-polylysine as an intradermal test of penicillin sensitivity. J.A.M.A., 189:599–604, 1964.

Brummett, R. E.: Drug induced ototoxicity. In, Nephrotoxicity and Ototoxicity of Drugs (Ficcastle, P., ed.). University of Rouen Press, Rouen, pp. 359–376, 1982.

Brummet, R. E.; and Fox, K. E.: Aminogylcoside-induced hearing loss in humans. Antimocrob. Agents Chemother., 33:797–800, 1989a.

Brummet, R. E.; and Fox, K. E.: Vancomycin- and erythromycin-induced hearing loss in humans. Antimicrob. Agents Chemother., 33:791–796, 1989b.

Brunton, L. L.: Laxatives. In, Goodman and Gilman's The Pharmacological Basis of Therapeutics, 7th ed. (Gilman, A. G.; Goodman, L. S.; Rall, T. W.; and Murad, F.; eds.). MacMillan, New York, pp. 994–1003, 1985.

Cal, J. C.; Bourdalle-Badie, M.; Croizet, G.; Janvier, P.; Erny, P.; Saric, J.; and Cambar, J.: The relationship between plasma cyclosporin levels and renal tubulotoxicity assessed by enzymuria after liver transplantation. Arch. Toxicol., 12(suppl.):175–178, 1988.

Chapman, P.: Rapid onset hearing loss after cisplatinum therapy: Case reports and literature review. J. Laryngol. Otol., 96:159–162, 1982.

Citron, K. M.: Ethambutol: A review with special reference to ocular toxicity. Tubercle, 50(suppl.):32–26, 1969.

Condemi, J. J.: Hypersensitivity reactions; disorders due to hypersensitivity. In, The Merck Manual, 15th ed. (Berkow, R.; and Fletcher, A. J.; eds.). Merck, Sharp & Dohme Research Labs., Rahway, N.J., pp. 294–322, 1987.

Cooper, J. A. D. Jr.; White, D. A.; and Matthay, R. A.: Drug-induced pulmonary disease: 1. Cytotoxic drugs. Am. Rev. Respir. Dis., 133:321–240, 1986a.

Cooper, J. A. D. Jr.; White D. A.; and Matthay, R. A.: Drug-induced pulmonary disease: 2. Non-cytotoxic drugs. Am. Rev. Respir. Dis., 488–505, 1986b.

Cousins, M. J.; Plummer, J. L. W.; and Hall, P. M.: Toxicity of volatile anesthetic agents. Can. Anaesth. Soc. J., 32:S52–S55, 1985.

Cove-Smith, J. R.; and Knapp, M. S.: Analgesic nephropathy: An important cause of chronic renal failure. Q. J. Med., 47:49–69, 1978.

Critchley, J. A. J. H.; Smith, M. F.; and Prescott, L. F.: Distalgesic abuse and retroperitoneal fibrosis. Br. J. Urol., 57:486–487, 1985.

Crombie, A. L.: Cataract formation associated with the use of phenothiazine derivatives. Prescriber's J., 21:222, 1981.

DeGrunchy, C. C.: Drug-induced Blood Disorders. Blackwell Scientific Publications, Oxford, 1975.

Dickinson, D. S.; Bailey, W. C.; Hirschowitz, B. I.; Soong, S. J.; Eidus, L.; and Hodgkin, M. M.: Risk factors of isoniazid (INH)-induced liver dysfunction. J. Clin. Gastroenterol., 3:271–279, 1981.

Drug and Therapeutics Bulletin. Consumer's Association, London, 1983.

Drug and Therapeutics Bulletin. Consumer's Association, London, 1980.

Edson, R. S.; and Terrell, C. L.: The aminoglycosides: Streptomycin, kanamycin, gentamicin, tobramycin, amikacin, netilmicin, and sisomicin. Mayo Clin. Proc., 62:916–920, 1987.

Ehrenfeld, M.; Nesher, R.; and Merin, S.: Delayed onset chloroquine retinopathy. Br. J. Ophthalmol., 70:281–283, 1986.

Elman, A.; Gullberg, R.; Nilsson, E.; Rendahl, I.; and Wachtmeister, L.: Chloroquine retinopathy in patients with rheumatoid arthritis. Scand. J. Rheumatol., 5:161–166, 1976.

Ettinger, B.; Norman, O.; and Sörgel, F.: Triamterene nephrolithiasis. J.A.M.A., 244:2443–2445, 1980.

Faber, B. F.; and Moellering, R. C. Jr.: Retrospective study of the toxicity of preparations of vancomycin from 1978 to 1981. Antimicrob. Agents Chemother., 23:138–141, 1983.

Food Advisory Committee, FDAC/REP/4, London, H.M. Stationery Office, 1987.

Fenoglio, J. J. Jr.; and Wagner, B. M.: Endomyocardial biopsy approach to drug-related heart disease. In, Principles and Methods of Toxicology, 2nd ed. (Hayes, A. W., ed.). Raven Press, New York, pp. 649–658, 1989.

Fillastre, J. P.; Raguenex-Viotte, G.; and Moulin, B.: Nephrotoxicity of antitumoral agents. Arch. Toxicol., 12(suppl.):117–124, 1988.

Fong, L. P.; Karpman, D. V.; and Goldblatt, J. E. K.: Ocular toxicity of quinine. Med. J. Aust., 141:528–529, 1984.

Franke, E. L.; and Neu, H. C.: Chloramphenicol and tetracycline. Med. Clin. North Am., 71:1155–1168, 1987.

Fraunfelder, F. T.: Transdermal scopolamine precipitating narrow angle glaucoma. N. Engl. J. Med., 307:1079, 1982.

French, A. J.; and Weller, C. V.: Interstitial myocarditis following the clinical and experimental use of sulfonamide drugs. Am. J. Pathol., 18:109–122, 1942.

Gallager, K. I.; and Jones, J. K.: Furosemide-induced ototoxicity. Ann. Intern. Med., 91:744–745, 1979.

Gibaldi, Milo: Nonoral medication. In, Biopharmaceutics and Clinical Pharmacokinetics, 3rd ed. (Milo Gibaldi) (ed.). Lea & Febiger, Philadelphia, pp. 85–112, 1984.

Giles, T. D.; and Modlin, R. K.: Death associated with ventricular arrhythmia and thioridazine hydrochloride. J.A.M.A., 205:108–110, 1968.

Gimenez-Camarasa, J. M.; Garcia-Calderon, P.; and deMoragas, J. M.: Lymphocyte transformation test in fixed drug eruption. N. Engl. J. Med., 292:819–821, 1975.

Girdwood, R. H.: Drug-induced anaemias. Drugs, 11:394–404, 1976.

Glazener, F.; Blake, K.; and Gradman, M.: Bradycardia, hypotension, and near syncope associated with Afrin (oxymetazoline) nasal spray. N. Engl. J. Med., 309:731, 1983.

Goldberger, M. J.: Antituberculous agents. Med. Clin. North Am., 72:661–668, 1988.

Greenberger, P. A.: Contrast media reactions. J. Allergy Clin. Immunol., 74:600–605, 1984.

Harber, L. C.; and Levine, G. M.: Photosensitivity dermatitis from household products. Gen. Pract., 39:95–101, 1969.

Harris, R. T.: Bulimarexia and related serious eating disorders with medical complications. Ann. Intern. Med., 99:800–807, 1983.

Haydon, R. C.; Thelin, J. W.; and Davis, W. E.: Erythromycin ototoxicity: Analysis and conclusions based on 22 case reports. Otolaryngol. Head Neck Surg., 99:678–684, 1984.

Hermans, P. E.; and Wilheim, M. P.: Vancomycin. Mayo Clin. Proc., 62:901–905, 1987.

Hewlett, W. R.; Bugelski, P. J.; Silver, A. C.; Klinker, A.; and Morgan, D. G.: In vivo and in vitro assessment of vancomycin-induced nephrotoxicity. Arch. Toxicol., 12(suppl.):129–136, 1988.

Idsoe, O.; Guthe, T.; and Willcox, R. R.: Nature and extent of penicillin side-reactions, with particular reference to fatalities from anaphylactic shock. Bull. W.H.O., 38:159–188, 1968.

Inman, W. H. W.; and Adelsteen, A. M.: Rise and fall of asthma mortality in England and Wales in relation to use of pressurized aerosols. Lancet, 2:279–285, 1969.

Jackson, G. G.; and Arcieri, G.: Ototoxicity of gentamicin in man: A survey and controlled analysis of clinical experience in the United States. J. Infect. Dis., 124(suppl.):130–137, 1971.

Jick, H.: Drug surveillance: the Boston collaborative program. Hosp. Pract., 9:145–153, Oct. 1974.

Joist, J. H.: Bleeding due to vascular and platelet disorders. In, Current Diagnosis (Conn, R. B., ed.). W. B. Saunders, Philadelphia, pp. 605–624, 1985.

Kahan, B. D.: Cyclosporin nephrotoxicity: Pathogenesis, prophylaxis, therapy, and prognosis. Am. J. Kidney Dis., 8:323–331, 1986.

Kaplowitz, N.; Tak Yee, A. W.; Simon, F. R.; and Stolz, A.: Drug-induced hapatoxicity. Ann. Intern. Med., 104:826–839, 1986.

Karch, F. E.; and Lasagna, L.: Toward the operational identification of adverse drug reactions. Clin. Pharmacol. Ther., 21:247–254, 1977.

Karch, F. E.; and Lasagna, L.: Adverse drug reactions—a critical review. J.A.M.A., 234:1236–1241, 1975.

Kerr, R. O.; Cardamone, J.; Dalmasso, A. P.; and Kaplan, M. E.: Two mechanisms of erythrocyte destruction in penicillin-induced hemolytic anemia. N. Engl. J. Med., 287:1322–1325, 1972.

Koch-Weser, J.: Definition and classification of adverse drug reactions. Drug Inform. Bull., 2:72–78, 1968.

Koch-Weser, J.; Sidel, V. W.; Sweet, R. H.; Kanarek, P.; and Eaton, A. E.: Factors determining physician reporting of adverse drug reactions: Comparison of 2000 spontaneous reports with surveillance studies at the Massachusetts General Hospital. N. Engl. J. Med., 280:20–26, 1969.

Koegel, L.: Ototoxicity: A contemporary review of aminoglycosides, loop diuretics, acetylsalicylic acid, quinine, erythromycin, and cisplatinum. Am. J. Otol., 6:190–199, 1985.

Kondo, J. J.; and Blaschke, T. F.: Drug-drug interactions in geriatric patients. In, Gerontology, 4th International Symposium (Platt, D., ed.). Heidelberg, pp. 257–269, 1989.

Kostenbauder, H. B.; Rapp, R. P.; McGoveen, J. P.; Foster, T. S.; Perrier, D. G.; Blacker, H. M.; Huylon, W. C.; and Kinkel, A. W.: Bioavailability and single dose pharmacokinetics of intramuscular diphenylhydantoin. Clin. Pharmcol. Ther., 18:449–456, 1975.

Kovotzer, J.; and Haddad, Z.: In vitro detection of human IgE mediated immediate hypersensitivity reaction to pollens and penicillin by a modified rat mast cell degranulation technique. J. Allergy, 45:126, 1970.

Küng, L. G.: Hypernephroides Karzinom und Karzinome der ableitenden Harnwege nach Phenacetinabusus. Schweiz. Med. Wschr., 106:47–50, 1976.

LaDelfa, I.; and Melmon, K. L.: Drug therapy and gastrointestinal diagnostic imaging. Specific pharmacologic effects of iodine-containing radio-contrast agents. In, Alimentary Tract Radiology (Marellis, A. R.; and Burheme, H. J.; eds.). C. V. Mosby, Baltimore, pp. 122–123, 1989.

Legha, S. S.; Benjamin, R. S.; MacKay, G.; Ewer, M.; Wallace, S.; Valdivieso, M.; Rasmussen, S. L.; Blumenschein, G. R.; and Freireich, E. J.: Reduction of doxorubicin cardiotoxicity by prolonged continuous intravenous infusion. Ann. Intern. Med., 96:133–139, 1982.

Lennard, H. L.; Epstein, L. J.; Bernstein, A.; and Ransom, D. C.: Hazards implicit in prescribing psychoactive drugs. Science, 169:438–441, 1970.

Len Tseng, H.: Interstitial myocarditis probably related to lithium carbonate intoxication. Arch. Pathol., 92:444–448, 1971.

Levine, B. B.: Immunologic mechanisms of penicillin allergy. N. Engl. J. Med., 275:115–125, 1966.

Levine, B. B.; and Zolov, D.: Prediction of penicillin allergy by immunological tests. J. Allergy, 43:231–244, 1969.

Levine, J. F.: Vancomycin: A review. Med. Clin. North Am., 71:1135–1145, 1987.

Lewis, J. H.: Acute drug-induced hepatic injury. In, Current Perspectives in Hepatology (Seef, L. B.; and Lewis, J. H.; eds.). Plenum Medical Book, New York, pp. 219–242, 1989.

Lewis, J. H.; and Zimmerman, H.: Drug-induced liver disease. Med. Clin. North Am., 73:775–792, 1989.

Lien, E. J.: Chemical structure and side effects. In, Side Effects and Drug Design. Marcel Dekker, New York, pp. 183–315, 1987a.

Lien, E. J.: Side Effects and Drug Design. Marcel Dekker, New York, 1987b.

Lien, E. J.; Lipsett, L. R.; and Lien, L. L.: Structure side effect sorting of drugs: VI. Ototoxicities. J. Clin. Hosp. Pharm., 8:15–33, 1983.

Lockey, S. D.: Reactions to hidden agents in foods, beverages, and drugs. Ann. Allergy, 29:461–466, 1971.

Lopez-Berestein, M. D.: Liposomal amphotericin B in the treatment of fungal infections. Ann. Intern. Med., 105:130–131, 1986.

Mackenzie, A. H.: Antimalarial drugs for rheumatoid arthritis. Am. J. Med., 75:48–58, 1983.

McDevitt, H. O.; and Benacerraf, B.: Genetic control of specific immune responses. Adv. Immunol., 11:31–74, 1969.

McQueen, E. G.: Pharmacological Basis of Adverse Drug Reactions. In, Avery's Drug Treatment, 3rd ed. (Speight, T. M., ed.). Adis Press, Hong Kong, pp. 223–254, 1987.

Melmon, K. L.; and Morrelli, H. F.: Drug reactions. Hypersensitivity. In, Clinical Pharmacology: Basic Principles in Therapeutics, 2nd ed. (Melmon, K. L.; and Morrelli, H. F.; eds.). Macmillian, New York, pp. 957–963, 1978.

Melville, A.: Set and serendipity in the detection of drug hazards. Soc. Sci. Med., 19:391–396, 1984.

Meyer, R. D.: Risk factors and comparisons of nephrotoxicity of aminoglycosides. Am. J. Med., 80(suppl. 6B):119–125, 1986.

Michaelson, G.: Urticaria induced by preservatives and dye in food and drugs. Br. J. Dermatol., 88:525–535, 1973.

Meischer, P. A.: Drug-induced thrombocytopenia. Semin. Hematol., 10:311–325, 1973.

Migasena, S.: Transient total blindness from quinine. Ann. Trop. Med. Parositol., 311:699–701, 1984.

Mitchell, J. R.; Potter, W. Z.; Hinson, J. A.; Snodgrass, W. R.; Timbrell, J. A.; and Gillette, J. R.: Toxic drug reactions. Handb. Exp. Pharmacol., 28:383–419, 1975.

Mitchell, J. R.; Thorgeirsson, S. S.; Potter, W. Z.; Jollow, D. J.; and Keiser, H.: Acetaminophen induced hepatic injury: Protective role of glutathione and rationale for therapy. Clin. Pharmacol. Ther., 16:676–684, 1974.

Mitchell, J. R.; Jollow, D. J.; Gilette, J. R.; and Brodie, B. B.: Drug metabolism as a cause of drug toxicity. Drug Metab. Dispos., 1:418–423, 1973a.

Mitchell, J. R.; Jollow, D. J.; Potter, W. Z.; Gilette, J. R.; and Brodie, B. B.: Acetaminophen induced hepatic necrosis: IV. Protective role of glutathione. J. Pharmacol. Exp. Ther., 187:211–217, 1973b.

Mongan, E.; Kelly, P.; Nies, K.; Porter, W. W.; and Paulus, H. E.: Tinnitus as an indicator of therapeutic serum salicylate level. J.A.M.A., 226:142–145, 1973.

Morris, T. W.; and Fischer, H. W.: The pharmacology of intravascular radiocontrast media. Annu. Rev. Pharmacol. Toxicol., 26:143–160, 1986.

Mullick, F. G.: Acute and chronic hepatotoxicity: Pathological aspects. In, Current Perspectives in Hepatology (Seeff, L. B.; and Lewis, J. H.; eds.). Plenum Medical Book, New York, pp. 253–268, 1987.

Murphy, M. L.; Bullock, R. T.; and Pearce, M. B.: The correlation of metabolic and ultrastructural changes in emetine myocardial toxicity. Am. Heart J., 87:105–108, 1974.

Mushlin, P. S.; and Olson, R. D.: Anthracycline cardiotoxicity: New insights. Ration. Drug Ther., 12:1–8, 1988.

Nierenberg, D. W.; and Glazener, F. S.: Aminophylline-induced exfoliative dermatitis: Cause and implications. West. J. Med., 137:328–331, 1982.

Oppelt, W. W.; White, E. D.; and Halpert, E. S.: The effect of corticosteroids on aqueous humor formation rate and outflow facility. Invest. Ophthalmol., 8:535–541, 1969.

O'Reilly, R. A.: Anticoagulant, antithrombin, and thrombolytic drugs. In, Goodman and Gilman's The Pharmacological Basis of Therapeutics (Gilman, A. G.; Goodman, L. S.; Rall, T. W.; and Murad, F.; eds.). MacMillian, New York, pp. 1138–1359, 1985.

Palmer, E. P.; and Guay, A. T.: Reversible myopathy secondary to abuse of ipecac in patients with major eating disorders. N. Engl. J. Med., 313:1457–1459, 1985.

Palmer, R. F.: Drug misuse and physician education. Clin. Pharmacol. Ther., 10:1–4, 1969.

Panacoast, S. J.: Aminoglycoside antibiotics in clinical use. Med. Clin. North Am., 72:581–612, 1988.

Parker, C. W.: Drug allergy. N. Engl. J. Med., 292:511–514, 726–732, 957–960, 1975.

Parker, C. W.; deWeck, A. L.; Kern, M.; and Eisen, H. N.: The preparation and some properties of penicillenic acid derivatives revelant to penicillin hypersensitivity. J. Exp. Med., 115:803–819, 1962.

Parry, M. F.: The penicillins. Med. Clin. North Am., 71:1093–1112, 1987.

Pead, P. J.; Saeed, A. A.; Hewitt, W. G.; and Brownfield, R. N.: Low immune responses to hepatitis B vaccine among healthy subjects. Lancet, 1:1152, 1985.

Pisciotta, A. V.: Drug-induced agranulocytosis. Drugs, 15:132–143, 1978.

Pohl, L. R.; Satoh, H.; Christ, D. D.; and Kenna, J. G.: The immunologic and metabolic basis of drug hypersensitivities. Annu. Rev. Pharmacol. Toxicol., 28:367–387, 1988.

Porter, J.; and Jick, H.: Drug-induced anaphylaxis, convulsions, deafness, and extrapyramidal symptoms. Lancet, 1: 587–588, 1977.

Post, J.: Yellow vision in patient taking chlorothiazide. N. Engl. J. Med., 263:398–399, 1960.

Pratt, W. B.; and Fekety, R.: The Antimicrobial Drugs. Oxford University Press, New York, 1986.

Prescott, L. F.: Analgesic nephropathy: A reassessment of the role of phenacetin and other analgesics. Drugs, 23:75–149, 1982.

Prescott, L. F.; Newton, R. W.; Swainson, C. P.; Wright, N.; Forrest, A. R. W.; and Matthew, H.: Successful treatment of severe paracetamol over-dosage with cysteamine. Lancet, 1:588–592, 1974.

Prien, R. F.; DeLong, S.; Cole, J. O.; and Levine, J.: Ocular changes occurring with prolonged high dose chlorpromazine therapy. Arch. Gen. Psychiatry, 23:464–468, 1970.

Rab, S. M.: Optic atrophy during chlorpromazine therapy. Br. J. Ophthalmol., 53:208–209, 1969.

Reid, J. L.; Rubin, P. C.; and Whiting, B.: Lecture Notes on Clinical Pharmacology, 3rd ed. Blackwell Scientific Publications, London, 1989.

Reid, W. H.; Blouin, P.; and Schermer, M.: A review of psychiatric medication and the glaucomas. Int. Pharmcopsychiatry, 11:163–176, 1976.

Reidenberg, M. M.; and Caccese, R. W.: Lymphocytic transformation tests and suggested drug allergy. J. Lab. Clin. Med., 86:997–1002, 1975.

Ries, F.; and Klastersky, J.: Nephrotoxicity induced by cancer chemotherapy with special emphasis on cisplatin toxicity. J. Kidney Dis., 8:368–379, 1986.

Roder, F.; Cottin, C.; and Jouglard, J.: Scopolamine transdermique et mydriase. Therapie, 44:447–448, 1989.

Rosenblum, A. H.: Penicillin allergy. J. Allergy, 42:309–318, 1968.

Rosketh, R.; and Storstein, O.: Quinidine therapy of chronic auricular fibrillation. Arch. Intern. Med., 111:184–189, 1963.

Rybak, L. P.: Drug ototoxicity. Annu. Rev. Pharmcol. Toxicol., 26:79–99, 1986.

Rybak, L. P.: Pathophysiology of furosemide ototoxicity. J. Otolaryngol., 11:127–133, 1982.

Schimmel, E. M.: The hazards of hospitalization. Ann. Intern. Med., 60:100–110, 1964.

Schweitzer, V. G.; and Olson, N. R.: Ototoxic effect of erythromycin therapy. Arch. Otolaryngol., 110:258–260, 1984.

Shaffer, R. N.; and Hetherington, J.: Anti-cholinesterase drugs and cataracts. Am. J. Opthalmol., 62:613–618, 1966.

Shaw, R. K.; Raitt, J. W.; and Glazener, F. S.: Agranulocytosis associated with thioridazine administration. J.A.M.A., 187: 614–615, 1964.

Sheffer, A. L.: Therapy of anaphylaxis. N. Engl. J. Med., 275: 1059–1061, 1966.

Sheffer, A. L.; and Pennoyer, D. S.: Management of adverse drug reactions. J. Allergy Clin. Immunol., 74:580–588, 1984.

Singer, I.; Rotenberg, D.; and Preschett, J. B.: Lithium-induced nephrogenic diabetes insipidus: In vivo and in vitro studies. J. Clin. Invest., 51:1081–1091, 1972.

Smidt, N. A.; and McQueen, E. G.: Adverse reactions to drugs: A comprehensive hospital in-patient survey. N.Z. Med. J., 76:397–401, 1972.

Smilkstein, M. J.; Knapp, G. L.; Kulig, K. W.; and Rumack, B. H.: Efficacy of oral N-acetyl cysteine in the treatment of acetaminophen overdosage: Analysis of the national multicenter study (1976–1985). N. Engl. J. Med., 319:1157–1162, 1988.

Smith, P. L.; Kagey-Sobotka, A.; Bleecker, E. R.; Traystman, R.; Kaplan, A. P.; Gralnick, H.; Valentine, M. D.; Permutt, S.; and Lichtenstein, L. M.: Physiologic manifestations of human anaphylaxis. J. Clin. Invest., 66:1072–1080, 1980.

Sogn, D. D.: Penicillin allergy. J. Allergy Clin. Immunol., 74: 589–593, 1984.

Solley, G. O.; Gleich, G. J.; and VanDellen, R. E.: Penicillin allergy: Clinical experience with a battery of skin-test reagents. J. Allergy Clin. Immunol., 69:238–244, 1982.

Spiteri, M. A.; and James, D. G.: Adverse ocular reaction to drugs. Postgrad. Med., 59:343–349, 1983.

Steel, K.; Gertman, P. M.; Crescenzi, C.; and Anderson, J.: Iatrogenic illness on a general medical service at a university hospital. N. Engl. J. Med., 304:638–642, 1981.

Stempel, E.; and Stempel, R.: Drug-induced photosensitivity. J. Am. Pharm. Assoc., 13:200–204, 1973.

Stewart, C. J.; Nunn, A. J.; Stableforth, D.; and Somner, A. R.: Death in asthma: disease or treatment? Lancet, 2:747, 1981.

Stewart, G. T.: Macromolecules residues contributing to the allergenicity of penicillins and cephalosporins. Antimicrob. Agents Chemother., 49:543–549, 1967.

Stewart, G. T.; and McGovern, J. P.: Penicillin Allergy—Clinical and Immunological Aspects. Charles C. Thomas, Springfield, Ill., 1970.

Stillman, M. T.; Napier, J.; and Blackshear, J. L.: Adverse effects of nonsteroidal anti-inflammatory drugs on the kidney. Med. Clin. North Am., 68:371–385, 1984.

Stolley, P. D.; and Lasagna, L.: Prescribing patterns of physicians. J. Chronic Dis., 22:395–405, 1969.

Stuart, J. J.: Ticarcillin-induced hemorrhage in a patient with thrombocytosis. South. Med. J., 73:1084–1085, 1980.

Swanson, D. P.; Thrall, J. H.; and Shetty, P. C.: Evaluation of intravascular low-osmolality contrast agents. Clin. Pharmacol., 5:877–891, 1986.

Swerlick, R. A.; and Lawley, T. J.: Cutaneous vasculitis: Its relationship to systemic disease. Med. Clin. North Am., 73: 1221–1235, 1989.

Taliercio, C. P.; Olney, B. A.; and Lie, J. T.: Myocarditis related to drug hypersensitivity. Mayo Clin. Proc., 60:463–468, 1985.

Theofilopoulos, A.; and Dixon, F. J.: The biology and detection of immune complexes. Adv. Immunol., 28:89–220, 1979.

Thorstrand, C.: Clinical features in poisonings by tricylic anti-depressants, with special reference to the ECG. Acta Med. Scand., 199:337–344, 1976.

Toone, E. C.: Ototoxicity of chloroquine. Arthritis Rheum., 8: 475–476, 1965.

Trowbridge, A. A.; Caraveo, J.; Green, J. B. III; Amaral, B.; and Stone, M. J.: Heparin-related thrombocytopenia: Studies of antibody-heparin specificity. Am. J. Med., 65:277–283, 1978.

Tsuji, A.; Yamana, T.; Miyamoto, E.; and Kiya, E.: Chemical reactions involved in penicillin allergy: Kinetics and mechanisms of penicillin aminolysis. J. Pharm. Pharmacol., 27: 580–587, 1975.

Turk, J. L.; and Baker, H.: Drug reactions: III. Immunoglobulin class E-anaphylactic antibodies. Br. J. Dermatol., 80:622–624, 1968.

Ukena, T.; Esber, H.; Bessette, R.; Park, T.; Crocker, B.; and Shaw, F. E. Jr.: Site of injection and response to hepatitis B vaccine. N. Engl. J. Med., 313:579–580, 1985.

Van Scoy, R. E.; and Wilson, W. R.: Antimicrobial agents in patients with renal insufficiency: Initial dosage and general recommendations. Mayo Clin. Proc., 62:1142–1145, 1987.

Venulet, J.: Increasing threat to man as a result of frequently uncontrolled and widespread use of various drugs. Int. J. Clin. Pharmacol., 12:389–394, 1975.

Verdier, D. D.; and Kennerdall, J. S.: Fixed, dilated pupil resulting from transfermal scopolamine. Am. J. Ophthalmol., 93:803–804, 1982.

Verstraete, M.; and Boogaerts, M. A.: Drug-induced hematological disorders. In, Avery's Drug Treatment, 3rd ed. (Speight, T., ed.). Adis Press, Hong Kong, pp. 1007–1022, 1987.

Vesell, E. S.; Passananti, G. T.; and Greene, F. E.: Impairment of drug metabolism in man by allopurinol and nortriptyline. N. Engl. J. Med., 283:1484–1488, 1972.

Volpe, B. T.; and Soave, R.: Formed visual hallucinations as digitalis toxicity. Ann. Intern. Med., 19:865–866, 1979.

von Voss, H.; Petrich, C.; Karch, D.; Shulz, H. C.; and Göbel, W.: Sodium valproate and platelet function. Br. Med. J., 2: 179, 1976.

Voss, H. E.; Redmond, A. P.; and Levine, B. B.: Clinical detection of the potential allergic reactor to penicillin by immunologic tests. J.A.M.A., 196:679–683, 1966.

Webster, L. T.: Drugs used in the chemotherapy of protozoal infections. In, Goodman and Gilman's the Pharmacologic Basis of Therapeutics, 8th ed. (Gilman, A. G.; Rall, T. W.; Nies, A. S.; and Taylor, P.; eds.). Pergamon Press, Elmsford N.Y., pp. 978–998, 1990.

Weiner, M.; and Bernstein, I. L.: Adverse Reactions to Drug Formulation Agents. Marcel Dekker, New York, 1989.

White, P. D. (citing Withering): Important toxic effect of digitalis overdosage on vision. N. Engl. J. Med., 272:904–905, 1965.

Wiemann, M. C.; and Calabresi, P.: Pharmacology of neoplastic agents. In, Medical Oncology (Calabresi, P.; Schein, P. S.; and Rosenberg, S. A.; eds.). MacMillan, New York, pp. 293–362, 1985.

Willetts, G. S.: Occular side effects of drugs. Br. J. Ophthalmol., 53:252–262, 1969.

Williams, D. M.; Lynch, R. E.; and Cartwright, G. E.: Drug-induced aplastic anemia. Semin. Hematol., 10:195–223, 1973.

Williamson, J.; Paterson, R. W. W.; McGavin, D. D. M.; Jasani, M. K.; Boyl, J. A.; and Doig, W. M.: Posterior subcapsular cataracts and glaucoma associated with long-term oral corticosteroid therapy. Br. J. Ophthalmol., 53:361–372, 1969.

Wilson, A. J.; and Mielke, C. H. Jr.: Neutropenia/agranulocytosis. In, Clinical Management of Poisoning and Drug Overdose (Haddard, L. M.; and Winchester, J. F.; eds.). W. B. Saunders, Philadelphia, pp. 897–899, 1983.

Wilson, K.: Sex-related differences in drug disposition in man. Clin. Pharmacokinet., 9:189–202, 1984.

Wilson, W. R.; and Cockerill, F. R. III: Tetracyclines, chloramphenicol, erythromycin, and clindamycin. Mayo Clin. Proc., 62:906–915, 1987.

Wright, A. J.; and Wilkowske, C. J.: The penicillins. Mayo Clin. Proc., 62:806–820, 1987.

Yamana, T.; Tsuji, A.; Miyamoto, E.; and Kiya, E.: Kinetics and mechanisms of penicillin aminolysis involved in penicillin allergy. J. Pharm. Pharmacol., 27:56–58, 1975.

Yunis, A. A.: Chloramphenicol: Relation of structure to activity and toxicity. Annu. Rev. Pharmacol. Toxicol., 28:83–100, 1988.

Yunis, A. A.; Miller, A. M.; Salem, Z.; Corbett, M. D.; and Arimura, G. K.: Nitrosochloramphenicol: Possible mediator in chloramphenicol-induced aplastic anemia. J. Lab. Clin. Med., 96:36–46, 1980.

Zollinger, H. U.; and Spühler, O.: Die nichteirige, chronische interstitielle Nephritis. Schweiz. Z. Allerg. Pathol. Bakteriol., 13:807–811, 1950.

40

Drug Interactions

J. M. Wright

A number of books and recent reviews on the subject of drug interactions (listed under "Suggested Reading" at the end of this chapter) provide information on the prevalence and mechanisms of such interactions, plus extensive lists of reported drug interactions. Most of these books are well referenced, making it possible to examine the evidence upon which the interaction is based. The interactions also are rated according to their likely clinical relevance, based on the magnitude or severity of the consequences of the interaction. The following section offers the practicing clinician a perspective on potential problems of drug interactions. Clinically important examples have been chosen to demonstrate the possible mechanisms of interactions.

DEFINITION OF DRUG INTERACTIONS

A drug interaction can be defined as a measurable modification (in magnitude or duration) of the action of one drug by prior or concomitant administration of another substance (including prescription and nonprescription drugs, food, or alcohol). The effect of the interaction can be desirable, adverse, or inconsequential. In a recent review article, McInnes and Brodie (1988) have suggested that the definition be changed to a "mathematical" definition; only when the combined effects of interacting drugs are greater or less than the arithmetic sum of their individual actions can the event be considered a true interaction. Unfortunately, our present methods for measuring clinical end points are not precise enough to apply this definition for most drug interactions. The best that can be done to simplify the complexity in the area is to distinguish between "potential" drug interactions and clinically important drug interactions. This chapter will focus on clinically important *adverse* drug interac-

tions. Clinically desirable drug interactions have been reviewed elsewhere (Caranasos et al., 1985) and are part of any good therapeutic regimen when multiple drugs with different mechanisms of efficacious effects are available for the same indication, for example, in the treatment of hypertension.

When describing an adverse drug interaction ordinarily there is an index drug the effect of which is enhanced or canceled by an interacting drug. In some cases two drugs having similar therapeutic or adverse effects, when combined, produce an adverse reaction through an addition of their effects. In such cases, there is no simple distinction between the index and the interacting drug. These interactions are easily recognized. Occasionally both drugs interact with each other. In such cases both drugs are index and both are interacting; a double drug interaction is the result (Wright et al., 1982).

CLINICAL IMPORTANCE OF DRUG INTERACTIONS

In order to understand the clinical importance of adverse drug interactions, we must have a measure of their prevalence. The best estimate comes from the Boston Collaborative Drug Surveillance Program; drug interactions were determined to account for 7% of in-hospital adverse drug reactions (Boston Collaborative Drug Surveillance Program, 1972). If approximately 30% of patients experience an adverse drug reaction while in the hospital (Jick, 1974), then in approximately 2% of inpatients (receiving an average of nine different drugs per hospitalization) the adverse drug reaction would be secondary to a drug interaction. However, it must be remembered that most of these reactions are transient and of minor discomfort to the patient. Serious life-threatening adverse drug reactions occur in 3% of hospital patients (Jick, 1974), and if drug interactions cause 7% of these, then the risk of a serious adverse drug interaction is 0.2%.

The risk in outpatients is probably less, primarily because most of them are exposed to fewer drugs. In one study (Puckett and Visconti, 1971), 2422 outpatients were studied prospectively for 2 months. Of these, 113 (4.7%) were taking combinations of drugs with a potential for interaction, but only 7 (0.3%) showed clinical evidence of an adverse interaction. This again is a relatively low risk. It is, of course, probable that many adverse drug interactions go unrecognized and the risks are higher than the minimum estimates. Although *life-threatening* drug reactions as a result of an interaction are not common and the average practitioner will not be challenged by such cases frequently, skillful clinicians can detect less obvious problems resulting from the interactions.

Potential drug interactions occur frequently. In order to estimate the frequency we need an index drug in which the action can be measured precisely. The oral anticoagulant drugs best fit this description; the effect can be closely measured by the prothrombin time. These drugs also have the longest list of potential interacting drugs (see Appendix II). In a study of 277 patients attending an anticoagulation clinic, 94 (23%) out of 413 treatment courses were likely, theoretically, to interact with anticoagulant therapy. This may be an underestimate of the potential for interaction as the prescribing clinicians may have deliberately avoided drugs well known to interact. How can we explain that potential interactions occur as frequently as 23% and yet clinically detectable adverse drug interactions occur as infrequently as 0.3 to 2%? The best explanation is that in most patients the effect of the interaction must be of small magnitude or the index drug affected must have a wide safety margin. Most potential drug interactions are thus clinically inconsequential.

An example is a recently described interaction between acetaminophen and isoniazid (Epstein et al., 1991). Isoniazid administered at a dose of 300 mg/day for 7 days markedly inhibited the microsomal oxidation of acetaminophen by an average of 70%. Because oxidative metabolism is only a minor component of the elimination of acetaminophen, this resulted in only a 15% decrease in the total body clearance of acetaminophen. The effect on the patient is equivalent to increasing the dose of acetaminophen by 18%, an effect unlikely to be clinically detectable at therapeutic or toxic doses. Even in the event of an acetaminophen overdose, isoniazid, by inhibiting the oxidative metabolism of acetaminophen, would potentially protect the patient from hepatotoxicity, the major toxic effect of acetaminophen.

Many drugs have flat dose–response curves and a high therapeutic index. Such drugs may interact with other drugs, but the interaction is unlikely to lead to an adverse effect.

In most situations in which more than one drug is prescribed, the risk of a clinically important adverse drug interaction is small. However, there are identifiable clinical settings, described later in the chapter, in which the risk is significantly greater. Unrecognized adverse drug interactions are most likely to occur in these high-risk clinical settings. In order to increase the likelihood of identifying an adverse drug interaction the clinician must be aware of the mechanisms by which they may occur. ***Principle: Knowing that two needed drugs can or will interact does not necessarily contraindicate their use. When they are used, dosage adjustments may be needed to obtain appropriate effects. If adversity appears when drugs are being used together, adjusting doses may be more appropriate than discontinuing needed therapy, even if a possible interaction has not yet been reported. Do not deny the possibility that you could be among the first to identify an unsuspected drug interaction*** (see chapters 1 and 41).

MECHANISMS OF DRUG INTERACTIONS

Mechanisms of drug interactions can be divided into those involving the pharmacokinetics and those involving the pharmacodynamics of the index drug. The end result is a significant increase or decrease in the magnitude or duration of one or more effects of the drug.

Pharmacokinetic Drug Interactions

Chemical or Pharmaceutic Interactions. Drugs can react physically or chemically with each other before they are administered to the patient or, in the case of oral preparations, before they are absorbed. The pharmaceutic companies are usually very careful to ensure that interactions affecting the chemical activity of mixtures do not occur in tablets or oral suspensions. When drugs are mixed prior to parenteral administration, they may interact and significantly decrease the activity of one or of each other (see Smith, 1984). As a general rule, drugs should not be mixed prior to parenteral administration unless they have been proved by rigorous testing to be chemically compatible.

Chemical interactions are very unlikely to occur once drugs reach the systemic circulation because the concentrations in plasma are low. However, such is not the case for orally administered drugs prior to absorption. The best known example of a chemical interaction in the GI tract is the chelation of calcium, magnesium, aluminum, or iron by tetracyclines, resulting in partial or complete failure of absorption of the cation–tetracycline complex. In this case, the effects of the bonded drugs are nullified. Cholestyramine and colestipol also can bind a number of anionic drugs and decrease their absorption. Except for tetracyclines, the magnitude of these interactions has not been associated with complete loss of efficacy. Once again, the demonstration that such a chemical interaction occurs does not mean that the medications cannot be given concomitantly. The magnitude of the interaction and the dose–response relationship of the drug must be taken into account. In one case it might be best to give the index drug 1 hour before or 2 hours after the interacting drug. In another case, it may be more convenient and enhance compliance to give the index drug along with the interacting drug. As in all cases, the dose of the drug must be titrated to the desired clinical end point. *Principle: When a fundamental mechanism of a drug reaction has been demonstrated with a given agent, look for that agent to interact with other drugs of similar chemical makeup even if the additional drugs are not used for the same indication and even if the interaction has not yet been described.*

Interactions Affecting Oral Bioavailability. Chemical interaction in the GI tract, described above, can decrease oral bioavailability. The other important steps necessary for a drug (taken orally) to reach the systemic circulation include gastric emptying, absorption across the intestinal wall, and passage from the portal circulation through the liver into the systemic circulation. Interactions can occur at these sites.

Gastric Emptying. Affects on rate of gastric emptying generally alter the rate but not the extent of absorption (bioavailability) of drug. The rate of gastric emptying is important when a rapid onset of effect of the drug is desired. Such is the case when rapid relief from pain or onset of sedation are required and parenteral administration is not possible. The best way to enhance the rate of gastric emptying is for the patient to take the drug on an empty stomach with a volume of water (at least 200 ml) and to remain in an upright position. Factors that slow gastric emptying include food (calories), recumbency, heavy exercise, autonomic neuropathy, and a number of drugs, including antacids, anticholinergic drugs, and narcotics (see Nimmo, 1976). Drugs that enhance gastric emptying, such as metoclopramide and domperidone, may result in earlier and higher peak concentrations of index drugs. In instances when the rate of onset of effect of the index drug is not important, effects on gastric emptying time do not generally result in clinically significant events. The exception to this rule is in using drugs that are inacti-

vated in the acid milieu of the stomach. In such cases (e.g., in using penicillin G and L-dopa) factors that delay gastric emptying can decrease bioavailability. In contrast, an increased rate of GI transit may decrease absorption of drugs with low dissolution rates or drugs that are very poorly absorbed (e.g., griseofulvin). It is not uncommon for patients with short GI transit times or the short-bowel syndrome to report the passage by rectum of intact enteric-coated tablets. Embarrassment should result if such a history were the first hints to the therapist that a regimen was not working.

Absorption. Most drugs are absorbed in the small intestine by a process of passive diffusion. Other drugs are unlikely to interfere with this process. Drugs can, however, damage the intestinal absorptive surface (e.g., oral neomycin, antineoplastic drugs) and potentially result in decreased absorption of otherwise poorly absorbed drugs.

Food that is taken in large quantities has a much greater potential for affecting drug absorption (Toothaker and Welling, 1980). Food can decrease, increase, or have no effect on the oral bioavailability of drugs. Two generalizations about drug–food interactions can be made. First (if the issue of lack of efficacy is omitted), there are very few instances of drug–food interactions having been proved to cause clinically adverse events. Therefore, they seldom justify the inconvenience to the patient of attempting to take the drug on an empty stomach. Second, the mechanism of the interaction is complex and not proved for most of the documented drug–food interactions (Carr, 1982).

Presystemic Elimination. Many drugs are extracted or metabolized during transit across the intestinal epithelium or during the first pass through the liver. This phenomenon (see chapter 37) has been called *presystemic elimination*, or *first-pass effect* (Routledge and Shand, 1979). A large number of commonly prescribed drugs are subject to significant presystemic hepatic elimination and thus have low oral bioavailability (e.g., propranolol, metoprolol, labetalol, verapamil, hydralazine, chlorpromazine, amitriptyline, imipramine, and morphine). These drugs have a high extraction ratio and high intrinsic hepatic clearance that varies inversely with liver blood flow, that is, their clearance is liver-blood-flow dependent. Therefore, oral bioavailability can be increased or decreased by drugs that increase or decrease liver blood flow, respectively; for example, propranolol and cimetidine directly reduce liver blood flow and would be expected to raise the steady-state concentration of the above drugs given at constant dosage before and after the administration of either interacting drug. The drugs listed above can also compete with each other and augment each other's bioavailability, for example, chlorpromazine and propranolol (Vestal et al., 1979; Peet et al., 1981). In addition, drugs that induce or inhibit liver microsomal metabolism (see Table 40–1) can respectively decrease or increase the bioavailability of drugs with high presystemic hepatic elimination (Daneshmend and Roberts, 1984). Another point to remember is that ingestion of these drugs with food generally increases their bioavailability; the mechanism is complex but probably involves transient increase in hepatic blood flow and transient inhibition of drug metabolism associated with eating (Liedholm and Melander, 1986).

The food–drug interactions while using monoamine oxidase inhibitors (MAOIs) are partly the result of inhibition of presystemic elimination. The nonselective MAOIs, such as phenelzine and tranylcypromine, inhibit MAO A in the intestinal wall and liver. Thus, tyramine, which is found in certain foods, and sympathomimetic drugs, particularly in over-the-counter decongestant mixtures, are not completely metabolized during absorption and the first pass through the liver. When these agents reach the systemic circulation, they can act directly on vessels or indirectly to release noradrenaline, causing the well-known syndrome of sympathetic hyperactivity. The selective MAO B inhibitors (e.g., selegiline, also known as deprenyl) are less likely to cause this interaction (Schulz et al., 1989).

Protein-Binding-Drug Interactions. Once a drug reaches the systemic circulation after parenteral or oral administration, it is distributed throughout the body. This distribution is dependent upon the ionic composition, lipid solubility, and protein-binding characteristics of the drug (see chapters 1 and 37). Protein binding occurs primarily to albumin or α_2-acid glyprotein in the plasma or to tissue proteins. Only free drug can exert a pharmacologic effect, and the serum concentration of measured drug usually reflects the total drug in the plasma, free plus bound. Drugs that are highly bound in plasma are potentially subject to displacement from this carrier protein by another drug with affinity for the same protein. When another highly bound drug is added, competitive displacement may occur, resulting in a *transient* increase in the free concentration of the index drug. This is followed by rapid redistribution and an increase in clearance, creating a new equilibrium of both drugs. The effect is likely to produce a clinically significant effect only if the index drug has a small volume of distribution, a narrow therapeutic ratio, and a rapid onset of action in relation to its concentration in plasma. Assessment of the role of displacement in drug interactions has been hampered by the difficulties in measuring free-drug concentrations. Many of the drug interactions formerly classified as displacement interactions were probably primarily the result of the interacting drug's also decreasing the clearance of the index drug (Koch-Weser and Sellers, 1976; MacKichan, 1989). *Principle: Knowing one mechanism of interaction between two drugs is not the same as knowing all the mechanisms that operate to produce the clinical effect. As settings vary, the net effect of the interaction can vary.*

Drug Interactions Due to Altered Biotransformation. Drug metabolism most often occurs in the liver and involves the conversion of an active, nonpolar drug to polar metabolites (generally less active or inactive) that are cleared by the kidneys. Occasionally, metabolites are pharmacologically active in similar or dissimilar ways from the progenitor or may be themselves toxic. The steady-state concentration of the drug in plasma is dependent on the volume of distribution and the clearance (chapter 1). Drugs that are extensively metabolized (i.e., only a small proportion of the dose administered is excreted unchanged in the urine) are susceptible to interactions affecting drug metabolism. Most drugs are metabolized by a number of different pathways, making prediction of the consequences of metabolic interactions difficult if not impossible. In fact, the metabolism of an index drug can be inhibited or induced by another drug or even by itself.

Many commonly prescribed drugs have the potential to inhibit the metabolism of other drugs. Whether this effect leads to a clinically significant interaction is dependent upon the magnitude of the decrease in clearance of the index drug and the consequences of the resulting increase in

Table 40–1. COMMONLY USED DRUGS THAT ALTER MICROSOMAL ENZYME ACTIVITY

Inhibitors of Enzyme Activity

Amiodarone	Metronidazole
Chloramphenicol	Miconazole
Cimetidine	Oral contraceptives
Disulfiram	Phenothiazines
Ethanol (acute)	Phenylbutazone
Erythromycin	Sulfinpyrazone
Isoniazid	Sulfonamides
Ketaconazole	Tricyclic antidepressants
Methylphenidate	Valproate

Inducers of Enzyme Activity

Barbiturates	Meprobamate
Carbamazepine	Phenytoin
Ethanol (chronic)	Phenobarbital
Ethchlorvynol	Primidone
Glutethimide	Rifampin
	Tobacco smoke

steady-state serum concentration of the index drug. Most clinically significant inhibitory interactions involve the hepatic microsomal oxidative enzymes. The magnitude of the effect is largely unpredictable because it depends on the specific enzyme or enzymes inhibited and the quantitative importance of that pathway in the overall clearance of the index drug. For example, isoniazid is a potent inhibitor of the microsomal oxidation of both carbamazepine and acetaminophen. With acetaminophen, conjugative metabolic pathways (type II) predominate, and this results in a clinically insignificant 15% decrease in total plasma clearance of acetaminophen (Epstein et al., 1991). In the case of carbamazepine, oxidative metabolic pathways (type I) predominate, and isoniazid inhibits total plasma clearance by as much as 45%, resulting in an increase in steady-state serum concentration of 85% and a significant risk of toxic effects (Wright et al., 1982). The time course of the change in serum concentration is dependent on the new half-life of the index drug (requiring 4–5 half-lives) to reach a new steady state (Rogge et al., 1989) (see chapters 1 and 36).

Enzyme inhibition can be produced by a number of different mechanisms (Testa and Jenner, 1981). Irreversible destruction or inactivation of an enzyme can lead to the longest-lasting effects (DeMontellano and Correia, 1983) (e.g., prolonged effect produced by the MAOIs). Another factor leading to the unpredictability of these interactions is that most microsomal inhibitors also have the capacity to induce microsomal enzymes (e.g., ethanol).

Commonly prescribed drugs that have been implicated in inhibitory drug interactions are listed in Table 40–1. Inhibitory interactions seldom contraindicate the concomitant use of the two drugs. The clinician must be aware of the interaction and decrease, if required, the dose of the index drug to prevent toxicity.

Drug Interactions Due to Altered Renal Excretion of Drugs. Water-soluble drugs are eliminated largely unchanged by the kidneys. The clearance of drugs that are excreted entirely by glomerular filtration is unlikely to be affected by other drugs. However, the clearance of drugs that are actively transported into the tubular lumen can be significantly inhibited by other drugs. This interaction can be used to advantage (e.g., probenecid decreases the clearance of penicillin) but occasionally may lead to toxicity (e.g., methotrexate toxicity can be caused by inhibition of its tubular secretion by salicylate) (Zuik and Mandel, 1975). *Principle: There is hardly a class of adverse drug interaction that cannot be used to therapeutic advantage.*

Lithium carbonate is a special case, because it is an ion that is excreted primarily by the kidney. As a univalent cation, it is affected by changes that alter total body balance of sodium. Renal clearance of lithium is significantly decreased by thiazide and loop diuretics (Mehta and Robinson, 1980); the sodium loss caused by the diuretic is associated with increased proximal tubular sodium and lithium reabsorption. Some NSAIDs also decrease renal elimination of lithium (Ragheb et al., 1980). Because of its low toxic/therapeutic ratio, lithium is one of the index drugs (see Table 40–2) with a high risk of adverse drug interactions.

Interactions Involving Enzyme Induction

The microsomal enzyme systems in the liver and other tissues are notable in that their activity can be induced by many drugs and chemicals. The process of induction involves increased protein synthesis, increased amounts of the enzyme, and consequently an increase in the V_{max} of the reaction. Because of the requirement for producing new proteins, the time course of induction is considerably longer than inhibition and may take 2 to 3 weeks to reach a maximal effect in humans. Drugs that induce metabolizing enzymes may be classified depending on the specific P450 enzymes that are induced. Inducible families of enzymes include the phenobarbital type, polycyclic hydrocarbon type, steroid type, and alcohol type. Commonly used drugs that are microsomal enzyme inducers are listed in Table 40–1.

Enzyme induction can enhance the metabolism of the inducing agent (autoinduction) and/or a variety of other drugs and some endogenous compounds, such as cortisol and bilirubin. Induction may be associated with marked increases in clearance of index drugs, resulting in loss of efficacy. For example, rifampin has been implicated as a cause of graft rejection in patients receiving otherwise adequate doses of cyclosporine and prednisone (Langhoff and Madsen, 1983) and as a cause of failure of effect of oral contraceptives (Breckenridge et al., 1979). Furthermore, in patients on a methadone maintenance program, the introduction of phenytoin has precipitated withdrawal

Table 40–2.   INDEX DRUGS WITH LOW THERAPEUTIC INDICES

Oral anticoagulants
Anticancer and immunosuppressive drugs
Antidysrhythmic drugs
Lithium carbonate
Oral hypoglycemic drugs
Anticonvulsants
Theophylline
Digoxin
Aminoglycosides

symptoms (Tong et al., 1981). If the induction interaction is recognized, the dose of the index drug can be increased appropriately. If the inducing drug is later stopped, the dose of the index drug may have to be decreased to prevent toxicity.

In some cases, induction of the increased rate of metabolism can result in increased formation of a toxic metabolite with serious consequences. For example, administration of carbamazepine may increase the risk of isoniazid-induced hepatotoxicity by increasing the formation of a toxic metabolite of isoniazid (Wright et al., 1982; Barbare et al., 1986).

Pharmacodynamic Drug Interactions

Pharmacodynamic mechanisms are difficult to classify. Any drug interaction that cannot be explained by a measurable pharmacokinetic alteration is basically attributed to a pharmacodynamic mechanism.

Receptor Interactions. A few adverse drug interactions are understandable and predictable based on their well-known pharmacologic effects. For example, β_2-adrenergic blocking drugs antagonize the effects of β_2-adrenergic agonists such as salbutamol and can significantly interfere with the clinical management of patients with asthma. Similarly, the antiparkinsonian action of L-dopa can be antagonized by the dopamine-blocking drugs haloperidol and metoclopramide. An understanding of the mechanism of action of the drug allows the clinician to predict and avoid such adverse interactions.

Drugs also can inhibit transport processes and thus affect the action of other drugs. The tricyclic antidepressants, through their action to block the reuptake of amines can potentiate the action of epinephrine and norepinephrine (Boakes et al., 1973b). For this reason, it is recommended that local anesthetics without sympathomimetics be used for patients taking tricyclic antidepressants (Boakes et al., 1973a). The tricyclic antidepressants also antagonize the antihypertensive action of clonidine; the suggested mechanism is by the α-receptor-antagonist action of the tricyclic compounds in the CNS (Briant et al., 1973).

It must be remembered that many drugs (antihistamines, antinauseants, phenothiazines, and tricyclic antidepressants) share with atropine the ability to block muscarinic receptors. These drugs alone may have mild anticholinergic effects. However, in combination they can produce a full-blown anticholinergic syndrome causing confusion and memory loss; the elderly are particularly at risk.

Other drugs (aminoglycosides, polymyxins, lo-cal anesthetics) have weak inhibiting effects on neuromuscular transmission, either by decreasing release of acetylcholine or by blocking nicotinic receptors. These drugs have no discernible effect in the patient with normal neuromuscular transmission, where a wide safety margin is present. However, in patients who have lost this safety margin (e.g., postsurgical patients who have received neuromuscular blocking drugs, or patients with myasthenia gravis), these drugs may produce neuromuscular paralysis and apnea (Sanders and Sanders, 1979).

Additive and Antagonistic Pharmacodynamic Interactions. Most of these interactions are intuitively evident. It should not be surprising that two drugs with sedative properties, for example, benzodiazepines and alcohol, can add to or potentiate each other's sedative action. This is equally so whether the sedative property of the drug is the primary action or whether it is a potential side effect, for example, methyldopa, propranolol, antihistamines, and so forth. It is important that physicians and patients be constantly reminded of the dangers of driving a motor vehicle while under the influence of drugs and/or alcohol. The additive effect of drugs affecting coagulation at two different steps, for example, warfarin and salicylates, also has been associated with severe adverse consequences.

Equally preventable interactions are those whose additive effects are undesirable adverse effects associated with each of the drugs, for example, both the hyperglycemia and the hypokalemia secondary to either hydrocortisone or hydrochlorothiazide or their combination. Another example is supplemental potassium, potassium-sparing diuretics, and angiotensin-converting enzyme inhibitors; each alone may occasionally cause hyperkalemia, but when they are used together in the hypertensive patient, the risk of causing clinically important hyperkalemia is greatly increased.

Potentiation of risk of toxicity through a pharmacodynamic mechanism is more difficult to establish and remember. Most physicians monitor and maintain potassium concentrations in patients taking digoxin because they are aware of the potentiation of digitalis toxicity by diuretic-induced hypokalemia. Physicians are less likely to be aware of the increased risk of ototoxicity and nephrotoxicity with the combination of aminoglycosides and furosemide.

Antagonistic pharmacodynamic interactions are more likely to go unrecognized, as it is easy to miss the fact that a chronically administered drug is no longer effective. *Principle: Unless the physician is particularly concerned about a drug interaction nullifying efficacy, he or she may attribute worsening of the disease to the disease process. In such a situation, the physician can come to believe that the disease is worsening in spite of therapy rather than because of it. Furthermore, many adverse drug interactions can mimic aspects of disease that were the indications for using the drugs in the first place.* The NSAIDs have potent antagonistic actions. These drugs are very commonly prescribed and are available to the public without prescription, for example, salicylates and ibuprofen. As a group, these drugs have renal effects that may cause clinically significant salt and water retention or reversible renal failure. These drugs, therefore, are frequently associated with loss of therapeutic effect of other drugs in patients with congestive heart failure or hypertension (Webster, 1985).

Unrecognized Drug Interactions. There always is concern about the possibility of dangerous unrecognized drug interactions that could cause preventable deaths. One such cause of death is the setting classified as *sudden death*. Adverse drug interactions leading to this type of sudden death certainly are possible. For instance, drugs that prolong the QT interval may cause lethal ventricular dysrhythmias. Class IA antiarrhythmic agents, including quinidine, procainamide, and disopyramide, have a potential proarrhythmic effect. Less well known is that the class III drugs amiodarone, bretylium, and sotalol, and the psychoactive drugs, tricyclic antidepressants, and phenothiazines, also can prolong the QT interval. If one adds to this the possibility that hypokalemia may increase the risk of ventricular dysrhythmia in the presence of a prolonged QT interval, there exists a potential for a number of dangerous interactions with combination of drugs that prolong the QT interval and drugs causing hypokalemia (McKibbin et al., 1984).

Drug Interactions Involving Multiple Mechanisms. Many drug–drug interactions involve more than one mechanism. The complexity of the problem is exemplified by the interaction of quinidine and digoxin; the administration of quinidine to patients receiving digoxin results in two- to threefold increase in steady-state concentration of digoxin. At least three different pharmacokinetic effects caused by quinidine have been described: (1) quinidine decreases the renal clearance of digoxin, (2) quinidine decreases the extrarenal clearance of digoxin, and (3) quinidine decreases the volume of distribution of digoxin. A number of careful studies produced conflicting data on the quantitative importance of each of these mechanisms (Fichtl and Doering, 1983). Moreover, there are questions whether the increase in the serum concentration of digoxin reflects an equivalent increase at the sites of action on the heart.

Despite best efforts, a precise measure of the clinical significance of this complex interaction is still lacking. However, the evidence suggesting that these changes may contribute to an increased risk of digoxin toxicity is sufficient to warrant decreasing the dose of digoxin by one half when quinidine is added.

The combination of verapamil and propranolol is another example of a complex interaction. This combination has been associated with congestive heart failure, severe bradycardia, AV block, and even ventricular asystole. However, others have advocated the efficacy and safety of the combination. In a recent study of this interaction in eight healthy young men, during exercise the combination of the two drugs produced clinically important fatigue that was not seen with the individual drugs (Carruthers et al., 1989). The combination significantly reduced heart rate and prolonged the exercise PR interval. These effects could only partially be explained by the two pharmacokinetic interactions that were demonstrated. The study raises doubt about the safety of the combination and again emphasizes the multiple mechanisms and complexity of many interactions.

HIGH-RISK CLINICAL SETTINGS

A physician cannot and should not try to remember all the documented or potential drug interactions. Since the risk is small in most clinical settings, there is no incentive to learn them by heart. The astute clinician can decrease the risk of adverse consequences of drug interactions by being aware of the clinical settings in which the risk of adverse drug interactions is increased.

The most common high-risk clinical setting occurs when the physician prescribes index drugs that have both low toxic/therapeutic ratios (therapeutic indices) and a relatively steep dose-response relationship (see Table 40-2). The classic example of such drugs is warfarin and the other oral anticoagulants. The effect of warfarin is dependent on a competitive equilibrium between warfarin and vitamin K_1 in the liver. Any perturbation in the pharmacokinetics of warfarin or vitamin K or in the turnover of the vitamin K-dependent clotting factors causes a change in the prothrombin time and necessitates a change in warfarin dose. The chance of an interaction is great enough with warfarin that most clinicians warn the patient not to start or stop any other drug (including OTC drugs), except when this can be done in a setting in which the effect on the prothrombin time can be monitored. By careful monitoring and adjustment of the dose of warfarin, adverse consequences due to bleeding or loss of effect can be prevented.

The other index drugs listed in Table 40-2 are

also at higher risk of adverse drug interactions than the average drug. These drugs have a defined narrow therapeutic index, and the concentration or effect of the drug can be monitored. Fortunately, most drugs have a wide safety margin and do not require the vigilance and frequent monitoring of the drugs listed in Table 40–2.

A patient receiving large numbers of drugs also is at high risk. As the number of drugs increases, the risk of an adverse drug reaction increases disproportionately (Smith et al., 1966; May et al., 1977; Nolan and O'Malley, 1988a,b). This disproportionate increase, most prevalent in patients taking 10 or more drugs, is most likely a result of drug interaction(s).

A third clinical setting with an increased risk of adverse drug reactions is the critically ill patient. These patients have lost their physiologic reserve in one or more systems and often are dependent on the actions of one or more drugs to function. Examples include patients with renal, hepatic, respiratory, heart, or autonomic failure, Alzheimer's dementia, and myasthenia gravis. In these patients, giving drugs with a narrow therapeutic window creates a particularly high risk setting. Further, the physician should not be lulled into a false sense of security simply because a drug has a large therapeutic index when given to a relatively healthy individual. The same drug given to some patients with a different disease may have a surprisingly narrow therapeutic index. For example, propranolol given to a patient with uncomplicated hypertension is relatively safe, but the risk would be quite different for a patient with congestive heart failure. Similarly, narcotics may be safe given to healthy patients with a toothache but not to patients with respiratory failure. In such patients relatively small change in the effect of a drug as a result of a drug interaction could have a significant clinical impact. Yet these patients are precisely those in whom the adverse drug interactions are most likely to go unrecognized. Their deterioration is most often attributed to their underlying disease and not to drug therapy. The newest group of patients at high risk are those with AIDS. They not only develop organ failure from a multitude of infections but receive large numbers of toxic drugs and have a propensity to immunologically mediated drug reactions.

A fourth setting for particularly high risk therapy is in prescribing for a passive patient. Most outpatients have a low risk of adverse drug interactions, probably because they take few drugs and they want an active role in their therapy. Active patients demand that the benefit/risk ratio of any medication is substantially in their favor. Passive patients are at significantly higher risk and often do not know the reason for taking or trying not to take many of their medications. Psy-

chiatric patients and the elderly constitute a large proportion of such passive patients. Most important, they *are more prone to receive many medications simultaneously and for indefinite periods.* The elderly also are prone to adverse drug interactions because of the deterioration in their physiologic functions that ordinarily compensate for the severe effects of drugs (e.g., compensation via the autonomic nervous system for insulin-induced hypoglycemia). Deterioration of homeostatic mechanisms leads to a lowering of the margin of safety of many drugs. Clinicians have a responsibility to be particularly thoughtful when treating such patients by minimizing the number of their medications.

A final group of patients who are prone to adverse drug interactions are drug abusers. These individuals are likely to be addicted to tobacco and alcohol, take illegal recreational drugs, and consume OTC drugs. They also are more likely to take excessive amounts of prescription drugs and to be erratic in their drug-taking behavior. Because of the large numbers of drugs being taken simultaneously and in large doses, the margin of safety is lost and drug interactions are more likely to result in adverse events.

In the high-risk clinical settings listed, recognition of a clinically important adverse drug interaction is extremely difficult. Unrecognized adverse drug interactions, both previously documented and previously undocumented, occur (see chapters 34, 36, and 41). The most likely adverse drug interaction to go unrecognized involves an interacting drug's diminishing the effectiveness of an index drug. For example, in a patient taking eight medications for the management of coronary insufficiency, high blood pressure, and congestive heart failure, the clinician has a difficult time proving the efficacy and necessity of each agent. One effective drug could readily cancel the effectiveness of another. Only by withdrawing drugs and careful clinical assessment can the necessity of each agent then be ensured. *Principle: When therapy in a high-risk patient is initiated, it probably is more appropriate for the patient's health to assess the efficacy and toxicity of each drug as it is added to a regime, rather than halt all drugs in order to regain efficacy or reverse toxicity.*

Computerized Drug-Interaction Systems. Computerized systems for identifying potential drug interactions have been available for many years (Cohen et al., 1974) but are not widely used today. Pharmacy-based computer systems (Kirking et al., 1986) are more widely used than physician-based systems (Davidson et al., 1987); however, neither has proved to be indispensable. The problems with computer systems reflect the problems of drug-interaction detection outlined above. These include a complex, uncertain data base, often dependent on single case reports; potential drug interactions that greatly outnumber the clinically important adverse interactions; a need for each potential drug interaction detected to be interpreted in the clinical setting of the individual patient; time required for data entry and decision making; and the characteristics of various computer systems that enhance or detract from their acceptability (Kirking et al., 1986). If these problems can be overcome and more efficient interactive systems can be developed, a computerized drug-interaction system specifically for use in high-risk clinical settings could be quite cost-effective.

PRINCIPLES OF PREVENTION OF ADVERSE DRUG INTERACTIONS

Following are straightforward principles that a clinician can employ to minimize the risk of causing an adverse drug interaction:

Principles:

1. Document and record all drugs, including OTC and recreational drugs, that your patient is consuming. This list must be carefully reviewed before a new medication is prescribed, for either outpatients or inpatients.

2. Learn about the pharmacodynamics and as much of the pharmacokinetics of the drugs you prescribe as possible, also keeping in mind the mechanisms of potential drug interactions.

3. Minimize the number of drugs given to any patient and try to ensure that the benefit/risk ratio of each is significantly greater than 1. This means being certain that each drug has the potential of identifiable benefit based on its known pharmacology or excellent empirical data. This principle of therapy is difficult to follow but can be met by careful assessment of clinical end points.

4. Be particularly vigilant with patients taking high-risk index drugs.

5. Be cautious in high-risk clinical settings. Intensive care specialists must be particularly cognizant of the risk of adverse drug interactions, both when they are using drugs for indications outside their specialty and when using drugs with which they have become overly familiar and perhaps complacent.

6. Look carefully for the possibility of an adverse drug interaction whenever a patient's course deteriorates. If the deterioration is due to drug therapy, it probably is reversible. Use of textbooks of drug interactions or adverse-drug-interaction computer programs in such settings may be valuable to detect something you have not considered.

7. Always look for previously undescribed interactions, particularly when prescribing new drugs or those with which you are not familiar. New drugs on the market will have had little or no testing in combination with most other drugs. The combination that you prescribe may represent a novel experiment. A positive development is that some, but not fully adequate, interaction data are now being generated prior to a new drug is becoming widely available (see Rogge et al., 1989).

In conclusion, the potential for measurable interactions to occur when two or more drugs are prescribed to a patient is considerable. The mechanisms of these interactions are complex, often multiple, and at present incompletely understood for many combinations. Fortunately, primarily because of the wide margin of safety of most drugs in most clinical settings, the risk of serious adverse drug interactions is low, but the morbidity of an interaction is not defined in terms of mortality alone. The physician must remain vigilant to detect or avoid these problems which may have deleterious effects on therapy.

SUGGESTED READING

Aronson, J. K.; and Grahame-Smith, D. G.: Clinical pharmacology. Adverse drug interactions. Br. Med. J., 282:288–291, 1981.

Brodie, M. J.; and Feely, J.: Adverse drug interaction. Br. Med. J., 296:845–849, 1988.

Griffin, J. P.; D'Arcy, P. F.; and Speirs, C. J. (eds.): A Manual of Adverse Drug Interactions, 4th ed. Wright, London, 1988.

Hansten, P. D. (ed.): Drug Interactions, 5th ed. Lea & Febiger, Philadelphia, 1985.

Hansten, P. D. (ed.): Drug Interactions Newsletter, Applied Therapeutics, San Francisco, monthly.

McInnes, G. T.; and Brodie, M. J.: Drug interactions that matter. A critical reappraisal. Drugs, 36:83–110, 1988.

The Mediphor Editorial Group, Division of Clinical Pharmacology, Stanford University School of Medicine. Drug Interaction Facts (Mangini, R. J., ed.). Lippincott, St. Louis, 1983.

Rizack, M. A.; and Hillman, C. D. M. (eds.): The Medical Letter Handbook of Adverse Drug Interactions. The Medical Letter, New Rochelle, N.Y., 1985.

Rosenberg, J. M.; and Rosenberg-Rosen, M. S. (eds.): Prescriber's Guide to Drug Interactions. Medical Economics Books, Oradell, N. J., 1989.

Shinn, A. F.; and Shewsbury, R. P. (eds.): Evaluations of Drug Interactions, 3rd ed. Mosby, St. Louis, 1985.

Weibert, R. T.; and Norcross, W. A. (eds.): Drug Interactions Index, 2nd ed. Medical Economics Books, Oradell, N.J., 1988.

REFERENCES

Barbare, J. C.; Lallement, P. Y.; Vorhauer, W.; and Veyssier, P.: Hépatotoxicité de l'isoniazide: Influence de la carbamazépine? Gastroenterol. Clin. Biol., 10:523–524, 1986.

Boakes, A. J.; Laurence, D. R.; Lovel, K. W.; O'Neil, R.; and Verrill, P. J.: Adverse reactions to local anaesthetic/vasoconstrictor preparations. Br. Dent. J., 133:137–140, 1973a.

Boakes, A. J.; Laurence, D. R.; Teoh, P. C.; Barar, F. S. K.; Benedikter, L. T.; and Prichard, B. N. C.: Interactions between sympathomimetic amines and antidepressant agents in man. Br. Med. J., 1:311–315, 1973b.

Boston Collaborative Drug Surveillance Program: Adverse drug interactions. J.A.M.A., 220:1238–1239, 1972.

Breckenridge, A. M.; Back, D. J.; and Orme, M.: Interactions between oral contraceptives and other drugs. Pharmacol. Ther., 7:617–626, 1979.

Briant, R. H.; Reid, J. L.; and Dollery, C. T.: Interaction between clonidine and desipramine in man. Br. Med. J., 1: 522–523, 1973.

Caranasos, G. J.; Stewart, R. B.; and Cluff, L. E.: Clinically desirable drug interactions. Annu. Rev. Pharmacol. Toxicol., 25:67–95, 1985.

Carr, C. J.: Food and drug interactions. Annu. Rev. Pharmacol. Toxicol., 22:19–29, 1982.

Carruthers, S. G.; Freeman, D. J.; and Bailey, D. G.: Synergistic adverse hemodynamic interaction between oral verapamil and propranolol. Clin. Pharmacol. Ther., 46:469–477, 1989.

Cohen, S. N.; Armstrong, M. F.; Briggs, R. L.; Feinberg, L. S.; Hannigan, J. F.; Hansten, P. D.; Hunn, G. S.; Moore, T. N.; Nishimura, T. G.; Podlone, M. D.; Shortliffe, E. H.; Smith, L. A.; and Yosten, L.: A computer-based system for the study and control of drug interactions in hospitalized patients. In, Drug Interactions (Morselli, P. L.; Garanttini, S.; and Cohen, S. N.; eds.). Raven Press, New York, 363–374, 1974.

Daneshmend, T. K.; and Roberts, C. J. C.: The effects of enzyme induction and enzyme inhibition on labetalol pharmacokinetics. Br. J. Clin. Pharmacol., 18:393–400, 1984.

Davidson, K. W.; Kahn, A.; and Price, R. D.: Reduction of adverse drug reactions by computerized drug interaction screening. J. Fam. Pract., 25:371–375, 1987.

Dollery, C.; and Brennan, P. J.: The Medical Research Council Hypertension Trial: The smoking patient. Am. Heart J., 115: P276–P281, 1988.

DeMontellano, P. R. O.; and Correia, M. A.: Suicidal destruction of cytochrome P-450 during oxidative drug metabolism. Annu. Rev. Pharmacol. Toxicol., 23:481–503, 1983.

Epstein, M. M.; Nelson, S. D.; Slattery, J. T.; Kalhorn, T. F.; Wall, R. A.; and Wright, J. M.: Inhibition of the metabolism of acetaminophen by isoniazid. Br. J. Clin. Pharmacol., 31: 139–142, 1991.

Fichtl, B.; and Doering, W.: The quinidine-digoxin interaction in perspective. Clin. Pharmacokinet., 8:137–154, 1983.

Jick, H.: Drugs—Remarkably nontoxic. N. Engl. J. Med., 291: 824–828, 1974.

Kirking, D. M.; Thomas, J. W.; Ascione, F. J.; and Boyd, E. L.: Detecting and preventing adverse drug interactions: The potential contribution of computers in pharmacies. Soc. Sci. Med., 22:1–8, 1986.

Koch-Weser, J.; and Sellers E. M.: Drug Therapy: Binding of drugs to serum albumin (second of two parts). N. Engl. J. Med., 294:311–316, 526–531, 1976.

Langhoff, E.; and Madsen, S.: Rapid metabolism of cyclosporin and prednisone in kidney transplant patient receiving tuberculostatic treatment. Lancet, 2:1031, 1983.

Liedholm, H.; and Melander, A.: Concomitant food intake can increase the bioavailability of propranolol by transient inhibition of its presystemic primary conjugation. Clin. Pharmacol. Ther., 40:29–36, 1986.

MacKichan, J. J.: Protein binding drug displacement interactions. Fact or fiction? Clin. Pharmacol., 16:65–73, 1989.

McKibbin, J. K.; Pocock, W. A.; Barlow, J. B.; Miller, R. M. S.; and Obel, I. W. P.: Sotalol, hypokalaemia, syncope, and torsade de pointes. Br. Heart J., 51:157–162, 1984.

May, F. E.; Stewart, R. B.; and Cluff, L. E.: Drug interactions and multiple drug administration. Clin. Pharmacol. Ther., 22:322–328, 1977.

McInnes, G. T.; and Brodie, M. J.: Drug interactions that matter: A critical reappraisal. Drugs, 36:83–110, 1988.

Mehta, B. R.; and Robinson, B. H. B.: Lithium toxicity induced by triamterene-hydrochlorothiazide. Postgrad. Med. J., 56:783–784, 1980.

Nimmo, W. S.: Drugs, diseases and altered gastric emptying. Clin. Pharmacokinet., 1:189–203, 1976.

Nolan, L.; and O'Malley, K.: Prescribing for the elderly: I. Sensitivity of the elderly to adverse drug reactions. J. Am. Geriatrics, 36:142–149, 1988a.

Nolan, L.; and O'Malley, K.: Prescribing for the Elderly: II. Prescribing patterns: Differences due to age. J. Am. Geriatrics, 36:245–254, 1988b.

Peet, M.; Middlemiss, D. N.; and Yates, R. A.: Propranolol in schizophrenia: II. Clinical and biochemical aspects of combining propanolol with chlorpromazine. Br. J. Psychiatry, 139:112–117, 1981.

Puckett, W. H. Jr.; and Visconti, J. A.: An epidemiological study of the clinical significance of drug-drug interactions in a private community hospital. Am. J. Hosp. Pharm., 28:247–253, 1971.

Ragheb, M.; Ban, T. A.; Buchanan, D.; and Frolich, J. C.: Interaction of indomethacin and ibuprofen with lithium in manic patients under a steady-state lithium level. J. Clin. Psychiatry, 41:11:397–398, 1980.

Rogge, M. C.; Solomon, W. R.; Sedman, A. J.; Welling, P. G.; Koup, J. R.; and Wagner, J. G.: The theophylline-enoxacin interaction: II. Changes in the disposition of theophylline and its metabolites during intermittent administration of enoxacin. Clin. Pharmacol. Ther., 46:420–428, 1989.

Routledge, P. A.; and Shand, D. G.: Presystemic drug elimination. Annu. Rev. Pharmacol. Toxicol., 19:447–468, 1979.

Schulz, R.; Antonin, K.-H.; Hoffman, E.; Jedrychowski, M.; Nilsson, E.; Schick, C.; and Bieck, P. R.: Tyramine kinetics and pressor sensitivity during monoamine oxidase inhibition by selegiline. Clin. Pharmacol. Ther., 46:528–536, 1989.

Sanders W. E.; and Sanders C. C.: Toxicity of antibacterial agents: Mechanism of action on mammalian cells. Annu. Rev. Pharmacol. Toxicol., 19:53–83, 1979.

Smith, M.: Drug interactions involving infusion therapy. In, Nervous System, Endocrine System and Infusion Therapy (Petrie, J. C., ed.). Vol. 2. Elsevier Science, Amsterdam, pp. 329–355, 1984.

Smith, J. W.; Seidl, L. G.; and Cluff, L. E.: Studies on the epidemiology of adverse drug reactions: V. Clinical factors influencing susceptibility. Ann. Intern. Med., 65:629–640, 1966.

Testa, B.; and Jenner, P.: Inhibitors of cytochrome P-450s and their mechanism of action. Drug Metab. Rev., 12:1–117, 1981.

Tong, T. G.; Pond, S. M.; Kreek, M. J.; Jaffery, N. F.; and Benowitz, N. L.; Phenytoin-induced methadone withdrawal. Ann. Intern. Med., 94:349–351, 1981.

Toothaker, R. D.; and Welling, P. G.: The effect of food on drug bioavailability. Annu. Rev. Pharmacol. Toxicol., 20: 173–199, 1980.

Vestal, R. E.; Kornhauser, D. M.; Hollifield, J. W.; and Shand, D. G.: Inhibition of propranolol metabolism by chlorpromazine. Clin. Pharmacol. Ther., 25:19–24, 1979.

Webster, J.: Interactions of NSAIDs with diuretics and beta-blockers: Mechanisms and clinical implications. Drugs, 30: 32–41, 1985.

Wright, J. M.; Stokes, E. F.; and Sweeney, V. P.: Isoniazid-induced carbamazepine toxicity and vice versa. A double drug interaction. N. Engl. J. Med., 307:1325–1327, 1982.

Zuik, M.; and Mandel, M. A.: Methotrexate-salicylate interaction: A clinical and experimental study. Surg. Forum, 26: 567–569, 1975.

41

A Clinical Epidemiologic Approach to Therapeutics

Brian L. Strom

Chapter Outline

The Host: Patient Factors in Clinical
    Therapeutics
The Agent: Information Available on
    Therapeutic Options
    Sources of Information

Types of Study Designs
The Environment: Synthesizing Information
    to Make a Therapeutic Decision
Summary

Throughout this book, we have tried to provide an approach to rational therapeutics that is useful in all areas and applications of drug therapy. In this final chapter, we will discuss some of the difficulties encountered when the prescribing physician tries to use the best information available about the efficacy and toxicity of drugs in his or her patients.

All active scientific fields, including clinical pharmacology, are continually advancing, and new drugs continually appear. Practicing clinicians need to integrate the new information available on drugs in the context of the core principles of clinical pharmacology. Only then can the best possible therapeutic decisions be made. Unfortunately, the information necessary to make the optimal decision often is incomplete, especially for the newest drugs (see chapters 34 and 35). Despite this deficiency, a clinical decision must be made for the patient at hand.

Linking clinical pharmacology with epidemiology and, in particular, clinical epidemiology can help the clinician to make the best possible decisions. *Epidemiology* studies the distribution and determinants of diseases in populations (MacMahon and Pugh, 1970; Friedman, 1974; Lilienfeld and Lilienfeld, 1980; Ahlbom and Norell, 1984; Mausner and Kramer, 1985; Kelsey et al., 1986). It conventionally considers the determinants of diseases that relate to the host, the agent, or the environment. For a question of therapeutics, the *host* is the patient, with his or her unique characteristics that need to be taken into account to individualize therapy. The *agent* is the drug or drugs and whatever information may be known about their effects. The *environment* is the body of clinical pharmacologic principles, such as those which

are in this book. This chapter will be organized in this fashion.

The field of *clinical epidemiology* focuses on how to critically review the medical literature and how to apply the principles of epidemiology to clinical medicine (Sackett et al., 1985; Schuman, 1986; Rothman, 1986; Weiss, 1986; Hennekens and Buring, 1987; Fletcher et al., 1988; Hulley and Cummings, 1988). Clinical epidemiology also has been conceptualized as involving four central aspects of disease: (1) burden of disease, including frequency and prognosis, (2) etiology of disease, (3) diagnosis, and (4) treatment of disease. All these are highly relevant to individual therapeutic decisions for a patient. This chapter presents a clinical epidemiologic approach to therapeutics by first discussing the information about the patient that must be taken into account, then the information about the drug, and finally placing these in context with selected core principles of clinical pharmacology. The chapter attempts to synthesize all three. Reference sources in which each of these topics is discussed in more detail are provided.

Finally, *pharmacoepidemiology* is the study of drug use and drug effects in populations (Strom, 1989a). In a sense, this chapter discusses clinical pharmacoepidemiology, that is, pharmacoepidemiology as it applies to the individual patient.

THE HOST: PATIENT FACTORS IN CLINICAL THERAPEUTICS

By now it should be clear that clinical therapeutics involves the use and choice of drugs tailored to the needs of the patient at hand. To tailor therapy to an individual patient's needs, one obviously has to explore the characteristics of the patient. Taking a traditional history and performing a physical examination (Bates, 1979) represent the first steps in making a therapeutic decision and are critical in making a correct diagnosis (Griner et al., 1981). The severity and prognosis of the disease must then be assessed. The severity of the disease partially determines the need for drug treatment. A severe disease and/or a poor prognosis are more compelling indications for drug treatment than the amelioration of symptoms of an inconsequential medical problem. In the former one should be more willing to incur known or unknown risks of toxicity. In contrast, a disease that is mild and self-limited should not, in general, be treated unless the treatment is both very effective and very benign.

The severity of the disease generally is determined by a clinical judgment, based on a clinician's observation of the individual patient. Determination of the prognosis of the disease, in contrast, is almost always a decision based on the available literature about the disease. While one may have sufficient clinical experience with a given disease to have a sense of its prognosis, reviewing the literature almost always adds further useful information. Studies of large populations of patients with the disease (case series — see below), preferably including a comparison with a control group of patients without that disease (cohort studies — see below), are needed to truly evaluate a disease's prognosis. When detailed information is available on the determinants of a good or poor prognosis, one can determine whether an individual patient has a prognosis similar to or different from others who have the same disease, for example, the stage of cancer.

In addition to the details of a patient's illness, one must pay careful attention to other factors in making a therapeutic decision. In particular, determining whether a patient is receiving other drugs is necessary to avoid drug interactions. Knowledge of past drug allergies can be used to avoid preventable adverse drug reactions (see chapter 39). Finally, awareness of other diseases from which the patient suffers, particularly those affecting renal and liver functions, allows perspective on how to avoid drug–disease interactions (see chapter 1). When all these factors can be considered, one can approach a therapeutic decision armed with sufficient detail about a possible indication for drug use in the patient.

THE AGENT: INFORMATION AVAILABLE ON THERAPEUTIC OPTIONS

Once one has decided that a patient has a disease that should be treated, one needs to consider the available options in choice of drug and drug regimen for the patient. In particular, a clinician must understand the clinical pharmacology of the therapeutic options available in this situation. For this decision, information on both the pharmacokinetics and the pharmacodynamics of the drug is needed.

Sources of Information

The primary source of this information is the medical literature. Textbooks often can provide a useful synthesis of the information available in the medical literature, easing the practitioner's task of analyzing the data and providing expert judgment. Section II of this book was intended to provide just such a service for many clinical situations. Other good sources of drug information are the U.S. Pharmacopoeia *Drug Information* series, the American Medical Association's *Drug Evaluations*, and so forth (United States Pharmacopoeia, 1988; American Medical Association, 1971). Clinical textbooks also may be useful.

Despite these sources, there will undoubtedly be many times when one needs to resort to the primary medical literature, either because the textbooks do not provide exactly the information needed or because the opinions expressed in the texts are incomplete, contradict each other, or need validation. Given the continual development of new drugs and the rapid acquisition of new data on old drugs, most textbooks risk being out of date on some topics almost as soon as they are published. It is for this reason that this book has stressed principles that should be applicable in many diseases, not just the examples given.

Clinicians must develop skills to investigate and properly interpret the medical literature themselves. Sometimes the information can be found in a physician's personal clinical files. However, even in the largest of practices, the incidence rates of a given drug- or disease-related event would have to be very high for personal experience to be sufficient for determining the best medical decisions.

Sometimes key references can be identified from references included in textbooks or in review articles. However, the results of different papers often are conflicting. Then critical evaluation of the medical literature depends on an individual's skills to validate and/or decide on the applicability of each paper to the patient at hand. A valid judgment cannot be made based on a selective literature search. Often the search must be comprehensive, even though abbreviated. Fortunately, this is now much easier with the advent of data bases such as Medline, and a number of commercial vendors of software that makes accessing Medline more user friendly to the individual clinician (e.g., Grateful Med and BRS Colleague). Some of these data bases even have the full text of the papers online, so the paper itself can be read without leaving the computer terminal. Of course this level of detailed literature search is not always necessary or feasible. One often is sufficiently aware of the literature in one's speciality that a computer search is unnecessary. What is important, however, is that one not be limited to selected or potentially biased sources of information such as isolated papers, a physician's personal experience, or the *Physicians' Desk Reference* (Physicians' Desk Reference, 1990).

Types of Study Designs

A major focus of clinical epidemiology is to enable clinicians to develop skills in interpreting the medical literature. There is a growing literature specifically aimed at how to read and critique the medical literature (e.g., Unknown, 1981a–1981e; Unknown, 1984a–1984c). To a degree, these skills develop as a function of practice, initially under supervision. However, one first has to understand the basic types of study designs used in clinical research and their advantages and disadvantages.

In Fig. 41–1 the various study designs are presented in hierarchical fashion. The least convinc-

Experimental Studies (Randomized Clinical Trials)

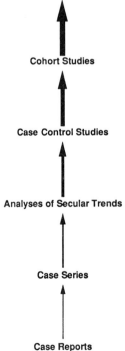

Cohort Studies

Case Control Studies

Analyses of Secular Trends

Case Series

Case Reports

Fig. 41–1. Study designs used in clinical research.

ing designs are on the bottom of the list and the most convincing designs (but hardest to do) on the top of the list. These are reviewed in more detail elsewhere (Strom, 1989b) and are thoroughly described in a number of clinical epidemiology texts (Sackett et al., 1985; Schuman, 1986; Rothman, 1986; Weiss, 1986; Hennekens and Buring, 1987; Fletcher et al., 1988; Hulley and Cummings, 1988). These designs are briefly reviewed here, especially as the methodology specifically applies to clinical pharmacology.

Case Reports. Much of the medical literature is composed of case reports. These describe an individual patient, his or her exposure to drugs, and the individual's clinical outcome. The drug exposures encountered by the individual may or may not have caused his or her clinical outcome. Most information on adverse drug effects comes, at least initially, from case reports sent either to the medical literature or to FDA's spontaneous reporting system (see chapter 34). This approach to uncovering the unknown effects of a drug is useful for raising hypotheses about possible drug effects. For example, oral contraceptives were first linked to venous thromboembolism in case reports (Ferguson, 1967). As another example, the fact that suprofen caused acute bilateral flank pain and renal failure was identified based on the spontaneous reporting system (Rossi et al., 1988). On the other hand, many case reports of possible adverse drug reactions in the literature subsequently are not confirmed to be due to the drug (Lauper, 1980). A causal relationship between drug and event is more likely when (1) one is studying a disorder that occurs extraordinarily rarely without the use of the drug, (2) one can compile a number of reports of individuals who had the same adverse outcome while taking the drug, or (3) one can compile a series of patients in whom the event appeared as the drug was given and then disappeared (i.e., the patient recovered) as the drug was discontinued, and finally recurred when the drug was restarted. Most case reports cannot be relied on to demonstrate whether a drug truly causes a given adverse outcome. These are very important limitations of the case report literature, even though those reports are common.

Case Series. Case series are reports of groups of patients who have either a common drug exposure or a common disease. These series focus on detecting subsequent disease outcome or antecedent exposures to drugs that can cause the disease, respectively. Case series are an improvement over case reports. Because these are groups of patients, they are more likely to be typical of those who have the exposure, or those who have the disease.

A case series can be useful, for example, for quantitating the incidence of an adverse event in a group of patients treated with a newly marketed drug. Absent a control group, however, they rarely can be used to conclude whether a drug causes a given outcome. Despite this shortcoming, case series frequently have been used to study the effects of marketed drugs, as so-called phase IV cohort studies. For example, a phase IV cohort study of prazosin was conducted to quantitate the frequency of first-dose syncope (Joint Commission on Prescription Drug Use, 1980).

Analyses of Secular Trends. Analyses of secular trends are studies that compare trends in exposures to drugs with trends in a given disease or event. The study looks to see whether the two trends coincide. The trends can be over time or across geographic areas. In studies relevant to clinical pharmacology, the exposures obviously are to drugs. The data on exposures generally come from marketing data about drug sales. The data on occurrences of disease usually come from publicly collected vital statistics. This approach is useful as a fast and easy method to provide support for or refutation of a hypothesis about a drug effect. Thus, the incidence of a disease in question can be explored to see whether it has increased since a new drug was released into the market, or whether the incidence of the disease differs in countries that have allowed the marketing of the drug versus those that have not. For example, the association between oral contraceptives and thromboembolism was confirmed by analyses of secular trends that confirmed coincident trends between increasing sales of oral contraceptives and increasing mortality rates from pulmonary embolism, trends that were present in women of reproductive age, but not in men or postmenopausal women (Markush and Seigel, 1969). However, usually there are many different exposures to drugs whose trends coincide with the trend in incidence of a disease. In addition, there are many exposures to factors other than drugs that also coincide with the changed incidence of the disease. These studies cannot generally differentiate which exposure is the causal factor in the events of interest.

Case Control Studies. Case control studies compare individuals with a disease to individuals without a disease. A search for differences in "exposures" antecedent to the disease is then undertaken (see Fig. 41–2). The case control approach can be very useful to explore any of a number of drugs as possible causes of a single disease, especially a very rare disease. The approach also is very useful for exploring diseases that take a long time to develop. For example, the association between oral contraceptives and thromboembolism was confirmed in case control studies (Sartwell et al., 1969). Case control studies can even be used to screen for beneficial drug effects. For example, the protective effect of aspirin on the development of myocardial infarction was suggested in a case control study (Rosenberg et al., 1982). This was confirmed in a randomized clinical trial, but not until many years later (Steering Committee of the Physicians' Health Study Research Group, 1989).

Case control studies are subject to a number of important problems, however. It is difficult to choose an undiseased control group that is properly comparable to the case group. Choosing the wrong control group can result in very misleading conclusions. Also, gathering drug histories retrospectively often is very difficult because patients and often clinicians are not aware of the drugs

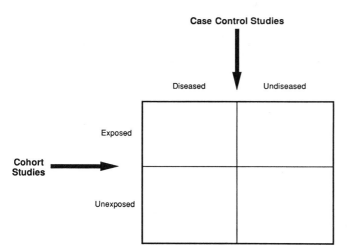

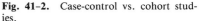

Fig. 41–2. Case-control vs. cohort studies.

the patients are taking now, let alone those that they took previously (Harlow and Linett, 1989). Examples of major errors in findings by case control studies include the studies linking reserpine to breast cancer (Heinonen et al., 1974; Armstrong et al., 1974; Boston Collaborative Drug Surveillance Program, 1974) and those linking coffee to pancreatic cancer (MacMahon et al., 1981).

Cohort Studies. Cohort studies compare exposed to unexposed patients and evaluate differences in outcome (see Fig. 41–2). Cohort studies are especially useful for the study of many possible outcomes from a single exposure, especially when it is a relatively uncommon exposure. This approach can be extremely useful in the study of a number of different effects caused by a single newly marketed drug. For example, a pair of large, long-term cohort studies of oral contraceptives performed in the United Kingdom were very useful in exploring the effects of these drugs (Royal College of General Practitioners, 1974; Vessey et al., 1976), including the risk of venous thromboembolism (Royal College of General Practitioners, 1978). However, cohort studies can be difficult and expensive to perform. Furthermore, even though they can show differences in the effects of the exposure in different groups, they still do not guarantee that the exposed and the unexposed groups are comparable.

Randomized Clinical Trials. Randomized clinical trials are studies in which the investigator has control of the therapy the patient receives. He or she randomly assigns the subjects of this study to receive the study drug, a control drug, or no drug at all (placebo). This is the "Cadillac" of study designs. It virtually guarantees that the groups being compared are similar; only the effects of the drug should cause differences between the two groups. For this reason, studies using this definitive design are required prior to marketing a drug. On the other hand, randomized clinical trials are not always feasible or ethical. For example, it would be impossible to perform a randomized clinical trial of oral contraceptives versus placebo, looking for differences in the risk of venous thromboembolism. This approach is particularly useful, and often necessary, when studying the expected beneficial effects of drugs, that is, drug efficacy. In contrast, the other techniques are usually sufficient to study the unexpected adverse or beneficial effects of drugs and sometimes can be used to study a drug's anticipated beneficial effects (Strom and Melmon, 1989).

Synthesis. When reviewing a paper on therapeutics, the reader should first determine which of the study designs is being used. That identification immediately reveals the advantages and disadvantages of the design and has major implications for the validity of the conclusions of the study. Each study design has an appropriate role in scientific progress. In general, science proceeds from the bottom of Fig. 41–1 upward, from case reports and case series suggesting an association to analyses of trends and case control studies exploring them. Finally, if a study question warrants the delay and investment, cohort studies and randomized clinical trials can be performed. A clinician must understand where in this process any given paper fits. Then the reader must evaluate how well the investigators carried out each study.

Finally, in addition to critically evaluating the design of the study, a clinician should pay attention to its size (Young et al., 1983; Strom, 1989c; Strom, 1989d). A study that does not show a statistically significant difference may be too small to detect an important difference, even if one is there. Such a "negative" conclusion does not represent evidence against the drug having the effect in question. As an analogy, the fact that one cannot find an amoeba when searching for it with a magnifying glass does not prove that the amoeba is not present.

THE ENVIRONMENT: SYNTHESIZING INFORMATION TO MAKE A THERAPEUTIC DECISION

At the point that the best available information about the patient's status and the effects of drugs under consideration for treatment are at hand, the last step is to synthesize the information about patient and therapy with the principles of clinical pharmacology to make a therapeutic decision.

First the clinician must decide on which, if any, drug to use. To do this, he or she must balance the efficacy of the drug with other factors, including its known toxicity, its novelty (remembering that a newer drug has as-yet-unknown toxicity), potential interactions with other drugs and with other illnesses the patient has, the cost of the drug, ease of administration, and so forth. The risk/benefit balance of a particular drug for a particular patient then needs to be compared with the risk/benefit balance for using other alternative drugs and procedures or leaving the patient untreated.

These comparisons need to be highly individualized for a given patient. For example, a physician confronted with a 20-year-old woman who appears to have sustained a pulmonary embolism while taking oral contraceptives will be likely to embark on heparin therapy, pending the results of more definitive diagnostic tests. If the patient were an 80-year-old man with known contraindications to heparin (e.g., bleeding ulcer, recent stroke), then there would be sensible reluctance to embark on anticoagulation, and other therapies would be chosen (see chapter 22). As another related example, after initiating anticoagulation with heparin in a patient with deep venous thrombosis, the physician would usually begin therapy with warfarin promptly. However, if the patient were a 20-year-old woman who had not taken her oral contraceptives and was pregnant, the oral anticoagulation would be contraindicated because of the teratogenic effects of warfarin (see chapter 22).

Once one chooses a drug, generally the choice of regimen is based on a similar risk/benefit judgment. Higher doses of a drug generally increase the likelihood of efficacy but also are more likely to result in toxicity.

One always should choose a specific therapeutic end point before starting a course of treatment: efficacy, toxicity, a target concentration, or a target dose. This end point must be chosen very overtly, or the patient is likely to receive continued therapy too long or to be removed from therapy prematurely. The optimal end point is a clinical one. The therapeutic end point for observation can include objective measures of drug effects as well as independent pharmacologic end points that define the risk/benefit balance of the drug in the individual patient. If one can observe the beneficial and toxic effects in the patient at hand, for example, digoxin used for treatment of atrial fibrillation, one should do so. Often such an end point is not available. In such a case, one should consider using a target concentration or, if necessary, even a target dose. For example, a physician treating an otherwise healthy young man with serious asthma with theophylline would be likely to "push" the drug regimen until a concentration of theophylline in plasma toward the upper end of its therapeutic range was obtained or until the patient recovered from bronchospasm or suffered from evident clinical toxicity (whichever came first). If the patient were a 70-year-old man with chronic obstructive pulmonary disease, arrhythmias, and little reversible lung disease, the potential risks of aggressive treatment with theophylline would be greater, while the potential benefits would be fewer.

Once a course of treatment is begun, monitoring its effects, stopping it, modifying it, or adding to it as needed are key decisions. The key parameters to be monitored are the chosen therapeutic end points. If the clinical effects of the drug are apparent in the patient, the clinician should observe them and change the regimen according to their presence. If the therapeutic end point is a plasma drug concentration, therapeutic drug monitoring still must be individualized. For example, while most patients do not become toxic with theophylline until the plasma concentration

exceeds 20 mg/l, some patients develop toxicity at lower concentrations. One should treat the patient rather than the laboratory test. Sometimes, if a clinical therapeutic end point is difficult to evaluate because of spontaneous variation in the course of the disease, it may be useful to perform an "N of 1 Trial" (see chapter 35).

In addition to monitoring end points of efficacy and toxicity, the clinician should monitor patient compliance. Generally, patients should be asked to bring all their medications with them on each visit. This makes it easier to be certain that the patient understands his or her regimen. The procedure allows clarification of the true regimen and permits informal or even formal pill counts to evaluate patient compliance (see chapter 33). Before abandoning a drug or adding a second drug for the same indication, the clinician should seek maximum benefit from the drug. This means ensuring maximum compliance and optimal and perhaps maximal dosing.

Finally, once the course of treatment is over, the physicians should examine whether there is anything unusual about the patient's reactions to the drug that deserves to be shared with colleagues. Only by sharing such experiences can we all learn more completely and more quickly about the effects of the drugs we use. In its simplest fashion, this could mean reporting adverse reactions to the drug to the FDA using the adverse drug reaction reporting form in the back of every *Physicians' Desk Reference* and FDA *Drug Bulletin*. It also could mean reporting the experience in the literature.

SUMMARY

This book presented general principles of rational therapeutics that required the physician to have the best information available concerning his or her patient and all available drugs. The practicing physician needs to make a decision in the best interest of his or her patient based on whatever information is available, even though that information is often inadequate. However, when the data are inadequate, it is even more important to be able to judge the validity and completeness of the limited information that is available. To quote Sir Austin Bradford Hill:

All scientific work is incomplete—whether it be observational or experimental. All scientific work is liable to be upset or modified by advancing knowledge. That does not confer upon us a freedom to ignore the knowledge we already have, or to postpone the action that it appears to demand at a given time.

Who knows, asked Robert Browning, but the world may end tonight? True, but on available evidence most of us make ready to commute on the 8:30 next day.

Sir Austin Bradford Hill (Hill, 1965)

REFERENCES

Ahlbom, A.; and Norell, S.: Introduction to Modern Epidemiology. Epidemiology Resources, Chestnut Hill, Massachusetts, 1984.

American Medical Association: Drug Evaluations, 6th ed. Philadelphia, 1971.

Armstrong, B.; Stevens, N.; and Doll, R.: Retrospective study of the association between use of rauwolfia derivatives and breast cancer in English women. Lancet, 2:672-675, 1974.

Bates, B.: A Guide to Physical Examination, 2nd ed. J. B. Lippincott, Philadelphia, Toronto, 1979.

Boston Collaborative Drug Surveillance Program: Reserpine and breast cancer. Lancet, 2:669-671, 1974.

Ferguson, J. N.: Pulmonary embolization and oral contraceptives. J.A.M.A., 200:560, 1967.

Fletcher, R. H.; Fletcher, S. W.; and Wagner, E. H.: Clinical Epidemiology. Williams & Wilkins, Baltimore, 1988.

Friedman, G.: Primer of Epidemiology. McGraw-Hill, New York, 1974.

Griner, P. F.; Mayewski, R. J.; Mushlin, A. I.; and Greenland, P.: Selection and interpretation of diagnostic tests and procedures. Ann. Intern. Med., 94:553-600, 1981.

Harlow, S. D.; and Linett, M. S.: Agreement between questionnaire data and medical records. The evidence for accuracy of recall. Am. J. Epidemiol., 129:233-248, 1989.

Heinonen, O. P.; Shapiro, S.; Tuominen, L.; and Turunen, M. I.: Reserpine use in relation to breast cancer. Lancet, 2: 675-677, 1974.

Hennekens, C. H.; and Buring, J. E.: Epidemiology in Medicine. Little Brown, Boston, 1987.

Hill, A. B.: The environment and disease: Association or causation? Proc. R. Soc. Med., 58:295-300, 1965.

Hulley, S. B.; and Cummings, S. R.: Designing Clinical Research. Williams & Wilkins, Baltimore, 1988.

Joint Commission on Prescription Drug Use: Final Report. Subcommittee on Health and Scientific Research, U.S. Senate, Washington, D.C., 1980.

Kelsey, J. L.; Thompson, W. D.; and Evans, A. S.: Methods in Observational Epidemiology. Oxford University Press, New York, 1986.

Lauper, R. D.: The medical literature as an adverse drug reaction early warning system. Report of the Joint Commission on Prescription Drug Use, Appendix VI, Subcommittee on Health and Scientific Research, United States Senate, Washington, D.C., 1980.

Lilienfeld, A. M.; and Lilienfeld, D. E.: Foundations of Epidemiology, 2nd ed. Oxford University Press, New York, 1980.

MacMahon, B.; and Pugh, T. F.: Epidemiology. Little Brown, Boston, 1970.

MacMahon, B.; Yen, S.; Trichopoulos, D.; Warren, K.; and Nardi, G.: Coffee and cancer of the pancreas. N. Engl. J. Med., 304:630-633, 1981.

Markush, R. E.; and Seigel, D. G.: Oral contraceptives and mortality trends from thromboembolism in the United States. Am. J. Public Health, 59:418-434, 1969.

Mausner, J. S.; and Kramer, S.: Mausner and Bahn—Epidemiology: An Introductory Text. W B Saunders, Philadelphia, 1985.

Physicians' Desk Reference: Medical Economics, Oradell, N.J., 1990.

Rosenberg, L.; Slone, D.; Shapiro, S.; Kaufman, D. W.; Miettinen, O. S.; and Stolley, P. D.: Aspirin and myocardial infarction in young women. Am. J. Public Health, 72:389-391, 1982.

Rossi, A. C.; Bosco, L.; Faich, G. A.; Tanner, A.; and Temple, R.: The importance of adverse reaction reporting by physicians. Suprofen and the flank pain syndrome. J.A.M.A., 259:1203-1204, 1988.

Rothman, K. J.: Modern Epidemiology. Little Brown, Boston, 1986.

Royal College of General Practitioners: Oral contraceptives, venous thrombosis, and varicose veins. J. R. Coll. Gen. Pract., 28:393-399, 1978.

Royal College of General Practitioners: Oral Contraceptives and Health. Pitman Publishing, London, chap. 7, 1974.

Sackett, D. L.; Haynes, R. B.; and Tugwell, P.: Clincal Epidemiology: A Basic Science for Clinical Medicine. Little Brown, Boston, 1985.

Sartwell, P. E.; Masi, A. T.; Arthes, F. G.; Greene, G. R.; and Smith, H. E.: Thromboembolism and oral contraceptives: An epidemiologic case-control study. Am. J. Epidemiol., 90: 365-380, 1969.

Schuman, S. H.: Practice-Based Epidemiology. Gordon and Breach, New York, 1986.

Steering Committee of the Physicians' Health Study Research Group: Final report on the aspirin component of the ongoing Physicians' Health Study. N. Engl. J. Med., 321:129-135, 1989.

Strom, B. L. (ed.): Pharmacoepidemiology. Churchill Livingstone, New York, 1989a.

Strom, B. L.: Study designs available for pharmacoepidemiology studies. In, Pharmacoepidemiology (Strom, B. L., ed.). Churchill Livingstone, New York, pp. 13-26, 1989b.

Strom, B. L.: Sample size considerations for pharmacoepidemiology studies. In, Pharmacoepidemiology (Strom, B. L., ed.). Churchill Livingstone, New York, pp. 27-37, 1989c.

Strom, B. L.: Sample size tables. In, Pharmacoepidemiology (Strom, B. L., ed.). Churchill Livingstone, New York, pp. 373-406, 1989d.

Strom, B. L.; and Melmon, K. L.: Using pharmacoepidemiology to study beneficial drug effects. In, Pharmacoepidemiology (Strom, B. L., ed.). Churchill Livingstone, New York, pp. 307-324, 1989.

Unknown: How to read clinical journals: I. Why to read them and how to start reading them critically. Can. Med. Assoc. J., 124:555-558, 1981a.

Unknown: How to read clinical journals: II. To learn about a diagnostic test. Can. Med. Assoc. J., 124:703-710, 1981b.

Unknown: How to read clinical journals: III. To learn the clinical course and prognosis of disease. Can. Med. Assoc. J., 124:869-872, 1981c.

Unknown: How to read clinical journals: IV. To determine etiology or causation. Can. Med. Assoc. J., 124:985-990, 1981d.

Unknown: How to read clinical journals: V. To distinguish useful from useless or even harmful therapy. Can. Med. Assoc. J., 124:1156-1162, 1981e.

Unknown: How to read clinical journals: VI. To learn about the quality of clinical care. Can. Med. Assoc. J., 130:377-381, 1984a.

Unknown: How to read clinical journals: VII. To understand an economic evaluation (part A). Can. Med. Assoc. J., 130: 1428-1434, 1984b.

Unknown: How to read clinical journals: VII. To understand an economic evaluation (part B). Can. Med. Assoc. J., 130: 1542-1549, 1984c.

United States Pharmacopoeia: Drug Information for the Health Care Professional. Volume IA. USP, Rockville, Md., 1988.

Vessey, M.; Doll, R.; Peto, R.; Johnson, B.; and Wiggins, P.: A long-term follow-up study of women using different methods of contraception—an interim report. J. Biosoc. Sci., 8:373-427, 1976.

Weiss, N.: Clinical Epidemiology. Oxford University Press, New York, 1986.

Young, M. J.; Bresnitz, E. A.; and Strom, B. L.: Sample size nomograms for interpreting negative clinical studies. Ann. Intern. Med., 99:248-251, 1983.

Appendix I

Pharmacokinetic Data for Commonly Used Drugs

Gregory Scott and David Nierenberg

The drugs included in this table were selected using several criteria. Each drug is commonly prescribed, administered either orally or parenterally, has recognized clinical utility, and has solid pharmacokinetic data readily available in accessible medical literature. Trade names, when supplied, are listed in parentheses. Several drugs recently approved by the U.S. Food and Drug Administration have been included, even though they have not yet attained the prescribing frequency of some of the more well-established agents. These drugs were included since it is probable that their clinical importance will rapidly increase.

The data were obtained from a variety of sources. For each drug, we first searched two recognized reference sources (McEvoy, 1989; *Physicians' Desk Reference*, 1989). For data on patients with end-stage renal disease, two other general reference sources were utilized (Bennett, 1988; Keller et al., 1982). These four references are cited below. Detailed information about most drugs was obtained from peer-reviewed articles in the recent medical literature, as cited at the end of the table. Although a reasonable effort was made by the authors to cite studies with sound scientific design, no guarantee as to the quality of the data can be made.

The investigators writing the reference articles used a variety of methods to calculate kinetic parameters and studied different patient populations. Thus, there was inevitably a range of values for each pharmacokinetic parameter reported. The values listed in this table represent a range of values from the best studies found. These values are usually internally consistent; for example, in most cases $t_{1/2} = 0.7 \times V_d/Cl$. In situations where the consistency is not apparent, values were usually obtained from several different studies.

Since there is considerable interindividual variability, a range is generally given, and although the majority of otherwise healthy individuals will have values for parameters that fall within this range, some will not. The comments should be useful to identify patient characteristics for which considerable variability is to be expected.

It is important to remember that the information included in the table applies to adults as reported in the literature. Analagous data are sometimes available for children but are not included in this table.

The following comments apply to the columns of the table:

Oral Bioavailability and T_{max}

Oral bioavailability (F) is the fraction of the dose administered orally that is absorbed and reaches the systemic circulation as active drug. F therefore takes on a value between 0 and 1.0. The time to maximum concentration in blood (T_{max}) applies only to orally administered prompt-release tablets or capsules. Data for solutions, suspensions, elixirs, and so forth, as well as sustained-release preparations, are not included. Oral suspensions and elixirs usually are more promptly absorbed, while sustained-release products usually are more slowly absorbed. Also, there may be some variability for the same generic drug produced by different manufacturers.

Volume of Distribution (V_d)

We list all volumes of distribution in units of liters per kilogram. While some sources normalize this value to an idealized patient of 70 kg, we have maintained the units of liters per kilogram to stress that the volume of distribution is extremely variable and related to the patient's weight and body habitus.

Protein Binding

The percentage protein binding is that percentage of the drug present in plasma that is bound to a plasma protein under physiologic conditions. Many drugs, especially acidic drugs, are bound to albumin, while some basic drugs may bind extensively to α_1-acid glycoprotein. Disease states that significantly affect the degree of protein binding generally are included in the comments column.

Clearance

The clearance (*Cl*) refers to the volume of plasma completely cleared of drug per unit time. We have listed clearance in the units milliliters per minute to allow the reader to relate this value easily to the creatinine clearance. Also, physicians are used to thinking of plasma flow to the liver (900 ml/min) and kidneys (725 ml/min) in these units.

For some calculations, thinking of clearance in units of liters per hour facilitates calculations. The reader can easily convert units of milliliters per minute to liters per hour by multiplying the former by a factor of 0.06.

Although clearance generally varies with ideal body weight, the value in the table has been normalized to a 70-kg person. Drug clearance in a patient with a weight that significantly deviates from 70 kg should be adjusted accordingly. The "% renal" refers to that percentage of the drug administered IV that is eventually cleared (excreted) by the kidneys as unchanged drug.

Half-Lives

Two half-lives are provided. The first is the distribution half-life ($t_{1/2\alpha}$) that represents the time over which the concentration of drug in the plasma is reduced by one half as a result of redistribution to other compartments. It does not include elimination. Since this redistribution half-life is usually short, the units are in minutes.

The elimination half-life ($t_{1/2\beta}$) is the time over which the concentration of drug in the body decreases by one half as a result of clearance of the parent compound. Unless otherwise noted, elimination half-life is reported in hours.

Therapeutic Range

The therapeutic range is the concentration of drug in plasma that usually provides a therapeutically desirable response in the majority of individuals without undue toxicity. The target concentration for an individual patient is usually chosen from within the therapeutic range. For anti-infective and anticancer agents, the therapeutic ranges are listed as variable since the drug concentrations necessary for therapeutic efficacy are so disease-dependent.

Drugs for which the clinical value of therapeutic drug monitoring has been clearly established have the therapeutic range boxed with a solid line. Drugs for which the clinical value of therapeutic drug monitoring is possibly established are enclosed by dotted lines. For most other drugs, routine therapeutic drug monitoring has not been clearly established to be necessary or useful.

For several drugs, peak (Pk) and trough (Tr) concentrations are listed if both have been shown to be useful.

Kinetics in End-Stage Renal Disease (ESRD)

For many drugs, severe renal dysfunction alters the drug's volume of distribution or elimination half-life. When such data are available, they are recorded in this column for patients with a creatinine clearance < 5 ml/min who are not receiving dialysis.

Supplement After Dialysis

For some drugs, hemodialysis (HD) or peritoneal dialysis (PD) removes a significant amount of drug from the body. In these situations, a supplemental dose after dialysis may be necessary (recorded as Yes). For a few drugs, quantitative estimates are made of the percentage of the total body burden removed by hemodialysis under the following conditions: duration of dialysis = 6 hours, flow rate = 200 ml/min, dialyzer area = 1 m², and pore size = 3 nm. From this table, the amount of drug to be administered after hemodialysis to maintain a therapeutic level may be calculated. Supplementation prior to dialysis is not recommended since distribution out of the central compartment will likely be incomplete, and thus a significant proportion of the supplementary dose will be removed. It should be remembered that drugs with a high degree of protein binding or large volume of distribution, or those that are sequestered outside the vascular compartment, are likely to have only a small amount of drug removed.

Other Comments

Patient or drug product characteristics that affect the pharmacokinetic values in the table are included under the "Comments" section.

Abbreviations

NR means "not relevant." For example, if a drug such as gentamicin is always administered IV, the oral bioavailability is not relevant. A dash (−) means that the data would be useful to know, but reliable data were not available.

REFERENCES

Bass, N. M.; and Williams, R. L.: Guide to drug dosage in hepatic disease. Clin. Pharmacokinet., 15:396–420, 1988.
Bennett, W. M.: Guide to drug dosage in renal failure. Clin. Pharmacokinet., 15:326–354, 1988.
Keller, F.; Offermann, G.; and Lode, H.: Supplementary dose after hemodialysis. Nephron, 30:220–227, 1982.
Lee, C. C.; and Marbury, T. C.: Drug therapy in patients un-

dergoing haemodialysis. Clinical pharmacokinetic considerations. Clin. Pharmacokinet., 9:42–66, 1984.

Manuel, M. A.; Paton, T. W.; and Cornish, W. R.: Drugs and peritoneal dialysis. Peritoneal Dialysis Bull., July–Sept.:117–125, 1983.

McEvoy, G. K. (ed.): AHFS Drug Information 89. American Society of Hospital Pharmacists, Bethesda, Md., 1989.

Paton, T. W.; Cornish, W. R.; Manuel, M. A.; and Hardy, B. G.: Drug therapy in patients undergoing peritoneal dialysis. Clinical pharmacokinetic considerations. Clin. Pharmacokinet., 10:404–426, 1985.

Physicians' Desk Reference, 43rd ed. Medical Economics Company, Oradell, N.J., 1989.

Vozeh, S.; Schmidlin, O.; and Taeschner, W.: Pharmacokinetic drug data. Clin. Pharmacokinet., 15:254–282, 1988.

Winchester, J. F.; Gelfand, M. C.; Knepshield, J. H.; and Schreiner, G. E.: Dialysis and hemoperfusion of poisons and drugs—An update. Trans. Am. Soc. Artif. Intern. Organs, 23:762–808, 1977.

Winek, C. L.: Drug and Chemical Blood-Level Data 1989. Fisher Scientific, Pittsburgh, PA, September, 1988.

GENERIC DRUG (TRADE)	F [T_{max}]	V_d (L/KG)	PROTEIN BINDING (%)	Cl (ML/MIN) [% RENAL]	$T_{1/2}$ α (MIN)	$T_{1/2}$ β (H)
Acetaminophen (Paracetamol, Tylenol)	0.8–0.95 [0.17–1]	0.94	25	250–450 [<10]	NR	1.3–3
Acetazolamide (Diamox)	— [2–4]	0.2	95	45 [90]	NR	4–8
Acyclovir (Zovirax)	0.15–0.3 [1.5–2.5]	0.46–0.88	9–33	250–350 [62–91]	20	2.1–3.5
Alfentanil (Alfenta)	NR	0.3–1.0	88–95	210–525 [<1]	0.4–3.1	0.75–3.5
Allopurinol (Lopurin, Zyloprim)	0.8–0.9 [2–6]	0.6–1.6	<1	760 [<10]	NR	1–3
Alprazolam (Xanax)	>0.8 [1–2]	1.0	70	85–100 [20]	NR	12–15
Alteplase (Activase, r-TPA)	NR	—	—	550–680 [—]	3.5–7	0.4–1
Amantadine (Symmetrel)	— [1–4]	8	60	275 [100]	NR	9–37
Amikacin (Amikin)	NR	0.25	<10	100 [94–98]	NR	2–3
Amiloride (Midamor)	0.5 [3–4]	5.0–5.4	—	500 [50]	NR	6–9
Amiodarone (Cordarone)	0.22–0.86 [3–7]	18–148	96	100–175 [<1]	NR	2.5–10 d[1] 40–55 d[2]
Amitriptyline (Elavil, Endep)	0.4–0.6 [2–12]	15.5	96	700–1000 [<5]	NR	9–25
Amoxicillin (Amoxil, Polymox, Trimox)	0.74–0.92 [1–2]	0.4	20	250–450 [60]	NR	1.0
Amphotericin B (Fungizone)	NR	4	90–95	30 [2–5]	24–48 h	15 d[1]
Ampicillin (Omnipen, Polycillin, Principen)	0.3–0.55 [1–2]	0.27–0.32	15–25	259 [20–64]	NR	0.7–1.4
Amrinone (Inocor)	0.9 [0.5–3]	1–1.6	35–49	200–500 [26]	2	3–6
Aspirin (Acetylsalicylic acid)	0.9[1] [0–1]	0.14–0.18	80–90	575–725 [<2]	NR	0.2–0.3

| THERAPEUTIC RANGE (MG/L) | ESRD | | SUPPLEMENT AFTER | | COMMENTS |
	$T_{1/2}$ (H)	V_d (L/KG)	HD (%)	PD (%)	
10–20	1.5–3.5	—	Yes	—	Cl reduced with hepatic dysfunction, increased with hyperthyroidism (and with toxic levels).
10–15	—	—	—	—	—
Variable	19.5	—	Yes	No	—
—	—	—	—	—	Cl reduced with cirrhosis, age >65.
—	—	—	—	—	Cl reduced with renal dysfunction; active metabolite (oxipurinol) has a $t_{1/2\beta}$ of 18–30 h.
0.2	—	—	No	—	Protein binding increased with cirrhosis; Cl reduced with cirrhosis, age >65 (males).
NR	—	—	-	—	—
—	3–8 d	—	No	No	Cl reduced with age >65.
5–10 (Tr) 20–30 (Pk)	30–86	0.35	50	Yes	V_d reduced with obesity; Cl increased in severely burned patients, obesity.
—	140	—	—	—	Food reduces F (0.3).
1–2.5	No change	—	No	No	[1]Initial $t_{1/2\beta}$. [2]Terminal $t_{1/2\beta}$.
0.05–0.20	—	—	No	No	V_d and $t_{1/2\beta}$ increased with age >65; nortriptyline is an active metabolite.
Variable	5–20	—	100	No	Cl decreased with uremia.
Variable	No change	—	No	No	[1]Multiple dosing.
Variable	7–20	—	35	No	V_d increased with cirrhosis; Cl reduced with severe hepatic dysfunction and age >65.
—	—	—	—	—	Cl reduced with CHF (140–210 ml/min).
20–250[2]	No change	—	50	Yes	[1]Enteric-coated (t_{max} 4–6 h). [2]Analgesic use is at the lower end and rheumatoid arthritis at the higher end of the therapeutic range. Protein binding is decreased with uremia.

GENERIC DRUG (TRADE)	$F\,[T_{max}]$	V_d (L/KG)	PROTEIN BINDING (%)	Cl (ML/MIN) [% RENAL]	$T_{1/2}$ α (MIN)	$T_{1/2}$ β (H)
Atenolol (Tenormin)	0.5 [2–4]	1.1	6–16	180 [85–100]	NR	6–7
Atracurium (Tracrium)	NR	0.12–0.19	82	300–425 [<20]	2–3	0.33
Atropine	0.9 [1]	3.3	18	— [30–50]	NR	2–3
Auranofin (Ridaura)	0.2–0.25 [2–4]	—	60	— [−]	4 h	21–31 d
Aurothioglucose (Solganol)	NR	—	85–95	— [50–90]	43	3–27 d
Azathioprine (Imuran)	0.3–0.9 [1–2]	0.2–1.4	30	1800–6100 [<2]	NR	0.1–0.2
Aztreonam (Azactam)	NR	0.11–0.22	46–60	65–120 [58–74]	12–40	1.3–2.2
Bretylium (Bretylol)	NR	5–6.5	<10	550–850 [60–90]	NR	7–10.5
Bromocriptine mesylate (Parlodel)	0.06 [1–1.5]	3.4	90–96	900 [<5]	NR	4–4.5[1]
Bumetanide (Bumex, Burinex)	0.85–0.95 [0.5–2]	0.14–0.28	94–97	120–250 [50–60]	0.1	1–1.5
Bupivacaine (Marcaine, Sensorcaine)	NR	0.5–1	82–96	470 [5]	NR	1.5–5.5
Bupropion (Wellbutrin)	— [<3]	19–21	82–88	— [<4]	72–84	10.7–13.8
Buspirone (Buspar)	0.02–0.13 [0.7–1.5]	5.3	95	2000 [<1]	NR	2–4
Captopril (Capoten)	0.75 [1]	0.7	25–30	675–1100 [40–50]	NR	1.5–2
Carbamazepine (Tegretol)	>0.7 [2–8]	1.2	75–90	50–125 [1–3]	NR	12–17
Cefaclor (Ceclor)	0.5 [0.5–2]	0.37–0.5	25	370–455 [60–85]	NR	0.6
Cefadroxil (Duricef)	0.85 [1.5]	0.16–0.4	20	200–310 [90]	NR	1.3–1.6
Cefazolin (Ancef, Kefzol)	NR	0.15	80	53–65 [75]	NR	1.8
Cefixime (Suprax)	0.4–0.5 [2–6]	—	65	— [50]	—	3–4

| THERAPEUTIC RANGE (MG/L) | ESRD | | SUPPLEMENT AFTER | | COMMENTS |
	$T_{1/2}$ (H)	V_d (L/KG)	HD (%)	PD (%)	
Variable	15–35	0.45	33	No	—
—	No change	—	—	—	Cl is increased slightly with renal dysfunction or hepatic dysfunction.
0.035–0.2	—	—	—	—	—
0.3–1.0	—	—	No	—	—
1–10	—	—	No	—	$t_{1/2\beta}$ increases up to 168 d after prolonged weekly use; data are for IM administration.
Variable	—	—	50	—	Mercaptopurine is an active metabolite.
Variable	8.4–8.7	—	27–58	10	$t_{1/2\beta}$ is decreased (1–1.3 h) with cystic fibrosis.
Variable	31–34	—	72	—	Cl reduced with uremia.
Variable	—	—	—	—	[1]$t_{1/2\beta}$ for the terminal phase is 45–50 h.
40–80[1]	No change	—	—	—	[1]ng/ml. Cl reduced with renal dysfunction.
0.22–3.45	—	—	—	—	—
—	—	—	—	—	—
0.09–0.15	6.1	—	No	—	Food increases F (decreases the first-pass effect); $t_{1/2\beta}$ increased with hepatic dysfunction; active metabolite.
—	20–40	—	Yes	—	F reduced 30%–40% by food; protein binding reduced with uremia.
4–12	—	—	No	—	Enhances its own metabolism (initial $t_{1/2\beta} = 25$–65 h).
Variable	2.9	—	30	Yes	—
Variable	20–25	—	75	No	—
Variable	40–57	0.1	45	No	V_d increased with uremia; protein binding and Cl reduced with uremia.
Variable	—	—	—	No	Food slows absorption; Cl reduced with age >65.

GENERIC DRUG (TRADE)	F $[T_{max}]$	V_d (L/KG)	PROTEIN BINDING (%)	Cl (ML/MIN) [% RENAL]	$T_{1/2}$ α (MIN)	$T_{1/2}$ β (H)
Cefonicid (Monocid)	NR	0.15	98	27 [>95]	NR	4.4
Cefoperazone (Cefobid)	NR	0.2	90	80 [30]	NR	2.0
Cefotaxime (Claforan)	NR	0.4	30–40	260 [70]	NR	1.2
Cefotetan (Cefotan)	NR	0.15	90	33–37 [80]	NR	3–4.6
Cefoxitin (Mefoxin)	NR	0.17	70	240–330 [85]	NR	0.7–1.0
Ceftazidime (Fortaz, Tazicef, Tazidime)	NR	0.23	17	100 [80–90]	NR	1.8
Ceftizoxime (Cefizox)	NR	0.26	30	130–160 [>95]	NR	1.6
Ceftriaxone (Rocephin)	NR	0.14–0.2	83–96	20 [65]	NR	7–8.5
Cefuroxime (Ceftin, Zinacef)	0.4–0.5 [2]	0.13–0.23	33–50	90 [90–100]	NR	1–2
Cephalexin (Keflex)	0.90 [1–2]	0.2–0.3	10–15	250–380 [>90]	NR	0.8–1.0
Chlorambucil (Leukeran)	— [−]	0.1–1.6	—	12–65 [−]	NR	0.6–1.3
Chloramphenicol base (Chloromycetin)	0.76–0.93 [1–3]	0.8	60	150–180 [5–30[1]]	NR	1.5–4.1
Chlordiazepoxide (Librium)	0.95 [1–2]	0.3	95	4–70 [<1]	NR	7–13
Chloroquine	0.7–0.95 [1–2]	116–285	50–65	625–850 [70]	NR	72–120
Chlorpheniramine maleate (Chlortrimeton)	0.25–0.45 [2–6]	2.5–6	69–72	100 [5–20]	NR	12–43
Chlorpromazine (Largactil, Thorazine)	0.2–0.4 [2.5–4]	21	92–97	375–800 [<1]	NR	30
Chlorpropamide (Diabinese)	0.9 [2–4]	0.15	90	2 [20]	NR	25–60

THERAPEUTIC RANGE (MG/L)	ESRD		SUPPLEMENT AFTER		COMMENTS
	$T_{1/2}$ (H)	V_d (L/KG)	HD (%)	PD (%)	
Variable	58–102	—	No	No	Cl reduced with uremia.
Variable	No change	—	No[1]	No	[1]Give dose after dialysis. V_d increased with cirrhosis; Cl reduced with hepatitis; $t_{1/2\beta}$ increased with cirrhosis.
Variable	4.2–11.5	—	37	No	Desacetylcefotaxime is the active metabolite.
Variable	13–35	—	50	No	—
Variable	13–22	—	30	No	—
Variable	12–35	—	50	25	—
Variable	30	—	100	—	—
Variable	15–57	—	No	No	—
Variable	15–22	—	75	No	F and t_{max} are for the axetil salt.
Variable	10–15	—	50	Yes	Cl decreased with uremia.
Variable	—	—	—	—	—
Variable[2]	3–7	—	No	No	[1]% renal for oral is at the lower end and for IV at the upper end. [2]Gray syndrome may occur in premature and newborn infants due to high levels. Protein binding, Cl, and $t_{1/2\beta}$ reduced with cirrhosis.
1–3	No change	—	No	—	V_d increased with age >65, female sex; V_d may be increased with cirrhosis, acute viral hepatitis; Cl reduced with age >65, female sex, cirrhosis, acute viral hepatitis.
0.01–0.40	5–50 d	—	No	—	Cl increased with acidic urine, decreased with alkaline urine.
0.017	280–330	—	Yes	No	Cl decreased with alkaline urine.
0.01–0.05	No change	—	No	No	—
30–363	50–200	—	—	No	Food delays absorption, but does not affect F; Cl increased with alkaline urine, decreased with acidic urine.

GENERIC DRUG (TRADE)	F [T_{max}]	V_d (L/KG)	PROTEIN BINDING (%)	Cl (ML/MIN) [% RENAL]	$T_{1/2}$ α (MIN)	$T_{1/2}$ β (H)
Chlorthalidone (Hygroton)	0.6 [1.5–6]	4.2	75	90–110 [60]	NR	40–50
Cimetidine (Tagamet)	0.6–0.7 [0.75–1.5]	1.3	15–20	425–650 [50–73]	NR	2
Ciprofloxacin (Cipro)	0.5–0.85 [0.5–2.3]	1.7–2.7	16–43	300–480 [15–50]	11–22	3–5
Cisplastin (Platinol)	NR	0.3–1.15	90	1200 [−]	24–48	1–1.2
Clindamycin (Cleocin)	0.9 [0.75–1]	9.8	0.93	200 [<10]	6	2–3
Clofibrate (Atromid S)	>0.9 [3–6]	5.2–5.7	95–98	8 [5]	NR	12–16
Clomipramine (Anafranil)	0.2–0.8 [1.5–4]	7–20	97	− [−]	NR	19–37
Clonidine (Catapres)	0.95 [3–5]	3.45	20	140–300 [40–60]	NR	12–16
Codeine	0.6 [1–2]	3–4	−	− [3–16]	NR	2.5–3.5
Co-trimoxazole (Bactrim, Septra)	S: 0.87 T: 0.98 [1–4]	S: 0.15–0.25 T: 1.4–1.7	S: 70 T: 44	− [S: 10, T: 30]	NR	S: 10–13 T: 8–10
Cyclophosphamide (Cytoxan)	0.75 [1]	0.7	0–10	60–125 [30]	NR	4–6.5
Cyclosporine (Sandiummune)	0.3 [3.5]	4–9	90	200–300 [<1]	72	19–27
Cytarabine (Ara-C, Cytosar-U)	0.2 [−]	1–5	13	600–1200 [<20]	NR	2–3
Desipramine (Norpramin)	0.5 [4–6]	15–37	90	1600–2100 [<30]	NR	14–25
Dezocine (Dalgan)	NR	8–15	−	2900–3600 [−]	NR	2.0–2.8
Diazepam (Valium)	0.8–1.0 [1]	2	98	25 [<1]	30	20–50

THERAPEUTIC RANGE (MG/L)	ESRD		SUPPLEMENT AFTER		COMMENTS
	$T_{1/2}$ (H)	V_d (L/KG)	HD (%)	PD (%)	
0.21–1.4	–	–	–	–	Cl decreased with age >65.
0.5–4.5	3.5–5	–	10	No	Cl decreased with age >65, uremia.
Variable	6–9	–	2–30	No	F reduced by Al^{2+}, Ca^{2+}, Mg^{2+} antacids; food slows rate but not extent of absorption.
Variable	< 10 d	–	–	–	–
Variable	1.5–3.5	0.6	No	No	Oral form is the HCl salt; IV form is the PO_4 salt; Cl is significantly affected only with severe renal or hepatic dysfunction.
122	29–88	–	No	–	V_d increased with cirrhosis, uremia; protein binding reduced with renal dysfunction, cirrhosis; Cl increased with nephrotic syndrome, decreased with uremia.
–	–	–	–	–	Cl may be dose-dependent; the active metabolite has a $t_{1/2\beta}$ of 54–77 h.
0.3–2.0[1]	39–42	–	No	–	[1]ng/ml.
0.03–0.12	No change	–	–	–	–
Variable	26	–	–	No	S = sulfamethoxazole; T = trimethoprim.
Variable	14	–	67	–	–
Variable	No change	–	No	No	Cl reduced with cirrhosis, renal dysfunction.
Variable	–	–	–	–	–
75–150[1]	–	–	No	No	[1]ng/ml. Cl decreased with age >65.
NR	–	–	–	–	V_d increased in hepatic cirrhosis; clearance unchanged in hepatic cirrhosis.
0.02–2.0	65	–	No	–	V_d increased with age >65, hypoalbuminemia; protein binding decreased with renal dysfunction, cirrhosis; $t_{1/2\beta}$ increased with age >65; three active metabolites.

GENERIC DRUG (TRADE)	$F\,[T_{max}]$	V_d (L/KG)	PROTEIN BINDING (%)	Cl (ML/MIN) [% RENAL]	$T_{1/2}$ α (MIN)	$T_{1/2}$ β (H)
Dicloxacillin sodium (Dynapen)	0.35–0.76 [0.5–2]	0.2	95–99	90–140 [60]	NR	0.6–0.8
Diflunisal (Dolobid)	>0.95 [2–3]	7.5	>98	65 [<5]	NR	8–12
Digoxin (Lanoxin)	0.6–0.85[1] [−]	5–7.3	20–30	75 [50–70]	30[2]	34–44
Diltiazem (Cardizem)	0.38–0.42 [2.8–4.0]	4.5	98	1000 [<4]	NR	5.1
Diphenhydramine (Benadryl)	0.4–0.6 [1–4]	2.5–4.7	80–85	700–770 [2]	NR	3–5
Disopyramide (Norpace)	0.6–0.83 [2–2.5]	0.6–1.4	50–65	1.3–1.4 [40–60]	2–4	4–10
Doxepin (Adapin, Sinequan)	0.2–0.4 [0.5–1]	20	80	75–110 [<1]	NR	6–8
Doxycycline (Vibramycin)	0.9–1.0 [1.5–4]	0.4–1.0	90	25–50 [20–26]	NR	22–24
Enalapril (Renitec, Vasotec)	0.55–0.75 [3–4]	–	50–60	100–158 [43–56]	NR	11
Encainide (Enkaid)	0.25–0.30[1] [0.5–1.5]	3.6–4	70–78	11,500[1] 230[2] [−]	NR	0.3–5.6[1] 8–13[2]
Epoetin α (Epogen, Human Erythropoietin)	NR	0.02–0.06	–	7–10 [−]	NR	4–13[1]
Erythromycin base (E-Mycin, ERYC, Ilotycin)	0.1–0.6 [1–4]	0.5–1	73–81	350–900 [<5]	NR	1.5–2
Esmolol (Brevibloc)	NR	1.2	55	20,000–23,000 [<2]	0.03	0.15
Ethacrynic acid (Edecrin)	– [<2]	0.1	90	– [−]	NR	2–4
Ethambutol (Myambutol)	0.75–0.80 [2–4]	2.5	8–22	550–650 [50]	NR	3.3

THERAPEUTIC RANGE (MG/L)	ESRD		SUPPLEMENT AFTER		COMMENTS
	$T_{1/2}$ (H)	V_d (L/KG)	HD (%)	PD (%)	
Variable	1–2.2	—	No	No	Protein binding decreased with uremia; Cl decreased with uremia, cirrhosis, increased with cystic fibrosis.
9–90	68–138	—	No	—	Plasma concentration increases more than proportionately with increased dose or multiple dose.
0.5–2.0[3]	4.5–6	4.6	5	No	[1]Tablet. [2]IV. [3]ng/ml. Protein binding decreased with uremia; V_d and Cl increased with hyperthyroidism, decreased with hypothyroidism; Cl decreased with uremia, CHF.
Variable	—	—	—	—	—
0.01–0.1	—	—	—	—	V_d increased in Orientals; protein binding decreased with cirrhosis; $t_{1/2\beta}$ increased with cirrhosis.
2–4	15	—	Yes	—	V_d decreased with uremia; protein binding increased with age >65; Cl decreased with CHF, uremia; $t_{1/2\beta}$ increased with hepatic dysfunction.
0.03–0.17	No change	—	No	No	Active metabolite.
Variable	15–36	—	No	No	F reduced by food, milk, divalent or trivalent cations; protein binding decreased with uremia.
—	40–60	—	Yes	Yes	Data (except F, T_{max}) are for enalaprilat, the active metabolite.
0.1–0.3	—	—	—	—	[1]Extensive and [2]poor metabolizer (90% and 10%, respectively); in poor metabolizers $F = 0.8–0.9$; in extensive metabolizers, Cl reduced in renal dysfunction. Two active metabolites.
—	—	—	—	No	[1]Chronic renal failure.
Variable	4–6	—	No	No	V_d increased with uremia; $t_{1/2\beta}$ increased with cirrhosis.
0.3–1.0	—	—	24	21	Elimination occurs primarily via metabolism in erythrocytes.
—	—	—	No	—	—
Variable	8–10	0.8	34	Yes	$t_{1/2\beta}$ increased with hepatic dysfunction.

GENERIC DRUG (TRADE)	F [T_{max}]	V_d (L/KG)	PROTEIN BINDING (%)	Cl (ML/MIN) [% RENAL]	$T_{1/2}$ α (MIN)	$T_{1/2}$ β (H)
Ethinyl estradiol (Estinyl)	0.4 [1–2;12]	1.5–4.3	98	380 [−]	NR	6–20
Ethosuximide (Zarontin)	— [1–4]	0.7	<10	3 [20]	NR	60
Etidronate (Didronel)	0.01–0.06 [−]	1.4	—	— [40–60]	NR	4.8–6.9[1] 12 d[2]
Famotidine (Pepcid)	0.4–0.5 [1–3]	1.1–1.4	15–20	381–483 [60–80]	11	2.5–4
Fentanyl (Sublimaze)	NR	4	84	850 [<10]	NR	2–6.5
Flecainide (Tambocor)	0.85–0.90 [1–6]	5.5–10	40–50	210–850 [25–40]	3–6	11.5–16
Fluconazole (Diflucan)	>0.9 [1–2]	0.7	11–12	— [80]	NR	20–50
Flucytosine (Ancobon, 5-FC)	0.75–0.90 [<6]	0.68	2–4	120 [75–90]	NR	2.5–6
Fluoxetine (Prozac)	<0.9 [4–8]	14–100	94	94–704 [<5]	NR	48–72
Fluphenazine (Prolixin)	— [2]	20	—	— [−]	NR	14.7–15.3
Flurazepam (Dalmane)	— [0.5–1.0]	3.4	97	150–475 [<1]	NR	2.3[1]
Flurbiprofen (Ansaid)	— [1.5–2]	0.07–0.13	99	20 [<10]	NR	4–7
Furosemide (Lasix)	0.64 [1–1.1]	0.2–0.3	91–99	130–210 [40–50]	10	1–2
Ganciclovir (Cytovene)	NR	0.4–0.6	1–2	100–250 [94–99]	7–24	2.5–4.2
Gentamicin sulfate (Garamycin)	NR	0.22–0.3	<10	60 [>95]	6–15	1.5–4
Glipizide (Glucotrol)	0.8–1.0 [1–3]	0.16	92–99	1400–2660 [<10]	8–36	3–4.7
Glyburide (DiaBeta, Micronase)	>0.9 [2–4]	0.13	99	91 [<1]	NR	1.4–1.8
Griseofulvin (Grisactin)	>0.9 [4–8]	1.5	—	— [<1]	NR	9–24

| THERAPEUTIC RANGE (MG/L) | ESRD | | SUPPLEMENT AFTER | | COMMENTS |
	$T_{1/2}$ (H)	V_d (L/KG)	HD (%)	PD (%)	
Variable	—	—	—	—	—
40–100	55	—	Yes	—	—
—	—	—	—	—	[1]IV. [2]chronic oral dosing. Food reduces F.
13–50[1]	24	—	No	—	[1]ng/ml.
Variable	—	—	—	—	—
0.2–1.0	19–26	—	No	—	Cl increased with acidic urine; active metabolites prolong duration of action.
Variable	—	—	50	—	—
25–120	30	—	80	Yes	—
—	86	—	No	—	Food slows rate but not extent of absorption; active metabolite.
0.9–17[1]	—	—	—	—	[1]ng/ml.
0.9–28	No change	—	No	—	[1]ng/ml. Two active metabolites prolong duration of action.
NR	—	—	—	—	Food slows rate but not extent of absorption.
1–10	2–4	—	No	—	V_d increased with nephrotic syndrome, cirrhosis; protein binding decreased with renal dysfunction, cirrhosis, hypoalbuminemia; Cl decreased with uremia, CHF.
Variable	—	—	50	—	Cl reduced with renal dysfunction.
0.5–2.0 (Tr) 4–8 (Pk)	24–48	—	60	Yes	V_d decreased with obesity; Cl decreased with renal dysfunction, edema, increased with cystic fibrosis.
Variable	—	—	—	—	—
30–50[1]	11	—	No	—	[1]ng/ml.
Variable	—	—	—	—	—

GENERIC DRUG (TRADE)	$F\,[T_{max}]$	V_d (L/KG)	PROTEIN BINDING (%)	Cl (ML/MIN) [% RENAL]	$T_{1/2}$ α (MIN)	$T_{1/2}$ β (H)
Growth hormone, recombinant (Humatrope, Protropin)	NR	0.03–0.07	–	120–200 [<1]	NR	0.1–0.4
Guanabenz (Wytensin)	0.7–0.8 [2–5]	93–147	90	7–13 [<1]	NR	4–14
Haloperidol (Haldol)	0.6 [2–6]	20	92	625–1025 [<10]	NR	10–20
Heparin	NR	0.07	–	35–45 [<10]	NR	0.7–1.5
Hydralazine (Apresoline)	0.26–0.55 [0.5–2]	1.3–7.7	88–90	2100–5000 [3–14]	NR	0.7–2.4
Hydrochlorothiazide (Esidrix, HCTZ, HydroDiuril)	0.6–0.7 [1.5–2.5]	3	40	250–425 [95]	NR	9.5–19
Hydrocortisone (Hydrocortone, SoluCortef)	– [–]	–	90–95	– [<1]	NR	1–2
Hydromorphone (Dilaudid)	0.6 [1]	1.2	–	– [1–13]	NR	2.5
Ibuprofen (Motrin)	0.8 [1–2]	0.14	90–99	40–70 [<10]	NR	1.8–2.0
Imipenem	NR	0.23–0.35	13–21	165–207 [70′]	14–19	0.85–1.3
Imipramine (Tofranil)	1.0 [1–2]	21	89	750–1300 [<1]	NR	8–16
Indapamide (Lozol)	>0.95 [2–2.5]	0.3	71–79	22 [7]	NR	14–18
Indomethacin (Indocin)	1.0 [0.5–2]	0.3–1.6	99	85–135 [5–10]	60	2.6–11.2
Insulin, regular human (Humulin R, Novolin R, Velosulin)	NR	0.08	5	800–2500 [<2]	NR	0.1–0.3
Interferon α_{2a} (Roferon-A)	NR	0.2–0.7[1] 5–10[2]	–	46–93[1] 157–272[2] [–]	NR	5.1[1] 4.6–9.8[2]
Interleukin-2	– NR	0.09–0.15	–	65–165 [–]	NR	0.5–1
Isoniazid (INH)	0.9 [1–2]	0.6	10–15	175–325[1] 375–650[2] [20[1], 5[2]]	NR	2.3–3.5[1] 0.75–2[2]

THERAPEUTIC RANGE (MG/L)	ESRD		SUPPLEMENT AFTER		COMMENTS
	$T_{1/2}$ (H)	V_d (L/KG)	HD (%)	PD (%)	
–	–	–	–	–	–
–	–	–	–	–	Cl decreased with hepatic dysfunction.
$6-10^1$	–	–	No	No	[1]ng/ml.
–	0.5–3	–	No	No	Cl decreases as dose increases; (dose-dependent kinetics.
0.2–0.9	11	–	No	No	F is at the low end for fast acetylators and the high end for slow acetylators; $t_{1/2\beta}$ doubles with CHF.
0.07–0.45	–	–	–	–	Cl decreased with uremia, CHF.
Variable	–	–	–	–	Diurnal variation in clearance with a slightly longer $t_{1/2\beta}$ in the morning; biologic $t_{1/2}$ is 8–12 h.
0.008–0.032	–	–	–	–	–
5–49	No change	–	–	–	Food delays absorption; dose-dependent kinetics.
Variable	2.7–3.7	–	Yes	No	% renal of imipenem is 70% when administered with cilastatin.
0.01–0.13	–	–	No	No	Cl decreased with age >65; desipramine is an active metabolite.
–	No change	–	No	–	–
0.5–3.0	No change	–	No	–	–
–	–	–	–	–	Cl decreased with increasing dose (nonlinear kinetics).
–	–	–	No	–	[1]Intermittent infusion. [2]Continuous infusion.
–	–	–	–	–	–
Variable	5^2, 12^1	–	67^2	Yes	[1]Slow acetylator. [2]Rapid acetylator. $t_{1/2\beta}$ increased with severe hepatic dysfunction; no difference in clinical response between rapid and slow acetylators when administered daily.

GENERIC DRUG (TRADE)	$F\,[T_{max}]$	V_d (L/KG)	PROTEIN BINDING (%)	Cl (ML/MIN) [% RENAL]	$T_{1/2}$ α (MIN)	$T_{1/2}$ β (H)
Isosorbide dinitrate (Isordil, Sorbitrate)	0.3 [0.5–1]	0.6–3	16–40	3100 [<10]	NR	4
Ketoconazole (Nizoral)	— [1–2]	—	84–99	— [2–4]	120	8
Ketoprofen (Orudis)	0.9 [0.5–2]	0.1	99	70–90 [<1]	NR	1.1–4
Ketorolac tromethamine (Toradol)	— [0.8–0.9]	0.1–0.25	99	25–38 [60]	—	5–6
Labetalol (Normodyne, Trandate)	0.25 [0.7–2]	9.4	50	1500 [<5]	6–42	2.5–8
Levodopa	— [1.4]	0.8–1.1	—	460–800 [−]	7	2.2
Levothyroxine (Levothroid, Synthroid)	0.5–0.8 [2–4]	0.2	99	— [−]	NR	156–168
Lidocaine (Xylocaine)	NR	3	60–80	700 [<10]	7–18	1.5–2.0
Lithium carbonate (Eskalith, Lithobid)	0.95–1.0 [0.5–3]	0.7–1	0	20–40 [95–99]	48–72	20–27
Lorazepam (Ativan)	0.90 [1–2]	1.5	85	50–70 [<1]	NR	10–20
Lovastatin (Mevacor)	0.05 [2–4]	—	95	300–1250 [<10]	NR	1.1–1.7
Maprotiline (Ludiomil)	>0.95 [8–24]	22–52	88	1060 [<10]	NR	27–58
Melphalan (Alkeran)	0.25–0.9 [2]	0.4–0.8	80–90	160–560 [10]	NR	1.5
Meperidine (Demerol, Pethidine)	0.5 [−]	4–5	60–80	800–1000 [5]	4–12	3.2–3.7
Metformin	0.6 [1.9]	0.8–1	0	400–480 [−]	NR	1.5–1.7
Methadone (Dolophine)	0.6–1.0 [1–5]	3–4.3	60–90	65–125 [20]	120–180	23–38
Methotrexate (Folex, Mexate)	0.6–0.9[1] [1–4]	0.4–0.8	50	30–200 [80−90]	45	3–10 8–15[2]

THERAPEUTIC RANGE (MG/L)	ESRD		SUPPLEMENT AFTER		COMMENTS
	$T_{1/2}$ (H)	V_d (L/KG)	HD (%)	PD (%)	
3–18[1]	No change	—	—	—	[1]ng/ml. Cl decreased with cirrhosis; active metabolites.
—	No change	—	No	No	F reduced with increased gut pH.
—	—	—	—	—	Food delays absorption; Cl reduced with renal dysfunction and age >65.
Variable	—	—	—	—	Food slows absorption.
—	No change	—	No	No	F increased with food, age >65, and cirrhosis.
—	—	—	—	—	
4–12[1]	—	—	—	—	[1]ng/ml.
1–5	1.3–3	—	No	—	V_d decreased with CHF, increased with cirrhosis; protein binding increased with age >65, uremia; Cl decreased with CHF, shock, therapy >24 h, increased with smoking.
0.4–1.3[1] 1.0–1.4[2]	—	—	Yes	Yes	[1]Affective, schizoaffective disorder. [2]Mania. Cl decreased with uremia, age >65; $t_{1/2\beta}$ increased with chronic dosing (>1 y).
0.02–0.24	32–70	—	No	—	V_d increased, protein binding decreased, and $t_{1/2\beta}$ increased with cirrhosis.
—	—	—	—	—	F increased 50% by food.
0.05–0.35	—	—	—	—	Active metabolite.
Variable	4–6	—	—	—	—
0.07–0.8	No change	—	—	—	F = 0.8–0.9 with cirrhosis; V_d increased with age >65; protein binding decreased with age >65, uremia; Cl = 390–570 with cirrhosis; % renal = 25% with acidic urine.
1–4	3.8–6	—	—	—	Cl = 75–100 with end-stage renal disease.
—	—	—	No	No	$t_{1/2\beta}$ increased with severe chronic liver disease.
Variable	—	—	Yes	No	[1]F may be as low as 0.2–0.3 with high doses. [2]Terminal $t_{1/2\beta}$; Cl decreased with uremia.

GENERIC DRUG (TRADE)	F [T_{max}]	V_d (L/KG)	PROTEIN BINDING (%)	Cl (ML/MIN) [% RENAL]	$T_{1/2}$ α (MIN)	$T_{1/2}$ β (H)
Methyldopa (Aldomet)	0.3–0.5 [3–6]	0.6	<15	150–300 [24–45]	12–18	1.3–1.7
Methylergonovine (Methergine)	0.6 [3]	0.2	—	120–240 [<3]	1.2–5	0.5–2
Methylprednisolone (Medrol, SoluMedrol)	0.7–0.9 [−]	0.85	40–60	250 [5]	NR	2.75
Metoclopramide (Maxdon, Reglan)	0.3–1.0 [1–2]	2.2–3.4	13–22	770 [20]	5	2.5–5
Metolazone (Diulo, Zaroxolyn)	0.4–0.9 [2–8]	1.6	33	110 [70–95]	NR	14
Metoprolol (Lopressor)	0.5 [1.5]	5.5	12	800–1300 [5–10]	—	3–7
Metronidazole (Flagyl)	0.8 [0.5–2]	0.7	10	70–100 [20]	NR	6–8
Mexiletine (Mexitil)	0.8–0.9 [2–4]	5.4	75	500–850 [15]	NR	8–10
Mezlocillin (Mezlin)	NR	0.14–0.31	16–42	161–202 [39–72]	7–16	1.0–1.2
Midazolam (Hypnovel, Versed)	NR	0.8–2.5	94–97	175–900 [<1]	6–18	1–4
Misoprostil (Cytotec)	— [0.25–0.5]	—	81–89	— [−]	NR	0.3
Moricizine (Ethmozine)	0.3–0.4 [1.5]	8.3–11	92–95	— [<1]	NR	6.4–13
Morphine sulfate	0.15–0.7 [0.7–4]	1–3.8	20–30	560–2400 [10]	NR	1–7
Nadolol (Corgard)	0.3–0.4 [2–4]	1.9	30	150–225 [<25]	NR	10–24
Nafcillin (Nafcil, Unipen)	NR	0.57–1.55	70–90	410–585 [20–30]	12	0.5–1.5
Naloxone (Narcan)	NR	3	—	1750 [<35]	5	1.0–1.5
Naproxen (Naprosyn)	1.0 [2–4]	0.12	99	10 [10]	NR	10–20
Nicardipine (Cardine)	0.15–0.4[1] [0.3–2]	0.64	>98	1900–9000 [<1]	NR	2–8

THERAPEUTIC RANGE (MG/L)	ESRD		SUPPLEMENT AFTER		COMMENTS
	$T_{1/2}$ (H)	V_d (L/KG)	HD (%)	PD (%)	
1–7.5	6–16	—	60	Yes	Cl reduced with uremia.
—	—	—	—	—	—
Variable	3	—	90	—	—
—	14	—	No	No	Extensive but variable first-pass effect.
—	—	—	No	—	Great variability in F and T_{max} among generic products.
0.02–0.34	No change	—	Yes	—	$t_{1/2\beta} = 7.6$ h in poor hydroxylators; $t_{1/2\beta}$ highly variable with age >65.
Variable	8–15	—	Yes	No	V_d may be reduced with age >65; Cl decreased with cirrhosis.
0.7–2.0	16	—	Yes	No	Cl decreased with uremia; renal clearance increased with acidic urine; $t_{1/2\beta}$ increased with CHF.
Variable	1.6–6	0.15	25	No	Cl decreased with hepatic dysfunction, uremia.
0.03–0.1[1] >0.1[2]	—	—	No	—	[1]Sedation. [2]Hypnosis. Cl may be decreased with chronic hepatitis, renal dysfunction; one active metabolite.
—	—	—	—	—	Undergoes rapid de-esterification to the active form.
NR	—	—	—	—	Extensive first-pass effect.
0.1	No change	—	No	—	Protein binding decreased with hepatic dysfunction; V_d and Cl decreased with age >65.
—	45	—	Yes	—	Cl decreased with renal dysfunction.
Variable	1.8–2.8	0.70	No	No	V_d and Cl decreased and % renal increased with cirrhosis.
Variable	—	—	—	—	—
30–90	No change	—	No	—	V_d increased with uremia, cirrhosis; protein binding increased with uremia, age >65, cirrhosis; Cl decreased with uremia.
—	—	—	—	—	[1]F increased with renal dysfunction and with increasing dose. Cl decreased with renal dysfunction.

GENERIC DRUG (TRADE)	$F\ [T_{max}]$	V_d (L/KG)	PROTEIN BINDING (%)	Cl (ML/MIN) [% RENAL]	$T_{1/2}$ α (MIN)	$T_{1/2}$ β (H)
Nifedipine (Adalat, Procardia)	0.45–0.6 [0.5–1.5]	0.6–1.1	96–98	450–750 [10]	NR	4–5.5
Nimodipine (Nimotop)	0.06 [1]	0.9	>95	980 [<10]	–	1–2
Nitroglycerin	0.4 [–]	3	60	5500–7100 [<1]	–	0.3–0.5
Norethindrone (Norlutin)	0.65 [0.5–4]	1.5–4.3	80	– [–]	NR	5–14
Norfloxacin (Noroxin)	0.3–0.5 [1–2]	–	10–15	– [25–40]	NR	2.3–4
Nortriptyline (Pamelor)	0.6 [7–8.5]	21–27	93	375–625 [<2]	NR	18–35
Omeprazole (PriLosec)	– [0.5–7]	0.19–0.48	95	– [<1]	3–7	1^1 2.3^2
Ondansetron (Zofran)	0.6 [1–1.5]	2.3	70–76	600–700 [<10]	NR	3–3.5
Oxacillin (Bactocill, Prostaphlin)	0.30–0.35 [0.5–2]	0.39–0.43	89–94	380 [50]	NR	0.3–0.8
Oxazepam (Serax)	>0.9 [3]	0.6–0.9	>95	130–160 [<1]	NR	5.7–10.9
Pancuronium (Pavulon)	NR	0.24	20	70–120 [35–45]	10–12	2.0–2.5
Pefloxacin (Floxin)	1.0 [1–1.5]	1.5–1.9	20–30	135 [<10]	NR	7–14
Penicillin G, aqueous (Benzylpenicillin, Pentids, Pfizerpen)	0.15–0.3 [0.5–1]	0.5–0.7	45–68	– [20]	NR	0.4–0.9
Penicillin V (Pen Vee K, Phenoxymethylpenicillin, Veetids)	0.6–0.73 [0.5–1]	0.5	75–89	– [26–65]	NR	0.5
Pentazocine (Talwin)	0.2 [1–3]	5.6	60	– [<10]	NR	2–3
Pentobarbital (Nembutal)	>0.9 [0.5–1]	1	35–45	50 [<1]	4	35–50
Perphenazine (Trilafon)	0.2 [4–8]	10–34	–	1600 [–]	NR	8–12
Phenobarbital (Phenobarbitone)	0.7–0.9 [8–12]	0.6–0.7	20–45	4 [25]	–	2–6 d

| THERAPEUTIC RANGE (MG/L) | ESRD | | SUPPLEMENT AFTER | | COMMENTS |
	$T_{1/2}$ (H)	V_d (L/KG)	HD (%)	PD (%)	
—	—	—	No	No	Cl decreased with cirrhosis.
—	—	—	—	—	Cl decreased with cirrhosis.
1.2–11[1]	—	—	—	—	[1]ng/ml. Cl may decrease over time (IV).
—	—	—	—	—	—
Variable	7.6	—	No	—	—
0.05–0.15	23	—	No	No	Cl decreased with age >65.
—	—	—	No	—	[1]IV. [2]p.o. F increased with repeated dosing, but stabilizes within 3–5 days; food delays absorption.
—	—	—	—	—	—
Variable	0.5–2	—	5	No	Food reduces extent of and delays absorption.
0.15–1.4	25	—	No	—	V_d and protein binding increased with uremia; Cl increased with uremia, hyperthyroidism, smoking.
0.09–1	4.3	—	—	—	Cl decreased age >65, uremia.
Variable	—	—	No	No	Food slows rate but not extent of absorption.
Variable	6–20	—	15	No	Cl decreased with hepatic dysfunction.
Variable	—	—	—	—	—
0.03–1.0	—	—	Yes	—	$F = 0.6–0.7$ with cirrhosis.
1–5[1] 5–15[2]	No change	—	No	—	[1]Sedation. [2]Hypnosis.
0.4–30[1]	—	—	—	—	[1]ng/ml.
<10[1] 10–20[2] 40[3]	117–160	—	Yes	Yes	[1]Sedation. [2]Anticonvulsant. [3]Hypnosis. Cl increased with alkaline urine; $t_{1/2\beta}$ increased with cirrhosis, age >65.

GENERIC DRUG (TRADE)	$F\,[T_{max}]$	V_d (L/KG)	PROTEIN BINDING (%)	Cl (ML/MIN) [% RENAL]	$T_{1/2}$ α (MIN)	$T_{1/2}$ β (H)
Phenytoin (Dilantin)	0.2–0.9 [1.5–3]	0.4–0.8	88–93	— [<5]	36	7–26
Pimozide (Orap)	— [6–8]	—	99	— [<1]	NR	55
Piperacillin (Pipracil)	NR	0.14–0.31	16–22	153–297 [42–90]	10–20	0.7–1.0
Piroxicam (Feldene)	>0.95 [3–5]	0.12–0.14	>99	2 [<5]	NR	30–86
Prazosin (Minipress)	0.4–0.8 [2–3]	0.5–0.6	97	190–225 [5–11]	NR	2–4
Prednisolone	0.7–0.95 [−]	1.3–1.7	90–95	500–700 [10–20]	NR	1.7–2.7
Prednisone (Deltasone)	0.9–1.0 [1–3]	1	70	200–300 [3]	NR	3–3.5
Primidone (Mysoline)	0.6–0.8 [3–4]	0.6	<20	45–100 [15–25]	NR	10–12
Probenecid (Benemid)	0.9 [2–4]	0.16	75	15–110[1] [5–11]	NR	4–17
Procainamide (Pronestyl)	0.75–0.95 [0.75–2.5]	2.2	14–23	470–600[1] [40–70]	4–6	2.5–4.7[1]
Prochlorperazine (Compazine, Stemetril)	— [−]	20	—	— [−]	—	3–5[1] 6.9[2]
Promethazine (Phenergan)	— [−]	13	76–80	110 [−]	NR	12
Propafenone (Rythmol)	0.03–0.4 [3]	—	97	— [<1]	NR	3–8[1] 9–25[2]
Propofol (Diprivan)	NR	2.5–5	97–99	1500–2300 [<1]	2–8	3–5

THERAPEUTIC RANGE (MG/L)	ESRD		SUPPLEMENT AFTER		COMMENTS
	$T_{1/2}$ (H)	V_d (L/KG)	HD (%)	PD (%)	
10–20[1]	8	1.4	No	No	[1]Lower with chronic renal failure due to decreased protein binding. V_d increased with uremia; Cl dose-dependent; Cl may be substantially reduced with cirrhosis.
—	—	—	—	—	—
Variable	2–6	—	48	No	V_d decreased and Cl increased with cystic fibrosis; Cl decreased with renal and hepatic dysfunction.
0.85–2[1] 5–13.5[2]	—	—	—	—	[1]Analgesia. [2]Anti-inflammatory. Food delays absorption.
—	—	—	No	No	Protein binding decreased with cirrhosis, hypoalbuminemia; Cl decreased with CHF.
Variable	No change	—	No	No	Protein binding decreased with hypoalbuminemia; Cl increased with increasing dose.
Variable	—	—	Yes	—	Biologic $t_{1/2}$ is 18–36 h.
5–12	14	—	Yes	—	Cl decreased with uremia; 15%–25% metabolized to phenobarbital.
40–60[2] 100–200[3]	—	—	—	—	[1]Dose-dependent. [2]Maximal inhibition of penicillin secretion. [3]Uricosuria. $t_{1/2\beta}$ increases as the dose increases.
4–8	10[2]; 20[3]	—	12[2]	No	[1]Slow acetylator at the low end, fast acetylator at the high end. [2]Fast acetylator. [3]Slow acetylator. V_d increased with CHF, obesity; Cl reduced with MI, CHF.
—	—	—	—	—	[1]Oral. [2]IV.
3–23[1]	—	—	—	—	[1]ng/ml.
—	—	—	—	—	[1]Extensive (90%) vs. [2]poor (10%) metabolizers. Nonlinear kinetics; F (mean 0.7) increased in severe hepatic dysfunction; two active metabolites.
—	—	—	—	—	Terminal $t_{1/2\beta} = 11$–12 h.

GENERIC DRUG (TRADE)	F [T_{max}]	V_d (L/KG)	PROTEIN BINDING (%)	Cl (ML/MIN) [% RENAL]	$T_{1/2}$ α (MIN)	$T_{1/2}$ β (H)
Propranolol (Inderal)	0.65 [1–1.5]	2.8	>90	625–1000 [<1]	10	3.4–6
Quinidine sulfate (Quinora)	0.65–0.95 [1–2]	2	80	180–300 [10–20]	NR	6–8
Quinine	— [1–3]	2.7	70	100–150 [<5]	NR	7–12
Ranitidine (Zantac)	0.4–0.6 [2–3]	1.2–1.9	10–19	650–800 [16–36]	—	1.7–3.2
Rifampin (Rifadin, Rimactane)	0.9[1] [2–4]	1	84–91	150–350 [<5]	NR	1.7–3
Spironolactone (Aldactone)	0.9 [1–2]	—	98	— [0]	NR	1.3–2
Streptokinase (Kabikinase, Streptase)	NR	—	—	— [—]	NR	0.3–1.4[1]
Sufentanil (Sufenta)	NR	2.4	92	780 [—]	—	1.5–5.5
Sulindac (Clinoril)	0.9 [1–2]	—	94	— [<20]	NR	7
Temazepam (Restoril)	>0.90 [2–3]	1	96	50–75 [<1]	24–36	9.5–12.4
Terfenadine (Seldane)	0.01 [1–2]	—	97	— [<10]	3.5 h	16–23
Tetracycline (Achromycin, Sumycin)	0.6–0.8 [2–3]	2	20–67	100–135 [60]	NR	6–12
Theophylline, anhydrous (SloPhyllin, Theolair)	>0.9 [2–4]	0.3–0.7	60	36–50 [<10]	—	4–16
Thioridazine (Mellaril)	— [—]	18	99	— [<10]	NR	20–24
Ticarcillin (Ticar)	NR	0.34–0.42	45–65	130–250 [80–93]	6–11	0.9–1.3
Tobramycin (Nebcin)	NR	0.25–0.30	<10	70 [>95]	—	2–4

THERAPEUTIC RANGE (MG/L)	ESRD		SUPPLEMENT AFTER		COMMENTS
	$T_{1/2}$ (H)	V_d (L/KG)	HD (%)	PD (%)	
0.01–0.34	8	3	No	—	V_d increased with hepatitis, hyperthyroidism; Cl increased with hyperthyroidism, smoking, decreased with hepatitis.
0.3–6.0	12	—	No	No	V_d decreased with CHF, increased with cirrhosis; protein binding decreased with hepatic dysfunction; Cl decreased with CHF, age >65, alkaline urine.
1.7–9.7	No change	—	Yes	No	V_d and Cl decreased with malaria; Cl increased with acidic urine.
35–100[1]	10	—	Yes	—	[1]ng/ml. Cl decreased with age >65, uremia; % renal decreased with uremia.
Variable	1.8–11	—	No	No	[1]Decreased with chronic use due to enzyme induction. Cl decreased with uremia; $t_{1/2\beta}$ increased with hepatic dysfunction.
—	No change	—	—	—	Food increases rate and extent of absorption; active metabolites.
—	—	—	—	—	[1]The lower value is seen in patients with streptokinase antibodies.
—	—	—	—	—	—
—	—	—	—	—	Food decreases the rate and extent of absorption.
0.4–0.9	—	—	No	—	—
—	—	—	—	—	Active metabolite.
Variable	57–120	—	No	No	F drastically decreased by food, dairy products, antacids; Cl decreased with hepatic dysfunction.
5–20	5–9	—	40	Yes	V_d decreased with obesity; Cl decreased with COPD, cor pulmonale, CHF, hepatic dysfunction, prolonged fever, increased with smoking.
0.1–2.6	—	—	—	—	Mesoridazine is an active metabolite.
Variable	13–16	—	Yes	No	Cl decreased with uremia.
0.5–2.0 (Tr) 4–8 (Pk)	27–56	—	50	Yes	V_d decreased with obesity; Cl increased with cystic fibrosis, decreased with uremia.

GENERIC DRUG (TRADE)	F [T_{max}]	V_d (L/KG)	PROTEIN BINDING (%)	Cl (ML/MIN) [% RENAL]	$T_{1/2}$ α (MIN)	$T_{1/2}$ β (H)
Tolazamide (Tolinase)	— [2–6]	—	94	— [7]	NR	4–7
Tolbutamide (Orinase)	0.85–1.0 [3–5]	0.15	95	20 [0]	NR	4.5–6.5
Tolmetin (Tolectin)	>0.95 [0.5–1]	0.13	99	50–125 [20]	1–2 h	1
Trazodone (Desyrel)	>0.90 [1–2]	—	89–95	— [<1]	3–6 h	5–9
Triamterene (Dyrenium)	0.3–0.7 [2–4]	8–18	67	1600 [5–10]	NR	1.7–2.5
Triazolam (Halcion)	0.5 [2]	1	80	450–700 [2]	NR	1.6–5.4
Valproic acid (Depakene, Epilim)	0.9–1.0 [1–4]	0.15	80–95	7 [<10]	NR	5–20
Vancomycin (Vancocin, Vancoled)	<0.2	0.4–1.0	52–60	65 [85]	7	4–6
Vecuronium (Norcuron)	NR	0.2–0.4	60–90	200–450 [<15]	4–9	0.5–1.3
Verapamil (Calan, Isoptin)	0.18–0.27 [1–2.5]	3.4–4.4	93	500–2600 [<3]	4	2.7–4.8
Warfarin sodium (Coumadin)	>0.90 [2–6]	0.15	97	3 [0]	6–12 h	0.5–3 d
Zidovudine (AZT, Retrovir)	0.5–0.76 [0.5–1.5]	1.4–1.6	34–38	1900 [14–18]	10	0.8–1.9

| THERAPEUTIC RANGE (MG/L) | ESRD | | SUPPLEMENT AFTER | | COMMENTS |
	$T_{1/2}$ (H)	V_d (L/KG)	HD (%)	PD (%)	
—	—	—	—	—	Active metabolites.
43–96	No change	—	No	—	F increased with fasting state, decreased with malabsorption syndrome; protein binding decreased with acute viral hepatitis, age >65; Cl increased with acute viral hepatitis.
37	—	—	—	—	F decreased up to 16% by food; protein binding decreased with uremia; Cl increased with alkaline urine.
0.7–1.6	—	—	—	—	Food delays, but increases the extent (up to 20%) of absorption.
—	10	—	—	—	F varies greatly between generic products; % renal increased with cirrhosis; active metabolite.
0.01	—	—	No	—	V_d decreased with obesity; Cl decreased with obesity, age >65.
50–100	—	—	—	—	Food delays absorption; V_d increased with cirrhosis; protein binding decreased with uremia, cirrhosis, burns, age >65; Cl decreased with age >65.
5–10 (Tr) 25–35 (Pk)	44–180	—	No	No	F minimal except in colitis; V_d decreased with obesity; Cl decreased with age >65, uremia.
—	15	—	—	—	Cl decreased with renal dysfunction (170–310 ml/min) and hepatic dysfunction (70–170 ml/min).
0.12–0.40	2.4–4	—	No	—	V_d, protein binding increased with cirrhosis; Cl decreased with cirrhosis, and after dosing for several days ($t_{1/2\beta}$ = 4.5–12 h).
1–11.8	30	—	—	No	Protein binding decreased with uremia; active metabolites.
—	—	—	—	—	—

GENERIC AND TRADE NAMES FOR DRUGS IN APPENDIX 1

Drug Name	Cross Reference
Acetaminophen	
Acetazolamide	
Acetylsalicylic acid	See **aspirin**
Achromycin™	See **tetracycline**
Activase™	See **alteplase**
Acyclovir	
Adalat™	See **nifedipine**
Adapin™	See **doxepin**
Aldactone™	See **spironolactone**
Aldomet™	See **methyldopa**
Alfenta™	See **alfentanil**
Alfentanil	
Alkeran™	See **melphalan**
Allopurinol	
Alprazolam	
Alteplase	
Amantadine	
Amikacin	
Amikin™	See **amikacin**
Amiloride	
Amiodarone	
Amitriptyline	
Amoxicillin	
Amoxil™	See **amoxicillin**
Amphotericin B	
Ampicillin	
Amrinone	
Anafranil™	See **clomipramine**
Ancef™	See **cefazolin**
Ancobon™	See **flucytosine**
Ansaid™	See **flurbiprofen**
Apresoline™	See **hydralazine**
Ara-C	See **cytarabine**
Aspirin	
Atenolol	
Ativan™	See **lorazepam**
Atracurium	
Atromid S™	See **clofibrate**
Atropine	
Auranofin	
Aurothioglucose	
Azactam™	See **aztreonam**
Azathioprine	
AZT	See **zidovudine**
Aztreonam	
Bactocil™	See **oxacillin**
Bactrim™	See **co-trimoxazole**
Benadryl™	See **diphenhydramine**
Benemid™	See **probenecid**
Benzylpenicillin™	See **penicillin G, aqueous**
Bretylium	
Bretylol™	See **bretylium**
Brevibloc™	See **esmolol**
Bromocriptine mesylate	
Bumetanide	
Bumex™	See **bumetanide**
Bupivacaine	
Bupropion	
Burinex™	See **bumetanide**
Buspar™	See **buspirone**
Buspirone	

Drug Name	Cross Reference
Calan™	See **verapamil**
Capoten™	See **captopril**
Captopril	
Carbamazepine	
Cardine™	See **nicardipine**
Cardizem™	See **diltiazem**
Catapres™	See **clonidine**
Ceclor™	See **cefaclor**
Cefaclor	
Cefadroxil	
Cefazolin	
Cefixime	
Cefizox™	See **ceftizoxime**
Cefobid™	See **cefoperazone**
Cefonicid	
Cefoperazone	
Cefotan™	See **cefotetan**
Cefotaxime	
Cefotetan	
Cefoxitin	
Ceftazidime	
Ceftin™	See **cefuroxime**
Ceftizoxime	
Ceftriaxone	
Cefuroxime	
Cephalexin	
Chlorambucil	
Chloramphenicol base	
Chlordiazepoxide	
Chloromycetin™	See **chloramphenicol base**
Chloroquine	
Chlorpheniramine maleate	
Chlorpromazine	
Chlorpropamide	
Chlorthalidone	
Chlortrimeton™	See **chlorpheniramine maleate**
Cimetidine	
Cipro™	See **ciprofloxacin**
Ciprofloxacin	
Cisplatin	
Claforan™	See **cefotaxime**
Cleocin™	See **clindamycin**
Clindamycin	
Clinoril™	See **sulindac**
Clofibrate	
Clomipramine	
Clonidine	
Codeine	
Compazine™	See **prochlorperazine**
Cordarone™	See **amiodarone**
Corgard™	See **nadolol**
Co-trimoxazole	
Coumadin™	See **warfarin sodium**
Cyclophosphamide	
Cyclosporine	
Cytarabine	
Cytosar-U™	See **cytarabine**
Cytotec™	See **misoprostil**
Cytovene™	See **ganciclovir**
Cytoxan™	See **cyclophosphamide**

Drug Name	Cross Reference
Dalgan™	See **dezocine**
Dalmane™	See **flurazepam**
Deltasone™	See **prednisone**
Demerol™	See **meperidine**
Depakene™	See **valproic acid**
Desipramine	
Desyrel™	See **trazodone**
Dezocine	
DiaBeta™	See **glyburide**
Diabinese™	See **chlorpropamide**
Diamox™	See **acetazolamide**
Diazepam	
Dicloxacillin sodium	
Didronel™	See **etidronate**
Diflucan™	See **fluconazole**
Diflunisal	
Digoxin	
Dilantin™	See **phenytoin**
Dilaudid™	See **hydromorphone**
Diltiazem	
Diphenhydramine	
Diprivan™	See **propofol**
Disopyramide	
Diulo™	See **metolazone**
Dolobid™	See **diflunisal**
Dolophine™	See **methadone**
Doxepin	
Doxycycline	
Duricef™	See **cefadroxil**
Dynapen™	See **dicloxacillin sodium**
Dyrenium™	See **triamterene**
Edecrin™	See **ethacrynic acid**
Elavil™	See **amitriptyline**
Enalapril	
Encainide	
Endep™	See **amitriptyline**
Enkaid™	See **encainide**
Epilim™	See **valproic acid**
Epoetin α	
Epogen™	See **epoetin** α
ERYC™	See **erythromycin base**
Erythromycin base	
Esidrix™	See **hydrochlorothiazide**
Eskalith™	See **lithium carbonate**
Esmolol	
Estinyl™	See **ethinyl estradiol**
Ethacrynic acid	
Ethambutol	
Ethinyl estradiol	
Ethmozine™	See **moricizine**
Ethosuximide	
Etidronate	
E-Mycin™	See **erythromycin base**
Famotidine	
5-FC	See **flucytosine**
Feldene™	See **piroxicam**
Fentanyl	
Flagyl™	See **metronidazole**
Flecainide	
Floxin™	See **pefloxacin**
Fluconazole	
Flucytosine	
Fluoxetine	

Drug Name	Cross Reference
Fluphenazine	
Flurazepam	
Flurbiprofen	
Folex™	See **methotrexate**
Fortaz™	See **ceftazidime**
Fungizone™	See **amphotericin B**
Furosemide	
Ganciclovir	
Garamycin™	See **gentamicin sulfate**
Gentamicin sulfate	
Glipizide	
Glucotrol™	See **glipizide**
Glyburide	
Grisactin™	See **griseofulvin**
Griseofulvin	
Growth hormone, recombinant	
Guanabenz	
Halcion™	See **triazolam**
Haldol™	See **haloperidol**
Haloperidol	
HCTZ	See **hydrochlorothiazide**
Heparin	
Human erythropoietin	See **epoetin** α
Humatrope™	See **growth hormone, recombinant**
Humulin R™	See **insulin, regular human**
Hydralazine	
Hydrochlorothiazide	
Hydrocortisone	
Hydrocortone™	See **hydrocortisone**
HydroDiuril™	See **hydrochlorothiazide**
Hydromorphone	
Hygroton™	See **chlorthalidone**
Hypnovel™	See **midazolam**
Ibuprofen	
Ilotycin™	See **erythromycin base**
Imipenem	
Imipramine	
Imuran™	See **azathioprine**
Indapamide	
Inderal™	See **propranolol**
Indocin™	See **indomethacin**
Indomethacin	
INH	See **isoniazid**
Inocor™	See **amrinone**
Insulin, regular human	
Interferon α_{2a}	
Interleukin-2	
Isoniazid	
Isoptin™	See **verapamil**
Isordil™	See **isosorbide dinitrate**
Isosorbide dinitrate	
Kabikinase™	See **streptokinase**
Keflex™	See **cephalexin**
Kefzol™	See **cefazolin**
Ketoconazole	
Ketoprofen	
Ketorolac tromethamine	

Drug Name	Cross Reference
Labetalol	
Lanoxin™	See **digoxin**
Largactil™	See **chlorpromazine**
Lasix™	See **furosemide**
Leukeran™	See **chlorambucil**
Levodopa	
Levothroid™	See **levothyroxine**
Levothyroxine	
Librium™	See **chlordiazepoxide**
Lidocaine	
Lithium carbonate	
Lithobid™	See **lithium carbonate**
Lopressor™	See **metoprolol**
Lopurin™	See **allopurinol**
Lorazepam	
Lovastatin	
Lozol™	See **indapamide**
Ludiomil™	See **maprotiline**
Maprotiline	
Marcaine™	See **bupivacaine**
Maxdon™	See **metoclopramide**
Medrol™	See **methylprednisolone**
Mefoxin™	See **cefoxitin**
Mellaril™	See **thioridazine**
Melphalan	
Meperidine	
Metformin	
Methadone	
Methergine™	See **methylergonovine**
Methotrexate	
Methyldopa	
Methylergonovine	
Methylprednisolone	
Metoclopramide	
Metolazone	
Metoprolol	
Metronidazole	
Mevacor™	See **lovastatin**
Mexate™	See **methotrexate**
Mexiletine	
Mexitil™	See **mexiletine**
Mezlin™	See **mezlocillin**
Mezlocillin	
Micronase™	See **glyburide**
Midamor™	See **amiloride**
Midazolam	
Minipress™	See **prazosin**
Misoprostil	
Monocid™	See **cefonicid**
Moricizine	
Morphine sulfate	
Motrin™	See **ibuprofen**
Myambutol™	See **ethambutol**
Mysoline™	See **primidone**
Nadolol	
Nafcillin	
Nafcil™	See **nafcillin**
Naloxone	
Naprosyn™	See **naproxen**
Naproxen	
Narcan™	See **naloxone**
Nebcin™	See **tobramycin**

Drug Name	Cross Reference
Nembutal™	See **pentobarbital**
Nicardipine	
Nifedipine	
Nimodipine	
Nimotop™	See **nimodipine**
Nitroglycerin	
Nizoral™	See **ketoconazole**
Norcuron™	See **vecuronium**
Norethindrone	
Norfloxacin	
Norlutin™	See **norethindrone**
Normodyne™	See **labetalol**
Noroxin™	See **norfloxacin**
Norpace™	See **disopyramide**
Norpramin™	See **desipramine**
Nortriptyline	
Novolin R™	See **insulin, regular human**
Omeprazole	
Omnipen™	See **ampicillin**
Ondansetron	
Orap™	See **pimozide**
Orinase™	See **tolbutamide**
Orudis™	See **ketoprofen**
Oxacillin	
Oxazepam	
Pamelor™	See **nortriptyline**
Pancuronium	
Paracetamol	See **acetaminophen**
Parlodel™	See **bromocriptine mesylate**
Pavulon™	See **pancuronium**
Pefloxacin	
Penicillin G, aqueous	
Penicillin V	
Pentazocine	
Pentids™	See **penicillin G, aqueous**
Pentobarbital	
Pen Vee K™	See **penicillin V**
Pepcid™	See **famotidine**
Perphenazine	
Pethidine™	See **meperidine**
Pfizerpen™	See **penicillin G, aqueous**
Phenergan™	See **promethazine**
Phenobarbital	
Phenobarbitone	See **phenobarbital**
Phenoxymethylpenicillin	See **penicillin V**
Phenytoin	
Pimozide	
Piperacillin	
Pipracil™	See **piperacillin**
Piroxicam	
Platinol™	See **cisplatin**
Polycillin™	See **ampicillin**
Polymox™	See **amoxicillin**
Prazosin	
Prednisolone	
Prednisone	
PriLosec™	See **omeprazole**
Primidone	
Principen™	See **ampicillin**
Probenecid	

Drug Name	Cross Reference	Drug Name	Cross Reference
Procainamide		**Temazepam**	
Procardia™	See **nifedipine**	Tenormin™	See **atenolol**
Prochlorperazine		**Terfenadine**	
Prolixin™	See **fluphenazine**	**Tetracycline**	
Promethazine		Theolair™	See **theophylline, anhy-drous**
Pronestyl™	See **procainamide**		
Propafenone		**Theophylline, anhydrous**	
Propofol		**Thioridazine**	
Propranolol		Thorazine™	See **chlorpromazine**
Prostaphlin™	See **oxacillin**	**Ticarcillin**	
Protropin™	See **growth hormone, re-combinant**	Ticar™	See **ticarcillin**
		Tobramycin	
Prozac™	See **fluoxetine**	Tofranil™	See **imipramine**
		Tolazamide	
		Tolbutamide	
Quinidine sulfate		Tolectin™	See **tolmetin**
Quinine		Tolinase™	See **tolazamide**
Quinora™	See **quinidine sulfate**	**Tolmetin**	
		Toradol™	See **ketorolac trometha-mine**
Ranitidine			
Reglan™	See **metoclopramide**	TPA	See **alteplase**
Renitec™	See **enalapril**	Tracrium™	See **atracurium**
Restoril™	See **temazepam**	Trandate™	See **labetalol**
Retrovir™	See **zidovudine**	**Trazodone**	
Ridaura™	See **auranofin**	**Triamterene**	
Rifadin™	See **rifampin**	**Triazolam**	
Rifampin		Trilafon™	See **perphenazine**
Rimactane™	See **rifampin**	Trimox™	See **amoxicillin**
Rocephin™	See **ceftriaxone**	Tylenol™	See **acetaminophen**
Roferon-A™	See **interferon α_{2a}**		
Rythmol™	See **propafenone**	Unipen™	See **nafcillin**
Sandimmune™	See **cyclosporine**	Valium™	See **diazepam**
Seldane™	See **terfenadine**	**Valproic acid**	
Sensorcaine™	See **bupivacaine**	Vancocin™	See **vancomycin**
Septra™	See **co-trimoxazole**	Vancoled™	See **vancomycin**
Serax™	See **oxazepam**	**Vancomycin**	
Sinequan™	See **doxepin**	Vasotec™	See **enalapril**
SloPhyllin™	See **theophylline, anhy-drous**	**Vecuronium**	
		Veetids™	See **penicillin V**
Solganol™	See **aurothioglucose**	Velosulin™	See **insulin, regular human**
SoluCortef™	See **hydrocortisone**		
SoluMedrol™	See **methylprednisolone**	**Verapamil**	
Sorbitrate™	See **isosorbide dinitrate**	Versed™	See **midazolam**
Spironolactone		Vibramycin™	See **doxycycline**
Stemetril™	See **prochlorperazine**		
Streptase™	See **streptokinase**	**Warfarin sodium**	
Streptokinase		Wellbutrin™	See **bupropion**
Sublimaze™	See **fentanyl**	Wytensin™	See **guanabenz**
Sufentanil			
Sufenta™	See **sufentanil**	Xanax™	See **alprazolam**
Sulindac		Xylocaine™	See **lidocaine**
Sumycin™	See **tetracycline**		
Suprax™	See **cefixime**	Zantac™	See **ranitidine**
Symmetrel™	See **amantadine**	Zarontin™	See **ethosuximide**
Synthroid™	See **levothyroxine**	Zaroxolyn™	See **metolazone**
		Zidovudine	
Tagamet™	See **cimetidine**	Zinacef™	See **cefuroxime**
Talwin™	See **pentazocine**	Zofran™	See **ondansetron**
Tambocor™	See **flecainide**	Zovirax™	See **acyclovir**
Tazicef™	See **ceftazidime**	Zyloprim™	See **allopurinol**
Tazidime™	See **ceftazidime**		
Tegretol™	See **carbamazepine**		

SUGGESTED READING

Acetaminophen

1. Forrest, J. A. H.; Clements, J. A.; and Prescott, L. F.: Clinical pharmacokinetics of paracetamol. Clin. Pharmacokinet., 7:93–107, 1982.

Acetazolamide

1. Chapron, D. J.; Sweeney, K. R.; Feig, P. U.; and Kramer, P. A.: Influence of advanced age on the disposition of acetazolamide. Br. J. Clin. Pharmacol., 19:363–371, 1985.
2. Sweeney, K. R.; Chapron, D. J.; Brandt, J. L.; Gomolin, I. H.; Feig, P. U.; and Kramer, P. A.: Toxic interaction between acetazolamide and salicylate: Case reports and a pharmacokinetic explanation. Clin. Pharmacol. Ther., 40: 518–524, 1986.

Acyclovir

1. Laskin, O. L.: Clinical pharmacokinetics of acyclovir. Clin. Pharmacokinet., 8:187–201, 1983.
2. de Miranda, P.; Good, S. S.; Krasny, H. C.; Connor, J. D.; Laskin, L. L.; and Lietman, P. S.: Metabolic fate of radioactive acyclovir in humans. Am. J. Med., 73(suppl.): 215–220, 1982.

Alfentanil

1. Davis, P. J.; and Cook, D. R.: Clinical pharmacokinetics of the newer intravenous anesthetic agents. Clin. Pharmacokinet., 11:18–35, 1986.

Allopurinol

1. Murrell, G. A. C.; and Rapaport, W. G.: Clinical pharmacokinetics of allopurinol. Clin. Pharmacokinet., 11:343–353, 1986.

Alprazolam

1. Greenblatt, D. J.; Divoll, M.; Abernethy, D. R.; Ochs, H. R.; and Shader, R. I.: Clinical pharmacokinetics of the newer benzodiazepines. Clin. Pharmacokinet., 8:233–252, 1983.
2. Evans, R. L.: Alprazolam. Drug. Intell. Clin. Pharm., 15: 633–638, 1981.

Alteplase

1. Verstraete, M.; Su, C. A. P. F.; Tanswell, P.; Feuerer, W.; and Collen, D.: Pharmacokinetics and effects on fibrinolytic and coagulation parameters of two doses of recombinant tissue-type plasminogen activator in healthy volunteers. Thromb. Haemost., 56:1–5, 1986.
2. Garabedian, H. D.; Gold, H. K.; Leinbach, R. C.; Yasuda, T.; Johns, J. A.; and Collen, D.: Dose-dependent thrombolysis, pharmacokinetics and hemostatic effects of recombinant human tissue-type plasminogen activator for coronary thrombosis. Am. J. Cardiol., 58:673–679, 1986.

Amantadine

1. Aoki, F. Y.; and Sitar, D. S.: Clinical pharmacokinetics of amantadine hydrochloride. Clin. Pharmacokinet., 14:35–51, 1988.

Amikacin

1. Sarubbi, F. A.; and Hull, J. H.: Amikacin serum concentrations: Predictions of levels and dosage guidelines. Ann. Intern. Med., 89(part 1):612–618, 1978.

Amiloride

1. Grayson, M. J.; Smith, A. J.; and Smith, R. N.: Absorption, distribution, and elimination of ^{14}C-amiloride in normal human subjects. Br. J. Pharmacol., 43:473P–474P, 1971.

Amiodarone

1. Gillis, A. M.; and Kates, R. E.: Clinical pharmacokinetics of the newer antiarrhythmic agents. Clin. Pharmacokinet., 9:375–403, 1984.
2. Latini, R.; Tognoni, G.; and Kates, R. E.: Clinical pharmacokinetics of amiodarone. Clin. Pharmacokinet., 9:136–156, 1984.

Amitriptyline

1. Breyer-Pfaff, U.; Gaertner, H. J.; Kreuter, F.; Scharek, G.; Brinkschulte, M.; and Wiatr, R.: Antidepressive effect and pharmacokinetics of amitriptyline and 10-hydroxynortriptyline plasma levels. Psychopharmacol., 76:240–244, 1982.

Amoxicillin

1. Zarowny, D.; Ogilvie, R.; Tamblyn, D.; MacLeod, C.; and Ruedy, J.: Pharmacokinetics of amoxicillin. Clin. Pharmacol. Ther., 16:1045–1051, 1974.
2. Wright, A. J.; and Wilkowske, C. J.: The penicillins. Mayo Clin. Proc., 58:21–32, 1983.
3. Bergan, T.: Pharmacokinetics of beta-lactam antibiotics. Scand. J. Infect. Dis., 42(suppl.):83–98, 1984.

Amphotericin

1. Daneshmend, T. K.; and Warnock, D. W.: Clinical pharmacokinetics of systemic antifungal drugs. Clin. Pharmacokinet., 8:17–42, 1983.

Ampicillin

1. Wright, A. J.; and Wilkowske, C. J.: The penicillins. Mayo Clin. Proc., 58:21–32, 1983.
2. Bergan, T.: Pharmacokinetics of beta-lactam antibiotics. Scand. J. Infect. Dis., 42(suppl.):83–98, 1984.

Amrinone

1. Rocci, M. L.; and Wilson, H.: The pharmacokinetics and pharmacodynamics of newer inotropic agents. Clin. Pharmacokinet., 13:91–109, 1987.

Aspirin

1. Needs, C. J.; and Brooks, P. M.: Clinical pharmacokinetics of the salicylates. Clin. Pharmacokinet., 10:164–177, 1985.

Atenolol

1. Nattel, S.; Gagne, G.; and Pineau, M.: The pharmacokinetics of lignocaine and β-adrenoceptor antagonists in patients with acute myocardial infarction. Clin. Pharmacokinet., 13: 293–316, 1987.

Atracurium

1. Weatherley, B. C.; Williams, S. G.; and Neill, E. A. M.: Pharmacokinetics, pharmacodynamics and dose-response relationships of atracurium administered IV. Br. J. Anaesth., 55(suppl. 1):39S–45S, 1983.
2. Miller, R. D.; Rupp, S. M.; Fisher, D. M.; Cronnelly, R.; Fahey, M. R.; and Sohn, Y. J.: Clinical pharmacology of vecuronium and atracurium. Anesthesiology, 61:444–453, 1984.

Atropine

1. Virtanen, R.; Kanto, J.; Iisalo, E.; Iisalo, E. U. M.; Salo, M.; and Sjövall, S.: Pharmacokinetic studies on atropine with special reference to age. Acta Anaesth. Scand., 26:297–300, 1982.

Auranofin

1. Blocka, K. L. N.; Paulus, H. E.; and Furst, D. E.: Clinical pharmacokinetics of oral and injectable gold compounds. Clin. Pharmacokinet., 11:133–143, 1986.

Aurothioglucose

1. Blocka, K. L. N.; Paulus, H. E.; and Furst, D. E.: Clinical pharmacokinetics of oral and injectable gold compounds. Clin. Pharmacokinet., 11:133–143, 1986.

Azathioprine

1. Ding, T. L.; Gambertoglio, J. G.; Amend, W. J. C.; Birnbaum, J.; and Benet, L. Z.: Azathioprine bioavailability and pharmacokinetics in kidney transplant patients (abstract). Clin. Pharmacol. Ther., 27:250, 1980.

Aztreonam

1. Mattie, H.: Clinical pharmacokinetics of aztreonam. Clin. Pharmacokinet., 14:148–155, 1988.

Bretylium

1. Garrett, E. R.; Green, J. R.; and Bialer, M.: Bretylium pharmacokinetics and bioavailabilities in man with various doses and modes of administration. Biopharm. Drug Dispos., 3: 129–164, 1982.

Bromocriptine

1. Cedarbaum, J. M.: Clinical pharmacokinetics of antiparkinsonian drugs. Clin. Pharmacokinet., 13:141–178, 1987.

Bumetanide

1. Beermann, B.; and Groschinsky-Grind, M.: Clinical pharmacokinetics of diuretics. Clin. Pharmacokinet., 5:221–245, 1980.

Bupivacaine

1. Mather, L. E.; Long, G. J.; and Thomas, J.: The intravenous toxicity and clearance of bupivacaine in man. Clin. Pharmacol. Ther., 12:935–943, 1971.

Bupropion

1. Findlay, J. W. A; van Wyck Fleet, J.; Smith, P. G.; Butz, R. F.; Hinton, M. L.; Blum, M. R.; and Schroeder, D. H.: Pharmacokinetics of bupropion, a novel antidepressant agent, following oral administration to healthy subjects. Eur. J. Clin. Pharmacol., 21:127–135, 1981.

Buspirone

1. Gammans, R. E.; Mayol, R. F.; and LaBudde, J. A.: Metabolism and disposition of buspirone. Am. J. Med., 80(suppl. 3B):41–51, 1986.
2. Mayol, R. F.; Adamson, D. S.; Gammans, R. E.; and LaBudde, J. A.: Pharmacokinetics and disposition of ^{14}C-buspirone HCl after intravenous and oral dosing in man (abstract). Clin. Pharmacol. Ther., 37:210, 1985.

Captopril

1. Duchin, K. L.; McKinstry, D. N.; Cohen, A. I.; and Migdalof, B. H.: Pharmacokinetics of captopril in healthy subjects and in patients with cardiovascular diseases. Clin. Pharmacokinet., 14:241–259, 1988.
2. Kubo, S. H.; and Cody, R. J.: Clinical pharmacokinetics of the angiotensin converting enzyme inhibitors: A review. Clin. Pharmacokinet., 10:377–391, 1985.

Carbamazepine

1. Bertilsson, L.; and Tomson, T.: Clinical pharmacokinetic and pharmacological effects of carbamazepine and carbamazepine-10,11-epoxide. An update. Clin. Pharmacokinet., 11:177–198, 1986.

Cefaclor

1. Bergan, T.: Pharmacokinetic properties of the cephalosporins. Drugs, 34(suppl. 2):89–104, 1987.

Cefadroxil

1. Bergan, T.: Pharmacokinetic properties of the cephalosporins. Drugs, 34(suppl. 2):89–104, 1987.

Cefazolin

1. Bergan, T.: Pharmacokinetic properties of the cephalosporins. Drugs, 34(suppl. 2):89–104, 1987.

Cefixime

1. Faulkner, R. D.; Bohaychuk, W.; Desjardins, R. E.; Look, Z. M.; Haynes, J. D.; Weiss, A. I.; and Silber, B. M.: Pharmacokinetics of cefixime after once-a-day and twice-a-day dosing to steady state. J. Clin. Pharmacol., 27:807–812, 1987.
2. Guay, D. R. P.; Meatherall, R. C.; Harding, G. K.; and Brown, G. R.: Pharmacokinetics of cefixime (CL 284,635; FK 027) in healthy subjects and patients with renal insufficiency. Antimicrob. Agents Chemother., 30:485–490, 1986.

Cefonicid

1. Bergan, T.: Pharmacokinetic properties of the cephalosporins. Drugs, 34(suppl. 2):89–104, 1987.

Cefoperazone

1. Bergan, T.: Pharmacokinetic properties of the cephalosporins. Drugs, 34(suppl. 2):89–104, 1987.
2. Balant, L.; Dayer, P.; and Auckenthaler, R.: Clinical pharmacokinetics of the third generation cephalosporins. Clin. Pharmacokinet., 10:101–143, 1985.

Cefotaxime

1. Bergan, T.: Pharmacokinetic properties of the cephalosporins. Drugs, 34(suppl. 2):89–104, 1987.
2. Balant, L.; Dayer, P.; and Auckenthaler, R.: Clinical pharmacokinetics of the third generation cephalosporins. Clin. Pharmacokinet., 10:101–143, 1985.

Cefotetan

1. Bergan, T.: Pharmacokinetic properties of the cephalosporins. Drugs, 34(suppl. 2):89–104, 1987.

Cefoxitin

1. Bergan, T.: Pharmacokinetic properties of the cephalosporins. Drugs, 34(suppl. 2):89–104, 1987.

Ceftazidime

1. Bergan, T.: Pharmacokinetic properties of the cephalosporins. Drugs, 34(suppl. 2):89–104, 1987.
2. Balant, L.; Dayer, P.; and Auckenthaler, R.: Clinical pharmacokinetics of the third generation cephalosporins. Clin. Pharmacokinet., 10:101–143, 1985.

Ceftizoxime

1. Bergan, T.: Pharmacokinetic properties of the cephalosporins. Drugs, 34(suppl. 2):89–104, 1987.
2. Balant, L.; Dayer, P.; and Auckenthaler, R.: Clinical pharmacokinetics of the third generation cephalosporins. Clin. Pharmacokinet., 10:101–143, 1985.

Ceftriaxone

1. Bergan, T.: Pharmacokinetic properties of the cephalosporins. Drugs, 34(suppl. 2):89–104, 1987.
2. Balant, L.; Dayer, P.; and Auckenthaler, R.: Clinical pharmacokinetics of the third generation cephalosporins. Clin. Pharmacokinet., 10:101–143, 1985.

Cefuroxime

1. Bergan, T.: Pharmacokinetic properties of the cephalosporins. Drugs, 34(suppl. 2):89–104, 1987.

Cephalexin

1. Bergan, T.: Pharmacokinetic properties of the cephalosporins. Drugs, 34(suppl. 2):89–104, 1987.

Chlorambucil

1. Ehrsson, H.; Wallin, I.; Nilsson, S. O.; and Johansson, B.: Pharmacokinetics of chlorambucil in man after administration of the free drug and its prednisolone ester. Eur. J. Clin. Pharmacol., 24:251–253, 1983.

Chloramphenicol base

1. Ambrose, P. J.: Clinical pharmacokinetics of chloramphenicol and chloramphenicol succinate. Clin. Pharmacokinet., 9:222–238, 1984.

Chlordiazepoxide

1. Greenblatt, D. J.; Shader, R. I.; and Divoll, M.: Benzodiazepines: A summary of pharmacokinetic properties. Br. J. Clin. Pharmacol., 11:11S–16S, 1981.

Chloroquine

1. White, N. J.: Clinical pharmacokinetics of antimalarial drugs. Clin. Pharmacokinet., 10:187–215, 1985.

Chlorpheniramine maleate

1. Paton, D. M.; and Webster, D. R.: Clinical pharmacokinetics of H_1-receptor antagonists (the antihistamines). Clin. Pharmacokinet., 10:477–497, 1985.

Chlorpromazine

1. Loo, J. C. K.; Midha, K. K.; and McGilveray, I. J.: Pharmacokinetics of chlorpromazine in normal volunteers. Commun. Psychopharmacol., 4:121–129, 1980.

Chlorpropamide

1. Ferner, R. E.; and Chaplin, S.: The relationship between the pharmacokinetic and pharmacodynamic effects of oral hypoglycaemic drugs. Clin. Pharmacokinet., 12:379–401, 1987.

Chlorthalidone

1. Beermann, B.; and Groschinsky-Grind, M.: Clinical pharmacokinetics of diuretics. Clin. Pharmacokinet., 5:221–245, 1980.

Cimetidine

1. Somogyi, A.; and Gugler, R.: Clinical pharmacokinetics of cimetidine. Clin. Pharmacokinet., 8:463–495, 1983.

Ciprofloxacin

1. Neuman, M.: Clinical pharmacokinetics of the newer antibacterial 4-quinolones. Clin. Pharmacokinet., 14:96–121, 1988.

Cisplatin

1. Balis, F. M.; Holcenberg, J. S.; and Bleyer, W. A.: Clinical pharmacokinetics of commonly used anticancer drugs. Clin. Pharmacokinet., 8:202–232, 1983.

Clindamycin

1. DeHaan, R. M.; Metzler, C. M.; and Schellenberg, D.: Pharmacokinetic studies of clindamycin phosphate. J. Clin Pharmacol., 13:190–209, 1973.

Clofibrate

1. Gugler, R.: Clinical pharmacokinetics of hypolipidaemic drugs. Clin. Pharmacokinet., 3:425–439, 1978.

Clomipramine

1. Nagy, A.; and Johansson, R.: The demethylation of imipramine and clomipramine as apparent from their plasma kinetics. Psychopharmacol., 54:125–131, 1977.
2. Kuss, H. J.; and Jungkunz, G.: Nonlinear pharmacokinetics of clomipramine after infusion and oral administration in patients. Prog. Neuro-Psychopharmacol. Biol. Psychiatry, 10:739–748, 1986.

Clonidine

1. Lowenthal, D. T.; Matzek, K. M.; and MacGregor, T. R.: Clinical pharmacokinetics of clonidine. Clin. Pharmacokinet., 14:287–310, 1988.

Codeine

1. Guay, D. R. P.; Awni, W. M.; Findlay, J. W. A.; Halstenson, C. E.; Abraham, P. A.; Opsahl, J. A.; Jones, E. C.; and Matzke, G. K.: Pharmacokinetics and pharmacodynamics of codeine in end-stage renal disease. Clin. Pharmacol. Ther., 43:63–71, 1988.
2. Adler, T. K.; Fujimoto, J. M.; Way, E. L.; and Baker, E. M.: Metabolic fate of codeine in man. J. Pharmacol. Exp. Ther., 114:251–262, 1955.

Co-trimoxazole

1. Walker, S. E.; Paton, T. W.; Churchill, D. N.; Ojo, B.; Manuel, M. A.; and Wright, N.: Trimethoprim-sulfamethoxazole pharmacokinetics during continuous ambulatory peritoneal dialysis (CAPD). Peritoneal Dialysis Int., 9:51–55, 1989.
2. Patel, R. B.; and Welling, P. G.: Clinical pharmacokinetics of co-trimoxazole (trimethoprim-sulphamethoxazole). Clin. Pharmacokinet., 5:405–423, 1980.

Cyclophosphamide

1. Balis, F. M.; Holcenberg, J. S.; and Bleyer, W. A.: Clinical pharmacokinetics of commonly used anticancer drugs. Clin. Pharmacokinet., 8:202–232, 1983.
2. Wiebe, V. J.; Benz, C. C.; and DeGregorio, M. W.: Clinical pharmacokinetics of drugs used in the treatment of breast cancer. Clin. Pharmacokinet., 15:180–193, 1988.

Cyclosporine

1. Ptachcinski, R. J.; Venkataramanan, R.; and Burckart, R. J.: Clinical pharmacokinetics of cyclosporine. Clin. Pharmacokinet., 11:107–132, 1986.

Cytarabine

1. Balis, F. M.; Holcenberg, J. S.; and Bleyer, W. A.: Clinical pharmacokinetics of commonly used anticancer drugs. Clin. Pharmacokinet., 8:202–232, 1983.
2. van Prooijen, R.; van der Kleijn, E.; and Haanen, C.: Pharmacokinetics of cytosine arabinoside in acute myeloid leukemia. Clin. Pharmacol. Ther., 21:744–750, 1977.

Desipramine

1. DeVane, C. L.; Savett, M.; and Jusko, W. J.: Desipramine and 2-hydroxydesipramine pharmacokinetics in normal volunteers. Eur. J. Clin. Pharmacol., 19:61–64, 1981.

Dezocine

1. Locniskar, A.; Greenblatt, D. J.; and Zinny, M. A.: Pharmacokinetics of dezocine, a new analgesic: Effect of dose and route of administration. Eur. J. Clin. Pharmacol., 30: 121–123, 1986.
2. O'Brien, J. J.; and Benfield, P.: Dezocine: A preliminary review of its pharmacodynamic and pharmacokinetic properties, and therapeutic efficacy. Drugs, 38:226–248, 1989.

Diazepam

1. Kaplan, S. A.; Jack, M. L.; Alexander, K.; and Weinfeld, R. E.: Pharmacokinetic profile of diazepam in man following single IV and PO and chronic PO administration. J. Pharmacol. Sci., 62:1789–1796, 1973.
2. Kanto, J. H.: Use of benzodiazepines during pregnancy, labour, and lactation, with particular reference to pharmacokinetic considerations. Drugs, 23:354–380, 1982.
3. Hillestad, L.; Hansten, T.; and Melsom, H.: Diazepam metabolism in man: Part I. Clin. Pharmacol. Ther., 16:479–484, 1974.
4. Hillestad, L.; Hansten, T.; and Melsom, H.: Diazepam metabolism in normal man: II. Serum concentration and clinical effect after oral administration and cumulation. Clin. Pharmacol. Ther., 16:485–489, 1974.

Dicloxacillin sodium

1. Nauta, E. H.; and Mattie, H.: Dicloxacillin and cloxacillin: Pharmacokinetics in healthy and hemodialysis patients. Clin. Pharmacol. Ther., 20:98–108, 1976.
2. Bergan, T.: Pharmacokinetics of beta-lactam antibiotics. Scand. J. Infect. Dis., 42(suppl.):83–98, 1984.

Diflunisal

1. Woodhouse, K. W.; and Wynne, H.: The pharmacokinetics of nonsteroidal antiinflammatory drugs in the elderly. Clin. Pharmacokinet., 12:111–122, 1987.
2. Verbeek, R. K.; Blackburn, J. L.; and Loewen, G. R.: Clinical pharmacokinetics of non-steroidal antiinflammatory drugs. Clin. Pharmacokinet., 8:297–331, 1983.

Digoxin

1. Mooradian, A. D.: Digitalis. An update of clinical pharmacokinetic, therapeutic monitoring techniques and treatment recommendations. Clin. Pharmacokinet., 15:165–179, 1988.

Diltiazem

1. Echizen, H.; and Eichelbaum, M.: Clinical pharmacokinetics of verapamil, nifedipine, and diltiazem. Clin. Pharmacokinet., 11:425–449, 1986.
2. Smith, M. S.; Verghese, C. P.; Shand, D. G.; and Pritchett, E. L. C.: Pharmacokinetics and pharmacodynamic effects of diltiazem. Am. J. Cardiol., 51:1369–1374, 1983.

Diphenhydramine

1. Paton, D. M.; and Webster, D. R.: Clinical pharmacokinetics of H_1-receptor antagonists (the antihistamines). Clin. Pharmacokinet., 10:477–497, 1985.

Disopyramide

1. Hinderling, P. H.; and Garrett, E. R.: Pharmacokinetics of the antiarrhythmic disopyramide in healthy humans. J. Pharmacokinet. Biopharm., 4:199–230, 1976.

Doxepin

1. Faulkner, R. D.; Pitts, W. M.; Lee, C. S.; Lewis, W. A.; and Fann, W. E.: Multiple dose doxepin kinetics in depressed patients. Clin. Pharmacol. Ther., 34:509–515, 1983.

2. Ziegler, V. E.; Biggs, J. T.; Wylie, L. T.; Rosen, S. H.; Hawf, D. J.; and Coryell, W. H.: Doxepin kinetics. Clin. Pharmacol. Ther., 23:573–579, 1978.

Doxycycline

1. Saivin, S.; and Houin, G.: Clinical pharmacokinetics of doxycycline and minocycline. Clin. Pharmacokinet., 15:355–366, 1988.

Enalapril

1. Kubo, S. H.; and Cody, R. I.: Clinical pharmacokinetics of the angiotensin converting enzyme inhibitors: A review. Clin. Pharmacokinet., 10:377–391, 1985.

Encainide

1. Roden, D. M.; and Woosley, K. L.: Clinical pharmacokinetics of encainide. Clin. Pharmacokinet., 14:141–147, 1988.
2. Wang, T.; Roden, D. M.; Wolfenden, H. T.; Woosley, R. L.; Wood, A. J. J.; and Wilkinson, G. R.: Influence of genetic polymorphism on the metabolism and disposition of encainide in man. J. Pharmacol. Exp. Ther., 228:605–611, 1984.
3. Wang, T.; Roden, D. M.; Wolfenden, H. T.; Woosley, R. L.; Wilkinson, G. R.; and Wood, A. J. J.: Pharmacokinetics of encainide and its metabolites in man (abstract). Clin. Pharmacol. Ther., 31:278, 1982.
4. Gillis, A. M.; and Kates, R. F.: Clinical pharmacokinetics of the newer antiarrhythmic agents. Clin. Pharmacokinet., 9: 375–403, 1984.

Epoetin

1. Lim, V. S.; DeGowin, R. L.; Zavala, D.; Kirchner, P. T.; Abels, R.; Perry, P.; and Fangman, J.: Recombinant human erythropoietin treatment in pre-dialysis patients. Ann. Intern. Med., 110:108–114, 1989.
2. MacDougall, I. C.; Roberts, D. E.; Neubert, P.; Dharmasena, A. D.; Coles, G. A.; and Williams, J. D.: Pharmacokinetics of recombinant human erythropoietin in patients on continuous ambulatory peritoneal dialysis. Lancet, 1:425–427, 1989.
3. Egrie, T. C.; Eschbach, T. W.; McGuire, T.; and Adamson, J. M.: Pharmacokinetics of recombinant human erythropoietin (r-HuEPO) administered to hemodialysis (HD) patients (abstract). Kidney Int., 33:262, 1988.

Erythromycin base

1. Chow, M. S.; and Ronfield, R. A.: Pharmacokinetic data and drug monitoring: Antibiotics and antiarrhythmics. J. Clin. Pharmacol., 15:405–418, 1975.

Esmolol

1. Riddell, J. G.; Harron, D. W. G.; and Shanks, R. G.: Clinical pharmacokinetics of β-adrenoceptor antagonists: An update. Clin. Pharmacokinet., 12:305–320, 1987.

Ethacrynic acid

1. Kim, K. E.; Onesti, G.; Moyer, J. H.; and Swartz, C.: Ethacrynic acid and furosemide. Am. J. Cardiol., 27:407–415, 1971.

Ethambutol

1. Holdiness, M. R.: Clinical pharmacokinetics of the antituberculosis drugs. Clin. Pharmacokinet., 9:511–544, 1984.

Ethinyl estradiol

1. Orme, M. L. E.; Back, D. J.; and Breckenridge, A. M.: Clinical pharmacokinetics of oral contraceptive steroids. Clin. Pharmacokinet., 8:95–136, 1983.

Ethosuximide

1. Avidberg, E. F.; and Dam, M.: Clinical pharmacokinetics of anticonvulsants. Clin. Pharmacokinet., 1:161–188, 1976.

Etidronate

1. Powell, J. H.; and DeMark, B. R.: Clinical pharmacokinetics of diphosphonates. In, Bone Resorption, Metastasis, and Diphosphonates (Garattini, S., ed.). Monographs of the Mario Negri Institute for Pharmacological Research, Milan, Italy: Based on a symposium held June 1984. Raven Press, New York, pp. 41–49, 1985.

Famotidine

1. Krishna, D. R.; and Klotz, U.: Newer H_2-receptor antagonists. Clinical pharmacokinetics and drug interaction potential. Clin. Pharmacokinet., 15:205–215, 1988.

Fentanyl

1. Mather, L. E.: Clinical pharmacokinetics of fentanyl and its newer derivatives. Clin. Pharmacokinet., 8:422–446, 1983.
2. McClain, D. A.; and Hug, C. L.: Intravenous fentanyl kinetics. Clin. Pharmacol. Ther., 28:106–114, 1980.

Flecainide

1. Gillis, A. M.; and Kates, R. E.: Clinical pharmacokinetics of the newer antiarrhythmic agents. Clin. Pharmacokinet., 9:375–403, 1984.

Fluconazole

1. Humphrey, M. J.; Jevons, S.; and Tarbit, M. H.: Pharmacokinetic evaluation of UK-49,858, a metabolically stable triazole antifungal drug in animals and humans. Antimicrob. Agents Chemother., 28:648–653, 1985.
2. Tucker, R. M.; Williams, P. L.; Arathoon, E. G.; Levine, B. E.; Haristein, A. I.; Hanson, L. H.; and Stevens, D. A.: Pharmacokinetics of fluconazole in cerebrospinal fluid and serum in human coccidioidal meningitis. Antimicrob. Agents Chemother., 32:369–373, 1988.

Flucytosine

1. Daneshmend, T. K.; and Warnock, D. W.: Clinical pharmacokinetics of systemic antifungal drugs. Clin. Pharmacokinet., 8:17–42, 1983.

Fluoxetine

1. Benfield, P.; Heel, R. C.; and Lewis, S. P.: Fluoxetine. A review of its pharmacodynamic and pharmacokinetic properties, and therapeutic efficacy in depressive illness. Drugs, 32: 481–508, 1986.

Fluphenazine

1. Balant-Gorgia, A. E.; and Balant, L.: Antipsychotic drugs. Clinical pharmacokinetics of potential candidates for plasma concentration monitoring. Clin. Pharmacokinet., 13:65–90, 1987.

Flurazepam

1. Cooper, S. F.; and Drolet, D.: Protein binding of flurazepam and its major metabolites in plasma. Curr. Ther. Res., 32: 757–760, 1982.
2. Greenblatt, D. J.; Divoll, M.; Harmatz, J. S.; MacLaughlin, D. S.; and Shader, R. I.: Kinetics and clinical effects of flurazepam in young and elderly noninsomniacs. Clin. Pharmacol. Ther., 30:475–486, 1981.

Flurbiprofen

1. Kaiser, D. G.; Brooks, C. D.; and Lomen, P. L.: Pharmacokinetics of flurbiprofen. Am. J. Med., 80(suppl. 3A):10–15, 1986.

Furosemide

1. Beermann, B.; and Groschinsky-Grind, M.: Clinical pharmacokinetics of diuretics. Clin. Pharmacokinet., 5:221–245, 1980.

Ganciclovir

1. Sommadossi, J. P.; Bevan, K.; Ling, T.; Lee, F.; Mastre, B.; Chaplin, M. D.; Nerenberg, C.; Koretz, S.; and Buhles, W. C.: Clinical pharmacokinetics of ganciclovir in patients with normal and impaired renal function. Rev. Infect. Dis., 10(suppl. 3):S507–S514, 1988.
2. Lake, K. D.; Fletcher, C. V.; Love, K. R.; Brown, D. C.; Joyce, L. D.; and Pritzker, M. D.: Ganciclovir pharmacokinetics during renal impairment. Antimicrob. Agents Chemother., 32:1899–1900, 1988.

Gentamicin sulfate

1. Sawchuk, R. J.; Zaske, D. E.; Cipolle, R. J.; Wargin, W. A.; and Strate, R. G.: Kinetic model for gentamicin dosing with the use of individual patient parameters. Clin. Pharmacol. Ther., 21:362–369, 1977.

Glipizide

1. Ferner, R. E.; and Chaplin, S.: The relationship between the pharmacokinetic and pharmacodynamic effects of oral hypoglycaemic drugs. Clin. Pharmacokinet., 12:379–401, 1987.

Glyburide

1. Ferner, R. E.; and Chaplin, S.: The relationship between the pharmacokinetic and pharmacodynamic effects of oral hypoglycaemic drugs. Clin. Pharmacokinet., 12:379–401, 1987.

Griseofulvin

1. Rowland, M.; Riegelman, S.; and Epstein, W. L.: Absorption kinetics of griseofulvin in man. J. Pharm. Sci., 57:984–989, 1968.

Growth hormone, human

1. Ho, K. Y.; Weissberger, A. J.; Stuart, M. C.; Day, R. O.; and Lazarus, L.: The pharmacokinetics, safety and endocrine effects of authentic biosynthetic human growth hormone in normal subjects. Clin. Endocrinol., 30:335–345, 1989.
2. Hindmarsh, P. C.; Matthews, D. R.; Brain, C. E.; and Pringle, P. J.: The half-life of exogenous growth hormone after suppression of endogenous growth hormone secretion with somatostatin. Clin. Endrocinol., 30:443–450, 1989.
3. Jorgensen, J. O.; Flyvbjerg, A.; and Christiansen, J. S.: The metabolic clearance rate, serum half-time and apparent distribution space of authentic biosynthetic human growth hormone in growth hormone-deficient patients. Acta Endocrinol., 120:8–13, 1989.

Guanabenz

1. Meacham, R. H.; Emmett, M.; Kyriakopoulos, A. A.; Chiang, S. T.; Ruelius, H. W.; Walker, B. R.; Narins, R. G.; and Goldberg, M.: Disposition of C-guanabenz in patients with essential hypertension. Clin. Pharmacol. Ther., 27:44–52, 1980.

Haloperidol

1. Balant-Gorgia, A. E.; and Balant, L.: Antipsychotic drugs. Clinical pharmacokinetics of potential candidates for plasma concentration monitoring. Clin. Pharmacokinet., 13:65–90, 1987.
2. Forsman, A.; Folsch, G.; Larsson, M.; and Ohman, R.: On the metabolism of haloperidol in man. Curr. Ther. Res., 21:606–617, 1977.

Heparin

1. Estes, J. W.: Clinical pharmacokinetics of heparin. Clin. Pharmacokinet., 5:204–220, 1980.

Hydralazine

1. Shammas, F. V.; and Dickstein, K.: Clinical pharmacokinetics in heart failure. An updated review. Clin. Pharmacokinet., 15:94–113, 1988.
2. Ludden, T. M.; McNay, J. L.; Shepherd, A. M. M.; and Lin, M. S.: Clinical pharmacokinetics of hydralazine. Clin. Pharmacokinet., 7:185–205, 1982.

Hydrochlorothiazide

1. Beermann, B.; and Groschinsky-Grind, M.: Clinical pharmacokinetics of diuretics. Clin. Pharmacokinet., 5:221–245, 1980.

Hydrocortisone

1. Morselli, P. L.; Marc, V.; Garattini, S.; and Zaccala, M.: Metabolism of exogenous cortisol in humans: I. Diurnal variation in plasma disappearance rate. Biochem. Pharmacol., 19:1643–1647, 1970.

Hydromorphone

1. Vallner, J. J.; Stewart, J. T.; Kotzan, J. A.; Kirsten, E. B.; and Honigberger, I. L.: Pharmacokinetics and bioavailability of hydromorphone following intravenous and oral administration to human subjects. J. Clin. Pharmacol., 21:152–156, 1981.

Ibuprofen

1. Woodhouse, K. W.; and Wynne, H.: The pharmacokinetics of nonsteroidal antiinflammatory drugs in the elderly. Clin. Pharmacokinet., 12:111–122, 1987.

Imipenem

1. Somani, P.; Freimer, E. H.; Gross, M. L.; and Higgins, J. T.: Pharmacokinetics of imipenem-cilastatin in patients with renal insufficiency undergoing continuous peritoneal dialysis. Antimicrob. Agents Chemother., 32:530–534, 1988.

Imipramine

1. Brosen, K.; Gram, L. F.; Klysner, R.; and Bech, P.: Steady state levels of imipramine and its metabolites: Significance of dose-dependent kinetics. Eur. J. Clin. Pharmacol., 30:43–49, 1986.

Indapamide

1. Beermann, G.; and Grind, M.: Clinical pharmacokinetics of some newer diuretics. Clin. Pharmacokinet., 13:254–266, 1987.

Indomethacin

1. Woodhouse, K. W.; and Wynne, H.: The pharmacokinetics of non-steroidal antiinflammatory drugs in the elderly. Clin. Pharmacokinet., 12:111–122, 1987.
2. Verbeek, R. K.; Blackburn, J. L.; and Loewen, G. R.: Clinical pharmacokinetics of non-steroidal antiinflammatory drugs. Clin. Pharmacokinet., 8:297–331, 1983.

3. Helleberg, L.: Clinical pharmacokinetics of indomethacin. Clin. Pharmacokinet., 6:245–258, 1981.

Insulin, regular human

1. Brogden, R. N.; and Heel, R. C.: Human insulin. A review of its biological activity, pharmacokinetics, and therapeutic use. Drugs, 34:350–371, 1987.

Interferon α_{2a}

1. Wills, R. J.; Dennis, S.; Spiegel, H. E.; Gibson, D. M.; and Nadler, P. I.: Interferon kinetics and adverse reactions after intravenous, intramuscular, and subcutaneous injection. Clin. Pharmacol. Ther., 35:722–727, 1984.
2. Wills, R. J.; and Spiegel, H. E.: Continuous intravenous infusion pharmacokinetics of interferon to patients with leukemia. J. Clin. Pharmacol., 25:616–619, 1985.

Interleukin-2

1. Gustavson, L. E.; Nadeau, R. W.; and Oldfield, N. F.: Pharmacokinetics of teceleukin (recombinant human interleukin-2) after intravenous or subcutaneous administration to patients with cancer. J. Biol. Resp. Mod., 8:440–449, 1989.

Isoniazid

1. Holdiness, M. R.: Clinical pharmacokinetics of the antituberculosis drugs. Clin. Pharmacokinet., 9:511–544, 1984.

Isosorbide dinitrate

1. Straehl, P.; and Galeazzi, R. L.: Isosorbide dinitrate bioavailability, kinetics, and metabolism. Clin. Pharmacol. Ther., 38:140–149, 1985.

Ketoconazole

1. Daneshmend, T. K.; and Warnock, D. W.: Clinical pharmacokinetics of systemic antifungal drugs. Clin. Pharmacokinet., 8:17–42, 1983.
2. Daneshmend, T. K.; and Warnock, D. W.: Clinical pharmacokinetics of ketoconazole. Clin. Pharmacokinet., 14:13–34, 1988.

Ketoprofen

1. Woodhouse K. W.; and Wynne, H.: The pharmacokinetics of non-steroidal antiinflammatory drugs in the elderly. Clin. Pharmacokinet., 12:111–122, 1987.
2. Verbeek, R. K.; Blackburn, J. L.; and Loewen, G. R.: Clinical pharmacokinetics of non-steroidal antiinflammatory drugs. Clin. Pharmacokinet., 8:297–331, 1983.

Ketorolac tromethamine

1. Mroszczak, E. J.; Lee, F. W.; Combs, D.; Sarnquist, F. H.; Huang, B. L.; Wu, A. T.; Tokes, L. G.; Maddox, M. L.; and Cho, D. K.: Ketorolac tromethamine absorption, distribution, metabolism, excretion, and pharmacokinetics in animals and humans. Drug Metab. Dispos., 15:618–626, 1987.
2. Mroszczak, E. J.; Ling, T.; Yee, J.; Massey, I.; and Sevelius, H.: Ketorolac tromethamine (KT) absorption and pharmacokinetics in humans (abstract). Clin. Pharmacol. Ther., 37:215, 1985.

Labetalol

1. McNeil, J. J.; and Louis, W. J.: Clinical pharmacokinetics of labetalol. Clin. Pharmacokinet., 9:157–167, 1984.

Levodopa/carbidopa

1. Cedarbaum, J. M.: Clinical pharmacokinetics of antiparkinsonian drugs. Clin. Pharmacokinet., 13:141–178, 1987.

2. Nu, H. J. G.; Woodward, W. R.; and Anderson, J. L.: The effect of carbidopa on the pharmacokinetics of intravenously administered levodopa: The mechanism of action in the treatment of parkinsonism. Ann. Neurol., 18:537–543, 1985.

Levothyroxine

1. Schussler, G. C.: The extravascular circulation and metabolism of thyroxine (abstract). Clin. Res., 16:274, 1968.
2. Nicoloff, J. T.; Low, J. C.; Dussault, J. H.; and Fisher, D. A.: Simultaneous measurement of thyroxine and triiodothyronine peripheral turnover kinetics in man. J. Clin. Invest., 51:473–483, 1972.

Lidocaine

1. Anderson, J. L.: Current understanding of lidocaine as an antiarrhythmic agent: A review. Clin. Ther., 6:125–141, 1984.

Lithium carbonate

1. Fyro, B.; Petterson, U.; and Sedvall, G.: Pharmacokinetics of lithium in manic-depressive patients. Acta. Psychiatry Scand., 49:237–247, 1973.
2. Goodnick, P. J.; Fieve, R. D.; Meltzer, H. L.; and Dunner, D. L.: Lithium elimination half-life and duration of therapy. Clin. Pharmacol. Ther., 29:47–50, 1981.

Lorazepam

1. Greenblatt, D. J.; Divoll, M.; Abernethy, D. R.; Ochs, H. R.; and Shader, R. F.: Clinical pharmacokinetics of the newer benzodiazepines. Clin. Pharmacokinet., 8:233–252, 1983.
2. Greenblatt, D. J.: Clinical pharmacokinetics of oxazepam and lorazepam. Clin. Pharmacokinet., 6:89–105, 1981.

Lovastatin

1. Stubbs, R. J.; Schwartz, M.; and Bayne, W. F.: Determination of mevinolin and mevinolinic acid in plasma and bile by reversed-phase high-performance liquid chromatography. J. Chromatog., 383:438–443, 1986.

Maprotiline

1. Riess, W.; Dubey, L.; Funfgeld, E. W.; Imhof, P.; Hurzeler, H.; Matussek, N.; Rajagopalan, T. G.; Raschdorf, F.; and Schmid, K.: The pharmacokinetic properties of maprotiline (Ludiomil) in man. J. Int. Med. Res., 3(suppl. 2):16–41, 1975.

Melphalan

1. Bosanquet, A. G.; and Gilby, E. D.: Pharmacokinetics of oral and intravenous melphalan during routine treatment of multiple myeloma. Eur. J. Clin. Oncol., 18:355–362, 1982.

Meperidine

1. Edwards, D. J.; Svensson, C. K.; Visco, J. P.; and Lalka, D.: Clinical pharmacokinetics of pethidine: 1982. Clin. Pharmacokinet., 7:421–433, 1982.

Metformin

1. Sirtori, C. R.; Franceschini, G.; Gulli-Kienle, M.; Cighetti, G.; Galli, G.; Bondioli, A.; and Conti, F.: Disposition of metformin (N,N-dimethylbiguanidine) in man. Clin. Pharmacol. Ther., 24:683–693, 1978.
2. Pentikainen, P. J.; Neuvonen, P. J.; and Penttila, A.: Pharmacokinetics of metformin after intravenous and oral administration to man. Eur. J. Clin. Pharmacol., 16:195–202, 1979.

Methadone

1. Anggard, E.; Gunne, L. M.; Holmstrand, J.; McMahon, R. E.; Sandberg, C. G.; and Sullivan, H. R.: Disposition of methadone in methadone maintenance. Clin. Pharmacol. Ther., 17:258–266, 1975.
2. Inturrisi, C. E.; Colburn, W. A.; Kaiko, R. F.; Houde, R. W.; and Foley, K. M.: Pharmacokinetics and pharmacodynamics of methadone in patients wtih chronic pain. Clin. Pharmacol. Ther., 41:392–401, 1987.

Methotrexate

1. Strother, D. R.; Glynn-Barnhart, A.; Kovnar, E.; Gregory, R. E.; and Murphy, S. B.: Variability in the disposition of intraventricular methotrexate: A proposal for rational dosing. J. Clin. Oncol., 7:1741–1747, 1989.
2. Dawson, A. H.; and Grygiel, J. J.: Variability of methotrexate pharmacokinetics and pharmacodynamics. Agents Actions, 24(suppl.):226–235, 1988.

Methyldopa

1. Myhre, E.; Rugstad, H. E.; and Hanson, T.: Clinical pharmacokinetics of methyldopa. Clin. Pharmacokinet., 7:221–233, 1982.

Methylergonovine

1. Mantyla, R.; Kleimola, T.; and Kanto, J.: Pharmacokinetics of methylergometrine (methylergonovine) in the rabbit and man. Acta. Pharmacol. Toxicol., 40:561–569, 1977.

Methylprednisolone

1. Stjernholm, M. R.; and Katz, F. H.: Effects of diphenylhydantoin, phenobarbital, and diazepam on the metabolism of methylprednisolone and its sodium succinate. J. Clin. Endocrinol. Metab., 41:887–893, 1975.

Metocloramide

1. Bateman, D. N.: Clinical pharmacokinetics of metoclopramide. Clin. Pharmacokinet., 8:523–529, 1983.

Metolazone

1. Tilstone, W. J.; Dargie, H.; Dargie, E. N.; Morgan, H. G.; and Kennedy, A. C.: Pharmacokinetics of metolazone in normal subjects and in patients with cardiac or renal failure. Clin. Pharmacol. Ther., 16:322–329, 1974.
2. Modi, K. N.; Iberra, L.; and Nodine, J. H.: Human pharmacokinetic studies with 14C-Zaroxolyn, a new type of diuretic agent (abstract). Fed. Proc., 29:276, 1970.

Metoprolol

1. Nattel, S.; Gagne, G.; and Pineau, M.: The pharmacokinetics of lignocaine and β-adrenoceptor antagonists in patients with acute myocardial infarction. Clin. Pharmacokinet., 13:293–316, 1987.

Metronidazole

1. Ralph, E. D.: Clinical pharmacokinetics of metronidazole. Clin. Pharmacokinet., 8:43–62, 1983.

Mexiletine

1. Gillis, A. M.; and Kates, R. E.: Clinical pharmacokinetics of the newer antiarrhythmic agents. Clin. Pharmacokinet., 9:375–403, 1984.

Mezlocillin

1. Wright, A. J.; and Wilkowske, C. J.: The penicillins. Mayo Clin. Proc., 58:21–32, 1983.
2. Bergan, T.: Pharmacokinetics of beta-lactam antibiotics Scand. J. Infect. Dis., 42(suppl.):83–98, 1984.

Midazolam

1. Davis, P. J.; and Cook, D. R.: Clinical pharmacokinetics of the newer intravenous anesthetic agents. Clin. Pharmacokinet., 11:18–35, 1986.
2. Greenblatt, D. J.; Divoll, M.; Abernethy, D. R.; Ochs, H. R.; and Shader, R. I.: Clinical pharmacokinetics of the newer benzodiazepines. Clin. Pharmacokinet., 8:233–252, 1983.

Misoprostol

1. Karim, A.: Antiulcer prostaglandin misoprostol: Single and multiple-dose pharmacokinetic profile. Prostaglandins, 33 (suppl.):40–50, 1987.

Moricizine

1. Salerno, D. M.; Sharkey, P. J.; Granrud, G. A.; Asinger, R. W.; and Hodges, M.: Efficacy, safety, hemodynamic effects, and pharmacokinetics of high-dose moricizine during short- and long-term therapy. Clin. Pharmacol. Ther., 42: 201–209, 1987.
2. Woosley, R. L.; Morganroth, J.; Fogoros, R. N.; McMahon, F. G.; Humphries, J. O.; Mason, D. T.; and Williams, R. L.: Pharmacokinetics of moricizine HCl. Am. J. Cardiol., 60:35F–39F, 1987.

Morphine sulfate

1. Sawe, J.; Dahlstrom, B.; Paalzow, L.; and Rane, A.: Morphine kinetics in cancer patients. Clin. Pharmacol. Ther., 30: 629–635, 1981.
2. Brunk, S. F.; and Delle, M.: Morphine metabolism in man. Clin. Pharmacol. Ther., 16:51–57, 1974.

Nadolol

1. Nattel, S.; Gagne, G.; and Pineau, M.: The pharmacokinetics of lignocaine and β-adrenoceptor antagonists in patients with acute myocardial infarction. Clin. Pharmacokinet., 13: 293–316, 1987.

Nafcillin

1. Wright, A. J.; and Wilkowske, C. J.: The penicillins. Mayo Clin. Proc., 58:21–32, 1983.
2. Bergan, T.: Pharmacokinetics of beta-lactam antibiotics. Scand. J. Infect. Dis., 42(suppl.):83–98, 1984.

Naloxone

1. Fishman, J.; Roffwang, H.; and Hellman, L.: Disposition of naloxone-7,8-3H in normal and narcotic dependent men. J. Pharmacol. Exper. Ther., 187:575–580, 1973.

Naproxen

1. Woodhouse, K. W.; and Wynne, H.: The pharmacokinetics of non-steroidal antiinflammatory drugs in the elderly. Clin. Pharmacokinet., 12:111–122, 1987.
2. Verbeek, R. K.; Blackburn, J. L.; and Loewen, G. R.: Clinical pharmacokinetics of non-steroidal antiinflammatory drugs. Clin. Pharmacokinet., 8:297–331, 1983.

Nicardipine

1. Abernethy, D. R.; and Schwartz, J. B.: Pharmacokinetics of calcium antagonists under development. Clin. Pharmacokinet., 15:1–14, 1988.

Nifedipine

1. Echizen, H.; and Eichelbaum, M.: Clinical pharmacokinetics of verapamil, nifedipine, and diltiazem. Clin. Pharmacokinet., 11:425–449, 1986.
2. Foster, T. S.; Hamann, S. R.; Richards, V. R.; Bryant, P. J.; Graves, D. A.; and McAllister, R. G.: Nifedipine ki-

netics and bioavailability after single intravenous and oral doses in normal subjects. J. Clin. Pharmacol., 23:161–170, 1983.

Nimodipine

1. Abernethy, D. R.; and Schwartz, J. B.: Pharmacokinetics of calcium antagonists under development. Clin. Pharmacokinet., 15:1–14, 1988.

Nitroglycerin

1. Bogaert, M. G.: Clinical pharmacokinetics of glyceryltrinitrate following the use of systemic and topical preparations. Clin. Pharmacokinet., 12:1–11, 1987.

Norethindrone

1. Orme, M. L. E.; Back, D. J.; and Breckenridge, A. M.: Clinical pharmacokinetics of oral contraceptive steroids. Clin. Pharmacokinet., 8:95–136, 1983.

Norfloxacin

1. Neuman, M.: Clinical pharmacokinetics of the newer antibacterial 4-quinolones. Clin. Pharmacokinet., 14:96–121, 1988.

Nortriptyline

1. Alexanderson, B.: Pharmacokinetics of desmethylimipramine and nortriptyline in man after single and multiple oral doses—A crossover study. Eur. J. Clin. Pharmacol., 5:1–10, 1972.

Omeprazole

1. Regardh, G. C.: Pharmacokinetics and metabolism of omeprazole in man. Scand. J. Gastroenterol., 21:99–104, 1986.

Ondansetron

1. Blackwell, C. P.; and Harding, S. M.: The clinical pharmacology of ondansetron. Eur. J. Cancer Clin. Oncol., 25 (suppl. 1):S21–S24, 1989.
2. Colthup, P. V.; and Palmer, J. L.: The determination in plasma and pharmacokinetics of ondansetron. Eur. J. Cancer Clin. Oncol., 25(suppl. 1):S71–S74, 1989.

Oxacillin

1. Chow, M. S.; and Ronfeld, R. A.: Pharmacokinetic data and drug monitoring. J. Clin. Pharmacol., 15:405–418, 1975.

Oxazepam

1. Greenblatt, D. J.: Clinical pharmacokinetics of oxazepam and lorazepam. Clin. Pharmacokinet., 6:89–105, 1981.

Pancuronium

1. Somogyi, A. A.; Shanks, C. A.; and Triggs, E. J.: Clinical pharmacokinetics of pancuronium bromide. Eur. J. Clin. Pharmacol., 10:367–372, 1976.

Pefloxacin

1. Bergeron, M. G.: The pharmacokinetics and tissue penetration of the fluoroquinolones. Clin. Invest. Med., 12:20–27, 1989.
2. Gonzalez, J. P.; and Henwood, J. M.: Pefloxacin: A review of its antibacterial activity, pharmacokinetic properties, and therapeutic use. Drugs, 37:628–668, 1989.

Penicillin G, aqueous

1. Wright, A. J.; and Wilkowske, C. J.: The penicillins. Mayo Clin. Proc., 58:21–32, 1983.

2. Bergan, T.: Pharmacokinetics of beta-lactam antibiotics. Scand. J. Infect. Dis., 42(suppl.):83–98, 1984.

Penicillin V

1. Wright, A. J.; and Wilkowske, C. J.: The penicillins. Mayo Clin. Proc., 58:21–32, 1983.
2. Bergan, T.: Pharmacokinetics of beta-lactam antibiotics. Scand. J. Infect. Dis., 42(suppl.):83–98, 1984.
3. Hellstrom, K.; Rosen, A.; and Swahn, A.: Absorption and decomposition of potassium-35-S-phenoxymethyl penicillin. Clin. Pharmacol. Ther., 16:826–833, 1974.

Pentazocine

1. Bullingham, R. E. S.; McQuay, H. J.; and Moore, R. A.: Clinical pharmacokinetics of narcotic agonist-antagonist drugs. Clin. Pharmacokinet., 8:332–343, 1983.

Pentobarbital

1. Smith, R. B.; Dittert, L. W.; Griffen, W. O.; and Doluisio, J. T.: Pharmacokinetics and distribution of pentobarbital after IV and oral administration. J. Pharmacokinet. Biopharm., 1:5–16, 1973.
2. Ehrenbo, M.: Pharmacokinetic and distribution properties of pentobarbital. J. Pharm. Sci., 63:1114–1118, 1974.
3. Breimer, D. D.: Clinical pharmacokinetics of hypnotics. Clin. Pharmacokinet., 2:93–109, 1977.

Perphenazine

1. Balant-Gorgia, A. E.; and Balant, L.: Antipsychotic drugs. Clinical pharmacokinetics of candidates for plasma concentration monitoring. Clin. Pharmacokinet., 13:65–90, 1987.
2. Bahl-Puustinen, M. L.; Liden, A.; Alm, C.; Nordin, C.; and Bertilsson, L.: Disposition of perphenazine is related to polymorphic debrisoquin hydroxylation in human beings. Clin. Pharmacol. Ther., 46:78–81, 1989.

Phenobarbital

1. Browne, T. R.; Evans, J. E.; Szabo, G. K.; Evans, B. A.; and Greenblatt, D. J.: Studies with stable isotopes: II. Phenobarbital pharmacokinetics during monotherapy. J. Clin. Pharmacol., 25:51–58, 1985.

Phenytoin

1. Richens, A.: Clinical pharmacokinetics of phenytoin. Clin. Pharmacokinet., 4:153–169, 1979.
2. Grasela, T. H.; Sheiner, L. B.; Rambeck, B.; Boenigk, H. E.; Dunlop, A.; Mullen, P. W.; Wadsworth, J.; Richens, A.; Ishizaki, T.; Chiba, K.; Miura, H.; Minagawa, K.; Blain, P. G.; Mucklow, J. C.; Bacon, C. T.; and Rawlins, M.: Steady-state pharmacokinetics of phenytoin from routinely collected patient data. Clin. Pharmacokinet., 8:355–364, 1983.

Pimozide

1. Pinder, R. M.; Brogden, R. N.; Sawyer, P. R.; Speight, T. M.; Spencer, R.; and Avery, G. S.: Pimozide: A review of its pharmacological properties and therapeutic uses in psychiatry. Drugs, 12:1–40, 1976.
2. McCreadie, R. G.; Heykants, J. J. P.; Chalmers, A.; and Anderson, A. M.: Plasma pimozide profiles in chronic schizophrenics. Br. J. Clin. Pharmacol., 7:533–534, 1979.

Piperacillin

1. Wright, A. J.; and Wilkowske, C. J.: The penicillins. Mayo Clin. Proc., 58:21–32, 1983.
2. Bergan, T.: Pharmacokinetics of beta-lactam antibiotics. Scand. J. Infect. Dis., 42(suppl.):83–98, 1984.

Piroxicam

1. Woodhouse, K. W.; and Wynne, H.: The pharmacokinetics of non-steroidal antiinflammatory drugs in the elderly. Clin. Pharmacokinet., 12:111–122, 1987.
2. Verbeek, R. K.; Blackburn, J. L.; and Loewen, G. R.: Clinical pharmacokinetics of nonsteroidal antiinflammatory drugs. Clin. Pharmacokinet., 8:297–331, 1983.

Prazosin

1. Vincent, J.; Meredith, P. A.; Reid, J. L.; Elliott, H. L.; and Rubin, P. C.: Clinical pharmacokinetics of prazosin–1985. Clin. Pharmacokinet., 10:144–154, 1985.

Prednisolone

1. Rose, J. Q.; Yurchak, A. M.; and Jusko, W. J.: Dose-dependent pharmacokinetics of prednisone and prednisolone in man. J. Pharmacokinet. Biopharm., 9:389–417, 1981.

Prednisone

1. Rose, J. Q.; Yurchak, A. M.; and Jusko, W. J.: Dose-dependent pharmacokinetics of prednisone and prednisolone in man. J. Pharmacokinet. Biopharm., 9:389–417, 1981.

Primidone

1. Huidberg, E. F.; and Dam, M.: Clinical pharmacokinetics of anticonvulsants. Clin. Pharmacokinet., 1:161–188, 1976.

Probenecid

1. Cunningham, R. F.; Isralli, Z. H.; and Dayton, P. G.: Clinical pharmacokinetics of probenecid. Clin. Pharmacol., 6:135–151, 1981.

Procainamide

1. Grasela, T. H.; and Sheiner, L. B.: Population pharmacokinetics of procainamide from routine clinical data. Clin. Pharmacokinet., 9:545–554, 1984.
2. Connolly, S. J.; and Kates, R. E.: Clinical pharmacokinetics of N-acetylprocainamide. Clin. Pharmacokinet., 7:206–220, 1982.

Prochlorperazine

1. Taylor, W. B.; and Bateman, D. N.: Preliminary studies of the pharmacokinetics and pharmacodynamics of prochlorperazine in healthy volunteers. Br. J. Clin. Pharmacol., 23:137–142, 1987.

Promethazine

1. Taylor, G.; Houston, J. B.; Shaffer, J.; and Mawer, G.: Pharmacokinetics of promethazine and its sulphoxide metabolite after intravenous and oral administration to man. Br. J. Clin. Pharmacol., 15:287–294, 1983.

Propafenone

1. Giani, P.; Landolina, M.; Giudici, G.; Bianchini, C.; Ferrario, G.; Marchi, S.; Riva, E.; and Latini, R.: Pharmacokinetics and pharmacodynamics of propafenone during acute and chronic administration. Eur. J. Clin. Pharmacol., 34:187–194, 1988.

Propofol

1. Cockshott, I. D.; Briggs, L. P.; Douglas, E. J.; and White, M.: Pharmacokinetics of propofol in female patients. Br. J. Anaesth., 59:1103–1110, 1987.
2. Kay, N. H.; Sear, J. W.; Uppington, J.; Cockshott, I. ⌐ and Douglas, E. J.: Disposition of propofol in patients dergoing surgery. Br. J. Anaesth., 58:1075–1079, 1986

Propranolol

1. Nattel, S.; Gagne, G.; and Pineau, M.: The pharmacokinetics of lignocaine and β-adrenoceptor antagonists in patients with acute myocardial infarction. Clin. Pharmacokinet., 13: 293–316, 1987.

Quinidine sulfate

1. Ochs, H. R.; Greenblatt, D. J.; and Woo, E.: Clinical pharmacokinetics of quinidine. Clin. Pharmacokinet., 5:150–168, 1980.

Quinine

1. White, N. J.: Clinical pharmacokinetics of antimalarial drugs. Clin. Pharmacokinet., 10:187–215, 1985.

Ranitidine

1. Roberts, C. J. C.: Clinical pharmacokinetics of ranitidine. Clin. Pharmacokinet., 9:211–221, 1984.
2. Krishna, D. R.; and Klotz, U.: Newer H_2-receptor antagonists. Clinical pharmacokinetic and drug interaction potential. Clin. Pharmacokinet., 15:205–215, 1988.

Rifampin

1. Holdiness, M. R.: Clinical pharmacokinetics of the antituberculosis drugs. Clin Pharmacokinet., 9:511–544, 1984.

Spironolactone

1. Karim, A.; Zagarella, J.; Hribar, J.; and Dooley, M.: Spironolactone: I. Disposition and metabolism. Clin. Pharmacol. Ther., 19:158–169, 1976.
2. Karim, A.; Zagarella, J.; Hutsell, T. C.; Chao, A.; and Baltes, B. J.: Spironolactone: II. Bioavailability. Clin. Pharmacol. Ther., 19:170–176, 1976.

Streptokinase

1. Col, J. J.; Col-De Beys, C. M.; Renkin, J. P.; and Lavenne-Pardonge, E. M.: Pharmacokinetics, thrombolytic efficacy and hemorrhagic risk of different stretokinase regimens in heparin-treated acute myocardial infarction. Am. J. Cardiol., 63:1185–1192, 1989.

Sufentanil

1. Davis, P. J.; and Cook, D. R.: Clinical pharmacokinetics of the newer intravenous anesthetic agents. Clin. Pharmacokinet., 11:18–35, 1986.

Sulindac

1. Verbeek, R. K.; Blackburn, J. L.; and Loewen, G. R.: Clinical pharmacokinetics of non-steroidal antiinflammatory drugs. Clin. Pharmacokinet., 8:297–331, 1983.

Temazepam

1. Greenblatt, D. J.; Divoll, M.; Abernethy, D. R.; Ochs, H. R.; and Shader, R. I.: Clinical pharmacokinetics of the newer benzodiazepines. Clin. Pharmacokinet., 8:233–252, 1983.

Terfenadine

1. Garteiz, D. A.; Hook, R. H.; Walker, B. J.; and Okerholm, R. A.: Pharmacokinetic and biotransformation studies of terfenadine in man. Arzneimittelforsch., 32:1185–1190, 1982.

Tetracycline

1. Barza, M.; and Scheife, R. T.: Antimicrobial spectrum, pharmacology, and therapeutic use of antibiotics: 1. Tetracyclines. Am. J. Hosp. Pharm., 34:49–57, 1977.

Theophylline, anhydrous

1. Hendeles, L.; and Weinberger, M.: Theophylline. A "state of the art" review. Pharmacotherapy, 3:2–44, 1983.
2. Vree, T. B.; Martea, M.; Tiggeler, R. G. W. L.; Hekster, Y. A.; and Hafkenscheid, J. C. M.: Pharmacokinetics of theophylline and its metabolites in a patient undergoing continuous ambulatory peritoneal dialysis. Clin. Pharmacokinet., 15:390–395, 1988.

Thioridazine

1. Axelsson, R.: On the serum concentrations and antipsychotic effects of thioridazine, thioridazine side-chain sulfoxide and thioridazine side-chain sulfone, in chronic psychotic patients. Curr. Ther. Res., 21:587–605, 1977.

Ticarcillin

1. Libke, R. D.; Clarke, J. T.; Ralph, E. D.; Luthy, R. P.; and Kirby, W. M. M.: Ticarcillin vs. carbenicillin: Clinical pharmacokinetics. Clin. Pharmacol. Ther., 17:441–446, 1975.

Tobramycin

1. Counts, G. W.; Blair, A. D.; Wagner, K. F.; and Turck, M.: Gentamicin and tobramycin kinetics. Clin. Pharmacol. Ther., 31:662–668, 1982.
2. Matzke, G. R.; Burkle, W. S.; and Lucarotti, R. L.: Gentamicin and tobramycin dosing guidelines: An evaluation. Drug Intell. Clin. Pharm., 17:425–432, 1983.

Tolazamide

1. Ferner, R. E.; and Chaplin, S.: The relationship between the pharmacokinetic and pharmacodynamic effects of oral hypoglycaemic drugs. Clin. Pharmacokinet., 12:379–401, 1987.

Tolbutamide

1. Balant, L.: Clinical pharmacokinetics of sulphonylurea hypoglycaemic drugs. Clin. Pharmacokinet., 6:215–241, 1981.
2. Ferner, R. E.; and Chaplin, S.: The relationship between the pharmacokinetic and pharmacodynamic effects of oral hypoglycaemic drugs. Clin. Pharmacokinet., 12:379–401, 1987.

Tolmetin

1. Verbeek, R. K.; Blackburn, J. L.; and Loewen, G. R.: Clinical pharmacokinetics of non-steroidal antiinflammatory drugs. Clin. Pharmacokinet., 8:297–331, 1983.

Trazodone

1. Rawls, W. N.: Trazodone. Drug Intell. Clin. Pharm., 16:7–13, 1982.

Triamterene

1. Pruitt, A. W.; Winkel, J. S.; and Dayton, P. G.: Variations in the fate of triamterene. Clin. Pharmacol. Ther., 21:610–619, 1977.

Triazolam

1. Greenblatt, D. J.; Divoll, M.; Abernethy, D. R.; Ochs, H. R.; and Shader, R. I.: Clinical pharmacokinetics of the newer benzodiazepines. Clin. Pharmacokinet., 8:233–252, 1983.

Valproic acid

1. Zaccara, G.; Messori, A.; and Moroni, F.: Clinical pharmacokinetics of valproic acid – 1988. Clin. Pharmacokinet., 15: 367–389, 1988.

Vancomycin

1. Matzke, G. R.; Zhanel, G. G.; and Guay, D. R. P.: Clinical pharmacokinetics of vancomycin. Clin. Pharmacokinet., 11: 257–282, 1986.

Vecuronium

1. Miller, R. D.; Rupp, S. M.; Fisher, D. M.; Cronnelly, R.; Fahey, M. R.; and Sohn, Y. J.: Clinical pharmacology of vecuronium and atracurium. Anesthesiology, 61:444–453, 1984.

Verapamil

1. Echizen, H.; and Eichelbaum, M.: Clinical pharmacokinetics of verapamil, nifedipine, and diltiazem. Clin. Pharmacokinet., 11:425–449, 1986.
2. Eichelbaum, M.; Somogyi, A.; von Unruh, G. E.; and Dengler, H. J.: Simultaneous determination of the intravenous and oral pharmacokinetic parameters of D,L-verapamil using stable isotope-labelled verapamil. Eur. J. Clin. Pharmacol., 19:131–137, 1981.

Warfarin sodium

1. Holford, N. H. G.: Clinical pharmacokinetics and pharmacodynamics of warfarin. Understanding the dose-effect relationship. Clin. Pharmacokinet., 11:483–504, 1986.

Zidovudine

1. Blum, M. R.; Liao, S. H. T.; Good, S. S.; and de Miranda, P.: Pharmacokinetics and bioavailability of zidovudine in humans. Am. J. Med., 85(suppl. 2A):189–194, 1988.
2. Langtry, H. D.; and Campoli-Richards, D. M.: Zidovudine: A review of its pharmacodynamic and pharmacokinetic properties, and therapeutic efficacy. Drugs, 37:408–450, 1989.

Appendix II

Drug Interactions

Gregory Scott and David Nierenberg

The number of potential drug interactions is enormous and increasing each year. Entire books have been devoted to this subject. However, many such potential drug interactions have not been observed clinically, or current reports are tentative and inconclusive. Some drug interactions occur, but are of minor or trivial clinical importance. Many important drug interactions are clear and obvious to the clinician from his knowledge of the primary pharmacologic actions of the drugs involved. For example, ethanol can potentiate the central nervous system (CNS) depressant effects of essentially any benzodiazepine, opioid, or other drug with CNS-depressant properties.

This table summarizes current knowledge of well-documented drug interactions (cited in two or more clinical reports), that have the potential to be clinically important (cause the physician to alter drug therapy), and that are not obvious from inspection of the most important pharmacologic properties of both drugs involved. The basis for the drug interaction, either pharmacokinetic or pharmacodynamic, is discussed in Chapters 1 and 28. Although drugs from the same pharmacologic class might be expected to cause the same interaction, only those specific drugs that have been shown to cause the interaction are listed. The only exception to this is where all the drugs most commonly used from a particular pharmacologic class have been shown to cause the interaction and the less commonly used agents may not have been studied; in this case, the name of the class appears rather than each individual drug. (Note, however, that the Cross-Reference Key lists not only the class, but individual drugs within that class as well.)

It is essential that the physician using this table understand two important points: *the listing of a drug interaction in the table does* not *mean that such an interaction will occur in every patient, and, the absence of a drug interaction in this table does* not *guarantee that such an interaction could not occur.* It is possible that the drug interaction has not yet been described. In some cases, the drug interaction has been described, but only by one anecdotal report; additional study is lacking. In other cases, especially for many pharmacody-

namic interactions, the interaction is so obvious (e.g., propranolol blocking the bronchodilatory effects of albuterol; atropine and benztropine causing increased antimuscarinic effects; hydrochlorothiazide and methyldopa causing enhanced hypotensive effects) that the interaction is not included in the table.

Finally, the primary drugs included in this table are those commonly prescribed drugs, as listed in Appendix I, that in addition have a narrow therapeutic index. Such drugs include hypoglycemic agents, anticancer drugs, antiarrhythmics, antihypertensives, anticonvulsants, some antimicrobial drugs, antidepressants, lithium, theophylline, and warfarin. For such drugs, relatively small pharmacokinetic or pharmacodynamic interactions can cause relatively large and important clinical effects that may lead to diminished efficacy or increased toxicity. Other drugs with a narrow therapeutic index, but which are not commonly used (e.g., cyclosporine) are not included as primary drugs in this table. On the other hand, the secondary drugs found in this table include any drug that interacts with the primary drug to cause a clinically important drug interaction.

Each interaction consists of two drugs, the *primary drug* and the *secondary drug*. The table is constructed to describe the effect (either pharmacokinetic or pharmacodynamic) of the secondary drug on the primary drug. The secondary drug acts to either enhance $(+)$ or diminish $(-)$ the intended or toxic effects of the primary drug.

The column labeled *severity* provides an estimate of the potential clinical importance and severity of the drug interaction. One (1) indicates that although the interaction results in a clinically important outcome, patient morbidity is usually minimal and is easily managed (e.g., a slight increase in oral bioavailability of digoxin due to an alteration of gastrointestinal (GI) flora by erythromycin). Two (2) implies that patient morbidity may be significant and that palliative measures may be required (e.g., phenytoin toxicity caused by the administration of valproic acid). Three (3) indicates that the interaction may result in severe toxicity and that aggressive management may be required (e.g., a hypertensive crisis precipitated by the administration of epinephrine to a patient already receiving propranolol).

The column labeled *comments* describes the pharmacokinetic and/or pharmacodynamic mechanism(s) and outcomes of the interaction. Where appropriate, the outcome is expressed in terms of a pharmacokinetic variable.

The factual information included in this table was gathered from the four major reference texts listed below, as well as primary reports cited in these texts. However, the choice of drugs to be included in this table, the assignment of scores for severity, and the summary comments were

prepared by the authors using their best judgment from information included in these and other sources.

REFERENCES

1. Tatro, D. S. (ed.): Drug Interaction Facts. Facts and Comparisons Division, J. B. Lippincott Company, St. Louis, Mo., 1990.
2. Hansten, P. D.: Drug Interactions (5th ed.). Lea & Febiger, Philadelphia, Pa., 1985.
3. Shinn, A. F.; and Shrewsbury, R. P.: Evaluations of Drug Interactions (3rd ed.). C. V. Mosby Company, St. Louis, MO., 1985.
4. McEvoy, G. K. (ed.): AHFS Drug Information 90. American Society of Hospital Pharmacists, Bethesda, Md., 1990.

PRIMARY DRUG	SECONDARY DRUG	EFFECT ON PRIMARY DRUG	POTENTIAL SEVERITY	COMMENTS (EFFECT OF SECONDARY DRUG ON PRIMARY DRUG)
Acetohexamide	MAO inhibitors	+	2	Potential interference in compensatory adrenergic response to hypoglycemia.
	Phenylbutazone	+	2	Renal excretion of active metabolite (hydroxyhexamide) reduced.
Amikacin	Penicillins	−	2	Chemical inactivation of amino group in patients with renal failure (and in vitro) resulting in microbiologic inactivity.
Amitriptyline	Cimetidine	+	2	Decreased first pass effect resulting in increased bioavailability; decreased rate of metabolism, thereby decreasing clearance; decreased volume of distribution.
	MAO inhibitors	+	2	Inhibition of microsomal enzymes leading to decreased clearance.
Captopril	Indomethacin	−	2	Decreased production of renal prostaglandins leading to loss of hypertension control.
Carbamazepine	Cimetidine	+	2	Inhibition of hepatic metabolism leading to decreased clearance.
	Danazol	+	2	Inhibition of hepatic metabolism leading to decreased clearance.
	Erythromycin	+	3	Inhibition of hepatic metabolism leading to decreased clearance.
	Isoniazid	+	2	Probable inhibition of hepatic metabolism leading to decreased clearance.
	Phenytoin	−	2	Induction of microsomal enzymes leading to increased clearance.
	Primidone	+	2	Inhibition of hepatic metabolism leading to decreased clearance.
	Propoxyphene	+	1	Possible inhibition of hepatic metabolism leading to decreased clearance.
	Troleandomycin	+	3	Inhibition of hepatic metabolism leading to decreased clearance.
	Verapamil	+	2	Inhibition of hepatic metabolism leading to decreased clearance.
Carmustine	Cimetidine	+	3	Possible inhibition of hepatic metabolism leading to decreased clearance.
Chlorpropamide	Ammonium chloride	+	1	Increased bioavailability.
	Chloramphenicol	+	2	Decrease in hepatic metabolism leading to decreased clearance.
	Clofibrate	+	1	Unknown mechanism leading to decreased clearance.
	Diazoxide	−	2	Possible decrease in insulin release or increase in catecholamine release leading to increased serum glucose.
	Dicumarol	+	2	Decrease in hepatic metabolism leading to decreased clearance.
	Levothyroxine	−	1	Unknown mechanism leading to hyperglycemia.

PRIMARY DRUG	SECONDARY DRUG	EFFECT ON PRIMARY DRUG	POTENTIAL SEVERITY	COMMENTS (EFFECT OF SECONDARY DRUG ON PRIMARY DRUG)
	MAO inhibitors	+	2	Potential interference in the compensatory adrenergic response to hypoglycemia.
	Phenylbutazone	+	2	Unknown mechanism leading to hypoglycemia.
	Rifampin	−	2	Induction of hepatic microsomal enzymes leading to increased clearance.
	Salicylates	+	2	Displacement from plasma proteins; decreased renal tubular secretion thus decreasing clearance.
	Sodium bicarbonate	−	2	Increased renal clearance.
	Sulfonamides	+	2	Decrease in hepatic metabolism leading to decreased clearance.
	Thiazides	+	2	Decreased tissue sensitivity to insulin, decreased insulin secretion, or increased potassium loss leading to hyperglycemia.
Desipramine	Cimetidine	+	2	Decreased first pass effect resulting in increased bioavailability; decreased rate of metabolism, thereby decreasing clearance; decreased volume of distribution.
	Fluoxetine	+	2	Potential inhibition of hepatic metabolism leading to decreased clearance.
	MAO inhibitors	+	2	Inhibition of microsomal enzymes leading to decreased clearance.
Digoxin	Amiodarone	+	2	Reduction in volume of distribution, renal and non-renal clearance, displacement from plasma proteins, thus reducing clearance; additive inhibition of atrioventricular node conduction.
	Antacids, oral	−	2	Decreased GI absorption due to adsorption leading to decreased bioavailability.
	Antineoplastics	−	2	Decreased GI absorption leading to decreased bioavailability.
	Cholestyramine	−	2	Decreased GI absorption and enterohepatic recirculation.
	Colestipol	−	2	Decreased GI absorption and enterohepatic recirculation.
	Cyclosporine	+	3	Decrease in volume of distribution and clearance.
	Diuretics	+	2	Hypokalemia and metabolic alkalosis augment myocardial depolarization, thus increasing risk of digoxin toxicity.
	Erythromycin	+	1	Metabolism by GI bacteria (occurs in about 10%) may be reduced through alteration in GI flora, thereby increasing bioavailability.
	Metoclopramide	−	2	Decreased GI absorption due to increased GI motility leading to decreased bioavailability.

PRIMARY DRUG	SECONDARY DRUG	EFFECT ON PRIMARY DRUG	POTENTIAL SEVERITY	COMMENTS (EFFECT OF SECONDARY DRUG ON PRIMARY DRUG)
	Penicillamine	−	2	Unknown mechanism leading to reduced plasma levels.
	Quinidine	+	3	Reduced volume of distribution and clearance.
	Quinine	+	2	Decreased nonrenal clearance.
	Tetracycline	+	3	Metabolism by GI bacteria (occurs in about 10%) may be reduced through alteration in GI flora, thereby increasing bioavailability.
	Verapamil	+	3	Decreased total body clearance and possibly volume of distribution; additive decrease in conduction and heart rate.
Disopyramide	Phenytoin	−	2	Increased rate of metabolism leading to increased clearance.
	Rifampin	−	2	Increased rate of metabolism leading to increased clearance.
Doxepin	Cimetidine	+	2	Decreased first pass effect leading to increased bioavailability; decreased rate of metabolism, thereby decreasing clearance; decreased volume of distribution.
	Propoxyphene	+	1	Inhibition of hepatic metabolism, thereby decreasing clearance.
Gentamicin	Ethacrynic acid	+	3	Possible additive auditory toxicity.
	Furosemide	+	3	Possible additive auditory toxicity.
	Penicillins	+, −	2	Chemical inactivation of the amino group in patients with renal failure (and in vitro) resulting in microbiologic inactivity; antimicrobial synergy against enterococci.
Glipizide	Ethanol	+	2	Delay in absorption and elimination, thereby prolonging activity.
Imipramine	Cimetidine	+	2	Decreased first pass effect leading to increased bioavailability; inhibition of microsomal enzymes, thereby decreasing clearance; decreased volume of distribution.
	Fluoxetine	+	2	Potential inhibition of hepatic metabolism leading to decreased clearance.
	MAO inhibitors	+	2	Inhibition of microsomal enzymes leading to decreased clearance.
Levothyroxine	Cholestyramine	−	1	Binding in gut may lead to decreased bioavailability.
	Phenytoin	−	2	Induction of hepatic metabolism and displacement from plasma proteins leading to increased clearance.
Lidocaine	Cimetidine	+	2	Inhibition of microsomal enzymes, reduced hepatic blood flow leading to decreased clearance.

PRIMARY DRUG	SECONDARY DRUG	EFFECT ON PRIMARY DRUG	POTENTIAL SEVERITY	COMMENTS (EFFECT OF SECONDARY DRUG ON PRIMARY DRUG)
	Metoprolol	+	2	Reduced hepatic blood flow, inhibition of microsomal enzymes leading to decreased clearance.
	Nadolol	+	2	Reduced hepatic blood flow, inhibition of microsomal enzymes leading to decreased clearance.
	Propranolol	+	2	Reduced hepatic blood flow, inhibition of microsomal enzymes leading to decreased clearance.
Lithium	Diclofenac	+	2	Decreased renal clearance.
	Ibuprofen	+	2	Decreased renal clearance.
	Indomethacin	+	2	Decreased renal clearance.
	Naproxen	+	2	Decreased renal clearance.
	Piroxicam	+	2	Decreased renal clearance.
	Sodium bicarbonate	−	2	Increased renal clearance.
	Sulindac	+	2	Decreased renal clearance.
	Thiazides	+	2	Decreased renal clearance.
Methotrexate	Nonsteroidal anti-inflammatory drugs	+	3	Unpredictable decrease in renal clearance due to diminished renal function and/or inhibition of tubular secretion.
	Probenecid	+	3	Decreased renal clearance due to inhibition of tubular secretion.
	Salicylates	+	3	Decreased renal clearance due to inhibition of tubular secretion; possible displacement from plasma proteins leading to an increase in free fraction.
Mexiletine	Phenytoin	−	2	Stimulation of hepatic metabolism leading to increased clearance.
Nortriptyline	Cimetidine	+	2	Decreased first pass effect leading to increased bioavailability; decreased rate of metabolism, thereby decreasing clearance; decreased volume of distribution.
	Fluoxetine	+	2	Potential inhibition of hepatic metabolism leading to decreased clearance.
Phenobarbital	Ethanol	+, −	3	Acute ingestion may decrease hepatic metabolism, thus reducing clearance. Chronic ingestion may induce hepatic enzymes, thereby increasing clearance.
	Valproic acid	+	2	Inhibition of hepatic metabolism leading to decreased clearance.
Phenytoin	Amiodarone	+	2	Inhibition of hepatic metabolism leading to decreased clearance.
	Bleomycin	−	2	Decreased absorption or increased hepatic metabolism.
	Carbamazepine	+, −	2	Variable effect on hepatic metabolism leading to increased or decreased plasma levels.

PRIMARY DRUG	SECONDARY DRUG	EFFECT ON PRIMARY DRUG	POTENTIAL SEVERITY	COMMENTS (EFFECT OF SECONDARY DRUG ON PRIMARY DRUG)
	Carmustine	−	2	Decreased absorption or increased hepatic metabolism.
	Chloramphenicol	+	2	Probably inhibition of hepatic metabolism leading to decreased clearance.
	Cimetidine	+	2	Inhibition of microsomal enzymes leading to decreased clearance.
	Cisplatin	−	2	Decreased absorption or increased hepatic metabolism.
	Diazoxide	−	2	Unknown mechanism leading to increased clearance.
	Dicumarol	+	2	Increased serum concentration and elimination half-life.
	Disulfiram	+	2	Inhibition of microsomal enzymes leading to decreased clearance.
	Isoniazid	+	2	Inhibition of microsomal enzymes leading to decreased clearance.
	Methotrexate	−	2	Decreased absorption or increased hepatic metabolism.
	Phenylbutazone	+	2	Displacement from protein binding sites; inhibition of hepatic metabolism leading to decreased clearance.
	Rifampin	−	2	Stimulation of microsomal enzymes leading to increased clearance.
	Sucralfate	−	2	Decreased GI absorption.
	Sulfadiazine	+	2	Inhibition of microsomal enzymes leading to decreased clearance.
	Sulfamethizole	+	2	Inhibition of microsomal enzymes leading to decreased clearance.
	Theophylline	−	2	Increased hepatic metabolism leading to increased clearance.
	Trimethoprim	+	2	Inhibition of hepatic metabolism leading to decreased clearance.
	Valproic acid	+	2	Increased free fraction and possible inhibition of hepatic metabolism.
	Vinblastine	−	2	Decreased absorption or increased hepatic metabolism.
	Warfarin	+	2	Increased serum concentration and elimination half-life.
Primidone	Carbamazepine	−	2	Increased hepatic metabolism leading to increased clearance.
	Ethosuximide	−	2	Unknown mechanism may lead to lower primidone and/or phenobarbital plasma levels.
	Methsuximide	−	2	Unknown mechanism may lead to lower primidone and/or phenobarbital plasma levels.
	Phenytoin	+	2	Probable decrease in hepatic metabolism leading to increased plasma levels.
Procainamide	Amiodarone	+	2	Unknown mechanism leading to decreased clearance.

PRIMARY DRUG	SECONDARY DRUG	EFFECT ON PRIMARY DRUG	POTENTIAL SEVERITY	COMMENTS (EFFECT OF SECONDARY DRUG ON PRIMARY DRUG)
	Cimetidine	+	2	Reduced renal clearance (including the active metabolite) possibly by inhibition of tubular secretion.
Propranolol	Ampicillin	−	2	Impaired GI absorption leading to decreased bioavailability.
	Chlorpromazine	+	2	Decreased hepatic metabolism resulting in a decreased first-pass-effect, thereby increasing bioavailability.
	Cimetidine	+	2	Inhibition of hepatic metabolism leading to decreased clearance and decreased first-pass effect.
	Epinephrine	−	3	Pharmacologic antagonism of beta-blockade leading to decreased pharmacodynamic effects. Unopposed alpha$_1$ effects (from epinephrine) lead to vasoconstriction and increased blood pressure.
	Hydralazine	+	2	Decreased first-pass effect leading to increased bioavailability.
	Ibuprofen	−	2	Decreased production of renal prostaglandins which may lead to increased blood pressure.
	Indomethacin	−	2	Decreased production of renal prostaglandins which may lead to increased blood pressure.
	Pentobarbital	−	2	Induction of hepatic enzymes leading to increased clearance; increased first pass-effect leading to decreased bioavailability.
	Phenobarbital	−	2	Induction of hepatic enzymes leading to increased clearance; increased first pass-effect leading to decreased bioavailability.
	Piroxicam	−	2	Decreased production of renal prostaglandins which may lead to increased blood pressure.
	Rifampin	−	2	Induction of hepatic enzymes leading to increased clearance.
	Sulindac	−	2	Decreased production of renal prostaglandins which may lead to increased blood pressure.
	Thioridazine	+	2	Decreased hepatic metabolism leading to a decreased first-pass-effect thereby increasing bioavailability.
Quinidine	Amiodarone	+	2	Unknown mechanism causing increased plasma level.
	Cimetidine	+	2	Increased GI absorption or decreased hepatic metabolism leading to increased plasma level and decreased clearance.
	Pentobarbital	−	2	Increased metabolic clearance.
	Phenobarbital	−	2	Increased metabolic clearance.
	Phenytoin	−	2	Stimulation of microsomal enzymes leading to increased clearance.

PRIMARY DRUG	SECONDARY DRUG	EFFECT ON PRIMARY DRUG	POTENTIAL SEVERITY	COMMENTS (EFFECT OF SECONDARY DRUG ON PRIMARY DRUG)
	Primidone	−	2	Increased hepatic clearance.
	Rifampin	−	2	Induction of hepatic microsomal enzymes.
	Verapamil	+	3	Reduced clearance; potential pharmacodynamic effects at the sinoatrial and atrioventricular nodes.
Theophylline	Cimetidine	+	3	Decreased hepatic metabolism leading to decreased clearance.
	Ciprofloxacin	+	2	Inhibition of microsomal enzymes leading to decreased clearance.
	Contraceptives, oral	+	2	Decreased hepatic metabolism leading to decreased clearance — rare interaction.
	Erythromycin	+	2	Decreased hepatic metabolism leading to decreased clearance.
	Norfloxacin	+	2	Inhibition of microsomal enzymes leading to decreased clearance.
	Pentobarbital	−	2	Induction of microsomal enzymes leading to increased clearance.
	Phenobarbital	−	2	Induction of microsomal enzymes leading to increased clearance.
	Phenytoin	−	2	Increased hepatic metabolism leading to increased clearance.
	Propranolol	+	2	Inhibition of hepatic metabolism leading to decreased clearance.
	Rifampin	−	2	Induction of hepatic metabolism leading to increased clearance.
	Secobarbital	−	2	Induction of microsomal enzymes leading to increased clearance.
	Ticlopidine	+	2	Unknown mechanism causing decreased clearance.
	Troleandomycin	+	2	Decreased hepatic metabolism leading to decreased clearance.
Tobramycin	Ethacrynic acid	+	3	Possible additive auditory toxicity.
	Furosemide	+	3	Possible additive auditory toxicity.
	Penicillins	−	2	Chemical inactivation of amino group in patients with renal failure (and in vitro) leading to microbiologic inactivity.
Tolbutamide	Chloramphenicol	+	1	Decrease in hepatic metabolism leading to decreased clearance.
	Diazoxide	−	2	Possible decrease in insulin release or increase in catecholamine release leading to increased serum glucose.
	Dicumarol	+	2	Decrease in hepatic metabolism leading to decreased clearance.
	Ethanol	−	2	Elimination half-life decreased.
	MAO inhibitors	+	2	Potential interference in compensatory adrenergic response to hypoglycemia.

PRIMARY DRUG	SECONDARY DRUG	EFFECT ON PRIMARY DRUG	POTENTIAL SEVERITY	COMMENTS (EFFECT OF SECONDARY DRUG ON PRIMARY DRUG)
	Phenylbutazone	+	3	Displacement from plasma proteins, reduction in rate of oxidation, or decrease in renal excretion.
	Salicylates	+	2	Displacement from plasma proteins leading to increased free fraction.
	Sulfinpyrazone	+	2	Decrease in hepatic metabolism leading to decreased clearance.
	Sulfonamides	+	2	Decreased hepatic metabolism leading to decreased clearance.
	Thiazides	−	2	Decreased tissue sensitivity to insulin, decreased insulin secretion, or increased potassium loss.
Valproic acid	Aspirin	+	2	Displacement from plasma proteins leading to increased free fraction.
	Carbamazepine	−	2	Induction of microsomal enzymes leading to increased clearance.
	Phenytoin	−	1	Increased hepatic metabolism leading to increased clearance.
Verapamil	Quinidine	+	3	Unknown mechanism leading to decreased clearance.
	Rifampin	−	2	Reduced oral bioavailability due to increased first-pass effect.
Warfarin	Allopurinol	+	1	Possible inhibition of hepatic metabolism leading to decreased clearance.
	Aminoglutethimide	−	2	Probable stimulation of microsomal enzymes leading to increased clearance.
	Amiodarone	+	3	Inhibition of hepatic metabolism leading to decreased clearance.
	Amobarbital	−	3	Induction of microsomal enzymes leading to increased clearance.
	Androgens, 17-alkyl	+	3	Unknown mechanism leading to enhanced effect.
	Aspirin	+	3	Inhibition of platelet aggregation, hypoprothrombinemia, displacement from plasma proteins leading to an enhanced effect.
	Carbamazepine	−	2	Possible induction of microsomal enzymes leading to increased clearance.
	Chloral hydrate	+	1	Displacement from plasma proteins leading to increased free fraction.
	Cholestyramine	−	2	Reduced oral bioavailability due to decreased GI absorption.
	Cimetidine	+	3	Decreased hepatic metabolism leading to decreased clearance.
	Clofibrate	+	3	Unknown mechanism leading to enhancement of vitamin K clotting factors.
	Co-trimoxazole	+	3	Decreased hepatic metabolism leading to decreased clearance.
	Disulfiram	+	2	Unknown mechanism leading to increase in pharmacodynamic response.

PRIMARY DRUG	SECONDARY DRUG	EFFECT ON PRIMARY DRUG	POTENTIAL SEVERITY	COMMENTS (EFFECT OF SECONDARY DRUG ON PRIMARY DRUG)
	Erythromycin	+	3	Potential inhibition of metabolism leading to decreased clearance.
	Ethacrynic acid	+	1	Displacement from plasma proteins leading to increased free fraction.
	Glutethimide	−	2	Possible induction of microsomal enzymes leading to increased clearance.
	Griseofulvin	−	2	Possible induction of metabolism leading to increased clearance.
	Metronidazole	+	3	Decreased hepatic metabolism leading to decreased clearance.
	Nalidixic acid	+	2	Displacement from plasma proteins leading to increased effect — rare interaction.
	Phenobarbital	−	3	Induction of microsomal enzymes leading to increased clearance.
	Phenylbutazone	+	3	Displacement from plasma proteins, decreased hepatic metabolism leading to decreased clearance.
	Ranitidine	+	2	Decreased hepatic metabolism leading to decreased clearance.
	Rifampin	−	2	Induction of microsomal enzymes leading to increased clearance.
	Secobarbital	−	3	Induction of microsomal enzymes leading to increased clearance.
	Sulfinpyrazone	+	3	Decreased hepatic metabolism, possible displacement from plasma proteins, and inhibition of platelet aggregation leading to enhanced effect.

GENERIC AND TRADE NAMES FOR DRUGS IN APPENDIX II

Drug Name	Comments
ACETOHEXAMIDE	Primary drug
Achromycin™	See tetracycline
Adapin™	See DOXEPIN
Adrenalin™	See epinephrine
Adriamycin™	See doxorubicin
Advil™	See ibuprofen
Allopurinol	Affects WARFARIN
Alternagel™	See aluminum salts
Aluminum salts	Affects DIGOXIN
AMIKACIN	Primary drug
Amikin™	See AMIKACIN
Aminoglutethimide	Affects WARFARIN
Amiodarone	Affects DIGOXIN, PHE-NYTOIN, PROCAIN-AMIDE, QUINIDINE, WARFARIN
AMITRIPTYLINE	Primary drug
Ammonium chloride	Affects CHLORPROPA-MIDE
Amobarbital	Affects WARFARIN
Amphojel™	See aluminum salts
Ampicillin	Affects AMIKACIN, GENTAMICIN, PROPRANOLOL, TOBRAMYCIN
Anadrol-50™	See oxymetholone
Androgens, 17-alkyl	Affects WARFARIN
Antabuse™	See disulfiram
Antacids, oral	Affects DIGOXIN
Antineoplastics	Affects DIGOXIN
Apresoline™	See hydralazine
Aquatag™	See benzthiazide
Aspirin	Affects CHLOR-PROPAMIDE, METHOTREXATE, TOLBUTAMIDE, VALPROIC ACID, WARFARIN
Atromid S™	See clofibrate
Azlin™	See azlocillin
Azlocillin	Affects AMIKACIN, GENTAMICIN, TOBRAMYCIN
Bactrim™	See co-trimoxazole
Basaljel™	See aluminum salts
Benzthiazide	Affects CHLORPRO-PAMIDE, LITHIUM, TOLBUTAMIDE
BiCNU™	See CARMUSTINE
Bleomycin	Affects DIGOXIN, PHENYTOIN
Bronkodyl™	See THEOPHYLLINE
Bumetanide	Affects DIGOXIN
Bumex™	See bumetanide
Calan™	See VERAPAMIL
Capoten™	See CAPTOPRIL
CAPTOPRIL	Primary drug
Carafate™	See sucralfate

Drug Name	Comments
CARBAMAZEPINE	Primary drug; also af-fects PHENYTOIN, PRIMIDONE, VAL-PROIC ACID, WAR-FARIN
Carbenicillin	Affects AMIKACIN, GENTAMICIN, TOBRAMYCIN
CARMUSTINE	Primary drug; also af-fects DIGOXIN, PHE-NYTOIN
Celontin™	See methsuximide
Chloral hydrate	Affects WARFARIN
Chloramphenicol	Affects CHLORPRO-PAMIDE, PHENY-TOIN, TOLBUTA-MIDE
Chloromycetin™	See chloramphenicol
Chlorothiazide	Affects DIGOXIN
Chlorpromazine	Affects PROPRAN-OLOL
CHLORPROPAMIDE	Primary drug
Cholestyramine	Affects DIGOXIN, LEV-OTHYROXINE, WAR-FARIN
Cimetidine	Affects AMITRIPTY-LINE, CARBAMAZE-PINE, CARMUSTINE, DESIPRAMINE, DOXEPIN, IMIPRA-MINE, LIDOCAINE, NORTRIPTYLINE, PHENYTOIN, PROCAINAMIDE, PROPRANOLOL, QUINIDINE, THEO-PHYLLINE, WAR-FARIN
Ciprofloxacin	Affects THEOPHYL-LINE
Cipro™	See ciprofloxacin
Cisplatin	Affects PHENYTOIN
Clinoril™	See sulindac
Clofibrate	Affects CHLORPROPA-MIDE, WARFARIN
Colestid™	See colestipol
Colestipol	Affects DIGOXIN
Contraceptives, oral	Affects THEOPHYL-LINE
Cordarone™	See amiodarone
Corgard™	See nadolol
Coumadin™	See WARFARIN
Co-trimoxazole	Affects PHENYTOIN, WARFARIN
Cuprimine™	See penicillamine
Cyclophosphamide	Affects DIGOXIN
Cyclosporine	Affects DIGOXIN
Cytadren™	See aminoglutethimide
Cytarabine	Affects DIGOXIN
Cytosar-U™	See cytarabine
Cytoxan™	See cyclohosphamide

Drug Name	Comments	Drug Name	Comments
Danazol	Affects CARBAMAZE-PINE, WARFARIN	Furosemide	Affects DIGOXIN, GEN-TAMICIN, TOBRA-MYCIN
Danocrine™	See danazol		
Darvon™	See propoxyphene	Gantrisin™	See sulfisoxazole
Demulen™	See contraceptives, oral	Garamycin™	See GENTAMICIN
Depakene™	See VALPROIC ACID	GENTAMICIN	Primary drug
Depakote™	See VALPROIC ACID	Geopen™	See carbenicillin
DESIPRAMINE	Primary drug	GLIPIZIDE	Primary drug
Diabinese™	See CHLORPROPA-MIDE	Glucotrol™	See GLIPIZIDE
		Glutethimide	Affects WARFARIN
Dialume™	See aluminum salts	Grifulvin™	See griseofulvin
Diazoxide	Affects CHLORPRO-PAMIDE, PHENY-TOIN, TOLBUTA-MIDE	Grisactin™	See griseofulvin
		Griseofulvin	Affects WARFARIN
		Hydralazine	Affects PROPRAN-OLOL
Diclofenac	Affects LITHIUM, METHOTREXATE	Hydrochlorothiazide	Affects CHLORPRO-PAMIDE, DIGOXIN, LITHIUM, TOLBU-TAMIDE
Dicumarol	Affects CHLORPRO-PAMIDE, PHENY-TOIN, TOLBUTA-MIDE		
		HydroDiuril™	See hydrochlorothiazide
		Hydroflumethiazide	Affects CHLORPRO-PAMIDE, LITHIUM, TOLBUTAMIDE
DIGOXIN	Primary drug		
Dilantin™	See PHENYTOIN	Hyperstat™	See diazoxide
DISOPYRAMIDE	Primary drug		
Disulfiram	Affects PHENYTOIN, WARFARIN	Ibuprofen	Affects LITHIUM, PRO-PRANOLOL
Diuretics	Affects DIGOXIN	Ilosone™	See erythromycin
Diuril™	See chlorothiazide	Ilotycin™	See erythromycin
Doriden™	See glutethimide	IMIPRAMINE	Primary drug
DOXEPIN	Primary drug	Inderal™	See PROPRANOLOL
Doxorubicin	Affects DIGOXIN	Indomethacin	Affects CAPTOPRIL, LITHIUM, METHO-TREXATE, PRO-PRANOLOL
Dymelor™	See ACETOHEXAMIDE		
Edecrin™	See ethacrynic acid		
EES™	See erythromycin	Isocarboxazid	Affects CHLORPROPA-MIDE, AMITRIPTY-LINE, DESIPRA-MINE, IMIPRAMINE, TOLBUTAMIDE
Elavil™	See AMITRIPTYLINE		
Elixophyllin™	See THEOPHYLLINE		
Emycin™	See erythromycin		
Endep™	See AMITRIPTYLINE		
Epinephrine	Affects PROPRAN-OLOL	Isoniazid	Affects CARBAMAZE-PINE, PHENYTOIN
ERYC™	See erythromycin	Isoptin™	See VERAPAMIL
Erythrocin™	See erythromycin		
Erythromycin	Affects CARBAMAZE-PINE, DIGOXIN, THEOPHYLLINE, WARFARIN	Kaopectate™	See aluminum salts
		Ketoprofen	Affects METHOTREX-ATE
Ery-Tab™	See erythromycin	Lanoxin™	See DIGOXIN
Esidrix™	See hydrochlorothiazide	Lasix™	See furosemide
Ethacrynic acid	Affects DIGOXIN, GEN-TAMICIN, TOBRA-MYCIN, WARFARIN	Levothroid™	See LEVOTHYROXINE
		LEVOTHYROXINE	Primary drug; also af-fects CHLORPROPA-MIDE
Ethanol	Affects GLIPIZIDE, PHENOBARBITAL, TOLBUTAMIDE		
		LIDOCAINE	Primary drug
Ethosuximide	Affects PRIMIDONE	LITHIUM	Primary drug
Eutonyl™	See pargyline	Lopressor™	See metoprolol
Feldene™	See piroxicam	Maalox™	See aluminum salts, mag-nesium salts
Flagyl™	See metronidazole		
Fluoxetine	Affects DESIPRAMINE, IMIPRAMINE, NOR-TRIPTYLINE	Magnesium salts	Affects DIGOXIN
Fulvicin™	See griseofulvin		

Drug Name	Comments	Drug Name	Comments
MAO inhibitors	Affects ACETOHEXA-MIDE, AMITRIPTYLINE, DESIPRAMINE, IMIPRAMINE, TOLBUTAMIDE	Parnate™	See tranylcypromine
		Pediazole™	See erythromycin
		Penicillamine	Affects DIGOXIN
		Penicillin G	Affects AMIKACIN, GENTAMICIN, TOBRAMYCIN
Marplan™	See isocarboxazid		
Matulane™	See procarbazine	Penicillins	Affects AMIKACIN, GENTAMICIN, TOBRAMYCIN
Mellaril™	See thioridazine		
Metandren™	See methyltestosterone		
Methandroid™	See methandrostenolone	Pentobarbital	Affects PROPRANOLOL, QUINIDINE, THEOPHYLLINE
Methandrostenolone	Affects WARFARIN		
METHOTREXATE	Primary drug; also affects DIGOXIN, PHENYTOIN		
		Pertofrane™	See DESIPRAMINE
		Phenelzine	Affects ACETOHEXA-MIDE, AMITRIPTYLINE, DESIPRAMINE, IMIPRAMINE, TOLBUTAMIDE
Methsuximide	Affects PRIMIDONE		
Methyltestosterone	Affects WARFARIN		
Metoclopramide	Affects DIGOXIN		
Metoprolol	Affects LIDOCAINE		
Metronidazole	Affects WARFARIN	PHENOBARBITAL	Primary drug; also affects PROPRANOLOL, QUINIDINE, THEOPHYLLINE, WARFARIN
MEXILETINE	Primary drug		
Mexitil™	See MEXILETINE		
Mezlin™	See mezlocillin		
Mezlocillin	Affects AMIKACIN, GENTAMICIN, TOBRAMYCIN	Phenylbutazone	Affects ACETOHEXAMIDE, CHLORPROPAMIDE, PHENYTOIN, TOLBUTAMIDE, WARFARIN
Milk of Magnesia™	See magnesium salts		
Motrin™	See ibuprofen		
Mylanta™	See aluminum salts, magnesium salts	PHENYTOIN	Primary drug; also affects CARBAMAZEPINE, DISOPYRAMIDE, LEVOTHYROXINE, MEXILETINE, PRIMIDONE, QUINIDINE, THEOPHYLLINE, VALPROIC ACID
Mysoline™	See PRIMIDONE		
Nadolol	Affects LIDOCAINE		
Nalidixic acid	Affects WARFARIN		
Naprosyn™	See naproxen		
Naproxen	Affects LITHIUM, METHOTREXATE		
Nardil™	See phenelzine	Piperacillin	Affects AMIKACIN, GENTAMICIN, TOBRAMYCIN
Nebcin™	See TOBRAMYCIN		
NegGram™	See nalidixic acid	Pipracil™	See piperacillin
Nembutal™	See pentobarbital	Piroxicam	Affects LITHIUM, PROPRANOLOL
Noctec™	See chloral hydrate		
Norfloxacin	Affects THEOPHYLLINE	Platinol™	See cisplatin
		Polycillin™	See ampicillin
Norinyl™	See contraceptives, oral	PRIMIDONE	Primary drug; also affects CARBAMAZEPINE, QUINIDINE
Norlestrin™	See contraceptives, oral		
Noroxin™	See norfloxacin		
Norpace™	See DISOPYRAMIDE	Principen™	See ampicillin
Norpramin™	See DESIPRAMINE	Probenecid	Affects METHOTREXATE
NORTRIPTYLINE	Primary drug		
Nuprin™	See ibuprofen	PROCAINAMIDE	Primary drug
		Procan SR™	See PROCAINAMIDE
Oncovin™	See vincristine	Procarbazine	Affects DIGOXIN
Orinase™	See TOLBUTAMIDE	Proloprim™	See trimethoprim
Ortho-Novum™	See contraceptives, oral	Pronestyl™	See PROCAINAMIDE
Orudis™	See ketoprofen	Propoxyphene	Affects CARBAMAZEPINE, DOXEPIN
Ovral™	See contraceptives, oral		
Oxymetholone	Affects WARFARIN	PROPRANOLOL	Primary drug; also affects LIDOCAINE, THEOPHYLLINE
Pamelor™	See NORTRIPTYLINE		
Pargyline	Affects ACETOHEXA-MIDE, AMITRIPTYLINE, DESIPRAMINE, IMIPRAMINE, TOLBUTAMIDE	Prozac™	See FLUOXETINE

Drug Name	Comments	Drug Name	Comments
Questran™	See cholestyramine	Sumycin™	See tetracycline
Quibron™	See THEOPHYLLINE	Synthroid™	See levothyroxine
Quinaglute™	See QUINIDINE		
Quinidex™	See QUINIDINE	Tagamet™	See cimetidine
QUINIDINE	Primary drug; also affects DIGOXIN, VERAPAMIL	TAO™	See troleandomycin
		Tegretol™	See CARBAMAZEPINE
		Tetracycline	Affects DIGOXIN
Quinine	Affects DIGOXIN	Theodur™	See THEOPHYLLINE
		Theolair™	See THEOPHYLLINE
Ranitidine	Affects WARFARIN	THEOPHYLLINE	Primary drug; also affects PHENYTOIN
Reglan™	See metoclopramide		
Rheumatrex™	See METHOTREXATE	Thiazides	Affects CHLORPROPAMIDE, LITHIUM, TOLBUTAMIDE
Rifadin™	See rifampin		
Rifampin	Affects CHLORPROPAMIDE, DISOPYRAMIDE, PHENYTOIN, PROPRANOLOL, QUINIDINE, THEOPHYLLINE, VERAPAMIL, WARFARIN	Thioridazine	Affects PROPRANOLOL
		Thiosulfil Forte™	See sulfamethizole
		Thorazine™	See chlorpromazine
		Ticar™	See ticarcillin
		Ticarcillin	Affects AMIKACIN, GENTAMICIN, TOBRAMYCIN
Rimactane™	See rifampin		
Riopan™	See magnesium salts	Ticlopidine	Affects THEOPHYLLINE
Salicylates	Affects CHLORPROPAMIDE, METHOTREXATE, TOLBUTAMIDE	TOBRAMYCIN	Primary drug
		Tofranil™	See Imipramine
		TOLBUTAMIDE	Primary drug
Saluron™	See hydroflumethiazide	Tranylcypromine	Affects ACETOHEXAMIDE, AMITRIPTYLINE, DESIPRAMINE, IMIPRAMINE, TOLBUTAMIDE
Sandimmune™	See cyclosporine		
Secobarbital	Affects THEOPHYLLINE, WARFARIN		
Septra™	See co-trimoxazole		
Sinequan™	See DOXEPIN	Trimethoprim	Affects PHENYTOIN, WARFARIN
Slobid™	See THEOPHYLLINE		
Slo-Phyllin™	See THEOPHYLLINE	Trimpex™	See trimethoprim
Sodium bicarbonate	Affects CHLORPROPAMIDE, LITHIUM	Troleandomycin	Affects CARBAMAZEPINE, THEOPHYLLINE
Sodium salicylate	Affects CHLORPROPAMIDE, METHOTREXATE, TOLBUTAMIDE, VALPROIC ACID, WARFARIN		
		Uniphyl™	See THEOPHYLLINE
Stanozolol	Affects WARFARIN	VALPROIC ACID	Primary drug; also affects PHENOBARBITAL, PHENYTOIN
Sucralfate	Affects PHENYTOIN		
Sulfadiazine	Affects PHENYTOIN	Verapamil	Affects CARBAMAZEPINE, DIGOXIN, QUINIDINE
Sulfamethizole	Affects CHLORPROPAMIDE, PHENYTOIN, TOLBUTAMIDE		
		Vinblastine	Affects PHENYTOIN
Sulfamethoxazole	Affects CHLORPROPAMIDE, TOLBUTAMIDE, WARFARIN	Vincristine	Affects DIGOXIN
		Voltaren™	See diclofenac
Sulfinpyrazone	Affects TOLBUTAMIDE, WARFARIN	WARFARIN	Primary drug; also affects PHENYTOIN
Sulfisoxazole	Affects CHLORPROPAMIDE, TOLBUTAMIDE	Winstrol™	See stanozolol
Sulfonamides	Affects CHLORPROPAMIDE, TOLBUTAMIDE	Xylocaine™	See LIDOCAINE
Sulindac	Affects LITHIUM, PROPRANOLOL	Zantac™	See ranitidine
		Zarontin™	See ethosuximide
		Zyloprim™	See allopurinol

Index*

* In this index all trade names (proprietary names) are capitalized.